Autonomic Failure

Autonomic Failure

A Textbook of Clinical Disorders of the Autonomic Nervous System

FIFTH EDITION

Edited by

Professor Christopher J. Mathias
DPhil DSc FRCP FMedSci

Professor of Neurovascular Medicine, Imperial College London and Institute of Neurology, University College London; Director, Autonomic & Neurovascular Medicine Unit at St Mary's Hospital and the Autonomic Unit, National Hospital for Neurology and Neurosurgery, Queen Square, London; Consultant Physician at St Mary's Hospital, National Hospital for Neurology and Neurosurgery, and Hospital of St John & St Elizabeth, London.

and

Sir Roger Bannister
MSc DM FRCP

Former Master, Pembroke College Oxford; Honorary Consultant Physician, National Hospital for Neurology and Neurosurgery, Queen Square, London; Honorary Consultant Neurologist, St. Mary's Hospital, London, Oxford; District Health Authority and Oxford Regional Health Authority, Oxford.

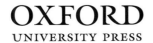

OXFORD
UNIVERSITY PRESS

OXFORD

UNIVERSITY PRESS

Great Clarendon Street, Oxford ox2 6DP
United Kingdom

Oxford University Press is a department of the University of Oxford.
It furthers the University's objective of excellence in research, scholarship,
and education by publishing worldwide. Oxford is a registered trade mark of
Oxford University Press in the UK and in certain other countries

Fifth Edition published in 2013

Impression: 1

British Library Cataloguing in Publication Data

Data available

Library of Congress Cataloging in Publication Data

Data available

ISBN 978–0–19–856634–2

Printed in Slovakia by Neografia

Oxford University Press makes no representation, express or implied, that the
drug dosages in this book are correct. Readers must therefore always check
the product information and clinical procedures with the most up-to-date
published product information and data sheets provided by the manufacturers
and the most recent codes of conduct and safety regulations. The authors and
the publishers do not accept responsibility or legal liability for any errors in the
text or for the misuse or misapplication of material in this work. Except where
otherwise stated, drug dosages and recommendations are for the non-pregnant
adult who is not breast-feeding.

Foreword

As a practising clinician and surgeon it is evident that the autonomic nervous system plays an essential role, not only in individual organ function but in a variety of processes needed for human survival, such as the integrated control of blood pressure and body temperature. The role of the autonomic nervous system was recognized over 100 years ago, but there has been a gap in translation of the steadily increasing fundamental knowledge into sound clinical practice. My colleagues, Professor Christopher Mathias and Sir Roger Bannister, along with others around the world, have reversed this. They have been at the forefront of advancing understanding of autonomic function in normal subjects and in a variety of autonomic disorders, localized and generalized, that affect both young and old. In this Textbook, they present an intertwining of fundamental and basic principles with detailed description of autonomic diseases, conditions and complications, linked to underlying pathophysiology, forming the platform for evidence and investigation based treatment. The autonomic field has embraced recent technological advances, and this has lead to improved diagnostic techniques and different forms of intervention, with the ability to safely, reproducibly and non-invasively monitor the effects of treatment that prevent, halt or reverse autonomic dysfunction.

Of additional importance is the increased awareness that autonomic disorders and ensuing complications need to be considered in planning health policy, as they can substantially influence the management of many associated disorders and their outcome. Autonomic complications significantly impair management of common disorders such as Parkinson's Disease and diabetes mellitus. Faints, syncope and falls are prevalent across different age groups and are a common cause of attendance at Accident and Emergency Departments. An autonomic cause is responsible in many of these patients. Syncope has many implications, with consequences for the individual and the family, especially if employment and driving issues arise, amongst others. Injuries resulting from falls substantially escalate surgical and medical costs, especially in the elderly. The Postural Tachycardia Syndrome, whose phenotype recently has been described along with its close association with another common inherited disorder, the Joint Hypermobility Syndrome/Ehlers Danlos III, raises additional issues. This condition is common in young individuals, with multiple features affecting cardiovascular, gastrointestinal and urinary bladder function, and thus may present to a wide spectrum of specialists, with doubts about the diagnosis resulting at times in unnecessary investigation and costs. Autonomic dysfunction and failure affecting various organs and systems increasingly occurs with increasing age, and this poses major national and global concerns with effectively planning healthcare in an expanding elderly population.

I therefore am delighted to write the foreword to this Textbook of Clinical Disorders of the Autonomic Nervous System, which provides crucial information crossing different specialties and disciplines, to physicians, surgeons or other specialist healthcare workers in the medical profession. Knowledge of the autonomic nervous system and its function will result in the early recognition, prompt diagnosis, and appropriate treatment of the many disorders and conditions causing or contributing to autonomic dysfunction. This should further improve the highest quality of healthcare provision that we continuously strive to provide for our patients.

Professor Lord Ara Darzi PC KBE HonFREng FMedSci
Professor of Surgery
Imperial College London & Imperial College Healthcare NHS Trust

Preface to the fifth edition

The autonomic field has evolved and expanded considerably, especially in the latter part of the last decade, and the Fifth Edition has endeavoured to encompass the many advances that have been achieved since the last edition. In the 1970's, when the first dedicated autonomic laboratories were started, the major emphasis was on disorders of the autonomic nervous system caused by damage, mainly irreversible, that often resulted in autonomic failure and orthostatic hypotension. This has changed substantially in the last two decades with advances in technology, such as non-invasive and continuous measurements that reproducibly record blood pressure, heart rate and other indices of autonomic function. This has increased awareness and understanding of pathophysiological processes, aided earlier diagnosis and improved treatment, especially of common conditions with intermittent autonomic dysfunction that result in orthostatic intolerance. These include the various forms of autonomic mediated syncope (AMS). In the new millennium another disorder, the Postural Tachycardia Syndrome (PoTS) has been increasingly recognized as a major cause of orthostatic Intolerance. PoTS is now considered an autonomic biomarker and part of an autonomic cluster, along with AMS and at times visceral involvement (mainly of the gastro-intestinal tract and bladder), in association with a common genetic connective tissue disorder, the Joint Hypermobility Syndrome/Ehlers Danlos III (*Nature Reviews Neurology* 2012, 8, 22–34). There is increasing realization that patients with such disorders should be investigated and managed by Autonomic Units because of their established experience in dealing with disorders affecting many systems, such as in Multiple System Atrophy. Increasing awareness of non-motor and mainly autonomic aspects in neurological diseases such as Parkinson's disease, autonomic neuropathy in medical disorders such as diabetes mellitus, and autonomic disturbances in the increasing elderly population are further examples of common conditions complicated by autonomic impairment. Autonomic Units are now an integral part of neurological centres and also of major hospitals, and contribute substantially to the diagnosis and treatment of an increasing range of neurological and medical disorders.

The Fifth Edition has been revised substantially with the addition of new chapters. It has incorporated the many advances that have occurred, with description of newer disorders and the impact of technological and therapeutic advances. We remain immensely grateful to our contributors who are leaders in the field, and who have so generously shared their expertise.

This new edition begins with classification of autonomic disorders, to include localized and generalized disorders, those with irreversible and reversible damage to autonomic centres and pathways, and those that result from intermittent autonomic dysfunction. This is followed by a history of the autonomic nervous system, covering the 100 plus years since Langley introduced the term "autonomic".

The first section provides the scientific basis needed for the recognition, diagnosis, investigation and treatment of autonomic disorders. This includes new chapters on surgical neuro-anatomy, vestibular-autonomic interaction and the autonomic neuroscience of sexual function. This is followed by the second section, on physiology and pathophysiology relevant to autonomic dysfunction, with new chapters on advances in understanding central autonomic control with functional neuroimaging, altitude and the autonomic nervous system, and renal-sympathetic relationships.

The third section provides details on clinical autonomic testing, with extensive revisions that emphasize the impact technological advances have made towards safe, non-invasive, accurate and reproducible investigation of autonomic nervous system function. It also includes a critical interpretation of complex abnormalities related to associated pathology enabling deeper understanding, and thus contributing to more precise, strategic and effective treatment. There are new chapters on measurement of catecholamines and their metabolites *in vivo*, the pressor effects of water ingestion in autonomic failure, exercise induced hypotension, the interaction and overlap between vestibular disorders, epilepsy and the autonomic nervous system, and the investigation and treatment of sexual dysfunction.

The fourth section provides the latest information on primary autonomic failure syndromes that include Multiple System Atrophy, Pure Autonomic Failure and Lewy body disease, along with neuroimaging, neuropathology and treatment of the motor and non-motor manifestations, especially orthostatic hypotension. There is a new chapter on experimental models of Multiple System Atrophy; this may accelerate progress in understanding and treatment of this devastating disease. Non-motor manifestations in Parkinson's disease are now recognized as a major clinical management problem and there are two new chapters, one on the neuropathological basis of autonomic involvement, and another on clinical aspects of autonomic dysfunction. This is followed by the fifth section with major revision of chapters on peripheral autonomic neuropathies and allied disorders, which include common disorders such as diabetes mellitus, rare disorders such as dopamine beta-hydroxylase deficiency, and other peripheral neuropathies including hereditary amyloid neuropathy. There is a new chapter on immune-mediated autonomic neuropathies, using intervention that in some have resulted in reversal of autonomic failure, which previously was not possible.

The sixth and final section includes revision of existing chapters, covering neuro-cardiovascular aspects, migraine, drugs, chemicals and toxins causing autonomic failure, and ageing. New chapters include transient loss of consciousness and the various causes of AMS, now recognized as causing > 50% of syncopal episodes, with a higher incidence in certain age groups such as teenagers. There is a new chapter on PoTS, in addition to other aspects of PoTS such as investigations described in Chapter 22. There are new chapters on shock, phaeochromocytoma, complex regional pain syndromes, and on surgery related to the autonomic nervous system.

Advances in the clinical management of autonomic disorders remain critically dependent on the bridge between basic and applied/translational science, and on blending clinical skills with information from appropriate investigation. It is intended that different sections of this book will make diagnosis more precise by fully evaluating the underlying anatomical and physiological deficits, thus leading to more effective management. Although a focussed and super-specialized approach is required, this has to be in the context of a broad and holistic base, which especially is needed with the even stronger interaction with different specialties, that include neurology, cardiology, geriatric medicine, endocrinology, internal medicine and rheumatology. The Fifth Edition is intended, as before, to provide clinicians, scientists, healthcare practitioners and therapists in different specialties and disciplines, with a rational guide to aid them in the recognition, diagnosis, evaluation and treatment of autonomic disorders.

CJM
RB

Contents

Acknowledgements

This Fifth Edition of Autonomic Failure owes very much to very many. We are especially grateful to our patients who have enabled us to continue to learn about, and at times unravel complex autonomic conditions, some listed previously under medically unexplained symptoms. We thank the clinical practitioners from across the United Kingdom and also worldwide who have referred patients to us. We remain indebted to our research, clinical and support staff within the Autonomic and Neurovascular Medicine Units at St Mary's Hospital and the National Hospital for Neurology and Neurology.

Advances in the autonomic field have been strongly underpinned by research, and we express our particular thanks to the many research fellows from the UK and worldwide with whom we have had the fortune to work with over the decades. We are particularly delighted that many have senior academic and clinical appointments, with some in Professorial positions, directing highly regarded autonomic and allied departments in the UK and abroad.

In 1989 we pioneered the role of Clinical Autonomic Scientists, who through their clinical service bring together innovation, research and technological advances, that have enabled us to substantially improve diagnosis, investigation and treatment of many autonomic disorders. They include Katharine Bleasdale-Barr, Madeline Tippetts, Lydia Mason and Laura Watson. We remain grateful to many other colleagues and collaborators at St Mary's Hospital and Imperial College London, and the National Hospital for Neurology and Neurosurgery at Queen Square and Institute of Neurology, University College London, who have been steadfastly supportive. CJM also thanks colleagues in the Hypermobility Units at the Hospital of St John and St Elizabeth and University College London Hospitals Trust for their collaboration and support.

Research into autonomic function and its disorders would not have been possible without the support of many Charities and Trusts, that over the last 3 decades have included the Wellcome Trust (who supported CJM from 1979 to 1992, initially as a Wellcome Senior Clinical Research Fellow and then as a Wellcome Senior Lecturer), the Sarah Matheson Trust (now the Multiple System Atrophy Trust), the Syncope Trust and Reflex Anoxic Seizures (STARS), the St Mary's Hospital Development Trust, the International Spinal Research Trust and the UK-India Education and Research Initiative. The Autonomic Charitable Trust, registered in 2012, will further promote increased awareness, recognition, understanding of mechanisms and treatment of autonomic disorders.

Finally, the task of co-ordinating the many aspects of this Fifth Edition with a large number of new authors and extensively revised chapters has been aided by Gemma Brennan, Andrew Owens and David Low in our departments, along with Pete Stevenson and Richard Martin at Oxford University Press, each of whom have been particularly supportive, and to whom we remain most grateful.

CJM
RB

List of contributors

Paul L. R. Andrews Department of Physiology, St. George's Hospital Medical School, London, UK

Felicia B. Axelrod New York University Medical Centre, New York, USA

Omer Aziz Honorary Clinical Research Fellow, Department of Surgery & Cancer, Imperial College London, UK

Abhay Bajpai Division of Cardiac and Vascular Sciences, St. George's University of London, London, UK

Roger Bannister Former Master, Pembroke College Oxford. Honorary Consultant Physician, National Hospital for Neurology and Neurosurgery, Queen Square, London. Honorary Consultant Neurologist, St. Mary's Hospital, London, Oxford. District Health Authority and Oxford Regional Health Authority, Oxford

Peter J. Barnes Professor of Thoracic Medicine, National Heart and Lung Institute, Imperial College School of Medicine, London, UK

Ralf Baron Department of Neurology, University of Kiel, Germany

Anne E. Bishop Emeritus Reader in Tissue Engineering & Regenerative Medicine, Department of Experimental Medicine & Toxicology, Imperial College Faculty of Medicine, Hammersmith Hospital, London, UK

Eduardo E. Benarroch Professor of Neurology, Mayo Graduate School of Medicine, Mayo Clinic, Rochester, MN, USA

Heiko Braak Clinical Neuroanatomy Section, Department of Neurology/Center for Clinical Research, University of Ulm, Ulm, Germany

F.D. Bremner Department of Neuro-ophthalmology, National Hospital for Neurology and Neurosurgery, London, UK

Adolfo Bronstein Neuro-otology Unit (Centre for Neuroscience), Imperial College London, Charing Cross Hospital, London, UK

David J. Brooks MRC Cyclotron Unit, Royal Postgraduate Medical School, Hammersmith Hospital, London, UK

Geoffrey Burnstock President, Autonomic Neuroscience Centre, University College Medical School, London, UK

A. John Camm Division of Cardiac and Vascular Sciences, St. George's University of London, London, UK

P. Castiglioni Fondazione Don C Gnocchi Centro di Bioingegneria, Milan, Italy

Sudhansu Chokroverty Departments of Neurology & Neurophysiology, Saint Vincent's Hospital & Medical Center, New York, USA

Victoria E. Claydon Assistant Professor, Cardiovascular Physiology Laboratory, Florida State University, USA

Jay N. Cohn Cardiovascular Division, Department of Medicine, University of Minnesota Medical School, USA

Kenneth J. Collins Honorary Senior Clinical Lecturer in Geriatric Medicine, Department of Geriatric Medicine, University College and Middlesex School of Medicine, St Pancras Hospital, London

Pietro Cortelli Dipartimento di Scienze Neurologiche, Alma Mater Studiorum-Universita'di Bologna

Hugo D. Critchley Autonomic Unit National Hospital for Neurology and Neurosurgery, University College London Hospitals, London, UK

Helen J. Cross National Centre for Young People with Epilepsy, Institute of Child Health, UCL, Great Ormond St Hospital for Children

Ara W. Darzi Professor of Surgery, Imperial College London & Imperial College Healthcare NHS Trust, London, UK

Soumendra N. Datta Department of Uro-Neurology, National Hospital for Neurology & Neurosurgery, UCLH, London, UK

William C. de Groat Distinguished Professor, Department of Pharmacology & Chemical Biology, University of Pittsburgh, PA, USA

Kelly Del Tredici-Braak Clinical Neuroanatomy Section, Department of Neurology/Center for Clinical Research, University of Ulm, Ulm, Germany

M. Di Rienzo La RC Centro di Bioingeneria, Fondazione Pro Juventute, Milan, Italy

Michael Donaghy Reader in Clinical Neurology and Consultant Neurologist, Department of Clinical Neurology, John Radcliffe Hospital, Oxford, UK

Mark Drinkhill Senior Lecturer, Cardiovascular and Diabetes Research, Leeds Institute of Genetics, Health and Therapeutics, University of Leeds, UK

Peter D. Drummond Division of Psychology, Murdoch University, Western Australia

John S. Duncan National Society for Epilepsy, Institute of Neurology, UCL; National Hospital for Neurology and Neurosurgery, London, UK

Michael Edmonds Diabetic Department, King's College Hospital, Denmark Hill, London, UK

Graeme Eisenhofer Clinical Neurocardiology Section, National Institute of Neurological Disorders and Stroke, National Institutes of Health, Bethesda, MD, USA

Stacy Elliott Sexual Medicine Consultant, Vancouver Coastal Health, BC Center for Sexual Medicine, Vancouver, Canada

Murray Esler Associate Director, Baker IDI Heart and Diabetes Institute, Melbourne, Victoria, Australia

Robert D. Fealey Department of Neurology, Mayo Clinic, Minnesota, USA

J. Anthony Firth Department of Surgical Oncology and Technology, Imperial College London, St Mary's Hospital, London, UK

Clare J. Fowler Department of Uro-Neurology, National Hospital for Neurology & Neurosurgery, UCLH, London, UK

Gary S. Francis Cardiovascular Division, Department of Medicine, University of Minnesota Medical School, USA

Hans L. Frankel National Spinal Injuries Centre, Stoke Mandeville Hospital, Aylesbury, Bucks, UK

Derek B. Frewin Department of Clinical and Experimental Pharmacology, The University of Adelaide, Australia

Peter J. Goadsby UCL Institute of Neurology, National Hospital for Neurology & Neurosurgery, Queen Square, London, UK

Blair Grubb Department of Cell Physiology and Pharmacology, University of Leicester, Leicester, UK

Roger Hainsworth Institute for Cardiovascular Research, University of Leeds, UK

Janice L. Holton Institute of Neurology, University College London, London, UK

Valeria Iodice Clinical Research Fellow, Autonomic and Neurovascular Medicine Unit, St Mary's Hospital, Imperial College London, UK

Wilfred Jänig Physiologisches Institut, Christian-Albrechts-Universität zu Kiel, Germany

Edward J. Johns Emeritus Professor, Physiology, University College Cork, Ireland

Karen Jones NH&MRC/Diabetes Australia Senior Research Fellow, Discipline of Medicine, University of Adelaide, Australia

John M. Karemaker Department of Physiology, University of Amsterdam, the Netherlands

Rose Anne Kenny Trinity College Institute for Neuroscience, Trinity College, College Green, Dublin, Ireland

C.T. Paul Krediet Department of Medicine, University of Amsterdam, the Netherlands

Gavin Lambert Human Autonomic Function Laboratory, Baker Medical Research Institute, Victoria, Australia

Andrew J. Lees National Hospital for Neurology & Neurosurgery, London, UK

Jacques W. M. Lenders Department of Internal Medicine, Division of General Internal Medicine, Radboud University Nijmegen Medical Center, Nijmegen, the Netherlands

Lewis A. Lipsitz Hebrew Rehabilitation Center for the Aged, Boston, USA

David A. Low Research Associate Fellow, Imperial College London, UK

Phillip A. Low Department of Neurology, Mayo Clinic, Minnesota, USA

Linda Luxon UCL Ear Institute, University College London, UK

Ian A. Macdonald The University of Nottingham Medical School, Queen's Medical Centre, Nottingham, UK

Robert Macfarlane Department of Neurosurgery, Addenbrooke's Hospital, Cambridge, UK

Giuseppe Mancia Divisione di Medicina, Ospedale San Gerardo dei Tintori, Monza, Italy

William M. Manger National Hypertension Association, New York, USA

Christopher J. Mathias Professor of Neurovascular Medicine, Imperial College London and Institute of Neurology, University College London. Director, Autonomic & Neurovascular Medicine Unit at St Mary's Hospital and the Autonomic Unit, National Hospital for Neurology and Neurosurgery, Queen Square, London. Consultant Physician at St Mary's Hospital, National Hospital for Neurology and Neurosurgery, and Hospital of St John & St Elizabeth, London

Margaret R. Matthews Department of Human Anatomy, University of Oxford, UK

Kevin E. McKenna Departments of Physiology and Urology, Northwestern University Feinberg School of Medicine, Chicago, IL, USA

Elspeth M. McLachlan Prince of Wales Medical Research Institute, Randwick, Australia

Michael A. Moskowitz Harvard Medical School, Massachusetts General Hospital, USA

Sinéad M. Murphy MRC Centre for Neuromuscular Diseases, Department of Molecular Neurosciences, UCL Institute of Neurology, London, UK

Uday Muthane Medical Director, Parkinson's & Aging Research Foundation, Bangalore, India

Krysztof Narkiewicz Cardiovascular Neurophysiology Laboratory, Cardiovascular Division, Department of Medicine, University of Iowa College of Medicine, Iowa City, USA

Markus Naumann Professor and Head of the Department of Neurology and Clinical Neurophysiology, Academic Hospital of the Ludwigs-Maximilians-University Munich, Klinikum Augsburg, Germany

Marios Nicolaou Honorary Clinical Lecturer, Department of Surgery & Cancer, Imperial College London, UK

Antonio Claudio Lucas da Nóbrega Department of Physiology and Pharmacology, Fluminense Federal University, Niterói, Brazil

Vera Novak Beth Israel Deaconess Med Center, Division of Gerontology, Boston, MA, USA

Jes Oleson Department of Neurology, Glostrup Hospital, Glostrup, Denmark

Karel Pacak Reproductive Biology and Medicine Branch, National Institute of Child Health and Human Development, National Institutes of Health, Bethesda, MD, USA

Waheeda Pagarkar Nuffield Hearing and Speech Centre, Royal National Throat Nose and Ear Hospital, London, UK

G. Parati Istituto Scientifico, Ospedale S Luca, Istituto Auxologico Italiano, Milan, Italy

Julian F.R Paton School of Physiology and Pharmacology University of Bristol

Stephen J. Peroutka Vice President, Scientific Affairs, PRA, USA

Julia M. Polak Emeritus Professor of Endocrine Pathology, Imperial College Faculty of Medicine, London, UK

Sanjay Purkayastha Honorary Clinical Lecturer, Department of Surgery & Cancer, Imperial College Faculty of Medicine, London, UK

Mary M. Reilly MRC Centre for Neuromuscular Diseases, Department of Molecular Neurosciences, UCL Institute of Neurology, London, UK

Tamas Revesz Institute of Neurology, University College London, London, UK

Maria Rivera-Ch Laboratory of High Altitude Adaptation, Laboratorios de Investigación y Desarrollo, Facultad de Ciencias y Filosofía, Universidad Peruana Cayetano Heredia, Lima, Peru

Martin A. Samuels Department of Neurology, Brigham & Women's Hospital, Boston, USA

Mike Schachter Senior Lecturer in Clinical Pharmacology, Department of Clinical Pharmacology, National Heart & Lung Institute, Imperial College Faculty of Medicine, London, UK

Niels H. Secher Perinatal Epidemiological Research Unit, Department of Obstetrics and Gynaecology, Aarhus University Hospital, Denmark

Melanie C. Sharp Department of Neurosurgery, Nottingham University Hospitals NHS Trust, Queen's Medical Centre Campus, Nottingham, UK

S.E. Smith Department of Neuro-ophthalmology, National Hospital for Neurology and Neurosurgery, London, UK

Virend K. Somers Cardiovascular Neurophysiology Laboratory, Cardiovascular Division, Department of Medicine, University of Iowa College of Medicine, Iowa City, USA

K. Michael Spyer Neuroscience, Physiology and Pharmacology, University College London, London, UK

Nadia Stefanova Section of Clinical Neurobiology, Department of Neurology, Medical University Innsbruck, Innsbruck, Austria

John B.P. Stephenson Fraser of Allander Neurosciences Unit, Royal Hospital for Sick Children, Glasgow, UK

Tilli Tansey Professor of the History of Modern Medical Sciences, Department of History, Queen Mary University of London, London, UK

David G. Thompson Professor of Gastroenterology, University of Manchester, Manchester, UK

Lars Lykke Thomsen Department of Neurology, Glostrup Hospital, Glostrup, Denmark

Anne L. Tonkin Department of Clinical and Experimental Pharmacology, The University of Adelaide, Australia

J. Gert van Dijk Leiden University Medical Centre, Department of Neurology and Clinical Neurophysiology, Leiden, the Netherlands

Johannes. J. Van Lieshout Department of Internal Medicine, Academic Medical Centre, University of Amsterdam, the Netherlands

P.A van Zwieten Departments of Pharmacotherapy and Cardiology, Academic Medical Centre, University of Amsterdam, Amsterdam, the Netherlands

Steven Vernino Department of Neurology, UT Southwestern Medical Center, Dallas, Texas, USA

Ekawat Vichayanrat Clinical Research Fellow, Autonomic and Neurovascular Medicine Unit, St Mary's Hospital, Imperial College London, UK

Angela Vincent Nuffield Department of Clinical Neurosciences, University of Oxford, John Radcliffe Hospital, Oxford, UK

B. Gunnar Wallin Institute of Neuroscience and Physiology, Sahlgrenska Academy at Göteborg University, Göteborg, Sweden

Gregor K. Wenning Department of Neurology, Medical University Innsbruck, Innsbruck, Austria

Wouter Wieling Department of Medicine, University of Amsterdam, the Netherlands

David L. Wingate Centre for Digestive Diseases, Barts and The London School of Medicine and Dentistry, The Wingate Institute, London, UK

Bill J. Yates University of Pittsburgh, Department of Otolaryngology, Eye and Ear Institute, Pittsburgh, PA, USA

Tim M. Young Neurovascular Medicine Unit, Faculty of Medicine, Imperial College London, St Mary's Hospital, UK

List of abbreviations

1-NMMA	l-NG-monomethyl-arginine
1-NOARG	l-NG nitro-arginine
3-NP	3-nitropropionic acid
4-DAMP	4-diphenyl-acetoxy-N-methyl-piperidine
5-HIAA	5-hydroxyin-doleacetic acid
5-HT	5-hydroxytryptamine, serotonin
6F-DOPA	6-[^{18}F]fluorodopamine
6-OHDA	6-hydroxydopamine
^{18}F-FDG	^{18}F-fluorodeoxyglucose
α-MSH	α-melanocyte stimulating hormone
AAAS	achalasia-addisonianism-alacrima syndrome gene
AADC	aromatic l-amino acid decarboxylase
AAG	autoimmune autonomic ganglionopathy
AASM	American Academy of Sleep Medicine
ABCD	albinism, black lock, cell migration disorder
ABP	arterial blood pressure
ACALD	adult cerebral adrenoleukodystrophy
ACE	angiotensin-converting enzyme
ACh	acetylcholine
AChE	acetylcholinesterase
AChR	acetylcholine receptor
ACTH	adrenocorticotropic hormone
AD	autonomic dysreflexia
ADC	apparent diffusion coefficient
ADRA2B	alpha-2B-adrenergic receptor
AF	autonomic failure
ALADIN	**A**lacrima, **A**chalasia, **A**drenal **I**nsufficiency, **N**eurological disorder
ALD	adrenoleukodystrophy
AMN	adrenomyeloneuropathy
AMP	adenosine monophosphate
AMPA	alpha-amino-3-hydroxy-5-methyl-4-isoxazole propionic acid
AMS	autonomic (neurally) mediated syncope
AngII	angiotensin II
ANNA-1	antineuronal nuclear antibody type 1
ANP	atrial natriuretic peptide
ANS	autonomic nervous system
AR	autoregressive modelling
ARIC	Atherosclerosis Risk in Communities study
ARMA	autoregressive moving average
AS	autonomic symptoms
ASIA	American Spinal Injury Association
ATP	adenosine triphosphate
AV	atrioventricular
AVNRT	atrioventricular nodal re-entrant tachycardia
AVRT	atrioventricular re-entrant tachycardia
AVP	argenine-vasopressin
BC	bulbocavernosus
BCR	bulbocavernosus reflex
BHS	breath-holding spells
BiPAP	bilevel positive airway pressure
BMI	body mass index
BMR	basal metabolic rate
BNST	bed nucleus of the stria terminalis
BOLD	blood oxygenation level dependent
BoNT/A	botulinum neurotoxin type A
BötC	Bötzinger Complex
BP	blood pressure
bpm	beats per minute
BPPV	benign paroxysmal positional vertigo
BPV	blood pressure variabilities
BRS	baroreflex sensitivity
CABG	coronary artery bypass grafting
cAMP	cyclic adenosine monophosphate
CAN	central autonomic network
CARP I	peripheral complex regional pain syndrome
CART	cocaine and amphetamine regulated transcript
CASS	composite autonomic scoring scale
CBD	corticobasal degeneration
CBF	cerebral blood flow
CBHS	cyanotic breath-holding spells
CBV	cerebral blood volume
CBV	central blood volume
CCEMG	corpus cavernosum electromyography
CCK	cholecystokinin
CCS	carotid sinus syndrome
CeNA	central nucleus of the amygdala
CG	coeliac ganglion
cGMP	cyclic guanosine monophosphate
CGRP	calcitonin-gene-related peptide
ChAT	choline acetyltransferase

CHF	congestive heart failure		DWI	diffusion-weighted imaging
CI	cardioinhibitory		DYN	dynorphin
CIPA	congenital insensitivity to pain with anhidrosis		EAAG	experimental autoimmune autonomic ganglionopathy
CISC	clean intermittent self-catheterization		ECA	evoked cavernous activity
CLQTS	congenital long QT syndrome		ECE1	endothelin-converting enzyme-1
CNP	2', 3'-cyclic nucleotide 3'-phosphodiesterase		ECG	electrocardiography/gram
CNS	central nervous system		ED	erectile dysfunction
cNTS	caudal nucleus tractus solitarii		EDA	electrodermal activity
CNV	contingent negative variation		EDRF	endothelium-derived relaxant factor
CO	cardiac output		EDN1	endothelin-1
COMT	catechol-O-methyltransferase		EDN3	endothelin-3
COPD	chronic obstructive pulmonary disease		EDNRB	endothelin receptor type B
COX-2	cyclooxygenase-2		EDRF	endothelium-derived relaxing factor
CPA	caudal pressor area		EDS	excessive daytime sleepiness
CPAP	continuous positive airway pressure		EEG	electroencephalography/gram
CPHPC	R-1-[6-[R-2-carboxy-pyrrolidin-1-yl]-6-oxo-hexanoyl]-pyrrolidine-2-carboxylic acid		EEMG	evoked electromyography/gram
			EGCG	epigallocatechin gallate
CRF	corticotropin releasing factor		EGG	electrogastrogram
CRH	corticotrophin releasing hormone		EGTA	[ethylene-bis(oxy-ethylenenitrilo)] tetraaceic acid
CRMP-5	collapsin response-mediated protein 5		EH	essential hypertension
CRPS I	complex regional pain syndrome type I		EIH	exercise-induced hypotension
CRPS	complex regional pain syndrome		EJP	excitatory junction potential
CS	carotid sinus		EM	electron microscopy
CSD	cortical spreading depression		EMG	electromyography
CSF	cerebrospinal fluid		e-NANC	excitatory non-adrenergic non-cholinergic nerves
CSH	carotid sinus hypersensitivity		ENCC	enteric neural crest-derived cells
CSM	carotid sinus massage		ENK	enkephalin
CSMG	coeliac–superior mesenteric		eNOS	endothelial nitric oxide synthase
CSN	carotid sinus nerve		ENS	enteric nervous system
CSP	carotid sinus pressure		EOG	electrooculography
CSS	carotid sinus syndrome		EPI	echoplanar imaging
CT	computerized tomography		EPSP	excitatory postsynaptic potential
CTZ	chemoreceptor trigger zone		ESCN	electrolyte-steroid-cardiopathy with necroses
CURS	Columbia University Rating Scale		ETS	endoscopic transthoracic sympathectomy
CVC	cutaneous vasoconstrictor		EUS	external urethral sphincter
CVLM	caudal ventrolateral medulla		FAP	familial amyloid polyneuropathy
DAT	dopamine active transporter		FAPWTR	Familial Amyloidotic Polyneuropathy World Transplant Registry
DBH	dopamine-beta-hydroxylase			
DBN	down-beat nystagmus		FEV_1	forced expiratory volume in one second
DBS	deep brain stimulation		FFI	fatal familial insomnia
DCCT	Diabetes Control and Complications study		FFT	fast Fourier transform
DDAVP	desmopressin		fMRI	functional magnetic resonance imaging
DEKAN	Deutsche Kardiale Autonome Neuropathie study		FRC	functional residual capacity
DHPG	dihydroxyphenylglycol		FVC	forced vital capacity
DIAD	Detection of Ischemia in Asymptomatic Diabetics study		GABA	γ-aminobutyric acid
			GAD	glutamic acid decarboxylase
DLBD	diffuse Lewy body disease		GCI	glial cytoplasmic inclusion
DLQI	Dermatology Life Quality Index		GDNF	glial cell line-derived neurotrophic factor
DM	diabetes mellitus		GEF	gastro-oesophageal reflux
DMH	dorsomedial hypothalamus		GHRF	growth hormone releasing factor
DMPP	dimethylphenylpiperazine		GIP	glucose-dependent insulinotropic peptide
DNP	dinitrophenol		GLP-1	glucagon-like peptide-1
DOCA salt	deoxycorticosterone acetate		GMP	guanosine monophosphate
DOPA	dihydroxyphenylalanine		GPi	globus pallidum interna
DOPAC	dihydroxyphenylacetic acid		GRP	gastrin-releasing peptide
DOPS	dihydroxyphenylserine		g-SSR	genital region sympathetic skin responses
DRD4	dopamine D4 receptor		GTN	glyceryl trinitrate
DRG	dorsal root ganglia		GTP	guanosine triphosphate
DTPA	diethylenetriamine pentaacetic acid			

HCM	hypertrophic cardiomyopathy	LN	Lewy neurite
HDL	high-density lipoprotein	L-NAME	NG-nitro-L-arginine-methyl-ester
HDR	head down rotation	LPL	lipoprotein lipase
HED	hydroxyephedrine	LQTS	long QT syndrome
HF	high frequency	Lst	lumbar spinothalamic
HGN	hypogastric nerve	LUT	lower urinary tract
HHIQ	Hyperhidrosis Impact Questionnaire©	LV	left ventricular
HLE	heat loss effectors	LVH	left ventricular hypertrophy
HPE	heat production effectors	MAO	monoamine oxidase
HR	heart rate	MAP	mean arterial blood pressure
HRV	heart rate variability	MARD	migraine anxiety related dizziness
HSAN	hereditary sensory and autonomic neuropathy	MBP	myelin basic protein
HSAN1	hereditary sensory and autonomic neuropathy type 1	MCA	middle cerebral artery
		mCPP	*meta*-chloro-phenylpiperazine
HSAN2	hereditary sensory and autonomic neuropathy type 2	MCP	middle cerebellar peduncle
		MD	Menière's disease
HSAN3	hereditary sensory and autonomic neuropathy type 3	MDD	major depressive disorder
		MDE	3,2-methylenedioxyethyamphetamine
HSAN4	hereditary sensory and autonomic neuropathy type 4	MDMA	3,4-methylenedioxymethamphetamine
		MEG	magnetic encephalographic
HSN1	hereditary sensory neuropathy type 1	MELAS	mitochondrial encephalomyopathy with lactic acidosis and stroke-like episodes
HSN2	hereditary sensory neuropathy type 2		
HSN3	hereditary sensory neuropathy type 3	MEN	multiple endocrine neoplasia
HSN4	hereditary sensory neuropathy type 4	MFB	medial forebrain bundle
HUT	head-up tilt	mGluR	metabotropic glutamate receptors
HVA	homovanillic acid	MHPG	3-methoxy-4-hydroxyphenylglycol
IC	ischiocavernosus	MIBG	meta-iodobenzyl guanidine
ICC	interstitial cells of Cajal	MMC	migrating motor complex
ICD	implantable cardioverter defibrillator	MPAP	mean pulmonary artery pressure
ICD	International Classification of Diseases	MPOA	medial preoptic area
IDDM	insulin-dependent diabetes mellitus	MPP+	1-methyl-4-phenylpyridinium ion
IEF	incontinence episode frequency	MPTP	1-methyl-4-phenyl-1,2,3,6-tetrahydropyridine
IGF-1	insulin-like growth factor-1	MR	motility regulating
IHD	ischaemic heart disease	MRA	magnetic resonance angiography
IJP	inhibitory junction potential	MRF	medullary reticular formation
IKBKAP	inhibitor of kappa light polypeptide gene enhancer in B cells, kinase complex-associated protein	MRI	magnetic resonance imaging
		MRS	magnetic resonance spectroscopy
ILAE	International League Against Epilepsy	MRV	magnetic resonance volumetry
ILR	implantable loop recorder	ms	milliseconds
IMG	inferior mesenteric ganglion	MSA	multiple system atrophy
IML	intermediolateral	MSH	melanocyte-stimulating hormone
IMN	intermesenteric nerves	MSLT	multiple sleep latency test
i-NANC	inhibitory non-adrenergic non-cholinergic	MSNA	muscular sympathetic nerve activity
interleukin-1	IL-1	MTR	magnetic transfer ratios
IP3	inositol triphosphate	MV	migrainous vertigo
IPD	idiopathic Parkinson's disease	MVC	muscle vasoconstrictor
IPPV	intermittent positive pressure ventilation	MWT	maintenance of wakefulness test
IPSP	inhibitory postsynaptic potential	NAA	N-acetyl aspartate
ISN	inferior splanchnic nerves	NAD	neuroaxonal dystrophy
KA	kainate	NANC	non-adrenergic, non-cholinergic
L-DOPA	L-3,4-dihydroxyphenylalanine	NCAM	neural cell adhesion molecule
LB	Lewy bodies	NE	norepinephrine
LBD	Lewy body disorders	NEAD	non-epileptic attack disorder
LBNP	lower body negative pressure	NEFA	non-esterified fatty acids
LDS	labyrinthine defective subjects	NEP	neutral endopeptidase
LEMS	Lambert–Eaton myasthenic syndrome	NES	non-epileptic seizures
LF	low frequency	NF 1	neurofibromatosis type 1
LMD/MS	liquid chromatography tandem mass spectrometry with laser dissection	NGF	nerve growth factor
		NGFB	nerve growth factor, beta S subunit

NHE	sodium/hydrogen exchanger	PGP9.5	protein gene product 9.5
NIDDM	non-insulin-dependent diabetes mellitus	PHI	peptide histidine isoleucine
NIR	near-infrared	PHM	peptide histidine methionine
NK-1	neurokinin 1	PHOX2B	paired-like homeobox 2B
NK-1-L-I	neurokinin-1 receptor-like-immunoreactive	PKA	protein kinase A
NKA	neurokinin A	PKC	protein kinase C
NMB	neuromedin B	PLMS	periodic limb movements in sleep
NMB-IR	neuromedin B immunoreactive	PLP	proteolipid protein
NMDA	N-methyl-D-aspartate	PMC	pontine micturition centre
NMN	normetanephrine	PNES	psychogenic non-epileptic seizures
NMS	non-motor symptoms	PNMT	phenylethanolamine-N-methyltransferase
nNOS	neuronal nitric oxide synthase	PNS	parasympathetic nervous system
nNOS	neuronal nitric oxide synthase	POAH	preoptic area, anterior hypothalamus and septum
NNP	nucleated neuronal profiles		
NO	nitric oxide	POTS	postural orthostatic tachycardia syndrome
NOS	nitric oxide synthase	PPH	postprandial hypotension
NPT	nocturnal penile tumescence	PPS	plasma protein solutions
NPY	neuropeptide Y	PRA	plasma renin activity
NREM	non-rapid eye movement (sleep)	PRF	pontine reticular formation
NRS	numerical rating scale	PRV	pseudorabies virus
NSAID	non-steroidal anti-inflammatory drug	PSD	power spectral density
NST	non-shivering thermogenesis	PSG	polysomnography
NT- proBNP	N-terminal pro-brain natriuretic peptide	PSOI	post-spaceflight orthostatic intolerance
NTRK1	neurotrophic tyrosine kinase receptor type 1	PSP	progressive supranuclear palsy
NTS	nucleus tractus solitarius; nucleus of the solitary tract	PSSR	penile sympathetic skin response
		PTCA	percutaneous transluminal coronary angioplasty
OBT	octanoid acid breath test	PVN	paraventricular nucleus
ODQ	1H-[1,2,4]-oxadiazolo[4,3-a]quinoxalin-l-one	QA	quinolinic acid
OGD	oesophago-gastric-duodenoscopy	QOL	quality of life
OH	orthostatic hypotension	QSART	quantitative sudomotor axon reflex test
OLMA	oculoleptomeningeal amyloidosis	RAGE	receptor for advanced glycation end products
OPC	olivopontocerebellar	RAR	rapidly adapting receptors
OPCA	olivopontocerebellar atrophy	RAS	reflex anoxic seizures/ reflex asystolic syncope
OSA	obstructive sleep apnoea	RBD	REM behaviour disorder
OSAS	obstructive sleep apnoea syndrome	rCBF	regional cerebral blood flow
OVAR	off-vertical axis rotation	rCMRGlc	resting regional cerebral glucose metabolism
OVLT	organum vasculosum laminae terminalis	RCSM	right carotid sinus massage
PA	primary aldosteronism	RET	rearranged during transfection proto-oncogene
PACAP	pituitary adenylate cyclase-activating peptide	RF	radiofrequency
PAF	pure autonomic failure	RGC	retrograde giant contraction
PAG	periaqueductal grey matter	ROI	region-of-interest
PAWP	pulmonary artery wedge pressure	RSNA	renal sympathetic nerve activity
PBN	parabrachial nucleus	RTPCR	reverse transcriptase polymerase chain reaction
pCO_2	arterial carbon dioxide partial pressure	RTX	resiniferatoxin
PCR	polymerase chain reaction	RV	residual volume
PD	Parkinson's disease	RVH	renovascular hypertension
PDE5	phosphodiesterase V	RVLM	rostral ventrolateral medulla
PDE5i	phosphodiesterase V inhibitors	SAECG	signal-averaged electrocardiogram
PE	phase encoding	SAP	serum amyloid protein
PEA	prolonged expiratory apnoea	SAR	slowly adapting receptors
PEEP	positive end-expiratory ventilation	SCA	spinocerebellar ataxias
PEP	pudendal evoked potentials	SCD	sudden cardiac death
PEPD	paroxysmal extreme pain disorder	SCG	superior cervical ganglia
PET	positron emission tomography	SCG	sympathetic chain ganglia
PEV	posturally evoked vomiting	SCI	spinal cord injury
PFT	pulmonary function tests	SCL	skin conductance leve
PGAD	persistent genital arousal disorder	SCLC	small-cell lung carcinoma
PGE1	prostaglandin E1	SCN	suprachiasmatic nucleus
PGE2	prostaglandin E2	SCR	skin conductance response

SDAAM	standard deviation of 5-minute median atrial-atrial intervals
SDB	sleep-disordered breathing
SDH	succinate dehydrogenase
SDNN	standard deviation of normal-to-normal interval
SDS	Shy–Drager syndrome
SDS	sodium dodecyl sulphate
SERT	serotonin reuptake transporter
SFO	subfornical organ
SHR	spontaneously hypertensive rat
SIDS	sudden infant death syndrome
SIF	small intensely fluorescent
SIP	sympathetically independent pain
SKP	skin potential
SkSNA	skin sympathetic nerve activity
SKT	skin temperature
SkVR	skin vasomotor reflex
SLC6A2	solute carrier family 6 (neurotransmitter transporter, noradrenaline), member 2
SLD	sublaterodorsal
SM	sudomotor
SMC	smooth muscle cell
SMD	space and motion discomfort
SMG	superior mesenteric ganglion
SMP	space and motion phobia
SMP	sympathetically maintained pain
SMS	space motion sickness
SNA	sympathetic nerve activity
SNc	substantia nigra pars compacta
SND	striatonigral degeneration
SND	sympathetic nerve discharge
SNS	sympathetic nervous system
SOX10	SRY-Box 10
SP	substance P
SPACE	single potential analysis of cavernosal EMG
SPECT	single photon emission computed tomography
SplSNA	splanchnic sympathetic nerve activity
SPN	sympathetic preganglionic neuron
SPTLC1	serine palmitoyltransferase, long-chain base subunit 1
SSNA	skin sympathetic nerve activity
SSR	sympathetic skin responses
SSRI	selective serotonin reuptake inhibitors
SSTR2	somatostatin receptor type 2
STN	subthalamic nucleus
StrN	striatonigral

SUD	sudden unexpected death
SUNCT	short-lasting unilateral neuralgiform headache attacks with conjunctival injection and tearing
SUNDS	sudden unexplained nocturnal death syndrome
SVT	supraventricular tachycardia
TCD	transcranial Doppler
TCS	transcranial sonography
TDP	torsade de pointes
TH	tyrosine hydroxylase
TIA	transient ischaemic attack
TLC	total lung capacity
TLOC	transient loss of consciousness
TNC	trigeminal nucleus caudalis
TPPP	tubulin polymerization promoting protein
TSH	thyroid stimulating hormone
TST	thermoregulatory sweat test
TTR	transthyretin
UAER	urinary albumin excretion rate
UCP1	uncoupling protein 1
UG	urogenital
UKPDS	UK Prospective Diabetes Study
UPDRS	Unified Parkinson's Disease Rating Scale
UPSIT	University of Pennsylvania Smell Inventory Test
VATS	video-assisted thorascopic surgery
VATS	video-assisted thorascopic sympathectomy
VBM	voxel based morphometry
VGKC	voltage-gated potassium channels
VGLUT	vesicular glutamate transporter
VHF	very high frequency
VHL	von Hippel-Lindau
VIP	vasoactive intestinal peptide
VLCFA	very long-chain fatty acids
VLM	ventrolateral medulla
VLPO	ventrolateral preoptic
VMA	vanillylmandelic acid
VPA	vaginal pulse amplitude
VPpc	ventroposterior medial parvicellular
VRG	ventral respiratory group
VT	ventricular tachyardia
VVC	visceral vasoconstrictor
WISC	Wechsler Intelligence Scale for Children
WPRL	Wellcome Physiological Research Laboratories
W-P-W	Wolff–Parkinson–White syndrome
X-ALD	X-linked adrenoleukodystrophy
XE^{133}	xenon-133

Introduction

Introduction and classification of autonomic disorders

Roger Bannister and Christopher J. Mathias

The autonomic nervous system innervates every organ in the body, creating, as Galen suggested, 'sympathy' between the various parts of the body. It has as complex a neural organization in the brain, spinal cord, and periphery as the somatic nervous system, but remains largely involuntary or automatic. Claude Bernard wrote 'nature thought it provident to remove these important phenomena from the capriciousness of an ignorant will'. Langley, who in 1898 first proposed the term 'autonomic nervous system', based his experiments on the blocking action of nicotine at synapses in ganglia. In 1921 Loewi discovered 'Vagusstoff', which was released by stimulation of the vagus nerve and proved to be acetylcholine. In the same year Cannon discovered that 'sympathin', later shown to be noradrenaline, was produced by stimulation of the sympathetic trunk. The basis was laid, therefore, for Dale's distinction between cholinergic and adrenergic transmission in the autonomic nervous system. A detailed history of the autonomic nervous system is provided after this chapter.

Peripheral autonomic function

The peripheral autonomic nervous system, an efferent system, is made up of neurons that lie outside the central nervous system and are concerned with visceral innervation. Both sympathetic and parasympathetic systems have preganglionic neurons in the brain and spinal cord arranged as shown in Fig. 1. The afferent limbs of autonomic reflexes may lie in any afferent nerve. The preganglionic sympathetic fibres are myelinated and leave the spinal roots as white rami communicantes and synapse in the ganglia of the sympathetic. Unmyelinated postganglionic fibres rejoin the anterior spinal roots by the arrangement shown in Fig. 2, although some sympathetic fibres traverse the paravertebral ganglia and synapse in more peripheral ganglia.

The transmitter at all preganglionic terminals is acetylcholine, which is not blocked by atropine (the nicotinic effect), whereas the action of acetycholine at the distal end of the cholinergic postganglionic fibres is blocked by atropine (the muscarinic effect). Muscarinic receptors are now subdivided into at least three subtypes. Noradrenaline is the principal transmitter for postganglionic sympathetic nerves, but there are a few areas where there is cholinergic transmission. These exceptions include sudomotor nerves, putative vasodilator fibres to muscle, and the adrenal medulla, which is innervated by preganglionic (cholinergic) fibres and which itself secretes both adrenaline and noradrenaline. Noradrenaline is stored in the postganglionic nerve terminals and is released by nerve activity or by sympathomimetic drugs, which may act partly indirectly on the ganglia or more centrally (e.g. ephedrine and amphetamine), or on the terminals (e.g. phenylephrine or tyramine). The different actions of noradrenaline and adrenaline are caused by relative effects on different receptors. α-adrenoceptors may be either postsynaptic (α_1) or presynaptic (α_2); the latter when stimulated decrease the release of the transmitter. α_2-adrenoceptors are also present at the postsynaptic level and cause vasoconstriction when stimulated with agonists. β-adrenoceptors mediate vasodilatation (especially in skeletal muscles), increase the rate and force of the heart (with a tendency to arrhythmias), and cause bronchial relaxation. They are further subdivided into β_1-adrenoceptors, mediating the chronotropic cardiac action of isoprenaline, and β_2-adrenoceptors, which are responsible for most of the peripheral effects of β-adrenergic stimulation. Though autonomic sensitivity phenomena were first described more than a century ago, and the research was summarized by Cannon and Rosenblueth in 1949 under the title, *The supersensitivity of denervated structures: a law of denervation*. Attention since then has concentrated on the 'up' and 'down' regulation of receptor function depending on the availability of the transmitter.

The cells of the autonomic nervous system tend to act in conjunction and this is achieved mainly by specialized intercellular junctions at the ganglion cells, which have been demonstrated by electron microscopy and freeze fracture techniques. The autonomic ganglia also contain small intensely fluorescent cells (SIF cells) that contain many peptides, thought to act as modulators and transmitters at synaptic sites. Substance P, vasoactive intestinal peptide (VIP), encephalins, and somatostatin have all been identified in autonomic ganglia although their precise role in control of nerve transmission is not yet known.

The previously held distinction between cholinergic and catecholaminergic cells, underlying the dual hypothesis of antagonism in the autonomic nervous system, is no longer tenable. Immature ganglion cells in culture contain both acetylcholine and catecholamines. Sympathetic ganglia have about 45% of acetylcholine-containing neurons in which non-adrenergic, non-cholinergic (NANC) transmission is now accepted. Within any central pathway

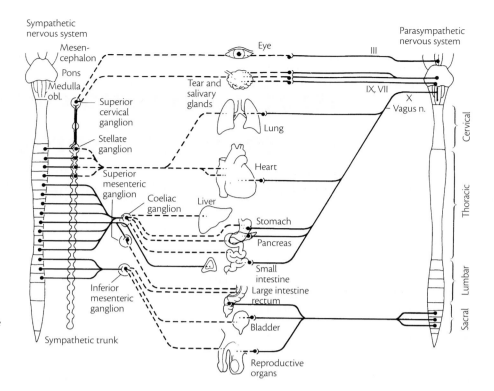

Fig. 1 Scheme outlining details of the cranio-sacral parasympathetic and thoraco-lumbar sympathetic outflow to various target organs (from Jänig 1995).

there is no simple consistency of a single transmitter and some cells have multiple transmitters: posterior root ganglion cells, for example, have been found to have as many as 10 neuropeptides and putative transmitters. After birth, sweat glands change from adrenergic to cholinergic sympathetic innervation, whereas innervation of some gut structures is switched from sympathetic to cholinergic mechanisms. Presynaptic cholinergic endings may affect noradrenergic sympathetic transmission, and noradrenaline may act not only directly as a transmitter but indirectly by modulating the effect of acetylcholine, as has been shown peripherally

where small doses of adrenaline and noradrenaline facilitate transmission but larger doses inhibit it.

Central control of the autonomic nervous system

The past decade has seen considerable advances in our understanding of the central autonomic network, because of a variety of advances mainly relating to non-invasive neuroimaging. These have enabled precise assessment of the central lesion in various disorders, thus enabling the linkage of specific lesions with functional deficits. Positron emission tomography (PET) and functional magnetic resonance imaging (fMRI) studies in normal healthy individuals have further aided delineation of the neural substrates subserving autonomic function (Critchley et al., 2011). This will be described further in Chapter 12, with description below of the functions of the hypothalamus.

The hypothalamus can be considered the 'highest' level of integration of autonomic function. It remains under the influence of the cortex and the group of structures known as the 'limbic system', which includes the olfactory areas, the hippocampus and amygdaloid complex, the cingulate cortex, and the septal area. These regions of the brain regulate the hypothalamus and are critical for emotional and affective expression. In phylogenetic development the limbic system represents the older or palaeomammalian cortex as opposed to the neomammalian cortex. Its function is thought to be concerned with levels below cognitive behaviour and inductive and deductive reasoning, though it nevertheless is concerned with a feeling of individuality and identity. It analyses the significance of the input of sensation to the organism in relation to the instinctive drives that promote the perpetuation of the individual by satisfying hunger, thirst, and sexual needs.

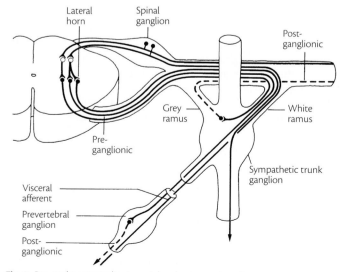

Fig. 2 Pre- and post-ganglionic peripheral autonomic pathways.

The hypothalamus is also concerned with maintaining homeostasis against a changing environment and ensures the propagation of the species by sexual and parental drives, which can at times override the more selfish self-perpetuating drives of the individual. The essence of its function is choice of patterns of behaviour based on sensory information. As it overlaps both with sensory and motor systems it is essential for many aspects of memory and learning. The autonomic nervous system and many metabolic functions are under the control of the limbic system by means of nerve centres, many of which are situated in the hypothalamus, lying ventrally to the thalamus and constituting the floor of the third ventricle. The hypothalamus contains a large number of scattered ganglion cells, which have been differentiated into a number of nuclei (Appenzeller and Oribe 1997).

The hypothalamus controls the autonomic nervous system in two ways, by means of the pituitary and hence other endocrine glands and by direct descending nervous pathways. Despite these descending pathways, some regions of the brainstem are to some extent autonomous and function in animals after pontine section of the brainstem. These include cardiac and respiratory function and 'centres' for vomiting and micturition, but under natural circumstances cardiovascular responses never occur in isolation but accompany the processes of exercise, digestion, sexual function, and temperature regulation. The integration of these changes takes place in the hypothalamus. The main course taken by descending sympathetic fibres from the hypothalamus is uncrossed and by way of the lateral tegmentum of the brainstem and lateral medullary formation. Some fibres end directly on the intermediolateral column cells, while others synapse in the reticular formation.

Diseases of the autonomic nervous system

The lesions of the nervous system in autonomic failure, with their widespread consequences, are, in Claude Bernard's terms, 'real experiments by which physicians and physiologists profit'. Some may complain that nature is an imprecise experimentalist! The study of individuals with rare disorders can sometimes throw much light on the subtle and complex integration of the autonomic nervous system (Mathias 1995, 2010). An example is the disease with a specific enzyme fault, dopamine-beta-hydroxylase deficiency (Chapter 49), which in addition to aiding our understanding of the specific role of noradrenaline in autonomic function, has also resulted in specific therapy of this disease (L-threo-dihydroxy-phenylserine, L-DOPS, Droxidopa), which also has now been used successfully in patients with other forms of neurogenic orthostatic hypotension, such as due to pure autonomic failure, multiple system atrophy, and also autonomic failure associated with Parkinson's disease (PD) (Mathias 2008). Advances in neuroimmunology have lead to the identification of antibodies directed specifically to nicotinic acetylcholine receptors, leading to successful treatments that reverse autonomic failure (Chapter 52). The syndromes of chronic autonomic failure also offer an example of the system degenerations that are so common in neurology and are yet so baffling. We need to find some common biological basis for this curious selective vulnerability. If we can do this, we shall be closer to finding an effective treatment, not only for these particular diseases but possibly also for a wider range of disabling progressive degenerative diseases of the nervous system.

The systematic application of physiological techniques of study to patients with autonomic failure started in the 1960s. Research interest in postural hypotension, the usual presenting symptom of autonomic failure, was stimulated by its occurrence after the weightlessness of space travel. Since then there have been striking advances in the investigation and classification of the syndromes of autonomic failure that were until recently both confused and confusing. Peripheral neuropathies with an autonomic component have long been recognized, particularly in diabetes, alcoholism, and amyloidosis. Sharpey-Schafer and Taylor (1960) showed that the sympathetic vasoconstrictor pathway to the hands was intact in diabetic autonomic neuropathy, and they therefore attributed the absence of circulatory reflexes and the postural hypotension to an afferent lesion. Though an afferent lesion could not be excluded, their interpretation was probably incorrect because the sympathetic efferent pathway to resistance vessels is often defective in patients with diabetes and the patchiness of lesions on the efferent side is now appreciated.

A large section of this book is concerned with the chronic or primary neurological disorders in which the autonomic nervous system is selectively involved by both preganglionic and postganglionic neuronal degeneration (Shy and Drager 1960, Johnson et al. 1966, Bannister et al. 1967). Some might doubt the worth of such serious attention given to rare diseases but there are many precedents to show that just such studies of rare disease often lead to the recognition of an entirely new group of disorders of which other examples then are found. It is certain that the detailed study of these diseases by the extensive biochemical, physiological and histochemical techniques now available has yielded a rich harvest of knowledge, much of it unexpected, which can now be applied more widely.

The detailed studies of autonomic failure are complemented by sections of the book that are devoted to particular diseases, such as diabetes mellitus (Chapter 53) in which autonomic disturbances occur sooner or later. Diabetes is overwhelmingly more common than other forms of autonomic dysfunction, and rapid advances have now been made such that the methods of testing, most of which were pioneered in relation to autonomic failure, are being applied to the even more complex disturbances in diabetes. There are also other large groups of patients with autonomic symptoms; first, patients with parkinsonian symptoms who may have multiple system atrophy (MSA); second, the elderly; and third, patients taking drugs that affect autonomic function.

In this edition there are more detailed descriptions of autonomic disorders in which there are no fixed or irreversible autonomic lesions, but where the clinical features result from a usually short-lived, intermittent dysfunction with no residual autonomic abnormalities detectable between episodes. These now account for a large proportion of patients referred to our two London Autonomic Units and include the different varieties of autonomic (neurally) mediated syncope (AMS), the postural tachycardia syndrome (PoTS) and essential hyperhidrosis (Chapters 32, 56, and 61), some of which affect younger individuals.

First symptoms of autonomic failure

Most forms of autonomic failure are insidious in their onset, with mild symptoms that are concealed for years because of autonomic or other compensatory mechanisms. As Cannon (1929) pointed out, this system can respond to many and varied stresses from the internal and external environment in ways that conceal its dysfunction. When man first took it upon himself millions of years ago to stand on his two legs he imposed great strains on the cardiovascular control needed to protect him against the effect of pooling of blood in the lower extremities. Postural hypotension occurring in emotional syncope raises the intriguing teleological question of whether it has evolutionary significance in avoiding danger by a sudden fall into the horizontal position and the simulation of death. However, a true fainting attack such as vasovagal syncope, as opposed to other causes of transient loss of consciousness, requires an intact autonomic nervous system, although persistent postural hypotension is the cardinal feature of autonomic failure (Mathias and Galizia 2010). Patients may start with mild symptoms of vague weakness, postural dizziness, or faintness, which can very easily be overlooked, or result in erroneous referral to a psychiatrist or cardiologist. The crux of the diagnosis is the measurement of blood pressure when standing rather than lying, still often neglected, which can, like the tip of an iceberg, reveal a much more complex underlying autonomic disturbance. In certain circumstances postural hypotension may be unmasked by food, alcohol, or exercise (Chapter 28). The blood pressure control mechanisms at the lower end of the scale are just as elaborate and fascinating as those that cause the more commonly studied problems of hypertension, though the study of these patients with *hypotension* has in fact thrown light on the mechanisms of *hypertension*.

Some patients with autonomic failure first have urinary bladder symptoms or impotence, not postural hypotension. In addition to the group of patients with autonomic failure alone, 'pure autonomic failure', there is a second group of patients that may present with symptoms of autonomic failure but within months also develop other neurological symptoms, usually with parkinsonism or cerebellar manifestations. However, there may be subtle features that suggest that the parkinsonism is atypical, with a predominance of rigidity and akinesis over tremor, or the presence of mild pyramidal signs. Such parkinsonian patients may develop marked postural hypotension when treated with levodopa or may fail to respond to this drug. Some may have additional bulbar involvement. These features raise the possibility of more widespread involvement of the central nervous system and point to the diagnosis of MSA.

Presentation in intermittent autonomic dysfunction

AMS may present at any age, with an increased incidence of vasovagal syncope around the teenage years; thus the vasovagal variety of AMS often occurs during teenage years, unlike carotid sinus hypersensitivity, which is more likely in individuals over 50 years of age (Thijs et al. 2004, Humm and Mathias 2006, Low and Mathias 2009). The symptoms can vary, with little warning in some but not so in others, enabling the latter to take corrective action. There is a female predominance in vasovagal syncope, similar to that in the increasingly recognized group with PoTS, where the onset may be linked to infection, surgery, physical trauma or to stress. These patients often are young (<40 years of age) and fainting as a feature of orthostatic intolerance often occurs initially, but is less of a problem later as there are recognizable warning signs, often palpitations, especially when upright, after exercise, and sometimes in response to food. A number of individuals with PoTS

also have the joint hypermobility syndrome/Ehlers Danlos III and in a subset of this group there are associated features such as posturally induced headache, bladder involvement (inadequate emptying or retention, frequency and polyuria), and gastrointestinal disturbances (acid regurgitation, abdominal distension, and diarrhoea or constipation) that are often labelled as the irritable bowel syndrome (Mathias et al. 2012). Further details are in Chapter 61.

Classification

In this chapter an historical approach to classification with further stratification into two major groups, autonomic disorders that result from damage to the autonomic pathways that are often but not necessarily irreversible, and the intermittent disorders where the autonomic nervous system is essentially normal except for malfunction at particular times (Mathias, 2009). A further approach to classification is added based upon the natural history of the autonomic disorder.

Accurate diagnosis is essential for proper management of autonomic failure (AF) but in attempting to classify autonomic disease there is a philosophical point to be borne in mind. As in much of medicine, we use a mixed diagnostic classification. There are localized disorders (Table 1) and more generalized disorders (Tables 2a and 2b); drugs are an important cause of autonomic dysfunction (Table 3). We have a list of diseases of largely known pathology, such as diabetes, and we make a diagnosis of 'secondary' AF when abnormal tests in life point to a structural disturbance of autonomic reflexes and pathways in patients with a specific disease. Other patients, without certainly known pathology in common, share certain autonomic symptoms and, from tests in life and observation of similar patients after death, we choose to use the word 'primary' disease (Table 2). In such patients tests can hardly be said to prove a disease but this is the only way we can place patients in different categories and hope, by research, to locate the lesions more precisely and hence improve their treatment.

Autonomic fibres are also damaged secondarily in a variety of medical disorders, most commonly in diabetes and alcoholism, but also in a wide range of acute, subacute, and chronic peripheral neuropathies (Table 2a). This is discussed later (Chapter 51).

Table 1 Examples of localized autonomic disorders

◆ Horner syndrome
◆ Holmes–Adie pupil
◆ Crocodile tears (Bogorad syndrome)
◆ Gustatory sweating (Frey's syndrome)
◆ Reflex sympathetic dystrophy
◆ Idiopathic palmar or axillary hyperhidrosis
◆ Chagas disease (*Trypanosoma cruzi*)*
◆ Surgical procedures#
◆ Sympathectomy (regional)
◆ Vagotomy and gastric drainage procedures in 'dumping' syndrome
◆ Organ denervation following transplantation (heart, lungs)

* Listed here because the disease targets specifically intrinsic cholinergic plexuses in the heart and gut.

Surgery also may cause other localized disorders, such as Frey syndrome after parotid surgery.

Table 2a Outline classification of autonomic disorders

Primary
Acute/subacute dysautonomias
◆ Pure pan-dysautonomia
◆ Pan-dysautonomia with neurological features
◆ Pure cholinergic dysautonomia
Chronic autonomic failure syndromes
◆ Pure autonomic failure
◆ Multiple system atrophy (Shy–Drager syndrome)
◆ Parkinson's disease with autonomic failure
◆ Lewy body disease
Secondary
Congenital
◆ Nerve growth factor deficiency
Hereditary
◆ Autosomal dominant trait
◆ Familial amyloid neuropathy
Autosomal recessive trait
◆ Familial dysautonomia—Riley–Day syndrome
◆ Dopamine-beta-hydroxylase deficiency
Metabolic diseases
◆ Diabetes mellitus
◆ Chronic renal failure
◆ Chronic liver disease
◆ Alcohol-induced
Inflammatory
◆ Guillain–Barré syndrome
◆ Transverse myelitis
Infections
◆ Bacterial—tetanus
◆ Viral—HIV infection
Neoplasia
◆ Brain tumours—especially of third ventricle or posterior fossa
◆ Paraneoplastic—especially adenocarcinoma of lung and pancreas
Surgery
◆ Vagotomy and drainage procedures—'dumping syndrome'
Trauma
◆ Cervical and high thoracic spinal cord transection
Intermittent autonomic dysfunction (see also Table 2b)
Drugs, chemical toxins (see also Table 3)
◆ By direct effects
◆ By causing a neuropathy

Table 2b Examples of intermittent autonomic dysfunction

Autonomic mediated syncope (AMS)
◆ Vasovagal syncope
◆ Carotid sinus hypersensitivity
◆ Situational syncope
Postural tachycardia syndrome (PoTS)
Initial orthostatic hypotension
Autonomic dysfunction in spinal cord injury
Essential (idiopathic) hyperhidrosis

Table 3 Drugs, chemicals, poisons and toxins causing autonomic dysfunction

Decreasing sympathetic activity
Centrally acting
◆ Clonidine
◆ Methyldopa
◆ Reserpine
◆ Barbiturates
◆ Anaesthetics
Peripherally acting
◆ Sympathetic nerve ending (guanethidine, bethanadine)
◆ α-adrenoceptor blockade (phenoxybenzamine)
◆ β-adrenoceptor blockade (propranolol)
Increasing sympathetic activity
◆ Amphetamines
◆ Releasing noradrenaline (tyramine)
◆ Uptake blockers (imipramine)
◆ Monoamine oxidase-A inhibitors (tranylcypromine)
◆ β-adrenoceptor stimulants (isoprenaline)
Decreasing parasympathetic activity
◆ Antidepressants (imipramine)
◆ Tranquillizers (phenothiazines)
◆ Antidysrhythmics (disopyramide)
◆ Anticholinergics (atropine, probanthine, benztropine)
◆ Toxins (botulinum)
Increasing parasympathetic activity
◆ Cholinomimetics (carbachol, bethanechol, pilocarpine, mushroom poisoning)
◆ Anticholinesterases
◆ Reversible carbonate inhibitors (pyridostigmine, neostigmine)
◆ Organophosphorus inhibitors (parathion)
Miscellaneous
◆ Alcohol, thiamine (vitamin B_1 deficiency)
◆ Vincristine, perhexiline maleate
◆ Thallium, arsenic, mercury
◆ Mercury poisoning (pink disease)
◆ Ciguatera toxicity
◆ Jellyfish and marine animal venoms, scombroid poisoning
◆ First dose of certain drugs (prazosin, captopril, propranolol)
◆ Withdrawal of chronically used drugs (clonidine, opiates, alcohol)

Adapted from Mathias (2010). See also Chapter 71.

We can now consider the more complex problem of the classification of the group of patients in whom AF appears to result from a primary or unexplained selective neuronal degeneration. This may occur in a 'pure' form without any other neurological signs. Or it may occur in association with two quite different degenerations of the nervous system, MSA, and PD.

Historically, the first reported cases of AF were described by Bradbury and Eggleston (1925) as 'idiopathic orthostatic hypotension' because of their presenting feature. This term is misleading because it stresses only one feature of AF and ignores the more usually associated neurological disturbances of urinary bladder control, sexual function, and sweating, and also because the word 'idiopathic' implies that it is a single disease entity, which though probable is not proven. The term 'pure autonomic failure' (PAF) is now generally accepted for this syndrome.

Two cases now recognized as AF with MSA were described by Shy and Drager in 1960 and it is appropriate to quote from their original description.

> "The full syndrome comprises the following features: orthostatic hypotension, urinary and rectal incontinence, loss of sweating, iris atrophy, external ocular palsies, rigidity, tremor, loss of associated movements, impotence, the findings of an atonic bladder and loss of rectal sphincter tone, fasciculations, wasting of distal muscles, evidence of a neuropathic lesion in the electromyogram that suggests involvement of the anterior horn cells, and the finding of a neuropathic lesion in the muscle biopsy. The date of onset is usually in the 5th to 7th decade of life."

Though they noted degeneration of the intermediolateral column cells in their pathological report, credit for first specifically linking this with the presenting features of postural hypotension rests with Johnson et al. (1966). At this stage olivopontocerebellar atrophy had not been linked with AF.

AF was also described in patients with otherwise apparently typical PD (Fichefet et al. 1965, Vanderhaegen et al. 1970, Muthane and Mathias 2011, Iodice et al. 2011). Such cases pathologically had hyaline eosinophilic cytoplasmic neuronal inclusions known as Lewy bodies, also present in PD (Chapters 41, 42, 44 and 45). It is an important fact that Lewy bodies, some of which may contain, apart from neurofilament proteins and ubiquitin, catecholamine degeneration products, are usually also found in the brains of patients with PAF, without parkinsonian features, but very rarely in patients with MSA. This evidence, discussed below, tends to separate patients with AF into two groups: first, pathologically proven-MSA without Lewy bodies and second, PAF, and AF with PD, with Lewy bodies.

It must be recognized that at an early stage an accurate prognosis of primary AF cannot be given. It may remain as PAF for a few years, relatively static, or in time it may also come to be associated either with PD or MSA; with care the earliest features of the other condition may be detected clinically. Conversely, the earliest features of AF may be detected later in some patients with PD or MSA. For example, Miyazaki (1978) has shown that careful study of cases of non-familial olivopontocerebellar atrophy with significant postural hypotension shows a high incidence of urinary, pyramidal, and extrapyramidal symptoms and signs, whereas familial cases, without postural hypotension, very rarely have these additional features.

There is evidence that virtually all patients with primary AF as opposed to secondary AF, studied at post-mortem, have severe loss of intermediolateral column cells, the final common pathway cell for the sympathetic nervous system (Chapter 41). It is becoming more probable that the pathological process, whether viral, biochemical, immunological, or of some other kind, that leads to this loss of intermediolateral column cells differs significantly in PAF (and probably in AF with PD), from that in AF with MSA. In PAF there appears to be an additional loss of ganglionic neurons (Chapter 42) that are relatively intact in MSA. This suggests the existence of a more distal process in PAF than in MSA. The hypothesis that at least one of the lesions in PAF is also more distal accords with the evidence that, in

general, plasma noradrenaline levels are lower in PAF than in MSA (Chapter 22). This view now finds support from neuroendocrine studies (Kimber et al. 1997) and MRI and PET brain scans of patients with PAF, which have failed to show evidence of lesions of the central autonomic nervous system (Chapter 40).

When considering the effects of treatment, so that like is compared with like, it is vital to diagnose patients as precisely as possible on the basis of physiological, pharmacological, biochemical, and neuro-imaging findings, even though the ultimate criterion of diagnosis is the post-mortem pathological findings. Moreover, it seems probable that there are a number of different types of sympathetic terminal dysfunction in AF, which may be the consequence of pathological processes that differ in degree or kind (Nanda et al. 1977, Bannister et al. 1979, Man in't Veld et al. 1987, Mathias et al. 1990). Just as the defects of nicotinic and muscarinic receptors in human disease have proved to be far more complex than ever was expected (Bannister and Hoyes 1981), it is probable that disturbances of sympathetic receptors will also prove at least as complex (Fraser et al. 1981).

The evaluation and accurate diagnosis of the cause of autonomic symptoms is necessary in order to plan treatment. Even if specific treatment is not available this evaluation will make it easier to manage the patient in such a way that the quality of life can be maintained for as long as possible.

Intermittent autonomic disorders may present to a wide variety to specialities and disciplines. Patients with AMS may initially be seen by paediatricians (if vasovagal syncope), geriatricians (if carotid sinus hypersensitivity) or cardiologists (Low and Mathias 2009, Mathias 2010). A newer entity, initial orthostatic hypotension, has recently been described (Wieling et al. 2007); it remains to be determined to what extent this entity can be separated from the others with orthostatic intolerance. Patients with PoTS (Mathias et al. 2012) may be referred to cardiologists, and as no structural cardiac abnormality or arrhythmia is found may then be considered to have panic attacks. Patients with essential hyperhidrosis are often referred to endocrinologists, to exclude secondary and in particular hormonal causes of excessive sweating.

Table 4 Classification based on natural history and intervention

◆ Fixed and irreversible— pure autonomic failure, spinal cord injury
◆ Progressive and irreversible—multiple system atrophy
◆ Progressive but stoppable— familial amyloid polyneuropathy, diabetes mellitus
◆ Reversible—immune mediated autonomic neuropathies

Classification of disorders causing damage to the autonomic nervous system may also be considered as outlined in Table 4, which relates to prognosis based on their natural history and/or possible interventional measures.

References

Appenzeller, O. and Oribe, E. (1997). *The autonomic nervous system* (5th edn). Elsevier, Amsterdam.

Bannister, R., Ardill, L., and Fentem, P. (1967). Defective autonomic control of blood vessels in idiopathic orthostatic hypotension. *Brain* **90**, 725–46.

Bannister, R., Davies, I. B., Holly, E., Rosenthal, T., and Sever, P. (1979). Defective cardiovascular reflexes and supersensitivity to sympathomimetic drugs in autonomic failure. *Brain* **102**, 163–76.

Bannister, R., and Hoyes, A. D. (1981). Generalised smooth-muscle disease with defective muscarinic receptor function. *Br. Med. J.* **282**, 1015–18.

Bradbury, S., and Eggleston, C. (1925). Postural hypotension: a report of three cases. *Am. Heart J.* **1**, 73–86.

Cannon, W. B. (1929). Organisation for physiological homeostasis. *Physiol. Rev.* **9**, 399–431.

Cannon, W. B., and Rosenblueth, A. (1949). *The supersensitivity of denervated structures: a law of denervation.* MacMillan, New York.

Consensus statement on the definition of orthostatic hypotension, pure autonomic failure and multiple system atrophy. (1996). *Clin. Aut. Res.* **6**, 125–6.

Critchley, H. D., Nagai, Y., Gray, M. A., and Mathias C. J. (2011). Dissecting axes of autonomic control in humans: Insights from neuroimaging. *Auton Neurosci.* **26**, 34–42.

Fichefet, J. P., Sternon, J. E., Franken, L., Demanet, J. C., and Vanderhaegen, J. J. (1965). Etude anatomo-clinique d'un cas d'hypotension orthostatique 'idiopathique'. Considerations pathogenique. *Acta Cardiol.* **20**, 332–48.

Fraser, C. M., Venter, J. C., and Kaliner, M. (1981). Autonomic abnormalities and auto-antibodies to beta-adrenergic receptors. *New Engl. J. Med.* **305**, 1165–70.

Jänig, W. (1995). In *Physiologie des menschen* (Ed. R. F. Schmidt and G. Thews), 26th edn, pp. 340–69, Springer Verlag, Heidelberg, Berlin.

Humm, A., and Mathias, C. J. (2006). Unexplained syncope—is screening for carotid sinus hypersensitivity indicated in all patients aged over 40 years? *Journal of Neurology, Neurosurgery and Psychiatry*, **77**: 1267–70.

Iodice, V., Low, D. A., Vichayanrat, E., Mathias, C. J. (2011). Cardiovascular Autonomic Dysfunction in Parkinson's Disease and Parkinsonian Syndromes. In: Ebadi, M., Pfeiffer, R. F. (eds). *Parkinson's Disease.* CRC Press, Florida.

Johnson, R. H., Lee, G. de J., Oppenheimer, D. R., and Spalding, J. M. K. (1966). Autonomic failure with orthostatic hypotension due to intermediolateral column degeneration. *Quart. J. Med.* **35**, 276–92.

Kimber, J. R., Watson, L., and Mathias, C. J. (1997). Distinction of idiopathic Parkinson's disease from multiple system atrophy by stimulation of growth hormone release with clonidine. *Lancet* **349**, 1877–81.

Low, D. A. and Mathias, C. J. (2009). Syncope: Physiology, Pathophysiology and Aeromedical Implications. In: Nicholson, A. *The Neurosciences and the Practice of Aviation Medicine.* Farnham: Ashgate Publishing Ltd., Farnham.

Man in't Veld, A. J., Boomsa, H., Moleman, P., and Schalekamp, M. A. D. H. (1987). Congenital dopamine-beta-hydroxylase deficiency: a novel orthostatic syndrome. *Lancet* **i**, 183–7.

Mathias, C. J., Bannister, R., Cortelli, P., Heslop, K., Polak, J. M., Raimbach, S., Springall, D. R., and Watson, L. (1990). Clinical, autonomic and therapeutic observations in two siblings with postural hypotension and sympathetic failure due to an inability to synthesize noradrenaline from dopamine because of a deficiency of dopamine beta hydroxylase. *Quart. J. Med.*, New Series **75**, 617–33.

Mathias, C. J. (1995). The classification and nomenclature of autonomic disorders—ending chaos, resolving conflict and hopefully achieving clarity. *Clin. Aut. Res.* **5**, 307–10.

Mathias, C. J. (2008). L-dihydroxyphenylserine (Droxidopa) in the treatment of orthostatic hypotension: the European experience. *Clin Auton Res.* **18**, 25–9.

Mathias, C. J. (2009). Autonomic Dysfunction. In Clarke, C., Howard, R., Rossor, M., Shorvon, S. (eds). *Neurology: A Queen Square Textbook.* 1st Edition ed. Chichester: Wiley Blackwell. p. 871–92.

Mathias, C. J. (2010). Disorders of the Autonomic Nervous System. In Warrell, D. A., Cox, T. M., Firth, J. D. (eds). *Oxford Textbook of Medicine.* 5th Edition. Oxford: Oxford University Press.

Mathias C. J., Galizia G. (2010). Orthostatic hypotension and orthostatic intolerance. In: Jameson, J. L., De Groot, L. J. (eds) *Endocrinology Adult and Pediatric*, 6th Edition. Saunders Elsevier, Philadelphia. p. 2063–82.

Mathias, C. J., Low, D. A., Iodice, V., Owens, A. P., Kirbis, M. and Grahame R. (2012). The Postural Tachycardia Syndrome (PoTS)—Current experiences and concepts. *Nature Reviews Neurology*, **8**, 22–34.

Miyazaki, M. (1978). Shy-Drager syndrome-a nosological entity? In *International symposium on spinocerebellar degenerations.* Medical Research Foundation, Tokyo.

Muthane, U. and Mathias, C. J. (2011). Orthostatic hypotension in Parkinson's Disease. In: Olanow, C. W., Stocchi, F., Lang, A. E. (eds). *Parkinson's Disease: non-motor and non-dopaminergic features.* Wiley-Blackwell. p. 284–95.

Nanda, R. N., Boyle, R. C., Gillespie, J. S., Johnson, R. H., Keogh, H. J. (1977). Idiopathic orthostatic hypotension from failure of noradrenaline release in a patient with vasomotor innervation. *J. Neurol. Neurosurg. Psychiat.* **40**, 11–19.

Sharpey-Schafer, E. P., and Taylor, P. J. (1960). Absent circulatory reflexes in diabetic neuritis. *Lancet* **i**, 559–62.

Shy, G. M., and Drager, G. A. (1960) A neurological syndrome associated with orthostatic hypotension. *Arch. Neurol., Chicago* **3**, 5511–27.

Thijs, R. D., Wieling, W., Kaufmann, H., and van Dijk G. (2004). Defining and classifying syncope. *Clin Auton Res.* **14**, 4–8.

Vanderhaegen, J. J., Perier, O., and Sternon, J. E. (1970). Pathological findings in idiopathic orthostatic hypotension: its relationship with Parkinson's disease. *Arch. Neurol., Chicago* **22**, 207–14.

Wieling, W., Krediet, C. T., van Dijk, N., Linzer, M., Tschakovsky, M. E. (2007). Initial orthostatic hypotension: review of a forgotten condition. *Clin. Sci. (Lond)* **112**, (3) 157–65.

Historical perspectives on the autonomic nervous system

with a particular emphasis on chemical neurotransmission

Tilli Tansey

Understanding what we now call the autonomic nervous system, its normal functioning, and the role of its various components, is clearly fundamental to the investigation and treatment of the dysfunctions of that system. This chapter will briefly review how our present day knowledge developed, focussing particularly on the discovery of the mechanisms of chemical neurotransmission in the autonomic nervous system.

Firstly, a note about terminology. The creation, and use, of new words, new definitions and new classifications are proper, and important, parts of scientific endeavour and exemplify the discovery of new facts and the development of fresh concepts. The autonomic nervous system is no exception, indeed the very expression 'autonomic nervous system' was not known before 1898, when, in a paper about the superior cervical ganglion (Fig. 1), the Cambridge physiologist J N Langley (Fig. 2), wrote:

> I propose to substitute the word 'autonomic' [for the word visceral]... The word implies a certain degree of independent action, but exercised under control of a higher power. The 'autonomic' nervous system means the nervous system of the glands and of the involuntary muscle; it governs the 'organic' functions of the body.

The term did not receive immediate or overwhelming acceptance, and for some years other expressions were current. As will be noted below, the words 'sympathy' and 'sympathetics', often used for the entire autonomic system, have a long history, and 'vegetative' and 'involuntary' were used well into the twentieth century. Throughout the present chapter, unless clearly contraindicated, the expression 'autonomic nervous system' will be used, although its use to refer to the system before 1898 is clearly anachronistic.

Sympathy and the sympathetics

Before the nineteenth century, knowledge about the autonomic nervous system was almost completely derived from anatomical studies of animals, and after the Renaissance also increasingly from human dissections. From dissections of apes and pigs, and possibly from observations on the wounded gladiators he attended as a physician, Galen (129–216) described a ganglionic (sympathetic)

chain, which he thought arose from the brain, and the white rami communicantes. For over a thousand years his account, rigidly maintained by medical and religious authorities, was accepted. Challenges and additions by later anatomists included those by Thomas Willis (1621–1675) who described the vagus or 'wandering nerves', and named the ganglionic nerves the 'intercostal nerves', and by Jacobus Winslow (1669–1760) who agreed with Willis that the ganglia were 'small brains', although he introduced the term 'great sympathetic nerve' instead of 'intercostal nerves'. The French anatomist François Xavier Bichat (1771–1802) distinguished between the somatic and visceral functions of the nervous system, and also acknowledged the influence of emotions on the visceral system. However, elucidation of the function of these components was patchy: Willis sectioned the vagus of a dog and observed that the heart fluttered; the French surgeon François Poerfour de Petit (1664–1741) noted that cutting the cervical sympathetic nerves affected pupil size and the nictating membrane; and the dedication

ON THE UNION OF CRANIAL AUTONOMIC (VISCERAL) FIBRES WITH THE NERVE CELLS OF THE SUPERIOR CERVICAL GANGLION. By J. N. LANGLEY, D.Sc., F.R.S., *Fellow of Trinity College, Cambridge.*

CONTENTS.

1. Introduction.
2. Union of the Central End of the Vagus with the Peripheral End of the Cervical Sympathetic.
   (i) General nature of the experiments.
   (ii) Evidence of connection of efferent fibres of the vagus with the cells of the superior cervical ganglion obtained by stimulating the nerves.
   (iii) Experimental evidence of growth of the afferent fibres of the vagus into the peripheral end of the sympathetic.
   (iv) Histological observations.
   (v) Tonic and reflex sympathetic actions by way of the vagus.
3. Union of the Central End of the Lingual Nerve with the Peripheral End of the Cervical Sympathetic.
4. Summary of Chief Results and Conclusions.

Fig. 1 Title of the article in which the word 'autonomic' was first used, from J N Langley (1898). With permission from Langley, J. N., On the union of cranial autonomic (visceral) fibres with the nerve cells of the superior cervical ganglion, *Journal of Physiology*, Wiley.

of his later compatriots to the guillotine permitted Albert Regnard and Paul Loye (1861–1890) to stimulate the vagus of a decapitated criminal and observe the appearance, 45 minutes after execution, of gastric juice on the inner surface of the stomach.

Nerves and nets

By the middle of the nineteenth century more elaborate anatomical and functional studies were underway. The development and informed use of microscopes encouraged the examination of numerous organs and tissues, including those of the autonomic nervous system. Robert Remak (1815–1865), discovered unmyelinated sympathetic fibres and that nerve fibres arose from ganglion cells, collections of which he found in the heart and bladder. The laborious quantitative work of Friedrich Bidder (1810–1894) and Alfred Wilhelm Volkmann (1800–1877), revealed that postganglionic fibres were more numerous than preganglionic fibres. Physiological experiments increasingly revealed functional aspects of the system: Bidder showed that curare did not inhibit autonomic control of the heart or intestine; Benedict Stilling (1810–1879) coined the expression 'vasomotor system' for the autonomic fibres to the muscle fibres in vessel walls; Claude Bernard (1813–1878) produced vasodilation by sectioning the sympathetic nerve; and Edouard Brown-Séquard (1817–1894) stimulated the cut-end to obtain vasoconstriction. Perhaps more startling were the experiments of Ernst Heinrich Weber (1795–1878) and his brother Eduard (1806–1871) who reported that vagal stimulation stopped the heart, thus introducing into neurophysiology the concept of inhibition.

Critical debates raged in the final decades of the nineteenth century about the detailed structure of the nervous system. The Italian anatomist Camillo Golgi (1844–1926) maintained that the nervous system was a complex net-like structure, a reticuluum; while the Spaniard Santiago Ramon y Cajal (1852–1934) proposed that each nerve cell was an independent unit, the neuron. The two men shared the Nobel Prize for Physiology or Medicine in 1906, both firmly wedded to their irreconcilable views. Improvements in histological techniques produced a mounting body of evidence supporting the neuron theory, which posed problems about the transfer of information between nerve cells, and between nerve and effector cells. The physiological implications of this were clearly recognized by Charles Sherrington (1857–1952), then investigating reflex activities of the nervous system, and in 1897 he proposed the word 'synapse' to describe the region between functional units of the nervous system. Physiological investigations of the autonomic nervous system were to reveal much about the properties of synapses.

'Like reading an account of the circulation before Harvey'

Just before the Second World War, the eminent neurologist Walter Langdon-Brown (1870–1946) declared that:

> to read an account of [the autonomic nervous] system before Gaskell is like reading an account of the circulation before Harvey.

Who then was Gaskell, and what were his contributions? Walter Gaskell (1847–1914, Fig. 3) was a Cambridge physiologist whose work elucidated much of the anatomical complexity of the system, his outstanding contribution being the clear delineation, both morphologically and functionally, of the two major nervous

outflows, the thoracolumbar (sympathetic) and craniosacral (parasympathetic). In 1886 he wrote, somewhat prophetically:

> The evidence is becoming daily stronger that every tissue is innervated by two sets of nerve fibres of opposite characters so that I look forward hopefully to the time when the whole nervous system shall be mapped out … into two great divisions of the nervous system which are occupied with chemical changes of a synthetical and analytical character respectively, which therefore in their actions must show the characteristic signs of such opposite chemical processes.

His work provided the morphological base for all subsequent studies on what Gaskell himself continued to call the 'visceral' or 'involuntary' nervous system. His close colleague J N Langley (1852–1925), quoted at the beginning of this chapter, devoted a substantial part of his career to investigating the distribution and function of the system, largely accepting Gaskell's differentiation although he regarded the nerve cells of the gastrointestinal tract's plexuses as a distinct, third, component of the autonomic nervous system, the 'enteric nervous system'.

In 1878 Langley started to use drugs as investigative tools, examining the effects of pilocarpine and atropine on the secretion of saliva from the submaxillary gland. Their opposing effects, stimulatory and inhibitory, suggested to him that there was a mutual exclusivity in their action that came about through some form of chemical interaction. He proposed:

> …there is some substance or substances in the nerve endings or gland cells with which both atropine and pilocarpine are capable of forming compounds.

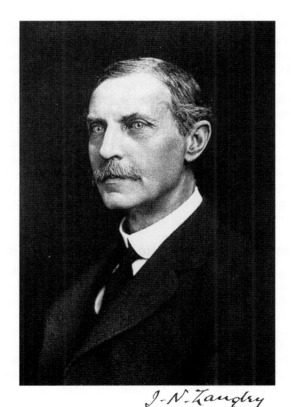

Fig. 2 J N Langley (1852–1925). With permission from the Physiological Society, from *Journal of Physiology* (1926), Wiley.

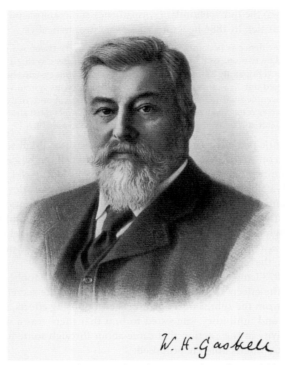

W. H. Gaskell

Fig. 3 Walter H Gaskell (1847–1914). With permisson from *The Cambridge Medical School: a biographical history*, Cambridge University Press (1932), facing page 95.

Langley also applied chemicals directly to autonomic ganglia with a paint brush, and discovered that nicotine caused facilitation of the neural impulse, closely followed by paralysis. This became a useful tool for dissecting out what he was able to distinguish, physiologically, as the preganglionic and postganglionic components of the system, and the results accelerated his interest in the specific and selective actions of the drugs *per se*. Langley provided pharmacological confirmation of Gaskell's anatomical divisions of the system, and he developed a theoretical account of the interactions between ganglion cells and chemicals. In 1905 he postulated the existence of 'receptive substances' between the nerve and the cell of the effective organ, activated by the arrival of the neural impulse at the nerve ending, thus, Langley argued, making the presynaptic release of specific chemicals unnecessary for the transmission of the neural effect.

From ergot to acetylcholine, via adrenaline

It was two of Gaskell and Langley's students, Henry Dale (1875–1968) and Thomas Elliott (1877–1961) who made the next set of important observations, although the significance of their findings was not recognized at the time. Elliott showed that stimulation of the hypogastric nerve could be mimicked by the application of adrenaline, and when, in 1904, he presented his results to the Physiological Society (Fig. 4), he suggested 'adrenaline might then be the substance liberated when the nervous stimulus reaches the periphery'. Precisely *what* he meant by this ambiguous statement is unclear, although it has been interpreted as the first definitive proposal of chemical neurotransmission. It can be understood, with the benefit of hindsight, to suggest that adrenaline might be released from the

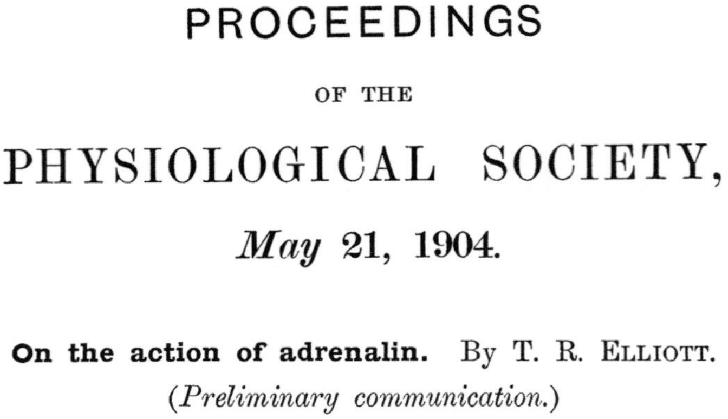

PROCEEDINGS

OF THE

PHYSIOLOGICAL SOCIETY,

May 21, 1904.

On the action of adrenalin. By T. R. ELLIOTT.
(Preliminary communication.)

Fig. 4 Title of T R Elliott's 1904 Communication to the Physiological Society, showing that stimulation of the hypogastric nerve could be mimicked by the application of adrenaline. With permission from *Journal of Physiology* (1904), Wiley, **31**:xx–xxi.

nerve endings in response to the passage of a nervous impulse. At the same time his Cambridge contemporary Henry Dale (Fig. 5) was at the Wellcome Physiological Research Laboratories (WPRL), working, at the suggestion of Henry Wellcome, on the pharmacology of extracts of ergot, then used in obstetric practice to reduce post-partum haemorrhage. Doing similar physiological experiments to those of Elliott, Dale observed that his preparation of ergot reversed the effects of splanchnic nerve stimulation *and* reversed the effect of adrenaline. This evidence corroborated Elliott's findings of close similarities between sympathetic nerve stimulation and the application of adrenaline. Dale recognized that his ergot derivative had, somehow, paralysed 'the structures which

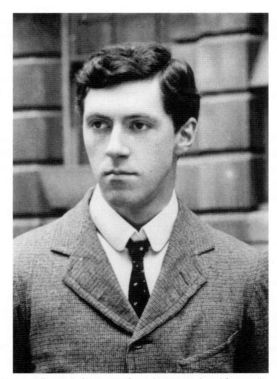

Fig. 5 Henry Hallett Dale (1876–1968), aged 27. Reproduced from a photograph of the medical firm of Dr Samuel Gee, St Bartholomew's Hospital, 1902. By permission of the Royal College of Physicians.

adrenaline stimulates', although like Elliott he was unable, or unwilling, to provide a hypothesis to explain the phenomenon. The experiments encouraged Dale, however, to investigate the action of chemicals on the autonomic nervous system further, which he continued to do for the rest of his scientific career. With the chemist George Barger (1878–1939), he started a detailed chemical and physiological study of chemicals structurally related to adrenaline. Barger synthesized the amines in his lab, and Dale tested their physiological effects. Over a period of nearly 3 years the two men examined more than 50 compounds, for many of which they invented the word 'sympathomimetic' to indicate mimicry of the effects of stimulation of the sympathetic nervous system. In 1913 Dale published an elegant dissection, and discussion, of the two major actions of adrenaline: vasoconstriction, the normally predominating effect that accounted for the pressor response; and the contrary effect of vasodilation when a lower dose was applied, but he was unable to clarify this difference. In private correspondence, Dale referred to this as 'the central mystery' of the sympathetic nervous system, and it was to plague investigators, and investigations, for many years. Efforts to explain how one chemical could bring about such apparently opposite effects gave rise to at least one convoluted theoretical account, the sympathin E and sympathin I story, as will be described below. That paper marked Dale's final major contribution to the study of transmitter candidates in the sympathetic nervous system, and it was his change of research direction, towards the parasympathetic nervous system, especially after the First World War, that was ultimately to provide a substantial body of evidence for chemical neurotransmission.

Acetylcholine comes to the fore

Dale's personal research work concentrated on the identification of acetylcholine as the chemical neurotransmitter in the parasympathetic system, and later at the neuromuscular junction of the peripheral nervous system. Acetylcholine was first synthesized in 1867, but not until 40 years later was a detailed study made of its pharmacological activities by Reid Hunt (1870–1948). Hunt investigated choline, which caused a lowering of blood pressure in the experimental animal, and several of its chemical derivatives, and demonstrated that of a range of 19 synthetic chemicals, *acetyl* choline had an even more effective depressor activity than choline. Writing in 1906, Hunt suggested:

> [Acetylcholine] is a substance of extraordinary activity. In fact, I think it safe to state that, as regards its effect upon the circulation, it is the most powerful substance known. It is one hundred thousand times more active than choline, and hundreds of times more active than nitroglycerine; it is a hundred times more active in causing a fall of blood pressure than is adrenaline in causing a rise.

He never succeeded in isolating the compound from any animal tissue, and acetylcholine was known only as an artificial, synthetic, compound for many years. Even the therapeutic possibilities of using this effective chemical were severely limited because its depressor effects, although profound, were extremely transitory. This problem, of acetylcholine's powerful but evanescent activity, was to cause both experimental and interpretative difficulties for many years.

Naturally occurring acetylcholine was first isolated by Henry Dale in 1913, in what he considered to be one of the luckiest incidents of his career. A sample of an obstetric ergot preparation was sent to Dale for routine physiological investigation. Injection into the vein of an anaesthetized cat caused immediate and intense inhibition of the heartbeat, from which the animal rapidly recovered. A further demonstration convinced Dale that the ergot was contaminated with an unusual depressor constituent that resembled the effects of muscarine. Muscarine, from the mushroom *Amanita muscaria*, caused slowing of the heart beat, similar to vagal stimulation. The effects Dale observed were, however, unlike those of muscarine, very short lasting and, recalling Hunt's work, Dale suggested to a chemist colleague, Arthur Ewins (1882–1957), that the mystery substance might be acetylcholine. Ewins rapidly confirmed that identification, and isolated acetylcholine from ergot, an important impetus to further work on its actions. Dale himself started a detailed physiological study in which he clearly distinguished the two principal effects of acetylcholine: one that could be reproduced by injections of muscarine; and one imitated by nicotine.

Writing in 1938, Dale summed up the situation as it had been just before the First World War:

> Such was the position in 1914. Two substances [adrenaline and acetylcholine] were known, with actions very suggestively reproducing those of the two main divisions of the autonomic nervous system; both, for different reasons, were very unstable in the body, and their actions were in consequence of a fleeting character; and one of them [adrenaline] was already known to occur as a natural hormone. These properties would fit them very precisely to act as mediators of the effects of autonomic impulses to effector cells, if there were any acceptable evidence of liberation at the nerve endings. The actors were named, and the parts allotted; a preliminary hint of the plot had, indeed, been given 10 years earlier, and almost forgotten; but only direct and unequivocal evidence could ring up the curtain, and this was not to come till 1921.

Adrenalin(e) and epinephrin(e) and their nor-derivatives

Here we must divert to a consideration of the terminology of the first endogenous chemical substances shown to affect the autonomic nervous system. The discovery of the physiological effects of an adrenal (suprarenal) gland extract was first reported in 1894 by George Oliver (1841–1915) and Edward Schäfer (1899–1933), who demonstrated its constrictor (pressor) effect on the arterial system, causing raised blood pressure. This stimulated a search to identify the chemical composition of the active principle, particularly in Britain, Germany and the USA. In 1899 John Abel (1857–1938) from Johns Hopkins announced his successful extraction of what he called 'epinephrin', although this was physiologically inert. Further chemical modifications produced similarly inert extracts, each of which was, confusingly, also called epinephrine. Finally, an early example of industrial espionage by Jokichi Takamine (1854–1922) resulted in Abel's technique being modified in the laboratories of Parke, Davis and Co. to produce a physiologically effective substance that was marketed under the trade name of 'Adrenalin', with a capital 'A' and no terminal 'e'. However, in Britain the word appears never to have been registered as a trademark, and was freely used, in the scientific community, either with or without the final 'e'. This was the word used by both Dale and Elliott in their seminal papers.

The discovery of the pronounced physiological activity of the *nor*-derivative of adrenaline, initially known only as a synthetic molecule, was to take many decades. As with acetylcholine, noradrenaline was known as a synthetic derivative at the beginning of the twentieth century, and when Barger and Dale undertook their extensive analysis of amine actions, published in 1910, noradrenaline was readily available from the Hoechst Dye Company, under the name 'arterrenol'. They noted its strong sympathomimetic activity, but, as Dale recalled in 1953, he was at that time concerned about the difficulty for Elliott's theory of adrenaline as the sympathetic transmitter that this synthetic derivative was 'more accurately sympathomimetic'. His recollections continue:

> Doubtless I ought to have seen that noradrenaline might be the main transmitter – that Elliott's theory might be right in principle and faulty only in this detail. If I had had so much insight, I might even then have stimulated my chemical colleagues to look for noradrenaline in the body; but they would almost certainly have failed to find it, with the methods that were then available. It is easy, of course [he commented ruefully] to be wise in the light of facts recently discovered [that of endogenous noradrenaline]; lacking them I failed to jump to the truth, and I can hardly claim credit for having crawled so near and then stopped short of it.

Vagusstoff and acceleransstoff

There were two main approaches to the further identification of a likely transmitter candidate: the type of work that Dale and Elliott had performed at the beginning of the century, observing the effects of applied chemicals and noting their correlation with endogenous neural stimulation. The second method was to attempt to recover and characterize a chemical after neural stimulation. Both techniques were adopted by the Austrian pharmacologist

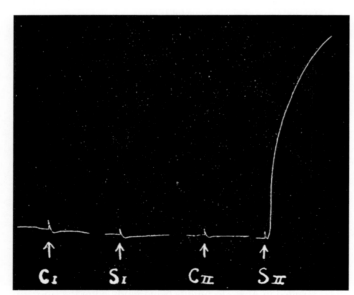

Fig. 6 Eserinized leech muscle as a measure of acetylcholine in an experiment to verify the connection between the output of acteylcholine and the transmission of nerve impulses to the sweat glands of an anaesthetized cat. CI and SI are measurements of acetylcholine in the venous outflow from the right foot of the anaesthetized cat, with the hairless pads which contain the sweat glands ligatured, CI being a control period of no stimulation, SI a period of stimulation of the right sympathetic chain. CII is a measurement of a similar control period from the left foot, with the hairless pads intact, and SII from a period of stimulation of the left sympathetic chain, which caused secretion of sweat and also the release of acetylcholine, as shown by the leech muscle response. Taken with permission of the Physiological Society, from Dale & Feldberg, *Journal of Physiology* (1934) **82**: p124, paper in Dale (1965).

Otto Loewi (1873–1961), who, in 1921 reported the results of the experiment that, to use Dale's analogy, 'could ring up the curtain'. It is now regarded as a classic experiment in the history of neurotransmission, and was seemingly simple. The beating hearts were removed from two frogs, and placed in separate irrigation chambers. Electrical stimulation of the vagal nerves to one heart caused a slowing, then a cessation, of the heart beat. Using a syringe, the fluid bathing the first heart was transferred into the chamber surrounding the second, still beating, heart, causing this too to slow and stop. Loewi claimed that this was strong evidence for the transfer of a chemical substance, released upon neural stimulation of the first heart, into the chamber containing the second heart. Similar experiments, stimulating sympathetic nerves to the first heart produced a stimulatory effect that was transferable with the surrounding fluid. Loewi proposed the release, by neural stimulation, of two substances—Vagusstoff (released by vagal, parasympathetic stimulation) and Acceleransstoff (released by sympathetic stimulation). These experiments were not, however, uncontroversial, and critics pointed to several inconsistencies and difficulties. Loewi began detailed chemical examinations and gradually the similarity of the Acceleransstoff to adrenaline was recognized, and further evidence was accrued that Vagusstoff was a choline ester, similar to acetylcholine, and rapidly inactivated by a blood-borne esterase. But acetylcholine had still not been identified as a normal constituent of the animal body, and it was to be some time before the positive identification of the postganglionic parasympathetic transmitter as acetylcholine. It was to come from Henry Dale who was searching for histamine.

Histamine

During the 1920s Dale was working for the Medical Research Council at its National Institute for Medical Research, and was principally occupied with experiments on the physiology and pharmacology of histamine, and its role in shock, allergy and anaphylaxis. Histamine was another substance not then generally acknowledged to occur naturally, because although Barger and Dale had isolated it from the fungus ergot of rye in 1910, there was little evidence for its presence in higher plants or animals. In 1911 Barger and Dale did report finding histamine in ox intestinal mucosa, although its production by contaminating bacteria could not be dismissed. Histamine had also attracted the attention of the noted cardiologist, Sir Thomas Lewis (1881–1945, Fig. 8). Lewis, who had actually shared rooms with Thomas Elliott for many years when both were bachelors, had worked extensively on mechanisms of the heart and its disorders during the first two decades of the twentieth century. By the mid-1920s he was becoming increasingly interested in the physiology of blood vessels, especially cutaneous vessels and their cellular responses to injuries. He described the 'triple response', the typical visible skin response to cellular injury, and Dale suggested to him that subcutaneous injection of histamine might produce a similar response, which it did. Like Dale, Lewis was reluctant to consider histamine, still then unknown as a natural constituent of the tissues, as an endogenous mediator of such injury. He used the expression 'H-substance' for a histamine-like substance that might be released from injured cells upon injury, although he stressed:

> … it is difficult to refrain from stating without reserve the simple conclusion that the vasodilator substance considered and the H-substance are one and the same, and that this substance is histamine, free or

held in loose combination. This conclusion would harmonize with the chief evidence at all points.

By the late 1920s there was much evidence that histamine, or a histamine-like substance, played important physiological mediator roles. Thus Dale and Harold Dudley (1887–1935) made a determined effort to find histamine in a 'clean' tissue (i.e. one without the risk of bacterial contamination). Ironically they found not only histamine, but finally also found convincing evidence for the presence of acetylcholine in the mammalian spleen. This important breakthrough stimulated further research on the role of acetylcholine, as Dale and Dudley suggested:

> … there has been a natural and proper reluctance to assume, in default of chemical evidence, that the chemical agent concerned in these effects, or in the humoral transmission of vagus action, was a substance known, hitherto, only as a synthetic curiosity, or as an occasional constituent of certain plant extracts…
>
> It appears to us that the case for acetylcholine as a physiological agent is now materially strengthened by the fact that we have now been able to isolate it from an animal organ and thus to show that it is a natural constituent of the body.

Acetylcholine again

The major problem that continued to complicate further research work on acetylcholine was the extreme transiency of its effects. Experiments to show its release after nervous stimulation were unsuccessful—if it was released it was so quickly hydrolysed by circulating cholinesterases that there was nothing left to measure. In 1933 a new arrival in Dale's laboratory, the pharmacologist Wilhelm Feldberg (1900–1993), a refugee from Nazi Germany, brought with him two valuable techniques:

- to increase the measurable levels of circulating acetylcholine by inhibiting the hydrolysing enzyme with eserine
- the use of a bioassay, of the ventral muscle of the leech, also treated with eserine, to measure acetylcholine.

These methods were immediately incorporated into the experiments in Dale's lab, and evidence began to accrue of the role of acetylcholine in ganglionic transmission in the autonomic nervous system, at the parasympathetic postganglionic junction and at the neuromuscular junction of the voluntary nervous system. In 1936 Henry Dale and Otto Loewi shared the Nobel Prize in Physiology or Medicine 'for their discoveries relating to the chemical transmission of nerve impulses'.

COMMENTARY

DO SOME NERVE CELLS RELEASE MORE THAN ONE TRANSMITTER?

GEOFFREY BURNSTOCK
Department of Anatomy and Embryology, University College, London, WC1E 6BT

Abstract—The concept that each nerve cell makes and releases only one nerve transmitter (widely known as Dale's Principle) has been re-examined. Experiments suggesting that some nerve cells store and release more than one transmitter have been reviewed. Developmental and evolutionary factors are considered. Conceptual and experimental difficulties in investigating this problem are discussed. It is suggested that the term 'transmitter' should be applied to any substance that is synthesised and stored in nerve cells, is released during nerve activity and whose interaction with specific receptors on the postsynaptic membrane leads to changes in postsynaptic activity. Expressed in this way, it seems likely that while many nerves do have only one transmitter, others in some species, during development or during hormone-dependent cycles, employ multiple transmitters.

Fig. 7 Title of Geoffrey Burnstock's 1976 paper, proposing that 'Dale's principle' of one-neuron, one transmitter' was no longer valid. With permission from *Neuroscience*, **1**, G Burnstock, Do some nerve cells release more than one transmitter?, 239–248, Copyright 1976, with permission from Elsevier.

One of the most significant developments of the period was not a laboratory finding, but the suggestion, by Dale, of the words 'cholinergic' and 'adrenergic', to describe nerve fibres by the nature of the chemical that they used, or might use, as a transmitter, rather than by the then accepted anatomical classification of fibres as sympathetic or parasympathetic. Dale's reasoning was straightforward; he wrote in 1934:

> I think such a usage would assist clear thinking, without committing us to precise chemical identifications, which may be long in coming.

The distinction was important, as it acknowledged that chemical neurotransmitters might be 'adrenaline-like' and 'acetylcholine-like' but were not necessarily either of those two chemicals. See also Fig. 6.

Cannon's sympathins and Ahlquist's receptors

While Dale and his colleagues focussed their attention on the parasympathetic nervous system, others were concentrating on chemically identifying the endogenous transmitter in the sympathetic branch. Shortly after Loewi's demonstration of Acceleransstoff in 1921, the American physiologist Walter Cannon (1871–1945) provided complementary evidence that in adrenalectomized animals stimulation of the hepatic nerve produced a chemical that caused acceleration of the heart beat. The word 'sympathin' was used for this unidentified substance, which was similar to, but not identical with, adrenaline. Further experiments by Cannon and Arturo Rosenblueth (1900–1970) suggested that the different effects observed after sympathetic nervous stimulation indicated the presence of two distinctly separate endogenous sympathin complexes, sympathin E (excitatory) and sympathin I (inhibitory). This theoretical account achieved quite successful currency in contemporary scientific literature, and by the late 1930s and 1940s the theory had almost achieved the status of a 'law', especially in American pharmacology. Cannon and Rosenblueth's major work *Autonomic neuro-effector systems* promoted their sympathin theory to the exclusion of all else, and in Britain, where the concept was less well received, one reviewer, John Gaddum (1900–1965), echoed the views of several colleagues when he suggested that it was 'unnecessarily complicated'. A former co-worker of Cannon's, the Belgian pharmacologist Zenon Bacq (1903–1984) went some way to clearing away the confusion sown by Cannon and Rosenblueth, by suggesting that 'sympathin I' was adrenaline and 'sympathin E' could be noradrenaline, although overall he remained sceptical of the sympathin scheme. By this time many other investigators were emphasizing the point made by Barger and Dale in 1910, that noradrenaline was a closer mimic of sympathetic activity than was adrenaline.

Two major boosts to the understanding of the sympathetic nervous system and the chemical identification of its transmitter(s) came shortly after the Second World War. Ulf von Euler (1905–1983) showed that extracts of sympathetic nerves and some of their end organs contained appreciable amounts of noradrenaline. This evidence effectively removed the long-standing refusal to consider noradrenaline as a transmitter because it was not known to occur naturally. An equally important theoretical contribution was made by Raymond Ahlquist (1914–1983) who resolved, and finally offered an adequate explanation for, some of the apparently paradoxical experimental differences observed by Dale and others.

Using a range of different adrenergic agonists, Ahlquist defined two major classes of adrenoceptors, with a range of differential potencies for catecholamines. He postulated *alpha-receptors*, which were more sensitive to noradrenaline than to adrenaline and isoprenaline, while *beta-receptors* were preferentially sensitive to isoprenaline, then to adrenaline and least responsive to noradrenaline. The awkward results reported by many investigators, including, of course, Cannon and Rosenblueth's observations, but not their theories, of both excitation and inhibition in the sympathetic system, could now be re-interpreted in the light of Ahlquist's scheme.

Consolidation and diversification

The increasing confirmation, and acceptance, of chemical transmission, of adrenergic nerves releasing noradrenaline, and cholinergic nerves releasing acetylcholine, became, in their turn, codified into a 'law'. This was largely influenced by John Eccles (1903–1997), who believed that the long latency at the terminals of the parasympathetic nervous system, such as those in the heart, contrasted markedly with much shorter latencies, at sites such as sympathetic ganglia and the voluntary neuromuscular junction, and proposed that electrical impulses were solely responsible for these faster responses. After formally announcing his 'conversion' to chemical mechanisms, he formulated what became known as 'Dale's Law' which stipulated 'one neuron, one transmitter'. As the concept of chemical neurotransmission achieved widespread acceptance it became the new orthodoxy, and it was widely assumed that only a few specific chemicals, including acetylcholine and noradrenaline, were involved in the process.

The idea of a simple duality, a sympathetic/adrenergic system countered by a parasympathetic/cholinergic system was gradually modified as evidence of new transmitter candidates and neuro-modulaters, emerged. During the 1950s and 1960s it became increasingly obvious that many autonomic nerve fibres were neither adrenergic nor cholinergic. Prime among those postulating more complex chemical mechanisms at autonomic neuroeffector junctions was Geoffrey Burnstock, [b. 1929, Figs 7 and 9] who, in 1963, first suggested that the myenteric plexus of the guinea pig intestine contained non-adrenergic, non-cholinergic (NANC) neurons, thus providing a pharmacological distinction for the 'enteric nervous system' postulated by Langley at the beginning of the century. By the late 1960s Burnstock and his group had provided extensive evidence for the existence of such neurons, and postulated that adenosine triphosphate (ATP) was the neurotransmitter at these neuronal terminals. This view, challenging contemporary dogma, received little sympathy, as one witness has recalled, 'Burnstock', wrote Michael Rand 'faced a considerable amount of tough opposition, not always in the spirit of scientific criticism.'

Chemical coding, and into the clinic

During the following decade, however, the hypothesis of ATP as a neurotransmitter, or as Burnstock proposed, echoing Dale's classification of 40 years earlier, purinergic transmission, gained considerable support. Increasing acceptance of ATP encouraged the investigation of other possible neurotransmitter candidates,

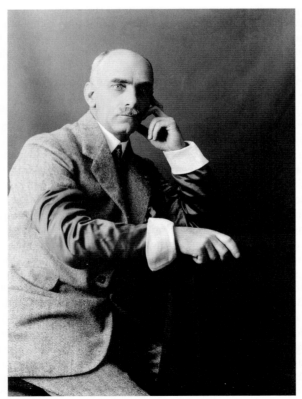

Fig. 8 Sir Thomas Lewis (1881–1945). With permission from Wellcome Images.

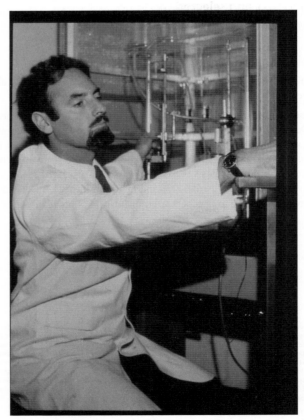

Fig. 9 Professor Geoff Burnstock in his laboratory in Melbourne in 1972 carrying out pharmacological studies of purinergic neurotransmission in guinea pig bladder and taenia coli. Reproduced with permission of Professor Geoffrey Burnstock.

including biologically active polypeptides such as somatostatin, vasoactive intestinal peptide (VIP), substance P and neurotensin. By the beginning of the twenty-first century purinergic signalling in the physiology and pathophysiology of neurotransmission and neuromodulation is a burgeoning field of enquiry.

This diversity of chemical mediators stimulated a further revolutionary hypothesis from Burnstock in 1976: that nerve cells might release more than one transmitter. The coexistence and co-release of transmitters from nerves has opened up an entirely new field of research on the autonomic nervous system. Understanding the details of these combinations of transmitters, known as 'chemical coding', has led to detailed physiological and pharmacological investigations into the effects of disease at the autonomic neuroeffector junction, and to the development of sophisticated pharmaceutical responses to those disease processes. Thus, since 1898 when Langley coined the word, basic scientific studies of the autonomic nervous system have continued to elucidate functional mechanisms that underlie all nervous system activity and the clinical application of such research, in diagnosis and therapeutics, has evolved in numerous directions, as other chapters in this volume will illustrate.

Acknowledgements

I am grateful to Mrs Wendy Kutner for secretarial help, to the Wellcome Photographic Library for supplying the illustrations, and to the Wellcome Trust for financial support.

References and selected further reading

Ackerknecht, E. H. (1974). The history of the discovery of the vegetative (autonomic) nervous system. *Medical History* **18**, 1–8.

Ahlquist, R. P. (1948). A study of the adrenotropic receptors. *American Journal of Physiology* **153**, 586–99.

Ahlquist, R. P. (1973). Adrenergic receptors: a personal and practical view. *Perspectives in Biology and Medicine* **16**, 119–22.

Aronson, J. K. (2000). "When name and image meet"—the argument for "adrenaline". *British Medical Journal* **320**, 506.

Barger, G. & Dale, H. H. (1910). Chemical structure and sympathomimetic action of amines. *Journal of Physiology* **41**, 19–59.

Burnstock, G. (1976). Do some nerve cells release more than one neurotransmitter? *Neuroscience* **1**, 239–48.

Burnstock, G. (2007). Physiology and pathophysiology of purinergic neurotransmission. *Physiological Reviews* **87**, 659–797.

Cannon, W. B. & Rosenblueth A. (1937). *Autonomic Neuro-Effector Systems*. Macmillan, New York.

Dale, H. H. (1965). *Adventures in Physiology, with Excursions into Autopharmacology*. The Wellcome Trust, London [a selection of Dale's papers, annotated by the author, including all the work referred to in this chapter].

Elliott, T. R. (1904). The reaction of the ferret's bladder to adrenalin. *Journal of Physiology* **31**, lix.

Euler, U. S von (1946). A specific sympathomimetic ergone in adrenergic nerve fibres (sympathin) and its relations to adrenaline and noradrenaline. *Acta Physiologica Scandinavica* **12**, 73–97.

Gaskell, W. H. (1886). On the structure, distribution, and function of the nerves which innervate the visceral and vascular systems. *Journal of Physiology* **7**, 1–80.

Gaskell, W. H. (1916). *The Involuntary Nervous System*. Longmans, Green & Co, London.

Hunt, R. & Taveau, M. (1906). On the physiological action of certain cholin derivitives and new methods for detecting choline. *British Medical Journal* **ii**, 1788–89.

Langley, J. N. (1898). On the union of cranial autonomic (visceral) fibres with the nerve cells of the superior cervical ganglion. *Journal of Physiology* **23**, 240–70.

Langley, J. N. (1921). *The Autonomic Nervous System. Part 1*. Heffer & Sons, Cambridge.

Lewis, T. (1912). *Clinical Disorders of the Heart Beat*. Shaw, London.

Lewis, T. (1927). *The Blood Vessels of the Human Skin and their Responses*. Shaw & Sons, London.

Pick, J. (1970). *The Autonomic Nervous System. Morphological, Comparative, Clinical and Surgical Aspects*. J B Lippincott Co, Philadelphia.

Rand, M. J. & Mitchelson, F. (1986) The guts of the matter: contribution of studies on smooth muscle to discoveries in pharmacology. In: Parham, M. J. & Bruinvels, J. (eds) *Discoveries in Pharmacology Volume 3: Pharmacological Methods, Receptors & Chemotherapy*. Elsevier, Amsterdam.

Sheehan, D. (1941) The autonomic nervous system prior to Gaskell. *New England Journal of Medicine* **224**, 457–60.

Tansey, E. M. (1995). What's in a name: Henry Dale and adrenaline, 1906. *Medical History* **39**, 459–76.

PART I

Scientific Aspects of Structure and Function

CHAPTER 1

Neurobiology of the autonomic nervous system

Wilfrid Jänig and Elspeth M. McLachlan

Introduction

Motor activity and patterned behaviours originating in the brain are only possible when the cells, tissues, and organs of the body are maintained in an optimal environment, so as to enable continuous adjustments to the varying internal and external demands that are placed on the organism, both in the short term and long term. Short-term control includes control of blood flow, body fluid volume and osmotic pressure, body temperature, gastrointestinal and pelvic organ function, and metabolism. Long-term control includes the growth and maintenance of body tissues and organs, sleep and wakefulness, protection and defence from the cellular level to the whole organism.

Just as motor actions are controlled by the brain, so are all other body functions. To perform these functions, the brain acts on peripheral target tissues of diverse composition (smooth muscle, cardiac muscle, exocrine and endocrine glands, metabolic tissues, immune cells, etc.). The *efferent systems* are neural (the autonomic nervous system) and hormonal (the neuroendocrine system). The timescales of these controls differ by orders of magnitude: autonomic regulation normally occurs in seconds to minutes whereas neuroendocrine regulation occurs over tens of minutes, hours, or even days. The *afferent signals* that lead to changes in these outputs are neural, hormonal, and humoral (e.g. blood glucose concentration, blood temperature). As with the somatomotor system, autonomic and endocrine regulations are represented in the brain (in the hypothalamus, brainstem, and spinal cord). Thus, the brain contains the 'sensorimotor programmes' for the coordinated regulation of the body's tissues and organs as well as its skeletal muscles. There is considerable integration within the brain, between not only the different areas that are involved with the outputs of autonomic and endocrine signals, but also between these and the somatomotor control systems.

The precision and biological importance of the control of peripheral target organs by the autonomic nervous system becomes most obvious (see chapters of this book):

- when the autonomic nervous system fails to function (e.g. during extreme physical stress, haemorrhagic shock, severe infectious diseases)
- when many peripheral autonomic neurons are damaged by injury, toxins or a metabolic disease (such as diabetic autonomic neuropathy)

- when particular groups of autonomic neurons are absent (such as in Hirschsprung's disease), or when dopamine-beta-hydroxylase, an enzyme for noradrenaline synthesis, is congenitally deficient
- when the spinal cord is lesioned (interrupting supraspinal connections with the spinal autonomic outflow)
- in old age when the components of the autonomic systems may degenerate so that neural control is less effective.

Under these circumstances, blood flow to active organs can be compromised, temperature regulation inadequate, and the storage functions of bladder and bowel poorly controlled. Even the simplest actions, such as standing up, may become a burden because of inadequate adjustments to maintain the pressure perfusing the brain, potentially leading to loss of consciousness.

This chapter describes the neuronal basis for the precise control of the peripheral target organs. It also discusses how autonomic neurons in the central nervous system (CNS) and in the periphery are organized and how, in normal health, these neurons integrate and transmit centrally derived signals to their peripheral targets. Understanding the biology of these nerve pathways should lead to a better understanding of both primary disorders of the autonomic nervous system and autonomic dysfunction that is secondary to disease. For the physiology of the various autonomic control systems, we refer the reader to the chapters in this book, to Jänig (2006), Llewellyn-Smith and Verbene (2011), and to Robertson et al. (2012).

Divisions of the autonomic nervous system

Langley (1921) originally proposed the generic term *autonomic nervous system* for mammals to describe the innervation of all tissues and organs except striated muscle fibres. Langley's division of the autonomic nervous system into the sympathetic, parasympathetic, and enteric nervous systems is now universally applied. The definition of the *sympathetic* and *parasympathetic nervous systems* is primarily anatomical. The outflow from the CNS is separated into systems originating from tectal, bulbar and sacral regions (the craniosacral or parasympathetic system) and a thoracolumbar system in the spinal cord (the sympathetic system). These correspond to the somitic levels from which neural crest cells migrate to become parasympathetic neurons and sympathetic neurons, respectively. The other main feature distinguishing the outflows is their separation by the cervical and lumbar enlargements (supplying the innervation of the limbs).

Both the sympathetic and parasympathetic systems consist of two populations of neurons in series that are connected synaptically. The sympathetic and parasympathetic neurons that innervate the target organs lie entirely outside the CNS. Their cell bodies are grouped in *autonomic ganglia*. Their axons are unmyelinated and project from these ganglia to the target organs in peripheral nerves. These neurons are called autonomic (sympathetic or parasympathetic) *ganglion cells* or *postganglionic neurons*. The neurons that connect the CNS to these postganglionic neurons are the *preganglionic neurons* that have cell bodies that lie in the spinal cord and brain stem. They send axons from the CNS into the ganglia where they form synapses on the dendrites and somata of the postganglionic neurons. Their axons are either thinly myelinated (conduction velocity 1–15 m/s; B-fibres) or unmyelinated (conduction velocity 0.1–1 m/s; C-fibres).

The *enteric nervous system,* which arises from neural crest cells of primarily vagal origin, is intrinsic to the wall of the gastrointestinal tract and consists of interconnecting plexuses along its length. These are responsible for the reflex activity involved in peristalsis and segmentation, and also secretory/absorptive activity during transit of food along the bowel (Furness 2006, Jänig 2006).

Organization of preganglionic neurons in the spinal cord and brainstem

Langley showed, by stimulating individual ventral roots, that the control of each target organ arises from preganglionic neurons in a few adjacent segments of the spinal cord. Within the spinal cord and brainstem, the preganglionic somata are topographically organized and form functionally distinct columns resembling those of the motoneuron pools supplying particular skeletal muscles. Retrograde labelling techniques have been used in experimental animals to demonstrate this, in particular for the dorsal motor nucleus of vagus (Undem and Weinreich 2005, Jänig 2006) and the lumbar (Jänig and McLachlan 1987), and sacral segments of the spinal cord (Chapter 9).

Thoracolumbar (sympathetic) system

The cell bodies of the sympathetic preganglionic neurons lie in the spinal cord, extending from segments T1 to the rostral part of L3 in humans. They are mainly clustered together in clumps at the edge of the intermediate grey matter, forming the intermediolateral columns. During development, the neurons migrate dorsolaterally from the central canal; a few cells end up in the dorsolateral funiculus (the lateral horn) whereas others remain in bands crossing the midline. Overall, there is a ladder-like arrangement of cells throughout the thoracolumbar segments. The neurons receive inputs from interneurons in the dorsal horn and intermediate zone as well as direct projections from the medulla, pons and hypothalamus, and other spinal segments (propriospinal inputs).

The preganglionic axons project ipsilaterally from the cord via the segmental ventral root and spinal nerve, and thence in the white ramus to the paravertebral chain where they synapse with postganglionic neurons in the same and several adjacent segmental ganglia. Most of the functional (i.e. effective) connections occur segmentally, consistent with Langley's functional definitions. However, neurons in the upper thoracic segments project rostrally to regulate targets in the head, whereas many lumbar preganglionic neurons project caudally to regulate targets in the lower trunk and hind limbs. Some preganglionic axons project across the chain into the splanchnic nerves (major, minor, and lumbar) and synapse in the *prevertebral ganglia* (coeliac, superior mesenteric, and inferior mesenteric), which supply the abdominal and pelvic viscera.

The *paravertebral ganglia* are interconnected to form a chain on either side of the vertebral column, extending from the base of the skull to the sacrum. There is usually one pair of ganglia per segment, except for the superior cervical ganglia (SCG) at the rostral end of the cervical sympathetic trunk and the stellate ganglia at the rostral end of the thoracic sympathetic chain, both of which represent several segmental ganglia fused together. Paravertebral ganglion cells project to the somatic territories in all parts of the body and innervate blood vessels, pilomotor muscles, and sweat glands. Most of the paravertebral neurons project through the grey rami to their respective spinal nerves and then via peripheral nerve trunks to the effector cells of trunk and limbs. There is no significant projection of paravertebral neurons to the extremities along blood vessels. Most postganglionic neurons in the SCG send their axons via the internal carotid nerve to join the nerves to target organs in the head; some postganglionic neurons in the SCG project to the upper two or three cervical segments. More than 50% of SCG neurons are vasoconstrictor innervating various vascular beds (skin, skeletal muscle, salivary and mucosal glands, intracranial) and the rest mainly pilomotor, sudomotor or secretomotor to salivary glands and mucosal glands. A subpopulation supplies targets in and around the eye and a few innervate the pineal gland. Postganglionic neurons in the stellate ganglia project through nerve branches to the heart and lungs and through grey rami to C4–T2 spinal nerves to supply the neck and upper limbs. Some paravertebral neurons project via the splanchnic nerves (including the pelvic nerves) to the viscera, where they mainly innervate blood vessels.

The *prevertebral ganglia* lie around the base of the large arterial branches from the abdominal aorta and contain, as well as vasoconstrictor neurons, neurons that regulate both motility and secretion. They project in nerve bundles accompanying the vascular supply to the abdominal organs or in specialized nerves (e.g. the mesenteric, colonic or hypogastric nerves to the pelvic organs). They receive preganglionic inputs from the mid to lower thoracic and upper lumbar segments. Some sympathetic postganglionic cell bodies are also found in the ganglia of the pelvic or hypogastric plexus, which contains both sympathetic and parasympathetic postganglionic neurons. The hypogastric nerve therefore also contains sympathetic preganglionic axons. These sympathetic neurons supply the internal reproductive organs, bladder and distal bowel.

The responses in effector cells and organs elicited by activity in sympathetic nerves are listed in Table 1.1.

Craniosacral (parasympathetic) system

The cell bodies of the parasympathetic preganglionic neurons lie in the brainstem and in sacral spinal cord segments S1–S3. In the brainstem, they are grouped in distinct nuclei (e.g. dorsal motor nucleus of the vagus, nucleus ambiguus, salivary nuclei, Edinger–Westphal nucleus) and project via distinct cranial nerves. They pass via III (oculomotor) nerve to the ocular smooth muscles and glands, via VII (facial) and XI (glossopharyngeal) nerves to the nasal and palatal glands, and many via X (vagus) nerve to the thoracic and abdominal viscera. In the sacral cord, the preganglionic neurons lie in clusters across the intermediate zone and around the

Table 1.1 Effects of activation of sympathetic and parasympathetic neurons on autonomic target organs

Organ and organ system	Activation of parasympathetic nerves	Activation of sympathetic nerves
Cardiac muscle	Decreased heart rate	Increased heart rate
	Decreased contractility (only atria)	Increased contractility (atria, ventricles)
Blood vessels		
Arteries		
In skin of trunk and limbs	0	Vasoconstriction
In skin and mucosa of face (nose, mouth, etc)	Vasodilation	Vasoconstriction
In visceral domain		Vasoconstriction
In skeletal muscle	0	Vasoconstriction
		Vasodilation (cholinergic)[1]
In heart (coronary arteries)		Vasoconstriction
In erectile tissue (helical arteries and sinusoids in penis and clitoris)	Vasodilation	Vasoconstriction
In vagina, cervix, uterus	Vasodilation	? (either vasodilation or vasoconstriction or both)
In cranium	Vasodilation	Vasoconstriction
Veins	0	Vasoconstriction
Gastrointestinal tract		
Longitudinal and circular muscle	Increased motility	Decreased motility
Sphincters	Relaxation	Contraction
Capsule of spleen	0	Contraction
Kidney		
Juxtaglomerula cells	0	Release of renin
Tubuli	0	Sodium resorption increased
Urinary bladder		
Detrusor vesicae	Contraction	Relaxation (minor)
Trigone, internal urinary sphincter	0	Contraction
Urethra	Relaxation	Contraction
Reproductive organs		
Seminal vesicle, prostate	0	Contraction
Vas deferens	0	Contraction
Uterus	0	Contraction
		Relaxation (depends on hormonal state)
Eye		
Dilator muscle of pupil	0	Contraction (mydriasis)
Sphincter muscle of pupil	Contraction (miosis)	0
Ciliary muscle	Contraction (accommodation)	
Tarsal muscle	0	Contraction (lifting of lid)
Orbital muscle	0	Contraction (protrusion of eye)
Tracheobronchial muscles	Contraction	Relaxation (mainly by circulating adrenaline)
Piloerector muscles	0	Contraction
Exocrine glands[2]		
Salivary glands	Copious serous secretion	Weak serous secretion (submandibular gland)
		Mucous secretion
Lacrimal glands	Secretion	0
Nasopharyngeal glands	Secretion	
Bronchial glands	Secretion	?

(Continued)

Table 1.1 (*Continued*)

Organ and organ system	Activation of parasympathetic nerves	Activation of sympathetic nerves
Sweat glands	0	Secretion (cholinergic)
Digestive glands (stomach, pancreas)	Secretion	Decreased secretion or 0 (depends also on changes of blood flow)
Mucosa (small, large intestine)	Secretion (mainly in large intestine)	Decreased secretion or reabsorption
Pineal gland	0	Increased synthesis of melatonin
Brown adipose tissue	0	Heat production
Metabolism		
Liver	0	Glycogenolysis, Gluconeogenesis
Fat cells	0	Lipolysis (free fatty acids in blood increased)
β-cells in islets of pancreas	Secretion	Decreased secretion
α-cells in islets of pancreas	0	Secretion of glucagon
Adrenal medulla[3]	0	Secretion of adrenaline and noradrenaline
Lymphoid tissue	0	Depression of immune response

[1] Only in some species.

[2] Secretion of exocrine glands by activation of secretomotor neurons accompanied by dilatation of associated vasculature.

[3] Cells in the *adrenal medulla* are ontogenetically homologous to sympathetic postganglionic neurons. When activated by their preganglionic axons, subgroups of medullary cells release either adrenaline or noradrenaline directly into the circulation. In humans, 85% of adrenal medullary output is adrenaline. Most of the effects of circulating catecholamines are mediated through adrenaline's actions on β-adrenoceptors.

lateral part of the ventral horn, and project via the sacral ventral roots and pelvic splanchnic nerves to supply the pelvic organs. Like the sympathetic preganglionic neurons, they receive inputs from local spinal interneurons as well as supraspinal and propriospinal projections (Jänig 2006).

Parasympathetic preganglionic neurons project their axons directly to the organs they supply, where the postganglionic neurons are located in small ganglia (often interconnected in a network or plexus) just outside, or even within the wall of the target organ. *Parasympathetic ganglia* are found in the head (ciliary ganglia to eye; pterygopalatine ganglia to lachrymal, nasal, and palatal glands; otic and submandibular ganglia to salivary glands) and near or in the wall of various effector organs (heart, airways, pancreas, gall bladder, pelvic organs). The cranial parasympathetic ganglia receive preganglionic innervation from brainstem nuclei and are generally larger aggregations of neurons than the parasympathetic ganglia of the trunk. Preganglionic neurons that project to the gastrointestinal tract synapse with neurons that are part of the enteric nervous system. This may not always be the case as some preganglionic neurons of pathways to the colon/rectum synapse with postganglionic neurons in the pelvic plexus, which in turn synapse with enteric neurons.

The responses in effector cells and organs elicited by activity in parasympathetic nerves are listed in Table 1.1. Most activity in parasympathetic neurons increases motility of visceral organs and generates secretion in the mucosae.

Enteric nervous system

Within the wall of the gastrointestinal tract, a complexly interconnected neuronal system extends from the oesophagus to the rectum. Two interconnected plexuses of ganglia are located:

◆ between the longitudinal and circular muscle layers (myenteric or Auerbach's plexus)

◆ in the submucosa (submucosal or Meissner's plexus).

Neurons of the myenteric ganglia project into the external longitudinal and internal circular muscle layers, whereas many in submucosal plexus extend into the mucosa. Some neurons of both enteric plexuses have processes that project circumferentially, orally, or anally for up to many centimetres (Furness and Costa 1987, Furness 2006).

Functionally, both plexuses contain afferent (sensory) neurons, interneurons, and motor neurons which bring about complex reflex changes in motility (peristalsis, segmentation, etc.) via excitatory or inhibitory actions on the smooth muscle layers, regulate secretion and absorption by the mucosal epithelial cells, and regulate protective reflexes involving the gut-associated lymphoid tissue. Mechanical and chemical stimuli excite afferent endings in the mucosa or within the muscle. Sets of neurons mediating specific reflexes are repeated at regular intervals along the tract, their properties being adapted progressively to the changing functions at different levels. The enteric nervous system, together with the gut tissues, behaves as an effector tissue, which is regulated via sympathetic and parasympathetic pathways from the CNS.

Propulsive (oral-aboral) peristalsis and the effects of the excitatory and inhibitory motor neurons on the muscle layers in some parts of the gastrointestinal tract (e.g. circular muscles of small intestine, colon and stomach) are also dependent on the so-called 'interstitial cells of Cajal'. These cells are of mesenchymal origin, as are smooth muscle cells. They form networks of electrically coupled pacemaker cells and are coupled electrically to the contractile smooth muscle cells. The electrical activity of these cells is responsible for generation and propagation of the rhythmic movements of the stomach and small intestine. Furthermore, they mediate some excitatory and inhibitory synaptic activity of enteric motor neurons to the circular musculature (Ward SM et al. 2004, Furness 2006, Jänig 2006). The interstitial cells of Cajal are also present in a number of other smooth muscle effector tissues but their role in mediating neurally evoked responses has not been clarified.

Autonomic effector responses to activation of sympathetic and parasympathetic axons

Table 1.1 describes the overall responses of the peripheral targets to activity in sympathetic and parasympathetic neurons. These responses have been defined by reflex activation or by electrical stimulation of the respective nerves. In some cases, the effects of nerve activity have been deduced by the absence of an organ function following transection of the nerve supply. It should be noted, however, that this may not be appropriate as the behaviour of some organs is significantly modified after denervation. The Table shows that:

◆ Most target tissues react predominantly to only *one* of the autonomic systems (the pacemaker cells in the heart are one exception).

◆ A few target organs react to activity in both autonomic systems (e.g. iris, heart, urinary bladder).

◆ Opposite reactions to activity in sympathetic and parasympathetic neurons are more the exception than the rule.

◆ Most responses are excitatory, that is inhibition (e.g. relaxation of muscle, decrease of secretion) is rare.

The Table shows that the idea of antagonism between the parasympathetic and sympathetic nervous systems is largely a misconception. Where there are reciprocal effects on the target organs, it can usually be shown either that the systems work synergistically or that they exert their influence under different functional conditions. For example, in larger mammals, fast changes of heart rate during changes of body position or mental arousal are generated via changes in the activity of parasympathetic neurons to the pacemaker cells; the sustained increase of heart rate during exercise is mainly generated by increased activity of sympathetic neurons.

It is important to note that the effects of nerve activity are not necessarily the same as the responses of the effector tissues to the application of exogenous transmitter.

Visceral afferent neurons

About 85% of the axons in the vagus nerve and about 50% of those in the splanchnic nerves (greater, lesser, least, lumbar, and pelvic) are afferent. These visceral afferents come from sensory receptors in the internal organs. Their cell bodies lie in the ganglia of nerves X and XI and in the dorsal root ganglia of the segments corresponding to the autonomic outflow (spinal visceral afferents). Most visceral afferent axons are unmyelinated, some are thinly myelinated. Spinal visceral afferents project through the *white rami* to the respective spinal segments. It is unlikely that peripheral axons of spinal afferent neurons project along the sympathetic chain and blood vessels to the extremities and to the head although some supply the ventral compartment of the vertebral column and parietal tissues directly from the sympathetic chain. Sometimes thoracolumbar and sacral afferents are labelled 'sympathetic' or 'parasympathetic' but this nomenclature is misleading. There is no reason to associate any of these visceral afferent neurons with only one of the autonomic systems (Jänig 2006).

Vagal and sacral visceral afferents

Visceral afferents from the lungs, cardiovascular system, gastrointestinal tract, evacuative, and reproductive organs project to the nucleus of the solitary tract in the brainstem or to the sacral spinal cord. Most of these afferents react to distension and contraction of the organs. Their activity encodes intraluminal pressure (e.g. arterial baroreceptor afferents, afferents from the urinary bladder) or volume (afferents from the gut, atria, and lungs). Some are chemosensitive (arising from arterial chemoreceptors in the carotid bodies, chemosensors in the gut mucosa, and osmosensors in the liver). Most vagal visceral afferents do not signal noxious events. Pelvic visceral afferents signal noxious events as well as distension and contraction; pain arises during strong contractions and distensions of the pelvic organs as well as after inflammation of the organ (Ritter et al. 1992, Jänig and Koltzenburg 1993, Jänig 2006, Undem and Weinreich 2005).

Thoracolumbar spinal visceral afferents

The sensory receptors of thoracolumbar visceral afferents are situated in the serosa, the mesenteries, and the walls of some organs. Many more of these afferents are associated with the pelvic organs than with the abdominal organs. Most are mechanosensitive and some are active only during tissue inflammation and ischaemia. These afferents are involved in:

◆ organ-specific spinal reflexes (e.g. cardio-cardiac, reno-renal)

◆ pain of all visceral organs (Cervero 1994, Jänig 2006).

Functional autonomic motor pathways

Many individual sympathetic preganglionic and postganglionic neurons are spontaneously active *in vivo* and/or can be activated or inhibited by appropriate physiological stimuli. This has been shown in anaesthetized animals for neurons of the lumbar sympathetic outflow to skeletal muscles, skin and pelvic viscera, and for neurons of the thoracic sympathetic outflow to the head and neck, as well as in unanaesthetized humans for the sympathetic outflow to skeletal muscles and skin. The reflexes observed correspond to the effector responses that are induced by changes in activity in these neurons. The reflex patterns elicited by stimulation of various afferent input systems are characteristic for each functional sympathetic pathway and therefore represent physiological 'fingerprints' for each pathway (Jänig 1985, 1996, Jänig and McLachlan 1992a). Reflex patterns for muscle vasoconstrictor (MVC), visceral vasoconstrictor (VVC), cutaneous vasoconstrictor (CVC), and sudomotor (SM) neurons and for one type of motility regulating (MR) neuron in anaesthetized animals are shown in Figs 1.1–1.3:

◆ Discharge patterns in MVC and VVC neurons consist of inhibition by arterial baroreceptors (Fig. 1.2a) but excitation by arterial chemoreceptors, cutaneous nociceptors, and spinal visceral nociceptors (Fig. 1.1a,b).

◆ Most CVC neurons are inhibited by stimulation of cutaneous nociceptors, spinal visceral afferents, arterial chemoreceptors, and central warm-sensitive neurons in the spinal cord and hypothalamus (Fig. 1.1). In humans most of these reflexes are difficult to see because of the strong influence of cortical emotional and cognitive activity on the cutaneous vasoconstrictor system (Chapter 25).

◆ SM neurons are activated by stimulation of Pacinian corpuscles in skin (Fig. 1.1c). In humans this reflex may be important to keep the glabrous skin elastic for proper sensory discrimination. Furthermore, in primates, sudomotor neurons are specifically activated during body warming.

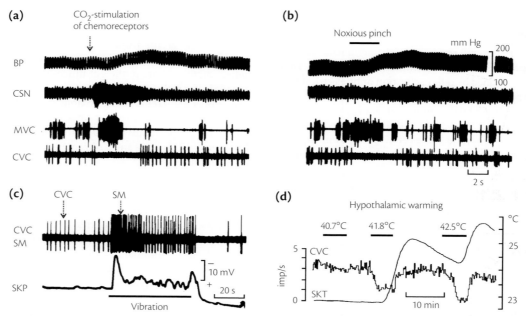

Fig. 1.1 Reflexes in muscle (MVC) and cutaneous (CVC) vasoconstrictor and sudomotor (SM) neurons recorded from postganglionic axons in anaesthetized cats. **(a)** Stimulation of carotid chemoreceptors by a bolus injection of CO_2-enriched saline into the carotid artery (at arrow) activated the MVC neurons and inhibited the CVC neuron (recorded simultaneously). Increased afferent activity in the carotid sinus nerve (CSN) was monitored. The increase of blood pressure evoked by chemoreceptor stimulation led to a baroreceptor-mediated inhibition of MVC activity but not of CVC activity. **(b)** Stimulation of cutaneous nociceptors by pinching the ipsilateral hind paw (indicated by bar) also excited the MVC neurons and inhibited the CVC neuron. **(c)** Simultaneous recording of a single CVC neuron (small signal) and a single SM neuron (larger signal) and the skin potential (SKP) from the central paw pad. Stimulation of Pacinian corpuscles by vibration excited the SM neuron and inhibited the CVC neuron. SM activation was correlated with the changes in the SKP. **(d)** Inhibition of CVC neurons to warming of the anterior hypothalamus. Note the increase of skin temperature (SKT) on the central paw pad followed the depression of CVC activity. (Data for **(a)** to **(c)** from Jänig and Kümmel, unpublished; **(d)** from Grewe et al. 1995. *J Physiol* **448**:139–2. With permission from W. Grewe, W. Janig and H. Kiimmel, Effects of hypothalamic thermal stimuli on sympathetic neurones innervating skin and skeletal muscle of the cat hindlimb, *Journal of Physiology*, Wiley.

- MR neurons are excited or inhibited by stimulation of sacral afferents from the urinary bladder, hindgut, or anal canal (Fig. 1.3), but are not affected by arterial baroreceptor activation (Fig. 1.2b). Functionally different types of MR neurons can be discriminated by way of their reflex pattern.

So far 12 different functional groups of postganglionic and preganglionic sympathetic neurons have been identified (Table 1.2). The neurons in eight of these pathways have ongoing activity under anaesthesia whereas in four pathways they are normally silent. Experimental studies (Fig. 1.4) show that:

- the reflex patterns observed in each group of sympathetic neurons are the result of integrative processes in spinal cord, brainstem, and hypothalamus

- functionally similar preganglionic and postganglionic neurons are synaptically connected in the sympathetic ganglia, probably with little or no 'cross-talk' between different peripheral pathways so that the centrally derived signals are relayed with little or no modulation through most ganglia

- the messages in these functional pathways are transmitted to the autonomic effector cells by distinct neuroeffector mechanisms.

In contrast, relatively few systematic studies have been made on the functional properties of parasympathetic preganglionic and postganglionic neurons. However, there are good reasons to assume that the principle of organization into functionally discrete pathways is the same as in the sympathetic nervous system, the main difference being that many targets of the sympathetic system are widely distributed throughout the body (e.g. blood vessels, sweat glands, erector pili muscles, fat tissue) (Jänig and McLachlan 1992a,b, Jänig 2006).

Organization and function of autonomic ganglia

A major function of the peripheral ganglia is to distribute the centrally integrated signals by connecting each preganglionic axon with several postganglionic neurons. The extent of divergence varies significantly, the ratio of preganglionic to postganglionic axons being, in pathways such as in the ciliary ganglion to the iris and ciliary body, as low as 1:4 and in others, such as in the superior cervical ganglion with many vasoconstrictor neurons, as high as 1:200 or more. It is clear, however, that limited divergence and much divergence, are not characteristic of the parasympathetic and sympathetic systems, respectively, although this has often been stated (Wang et al. 1995). Probably, by analogy with somatic motor units, limited divergence is common in pathways to small targets with discrete functions whereas widespread divergence is a feature of pathways to anatomically extensive effectors that act more or less simultaneously. Such effectors may be innervated by either system (McLachlan 1995).

Sympathetic ganglia

Structurally, sympathetic postganglionic neurons have several dendrites, the number of which is correlated with the number of preganglionic inputs (Purves et al. 1986, Boyd et al. 1996).

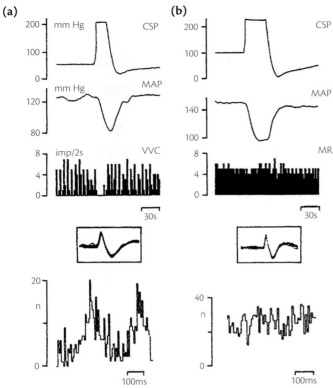

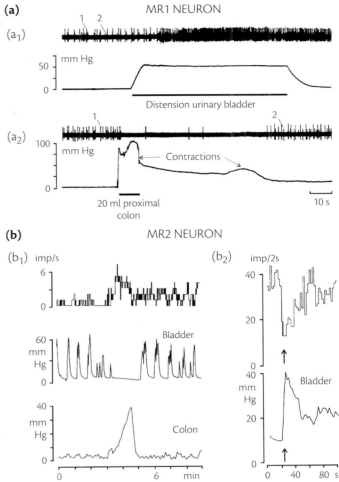

Fig. 1.2 Baroreceptor reflexes in sympathetic preganglionic neurons of the cat. Responses of **(a)** a single visceral vasoconstrictor (VVC) neuron, **(b)** a single motility regulating (MR) neuron and blood pressure to step pressure changes at the carotid sinus baroreceptors. Traces (from above, down) show carotid sinus pressure (CSP), mean arterial blood pressure (MAP) and neuronal activity in the VVC neuron and the MR neuron (peristimulus histograms). The activity of the neurons was recorded from the axons isolated from one of the lumbar splanchnic nerves in anaesthetized cats. Insets show the form of the action potentials of each unit. Post-R-wave histograms (below) from 500 superimposed sweeps over two cardiac cycles show the absence of cardiac rhythmicity in the activity of the MR neuron. With permission from the *Journal of the Autonomic Nervous System*, **42**, M. Michaelis, A. Boczek-Funcke, H.-J. Habler, W. Janig.

Fig. 1.3 Reflexes in motility-regulating neurons in response to stimulation of the urinary bladder or colon in the cat. Recordings from postganglionic axons isolated from the hypogastric nerve. **(a)** Two motility-regulating neurons type 1: Activation during distension of the urinary bladder (a1, filling with 20 ml saline) and inhibition during distension/contraction of the colon (a2, filling with 20 ml saline); during filling and after emptying the colon contracted. **(b)** Motility-regulating neuron type 2: Activation during contraction of the colon (b1) and inhibition during contraction of the urinary bladder (b1, b2). In b2 20 contractions are superimposed. This neuron was activated or inhibited during distension of the colon or bladder, respectively. With permission from W. Janig, M. Schmidt, A. Schnitzler and Ursula Wtesselmann, Differentiation of Sympathetic Neurones Projecting in the Hypogastric Nerves in Terms of their Discharge Patterns in cats, *Journal of Physiology*, Wiley.

Each convergent preganglionic axon produces an excitatory postsynaptic potential (EPSP) by releasing acetylcholine that activates nicotinic receptor-channels. The mode of transmission differs from that of excitatory transmission in the CNS. The amplitude of the potential produced by one quantum of acetylcholine released from a synaptic vesicle is ~0.5–1 mV. The amplitude of the multiquantal EPSP evoked by the action potential in a single preganglionic axon varies between inputs, ranging from a few to many tens of millivolts, with >15 mV usually being suprathreshold. In most postganglionic neurons, one input (sometimes two, rarely more) has, like the skeletal neuromuscular junction, a high safety factor and always initiates an action potential (Fig. 1.5). Thus the ganglion cell relays the incoming impulses of only one or a few of its preganglionic inputs that probably arise in one spinal segment. As a result, postganglionic axons with ongoing activity (mostly vasoconstrictor) discharge at only about 1 Hz (Chapter 25) (Jänig 1995, 2006), which is comparable to the rate of firing of individual preganglionic axons. When activity increases during reflex activation or arousal, postganglionic neurons can discharge in short bursts at up to 5–10 Hz, more often by increased discharge of the suprathreshold preganglionic inputs than by summation of EPSPs.

The function of the sub-threshold synapses in ganglia of paravertebral (mainly vasoconstrictor) pathways is not clear; they may simply be redundant. The larger subthreshold EPSPs may sometimes reach threshold (Bratton et al. 2010) either because of quantal variation or because of summation with smaller inputs. In addition, modifications of ion channels (and so membrane conductance) during the afterhyperpolarization or by some local or circulating substances may change the effectiveness of EPSPs. However, if the strong input is lost, a new strong input rapidly develops, probably from an existing weak input, suggesting a preference for the maintenance of particular transganglionic pathways (Ireland 1999, McLachlan 2003).

Sympathetic *paravertebral neurons* have relatively uniform cell properties. At least one of these inputs is suprathreshold and relays

Table 1.2 Functional classification of sympathetic neurons based on reflex behaviour in vivo[a]

Likely function	Location	Target organ	Likely target tissue	Major identifying stimulus[b]	Ongoing activity
Vasoconstrictor					
Muscle	Lumbar[c]	Hind limb muscle	Resistance vessels	Baro-inhibition[d]	Yes
	Cervical[e]	Head and neck muscle	Resistance vessels	Baro-inhibition	Yes
Cutaneous	Lumbar	Hind limb skin vessels	Thermoregulatory vessels	Inhibited by CNS warming	Yes
	Cervical	Head and neck skin	Thermoregulatory vessels	Inhibited by CNS warming	Yes
Visceral	Lumbar splanchnic	Pelvic viscera	Resistance vessels	Baro-inhibition	Yes
Vasodilator					
Muscle	Lumbar	Hind limb muscle	Muscle arteries	Hypothalamic stimulation	No
Cutaneous	Lumbar	Hind limb skin	Skin vasculature	?	No
Sudomotor	Lumbar	Paw pads	Sweat glands	Vibration (in cat), central warming (human)	Yes, some
Pilomotor	Lumbar	Tail	Piloerector muscles	Hypothalamic stimulation	No
Inspiratory	Cervical	Airways?	Nasal mucosal vasculature	Inspiration	Yes
Pupillomotor	Cervical	Iris	Dilator pupillae muscle	Inhibition by light	Yes, some
Motility regulating					
Type 1	Lumbar splanchnic	Hindgut, urinary tract	Visceral smooth muscle	Bladder distension	Yes
Type 2	Lumbar splanchnic	Hindgut, urinary tract	Visceral smooth muscle	Inhibited by bladder distension	Yes
Reproduction	Lumbar splanchnic	Internal reproductive organs	Visceral smooth muscle, other?	?	No

[a] Experimental data from anaesthetized cats (Jänig 1985, 1996, Jänig and McLachlan 1987).
[b] Excitation by stimulus unless inhibition specified.
[c] 'Lumbar' refers to preganglionic and postganglionic axons in lumbar outflow.
[d] 'Baro-inhibition' indicates inhibition by stimulation of arterial baroreceptors.
[e] 'Cervical' refers to preganglionic axons in the cervical sympathetic trunk.

CNS-derived signals directly (Fig. 1.5a). In contrast, *prevertebral neurons* do not have uniform properties. In several species of experimental animal, three broad groups of sympathetic neuron have been shown to differ electrophysiologically (by their resting K[+] channels and the voltage-dependent and Ca[2+]-dependent K[+] channels that control their excitability), morphologically (by their size and dendritic branching), and neurochemically (by their neuropeptide content) (Boyd et al. 1996). Two groups, including most paravertebral neurons, have suprathreshold preganglionic connections, but the mode of synaptic transmission in the third group is different. These neurons are mainly found in prevertebral ganglia; they receive preganglionic inputs that do not necessarily activate them. However, they also receive many small amplitude nicotinic inputs from intestino-fugal neurons that are activated by distension of the intestine. Summation of the EPSPs arising from the intestine with those from preganglionic inputs is necessary to initiate their discharge. These neurons also depolarize slowly when the intestine is distended (Kreulen and Peters 1986) so that the small nicotinic responses are brought closer to threshold for firing. The slow depolarizations arise from the release of neuropeptides such as substance P (SP) from spinal primary afferent neuron collaterals (see Fig. 1.7). These prevertebral neurons therefore depend on temporal and spatial integration of incoming excitatory signals, unlike neurons in paravertebral ganglia. The function of these connections is discussed below.

Muscarinic and/or peptidergic contributions to ganglionic transmission may follow high-frequency activation of preganglionic inputs, as has been shown in muscle vasoconstrictor pathways in anaesthetized cats (Jänig 1995, 2006) and in some prevertebral neurons, but such contributions to ganglionic transmission have not been demonstrated in humans.

Parasympathetic ganglia

The structure of many parasympathetic ganglion cells, with few or no dendrites, is simpler than that of sympathetic postganglionic neurons. The preganglionic input is correspondingly simple, often consisting of a single suprathreshold input. However, some parasympathetic ganglia in the trunk contain, as well as postganglionic neurons, neurons that behave as primary afferent neurons and interneurons, i.e. they have the potential for reflex activity independent of the CNS, like the enteric nervous system (see 'Enteric nervous system', p.24). For example, in the intracardiac ganglia (Edwards et al. 1995; Fig. 1.6), only a subgroup of the ganglion cells receives an input from preganglionic axons and projects to cardiac muscle. A sub-population of neurons that cannot be activated synaptically may be afferent neurons (A in Fig. 1.6). These cells have intrinsic-like ongoing activity, which might be responsible for ongoing synaptic activity recorded in other neurons within the ganglia. A third group of smaller neurons receives local synaptic inputs and may also terminate on cardiac muscle (S in Fig. 1.6). Although both the location of the endings of the putative afferent neurons and the adequate stimuli that excite them remain mysteries, these peripheral connections are a feature of several parasympathetic ganglia (e.g. pancreatic, see McLachlan 1995). Transmission in intramural

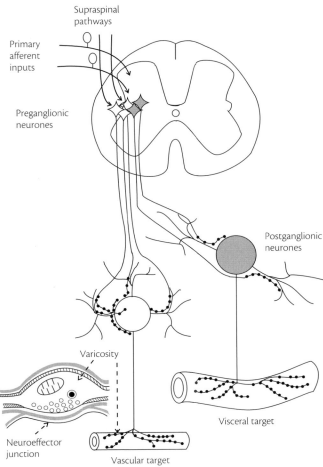

Fig. 1.4 Organization of the sympathetic nervous system into building blocks. Separate functional pathways extend from the CNS to the effector organs. Preganglionic neurons located in the intermediate zone integrate signals descending from brainstem and hypothalamus and arising segmentally from primary afferent axons. The preganglionic neurons project to peripheral ganglia and converge onto postganglionic neurons. The postganglionic axons form multiple neuroeffector junctions with their target cells (see Figs 1.8 and 1.9). With permission from *Trends in Neurosciences*, **15**, W. Jänig, E. M. McLachlan, Characteristics of function-specific pathways in the sympathetic nervous system, 475–481, Copyright (1992), with permission from Elsevier.

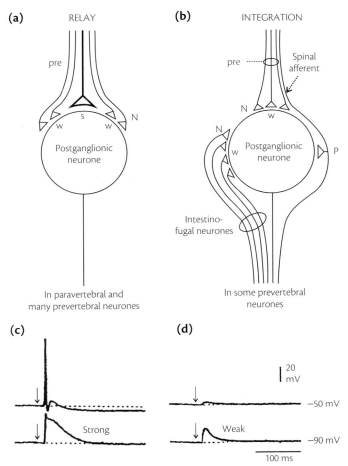

Fig. 1.5 Two types of transmission in autonomic ganglia. **(a)** Most ganglion cells receive one or a few preganglionic inputs that, when activated, produce a suprathreshold ('strong', S) response. Most also receive several weak (w) convergent inputs that evoke only a subthreshold (ineffective) synaptic potential. Transmission occurs via the S input, which relays its signals directly to the postganglionic neuron. Summation of weak responses is rare. **(b)** In some sympathetic prevertebral neurons, the preganglionic inputs are of the weak type but other cholinergic inputs that arise in the enteric nervous system also converge on the cell. Activation occurs by temporal and/or spatial summation. Peptides released from spinal afferent neurons (P) may potentiate transmission (see Fig. 1.7) **(c, d)** Synaptic potentials recorded in postganglionic neurons at resting membrane potential (upper traces) and with the membrane hyperpolarized to block action potential initiation (lower traces). Preganglionic axons were electrically stimulated (arrows; the stimulus artefacts were removed for clarity). When a single strong input is stimulated **(c),** the response is suprathreshold at resting membrane potential and a large amplitude excitatory synaptic potential is evoked at –90 mV. In response to stimulation of a single weak preganglionic axon **(d),** a small subthreshold excitatory synaptic potential is evoked that increases in amplitude with hyperpolarization. The differences in amplitude between strong and weak inputs reflect differences in the number of quanta of acetylcholine released from each preganglionic input.

ganglia shows some similarities to sympathetic ganglia and some to the enteric system. No evidence of either interneurons or intrinsic-like ongoing activity has yet been detected in cranial ganglia.

The pelvic or hypogastric plexuses contain the neurons that innervate the pelvic organs. Some of these ganglion cells are noradrenergic and are innervated by lumbar preganglionic axons; others are cholinergic and receive sacral inputs (Keast 1995). A substantial proportion of pelvic neurons receive synaptic connections from both hypogastric and pelvic nerves.

Peripheral reflexes

Spinal visceral afferent neurons are not only involved in reflexes at spinal and supraspinal levels but probably also in peripheral reflexes that do not involve the CNS. In addition, neurons within the enteric nervous system (and possibly other effector tissues) have axons that project back into autonomic prevertebral ganglia through the mesenteric nerves and initiate reflex activity in postganglionic neurons. These latter are known as *intestino-fugal*

neurons of the enteric nervous system (i.e. they project out of the gastrointestinal tract from cell bodies within the enteric ganglia and do not enter the central nervous system). Distension activates mechanosensitive endings of enteric afferent neurons that activate the intestino-fugal neurons (Fig. 1.7). Afferent axons of intestino-fugal neurons from a considerable length of the intestine converge on each ganglion cell although the majority probably arise in the proximal colon. Summation of the synaptic effects of enteric

INTRACARDIAC GANGLIA

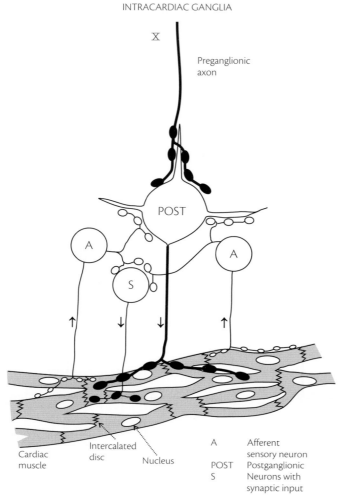

Fig. 1.6 Some parasympathetic ganglia are not simple relays. Diagram of the component neurons of intracardiac ganglia. Only one neuron type (POST) receives vagal synaptic inputs. SAH cells and another neuron type (S, synaptic) receive synaptic inputs with ongoing activity arising from the third neuron type which is spontaneously active (A, afferent). A cells may be sensory neurons with afferent terminals within the heart. With permission from Edwards, F. R., Hirst, G. D., Klemm, M. F., and Steele, P. A., Different types of ganglion cell in the cardiac plexus of guinea-pigs, *J. Physiol.*, Wiley.

neurons triggers discharges in postganglionic neurons and leads to the release of noradrenaline and thus relaxation of other parts of the intestine. These peripheral reflexes presumably contribute to the storage function of the large bowel aiding to reabsorb fluid and electrolytes. Peptides released in sympathetic prevertebral ganglia from collaterals of spinal visceral afferent neurons activated by distension can enhance cholinergic synaptic transmission from both preganglionic axons and enteric neurons (Fig. 1.7b).

Transmitter substances in autonomic neurons

The principles of chemical transmission were defined in the autonomic nervous system based on the release of the 'conventional' neurotransmitters, acetylcholine and noradrenaline. However, it is now clear that several chemical substances are often contained

within individual autonomic neurons, can be released by action potentials, and can have multiple actions on effector tissues (Furness et al. 1989, Morris and Gibbins 1992; see Chapter 5).

◆ Acetylcholine is released by all preganglionic axons at their synapses in ganglia, and the effects of nerve activity are normally completely antagonized by blockade of nicotinic acetylcholine receptors. Under some experimental conditions, repetitive activation of preganglionic axons can release enough acetylcholine to activate muscarinic receptors that are presumably located extrasynaptically (Jänig 1995, 2006).

◆ Most sympathetic postganglionic axons release noradrenaline, but sudomotor and muscle vasodilator axons are cholinergic. Most, but not all, nerve-mediated effects can be antagonized by blockade of adrenoceptors or muscarinic acetylcholine receptors.

◆ Although parasympathetic postganglionic neurons in many tissues release ACh, not all effects of stimulating parasympathetic nerves are blocked by muscarinic antagonists (Table 1.3) and so must be mediated by other transmitters. Whereas recent evidence confirms that all parasympathetic neurons are cholinergic (Keast 1995), many also release other substances.

The role of non-conventional transmitters has been studied extensively. Often several transmitters seem to be involved in producing the same neurally evoked response, e.g. in the enteric nervous system, nitric oxide (NO) and VIP, possibly together with adenosine 5′-triphosphate (ATP), are thought to mediate inhibition of gastrointestinal smooth muscle by enteric neurons. 'Nitrergic' nerves (containing the enzyme neuronal nitric oxide synthase) are vasodilator or relaxant in several tissues (Table 1.3). Their action is demonstrated by the absence of responses after blockade of NO synthesis with, for example L-NAME. Currently, various peptides, ATP and NO appear to act as co-transmitters.

Responses of tissues to nerve-released noradrenaline and acetylcholine may be hard to detect except by repetitive activation of many axons. High-frequency stimuli, particularly in bursts, may produce effector responses due to the concomitant release of a neuropeptide. Immunohistochemistry has revealed the presence of many neuropeptides, although only a few of these have been demonstrated to modify function after release from nerve terminals *in vivo*. Examples are:

◆ Neuropeptide Y (NPY) in sympathetic vasoconstrictor axons potentiates the contractile effects of nerve-released noradrenaline on adrenoceptors. In the heart, NPY released by sympathetic postganglionic axons inhibits vagal slowing generated by parasympathetic cardiomotor neurons.

◆ VIP is released from cholinergic vasodilator or secretomotor neurons. It is thought to contribute to vasodilation in for example erectile tissue (where NO seems to be the primary transmitter), to vasodilation generated around sweat glands by activation of sudomotor neurons and to vasodilation generated within salivary glands by activation of secretomotor neurons.

◆ Sympathetic axons and primary afferent neurons that express SP and calcitonin-gene-related peptide (CGRP) interact in the regulation of some vascular beds, such as skin and mesentery. This interaction occurs postjunctionally, and not between the nerve terminals. CGRP, thought to be released by axon reflex activation of afferent terminals during inflammation, is a potent vasodilator.

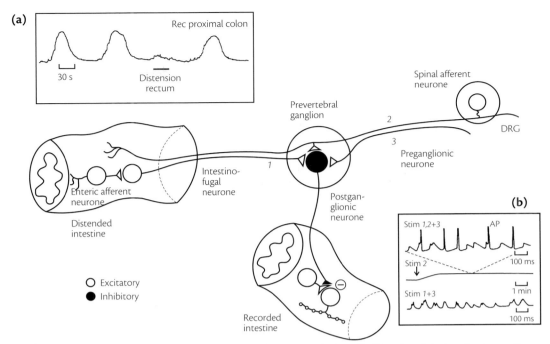

Fig. 1.7 Peripheral reflexes involving enteric and dorsal root afferents and sympathetic prevertebral ganglia. Distension of the bowel activates afferent terminals of local enteric neurons, which connect with intestino-fugal neurons (neuron 1) that project to the prevertebral ganglia. Visceral primary afferent neurons (neuron 2) with cell bodies in the dorsal root ganglia (DRG) are also activated. The intestino-fugal neurons excite postganglionic neurons projecting to another part of the bowel. This leads to inhibition (-) of enteric excitatory muscle motor neurons and relaxation. Collateral branches of primary afferent neurons (neuron 2) activated by the same stimulus release substance P around the same postganglionic neuron producing a slow depolarization. When 1 and 2 occur together with the ongoing inputs from preganglionic (3) neurons (1 + 2 + 3), they summate and action potentials are initiated. **Inset (a)**: Recording of the intraluminal pressure in an isolated proximal segment of the colon and distension of the rectum in an anaesthetized cat. The inferior mesenteric ganglion (IMG) was decentralized by section of the preganglionic axons in the lumbar splanchnic nerves. The regular contraction waves of the proximal colon were inhibited during distension of the rectum. This inhibition was mediated by the IMG. From Kuntz, A. *J. Comp. Neurol.* **72**, 371–382 (1940). **Inset (b)**: Lower trace, subthreshold cholinergic postsynaptic potentials (1 + 3) elicited in a prevertebral postganglionic neuron during activity in intestino fugal (neuron 1) and preganglionic neurons (neuron 3). Middle trace, slow depolarization generated by activity in peptidergic spinal visceral afferent neuron (neuron 2). Upper trace, enhancement of nicotinic postsynaptic potentials by slow depolarization leads to generation of action potentials. Idealized in vivo behaviour derived from in vitro experiments. W. Jänig, *The Integrative Action*, © Jänig 2006, published by Cambrige University Press, reproduced with permission.

Table 1.3 Possible transmitter substances in autonomic neurons

System	Neuron	Transmitter	Co-transmitters
Parasympathetic	Preganglionic	ACh	
	Postganglionic	ACh	VIP and/or NO
Sympathetic	Preganglionic	ACh	
	Postganglionic	NAd,	ATP and/or NPY
		some ACh	VIP and/or NO
Enteric	[Vagal and pelvic inputs	ACh]	
	[Sympathetic inputs	NAd]	
	Intrinsic afferent neurons	Substance P (tachykinins)	
	Interneurons	ACh	Some ATP
	Motor		
	Excitatory	ACh	Substance P (tachykinins)
	Inhibitory	NO/?VIP/PACAP/?ATP	
	Secretomotor	ACh	VIP

ACh, acetylcholine; NAd, noradrenaline; ATP, adenosine 5'-triphosphate; NO, nitric oxide; NPY, neuropeptide Y; VIP, vasoactive intestinal polypeptide; PACAP, pituitary adenylate cyclase-activating peptide.

Thus, in peripheral tissues, the effects of activity in autonomic nerve terminals can be due to the release of several different compounds. However, when the effects of nerve activity are not blocked completely by an adrenoceptor or muscarinic antagonist at a concentration that entirely abolishes the response to exogenous transmitter, it may be that the receptors rather than the transmitters are not conventional ones.

Mechanisms of neuroeffector transmission

The effects of exogenous transmitter substances on cellular effector functions are known for many tissues but the consequences of activation of postjunctional receptors by neurally released transmitters have been investigated surprisingly rarely. When they have, the mechanisms of neuroeffector transmission have been found to be diverse. Excitation or inhibition may involve a range of cellular events, including:

- brief openings of ligand-gated channels (as at many neuronal synapses) or slower conductance changes mediated by second messenger systems

- the ensuing depolarization may open voltage-dependent Ca^{2+} channels, leading to Ca^{2+} influx

- receptor activation, which may lead, after G-protein activation, to release of Ca^{2+} from intracellular Ca^{2+} stores or modulation of the Ca^{2+} sensitivity of the contractile/secretory mechanism

- β-adrenoceptors linked to adenylate cyclase modify cell function by changing intracellular levels of cyclic adenosine monophosphate (AMP)

- inhibition (relaxation) often involves the activation of cyclic guanosine monophosphate (GMP)-dependent protein kinases.

Other intracellular pathways may also be involved. *One important concept has emerged: the mechanism utilized by endogenously released transmitter appears generally to differ from that activated by exogenous transmitter substances or their analogues* (Hirst et al. 1996). The following examples illustrate this point.

Innervation of the cardiac pacemaker

Vagal stimulation slows action potential firing in atrial pacemaker cells. During nerve stimulation, the action potentials slow without any change in their configuration and without membrane hyperpolarization (Fig. 1.8b). Exogenous acetylcholine, in contrast, slows firing by hyperpolarizing the membrane and reducing the amplitude and duration of the action potentials, consistent with an increase in K^+ conductance (Fig. 1.8c). Both responses are blocked by atropine but, as the postreceptor conductance changes clearly differ, the muscarinic receptors activated by vagal acetylcholine cannot be the same as those to which exogenous acetylcholine binds.

Similar data have been obtained for the sympathetic innervation, which increases the rate of pacemaking. Both neurally released and exogenous noradrenaline activate β-adrenoceptors but neural noradrenaline modifies the pacemaker current independently of the rise in cyclic AMP levels produced by exogenous noradrenaline. Because both noradrenergic and cholinergic axons form close neuromuscular junctions on cardiac pacemaker cells and these junctions cover ≤1% of the pacemaker cell surface (Fig. 1.8a), it seems likely that neurally released transmitters act on junctional receptors that differ from those at extrajunctional sites. The latter would most readily be activated by exogenous compounds. Junctional and extrajunctional receptors are most likely connected

by different intracellular pathways to the cellular effectors (ion channels).

Cholinergic innervation of the ileum

The longitudinal muscle of the ileum is innervated by cholinergic neurons that lie in the myenteric plexus. Nerve-evoked contractions and contractions to exogenous acetylcholine are both abolished by atropine. Nerve-evoked contractions are reduced but not abolished by blockade of voltage-dependent Ca^{2+} channels. Depolarizations evoked by nerve stimulation are associated with increases in intracellular Ca^{2+}. Both the depolarizations (and the

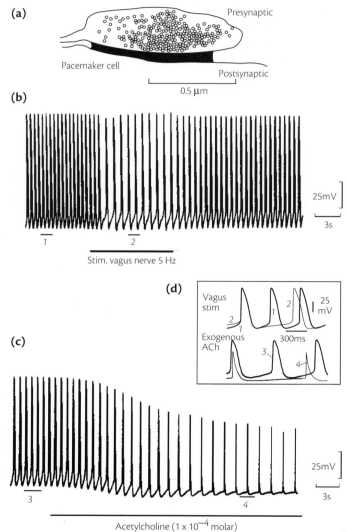

Fig. 1.8 Innervation of the cardiac pacemaker. **(a)** Tracings of a cholinergic varicosity forming a neuromuscular junction on a cell of the guinea pig sinoatrial node. From Choate et al. 1993. J Auton Nerv Syst 44:1–12. Membrane effects of **(b)** acetylcholine (ACh) released by parasympathetic cardiomotor axons and **(c)** exogenously applied ACh differ. **(d)** Nerve-mediated responses show no change in action potential configuration but a reduced slope of the pacemaker potential (upper records in inset), whereas exogenous ACh hyperpolarizes the membrane and shunts the action potential, reducing its amplitude and duration, due to opening of potassium channels and subsequent decrease in membrane resistance (lower records in inset). 1 to 4 refer to the time periods marked in **(b)** and **(c)**. With permission from Campbell G D, Edwards F R, Hirst G D and O'Shea J E, Effects of vagal stimulation and applied acetylcholine on pacemaker potentials in the guinea-pig heart, *Journal of Physiology*, Wiley.

accompanying contraction) are blocked by calcium-channel antagonists that do not affect the depolarization and contraction produced by exogenous acetylcholine. Figure 1.9 summarizes the cellular mechanisms that seem to be involved in these responses. Close junctions between varicose terminals and smooth muscle also exist in this tissue. These findings suggest that muscarinic receptors involved in transmission from cholinergic nerves to this muscle are restricted to the junctional membrane and differ from those activated by exogenous acetylcholine.

Sympathetic innervation of blood vessels

Blood vessels are innervated by sympathetic nerve terminals containing noradrenaline, ATP and in most cases also NPY. Most blood vessels constrict when exogenous noradrenaline is applied to them. This pharmacological action of noradrenaline is mediated by α_1-adrenoceptors or α_2-adrenoceptors, or sometimes both. Constriction may depend on the entry of extracellular Ca^{2+} through voltage-dependent channels, but much of the Ca^{2+} triggering vasoconstriction is released from intracellular stores by second messengers.

Many of the sympathetic varicosities on small arterial vessels of less than 0.5 mm diameter form close neuromuscular junctions (Luff and McLachlan 1989), the proportion that do not form

junctions varying between vessels at different sites throughout the circulation and between species. In vessels with neuromuscular junctions, nerve stimulation evokes brief depolarizations due to the action of ATP on P_{2X} purinoceptors and/or slow depolarizations due to the actions of noradrenaline on α_1-adrenoceptors or α_2-adrenoceptors (Hirst et al. 1996). Constriction of small arteries during ongoing sympathetic nerve activity is abolished by various combinations of α-adrenoceptor antagonists but is partly dependent on membrane depolarization (Brock et al. 1997). However, this is not always the case. Nerve-evoked vasoconstriction is resistant to α-adrenoceptor antagonists in arterioles of the intestinal submucosa and the basilar artery where it is mediated solely by P_{2X} purinoceptors. P_{2X} receptors synergize with $\alpha1$-adrenoceptors to elicit nerve-evoked responses in small mesenteric, median and saphenous arteries but not tail arteries (Brock et al., 2007). The purinergic contribution in small mesenteric arteries is greater at higher distending pressures (Rummery et al., 2007). Further, the mechanisms underlying neurally evoked constriction of veins differs in different tissues. Thus neural control of vasoconstriction can involve distinct transmitters and postjunctional receptors and both voltage-dependent and voltage-independent mechanisms in different parts of the vascular tree and even between levels in a single vascular bed.

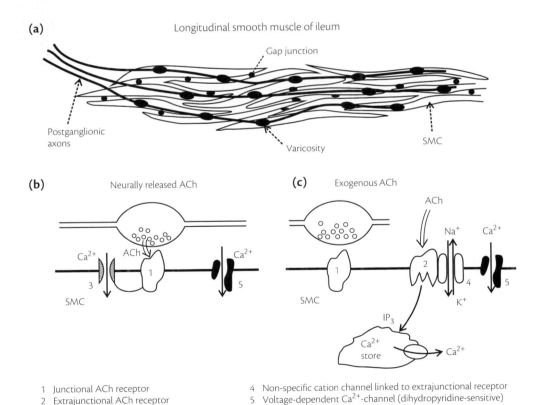

1 Junctional ACh receptor
2 Extrajunctional ACh receptor
3 Cation channel (possibly Ca^{2+} selective) linked to junctional receptor

4 Non-specific cation channel linked to extrajunctional receptor
5 Voltage-dependent Ca^{2+}-channel (dihydropyridine-sensitive)

Fig. 1.9 Neuroeffector transmission to the longitudinal muscle of the ileum. **(a)** The varicosities of cholinergic nerve terminals form close synaptic contacts with the longitudinal smooth muscle cells. **(b)** Acetylcholine (ACh) released by nerve impulses from the varicosities activates junctional muscarinic receptors (1) leading to depolarization by activation of Ca^{2+} selective ion channels (3). This depolarization opens voltage-activated Ca^{2+} channels (5). **(c)** In contrast, ACh applied by superfusion activates extrajunctional muscarinic receptors (2) linked to non-selective cation channels (4), leading to depolarization and activation of voltage-activated Ca^{2+} channels (5). In addition, exogenous ACh releases Ca^{2+} from intracellular stores via the inositol triphosphate (IP3) pathway. Increased intracellular Ca^{2+} from both sources contributes to muscle contraction. SMC, smooth muscle cell. Gap junction channels allow electrical and chemical signals to pass directly between neighbouring cells. With permission from *Neuroscience*, **65**, H. M. Cousins, F. R. Edwards, G. D. S. Hirst, Neuronally released and applied acetylcholine on the longitudinal muscle of the guinea-pig ileum, 193–207, Copyright (1995), with permission from Elsevier.

Other effectors

The examples given above indicate the diversity of mechanisms for neuroeffector transmission in different targets. As the responses of other tissues to nerve stimulation are studied, our traditional ideas about the ability of conventional transmitters to mimic the effects of nerve activity must be reconsidered. If the intention is to interfere with ongoing nerve-mediated effects *in vivo*, it is more useful to determine which antagonists reduce or abolish the effects of nerve activity than to know which receptor subtypes are present on the tissue.

Conclusion

The autonomic nervous system supplies each target organ and tissue via a separate pathway which consists of sets of preganglionic and postganglionic neurons with distinct patterns of reflex activity. This has been established for the lumbar sympathetic outflow to skin, skeletal muscle and viscera, for the thoracic sympathetic outflow to the head and neck, in experimental animals and probably applies to all autonomic systems. The specificity of the messages that these pathways transmit from the CNS arises from integration within precisely organized pathways in the spinal cord, brainstem and hypothalamus. The messages travel along discrete functional pathways and are transmitted to the target tissues often via organized neuroeffector junctions. Modulation in the periphery may occur within each pathway, sometimes in ganglia and sometimes at the level of the effector organs. Much remains to be discovered about the neural control of the diverse functions of the vasculature, glands, and viscera.

Acknowledgements

The authors were supported by the Deutsche Forschungsgemeinschaft, Germany, and the National Health Medical Research Council of Australia.

References

Boyd, H., McLachlan, E. M., Keast, J. R., and Inokuchi, H. (1996). Three electrophysiological classes of guinea pig sympathetic neuron have distinct morphologies. *J. Comp. Neurol.* **369**, 372–87.

Bratton, B., Davies, P., Jänig, W., and McAllen, R. (2010). Ganglionic transmission in a vasomotor pathway studied in vivo. *J. Physiol.(Lond.)* **588**, 1647–59.

Brock, J. A., McLachlan, E. M., and Rayner, S. E. (1997). Contribution of α-adrenoceptors to depolarization and contraction evoked by continuous asynchronous sympathetic nerve activity in rat tail artery. *Br. J. Pharmacol.* **120**, 1513–21.

Cervero, F. (1994). Sensory innervation of the viscera: peripheral basis of visceral pain. *Physiol. Rev.* **75**, 95–138.

Edwards, F. R., Hirst, G. D., Klemm, M. F., and Steele, P. A. (1995). Different types of ganglion cell in the cardiac plexus of guinea-pigs. *J. Physiol.(Lond.)* **486**, 453–71.

Furness, J.B. (2006). *The enteric nervous system.* Blackwell Science Ltd, Oxford.

Furness, J. B., Morris, J. L., Gibbins, I. L., and Costa., M. (1989). Chemical coding of neurons and plurichemical transmission. *Ann. Rev. Pharmacol. Toxicol.* **29**, 289–306.

Furness, J. B. and Costa, M. (1987). *The enteric nervous system.* Churchill Livingstone, Edinburgh.

Hirst, G. D., Choate, J. K., Cousins, H. M., Edwards, F. R., and Klemm, M. F. (1996). Transmission by post-ganglionic axons of the autonomic nervous system: the importance of the specialized neuroeffector junction. *Neuroscience* **73**, 7–23.

Ireland, D. R. (1999). Preferential formation of strong synapses during re-innervation of guinea pig sympathetic ganglia. *J. Physiol.* **520**, 827–37.

Jänig, W. (1985). Organization of the lumbar sympathetic outflow to skeletal muscle and skin of the cat hindlimb and tail. *Rev. Physiol. Biochem. Pharmacol.* **102**, 119–213.

Jänig, W. (1995). Ganglionic transmission *in vivo*. In *Autonomic ganglia*, (ed. E.M. McLachlan), pp. 349–95. Harwood Academic Publishers, Luxembourg.

Jänig, W. (1996). Spinal cord reflex organization of sympathetic systems. In *The emotional motor system*, (ed. R. Bandler, G. Holstege, and C. B. Saper). *Prog. Brain Res.* **107**, 43–77.

Jänig, W. (2006). *The integrative action of the autonomic nervous system. Neurobiology of homeostasis.* Cambridge University Press, Cambridge.

Jänig, W. and Koltzenburg, M. (1993). Pain arising from the urogenital tract. In *The autonomic nervous system*, (ed. G. Burnstock), Vol. 2 *Nervous control of the urogenital system* (ed. C. A. Maggi), pp. 523–76. Harwood Academic Publishers, Chur, Switzerland.

Jänig, W. and McLachlan, E. M. (1987). Organization of lumbar spinal outflow to the distal colon and pelvic organs. *Physiol. Rev.* **67**, 1332–1404.

Jänig, W. and McLachlan, E. M. (1992a). Characteristics of function-specific pathways in the sympathetic nervous system. *Trends Neurosci.* **15**, 475–81.

Jänig, W. and McLachlan, E. M. (1992b). Specialized functional pathways are the building blocks of the autonomic nervous system. *J. Autonom. Nerv. Syst.* **41**, 3–14.

Keast, J. R. (1995). All pelvic neurons in male rats contain immunoreactivity for the synthetic enzymes of either noradrenaline or acetylcholine. *Neurosci. Lett.* **196**, 209–12.

Kreulen, D.L. and Peters, S. (1986). Non-cholinergic transmission in a sympathetic ganglion of the guinea- pig elicited by colon distension. *J. Physiol. (Lond)* **374**, 315–34.

Langley, J. N. (1921). *The autonomic nervous system*, part 1. Heffer, Cambridge.

Llewellyn-Smith, I. J. and Verbene, A. J. M. (eds.) (2011). *Central regulation of autonomic functions.* 2nd edition. Oxford University Press, New York.

Luff, S. E. and McLachlan, E. M. (1989). Frequency of neuromuscular junctions on arteries of different dimensions in the rabbit, guinea-pig and rat. *Blood Vessels* **26**, 95–106.

McLachlan, E. M. (ed.) (1995). *Autonomic ganglia.* Harwood Academic Publishers, Luxembourg.

McLachlan, E. M. (2003). Transmission of signals through sympathetic ganglia: modulation, integration or simply distribution? *Acta Physiol. Scand.* **177**, 227–35.

Morris, J. L. and Gibbins, I. L. (1992). Co-transmission and neuromodulation. In *Autonomic neuroeffector mechanisms*, (ed. G. Burnstock and C.H.V. Hoyle), pp. 33–119. Harwood Academic Publishers, Chur, Switzerland.

Purves, D., Rubin, E., Snider, W. D., and Lichtman, J. (1986). Relation of animal size to convergence, divergence, and neuronal number in peripheral sympathetic pathways. *J. Neurosci.* **6**, 158–63.

Ritter, S., Ritter, R. C., and Barnes, C. D. (ed.) (1992). *Neuroanatomy and physiology of abdominal vagal afferents.* CRC Press, Boca Raton.

Robertson, D., Biaggio, I., Burnstock, G., Low, P. A., and Paton, J. F. R. (eds.) (2012). *Primer on the autonomic nervous system.* 3rd edition. Elsevier, Academic Press Amsterdam Boston.

Rummery, N. M., Brock, J. A., Pakdeechote, P., Ralevic, V., and Dunn, W. R. (2007). ATP is the predominant sympathetic neurotransmitter in rat mesenteric arteries at high pressure. *J. Physiol.* **582**, 745–754.

Undem, B. and Weinreich, D. (eds.)(2005). *Advance in vagal afferent neurobiology.* CRC Press, Boca Raton.

Wang, F. B., Holst, M. C., and Powley, T. L. (1995). The ratio of pre- to postganglionic neurons and related issues in the autonomic nervous system. *Brain Res. Rev.* **21**, 93–115.

Ward, S. M., Sanders, K. M., and Hirst G. D. S. (2004). Role of interstitial cells of Cajal in neural control of gastrointestinal smooth muscles. *Neurogastroenterol. Motil.* **16**, Suppl 1, 112–117.

CHAPTER 2

Central nervous control of the cardiovascular system

J.F.R. Paton and K.M. Spyer

Introduction

The central neuronal networks within the spinal cord, brainstem and hypothalamus that are responsible for controlling cardiovascular autonomic outflows have been identified. This provides a basis for understanding the role of the central nervous system (CNS) in homeostatic regulation of circulation and the changes that accompany pathologies of the cardiovascular system. This chapter will highlight progress that has been made in our understanding of the central control of the cardiovascular autonomic nervous system in both health and disease states, such as hypertension and heart failure. We shall start by reflecting on the main aim of the CNS in regards to controlling the circulation.

Overall aim of central nervous control of the cardiovascular system

The cardiovascular system has a major role in homeostasis. It achieves this largely by adjusting blood flow to different vascular beds in proportion to the level of their metabolic activity. Not enough emphasis can be given to the importance of the control of blood flow; arterial pressure is simply a means to drive flow. The CNS achieves adequate perfusion of organs by maintaining arterial pressure within relatively fine limits. This is achieved by controlling both cardiac output and arterial vascular resistance in the face of different demands put on the cardiovascular system. Such demands include digestion (blood flow increase to gastrointestinal tract) or exercise (increase blood flow to skeletal muscle). The fine regulation is achieved through the interplay of reflex inputs from bodily organs providing feedback (arterial pressure, blood gas levels) and central autonomic drives. In order to achieve this regulation, the autonomic outflows are patterned, and these patterns are specific and appropriate dependent on the different behavioural state of the organism. From studies in man and animals, much has now been learned of the cardiovascular pattern of response that accompany sleep, exercise, and emotional responses, yet it is only with respect to affective behaviour that we have a detailed description of the central structures and neural pathways that are involved in mediating these complex autonomic changes (Jordan 1990, Spyer 1994). The classic investigations on the defence reaction of the cat by Hilton and his colleagues (reviewed by Jordan 1990), and the playing-dead or freezing response of the rabbit,

have shed considerable light on the role of the amygdala and hypothalamus in organizing these responses. These two distinct animal models of behaviour have provided information of considerable significance in understanding the human adaptations to environmental and emotional stress—but it is the downstream neuronal machinery within the medulla oblongata and spinal cord that provides the neuronal substrate that plays out these cardiovascular adjustments and it is these mechanisms that we consider here. We shall work backwards into the CNS by first considering the preganglionic autonomic neurons.

Cardiovascular autonomic neurons

The sympathetic and vagal preganglionic neurons are the final common pathway within the CNS through which control can be exerted. Sympathetic preganglionic neurons are localized segmentally within the intermediolateral cell column of the thoracic and upper lumbar spinal cord (Gilbey 1997, Jänig 2006). 'Vasomotor' neurons are distributed throughout the extent of the column. Sympathetic neurons that influence cardiac activity, both chronotropic and inotropic, are restricted to the upper thoracic segments of the cord (T1–T4). The postganglionic neurons are located outside the CNS in paravertebral chains. Each preganglionic neuron can innervate up to 10 postganglionic neurons. The vagal preganglionic neurons that affect the heart are located within both the external formation of the nucleus ambiguus located in the ventrolateral medulla (VLM) and the dorsal vagal nucleus (Izzo and Spyer 1997, Standish et al. 1994). The latter are likely to control coronary blood flow in addition to other cardiac influences. Evidence exists that vagal preganglionic neurons subserving chronotropic and dromotropic function are separated spatially within the nucleus ambiguus of the cat (Gatti et al. 1996) and that this organization is reflected by separate cardiac ganglia containing postganglionic neurons capable of altering beat rate, contractility or conduction speed (cat: Gatti et al. 1995, rat: Sampaio et al. 2003). This level of organization within both the medulla and the cardiac ganglia suggest a highly organized level of neural control. We shall return to this when we discuss the rostral ventrolateral medulla, cardiovagal motoneurons and the nucleus tractus solitarii (NTS) where evidence again indicates a high degree of organization based on cardiovascular autonomic function.

Connectivity and organization of sympathetic neurons: from pre-motor to postganglionic

From both the ongoing and reflexly evoked patterns of activity of sympathetic postganglionic nerve fibres established in animals, but also found in humans, sympathetic postganglionic fibres have been classified functionally as, for example: skeletal muscle vasoconstrictor, cutaneous vasoconstrictor, pseudomotor and piloerector neurons (e.g. Jänig and Häbler 2003, Wallin and Elam 1994). This suggests the possibility of highly organized patterns of innervation of postganglionic neurons from distinct subsets of preganglionic sympathetic neurons. Indeed, based on intracellular recordings of sympathetic preganglionic neurons it is evident that they do display differences in their ongoing discharge patterns and intrinsic membrane properties (Dembowsky et al. 1986, Spanswick and Logan 1990), which is consistent with the notion of functionally distinct classes but requires further validation. The question of whether functionally diverse preganglionic neurons receive descending drives from specific subsets of supraspinal sympathetic pre-motor neurons remains a possibility. The origins of pre-motor sympathetic neurons has been well documented anatomically using both conventional neuroanatomical approaches (e.g. retrograde and anterograde tracers) and retrograde trans-synaptic viral tracers (e.g. Jansen et al. 1995, Strack et al. 1989a, see Jänig 2006, for review). Loewy and colleagues used trans-synaptic retrograde labelling with a reduced virulent strain of pseudorabies virus and demonstrated a range of descending pathways that innervate sympathetic preganglionic neurons destined for the adrenal medulla (Strack et al. 1989b) and kidney (Schramm et al. 1993). These inputs originate from hypothalamic, midbrain, pontine, and medullary cell groups (Fig. 2.1) but show no obvious neuroanatomical differences. However, the phenotypes of the spinally projecting neurons based on their neurochemical content are distinct and this may subserve specific functions.

There is a vast array of transmitter substances in terminals forming close appositions with preganglionic sympathetic neurons (e.g. glutamate, γ-aminobutyric acid [GABA], glycine, noradrenaline, adrenaline, dopamine, serotonin, substance P, encephalin, oxytocin, vasopressin, and purines), which may be co-released (reviewed by Pilowsky and Goodchild 2002). Llewellyn-Smith and colleagues attempted to isolate transmitters involved in mediating baroreflex sympathoexcitatory responses using the immediate early gene c-*fos* and choline acetyltransferase to identify the sympathetic preganglionic neurons recruited during hypotension. They found terminal appositions containing immunoreactivity for tyrosine hydroxylase, serotonin, substance P, enkephalin, neuropeptide Y (NPY), phenylethanolamine-N-methyltransferase (PNMT), and galanin with some segmental distribution (Minson et al. 2002). The physiological significance of these diverse phenotypically distinct innervations may provide the substrate for activating specific populations of preganglionic neurons allowing differential control of blood flow appropriate for different behavioural states. For example, during exercise catecholaminergic innervation might be essential for activating renal vasoconstrictors but not other vascular beds. Next, we will consider innervation of sympathetic preganglionic neurons that arise from the glutamatergic, adrenaline/noradrenaline and serotonin containing neurons of the ventral medulla as these have been most well investigated.

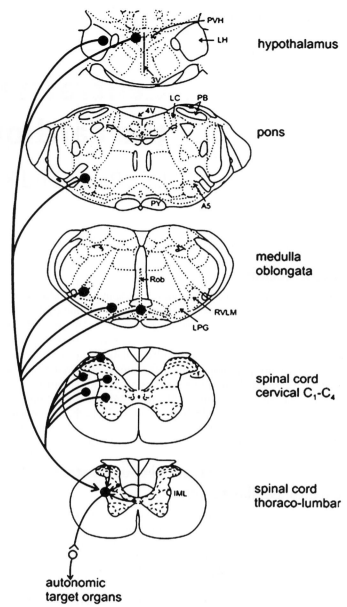

Fig. 2.1 Location of pre-motor sympathetic neurons. Descending drives to the sympathetic preganglionic motor neurons (located within the intermediolateral [IML] cell column) originate from the lateral (LH) and paraventricular hypothalamic nuclei (PVN), the A5 noradrenergic cell group in the caudal ventrolateral pons, the rostral ventrolateral medulla (RVLM), the rostral medial medulla or midline raphe (pallidus, magnus and obscurus, Rob) as well as spinal segmental interneurons within laminae of the dorsal horn at cervical, thoracic and lumbar levels. See text for discussion. Other abbreviations: LC, locus coeruleus; LF, lateral funiculus; LPG, lateral paragigantocellular nucleus; PB, parabrachial nucleus; PY, pyramid; sp5, spinal trigeminal tract; 3V and 4V, third and fourth ventricle respectively. Reprinted from *Brain Research*, **683**, Jansen, A.S., Wessendorf, M.W., and Lowey, A.D., Transneuronal labeling of CNS neuropeptide and monoanime neurons after pseudorabies virus injections into the stellate ganglion, 1–24, Copyright 1995, with permission from Elsevier and also reprinted from *Neuroscience*, **77**, Jansen, A.S., and Lowey, A.D., Neurons lying in the white matter of the upper cervical spine cord project to the intermediolateral cell column, 889–898, Copyright 1997, with permission from Elsevier.

Pre-motor sympathetic neurons

A major source of excitatory input to sympathetic preganglionic neurons under anaesthetized conditions originates from the rostral ventrolateral medulla (RVLM) (Fig. 2.1). Indeed, there is a belief that these neurons represent the classical 'vasomotor' centre (Guyenet 1990). Although the RVLM provides significant drive, it should be emphasized that it is not the only means by which the CNS regions can influence levels of sympathetic activity (see the retrograde tract tracing data reviewed above). By example we discuss later the contribution of midline raphe as another driver of sympathetic activity (Fig. 2.1). As the reader will see, what effects sympathetic activity depends very much on the state of the animal, leaving us to suggest that different descending controls may be more or less important, depending on the behavioural state.

The pre-motor sympathetic neurons of the RVLM

The following discussion summarizes some of the evidence supporting a major role of the RVLM in sympathetic nerve activity generation. Spinally projecting RVLM neurons form a relatively discrete group of cells caudal to the facial nucleus extending caudally towards the obex in the rat. They comprise both glutamate (i.e. express vesicular glutamate transporter 2 [VGLUT 2] messenger RNA [mRNA]) and adrenaline-containing neurons (e.g. are immunopositive for tyrosine hydroxylase or PNMT; the C1 group; see Guyenet 2006, for review). It has been estimated that 50–70% of RVLM neurons are C1 cells but that 80% of C1 neurons also express VGLUT 2 mRNA (Guyenet 2006). It should be stressed that spinally projecting neurons does not necessarily mean that they innervate directly the preganglionic sympathetic neurons in the intermediolateral cell column. However, complementary ultrastructural evidence has shown direct monosynaptic connections of RVLM neurons with both the soma and dendrites of sympathetic preganglionic neurons (Zagon and Smith 1993). Moreover, there is a wealth of information suggesting that the RVLM region and the spinally projecting neurons contained within it have a sympathoexcitatory function. Classically, application of glycine on to the rostroventrolateral medullary surface produced profound falls in arterial pressure (Guertzenstein and Silver, 1974) whereas direct intraparenchymal injection of neuronal excitants (e.g. glutamate) caused pressor responses in anaesthetized animals (Dampney et al. 1982). However, the level of arterial pressure following RVLM lesions can return back to control under certain circumstances (Cochrane and Nathan 1994) supporting the importance of multiple descending pathways affecting sympathetic activity as well as spinal mechanisms and other pressor systems (e.g. vasopressin, angiotensin II). Incidentally, in chronically spinalized rats sympathetic discharge is well maintained and correlated with dorsal horn neuron activity (Chau et al. 2000) and capable of generating substantial excitatory responses to afferent inputs (Bravo et al. 2004) and ischaemia (Braga et al. 2007). Indeed, in quadriplegic humans hypertension involves diffuse sympathetic discharge (Wallin 1986). These studies support the ability of the isolated spinal cord in generating sympathetic nerve activity.

At the single cell level, RVLM spinally projecting neurons have properties indicative of a sympathoexcitatory function (Fig. 2.2):

- They have a strong cardiac rhythm in their ongoing discharge, which originates from an inhibitory input generated by the arterial baroreceptor reflex.

- They fire at around 20 Hz in the rat and this discharge rate is directly related to the level of arterial blood pressure (Fig. 2.2).

- Spike-triggered averaging shows a strong correlation with postganglionic sympathetic nerve activity (see Guyenet 2006 and Sun 1996, for reviews).

Guyenet's group have studied the functional role of the C1 neurons using a selective neurotoxin. This resulted in a slight fall in arterial pressure and reduced evoked pressor responses from the RVLM (Schreihofer et al. 2000) underpinning a role for this cell group in maintenance of arterial pressure, at least in the anaesthetized rat. Using photostimulation to activate C1 neurons selectively arterial pressure increased modestly in both anaesthetized (~15 mmHg; Abbott et al. 2009) and conscious rats (~4 mmHg; Kanbar et al. 2010).

As implicated above there is evidence supporting a high degree of organization based on cardiovascular function at both the preganglionic and postganglionic sympathetic levels (e.g. cardiac ganglia regulating chronotropism vs dromotropism). Considering this specificity, highly discrete loci could be identified within the RVLM that affected different sympathetic motor outflows/vascular beds in the cat (Dampney and McAllen 1988). This was consistent with the idea of a viscerotopographical representation within the RVLM, which was rather analogous to the motor homunculus in the cerebral cortex. The idea of RVLM viscerotopography is provocative and begs the question of whether functional specificity exists within other nuclei that connect to the RVLM. Indeed, we shall return to this when we consider the NTS.

Origin(s) of activity of RVLM pre-motor sympathetic neurons

A question that has arisen is the origin of the activity of RVLM neurons. In an *in vitro* slice preparation made from immature rats, spinally projecting RVLM cells exhibit tonic beating activity due to an intrinsic pacemaker property. For example, their discharge is not silenced in the presence of kynurenic acid, the non-selective inotropic receptor antagonist of glutamate (Guyenet 1990). While this is suggestive of intrinsically generated activity, one cannot rule out the presence of non-glutamatergic excitatory drive. Lipski et al. (1996) have provided a contrary view with regard to generation of their discharge, questioning the absence of synaptic drive as a basis for rhythmic activity. Their studies were performed in anaesthetized adult rats *in vivo* where they noted that each action potential was preceded by a fast excitatory postsynaptic potential. This is consistent with the evidence that antagonism of NMDA and non-NMDA receptors produces falls in arterial pressure and reductions in sympathetic motor activity (once inhibition is blocked within the RVLM; Ito and Sved 1997, Miyawaki et al. 2002). All said, RVLM neurons clearly do have the capability to pacemake; the question is, under what conditions is this expressed as this does not seem to be present in the *in vivo* anaesthetized rat. This may occur under conditions of brain ischemia when synaptic transmission is known to fail. Such a mechanism would assist in maintaining adequate arterial pressure in conditions when oxygen supply is reduced thereby promoting animal survival.

There are a number of possible origins for excitatory drive to the RVLM including pontine structures, hypothalamic and amygdaloid regions essential for the coordination of a behavioural response (fight and flight vs play dead; see Spyer 1994, for review) with an

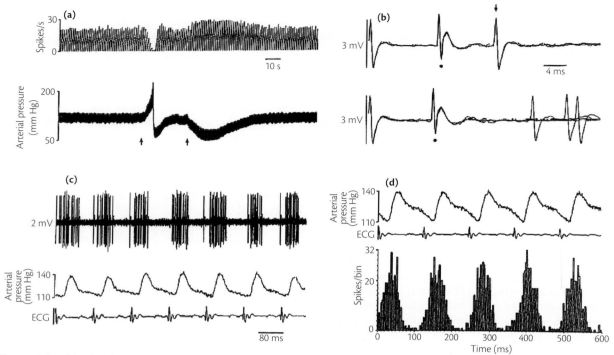

Fig. 2.2 Characteristics of the identified rostral ventrolateral spinal 'vasomotor' neurons. **(a)** Effect of change in arterial pressure on the neuronal discharge rate. Neuronal activity is represented in the form of an integrated rate histogram. Arterial pressure was elevated via descending aortic constriction (started at the first arrow and stopped when the neuron become silent) and reduced by intravenous injection of 0.1–0.2 mg sodium nitroprusside (at the second arrow). **(b)** Spinal projection of the neuron. The evoked antidromic spikes (arrow) by the spinal cord stimulation (asterisks) collided with spontaneously occurring spikes and failed to occur at recording site when the stimulation was applied within a critical period after spontaneously occurring spikes (bottom trace). **(c)** Pulse-synchronous discharge of the rostral ventrolateral spinal 'vasomotor' neuron. The arterial pressure trace (middle) and ECG signal (bottom) represent a single sweep, whereas the trace of neuronal discharge represents 12 consecutive sweeps, all triggered on ECG signals. **(d)** ECG-triggered time histograms of the neuronal activity (300 sweeps, 3 ms/bin). The top and middle traces represent averaged arterial pressure and ECG signals, respectively (50 sweeps each). Sun, M.-K. and Spyer, K. M., Nociceptive inputs into rostral ventrolateral medulla-spinal vasomotor neurones in rats, *J. Physiol.*, Wiley.

appropriate change in cardiovascular system. In addition, angiotensin II acting on angiotensin II type 1 receptors has been shown to exert a powerful sympathoexcitatory effect from the RVLM whereas antagonizing this receptor subtype only reduces arterial pressure in the spontaneously hypertensive rat. This is indicative of a tonic angiotensinergic drive unique to the SHR (Ito et al. 2002). Moreover, a source of this tonic drive may descend from the hypothalamic paraventricular nucleus (PVN; Ito et al. 2002). The possibility remains that the sympathoexcitation seen during a hypothalamically mediated defence response is mediated, in part, by angiotensin II acting at the level of the RVLM. An additional excitatory input comes from the respiratory network which is partially interwoven spatially with the RVLM. Given their close proximity, the expiratory Bötzinger cells and inspiratory pre-Bötzinger cells are likely to contribute to the central respiratory modulation of RVLM neurons and hence provide the substrate for central cardiorespiratory coupling that undermines the matching of cardiac output with minute ventilation.

RVLM-spinal signalling: a choice of transmitters

With evidence of glutamatergic and catecholaminergic RVLM premotor sympathetic neurons one would predict that both glutamate and adrenaline/noradrenaline would activate sympathetic preganglionic neurons. First, activating the RVLM either electrically or with the application of excitant amino acids resulted in monosynaptically evoked excitatory postsynaptic potentials in sympathetic

preganglionic motoneurons that were mediated by both non-NMDA- and NMDA-type receptors, providing support for glutamate as a primary transmitter (Deuchers et al. 1995). In terms of the catecholaminergic drive from RVLM, Sved has questioned whether C1 neurons actually release adrenaline in the intermediolateral cell column since there appears a paucity of this amine whereas noradrenaline is abundant (Sved, 1989) leaving open the question of whether C1 neurons actually release adrenaline onto preganglionic sympathetic neurons. In terms of the effects of catecholaminergic ligands acting on preganglionic sympathetic neurons, this is complex and depends on the receptor subtype activated as both α_1- and α_2-adrenergic receptors are present. Iontophoretic application of adrenaline and noradrenaline inhibit sympathetic preganglionic neuron activity *in vitro* (Coote and Lewis 1995), which is contrary to the proposed role of C1 neurons being sympathoexcitatory. However, the inhibitory influence of noradrenaline can be reversed by applying glutamate supporting the notion that catecholamine release may act to boost glutamatergic excitatory drive. Indeed, Marks et al. (1990) have shown that α_2-adrenoceptor stimulation excites preganglionic neurons in cats and rats *in vivo* where presumably glutamatergic excitatory drive is higher.

In summary, RVLM neurons have a pivotal role in the command of sympathetic outflow based on both their ongoing activity, the integration of synaptic drives from many other CNS regions regulating cardiovascular activity as well as reflex pathways such as baroreceptor, peripheral chemoreceptor and nociceptive inputs (see Guyenet 2006). We reviewed the action of a viscerotopography within RVLM and that downstream transmission to sympathetic preganglionic neurons involves multiple transmitters released from RVLM axonal terminals. The transmitter released may be vascular bed specific but is also likely to be state-dependent and undoubtedly susceptible to modulation by transmitter substances released endogenously at the level of the intermediolateral cell column. Finally, a major input to the RVLM neuron must include arterial baroreceptors, which provide a major restraining control over cardiovascular sympathetic nerve activity. The caudal VLM (CVLM) relays this information to the RVLM and is discussed below.

Caudal ventrolateral medulla and the baroreceptor reflex

A major source of the inhibitory input to RVLM sympathoexcitatory neurons that is evoked by the arterial baroreceptors originates from a group of GABA-containing neurons in the caudal ventrolateral medulla (Fig. 2.3). The CVLM projects to the RVLM and is a target of an efferent projection from baroreceptor activated glutamatergic neurons within the NTS, the nucleus that contains the baroreceptor afferent terminals (Weston et al. 2003, Izzo and Spyer 1997). The NTS also mediates the peripheral chemoreceptor reflex which produces sympathoexcitation and depends on an excitatory projection from NTS to RVLM thereby bypassing the CVLM (Koshiya and Guyenet 1996).

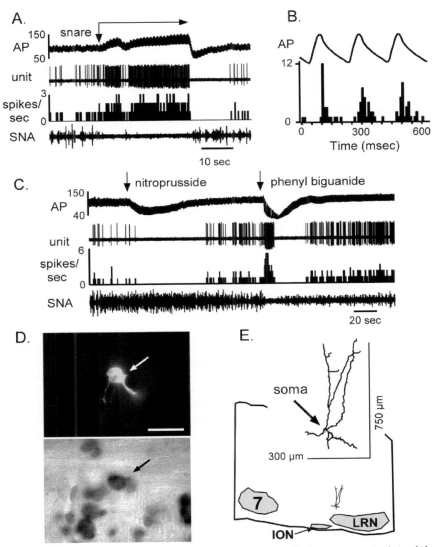

Fig. 2.3 Characteristics of a caudal ventrolateral medullary GABAergic neuron. The neuron is activated by baroreceptor stimulation **(A)** achieved by raising arterial pressure (AP) by tightening a snare around the abdominal aorta. Note concurrent inhibition of sympathetic nerve activity (SNA). Caudal ventrolateral medulla (CVLM) neurons have ongoing activity that is pulse modulated **(B)**, suggestive of a beat-by-beat baroreceptor input, and inhibited when arterial pressure is lowered either by sodium nitroprusside or activation of cardiopulmonary receptors with phenylbiguanide **(C)**. The phenotype of this cell was GABAergic (see panel **D**) as demonstrated by labelling the cell with biotinamide juxtacellularly and revealed with streptavidin Cy3 (white arrow) and subsequent processing for GAD67 mRNA by *in situ* hybridization (black arrow; same neuron). The location of the cell is shown in **(E)** and was 1.35 mm caudal to the facial nucleus and 1.9 mm lateral to midline. Not shown here, but discussed in text, is that many CVLM neurons have respiratory modulated discharge (see Mandel and Schreihofer 2006) and are therefore a potential site at which respiratory modulation of sympathetic activity occurs. Schreihofer, A.M., and Guyenet, P.G. (2002) *Clin. Exp. Pharmacol. Physiol.* **29**, 514–521, with permission from Wiley.

The role of baroreceptors in long-term control of arterial pressure has been debated. Arterial baroreceptors have long thought to buffer arterial pressure on a moment by moment basis (Cowley et al. 1973) but not determine the set point of arterial pressure. However, data from Thrasher (2004) has shown that baroreceptor unloading causes a persistent pressor response that is well maintained for 2 weeks and remains above control levels by week 5 (Thrasher 2005). Additionally, electrical stimulation of the carotid sinus region in the conscious dog results in a maintained lower level of arterial pressure for 3 weeks (Lohmeier et al. 2010). The latter experiment has led to a clinical trial for alleviating the symptoms of essential hypertension (Heusser et al. 2010). Conversely, Barrett et al. (2003) has raised systemic arterial pressure chronically with intravenous infusions of angiotensin II and found that renal sympathetic nerve is depressed (via the baroreceptor reflex) and that this remains for days in instrumented conscious rabbits. Therefore, we can conclude that studies of chronic baroreceptor reflex function remain essential in furthering our understanding of the regulation of arterial pressure in the long term, which now becomes highly relevant in disease states such as hypertension.

The following is a synopsis of some evidence supporting the role of the CVLM in sympathetic activity regulation and pattern formation. Blessing (1988) demonstrated that stimulation of the CVLM produced profound depressor responses dependent upon GABAergic transmission in the RVLM. Later, Jeske et al. (1993) demonstrated that CVLM neurons with projections to RVLM were excited by baroreceptor stimulation thereby completing the central arc of the baroreflex. CVLM neuron activity has been shown to be pulse modulated, presumably by baroreceptors, tightly coupled to arterial pressure and inversely coupled to sympathetic discharge (Schreihofer and Guyenet 2002) (Fig. 2.3). These cells express an enzyme necessary for production of GABA (i.e. contain GAD67 mRNA) (Schreihofer and Guyenet 2003) (Fig. 2.3) and therefore fulfil the criterion for a sympathoinhibitory CVLM neuron. Many CVLM neurons also show respiratory modulation (Mandel and Schreihofer 2006, Schreihofer and Guyenet 2002), which could explain the respiratory related discharge of RVLM neurons and, as such, provides another access point for coupling of sympathetic and respiratory activity.

Midline raphe: thermoregulation, metabolism and obesity

Evidence exists for direct connections, via small myelinated axons, originating from the raphe complex (e.g. the raphe magnus and pallidus) to sympathetic preganglionic neurons (Zagon and Bacon 1991) (Fig. 2.4) including those that innervate the adrenal medulla (Bacon et al. 1990). When delivered by iontophoresis on to sympathetic preganglionic neurons (thoracic and lumbar), 5-hydroxytrymptamine (5-HT) evokes excitation in most cases but inhibition in some (Gilbey and Stein 1991). Interestingly, sympathetic neurons excited by 5-HT were invariably inhibited by noxious input, whereas those few that were inhibited by 5-HT were excited by the equivalent noxious input. The basis for these actions may reflect the heterogeneity of 5-HT receptor subtypes located on sympathetic preganglionic neurons but equally could underlie the distinct patterning of sympathetic activity that is evoked to noxious inputs and, hence, to the cardiovascular adjustments made during pain.

While the 5-HT system may be involved in coordinating appropriate sympathetic responses to noxious stimulation, it has become

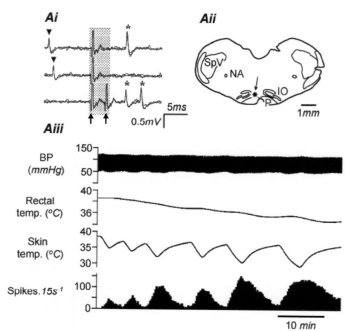

Fig. 2.4 Cold-sensitive raphe spinal neuron. **Ai:** demonstrates that the neuron was spinally projecting as it followed the antidromic collision test (upper two traces) and high frequency stimulation (paired pulses, 3 ms separation). The arrow heads indicate ongoing spikes and the asterisks indicate antidromic spikes. Stimuli were applied to the lumbar cord and are arrowed. **Aii:** location of recording site indicates neuron was within raphe pallidus. Lowering skin and rectal temperature excited the neuron and this could be shown repeatedly (**Aiii**). These neurons are likely responsible for driving sympathetic neurons innervating the cutaneous vascular bed as well as brown fat for stimulatory thermogenic and metabolic effects. See text for discussion. From Rathner, J.A., Owens, N.C., and McAllen, R.M. (2001) *J. Physiol.* **535**, 841–854, with permission from Wiley.

clear that it plays a role in thermoregulation. Indeed, intrathecal application of 5-HT to the spinal cord evoked a highly coordinated rhythmic pattern of sympathetic activity, so called T-rhythm (~1 Hz), which is known to be present in sympathetic neurons innervating the tail—a major thermoregulatory organ (Marina et al. 2006). Inhibition of raphe nuclei (magnus and pallidus) lowers discharge in sympathetic vasoconstrictor fibres supplying the tail but not those in the splanchnic bed or to the heart (Marina et al. 2006) indicating that these raphe neurons affect a functionally specific sub-population of sympathetic preganglionic neurons. Prostaglandin E2 administration, given to evoke thermogenesis, produces activation of sympathetic nerves innervating brown adipose fat (and those to the tail) (Marina et al. 2006) that is mediated via raphe magnus (Morrison 2003). Indeed, raphe magnus neurons are stimulated when body temperature is lowered (Rathner et al. 2001) (Fig. 2.4). Some serotonergic neurons also responded to noxious stimulation (Rathner et al. 2001) providing a nodal point for the integration of pain and fever.

Cao and Morrison (2006) have demonstrated that a major driver of raphe magnus descends from the dorsomedial hypothalamic region (pre-optic nuclei) which may, in part, mediate the response to cooling. With the worldwide problems of obesity bodily mechanisms of energy expenditure have driven both clinical and pharmaceutical interest. Normally leptin, released from adipose tissues, provides a feedback mechanism controlling adiposity (see Morrison 2004, for review). Leptin increases sympathetic activity to brown adipose tissue to initiate thermogenesis and energy expenditure. It is known to act on the arcuate nucleus, which releases α-melanocyte stimulating hormone that acts on melanocortin-4 receptors; the latter are located within a variety of hypothalamic nuclei known to affect sympathetic activity. Indeed, melanocortin-4 receptor agonist produces the same response as leptin. The precise details of the central pathways involved are as yet unknown but conditional transgenic animals indicate that:

◆ an absence of either melanocortin-4 or leptin receptors causes obesity (mice and man)

◆ melanocortin-4 receptors in the paraventricular hypothalamus and/or amygdala are sufficient to control food intake, but the presence of these receptors elsewhere control energy expenditure, suggesting a functional divergence in the role of these receptors (Balthasar 2006).

In conclusion, the central pathways regulating thermogenesis and energy expenditure engage the medullary raphe serotonergic system that selectively drives sympathetic outflows for controlling body heat and energy expenditure (Fig. 2.4). Superimposed onto this serotonergic system is a hypothalamic neuronal circuit that clearly regulates temperature and energy requirements. It is this circuit that requires further interrogation to understand the integrative aspects of obesity, diabetes and hypertension—all contributors to the metabolic syndrome.

Vagal preganglionic cardiomotor neurons

There are two spatially separate pools of cardiac vagal motoneurons. Those motoneurons located in the nucleus ambiguus have B-fibre axons that effect chronotropism (Jones et al. 1994, 1995). However, there appears to be spatially distinct subgroups of ambiguual neurons with distinct cardiac function (e.g. chrono-, dromo- and iono- tropism; see Gatti et al. 1996) but whether all these functions are mediated by B-fibres is not known. A second group of cardiac vagal motoneurons are located in the dorsal vagal nucleus (Izzo and Spyer 1997, Standish et al. 1994). These neurons have C-fibre axons in most species but in rabbit B-fibres also arise from these vagal motoneurons. While activation of cardiac vagal motor cells with C-fibres produces bradycardia, this effect is smaller than activating B-fibre axons originating from the nucleus ambiguus and with a different time course and pharmacology of action within the cardiac ganglion (Jones et al. 1994). Thus, C-fibre cardiac vagal motoneurons may also control cardiac functions other than chronotropism, which could include coronary blood flow, for example. Unlike B-fibre type cardiac vagal motoneurons, the majority with C-fibres appear not to be modulated by baroreceptor, lung inflation or central respiratory inputs (Jones et al. 1998). However, they receive a powerful excitatory input from unmyelinated vagal afferents with endings in the pulmonary vascular bed that are sensitive to oedema, and experimentally stimulated with a serotonergic type 3 receptor agonist (phenylbiguanide), and hence appear to participate in a C-fibre-to-C-fibre vagal reflex. Based on the idea that this reflex may be triggered in heart failure when pulmonary congestion is prevalent, a coronary vasodilating role for the C-fibre dorsal vagal motoneurons innervating the heart is a plausible suggestion and one that requires testing.

There are multiple inputs to the nucleus ambiguus but these are not exclusive to this region as they also innervate the RVLM and include: bed nucleus of the stria terminalis; substantia innominata; central nucleus of the amygdala; paraventricular hypothalamic nucleus; dorsomedial hypothalamic nucleus; lateral hypothalamic area; zona incerta; posterior hypothalamus; mesencephalic central grey; mesencephalic reticular formation; the parabrachial nucleus, including the Kölliker–Fuse nucleus; the NTS and the medullary reticular formation. A particularly powerful source of afferent input to the nucleus ambiguus arises from the caudal NTS (cNTS), and ultrastructural studies, using the anterograde transport of biocytin, have shown monosynaptic connections being made from the NTS on to vagal neurons of the nucleus ambiguus (Izzo and Spyer 1997). Similarly, evidence has been derived to show that cardiomotor vagal neurons are contacted by synaptic boutons containing 5-HT (Izzo et al. 1993). Subsequent studies showed that serotonin applied iontophoretically excite cardiac vagal motoneurons mediated by a 5-HT$_{1a}$ receptor (Wang and Ramage 2001). Moreover, blockade of this serotonin receptor subtype prevented the reflex activation of cardiac vagal motoneurons evoked by stimulation of pulmonary C-fibre afferents (Wang and Ramage 2001). All said, serotonin plays a major role in the reflex activation of cardiac vagal motoneurons. A question for the future would be under what circumstances is 5-HT released and where is it coming from? Based on the discussion above, perhaps it is switched on under conditions of thermogenesis (see p.40).

Sinus arrhythmia: a classic case of cardiorespiratory coupling

In the early 1930s, Anrep and his colleagues demonstrated that sinus arrhythmia was the consequence of respiratory influences of the vagal outflow to the heart (Anrep et al. 1936a, 1936b) (Figs 2.5 and 2.6). They identified a central origin and a peripheral source dependent on reflexes evoked during respiratory movements, such as lung inflation inputs. Electrophysiological studies in the cat show that the central mechanism involves a direct synaptic regulation of cardiac vagal motoneurons exerted by a subset of those brainstem neurons that are responsible for generating the respiratory rhythm (Richter and Spyer 1990). Identified cardiac vagal preganglionic motoneurons are actively hyperpolarized during inspiration by a wave of chloride-dependent inhibitory postsynaptic potentials (Gilbey et al. 1984). Hence, any influence that increases inspiratory drive will lead, by this process, to both a suppression of vagal efferent discharge and a reduced sensitivity of these neurons to other excitatory inputs, whether central or reflex in origin. The outcome is a tachycardia in inspiration, sinus arrhythmia. Both the pattern of discharge and membrane potential trajectory of cardiac vagal motoneurons during the respiratory cycle indicates that they have close similarities to one type of respiratory neuron, the post-inspiratory neuron (Fig. 2.5). Functionally post-inspiratory neurons provide the off-switch to inspiration and as such form an essential component of the respiratory rhythm generator, which has led to the idea that breathing comprises three phases: inspiration, post-inspiration and expiration (Fig. 2.5) (Richter and Spyer 1990). Intriguingly, both cardiac vagal and post-inspiratory neurons discharge during the first part of the expiratory phase, a time when heart rate falls, which is an important component of sinus arrhythmia (Fig. 2.5). Such cells could form a common cardiorespiratory neuron (Fig. 2.5) (Richter and Spyer 1990). It should be realised that this central coupling is also geared precisely with control of the larynx, such that the glottis

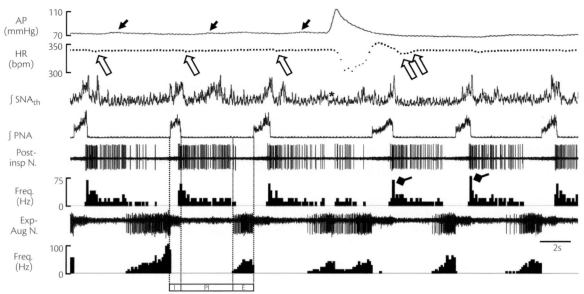

Fig. 2.5 Common cardiorespiratory neurons in the medulla. Simultaneous recordings of arterial pressure (AP), heart rate (HR) in beats per minute (bpm), integrated thoracic sympathetic chain activity (SNA$_{th}$), integrated phrenic nerve activity (PNA) and two ventrolateral medullary expiratory neurons from the Bötzinger complex together with their corresponding firing rates in steady state conditions and during a baroreceptor reflex. The three phases of breathing are clearly demarked (horizontal lines) as inspiration (I), post-inspiration (PI) and expiration (E) based on the firing of PNA and the two respiratory cells. Note the sinus arrhythmia (open arrow) as well as the Hering–Traub waves in the arterial pressure trace (solid arrow); the latter are mediated by the respiratory-related increases in sympathetic discharge (coincident with the inspiratory-expiratory transition). During the transient rise in arterial pressure, to stimulate the baroreceptor reflex, both heart rate and SNA are reduced (*). This also activates the post-inspiratory neuron (Post-Insp N.) and inhibition of the expiratory augmenting neuron (Exp-Aug N.), reflecting an inhibitory connection between these cells. Note the accentuated sinus arrhythmia (double open arrows) after the stimulus, which reflects an increased excitability of cardiac vagal motoneurons; the post-inspiratory neuron also exhibits heightened excitability reflected by its higher peal discharge frequency (square head arrows). The pattern and phase of firing of the post-inspiratory neuron is similar to ambiguual cardiac vagal motoneurons with B-fibre axons (Gilbey et al. 1984; Wang and Ramage 2001), which are also excited by baroreceptor reflex activation forming the idea of common cardiorespiratory neurons (Richter and Spyer 1990). Unpublished data from D. Baekey, T. Dick and JFR Paton.

opens during inspiration (abduction) but exhibits adduction in early expiration (Fig. 2.6) (Paton and Nolan 2000). Indeed, laryngeal motoneurons show similar discharge profiles to cardiac vagal motoneurons and post-inspiratory cells. This respiratory patterning of cardiac vagal and laryngeal motor outflows is mirrored by similar changes in the excitability of sympathetic preganglionic motoneurons (Figs 2.5 and 2.6) (Richter and Spyer 1990). Studies in the rat and cat have shown that sympathetic preganglionic neurons show distinct phases of activity correlating with the central respiratory cycle (Figs 2.5 and 2.6), which causes respiratory related waves in arterial pressure (Hering Traub waves; Simms et al. 2009) (Fig. 2.5). As mentioned earlier, there is evidence that neurons in the CVLM and RVLM have their activity modulated by respiratory activity, which could account for the respiratory related discharge of postganglionic sympathetic nerves, but it also remains a distinct possibility that a portion of the respiratory discharge of sympathetic preganglionic neurons is mediated by direct connections from spinally projecting medullary respiratory neurons (Richter and Spyer 1990).

With cardiac vagal motoneuron activity being modulated by the respiratory cycle, it is unsurprising that the efficacy of the baroreceptor reflex efficacy is respiratory phase-dependent (Baekey et al. 2010). Experimental and computational modelling studies also reveal that baroreceptor activation also prolongs expiration by activating post-inspiratory neurons and inhibiting augmenting expiratory neurons of the Bötzinger Complex (BötC) Baekey et al. 2010). It is likely that these BötC neurons are also involved in the respiratory modulation of sympathetic activity and contribute to the respiratory modulation of the sympathetic baroreceptor reflex.

It is necessary to return to pulmonary stretch receptors, which depress both cardiac vagal motoneuron excitability and reflexes that evoke vagal bradycardia (see Daly 1997). But the central site at which slowly adapting vagal lung stretch afferents act has yet to be discerned. Detailed neurophysiological studies have *not* revealed an inhibitory action of this input on NTS neurons receiving baroreceptor or chemoreceptor inputs, although there is no doubt that lung inflation modulates the sensitivity of cardiac vagal preganglionic motoneurons to these reflex inputs. It is notable that the effects of lung inflation inputs are not of similar magnitude on all reflexes. Reflex activation of those pulmonary receptors excited by phenylbiguanide is much less affected by lung inflation than are either baroreceptor, chemoreceptor, or cardiac afferent inputs (Daly 1997). Nevertheless, it is clear that changes in respiratory state will exert an enormous direct influence on the sensitivity of both vagal and sympathetic neurons to other inputs. For example, in conditions of apnoea (e.g. breath-hold diving, sleep apnoea, sudden infant death syndrome [SIDS]) the absence of pulmonary stretch receptor activity presents a potential source of hazard as at this time, cardiac vagal motoneurons are highly sensitive to other concomitant excitatory inputs thereby enhancing the possibility of fatal bradycardia (Daly 1997).

Physiological relevance of respiratory sinus arrhythmia

The functional relevance of respiratory modulation of cardiac vagal activity and sympathetic vasomotor discharge has been reviewed (Simms et al. 2010). It may optimize oxygen delivery and carbon dioxide removal by precise matching of pulmonary perfusion to

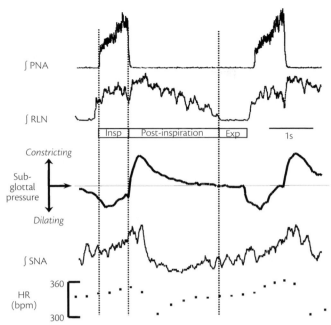

Fig. 2.6 Cardio-laryngo-sympathetic-respiratory coupling. A montage showing integrated activities of the phrenic (PNA), recurrent laryngeal nerve (RLN) and sympathetic nerve activity (SNA; thoracic chain) to show coordination of cranial and spinal cardiorespiratory motor outflows in a perfused rat preparation without pulmonary stretch receptor feedback (see Paton and Nolan 2000). During central inspiration (increased PNA; Insp) heart rate (HR) increases (due to central synaptic inhibition of cardiac vagal motoneurons and increasing sympathetic discharge) and the glottis dilates due to activation of laryngeal abductors. During early expirations (so called, post-inspiration), heart rate falls as the inspiratory related inhibition of the cardiac vagal motoneurons is removed. At this time the laryngeal adductors fire causing a transient constriction of the glottis; the latter stalls expiratory air flow so giving adequate time for gas exchange. Note also, that the SNA is respiratory phase locked and peaks in the post-inspiratory phase. With permission from Paton, J.F.R., and Nolan P.J. (2000). *Respir. Physiol.* **119**, 101–111.

ventilation with a consequent reduction in intrapulmonary shunt (Hayano et al. 1996). Coupling may provide a mechanism to reduce fluctuations in blood pressure due to respiratory phase-related changes in venous return. During expiration venous blood flow to the heart is reduced by the relative increase in intrathoracic pressure, whereas during inspiration venous return is enhanced due to both the negative intrathoracic pressure and increased abdominal pressure as the diaphragm moves downwards. During expiration when venous return is reduced, the cycle of respiratory sinus arrhythmia produces a slowing of heart rate that allows longer ventricular filling time helping to maintain stroke volume and hence blood pressure. This vagally mediated bradycardia during expiration also assists with coronary blood flow by prolonging diastole and also perhaps by reducing ventricular contractility and producing coronary dilatation (reviewed in Simms et al. 2010).

The NTS and reflex control of the cardiovascular system

The NTS itself makes extensive connections with regions of the lower brainstem, including the nucleus ambiguus, CVLM and RVLM, and with the various pontine nuclei that are concerned with cardiorespiratory regulation, and with forebrain structures. The ascending pathways from the NTS may control neuroendocrine

function, such as regulation of vasopressin release from the neurohypophysis during hypotension (i.e. baroreceptor unloading). Notwithstanding, the basic reflex is accomplished within the medulla (Fig. 2.7) and involves the cardiomotor neurons of the nucleus ambiguus and the neurons of the CVLM and RVLM. Interestingly, it appears that the baroreceptor reflex is the only reflex that produces a reciprocal response in parasympathetic and sympathetic motor outflows to the heart; all other visceral reflex responses appear to co-activate both autonomic limbs irrespective of the polarity of the heart rate change (see Andresen and Paton 2011; Paton et al. 2005 for reviews).

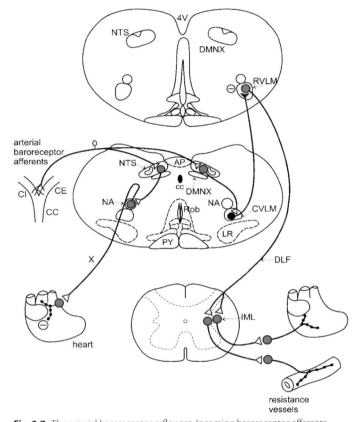

Fig. 2.7 The arterial baroreceptor reflex arc. Incoming baroreceptor afferents terminate in the nucleus tractus solitarii (NTS). Glutamate is an important transmitter here. Whether these same neurons project out of NTS directly to the nucleus ambiguus (NA) and caudal ventrolateral medulla (CVLM) is not known (but see text and Deuchars et al. 2000). It is likely that there are separate NTS neurons projecting to the NA and CVLM (see text and Simms et al. 2007). Both the latter projections are excitatory and involve glutamate acting on ionotropic receptors. The CVLM sends inhibitory GABAergic projections to the rostral ventrolateral medulla (RVLM) (Schreihofer and Guyenet 2002) which is a pre-motor site driving sympathetic preganglionic neurons located in the intermediolateral cell column (IML). From here, projections pass out of the ventral root targeting relevant postganglionic neurons that innervate target organs. Increased arterial pressure excites NTS causing inhibition of sympathetic activity and excitation of cardiac vagal outflows. This reflexly evoked reciprocal pattern of autonomic activity is unique to the baroreceptor reflex (see Paton et al. 2005). Other abbreviations: AP, area postrema; CC, CE and CI, common, external and internal carotid arteries; DLF, dorsolateral funiculus; DMNX, dorsal vagal motor nucleus; PY, pyramid; Rob, rahe obscurus; X, vagus. 4V, fourth ventricle. Reproduced form Guyenet, P. G. (1990). Role of the ventral medulla oblongata in blood pressure regulation. In 'Central Regulation of Autonomic Functions', ed. A.D. Lowey and K.M. Spyer. With permission of Oxford University Press.

It is well documented that several groups of peripheral receptors contribute to the reflex control of circulation. Probably the most important of these include the arterial baroreceptor and peripheral chemoreceptors, and receptors within the heart as well as the airways and lungs (Daly 1997, Hainsworth 1991, Spyer 1990, 1994). The primary site of termination and interaction of these afferents is at the level of the NTS (Fig. 2.7), and as such this structure provides a most powerful site for modulation (Spyer 1994, Paton 1999). For brevity, we consider here the baroreceptor reflex.

Neurophysiological studies have shown that specific areas of the NTS (dorsolateral and dorsomedial) receive innervation from the arterial baroreceptors (myelinated and unmyelinated fibres), and that these same regions also receive innervation from other afferents such as the arterial chemoreceptors and gastro-intestinal afferents (Fig. 2.8). Thus, it would appear that within a sub-region of the NTS, neurons receiving inputs from functionally distinct afferent inputs (baroreceptor, chemoreceptors and gastrointestinal receptors) all reside as neighbours (Fig. 2.8). This should not imply a lack of functional organization as it now appears, as discussed below, that this does exist but does not depend on spatial organization (Andresen and Paton 2011, Paton 1999).

The importance of the NTS in cardiovascular control should not be underestimated. Destruction of the NTS (or a stroke in this region) leads acutely to fulminating hypertension with concomitant pulmonary oedema, and chronically to maintained hypertension (Doba and Reis 1973). This suggests a major role for the NTS in:

♦ regulation of reflex gain

♦ determination of the set-point of arterial pressure.

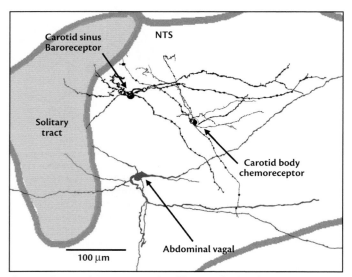

Fig. 2.8 Absence of viscerotopography of functionally identified nucleus tractus solitarii (NTS) neurons in the NTS. Montage of whole cell recorded and labelled NTS neurons that were activated by baroreceptor, chemoreceptor and abdominal vagus nerve afferent inputs, and monosynaptic inputs from the solitary tract (not shown). Despite their different functions these cells are neighbours suggesting an absence of viscerotopography at the neuronal level in NTS. However, afferent fibre termination does show some viscerotopography (Spyer 1990) suggesting that some inputs land on dendrites some distance away from the cell body. The baroreceptor responsive neurons mostly projected out of NTS to the ventrolateral medulla with some exhibiting axonal collaterals within NTS (see Deuchars et al. 2000). Paton, J.F.R. (1999). *Exp. Physiol.* **84**, 815–833, with permission from Wiley.

Importantly, with data supporting a role for baroreceptors in the long-term regulation of arterial pressure (Barrett et al. 2003, Lohmeier et al. 2010, Thrasher 2005), any down-regulation of the gain of this reflex is likely to contribute to arterial hypertension.

There is now good evidence that NTS neurons that are excited by stimulation of the arterial baroreceptors (Fig. 2.9) also receive convergent excitatory inputs form other reflex inputs that exert qualitatively similar reflex response patterns (Dawid-Milner et al. 1995, Deuchars et al. 2000, Paton 1998). Furthermore, many NTS neurons that are excited by baroreceptor stimulation are inhibited by chemoreceptor afferent inputs (Paton et al. 2001a, Silva-Carvalho et al. 1995a). One interpretation of this is a functional organization of neurons within the NTS based on their projection targets to, for example, cardiac vagal versus CVLM versus RVLM neurons. Indeed, intracellular labelling of baroresponsive NTS neurons showed that the majority (including those shown to receive direct afferent inputs) project out of the NTS into ventrolateral medullary regions including ambiguus and CVLM (Fig. 2.8) (Deuchars et al. 2000).

Studies in a arterially perfused decerebrate rat preparation, which allows finite control of systemic pressure and flow, demonstrate distinct pressure thresholds for baroreceptor reflex mediated vagal bradycardia (~83 mmHg) versus sympathoinhibition (~65 mmHg) (Simms et al. 2007) (Fig. 2.10). This supports the idea of separate channels of information leaving NTS destined for each limb of the autonomic nervous system. It may be that these separate channels of communication exist within the baroreceptor afferents themselves and are already dedicated to driving vagal versus sympathetic outflows at this level. This degree of organization is supported by the observation that numerous neuromodulators acting within the NTS affect preferentially the cardiac vagal component of the baroreceptor reflex and not the sympathetic component (Pickering et al. 2003). Thus, these data lead to the prediction that within the NTS there are dedicated pre-motor cardiac vagal neurons and pre-CVLM neurons and that these form completely separate entities that provides flexibility for independent modulation as is seen, for example, during exercise (e.g. Raven et al. 2006).

Similar observations have been found in humans in which muscle vasoconstrictor sympathetic nerve activity is sensitive to increases in arterial pressure that are without effect on heart rate (Eckberg et al. 1988). Interestingly, the baroreceptor control of sympathetic nerve activity is better correlated to cardiac output rather than to the absolute level of arterial pressure in humans (Charkoudian et al. 2005), suggesting that baroreceptors are designed to detect changes in blood flow. Indeed, it has been previously shown that carotid sinus baroreceptors are sensitized under conditions of altered flow and pressure rather than static pressure changes alone such that they exhibit lower thresholds for discharge (Hajduczok et al. 1988). Ultimately it is blood flow that organs care about and it would now appear that baroreceptor modulation of vascular resistance is providing a means to accurately control this.

NTS: a site for effective modulation

There is substantial evidence that GABA transmission at the level of the NTS plays a key role in the regulation of the sensitivity of the baroreceptor reflex and appears to be tonically active acting on $GABA_A$ receptors (Fig. 2.9). Numerous central and peripheral pathways as well as endogenous and exogenously applied modulators act to depress the baroreceptor reflex through enhanced GABA

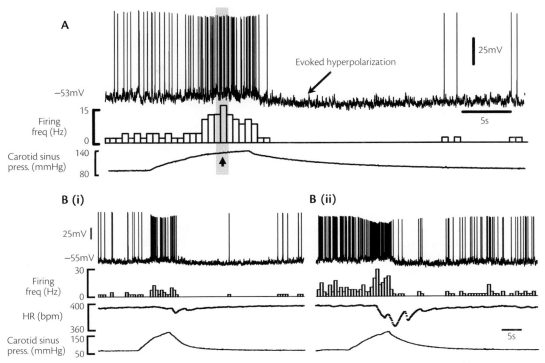

Fig. 2.9 Baroreceptive neurons in the nucleus tractus solitarii (NTS) are under a restraining inhibitory tone. Whole cell recordings of baroreceptive neurons from rat. **A:** A typical 'adaptive' response where the peak depolarization and firing response occurs before the maximal stimulus, in this case a rise in carotid sinus pressure (arrowed). Note the after hyperpolarization that reduces the electrical excitability of the neuron to subsequent baroreceptor inputs. **B**: The firing response of another baroreceptive neuron showing an adaptive response in control **(i)** and after bicuculline **(ii)**, a $GABA_A$ receptor antagonist. A mechanism for driving this inhibition is from angiotensin II and nitric oxide (see Fig. 2.11 and text for discussion). Paton, J.F.R. (1999). *Exp. Physiol.* **84**, 815–833 and Paton, J.F.R., Li, Y.-W. & Schwaber, J.S (2001c) *Ann. New York Acad. Sci.* **940**, 157–168, with permission from Wiley.

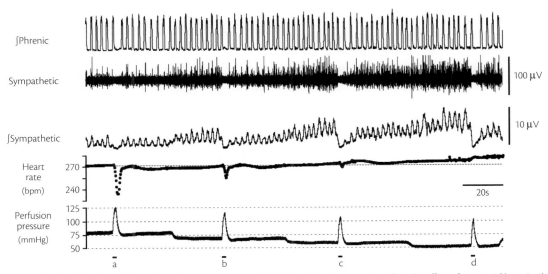

Fig. 2.10 Distinct pressure threshold for the cardiac vagal and vasomotor sympathetic limbs of the baroreceptor reflex. The effect of sequential lowering baseline perfusion pressure (i.e. arterial pressure) on the responses (heart rate and lower thoracic sympathetic nerve activity) to transient rises in perfusion pressure to stimulate arterial baroreceptors is depicted. **(a)** From an initial baseline pressure the pressure challenge evokes a baroreflex mediated bradycardia and sympathoinhibition. The subsequent equivalent perfusion ramps from the lowered baselines **(b–d)** produce striking baroreflex sympathoinhibition but a progressive attenuation **(b, c)** and then complete loss of the baroreflex bradycardia **(d).** Note that the progressive reductions in baseline pressure were associated with a marked increase in the ongoing sympathetic nerve activity but comparatively little change in heart rate. Fluctuations in sympathetic activity are respiratory modulated. Simms, A.E., Paton, J.F.R., and Pickering, A.E. (2007) *J. Physiol.* **579**, 473–486, with permission from Wiley.

transmission. In most cases this acts on GABA$_A$ receptors. Here, we consider a number of examples.

Defence response

One of the most striking features of the defence reaction elicited on electrical stimulation of either the hypothalamus or the amygdala is the concomitant rise in arterial blood pressure and heart rate. This suggests a central suppression of the baroreceptor reflex (Spyer 1990, 1994). In part, this resetting could be seen as a consequence of increased inspiratory activity, which, on the basis of our review, would be expected to exert a profound inhibition of cardiac vagal efferent activity. However, both vascular and cardiac components of the reflex appear to be affected. Since the descending output from both amygdala and hypothalamus appears to target the NTS, it is probable that this is the site of major interaction between reflex and central drives. Indeed, NTS neurons that are excited by baroreceptor stimulation receive an inhibitory input on stimulating within the hypothalamic defence area. The inhibitory action is mediated by GABA acting at GABA$_A$ receptors and may be antagonized by the iontophoretic application of bicuculline (Spyer 1994). The descending pathways are likely to be glutamatergic and converge on intrinsic GABAergic neurons of the NTS, since there is no evidence that descending GABAergic pathways are involved (Silva-Carvalho et al. 1995b). Direct inhibition of NTS neurons mediating the baroreceptor reflex no doubt contribute to the profound tachycardia and pressor response that characterizes the fight or flight response.

Nociceptive response

Activation of nociceptors produces reflex tachycardia and sympathoexcitation; the former is mediated in most part through the NTS (Boscan and Paton 2001). Based on latency of synaptic inputs, nociceptors project via relatively direct pathways to the NTS (Boscan et al. 2002). This nociceptor reflex response is concurrent with an inhibition of the cardiac vagal component of the baroreceptor reflex (Pickering et al. 2003). This is again dependent upon GABAAA receptor activation: Boscan et al. (2002) showed that substance P acting on neurokinin type 1 (NK-1) receptors appears to drive the local NTS inhibitory interneurons that depress the baroreceptor reflex. It is likely that inhibition of this component of the baroreceptor reflex contributes to the manifestation of the noxious evoked tachycardia as the latter is attenuated after NTS NK-1 receptors are antagonized (Pickering et al. 2003). It appears that a similar mechanism operates for resetting of the baroreceptor reflex and reflex tachycardia observed during exercise (see Potts et al. 2003).

Angiotensin II and nitric oxide

Much attention has been given to the actions of angiotensin II (AngII) within the NTS because of its potential central role underpinning neurogenic hypertension. AngII acting in the NTS inhibits the baroreceptor reflex. This takes the form of depressing both the cardiac vagal and cardiac sympathetic components (Boscan et al. 2001, Paton and Kasparov 1999). The revelation that the effects of AngII were caused by activation of endothelial nitric oxide synthase (eNOS), which released NO and subsequently stimulated soluble guanylyl cyclase (Paton et al. 2001b, 2006), led to the proposal of *vascular-neuronal signaling* in the NTS (Fig. 2.11) (Paton et al. 2002). Moreover, chronic inhibition of eNOS using virally mediated gene transfer to knock down eNOS activity specifically in

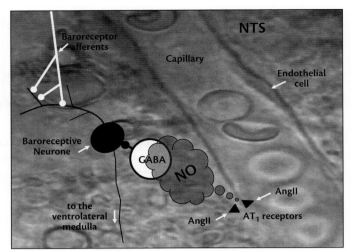

Fig. 2.11 Vascular-neuronal signalling in the nucleus tractus solitarii (NTS) regulates cardiovascular function. A differential interference contrast image of living NTS depicting a capillary full of erythrocytes. Findings indicate that angiotensin II (AngII) (blood-borne or of central origin) acting on angiotensin II type 1 (AT$_1$) receptors anchored to the endothelium activates endothelial nitric oxide synthase (eNOS) to release nitric oxide (NO) from the endothelium that diffuses into the NTS to enhance release of -aminobutyric acid (GABA), which depresses baroreceptor reflex function (see Paton et al. 2001b, 2002, 2006, Wang et al. 2006, 2007). Further, chronic blockade of eNOS in the NTS of conscious rats increases baroreceptor reflex gain and in the spontaneously hypertensive rat also lowers arterial pressure (Waki et al. 2006). Thus, eNOS activity plays a chronic role in the regulation of baroreflex gain and the set-point of arterial pressure.

NTS, improved baroreceptor reflex gain in conscious rats (Waki et al. 2006) suggesting that NO (perhaps driven by endogenous AngII) tonically restrains the baroreceptor reflex at the level of the NTS. The idea that bioactive molecules circulating within the blood vessels in NTS can stimulate to release signaling molecules from the endothelium that affect neuronal transmission (Fig. 2.11) has now been suggested by others for immune to brain signalling during fever (Schiltz and Sawchenko 2003). Regarding NO and the baroceptor reflex, it appears that this acts on the axons and terminals of GABAergic NTS interneurons via activation of cyclic adenosine diphosphate ribose ryanodine-sensitive calcium stores leading to an increased release of GABA and hence enhanced evoked inhibitory postsynaptic potentials (Wang et al. 2006, 2007).

Central control of arterial pressure is altered in hypertension and heart failure

There is growing evidence from both animal and human studies that sympathetic activity is heightened in hypertension, heart failure, obesity, and diabetes. The big question is whether raised sympathetic discharge precedes the pathology and, if it does, is there a causal link? Grassi has stated that the elevated levels of sympathetic nerve discharge are important in the development and maintenance of hypertension (Grassi 2004). Intriguingly, raised levels of muscle vasoconstrictor sympathetic nerve activity have been observed in the progeny of parents who were both hypertensive as well as borderline and white coat hypertensive patients. This suggests that, from its onset, hypertension is associated with sympathetic overactivity. In the neonatal spontaneously hypertensive rats (SHR), sympathetic nerve activity is already raised before hypertension has developed, and contributes to higher vascular resistance (Simms et al. 2009). To prove causality is scientifically challenging and will require further investigation but any data will have wider implications for numerous diseases associated with high sympathetic activity. In animal models of cardiovascular disease there are changes within central nervous cardiovascular control networks which, if corrected, have been found to reduce the pathological phenotype. We will briefly review some examples based on the SHR and animals with induced heart disease to make the point for a significant involvement of the autonomic nervous system in cardiovascular pathology:

◆ *Up-regulation of eNOS in the NTS of the SHR:* As described above, eNOS generated NO appears to increase GABA transmission to depress the baroreceptor reflex. In the NTS of the SHR, eNOS was up-regulated compared with normotensive control rats (Fig. 2.12) (Waki et al. 2006). This led to the prediction that its knock down might increase baroreflex function and heart rate variability both of which are depressed in this animal model. Chronic over expression of a dominant negative protein to block eNOS activity in the NTS not only elevated both baroreceptor reflex gain and heart rate variability but also lowered arterial pressure (Fig. 2.12) (Waki et al. 2006). The inference from these data is that excessive eNOS activity in NTS contributes to the maintenance of the cardiovascular autonomic dysfunction of the SHR. Whether this involves NO signaling itself or oxidized products from NO, such as peroxynitrite, remains to be resolved.

◆ *Up-regulation of PI3 kinase in the RVLM:* AngII acting on AT_1 receptors has been shown to exert a powerful sympathoexcitatory effect from the RVLM. However, antagonizing this receptor

subtype in the SHR alone reduces arterial pressure indicative of a tonic angiotensinergic drive to the RVLM that may be unique to the SHR (Ito et al. 2002). This additional tonic drive may descend from the PVN (Ito et al. 2002, Sved et al. 2003). In this context, Raizada's group have shown that in presympathetic motor areas of the brain of the SHR (e.g. PVN and RVLM) there appears to be an additional signalling pathway involving PI3 kinase that is driven by AngII acting on AT_1 receptors (Veerasingham et al. 2005). Antagonizing this signalling pathway should reduce arterial pressure in the SHR and, indeed, acute blockade of PI3 kinase signalling in the RVLM reduced arterial pressure in the SHR but was without effect in the normotensive control rat (Seyedabadi et al. 2001). The acid test will be to assess the chronic effect of blocking PI3 kinase signalling in RVLM on arterial pressure levels in the conscious SHR.

◆ *Up-regulation of PI3 kinase in the NTS:* In the NTS of SHR there is an elevated mRNA levels of p110beta and p110delta—two catalytic subunits of PI3K relative to normotensive rats (Zubcevic et al. 2009). Chronic blockade of PI3K signalling by lentiviral-mediated expression of a mutant form of p85alpha in the NTS lowered arterial pressure in SHR but not the Wistar-Kyoto rats (Zubcevic et al. 2009). This suggests that PI3K signaling in the NTS of SHR restrains arterial pressure. In addition, PI3K in the NTS of the SHR may also be selectively involved in AngII-mediated signalling that includes a reduction in baroreceptor reflex function via a NADPH-ROS mediated pathway (Sun et al. 2009).

◆ *Down-regulation of NO and GABA signalling in the PVN of animals in heart failure:* In heart failure-induced animals there

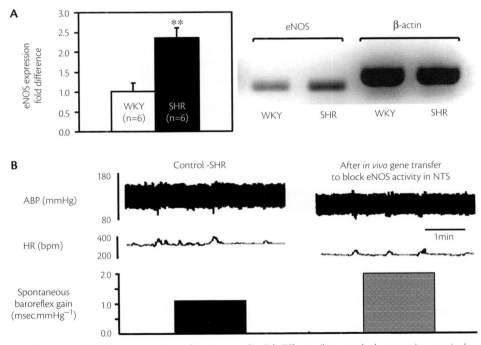

Fig. 2.12 Endothelial nitric oxide synthase (eNOS) activity in the nucleus tractus solitarii (NTS) contributes to the hypertensive state in the spontaneously hypertensive rat (SHR). **A:** Using real-time quantitative polymerase chain reaction, the level of eNOS messenger RNA in the SHR was greater than that in the normotensive, Wistar Kyoto rat (WKY). **B:** Original recordings from a single representative SHR to show that chronic blockade of eNOS activity in the NTS lowered blood pressure and heart rate but improved the spontaneous baroreceptor reflex gain. Cardiovascular variables were recorded using radiotelemetry. eNOS activity was reduced by adenoviral mediated expression of a dominant negative ('truncated' eNOS) protein. ABP, arterial blood pressure; HR, heart rate; Data with permission from Waki et al. 2006.

are a number of changes within the PVN that contribute to the raised levels of sympathetic activity (see Benarroch 2005, Zucker 2006, for reviews). These changes include a reduction in neuronal nitric oxide synthase (nNOS) and presumed production of NO. As with the NTS (see p.44), NO has been implicated in driving GABA transmission in the PVN. Its apparent diminution in the PVN in heart failure excites pre-motor sympathetic neurons through dis-inhibition contributing to the sympathoexcitatory state (Zucker 2006). What remains unresolved is whether other regions of the brainstem are also affected and how the failing, ischaemic heart signals to the brain and induces sympathoexcitation. Studies have suggested both afferent signalling via the vagus nerve as well as actions via enhanced levels of proinflammatory cytokines; the latter may act directly within the PVN or via subfornical organs, which then project to PVN pre-motor sympathetic neurons (e.g. Francis et al. 2004).

- *Beneficial effect of beta-blockers in heart failure include an action on the brainstem:* Heart failure is treated effectively with β-adrenoceptor blockers. What remains uncertain is the site at which these drugs act. Since they cross the blood–brain barrier it is of interest to note that blockade of β-adrenoceptors directly in the brain (chronic intracerebroventricular administration of metoprolol) attenuated the progression of left ventricular remodelling in a rat model of myocardial infarction-induced heart failure (Gourine et al. 2008). These results suggest that beta-blockers act in the brain and contribute to the beneficial effect on the failing heart.

- *Brain perfusion as a major determinant of arterial blood pressure:* Cerebral vessels in the SHR are narrow compared with the normotensive rat and this occurs before hypertension occurs. This begs the question that cerebral perfusion may dictate the set point of arterial pressure. High cerebral vascular resistance and hypoperfusion of the brain leads to hypertension (Cates et al. 2010, Paton et al. 2007, 2009). In humans, vertebral vascular resistance correlated with mean arterial pressure supporting the idea that cerebral perfusion is a determinant of set point of arterial pressure (Thomson and Dickinson, 1960).

Taken together, these observations open numerous doors. First, they highlight the power of combining modern molecular approaches to systems physiology and pathophysiology. The ability to genetically intervene with viral vectors at a specific cardiovascular control sites within the brain and study changes in cardiovascular function chronically is powerful and has huge potential for the future. Second, the revelation and belief that cardiovascular diseases involves alterations within brainstem regions controlling autonomic function must prompt fresh approaches for finding novel therapeutic targets. Indeed, this supports the analysis of differentially expressed genes between normotensive and hypertensive rats. Third, although yet to be fully validated the possibility that changes within the autonomic nervous system precede cardiovascular pathology gives important insight into methods of diagnosis and preventative treatment. Finally, if the latter is true then designing ways to deliver new pharmacological or genetic intervention to the relevant brain regions presents a formidable challenge. With the alarming failure rate of current pharmacological regimens to normalize arterial pressure in hypertensive patients (50–60%) (Mann 2003) there is a clear mission is to gain a better understanding of the autonomic nervous system in the development and maintenance of cardiovascular pathology.

Conclusion

In endeavouring to provide a relatively contemporary analysis of the central nervous control of the cardiovascular system, this review has assessed the neural pathways by which the excitability of both vagal and sympathetic preganglionic motoneurons is regulated in health and disease. Emphasis has been placed on understanding the reflex and, particularly, the baroreflex control of these two groups of autonomic neurons. Further, attempts have been made to identify the central neural mechanisms by which these reflex inputs are modulated in different physiological and pathophysiological conditions. A fundamental design principle appears to involve a tight coupling of respiratory and cardiovascular regulation which provides a neat intrinsic way to elevated cardiac output and respiration that is appropriate to a change in behavioural state. However, it is not inconceivable that an inappropriate change in the strength of coupling between the respiratory rhythm generating network and sympathetic and cardiac vagal motoneurons could well contribute to pathology. Indeed, we have emphasized the role of the autonomic nervous system in the aetiology of some cardiovascular diseases giving examples of how changes in the balance of excitatory versus inhibitory synaptic transmission, intracellular signalling messengers and blood-to-brain communication can all lead to the generation of excessive sympathetic activity. The modification of reflex action, which can be exerted by rostral brainstem and subcortical areas, may provide an indication of potential mechanisms whereby stress and emotion can cause profound changes in the cardiovascular system. Whether these normally acute, and clearly reversible, changes may be converted, on repetition, to prolonged and irreversible alterations in gene expression and subsequent protein function remain to be determined.

Acknowledgements

The financial support of the British Heart Foundation, the Wellcome Trust and the National Institutes of Health (grant HL033610–18) is gratefully acknowledged. JFRP was in receipt of a Royal Society Wolfson Research Merit Award.

References

Abbott, S. B., Stornetta, R. L., Socolovsky, C. S., West, G. H. and Guyenet, P. G. (2009). Photostimulation of channelrhodopsin-2 expressing ventrolateral medullary neurons increases sympathetic nerve activity and blood pressure in rats. *J Physiol.* **587**, 5613–31.

Andresen, M. C. and Paton, J. F. R. (2011). Cardiovascular afferent processing in the nucleus of the solitary tract. In: *Central Regulation of Autonomic Functions*, Second Edition. Editors: I. Llewellyn-Smith & A. Verberne. Oxford University Press.

Anrep, G. V., Pascual, W., and Rössler, R. (1936a). Respiratory variations of the heart rate. I. The reflex mechanism of the sinus arrhythmia. *Proc. Roy.Soc.Lond.*, **119** (Series B), 191–217.

Anrep, G. V., Pascual, W., and Rössler, R. (1936b). Respiratory variations of the heart rate. II. The central mechanism of the sinus arrhythmia and the inter-relationship between central and reflex mechanism. *Proc.Roy. Soc.Lond.*, **119** (Series B), 218–30.

Bacon, S. J., Zagon, A., and Smith, A. D. (1990). Electron microscopic evidence of a monosynaptic pathway between cells in the caudal raphe nuclei and sympathetic preganglionic neurons in the rat spinal cord. *Exp. Brain Res.* **79**, 589–602.

Baekey, D. M., Molkov, Y. I., Paton, J. F. R., Rybak, I. A. and Dick, T. E. (2010). Effect of baroreceptor stimulation on the respiratory pattern: Insights into respiratory-sympathetic interactions. *Respiration Physiology & Neurobiology* **174**, 135–45.

Balthasar, N. (2006). Genetic dissection of neuronal pathways controlling energy homeostasis. *Obesity*, **14** Suppl 5:222S–7S.

Barrett, C. J., Ramchandra, R., Guild, S. J., Lala, A., Budgett, D. M. and Malpas, S. C. (2003). What sets the long-term level of renal sympathetic nerve activity: a role for angiotensin II and baroreflexes? *Circ. Res.* **92**, 1330–36.

Benarroch, E. E. (2005). Paraventricular nucleus, stress response, and cardiovascular disease. *Clin. Auton. Res.* **15**, 254–63.

Blessing, W. W. (1988). Depressor neurons in rabbit caudal medulla act via GABA receptors in rostral medulla. *Am. J. Physiol.* **254**, H686–92.

Boscan, P. Ch., Allen, A. M. and Paton, J. F. R. (2001). Baroreflex inhibition of cardiac sympathetic outflow is attenuated by angiotensin II in the solitary tract nucleus. *Neurosci.*, **103**, 153–60.

Boscan, P., Kasparov, S., and Paton J. F. R. (2002). Somatic nociception activates NK1 receptors in the nucleus tractus solitarii to attenuate the baroreceptor cardiac reflex. *Eur. J. Neurosci.* **16**, 907–20.

Boscan, P., and Paton, J. F. R. (2001). Role of the solitary tract nucleus in mediating nociceptive evoked cardiorespiratory responses. *Auton. Neurosci.* **86**, 170–82.

Braga, V. A., Paton, J. F. R. and Machado, B. M. (2007). Ischemia-induced sympathoexcitation in spinalyzed rats. *Neuroscience Letters*, (in press)

Bravo, G., Guizar-Sahagun, G., Ibarra, A., Centurion, D., and Villalon, C. M. (2004). Cardiovascular alterations after spinal cord injury: an overview. *Curr. Med. Chem. Cardiovasc. Hematol. Agents.* **2**, 133–48.

Cao, W. H., and Morrison, S. F. (2006). Glutamate receptors in the raphe pallidus mediate brown adipose tissue thermogenesis evoked by activation of dorsomedial hypothalamic neurons. *Neuropharm.* **51**, 426–37.

Cates, M. J., Abdala, A. P. L., Langton, P. D. and Paton, J. F. R. (2010). Elevated posterior cerebral artery resistance in pre-hypertensive spontaneously hypertensive rats: implications for sympathetic activity generation and vasomotor tone. *Hypertension* (in revision).

Charkoudian, N., Joyner, M. J., Johnson, C. P., Eisenach, J. H., Dietz, N. M., and Wallin, B. G. (2005). Balance between cardiac output and sympathetic nerve activity in resting humans: role in arterial pressure regulation. *J. Physiol.* **568**, 315–21.

Chau, D., Johns, D. G., and Schramm, L. P. (2000). Ongoing and stimulus-evoked activity of sympathetically correlated neurons in the intermediate zone and dorsal horn of acutely spinalized rats. *J. Neurophysiol.* **83**, 2699–2707.

Cochrane, K. L., and Nathan, M. A. (1994). Pressor systems involved in the maintenance of arterial pressure after lesions of the rostral ventrolateral medulla. *J. Auton. Nerv. Syst.* **46**, 9–18.

Coote, J. H., and Lewis, D. I. (1995). Bulbospinal catecholamine neurons and sympathetic pattern generation. *J. Physiol. Pharmacol.* **46**, 259–71.

Cowley, A. W. Jr., Liard, J. F., and Guyton, A. C. (1973). Role of baroreceptor reflex in daily control of arterial blood pressure and other variables in dogs. *Circ. Res.* **32**, 564–76.

Daly, M. de B. (1997). Peripheral arterial chemoreceptors and respiratory–cardiovascular integration. *Monographs of the Physiological Society*, Vol. 46. Clarendon Press, Oxford.

Dampney, R. A., Goodchild, A. K., Robertson, L. G., and Montgomery, W. (1982). Role of ventrolateral medulla in vasomotor regulation: a correlative anatomical and physiological study. *Brain Res.* **249**, 223–35.

Dampney, R. A., and McAllen, R. M. (1988). Differential control of sympathetic fibres supplying hindlimb skin and muscle by subretrofacial neurons in the cat. *J. Physiol.* **395**, 41–56.

Dawid-Milner, M. S., Silva-Carvalho, L., Goldsmith, G. E., and Spyer, K. M. (1995). Hypothalamic modulation of laryngeal reflexes in the anaesthetized cat; role of the nucleus tractus solitarii. *J. Physiol.* **487**, 739–49.

Dembowsky, K., Czachurski, J., and Seller, H. (1986). Three types of sympathetic preganglionic neurons with different electrophysiological properties are identified by intracellular recordings in the cat. *Pflugers Arch.* **406**, 112–20.

Deuchars, J., Li, Y. W., Kasparov, S., and Paton, J. F. R. (2000). Morphological and electrophysiological properties of neurons in the dorsal vagal complex of the rat activated by arterial baroreceptors. *J. Comp. Neurol.* **417**, 233–49.

Deuchars, S. A., Morrison, S. F., and Gilbey, M. P. (1995). Medullary stimulation elicits EPSPs in neonatal rat sympathetic preganglionic neurons *in vitro*. *J. Physiol.* **487.2**, 453–63.

Dickinson, C. J. and Thomson, A. D. (1960). A post mortem study of the main cerebral arteries with special reference to their possible role in blood pressure regulation. *Clin Sci.* **19**, 513–38.

Doba, N., and Reis, D. J. (1973). Acute fulminating neurogenic hypertension produced by brainstem lesions in the rat. *Circ Res.* **32**, 54–53.

Eckberg, D. L., Rea, R. F., Andersson, O. K., Hedner, T., Pernow, J., Lundberg, J. M., and Wallin, B. G. (1988). Baroreflex modulation of sympathetic activity and sympathetic neurotransmitters in humans. *Acta. Physiol. Scand.* **133**, 221–31.

Francis, J., Zhang, Z. H., Weiss, R. M., and Felder, R. B. (2004). Neural regulation of the proinflammatory cytokine response to acute myocardial infarction. *Am. J. Physiol.*, **287**, H791–97.

Gatti, P. J., Johnson, T. A., Phan, P., Jordan, I. K. 3rd, Coleman, W., and Massari, V. J. (1995). The physiological and anatomical demonstration of functionally selective parasympathetic ganglia located in discrete fat pads on the feline myocardium. *J. Auton. Nerv. Syst.* **51**, 255–59.

Gatti, P. J., Johnson, T. A., and Massari, V. J. (1996). Can neurons in the nucleus ambiguus selectively regulate cardiac rate and atrio-ventricular conduction? *J. Auton. Nerv. Syst.* **57**, 123–27.

Gilbey, M. P. (1997). Fundamental aspects of the control of sympathetic preganglionic neuronal discharge. In *Central nervous control of autonomic function. Series: The autonomic nervous system*, Vol. 11 (ed. D. Jordan), pp. 1–28. Harwood Academic Publishers, The Netherlands.

Gilbey, M. P., Jordan, D., Richter, D. W., and Spyer, K. M. (1984). Synaptic mechanisms involved in the inspiratory modulation of vagal cardio-inhibitory neurons in the cat. *J. Physiol., London* **356**, 65–78.

Gilbey, M. P., and Stein, R. D. (1991). Characteristics of sympathetic preganglionic neurons in the lumbar spinal cord of the cat. *J. Physiol.* **432**, 427–43.

Gourine, A., Bondar, S. I., Spyer, K. M. and Gourine, A. V. (2008). Beneficial effect of the CNS beta-adrenoceptor blockade on the failing heart. *Circ Res.* **102**, 633–36.

Grassi, G. (2004). Counteracting the sympathetic nervous system in essential hypertension. *Curr. Opin. Nephrol. Hypertens.* **13**, 513–519.

Guertzenstein, P. G., and Silver, A. (1974). Fall in blood pressure produced from discrete regions of the ventral surface of the medulla by glycine and lesions. *J. Physiol.* **242**, 489–503.

Guyenet, P. G. (1990). Role of the ventral medulla oblongata in blood pressure regulation. In *Central regulation of autonomic functions*, (ed. A. D. Loewy and K. M. Spyer), pp. 145–67. Oxford University Press, New York.

Guyenet, P. G. (2006). The sympathetic control of blood pressure. *Nat. Neurosci.Revs.* **7**, 335–46.

Hainsworth, R. (1991). Reflexes from the heart. *Physiol. Rev.* **71**, 617–58.

Hajduczok, G., Chapleau, M. W., and Abboud, F. M. (1988). Rheoreceptors in the carotid sinus of dog. *Proc. Natl. Acad. Sci.* **85**, 7399–7403.

Hayano, J., Yasuma, F., Okada, A., Mukai, S. and Fujinami, T., (1996). Respiratory sinus arrhythmia. A phenomenon improving pulmonary gas exchange and circulatory efficiency. *Circulation.* **94**, 842–47.

Heusser, K., Tank, J., Engeli, S., *et al.* (2010). Carotid baroreceptor stimulation, sympathetic activity, baroreflex function, and blood pressure in hypertensive patients. *Hypertension.* **55**, 619–26.

Ito, S., Komatsu, K., Tsukamoto, K., Kanmatsuse, K., and Sved, A. F. (2002). Ventrolateral medulla AT1 receptors support blood pressure in hypertensive rats. *Hypertension*, **40**, 552–59.

Ito, S., and Sved, A. F. (1997). Tonic glutamate-mediated control of rostral ventrolateral medulla and sympathetic vasomotor tone. *Am. J. Physiol.* **273**, R487–94.

Izzo, P. N., Deuchars, J., and Spyer, K. M. (1993). Localization of cardiac vagal preganglionic motoneurons in the rat: immunocytochemical evidence of synaptic inputs containing 5-hydroxytryptamine. *J. Comp. Neurol.* **327**, 572–83.

Izzo, P. N. and Spyer, K. M. (1997). The parasympathetic innervation of the heart. In *The autonomic nervous system*, Vol. 11, (ed. G. Burnstock), Harwood Academic Publishers, The Netherlands.

Jänig, W. (2006). *The integrative action of the autonomic nervous system.* Cambridge University Press.

Jänig, W. and Häbler, H. J. (2003). Neurophysiologicalanalysis of target related sympathetic pathways—from animal to humans: similarities and differences. *Acta. Physiol. Scand.* **177**, 255–74.

Jansen, A. S. P., Nguyen, X. V., Karpitskiy, V., Mettenleiter, T. C., and Loewy, A. D. (1995). Central command neurons of the sympathetic nervous system: Basis of the fight-or-flight response. *Science*, **270**, 644–6.

Jeske, I., Morrison, S. F., Cravo, S. L., and Reis, D. J. (1993). Identification of baroreceptor reflex interneurons in the caudal ventrolateral medulla. *Am. J. Physiol.* **264**, R169–78.

Jones, J. F. X., Wang, Y., and Jordan, D. (1994). Activity of cardiac vagal preganglionic neurons during the pulmonary chemoreflex in the anaesthetized cat. In *Arterial chemoreceptors cell to system: advances in experimental medicine and biology*, Vol. 360, (ed. R. G. O'Regan, P. Nolan, D. S. McQueen and D. J. Paterson), pp. 301–3. Plenum Press, New York.

Jones, J. F. X., Wang, Y., and Jordan, D. (1995). Heart rate responses to selective stimulation of cardiac vagal C fibres in anaesthetized cats, rats and rabbits. *J. Physiol.* **489**, 203–214.

Jones, J. F. X., Wang, Y., and Jordan, D. (1998). Activity of C fibre cardiac vagal efferents in anaesthetized cats and rats. *J. Physiol.* **507**, 869–80.

Jordan, D. (1990). Autonomic changes in affective behaviour. In *Central regulation of autonomic functions*, (ed. A. D. Loewy and K. M. Spyer), pp. 349–66. Oxford University Press, New York.

Kanbar, R., Stornetta, R. L., Cash, D.R., Lewis, S.J. and Guyenet, P. G. (2010). Photostimulation of Phox2b medullary neurons activates cardiorespiratory function in conscious rats. *Am J Respir Crit Care Med.* **182**, 1184–94.

Koshiya, N., and Guyenet, P. G. (1996). NTS neurons with carotid chemoreceptor inputs arborize in the rostral ventrolateral medulla. *Am. J. Physiol.* **270**, R1273–88.

Lipski, J., Kanjhan, R., Kruszewska, B., and Rong, W. (1996). Properties of presympathetic neurons in the rostral ventrolateral medulla in the rat: an intracellular study *in vivo. J. Physiol.* **490**, 729–44.

Llewellyn-Smith, I. J., Arnolda, L. F., Pilowsky, P. M., Chalmers, J. P., and Minson, J. B. (1998). GABA- and glutamate-immunoreactive synapses on sympathetic preganglionic neurons projecting to the superior cervical ganglion. *J. Auton. Nerv. Syst.* **71**, 96–110.

Lohmeier, T. E., Iliescu, R., Dwyer, T. M., Irwin, E. D., Cates, A. W. and Rossing, M. A. (2010). Sustained suppression of sympathetic activity and arterial pressure during chronic activation of the carotid baroreflex. *Am J Physiol.* **299**, H402–H409.

Mandel, D. A. and Schreihofer, A. M. (2006). Central respiratory modulation of barosensitive neurons in rat caudal ventrolateral medulla. *J. Physiol.* **572**, 881–96.

Mann, S. J. (2003). Neurogenic essential hypertension revisited: the case for increased clinical and research attention. *Am. J. Hypertens.* **16**, 881–88.

Marina, N., Taheri, M., and Gilbey, M. P. (2006). Generation of a physiological sympathetic motor rhythm in the rat following spinal application of 5-HT. *J. Physiol.* **571**, 441–50.

Marks, S. A., Stein, R. D., Dashwood, M. R., and Gilbey, M. P. (1990). [3H] prazosin binding in the intermediolateral cell column and the effects of iontophoresed methoxamine on sympathetic preganglionic neuronal activity in the anaesthetized cat and rat. *Brain Res.* **530**, 321–34.

Minson, J. B., Arnolda, L. F., and Llewellyn-Smith, I. J. (2002). Neurochemistry of nerve fibers apposing sympathetic preganglionic neurons activated by sustained hypotension. *J. Comp. Neurol.* **449**, 307–318.

Miyawaki, T., Goodchild, A. K., and Pilowsky, P. M. (2002). Evidence for a tonic GABA-ergic inhibition of excitatory respiratory-related afferents to presympathetic neurons in the rostral ventrolateral medulla. *Brain Res.* **924**, 56–62.

Morrison, S. F. (2003). Raphe pallidus neurons mediate prostaglandin E2-evoked increases in brown adipose tissue thermogenesis. *Neurosci.* **121**, 17–24.

Morrison, S. F. (2004). Central pathways controlling brown adipose tissue thermogenesis. *News Physiol Sci.* **19**, 67–74.

Paton, J. F. R. (1998). Convergence properties of solitary tract neurons driven synaptically by cardiac vagal afferents in the mouse. *J. Physiol.* **508**, 237–52.

Paton, J. F. R. (1999). The Sharpey-Schafer prize lecture: nucleus tractus solitarii: integrating structures. *Exp. Physiol.* **84**, 815–33.

Paton, J. F. R., Boscan, P., Pickering, A. E., and Nalivaiko, E. (2005). The yin and yang of cardiac autonomic control: vago-sympathetic interactions revisited. *Brain Res. Rev.* **49**, 555–65.

Paton J. F. R., Deuchars, J., Ahmad, Z., Wong, L.-F., Murphy, D. and Kasparov, S. (2001b). Adeno viral vector demonstrates that angiotensin II induced depression of the cardiac baroreflex is mediated by endothelial nitric oxide synthase in the nucleus tractus solitarii. *J Physiol.* **531.2**, 445–58.

Paton, J. F. R., Deuchars, J., Li, Y. W., and Kasparov, S. (2001a). Properties of solitary tract neurons responding to peripheral arterial chemoreceptors. *Neurosci.* **105**, 231–48.

Paton J. F. R. Dickinson, C.J. and Mitchell, G. (2009). Harvey Cushing and the regulation of blood pressure in giraffe, rats and man: introducing Cushing's mechanism. *Experimental Physiology*, **94**, 11–17.

Paton, J. F. R., Kasparov, S. and Paterson, D. J. (2002). Site-specific differential modulation of cardiac autonomic control by nitric oxide. *TINS*, **25**, 626–31.

Paton, J. F. R., and Kasparov, S. (1999). Differential effects of angiotensin II on cardiovascular reflexes mediated by nucleus tractus solitarii I. A microinjection study. *J.Physiol.* **521.1**, 213–25.

Paton, J. F. R., Li, Y.-W. & Schwaber, J. S. (2001c). Response properties of baroreceptive NTS neurons. *Ann. New York Acad. Sci.* **940**, 157–68.

Paton, J. F. R., Lonergan, T., Deuchars, J., James, P. E., and Kasparov, S. (2006). Detection of angiotensin II mediated nitric oxide release within the nucleus of the solitary tract using electron-paramagnetic resonance (epr) spectroscopy. *Auton.Neurosci.: Basic Clin.* **126–127**, 193–201.

Paton, J. F. R., and Nolan P. J. (2000). Similarities in reflex control of laryngeal and cardiac vagal motor neurons. *Respir. Physiol.* **119**, 101–111.

Paton, J. F. R., Waki, H., Abdala, A. P. L., Dickinson, C. J. and Kasparov, S. (2007). Vascular-brain signaling in hypertension: role of angiotensin ii and nitric oxide. *Current Hypertension Reports*, **9**, 242–47.

Pickering, A. E., Boscan, P., and Paton, J. F. R. (2003). Nociception attenuates parasympathetic but not sympathetic baroreflex via NK1 receptors in the rat nucleus tractus solitarii. *J. Physiol.* **551**, 589–99.

Pilowsky, P. M., and Goodchild, A. K. (2002). Baroreceptor reflex pathways and neurotransmitters: 10 years on. *J. Hypertens.* **20**, 1675–88.

Potts, J. T. (2006). Inhibitory neurotransmission in the nucleus tractus solitarii: implications for baroreflex resetting during exercise. *Exp. Physiol.* **91**, 59–72.

Potts, J. T., Paton, J. F. R., Mitchell, J. H., Garry, M. G., Kline, G., Anguelov, P. T., and Lee, S. M. (2003). Contraction-sensitive skeletal muscle afferents inhibit arterial baroreceptor signalling in the nucleus of the solitary tract: role of intrinsic GABA interneurons. *Neurosci.* **119**, 201–214.

Rathner, J. A., Owens, N. C., and McAllen, R. M. (2001). Cold-activated raphe-spinal neurons in rats. *J. Physiol.* **535**, 841–54.

Raven, P. B., Fadel, P. J., and Ogoh, S. (2006). Arterial baroreflex resetting during exercise: a current perspective. *Exp. Physiol.* **91**, 37–49.

Richter, D. W. and Spyer, K. M. (1990). In *Central regulation of autonomic functions*, (ed. A. D. Loewy and K. M. Spyer), pp. 189–207. Oxford University Press, New York.

Sampaio, K. N., Mauad, H., Spyer, K. M., and Ford, T. W. (2003). Differential chronotropic and dromotropic responses to focal stimulation of cardiac vagal ganglia in the rat. *Exp. Physiol.* **88**, 315–27.

Schiltz, J. C., and Sawchenko, P. E. (2003). Signaling the brain in systemic inflammation: the role of perivascular cells. *Front. Biosci.* **8**, 1321–29.

Schramm, L. P., Strack, A. M., Platt, K. B., and Loewy, A. D. (1993). Peripheral and central pathways regulating the kidney: a study using pseudorabies virus. *Brain Res.* **616**, 251–62.

Schreihofer, A. M., Stornetta, R. L., and Guyenet, P. G. (2000). Regulation of sympathetic tone and arterial pressure by rostral ventrolateral medulla after depletion of C1 cells in rat. *J. Physiol.* **529**, 221–36.

Schreihofer, A. M., and Guyenet, P. G. (2002). The baroreflex and beyond: control of sympathetic vasomotor tone by GABAergic neurons in the ventrolateral medulla. *Clin. Exp. Pharmacol. Physiol.* **29**, 514–21.

Schreihofer, A. M., and Guyenet, P. G. (2003). Baro-activated neurons with pulse-modulated activity in the rat caudal ventrolateral medulla express GAD67 mRNA. *J.Neurophysiol.* **89**, 1265–77.

Seyedabadi, M., Goodchild, A. K., and Pilowsky, P. M. (2001). Differential role of kinases in brain stem of hypertensive and normotensive rats. *Hypertension.* **38**, 1087–92.

Silva-Carvalho, L., Dawid-Milner, M. S., Goldsmith, G. E., and Spyer, K. M. (1995a). Hypothalamic modulation of the arterial chemoreceptor reflex in the anaesthetized cat: role of the nucleus tractus solitarii. *J. Physiol.* **487.3**, 751–60.

Silva-Carvalho, L., Dawid-Milner, M. S., and Spyer, K. M. (1995b). The pattern of excitatory inputs to the nucleus tractus solitarii evoked on stimulation in the hypothalamic defence area of the cat. *J. Physiol.* **487.3**, 727–37.

Simms, A. E., Paton, J. F. R., and Pickering, A. E. (2007). Hierarchical recruitment of the sympathetic and parasympathetic limbs of the baroreflex in normotensive and spontaneously hypertensive rats. *J. Physiol.* **579**, 473–86.

Simms, A. E., Paton, J. F. R., Pickering, A. E. and Allen, A. M. (2009). Amplified respiratory-sympathetic coupling in neonatal and juvenile spontaneously hypertensive rats: does it contribute to hypertension? *Journal of Physiology*, **587.3**, 597–610.

Simms, A. E., Paton, J. F. R., Pickering, A. E. and Allen, A. M. (2010). Is augmented central respiratory–sympathetic coupling involved in the generation of hypertension? *Respiration Physiology & Neurobiology*, **174**, 89–97.

Spanswick, D. and Logan, S. D. (1990). Sympathetic preganglionic neurons in neonatal rat spinal cord in vitro: electrophysiological characteristics and the effects of selective excitatory amino acid receptor agonists. *Brain Res.* **525**, 181–88.

Spyer, K. M. (1990). The central nervous organisation of reflex circulatory control. In *Central regulation of autonomic functions*, (ed. A. D. Loewy and K. M. Spyer), pp. 168–88. Oxford University Press, New York.

Spyer, K. M. (1994). Annual Review Prize Lecture: Central nervous mechanisms contributing to cardiovascular control. *J. Physiol.* **474**, 1–19.

Standish, A., Enquist, L. W., and Schwaber, J. S. (1994). Innervation of the heart and its central medullary origin defined by viral tracing. *Science.* **263**, 232–34.

Strack, A. M., Sawyer, W. B., Hughes, J. H., Platt, K. B., and Loewy, A. D. (1989a). A general pattern of CNS innervation of the sympathetic outflow demonstrated by transneuronal pseudorabies viral infections. *Brain Res.* **491**, 156–62.

Strack, A. M., Sawyer, W. B., Platt, K. B., and Loewy, A. D. (1989b). CNS cell groups regulating the sympathetic outflow to adrenal gland as revealed by transneuronal cell body labeling with pseudorabies virus. *Brain Res.* **491**, 274–96.

Sun, C., Zubcevic, J., Polson, J. W., Potts, J. T., Diez-Freire, C., Zhang, O., Raizada, M. K. and Paton, J. F. R. (2009). Shift to an involvement of PI3-kinase in angiotensin II actions on nucleus tractus solitarii neurons of the spontaneously hypertensive rat. *Circulation Research*, **105**: 1248–55.

Sun, M.-K. (1996). Pharmacology of reticulospinal vasomotor neurons in cardiovascular regulation. *Pharmacological Reviews*, **48**, (4), 465–94.

Sun, M.-K. and Spyer, K. M. (1991). Nociceptive inputs into rostral ventrolateral medulla-spinal vasomotor neurons in rats. *J. Physiol., London* **436**, 685–700.

Sved, A. F. (1989). PNMT-containing catecholaminergic neurons are not necessarily adrenergic. *Brain Res.* **481**, 113–118.

Sved, A. F., Ito, S., and Sved, J. C. (2003). Brainstem mechanisms of hypertension: role of the rostral ventrolateral medulla. *Curr. Hypertens Rep.* **5**, 262–68.

Thrasher, T. N. (2004). Baroreceptors and the long-term control of blood pressure. *Exp Physiol.* **89**, 331–35.

Thrasher, T. N. (2005). Effects of chronic baroreceptor unloading on blood pressure in the dog. *Am J Physiol Regul Integr Comp Physiol.* **288**, R863–71.

Veerasingham, S. J., Yamazato, M., Berecek, K. H., Wyss, J. M., and Raizada, M. K. (2005). Increased PI3-kinase in presympathetic brain areas of the spontaneously hypertensive rat. *Circ Res.* **96**, 277–89.

Waki, H., Murphy, D., Yao, S. T., Kasparov, S. and Paton, J. F. R. (2006). Endothelial nitric oxide synthase in the nucleus tractus solitarii contributes to the hypertension in the spontaneously hypertensive rat. *Hypertension,* **48**, 644–50.

Wallin, B. G. (1986). Abnormalities of sympathetic regulation after cervical cord lesions. *Acta Neurochir Suppl (Wien).* **36**, 123–34.

Wallin, B. G. and Elam, M. (1994). Insights from intraneural recordings of sympathetic nerve traffic in humans. *News Physiol.Sci.*, **9**, 203–207.

Wang, S., Paton, J. F. R., and Kasparov, S. (2007). Differential sensitivity of excitatory and inhibitory synaptic transmission to modulation by nitric oxide in the nucleus tractus solitarii. *Exp. Physiol.* (in press).

Wang, S., Teschemacher, A. G., Paton, J. F. R., and Kasparov, S. (2006). Mechanism of nitric oxide action on inhibitory GABAergic signaling within the nucleus tractus solitarii. *FASEB J.* **20**, 1537–49.

Wang, Y., and Ramage, A. G. (2001). The role of central 5-HT(1A) receptors in the control of B-fibre cardiac and bronchoconstrictor vagal preganglionic neurons in anaesthetized cats. *J. Physiol.* **536**, 753–67.

Weston, M., Wang, H., Stornetta, R. L., Sevigny, C. P., and Guyenet, P. G. (2003). Fos expression by glutamatergic neurons of the solitary tract nucleus after phenylephrine-induced hypertension in rats. *J Comp Neurol.* **460**, 525–41.

Zagon, A. and Bacon, S. J. (1991). Evidence of monosynaptic pathway between cells of the ventromedial medulla and the motoneuron pool of the thoracic spinal cord in rat: electron microscopic analysis of synaptic contacts. *Eur. J. Neurosci.* **3**, 55–65.

Zagon, A., and Smith, A. D. (1993). Monosynaptic projections from the rostral ventrolateral medulla oblongata to identified sympathetic preganglionic neurons. *Neurosci.* **54**, 729–43.

Zubcevic, J., Nikiforova, N., Raizada, M. K. and Paton J. F. R. (2009). Chronic blockade of phosphatidylinositol 3-kinase in the nucleus tractus solitarii is prohypertensive in the spontaneously hypertensive rat. *Hypertension.* **53**, 97–103.

Zucker, I. H. (2006). Novel mechanisms of sympathetic regulation in chronic heart failure. *Hypertension*, **48**, 1005–1011.

CHAPTER 3

Neurotransmitters and neuromodulators in the central nervous system and cardiovascular regulation

Eduardo E. Benarroch

Key points

- The areas of the central nervous system controlling cardiovascular function include the insular and anterior cingulate cortices, amygdala, paraventricular nucleus of the hypothalamus, periaqueductal gray, parabrachial nucleus, nucleus of the solitary tract, ventrolateral medulla, medullary raphe, vagal nuclei, and intermediolateral cell column.

- Rapid communication within these regions is mediated by the excitatory amino acid L-glutamate and the inhibitory amino acid γ-aminobutyric acid (GABA).

- Catecholamines, serotonin, histamine, acetylcholine, nitric oxide, purines, peptides, steroids, and cytokines modulate the activity of central autonomic neurons.

- Glutamatergic neurons of the rostral ventrolateral medulla are critical for control of sympathetic output and maintenance of blood pressure, and their activity is controlled by descending and propriobulbar influences mediated by glutamate, GABA glycine, nitric oxide, and several neuropeptides, including angiotensin II.

- Neurons of the nucleus of the solitary tract receive excitatory glutamatergic inputs from baroreceptor and cardiac afferents, are critical for cardiovascular reflexes, and their activity is controlled by complex neurochemical influences.

- The paraventricular nucleus integrates visceral, humoral, and limbic inputs and initiates sympathoadrenal and adrenocortical responses to stress; its function is controlled by glutamate, GABA, nitric oxide, catecholamines, and several neuropeptides.

- The central neurochemical systems involved in cardiovascular control have been implicated in mechanisms of orthostatic hypotension in neurodegenerative disorders and in cardiovascular disorders such as congestive heart failure and hypertension.

Introduction

The central neural circuits controlling arterial blood pressure (BP), heart rate (HR), and renal function are located throughout the neuraxis, have a complex neurochemical organization, and are highly interconnected (Loewy 1991, Spyer 1994, Dampney et al. 2003b, Saper 2002). These regions integrate central and peripheral commands to maintain a continuous level of activity of cardiovascular effectors, prevent wide variations of BP through compensatory reflexes, initiate integrated adaptive responses in response to external or internal stimuli, and provide appropriate adjustments of tissue blood flow to support specific behaviours.

Advances in anatomical, physiological, and pharmacological techniques have provided a wealth of information about the functional anatomy and neurochemistry of the central pathways controlling cardiovascular function. These techniques include, among others, anterograde, retrograde, and transneuronal transport methods to map central autonomic pathways (Strack et al. 1989) assessment of stimulus-dependent expression of immediate early genes (Dampney et al. 2003a); immunocytochemical identification of neurons and fibres (Koutcherov et al. 2000); localization of receptors by immunocytochemistry or *in situ* hybridization (Allen et al. 1988); local microinjection of selective agonists or antagonists combined with recording of BP, HR, and sympathetic nerve activity (Morrison 2001, Sun 1996); and, most recently, juxtacellular mRNA labelling of extracellularly recorded neurons *in vivo* (Guyenet et al. 2004).

The central autonomic circuits interact via a complex 'chemical coding' provided by two types of signals:

- fast, point-to-point excitation or inhibition mediated primarily by L-glutamate or γ-aminobutyric acid (GABA), respectively

- modulatory influences on neuronal excitability, mediated by acetylcholine; monoamines, including norepinephrine, epinephrine, serotonin (5-HT), and histamine; peptides, including cytokines; purines such as adenosine triphosphate (ATP); nitric oxide (NO); and steroids.

The complexity of this chemical coding stems from the coexistence of different neurotransmitters in single neurons, the presence of various receptors subtypes for a given neurotransmitter, the presynaptic and postsynaptic interactions among the various neurochemicals, and the plasticity of neurotransmitter expression or receptor function in response to activity and environmental factors.

Overview of the functional and neurochemical anatomy of central cardiovascular control

Central autonomic control areas

The areas of the central nervous system controlling cardiovascular function include the insular and anterior cingulate cortices; the central nucleus of the amygdala (CeNA) and bed nucleus of the stria terminalis; the paraventricular nucleus (PVN) and lateral hypothalamic area; the periaqueductal gray matter of the midbrain, the parabrachial nucleus of the pons, the nucleus of the solitary tract (NTS); the ventrolateral medulla (VLM) and the medullary raphe nuclei. The final outputs of these central regulatory circuits are mediated by the sympathetic preganglionic neurons (SPNs) of the intermediolateral cell column, cardiovagal neurons of the nucleus ambiguus, and vasopressin (AVP) secreting magnocellular neurons of the hypothalamus (Spyer 1994, Dampney et al. 2003b).

The insular cortex is the primary viscerosensory cortex and contains a viscerotropic map of taste and general visceral afferents. It is also the primary cortical area receiving inputs from nociceptors and thermoreceptors (Saper 2002). The anterior cingulate cortex, via its interconnections with the prefrontal cortex, insula, and amygdala, is involved in evaluation of the emotional and motivational value external or internal stimuli, including pain, and in generation of adaptive cardiovascular adjustments to support behaviours triggered by these stimuli (Critchley et al. 2003). The amygdala provides emotional significance to sensory stimuli and, via its output structure, the CeNA, generates the cardiovascular, endocrine, and motor responses associated with emotion (Henderson et al. 2002, LeDoux 1996). The PVN is an important site for integration of autonomic and neuroendocrine responses to stress (Sawchenko et al. 2000). The periaqueductal gray is a site of integration of autonomic, behavioural, and antinociceptive stress responses (Lovick 1993). The parabrachial nucleus consists of several subnuclei that integrate and relay of visceral, pain, and temperature information to rostral areas and regulate medullary reflexes (Saper 2002). The NTS is the first relay station for taste and general visceral afferents and has a viscerotopic organization (Loewy and Spyer 1990; Lawrence and Jarrot 1996). It has two main functions:

◆ relay of visceral information, either directly or via the parabrachial nucleus and VLM, to the hypothalamus, thalamus, and amygdala

◆ initiation of medullary reflexes controlling cardiovascular, respiratory, and gastrointestinal functions.

The rostral VLM contains neurons that activate the SPNs involved in maintenance of BP (Spyer 1994, Dampney et al. 2003b). Rostral VLM neurons mediate essentially all supraspinal reflex and behavioural influences controlling sympathetic activity, including responses to hypoxia (Makeham et al. 2005, Guyenet 2000). The caudal VLM is a site of integration of medullary reflexes via its connections with the NTS, rostral VLM, and hypothalamus (Dampney et al. 2003b). The caudal raphe nuclei provide inputs to SPNs controlling outputs to skin blood vessels involved in thermoregulation (Morrison 2001).

Chemical signalling in central autonomic pathways

Fast, point-to-point transmission of excitatory or inhibitory signals in central autonomic areas involves ligand-gated ion channel receptors. L-glutamate or in some cases adenosine triphosphate (ATP), serotonin (5-HT), or acetylcholine, elicit fast excitation by opening cation channels permeable to Na^+, Ca^{2+}, or both. Inhibitory amino acids, such as GABA or glycine, elicit fast inhibition by opening of Cl-channels. Modulatory signals initiated by glutamate, GABA, acetylcholine, monoamines, neuropeptides, and adenosine primarily involve activation of GTP-binding (G) protein-coupled receptors. Receptors coupled to G_s activate adenylyl cyclase and cyclic AMP formation and exert multiple effects on ion channels. Receptors coupled to $G_{i/o}$ inhibit adenylyl cyclase, increase K^+ channel permeability (thus reducing neuronal excitability), and decrease presynaptic Ca^{2+} channel permeability (thus reducing neurotransmitter release). Receptors coupled to $G_{q/11}$ increase intracellular Ca^{2+} and, in general, reduce K^+ channel permeability (thus increasing neuronal excitability). Nitric oxide (NO) and steroids have direct access of intracellular signalling mechanisms.

Neuropeptides, monoamines, NO, and steroids may diffuse through the extracellular fluid to act on targets distant from the site of release by a mechanism of 'volume transmission'. Angiotensin II, vasopressin (AVP), natriuretic peptides, opioids, corticotropin releasing factor (CRF; also called corticotrophin releasing hormone [CRH]), and cytokines (e.g. interleukin-1) control cardiovascular function by acting both as circulating signals and endogenous transmitters in central autonomic pathways. As circulating signals, they affect peripheral targets and exert central effects by acting via receptors in the circumventricular organs. These structures, which include the subfornical organ (SFO) and the area postrema, lack a blood–brain barrier and project to other brain autonomic regions, including the PVN and NTS (Sawchenko et al. 2000, McKinley et al. 2001).

Fast neurotransmission

L-glutamate

L-glutamate is the primary transmitter of all excitatory pathways connecting central autonomic regions. Glutamatergic neurons are identified by their expression of vesicular glutamate transporters (VGLUTs), particularly VGLUT1 and VGLUT2 (Guyenet et al. 2004). Fast excitatory transmission is mediated via three classes of ionotropic glutamate receptors; AMPA (alpha-amino-3-hydroxy-5-methyl-4-isoxazole propionic acid), kainate, and NMDA (N-methyl-D-aspartate) receptors. Most AMPA and kainate receptors are permeable to Na^+ whereas the NMDA receptor is a Ca^{2+} channel that is positively modulated by glycine and blocked by Mg^{2+} in a voltage-dependent manner. Activation of these ionotropic, as well as some metabotropic glutamate receptors (mGluRs) results in an increase in intracellular Ca^{2+}, which triggers several transduction cascades, including activation of neuronal nitric oxide synthase (NOS). Glutamate is the primary neurotransmitter of many critical central autonomic pathways, including baroreceptor afferents terminating in the NTS (Talman 1997); descending sympathoexcitatory inputs from the rostral VLM to SPNs (Morrison 2003); sympathoexcitatory projections from baroreceptive NTS neurons to cardiovagal neurons of the nucleus ambiguus (Wang et al. 2001); and descending excitatory inputs from the hypothalamus and other regions to vasomotor neurons of the rostral VLM (Dampney et al. 2003a).

GABA and glycine

GABA is the main neurotransmitter of local circuit inhibitory neurons present throughout the central autonomic regions. These neurons are identified by their expression of glutamic acid decarboxylase (GAD) (Guyenet et al. 2004). GABA produces both pre and postsynaptic inhibition, via $GABA_A$ and $GABA_B$ receptors. The $GABA_A$ receptors are Cl-channels that mediate fast inhibition and are allosterically potentiated by barbiturates, benzodiazepines, alcohol, general anaesthetics, and some steroids. The $GABA_B$ receptors are coupled to $G_{i/o}$ and mediate both postsynaptic and presynaptic inhibition. GABA is critically involved in circuits mediating the baroreflex at the level of the NTS (Callera et al. 2000, Chen and Bonham 2005), and rostral and caudal VLM (Guyenet et al. 2004, Dampney et al. 2003), as well as respiratory modulation of cardiovagal neurons of the nucleus ambiguus (Wang et al. 2003) and reflex inhibition of sympathoexcitatory and AVP secreting neurons of the PVN (Giuliano et al. 1989). Glycine is another inhibitory amino acid neurotransmitter that is present particularly in neurons of the medulla and spinal cord and exerts fast inhibition by glycine GlyR1 receptors, which are Cl-channels. Medullary cardiorespiratory neurons may co-express markers for GABA and glycine (Guyenet et al. 2004).

Neuromodulation

Acetylcholine

Acetylcholine is the primary neurotransmitter of the preganglionic sympathetic and parasympathetic neurons, as well as some local neurons of the NTS, VLM, and hypothalamus. These neurons are identified by their immunoreactivity for choline-acetyltransferase. Acetylcholine elicits fast postsynaptic excitation and increases neurotransmitter release via nicotinic receptors and modulates neuronal excitability and neurotransmitter release via different muscarinic receptor subtypes. In general, activation of muscarinic M_1 type receptors increases neuronal excitability, whereas M_2 receptors mediate presynaptic or postsynaptic inhibitory effects. Acetylcholine has been implicated in stimulation of secretion of AVP; activation of sympathoexcitatory neurons in the rostral VLM and intermediolateral cell column (Giuliano et al. 1989); regulation of the baroreflex at the level of the NTS; and inspiratory inhibition of cardiovagal neurons of the nucleus ambiguus (Spyer and Jordan 1987).

Catecholamines

Central catecholaminergic neurons synthesize dopamine, norepinephrine, or epinephrine and are identified by their immunoreactivity for tyrosine hydroxylase (TH) (Saper et al. 1991, Benarroch et al. 1998) (Fig. 3.1). Dopamine-beta-hydroxylase allows transformation of dopamine into norepinephrine, and phenylethanolamine-N-methyltransferase (PNMT) is a marker of epinephrine neurons (Gai et al. 1993). Norepinephrine and epinephrine neurons form two anatomically segregated but functionally integrated systems, the locus coeruleus and the lateral tegmental system. The lateral tegmental system includes neurons of the A5 group in the ventrolateral pons; a ventrolateral (A1/C1) group, close to the ventral medullary surface; and a dorsomedial (A2/C2) group in the region of the NTS (Guyenet 1991, Ruggiero et al. 1989) (Fig. 3.1). The A1, A2, and A5 groups synthesize norepinephrine; whereas the C1 and C2/3 groups synthesize epinephrine. Lateral tegmental catecholaminergic neurons have extensive interconnections with areas involved in autonomic and neuroendocrine control, including preganglionic autonomic neurons, autonomic brainstem nuclei, hypothalamus, and amygdala (Sawchenko et al. 2000, Arango et al. 1988).

The responses to catecholamines are complex and are mediated by three types of receptors:

◆ α_1 receptors, which in general mediate excitatory effects

◆ α_2 receptors, which mediate presynaptic and postsynaptic inhibition

◆ β receptors, which activate adenylyl cyclase.

Catecholamines have been implicated in modulation of SPNs (Guyenet 1991); facilitation of the baroreflex at the level of the NTS, presynaptic inhibition of C1 neurons; and stimulation of AVP and CRH secretion from the hypothalamus (Chen et al. 2004).

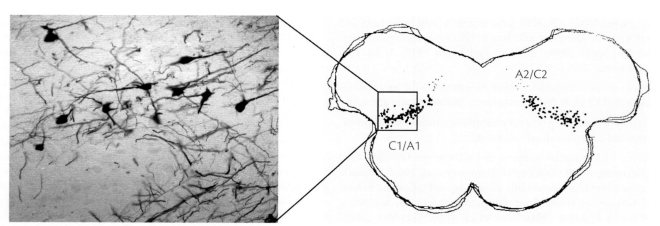

Fig. 3.1 Distribution of catecholaminergic neurons in the human medulla as identified by immunoreactivity to tyrosine hydroxylase.

Serotonin

Serotonin (5-hydroxytryptamine, 5-HT) is synthesized from L-tryptophan by action of tryptophan hydroxylase, which is thus the neurochemical marker of serotonergic neurons (Tork and Hornung 1990) (Fig. 3.1). Serotonergic innervation of central autonomic regions arises primarily from the medullary raphe nuclei, including the nucleus of raphe pallidus and raphe obscurus, as well as serotonergic neurons in the VLM (Fig. 3.1). Centrally administered serotonin elicits complex cardiovascular effects, which are mediated by several types of receptors. In general, 5-HT$_1$-type receptors mediate presynaptic or postsynaptic inhibition and 5-HT$_2$ receptors elicit increase in neuronal excitability; the 5-HT$_3$ receptors are action channels permeable to Ca^{2+} and mediate fast excitatory responses. Serotonin has been implicated in baroreflex modulation at the level of the NTS (Lawrence and Jarrott 1996), control of paraventricular CRH neurons, and both excitatory and inhibitory control of SPNs (Chalmers and Pilowsky 1991).

Neuropeptides

Neuropeptides and their receptors have a widespread but heterogenous distribution in the central autonomic network. The hypothalamus, amygdala, and NTS are among the areas of the brain richest in neuropeptides. Hypothalamic peptidergic neurons projecting to central autonomic areas are concentrated in the PVN and perifornical area of the lateral hypothalamus. These hypothalamic peptidergic systems integrate the control of cardiovascular with other homeostatic functions, including energy metabolism, response to stress, and sleep-wake cycle. The autonomic PVN neurons may utilize AVP, oxytocin, CRF (CRH), somatostatin, enkephalin, dynorphin, or angiotensin II, in addition to L-glutamate as their neurotransmitters (Hallbeck et al. 2001). At least some of these neurochemical transmitters mediate excitatory inputs from the PVN to the rostral VLM (Dampney et al. 2003a) or SPNs (Coote 2005).

A group of neurons of the posterior lateral hypothalamus (perifornical area) synthesize hypocretin (also called orexin) and send extensive projections to the hypothalamus, brain stem, and spinal cord, including nuclei involved in regulation of food intake, arousal, and autonomic function (Berthoud et al. 2005). For example, these neurons send excitatory projections to the PVN that increase sympathetic outflow (Date et al. 1999) and collateral inputs to the NTS and nucleus ambiguus (Ciriello et al. 2003), where they regulate baroreflex responses (Smith et al. 2002). These hypocretin/orexin neurons are inhibited by circulating leptin, a major anorexigenic signal secreted by adipose tissue. In contrast, leptin activates neurons of the hypothalamic arcuate nucleus that synthesize α-melanocyte stimulating hormone (α-MSH) and cocaine and amphetamine regulated transcript (CART) and project to the PVN and other autonomic regions, including the intermediolateral cell column (Elmquist 2001). Projections from these α-MSH neurons to the PVN may not only mediate the anorexigenic but also the central sympathoexcitatory effects of circulating leptin (Zhang and Felder 2004).

Several peptides, including angiotensin II, natriuretic peptides, AVP, endothelin, and cytokines can influence cardiovascular functions by several mechanisms. They may exert directly on cardiovascular target organs activate receptors in the circumventricular organs that project to central autonomic areas, or act as endogenous neurochemical signals released from central autonomic pathways.

A typical example of these multiple actions is that of angiotensin II (McKinley et al. 2003). Circulating angiotensin II elicits peripheral vasomotor, sympathoexcitatory, and aldosterone-releasing effects, and acts via receptors in the SFO to activate sympathoexcitatory and AVP-secreting neurons of the PVN. In addition, angiotensin II containing neurons or fibres are present in several regions involved in cardiovascular control and fluid homeostasis, including the PVN, NTS, VLM, and intermediolateral cell column (McKinley et al. 2003). The cardiovascular effects of angiotensin II are primarily mediated by AT$_1$ receptors, which are highly expressed in these regions (Allen et al. 1991, Benarroch and Schmeichel 1998, Ahmad et al. 2003). Activation of these receptors elicits sympathoexcitation and AVP release, resulting in increase in BP (Dampney et al. 2003a, McKinley et al. 2003). The sympathoexcitatory effects of angiotensin II may involve local production of superoxide (Lindley et al. 2004). Angiotensin II also exerts complex effects on baroreflex and chemoreflexes at the level of the NTS (Paton and Kasparov 1999).

Circulating AVP exerts a potent antidiuretic action via V$_2$ receptors in the renal tubules, and vasoconstrictor effects via vascular V$_1$ receptors. However, circulating AVP does not elicit hypertension because it also activates the baroreflex indirectly, via V$_1$ receptors in the area postrema (Hasser et al. 1997). AVP also present in projections from the PVN to other central autonomic regions, including the rostral VLM and intermediolateral cell column and may act via V1 receptors to mediate some of the central sympathoexcitatory effects of angiotensin II (Yang and Coote 2003). Natriuretic peptides and their receptors overlap in their brain distribution with the angiotensin system. Natriuretic peptides have complex intearctions with the sympathetic system both at peripheral and central levels (Luchner and Schunkert 2004).

Substance P is present in primary visceral afferents, in pathways from the amygdala and NTS, and in bulbospinal pathways from the raphe and VLM. It acts via depolarizing neurokinin 1 (NK-1) receptors and has been implicated in transmission of excitatory information from baroreceptor afferents to the NTS (Helke and Seagard 2004), activation of sympathetic chemoreflex at the level of the rostral VLM (Makeham et al. 2005, Li and Guyenet 1997), and excitatory inputs from the VLM to SPNs (Minson et al. 2002). Opioid peptides have been identified in virtually all central autonomic areas and have predominantly inhibitory action, both presynaptically and postsynaptically. The central cardiovascular effects of opioids are complex and vary with the site of application, receptor, species, and state of consciousness.

Nitric oxide

NO is a highly diffusible messenger that activates cytoplasmic guanylate cyclase and modulates responses to glutamate, GABA, or other transmitters. Brain NO is produced primarily by the constitutively expressed NOS, which is activated Ca^{2+}/calmodulin in response to glutamatergic inputs acting via NMDA receptors. Neurons containing NOS are identified by their reactivity for NADPH-diaphorase and include neurons in the PVN, NTS, and SPNs. Many of the effects of NO involve activation of cytoplasmic guanylate cyclase, leading to the production of cyclic GMP. Nitric oxide exerts complex effects on central circuits controlling cardiovascular function, as it may act both presynaptically, affecting the release of other neurotransmitters, or postsynaptically, affecting the responses of target neurons.

Specific circuits

Sympathetic preganglionic neurons

Functional overview

The SPNs are organized into functionally distinct units controlling the different vascular beds, heart, and adrenal gland. These neurons receive selective innervation from multiple sources and project to target-specific postganglionic neurons. Inputs to SPNs originate from two main sources, segmental visceral and somatic afferents and supraspinal pathways (Fig. 3.2). Several descending pathways, arising primarily from the hypothalamus and lower brainstem and containing a variety of neurotransmitters, exert a differential control on SPNs. The main supraspinal sources are the PVN, the periformical region of the lateral hypothalamus; noradrenergic A5 group; the rostral VLM, including the C1 group; and ventromedial medulla and caudal raphe nuclei (Strack et al. 1989). These pathways and their target SPNs are incorporated into pattern generator modules that differentially affect separate spinal sympathetic outflows (Saper 2002, Morrison 2001, Sved et al. 2001). For example, neurons of the rostral VLM projecting to SPNs

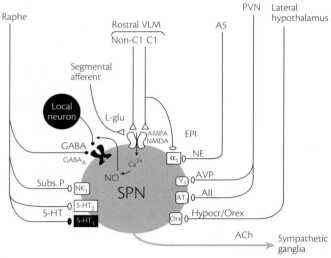

Fig. 3.2 Neurochemical influences on cardiovascular sympathetic preganglionic neurons (SPNs). The SPNs receive segmental inputs from somatic and visceral afferents and local neurons, and descending projections from the paraventricular hypothalamic nucleus (PVN), lateral hypothalamus, A5 group of the pons, rostral ventrolateral medulla (VLM), including the C1 and non-C1 groups, and ventromedial medulla, including the caudal raphe nuclei. Excitatory influences (white) increase sympathetic activity, blood pressure, and heart rate. Inhibitory influences (black) inhibit sympathetic activity. The SPNs are excited by glutamate, provided by segmental afferents and descending projections from C1 and non-C1 neurons of the rostral VLM, via activation of AMPA (alpha-amino-3-hydroxy-5-methyl-4-isoxazole propionic acid) and NMDA (N-methyl-D-aspartate) receptors. Local neurons and descending projections of the raphe release γ-aminobutyric acid (GABA), which inhibits SPNs via GABA$_A$ receptors. The SPNs also receive several modulatory influences. Epinephrine (EPI) and norepinephrine (NE) acting via α_1 receptors, arginine-vasopressin (AVP) acting via V$_1$ receptors, angiotensin II (AII) acting via AT$_1$ receptors, hypocretin/orexin (Hypocr/Orex) acting via Orexin (Orex) receptors; substance P (Subs P) acting via NK$_1$ receptors, increase SPN excitability. Serotonin (5-HT) increases SPN excitability via 5-HT$_2$ receptors and decrease excitability via 5-HT$_1$ receptors. Nitric oxide (NO), release in response to NMDA receptor activation, may act as a local regulatory signal increasing GABAergic transmission.

activating muscle and splanchnic vasoconstriction mediate baroreflex influences on BP. In contrast, neurons in the rostral medullary raphe projecting to SPNs controlling skin vasoconstriction are not affected by the baroreflex but rather activated by the hypothalamus (related to thermoregulation) and amygdala (related to emotion).

Neurochemical influences

The SPNs are activated by segmental and descending glutamatergic inputs. Glutamate arising from both C1 and non-C1 cells of the rostral VLM are critical for tonic and phasic excitation of SPNs, via activation of both NMDA and non-NMDA receptors (Morrison 2003). Glutamate release in the IML may be presynaptically inhibited by A1 receptors (Deuchars et al. 2001). Activation of NMDA receptors leads to the production of NO, which, in turn, may act as a negative feedback signal reducing NMDA-mediated excitatory response, acting as a local feedback signal (Arnolda et al. 2000). Fast inhibition of SPNs is mediated by GABA or glycine, which may be released from projections arising from the rostral ventromedial medulla (Stornetta et al. 2004) or local neurons in the central gray matter (Deuchars et al. 2005).

Monoaminergic and peptidergic inputs from the brain stem and hypothalamus may exert multiple modulatory effects on SPNs. For example, catecholaminergic inputs from the A5 and C1 groups produce both α_1-receptor mediated activation and α_2-receptor mediated inhibition of SPNs (Guyenet 1991). Serotonin, which is present in projections from the medullary raphe, may increase or decrease excitability of SPNs, via 5-HT$_2$ or 5-HT$_1$ receptors, respectively. These projections may also release substance P via NK-1 receptors (Burman et al. 2001).

Two important sources of hypothalamic projection to the SPNs are the PVN and the periformical area. The PVN projection to the intermediolateral cell column is neurochemically complex and may provide glutamate as well as multiple neuropeptides (Hallbeck et al. 2001), including AVP. This neuropeptide may activate SPNs via V1 receptors (Motawei et al. 1999, Kolaj and Renaud 1998). Neurons of the periformical area of the posterior lateral hypothalamus synthesizing hypocretin/orexin project to the intermediolateral cell column and excite SPNs (Berthoud et al. 2005, Llewellyn-Smith et al. 2003, Antunes et al. 2001). Excitability of SPNs is also controlled by local mechanisms, including production of hydrogen peroxide (Lin et al. 2003).

Rostral ventrolateral medulla

Role in vasomotor control

The rostral VLM contains tonically firing glutamatergic neurons and C1 neurons that may utilize glutamate, epinephrine, NPY, substance P, or CART as their neurotransmitters, in various combinations (Ruggiero et al. 1989, Chalmers and Pilowsky 1991). Glutamatergic rostral VLM neurons provide tonic monosynaptic excitation to SPNs and constitute the final common effectors of multiple reflexes and descending influences affecting sympathetic activity and BP. Neurons of the rostral VLM have a major role in maintenance of tonic background excitation of sympathetic vasomotor neurons. Stimulation of the rostral VLM produces increase in BP, HR, sympathetic nerve activity, and circulating adrenomedullary catecholamines. Impaired rostral VLM function in anaesthetized elicits a rapid fall in arterial pressure to levels comparable to those observed acutely after cervical spinal cord transection. Although in the chronic state there is gradual normalization of arterial pressure, some rapid sympathoexcitatory reflexes, such as the chemoreflex-elicited pressor response, are permanently impaired following rostral VLM lesions. The discharge of rostral VLM neurons, like that of the muscle SPNs neurons, is time-locked with the cardiac rhythm due to the influence from the baroreceptors. The tonic activity of glutamatergic vasomotor rostral VLM neurons does not appear to depend on intrinsic pacemaker properties but rather on tonic excitatory drive from one or several of the multiple afferents. These rostral VLM neurons may also act as chemosensors activated by hypoxia and mediate sympathoexcitatory and responses to hypoxia-ischaemia (Makeham et al. 2005, Guyenet 2000).

Neurochemical influences

The activity of the bulbospinal sympathoexcitatory rostral VLM neurons is regulated by many neurochemical influences (Fig. 3.3) (Sun 1996). Their resting activity is determined by the balance of powerful tonic excitatory and inhibitory synaptic inputs (Dampney et al. 2003a). Excitatory inputs are mediated by glutamate acting via AMPA and NMDA receptors and arise from several sources, including peripheral chemoreceptors; somatic receptors; tonically active neurons in the pontine reticular formation and lateral tegmental field of the medulla; and PVN. Activation of NMDA receptors may result in NO production by rostral VLM neurons. The effects of NO in the VLM are complex. Neuronally released NO may elicit sympathoexcitation, perhaps by potentiating glutamatergic mechanisms (Chan et al. 2003), whereas endothelial NO may elicit hypotension and bradycardia, perhaps by facilitating GABA release (Mayorov 2005).

The rostral VLM neurons receive powerful GABAergic inhibition mediated primarily by $GABA_A$ receptors. These inputs arise from neurons of the caudal VLM, including those mediating baroreflex-dependent and baroreflex-independent tonic inhibition of the rostral VLM sympathoexcitatory neurons (Guyenet et al. 2004). These sympathoinhibitory GABAergic caudal VLM neurons are, in turn, the target of inhibition from tonically active GABAergic neurons in the caudal pressor area, which may contribute to maintenance of basal sympathetic activity (Dampney et al. 2003a). NO, which can be synthesized by neurons in the caudal VLM, may participate in baroreflex control of rostral VLM neurons (Kantzides and Badoer 2005).

The sympathoexcitatory rostral VLM neurons are the target of many neuromodulatory influences. Activation of muscarinic,

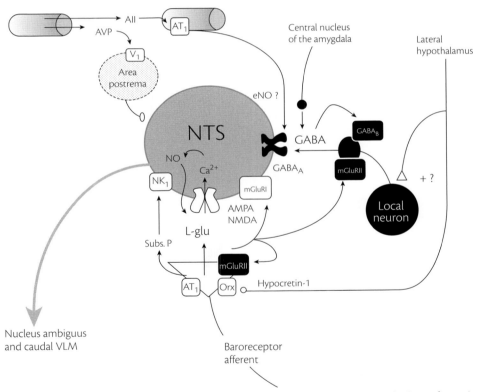

Fig. 3.3 Neurochemical influences on baroreceptive neurons of the nucleus of the solitary tract (NTS). These neurons receive inputs from primary baroreceptor afferents and project to the nucleus ambiguus and caudal ventrolateral medulla (VLM) to initiate cardiovagal excitation and sympathetic inhibition, respectively. Excitatory influences (white) produce a decrease in blood pressure, and heart rate. Inhibitory influences (black) inhibit the baroreflex and elicit hypertension and tachycardia. Primary baroreceptor afferents excite NTS neurons via release of L-glutamate, which acts via AMPA (alpha-amino-3-hydroxy-5-methyl-4-isoxazole propionic acid), NMDA (N-methyl-D-aspartate) and type 1 metabotropic receptors (nGluR1). These effects are potentiated by nitric oxide (NO), produced in response glutamate -triggered increase in intracellular Ca^{2+}, and substance P (subs P), which is co-released by the primary afferent and acts via neurokinin-1 (NK_1) receptors. Glutamate release by primary afferents may be facilitated by angiotensin II (acting via AT_1 receptors) and hypocretin-1, acting via orexin (Orx) receptors, and is inhibited by presynaptic type II metabotropic glutamate receptors (mGluRII). Baroreceptor responses are inhibited by γ-aminobutyric acid (GABA), released from local neurons and projections from the central nucleus of the amygdala and acting via $GABA_A$ receptors. Activation of presynaptic $GABA_B$ and mGluRII receptors inhibit local release of GABA. Circulating arginine vasopressin (AVP) acts via V_1 receptors in the area postrema to activate baroreceptive NTS neurons. In contrast, circulating AII inhibits the baroreflex, perhaps by AT_1 receptor mediated release of endothelial NO, which may potentiate GABAergic mechanisms.

β-adrenergic, vasopressin V_1, angiotensin AT_1, substance P NK-1, endothelin ET_1, or P_{2x} purinoreceptors in this region elicits sympathoexcitation and increase of BP and HR (Sun 1996). However, these influences do not appear to be critical for maintenance of resting sympathetic activity or BP (Dampney et al. 2003a). There has been increased interest in the role of angiotensin II in the rostral VLM, given its potential implications in the pathophysiology of arterial hypertension. Angiotensin II may be in part provided by projections from the PVN, and acts via AT_1 receptors that are highly concentrated in the rostral VLM. Activation of 5-HT_1 serotonergic, atrial natriuretic peptide-, opioid-, a_2-adrenergic-, or imidazoline I_1 receptors in the rostral VLM elicits sympathoinhibition and hypotension (Sun 1996). The C1 neurons appear to be the primary target of both excitation via AT_1 receptors and inhibition via a_2-receptors activated by clonidine. Clonidine also elicits sympathoinhibition via I_1 imidazoline receptors, which may be activated by the endogenous agonist, agmatine (Yang et al. 2005). A residual activity in sympathoexcitatory rostral VLM after blockade of all synaptic influences may reflect residual chemosensitivity to hypoxia, which directly activates O_2-sensitive Ca^{2+} channels or intrinsic 'pacemaker' activity of these neurons (Dampney et al. 2003a).

Nucleus of the solitary tract

Overview of the baroreflex circuit

The organization of the medullary baroreflex circuit has been extensively investigated (Spyer 1994, Dampney 1994). Baroreceptor-stimulated NTS neurons initiate a feedback loop that ultimately results in excitation of cardiovagal neurons and inhibition of sympathoexcitatory neurons in the rostral VLM. A currently accepted model is that sympathoinhibitory information from barosensitive NTS neurons is relayed through GABAergic neurons in the caudal VLM, which in turn inhibit sympathoexcitatory neurons of the rostral VLM; cardiovagal activation may involve direct excitatory projections from the NTS to the nucleus ambiguus (Spyer 1994, Dampney 1994). Barosensitive NTS neurons also give rise to an ascending projection that ultimately leads to local GABAergic inhibition of AVP-secreting magnocellular neurons of the hypothalamus (Dampney 1994, Dampney et al. 2003b, Spyer 1994).

Neurochemical control of NTS neurons

The baroreflex is regulated by severe neurochemical influences acting at the level of the NTS (Fig. 3.4). Baroreceptor afferents release L-glutamate, which activates NTS neurons via inotropic and metabotropic receptors (Lawrence and Jarrott 1996, Talman 1997,

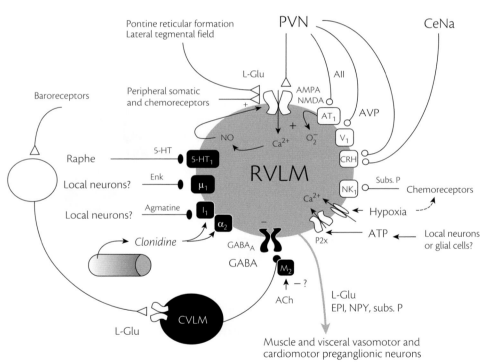

Fig. 3.4 Neurochemical influences on sympathoexcitatory neurons of the rostral ventrolateral medulla (RVLM). These neurons release L-glutamate, epinephrine, neuropeptide Y, and substance P to the intermediolateral cell column. The resting activity of RVLM neurons is determined by the balance of powerful tonic excitatory synaptic inputs mediated by L-glutamate and inhibitory inputs mediated by γ-aminobutyric acid (GABA). Excitatory influences (white) increase sympathetic activity, blood pressure, and heart rate. Inhibitory influences (black) inhibit sympathetic activity and elicit hypotension and bradycardia. Glutamatergic inputs may arise from peripheral chemoreceptors, somatic receptors, pontine reticular formation, lateral tegmental field of the medulla, and paraventricular nucleus (PVN), and act AMPA (alpha-amino-3-hydroxy-5-methyl-4-isoxazole propionic acid), NMDA (N-methyl-D-aspartate) receptors to elicit sympathoexcitation. Activation of NMDA receptors may result in nitric oxide (NO) production which potentiates these effects. GABAergic arise from neurons of the caudal VLM, which mediates baroreflex inhibition of RVLM neurons via $GABA_A$ receptors. These sympathoinhibitory GABAergic caudal VLM neurons are, in turn, the target of inhibition from tonically active GABAergic neurons in the caudal pressor area (CPA). Activation of muscarinic, β-adrenergic, vasopressin V_1, angiotensin AT_1, corticotrophin releasing hormone (CRH), substance P NK-1, endothelin ET_1 or P_{2x} purinoreceptors activates RVLM neurons resulting in sympathoexcitation. In contrast, activation of 5-HT_1 serotonergic, atrial natriuretic peptide-; opioid-, $α_2$-adrenergic- or imidazoline I_1 elicits sympathoinhibition and hypotension. The sympathoinhibitory drug clonidine acts via $α_2$ and I_1 receptors; the I_1 receptors are also the target of the endogenous agonist, agmatine. The RVLM are activated by hypoxia, which directly activates O_2-sensitive Ca^{2+} channels.

Van Giersbergen et al. 1992). Glutamate, acting via presynaptic metabotropic type II autoreceptors, inhibits its own release from baroreceptor afferents. Some barosensitive NTS neurons contain NOS (Chan and Sawchenko 1998) and may synthesize and release NO in response to increased intracellular levels of Ca^{2+} triggered by activation of glutamate receptors. Nitric oxide may thus mediate the effect of NMDA receptor activation in response to baroreflex inputs (Chianca et al. 2004) and facilitates the baroreflex at the level of the NTS (Dias et al. 2005). Primary baroreceptor afferents also release substance P, which, acting via NK_1 receptors, may stimulate barosensitive NTS neurons both directly and by potentiating the excitatory effects of glutamate (Helke and Seagard 2004).

Several neurochemical influences, arising from local neurons or other autonomic regions, may act at the level of the NTS to affect arterial pressure or baroreflex responses (Fig. 3.4) (Lawrence and Jarrott 1996;, Van Giersbergen et al. 1992). The NTS contains local GABAergic neurons that regulate baroreflex function via both pre- and postsynaptic mechanisms (Callera et al. 2000, Chen and Bonham 2005). Many NTS neurons activated during hypertension are GABAergic but do not project directly to the rostral VLM (Chan and Sawchenko 1998). Activation of local $GABA_A$ receptors in the NTS inhibits barosensitive neurons and results in increase of BP and heart rate (Spyer 1994). Glutamate, released from baroreceptive afferents, may activate presynaptic metabotropic type II heteroreceptors and inhibit GABA release from local inhibitory NTS neurons, thus potentiating baroreflex responses (Chen and Bonham 2005). Activation of $GABA_B$ receptors may also elicit presynaptic inhibition of release of GABA from local neurons in the NTS, resulting in depressor effects (Lawrence and Jarrott 1996). The NTS also receives descending GABAergic projections from the CeNA (Saha et al. 2000). These projections, together with descending projections from the lateral hypothalamus activating local GABAergic neurons, may mediate the inhibitory effects of emotion and stress on the gain of the baroreflex (Spyer 1994).

The NTS receives noradrenergic innervation from the A2, A1, and A5 areas (Lawrence and Jarrott 1996). Norepinephrine facilitates baroreflex responses via activation of local α_2-receptors. Neuropeptide Y and galanin coexist with norepinephrine in NTS neurons and afferents and may modulate the baroreflex both directly and via interactions with adrenergic mechanisms (Lawrence and Jarrott 1996). The NTS receives endorphin-containing inputs from the hypothalamus and contains enkephalin-producing neurons. Activation of opioid receptors in the NTS may inhibit baroreflex responses (Lawrence and Jarrott 1996).

Angiotensin II, AVP, natriuretic peptides, and endothelin may modulate baroreflex responses by acting either as circulating signals affecting receptors of the area postrema or as endogenous neurochemical mediators in intrinsic neurons and pathways innervating the NTS. Angiotensin II, acting via AT_1 receptors, can affect NTS neurons both directly and indirectly. There is evidence that angiotensin II inhibits the baroreflex (Matsumura et al. 1998). This may involve activation endothelial NO production and local GABAergic mechanisms. However, angiotensin II may also potentiate release of substance P from baroreceptor afferents (Barnes et al. 2003). Circulating AVP potentiates the baroreflex by acting via V_1 receptors in the area postrema (Hasser et al. 1997), whereas endogenous AVP (presumably released from PVN projections to the NTS) inhibits baroreflex responses (Lawrence and Jarrott 1996). The hypocretin/orexin neurons of the posterior lateral

hypothalamus send direct projections to the NTS, where hypocretin-1 presynaptically increases glutamate release from primary afferents (Smith et al. 2002) and increases sensitivity of NTS neurons to baroreceptor afferent input (de Oliveira et al. 2003).

Paraventricular nucleus

Functional organization

The PVN is a complex effector nucleus that is critical for coordinated autonomic and endocrine responses to stress (Swanson 1991; Benarroch 2005). The PVN consists of several cytoarchitectonically, neurochemically, and functional distinct subnuclei (Koutcherov et al. 2000). It contains:

♦ magnocellular neurons that project to the posterior pituitary and secrete AVP to blood stream

♦ parvicellular CRH neurons that project to the median eminence and activate the corticotrope cells of the anterior pituitary, leading to adrenocortical activation

♦ intermixed populations of neurochemically complex neurons that project to preganglionic sympathetic or parasympathetic neurons as well as the NTS, rostral VLM, and other brainstem regions.

Separate populations of PVN neurons selectively control functionally distinct subpopulations of preganglionic sympathetic or parasympathetic neurons (Saper 2002, Coote 2005). The PVN has been implicated in several aspects of cardiovascular control, including sympathoexcitatory responses to stress (Coote 2005, Badoer 2001). Stimulation of the PVN leads to an increase in blood pressure, heart rate, and renal sympathetic nerve activity. These effects involve direct PVN projections to cardiac, vasomotor, and renal SPNs, as well as inputs to premotor sympathetic neurons of the rostral VLM (Coote 2005). The excitatory input from the PVN to the rostral VLM may be mediated by glutamate, AVP (acting via V^1 receptors), or AII (via AT^1 receptors) (Dampney et al. 2003a).

Neurochemical influences on the paraventricular nucleus

The PVN receives and integrates four main types of inputs: interoceptive, humoral, limbic, and intra hypothalamic, and its neurochemical regulation are very complex (Fig. 3.5). Inputs from visceral receptors, nociceptors, and thermoreceptors are carried both by spinal afferents that synapse in the dorsal horn (particularly lamina I) and vagal afferents that terminate in the NTS and reach all subdivisions of the PVN via direct projections from the dorsal horn or NTS or via a relay in the parabrachial nucleus, the catecholaminergic cells of the A1/C1 groups of the VLM, or both (spinohypothalamic pathway) or NTS, or via a relay in the parabrachial nucleus, the A1/C1 groups, or both. The vagal afferents may also be activated by circulating cytokines. Circulating angiotensin II acts via AT_1 receptors of the SFO, which contains angiotensinergic neurons that project to the PVN (McKinley et al. 2003). Circulating cytokines may also act via the circumventricular organs or activate vagal afferents that terminate in the NTS and trigger signals conveyed to the PVN via the catecholaminergic neurons of the VLM (Sawchenko et al. 2000). The orbitomedial prefrontal cortex and amygdala, activated by external stressors, provide signals that are relayed to the PVN via the bed nucleus of the stria terminalis and the dorsomedial nucleus of the hypothalamus (Sawchenko et al. 2000).

The synaptic control of PVN neurons is complex. They receive excitatory inputs mediated by glutamate acting via NMDA and AMPA receptors and inhibitory inputs mediated by GABA acting

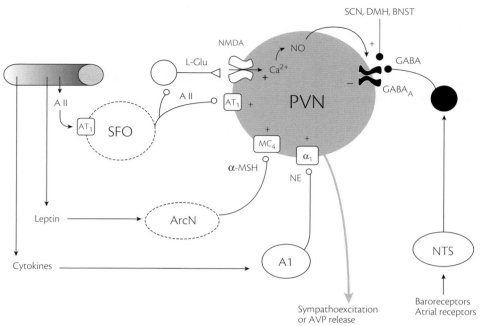

Fig. 3.5 Humoral and neural control of sympathoexcitatory or magnocellular vasopressin (arginine-vasopressin [AVP] neurons of the paraventricular nucleus (PVN). Excitatory influences (white) increase AVP release, sympathetic activity, or both. Inhibitory influence (black) may decrease AVP release, sympathetic output to the heart and kidneys, or both. PVN neurons are activated by glutamate, acting via N-methyl-D-aspartate (NMDA) receptors and inhibited by γ-aminobutyric acid (GABA), acting via GABA$_A$ receptors. Circulating angiotensin II (A II) acts via AT$_1$ receptors to activate neurons in the subfornical organ (SFO). The SFO sends excitatory AII projections and acts via local glutamatergic neurons that activate the PVN neurons. Activation of NMDA receptors leads to production of nitric oxide (NO), which potentiates the inhibitory effects of GABA. GABA mediates the inhibitory effects of baroreceptors and atrial receptors on sympathoexcitatory and AVP secreting PVN neurons. GABA also mediated inhibitory limbic influences mediated by the bed nucleus of the stria terminalis (BNST) and dorsomedial hypothalamus (DMH), as well as circadian influences from the suprachiasmatic nucleus (SCN). Norepinephrine (NE), released from A1 neurons of the caudal ventrolateral medulla activates PVN neurons via α$_1$ receptors and mediates the stimulating effects of endogenous stressors on these cells. Leptin acts via neurons of the arcuate nucleus (ArcN) that synthesize α-melanocyte stimulating hormone (α-MSH) and project to the PVN. These projections contribute to the sympathoexcitatory effects of leptin.

primarily via GABA$_A$ receptors. Activation of NMDA receptors lead to an increase in NO production in the PVN. NO inhibits PVN neurons, in part by potentiating the effects of GABA (Yang and Coote 2003, Li et al. 2004). Sources of GABAergic inputs to the PVN include those from local neurons relaying inhibitory influences from baroreceptors and atrial receptors on magnocellular AVP neurons (Jhamandas and Renaud 1987) or renal sympathoexcitatory neurons (Yang and Coote 2003) and inputs from the bed nucleus of the stria terminalis, which relay inhibitory limbic forebrain influences on responses to external stressors (Sawchenko et al. 2000).

The catecholaminergic inputs from the A1/C1 groups are critical for activation of the AVP secreting and sympathoexcitatory PVN neurons in response to internal stressors such as cytokines (Sawchenko et al. 2000). Norepinephrine, acting via presynaptic α$_1$-receptors, activates glutamatergic inputs to magnocellular AVP neurons (Boudaba et al. 2003); and via presynaptic α$_2$-receptors reduces release of GABA from inhibitory synapses on sympathoexcitatory PVN neurons (Li et al. 2005). Circulating AII, acting via AT$_1$ receptors, activates neurons of the SFO that send excitatory inputs to the magnocellular AVP neurons (McKinley et al. 2003), and renal sympathoexcitatory neurons (Jezova et al. 1998). The excitatory SFO input to the PVN is also mediated by AII, which acts both directly via AT$_1$ receptors on PVN neurons (Cato and Toney 2005) and indirectly via release of glutamate from local interneurons (Latchford and Ferguson 2004).

The PVN, together with the arcuate nucleus and the lateral hypothalamus, forms a network that mediates the effects of circulating leptin on food intake and sympathetic activity. The PVN receives inputs from α-MSH neurons in the lateral arcuate nucleus, which is activated by leptin and mediate its anorexigenic effect, and from NPY neurons of the medial arcuate nucleus and hypocretin/orexin neurons of the posterior lateral hypothalamus, both of which are inhibited by leptin (Elmquist 2001). Whereas α-MSH inputs activate sympathoexcitatory PVN neurons, NPY inputs inhibit them (Zhang and Felder 2004). Thus, the PVN may be a critical mediator of the sympathoexcitatory responses to circulating leptin.

Clinical correlations

Tetraplegia

Interruption of supraspinal inputs to SPNs produces severe abnormalities in control of sympathetic function in tetraplegic patients. Interruption of the tonic glutamatergic inputs from the rostral VLM may explain the low levels of supine BP, circulating catecholamines, and sympathetic nerve activity; and the profound orthostatic hypotension in response to tilt with no compensatory increase in sympathetic activity. Interruption of descending monoaminergic and peptidergic modulatory influences accounts for the unpatterned, generalized sympathetic activation triggered by somatic or visceral stimuli below the lesion in chronic tetraplegics (autonomic dysreflexia) and is characterized by acute hypertension, vasomotor changes, and bradycardia, together with other manifestations of autonomic hyperactivity. Patients with chronic tetraplegia have intact supraspinal reflex circuits controlling cardiovagal outflow and AVP release. They have a marked increase in AVP secretion in response to hypotension induced by tilt and have exaggerated pressor responses to circulating AVP (Puritz et al. 1983).

Multiple system atrophy and Lewy body disorders

Multiple system atrophy (MSA) and Lewy body disorders (LBD) including Parkinson's disease and dementia with Lewy bodies are neurodegenerative disorders that may manifest with prominent cardiovascular, gastrointestinal, urological, respiratory, and sleep disturbances. There is evidence that autonomic failure in MSA is primarily due to central mechanisms, whereas in LBD there is also involvement of autonomic ganglia. In MSA, there is a consistently severe depletion of catecholaminergic neurons in the rostral and caudal VLM (Benarroch et al. 1998) whereas these neurons are much less involved in LBD, despite the presence of Lewy bodies in this region and severe orthostatic hypotension (Benarroch et al. 2005). Loss of C1 neurons may deprive SPNs from their tonic excitatory input, thus explaining orthostatic hypotension, and may prevent baroreflex mediated sympathoinhibition, thus explained supine hypertension in patients with MSA. Loss of A1 neurons may explain the lack of reflex activation of AVP release in response to orthostatic hypotension, despite preserved AVP release in response to osmotic stimuli in these patients (Puritz et al. 1983). There is also loss of medullary serotonergic neurons in patients with MSA, which is much more severe than that seen in LBD (Benarroch et al. 2005). This may contribute to impaired thermoregulatory responses in patients with MSA.

Congestive heart failure

Abnormal neurochemical control of the PVN may have a critical role in the increased sympathetic output to the heart, blood vessels, and kidneys that occurs in congestive heart failure (Felder et al. 2003). This condition is characterized by impaired baroreceptor and atrial receptor triggered inhibition of renal sympathoexcitatory output and AVP-releasing PVN neurons, which may be due to impaired GABAergic and NO-mediated inhibition of these cells (Li and Patel 2003). Circulating angiotensin II, which is elevated in congestive heart failure, activates SFO neurons that send angiotensinergic inputs to the PVN. Angiotensin II, acting via AT1 receptors, excites PVN neurons, including a magnocellular AVP-secreting neurons and neurons that activate sympathoexcitatory outputs to the kidney (Coote 2005). Circulating angiotensin II also triggers secretion of aldosterone which, acting via mineralocorticoid receptors in the PVN, contributes to increased sympathetic activity (Weber et al. 2003). Thus, the PVN has a pivotal role in the feedforward relationship between the renin-angiotensin-aldosterone axis and the sympathetic output to the kidney.

Hypertension and metabolic syndrome

Activation of the PVN during stress may trigger endocrine and autonomic responses that give rise to the metabolic syndrome; consisting of hypertension, obesity, dyslipidaemia, insulin resistance, and glucose intolerance or type 2 diabetes mellitus (Hjemdahl 2002). Stress elicits significant sympathetically mediated cardiovascular changes leading to hypertension, one of the cardinal features of the metabolic syndrome. The role of the PVN in stress-induced hypertension has been demonstrated in several experimental models, including the spontaneously hypertensive rat (SHR). Angiotensin II, acting via AT_1 receptors in the SFO, is critical for activation of the sympathoadrenal response to acute stress. These responses are exaggerated in the SHR, involve the SFO, and are mediated by neurons of the PVN that send excitatory (possibly angiotensinergic) projections to sympathoexcitatory neurons of the rostral VLM (Ku and Li 2003). Activation of AT_1 receptors at the level of the rostral VLM is required for maintenance of increased sympathetic activity and hypertension in the setting of genetic or salt-induced hypertension (Ito et el. 2002). This sympathoexcitatory effect of AT_1 receptor activation in the rostral VLM may also involve local production of superoxide ion (Mayorov et al. 2004). Superoxide may interfere with NO-mediated inhibitory signals at the level of the rostral VLM leading to hypertension (Tai et al. 2005).

There are complex relationships between obesity, leptin resistance, and hypertension (Mark et al. 2002). Most cases of human obesity appear to be associated with leptin-induced increased sympathetic activity despite loss of the metabolic effects of leptin. Leptin may increase sympathetic activity by its actions at the level of the hypothalamus. These effects are indirect and may be mediated by leptin-responsive neurons projecting to the PVN (Zhang and Felder 2004). Leptin-activated α-MSH neurons of the medial portion of the arcuate nucleus activate sympathoexcitatory neurons of the PVN, whereas leptin-inhibited NPY neurons of the medial arcuate nucleus inhibit these sympathoexcitatory PVN neurons.

Summary

There is a complex central neurochemical control of cardiovascular function. It is exerted by several neurochemical transmitters, including L-glutamate, GABA, acetylcholine, catecholamines, 5-HT, a variety of neuropeptides, including angiotensin II, AVP, and hypocretin; and local signals such as NO and superoxide. These influences interact at pivotal central areas controlling sympathetic activity, including the intermediolateral cell column, VLM, NTS, and PVN, regulating tonic, reflex, and adaptive control of BP and heart rate. Disorders in these neurochemical mechanisms underlie abnormalities in cardiovascular regulation, including from those observed in acute nervous system injuries, neurodegenerative disorders, and primary cardiovascular disorders such as congestive heart failure and arterial hypertension. The increasing understanding of these mechanisms will likely provide further therapeutic targets for management of these conditions.

Acknowledgements

This study was supported by a grant from the National Institutes of Health (NS32352-P2) and Mayo Funds.

References

Ahmad, Z., Milligan, C. J., Paton, J.F., Deuchars, J. (2003). Angiotensin type 1 receptor immunoreactivity in the thoracic spinal cord. *Brain Research* **985**, 21–31.

Allen, A. M., Chai, S. Y., Clevers, J., McKinley, M. J., Paxinos, G., Mendelsohn, F. A. (1988). Localization and characterization of angiotensin II receptor binding and angiotensin converting enzyme in the human medulla oblongata. *J Compar. Neurol.* **269**, 249–64.

Allen, A. M., Paxinos, G., McKinley, M. J., Chai, S. Y., Mendelsohn, F. A. (1991). Localization and characterization of angiotensin II receptor binding sites in the human basal ganglia, thalamus, midbrain pons, and cerebellum. *J Compar. Neurol.* **312**, 291–8.

Antunes, V. R., Brailoiu, G. C., Kwok, E. H., Scruggs, P., Dun, N. J. (2001). Orexins/hypocretins excite rat sympathetic preganglionic neurons in vivo and in vitro. *Am. J Physiol. Regul. Integr. Comp. Physiol.* **281**, R1801–7.

Arango, V., Ruggiero, D. A., Callaway, J. L., Anwar, M., Mann, J. J., Reis, D. J. (1988). Catecholaminergic neurons in the ventrolateral medulla and nucleus of the solitary tract in the human. *J Compar. Neurol.* **273**, 224–40.

Arnolda, L. F., McKitrick, D. J., Llewellyn-Smith, I. J., Minson, J. B. (2000). Nitric oxide limits pressor responses to sympathetic activation in rat spinal cord. *Hypertension* **36**, 1089–92.

Badoer, E. (2001). Hypothalamic paraventricular nucleus and cardiovascular regulation. *Clin. Exp. Pharmacol. Physiol.* **28**, 95–9.

Barnes, K. L., DeWeese, D. M., Andresen, M. C. (2003). Angiotensin potentiates excitatory sensory synaptic transmission to medial solitary tract nucleus neurons. *Am. J Physiol. Regul. Integr. Comp. Physiol.* **284**, R1340–53.

Benarroch, E. E. (2005). Paraventricular nucleus, stress response, and cardiovascular disease. *Clin. Auton. Res.* in press.

Benarroch, E. E., Schmeichel, A. M. (1998). Immunohistochemical localization of the angiotensin II type 1 receptor in human hypothalamus and brainstem. *Brain Research* **812**, 292–6.

Benarroch, E. E., Schmeichel, A. M., Low, P. A., Boeve, B. F., Sandroni, P., Parisi, J. E. (2005). Involvement of medullary regions controlling sympathetic output in Lewy body disease. *Brain* **128**, 338–44.

Benarroch, E. E., Smithson, I. L., Low, P. A., Parisi, J. E. (1998). Depletion of catecholaminergic neurons of the rostral ventrolateral medulla in multiple systems atrophy with autonomic failure. *Ann. Neurol.* **43**, 156–63.

Berthoud, H. R., Patterson, L. M., Sutton, G. M., Morrison, C., Zheng, H. (2005). Orexin inputs to caudal raphe neurons involved in thermal, cardiovascular, and gastrointestinal regulation. *Histochem. Cell Biol.* **123**, 147–56.

Boudaba, C., Di, S., Tasker, J. G. (2003). Presynaptic noradrenergic regulation of glutamate inputs to hypothalamic magnocellular neurones. *J Neuroendocrinol.* 15, 803–10.

Burman, K. J., McKitrick, D. J., Minson, J. B., West, A., Arnolda, L. F., Llewellyn-Smith, I. J. (2001). Neurokinin-1 receptor immunoreactivity in hypotension sensitive sympathetic preganglionic neurons. *Brain Research* 915, 238–43.

Callera, J. C., Bonagamba, L. G., Nosjean, A., Laguzzi, R., Machado, B. H. (2000). Activation of GABA receptors in the NTS of awake rats reduces the gain of baroreflex bradycardia. *Auton. Neurosci.* **84**, 58–67.

Cato, M. J., Toney, G. M. (2005). Angiotensin II excites paraventricular nucleus neurons that innervate the rostral ventrolateral medulla: an in vitro patch-clamp study in brain slices. *J Neurophysiol.* **93**, 403–13.

Chalmers, J., Pilowsky, P. (1991). Brainstem and bulbospinal neurotransmitter systems in the control of blood pressure. *J Hypertens.* **9**, 675–94.

Chan, R. K., Sawchenko, P. E. (1998). Organization and transmitter specificity of medullary neurons activated by sustained hypertension: implications for understanding baroreceptor reflex circuitry. *J Neurosci.* **18**, 371–87.

Chan, S. H., Wang, L. L., Chan, J. Y. (2003). Differential engagements of glutamate and GABA receptors in cardiovascular actions of endogenous nNOS or iNOS at rostral ventrolateral medulla of rats. *Br. J Pharmacol.* **138**, 584–93.

Chen, C. Y., Bonham, A. C. (2005). Glutamate suppresses GABA release via presynaptic metabotropic glutamate receptors at baroreceptor neurones in rats. *J Physiol.* **562**, 535–51.

Chen, X. Q., Du, J. Z., Wang, Y. S. (2004). Regulation of hypoxia-induced release of corticotropin-releasing factor in the rat hypothalamus by norepinephrine. *Regul. Pept.* **119**, 221–8.

Chianca, D. A., Jr., Lin, L. H., Dragon, D. N., Talman, W. T. (2004). NMDA receptors in nucleus tractus solitarii are linked to soluble guanylate cyclase. *Am. J Physiol. Heart. Circ. Physiol.* **286**, H1521–7.

Ciriello, J., McMurray, J. C., Babic, T., de Oliveira, C. V. (2003). Collateral axonal projections from hypothalamic hypocretin neurons to cardiovascular sites in nucleus ambiguus and nucleus tractus solitarius. *Brain Research* **991**, 133–41.

Coote, J. H. (2005). A role for the paraventricular nucleus of the hypothalamus in the autonomic control of heart and kidney. *Exp. Physiol.* **90**, 169–73.

Critchley, H. D., Mathias, C. J., Josephs, O., *et al.* (2003). Human cingulate cortex and autonomic control: converging neuroimaging and clinical evidence. *Brain* **126**, 2139–52.

Dampney, R. A. (1994). Functional organization of central pathways regulating the cardiovascular system. *Physiological Reviews* **74**, 323–64.

Dampney, R. A., Horiuchi, J., Tagawa, T., Fontes, M. A., Potts, P.D., Polson, J. W. (2003a). Medullary and supramedullary mechanisms regulating sympathetic vasomotor tone. *Acta Physiologica Scandinavica* **177**, 209–18.

Dampney, R. A., Polson, J. W., Potts, P. D., Hirooka, Y., Horiuchi, J. (2003b). Functional organization of brain pathways subserving the baroreceptor reflex: studies in conscious animals using immediate early gene expression. *Cell. Mol. Neurobiol.* **23**, 597–616.

Date, Y., Ueta, Y., Yamashita, H., *et al.* (1999). Orexins, orexigenic hypothalamic peptides, interact with autonomic, neuroendocrine and neuroregulatory systems. *Proc. Natl. Acad. Sci. U S A* **96**, 748–53.

de Oliveira, C. V., Rosas-Arellano, M. P., Solano-Flores, L. P., Ciriello J. (2003). Cardiovascular effects of hypocretin-1 in nucleus of the solitary tract. *Am. J Physiol. Heart. Circ. Physiol.* **284**, H1369–77.

Deuchars, S. A., Brooke, R. E., Deuchars, J. (2001). Adenosine A1 receptors reduce release from excitatory but not inhibitory synaptic inputs onto lateral horn neurons. *J Neurosci.* **21**, 6308–20.

Deuchars, S. A., Milligan, C. J., Stornetta, R. L., Deuchars J. (2005). GABAergic neurons in the central region of the spinal cord: a novel substrate for sympathetic inhibition. *J Neurosci.* **25**, 1063–70.

Dias, A. C., Vitela, M., Colombari, E., Mifflin, S. W. (2005). Nitric oxide modulation of glutamatergic, baroreflex, and cardiopulmonary transmission in the nucleus of the solitary tract. *Am. J Physiol. Heart. Circ. Physiol.* **288**, H256–62.

Elmquist, J. K. (2001). Hypothalamic pathways underlying the endocrine, autonomic, and behavioral effects of leptin. *Int. J Obes. Relat. Metab. Disord.* **25** Suppl 5, S78–82.

Felder, R. B., Francis, J., Zhang, Z. H., Wei, S. G., Weiss, R. M., Johnson, A. K. (2003). Heart failure and the brain: new perspectives. *Am. J Physiol. Regul. Integr. Comp. Physiol.* **284**, 259–76.

Gai, W. P., Geffen, L. B., Denoroy, L., Blessing, W. W. (1993). Loss of C1 and C3 epinephrine-synthesizing neurons in the medulla oblongata in Parkinson's disease. *Ann. Neurol.* **33**, 357–67.

Giuliano, R., Ruggiero, D. A., Morrison, S., Ernsberger, P., Reis, D. J. (1989). Cholinergic regulation of arterial pressure by the C1 area of the rostral ventrolateral medulla. *J Neurosci.* **9**, 923–42.

Guyenet, P. G. (1991). Central noradrenergic neurons: the autonomic connection. *Prog. Brain. Res.* **88**, 365–80.

Guyenet, P. G. (2000). Neural structures that mediate sympathoexcitation during hypoxia. *Resp. Physiol.* **121**, 147–62.

Guyenet, P. G., Stornetta, R. L., Weston, M. C., McQuiston, T., Simmons, J. R. (2004). Detection of amino acid and peptide transmitters in physiologically identified brainstem cardiorespiratory neurons. *Auton. Neurosci.* **114**, 1–10.

Hallbeck, M., Larhammar, D., Blomqvist, A. (2001). Neuropeptide expression in rat paraventricular hypothalamic neurons that project to the spinal cord. *J Comp. Neurol.* **433**, 222–38.

Hasser, E. M., Bishop, V. S., Hay, M. (1997). Interactions between vasopressin and baroreflex control of the sympathetic nervous system. *Clin. Exp. Pharmacol. Physiol.* **24**, 102–8.

Helke, C. J., Seagard, J. L. (2004). Substance P. in the baroreceptor reflex: 25 years. *Peptides* **25**, 413–23.

Henderson, L. A., Macey, P. M., Macey, K. E., *et al.* (2002). Brain responses associated with the Valsalva maneuver revealed by functional magnetic resonance imaging. *J Neurophysiol.* **88**, 3477–86.

Hjemdahl, P. (2002). Stress and the metabolic syndrome: an interesting but enigmatic association. *Circulation* **106**, 2634–6.

Ito, S., Komatsu, K., Tsukamoto, K., Kanmatsuse, K., Sved, A. F. (2002). Ventrolateral medulla AT1 receptors support blood pressure in hypertensive rats. *Hypertension* **40**, 552–9.

Jezova, D., Ochedalski, T., Kiss, A., Aguilera, G. (1998). Brain angiotensin II modulates sympathoadrenal and hypothalamic pituitary adrenocortical activation during stress. *J Neuroendocrinol.* **10**, 67–72.

Jhamandas, J. H., Renaud, L. P. (1987). Neurophysiology of a central baroreceptor pathway projecting to hypothalamic vasopressin neurons. *Can. J Neurol. Sci.* **14**, 17–24.

Kantzides, A., Badoer, E. (2005). nNOS-containing neurons in the hypothalamus and medulla project to the RVLM. *Brain Res.* **1037**, 25–34.

Kolaj, M., Renaud, L. P. (1998). Vasopressin-induced currents in rat neonatal spinal lateral horn neurons are G-protein mediated and involve two conductances. *J Neurophysiol.* **80**, 1900–10.

Koutcherov, Y., Mai, J. K., Ashwell, K. W., Paxinos, G. (2000). Organization of the human paraventricular hypothalamic nucleus. *J Comp. Neurol.* **423**, 299–318.

Ku, Y. H., Li, Y. H. (2003). Subfornical organ-angiotensin II pressor system takes part in pressor response of emotional circuit. *Peptides* **24**, 1063–7.

Latchford, K. J., Ferguson, A. V. (2004). ANG II-induced excitation of paraventricular nucleus magnocellular neurons: a role for glutamate interneurons. *Am. J Physiol. Regul. Integr. Comp. Physiol.* **286**, R894–902.

Lawrence, A. J., Jarrott, B. (1996). Neurochemical modulation of cardiovascular control in the nucleus tractus solitarius. *Prog. Neurobiol.* **48**, 21–53.

LeDoux, J. (1996). Emotional networks and motor control: a fearful view. *Prog. Brain. Res.* **107**, 437–46.

Li, D. P., Atnip, L. M., Chen, S. R., Pan, H. L. (2005). Regulation of synaptic inputs to paraventricular-spinal output neurons by alpha2 adrenergic receptors. *J Neurophysiol.* **93**, 393–402.

Li, D. P., Chen, S. R., Finnegan, T. F., Pan, H. L. (2004). Signalling pathway of nitric oxide in synaptic GABA release in the rat paraventricular nucleus. *J Physiol.* **554**, 100–10.

Li, Y. F., Patel, K. P. (2003). Paraventricular nucleus of the hypothalamus and elevated sympathetic activity in heart failure: the altered inhibitory mechanisms. *Acta. Physiol. Scand.* **177**, 17–26.

Li, Y. W., Guyenet, P. G. (1997). Effect of substance P. on C1 and other bulbospinal cells of the RVLM in neonatal rats. *Am. J Physiol.* **273**, R805–13.

Lin, H. H., Chen, C. H., Hsieh, W. K., Chiu, T. H., Lai, C. C. (2003). Hydrogen peroxide increases the activity of rat sympathetic preganglionic neurons in vivo and in vitro. *Neuroscience* **121**, 641–7.

Lindley, T. E., Doobay, M. F., Sharma, R. V., Davisson, R. L. (2004). Superoxide is involved in the central nervous system activation and sympathoexcitation of myocardial infarction-induced heart failure. *Circulation Res.* **94**, 402–9.

Llewellyn-Smith, I. J., Martin, C. L., Marcus, J. N., Yanagisawa, M., Minson, J. B., Scammell, T. E. (2003). Orexin-immunoreactive inputs to rat sympathetic preganglionic neurons. *Neuroscience Letters* **351**, 115–9.

Loewy, A. D. (1991). Forebrain nuclei involved in autonomic control. *Prog. Brain Res.* **87**, 253–68.

Loewy, A. D., Spyer, K.M. (1990). *Central Regulation of Autonomic Functions*. Oxford: Oxford University Press.

Lovick, T. A. (1993). Integrated activity of cardiovascular and pain regulatory systems: role in adaptive behavioural responses. *Prog. Neurobiol.* **40**, 631–44.

Luchner, A., Schunkert, H. (2004). Interactions between the sympathetic nervous system and the cardiac natriuretic peptide system. *Cardiovasc. Res.* **63**, 443–9.

Makeham, J. M., Goodchild, A. K., Pilowsky, P. M. (2005). Nk1 receptor activation in rat ventrolateral medulla selectively attenuates somatosympathetic reflex while antagonism attenuates sympathetic chemoreflex. *Am. J Physiol. Regul. Integr. Comp. Physiol.* in press.

Mark, A. L., Correia, M. L., Rahmouni, K., Haynes, W. G. (2002). Selective leptin resistance: a new concept in leptin physiology with cardiovascular implications. *J Hypertension* **20**, 1245–50.

Matsumura, K., Averill, D. B., Ferrario, C. M. (1998). Angiotensin II acts at AT1 receptors in the nucleus of the solitary tract to attenuate the baroreceptor reflex. *Am. J Physiol.* **275**, R1611–9.

Mayorov, D. N. (2005). Selective sensitization by nitric oxide of sympathetic baroreflex in rostral ventrolateral medulla of conscious rabbits. *Hypertension* **45**, 901–6.

Mayorov, D. N., Head, G. A., De Matteo, R. (2004). Tempol attenuates excitatory actions of angiotensin II in the rostral ventrolateral medulla during emotional stress. *Hypertension* **44**, 101–6.

McKinley, M. J., Albiston, A. L., Allen, A.M., *et al.* (2003). The brain renin-angiotensin system: location and physiological roles. *Int. J Biochem. Cell. Biol.* **35**, 901–18.

McKinley, M. J., Allen, A. M., Mathai, M. L., *et al.* (2001). Brain angiotensin and body fluid homeostasis. *Jpn. J Physiol.* **51**, 281–9.

Minson, J. B., Arnolda, L. F., Llewellyn-Smith, I. J. (2002). Neurochemistry of nerve fibers apposing sympathetic preganglionic neurons activated by sustained hypotension. *J Compar. Neurol.* **449**, 307–18.

Morrison, S. F. (2001). Differential control of sympathetic outflow. *Am. J Physiol. Regul. Integr. Comp. Physiol.* **281**, 683–98.

Morrison, S. F. (2003). Glutamate transmission in the rostral ventrolateral medullary sympathetic premotor pathway. *Cell. Mol. Neurobiol.* **23**, 761–72.

Motawei, K., Pyner, S., Ranson, R. N., Kamel, M., Coote, J. H. (1999). Terminals of paraventricular spinal neurones are closely associated with adrenal medullary sympathetic preganglionic neurones: immunocytochemical evidence for vasopressin as a possible neurotransmitter in this pathway. *Exp. Brain. Res.* **126**, 68–76.

Paton, J. F., Kasparov, S. (1999). Differential effects of angiotensin II on cardiorespiratory reflexes mediated by nucleus tractus solitarii—a microinjection study in the rat. *J Physiol.* **521** Pt 1, 213–25.

Puritz, R., Lightman, S. L., Wilcox, C. S., Forsling, M., Bannister, R. (1983). Blood pressure and vasopressin in progressive autonomic failure. Response to postural stimulation, L-dopa and naloxone. *Brain* **106**, 503–11.

Ruggiero, D. A., Cravo, S. L., Arango, V., Reis, D. J. (1989). Central control of the circulation by the rostral ventrolateral reticular nucleus: anatomical substrates. *Prog. Brain. Res.* **81**, 49–79.

Saha, S., Batten, T. F., Henderson, Z. (2000). A GABAergic projection from the central nucleus of the amygdala to the nucleus of the solitary tract: a combined anterograde tracing and electron microscopic immunohistochemical study. *Neuroscience* **99**, 613–26.

Saper, C. B. (2002). The central autonomic nervous system: conscious visceral perception and autonomic pattern generation. *Ann. Rev. Neurosci.* **25**, 433–69.

Saper, C. B., Sorrentino, D. M., German, D. C., de Lacalle, S. (1991). Medullary catecholaminergic neurons in the normal human brain and in Parkinson's disease. *Ann. Neurol.* **29**, 577–84.

Sawchenko, P. E., Li, H. Y., Ericsson, A. (2000). Circuits and mechanisms governing hypothalamic responses to stress: a tale of two paradigms. *Prog. Brain. Res.* **122**, 61–78.

Smith, B. N., Davis, S. F., Van Den Pol, A. N., Xu, W. (2002). Selective enhancement of excitatory synaptic activity in the rat nucleus tractus solitarius by hypocretin 2. *Neuroscience* **115**, 707–14.

Spyer, K. M. (1994). Annual Review Prize Lecture: Central nervous mechanisms contributing to cardiovascular control. *J Physiol.* **474**, 1–19.

Spyer, K. M., Jordan, D. (1987). Electrophysiology of the nucleus ambiguus. In: Hainsworth, R., McWilliam, P. N., Mary, D. A. S. G., eds. *Cardiogenic Reflexes*, pp. 237–349. Oxford University Press, Oxford.

Stornetta, R. L., McQuiston, T. J., Guyenet, P. G. (2004). GABAergic and glycinergic presympathetic neurons of rat medulla oblongata identified by retrograde transport of pseudorabies virus and in situ hybridization. *J Compar. Neurol.* **479**, 257–70.

Strack, A. M., Sawyer, W. B., Hughes, J. H., Platt, K. B., Loewy, A. D. (1989). A general pattern of CNS innervation of the sympathetic outflow demonstrated by transneuronal pseudorabies viral infections. *Brain Res.* **491**, 156–62.

Sun, M. (1996). Pharmacology of reticulospinal vasomotor neurons in cardiovascular regulation. *Pharmacol. Rev.* **48**, 465–94.

Sved, A. F., Cano, G., Card, J. P. (2001). Neuroanatomical specificity of the circuits controlling sympathetic outflow to different targets. *Clin. Exp. Pharmacol. Physiol.* **28**, 115–9.

Swanson, L. W. (1991). Biochemical switching in hypothalamic circuits mediating responses to stress. *Prog. Brain. Res.* **87**, 181–200.

Tai, M. H., Wang, L. L., Wu, K. L., Chan, J. Y. (2005). Increased superoxide anion in rostral ventrolateral medulla contributes to hypertension in spontaneously hypertensive rats via interactions with nitric oxide. *Free Radic. Biol. Med.* **38**, 450–62.

Talman, W. T. (1997). Glutamatergic transmission in the nucleus tractus solitarii: from server to peripherals in the cardiovascular information superhighway. *Braz. J Med. Biol. Res.* **30**, 1–7.

Tork, I., Hornung, J. P. (1990). Raphe nuclei and the serotonergic system. In: Paxinos G, ed. *The Human Nervous System*, pp. 1001–22. Academic Press, New York.

Van Giersbergen, P. L., Palkovits, M., de Jong, W. (1992). Involvement of neurotransmitters in the nucleus tractus solitarii in cardiovascular regulation. *Physiol. Rev.* **72**, 789–824.

Wang, J., Irnaten, M., Neff, R. A., *et al.* (2001). Synaptic and neurotransmitter activation of cardiac vagal neurons in the nucleus ambiguus. *Ann. N Y Acad. Sci.* **940**, 237–46.

Wang, J., Wang, X., Irnaten, M., *et al.* (2003). Endogenous acetylcholine and nicotine activation enhances GABAergic and glycinergic inputs to cardiac vagal neurons. *J Neurophysiol* **89**, 2473–81.

Weber, K. T., Sun, Y., Wodi, L. A., *et al.* (2003). Toward a broader understanding of aldosterone in congestive heart failure. *JRRAS* **4**, 155–63.

Yang, J., Wang, W. Z., Shen, F. M., Su, D. F. (2005). Cardiovascular effects of agmatine within the rostral ventrolateral medulla are similar to those of clonidine in anesthetized rats. *Exp. Brain. Res.* **160**, 467–72.

Yang, Z., Coote, J. H. (2003). Role of GABA and NO in the paraventricular nucleus-mediated reflex inhibition of renal sympathetic nerve activity following stimulation of right atrial receptors in the rat. *Exp. Physiol.* **88**, 335–42.

Yang, Z., Coote, J. H. (2003). The influence of vasopressin on tonic activity of cardiovascular neurones in the ventrolateral medulla of the hypertensive rat. *Auton. Neurosci.* **104**, 83–7.

Zhang, Z. H., Felder, R. B. (2004). Melanocortin receptors mediate the excitatory effects of blood-borne murine leptin on hypothalamic paraventricular neurons in rat. *Am. J Physiol. Regul. Integr. Comp. Physiol.* **286**, R303–10.

CHAPTER 4

Adrenergic and cholinergic receptors

Mike Schachter and P. A. van Zwieten

Introduction

Since the discovery of the neurohumoral phenomena associated with the autonomic nervous system there has been a great deal of interest in the receptors that are the targets of the endogenous neurotransmitters, in particular noradrenaline/adrenaline in the sympathetic nervous system and acetylcholine in the parasympathetic nervous system. This field is of particular interest in a variety of physiological and pathophysiological processes involving virtually all organ systems. Much of our present, detailed knowledge of autonomic receptors has been obtained using pharmacological methods resulting from the availability of a large number of experimental compounds, which are more or less selective agonists or antagonists with respect to the numerous receptor subtypes associated with the autonomic nervous system. Conversely, the more detailed knowledge of the various receptor types has also allowed the discovery of new and more specific therapies for a variety of diseases, predominantly those involving the cardiovascular system. The adrenergic system and its receptors have been studied with great intensity, and a wealth of valuable information has been obtained during the past 2–3 decades. More recently, the field of cholinergic receptors has also received a strong impetus from the discovery that muscarinic receptors are heterogeneous and therefore should be subdivided into different subtypes with different spectra of biological functions and agonists/antagonists.

Adrenoceptors (adrenergic receptors)

Subdivision and classification

Adrenoceptors are the primary targets of the endogenous neurotransmitters noradrenaline and adrenaline, particularly in mediating sympathetic activation to peripheral organs, thus causing very well-known effects such as increased cardiac activity (heart rate and contractile force), vasoconstriction, and increased plasma glucose levels. In addition, the various adrenoceptors are also important as targets of several synthetic drugs, which can be used to mimic the effects of catecholamines or, conversely, to decrease their actions.

Ahlqvist (1948) postulated that the adrenoceptors are different in various organs and he proposed the subdivision into α- and β-subtypes, a classification which is now widely accepted.

There has since been further subdivision into β_1/β_2- and α_1/α_2-adrenoceptors (Lands et al. 1967). More recently, evidence has been put forward for the existence of a distinct β_3-adrenoceptor that may have a particularly important role in thermogenesis. Subsequently, a more sophisticated subdivision of α_1-adrenoceptors into α_{1A}, α_{1B}, α_{1D}, and possibly other subtypes, has been derived from radioligand binding studies. Similarly, the more refined subdivision of α_2-adrenoceptors into $\alpha_{2A}/\alpha_{2B}/\alpha_{2C}$ has been proposed. However, this has not been generally translated into therapeutic applications. The subdivision and classification into α/β, β_1/β_2 and α_1/α_2 are based upon functional pharmacological data, as reflected by a particular preference for certain agonists and antagonists at postsynaptic (postjunctional) sites with respect to the postganglionic sympathetic neurons and their adjacent synapses. Most of the α- and β-adrenoceptor subtypes have been isolated, and their chemical structures (amino acid sequences) have been analysed by molecular biological techniques. The distinction between the various subtypes, based upon functional studies with agonists and antagonists has been confirmed by the determination of receptor structures by means of cloning techniques.

The concept of *presynaptic and postsynaptic* receptors, which is not unique for α-adrenoceptors, was developed and substantiated in the 1970s predominantly by Langer, Starke, and their co-workers (Langer 1981, Starke 1981). The terminology pre/postsynaptic (or pre/postjunctional) refers to the anatomical position of the receptors and does not necessarily coincide with their functional pharmacological profile. Accordingly, presynaptic adrenoceptors belong to the α_2- and β_2- types, whereas in most blood vessels both α_1- and α_2-, but only β_2-adrenoceptors are found at postsynaptic sites. Postsynaptic adrenoceptors, located in the end-organs (Fig. 4.1) are the targets of neurotransmitters and synthetic drugs, and their stimulation or blockade will be translated into a variety of physiological and pharmacological effects. Presynaptic receptors are located at the membranes of the presynaptic vesicles, which are the stores of noradrenaline. The stimulation (or blockade) of presynaptic adrenoceptors modulates the release of noradrenaline from its vesicular storage (Fig. 4.1).

It is widely accepted that adenosine trisphosphate (ATP) and neuropeptide Y (NPY) are important co-transmitters, which are released from the nerve endings simultaneously with noradrenaline.

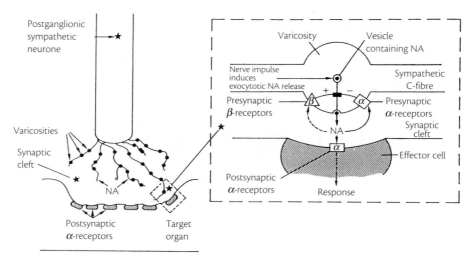

Fig. 4.1 Adrenergic synapse. Nerve activity releases the endogenous neurotransmitter noradrenaline (NA) and also adrenaline from the varicosities. Noradrenaline and adrenaline reach the postsynaptic α- (or β-) adrenoceptors on the cell membrane of the target organ by diffusion. Upon receptor stimulation, a physiological or analogous pharmacological effect is initiated. Presynaptic α_2-adrenoceptors on the membrane (see insertion), when activated by endogenous noradrenaline as well as by exogenous agonists, induce an inhibition and blockade a facilitation of the amount of transmitter noradrenaline released per nerve impulse. Conversely, the stimulation of presynaptic β_2-receptors enhances noradrenaline release from the varicosities. Once noradrenaline has been released, it crosses the synaptic cleft and reaches both α- and β-adrenoceptors at postsynaptic sites, thus causing physiological effects such as vasoconstriction or tachycardia.

The subdivision into α_1/α_2- or $\beta_1/\beta_2/\beta_3$-adrenoceptors implies that all sympathomimetic and sympatholytic drugs should be defined more precisely with respect to their receptor profile (Tables 4.1 and 4.2).

The endogenous catecholamines, noradrenaline and adrenaline, are fairly unselective since they can stimulate several receptor subtypes simultaneously. From a teleological point of view this seems plausible—the activation of a large number of different receptor subtypes can thus be realized by means of one or two neurotransmitters only, and there is no necessity for numerous different release systems for a large variety of humoral (neurotransmitter) systems. Conversely, there are now several synthetic compounds available that are selective stimulants or antagonists with respect to one particular adrenoceptor subtype.

α-Adrenoceptors

α-Adrenoceptors are found in particular in blood vessels and to a less important degree in the heart, as well as in other tissues and organs such as platelets, the vas deferens, the kidney, urethra, prostate, and the central nervous system (CNS). As a result of the development of cloning techniques much has been learned over the past few years concerning the structures of the various α-adrenoceptor subtypes. For the α_1- and α_2-adrenoceptor subtypes the amino acid sequence has now been elucidated, like so many receptors the various α-adrenoceptor subtypes appear to contain seven transmembrane helices. A great deal of information now exists with respect to the processes of signal transduction subsequent to α-adrenoceptor stimulation. All adrenoceptors are G-protein coupled. With respect to the α_1-adrenoceptor, a G_1-protein mediates the activation of phospholipase Cβ, leading to increased intracellular calcium levels through release from internal calcium stores and through influx. The α_2-adrenoceptor, when activated, will mediate the inhibition of adenylyl cyclase via a G_i-protein, indirectly raising intracellular calcium activity. The α_2-adrenoceptor is also coupled to ion channels, and therefore involved in the regulation of Ca^{2+} and K^+ ion fluxes.

Table 4.1 α-Adrenoceptor agonists and antagonists: characterization with respect to their selectivity for α_1- and α_2-adrenoceptors

Agents		Receptor stimulated or blocked
Agonists		
◆ Nordrenaline (neurotransmitter)		$\alpha_1 + \alpha_2 + \beta_1$
◆ Adrenaline (neurotransmitter)		$\alpha_1 + \alpha_2 + \beta_1 + \beta_2$
◆ Phenylephrine		$\alpha_1 > \alpha_2$
◆ Clonidine (Catapres, Catapresan)		$\alpha_2 > \alpha_1$
◆ Guanfacine		$\alpha_2 > \alpha_1$
◆ Azepexole (B-HT 933)		α_2
◆ B-HT 920		α_2
◆ UK-14,304		α_2
Antagonists		
◆ Phentolamine (Regitine)		$\alpha_1 + \alpha_2$
◆ Tolazoline		$\alpha_2 > \alpha_1$
◆ Prazosin		α_1
◆ Doxazosin		α_1
◆ Terazosin		α_1
◆ Trimazosin		α_1
◆ Tamsulosin		α_{1A}
◆ Labetalol		$\alpha_1 + \beta_1 + \beta_2$
◆ Corynanthine		α_1
◆ Rauwolscine	Diastereoisomers	α_2
◆ Yohimbine		α_2
◆ Idazoxan		α_2

Table 4.2 β-Adrenoceptor agonists and antagonists: characterization with respect to their selectivity for β_1- and β_2-adrenoceptors

Agents	Receptors stimulated or blocked
Agonists	
◆ Noradrenaline (neurotransmitter)	$\beta_1 + \alpha_1 + \alpha_2$
◆ Adrenaline (neurotransmitter)	$\beta_1 + \beta_2 + \alpha_1 + \alpha_2$
◆ Dobutamine	$\beta_1 > \beta_2 + \alpha_1$
◆ Isoprenaline	$\beta_1 + \beta_2$
◆ Orciprenaline	$\beta_1 + \beta_2$
◆ Fenoterol	$\beta_2 \gg \beta_1$
◆ Pirbuterol	$\beta_2 \gg \beta_1$
◆ Rimiterol	$\beta_2 \gg \beta_1$
◆ Ritodrine	$\beta_2 \gg \beta_1$
◆ Salbutamol	$\beta_2 \gg \beta_1$
◆ Terbutaline	$\beta_2 \gg \beta_1$
◆ BRL 37344	$\beta_3 > \beta_1$ and β_2
Antagonists	
◆ Propranolol	
◆ Alprenolol	
◆ Pindolol	And various other non-selective β-blockers $\beta_1 + \beta_2$
◆ Oxprenolol	
◆ Timolol	
◆ Sotalol	
◆ Atenolol	$\beta_1 > \beta_2$
◆ Metoprolol	$\beta_1 > \beta_2$
◆ Bisoprolol	$\beta_1 \gg \beta_2$
◆ ICI $_{11}8,55_1$	$\beta_2 > \beta_1$
◆ Carazolol	$\beta_3 > \beta_1$ and β_2

In blood vessels the postsynaptic α-adrenoceptors are of both the α_1- and α_2-subtypes, the former being more widely distributed. Their stimulation with an appropriate agonist causes vasoconstriction; this is so for both α_1- and α_2-adrenoceptor stimulation. Conversely, the blockade of both α_1- and α_2-adrenoceptors at postsynaptic sites causes vasodilatation. The stimulation of presynaptic α_2-adrenoceptors with an agonist induces the inhibition of noradrenaline from its vesicular stores, whereas α_2-adrenoceptor blockade enhances the release of noradrenaline. Since presynaptic α-adrenoceptors are virtually only of the α_2-type, the selective stimulation or inhibition of α_1-adrenoceptors does not interfere with the presynaptic release of noradrenaline. (Reviewed by Starke 1981, van Zwieten and Timmermans 1984, Insel 1996.)

Stimulation of myocardial α_1-adrenoceptors increases contractility which, in the human heart, is much weaker than that caused by β_1-adrenoceptor excitation. Platelet aggregation is enhanced by stimulation of the α_2-adrenoceptors. Stimulation of α_2-adrenoceptors in certain CNS regions, such as the nucleus tractus solitarii, vagal nucleus, and vasomotor centre, will cause a hypotensive response due to the reduction of peripheral sympathetic nervous activity. This mechanism is the basis of the antihypertensive activity of clonidine and -methyldopa (via its active metabolite—methylnoradrenaline), which are α_2-adrenoceptor stimulants. More recently it has been discovered that clonidine also owes an important part of its central antihypertensive activity to the stimulation of imidazoline (I_1) receptors in the rostral ventro-lateral medulla. Moxonidine and rilmenidine are somewhat more selective I_1-receptor stimulants, which have been introduced as centrally acting antihypertensives with a possibly lower incidence of adverse reactions such as sedation and dry mouth, which are known to be mediated by central α_2-adrenoceptors. However, their efficacy is also less impressive and their clinical use remains limited (reviewed by van Zwieten et al. 1984, van Zwieten 1997). The α_2-adrenoceptors in the brain are similar to, or most likely identical with, peripheral vascular α_2-receptors, both in radioligand-binding experiments and with respect to their preference for known selective agonists and antagonists (van Zwieten and Chalmers 1994).

The further subdivision of α_1-adrenoceptors into α_{1A}, α_{1B}, α_{1D}, and possible further subpopulations has so far not led to important functional insights or therapeutic improvements. It may be mentioned that the α_{1A}-adrenoceptor seems to be the functionally predominant subtype in urethral and prostate tissues, whereas its density and functional relevance in blood vessels appear to be much lower.

α-Adrenoceptor changes associated with disease

Hypertensive disease in an established phase has been reported to be associated with an increased density of α_2-adrenoceptors in thrombocytes, although this may be a secondary phenomenon. Changes in α_1-adrenoceptor density in hypertensives are usually very small and not relevant as a potential cause of hypertension. Several authors have established that there exists an exaggerated response to both α_1- and α_2-adrenoceptor agonists in hypertensives, which is probably not related to changes in α-receptor characteristics but rather the reflection of vascular hypertrophy.

Congestive heart failure is characterized by a decreased density of cardiac β-adrenoceptors, thus causing a relatively enhanced sensitivity of cardiac α_1-receptors.

α-Adrenoceptor agonists and antagonists as therapeutic agents

Vasoconstriction via α_1/α_2-adrenoceptor stimulation is an important physiological and pathophysiological process, although it is of limited therapeutic interest, as in the use of nasal and ophthalmic decongestants or the addition of adrenaline or noradrenaline to local anaesthetic agents. Attempts to use the α_1-agonist midodrine in autonomic dysfunction leading to postural hypotension have proved unsuccessful. α-Adrenoceptor antagonists (α-blockers) are the major example of therapeutic agents that owe their efficacy (and most of their side-effects) to their interaction with α-adrenoceptors. Prazosin and related selective α_1-adrenoceptor antagonists (e.g. the more therapeutically useful doxazosin or terazosin) are clearly preferable to non-selective ($\alpha_1 + \alpha_2$)-blockers such as phentolamine. The non-selective α-blockers enhance the release of endogenous noradrenaline as a result of presynaptic α_2-receptor blockade, and they are likely to cause pronounced reflex tachycardia. These problems are not encountered during the use of selective α_1-blockers, which do not interfere with the α_2-receptor-mediated presynaptic mechanisms and because of central effects cause even less tachycardia than one would expect. Prazosin and related drugs, especially doxazosin, are used as anti-hypertensives, and occasionally as vasodilators in the treatment of congestive heart failure. Vasodilatation, based on α_1-adrenoceptor blockade, readily explains the therapeutic efficacy of these compounds. Orthostatic hypotension, their major adverse reaction, is also caused by rapid vasodilatation, predominantly in the venous vascular bed. Owing to its slower onset of action, doxazosin causes less orthostatic hypotension and reflex tachycardia, and has therefore totally superseded prazosin: a modified-release formulation without a sharp initial peak in plasma level is now most commonly used. Even with the immediate-release, once-daily dose is adequate for treatment of hypertension, usually in combination therapy (van Zwieten et al. 1984, van Zwieten 1995).

Selective α_1-adrenoceptor antagonists have been introduced recently in the treatment of impaired micturition, associated with prostate hyperplasia. Tamsulosin and alfuzosin, both relatively selective α_{1A}-adrenoceptor antagonists, enhance micturition in these patients through a relaxant effect on the internal sphincter of the bladder, with a weaker effect on blood vessels, and, therefore a reduced (but not absent) risk of orthostatic hypotension when compared with doxazosin.

The older antihypertensive, α-methyldopa, still widely used in pregnancy-associated hypertension, owes its antihypertensive activity (via its active metabolite α-methylnoradrenaline) to the stimulation of α_2-adrenoceptors in the CNS. Clonidine exerts peripheral sympathoinhibition and central anti-hypertensive activity due to the stimulation of both α_2-adrenoceptors and imidazoline (I_1) receptors in the brainstem, specifically the ventrolateral medulla. The central α_2-adrenoceptors are very similar if not identical to their peripheral counterparts.

β-Adrenoceptors

β-Adrenoceptors are found in cardiac myocytes, in most blood vessels, in the bronchi and intestine, on lymphocytes, adipocytes, and in the CNS. Stimulation of postsynaptic β-adrenoceptors will cause a variety of physiological and pharmacological effects, as outlined in Table 4.3. β-Receptor blockade by β-adrenoceptor antagonists (β-blockers) suppresses these effects and this is the basis of their therapeutic efficacy and also of most of their adverse reactions. The molecular structure of β-receptors in several tissues and systems has been elucidated. As established for many receptor types, the structure of β-adrenoceptors is characterized by the classic structure of seven transmembrane helices, with particular areas/regions that are required for the combination with agonists and antagonists (in the extracellular part) or with coupling proteins at intracellular sites.

As for the α-adrenoceptors, much information is now available concerning the signal transduction processes that are triggered by adrenoceptor stimulation with appropriate agonists. β-Adrenoceptors are also G-protein coupled. Accordingly, β-receptor stimulation is associated with the activation of a G_s-protein, and, subsequently adenylyl cyclase. At postsynaptic sites, both β_1- and β_2-adrenoceptors are found, as summarized in Table 4.3.

β-Adrenoceptors at presynaptic sites are predominantly of the β_2-type. Their stimulation with an agonist causes enhanced release of endogenous noradrenaline from its vesicular stores. Conversely, the blockade of β_2-adrenoceptors with an appropriate antagonist will reduce the rate of release of endogenous noradrenaline from presynaptic storage sites. β-Adrenoceptors are present in various

Table 4.3 Effects on the stimulation and blockade by 1-, 2- and 3-adrenoceptors by means of appropriate agonists and antagonists

Receptor type	Tissue/organ	Stimulation (agonist)	Blockade (antagonist)
β_1	Cardiac pacemaker cells	Heart rate $\uparrow$	Heart rate $\downarrow$
	AV node	AV conduction $\uparrow$	AV conduction $\downarrow$
	Myocardium	Contractility $\uparrow$	Contractility $\downarrow$
	Intestine	Relaxation	—
β_2	Bronchi	Relaxation	Constriction
	Myocardium ($\beta_2 < \beta_1$)	Contractility $\uparrow$	Contractility $\downarrow$
	Blood vessels	Dilatation	Constriction
	Intestine	Relaxation	—
	Adenylyl cyclase	Hyperglycaemia	Hypoglycaemia
	Free	Fatty acids $\uparrow$	Free fatty acids $\downarrow$
β_3	Adipose tissues (brown)	Lipolysis	?
		Thermogenesis	
		Contractility $\downarrow$	
		Vasodilatation	

structures of the CNS, but their functional role and potential basis as a therapeutic target remain uncertain, though anti-depressants may modulate central β-adrenoceptor function. These receptors are very similar to, if not identical with, their peripheral counterparts.

More recently, a great deal of information concerning the β_3-adrenoceptor has become available. β_3-Adrenoceptors are found in brown adipose tissue, intestinal smooth muscle, and blood vessels. The role of these receptors in humans has not been defined in detail, but it has been demonstrated that when stimulated they enhance lipolysis and the generation of heat in adipose tissues. But possible cardiovascular functions for these receptors have recently been delineated: vasodilatation and, rather surprisingly, an inhibitory effect on cardiac contractility (Dessy and Balligand 2010).

β-Adrenoceptor changes associated with disease

With respect to the influence of disease on β-adrenoceptors, the most convincing results have been obtained in congestive heart failure (CHF). Various types of CHF, caused by severe coronary heart disease and valvular disease, are associated with a significant degree of down-regulation of both β_1- and β_2-adrenoceptors, as reflected by a reduction in the density of both receptor subtypes in the myocardium. In the myocardial tissue of patients with dilated cardiomyopathy the down-regulation remains limited to β_1-adrenoceptors, without changes in the density of β_2-adrenoceptors. The reduced density of β-adrenoceptors is most probably explained by the elevated plasma levels of noradrenaline reported in patients with advanced stages of CHF. The lowered density of cardiac β-receptors in CHF readily explains the well-known tachyphylaxis towards β-adrenoceptor agonists, which may be used in the treatment of CHF: partly for this reason their use is in fact very limited. β-receptor down-regulation may be reversed by treatment with β-blockers in very low doses and this may partly be the basis of the observation that low-dose β-blocker therapy may be beneficial in CHF, despite the risk of negative inotropic effects. It has also been shown that in congestive heart failure β_2-adrenoceptors are uncoupled, possibly as a result of an increase in G-protein receptor kinases. Reports on changes in β-adrenoceptor density (in particular the β$_2$-receptors on lymphocytes) in hypertension are controversial: increased, decreased, or unchanged β$_2$-receptor densities on lymphocytes from essential hypertensives have all been described.

β$_3$-Adrenoceptor changes may be involved in certain types of obesity, in particular those associated with non-insulin-dependent diabetes mellitus (NIDDM), as found in the Pima Indians, for example.

β-Adrenoceptor agonists and antagonists as therapeutic agents

β-Adrenoceptor agonists may be used to increase contractile force in patients with CHF, or as bronchodilators in patients with asthma or other types of obstructive airways disease. The use of β-agonists in CHF is associated with various side-effects: these inotropic agents may cause tachycardia, with an increased risk of tachyarrhythmias. None of the β-adrenoceptor agonists so far available can be used orally, making intravenous administration unavoidable. Chronic administration of these compounds leads to down-regulation and desensitization of β-adrenoceptors and hence to tachyphylaxis. Of the drugs available at present, dobutamine is the only one used at all frequently. Its use is limited to infusions of a few days' duration, and its beneficial effect is no more than palliative. It is more frequently utilized in stress echocardiography.

Salbutamol, salmeterol, terbutaline, and fenoterol are selective β$_2$-adrenoceptor stimulants. They are very well known as bronchodilators, which have replaced non-selective β$_1$ + β$_2$-agonists, such as isoprenaline and orciprenaline. These latter compounds cause a considerably greater degree of tachycardia (as a result of their β$_1$-component) than observed for the selective β$_2$-receptor stimulants.

β$_2$-Adrenoceptor stimulants, such as ritodrine, are used in obstetrics, with the aim of arresting premature labour, via relaxation of uterus smooth muscle.

β$_3$-Adrenoceptor agonists can be thought of as potential anti-obesity drugs, especially in patients with NIDDM, although clinical data on this potential treatment are hardly available, and in humans there is much less brown fat than in rodents.

β-Adrenoceptor antagonists (β-blockers) have obtained widespread therapeutic application, especially in the treatment of essential hypertension and angina pectoris. Their therapeutic efficacy is caused by the blockade of β$_1$-adrenoceptors, and so are most of their adverse reactions. This important subject has been reviewed extensively (Fitzgerald 1991, Bielecka-Dabrowa et al. 2010), but their role in hypertension is much less prominent than a decade ago However, it should be noted that the newer vasodilator β-blockers (carvedilol, nebivolol) do not have and almost certainly will not have comprehensive outcome data.

The use of beta-blockers in congestive heart failure has been mentioned. Starting from a low dose these drugs have to be carefully titrated. The beneficial effect in this condition is probably caused by a reduction of tachycardia (an expression of sympathetic hyperactivation in patients with CHF), and possibly also by the partial reversal of β-adrenoceptor down-regulation in the hearts of such patients.

Cholinergic receptors

Traditionally, cholinergic receptors have been subdivided into nicotinic and muscarinic subtypes, based predominantly on the classic work in this field by Sir Henry Dale and his co-workers in the 1930s. The nicotinic receptors are located in the autonomic ganglia (both sympathetic and parasympathetic) and in neuromuscular junctions. Muscarinic receptors are located in all target organs of the parasympathetic nervous system. More recently, muscarinic receptors have also been demonstrated in certain structures of peripheral sympathetic (adrenergic) neurons. The CNS also contains muscarinic receptors, which are involved in cognitive processes, extrapyramidal functions, and probably also in the central regulation of blood pressure and heart rate.

The distinction between nicotinic and muscarinic receptors was based initially on differential pharmacodynamic effects and preferences for agonists and antagonists. Molecular biological techniques have confirmed the different structures and amino acid sequences of both types of cholinergic receptors. As in numerous other receptors, both the nicotinic and muscarinic receptors contain the well-known pattern of seven helices. Both nicotinic and muscarinic cholinergic receptors are G-protein coupled.

Nicotinic cholinergic receptors

Nicotinic receptors are known to play a pivotal role in neurohumoral transmission in all autonomic ganglia (parasympathetic and sympathetic) as well as at neuromuscular junctions. It has been proposed that different subtypes of nicotinic receptors may exist but this hypothesis has not been as fully substantiated as for the muscarinic receptors.

Both agonists and antagonists for nicotinic receptors have been developed, though only a few of these are clinically useful. Nicotine (in low doses) and dimethylphenylpiperazine (DMPP) are classic stimulants of nicotinic receptors, both in the sympathetic and parasympathetic autonomic ganglia. Succinylcholine (suxamethonium) is an agonist, particularly with respect to the nicotinic receptors in neuromuscular junctions. Its muscle relaxant action, previously used in anaesthesiology, is based upon the permanent depolarization it causes so blocking neurotransmission.

All inhibitors of the enzyme cholinesterase, such as neostigmine, fysostigmine, pyridostigmine, and tacrine, but also the polyalkylphosphates such as fluostigmine, parathion, and sarin (a nerve gas), will cause the accumulation of endogenous acetylcholine, which is an agonist for both nicotinic and muscarinergic cholinergic receptors. The beneficial effect of neostigmine and related drugs in myasthenia gravis and related disorders of neuromuscular transmission is based upon the stimulation of nicotinic receptors in the neuromuscular junction due to increased levels of acetylcholine. Their main side-effects are caused by stimulation of parasympathetic muscarinic receptors. The polyalkylphosphates (some of them nerve gases or insecticides) are only of toxicological interest. Their extremely high toxicity is based predominantly upon a general activation of all cholinergic receptors (including those in the CNS) by accumulated endogenous acetylcholine after irreversible inhibition of acetylcholinesterase

Antagonists to nicotinic receptors in the autonomic ganglia are the ganglioplegic agents or ganglion blockers. Examples of these are pentolinium, hexamethonium, or trimetaphan. These compounds were among the first drugs used to treat hypertension. Their antihypertensive activity is based upon the blockade of transmission in sympathetic ganglia. These compounds were effective antihypertensives, but have long been obsolete because of their severe adverse reactions, which are largely based upon the simultaneous blockade of both sympathetic and parasympathetic ganglia. The most serious problem was severe and sometimes incapacitating postural hypotension.

A second group of nicotinic receptor antagonists are the compounds related to tubocurarine, such as gallamine, pancuronium, vecuronium, and rocuronium. They are muscle relaxants, widely used in anaesthesiology. Their beneficial effect is based upon blockade of transmission in the neuromuscular junction as a result of competitive antagonism at the level of nicotinic receptors.

Muscarinic cholinergic receptors

Muscarinic receptors are part of the parasympathetic nervous system as targets of the endogenous neurotransmitter acetylcholine and located on effector organs. Recent studies indicate that muscarinic receptors in various organs and tissues are heterogeneous. There are at least four subtypes (M_1, M_2, M_3, and M_4) and possibly more. By analogy with the sympathetic system, the existence of presynaptic muscarinic receptors in addition to those at postsynaptic sites has been demonstrated.

Furthermore, the classification of muscarinic receptor subtypes requires a more precise designation of receptor agonists/antagonists with respect to their preference for the various classes of muscarinic receptors. A major problem is the limited availability of highly selective agonists and antagonists, which are suitable as tools in the pharmacological analysis of the muscarinic receptor subtypes.

Subdivision and classification

The subdivision of muscarinic receptors into at least four subtypes is based predominantly upon radioligand-binding studies because of the availability of appropriate ligands and selective M-receptor antagonists. These four subtypes, M_1, M_2, M_3, and M_4, and the antagonists used are listed in Table 4.4, which also shows the tissues where these receptor subtypes can be demonstrated to exist. The introduction of pirenzepine, a selective antagonist to M_1 receptors, has been a major breakthrough in the modern classification of M receptors, though it is clinically obsolete as an acid suppressant drug in peptic ulcer. The concept of M_1, M_2, and M_3 receptors was formulated originally by Doods et al. (1987). Apart from these three well-established subtypes, a fourth type (M_4) has

been identified recently. The radioligand-binding studies that have been pivotal to the subclassification of M receptors have been followed up by functional experiments, the results of which are globally in line with the findings of the binding data. Table 4.4 shows the functional aspects of stimulation/blockade of the M-receptor subtypes (reviewed by Eglen 1995; Lambrecht et al. 1995).

Molecular biological cloning techniques on the other hand have led to the identification of at least five different muscarinic receptor species, the amino acid sequence and structure of which have been elucidated. Again, the model of seven transmembrane helices underlies the structure of these receptor species. These five muscarinic receptor species have been denominated as m_1, m_2, m_3, m_4, and m_5, respectively. The m_1, m_2, m_3, and m_4 types broadly coincide with the M_1-, M_2-, M_3-, and M_4-receptor subtypes established by means of radioligand-binding techniques (Table 4.4). The functional role of the m_5 species so far remains unknown (Bonner 1987, Ishii and Kurachi 2006).

Biochemical studies have indicated that muscarinic receptors are coupled to adenylyl cyclase via G-proteins. In contrast to β-adrenoceptors, the influence of muscarinic receptor stimulation is inhibitory (involving a G_i-protein), thus causing a decrease in the cellular concentration of cyclic adenosine monophosphate (cAMP) and therefore functionally increasing intracellular calcium activity, or linked via G_q to phospholipase C and therefore directly increasing intracellular calcium levels.

Muscarinic receptor agonists and antagonists: potential therapeutic agents

Acetylcholine, the endogenous neurotransmitter in the parasympathetic nervous system, is a non-selective agent that stimulates muscarinic receptors of the three subtypes, M_1, M_2, and M_3, in addition to nicotinic cholinergic receptors. Most of the classic synthetic muscarinic receptor agonists are non-selective with respect to the various muscarinic receptor subtypes. This lack of selectivity is known for muscarine, aceclidine, pilocarpine, bethanechol, carbachol, and arecoline. Carbachol and arecoline also stimulate ganglionic nicotinic receptors in addition to their agonistic effect on muscarinic receptors.

Methacholine appears to possess some selectivity towards the vascular muscarinic receptors, which may be of the M_2 or the M_3 type, depending on the vascular bed and animal species investigated. The experimental compounds McN-A 343 and xanomeline appear to display selectivity towards M_1 receptors, particularly those present in the brain and at the sympathetic ganglia. Virtually all other muscarinic receptor agonists available are non-selective with respect to the various M-receptor subtypes. In fundamental pharmacology the development of highly selective agonists for the muscarinic receptor subtypes would be most valuable.

Vascular muscarinic M_3 receptors are involved in the release of nitric oxide (NO) from endothelium. Consequently, the vasodilator action of acetylcholine is an indirect effect, mediated by NO. In endothelium-denuded vessels acetylcholine causes vasoconstriction, as a result of the stimulation of M-receptors on vascular smooth muscle. Atropine is a non-selective antagonist with a high affinity for all the muscarinic receptor subtypes. Pirenzepine is a selective M_1-receptor antagonist, with a much lower affinity for M_2 or M_3 receptors. AF-DX 116 is a cardioselective antagonist for M_2 receptors, as is methoctramine. 4-DAMP (4-diphenyl-acetoxy-N-methyl-piperidine) shows some selectivity for M_3-receptors as do

Table 4.4 Various types of muscarinic receptors in different tissues. The effects of receptor stimulation and blockade by appropriate agonists and antagonists are also shown

Receptor type	Tissue/organ	Stimulation (agonist)	Blockade (antagonist)
M_1	Neurons	Excitation	Depression
	Ganglia (sympathetic)	Noradrenaline release ↑	Noradrenaline release ↓
M_2	Heart	Bradycardia	Tachycardia
		Contractility ↓	Contractility ↑
	Smooth muscle	Contraction	Relaxation
M_3	Glands	Secretion ↑	Secretion ↓
	Ileum	Contraction	Relaxation
M_4	Striatum	?decreased locomotion	
	Lungs		

hexahydro-sila-difenidol and related compounds. Tropicamide and himbacine show moderate selectivity for the M_4 receptor.

The present muscarinic receptor classification is predominantly based upon the series of antagonists and agonists mentioned above. Since the number of experimental compounds is rapidly increasing, the receptor classification may be subject to future changes, though there has been little indication of this recently.

Therapeutic applications

Muscarinic receptor stimulants have traditionally been used for activation of the smooth muscle of the intestine and/or urinary bladder and for lowering elevated intraocular pressure in glaucoma. Carbachol and bethanechol, which are used to stimulate smooth muscle, are examples of the former. They display modest selectivity towards intestinal and urinary bladder smooth muscle as compared to that of the cardiovascular system and they have little clinical usefulness. Adverse reactions are related to stimulation of the peripheral parasympathetic nervous system. Pilocarpine, when applied locally to the eye, causes miosis and a reduction of intraocular pressure, a property clearly relevant in glaucoma treatment. Systemic side-effects do not usually occur, although the ocular adverse reactions are substantial. However, there is significant interference with vision and the clinical use of pilocarpine has greatly decreased with the introduction of newer agents.

Therapeutic applications of selective muscarinic receptor agonists are currently a matter of speculation. Highly cardioselective M_2-receptor agonists may be used to reduce heart rate in the treatment of angina pectoris or and supraventricular tachycardia. M_1-receptor stimulation in the CNS has been proposed as a therapeutic approach to treat Alzheimer's disease. This is currently achieved indirectly, by the use of acetylcholinesterase inhibitors (donepezil, galantamine, rivastigmine) though galantamine also has nicotinic receptor agonist activity.

Various non-selective M-receptor antagonists may be used in ophthalmology to provoke mydriasis, tropicamide being the one most commonly used because of its relatively short duration of action. Hyoscine may be used as a potent centrally acting anti-emetic agent, especially in motion sickness.

On theoretical grounds cardioselective M_2-receptor antagonists may benefit patients with impaired atrioventricular (AV) conduction in the period before a pacemaker is implanted, and may also have some use in conditions such as the sick sinus syndrome, digitalis intoxication, or arrhythmia caused by torsade de pointes (TDP). Finally, coronary spasm may involve a cholinergic component in certain patients and the beneficial effects of atropine have been demonstrated. A highly selective antagonist of vascular M_2 (or M_3) receptors, which appears to be involved in this type of spasm, may be preferable to a non-selective agent such as atropine.

Probably the most extensive therapeutic use of muscarinic receptor antagonists is in bladder disorders, specifically overactive bladder and associated incontinence. A large number of drugs have been developed for this indication (darifenacin, fesoterodine, propiverine, solifenacin, tolterodine, trospium), with $M_{2/3}$ antagonist properties (Hegde 2006). Oxybutynin has similar anticholinergic properties, with other muscle relaxant effects. These drugs have moderate efficacy in relieving symptoms but are not devoid of anticholinergic effects beyond the bladder, notably dry mouth and blurred vision.

References

Ahlqvist, R. P. (1948). A study of the adrenotropic receptors. *Am. J. Physiol.* **153**, 586–91.

Bielecka-Dabrowa A., Aronow W.S.,Rysz J., Banach M.(2010) Current place of beta-blockers in the treatment of hypertension. *Curr. Vasc. Pharmacol.* 8, 733–41.

Bonner, T. I. (1989). The molecular basis of muscarinic receptor diversity. *Trends Neurosci.* **12**, 148–51.

Dessy C., Balligand J. L. (2010). Beta3-adrenergic receptors in cardiac and vascular tissues : emerging concepts and therapeutic perspectives. *Adv. Pharmacol.* 59, 135–63.

Doods, H. N., Mathy, M.-J., Davidesko, D., van Charldorp, K. J., de Jonge, A., and van Zwieten, P. A. (1987). Selectivity of muscarinic antagonists in radioligand and *in vivo* experiments for the putative M_1, M_2 and M_3 receptors. *J. Pharmacol. Exp. Ther.* **246**, 929–34.

Eglen, R. M. (1995). Muscarinic M_2 and M_3 receptors in smooth muscle. *Exp. Opin. Invest. Drugs* **4**, 1167–71.

Fitzgerald, J. D. (1991). The applied pharmacology of beta-adrenoceptor agonists (beta blockers) in relation to clinical outcomes. *Cardiovasc. Drugs Ther.* **5**, 561–76.

Goyal, R. K. (1989). Muscarinic receptor subtypes. Physiology and clinical implications. *New Engl. J. Med.* **321**, 1022–8.

Hegde, S. S. (2006). Muscarinic receptors in the bladder: from basic research to therapeutics. *Br. J. Pharmacol.* **147** suppl 2, S80–87.

Insel, P. A. (1996). Adrenergic receptors—evolving concepts and clinical implications. *N. Engl. J. Med.* **334**, 580–5.

Ishii M., Kurachi Y. (2006). Muscarinic acetylcholine receptors. *Curr. Pharm. Design.* **12**, 3573–81.

Lambrecht, G., Gross, J., Hacksell, U. *et al.* (1995). The design and pharmacology of novel selective muscarinic agonists and antagonists. *Life Sci.* **56**, 815–22.

Lands, A. M., Arnold, A., McAuliff, J. P., Lunduena, F. P., and Brown, R. G. (1967). Differentiation of receptor systems activated by sympathomimetic amines. *Nature* **214**, 597–8.

Langer, S. Z. (1981). Presynaptic regulation of the release of catecholamines. *Pharmacol. Rev.* **32**, 337–62.

Starke, K. (1981). α-Adrenoceptor subclassification. *Rev. Physiol. Biochem. Pharmacol.* **88**, 199–236.

Van Zwieten, P. A. (1995). Alpha-adrenoceptor blocking agents in the treatment of hypertension. In *Hypertension: pathophysiology, diagnosis and management*, (ed. J. H. Laragh and B. M. Brenner), 2nd edn, pp. 2917–35, Raven Press, New York.

Van Zwieten, P. A. (1997). Central imidazoline (I_1) receptors as targets of centrally acting antihypertensives. *J. Hypertension*, **15**, 117–25.

Van Zwieten, P. A. and Chalmers, J. P. (1994). Different types of centrally acting antihypertensives and their targets in the central nervous system. *Cardiovasc. Drugs Ther.* **8**, 787–99.

Van Zwieten, P. A. and Timmermans, P. B. M. W. M. (1984). Central and peripheral α-adrenoceptors. Pharmacological aspects and clinical potential. *Adv. Drug Res.* **13**, 209–54.

Van Zwieten, P. A., Timmermans, P. B. M. W. M., and van Brummelen, P. (1984). Role of alpha-adrenoceptors in hypertension and in antihypertensive treatment. *Am. J. Med.* **77**, 17–25.

CHAPTER 5

Structural and chemical organization of the autonomic nervous system with special reference to non-adrenergic, non-cholinergic transmission

Geoffrey Burnstock

Key points

- The autonomic neuroeffector junction is non-synaptic with transmitter released 'en passage' from terminal fibre varicosities at variable distances from postjunctional sites, which do not show specialization.

- There is a multiplicity of autonomic neurotransmitters including, in addition to the classic transmitters acetylcholine and noradrenaline, adenosine triphosphate (ATP), nitric oxide (NO), various polypeptides, amino acids and monoamines.

- Cotransmission is common with combinations of acetylcholine or noradrenaline co-localized with peptides, NO and ATP, so that the terms 'cholinergic', 'adrenergic', peptidergic, 'purinergic' and 'nitrergic' nerves should no longer be used, although they are acceptable terms for describing neurotransmission. The proportions of cotransmitters varies between species, during development and aging and under different physiological and pathophysiological conditions.

- Neuromodulation involves both prejunctional modulation of transmitter release and postjunctional modulation of transmitter action.

- Changes in cotransmitter and receptor expression occur in autonomic disease. For example: there is significant increase in the purinergic component of parasympathetic cotransmission in the urinary bladder in interstitial cystitis, obstructed and neurogenic bladder; increase in sympathetic purinergic cotransmission in spontaneously hypertensive rats; and vasoactive intestinal peptide (VIP) levels are reduced in enteric nerves in idiopathic constipation and in nerves supplying diabetic blood vessels and corpus cavernosum.

Introduction

Within the past 30 years, new discoveries have changed our understanding of the organization of the autonomic nervous system, including the structure of the autonomic neuroeffector junction and the multiplicity of neurotransmitters that take part in the process of autonomic neuroeffector transmission, as well as cotransmission, neuromodulation, receptor expression and trophic factors (Burnstock 1986a, 2009). An outstanding feature of autonomic neurotransmission is the inherent plasticity afforded by its structural and neurochemical organization and the interaction between expression of neural mediators and environmental factors. In this way autonomic neurotransmission is matched to ongoing changes in demands and can sometimes be compensatory in pathophysiological situations. Selective neurochemical changes have been demonstrated in disorders of the autonomic nervous system. An understanding of the mechanisms governing the expression of neurotransmitters and their receptors will allow selective manipulation for the therapeutic treatment of diseases that feature autonomic dysfunction.

Autonomic neuroeffector junction

The autonomic neuroeffector junction between autonomic nerve fibres and smooth muscle cells differs in several ways from the neuromuscular junction in skeletal muscle and from the synapses in the central and peripheral nervous systems (Burnstock 1986b, 2008). A major difference is that the autonomic effector is a muscle bundle rather than a single cell. Only a certain percentage of smooth muscle cells are directly innervated and low resistance pathways between individual muscle cells allow electrotonic spread of activity within the effector muscle bundle. Morphologically, the sites of electrotonic coupling are represented by gap junctions or nexuses. These gap junctions vary in size from punctate junctions to junctional areas of more than 1 µm in diameter. Gap junctions are not static but undergo a continual process of formation and removal.

Another characteristic of the autonomic neuromuscular junction is that it does not have a well-defined structure with prejunctional and postjunctional specializations like the skeletal muscle motor end plate. Unmyelinated, highly branched, postganglionic autonomic nerve fibres reaching the effector smooth muscle become beaded or varicose (Fig. 5.1). These varicosities are not static in their relationships to smooth muscle, consistent with the lack of postjunctional specialization, characteristic of non-synaptic transmission (Burnstock 2008). They are 0.5–2 µm in diameter and about 1 µm in length and are packed with vesicles and mitochondria. Neurotransmitters and neuromodulators from autonomic nerve fibres are released from these varicosities that occur at intervals of 5–10 µm along axons. The minimum distance of the cleft between the varicosity and smooth muscle varies considerably depending on the tissue, from 20 nm in densely innervated structures such as the vas deferens to 1–2 µm in large elastic arteries. Thus prejunctional and postjunctional sites are particularly accessible for neuromodulatory influences, where local agents may reduce or increase the release of neurotransmitter or may alter the extent or time course of neurotransmitter action. During conduction of an impulse along an autonomic axon neurotransmitter is released en passage from varicosities at variable distances from effector cells. A given impulse evokes release from only some of the varicosities that it encounters.

Release of neurotransmitter causes a transient change in membrane potential of the postjunctional cell. If the result of a single pulse is a depolarization, the response is called an excitatory junction potential (EJP). EJPs summate and facilitate with repetitive stimulation and upon reaching sufficient amplitude, the threshold for the generation of an action potential is reached, which results in mechanical contraction. If the result of a single pulse of neurotransmitter release is a hyperpolarization, the response is called an inhibitory junction potential (IJP). IJPs prevent action potential discharge in spontaneously active smooth muscle and thus cause relaxation.

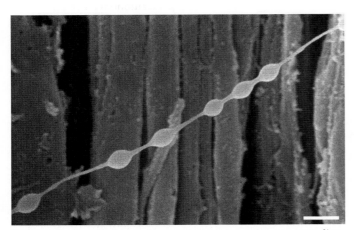

Fig. 5.1 A scanning electron micrograph of a single terminal varicose nerve fibre lying over smooth muscle of the small intestine of the rat. Scale bar = 3 µm. With permission from Burnstock (1988).

Multiplicity of neurotransmitters in the autonomic nervous system

A neurotransmitter is a chemical substance released from nerves upon electrical stimulation and which acts on specific receptors on adjacent effector cells to bring about a response, thus acting as a chemical messenger of neural activation. In early studies, acceptance of a substance as a neurotransmitter required satisfaction of the following criteria:

◆ The presynaptic neuron synthesizes and stores the transmitter.

◆ The transmitter is released in a calcium-dependent manner.

◆ There should be a mechanism for terminating the activity of the transmitter, either by enzymatic degradation or by cellular uptake.

◆ Local exogenous application of the substance should mimic its effects following release due to electrical nerve stimulation.

◆ Agents that block or potentiate the endogenous activity of the transmitter should also affect local exogenous application in the same way.

The classic view of autonomic nervous control as antagonistic actions of noradrenaline (NA) and acetylcholine (ACh) causing either constriction or relaxation, depending on the tissue, was changed in the early 1960s when clear evidence of a non-adrenergic, non-cholinergic (NANC) system was presented (Burnstock 1986a). About a decade later, studies of autonomic neurotransmission revealed a multiplicity of neurotransmitters in the autonomic nervous system (ANS). Neurally released substances, including monoamines, amino acids, neuropeptides, adenosine 5'-triphosphate (ATP) and nitric oxide (NO) were identified (Table 5.1). Since NO does not conform to the constraints of the criteria outlined above, although it certainly acts as a rapid chemical messenger in the ANS, a reappraisal of the criteria for defining a neurotransmitter has been proposed (Hoyle and Burnstock 1996), taking into account evidence for non-vesicular, Ca^{2+}-independent release of some classic neurotransmitters, and the intracellular site of action of NO. The rapid expansion of the number of proposed autonomic neurotransmitters in recent years, including endothelin, secretoneurin, pituitary adenylate cyclase-activating peptide (PACAP), which is similar in structure to vasoactive intestinal peptide (VIP), glutamate and carbon monoxide, makes it likely that the list is still incomplete.

Noradrenaline

The synthesis of NA is catalysed by three enzymes, tyrosine hydroxylase (TH), L-3,4-dihydroxyphenylalanine (L-dopa) decarboxylase, and dopamine-beta-hydroxylase (DBH). The rate limiting enzyme, TH, requires tyrosine, oxygen and the cofactor tetrahydrobiopterin, and is subject to multiple regulatory mechanisms mediated by phosphorylation by protein kinases in addition to regulation at the level of gene transcription (Fillenz 1995). NA exists in the neuronal cytosol, but is stored in small and large dense core vesicles together with other cotransmitters, chromogranins and DBH. Thus in sympathetic neurons, the vesicles are involved in not only storage and release of NA, but also with the last stage of its synthesis. Following electrical stimulation the vesicular contents are released by exocytosis, in a Ca^{2+}-dependent manner, into the extracellular space.

Table 5.1 Established and putative neurotransmitters/ neuromodulators in the autonomic nervous system

Noradrenaline (NA)
Acetylcholine (ACh)
Adenosine 5'-triphosphate (ATP) and other nucleotides
Nitric oxide (NO)
Carbon monoxide (CO)
5-Hydroxytryptamine (5-HT)
Dopamine (DA)
γ-Aminobutyric acid (GABA)
Glutamate (GLU)
Neuropeptides
Neuropeptide Y (NPY)/pancreatic polypeptide (PP)
Enkephalin (ENK)/endorphin (END)/dynorphin (DYN)
Vasoactive intestinal polypeptide (VIP) and related peptides PHI and PHM
Pituitary adenylate cyclase-activating peptide (PACAP)
Substance P (SP)/neurokinin A (NKA)/neurokinin B (NKB)
Calcitonin gene-related peptide (CGRP)
Somatostatin (SOM)
Galanin (GAL)
Gastrin releasing peptide (GRP) /bombesin (BOM)
Neurotensin (NT)
Cholecystokinin (CCK) /gastrin (GAS)
Angiotensin II (AII)
Adrenocorticotrophic hormone (ACTH)
Secretoneurin
Endothelin (ET)

After interaction with specific receptors, the action of NA is rapidly terminated by reuptake into the nerve varicosity or into non-neuronal cells, where it is metabolized by the intracellular enzymes, monoamine oxidase (MAO) and catechol-O-methyltransferase (COMT).

NA produces a variety of effects by interaction with a number of different adrenoceptor subtypes. Several subtypes of α_1-, α_2- and β-adrenoceptors have now been characterized and cloned (Chapter 3). There are many regulatory systems inherent to the adrenergic machinery, including autoinhibition of NA release via presynaptic α_2 receptors, regulation of NA synthesis and adreno-ceptor desensitization and supersensitivity dependent on agonist exposure. A schematic of noradrenergic transmission is presented in Fig. 5.2A.

Acetylcholine

The synthesis of ACh from choline and acetyl coenzyme A is cata-lysed by choline acetyltransferase (ChAT) and takes place in the neuronal cytoplasm. ACh is then pumped into small agranular vesicles, which have a specific ACh transporter in their membranes, and stored until Ca^{2+}-dependent exocytotic release upon electrical stimulation. ACh released during neurotransmission is inactivated by hydrolysis due to the action of acetylcholinesterase (AChE),

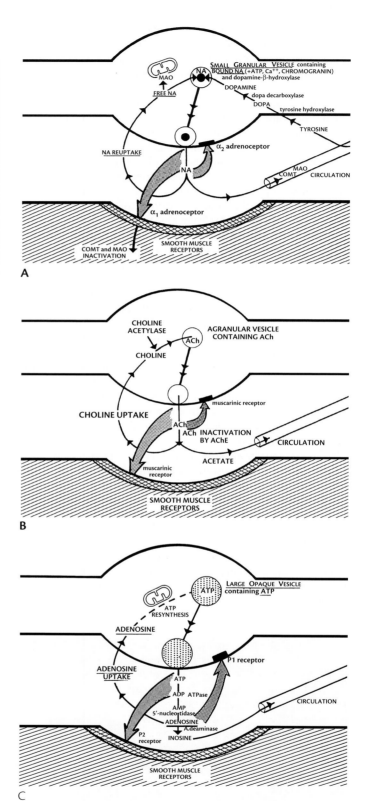

Fig. 5.2 Simplified schematic representation of synthesis, storage, release, receptor activation and neurotransmitter inactivation at neuromuscular junctions. **A:** Noradrenergic neurotransmission; **B:** cholinergic neurotransmission; **C:** purinergic neurotransmission. With permission from Burnstock G., Purinergic nerves, *Pharmacol. Rev.*, 1972, **24**: 509–81.

which is localized on both presynaptic and postsynaptic membranes. The choline that results from this breakdown is recycled by transport back into the nerve varicosities by a metabolically driven high affinity choline uptake mechanism for resynthesis and vesicular storage of ACh. Choline uptake into the presynaptic terminal is the rate limiting factor for ACh synthesis. A schematic of cholinergic autonomic neurotransmitters is present in Fig. 5.2B.

ACh acts on two different classes of receptors (Chapter 3). Nicotinic receptors are ionotropic receptors consisting of subunits that constitute multimeric ligand-gated Na^+ channels, which mediate fast responses. In the autonomic nervous system, nicotinic receptors (subtype N_2) are mainly found within ganglia. In contrast, muscarinic receptors are metabotropic receptors coupled with G proteins, with slower responses, and are widespread throughout autonomic effector tissues and smooth muscle.

ATP

The purine nucleotide, ATP, was the first substance that was found to best satisfy the criteria for a neurotransmitter in NANC nerves (Burnstock 1972). There is now substantial evidence to support widespread purinergic signalling in both neuronal and non-neuronal systems (Burnstock 1997, Burnstock and Knight 2004). ATP is a transmitter at neuroeffector junctions (Fig. 5.2C) and at synapses in peripheral autonomic ganglia and in the brain and spinal cord (Burnstock 2007a). ATP is also a major signalling molecule in the enteric nervous system (Burnstock 2001a) and on sensory nerves, where it is involved in both physiological reflexes and nociception (Burnstock 2001b). ATP is synthesized in nerve terminals and is stored in vesicles, often co-localized with other neurotransmitters. After its release and activation of purine receptors, ATP is rapidly broken down to adenosine by Mg^{2+}-activated ATPase (a ubiquitous membrane-bound ecto-ATPase) and ecto-5'-nucleotidase located at sites of ATP release. Ecto-5'-nucleotidase is strongly inhibited by ADP. Adenosine is transported into neurons and non-neuronal cells via a nucleoside carrier high-affinity uptake system and either phosphorylated to ATP and reincorporated into physiological stores or broken down by adenosine deaminase to inosine, which is inactive and leaks into the circulation. In addition to ATP, there is now evidence that small amounts of other nucleotides, such as ADP, AMP, GTP, UTP and diadenosine polyphosphates are stored in synaptic vesicles and may play neuromodulatory roles in signalling in the nervous system.

Based on the relative potencies of purine nucleosides and nucleotides and second messenger systems on a variety of tissues, two major types of purine receptor were distinguished (Burnstock 1978). P1 receptors are most sensitive to adenosine, and are competitively blocked by methylxanthines. P2 receptors are most sensitive to ATP, and their occupation may lead to prostaglandin synthesis. Pharmacological, biochemical, receptor binding and cloning studies, have enabled subdivision of these two types of receptor (Ralevic and Burnstock 1998). There are four subtypes of P1 receptors, namely A_1, A_{2A}, A_{2B} or A_3 subtypes: A_1-receptors are preferentially activated by N^6-substituted adenosine analogues, and their occupation leads to decreased cyclic adenosine monophosphate (cAMP) levels, whereas A_2-receptors show preference for 5'-substituted compounds and cAMP levels are increased; occupation of A_3 receptors does not lead to changes in adenylate cyclase. Selective agonists and antagonists for these P1 receptor subtypes have been identified.

Following expression cloning, transduction mechanism studies and the use of newly synthesized agonists and antagonists, in keeping with other neurotransmitters, P2 receptors have been divided into two major families, a P2X receptor family which are ligand-gated ion channel receptors mediating fast transmission and a P2Y receptor family which are G protein-coupled receptors mediating slower responses. Currently, seven P2X ($P2X_{1-7}$) subclasses and eight P2Y ($P2Y_{1,2,4,6,8,11,12,13,14}$) subclasses have been recognized (Burnstock 2007b). These incorporate the receptors that respond to the pyrimidine derivatives UTP and UDP, as well as to ATP and also receptors that respond to adenine dinucleotide polyphosphates.

Neuropeptides

Peptides involved in neurotransmission in the autonomic nervous system are a large and diverse group (Table 5.1). Like the classic neurotransmitters, they are stored in vesicles and are released on depolarization to act on specific receptors to produce an effector response. However, by virtue of their structure, there are important differences from classic neurotransmission in their mode and site of synthesis and in their inactivation after release: namely, they are synthesized and packaged into vesicles in the nerve cell body rather than in nerve varicosities and there are no mechanisms for reuptake and recycling of neuropeptides after receptor activation (Dockray 1995). Neuropeptides are stored in large electron-dense cored vesicles and released by exocytosis. The regulation of neuropeptide neurotransmission is quite different from the classic neurotransmitters, because replacement of neuropeptides after release is dependent on new synthesis in the nerve cell body and axonal transport, a relatively slow processes compared with local synthesis in nerve terminals by enzymatic activity and replacement by efficient reuptake mechanisms. Neuropeptide release is more easily exhausted by repeated or prolonged stimulation.

There is no known reuptake mechanism for removal of neuropeptides from the site of action; their action is terminated by internalization and degradation of the receptor-bound peptide but mainly by metabolism by proteolytic enzymes. A few key ectoenzymes, including endopeptidase 24.11 and angiotensin-converting enzyme are thought to account for the degradation of most neuropeptides. The regulation of expression of these ectopeptidases is another level of modulation of peptidergic neurotransmission. Neuropeptide receptors are G protein-coupled receptors that activate either adenylyl cyclase or phospholipase C as signal transducers.

Nitric oxide

NO has been added to the list of putative neurotransmitters in the autonomic nervous system. The nature of these molecules and their actions means that it has been necessary to amend the criteria for defining a neurotransmitter. NO is not stored within neurons because they can travel freely through membranes. Furthermore, NO does not act on extracellular receptors on the postjunctional membrane of the target, but rather at intracellular sites (Fig. 5.3).

NO is synthesized in a reaction in which L-arginine is converted to L-citrulline by nitric oxide synthase (NOS). The reaction is dependent on NADPH, which is a cosubstrate with molecular oxygen. NOS can exist in three main isoforms (types I–III). Type I is constitutively expressed and was first identified in neurons (Lincoln et al. 1997). Immunohistochemical studies have shown that type I NOS is present in a variety of autonomic neurons.

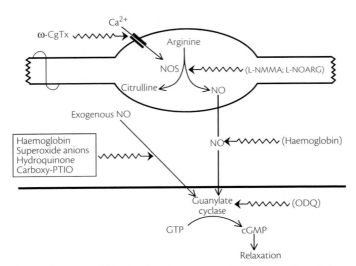

Fig. 5.3 Current model for the nitrergic neurotransmission process. The arrival of an action potential at the terminal region opens voltage-operated Ca^{2+} channels, allowing calcium to enter the neuronal cytoplasm and activate nitric oxide synthase (NOS). The enzyme converts l-arginine to l-citrulline, with the concomitant production of nitric oxide (NO). The NO rapidly diffuses out of the nerve cell, across the gap, and into the postjunctional cell (usually smooth muscle), where it binds to the haem group of soluble guanylate cyclase and consequently activates the conversion of guanosine triphosphate (GTP) to cyclic guanosine monophosphate (cGMP). Nitrergic transmission may be inhibited by ω-conotoxin (ω -CgTx; inhibits calcium channel), l-NG-monomethyl-arginine and l-NG nitro-arginine (l-NMMA and l-NOARG; inhibit NOS), haemoglobin (traps NO in the junctional gap), or 1H-[1,2,4]-oxadiazolo[4,3-a]quinoxalin-l-one (ODQ; inhibits soluble guanylate cyclase). Exogenous NO mimics the relaxant effect of nitrergic stimulation and is similarly inhibited by the presence of haemoglobin. However, several substances (superoxide anions; hydroquinone; carboxy-PTIO) strongly inhibit the relaxation to exogenous NO but have little effect on nitrergic responses, raising doubts about whether NO is released from the nerve as a free radical or in some other form. Reprinted from *Gen. Pharmacol.,* **28**, Gibson A. and Lilley E., Superoxide anions, free-radical scavengers, and nitrergic neurotransmission, 489–93, Copyright (1997), with permission from Elsevier.

Type I NOS only synthesizes small amounts of NO during conditions of raised intracellular Ca^{2+} such as occur during an action potential. This is of fundamental importance to the function of NO as a neurotransmitter. It is the synthesis of NO that is stimulated during transmission by a Ca^{2+}-dependent mechanism, not its release from intracellular stores. Analogues of l-arginine compete with l-arginine for binding of NOS and have been used as inhibitors of NOS in pharmacological studies. Such analogues have been instrumental in demonstrating NO-dependent responses in autonomic transmission.

Once NO has been synthesized, it can diffuse freely through membranes to the postjunctional target. Being a free radical, NO is unstable. Thus, for ending NO-dependent responses there is no need for the mechanisms such as degradative enzymes or reuptake that are required for other neurotransmitters. NO binds readily to the haem group of haemoglobin which can thus inhibit NO-dependent responses. Similarly, free radical generators such as hydroquinone and pyrogallol are frequently used to inhibit nitrergic transmission by the ability of free radicals to react with and inactivate NO. Conversely, superoxide dismutase, which removes superoxide anions, can enhance NO-dependent responses.

A variety of substances including sodium nitroprusside, S-nitroso-N-penicillamine and sydnonimins such as SIN-1 can

release NO. Such agents have been used as NO donors together with free NO to demonstrate that exogenous application of NO can mimic a nerve-mediated response. In autonomic transmission, NO produces its effects in the target predominantly by its interaction with intracellular guanylate cyclase.

Other neurotransmitters

Several other neurotransmitters have been identified in autonomic nerves (Robertson et al. 2004). 5-HT is an indolamine synthesized from tryptophan via 5-hydroxytryptophan by two enzymes, tryptophan hydroxylase and l-aromatic amino acid decarboxylase. Neuronal synthesis of 5-HT has been demonstrated in myenteric neurons, but it is also often regarded as false neurotransmitter as it is taken up and employed as a neurotransmitter by sympathetic nerves. 5-HT is taken up into small clear and large granular vesicles and is released in a Ca^{2+}-dependent manner. After release it is catabolized by MAO-A to 5-hydroxyindoleacetaldehyde and subsequently to 5-hydroxyindoleacetic acid. There are multiple 5-HT receptors (5-HT$_3$ ionotropic; 5-HT$_{1,2,4,5,6,7}$ metabotropic) in sympathetic, parasympathetic and sensory ganglia.

GABA, glutamate and dopamine, classical neurotransmitters in the central nervous system, are also autonomic neurotransmitters. GABA plays a role in enteric neurotransmission via excitatory GABA$_A$ and prejunctional inhibitory GABA$_B$ receptors. The GABA synthesizing and catabolizing enzymes (glutamate decarboxylase and 4-aminobutyrate:2-oxoglutarate transaminase, respectively), GABA itself, and high affinity GABA uptake sites have all been localized in gastrointestinal tissue.

After convincing evidence that NO can act as a neurotransmitter was presented, it was soon proposed that carbon monoxide (CO) could behave in an analogous way to NO as a neuronal messenger. There is recent evidence for endothelin in perivascular nerves in cerebral blood vessels.

Cotransmission/neuromodulation/ chemical coding

Cotransmission

The concept of cotransmission was first formulated by Burnstock in 1976 (Burnstock 1976) incorporating hints in the earlier literature from both vertebrate and invertebrate systems. It is now well established (Burnstock 1990a, 2004, Kupfermann 1991). Immunohistochemical evidence of coexistence of more than one neurotransmitter should not necessarily be interpreted as evidence of cotransmission since in order for substances to be termed cotransmitters it is essential to show that postjunctional actions to each substance occur via their own specific receptors. For example, many neuropeptides have slow trophic actions on surrounding tissues and this may be their primary role or they may act as neuromodulators. The relative contribution of each transmitter to neurogenic responses is dependent on the parameters of stimulation. For example, short bursts (1 second) of electrical stimulation of sympathetic nerves at low frequency (2–5 Hz) favour ATP release whereas longer periods of nerve stimulation (30 seconds or more) favour NA release.

Peptides, purine nucleotides and NO (identified by localization of NOS) are often found together with the classic neurotransmitters, NA and ACh. In fact, most, if not all, nerve fibres in the autonomic nervous system contain a mixture of different neurotransmitter

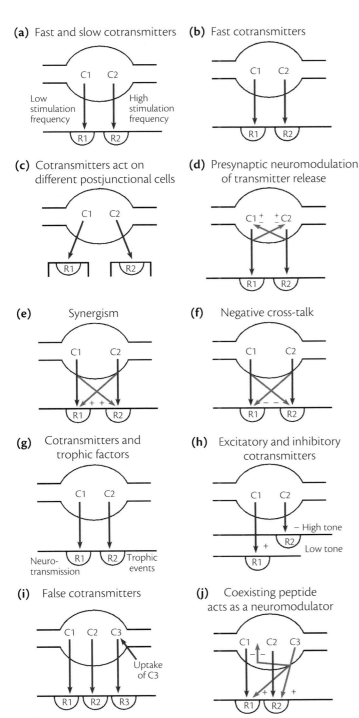

Fig. 5.4 Spectrum of signalling variations offered by cotransmission (blue arrows—neurotransmission; red arrows—prejunctional or postjunctional neuromodulation. **(a)** Fast transmission is usually produced by small molecules (C1) released at low frequency nerve stimulation acting on ionotropic receptors (R1), whereas slow transmission is usually produced by release of peptides (C2) or other molecules at high frequency stimulation acting on G protein-coupled receptors (R2). **(b)** Cotransmitters C1 and C2 can both be fast messengers acting via ionotropic receptors (R1 and R2). **(c)** Cotransmitters C1 and C2 act on receptors (R1 and R2) localized on different postjunctional cells. **(d)** Cotransmitters C1 and C2 not only act postjunctionally via R1 and R2 but can also act as prejunctional modulators to either inhibit (-) or enhance (+) the release of C1 and/or C2. **(e)** Cotransmitters C1 and C2 act synergistically to enhance the combined responses produced via R1 and R2 receptors. **(f)** Cotransmitters C1 and

substances that vary in proportion in different tissues and species and during development and disease. The widespread use of double and triple immunohistochemical labelling techniques has been critical to the demonstration of co-localization of potential cotransmitters within the same nerve fibre and has been invaluable when combined with electron microscopy. Different neurotransmitters within the same varicosity may be localized in the same or separate vesicular populations using postembedding colloidal gold techniques. In the gastrointestinal tract many neurons contain multiple transmitters (Furness and Sanger 2002). ATP is a cotransmitter with calcitonin gene-related peptide (CGRP) and substance P (SP) in many sensory-motor nerves and ATP, NO and vasoactive intestinal peptide (VIP) in enteric NANC inhibitory nerves. Transmitters with seemingly diverse and opposing effector action are sometimes co-localized in the same neuron, but generally they act in the same way and usually synergistically.

Neuromodulation

Some substances stored and released from nerves do not have direct actions on effector muscle cells but alter the release and/or the actions of other transmitters; these substances are termed neuromodulators. Many other substances (e.g. circulating neurohormones, locally released agents such as prostanoids, bradykinin, histamine and endothelin, and neurotransmitters from nearby nerves) are also neuromodulators in that they modify the process of neurotransmission. Many substances that are cotransmitters are also neuromodulators.

The wide and variable cleft characteristic of autonomic neuroeffector junctions makes them particularly amenable to the mechanisms of neural control mentioned above. The many different ways in which cotransmitters and neuromodulators interact to effect neurotransmission have been described (Burnstock 2004) and are outlined in Fig. 5.4.

Chemical coding

The precise combinations of neurotransmitters (and neuromodulators) contained in individual neurons and their projections and central connections, termed their 'chemical coding', has been defined in studies of the enteric nervous system (Furness and Costa 1987) and peripheral autonomic and sensory ganglia (Morris and Gibbins 1989).

C2 may act to inhibit the responses evoked via R1 and/or R2. **(g)** Cotransmitter C1 evokes neurotransmission via R1 receptors, while C2 evokes long-term (trophic) responses of postjunctional cells via R2 receptors. **(h)** Cotransmitter C1 produces excitation via R1 receptors when the postjunctional smooth muscle target has low tone, with C2 having little influence, but when the smooth muscle tone is high, the dominant response might be relaxation produced by C2 via R2 receptors. **(i)** Substance C3 is taken up by nerve terminals, rather than being synthesized and stored as is true for the cotransmitters C1 and C2. C3 may then be released on nerve stimulation to act on postjunctional R3 receptors. In these circumstances, C3 would be known as a 'false transmitter'. **(j)** A coexisting substance C3 (often a peptide) can be synthesized and stored in a nerve, but not act directly via a postjunctional receptor to produce changes in postjunctional cell activity. It may, however, act as a prejunctional inhibitor (−) of the release of the cotransmitters C1 and C2 or as a postjunctional enhancer (+) of the responses mediated by R1 and R2. Reprinted from *Int. Rev. Cytol.* **240**, Burnstock G. and Knight G., Cellular distribution and functions of P2 receptor subtypes in different systems, 31–304, Copyright (2004), with permission from Elsevier.

Neurotransmission at the sympathetic neuroeffector junctions: evidence for co-release and roles of NA, ATP and NPY

It is now recognized that the main neurotransmitters/neuromodulators in postganglionic sympathetic nerves are NA, ATP and neuropeptide Y (NPY) (Burnstock 1995, Lundberg 1996, Burnstock and Verkhratsky 2010). These substances are co-released in varying proportions, depending on the tissue and species, and also on the parameters of stimulation. Short bursts at low frequency particularly favour the purinergic component, whereas longer periods of nerve stimulation favour the adrenergic component and NPY release is optimal with high frequency intermittent bursts of stimulation. A considerable variability in the contribution of a purinergic component to sympathetic neurotransmission has been demonstrated in different blood vessels, for example, rabbit saphenous and mesenteric arteries have a substantial purinergic component, whereas in the rabbit ear artery the purinergic component is relatively small. In intestinal submucosal arteries the responses to sympathetic nerve stimulation are mediated solely by ATP with NA acting as a prejunctional modulator via α_2-adrenoceptors. The initial electrophysiological postjunctional response to sympathetic nerve stimulation is a rapid, transient EJP that is mediated by ATP. In some vessels the EJP is followed by a slow depolarization that is mediated by NA. Postjunctionally, the effects of ATP and NA released as sympathetic cotransmitters are generally synergistic. NA and ATP can depress sympathetic neurotransmission by prejunctional modulation, via α_2-adrenoceptors or predominantly via P1 receptors following extracellular breakdown to adenosine, but also via P2 receptors in some vessels. Prejunctional P2 receptor-mediated increase in NA release has also been reported.

In most tissues, including the vas deferens and many blood vessels, NPY does not act as a genuine neurotransmitter, having little direct postjunctional action, but rather acts as a neuromodulator, often by prejunctional attenuation of NA and ATP release and/or postjunctional potentiation of responses to adrenergic and purinergic components of sympathetic nerve responses. In tissues where NPY does have a direct vasoconstrictor effect, for example in blood vessels of the spleen and kidney and coronary and cerebral arteries, the response is characteristically slow in onset and long lasting.

Other substances localized within sympathetic nerves include 5-HT, which is largely taken up by sympathetic nerves and released as a false transmitter. Opioid peptides are also widely distributed in sympathetic neurons where their functional role appears to be related to their prejunctional inhibitory effects on sympathetic neurotransmission.

Neurotransmission at the parasympathetic neuroeffector junctions: the atropine-resistant components of parasympathetic neurotransmission

ACh, VIP, ATP and NO are cotransmitters commonly synthesized in and released from parasympathetic nerves (Lundberg 1996). As with sympathetic cotransmission, the relative functional importance of the cotransmitters in parasympathetic neurotransmission is variable in different tissues and species. For example, NO may be the main mediator of neurogenic vasodilatation in cerebral vessels, whereas VIP may be of more importance during neurogenic vasodilatation in the pancreas. The coordinated roles of VIP and ACh in parasympathetic neurotransmission were demonstrated in an elegant study of the cat exocrine salivary gland innervation. This showed that VIP and ACh were stored in separate vesicles in the

same nerve terminal, and were both released upon transmural nerve stimulation, but with different stimulation parameters. ACh was released during low frequency stimulation to increase salivary secretion from acinar cells and to elicit some minor dilatation of blood vessels in the gland. At high stimulation frequencies, VIP was released to produce marked dilatation of the blood vessels in the gland and to act as a neuromodulator postjunctionally on the acinar gland to enhance the actions of ACh, and prejunctionally on the nerve varicosities to enhance the release of ACh. ACh was also found to have an inhibitory action on the release of VIP. VIP has since been shown to have a direct vasodilatory action in the submandibular gland in man. PACAP also seems to be present in VIP-containing parasympathetic nerves. NOS is often colocalized with ACh and VIP in parasympathetic nerves innervating blood vessels. Postganglionic nerves from pelvic ganglia containing VIP, ACh and NOS project to the urethra, colon and penis. The human bladder body receives a dense parasympathetic innervation comprised predominantly of ACh-containing nerves. In the rodent bladder, ATP is a major cotransmitter in these nerves. However, only a small purinergic component is present in human bladder, except in pathological conditions.

Neurotransmission at sensory-motor neuroeffector junctions: the roles of SP, CGRP, and ATP

The motor function of sensory nerves, whereby antidromic impulses down collatoral fibres results in local release of sensory neurotransmitters, is widespread in autonomic effector systems and forms an important physiological component of autonomic control (Rubino and Burnstock 1996). To distinguish these nerves from the other subpopulation of afferent fibres that have an entirely sensory role and have terminals containing few vesicles and a predominance of mitochondria, they have been termed 'sensory-motor' nerves

SP and CGRP are cotransmitters in many unmyelinated, primary afferent nerves. They often coexist in the same large granular vesicles in capsaicin-sensitive nerve terminals. The proportions of coexistence of SP and CGRP varies with species; for example, in the guinea pig most sensory neurons containing CGRP also contain SP, but in the rat about 50% of CGRP-containing neurons do not contain SP. In the vasculature, unlike CGRP, SP does not appear to act directly on receptors of the vascular smooth muscle, but rather acts via occupation of receptors on endothelial cells lining the lumen to bring about NO release and consequent vasodilatation. This action of neurally released SP may be particularly important in the microvasculature, but access of neurally released SP to the endothelium in large vessels is questionable; it is largely released from endothelial cells to act on receptors on endothelial cells to release NO, resulting in vasodilation (Burnstock and Ralevic 1994). ATP is now also established as a cotransmitter with glutamate in small primary sensory nerves in the gut mediating mechanical and/or nociceptive signals (Burnstock 2001a).

Other neuropeptides and transmitters have been localized in sensory-motor nerves. For example, in the human urinary bladder, VIP, cholecystokinin (CCK) and dynorphin (DYN) are present together with SP and CGRP in the afferent projections to the lumbosacral spinal cord. In the guinea pig, dorsal root ganglia neurons containing SP, CGRP, CCK and DYN project to the epidermis and small dermal blood vessels. NOS has been localized in populations of primary sensory neurons of trigeminal and dorsal root ganglia.

Endothelin, a potent vasoconstrictor peptide with mitogenic actions is also localized in neurons of these sensory ganglia, often co localized with SP. There are increasing examples in the literature of cross-talk between sensory-motor, sympathetic and parasympathetic nerves. In the heart, SP has excitatory effects on cardiac parasympathetic innervation, in contrast to CGRP which is inhibitory.

Neurotransmission involving intrinsic neurons: special reference to neurotransmitters localized in nerve cell bodies in the heart, bladder, intestine, and lung

Many intrinsic neurons localized within autonomic neuroeffector tissues are part of the postganglionic parasympathetic system, but there are also intrinsic neurons derived from neural crest tissue that is different from that which forms sympathetic and parasympathetic neurons. For example, intrinsic neurons that are abundant in the gut and possibly subpopulations in the heart and airways.

The most extensive system of intrinsic neurons is in the myenteric and submucous plexuses of the gastrointestinal tract. These enteric neurons contain numerous neuroactive substances of which most are involved in neurotransmission or neuromodulation at the ganglion level and/or have a trophic role; only a small percentage are involved in neuromuscular transmission. The chemical coding of enteric neurons has been examined in detail, particularly in the guinea pig (Furness and Sanger 2002). ATP, NO and VIP mediate NANC inhibitory neurotransmission in the gut in varying proportions depending on the region. ACh and SP are cotransmitters in enteric excitatory neurons.

There are many intrinsic neurons in the heart, particularly in the right atrium. The neurochemical makeup of the intrinsic cardiac ganglia is heterogeneous and includes a variety of neurochemical markers. For example, subpopulations of atrial intrinsic neurons from newborn guinea pigs immunostain for NPY, 5-HT, haem oxygenase-2 and NOS, and these neurons probably also utilize ACh and ATP. Most airway intrinsic neurons contain ChAT, but NOS and VIP are also found in these neurons in humans. Intrinsic ganglia in the human urinary bladder wall contain a number of neuroactive substances (VIP, NOS, NPY, ATP, galanin and occasionally TH); in the bladder neck, a few intrinsic neurons contain enkephalin (ENK) and SP. Intramural ganglia containing NPY and VIP have been identified in human urethra.

Plasticity of the autonomic nervous system: some examples of altered expression of neurotransmitters/neuromodulators in autonomic nerves during development, ageing, following trauma, surgery, chronic exposure to drugs and in disease

Neurons possess the genetic potential to produce many neurotransmitters. The particular combination and quantity that results is partly pre-programmed and partly determined by 'trophic' factors and hormones that trigger the expression or suppression of the appropriate genetic machinery. A number of studies have demonstrated the plasticity of the autonomic nervous system in development and ageing, following trauma, surgery, and chronic exposure to drugs, and in disease (Milner and Burnstock 1994). The plasticity of expression of neural substances coordinated to environmental cues allows rapid and precise matching of neurotransmission to altered demands. Several neurotransmitters/neuromodulators are themselves trophic molecules, with mitogenic or growth-promoting/growth-inhibiting properties.

There are often remarkable changes in the organization and neurotransmitter expression in the autonomic nervous system as a result of pathophysiological situations such as trauma, surgery or disease (Burnstock 1990b). Some of this plasticity is of compensatory advantage, while some lead to altered neural control of effector tissues which is not beneficial. Manipulation of the ANS to encourage beneficial compensatory changes in nerve growth and the expression of neurotransmitters/neuromodulators and their receptors is an attractive approach to therapeutic manipulation of autonomic dysfunction.

Development and ageing

Vascular developmental innervation patterns vary considerably with the location and species. Developmental changes in the density of nerve fibres containing both NA and NPY supplying the basilar artery of the young rat do not proceed in synchrony; increased expression of NA occurs between 4–6 weeks, while increased expression of NPY occurs later, at 6–8 weeks.

During development, NA-containing sympathetic nerves innervating sweat glands acquire cholinergic and peptidergic function. When axons first contact the developing glands they exhibit only catecholamine fluorescence and immunoreactivity to TH. With maturation, cholinergic markers (AChE and ChAT) and VIP are detected, followed by CGRP-immunoreactivity several days later, while adrenergic markers disappear. Visceral targets specify neurotransmitter expression in sympathetic, parasympathetic and sensory nerves during development. There is plasticity too in the responses to cotransmitters during development: for example, during the transition from neonate to adult, the relative contribution of ATP and ACh to contractile responses of the urinary bladder changes; in the neonate rabbit, responses to ATP are significantly greater than in the adult, while those to ACh remain constant.

The innervation of autonomic target tissues varies considerably with increasing age. Age-related changes, in the pattern of innervation of blood vessels by sympathetic nerves, vary from one vessel to another (Cowen and Gavazzi 1998). For example, the adrenergic innervation of small arteries (mesenteric, femoral and basilar) of ageing rabbits changes only slightly while the larger elastic arteries (renal and carotid) show a significant reduction in nerve density in old age. Immunohistochemical studies have shown that there is a decrease in vasoconstrictor and increase in vasodilator neurotransmitters in cerebrovascular nerves in old age. In rat cerebral vessels there is a reduction in the density of nerve fibres containing NA with age, as in other vessels, and an increase in the density of CGRP and VIP-immunoreactive nerves. In the mesenteric arterial bed, decreased sensory nerve vasodilator function occurs in old age. In the femoral artery, CGRP levels are reduced, while NPY levels remain constant.

The responsiveness of sensory CGRP-positive neurons to nerve growth factor (NGF) does not vary with age, but sympathetic nerves require more NGF in old animals to increase nerve density. In the gastrointestinal tract, there is extensive loss of enteric neurons and extrinsic sympathetic innervation in old age. While the total number of myenteric neurons in the intestine declines with age, an increasing proportion that remain contain NOS.

Age-related up or down regulation of neurotransmitter receptor expression adds to overall changes in autonomic function.

For example, increased A_1 adenosine receptor density in the rabbit heart with ageing may explain the increased sensitivity of senescent heart to the negative inotropic action of adenosine. Decreased expression of this receptor in the testis of the aged rat may be related to deficiencies in spermatogenesis accompanying the ageing process.

Pregnancy

During pregnancy the uterine wall undergoes considerable hypertrophy and hyperplasia with profound changes in innervation, particularly in the fetus-bearing regions. There is a progressive loss of NA-containing nerves innervating the uterus leading to a disappearance of these sympathetic nerves in late pregnancy in parallel with a decrease in NPY- and VIP-containing nerves (Milner and Burnstock 1994). Afferent rather than motor responses of sensory-motor nerves may predominate in late pregnancy as the relaxant responses to CGRP are diminished or absent at term.

In late pregnancy, there is hypertrophy and hyperplasia of the smooth muscle of uterine artery, but the density of innervation of this vessel remains high because of the growth of many new axons. There is, however, a marked decrease of NA-containing nerves and NA content while, at the same time, there is an increase in NPY. 5-Hydroxydopamine is normally taken up by the high affinity NA uptake mechanism in sympathetic nerves. There is an increase in the proportion of 5-hydroxydopamine-labelled varicosities in the uterine artery during pregnancy. In late pregnancy, there is a switch from adrenergic to predominantly cholinergic responses in this vessel. In pregnant human uterine arteries, sympathetic responses to electrical field stimulation and endogenous NA levels are reduced and neuronally mediated dilatation, mediated in part by NO, is increased.

NPY, CGRP and SP perivascular expression in the kidney cortex is diminished in late pregnancy. Dysfunction of these mechanisms during pregnancy may contribute to the development of pre-eclampsia.

Trauma and surgery

In addition to surgical denervation, guanethidine and capsaicin are two neurotoxins that have been used as tools to study the effects of either selective long-term sympathectomy or sensory (primary afferent) denervation, respectively. Chemical denervation and selected ganglionectomy studies have shown that loss of sympathetic or sensory innervation induces remarkable changes in the nerves that remain. For example, in certain situations there may be a switch in phenotype from cholinergic to adrenergic following reinnervation after sympathectomy. Neonatal sensory denervation facilitates reinnervation of smooth muscle by sympathetic nerves and results in sympathetic hyperinnervation of selected tissues such as the small blood vessels in the rat lung.

Total denervation of extrinsic nerves to the gut provokes marked plasticity of enteric neurons. Submucosal arteries normally innervated by extrinsic sympathetic and sensory nerves are reinnervated by an abundance of SP- and VIP-containing nerves of intrinsic origin. Loss of extrinsic nerves to the gut is associated with an increase in NOS-containing neurons in the myenteric plexus and potentiation of inhibitory neurotransmission to longitudinal smooth muscle. Following extrinsic denervation of the human respiratory tract by heart–lung transplantation, there are significant changes to the neurochemical makeup of the intrinsic neurons that remain: namely, there is the appearance of NPY- and TH- positive neurons that are not found in non-transplanted respiratory tract. Following transection of preganglionic autonomic nerves or in spinal cord injury there are marked changes in the nerves that remain. Such changes can be manifested not only as nerve growth and changes in neurotransmitter expression but, remarkably, in reorganization of nerve pathways and their function. The most dramatic examples of such plasticity occur in the urogenital tract and it is probable that anatomical reorganization of nerve pathways in this region accounts for this.

Parasympathetic decentralization either by transection of the pelvic nerve or ventral roots in the cat has been shown to result in an increase of NA-containing nerves in the bladder and urethra. Similar changes have been found in human bladders from patients with sacral spinal cord lesions. Increased expression of NA-containing nerves has also been observed in the striated muscle of the external urethral sphincter in humans following sacral spinal cord injury.

Disease

Disorders of the urogenital tract can occur for a wide variety of reasons. Those involving the autonomic nervous system range from trauma and diseases such as multiple sclerosis that affect the preganglionic autonomic neurons in the spinal cord, to iatrogenic causes such as radical surgery or X-irradiation that can result in local nerve damage, and, finally, metabolic disorders such as diabetes that affect autonomic neuromuscular transmission. The most common cause of bladder dysfunction in males is obstruction resulting from benign prostatic hypertrophy. Receptor expression may be affected following obstruction. Increased expression of α-adrenoceptors has been observed in human bladder strips from patients with prostatic bladder obstruction and NA can cause contraction of the muscle, a response that does not usually occur in unobstructed bladder. Similarly, under normal conditions, the contractile response to nerve stimulation in human bladder does not contain a significant purinergic component indicated by atropine resistance. However, increased purinergic transmission can be demonstrated in patients with unstable obstructed bladders (Burnstock 2001c, 2006). Upregulation of purinergic receptors appears to occur in hyporeflexia, whether this is due to obstruction, interstitial cystitis or neurogenic bladders.

Penile erection is a vascular event and it is important to recognize that local vasodilatation in the penis is under dual control by autonomic nerves and the endothelium. In the periphery major causes of impotence are vascular disease and diabetic autonomic neuropathy. Both neurogenic and endothelium-dependent relaxation of erectile smooth muscle can be impaired in diabetic men with impotence and in experimental diabetes. Within the corpus cavernosum, reduced levels of NA and decreased innervation by VIP-containing and AChE-positive nerve fibres have been reported in diabetic patients with impotence.

VIP levels are reduced in the myenteric plexus and muscle layers of patients with idiopathic constipation, while levels of SP and NPY are normal. In constipation associated with idiopathic megacolon or megarectum, abnormalities in inhibitory systems may contribute to abnormal gut function and subsequent bowel dilatation: in the rectum of these patients the density of innervation by nerves containing VIP and NADPH-diaphorase (a marker for NOS) is increased in the muscularis mucosae and lamina propria, but decreased in the longitudinal muscle layer.

Irregularities of the sympathetic nervous system, renin-angiotensin system and endothelial factors have all been implicated in the development of hypertension.

Examination of sympathetic neurotransmission in the tail and mesenteric arteries of the spontaneously hypertensive rat (SHR) has revealed a greater cotransmitter role for ATP compared with NA. Decreased sensory-motor nerve innervation may contribute to the development of hypertension. In the mesenteric arterial bed, the density of CGRP-containing nerve fibres and sensory-motor vasodilatation is decreased in the SHR and plasma CGRP levels are decreased. Defective neurovascular sensory motor control as an early event is suggested by the reduction of CGRP-containing nerve fibre density around capillaries in dermal papillae in Raynaud's phenomenon and systemic sclerosis. Reduced sensory innervation may affect the endothelial expression of vasoconstrictor and vasodilator substances and contribute to the pathology of this disorder.

Diabetes is the most common cause of autonomic neuropathy. Diabetic autonomic neuropathy has been implicated in dysfunction of the cardiovascular, gastrointestinal, and urogenital systems. Not all autonomic nerves are affected in the same way by diabetes. Thus, in rat cerebral vessels, there is a reduction of VIP and 5-HT, but not NPY or NA in perivascular nerves in STZ-induced diabetes. In the proximal colon, intrinsic VIP-containing and extrinsic NA-containing nerves undergo degeneration in STZ-induced diabetes, while 5-HT, SP- and CGRP-containing nerves display altered levels of their neurotransmitters without undergoing degeneration. NPY-containing nerves appear to be unaffected by diabetes in this region.

Conclusion

A combination of the variety of neurotransmitters involved in autonomic neurotransmission and the interactions between sympathetic, parasympathetic, sensory-motor nerves, and those arising from intrinsic ganglia, via mechanisms of cotransmission, and prejunctional and postjunctional neuromodulation, indicate the complexity of peripheral autonomic control and the variety of ways by which autonomic dysfunction can occur. Recent advances in the unravelling of these mechanisms, together with molecular identification of specific receptor subtypes, and localization and characterization of their expression, and of the long-term effects of dysfunction, will bring advances towards the design of treatment regimens to combat autonomic failure.

References

Burnstock, G. (1972). Purinergic nerves. *Pharmacol. Rev.* **24**, 509–81.

Burnstock, G. (1976). Do some nerve cells release more than one transmitter? *Neuroscience* **1**, 239–48.

Burnstock, G. (1978). A basis for distinguishing two types of purinergic receptor. In R. W. Straub, L. Bolis, eds *Cell Membrane Receptors for Drugs and Hormones: A Multidisciplinary Approach*, pp. 107–18. Raven Press, New York.

Burnstock, G. (1986a). The changing face of autonomic neurotransmission (The first von Euler lecture in physiology). *Acta Physiol. Scand.* **126**, 67–91.

Burnstock, G. (1986b). Autonomic neuromuscular junctions: current developments and future directions. *J. Anat.* **146**, 1–30.

Burnstock, G. (1988). Autonomic neural control mechanisms, with special reference to the airways. In M. A. Kaliner, P.J. Barnes, eds *The Airways: Neural Control in Health and Disease*. Pp. 1–22. Marcel Dekker, New York.

Burnstock, G. (1990a). Co-transmission. The Fifth Heymans Lecture—Ghent, 17 February 1990. *Arch. Int. Pharmacodyn. Thér.* **304**, 7–33.

Burnstock, G. (1990b). Changes in expression of autonomic nerves in aging and disease. *J. Auton. Nerv. Syst.* **30**, S25–34.

Burnstock, G. (1995). Noradrenaline and ATP: cotransmitters and neuromodulators. *J. Physiol. Pharmacol.* **46**, 365–84.

Burnstock, G. (1997). The past, present and future of purine nucleotides as signalling molecules. *Neuropharmacology*, **36**, 1127–39.

Burnstock, G. (2001a). Purinergic signalling in gut. In M. P. Abbracchio, M. Williams, eds *Handbook of Experimental Pharmacology, Volume 151/II. Purinergic and Pyrimidinergic Signalling II—Cardiovascular, Respiratory, Immune, Metabolic and Gastrointestinal Tract Function*, pp. 141–238. Springer-Verlag, Berlin.

Burnstock, G. (2001b). Purine-mediated signalling in pain and visceral perception. *Trends Pharmacol. Sci.* 22, 182–88.

Burnstock, G. (2001c). Purinergic signalling in lower urinary tract. In M. P. Abbracchio, M. Williams, eds *Handbook of Experimental Pharmacology, Volume 151/I. Purinergic and Pyrimidinergic Signalling I—Molecular, Nervous and Urinogenitary System Function*, pp. 423–515. Springer-Verlag, Berlin.

Burnstock, G. (2004). Cotransmission. *Curr. Op. Pharmacol.* **4**, 47–52.

Burnstock, G. (2006) Pathophysiology and therapeutic potential of purinergic signaling. *Pharmacol. Rev.*, **58**, 58–86.

Burnstock, G. (2007a) Physiology and pathophysiology of purinergic neurotransmission. *Physiol. Rev.* **87**, 659–797.

Burnstock, G. (2007b) Purine and pyrimidine receptors. *Cell. Mol. Life Sci.* **64**, 1471–83.

Burnstock, G. (2008) Non-synaptic transmission at autonomic neuroeffector junctions. *Neurochem. Int.* **52**, 14–25.

Burnstock, G. (2009). Autonomic neurotransmission: 60 years since Sir Henry Dale. *Ann. Rev. Pharmacol. Toxicol.* **49**, 1–30.

Burnstock, G. and Knight, G. (2004). Cellular distribution and functions of P. 2 receptor subtypes in different systems. *Int. Rev. Cytol.* **240**, 31–304.

Burnstock, G. and Ralevic, V. (1994). New insights into the local regulation of blood flow by perivascular nerves and endothelium. *Br. J. Plastic Surg.* **47**, 527–43.

Burnstock, G. and Verkhratsky, A. (2010). Vas deferens—a model used to establish sympathetic cotransmission. *Trends Pharmacol. Sci.* **31**, 131–39.

Cowen, T. and Gavazzi, I. (1998). Plasticity in adult and ageing sympathetic neurons. *Prog. Neurobiol.* **54**, 249–88.

Dockray, G. J. (1995). Transmission: Peptides. In G. Burnstock, C. H. V. Hoyle, eds *Autonomic Neuroeffector Mechanisms*, pp. 409–64. Harwood Academic, Chur, Switzerland.

Fillenz, M. (1995). Transmission: Noradrenaline. In G. Burnstock, C. H. V. Hoyle, eds *Autonomic Neuroeffector Mechanisms*, pp. 323–65. Harwood Academic, Chur, Switzerland.

Furness, J. B. and Costa, M. (1987). *The Enteric Nervous System*. Churchill Livingstone, Edinburgh.

Furness, J. B. and Sanger, G. J. (2002). Intrinsic nerve circuits of the gastrointestinal tract: identification of drug targets. *Curr. Op. Pharmacol.* **2**, 612–22.

Gibson, A. and Lilley, E. (1997). Superoxide anions, free-radical scavengers, and nitrergic neurotransmission. *Gen. Pharmacol.* **28**, 489–93.

Hoyle, C. H. V. and Burnstock, G. (1996). Criteria for defining enteric neurotransmitters. In T. S. Gaginella, ed. *Handbook of Methods in Pharmacology*, pp. 123–40. CRC Press, London.

Kupfermann, I. (1991). Functional studies of cotransmission. *Physiol. Rev.* **71**, 683–732.

Lincoln, J., Hoyle, C. H. V. and Burnstock, G. (1997). *Nitric Oxide in Health and Disease*, pp. 1–355. Cambridge University Press, Cambridge.

Lundberg, J. M. (1996). Pharmacology of cotransmission in the autonomic nervous system: integrative aspects on amines, neuropeptides, adenosine triphosphate, amino acids and nitric oxide. *Pharmacol. Rev.* **48**, 113–78.

Milner, P. and Burnstock, G. (1994). Trophic factors and the control of smooth muscle development and innervation. Volume 1. In D. Raeburn, M. A. Giembycz, eds *Airways Smooth Muscle: Development and Regulation of Contractility,* pp. 1–39. Birkhauser Verlag, Switzerland.

Morris, J. L. and Gibbins, I. L. (1989). Co-localization and plasticity of transmitters in peripheral autonomic and sensory neurons. *Int. J. Dev. Neurosci.* **7**, 521–31.

Ralevic, V. and Burnstock, G. (1998). Receptors for purines and pyrimidines. *Pharmacol. Rev.* 50, 413–92.

Robertson, D., Biaggioni, I., Burnstock, G. and Low, P. (2004). *Primer on the autonomic nervous system, 2nd Edition,* pp. 1–459. Elsevier, San Diego.

Rubino, A. and Burnstock, G. (1996). Capsaicin-sensitive sensory-motor neurotransmission in the peripheral control of cardiovascular function. *Cardiovasc. Res.* **31**, 467–79.

CHAPTER 6

Autonomic surgical neuroanatomy

Sanjay Purkayastha, J. Anthony Firth and Ara W. Darzi

Key points

- The outflow nerves of the autonomic nervous system (ANS) are generally considered to be III, VII, IX, X and S2–S4 (craniosacral—parasympathetic) and T1–L2 (thoracolumbar—sympathetic).

- The two ANS divisions do not act in simple opposition; the parasympathetic is restricted to the viscera, and the distinction between sympathetic and parasympathetic is not sharp, particularly in the pelvic plexus.

- Sympathetic postganglionic neurons for the somatic area and the thoracic viscera reside in the paravertebral ganglia; those for the abdominal and pelvic viscera are mainly in the pre-aortic ganglia.

- In general enteroceptive (biofeedback) sensory fibres run with the parasympathetic and visceral pain fibres with the sympathetic.

- Surgery for regulatory problems of the ANS is most common for the sympathetic system.

- Conditions warranting surgery include hyperhidrosis, Frey's syndrome, chronic regional pain syndrome, refractory angina and cardiac arrhythmias, and Raynaud's syndrome.

- There are numerous approaches that may be used due to the diversity of the anatomy of the ANS, but in general the approaches may be local, open or laparoscopic.

- Avoidance of injury to the ANS during general surgical procedures is a concept that surgeons must be aware of to reduce operative morbidity.

Introduction

Autonomic neuroanatomy was studied closely along with its physiology, initially by Claude Bernard in France, during the mid-nineteenth century. Later in the same century, Ernst Heinrich Weber, a German physiologist noted that this functional neuronal unit was comprised of two opposing systems, the parasympathetic and sympathetic systems. It was not until the beginning of the twentieth century that the regulatory and involuntary functional aspects of the autonomic nervous system (ANS) were mapped and described by William Gaskell along with John Langley at Cambridge University.

Surgical treatment for conditions related to autonomic neuropathology or regulatory dysfunction date back to the late nineteenth century, when a form of cervical sympathectomy was performed as a treatment for epilepsy by Alexander, closely followed by stellectomies for exophthalmic goitre by Jaboulay and Jonnesco, treatment for glaucoma and surgery on the ANS related to visual function to name but a few of the early ANS surgical procedures. Such surgery relies on a precise understanding of not only the underlying neuroanatomy but also the general anatomy of the region involved in the surgical approach and the other structures in danger throughout the approach and definitive procedure. Due to the central nature of the core anatomical components of the ANS these approaches have varied not only in their delineation (e.g. anterior or posterior), but also in their region (e.g. supraclavicular, axillary, thoracic, lumbar) and their type (e.g. open, laparoscopic, and percutaneous).

Thus the understanding of surgical anatomy required for performing procedures on the ANS almost falls within the remit of the old fashioned 'general surgeon'. However with super-specialization and the increasing number of subspecialties within general surgery, it is more common for surgeons with 'regional' expertise to carry out such procedures (i.e. a thoracic surgeon for thoracic sympathectomies or a gastrointestinal surgeon carrying out lumbar sympathectomies). However 'generalists' are becoming apparent in the field of surgery on the ANS. These are usually one of two entities: firstly, surgeons with a specific interest in ANS surgery (tertiary referral) or, secondly, radiologists who carry out image-guided percutaneous procedures on any region of the ANS system.

Thus, taking into consideration all the possible approaches, procedures, and pathology that may be treated surgically, it is obvious that the ideal understanding of anatomy is that which covers the breadth of anatomical diversity involved. However, more specifically it is important to gain a general understanding of the anatomy of the ANS and an understanding of the benefits and pitfalls of the common approaches for the most common procedures carried out today. Finally it is also important to gauge when the ANS structures are at risk when other surgical procedures are being carried out. This chapter aims to provide an understanding of the aforementioned important concepts in anatomy related to autonomic surgery.

Following a description of the general anatomy of the ANS the anatomy relevant to the surgery for the following procedures will be discussed:

- surgery for hyperhidrosis
- treatment for Frey's syndrome
- treatment for chronic regional pain syndrome
- treatment for refractory angina and cardiac arrhythmias
- treatment of Raynaud's syndrome
- avoidance of injury to the ANS during general surgical procedures.

Autonomic anatomical basics

Strategy of the autonomic nervous system

The ANS has evolved in vertebrates to provide a mechanism for regulation of smooth and cardiac muscle, and of exocrine glands that is more rapid in action than a circulating endocrine signal. In addition the autonomic, being based on neuronal connections, has inbuilt anatomical specificity of targeting, unlike endocrine signals, the targeting of which is determined purely by which cells express appropriate receptors. Thus autonomic nerves are able to target a particular sector of those cells expressing acetylcholine (ACh), catecholamine or various other receptors.

This raises the question of why such neuronal control cannot be executed by motor neurons similar to those controlling skeletal muscle. Such a mechanism would be possible but would be very uneconomical in terms of the amount of central nervous space that would be required. Control of skeletal muscle requires precision of targeting, each neuron having exclusive control of a single motor unit comprising tens, hundreds or thousands of skeletal muscle cells so that activity of a muscle can be increased by increments of the size of single motor units. Skeletal muscle is completely dependent on its innervation and, in the absence of neuronal input, loses all tone and atrophies in the longer term. By contrast, the tissues innervated by the autonomic are frequently regulated by a variety of local, circulating, and synaptic inputs, so the ANS up-regulates or down-regulates this background activity. Usually there is no need for each cell to receive its own autonomic synapse because of the extensive electrical coupling of smooth and cardiac muscle, and epithelial cells through gap junctions. The lower dependence of autonomic target tissues on spatially precise innervation means that it is acceptable for a fairly small number of central neurons (the preganglionic cells) to synapse in autonomic ganglia with a much larger number of postganglionic neurons; this multiplies the numbers of neuroeffector synapses that can be formed without a large requirement for space within the central nervous system. Rapid response is only crucial for skeletal muscle, so the delay produced by the ganglionic synapse is not important for the autonomic target tissues.

Autonomic preganglionic neurons lie within the lateral column of spinal cord grey matter or its extension into the brainstem. Overall integration of autonomic function depends on the hypothalamus, often via reticular centres in the brainstem and descending reticular pathways in the spinal cord. In general, the rostral parts of the hypothalamus integrate the parasympathetic whereas the sympathetic depends on more caudal hypothalamic regions, though there is considerable overlap. Postganglionic sympathetic neurons,

like the sensory neurons of the dorsal root ganglia, develop from migrating neural crest cells rather than from the neural tube itself.

The name 'autonomic' suggests independence from regulation by other parts of the central nervous system. However, the limbic system provides substantial input into the hypothalamic autonomic centres; perhaps this is not surprising in view of the well-known responses of autonomic targets to emotional states. The fact that some degree of control of such responses can be learned may point to a reason for the significant inputs from various regions of the cerebral cortex.

Sympathetic and parasympathetic systems

The preganglionic neurons of the autonomic form a single discontinuous column consisting of the parasympathetic nuclei of the oculomotor, facial, glossopharyngeal and vagus nerves, the thoracolumbar sympathetic column and the sacral parasympathetic column. This strongly implies that a proto-autonomic system in the early vertebrates subsequently differentiated into sympathetic and parasympathetic components that came to overlap extensively in the distributions of their postganglionic components within the body (Butler and Hodos 1996, Gibbins 1993, Young 1981). It is thus not a surprise that both the sympathetic and the parasympathetic use cholinergic (nicotinic type) receptors at the ganglionic synapses between preganglionic and postganglionic neurons.

The common origin of the two divisions of the ANS may also account for the fact that the relationship of autonomic division to postganglionic transmitter is not clear-cut. In mature human sweat glands the sympathetic supply is unusual in being cholinergic, but in infants these synapses are adrenergic. In various species, such as horses, sweat gland innervation remains adrenergic throughout life. All this is a considerable simplification, as purinergic and peptidergic terminals can also be identified as components of the sympathetic supply to target organs (Kennedy et al. 1994, Lundberg 1996).

One of the most important distinctions between the craniosacral (parasympathetic) and the thoracolumbar (sympathetic) outflows is their distribution. The sympathetic distributes to target structures throughout the entire body, whereas the parasympathetic distributes only to visceral structures (broadly interpreted to include the optic globe). Autonomic targets in the body wall, limbs and skin receive a sympathetic outflow but no parasympathetic.

Two systems in opposition?

The concept of opposite actions of sympathetic and parasympathetic innervation is of rather limited usefulness.

- Sympathetic nerves distribute to the whole body whereas the parasympathetic supply is to visceral structures only. Thus somatic vascular smooth muscle, sweat glands and erector pili muscles lack any parasympathetic supply.

- Even if an organ receives both sympathetic and parasympathetic nerves, they may innervate different tissues and so not be opposite in action. In the heart, the sympathetic innervates the pacemaker and myocardium so increases both rate and force of contraction, whereas the vagal parasympathetic innervates the pacemaker only so affects rate but not force.

- Possibly the most 'classic' example of the often-cited opposition relationship between the sympathetic and parasympathetic is the alimentary tract, in which the parasympathetic generally increases secretion and transit whereas the sympathetic does the reverse. This example is somewhat atypical because both divisions of the autonomic regulate activity within the enteric nervous system, a complex local network that integrates local gut activity independently of the central nervous system. Thus a piece of intestine maintained in a physiological saline bath can generate integrated peristaltic movements that can be regulated by cholinergic or adrenergic drugs introduced into the bath.

A more useful distinction is that the sympathetic often functions as an integrated system, as in the 'fight-or-flight' response. The adrenal medulla consists of modified postganglionic neurons that secrete catecholamines into the blood circulation, so producing responses in all peripheral cells with appropriate receptors. The parasympathetic is more focussed. Generalized parasympathetic activation has been described as a 'rest-and-digest' response; however, as this would increase gut transit, constrict the pupils, produce tear and saliva secretion, erection and micturition, it can scarcely be seen as a functionally integrated response. Though the basis for this difference must lie mainly in central connection patterns, the more focussed nature of the parasympathetic distribution is reflected in its neuronal organization, with long preganglionic axons synapsing with ganglia that lie very close to, or even within, the target organs.

Principles of autonomic distribution

Detailed diagrams and descriptions of autonomic nerve pathways may be found in major anatomy and neuroscience textbooks (Snell 2001, Standring 2005). The following may be found useful as guiding principles before examining the detailed information. A key point is that anatomical nerves are merely bundles of axons that happen to be following the same route. Autonomic axons tend to follow any other nerve that is going their way.

- In the head and neck, the parasympathetic ganglia are connected to branches of the trigeminal nerve (a fairly ubiquitous sensory nerve), through which the postganglionic axons distribute to their target organs.

- Parasympathetic preganglionic axons supplying thoracic and most of the abdominal viscera follow the vagus nerve, a very mixed nerve also containing many non-autonomic axons, synapsing with postganglionic axons in the cardiac and pulmonary plexi.

- Parasympathetic preganglionic axons supplying the distal colon and the pelvic viscera leave the sacral spinal nerve roots to enter the pelvis through the anterior sacral foramina. As with the vagal supply to the abdomen, their ganglia are small, numerous, and close to or within the target organs.

- Preganglionic sympathetic neurons follow thoracic or upper lumbar spinal nerves, leaving (as bundles of myelinated axons called white rami) to synapse with postganglionic neurons in the closely adjacent ganglia of the paravertebral chains. Postganglionic axons supplying somatic targets return to their own or adjacent spinal nerves (through unmyelinated grey rami) and distribute through their branches. Although the sympathetic outflow from the spinal cord is T1–L2, the paravertebral chains and their ganglia extend from the cervical to the sacral regions to provide inputs to target organs in these regions, via the spinal nerves for somatic structures but following the branches of the carotid arterial system in the head.

- Preganglionic sympathetic axons destined for the viscera also follow the spinal nerves and white rami to the paravertebral chain ganglia. Those destined for the thoracic viscera mainly synapse within the chains, the postganglionic axons joining parasympathetic nerves to form the cardiac and pulmonary plexuses in the mediastinum. Those targeted on the abdominal viscera leave the paravertebral chains (without synapsing) as splanchnic nerves, which descend the posterior thoracoabdominal wall to synapse mainly in the pre-aortic ganglia around the coeliac and mesenteric arterial roots. Their postganglionic axons reach target organs though the mesenteries and other routes.

- Preganglionic axons supplying the adrenal medulla also pass through white rami, paravertebral chains and splanchnic nerves, passing through the coeliac plexus without synapsing to innervate the adrenal medullary chromaffin cells. These are postganglionic sympathetic neurons that lack axons but secrete catecholamines by the endocrine route into the systemic circulation.

The distribution of the thoracolumbar sympathetic outflow is broadly segmental. Spinal nerves T1–T2 supply the head and neck, T2–T8 the upper limbs, T2–T4 or T5 the thoracic viscera, T5–L2 the gastrointestinal system, T12–L2 the pelvic viscera and T10–L2 the lower limbs.

Autonomic sensory neurons

The autonomic nerves are involved in numerous reflexes at spinal and cranial levels, and are accompanied by many sensory axons.

Those associated with the parasympathetic are principally from visceral enteroceptors concerned with pressure, stretch, and chemical senses. These are very numerous; they form the largest single functional group of axons in the vagus.

Sensory axons running with the visceral sympathetic predominantly deal with pain, so understanding of the segmental distribution of the sympathetic is fundamental to the interpretation of referred visceral pain, and sympathectomy provides one therapeutic approach to intractable pain.

Hyperhidrosis and facial blushing

Surgery for hyperhidrosis and facial flushing involves sympathectomy. The main anatomical considerations are the following.

Sweat glands and cutaneous vascular smooth muscle receive their sympathetic supply through the spinal nerves. For the upper limb, the preganglionic axons leave the spinal cord mainly in T3–T6. These axons generally ascend within the paravertebral chains before synapsing, the postganglionic neurons arising from the T2 and T3 ganglia and leaving the sympathetic chain at the appropriate levels to join the roots of the brachial plexus (C5–T1) and T2–T3 for the axilla. The anatomy of the sympathetic is quite variable; the most important variation affecting the upper limb is the occurrence of a nerve of Kuntz, connecting T1 and T2 and so by-passing part of the paravertebral chain. The usual anatomical basis for denervation of the upper limb sweat glands targets the T2 and T3 ganglia and their rami, either directly or by interrupting the chain superior to the T2 ganglion so as to cut the outflow from

T2 and T3 to the grey rami entering the roots of the brachial plexus. An axillary transthoracic approach puts few important structures at risk; the main consideration is to avoid injury to the long thoracic nerve that descends on and supplies serratus anterior. A supraclavicular approach requires attention to a large number of structures near the thoracic inlet, including the internal jugular vein, subclavian vessels, phrenic nerve, brachial plexus, thoracic and other lymph ducts and the stellate ganglion. Injury to the stellate ganglion will compromise the T1 sympathetic supply to structures of the head, producing a Horner's syndrome.

Most of the lower limb receives its sympathetic supply from the L2 and L3 ganglia of the chain. Adjacent vulnerable structures are the inferior vena cava, the inferior pole of the kidney and the ureter. Some supply to the lower limb derives from the L1 ganglion; however, this also supplies the genital ducts so ablation or disconnection is likely to interfere with the smooth muscle responsible for seminal emission and so prevent the urethral dilation that triggers the ejaculation reflex.

Thoracic sympathectomy is the procedure of choice for palmar hyperhidrosis and facial blushing. The approach to surgery for such conditions can be divided into local and general procedures which can further be classified into open and laparoscopic.

A local surgical approach to the treatment of hyperhidrosis involves excision of the culprit glands. This is only possible if the hyperhidrosis is significantly localized (e.g. in the axilla or groin). Such excision of superficial tissues, however, are associated with potential complications of scarring, postoperative infection, and contractures in regions where skin folds are excised, and so extensive surgery of this type is rarely performed, especially without plastic surgical input.

More commonly sympathectomy is performed for the treatment of hyperhidrosis especially when the upper limbs are affected (hyperhidrosis palmaris). There are several approaches for a thoracic sympathectomy. These can be classified as for all surgical procedures into open and laparoscopic. The open approaches include the posterior, anterior thoracic and axillary transthoracic approaches and the supraclavicular approach.

Open posterior approach

The skin incision is made in the midline over the spinous processes of C6–T4 vertebrae. Variations of this include bilateral paramedian dorsal oblique incisions or paravertebral vertical incisions. The superficial muscles are laterally retracted or split to enable visualization of the costovertebral levels in question. This, the lateral process of the second thoracic vertebra and 2–3 cm of the ribs may be excised to expose the T2 and stellate ganglia. This approach enables access to the intercostals nerves, roots and ganglia as well as the sympathetic chain.

Open anterior thoracic approach

Open anterior thoracic approach consists of an oblique incision over one of the first three intercostal spaces starting over the sternum. Muscle splitting though pectoralis major and the intercostal muscles allow access to the pleura, which are then incised. The lung parenchyma is retracted inferiorly and the posterior pleura are then further incised to gain access to the sympathetic chain. Thus the upper ganglia may be resected without involving the stellate ganglion in the procedure.

Open axillary transthoracic approach

Open axillary transthoracic approach begins with an incision in the second intercostal space between pectoralis major and latisimus dorsi. Care must be taken to avoid the long thoracic nerve with this approach. This incision allows access to the thoracic cavity via serratus anterior and the intercostals muscles which are split in the process. The ribs may then be spread which enables visualization of the upper sympathetic chain, behind the parietal pleura. It is important to identify the first rib at this stage, before incision the sympathetic trunk and excision the appropriate ganglia.

Open supraclavicular approach

For the open supraclavicular approach, an approximately 7 cm incision is made 1 cm above and parallel to the clavicle, starting around the sternoclavicular joint. Once the clavicular head of the sternocleidomastoid muscle is identified and divided the internal jugular vein becomes apparent and must be preserved. Next the omohyoid is divided and retracted, thus revealing the anterior scalene muscle along with the phrenic nerve as its anterior relation. Care must be taken at this stage to avoid injuring the thoracic duct if operating on the left side. Medial retraction of the phrenic nerve and is followed by transaction of scalenus anterior to expose the subclavian artery which is retracted superiorly. The fascia between the brachial plexus and the subclavian artery is incised and opened, to expose the dome of the pleura, which is mobilized with blunt dissection to reveal the sympathetic chain behind it.

Thoracoscopic sympathectomy

Thoracoscopic sympathectomy consists in making a tiny incision (approximately 1 cm) behind the pectoralis-fold in the axilla (in the 5th intercostal space). Then a small amount of CO_2 is insufflated into the thoracic cavity (as for a diagnostic thoracoscopy) to allow access with an endoscopic instrument, specially modified for this operation. The lung on the side of the procedure is then deflated for the duration of the operation. It is possible for the surgeon to identify and severe the sympathetic nerves. A second port may be placed in the 5th intercostal space for the operating instrumentation. If a third port is needed then this may be placed in the 4th intercostal space. In facial hyperhidrosis and facial blushing, it is sufficient to sharply divide the fibres running from the second thoracic ganglion upward, leaving the 2nd ganglion almost intact. Treatment of palmar hyperhidrosis requires total destruction of the second ganglion, always taking great care not to cause any spreading of thermal energy along the nervous trunk in order to avoid damage to the stellate ganglion. Eventually, the CO_2 is re-aspirated and the incision closed. Finally, the procedure may be repeated on the other side.

Surgical anatomy for the treatment for Frey's syndrome

Frey's syndrome is also known as Baillarger's syndrome, Dupuy's syndrome, Frey–Baillarger syndrome, and auriculotemporal syndrome.

Description

Frey's syndrome is characterized by warmth and sweating over the malar region of the face (usually unilaterally) on eating or thinking about food, or is brought on by the consumption of foods that produce strong salivary stimuli. It may follow damage in the parotid region by trauma, mumps, purulent infection or parotidectomy. It is thought that autonomic fibres to salivary glands have become connected in error with the sweat glands when they become reconnected after the damage that originally caused their connection to be interrupted. It may be permanent. Some cases are congenital and probably due to birth trauma.

Anatomy

The parotid region is neuroanatomically complex. Parasympathetic secretomotor nerves to the parotid salivary gland originate in the glossopharyngeal nerve which is deeply placed, running close to the pharynx along the stylopharyngeus muscle. However, its preganglionic parasympathetic component travels by a complex path to the otic ganglion, suspended from the beginning of the auriculotemporal branch of the mandibular division of the trigeminal nerve. The auriculotemporal is principally the sensory nerve of the temporal and adjoining scalp skin, but also provides a direct route for postganglionic parasympathetic nerves from the otic ganglion to the parotid gland. Acid or spicy taste stimuli (reaching the brainstem mainly through the facial nerve) normally elicit reflex parotid salivation mediated by the glossopharyngeal-otic ganglion-auriculotemporal pathway. The sympathetic nerves in the head mainly follow the carotid tree reaching the auriculotemporal region largely as a plexus surrounding the superficial temporal artery, a terminal branch of the external carotid arising within the substance of the parotid gland. Injury in the parotid region followed by aberrant regeneration of damaged parasympathetic axons in the auriculotemporal may result in parasympathetic terminals being formed on sweat gland in the auriculotemporal region. Unfortunately human sweat glands use cholinergic (muscarinic) receptors, so the mis-innervation will be functional and taste stimulation will lead to inappropriate sweating. This may also extend to the post-auricular scalp as the auriculotemporal and great auricular nerves frequently anastomose.

The treatment of Frey's syndrome ultimately depends on how severely symptomatic patients are affected. Currently medical therapy is the treatment of choice, starting with simple topical agents such as antiperspirants, followed by anticholinergic agents and even injections of botulinum toxin into the affected area. Surgical treatments are very limited at present: prevention of the condition through precise anatomical approaches to parotid surgery or the use of musculocutaneous flaps to keep the skin and secretomotor nerves separate being useful techniques to avoid this essentially iatrogenic condition.

Surgical anatomy for the treatment for chronic regional pain syndrome

Pain fibres from the abdominal and pelvic viscera principally run along the sympathetic pathways. Potential sites of intervention for the treatment of chronic regional pain syndrome (CRPS) therefore include the coeliac, aorticorenal, superior and inferior groups of pre-aortic ganglia, the splanchnic nerves (converging from the paravertebral chains to an area anterior to the 12th thoracic vertebra) and the appropriate thoracic or upper lumbar segments of the paravertebral sympathetic chains (Arcidiacono and Rossi 2004).

The pre-aortic ganglia are anatomically fairly variable and the coeliac, aorticorenal and superior mesenteric ganglia often more or less coalesce to form a single complex in the T12–L2 vertebral segment of the pre-aortic and medial para-aortic region.

Classically, surgical control of CRPS involved thoracic or lumbar sympathectomies, which are described in the sections on hyperhidrosis and Raynaud's syndrome respectively. However, visceral abdominal pain is a major problem in CRPS, which may be treated by blocking or ablating the coeliac plexus. This must be differentiated from the splanchnic nerves, which lie above the diaphragm. The coeliac plexus may be approached surgically or percutaneously with radiological (computerized tomography [CT]) or endoscopic ultrasound guidance. The posterior approach used straight needles under CT guidance to deliver phenol or alcohol to the coeliac plexus. However, there have been a small number of reports of paraplegia as a complication of this approach and so in many centres it has been largely abandoned. The surgical approach is a straightforward transperitoneal abdominal approach, for both open and laparoscopic techniques, with port placements being variable depending on the surgeon's preference. Endoscopic ultrasound guided celiac plexus block or ablation is performed by placing the probe into the stomach in a similar fashion to performing an oesophago-gastric-duodenoscopy (OGD). The probe is then pushed towards the lesser curve in the subcardiac area. It is gently pressed against the gastric wall here to allow identification of the surrounding structures, especially the aorta, which is visualized using colour Doppler techniques. Careful evaluation allows identification of the origin of the celiac trunk off the aorta. Small hollow needled devices are passed through the posterior gastric wall to allow the celiac plexus to be sprayed with a neurolytic agent such as dehydrated alcohol.

Refractory angina and cardiac arrhythmias

Visceral pain fibres from the thoracic viscera run through the cardiac and pulmonary plexuses in the mediastinum through the T1–T4 paravertebral sympathetic ganglia to enter the spinal cord in the dorsal roots of spinal nerves T1–T5. Motor fibres to the heart arise from both divisions of the ANS. The parasympathetic component is vagal, is routed through the cardiac plexuses, and innervates only the pacemaker tissue of the heart so that it can slow heart rate but has no effect on the force of contraction. The sympathetic supply from spinal segments T1–T5 synapses in paravertebral chain ganglia T1–T4 and also reaches the heart through the cardiac plexuses.

The surgical treatment of refractory angina is only considered if the symptoms are severely debilitating and all efforts have been made to revascularize the myocardium, both endoluminally with angioplasty and surgically with coronary artery bypass grafting. These patients tend to have distal small vessel disease not amenable to therapies available at present, so surgical therapies for these patients involve sympathetic ablation at a thoracic level. However as many of these patients have already had sternotomies and or thoracotomies, the transthoracic approach may be complicated by multiple adhesions from their previous surgery. This especially hinders thorascopic approaches (as described above). Experienced thoracic surgeons, however, may use video-assisted thorascopic surgery (VATS) despite previous surgery. The open approach for this is identical to the open anterior thoracic technique for thoracic sympathectomy for the treatment of hyperhidrosis, unless another thoracic procedure is to be performed simultaneously, when a midline sternotomy would be the approach of choice.

Surgery has also been used for the treatment of cardiac arrhythmias, such as atrial fibrillation. Vagal ablation has been documented through many approaches including open sternotomy and thoracotomy, and minimally invasive techniques as well as transcatheter techniques. Ventral cardiac denervation has been used during coronary artery bypass grafting to reduce the incidence of post operative atrial fibrillation following revascularization.

Congenital long QT syndrome that is refractory to pharmacological therapies may be treated surgically by using left-sided cardiac sympathetic innervation. This is carried out via a left anterior thoracic approach but includes ablation of the lower portion of the stellate ganglion as well as the first five thoracic ganglia on the left side.

Surgical anatomy for the treatment of Raynaud's syndrome and ischaemic symptoms

Both these conditions may be treated surgically with the use of sympathectomy. Anatomical considerations are generally similar to hyperhidrosis, so approaches to thoracic sympathectomy are described above in the section on 'Surgical anatomy for the treatment of hyperhidrosis and facial blushing'. In this section, lumbar sympathectomy at its approaches will be described. Once again open and laparoscopic approaches may be used.

Open lumbar sympathectomy (oblique retroperitoneal approach)

Open lumbar sympathectomy may be performed using a small transverse incision positioned lateral to the rectus sheath placed halfway between the supracristal line and the inferior aspect of the costal margin. The layers are incised in order down to external oblique, which is opened the direction of its fibres. Internal oblique and the transverse abdominal muscles are then split and the anterior peritoneum visualized. This is then retracted medially to expose psoas muscle and the genitofemoral nerve. The sympathetic chain may then be palpated upon the vertebral column prior to dissection and destruction of the offending levels and ganglions necessary for symptomatic relief to the patient.

Laparoscopic lumbar sympathectomy

Retroperitoneal approach

For the retroperitoneal approach the patient is placed in the lateral position, with the table broken so as to maximize the space just below the 11th rib and the iliac crest. Two small 2 cm transverse incisions are made at the level of the umbilicus at the anterior and posterior axillary lines. Muscle splitting techniques are then used to dissect down to the peritoneum without incising this layer. The peritoneum is then manually pushed to one side to allow access to the anterior aspect of the retroperitoneum. This is then carefully incised to allow unsufflation with CO_2 to develop the retroperitoneal space. Two further port sites for assisting instruments or retractors may be created 4 cm below the initial two incisions

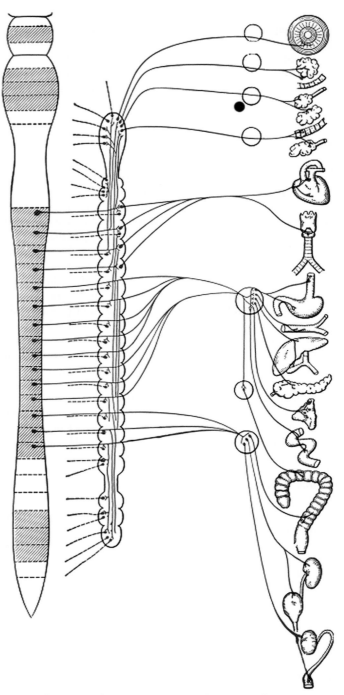

Fig. 6.1 Efferent sympathetic nervous system. With permission from *Gray's Anatomy* 39th edition, Susan Standring, Copyright Elsevier 2004.

in a similar manner. Once the retroperitoneal space is delineated, the sympathetic chain may be visualized between the inferior vena cava and the psoas muscle. This may be made clearer on the left side by gently moving the iliac vessels out of the way. Transection of the sympathetic ganglion may then be carried out at the appropriate level using different modalities including thermal and ultrasonic ablation or even the application of minimally invasive clips.

Anterior transperitoneal approach

Anterior transperitoneal approach may be used if the retroperitoneal approach is not possible or if an intraperitoneal procedure needs to be carried out simultaneously. Standard approaches to abdominal laparoscopy may be used with infra-umbilical positioning of the first 10 mm port through the linea alba and then port placement as required for the intraperitoneal procedure that is to be carried out first. The lateral attachments of the right or left colon may then be incised down from the hepatic or splenic flexures down to the pelvic inlet, to bring the respective sides of the colon to be reflected medially. The L2 lumbar ganglion may then be seen below the renal pedicle. Once the sympathetic chain is identified it may be ablated as described above in the retroperitoneal laparoscopic approach.

Avoidance of injury to the autonomic nervous system during general surgical procedures

Common surgical procedures that have autonomic dysfunction as a recognized complication are:

◆ oesophageal surgery—sympathetic chain and vagal injury

◆ thoracic surgery around the root of the lung—sympathetic chain and vagal injury

◆ rectal surgery (especially total mesorectal excision for rectal cancer)—impotence and sexual function

◆ radical prostatectomy—impotence and sexual function

◆ pelvic surgery—impotence and sexual function

The pelvic autonomic plexus contains both sympathetic and parasympathetic components, and is essential for normal bladder and bowel function and for sexual function.

The main sympathetic inputs are postganglionic neurons from the superior hypogastric plexus (derived from the last few roots of the sympathetic outflow through mainly the L1 ganglia). This plexus has bilateral extensions into the pelvis termed the hypogastric nerves, lying medial to the ureters on each side of the midsagittal plane, which communicate with the pelvic autonomic plexus (inferior hypogastric plexus). A second sympathetic input to the pelvic autonomic plexus is the sacral splanchnic nerves arising from the sacral extensions of the paravertebral trunks, mainly from its S2 ganglion. The parasympathetic input to the pelvic autonomic plexus consists of preganglionic nerves mainly from the roots of S2 and S3 (with varying amounts of S1, S4 and S5) entering the pelvis through the anterior sacral foramina. These elements combine to form the mixed pelvic autonomic plexus, which lies at the S4–S5 vertebral levels. In men the pelvic plexus is closely related to the prostate, seminal vesicles and the rectovesical peritoneal pouch, commonly extending to the para-rectal area on each side. It lies external to the fatty mesorectal sheath investing the rectum. In women the corresponding plexus is centred lateral to the cervix and vaginal fornix, extending to the lateral vaginal wall, the base of the bladder and posteriorly towards the para-rectal area. Branches to the pelvic organs extend from the nearest parts of the pelvic plexus. In general the plexus lies within the bowl-shaped surface defined by the main vascular plane of the internal iliac vessels (Baader and Herrmann 2003).

References

Arcidiacono, P. G., Rossi, M. (2004). Celiac plexus neurolysis. *Jop* **5**(4), 315–21.

Baader, B., Herrmann, M. (2003). Topography of the pelvic autonomic nervous system and its potential impact on surgical intervention in the pelvis. *Clin. Anat.* **16**(2),119–30.

Bandyk, D. F., Johnson, B. L., Kirkpatrick, A. F., Novotney, M. L., Back, M. R., Schmacht, D. C. (2002). Surgical sympathectomy for reflex sympathetic dystrophy syndromes. *J Vasc. Surg.* **35**(2), 269–77.

Butler, A. B., Hodos, W. *Comparative Vertebrate Neuroanatomy* 3rd Ed (1996), pp. 343–44. Wiley-Liss.

Gibbins, I. (1993). Comparative anatomy and evolution of the autonomic nervous system. In Comparative Physiology and Evolution of the Autonomic Nervous System, pp. 1–67 (ed. S. Nilsson & S. Holmgren) Chur, Switzerland: Harwood Academic Publications

Hashmonai, M., Kopelman, D. (2003). History of sympathetic surgery. *Clin. Auton. Res.* **13** Suppl 1, I6–9.

Hashmonai, M., Kopelman, D. (2003). The pathophysiology of cervical and upper thoracic sympathetic surgery. *Clin. Auton. Res.* **13** Suppl 1, I40–4.

Hsia, J. Y., Chen, C. Y., Hsu, C. P., Shai, S. E., Yang, S. S. (1999). Outpatient thoracoscopic limited sympathectomy for hyperhidrosis palmaris. *Ann. Thorac. Surg.* **67**(1), 258–9.

Kennedy, W. R., Wendelschafer-Crabb, G., Brelje, T. C. (1994). Innervation and vasculature of human sweat glands: an immunohistochemistry-laser scanning confocal fluorescence microscopy study. *J Neurosci.* **14**(11 Pt 2), 6825–33.

Kopelman, D., Hashmonai, M. (2003). Upper thoracic sympathetic surgery. Open surgical techniques. *Clin. Auton. Res.* **13** Suppl 1, I10–5.

Lundberg, J. M. (1996). Pharmacology of cotransmission in the autonomic nervous system: integrative aspects on amines, neuropeptides, adenosine triphosphate, amino acids and nitric oxide. *Pharmacol. Rev.* **48**(1), 113–78.

Schiller, Y. (2003). The anatomy and physiology of the sympathetic innervation to the upper limbs. *Clin. Auton. Res.* **13** Suppl 1, I2–5.

Snell, R. S. (2001). *Clinical Neuroanatomy for Medical Students* (5th Ed) Baltimore : Lippincott Williams & Wilkins.

Standring, S. (Ed) (2005). *Gray's Anatomy* (37th Ed). Edinburgh: Elsevier Churchill Livingstone.

Sverzut, C. E., Trivellato, A. E., Serra, E. C., Ferraz, E. P., Sverzut, A. T. (2004). Frey's syndrome after condylar fracture: case report. *Braz. Dent. J* **15**(2), 159–62.

Watarida, S., Shiraishi, S., Fujimura, M., *et al.* (2002). Laparoscopic lumbar sympathectomy for lower-limb disease. *Surg. Endosc.* **16**(3), 500–3.

Wronski, J. (1998). Lumbar sympathectomy performed by means of videoscopy. *Cardiovasc. Surg.* **6**(5), 453–6.

Young, J. Z. (1981). *The Life of Vertebrates* (3rd Ed) 1981. pp. 55, 86. Oxford: Clarendon.

CHAPTER 7

Autonomic and neurohumoral control of the cerebral circulation

Michael A. Moskowitz, Melanie C. Sharp and Robert Macfarlane

Key points

- Sensory and autonomic nerves influence cerebral blood flow under a variety of pathological conditions.

- The sensory innervation to the cranium (the trigeminovascular system) has a central role to play in many types of headache.

- Neurotransmitter release from sensory nerve endings in the dura mater causes neurogenic inflammation in the dura mater.

- A number of drugs efficacious in treating headache inhibit neurogenic inflammation.

- Cortical spreading depression may be one important mechanism for stimulating the trigeminovascular system in migraine.

- Selective prejunctional receptor antagonists are a key pharmaceutical target in the search for better headache treatments.

Introduction

There is considerable evidence to support the notion that the sensory and autonomic innervation to the cranium can influence cerebral blood flow (CBF) under a variety of pathological conditions, and that perivascular sensory nerves play a pivotal role in the development of certain types of head pain, including migraine and cluster headache. This chapter will explore current knowledge of the neural control of the cerebral circulation, and the circumstances under which modulation of the activity of these nerves may be of therapeutic benefit.

Vascular hypothesis of migraine

A vascular aetiology for migraine was first proposed in the 1930s. Accentuated pulsation was observed in the superficial temporal artery during the headache phase of migraine, and treatment with the vasoconstrictor ergotamine both relieved the headache and appeared to attenuate the arterial pulsation. Subsequent studies demonstrated that stimulation of dural arteries at craniotomy

provoked throbbing ipsilateral head pain, and that several other drugs efficacious in treating migraine were also vasoconstrictors. The fact that dilatation of cerebral arteries induced by either pharmacological means (e.g. glyceryl trinitrate [GTN] or histamine administration) or by mechanical distension (e.g. balloon angioplasty) results in head pain, and that sumatriptan, an effective antimigraine drug that has no known analgesic properties, reduces middle cerebral artery calibre, adds further weight to a direct association between cerebral vasodilatation and headache. Functional magnetic resonance imaging (fMRI) has shown a 10–35% reduction in CBF and cerebral blood volume (CBV) in the visual cortex during the aura phase of migraineurs who have a visual aura (Sanchez del Rio et al. 1999). During the headache phase a decrease in the mean transit time and an increase in regional CBF occurs, suggestive of hyperperfusion.

Indeed, having identified that cerebral blood vessels contain $5\text{-HT}_{1\beta}$ receptors that mediate constriction, sumatriptan was developed specifically as a selective agonist for this receptor, and has been shown to be efficacious in the treatment of migraine. Yet, compelling though the vascular hypothesis may at first sight appear, the link between vasodilatation and head pain cannot be that simple. Subarachnoid haemorrhage is a potent cause of headache yet is associated with vasoconstriction not vasodilatation, and a doubling of CBF by carbon dioxide inhalation is not painful at all. Furthermore, single photon emission computed tomography (SPECT) studies of regional CBF have failed to show a consistent relationship between headache and hyperaemia during the acute phase of migraine headache. Neither has perfusion-weighted MRI identified a good correlation between CBF, CBV, and headache (Cutrer et al. 1998). The same holds true for countless other studies spanning more than 50 years, which have been designed to validate cerebral vasodilatation as the fundamental basis for the headache in migraine.

The sensory innervation to the cranium is central to the appreciation of head pain. Not only do sensory fibres transmit nociceptive information, they promote a sterile inflammatory response within target tissues. As such the trigeminal nerve, its associated neuro-transmitters, and the pain-sensitive structures within the cranium are a logical focus for study in search of a better understanding of the pathophysiological basis for headache. Furthermore, pial sensory and autonomic nerve endings contain potent vasoactive neuropeptides that may influence CBF under a variety of other circumstances. Because sensitization of the sensory nerves follows chemical stimulation of dura mater, it has been proposed that meningeal afferents contribute to mechanical hypersensitivity (i.e. worsening of head pain by coughing, breath-holding or sudden movement) and the throbbing pain of migraine (Strassman et al. 1996).

Autonomic and sensory innervation of the cerebral vasculature: neurogenic influences on cerebral blood flow

Autonomic

Sympathetic

The sympathetic innervation to the cerebral vasculature is largely via the superior cervical ganglion. In addition to the catecholamines, sympathetic nerve terminals contain another potent vasoconstrictor, neuropeptide Y (NPY). This 36-amino-acid neuropeptide is found in abundance in both the central and peripheral nervous systems.

Only minor (5–10%) reductions in CBF accompany electrical stimulation of sympathetic nerves, far less than that seen in other vascular beds. Although feline pial arterioles vasoconstrict in response to topical noradrenaline and the response is blocked by the α-blocker phenoxybenzamine, application of the latter alone at the same concentration has no effect on vessel calibre. This and other observations from denervation studies indicate that the sympathetic nervous system does not exert a significant tonic influence on cerebral vessels under physiological conditions. Neither does the sympathetic innervation contribute to CBF regulation under conditions of hypotension or hypoxia. However, sympathetic stimulation does produce a profound fall in CBF if cerebral vessels have been dilated by hypercapnia. From this observation came the 'dual control' hypothesis, proposing that the cerebral circulation is comprised of two resistances in series. Extraparenchymal vessels are thought to be regulated largely by the autonomic nervous system, while intraparenchymal vessels are responsible for half the resistance under physiological conditions, and are governed primarily by intrinsic metabolic and myogenic factors.

As well as exerting a significant influence on CBV, the sympathetic innervation has been shown to protect the brain from the effects of acute severe hypertension. When blood pressure rises above the limits of autoregulation, activation of the sympathetic nervous system attenuates the anticipated rise in CBF, and reduces the plasma protein extravasation that follows breakdown of the blood–brain barrier. The autoregulatory curve is 'reset' such that both the upper and lower limits are raised. This is an important physiological mechanism by which the cerebral vasculature is protected from injury during surges in arterial blood pressure. Although cerebral vessels escape from the vasoconstrictor response to sympathetic stimulation under conditions of normotension, this does not occur during acute hypertension.

Sympathetic nerves are thought also to exert trophic influences upon the vessels that they innervate. Sympathectomy reduces the

hypertrophy of the arterial wall that develops in response to chronic hypertension. Denervation has been shown to increase the susceptibility of stroke-prone spontaneously hypertensive rats to bleed into the cerebral hemisphere that has been sympathectomized (Mueller and Heistad 1980).

Parasympathetic

The cerebrovascular parasympathetic innervation derives from multiple sources, including the sphenopalatine and otic ganglia, and small clusters of ganglion cells within the cavernous plexus, Vidian, and lingual nerves. Vasoactive intestinal peptide (VIP), a potent 28-amino-acid polypeptide vasodilator that is not dependent on endothelium-derived relaxing factor (EDRF), has been localized immunohistochemically within parasympathetic nerve endings, as has nitric oxide synthase (NOS), the enzyme that forms nitric oxide (NO) from L-arginine. The multiple sources of innervation and the lack of a suitable VIP antagonist have for some time hampered investigation of the role of the parasympathetic innervation on the cerebral circulation. However, lesioning experiments are now possible following identification of unique parasympathetic anatomy in the rat, where the fibres enter the cranium from the orbit via the ethmoidal foramen.

Although stimulation of parasympathetic nerves does elicit a rise in cortical blood flow, there is, like the sympathetic nervous system, little to suggest that cholinergic mechanisms contribute significantly to CBF regulation under physiological conditions. Nor are parasympathetic nerves involved in the vasodilatory response to hypercapnia. However, chronic parasympathetic denervation increases infarct volume by 37% in rats subjected to permanent middle cerebral artery occlusion, primarily because of a reduction in CBF under situations when perfusion pressure is reduced (Kano et al. 1991). This suggests that parasympathetic nerves may help to maintain cerebral perfusion at times of reduced blood flow, and may in part explain why patients with autonomic neuropathy, such as diabetics, are at increased risk of stroke.

Sensory

The sensory innervation to the brain and meninges is largely via unmyelinated nerve fibres, and has been studied with axonal tracing techniques using wheatgerm agglutinin and horseradish immunoperoxidase. The basic anatomy is remarkably similar in different mammalian species. The sensory innervation is confined to the dura mater, particularly the dural arteries and venous sinuses, and the larger intracranial arteries (>50 μm diameter). Structures within the supratentorial compartment and rostral third of the posterior fossa are supplied by the ophthalmic division of the trigeminal nerve, supplemented by a small contribution from the maxillary and mandibular divisions in primates. The more caudal elements in the posterior fossa are innervated principally by the C1–2 dorsal roots, but with a contribution from the vagal and trigeminal ganglia. The distribution is ipsilateral, with the exception of midline structures that receive a dual innervation. Each individual ganglion cell projects multiple axon collaterals that innervate both the larger branches of the circle of Willis and the overlying dura mater. The extracranial trigeminal innervation is distinct, and no individual neuron supplies both intracranial and extracranial structures. Centrally, however, there is convergence, with somatic afferents (innervating the extra-calvarial structures) and visceral afferents (innervating the meninges and cerebral vessels) synapsing onto single interneurons within the trigeminal nucleus caudalis.

Trigeminovascular fibres probably reach the internal carotid artery at the pericarotid plexus within the cavernous sinus, and enter the middle cranial fossa with it. The sensory C-fibres form a fine network on the adventitial surface of cerebral vessels, and at the junction between adventitia and media. The axons have multiple vesicle-containing *boutons en passant* which are in close proximity to vascular smooth muscle.

Trigeminovascular system

Contained within vesicles in the naked nerve endings are many different neuropeptides. The most important include calcitonin-gene-related peptide (CGRP), one of the three products of the calcitonin gene, together with the tachykinins, substance P (SP) and neurokinin A (NKA). SP and CGRP are co-localized within nerve terminals. All three, particularly CGRP, are vasodilators, whereas SP and NKA also promote plasma protein extravasation within dura mater (reviewed by Limmroth et al. 1996). Unlike the tachykinins, CGRP inhibits the vasoconstrictor response to sympathetic stimulation and shortens the constrictor response to noradrenaline.

Neurotransmitter release may follow either orthodromic or antidromic mechanisms. Electrical stimulation of the trigeminal ganglion elicits neurogenic vasodilatation in the facial skin and dura mater, and an increase in CGRP levels in the superior sagittal sinus. The cutaneous vasodilatation that accompanies reperfusion of a limb after a period of arterial occlusion is associated with an increase in venous SP, is diminished by chronic sensory denervation, and mimicked by intra-arterial infusion of substance P. The molecules released in response to tissue injury are likely to provide the stimulus for sensory depolarization during ischaemia.

Electrical stimulation of trigeminal afferents elicits a relatively small (17%) and short-lived increase in CBF. Denervation studies, primarily in cats and rats, have demonstrated that perivascular sensory nerves do not have a significant role to play in CBF regulation under physiological conditions. Basal CBF and the vasodilatory response to hypercapnia are unaffected by neurotransmitter depletion. This is in keeping with the nature of these neuropeptides, which have relatively long-lasting effects on the cerebral circulation, and are therefore unsuited for moment-to-moment regulation. However, trigeminal ganglionectomy diminishes the increase in CBF (around 30%) that accompanies acute severe hypertension or seizures in cats, and diminishes the extravasation of radiolabelled albumin that results from disruption of the blood–brain barrier (Sakas et al. 1989). Chronic sensory denervation also attenuates the increase in blood flow that occurs during the early phase of bacterial meningitis (Weber et al. 1996). The hyperaemic response to transient global cerebral ischaemia is reduced by around 50% in cortical grey matter following chronic sensory denervation, but not in the white matter or deep grey matter of the same vascular territory, both of which have a sparse sensory innervation (Moskowitz et al. 1989, Sakas et al. 1989). The pial arteriolar constrictor response to topical noradrenaline is also prolonged by trigeminal ganglionectomy. A number of putative substances have been implicated in sensory nerve fibre activation during these pathological processes, including bradykinin, potassium, hydrogen ions, adenosine, prostaglandins, leucotrienes, and arachidonate metabolites.

None of the changes in blood flow described above occur acutely after nerve section, i.e. before the nerve endings have been depleted of their neurotransmitters. Nor do they occur after section of the trigeminal nerve proximal to the Gasserian ganglion. The latter will block central transmission, but will not promote Wallerian degeneration as will sectioning of the distal nerve. This indicates that neurotransmitters are released in response to antidromic stimulation independent of central control, i.e. via axon reflex-like mechanisms.

There are several circumstances under which sensory nerve-mediated vasodilatation may be beneficial. It has been suggested that one role may be to provide a protective mechanism to enhance CBF early after subarachnoid haemorrhage, when there is excessive vasoconstriction of large arteries. Several days after subarachnoid haemorrhage there is depletion of neurotransmitters from sensory nerve endings and, in some experimental models, this coincides with the development of cerebral vasospasm. Experiments in the monkey have shown that instillation of CGRP into the basal cisterns significantly attenuates the development of delayed vasospasm after subarachnoid haemorrhage (Inoue et al. 1996). Secondly, the post-occlusive hyperaemia mediated by the trigeminovascular system may help to re-establish perfusion after a period of ischaemia, thereby reducing the risk that some areas of the brain will fail to reperfuse at all—the 'no-reflow' phenomenon (reviewed by Macfarlane et al. 1991). Thirdly, CGRP has been shown to have a trophic effect on cultured endothelial cells, suggesting a possible role for sensory nerves in angiogenesis (Haegerstrand et al. 1990).

Neurogenic inflammation and head pain

Neurogenic inflammation is thought to be an important immediate endogenous defence mechanism in response to real or threatened tissue injury (the nocifensor system). The inflammatory response is thought to sensitize the nerve endings, thereby perpetuating the pain after the injurious stimulus has been removed.

Cephalic blood vessels contain a number of nociceptive molecules, including histamine, serotonin, bradykinin, and prostaglandins. CGRP infusion promotes vasodilatation and causes headache. Intravenous infusion of SP and NKA, or electrical stimulation of the trigeminal ganglion, results in vasodilatation, platelet aggregation, mast cell degranulation, the formation of endothelial microvilli and vesicles in postcapillary venules, and an increase in plasma protein extravasation in the ipsilateral dura.

Mast cells are found in abundance in the dura mater, and are in close proximity to SP-containing nerve fibres. Unilateral sensory stimulation results in mast cell degranulation, indicating that neural mechanisms may play one important part in the development of neurogenic inflammation. Not only do mast cells secrete many vasoactive, nociceptive, and chemoactive substances, but these in turn are able to stimulate SP release from sensory nerves, thereby amplifying the process. Perivascular oedema, plasma protein extravasation, mast cell degranulation, platelet aggregation, and vasodilatation have all been observed microscopically in the dura following both electrical sensory stimulation and in response to noxious chemical irritation (Dimitriadou et al. 1991). In the dura mater, neurogenic inflammation is blocked by drugs efficacious in treating migraine, including sumatriptan, the ergot alkaloids, indometacin, aspirin, chronic administration of corticosteroids, and some non-steroidal anti-inflammatory drugs (NSAIDs) (Buzzi et al. 1989). However several failed clinical trials with NK-1 receptor antagonists, and a positive trial with a CGRP receptor antagonist, suggests that CGRP plays a more significant role in headache pathogenesis.

There is good evidence to suggest that serotonin receptors within the dura are a site of action for a number of antimigraine drugs. To date, 14 receptor subtypes have been identified, with marked species variability. Trigeminovascular axons innervating the dura mater possess $5-HT_{1D}$-like receptors, of which there are at least six receptor subtypes (reviewed by Moskowitz and Waeber 1996). The antimigraine drugs sumatriptan and the ergot alkaloids are $5-HT_{1B/D}$ agonists, and have been shown both to block neurogenic inflammation in response to trigeminal ganglion stimulation and to attenuate the concomitant increase in CGRP within the superior sagittal sinus. Pretreatment with the $5-HT_{1D}$ receptor antagonist GR-127,935 blocks the effects of sumatriptan on leakage of plasma protein in dura mater. The mechanism must occur via prejunctional mechanisms because the inflammatory response to exogenous SP and NKA is unaffected by sumatriptan, the sumatriptan analogue CP-122,288, or by dihydroergotamine. Neither can the mechanism of action of the antimigraine drugs be the result of vasoconstriction of meningeal arteries, since neither angiotensin nor phenylephrine are able to diminish neurogenic inflammation in the same animal model. A strain of knockout mice, deficient in the expression of the $5-HT_{1B}$ receptor, have helped to confirm the importance of this receptor subtype for the actions of sumatriptan, dihydroergotamine, and other $5-HT_1$ receptor agonists in this species (Yu et al. 1996). In rats, not only do the antimigraine drugs diminish plasma protein extravasation and attenuate CGRP levels within the superior sagittal sinus, but they reduce the ultrastructural changes seen in the endothelium, platelets, and mast cells as a result of sensory fibre stimulation. $5-HT_{1F}$ receptors are expressed in meningeal vascular smooth muscle, but are not coupled to vasoconstriction. The pharmacological profiles of human and guinea pig 5-HT receptors are almost identical (Zgombick et al. 1995). Guinea pig studies on the effects of PNU-109,291, a selective $5-HT_{1D}$ receptor agonist, have shown a dose-dependent reduction in dural plasma extravasation and c-*fos* expression within the trigeminal nucleus caudalis in response to electrical and chemical meningeal stimulation (Cutrer et al. 1999). This may offer a further therapeutic avenue for the treatment of migraine and related headaches because existing antimigraine drugs are relatively nonselective for 5-HT receptors (and hence constricting both cerebral and coronary arteries), but $5-HT_{1D}$ receptor messenger RNA and protein are expressed in trigeminal ganglia, but not vascular smooth muscle. Other prejunctional receptor types, including α_2, histamine H_3, u-opioid, somatostatin, GABA, L-glutamate, and adenosine A_1 receptors have also been identified (Sanchez del Rio and Moskowitz 2000).

Trigeminovascular system and headache

The anatomy of the cranial sensory innervation accounts for a number of the characteristics of headache which, in many respects, are no different to the types of pain experienced with inflammation in other organs. As well as the strictly unilateral distribution of some headaches, the convergence of trigeminal somatic and intracranial nerves onto single interneurons accounts for referral of pain to the forehead (or cervico-occipital region in the case of the caudal elements within the posterior fossa innervated by C1–2) and for the accompanying tension in the frontalis, temporalis, and

cervico-occipital musculature (analogous to referred pain and muscle rigidity in cholecystitis or appendicitis, for example). Because the innervation is sparse and with large receptive fields, the pain is poorly localized. Central projections to the nucleus of the tractus solitarius account for the autonomic responses (sweating, tachycardia, hypertension, and vomiting) that may accompany it. Following experimental subarachnoid haemorrhage, a potent cause of headache, peptide and messenger RNA synthesis increase within the trigeminal ganglion, consistent with elevated metabolic and neuronal activity. Clinically, an increase in levels of CGRP can be detected in the jugular vein of patients with migraine and subarachnoid haemorrhage, suggesting enhanced release from sensory nerves. Agents that either destroy sensory nerve fibres (e.g. neonatal capsaicin), block action potentials (local anaesthetics), or inhibit neuropeptide release ($5-HT_{1D}$-like agonists), all inhibit neurogenic inflammation in the dura mater. Elevated CGRP levels in the superior sagittal sinus in both animals and humans are decreased by treatment with the serotonin agonist sumatriptan (Goadsby and Edvinsson 1991).

NO has been implicated in migraine pathogenesis, based on the delayed development of typical migraine headache a few hours after administering GTN to migraineurs. Reuter et al. (2001) have shown a dose-dependent delayed inflammatory response within rat dura to GTN infusion. This occurs via induction of NOS, and is consistent with the notion that dural inflammation is an important substrate for headache. The delayed onset can be explained by the time taken for transcription and translation-dependent mechanisms to occur within macrophages. Parthenolide, an anti-inflammatory drug used to treat migraine, has been shown to attenuate the transcription factor nuclear factor κB (Reuter et al. 2002). This molecule plays a pivotal role in iNOS induction, and controls transcription of acute phase proteins associated with the inflammatory response (e.g. adhesion molecules, cytokines, antioxidant enzymes and cyclo-oxygenase-2).

Interactions between sensory and autonomic nerves

Neuropeptide receptors (found, among other places, in postganglionic sympathetic fibres innervating the dura mater) have been identified on trigeminovascular afferents, and NPY receptor agonists suppress plasma protein extravasation in response to trigeminal ganglion stimulation via prejunctional mechanisms (Yu and Moskowitz 1995, 1996).

Sensory and parasympathetic nerves may have synergistic effects on the meningeal plasma protein extravasation response. The GABA transaminase activator valproic acid (another drug useful for the prophylactic treatment of migraine), and the $GABA_A$ receptor agonist, muscimol, block neurogenic plasma extravasation. The GABA receptor does not reside on trigeminovascular fibres (Lee et al. 1995). Instead, its action depends upon the integrity of parasympathetic fibres emanating from the sphenopalatine ganglion (Cutrer et al. 1995). The potential therapeutic relevance of this will be discussed later.

Central neurogenic mechanisms

The central connections of the trigeminovascular system beyond the trigeminal nuclear complex are poorly understood, but relays project to the medial, ventral, posterior medial, and interlaminar nuclei of the thalamus and thence to the cerebral cortex. Some circumstantial evidence for central trigeminal activation has become available from studies using antisera directed against the product of the early immediate response gene, c-fos. The expression of this gene has been used widely as a marker of neural activation. Following meningeal stimulation by either experimental subarachnoid haemorrhage or chemical irritation, postsynaptic cells within rexed laminae I and II_0 of the trigeminal nucleus caudalis (a region analogous to the dorsal horn of the spinal cord and involved in the processing of nociceptive information) express the protein antigen in a dose-dependent fashion (Nozaki et al. 1992a). This response can be blocked by either sensory denervation or treatment with antimigraine drugs, as well as with analgesics such as morphine. However, sumatriptan does not decrease the c-fos response induced when a noxious stimulus is applied to the nasal mucosa, a trigeminally innervated structure that does not possess $5-HT_1$-like receptors. If sumatriptan were acting as an analgesic per se, both the response to noxious meningeal and nasal stimulation should be blocked.

Clinical implications

Neural mechanisms in migraine

The initiating event in migraine, and the mechanisms by which the trigeminovascular system might be activated, are unclear. Cortical spreading depression has been postulated as the initiating event in migraine, in which a propagating wave of neuronal and glial depolarization spreads across the hemisphere at a rate of approximately 2–6 mm/minute. This is followed by depressed neuronal bioelectrical activity, transient loss of membrane ionic gradients and a surge in extracellular potassium. MMPs are a gene family of neutral proteases that have been implicated in processes such as opening of the blood–brain barrier, ingress of immune cells, shedding of cytokines and causing direct cellular damage. Cortical spreading depression has been found to alter blood–brain barrier permeability by activating MMPs (Gursoy-Ozdemir et al. 2004). A number of substances are capable of inducing this phenomenon in animals, although it has not been well documented in the human brain in vivo. Spreading depression can be elicited experimentally by the microapplication of potassium chloride to the pial surface of the cortex. Moskowitz et al. (1993) have shown that spreading depression is capable of activating the trigeminovascular system, as evidenced by an increase in c-fos immunoreactivity within the trigeminal nucleus caudalis. Both chronic trigeminal denervation and the antimigraine drug sumatriptan suppress c-fos expression in the trigeminal nucleus caudalis in response to spreading depression, but neither inhibits spreading depression per se. Recent studies using blood oxygen-level dependent (BOLD) fMRI during the visual aura phase of migraine have lent support to the hypothesis that an electrophysiological event, such as cortical spreading depression, generates the aura in the visual cortex (Hadjikhani et al. 2001). However, some questions still remain about this association. The aura is not always contralateral to the head pain, aura without headache is common, and neither does the aura always precede it. Even if spreading depression proves not to be the initiating event in migraine, studies such as this are important in establishing that endogenous neurophysiological events within the cerebral cortex are capable of activating trigeminovascular fibres innervating the meninges and cortical vessels.

Unifying hypothesis for migraine

Although there is no direct evidence for neurogenic inflammation in human meninges, nor has it been observed during migraine, experimental headache in humans induced by histamine injection does not occur after trigeminal nerve section. We believe that some as yet unidentified trigger (likely to be a neurophysiologically driven ionic or metabolic mechanism within the brain) is responsible for depolarizing trigeminal perivascular sensory afferents on the surface of the cortex during migraine. Hydrogen ions, potassium, arachidonate metabolites, serotonin, histamine, and NO are all possible candidates for sensitizing unmyelinated trigeminal nerve endings.

Because of the anatomical arrangement of the trigeminal nerve fibres, axon collaterals are also depolarized in the ipsilateral dura mater. Perivascular release of neuropeptides results in vasodilatation, while in the dura mater there follows neurogenic inflammation. The latter sensitizes the nerve endings, hence perpetuating the headache. Central projections, specifically those to the trigeminal nucleus caudalis, superior salivatory nucleus and parasympathetic efferents via the sphenopalatine ganglia, are responsible for the vegetative symptoms that accompany the headache. The postganglionic parasympathetic fibres promote vasodilatation and augment blood flow via release of VIP, NO and acetylcholine into the dura (Bolay et al. 2002). Antimigraine drugs are effective not by directly altering vessel calibre, but by their prejunctional activity that blocks neurotransmitter release and neurotransmission. The effect is to suppress neurogenic inflammation and central transmission, thereby alleviating the headache. It follows that vasodilatation is a corollary of migraine headache, rather than the source, thus accounting for the sometimes paradoxical association between the two. Vasodilatation might modulate pain, but not if the meningeal vessels are not already sensitized. Recent clinical trials showing that a CGRP receptor antagonist aborts migraine headache is consistent with this view, although central mechanisms cannot be excluded entirely. Furthermore, the antimigraine drugs do not address the source of the head pain but act on the final common pathway, namely trigeminovascular activation within the dura mater. The action of $5-HT_{1D}$ agonists on receptor targets in brainstem remains a distinct possibility, although preclinical data remain unclear as to the extent of their CNS penetration. The possibility that there is a migraine 'generator' within the brainstem deserves further scrutiny. In this instance, ascending projecting fibres might modulate the threshold for cortical events or affect vascular tone as a mechanism for initiating an attack.

Pharmacological strategies for treating head pain

There are important benefits to be gained from a better understanding of the pathophysiology of migraine and of the precise mechanism of action of drugs beneficial in alleviating headache. The first is to develop an agent that is specific for the appropriate receptor subtype, thereby improving potency and reducing unwanted actions. Although sumatriptan is an effective antimigraine drug, it has significant unwanted vascular side-effects. These occur largely through postjunctional receptor activity mediating vasoconstriction, particularly in the coronary circulation. This effect on vascular smooth muscle can be particularly important in certain circumstances, for example subarachnoid haemorrhage, where vasoconstriction or hypotension may exacerbate cerebral ischaemia. Studies using reverse transcriptase polymerase chain reaction (RTPCR) and specific probes for 5H-HT$_{1D}$ and 5-HT$_{1\beta}$ gene sequences have found that, although 5-HT$_{1D}$ can be amplified selectively from human trigeminal ganglion, 5-HT$_{1D}$ messenger RNA was not expressed within vascular smooth muscle of pial arteries in one study, but was expressed in another (Bouchelet et al. 1996) although not coupled to vasoconstriction. This raises the possibility that drugs can be developed which will activate prejunctional receptors in the dura mater without also causing pial or coronary artery vasoconstriction (Rebeck et al. 1994). The pharmacological profiles of human and guinea pig 5-HT receptors are almost identical (Zgombick et al. 1995). Guinea pig studies on the effects of PNU-109,291, a selective 5-HT$_{1D}$ receptor agonist, have shown a dose-dependent reduction in c-*fos* expression within the trigeminal nucleus caudalis in response to electrical and chemical meningeal stimulation (Cutrer et al. 1999). This may offer a further therapeutic avenue for the treatment of migraine and related headaches because existing anti-migraine drugs are relatively nonselective for 5-HT receptors (and hence constricting both cerebral and coronary arteries). However, 5-HT$_{1D}$ receptor messenger RNA and protein are expressed in trigeminal ganglia, but not vascular smooth muscle. Moreover, if sumatriptan and the ergot alkaloids are acting on the final common pathway in headache, rather than the aetiology, they may help to alleviate pain caused by meningeal irritation from a variety of conditions, such as meningitis, head injury, or subarachnoid haemorrhage. This has been explored experimentally by looking at c-*fos* immunoreactivity within the trigeminal nucleus caudalis (TNC) after experimental subarachnoid haemorrhage and chemically-induced meningitis. Both surgical sensory deafferentation and sumatriptan suppressed the c-*fos* response (Nozaki et al. 1992a, b) in the TNC. The potential benefit of new drugs over conventional analgesics is their effectiveness in alleviating severe headache without depressing conscious level, impairing respiration, or compromising CBF. L-Glutamate is a major neuroexcitatory neurotransmitter in the mammalian nervous system, and plays an important role in primary afferent neurotransmission, including nociception. It coexists with substance P in trigeminal c-fibres. The NMDA receptor antagonist MK-801 also reduces c-*fos* expression in a rodent model (Mitsikostas et al. 1998). However, the use of NMDA receptor antagonists in humans may be limited by unwanted central side-effects (e.g. hypertension, paraesthesiae, motor retardation, perceptual disturbance). Modulation of non-NMDA glutamate receptors (AMPA [alpha-amino-3-hydroxy-5-methyl-4-isoxazole propionic acid] and metabotropic glutamate) is a further possibility to be explored (Mitsikostas et al. 1999).

However, the relevance of the c-*fos* and neurogenic plasma extravasation models as predictors of antimigraine efficacy is controversial. While several drugs effective in suppressing c-*fos* expression in the TNC in rodents are effective antimigraine drugs (e.g. sumatriptan, sodium valproate, NSAIDs and butalbital), others have not proved to be efficacious in human trials (including neurokinin 1 receptor antagonists such as RPR-100 893 and the sumatriptan analogue CP-122 288). It is possible that species differences exist in receptor subtypes and amino acid sequences, or in the relative role of released neuropeptides in trigeminovascular neurotransmission.

The GABA$_A$ receptor is another avenue of potential therapeutic importance. Although agonists of this receptor complex (such as valproate, neurosteroids, and benzodiazepines) block neurogenic plasma extravasation, the receptor complex cannot reside on trigeminovascular fibres because valproate remains effective in animals treated neonatally with capsaicin (which permanently depletes their C fibres). Instead, it requires the integrity of parasympathetic fibres emanating from the sphenopalatine ganglion; presumably those innervating the meninges. Hence, unlike the 5-HT$_1$-like family, this receptor complex lies outside the blood–brain barrier, probably acting through postjunctional receptors within the meninges (Lee et al. 1995).

Conclusion

Although much remains to be discovered about the neurophysiological basis for migraine, molecular pharmacology is contributing greatly to knowledge of neuropeptides and neurotransmitter receptors. Further drug discoveries may be possible even without full knowledge of the underlying pathophysiological mechanisms. The triggers for migraine, its neurophysiological basis, and the dissociation of vessel calibre from headache and its treatment, are important issues to be resolved over the next decade.

Acknowledgement

MAM is the recipient of the Bristol-Meyers Unrestricted Research Award in Neuroscience. National Institutes of Health, (1P01NS35611–01), Migraine Program Project, Michael Moskowitz, P.I.

References

Bolay, H., Reuter, U., Dunn, A. K., Huang, Z., Boas, D. A., Moskowitz, M. A. (2002). Intrinsic brain activity triggers trigeminal meningeal afferents in migraine model. *Nature Medicine* **8**, 136–42.

Bouchelet, I., Cohen, Z., Case, B., Seguela, P., and Hamel, E. (1996). Differential expression of sumatriptan-sensitive 5-hydroxytryptamine receptors in human trigeminal ganglia and cerebral blood vessels. *Mol. Pharmacol.* **50**, 219–23.

Buzzi, M. G., Sakas, D. E., and Moskowitz, M. A. (1989). Indomethacin and acetylsalicylic acid block neurogenic plasma protein extravasation in rat dura mater. *Eur. J. Pharmacol.* **165**, 251–8.

Cutrer, F. M., Limmroth, V., Ayata, G., and Moskowitz, M. A. (1995). Attenuation by valproate of c-*fos* immunoreactivity in trigeminal nucleus caudalis induced by intracisternal capsacin. *Br. J. Pharmacol.* **116**, 3199–204.

Cutrer, F. M., Sorensen, G., Weisskoff, R. M., *et al.* (1998) Perfusion-weighted imaging defects during spontaneous migrainous aura. *Ann. Neurol.* **43**, 25–31.

Cutrer, F. M., Yu, X-J., Ayata, G., Moskowitz, M. A., Waeber, C. (1999). Effects of PNU-109,291, a selective 5-HT$_{1D}$ receptor agonist, on electrically induced dural plasma extravasation and capsaicin-evoked c-fos immunoreactivity within trigeminal nucleus caudalis. *Neuropharmacology* **38**, 1043–53.

Dimitriadou, V., Buzzi, M. G., Moskowitz, M. A., and Theoharides, T. C. (1991). Trigeminal sensory fibre stimulation induces morphological changes reflecting secretion in rat dura mater mast cells. *Neuroscience* **44**, 97–112.

Goadsby, P. J. and Edvinsson, L. (1991). Sumatriptan reverses the changes in CGRP seen in the headache phase of migraine. *Cephalgia* **11**, (Suppl. 3).

Goadsby, P. J. and Edvinsson, L. (1993). The trigeminovascular system and migraine: studies characterizing cerebrovascular and neuropeptide changes seen in humans and cats. *Ann. Neurol.* **33**, 48–56.

Gursoy-Ozdemir, J., Qiu, J., Matsuoka, N., *et al.* (2004). Cortical spreading depression activates and upregulates MMP-9. *J. Clin. Invest.* 113, 1447–55.

Hadjikhani, N., Sanchez del Rio, M., Wu, O. *et al.* (2001). Mechanisms of migraine aura revealed by functional MRI in human visual cortex. *PNAS*, **98**, 4687–92.

Haegerstrand, A., Dalsgaard, C. J., Jonzon, B., Larsson, O., and Nilsson, J. (1990). Calcitonin gene-related peptide stimulates proliferation of human endothelial cells. *Proc. Natl Acad. Sci. USA* **87**, 3299–303.

Inoue, T., Shimizu, H., Kaminuma, T., Tajima, M., Watabe, K., and Yoshimoto, T. (1996). Prevention of cerebral vasospasm by calcitonin gene-related peptide slow-release tablet after subarachnoid hemorrhage. *Neurosurgery* **39**, 984–90.

Kano, M., Moskowitz, M. A., and Yokota, M. (1991). Parasympathetic denervation of rat pial vessels significantly increases infarction volume following middle cerebral artery occlusion. *J. Cereb. Blood Flow Metab.* **11**, 628–37.

Lee, W. S., Limmroth, V., Cutrer, F. M., Waeber, C., and Moskowitz, M. A. (1995). Peripheral GABA$_a$ receptor mediated effects of sodium valproate on dural plasma protein extravasation to substance P. and trigeminal stimulation. *Br. J. Pharmacol.* **116**, 1661–7.

Limmroth, V., Cutrer, F. M., and Moskowitz, M. A. (1996). Neurotransmitters and neuropeptides in headache. *Curr. Opin. Neurol.* **9**, 206–10.

Macfarlane, R., Moskowitz, M. A., Sakas D. E. *et al.* (1991). The role of neuroeffector mechanisms in hyperperfusion syndromes. *J. Neurosurg.* **75**, 845–55.

Mitsikostas, D. D., Sanchez del Rio, M., Waeber, C., Huang, Z., Cutrer, F. M., Moskowitz, M. A., (1999). Non-NMDA glutamate receptors modulate capsaicin induced c-fos expression within trigeminal nucleus caudalis. *Br. J. Pharmacol* **127**, 623–30.

Mitsikostas, D. D., Sanchez del Rio, M., Waeber, C., Moskowitz, M. A., Cutrer, F. M. (1998). *The NMDA receptor santagonist MK-801 reduces capsaicin-induced c-fos expression within rat trigeminal nucleus caudalis. Pain*, **76**, 239–48.

Moskowitz, M. A., Nozaki, K., and Kraig, R. P. (1993). Neocortical spreading depression provokes the expression of c-*fos* protein-like immunoreactivity within trigeminal nucleus caudalis via trigeminovascular mechanisms. *J. Neurosci.* **13**, 1167–77.

Moskowitz, M. A., Sakas, D. E., Wei, E. P., Buzzi, M. G., Ogilvy, C., and Kontos, H. A. (1989). Postocclusive hyperemia in feline cortical grey matter is mediated by trigeminal sensory axons. *Am. J. Physiol.* **257**, H1736–9.

Moskowitz, M. A. and Waeber, C. (1996). Migraine enters the molecular era. *Neuroscientist* **2**, 191–200.

Mueller, S. M. and Heistad, D. D. (1980). Effect of chronic hypertension on the blood–brain barrier. *Hypertension* **2**, 809–12.

Nozaki, K., Boccalini, P., and Moskowitz, M. A. (1992*a*). Expression of c-*fos*-like immunoreactivity in brainstem after meningeal irritation by blood in the subarachnoid space. *Neuroscience* **49**, 669–80.

Nozaki, K., Moskowitz, M. A., and Boccalini, P. (1992*b*). CP-93,129, sumatriptan, dihydroergotamine block c-*fos* expression within rat trigeminal nucleus caudalis caused by chemical stimulation of the meninges. *Br. J. Pharmacol.* **106**, 409–15.

Rebeck, G. W., Maynard, K. I., Hyman, B., and Moskowitz, M. A. (1994). Selective 5-HT$_{1D\alpha}$ receptor gene expression in trigeminal ganglia: implications for anti-migraine drug development. *Proc. Natl Acad. Sci. USA* **49**, 669–80.

Reuter, U., Bolay, H., Jansen-Olesen, I., *et al.* (2001). Delayed inflammation in rat meninges: implications for migraine pathophysiology. *Brain*, **124**, 2490–2502.

Reuter, U., Chiarugi, A., Bolay, H., Moskowitz, M.A. (2002) Nuclear factor-kB as a molecular target for migraine therapy. *Ann. Neurol.* **51**, 507–516.

Sakas, D. E., Moskowitz, M. A., Wei, E. P., Kontos, H. A., Kano, M., and Ogilvy, C. (1989). Trigeminovascular fibers increase blood flow in cortical grey matter by axon reflex-like mechanisms during acute severe hypertension and seizures. *Proc. Natl Acad. Sci. USA* **86**, 1401–5.

Sanchez del Rio, M., Bakker, D., Wu, O., Agosti, R. *et al.* (1999). Perfusion weighted imaging during migraine: spontaneous visual aura and headache. *Cephalgia*, **19**, 701–707.

Sanchez del Rio, M., Moskowitz, M.A. (2000). The trigeminal system. In: Olesen J., Tfelt-Hansen P., Welch K. M. A. eds. *The Headaches*, 2nd edn. Pp. 141–49. Lippincott Williams & Wilkins, Philadelphia.

Strassman, A. M., Raymond, S. A., and Burnstein, R. (1996). Sensitization of meningeal sensory neurons and the origin of headaches. *Nature* **834**, 560–4.

Weber, J. R., Angstwurm, K., Bove, G. M., *et al.* (1996). The trigeminal nerve and augmentation of regional cerebral blood flow during experimental bacterial meningitis. *J. Cereb. Blood Flow Metab.* **16**, 1319–24.

Yu, X.-J., Waeber, C., Castanon, N., *et al.* (1996). 5-carboxamido-tryptamine, CP-122,288 and dihydroergotamine but not sumatriptan, CP-93,129, and serotonin-5-O-carboxymethyl-glycyl-tyrosinamide block dural plasma protein extravasation in knockout mice that lack 5-hydroxytryptamine$_{1B}$ receptors. *Mol. Pharmacol.* **49**, 761–5.

Yu, X.-J. and Moskowitz, M. A. (1995). Neuropeptide Y inhibits neurogenic plasma extravasation in rat dura mater via prejunctional neuropeptide Y$_2$ receptor coupled to pertussis toxin-sensitive G protein. *Cephalgia* **15**, (Suppl. 14), 103.

Yu, X.-J. and Moskowitz, M. A. (1996). Neuropeptide Y Y$_2$ receptor-mediated attenuation of neurogenic plasma extravasation acting through pertussus toxin-sensitive mechanisms. *Br. J. Pharmacol.* **119**, 229–32.

Zgombick, J. M., Schechter, L. E., Kucharewicz, S., Weinshank, R. L., Branchek, T. A. (1995) Ketanserin and ritanserin discriminate between recombinant human 5-HT$_{1Da}$ and 5-HT$_{1DB}$ receptor subtypes. *Eur. J. Pharmacol*, **291**, 9–15.

CHAPTER 8

Vestibular system influences on respiratory muscle activity and cardiovascular functions

Bill J. Yates and Adolfo M. Bronstein

Key points

- Stimulation of vestibular receptors elicits alterations in sympathetic nervous system activity and blood pressure as well as changes in activity of both respiratory pump muscles and upper airway muscles.

- In animal models, changes in blood flow elicited by vestibular stimulation are patterned, and differ between vascular beds.

- Damage to the vestibular labyrinth of animal models results in an inability to decrease blood flow to the lower body during head-up postural alterations. This deficit in adjusting regional blood flow leads to blood pressure instability.

- Lesions within the central vestibular system (vestibular nuclei) of animal models can result in a persistent disturbance in the ability to adjust blood pressure during postural changes, as can lesions of the vestibulocerebellum when followed by peripheral vestibular damage.

- Bilateral labyrinthine damage in animal models results in an alteration in the resting activity of respiratory pump muscles, as well as a deficit in the ability to adjust respiratory activity during postural alterations.

- Vestibular influences on sympathetic nervous system activity are mediated through a neural circuit that includes cells in the rostral ventrolateral medulla and the medullary reticular formation. The neural pathway relaying vestibular signals to respiratory motoneurons has not been determined, but includes cells in addition to those in the medullary respiratory groups.

- A circumscribed region of the caudal vestibular nuclei mediates vestibular system influences on control of blood pressure and breathing. This region receives multiple types of sensory signals, including inputs from receptors in skin, muscle, the viscera, and the labyrinth.

- A number of studies on humans have revealed that stimuli that activate vestibular receptors elicit cardiovascular and respiratory responses. Many of these studies were confounded by the fact that the stimuli employed could have activated non-labyrinthine receptors. However, a few experiments that made use of labyrinthine defective subjects as controls have confirmed that vestibulo-autonomic responses are present in humans.

- Disturbances in cardiovascular and respiratory regulation are only prominent in patients in the acute phase of peripheral vestibular dysfunction, and dissipate rapidly as compensation occurs.

- Vestibular stimulation may exacerbate hyperventilation in patients with panic disorder. In addition, individuals in the acute phase of vestibular disease may be more susceptible to orthostatic hypotension, such that vasoactive drugs should be prescribed cautiously.

Introduction

Although it has been known for over a century that stimulation of receptors located in the vestibular labyrinth produces alterations in blood pressure and breathing, it has only been appreciated within the past 20 years that the vestibular system contributes significantly to autonomic regulation (see Biaggioni et al. 1998, Ray and Carter 2003, Ray and Monahan 2002, Yates 1992, Yates et al. 2002, 2000a, Yates and Kerman 1998, for reviews). This chapter will discuss recent data regarding the effects of stimulation of vestibular receptors on both respiratory and cardiovascular control, as well as findings demonstrating that damage to the peripheral or central vestibular system compromises the ability to adjust breathing and blood pressure during movement and changes in posture. Current knowledge regarding the neural circuitry responsible for relaying vestibular signals to the sympathetic nervous system and respiratory motoneurons will also be summarized. In addition, the clinical implications of deficits in regulating blood pressure and breathing after disruption of labyrinthine signals to the CNS will be discussed.

Physiological necessity for vestibular influences on autonomic regulation

Head-up tilts of quadrupeds, like standing in humans, typically leads to pooling of blood in the venous circulation, and an associated decrease in return of blood to the heart (Rushmer 1976). Starling's Law of the Heart stipulates that this decrease in venous return would result in a drop in blood pressure, unless simultaneous vasoconstriction also occurs in the arterial circulation to raise peripheral resistance (Guyton and Hall 2006). A number of mechanisms act to resist posturally related hypotension, which are discussed in other chapters of this book. However, these mechanisms, such as the baroreceptor reflex, typically do not begin to counteract orthostasis until a sizable drop in blood pressure has already occurred. Thus, although these feedback-regulated mechanisms help to prevent a long-term decrease in blood pressure following a change in posture, they have limited effects early during a movement. The existence of vestibulo-cardiovascular reflexes is not surprising, therefore, as the vestibular system rapidly detects when changes in body position, including those that can affect circulation, are occurring. In fact, it seems practical for the vestibular system to participate in cardiovascular adjustments, because it can act to stabilize the circulation during movement even before blood pressure has changed significantly.

Alterations in posture can also affect the resting length of respiratory pump muscles, requiring adjustments in the activity of these muscles if ventilation is to be unaffected. For example, nose-up tilt of quadrupeds or standing in humans from a supine position can produce diaphragm shortening (Newman et al. 1986). Compensation for the effects of gravity on diaphragm length during supine to head-up body tilts includes both an increase in diaphragm activity and a co-contraction of the abdominal muscles, although increases in abdominal muscle activity appear to be more important in this postural response (Cotter et al. 2001, Gorini and Estenne 1991). Activity of some upper airway muscles also increases during certain postural alterations. This increase in activity is most evident when humans assume a supine position or quadrupeds are tilted nose-up, as under these conditions the tongue tends to shift to the back of the throat and may obstruct the airway (Sauerland and Harper 1976). In particular, the tongue protruder muscle genioglossus and perhaps some pharyngeal muscles must be more active during these postural changes in order to maintain airway patency. Failure of this response in humans produces snoring and obstructive sleep apnoea. Thus, it is appropriate for the vestibular system to contribute to regulating respiratory muscle activity, to assure that rapid adjustments in this activity occur during postural alterations.

Vestibular system influences on the cardiovascular system: data from animal models

Effects of stimulating vestibular receptors on the cardiovascular system

Although most movements of the body activate both vestibular and non-labyrinthine sensory receptors, it is possible to independently elicit vestibular inputs under experimental conditions. One method to activate vestibular afferents selectively is through electrical stimulation of VIIIth cranial nerve branches in the labyrinth. While electrical stimulation of the vestibular nerve is non-physiological (in that firing of afferents that signal head movements in a variety of directions is simultaneously increased), this technique has been used to show that the vestibular system can affect cardiovascular regulation.

Electrical vestibular stimulation modulates the activity of sympathetic nerves that innervate targets distributed throughout the body, including blood vessels (Kerman and Yates 1998, Kerman et al. 2000b). In addition, prolonged electrical stimulation of vestibular afferents results in alterations in blood pressure and blood flow through vascular beds, as illustrated in Fig. 8.1A. Interestingly, electrical vestibular stimulation elicited distinct stereotyped changes in blood flow through different vascular beds (Kerman et al. 2000a), indicating that the vestibular system has coordinated influences on activity of the neural circuitry regulating vascular resistance, and does not just produce a generalized change in sympathetic nervous system outflow.

A Electrical vestibular stimulation

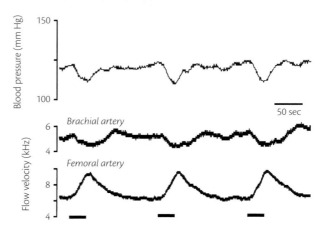

B Natural vestibular stimulation

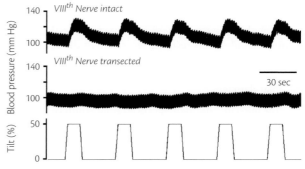

Fig. 8.1 Cardiovascular effects produced by stimulating vestibular receptors in a paralyzed and ventilated, baroreceptor-denervated feline model. **A:** Alterations in mean blood pressure and blood flow elicited by electrical stimulation of the vestibular portion of the VIIIth cranial nerve. In these examples, thick bars beneath the bottom trace designate when the ipsilateral nerve was stimulated using a 30 sec continuous train delivered at 333 Hz, with each pulse being 0.2 ms in duration. The stimulus intensity was 1.7 times the vestibulo-ocular reflex threshold. This stimulus produced depressor responses that were accompanied by increases in blood flow to the hindlimb and decreases in flow to the forelimb. Used with permission from The American Physiological Society (Kerman 2000). **B:** Changes in blood pressure during trapezoidal head rotations (on a fixed body) in cats with extensive denervations to eliminate non-labyrinthine inputs that could be produced by the movements. When innervation of the labyrinth was intact (top panel), large increases in blood pressure accompanied each head movement. However, transection of the VIIIth cranial nerves eliminated the changes in blood pressure during head rotation (bottom panel). With kind permission from Springer Science+Business Media: *Experimental Brain Research*, Pressor response elicited by nose-up vestibular stimulation in cats, **113**, 1997, 165–68, Woodring SF, Rossiter CD and Yates BJ.

In addition to electrically stimulating branches of the VIIIth cranial nerve, it is possible to selectively activate vestibular afferents by performing head rotations in an animal with extensive denervations to eliminate non-labyrinthine inputs that might be produced by this movement. The denervations performed in previous experiments included transection of the vagus and glossopharyngeal nerves to eliminate autonomic signals that might be elicited during head rotation, as well as a C_1–C_4 dorsal rhizotomy to remove inputs from the neck; in some animals the trigeminal nerve was also cut intracranially on both sides to ensure that alterations in somatosensory inputs from the face during head movement could not produce changes in sympathetic nervous system activity (Woodring et al. 1997, Yates and Miller 1994). In this preparation, head rotations in the pitch (sagittal) plane, but not the roll (lateral) or yaw (horizontal) planes, modulated sympathetic outflow. In particular, nose-up tilt of the head produced an increase in activity recorded from a sympathetic nerve, whereas nose-down pitch elicited a decrease in activity (Yates and Miller 1994). Sustained nose-up head rotations also evoked an increase in blood pressure (Woodring et al. 1997), as shown in Fig. 8.1B. It is noteworthy, however, that the animals used in these experiments had been rendered baroreceptor-denervated through transection of the IXth and X[th] cranial nerves, as large changes in blood pressure would be unlikely to occur in animals with an intact baroreceptor reflex. Nonetheless, these data show that activation of specific populations of vestibular afferents results in changes in activity of sympathetic nervous system fibres that regulate blood pressure.

Effects of vestibular system lesions on regulation of blood pressure

As would be predicted from the findings discussed earlier, a bilateral labyrinthectomy resulted in increased blood flow to the lower body and decreased lower body vascular resistance (Fig. 8.2) as well as instability in blood pressure (see panels A and B of Fig. 8.3) at the onset of head-up tilts in conscious animal models (Jian et al. 1999,Wilson et al. 2006). Head-up rotations additionally elicit an increase in vascular resistance in the forelimb, which likely aids in

preventing a drop in blood pressure during the postural alteration (Wilson et al. 2006). However, this increase in forelimb vascular resistance was not attenuated following a bilateral vestibular neurectomy, as occurs in the hindlimb (Wilson et al. 2006). This result indicates the existence of neural pathways that independently control sympathetic outflow to the forelimb and hindlimb, and which provide for distinct vestibular-elicited changes in blood flow in each vascular bed.

A severe impairment in the ability to regulate blood flow and blood pressure during postural alterations persisted for just 1 week, after which time blood pressure and hindlimb blood flow remained relatively stable during head-up tilts (Figs 8.2, 8.3A, and 8.3B). In contrast, lesions of the central vestibular system can produce a prolonged impairment in posturally related cardiovascular responses. Although ablation of the posterior cerebellar vermis did not affect regulation of blood pressure, the combination of damage to the cerebellar uvula along with a bilateral labyrinthectomy resulted in hypotension during head-up rotations, as shown in Fig. 8.3C (Holmes et al. 2002). The deficits in adjusting blood pressure were still present 1 month following the removal of vestibular inputs, when the experiment was terminated (Holmes et al. 2002). These findings led to the conclusion that plasticity within the CNS was responsible for the recovery of cardiovascular responses after damage to the peripheral vestibular system, and that the occurrence of this adaptation was dependent upon the cerebellar uvula remaining intact.

In another series of experiments, chemical lesions were placed bilaterally within the area of the vestibular nuclei that mediates autonomic responses (Mori et al. 2005). In a variety of species, this 'autonomic region' of the vestibular nucleus complex is comprised of portions of the medial and inferior vestibular nuclei located caudal to the lateral vestibular nucleus (Yates 1992). These vestibular nucleus lesions produced a permanent loss of the capacity to rapidly adjust blood pressure during head-up tilts of the animal, as shown in Fig. 8.3D (Mori et al. 2005). The differences between these data and the results collected subsequent to a bilateral vestibular neurectomy (Jian et al. 1999) suggest that the adaptive plasticity

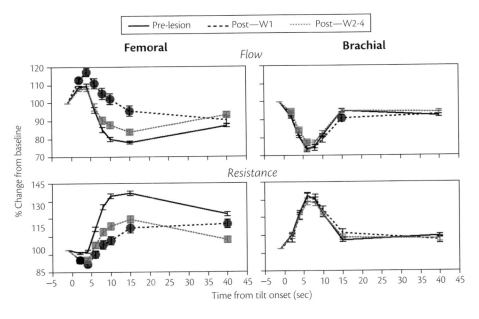

Fig. 8.2 The average effects of removal of vestibular inputs on femoral and brachial blood flow and vascular resistance relative to pre-tilt. Lines illustrate mean data recorded prior to vestibular lesion (pre-lesion), during the first week after the vestibular neurectomy (post-W1), and the following 3 weeks (post-W2–4). Symbols indicate post-lesion changes in blood flow and vascular resistance during tilt that were significantly different from those recorded when vestibular inputs were present. For points where no symbols are present, no significant differences were found. Error bars indicate one S.E.M. With permission from Wilson TD, Cotter LA, Draper JA, Misra SP, Rice CD, Cass SP and Yates BJ, Vestibular inputs elicit patterned changes in limb blood flow in conscious cats. *Journal of Physiology*, Blackwell.

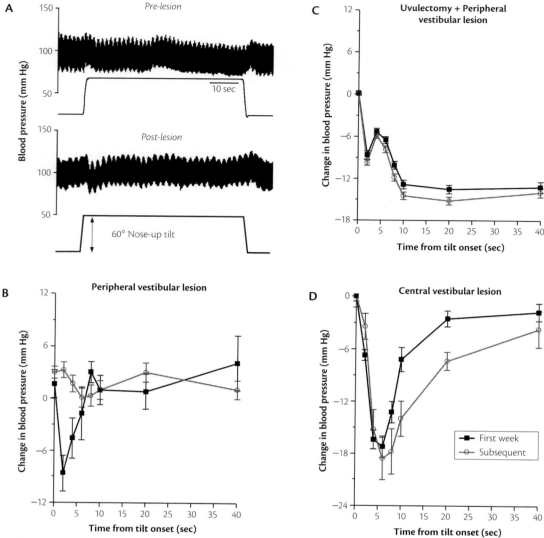

Fig. 8.3 Effects of vestibular system lesions on cardiovascular regulation in a conscious feline model. **A:** Blood pressure recordings made during 60° head-up rotations of a prone animal, both before (pre-lesion) and in the first week subsequent (post-lesion) to a bilateral vestibular neurectomy. In this animal, removal of vestibular inputs resulted in a decrease in blood pressure at onset of nose-up tilt. Used with permission from The American Physiological Society (Jian 1999). **B–D:** Changes in arterial blood pressure recorded in conscious cats during 60° head-up tilts subsequent to peripheral or central vestibular system lesions. Each panel shows averaged data from a single animal. To simplify comparisons, the blood pressure changes were plotted relative to those that occurred before lesions. Responses recorded in the first week following lesions are depicted by solid symbols, and those monitored during the subsequent three weeks are indicated by open symbols. Error bars represent one standard error. **B:** responses recorded following a bilateral labyrinthectomy; data are from Jian et al. 1999. **C:** responses recorded following a combined ablation of the cerebellar uvula and a bilateral labyrinthectomy; reprinted from *Brain Research*, **938**, Holmes MJ, Cotter LA, Arendt HE, Cass SP and Yates BJ, Effects of lesions of the caudal cerebellar vermis on cardiovascular regulation in awake cats, 62–72 Copyright 2002, with permission from Elsevier. **D:** responses recorded following placing chemical lesions bilaterally in the caudal vestibular nuclei; data are from Mori et al. 2005.

that is responsible for recovery of compensatory cardiovascular responses following removal of labyrinthine inputs is mediated through the caudal vestibular nuclei.

Vestibular system influences on respiration: data from animal models

As noted in earlier, changes in posture require alterations in the activity of respiratory muscles if ventilation is to be unaffected. A number of lines of evidence demonstrate that the vestibular system participates in eliciting these posturally related respiratory responses. Electrical vestibular stimulation evoked prominent changes in

activity of nerves innervating respiratory pump muscles and upper airway muscles at latencies < 15 ms (Siniaia and Miller 1996, Yates et al. 1993). Examples of such responses are illustrated in Fig. 8.4A. These responses were eliminated by inactivation of caudal portions of the medial and inferior vestibular nuclei, indicating that they were the result of stimulating vestibular afferents. The presence of vestibular inputs to respiratory muscles was confirmed by examining the effects of head rotations on a stable body in animals with extensive denervations to eliminate non-labyrinthine inputs that might be produced by the movement (Rossiter et al. 1996, Rossiter and Yates 1996). In particular, rotating the head nose-up elicited increases in respiratory muscle activity, as shown in Fig. 8.4B.

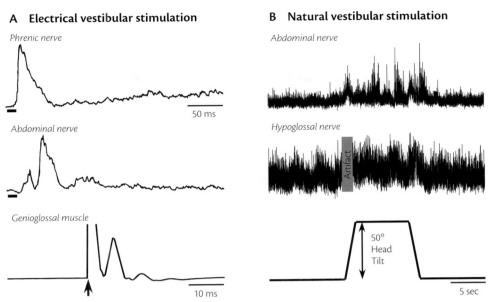

Fig. 8.4 Effects of stimulating vestibular receptors on respiratory muscles in a feline model. **A:** Alterations in activity of the phrenic nerve (top panel), abdominal nerve (middle panel), and the genioglossal muscle (bottom panel) elicited by electrical stimulation of the vestibular portion of the VIIIth cranial nerve. Thick bars beneath the top two traces designate when a vestibular nerve was stimulated using a train of five stimuli, 175 μA in intensity, that were delivered at 333 Hz. These two traces are the average of 54 sweeps. An arrow beneath the bottom trace indicates when a single electrical pulse of 300 μA intensity was delivered to the vestibular nerve; this waveform is the average of 33 sweeps. **B:** Activity recorded from the abdominal and hypoglossal nerves during trapezoidal head rotations (on a fixed body) in cats with extensive denervations to eliminate non-labyrinthine inputs that could be produced by the movements. Each trace is the average of 30 sweeps.

Alterations in the discharges of respiratory muscles could also be elicited by stimulation of brain areas processing vestibular inputs. Chemical stimulation of specific regions of the caudal vestibular nuclei produced large changes in the frequency and depth of breathing (Xu et al. 2002). Furthermore, a number of studies showed that stimulation of three regions of the cerebellum, the rostral fastigial nucleus, the anterior lobe (lobules I–V), and the uvula (located in the caudal cerebellar vermis), affected respiratory muscle activity (for review see Balaban 1996). Each of these cerebellar areas receives labyrinthine input and is connected directly or indirectly with regions of the vestibular nuclei that mediate vestibular influences on respiration, and thus may modulate these responses. These data show that multiple brain regions that process labyrinthine inputs participate in respiratory regulation.

Experiments conducted in conscious cats have also compared alterations in the activity of respiratory muscles during postural changes before and after removal of labyrinthine inputs. Electromyography (EMG) was used to record activity from the diaphragm, abdominal muscles, and the tongue protruder genioglossus of animals that were prone or tilted nose-up or ear-down at amplitudes up to 60°, both before and subsequent to a bilateral vestibular neurectomy (Cotter et al. 2004, Cotter et al. 2001). Examples of these data are shown in Fig. 8.5. Elimination of vestibular inputs greatly diminished the augmentation in abdominal muscle activity that previously occurred during nose-up tilt, and also resulted in a large increase in the spontaneous activity of this musculature (Cotter et al. 2001). The small enhancement of diaphragm activity during nose-up tilt was also diminished following removal of vestibular inputs, and the spontaneous discharges of this muscle related to breathing were significantly larger following the lesions (Cotter et al. 2001). More complex responses were recorded from genioglossus during whole-body tilts (Cotter et al. 2004). Both pitch

and roll body tilts produced modifications in muscle firing that were dependent on the amplitude of the rotation, but the relative effects of ear-down and nose-up tilts on genioglossal activity were variable from animal to animal. The response variability observed might reflect the fact that genioglossus is comprised of many compartments and participates in a variety of tongue movements; in each animal, EMG recordings presumably sampled the firing of different proportions of fibres in the various compartments and subcompartments of the muscle. Nonetheless, alterations in genioglossal muscle activity during body rotations were attenuated following a bilateral labyrinthectomy, demonstrating that the vestibular system contributes to producing these responses (Cotter et al. 2004).

A recent study determined the effects of bilateral destruction of the inner ear on the movement of air into and out of the lungs of conscious animals (Arshian et al. 2007). Removal of vestibular inputs resulted in a 15% reduction in breathing rate, a 13% decrease in minute ventilation, a 16% decrease in maximal inspiratory airflow rate, and a 14% decrease in the maximal expiratory airflow rate measured when the animals were in the prone position. However, the lesions did not appreciably affect phasic changes in airflow parameters related to alterations in posture. These results suggest that the role of the vestibular system in the control of breathing is to modify baseline respiratory parameters in proportion to the general intensity of ongoing movements, and not to rapidly alter ventilation in accordance with body position.

Although bilateral damage to the labyrinths altered the spontaneous activity of the respiratory muscles as well as their responses to tilt, recovery began within a few days after the lesions, presumably because of plasticity in the CNS (Cotter et al. 2001). These findings show that although labyrinthine inputs ordinarily contribute to regulation of respiration, other sensory signals can substitute for the vestibular inputs if they are lost.

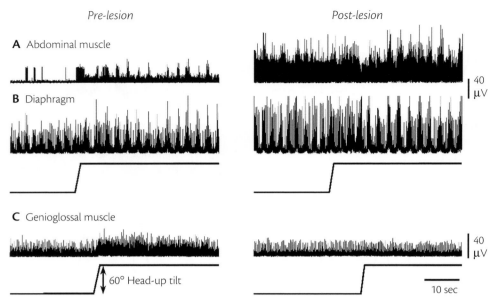

Fig. 8.5 Effects of removal of vestibular inputs on activity of respiratory muscles in conscious felines. The left column shows activity recorded from the abdominal muscle rectus abdominis (**A**), the diaphragm (**B**), and the genioglossal muscle (**C**) during a 60° head-up tilt of the animal's body. The change in posture elicited a large in increase in abdominal and genioglossal muscle activity, and a small increase in diaphragm discharges. The right column depicts activity recorded within the first week subsequent to a bilateral vestibular neurectomy. Removal of vestibular inputs resulted in an increase in baseline firing of both abdominal muscles and the diaphragm, but the modulation of muscle activity during changes in body position was attenuated. Although baseline genioglossal activity was not affected by the vestibular neurectomy, the procedure eliminated the increase in firing that previously occurred during head-up tilts. Used with permission from The American Physiological Society (Cotter 2004)..

Neural mechanisms mediating vestibular influences on autonomic regulation

The use of a variety of experimental approaches, including anatomic, neurophysiological, and ablation techniques, has established the minimal neural circuit through which the vestibular system contributes to cardiovascular regulation (Yates 1992, Yates and Kerman 1998, Yates et al. 1995). Neurons located in the 'pressor region' of the rostral ventrolateral medulla appear to be critical for relaying vestibular signals to sympathetic preganglionic neurons in the spinal cord (Yates et al. 1995). In turn, cells in the rostral ventrolateral medulla receive vestibular signals through a multisynaptic pathway that includes neurons in the reticular formation (Yates and Kerman 1998). Furthermore, bulbospinal neurons in the rostral ventrolateral medulla that respond to vestibular stimulation receive convergent baroreceptor inputs, suggesting that these neurons also mediate the baroreceptor reflex (Yates et al. 1991).

The neural pathway that relays vestibular signals to respiratory motoneurons is not as well established as the one mediating vestibular influences on the sympathetic nervous system. Historically, premotor respiratory neurons were thought to be mainly confined to two columns located in the lateral reticular formation of the caudal medulla, the so-called 'brainstem respiratory groups'. Although some respiratory group neurons receive vestibular signals (Miller et al. 1995), functional lesions that inactivate these cells or their axons do not eliminate vestibulo-respiratory responses (Yates et al. 1995). Furthermore, vestibular stimulation can produce an increase in activity of respiratory pump muscles without affecting the firing of respiratory group neurons (Yates et al. 2002). Thus, premotor neurons in addition to those in the respiratory groups must make synaptic contacts with diaphragm and abdominal motoneurons. We have determined the locations of these neurons

through studies in which a transneuronal tracer, pseudorabies virus, was injected into the diaphragm, abdominal musculature, and genioglossus. These experiments showed that additional premotor respiratory neurons are located in two regions: the medial medullary reticular formation (MRF) and the spinal gray matter (Billig et al. 2000, Shintani et al. 2003). Physiological studies have confirmed that some MRF neurons with projections to the phrenic motor pool have appropriate responses to vestibular stimulation to mediate labyrinthine influences on diaphragm motoneurons (Wilkinson et al. 2004). However, inactivation of the MRF using lidocaine or muscimol produced a large increase in spontaneous activity and responses to vestibular stimulation of respiratory muscles (Mori et al. 2001). These findings led to the hypothesis that MRF neurons receiving labyrinthine inputs inhibit respiratory motoneurons, whereas a population of cells located elsewhere mediates vestibular-induced increases in respiratory activity. Spinal interneurons constitute the other group of premotor respiratory neurons identified in transneuronal tracing studies, although it has not yet been determined whether these cells participate in mediating vestibulo-respiratory responses.

Lesions of a circumscribed caudal area of the vestibular nuclei eliminate vestibular influences on control of both respiration and blood pressure (Yates et al. 1993). A recent transneuronal tracing study revealed that this vestibular nucleus region receives substantial direct and/or polysynaptic input from the spinal gray matter and the gracile, cuneate, and solitary nuclei, indicating that the neurons located there process a variety of sensory signals (Jian et al. 2005). Physiological experiments have also shown that the firing of neurons in the 'autonomic region' of the vestibular nuclei is modulated by stimulation of nerves innervating the skin, muscle and viscera (Jian et al. 2002). This multisensory processing likely explains the observation that some vestibular nucleus neurons still respond to changes in body position in space following a bilateral labyrinthectomy (Yates et al. 2000b). Furthermore, these data account for the findings that autonomic disturbances subsequent to peripheral vestibular lesions dissipate quickly (Cotter et al. 2004, 2001, Jian et al. 1999), whereas those produced by vestibular nucleus lesions are persistent (Mori et al. 2005).

Studies in humans and clinical implications

Clinicians have long been aware of an important input from the vestibular system to the autonomic system. Clinical observations of some distressing symptoms in patients with acute vestibular lesions, such as nausea, vomiting, occasionally diarrhoea, sweatiness, tachycardia and palpitations, vividly illustrate the existence of vestibulo-autonomic projections. More recently, clinical researchers have raised important new issues, such as a possible connection between vestibular disorders, anxiety and autonomic symptoms, as well as putative neuroanatomical sites capable of mediating these interactions. Specifically, the parabrachial nucleus, in connection with limbic areas, appears to be ideally placed in the brain to mediate vestibular influences on the level of anxiety, as this nucleus is involved in vestibular, autonomic and neurobehavioural processes (Balaban and Thayer 2001). Finally, attention has been drawn to the possibility that some ill-defined symptoms in patients with a chronic vestibular lesion, such as orthostatic intolerance or light-headedness, may represent disordered vestibular-autonomic control (Furman et al. 1998). Thus, there are many reasons why diagnosis and management of vestibular patients would improve if we understood human vestibular-autonomic control better than we do at present. Herewith we discuss insights into vestibulo-autonomic interactions gained through studies in humans during the past 15 years.

Vestibulo-respiratory interactions

The respiratory system is a good candidate through which to study the complex vestibular-anxiety-autonomic interrelations. Patients with panic disorder hyperventilate and this makes them dizzy. The reciprocal also appears to be true, in that vestibular patients often hyperventilate and feel 'panicky'. The latter is often observed during caloric vestibular testing, and many patients cannot complete their vestibular tests due to anxiety-panic symptoms. As a starting point we have examined two questions:

1 Does hyperventilation affect balance and if so, how?

2 Does vestibular input affect breathing?

In order to investigate whether hyperventilation affects balance, Sakellari and Bronstein (Sakellari and Bronstein 1997) asked subjects to over-breathe voluntarily for specified lengths of time and then to stop. At this point (i.e. during the subsequent phase of normal breathing or hypopnoea), but with subjects still in hypocapnia, different variables were measured. It was found that normal subjects become posturally unstable, with large amplitude and low frequency body sway movements. Patients with bilateral severe loss of peripheral vestibular function (labyrinthine defective subjects or LDS) became equally unstable during hyperventilation, suggesting that the unsteadiness was more likely to be mediated by non-vestibular than by direct vestibular mechanisms (Sakellari and Bronstein 1997). Additional experiments, for instance measuring click-elicited, vestibular-evoked myogenic potentials that remained unchanged after hyperventilation, confirmed this view (Sakellari et al. 1997). Thus, hyperventilation mostly interferes with somatosensory mechanisms and central processes mediating vestibular compensation (Sakellari et al. 1997).

These experimental observations carry some implications for clinical practice. Therapists need to be vigilant of patients developing hyperventilation during rehabilitation since this, as discussed above, interferes with vestibular compensation. If hyperventilation does occur, compensatory breathing exercises should be prescribed. Another point concerns the diagnosis of dizziness due to hyperventilation. Many physicians, in the absence of clinical findings in a dizzy patient, ask the patient to hyperventilate in order to see if this induces dizziness or reproduces the patient's symptoms. It is our advice that physicians should not rely excessively on the voluntary hyperventilation test for diagnosis of hyperventilation-related dizziness. After all, voluntary hyperventilation induces dizziness and objective loss of balance in all individuals as well as nystagmus in patients with a pre-existing vestibular abnormality (Minor et al. 1999, Sakellari et al. 1997).

The question of whether vestibular stimulation influences breathing has been examined with the use of caloric and rotational stimuli. A general problem in this area of research is determining how much of an observed effect is actually vestibular in origin, although this can be partly overcome by incorporating LDS as controls. Both caloric (Jauregui-Renaud et al. 2000) and rotational stimuli (Jauregui-Renaud et al. 2001, Thurrell et al. 2003) induce a slight increase in respiratory frequency that is not detected in LDS. The findings could indicate that the vestibular organs, as specialized motion transducers, synchronize or 'entrain' body musculature, including respiratory muscles, to similar frequencies as the ongoing movement (Thurrell et al. 2003). More generally, body movements, particularly active movements, are likely to increase oxygen consumption, and the vestibular system could provide an early signal to the CNS to increase ventilation accordingly.

An important clinical implication is that these findings provide the physiological basis for 'vestibular induced' panic attacks, in which respiratory symptoms and hyperventilation can feature prominently. Indeed, vestibular patients reporting respiratory-autonomic symptoms do exhibit increased heart and respiration rate during head movements (Yardley et al. 1998). Physicians need to be aware that panic symptoms preceded by 'true' rotational vertigo may indicate an underlying vestibular disorder as a trigger for the panic episode. Similarly, it has been suggested that patients with vestibular lesions may suffer from a form of 'vestibulo-respiratory ataxia' (M.A. Gresty, personal communication) due to disruption of the vestibulo-respiratory drive. Although this is somewhat speculative and no clear definition of this putative syndrome yet exists, physical therapists need to be vigilant and, if in doubt, include breathing retraining during vestibular exercises.

Vestibulo-cardiovascular interactions

An important aspect of the experiments mentioned in the previous section was the demonstration that some vestibulo-cardiovascular effects are secondary to primary vestibulo-respiratory effects. For instance, caloric irrigation (Jauregui-Renaud et al. 2000) induced an increase in the high frequency (0.15–0.40 Hz) component of heart rate variability. This response, however, was only present if subjects breathed freely and disappeared if respiration was synchronized with a metronome. In this circumstance, changes in

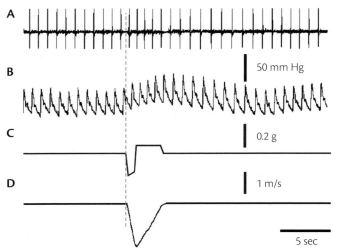

Fig. 8.6 Changes in heart rate and blood pressure in a human subject during forward linear acceleration, with the head restrained in the upright position. A vertical dashed line denotes the onset of the acceleration. **A:** recording of the electrocardiogram. **B:** non-invasive recording of blood pressure. **C:** stimulus acceleration profile, derived from accelerometer recordings. **D:** stimulus velocity. With kind permission from Springer Science+Business Media: *Experimental Brain Research*, Cardiovascular responses elicited by linear acceleration in humans, **125**, 1999, 476–84, Yates BJ, Aoki M, Burchill P, Bronstein AM and Gresty MA.

heart rate and blood pressure variability were apparently secondary to a caloric-elicited increase in respiration frequency. We will now review the evidence suggesting the presence of direct, non-respiratory mediated, vestibulo-cardiovascular responses in humans.

In experiments with individuals seated on a linear sled, facing the direction of motion, Yates et al. (Yates et al. 1999) observed an increase in blood pressure and heart rate soon after the onset of acceleration. The response occurred instantaneously, sometimes within one heartbeat, which is too rapid to be secondary to breathing changes (Fig. 8.6). This rapid effect was not observed in LDS. In order to more precisely determine the latency between head acceleration and cardiovascular responses, Radtke et al. (Radtke et al. 2000) devised an experiment in which the stimulus (head acceleration) was triggered by the R-spike of the subject's

electrocardiogram (ECG). The experimental design, illustrated in Fig. 8.7, employed the 'head drop' paradigm, in which the head is suddenly released into free fall. From previous experiments it was known that this sudden head acceleration, which stimulates both semicircular canals and otolith organs, is capable of activating short latency vestibulo-spinal mechanisms in normal individuals but not in LDS (Ito et al. 1995, Munchau et al. 2001). Head drops reduced the interval between the triggering R-wave and the next R-wave; by varying the delay between the R-wave and the head drop, the latency of the vestibulo-cardiac reflex was estimated to be approximately 500 ms The early modulation of heart rate was not consistently observed in LDS, confirming the view that vestibular inputs contribute to generating a fast cardiac response to rapid head-body reorientations. Changes in blood pressure and peripheral blood flow were observed 2–3 heartbeats later both in normal individuals and LDS (Radtke et al. 2003), indicating that non-vestibular signals contributed to producing these cardiovascular responses.

Other researchers have investigated the influence of vestibular activation on muscular sympathetic nerve activity (MSNA) in the lower limbs by performing microneurography. Caloric irrigation of the ear increases MSNA in a manner that is proportional to the intensity of the vestibular stimulus and the resulting nystagmus (Cui et al. 1997). Otolith activation also increases MSNA, and this has been demonstrated with two techniques. The first method is by inverting the normal upright position of the head, achieved by having subjects supine and then flexing their neck such that the top of the head points down to the ground (referred to as head down rotation [HDR]) by the authors of the study) (Hume and Ray 1999, Ray and Carter 2003, Ray and Monahan 2002). Recordings were performed when the head position was stable, however, and not during the dynamic component of the rotation that also activated semicircular canals. The increase in MSNA elicited by this manoeuvre was observed consistently, but two problems remain with these data:

♦ It is not known whether the findings were the result of selective activation of vestibular endorgans, as LDS have never been tested.

♦ The functional significance of such an otolith-sympathetic reflex is unclear.

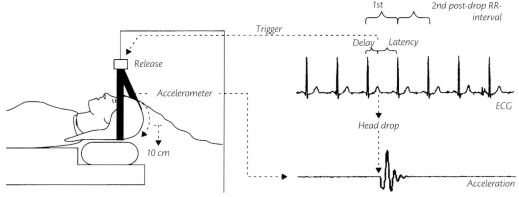

Fig. 8.7 Design of an experiment to determine the latency of vestibulo-cardiovascular influences in human subjects. Tests were done with subjects in a supine position with the head suspended 10 cm above a cushion in a sling with an electromechanical release. Release of the head was triggered at a predetermined delay after an R-spike of an ECG and resulted in an abrupt acceleration (about 0.8 g for about 140 ms) as the head returned to its normal alignment from a flexed posture with little neck extension. The latency of the effect of vestibular stimulation on the cardiac cycle length was estimated by considering the delays in the stimulus (time interval between a triggering R-spike and onset of the head drop) and the changes in the R-R interval. Reprinted from *The Lancet*, **356**, Radtke A, Popov K, Bronstein AM and Gresty MA, Evidence for a vestibulo-cardiac reflex in man, 736–7, Copyright 2000, with permission from Elsevier.

An increase in peripheral arterial vasoconstriction, presumably leading to an increase in cerebral blood flow, would not appear to be necessary when the head is upside down. In spite of these caveats the findings are of potential clinical relevance, as dysfunction in this reflex may partly explain orthostatic intolerance in vestibular patients or the elderly (Monahan and Ray 2002).

Kaufmann et al. (Kaufmann et al. 2002) studied the otolith-sympathetic reflex by measuring MSNA during off-vertical axis rotation (OVAR). The authors were able to estimate that the delay or latency at which this mechanism operates, particularly during the nose-up phase of rotation, is approximately 400 ms This latency is compatible with that determined by the experiments of Yates et al. (1999) and Radtke et al. (2000, 2003) during forward acceleration and 'head drop', respectively. Here again, however, the fact that LDS were not studied does not allow one to be confident as to whether the findings observed during OVAR were the result of stimulating vestibular receptors or other graviceptors such as visceral receptors (Mittelstaedt 1992, 1996).

Recovery from the effects of vestibular system dysfunction on autonomic regulation in patients

A considerable obstacle in understanding vestibular-autonomic control in humans is posed by the rapid development of vestibular compensation after acute peripheral lesions. A recent clinical study by Jauregui-Renaud et al. (2003) illustrates this point. In this study, a battery of simple clinical tests of autonomic cardiovascular control was applied to a group of patients with acute vertigo due to unilateral vestibular neuritis. These tests occurred within 48 hours of vertigo onset, and a complete semicircular canal paresis was documented in all cases. In the acute stage there was evidence of reduced vascular sympathetic reactivity during orthostatic challenges and during immersion of the hand in cold water, but these abnormalities had dissipated when tests were conducted again 2 weeks later (Fig. 8.8). A potentially important clinical implication

of this study (Jauregui-Renaud et al. 2003) is that dosages of vasoactive medications (e.g. antihypertensive drugs), may have to be reduced during the acute phase of an acute vestibular episode as patients may be prone to suffer orthostatic hypotension.

Whether these findings indicate a specific dysfunction of vestibulo-sympathetic mechanisms, or whether they just reflect a generalized loss of sympathetic reactivity during acute, distressing symptoms, needs further investigation. However, the fact that recovery of vestibulo-ocular and vestibulo-postural responses occurred over a similar time course as which deficiencies in autonomic responses resolved suggests that a common mechanism is involved (Jauregui-Renaud et al. 2003). Yet, little is known about the mechanisms responsible for potential recovery of autonomic responses following disease or damage of the vestibular system in humans. On the basis of animal experiments (Holmes et al. 2002), however, the cerebellar uvula and paraflocular region appear to be good candidates for mediating central vestibulo-autonomic compensation. It is interesting to note, therefore, that these cerebellar areas have been identified as possible sites for vestibular processing underlying motion sickness (Cohen et al. 2003).

As briefly discussed above, a major limitation of most studies of vestibulo-autonomic control is the fact that they were conducted in chronic, usually well-compensated, patients. According to the animal experiment literature and the only study in acute human patients (Jauregui-Renaud et al. 2003), the process of compensation for vestibulo-autonomic dysfunction is rapid and effective. Studies in patients with acute bilateral vestibular disorders (e.g. subsequent to ototoxicity or meningitis), would be particularly useful although most of these patients are too ill to undergo research experiments. Due to this limitation, we do not as yet know the magnitude of the contribution of the vestibular system to cardiorespiratory control in man. The experiments performed so far suggest that the contribution is small and variable but, as mentioned, this may be due to compensation processes. In contrast, vestibular input into gastric motility (Koch 1999) and nausea mechanisms seems large and, according to patients' reports, clinically relevant. However, apart from a consideration of motion sickness, little research effort has been devoted to this potentially important area.

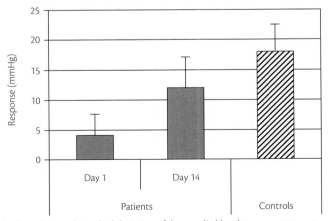

Fig. 8.8 Mean and standard deviation of the systolic blood pressure response to immersion of the hand in cold water (cold hand test) of seven patients with vestibular neuritis and seven age-matched healthy subjects. Patients were tested near the onset of vertigo (acute phase of their vestibular dysfunction) and at a 2-week follow up. Reprinted from *Archives of Medical Research*, **34**, Jauregui-Renaud K, Hermosillo AG, Gomez A, Marquez MF, Cardenas M and Bronstein AM, Vestibular function interferes in cardiovascular reflexes, 200–4, Copyright 2003, with permission from Elsevier.

Summary and conclusion

A number of lines of inquiry have demonstrated that the vestibular system contributes to adjusting blood distribution in the body as well as respiratory muscle activity during movement and postural adjustments. These vestibulo-autonomic responses apparently contribute to maintaining stable blood delivery to the tissues and stable blood oxygenation during movement and postural alterations. Accordingly, vestibular system lesions produce a number of deleterious effects, including a disruption in the ability to rapidly adjust blood pressure and respiratory muscle activity during movement and changes in posture. Following damage to the labyrinth or VIIIth cranial nerves, these deficits resolved over time. However, it should be noted that the testing conditions employed in the studies that produced these observations were somewhat artificial. It is probable that the animal and human subjects expected to undergo experimental procedures, and were particularly vigilant during data collection sessions. It is unlikely that such a high level of attention to environmental cues regarding body position in space was maintained outside of laboratory conditions. Thus, peripheral vestibular dysfunction could result in long-lasting deficits in correcting blood pressure that only become apparent when the level of alertness diminishes. Additional experiments will be required to examine this possibility. In animals, central vestibular system lesions can also produce pronounced and prolonged dysfunction of autonomic responses that are required during changes in posture, although analogous studies are yet to be performed in humans. Moreover, understanding the clinical implications of vestibulo-autonomic influences will require further studies of patients in the acute phase of recovery from vestibular dysfunction.

Acknowledgements

Dr Yates's research is supported by the National Institutes of Health (NIH) of the United States, grants R01-DC00693 and R01-DC03732. Core support for his laboratories is funded by NIH grants EY08098 and DC05205. A Programme Grant from the Medical Research Council (UK) supports Dr Bronstein's research.

References

Arshian, M., Holtje, R. J., Cotter, L. A., Rice, C. D., Cass, S. P. and Yates, B. J. (2007). Consequences of postural changes and removal of vestibular inputs on the movement of air in and out of the lungs of conscious felines. *J Appl. Physiol.*, **103**, 347–52.

Balaban, C. D. (1996). The role of the cerebellum in vestibular autonomic function. In B. J. Yates and A. D. Miller, eds. *Vestibular autonomic regulation*, pp. 127–44. CRC Press, Boca Raton, FL.

Balaban, C. D. and Thayer, J. F. (2001). Neurological bases for balance-anxiety links. *J Anxiety Disord.*, **15**, 53–79.

Biaggioni, I., Costa, F. and Kaufmann, H. (1998). Vestibular influences on autonomic cardiovascular control in humans. *J Vestibular Res.* **8**, 35–41.

Billig, I., Foris, J. M., Enquist, L. W., Card, J. P. and Yates, B. J. (2000). Definition of neuronal circuitry controlling the activity of phrenic and abdominal motoneurons in the ferret using recombinant strains of pseudorabies virus. *J Neurosci.* **20**, 7446–54.

Cohen, B., Dai, M. and Raphan, T. (2003). The critical role of velocity storage in production of motion sickness. *Annals of the New York Academy Scienc,* **1004**, 359–76.

Cotter, L. A., Arendt, H. E., Cass, S. P., *et al.* (2004). Effects of postural changes and vestibular lesions on genioglossal muscle activity in conscious cats. *J Appl. Physiol* **96**, 923–30.

Cotter, L. A., Arendt, H. E., Jasko, J. G., Sprando, C., Cass, S. P. and Yates, B. J. (2001) Effects of postural changes and vestibular lesions on diaphragm and rectus abdominis activity in awake cats. *J Appl. Physiol* **91**, 137–44.

Cui, J., Mukai, C., Iwase, S., *et al.* (1997). Response to vestibular stimulation of sympathetic outflow to muscle in humans. *J Auton. Nerv. Syst.* **66**, 154–62.

Furman, J. M., Jacob, R. G. and Redfern, M. S. (1998). Clinical evidence that the vestibular system participates in autonomic control. *J Vestibular Res.* **8**, 27–34.

Gorini, M. and Estenne, M. (1991) Effect of head-up tilt on neural inspiratory drive in the anesthetized dog. *Respiration Physiology* **85**, 83–96.

Guyton, A. C. and Hall, J. E. (2006). *Textbook of Medical Physiology, 11th ed.* Philadelphia, Saunders.

Holmes, M. J., Cotter, L. A., Arendt, H. E., Cass, S. P. and Yates, B. J. (2002). Effects of lesions of the caudal cerebellar vermis on cardiovascular regulation in awake cats. *Brain Research* **938**, 62–72.

Hume, K. M. and Ray, C. A. (1999). Sympathetic responses to head-down rotations in humans. *J Appl. Physiol.* **86**, 1971–76.

Ito, Y., Corna, S., von Brevern, M., Bronstein, A., Rothwell, J. and Gresty, M. (1995). Neck muscle responses to abrupt free fall of the head: comparison of normal with labyrinthine-defective human subjects. *Journal of Physiology* **489**, 911–6.

Jauregui-Renaud, K., Gresty, M. A., Reynolds, R. and Bronstein, A. M. (2001). Respiratory responses of normal and vestibular defective human subjects to rotation in the yaw and pitch planes. *Neuroscience Letters* **298**, 17–20.

Jauregui-Renaud, K., Hermosillo, A. G., Gomez, A., Marquez, M. F., Cardenas, M. and Bronstein, A. M. (2003). Vestibular function interferes in cardiovascular reflexes. *Arch. Med. Res.* **34**, 200–4.

Jauregui-Renaud, K., Yarrow, K., Oliver, R., Gresty, M. A. and Bronstein, A. M. (2000). Effects of caloric stimulation on respiratory frequency and heart rate and blood pressure variability. *Brain Research Bulletin* **53**, 17–23.

Jian, B. J., Acernese, A. W., Lorenzo, J., Card, J. P. and Yates, B. J. (2005). Afferent pathways to the region of the vestibular nuclei that participates in cardiovascular and respiratory control. *Brain Research* **1044**, 241–50.

Jian, B. J., Cotter, L. A., Emanuel, B. A., Cass, S. P. and Yates, B. J. (1999). Effects of bilateral vestibular lesions on orthostatic tolerance in awake cats. *J Appl. Physiol.* **86**, 1552–60.

Jian, B. J., Shintani, T., Emanuel, B. A. and Yates, B. J. (2002). Convergence of limb, visceral, and vertical semicircular canal or otolith inputs onto vestibular nucleus neurons. *Exp. Brain Res.* **144**, 247–57.

Kaufmann, H., Biaggioni, I., Voustianiouk, A., *et al.* (2002). Vestibular control of sympathetic activity. An otolith-sympathetic reflex in humans. *Exp. Brain Res.* **143**, 463–9.

Kerman, I. A., Emanuel, B. A. and Yates, B. J. (2000a). Vestibular stimulation leads to distinct hemodynamic patterning. *Am. J Physiol. Regul. Integr. Comp. Physiol.* **279**, R118–25.

Kerman, I. A., Yates, B. J. and McAllen, R. M. (2000b). Anatomic patterning in the expression of vestibulosympathetic reflexes. *Am. J Physiol. Regul. Integr. Comp. Physiol.* **279**, R109–17.

Kerman, I. A. and Yates, B. J. (1998). Regional and functional differences in the distribution of vestibulosympathetic reflexes. *Am. J Physiol. Regul. Integr. Comp. Physiol.* **275**, R824–R35.

Koch, K. L. (1999). Illusory self-motion and motion sickness—a model for brain-gut interactions and nausea. *Dig. Dis. Sci.* **44**, 53S–7S.

Miller, A. D., Yamaguchi, T., Siniaia, M. S. and Yates, B. J. (1995) Ventral respiratory group bulbospinal inspiratory neurons participate in vestibular-respiratory reflexes. *J Neurophysiol.* **73**, 1303–07.

Minor, L. B., Haslwanter, T., Straumann, D. and Zee, D. S. (1999). Hyperventilation-induced nystagmus in patients with vestibular schwannoma. *Neurology* **53**, 2158–68.

Mittelstaedt, H. (1992). Somatic versus vestibular gravity reception in man. *Annals of the New York Academy of Sciences* **656**, 124–39.

Mittelstaedt, H. (1996). Somatic graviception. *Biological Psychology* **42**, 53–74.

Monahan, K. D. and Ray, C. A. (2002). Vestibulosympathetic reflex during orthostatic challenge in aging humans. *Am. J Physiol. Regul. Integr. Comp. Physiol.* **283**, R1027–32.

Mori, R. L., Bergsman, A. E., Holmes, M. J. and Yates, B. J. (2001). Role of the medial medullary reticular formation in relaying vestibular signals to the diaphragm and abdominal muscles. *Brain Research* **902**, 82–91.

Mori, R. L., Cotter, L. A., Arendt, H. E., Olsheski, C. J. and Yates, B. J. (2005). Effects of bilateral vestibular nucleus lesions on cardiovascular regulation in conscious cats. *J Appl. Physiol.* **98**, 526–33.

Munchau, A., Corna, S., Gresty, M. A., *et al.* (2001). Abnormal interaction between vestibular and voluntary head control in patients with spasmodic torticollis. *Brain* **124**, 47–59.

Newman, S. L., Road, J. D. and Grassino, A. (1986). In vivo length and shortening of canine diaphragm with body postural change. *J Appl. Physiol.* **60**, 661–69.

Radtke, A., Popov, K., Bronstein, A. M. and Gresty, M. A. (2000). Evidence for a vestibulo-cardiac reflex in man. *Lancet* **356**, 736–7.

Radtke, A., Popov, K., Bronstein, A. M. and Gresty, M. A. (2003). Vestibulo-autonomic control in man: Short- and long-latency vestibular effects on cardiovascular function. *J Vestibular Res.* **13**, 25–37.

Ray, C. A. and Carter, J. R. (2003). Vestibular activation of sympathetic nerve activity. *Acta Physiologica Scandinavica* **177**, 313–9.

Ray, C. A. and Monahan, K. D. (2002). The vestibulosympathetic reflex in humans: neural interactions between cardiovascular reflexes. *Clin. Exp. Pharmacol. Physiol.* **29**, 98–102.

Rossiter, C. D., Hayden, N. L., Stocker, S. D. and Yates, B. J. (1996). Changes in outflow to respiratory pump muscles produced by natural vestibular stimulation. *J Neurophysiol* **76**, 3274–84.

Rossiter, C. D. and Yates, B. J. (1996). Vestibular influences on hypoglossal nerve activity in the cat. *Neuroscience Letters* **211**, 25–28.

Rushmer, R. F. (1976). *Cardiovascular Dynamics,* Philadelphia, Saunders.

Sakellari, V., Bronstein, A. M., Corna, S., Hammon, C. A., Jones, S. and Wolsley, C. J. (1997). The effects of hyperventilation on postural control mechanisms. *Brain* **120**, 1659–73.

Sakellari, V. and Bronstein, A. M. (1997). Hyperventilation effect on postural sway. *Arch. Phys. Med. Rehabil.* **78**, 730–6.

Sauerland, E. K. and Harper, R. M. (1976). The human tongue during sleep: electromyographic activity of the genioglossus muscle. *Exp. Neurol.* **51**, 160–70.

Shintani. T., Anker, A. R., Billig, I., Card, J. P. and Yates, B. J. (2003). Transneuronal tracing of neural pathways influencing both diaphragm and genioglossal muscle activity in the ferret. *J Appl. Physiol.* **95**, 1453–9.

Siniaia, M. S. and Miller, A. D. (1996). Vestibular effects on upper airway musculature. *Brain Research* **736**, 160–64.

Thurrell, A., Jauregui-Renaud, K., Gresty, M. A. and Bronstein, A. M. (2003). Vestibular influence on the cardiorespiratory responses to whole-body oscillation after standing. *Exp. Brain Res.* **150**, 325–31.

Wilkinson, K. A., Maurer, A. P., Sadacca, B. F. and Yates, B. J. (2004). Responses of feline medial medullary reticular formation neurons with projections to the C5-C6 ventral horn to vestibular stimulation. *Brain Research* **1018**, 247–56.

Wilson, T. D., Cotter, L. A., Draper, J. A., Misra, S. P., Rice, C. D., Cass, S. P. and Yates, B. J. (2006). Vestibular inputs elicit patterned changes in limb blood flow in conscious cats. *J Physiol.* **575**, 671–84.

Woodring, S. F., Rossiter, C. D. and Yates, B. J. (1997). Pressor response elicited by nose-up vestibular stimulation in cats. *Exp. Brain Res.* **113**, 165–68.

Xu, F., Zhuang, J., Zhou, T-R., Gibson, T. and Frazier, D. T. (2002). Activation of different vestibular subnuclei evokes differential respiratory and pressor responses in the rat. *J Physiol.* **544**, 211–23.

Yardley, L., Gresty, M., Bronstein, A. and Beyts, J. (1998). Changes in heart rate and respiration rate in patients with vestibular dysfunction following head movements which provoke dizziness. *Biological Psychology* **49**, 95–108.

Yates, B. J. (1992). Vestibular influences on the sympathetic nervous system. *Brain Research Reviews* **17**, 51–59.

Yates, B. J., Aoki, M., Burchill, P., Bronstein, A. M. and Gresty, M. A. (1999). Cardiovascular responses elicited by linear acceleration in humans. *Exp. Brain Res.* **125**, 476–84.

Yates, B. J., Billig, I., Cotter, L. A., Mori, R. L. and Card J. P. (2002). Role of the vestibular system in regulating respiratory muscle activity during movement. *Clin. Exp. Pharmacol. Physiol* **29**, 112–7.

Yates, B. J., Holmes, M. J. and Jian, B. J. (2000a). Adaptive plasticity in vestibular influences on cardiovascular control. *Brain Research Bulletin* **53**, 3–9.

Yates, B. J., Jakus, J. and Miller, A. D. (1993). Vestibular effects on respiratory outflow in the decerebrate cat. *Brain Research* **629**, 209–17.

Yates, B. J., Jian, B. J., Cotter, L. A. and Cass, S. P. (2000b). Responses of vestibular nucleus neurons to tilt following chronic bilateral removal of vestibular inputs. *Exp. Brain. Res.* **130**, 151–8.

Yates, B. J., Siniaia, M. S. and Miller, A. D. (1995). Descending pathways necessary for vestibular influences on sympathetic and inspiratory outflow. *Am. J Physiol. Regul. Integr. Comp. Physiol.* **268**, R1381–R85.

Yates, B. J., Yamagata, Y. and Bolton, P. S. (1991). The ventrolateral medulla of the cat mediates vestibulosympathetic reflexes. *Brain Research* **552**, 265–72.

Yates, B. J. and Kerman, I. A. (1998). Post-spaceflight orthostatic intolerance, possible relationship to microgravity-induced plasticity in the vestibular system. *Brain Research Reviews* 28, 73–82.

Yates, B. J. and Miller, A. D. (1994). Properties of sympathetic reflexes elicited by natural vestibular stimulation: implications for cardiovascular control. *Journal of Neurophysiology* **71**, 2087–92.

CHAPTER 9

Neural control of the urinary bladder

William C. de Groat

Key points

- The functions of the lower urinary tract to store and periodically release urine are regulated by a complex neural control system located in the brain and spinal cord.

- Information from the spinal cord is conveyed to the lower urinary tract by three sets of peripheral nerves (sympathetic, parasympathetic and somatic).

- The nervous system maintains a reciprocal relationship between the bladder and the urethral outlet.

- During urine storage the sympathetic and somatic nerves activate the urethral smooth and striated muscle, respectively, while the parasympathetic control of the bladder is inactive.

- During micturition parasympathetic nerves are activated to contract the bladder and relax the urethra, while sympathetic and somatic nerve activity is inhibited.

- Urine storage reflexes are organized in the spinal cord, whereas micturition reflexes are mediated by pathways in the brain.

- Electrophysiological studies in animals and functional brain imaging studies in humans have identified many neuronal populations in the frontal cortex, hypothalamus, limbic system, and pontine micturition centre involved in bladder control.

- Many neurotransmitters including glutamic acid, γ-aminobutyric acid, glycine, acetylcholine, norepinephrine, serotonin, and dopamine have been identified in the neural circuits controlling the lower urinary tract. Glutamic acid and acetylcholine are the major excitatory transmitters in the central and peripheral nervous system, respectively.

- Because the functions of the lower urinary tract are totally dependent on neural control, micturition can be affected by various diseases or injuries of the peripheral and central nervous system.

Introduction

The functions of the lower urinary tract to store and periodically release urine are dependent upon neural circuits located in the brain, spinal cord, and peripheral ganglia (Morrison et al. 2005).

This dependence on central nervous control distinguishes the lower urinary tract from many other visceral structures (e.g. the gastrointestinal tract and cardiovascular system) that maintain a certain level of activity even after elimination of extrinsic neural input. The lower urinary tract is also unusual in regard to its pattern of activity and the complexity of its neural regulation. For example, the urinary bladder has two principal modes of operation: storage and elimination. Thus many of the neural circuits controlling the bladder exhibit switch-like or phasic patterns of activity, in contrast to tonic patterns occurring in autonomic pathways to cardiovascular organs. In addition, micturition is under voluntary control and depends upon learned behaviour that develops during maturation of the nervous system, whereas many other visceral functions are regulated involuntarily. Micturition also depends on the integration of autonomic and somatic efferent mechanisms within the lumbosacral spinal cord (Morrison et al. 2005). This is necessary to coordinate the activity of visceral organs (the bladder and urethra) with that of urethral striated muscles. This chapter will review the peripheral and central neural mechanisms controlling the lower urinary tract and the disruption of this control by neural injury.

Innervation of the lower urinary tract

The storage and periodic elimination of urine is dependent upon the activity of two functional units in the lower urinary tract:

- a reservoir (the urinary bladder)

- an outlet, consisting of bladder neck, urethra, and striated muscles of the urethral sphincter (Morrison et al. 2005, Fry et al. 2005).

These structures are, in turn, controlled by three sets of peripheral nerves: sacral parasympathetic (pelvic nerves), thoracolumbar sympathetic (hypogastric nerves and sympathetic chain), and sacral somatic nerves (pudendal nerves) (Fig. 9.1) (Morrison et al. 2005).

Sacral parasympathetic pathways

The sacral parasympathetic outflow provides the major excitatory input to the urinary bladder. Cholinergic preganglionic neurons located in the intermediolateral region of the sacral spinal cord (Morgan et al. 1993) send axons via the pelvic nerves to ganglion

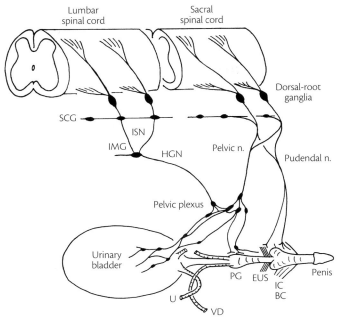

Fig. 9.1 Diagram showing the sympathetic, parasympathetic, and somatic innervation of the urogenital tract of the male cat. Sympathetic preganglionic pathways emerge from the lumbar spinal cord and pass to the sympathetic chain ganglia (SCG) and then via the inferior splanchnic nerves (ISN) to the inferior mesenteric ganglia (IMG). Preganglionic and postganglionic sympathetic axons then travel in the hypogastric nerve (HGN) to the pelvic plexus and the urogenital organs. Parasympathetic preganglionic axons which originate in the sacral spinal cord pass in the pelvic nerve to ganglion cells in the pelvic plexus and to distal ganglia in the organs. Sacral somatic pathways are contained in the pudendal nerve, which provides an innervation to the penis, the ischiocavernosus (IC), bulbocavernosus (BC), and external urethral sphincter (EUS) muscles. The pudendal and pelvic nerves also receive postganglionic axons from the caudal sympathetic chain ganglia. These three sets of nerves contain afferent axons from the lumbosacral dorsal root ganglia. U, ureter; PG, prostate gland; VD, vas deferens. Reprinted by permission from Macmillan Publishers Ltd: *Spinal Cord*, de Groat WC, copyright 1995.

Table 9.1 Receptors for putative transmitters in the lower urinary tract

Tissue	Cholinergic	Adrenergic	Other
Bladder body	$+ (M_2)$ $+ (M_3)$	$- (\beta_2)$ $- (\beta_3)$	$+$ Purinergic (P2X$_1$) $-$ VIP $+$ Substance P (NK$_2$)
Bladder base	$+ (M_2)$ $+ (M_3)$	$+ (\alpha_1)$	$-$ VIP $+$ Substance P (NK$_2$) $+$ Purinergic (P2X)
Urothelium	$+ (M_2)$ $+ (M_3)$	$+\alpha$ $+\beta$	$+$ TRPV1 $+$ TRPM8 $+$ P2X $+$ P2Y $+$ Substance P $+$ Bradykinin (B2)
Urethra	$+ (M)$	$+ (\alpha_1)$ $+ (\alpha_2)$ $- (\beta)$	$+$ Purinergic (P2X) $-$ VIP $-$ Nitric oxide
Sphincter striated muscle	$+ (N)$		
Adrenergic nerve terminals	$- (M_2)$ $+ (M_1)$	$- (\alpha_2)$	$-$ NPY
Cholinergic nerve terminals	$- (M_2)$ $+ (M_1)$	$+ (\alpha_1)$	$-$ NPY
Afferent nerve terminals			$+$ Purinergic (P2X$_{2/3}$) $+$ TRPV1
Ganglia	$+ (N)$ $+ (M_1)$	$+ (\alpha_1)$ $- (\alpha_2)$ $+ (\beta)$	$-$ Enkephalinergic (δ) $-$ Purinergic (P$_1$) $+$ Substance P

VIP, vasoactive intestinal polypeptide; NPY, neuropeptide Y; TRP, transient receptor potential. Letters in parentheses indicate receptor type (e.g. M (muscarinic) and N (nicotinic). + and − signs indicate excitatory and inhibitory effects.

cells in the pelvic plexus and in the wall of the bladder. Transmission in bladder ganglia is mediated by a nicotinic cholinergic mechanism, which can be modulated by activation of various receptors including muscarinic, adrenergic, purinergic, and peptidergic (Table 9.1) (de Groat and Booth 1993). Ganglia in some species (cats and rabbits) also exhibit a prominent frequency-dependent facilitatory mechanism that can amplify parasympathetic activity passing from the spinal cord to the bladder (de Groat and Booth 1993). The ganglion cells in turn excite bladder smooth muscle via the release of cholinergic (acetylcholine) and non-cholinergic, non-adrenergic transmitters. Cholinergic excitatory transmission in the bladder is mediated by muscarinic receptors, which are blocked by atropine (Morrison et al. 2005, Andersson 1993, Andersson and Arner 2004), whereas non-cholinergic transmission is mediated by the purinergic transmitter, adenosine triphosphate (ATP), acting on P2X purinergic receptors (Table 9.1) (Ralevic and Burnstock 1998, Burnstock 2001). Both M_2 and M_3 muscarinic receptor subtypes are expressed in bladder smooth muscle; however examination of subtype selective muscarinic receptor antagonists and studies of muscarinic receptor knockout mice have revealed that the M_3 subtype is the principal receptor involved in excitatory transmission (Matsui et al. 2000, Matsui

et al. 2002). Modulatory receptors are also present prejunctionally on parasympathetic nerve terminals. Activation of these receptors by acetylcholine can enhance (M_1 receptors) or suppress (M_4 receptors) transmitter release, depending upon the intensity of neural firing (Somogyi et al. 1996, de Goat and Yoshimura 2001). Inhibitory input to the urethral smooth muscle is mediated by nitric oxide released by parasympathetic nerves (Andersson 1993, Andersson and Arner 2004). Postganglionic neurons innervating the bladder also contain neuropeptides, such as vasoactive intestinal polypeptide (VIP) and neuropeptide Y (NPY). These substances are co-released with acetylcholine or ATP and may function as modulators of neuroeffector transmission.

Thoracolumbar sympathetic pathways

Sympathetic pathways to the lower urinary tract originate in the lumbosacral sympathetic chain ganglia as well as in the prevertebral inferior mesenteric ganglia. Input from the sacral chain ganglia passes to the bladder via the pelvic nerves, whereas fibres from the rostral lumbar and inferior mesenteric ganglia travel in the hypogastric nerves. Sympathetic efferent pathways in the hypogastric and pelvic nerves in the cat elicit similar effects in the bladder, consisting of:

- inhibition of detrusor muscle via β-adrenergic receptors
- excitation of the bladder base and urethra via α_1-adrenergic receptors (Morrison et al. 2005, Andersson and Arner 2004).
- inhibition and facilitation in bladder parasympathetic ganglia via α_2- and α_1-adrenergic receptors, respectively (Table 9.1) (de Groat and Booth 1993).

Somatic efferent pathways

The efferent innervation of the urethral striated muscles in various species originates from cells in a circumscribed region of the lateral ventral horn that is termed Onuf's nucleus (de Groat et al. 2001). Sphincter motoneurons send their axons into the pudendal nerve and excite sphincter muscles via the release of acetylcholine which stimulates postjunctional nicotinic receptors.

Afferent pathways

Afferent axons innervating the urinary tract are present in the three sets of nerves (Morrison et al. 2005). The most important afferents for initiating micturition are those passing in the pelvic nerve to the sacral spinal cord. These afferents are small myelinated (Aδ) and unmyelinated (C) fibres, which convey information from receptors in the bladder wall to second-order neurons in the spinal cord. Aδ bladder afferents in the cat respond in a graded manner to passive distension as well as active contraction of the bladder and exhibit pressure thresholds in the range of 5–15 mmHg, which are similar to those pressures at which humans report the first sensation of bladder filling. These fibres also code for noxious stimuli in the bladder. On the other hand, C-fibre bladder afferents in the cat have very high thresholds and commonly do not respond to even high levels of intravesical pressure (Habler et al. 1990). However, activity in some of these afferents is unmasked or enhanced by chemical irritation of the bladder mucosa. These findings indicate that C-fibre afferents in the cat have specialized functions, such as the signalling of inflammatory or noxious events in the lower urinary tract. In the rat, A-fibre and C-fibre bladder afferents cannot be distinguished on the basis of stimulus modality; thus both types of afferents consist of mechanosensitive and chemosensitive populations (Morrison et al. 2005). C-fibre afferents are sensitive to the neurotoxins, capsaicin and resiniferatoxin as well as to other substances such as tachykinins, nitric oxide, ATP, prostaglandins and neurotrophic factors released in the bladder by afferent nerves, urothelial cells and inflammatory cells (Morrison et al. 2005, Maggi 1993, Rong et al. 2002, Chuang et al. 2001). These substances can sensitize the afferent nerves and change their response to mechanical stimuli.

The properties of lumbosacral dorsal root ganglion cells innervating the bladder, urethra and external urethral sphincter in the rat have been studied with patch clamp recording techniques in combination with axonal tracing methods to identify the different populations of neurons (Yoshimura et al. 1996, Yoshimura and de Groat 1997, Yoshimura and de Groat 1999, Yoshimura et al. 2003). Based on responsiveness to capsaicin it is estimated that approximately 70% of bladder afferent neurons in the rat are of the C-fibre type. These neurons exhibit high threshold tetrodotoxin-resistant sodium channels and action potentials and phasic firing (one to

two spikes) in response to prolonged depolarizing current pulses. Approximately 90% of the bladder C-fibre afferent neurons also are excited by ATP, which induces a depolarization and firing by activating $P2X_3$ or $P2X_{2/3}$ receptors (Zhong et al. 2003). A-fibre afferent neurons are resistant to capsaicin and ATP, exhibit low threshold tetrodotoxin-sensitive sodium channels and action potentials and tonic firing (multiple spikes) to depolarizing current pulses. C-fibre bladder afferent neurons also express a slowly decaying A-type K^+ current that controls spike threshold and firing frequency (Yoshimura et al. 1996, Yoshimura et al. 2003). Suppression of this K^+ current by drugs or chronic bladder inflammation induces hyperexcitability of the afferent neurons (Yoshimura and de Groat 1999).

A large percentage of bladder afferent neurons contain peptides: calcitonin-gene-related peptide, VIP, pituitary adenylate cyclase-activating peptide (PACAP), tachykinins, galanin and opioid peptides (Morrison et al. 2005, Maggi 1993). Nerves containing these peptides are common in the bladder, in the submucosal and epithelial layers, and around blood vessels. Peptidergic bladder afferent neurons in the rat also express TrkA, a high affinity receptor for nerve growth factor (NGF) and receptors for tachykinins (NK-2 and NK-3 receptors) and endothelins (Morrison et al. 2005). These findings suggest that the neuropeptides may be important transmitters in the afferent pathways from the lower urinary tract.

Urothelium

The urothelium, which has been traditionally viewed as a passive barrier at the bladder lumenal surface (Lewis 2000, Apodaca 2004), also has specialized sensory and signalling properties that allows urothelial cells to respond to their chemical and physical environment and to engage in reciprocal chemical communication with neighbouring nerves in the bladder wall (Apodaca 2004, Ferguson et al. 1997, Birder et al. 1998, Birder et al. 2001, Birder et al. 2002). These properties include:

- expression of nicotinic, muscarinic, tachykinin, adrenergic and capsaicin (TRPV1) receptors
- responsiveness to transmitters released from afferent nerves,
- close physical association with afferent nerves
- ability to release chemical mediators such as ATP and nitric oxide that can regulate the activity of adjacent nerves and thereby trigger local vascular changes and/or reflex bladder contractions.

The role of ATP in urothelial-afferent communication has attracted considerable attention because bladder distension releases ATP from the urothelium (Ferguson et al. 1997, Sun et al. 2001, Birder et al. 2003) and intravesical administration of ATP induces bladder hyperactivity, an effect blocked by administration of P2X purinergic receptor antagonists that suppress the excitatory action of ATP on bladder afferent neurons (Morrison et al. 2005). Mice in which the $P2X_3$ receptor was knocked out exhibited hypoactive bladder activity and inefficient voiding (Cockayne et al. 2000) suggesting that activation of $P2X_3$ receptors on bladder afferent nerves by ATP released from the urothelium is essential for normal bladder function. In humans and cats with interstitial cystitis, a painful bladder condition, ATP release from urothelial cells is enhanced (Sun et al. 2001, Birder et al. 2003). Higher levels of ATP may induce abnormal afferent nerve firing and pain.

Reflex control of the lower urinary tract

The neural pathways controlling lower urinary tract function are organized as simple on–off switching circuits (Fig. 9.2) that maintain a reciprocal relationship between the urinary bladder and urethral outlet. The principal reflex components of these switching circuits are listed in Table 9.2 and illustrated in Fig. 9.3. Intravesical pressure measurements during bladder filling in both humans and animals reveal low and relatively constant bladder pressures when bladder volume is below the threshold for inducing voiding (Fig. 9.3a) (Morrison et al. 2005). The accommodation of the bladder to increasing volumes of urine is primarily a passive phenomenon dependent upon the intrinsic properties of the vesical smooth muscle and quiescence of the parasympathetic efferent pathway.

Table 9.2 Reflexes to the lower urinary tract

Afferent pathway	Efferent pathway	Central pathway
URINE STORAGE Low level vesical afferent activity (pelvic nerve)	◆ External sphincter contraction (somatic nerves) ◆ Internal sphincter contraction (sympathetic nerves) ◆ Detrusor inhibition (sympathetic nerves) ◆ Ganglionic inhibition (sympathetic nerves) ◆ Sacral parasympathetic outflow inactive	Spinal reflexes
MICTURITION High level vesical afferent activity (pelvic nerve)	◆ Inhibition of external sphincter activity ◆ Inhibition of sympathetic outflow ◆ Activation of parasympathetic outflow to the bladder	Spinobulbospinal reflexes
	◆ Activation of parasympathetic outflow to the urethra	Spinal reflex

In addition, in some species urine storage is also facilitated by sympathetic reflexes that mediate an inhibition of bladder activity, closure of the bladder neck, and contraction of the proximal urethra (Table 9.2, Fig. 9.3). During bladder filling the activity of the sphincter electromyogram (EMG) also increases (Fig. 9.2b), reflecting an increase in efferent firing in the pudendal nerve and an increase in outlet resistance that contributes to the maintenance of urinary continence.

The storage phase of the urinary bladder can be switched to the voiding phase either involuntarily (reflexly) or voluntarily (Fig. 9.2). The former is readily demonstrated in the human infant (Fig. 9.2a) when the volume of urine exceeds the micturition threshold. At this point, increased afferent firing from tension receptors in the bladder produces firing in the sacral parasympathetic pathways and inhibition of sympathetic and somatic pathways. The expulsion phase consists of an initial relaxation of the urethral sphincter (Fig. 9.2a) followed by a contraction of the bladder, an increase in bladder pressure, and flow of urine. Relaxation of the urethral outlet is mediated by activation of a parasympathetic reflex pathway to the urethra (Table 9.2) that triggers the release of nitric oxide, an inhibitory transmitter (Andersson 1993), as well as by removal of adrenergic and somatic excitatory inputs to the urethra.

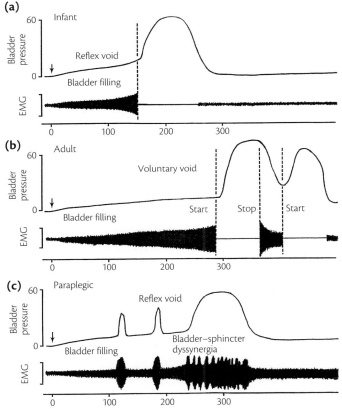

Fig. 9.2 Combined cystometrograms and sphincter electromyograms (EMG) comparing reflex voiding responses in an infant **(a)** and in a paraplegic patient **(c)** with a voluntary voiding response in an adult **(b)**. The abscissa in all records represents bladder volume in millilitres and the ordinates represent bladder pressure in cmH$_2$O and electrical activity of the EMG recording. On the left side of each trace the arrows indicate the start of a slow infusion of fluid into the bladder (bladder filling). Vertical dashed lines indicate the start of sphincter relaxation, which precedes by a few seconds the bladder contraction in **(a)** and **(b)**. In part **(b)** note that a voluntary cessation of voiding (stop) is associated with an initial increase in sphincter EMG followed by a reciprocal relaxation of the bladder. A resumption of voiding is again associated with sphincter relaxation and a delayed increase in bladder pressure. On the other hand, in the paraplegic patient **(c)** the reciprocal relationship between bladder and sphincter is abolished. During bladder filling, transient uninhibited bladder contractions occur in association with sphincter activity. Further filling leads to more prolonged and simultaneous contractions of the bladder and sphincter (bladder–sphincter dyssynergia). Loss of the reciprocal relationship between bladder and sphincter in paraplegic patients interferes with bladder emptying.

Anatomy of central nervous pathways controlling the lower urinary tract

The reflex circuitry controlling micturition consists of four basic components: spinal efferent neurons, spinal interneurons, primary afferent neurons and neurons in the brain that modulate spinal reflex pathways. New research methodologies, including transneuronal virus tracing (Figs. 9.4, 9.5) (Nadelhaft et al. 1992, Vizzard et al. 1995), measurements of gene expression (Fig. 9.5B) (Birder and de Groat 1993), and patch-clamp recording in spinal cord slice preparations (Araki and de Groat 1996), have recently provided new insights into the morphological and electrophysiological properties of these reflex components.

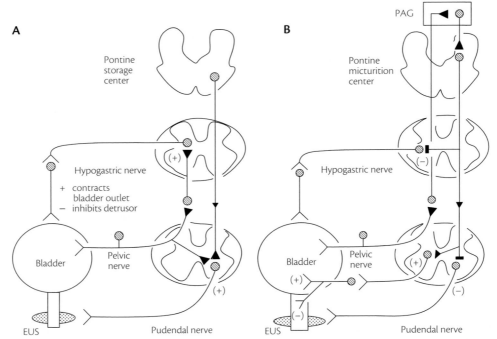

Fig. 9.3 Diagram showing neural circuits controlling continence and micturition. **(A)** Urine storage reflexes. During the storage of urine, distention of the bladder produces low level vesical afferent firing, which in turn stimulates (1) the sympathetic outflow to the bladder outlet (base and urethra) and (2) pudendal outflow to the external urethral sphincter. These responses occur by spinal reflex pathways and represent guarding reflexes, which promote continence. Sympathetic firing also inhibits detrusor muscle and modulates transmission in bladder ganglia. A region in the rostral pons (the pontine storage centre) increases external urethral sphincter activity. **(B)** Voiding reflexes. During elimination of urine, intense bladder afferent firing activates spinobulbospinal reflex pathways passing through the pontine micturition centre, which stimulate the parasympathetic outflow to the bladder and internal sphincter smooth muscle and inhibit the sympathetic and pudendal outflow to the urethral outlet. Ascending afferent input from the spinal cord may pass through relay neurons in the periaqueductal gray (PAG) before reaching the pontine micturition centre.

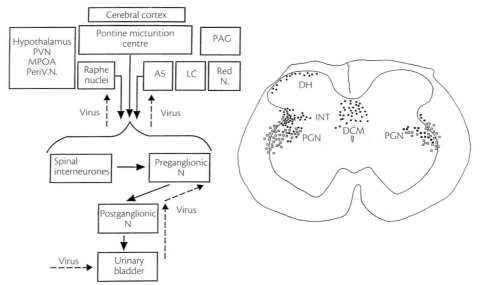

Fig. 9.4 Transneuronal virus tracing of the central pathways controlling the urinary bladder of the rat. Injection of pseudorabies virus into the wall of the urinary bladder leads to retrograde transport of virus (dashed arrows) and sequential infection of postganglionic neurons, preganglionic neurons, and then various central neural circuits synaptically linked to the preganglionic neurons. Normal synaptic connections are indicated by solid arrows. At long survival times virus can be detected with immunocytochemical techniques in neurons at specific sites throughout the spinal cord and brain, extending to the pontine micturition centre in the pons (i.e. Barrington's nucleus) and to the cerebral cortex. Other sites in the brain labelled by virus are: (1) the paraventricular nucleus (PVN), medial preoptic area (MPOA) and periventricular nucleus (Peri V.N.) of the hypothalamus; (2) periaqueductal grey (PAG); (3) locus coeruleus (LC) and subcoeruleus; (4) red nucleus; (5) medullary raphe nuclei; and (6) the noradrenergic cell group designated A5. L6 Spinal cord section, showing on the left side the distribution of virus-labelled parasympathetic preganglionic neurons (□) and interneurons (•) in the region of the parasympathetic nucleus, the dorsal commissure (DCM), and the superficial laminae of the dorsal horn (DH), 72 hours after injection of the virus into the bladder. The right side shows the entire population of preganglionic neurons (PGN) (□) labelled by axonal tracing with the fluorescent dye (fluorogold), injected into the pelvic ganglia and the distribution of virus-labelled bladder PGN (•). Composite diagram of neurons in 12 spinal sections (42 μm).

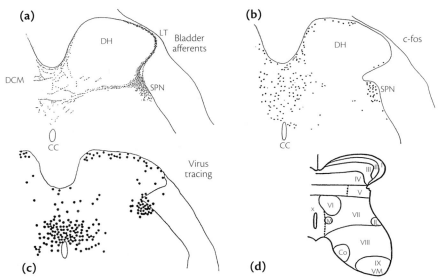

Fig. 9.5 Comparison of the distribution of bladder afferent projections to the L6 spinal cord of the rat **(a),** with the distribution of c-*fos*-positive cells in the L6 spinal segment following chemical irritation of the lower urinary tract of the rat **(b),** and the distribution of interneurons in the L6 spinal cord labelled by transneuronal transport of pseudorabies virus injected into the urinary bladder **(c)**. Afferents labelled by WGA-HRP injected into the urinary bladder. C-*fos* immunoreactivity is present in the nuclei of cells. DH, dorsal horn; SPN, sacral parasympathetic nucleus; CC central canal. Calibration represents 500 μm. **(d)** The laminar organization of the cat spinal cord. These data show that spinal interneurons involved in the reflex control of the urinary bladder are concentrated in specific regions of the spinal cord that receive afferent input from the lower urinary tract. Some of these interneurons provide excitatory input to the parasympathetic preganglionic neurons and represent an essential component of the spinal micturition reflex pathway.

Pathways in the spinal cord

The spinal cord grey matter is divided into three general regions:

- the dorsal horn, which contains interneurons that process sensory input

- the ventral horn, which contains motoneurons

- an intermediate region located between the dorsal and ventral horns, which contains interneurons and autonomic preganglionic neurons (Figs 9.4, 9.5).

These regions are further subdivided into layers or laminae that are numbered, starting with the superficial layer of the dorsal horn (lamina I) and extending to the ventral horn (lamina IX) and the commissure connecting the two sides of the spinal cord (lamina X) (Fig. 9.5d).

Efferent neurons

Parasympathetic preganglionic neurons are located in the intermediolateral grey matter (laminae V–VII) in the sacral segments of the spinal cord (Fig. 9.4), whereas sympathetic preganglionic neurons are located in medial (lamina X) and lateral sites (laminae V–VII) in the rostral lumbar spinal cord. External urethral sphincter (EUS) motoneurons are located in lamina IX in Onuf's nucleus (Morrison et al. 2005, de Groat et al. 2001). As shown in Fig. 9.6, parasympathetic preganglionic neurons and EUS motoneurons send dendrites to similar regions of the spinal cord, indicating that these sites contain important pathways for coordinating bladder and sphincter function.

Afferent projections in the spinal cord

Afferent pathways from the lower urinary tract (LUT) project to discrete regions of the dorsal horn that contain interneurons and efferent neurons innervating the LUT (Steers et al. 1991).

Afferent pathways from the urinary bladder project into Lissauer's tract at the apex of the dorsal horn and then pass rostrocaudally, giving off collaterals that extend laterally and medially through the superficial layer of the dorsal horn (lamina I) into the deeper layers (laminae V–VII and X) at the base of the dorsal horn (Fig. 9.5a). The lateral pathway terminates in the region of the sacral parasympathetic nucleus and also sends some axons to the dorsal commissure (Fig. 9.5a). Pudendal afferent pathways from the urethra and urethral sphincter exhibit a similar pattern of termination in the sacral spinal cord (de Groat et al. 2001). The overlap of bladder and urethral afferents in the lateral dorsal horn and dorsal commissure indicates that these regions are likely to be important sites of viscerosomatic integration and involved in coordinating bladder and sphincter activity.

Spinal interneurons

As shown in Figures 9.4 and 9.5, interneurons retrogradely labelled by injection of pseudorabies virus (PRV) into the urinary bladder or urethra of the rat are located in regions of the spinal cord receiving afferent input from the bladder (Nadelhaft et al. 1992, Vizzard et al. 1995). Large populations of interneurons are located just dorsal and medial to the preganglionic neurons as well as in the dorsal commissure and lamina I (Fig. 9.5c).

The spinal neurons involved in processing afferent input from the lower urinary tract have been identified by the expression of the immediate early gene, c-*fos* (Fig. 9.5b). In the rat, stimulation of the bladder and urethra increases the levels of Fos protein primarily in the dorsal commissure, the superficial dorsal horn, and in the area of the sacral parasympathetic nucleus (Fig. 9.5b) (Birder and de Groat 1993). Some of these interneurons send long projections to the brain, whereas others make local connections in the spinal cord and participate in segmental spinal reflexes

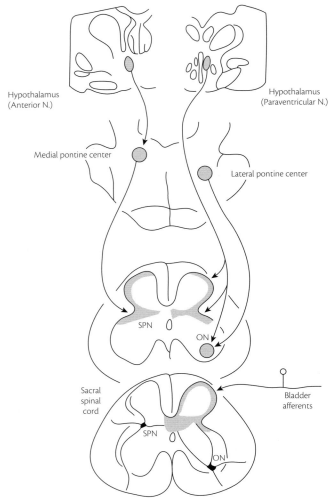

Fig. 9.6 Neural connections between the brain and the sacral spinal cord that may be involved in the regulation of the lower urinary tract in the cat. Lower section of spinal cord shows the location and morphology of a preganglionic neuron in the sacral parasympathetic nucleus (SPN), a sphincter motoneuron in Onuf's nucleus (ON), and the sites of central termination of afferent projections from the urinary bladder. Upper section of the spinal cord shows the sites of termination of descending pathways arising in the pontine micturition centre (medial), the pontine sphincter or urine storage centre (lateral), and the paraventricular nuclei of the hypothalamus. Section through the pons shows the projection from the anterior hypothalamic nuclei to the pontine micturition centre.

(Araki and de Groat 1996). The former are involved in transmitting sensory input to supraspinal centres for subsequent relay to the cerebral cortex or to micturition reflex circuits in the brainstem. Ascending axons terminate in several areas, including the periaqueductal grey (PAG) (Blok et al. 1995) and the gracile nucleus. It is believed that neurons in the PAG relay information to the pontine micturition centre and initiate the micturition reflex. Projections to the gracile nucleus carry nociceptive signals which are eventually routed to the thalamus and cortex.

Patch–clamp recordings from parasympathetic preganglionic neurons in the neonatal rat spinal slice preparation have revealed that interneurons located immediately dorsal and medial to the parasympathetic nucleus make direct monosynaptic connections with the preganglionic neurons (Araki and de Groat 1996).

Microstimulation of interneurons in both locations elicits glutamatergic, N-methyl-D-aspartate (NMDA), and non-NMDA excitatory postsynaptic currents in preganglionic neurons (Araki and de Groat 1996). Stimulation of a subpopulation of medial interneurons elicits GABAergic and glycinergic inhibitory postsynaptic currents. Thus local interneurons are likely to play an important role in both excitatory and inhibitory reflex pathways controlling the preganglionic outflow to the lower urinary tract

Pathways in the brain

In the rat, transneuronal virus tracing methods have identified many populations of neurons in the brain that are involved in the control of bladder, urethra, and the urethral sphincter, including Barrington's nucleus (the pontine micturition centre [PMC]); medullary raphe nuclei, which contain serotonergic neurons; the locus coeruleus, which contains noradrenergic neurons; PAG, and the A5 noradrenergic cell group (Fig. 9.4) (Nadelhaft et al. 1992, Vizzard et al. 1995). Several regions in the hypothalamus and the cerebral cortex also exhibited virus-infected cells. Neurons in the cortex were located primarily in the medial frontal cortex.

Other anatomical studies in which anterograde tracer substances were injected into brain areas and then identified in terminals in the spinal cord (Fig. 9.6) are consistent with the virus tracing data. Tracer injected into the paraventricular nucleus of the hypothalamus labelled terminals in the sacral parasympathetic nucleus as well as the sphincter motor nucleus. On the other hand, neurons in the anterior hypothalamus project to the PMC. Neurons in the PMC in turn project primarily to the sacral parasympathetic nucleus and the lateral edge of the dorsal horn and the dorsal commissure, areas containing dendritic projections from preganglionic neurons, sphincter motoneurons, and afferent inputs from the bladder. Conversely, projections from neurons in the lateral pons terminate rather selectively in the sphincter motor nucleus (Fig. 9.6). Thus the sites of termination of descending projections from the PMC are optimally located to regulate reflex mechanisms at the spinal level.

Organization of urine storage and voiding reflexes

Sympathetic storage reflex

Although the integrity of the sympathetic input to the lower urinary tract is not essential for the performance of micturition it does contribute to the storage function of the bladder. Surgical interruption or pharmacological blockade of the sympathetic innervation can reduce urethral outflow resistance, reduce bladder capacity, and increase the frequency and amplitude of bladder contractions recorded under constant volume conditions (Morrison et al. 2005).

Sympathetic reflex activity is elicited by a sacrolumbar intersegmental spinal reflex pathway that is triggered by vesical afferent activity in the pelvic nerves (Fig. 9.3). The reflex pathway is inhibited when bladder pressure is raised to the threshold for producing micturition. This inhibitory response is abolished by transection of the spinal cord at the lower thoracic level, indicating that it originates at a supraspinal site, possibly the pontine micturition centre. Thus, the vesicosympathetic reflex represents a negative feedback mechanism that allows the bladder to accommodate larger volumes (Fig. 9.3).

Urethral sphincter storage reflex

Motoneurons innervating the striated muscles of the urethral sphincter exhibit a tonic discharge that increases during bladder filling (Fig. 9.2). This activity is mediated in part by low-level afferent input from the bladder (Table 9.2, Fig. 9.3a). During micturition the firing of sphincter motoneurons is inhibited. This inhibition is dependent in part on supraspinal mechanisms (Fig. 9.3b), since it is less prominent in chronic spinal animals. Electrical stimulation of the pontine micturition centre induces sphincter relaxation, suggesting that bulbospinal pathways from the pons may be responsible for maintaining the normal reciprocal relationship between bladder and sphincter (Mallory et al. 1991).

Voiding reflexes

Spinobulbospinal micturition reflex pathway

Micturition is mediated by activation of the sacral parasympathetic efferent pathway to the bladder and the urethra as well as reciprocal inhibition of the somatic pathway to the urethral sphincter (Table 9.2) (Fig. 9.3b). Studies in cats using brain-lesioning techniques revealed that neurons in the brainstem at the level of the inferior colliculus have an essential role in the control of the parasympathetic component of micturition (Fig. 9.3b). Removal of areas of the brain above the inferior colliculus by intercollicular decerebration usually facilitates micturition by elimination of inhibitory inputs from more rostral centres (Morrison et al. 2005). However, transections at any point below the colliculi abolish micturition. Bilateral lesions in the rostral pons in the region of the locus coeruleus in cats, or Barrington's nucleus in rats, also abolishes micturition, whereas electrical or chemical stimulation at these sites suppresses urethral sphincter activity, triggers bladder contractions and release of urine (Morrison et al. 2005). These observations led to the concept of a spinobulbospinal micturition reflex pathway that passes through a centre in the rostral brainstem (the PMC) (Figs. 9.3b, 9.7). The pathway functions as an 'on–off' switch that is activated by a critical level of afferent activity arising from tension receptors in the bladder and is, in turn, modulated by inhibitory and excitatory influences from areas of the brain rostral to the pons (e.g. diencephalon and cerebral cortex) (Fig. 9.7).

Suprapontine control of micturition

Lesion and electrical stimulation studies in humans and animals indicate that voluntary control of micturition depends on connections between the frontal cortex, hypothalamus and other forebrain structures such as anterior cingulate gyrus, amygdala, bed nucleus of the stria terminalis and septal nuclei, where electrical stimulation elicits excitatory bladder effects. Damage to the cerebral cortex due to tumours, aneurysms or cerebrovascular disease, appear to remove inhibitory control of the pontine micturition centre resulting bladder overactivity.

Human positron emission tomography (PET) scan studies reveal that the inferior frontal cortical gyrus in addition to the hypothalamus, the PMC and the PAG are activated (i.e. exhibited increased blood flow) during bladder filling or voluntary micturition (Blok et al. 1997a, Blok et al. 1998, Athwal et al. 1999, Athwal et al. 2001). However, the anterior cingulate gyrus exhibited decreased activity. A PET study was also conducted in adult female volunteers to identify brain structures involved in voluntary control of pelvic

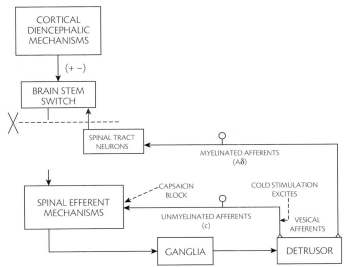

MICTURITION REFLEX PATHWAYS

Fig. 9.7 Diagram showing the organization of the parasympathetic excitatory reflex pathway to the detrusor muscle. Scheme is based on electrophysiological studies in cats. In animals with an intact spinal cord, micturition is initiated by a supraspinal reflex pathway passing through a centre in the brainstem. The pathway is triggered by myelinated afferents (A δ fibres), which are connected to the tension receptors in the bladder wall. Injury to the spinal cord above the sacral segments interrupts the connections between the brain and spinal autonomic centres and initially blocks micturition. However, over a period of several weeks following cord injury, a spinal reflex mechanism emerges, which is triggered by unmyelinated vesical afferents (C-fibres); the A-fibre afferent inputs are ineffective. The C-fibre reflex pathway is usually weak or undetectable in animals with an intact nervous system. Stimulation of the C-fibre bladder afferents by installation of ice water into the bladder (cold stimulation) activates voiding responses in patients with spinal cord injury. Capsaicin (20–30 mg, subcutaneously) blocks the C-fibre reflex in chronic spinal cats, but does not block micturition reflexes in intact cats. Intravesical capsaicin also suppresses detrusor hyperreflexia and cold-evoked reflexes in patients with neurogenic bladder dysfunction.

floor muscles. The results revealed that the superomedial precentral gyrus, the most medial portion of the motor cortex, is activated during pelvic floor contraction (Blok et al. 1997b). In addition the right anterior cingulate gyrus was activated during sustained pelvic floor straining.

Spinal micturition reflex pathway

Spinal cord injury rostral to the lumbosacral level eliminates voluntary and supraspinal control of voiding, leading initially to an areflexic bladder and complete urinary retention followed by a slow development of automatic micturition and bladder hyperactivity (Fig. 9.2c) mediated by spinal reflex pathways (de Groat 1995). However, voiding is commonly inefficient due to simultaneous contractions of the bladder and urethral sphincter (bladder–sphincter dyssynergia) (Fig. 9.2c). Electrophysiological studies in animals have shown that the micturition reflex pathways in spinal intact animals and in those with chronic spinal injuries are markedly different (Cheng et al. 1999). One change occurs in the afferent limb of the micturition reflex, which in cats with chronic spinal injuries consists of unmyelinated (C-fibre) axons (Fig. 9.7). However, in cats with an intact spinal cord, myelinated (A-δ) afferents activate the micturition reflex (Fig. 9.7). In normal cats, capsaicin did not block reflex contractions of the bladder or the

A-δ-fibre evoked bladder reflex. However, in cats with chronic spinal injury capsaicin, a neurotoxin known to disrupt the function of C-fibre afferents, completely blocked C-fibre-evoked bladder reflexes (de Groat 1995, Cheng et al. 1999).

Chronic spinal injury in humans also causes the emergence of an unusual bladder reflex that is elicited in response to infusion of cold water into the bladder (Geirsson et al. 1993). The response to cold water does not occur in normal adults but does occur in:

- infants
- patients with multiple sclerosis or Parkinson's disease
- elderly patients with hyperactive bladders.

Studies in animals indicate that cold temperature activates receptors in bladder C-fibre afferents and urothelial cells (Fig. 9.7) (Fall et al. 1990). The presence of the cold reflex in infants, its disappearance with maturation of the nervous system, and its re-emergence under conditions in which higher brain functions are disrupted suggests that it may reflect a primitive spinal involuntary voiding reflex activated by C-fibre afferents. Evidence of the contribution of C-fibre bladder afferents to bladder hyperactivity and involuntary voiding has been obtained in clinical studies in which capsaicin or resiniferatoxin, C-fibre afferent neurotoxins, were administered intravesically to patients with hyperreflexic bladders due to multiple sclerosis or spinal cord injuries. In these patients capsaicin increased bladder capacity and reduced the frequency of incontinence.

The emergence of C-fibre bladder reflexes seems to be mediated by several mechanisms including changes in central synaptic connections and alterations in the properties of the peripheral afferent receptors that lead to sensitization of the 'silent' C fibres and the unmasking of responses to mechanical stimuli (de Groat 1995). In rats it has been shown that bladder afferent neurons undergo both morphological (neuronal hypertrophy) and physiological changes (upregulation of TTX-sensitive Na^+ channels and downregulation of TTX-resistant Na^+ channels) following spinal cord injury. It has been speculated that this neuroplasticity is mediated by the actions of neurotrophic factors such as nerve growth factor (NGF) released within the spinal cord or the urinary bladder. The production of neurotrophic factors including NGF increases in the bladder after spinal cord injury (Vizzard 2006), and chronic administration of NGF into the bladder of rats induced bladder hyperactivity and increased the firing frequency of dissociated bladder afferent neurons. On the other hand, intrathecal application of NGF antibodies, which neutralized NGF in the spinal cord, suppressed detrusor hyperreflexia and detrusor-sphincter dyssynergia in spinal cord injured rats (Seki et al. 2004).

Neurotransmitters in central micturition reflex pathways

Excitatory neurotransmitters

Excitatory transmission in the central pathways to the lower urinary tract may depend on several types of transmitters, including; glutamic acid, neuropeptides (substance P), nitric oxide and ATP (Morrison et al. 2005, de Groat and Yoshimura 2001). Pharmacological experiments in rats have revealed that glutamic acid is an essential transmitter in the ascending, pontine, and descending limbs of the spinobulbospinal micturition reflex pathway and in spinal reflex pathways controlling the bladder and external urethral sphincter. NMDA and non-NMDA glutamatergic synaptic mechanisms appear to interact synergistically to mediate transmission in these pathways

Inhibitory neurotransmitters

Several types of inhibitory transmitters, including inhibitory amino acids (γ-aminobutyric acid [GABA], glycine) and opioid peptides (enkephalins) can suppress the micturition reflex when applied to the central nervous system. Experimental evidence in anaesthetized animals indicates that GABA and enkephalins exert a tonic inhibitory control in the PMC and regulate bladder capacity. GABA and enkephalins also have inhibitory actions in the spinal cord (Morrison et al. 2005, de Groat and Yoshimura 2001, Mallory et al. 1991).

Transmitters with mixed excitatory and inhibitory actions

Some transmitters (dopamine, 5-hydroxytryptamine, acetylcholine and non-opioid peptides including VIP, corticotropin-releasing factor) have both inhibitory and excitatory effects on reflex bladder activity depending on the type of receptor activated (Morrison et al. 2005, de Groat and Yoshimura 2001). For example, the inhibitory effects of dopamine are mediated by D_1-like receptor subtypes (D_1 and D_5) and the facilitatory effects are mediated by D_2-like (D_2, D_3 and D_4) receptor subtypes. Loss of forebrain dopaminergic mechanisms in patients with idiopathic Parkinson's disease is associated with bladder hyperactivity.

Activation of cholinergic receptors in the rat brain also elicits mixed effects. Nicotinic agonists administered intracerebroventricularly suppress voiding in awake or anaesthetized rats, whereas activation of muscarinic receptors stimulates bladder activity during bladder filling but suppress voluntary voiding. Atropine blocked both the inhibitory and excitatory effects of muscarinic agonists. Intracerebroventricular administration of atropine alone increased bladder capacity and reduced voiding efficiency indicating that muscarinic excitatory mechanisms in the brain are tonically active (Morrison et al. 2005, de Groat and Yoshimura 2001).

Conclusion

The functions of the lower urinary tract to store and periodically eliminate urine are regulated by a complex neural control system that performs like a simple switching circuit to maintain a reciprocal relationship between the bladder and urethral outlet. The switching circuit is modulated by several neurotransmitter systems and is therefore sensitive to a variety of drugs and neurological diseases. A more complete understanding of the neural mechanisms involved in bladder and urethral control will no doubt facilitate the development of new diagnostic methods and therapies for lower urinary tract dysfunction.

References

Andersson, K. E. (1993). Pharmacology of lower urinary tract smooth muscle and penile erection tissues. *Pharmacol Rev* **45**, 253–308.

Andersson, K. E., Arner, A. (2004). Urinary bladder contraction and relaxation: physiology and pathophysiology. *Physiol Rev* **84**, 935–86.

Apodaca, G. (2004) The uroepithelium: not just a passive barrier. *Traffic* **5**, 117–28.

Araki, I. and de Groat, W.C. (1996). Unitary excitatory synaptic currents in preganglionic neurons mediated by two distinct groups of interneurons in neonatal rat sacral parasympathetic nucleus. *J Neurophysiol* **76**, 215–26.

Athwal, B. S., Berkley, K. J., Brennan, A., *et al.* (1999). Brain activity associated with the urge to void and bladder fill volume in normal men: preliminary data from a PET study. *BJU Int* **84**,148–49.

Athwal, B. S., Berkley, K. J., Hussain, I., *et al.* (2001). Brain responses to changes in bladder volume and urge to void in healthy men. *Brain* **124**, 369–77.

Birder, L. A. and de Groat, W. C. (1993). Induction of c-fos expression in spinal neurons by nociceptive and nonnociceptive stimulation of LUT. *Am J Physiol* **265**, R326–33.

Birder, L. A., Apodaca, G., de Groat, W. C., Kanai, A. J. (1998). Adrenergic and capsaicin evoked nitric oxide release from urothelium and afferent nerves in urinary bladder. *Am J Physiol* **275**, F226–29.

Birder, L. A., Barrick, S., Roppolo, J. R., *et al.* (2003). Feline interstitial cystitis results in mechanical hypersensitivity and altered ATP release from bladder urothelium. *Am J Physiol* **285**, F423–249.

Birder, L. A., Kanai, A. J., de Groat, W. C., *et al.* (2001). Vanilloid receptor expression suggests a sensory role for urinary bladder epithelial cells. *Proc Natl Acad Sci U S A* **98**, 13396–13401.

Birder, L. A., Nakamura. Y., Kiss, S., *et al.* (2002). Altered urinary bladder function in mice lacking the vanilloid receptor TRPV1. *Nat Neurosci* **5**, 856–60.

Blok, B. F., De Weerd, H., Holstege, G. (1995). Ultrastructural evidence for a paucity of projections from the lumbosacral cord to the pontine micturition centre or M-region in the cat: a new concept for the organization of the micturition reflex with the periaqueductal gray as central relay. *J Comp Neurol* **359**, 300–309.

Blok, B. F., Sturms, L. M., Holstege, G. (1998). Brain activation during micturition in women. *Brain* **121**, 2033–42.

Blok, B. F., Willemsen, A. T., Holstege, G. (1997a). A PET study on brain control of micturition in humans. *Brain* **120**, 111–21.

Blok, B. F. M., Sturms, L. M., Holstege, G. (1997b). A PET study on cortical and subcortical control of the pelvic floor musculature in women. *J Comp Neurol* **389**, 535–44.

Burnstock, G. (2001). Purinergic signaling in the lower urinary tract. In: Abbracchio M.P., Williams M., eds. *Handbook of Experimental Pharmacology*. pp. 423–515. Springer Verlag, Berlin.

Cheng, C. L., Liu, J. C., Chang, S. Y., Ma, C. P., de Groat, W. C. (1999). Effect of capsaicin on the micturition reflex in normal and chronic spinal cord-injured cats. *Am J Physiol* **277**, R786–94.

Chuang, Y., Fraser, M. O., Yu, Y., Chancellor, M. B., de Groat, W. C., Yoshimura, N. (2001). The role of bladder afferent pathways in the bladder hyperactivity induced by intravesical administration of nerve growth factor. *J Urol* **165**, 975–79.

Cockayne, D. A., Hamilton, S. G., Zhu, Q. M., *et al.* (2000). Urinary bladder hyporeflexia and reduced pain-related behaviour in P2X3-deficient mice. *Nature* **407**, 1011–1015.

de Groat, W. C. (1995). Mechanisms underlying the recovery of lower urinary tract function following spinal cord injury. *Paraplegia* **33**, 493–505.

de Groat, W. C., Booth, A. M. (1993). Synaptic transmission in pelvic ganglia. In: Maggi C.A., editor. *The Autonomic Nervous System, Vol. 3, Nervous Control of the Urogenital System*. pp. 291–347. Harwood Academic Publishers, London.

de Groat, W. C., Yoshimura, N. (2001). Pharmacology of the lower urinary tract. *Ann Rev Pharmacol Toxicol* **41**, 691–721.

de Groat, W. C., Fraser, M.O., Yoshiyama, M., *et al.* (2001). Neural control of the urethra. *Scand J Urol Nephrol Suppl*: 35–43.

Fall, M., Lindstrom, S., Mazieres, L. (1990). A bladder-to-bladder cooling reflex in the cat. *J Physiol* **427**, 281–300.

Ferguson, D. R., Kennedy, I., Burton, T. J. (1997). ATP is released from rabbit urinary bladder cells by hydrostatic pressure changes- a possible sensory mechanism? *J. Physiol. (Lond.)* **505**, 503–11.

Fry, C. H., Brading, A. F., Hussain, M., *et al.* (2005) Cell Biology. In: Abrams, P., Cardozo, L., Khoury, S., and Wein, A., editors. *Incontinence*. Vol. 3, pp. 313–62. Health Publications, Ltd., Jersey, UK.

Geirsson, G., Fall, M., Lindstrom, S. (1993). The ice-water test—a simple and valuable supplement to routine cystometry. *Br J Urol* **71**, 681–85.

Habler, H. J., Janig, W., Koltzenburg, M. (1990). Activation of unmyelinated afferent fibres by mechanical stimuli and inflammation of the urinary bladder in the cat. *J Physiol* **425**, 545–62.

Lewis, S. A. (2000) Everything you wanted to know about the bladder epithelium but were afraid to ask. *Am J Physiol* **278**, 867–74.

Maggi, C.A. (1993) The dual sensory and efferent functions of the capsaicin-sensitive primary sensory neurons in the urinary bladder and urethra. In: Maggi, C.A. editor. *The Autonomic Nervous System, Vol. 3, Chapter 13, Nervous Control of the Urogenital System*. pp. 383–422. Harwood Academic Publishers, London.

Mallory, B. S., Roppolo, J. R., de Groat, W. C. (1991). Pharmacological modulation of the pontine micturition center. *Brain Res* **546**, 310–20.

Matsui, M., Motomura, D., Fujikawa, T., *et al.* (2002). Mice lacking M2 and M3 muscarinic acetylcholine receptors are devoid of cholinergic smooth muscle contractions but still viable. *J Neurosci* **22**, 10627–32.

Matsui, M., Motomura, D., Karasawa, H., *et al.* (2000). Multiple functional defects in peripheral autonomic organs in mice lacking muscarinic acetylcholine receptor gene for the M3 subtype. *Proc Nat Acad Sci* **97**, 9579–84.

Morgan, C. W., de Groat, W. C., Felkins, L. A., Zhang, S. J. (1993). Intracellular injection of neurobiotin or horseradish peroxidase reveals separate types of preganglionic neurons in the sacral parasympathetic nucleus of the cat. *J Comp Neurol* **331**, 161–82.

Morrison, J., Birder, L., Craggs, M., *et al.* (2005). Neural control. In: Abrams, P., Cardozo, L., Khoury, S., and Wein, A., editors. *Incontinence*. Vol. 3, pp. 363–422. Health Publications, Ltd., Jersey, UK.

Nadelhaft, I., Vera, P. L., Card, J. P., *et al.* (1992). Central nervous system neurons labelled following the injection of pseudorabies virus into the rat urinary bladder. *Neurosci Lett* **143**, 271–74.

Ralevic, V., Burnstock, G. (1998). Receptors for purines and pyrimidines. *Physiol Rev* **50**, 413–92.

Rong W., Spyer K. M., Burnstock, G. (2002). Activation and senstitization of low and high threshold afferent fibres mediated by P2X receptors in the mouse urinary bladder. *J Physiol Lond.* **541**, 591–600.

Seki, S., Sasaki, K., Nishizawa, O., *et al.* (2004). Suppression of detrusor-sphincter dyssynergia by immunoneutralization of nerve growth factor in lumbosacral spinal cord in spinal cord injured rats. *J Urol* **171**, 478–82.

Somogyi, G. T., Tanowitz, M., Zernova, G., *et al.* (1996) M1 muscarinic receptor facilitation of ACh and noradrenaline release in the rat urinary bladder is mediated by protein kinase C. *J Physiol (Lond)* **496**, 245–54.

Steers, W. D., Ciambotti, J., Etzel, B., Erdman, S., de Groat, W. C. (1991). Alterations in afferent pathways from the urinary bladder of the rat in response to partial urethral obstruction. *J Comp Neurol* **310**, 401–410.

Sun, Y., Keay, S., De Deyne, P. G., *et al.* (2001). Augmented stretch activated adenosine triphosphate release from bladder uroepithelial cells in patients with interstitial cystitis. *J Urol* **166**, 1951–56.

Szallasi, A., Fowler, C. J. (2002) After a decade of intravesical vanilloid therapy: still more questions than answers. *Lancet Neurology* **1**,167–72.

Vizzard, M. A., Erickson, V. L., Card, J. P., *et al.* (1995). Transneuronal labeling of neurons in the adult rat brain and spinal cord after injection of pseudorabies virus into the urethra. *J Comp Neurol* **355**, 629–40.

Vizzard, M. A. (2006). Neurochemical plasticity and the role of neurotrophic factors in bladder reflex pathways after spinal cord injury. In: Weaver L.C., Polosa C. (eds.): *Autonomic dysfunction after spinal cord injury: the problems and underlying mechanisms*. Chapter 31. Elsevier, The Netherlands, **152**, 97–155.

Yoshimura, N., de Groat, W. C. (1997). Plasticity of Na + channels in afferent neurones innervating rat urinary bladder following spinal cord injury. *J Physiol* **503**, 269–76.

Yoshimura, N., de Groat, W. C. (1999). Increased excitability of afferent neurons innervating rat urinary bladder after chronic bladder inflammation. *J Neurosci* 19, 4644–53.

Yoshimura, N., White, G., Weight, F. F., de Groat, W. C. (1996). Different types of Na + and A-type K + currents in dorsal root ganglion neurones innervating the rat urinary bladder. *J Physiol* **494**, 1–16.

Yoshimura, N., Seki, S., Erickson, K. A., Erickson, V. L., Chancellor, M. B., de Groat, W. C. (2003). Histological and electrical properties of rat dorsal root ganglion neurons innervating the lower urinary tract. *J Neurosci* **23**, 4355–61.

Zhong, Y., Banning, A. S., Cockayne, D. A., Ford, A. P., Burnstock, G., McMahon, S. B. (2003). Bladder and cutaneous sensory neurons of the rat express different functional P2X receptors. *Neurosci* **120**, 667–75.

CHAPTER 10

The autonomic neuroscience of sexual function

Kevin E. McKenna

Key points

- Sexual function requires spatial and temporal coordination between sympathetic, parasympathetic and somatic outflow to the pelvis.

- The neural regulation of sexual function show significant similarities in the two sexes.

- Sexual responses are largely organized at the lumbosacral level, and the spinal cord is under inhibitory and excitatory control from brainstem and diencephalic nuclei.

- The supraspinal nuclei involved in the control of sexual function are heavily interconnected, receive pelvic sensory input. Many of these nuclei are influenced by sex steroids.

Introduction

In recent years, there has been tremendous progress in our understanding of the neural control of sexual function. It was little over 15 years ago that the neural messenger mediating penile erection, nitric oxide, was identified, following a search of over 100 years. This discovery helped the development and introduction of effective oral treatments for erectile dysfunction, which has been a goal from ancient times. Less than 5 years ago, the spinal neurons responsible for generating ejaculation were identified. Less spectacular, but just as important, has been an accelerating accumulation of knowledge about the pathways and neurochemistry underlying a variety of sexual responses in both sexes. Recently, functional imaging studies have extended this advancement into humans. This chapter will summarize many of these findings, but also make clear that many very important questions remain to be answered in this field.

General principles of the organization of sexual function

Sexual differences and similarities

Despite the major differences in the internal and external sexual organs of males and females, the sexual physiology is remarkably similar in the two sexes. The similarities include the general organization of pelvic innervation, spinal and brainstem pathways, supraspinal nuclei which control sexual function, spinal reflexes, and major neurochemical systems. A pronounced similarity of male and female orgasm was emphasized by Kinsey and colleagues (Kinsey et al. 1953), and later by Masters and Johnson (1966). They noted that the descriptions by men and women of the subjective experiences of orgasm are indistinguishable. The rhythmic contractions of pelvic muscles displayed the same pattern of activity. The extragenital components of orgasm, heart rate, respiration, sweating, and secretion of oxytocin, are also equivalent. They argued that there was a strong implication that the neural substrates of sexual responses are the same in both sexes. Subsequent research has demonstrated this proposition largely true.

Some sex differences, both structural and functional, have been identified. Sexual dimorphism has been identified in a number of nuclei in both animals and humans, including lumbosacral autonomic (see Fig. 10.2) and motoneuronal pools and hypothalamic nuclei. The pudendal motoneurons express androgen receptors. Systemic exposure to androgens during critical perinatal periods leads to the development of a masculine phenotype (more and larger neurons) in either sex. Deprivation of androgens results in the feminine phenotype (Breedlove 1984). However, no major reflexive or cellular electrophysiological differences have been detected between the two phenotypes.

The developmental androgen-dependent sexual dimorphism was initially believed to be mediated by the androgen receptors within the motoneurons. However, further experiments revealed that the masculine phenotype of the pudendal motoneuronal nuclei is primarily due to the masculinization of their target muscles by androgens. The role of the motoneuronal androgen receptors is unknown. It is probable that the sexual dimorphism of autonomic spinal efferents is also a reflection of peripheral sex differentiation.

Hierarchy of control

A clear conclusion of animal experiments and clinical investigation is that sexual responses are organized at the level of the lumbosacral spinal cord. Penile erection, female genital sexual arousal, and sexual climax in both sexes, have all been demonstrated in animals and human subjects following complete spinal cord transection. The pattern and sequence of pelvic neural activity are comparable to those seen with an intact neuraxis. The substrates for this spinal control are discussed below.

Despite the spinal organization of sexual responses, spinal cord injury still results in significant sexual dysfunction. For example, penile erection may be relatively easy to initiate by genital stimulation, but is often very difficult to maintain without the use of erection-enhancing drugs. Ejaculation is often very difficult to elicit with typical sexual stimulation, such as vaginal intercourse. Vibratory ejaculation to collect semen for artificial insemination often requires the use of intense stimuli. Of course, spinal cord injury may result in devastating loss of sexual sensation.

Innervation of the sexual organs

Parasympathetic

The parasympathetic preganglionic neurons controlling the sexual organs (as well as the bladder and colon) are located in the intermediolateral cell column of the sacral spinal cord, in a nucleus called the sacral parasympathetic nucleus (SPN, Fig. 10.1). Their axons travel in the pelvic nerve (also called the pelvic splanchnic nerve) and innervate ganglion cells in the pelvic plexus (also called the inferior hypogastric plexus), which lies on the lateral aspect of the cervix in females and the prostate in males. The preganglionic fibers provide an excitatory input to the postganglionic neurons via a nicotinic cholinergic transmission. Postganglionic axons provide innervation to erectile tissue in the penis/clitoris and in the circumvaginal area; smooth muscle of the urethra, accessory sex glands, and vagina and uterus; secretory epithelium of glandular tissue; and the vasculature within the pelvis. Most of the postganglionic nerves form a relatively diffuse network of fibers extending from the pelvic plexus. The most prominent postganglionic nerve is the cavernous nerve, which provides the vasodilatory, erectile input to the penis and clitoris (Langworthy, 1965). In the rat, ganglion cells extend into the cavernous nervefor several millimeters. Thus, preganglionic neurons innervating the penis and clitoris can be labeled by application of tracer to the cavernous nerve (Fig. 10.2). The postganglionic neurons contain acetylcholine and a variety of other neurotransmitters, including nitric oxide and vasoactive intestinal polypeptide (VIP). In the penis and clitoris, nitric oxide is the primary neurotransmitter mediating erection. VIP is probably responsible for mediating vaginal vasodilation and lubrication. Pelvic glandular secretion is stimulated by acetylcholine.

Sympathetic

The sympathetic innervation of the sexual organs originates from the lower lumbar spinal segments. Preganglionic neurons are located in both the intermediolateral column (IML) and the dorsal commissural nucleus (DCN), also called the central autonomic cell group (CA). The IML preganglionic neurons preferentially project to the sympathetic chain ganglia and the DCN neurons to the prevertebral ganglia. IML neurons may be more likely to be vasoconstrictor and the DCN neurons related to visceral motility (Jänig and McLachlan, 1987). Some preganglionic axons innervate postganglionic neurons in the lower sympathetic chain ganglia. The postganglionic axons from the sympathetic chain reach pelvic organs via the pelvic or pudendal nerves. Other preganglionic axons travel in the lumbar splanchnic nerves. These axons either innervate postganglionic neurons in the inferior mesenteric ganglion or continue in the hypogastric nerve to the pelvic ganglia.

The sympathetic innervation stimulates contraction in smooth muscle of the internal sexual organs. It is essential for contraction of the ductus deferens, prostate and seminal vesicles during the emission phase of ejaculation, mediated primarily by noradrenergic mechanisms. Vaginal smooth muscle contracts in response to

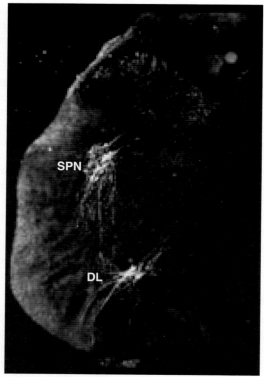

Fig. 10.1 Transverse section of the L6 spinal cord of the male rat showing parasympathetic preganglionic neurons in the sacral parasympathetic nucleus (SPN) and pudendal neurons in the dorsolateral nucleus (DL) following application of HRP to the pelvic and pudendal nerves. Labeled pelvic and pudendal afferents can be seen in the medial dorsal and intermediate parts of spinal gray matter. A similar pattern of labeling is seen in the female.

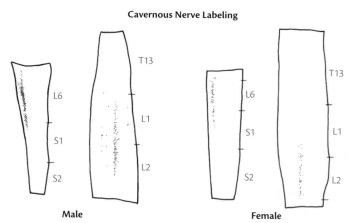

Cavernous Nerve Labeling

Male

Female

Fig. 10.2 Diagrams showing the number and location of parasympathetic (left) and sympathetic (right) preganglionic neurons labeled by application of HRP to the cavernous nerve in a male (top) and female (bottom) rat. Note the similarity of distribution, but strong difference in the number of neurons labeled. Reproduced with permission from: K.E. McKenna and L. Marson. Spinal and Brainstem Control of Sexual Function. In: *Central Control of Autonomic Function*, D. Jordan (ed.). Harwood Academic Publishers, Amsterdam, pp. 151–188, 1997.

adrenergic stimulation and stimulation of the hypogastric nerve elicits vaginal contractions. However, the role of the sympathetic innervation of the vagina during sexual arousal and climax are still unclear.

The penis and clitoris receive two distinct sympathetic inputs, via the pudendal nerve and the cavernous nerves. The dorsal nerve of the penis/clitoris, the primary sensory branch of the pudendal nerve, supplies most, if not all, of the noradrenergic, vasoconstrictor innervation of the penis and clitoris. These are derived from the caudal sympathetic chain. They mediate detumescence of the phallus following climax. The cavernous sympathetic fibers are derived from ganglion cells in the pelvic plexus, innervated by preganglionic fibers in the hypogastric nerve. The role of this innervation of the penis/clitoris remains unclear. These postganglionic neurons are not catecholaminergic and are not vasoconstrictor. Stimulation and lesion of the hypogastric nerve have yielded inconsistent effects on penile erection.

Somatic

The striated perineal muscles are innervated by the pudendal nerve. The motoneurons of the pudendal nerve are located in the ventral horn in lower lumbar and/or upper sacral segments of the spinal cord, depending on the species. In many species, including humans, these motoneurons are located in a single nucleus called Onuf's nucleus. In rodents, the motoneurons are located in two separate nuclei, the dorsolateral (DL) and dorsomedial (DM) nuclei (Fig. 10.3). The dorsolateral nucleus contains the motoneurons innervating the external urethral sphincter ans ischiocavernosus; the dorsomedial nucleus innervates the external anal sphincter and the bulbocavernosus muscle. The perineal muscles are rhythmically activated during sexual climax, and are important for penile rigidity.

Sensory

The sensory innervation of the sexual organs is provided by the pelvic, hypogastric and pudendal nerves. The pelvic and hypogastric nerves provide sensory innervation of the internal sexual organs. However, their role in sexual function is unclear.

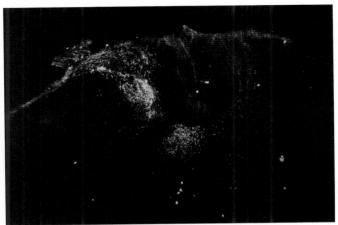

Fig. 10.4 Transverse section of the L6 spinal cord in the male rat showing afferent fibers labeled following unilateral application of HRP to the pudendal nerve. Note the restriction of labeling to the medial portion of the dorsal horn, dorsal gray commissure, and extending into the medial portion of the contralateral dorsal horn. The distribution of labeling in the female is similar, but fewer fibers are seen.

The pudendal nerve provides sensory innervation to the penis and clitoris and the perineal region. Stimulation of these afferents elicits reflexive sexual responses in both sexes, and they are responsible for the perception of sexual stimulation of the external genitals. The majority of pudendal sensory fibers form the dorsal nerve of the penis/clitoris. The central terminals of the pudendal afferents terminate in all layers of the medial dorsal horn, in the midline of the dorsal gray commissure, and in the contralateral medial dorsal horn (Fig. 10.4). Some of the afferent fibers ascend in the dorsal columns.

Penile and clitoral erectile mechanisms

Architecture of the erectile tissue

The shaft of the penis/clitoris consists of two corpora cavernosa, which are fused in the midline to form a dumbbell cross section. Proximally, the corpora separate into two tails, the crura, which are attached to the caudal surface of the ischium. Surrounding each crus is the isciocavernosus muscle. The corpora are surrounded by a fascial layer, the tunica albuginea. In the male, the tunica is extremely tough and inelastic. In the dorsal groove, there is the prominent dorsal vein, as well as the dorsal nerves. In the male, the corpus spongiosum lies in the ventral groove. The urethra runs in the center of the erectile tissue of the corpus spongiosum. At the base of the penis, the urethra and corpus spongiosum expands into the urethral bulb, which is surrounded by the bulbospongiosus muscle.

The penile and clitoral erectile tissue consists of sinusoids that are lined with endothelium and smooth muscle. These are collapsed, potential spaces in the flaccid state. The arterial supply of the sinusoids is from the helicine arteries, which are branches of the deep artery of the penis/clitoris. The venous drainage of the sinusoids is by way of the emissary veins, which penetrate the tunica albuginea (Fig. 10.6).

Dynamics of the erectile process

In the flaccid state, the smooth muscle of the arterioles and sinusoids of the penis and clitoris are maintained in a contracted state. Erection begins with active relaxation of this smooth muscle.

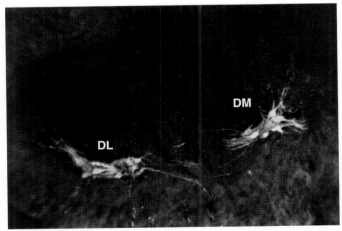

Fig. 10.3 Transverse section of the L6 segment of the male rat spinal cord showing pudendal motoneurons in the dorsolateral (DL, left) and the dorsomedial (DM, right) nuclei. In humans and many non-rodents, all pudendal neurons are located in a single nucleus, Onuf's nucleus.

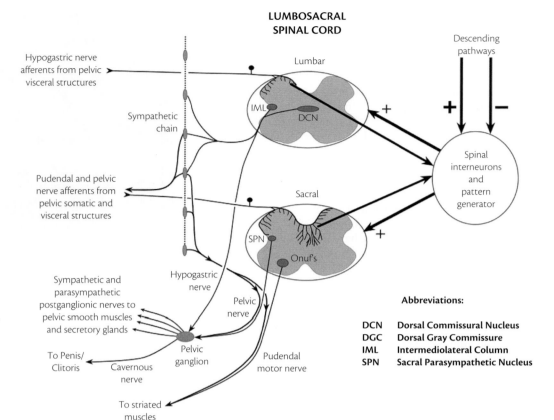

Fig. 10.5 Schematic diagram of the innervation of the the male and female sexual organs. The sympathetic, parasympathetic and somatic components together form a highly integrated system. Coordinated sexual outflow is organized at the spinal cord level and can be activated by reflex mechanisms, modulated by descending pathways, or directly activated by supraspinal sites.

Abbreviations:

DCN   Dorsal Commissural Nucleus
DGC   Dorsal Gray Commissure
IML   Intermediolateral Column
SPN   Sacral Parasympathetic Nucleus

Blood flow increases several-fold. This is also aided by sympathetically mediated vasoconstriction in pelvic vascular beds outside the penis/clitoris. The sinusoids fill with blood, swelling the erectile tissue, a process known as tumescence. The expansion of the sinusoids compresses the venous plexus under the tunica, and expands the tunica. The expansion of the tunica compresses the emissary veins, preventing outflow of blood from the corpora (Fig. 10.6). The intracorporal pressure at this point is typically at or just below mean arterial pressure. In the male, contraction of the ischiocavenosus muscle around the crura of the penis squeezes blood into the shaft. Because the tunica is inelastic, the pressure rises dramatically, reaching several hundred millimeters of mercury (Lue, 2000). Detumescence is an active process, especially following climax. Noradrenergic fibers innervating the erectile arterioles and sinusoids from the sympathetic chain, via the dorsal nerve, causes smooth muscle contraction. This decreases arterial flow and constricts the sinusoids, allowing venous drainage.

Biochemical mechanisms underlying erection

A large variety of messengers have been identified in nerve fibers in the sexual organs. The functions of many remain to be elucidated. The best studied is that responsible for penile (and clitoral erection). Eckhard first demonstrated that penile erection could be induced by electrical stimulation of the pelvic nerve in 1863. Since that time, numerous investigators attempted to identify the neurotransmitter. Because the erectile response could not be mimicked with agonists, or blocked with antagonists of the classical transmitters, noradrenaline and acetylcholine, the responsible mechanism

was referred to as non-adrenergic/non-cholinergic (NANC). Numerous candidates were proposed until the NANC neurotransmitter responsible for cavernosal smooth muscle relaxation was definitively identified as nitric oxide (Ignarro et al. 1990). Clitoral erection was subsequently shown to be mediated by nitric oxide, as well.

Two isoforms of nitric oxide synthase (NOS) are present in the penis, NOS I (also known as neural NOS, or nNOS) and NOS III (also known as endothelial NOS or eNOS). NOS I is found in the cavernous nerve parasympathetic fibers. NOS III is located in the endothelial cells. These appear to form an amplification cascade. Nitric oxide produced by NOS I in the nerve terminals relaxes smooth muscle and probably activates NOS III in the endothelium to produce nitric oxide, which further relaxes smooth muscle. Nitric oxide causes an activation of guanylate cyclese and increases of cGMP in smooth muscle. The increases in cGMP have several effects which contribute to smooth relaxation, mainly by reducing levels of intracellular calcium. These include activation of protein kinase G (PKG), sequestration of intracellular calcium, and hyperpolarization (Fig. 10.7). This nitric oxide erectile response is regulated by the breakdown of cGMP by phosphodiesterase type 5 (PDE5). Inhibition of PDE5 is the basis for effective oral treatment of erectile dysfunction (Rosen and McKenna, 2002). Note, however, that these drugs do not initiate erectile responses, but enhance and prolong the effects of nitric oxide. In conditions where the nitric oxide innervation is severely damaged, such as in advanced diabetes or following surgery for prostate cancer (which may damage the pelvic plexus or cavernous nerve), the effectiveness of PDE5 inhibitors is greatly reduced. Impairment of blood flow by severe

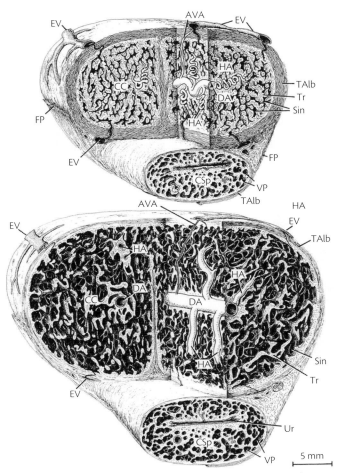

Fig. 10.6 The penis in the flaccid (top) and erect state (bottom). Blood flows into the penis through the deep arteries and into the helicine arteries. It leaves through either the efferent veins or arteriovenous anastamoses. In the erect state, the smooth muscle of the cavernous sinuses are relaxed, allowing them to fill with blood. The expansion of the erectile tissue compresses the drainage of blood through the efferent veins. CC, corpus cavernosus; CSp, corpus spongiosus; DA, deep arteries; HA, helicine arteries; EV, efferent veins; Sin, cavernous sinuses; AVA, arteriovenous anastomoses; TAlb, tunica albuginea; TR, trabeculae; FP, fascia penis; VP, venous plexus; Ur, urethra; IC, intima cushions. Reproduced with permission from: R.V. Krstic, *Human Microscopic Anatomy*, Springer-Verlag, Berlin, 1997).

atherosclerosis also causes severe dysfunction of the erectile response in the penis and clitoris.

Vaginal lubrication

Anatomy of the vaginal epithelium

The vagina is composed of three layers: a squamous epithelium mucous membrane, a smooth muscle layer (composed of inner circular and outer longitudinal muscle fibers), and an outer adventitia layer. This is surrounded by an extensive venous plexus that is more pronounced in the outer one-third of the vagina (Fig. 10.8). The vaginal mucosa is devoid of secretory glands. The vagina is estrogen dependent, and undergoes atrophy following menopause. The vaginal wall is endowed with a rich nerve supply that is more extensive in the distal part. A large variety of classical and peptidergic transmitters (norepinephrine, acetylcholine, dopamine,

serotonin, nitric oxide, VIP, substance P, NPY, TRH, CGRP, somatostatin, oxytocin, cholecystokinin and others) have been described, but their roles are unclear but the exact function of most of these is unknown (Hoyle et al. 1996).

Vascular mechanisms

Sexual arousal results in genital vasocongestion and vaginal lubrication, due to vasodilation of the vaginal vascular bed and increased blood flow. The vasocongestion may also be aided by a reduction of venous drainage. There is also relaxation of the vaginal smooth muscle. The vaginal lubrication is a transudate that originates from the subepithelial vascular bed and diffuses passively intercellularly through the mucosa and into the vaginal lumen. The transudate is produced by a Starling mechanism due largely to the increased capillary pressure resulting from the vasodilation (Levin, 1991).

The vaginal vasodilation and resulting lubrication are produced by activation of the sacral parasympathetic outflow. The identity of the neurotransmitter(s) mediating the vaginal vasodilation is still not certain. Cholinergic antagonists do not prevent vaginal lubrication. Unlike the clitoris, nitric oxide appears to play little role in the vagina, since there are very few nitric oxide synthase-containing fibers in the premenopausal vagina, and virtually none after menopause (Hoyle et al. 1996). The most likely candidate is VIP. VIP fibers are abundant in the vagina. Vaginal lubrication can be induced by injection of VIP into the vaginal wall in women. It remains to be determined if lubrication induced by sexual stimuli can be blocked by specific VIP antagonist (Levin, 1991).

Sexual climax

Nomenclature

The nomenclature of the culmination of the sex act is problematic. The term orgasm is commonly used. However, this refers to the pelvic responses, but also generally connotes the intense subjective pleasurable experience, as well. This subjective experience cannnot be verified in animal studies, and is therefore inappropriate. In males, the term ejaculation is often used. However, there are some experimental and clinical situations where sexual stimulation leads to the pelvic activity and/or subjective experience typically associated with ejaculation, but no ejaculate is produced. For example, in men who have undergone radical pelvic surgery for the treatment of cancer, sexual stimulation can elicit both the subjective sensation of orgasm, as well as the rhythmic striated pelvic muscle contractions characteristic of ejaculation. However, the surgical removal of the accessory sex glands makes ejaculation of semen impossible (Bergman et al. 1979).

The nomenclature is also problematic in females. Rhythmic pelvic contractions elicited by sexual stimulation can be elicited in women with spinal cord injury (Sipski et al. 2001). These were identical to orgasmic pelvic contractions in healthy women. However, the women with spinal cord injury had severely impaired or absent sensation of orgasm. Similarly, sexual responses can be elicited in anesthetized, spinalized rats (McKenna et al. 1991). In neither case is the term orgasm appropriate.

The term sexual climax appears to be the most appropriate for a variety of reasons. It has a long history as a term for the culmination of the sex act in both males and females. Therefore, it does not require ejaculation of semen. Nor does it appear to require the conscious perception of orgasmic pleasure (nor does it exclude it),

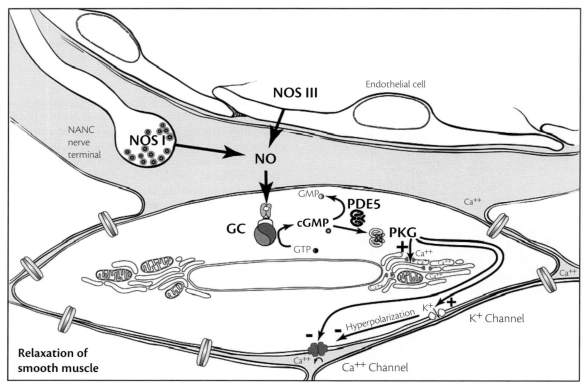

Fig. 10.7 Relaxation of Penile Smooth Muscle: cGMP Mechanisms. Nitric oxide (NO) produced by nitric oxide synthase Type I (NOS I) in NANC nerves and nitric oxide synthase Type III (NOS III) in endothlial cells activates guanylyl cyclase (GC) in smooth muscle cells. This results in the production of cGMP from GTP. cGMP is metabolized by phosphodiesterase type 5 (PDE5). cGMP causes the activation of protein kinase G (PKG). PKG causes an increased uptake of calcium (Ca++) into intracellular stores and a reduction of calcium entry into the cell through calcium channels. PKG also opens potassium (K+) channels, leading to hyperpolarization, which also closes the calcium channels. The resulting decrease in intracellular calcium concentration from these mechanisms leads to relaxation of the smooth muscle cell. Smooth muscle cells are connected with gap junctions, allowing spread of electrical and ionic activity throughout the tissue. Reproduced with permission from: R.C. Rosen and K.E. McKenna, PDE-5 inhibition and sexual response: Pharmacological mechanisms and clinical outcomes. *Annual Review of Sex Research* **13**:36–88, 2002.

which cannot be inferred in animals and may be diminished or absent in some clinical situations. This is the term that will be used in this review. In some experimental situations with anesthetized animals, physiological or neural activity, which closely resembles sexual climax, may be elicited by drugs, electrical stimulation of brain regions or peripheral nerves, or other stimuli. Because the sexual context of the stimuli may not be entirely clear, the term climax-like response appears most appropriate.

Phenomenology of sexual climax: females

Sexual climax is a response that involves the entire body, not confined to the genitals. The genital responses consist of rhythmic contractions of the smooth muscle of the vagina and uterus, and the pelvic striated muscles: the pelvic diaphragm, the external anal and urethral sphincters. The rhythmic contractions of the striated muscles are highly regular, with 8 to 20 synchronous contractions of all the pelvic muscles. The interval between contractions starts at 0.6 to 0.8 seconds and increases by approximately 100 milliseconds with each subsequent contraction (Fig. 10.8). Extragenital responses consist of a characteristic cardioacceleration, increases in blood pressure, and respiration. There is usually a generalized flushing of the skin and sweating. There are tonic muscular contractions throughout the body, followed by a profound relaxation. Plasma levels of prolactin, oxytocin, vasopressin, and epinephrine increase with orgasm. The increase in prolactin is perhaps the most

consistent endocrine response to climax (Kruger et al. 2005). Subjectively, climax is associated with intense pleasure, followed by a profound relaxation.

Phenomenology of sexual climax: males

The defining feature of male sexual climax is ejaculation. This is divided into two phases, emission and expulsion. Sexual stimulation causes stimulation of the smooth muscle of the accessory sex glands and ductus deferens to express seminal fluids into the urethra. This is accompanied by contraction of the bladder neck and the external urethral sphincter, creating an enclosed space for the seminal fluids in the prostatic urethra. The emission phase is a coordinated response induced by sympathetic activation, primarily the hypogastric nerve (Recker and Tscholl, 1993). Parasympathetic mechanisms may also be involved, primarily in the control of epithelial secretion. Pudendal activation contracts the external urethral sphincter.

The expulsion phase consists of rhythmic contractions of smooth muscle of the urethra and the striated pelvic muscles. These contractions are very similar to those seen in female climax (Fig. 10.8). The expulsion of semen from the urethral meatus is primarily due to the contraction of the bulbospongiosus muscle. Alternating relaxation and contraction of the external urethral sphincter propels seminal fluid from the prostatic urethra into the urethral bulb at the base of the penis. The bulbospongiosus muscle surrounds

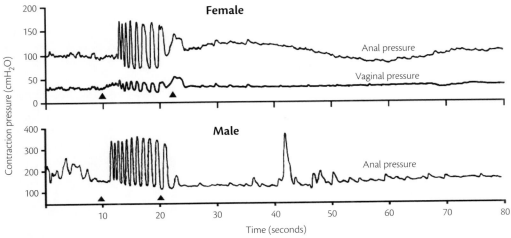

Fig. 10.8 Physiological recordings of the most common pattern of orgasm in male and female volunteers induced by masturbation. The pelvic contractions of orgasm were measured by the means of probes inserted into the anus and vagina and the contractions are indicated by increases in pressure around the probes. Note that the contractions are highly regular with a consistent increase in the interval between each contraction. The arrows indicate the beginning and end of subjectively recorded orgasm. Adapted with permission from J.G. Bohlen, J.P. Held, M.O. Anderson, and A. Ahlgren, The female orgasm: Pelvic contractions, Archives of Sexual Behavior 11, 367–386, 1984; and J.G. Bohlen, J.P. Held, and M.O. Anderson, The male orgasm: Pelvic contractions measured by anal probe, Archives of Sexual Behavior **9**, 503–521, 1980.

the urethral bulb. Rhythmic contractions expel the semen in spurts (Fig. 10.9).

The extragenital responses in the male are essentially the same as in the female. The cardiorespiratory, autonomic, muscular and endocrine responses show the same patterns as described above for the female. The major difference is that in the male, climax is followed by a prolonged refractory period. This includes a sympathetically mediated detumescence and suppression of erection, sensory changes in the genitals, and loss of interest in sexual activity. In the female, climax is not necessarily followed by a refractory period. Multiple orgasms without loss of arousal appear to be a general capability in the human female. No satisfactory explanation exists for this difference between the sexes.

Spinal pathways

Reflexive clitoral and penile erections

Sexual arousal responses are primarily organized at the spinal level and are under descending excitatory and inhibitory control. Sensory stimuli mediating sexual reflexes are conveyed primarily by the pudendal nerve. Reflexive efferent activity may be relatively restricted, or consist of highly complex coordinated sympathetic, parasympathetic and somatic activation, involving several organs, nerves and spinal segments.

One reflex is the activation of erectile fibers in the cavernous nerve by stimulation of the pudendal afferents innervating the penis. This is a long-latency polysynaptic response. The penile afferents are low threshold myelinated fibers (Fig. 10.10). The homologous reflex in females is presumed, but has not been directly demonstrated.

Vaginal vasodilation and lubrication

The exact mechanisms of vaginal vasodilation and lubrication are unknown. Stimulation of the pelvic nerve can induce vaginal vasodilation. It is likely, but has not been directly demonstrated, that stimulation of pudendal genital afferents can elicit this response, similar to the reflex activation of penile parasympathetic fibers.

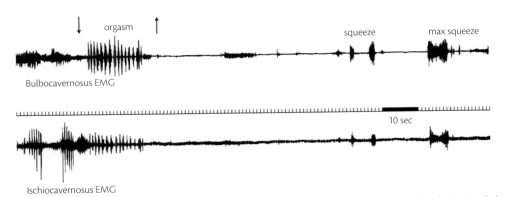

Fig. 10.9 The electromyographic (EMG) recording from the bulbocavernosus (bulbospongiosus) and ischiocavernosus muscles during ejaculation induced by masturbation in a healthy volunteer. Note that the activity in the two muscles is synchronized and consists of a series of highly regular rhythmic contraction. The arrows indicate the beginning and end of subjectively recorded orgasm (reproduced with permission from T.C. Gerstenberg, R.J. Levin, and G. Wagner, Erection and ejaculation in man. Assessment of the electromyography activity of the bulbocavernosus and ischiocavernosus muscles, *Br J Urol* **65**, 395–402, 1990).

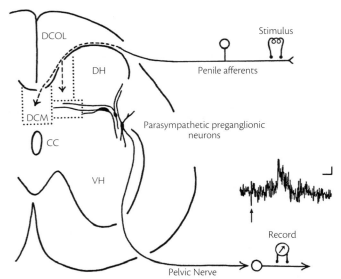

Fig. 10.10 The reflex pathway for inducing penile erection. Horseradish peroxidase axonal tracing studies in the cat and rat have shown the relationship between sacral parasympathetic preganglionic neurons and afferent projections from the penis. Penile afferents in the pudendal nerve project to interneurons in the medial side of the dorsal horn (DH) and the dorsal commissure (DCM) in the S2 segment of the spinal cord. Preganglionic neurons send dendrites into regions of afferent termination. In the rat, electrical stimulation of penile afferents in the dorsal nerve of the penis elicits polysynaptic reflex firing in efferent pathways to the penis. Inset is an example of a reflex discharge in parasympathetic postganglionic axons in penile nerves. The reflexes, which occur at a long latency (mean 75 ms), are present in normal and chronic spinal rats and are blocked by section of the pelvic nerve. Stimulus marked by arrow. DCOL, dorsal column; VH, ventral horn; CC, and central canal. Horizontal calibration 20 ms, vertical calibration 10 μV. Reproduced with permission from W.C. de Groat, Neural control of the urinary bladder and sexual organs. In: *Autonomic failure. A textbook of clinical disorders of the autonomic nervous system*, (4th edition). Edited by C.J. Mathias and R. Bannister, Oxford University Press, Oxford, 2002.

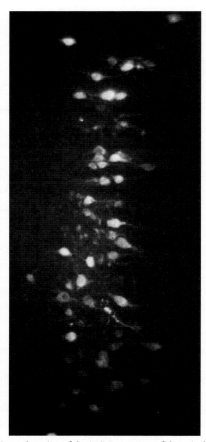

Fig. 10.11 Horizontal section of the L3/L4 segments of the spinal cord of a male rat. The section shows the midline of the spinal cord, dorsal to the central canal. The LSt cells responsible for generating ejaculation are shown immunohistochemically labeled for galanin.

Somatic reflexes

The bulbocavernosus reflex is a spinal segmental reflex. It is activated by light pressure or stroking of the penis and consists of a contraction of the perineal muscles. There is a simultaneous contraction of all of the muscles innervated by the pudendal nerve. The afferent limb is mediated by pudendal nerve sensory fibers and the efferents are pudendal nerve motoneuron axons. It has been demonstrated that this reflex involves spinal interneurons interposed between the sensory fibers and the motoneurons. The purpose of the bulbocavernosus is not definitely known. However, during sexual arousal, the contraction of the bulbocavernosus and ischiocavernosus muscles would cause an increased erection of the glans and shaft of the penis, respectively. The contraction of the external urethral sphincter may promote the buildup of seminal fluid in the posterior urethra.

Spinal organization of sexual climax

A major discovery in sexual medicine was made recently when the neurons which generate ejaculation were identified in rats (Truitt and Coolen 2002). These investigators were engaged in a program to identify CNS neurons that were activated following various components of male sexual behavior. Neurons which were activated by c-fos staining, the product of an early intermediate gene,

which is often activated by strong stimulation of a neuron. A column of neurons near the central canal of segments L3 and L4 were consistently stained following ejaculation, but not other components of sexual behavior. These neurons stain positively for the peptide galanin (Fig. 10.11). They project to the subparafascicular nucleus of the thalamus and are therefore referred to as lumbar spinothalamic (LSt) cells.

When the LSt were destroyed by a specific lesioning technique, the rats were completely unable to ejaculate, with no other impairment of sexual behavior. Subsequent studies demonstrated that LSt cells receive projections from pudendal sensory fibers, and project to sympathetic, parasympathetic and somatic efferent neurons projecting to the sexual organs. The LSt cells receive descending projections from supraspinal sites known to be involved in sexual function. Eliciting climax-like responses in anesthetized animals activate the LSt cells, and lesions of the LSt disrupted those reflexes. Taken together, these data strongly support the conclusion that the LSt cells are responsible for generating the neural activity that underlies ejaculation. Their thalamic projections probably transmit sensory signals to provide the pleasurable sensation of ejaculation. If this ejaculatory system is the same in the human, the thalamic projection provides an obvious explanation for the simultaneity of ejaculation and the conscious perception of orgasm (see Figs 10.8 and 10.9).

A column of LSt cells is also present in the female rat. This finding suggests that the LSt cells are responsible for generating female sexual climax. The similarity of climax in the two sexes has already been noted. However, the female LSt cells were not activated following copulatory behavior (Truitt et al. 2003). A possible explanation is that the copulatory testing used in the study did not fully mimic mating behavior of rats in the wild, and the female rats did not experience sexual climax. Evidence that the LSt cells in the female are functionally homologous to the male is provided by the observation that elicitation of climax-like responses in the female activates the LSt cells (Marson et al. 2003). Further experiments are needed to conclusively demonstrate that the LSt cells are responsible for generating sexual climax in both males and females.

A question that generates a very large amount of speculation in popular books and the lay press, but surprisingly little scientific discussion, is what triggers sexual climax? Clearly, the quality and duration of sexual stimulation, the degree of mental sexual arousal, levels of stress and anxiety all play some role. The organization of the LSt cells suggests a possible theory. The LSt cells receive segmental sensory input from the genitals. Much of this genital input is probably excitatory to the LSt cells. It is also possible that the LSt receive some inhibitory spinal sensory input (eg. pain). The LSt cells are also the targets of descending projections, both inhibitory and excitatory. Perhaps there is no specific trigger for sexual climax. Instead, it may be activated when the sum of all the excitatory (spinal and descending) inputs minus the sum of all the inhibitory (spinal and descending) to the LSt cells reaches some threshold. This theory is consistent with the fact that climax can be elicited with little or no genital sensory input, for example by fantasy, sleep-related, some extreme cases of premature ejaculation, and some drug-induced climax. On the other hand, it also suggests that with the loss of descending inputs to the LSt cells in spinal cord injury, significantly greater genital stimuli are required. Further research is required to test this idea.

Supraspinal control of sexual functions

Although the preceding review demonstrates that complex sexual functions are organized at the spinal level, supraspinal mechanisms are crucial for the control of sexual responses and integration with behavioral and neuroendocrine states. Some supraspinal sites have been identified as critical for control of sexual function. The majority of this work has focused on male sexual function. The supraspinal control of female sexual function requires more investigation. In addition, anatomical studies have identified supraspinal nuclei with connections to spinal sites relevant to sexual function, but the functional significance of these connections is currently unknown.

Brainstem nuclei and pathways

Normally, spinal sexual reflexes are suppressed by a tonic descending inhibition. Lesion and tract tracing experiments have identified the source of this inhibition as the rostral pole of the nucleus paragigantocellularis (nPGi) in the rostral ventrolateral medulla. Acute and chronic neurotoxic lesions enable the elicitation of spinal sexual reflexes equivalent to spinal transection (McKenna, 1999). Several lines of evidence indicate that serotonin is the inhibitory neurotransmitter: A large majority of nPGi neurons projecting to the lumbosacral spinal cord are serotonergic; nPGi neurons transneuronally labeled from genital organs stain positively for serotonin; serotonergic neurotoxic lesions attenuate, but do not abolish the descending inhibition; intrathecal serotonin is inhibitory to sexual reflexes in spinalized rats; and drugs that raise CNS serotonin levels, such as SSRI antidepressants, are inhibitory to sexual function in humans. However, definitive proof that serotonin mediates the descending inhibition is lacking. Most importantly, spinal application of serotonergic antagonists has thus far been ineffective in abolishing the descending inhibition. Further studies are necessary to resolve this question.

An important point to note is that the nPGi is probably exerting its control of sexual reflexes in the context of a more general descending homeostatic control. The nPGi and nearby regions have been shown to be involved in cardiovascular, nociceptive, and urinary functions, in addition to sexual function (Mason, 2005). Thus, the role of the nPGi on sexual function may be reflective of a broader control of spinal somatic, autonomic and sensory systems appropriate to particular behavioral states.

Retrograde, anterograde and viral transneuronal studies in both males and females have consistently identified several brainstem regions as involved in control of sexual function. These include the noradrenergic A5 cell group in the venrolateral medulla and the locus ceruleus in the pons, the serotonergic raphe pallidus and magnus, and Barrington's nucleus in the parabrachial complex. However, the functional role of these descending projections is unknown. A specific role for these nuclei in sexual function is questionable, given that these same nuclei are also labeled following viral injections in a large number of visceral organs, including urinary organs, the adrenal, kidney, pancreas and the airway. As with the nPGi, it is likely that these brainstem nuclei mediate a broad descending modulation of homeostasis, and not a specific control of sexual function alone.

The periaqueductal gray (PAG) in the midbrain has been shown in numerous studies to have an important role in both male and female sexual function. PAG lesions severely impair male and female sexual behavior. Neurons in the PAG are activated (as indicated by Fos staining) following sexual behavior. PAG neurons receive lumbosacral afferent input. Viral injections into male and female genital organs result in transneuronal labeling of PAG neurons. Both estrogen and androgen receptors have been identified in PAG neurons. Stimulation of the PAG elicits sexual responses. In addition, the PAG receives inputs from hypothalamic regions involved in sexual function, and in turn projects to the nPGi (Fig. 10.12). Specific lesions of the PAG have been shown to block sexual responses induced by hypothalamic stimulation. Thus, the PAG appears to represent a major relay for both ascending and descending aspects of sexual function, as well as a site of hormonal modulation. However, once again, it must be stressed that this control is probably exerted by the PAG in the context of its role in mediating the somatic and autonomic expression of behavioral states.

Diencephalic nuclei and pathways

The central role of the hypothalamus in sexual function is indisputable. The hypothalamus is the critical integrative site for sexual behavior in both sexes and is a major site for the endocrine control of sexual behavior. The most important nuclei are the medial preoptic area (MPOA), the ventromedian nucleus (VMN) and the paraventricular nucleus (PVN). The MPOA is essential for male sexual behavior (Dominguez and Hull, 2005). MPOA stimulation

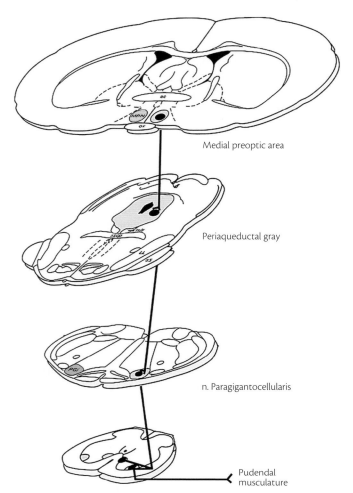

Medial preoptic area

Periaqueductal gray

n. Paragigantocellularis

Pudendal musculature

Fig. 10.12 Summary figure showing the MPOA-PAG-nPGi-spinal cord circuit. MPOA projections to the periaqueductal gray (PAG) terminate preferentially among PAG neurons projecting to the nucleus paragigantocellularis (nPGi). Descending projections from the nPGi terminate within the dorsomedial and dorsolateral motor pools of the ventral horn of the lumbosacral spinal cord. Motoneurons from these pools innervate the bulbospongiosus and ischiocavernosus muscles, which are essential for penile erection and ejaculation. Reproduced with permission from: A.Z. Murphy and G.E. Hoffman, Distribution of gonadal steroid receptor-containing neurons in the preoptic-periaqueductal gray-brainstem pathway: a potential circuit for the initiation of male sexual behavior. *Journal of Comparative Neurology* **438**: 191–212, 2001.

facilitates sexual behavior in unanesthetized animals and activates erectile and ejaculatory responses in anesthetized animals. Lesions of the MPOA abolish male copulatory behavior in every species tested. Implantation of testosterone into the MPOA of castrated animals restores sexual behavior, indicating that this is the primary site for androgen control of male sexual behavior. Despite the severe impairment of copulatory behavior following MPOA lesions, animals are still capable of sexual response (for example, monkey may still exhibit erection and ejaculation from masturbation). Further, sexual motivation remains relatively intact following MPOA lesions. The copulatory deficits from lesions appear to be due to a severe impairment in animals' ability to recognize the estrous females as sexual targets. They will investigate females and work for access to them, but do not mount or copulate with them.

These effects are consistent with the concept that the MPOA integrates hormonal and complex sensory and social cues to activate sexual behavior.

The role of the MPOA in females is more complex. Stimulation of the MPOA increases vaginal blood flow, but it also decreases receptive behavior. Lesions of the MPOA increase female receptive behavior. Interestingly, MPOA lesions in the rat also lengthen the amount of time the female stays away from the male in paced mating behavior (where the female can control the timing and frequency of sexual contact). MPOA lesions thus appear to result in impairment of mate selection or social interaction necessary for sexual function in both sexes.

The MPOA does not project directly to the spinal cord to affect sexual responses. It does have major projections to the PAG, and in turn the PAG projects to the nPGi (Fig. 10.12), as well as other descending neurons in the medullary reticular formation. In addition, lesions of the PAG block the activation of ejaculatory-like responses induced by MPOA stimulation. Thus, the facilitatory control of sexual function by the MPOA is mediated by midbrain and brainstem relays.

The ventromedian nucleus has been shown to be crucial site for female sexual behavior. Estrogen- and progesterone-sensitive neurons in the PVN mediate the receptive components of female sexual behavior. The VMN receives projections from the MPOA, and in turn projects to the PAG. PAG lesions block receptivity induced by VMN stimulation. VMN control of receptive behavior is relayed through the PAG and the medullary reticular formation. The VMN is also transneuronally labeled from the clitoris and vagina, indicating it may also be involved in genital responses.

The paraventricular nucleus has been the subject of many studies of male sexual function, primarily erection. It is reciprocally connected with the MPOA. It receives sensory input from the genitals. Its parvocellular division has direct projections to brainstem autonomic nuclei, including the nPGi. It also projects directly to sacral parasympathetic preganglionic neurons innervating the penis. Electrical and chemical stimulation of the PVN elicits penile erection. Lesions of the PVN impair erectile function.

The neurochemistry of PVN has been extensively investigated (Argiolas and Melis, 2004). Some of the spinally-projecting PVN neurons contain oxytocin. Oxytocin synapses are present on sacral parasympathetic neurons. Intrathecal oxytocin induces penile erection and this effect is blocked by a specific oxytocin antagonist. Within the PVN, glutamate, dopamine, nitric oxide and oxytocin itself are all excitatory to erection. Opioids and GABA are inhibitory to erection (Fig. 10.13). The functional role of the PVN in female sexual function is unknown. However, PVN neurons are transneuronally labeled from the clitoris and vagina, and oxytocinergic projections from the PVN to the lumbosacral cord have been identified. These anatomical findings suggest that the PVN is likely to facilitate female genital arousal.

Ejaculation induces the expression of Fos in neurons in the suparafascicular nucleus of the thalamus. This effect is specific to ejaculation, and not to erection or copulation without ejaculation. These neurons receive projections from the LSt cells in the lumbar spinal cord, which are also specifically activated by ejaculation. The subparafascicular nucleus is reciprocally connected with the MPOA. The MPOA is in turn reciprocally connected with the bed nucleus of the stria terminalis (BNST) and the medial amygdala. This densely interconnected set of nuclei (Fig. 10.14) probably

Paraventricular Nucleus

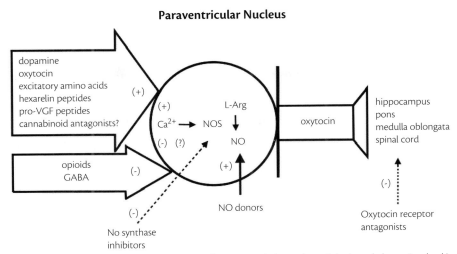

Fig. 10.13 A schematic representation of oxytocinergic neurons originating in the paraventricular nucleus of the hypothalamus involved in sexual activity. These neurons are activated by dopamine, excitatory amino acids, oxytocin itself and hexarelin analogue peptides facilitates penile erection and sexual activity. The activation of these neurons and the facilitatory effects on penile erection and sexual activity can be reduced and/or abolished by the stimulation of opioid and GABAergic receptors. The activation of oxytocinergic neurons mediating sexual activity is mediated by the activation of NO-synthase present in the cell bodies of these neurons. These neurochemical mechanisms are involved when penile erection occurs in physiological contexts. Reproduced with permission from: A. Argiolas and M.R. Melis, The role of oxytocin and the paraventricular nucleus in the sexual behaviour of male mammals, *Physiology & Behavior* **83**, 309–17, 2004.

mediates the rewarding sensation of ejaculation (Coolen, 2005). It remains to be determined if this circuit is involved in female sexual climax.

Forebrain mechanisms

In rodents, the medial amygdala is a key region for integration of chemosensory, somatosensory and hormonal stimuli in male sexual function. Rodent sexual behavior is highly dependent on olfactory stimuli, and the medial amygdala relays information from the olfactory bulbs to the medial hypothalamus. Medial amygdala neurons contain androgen receptors and this region shows a significant sexual dimorphism, the male being considerably larger. Testosterone implants in the medial amygdala restores copulatory behavior of castrated males. Sexual behavior induces Fos activation

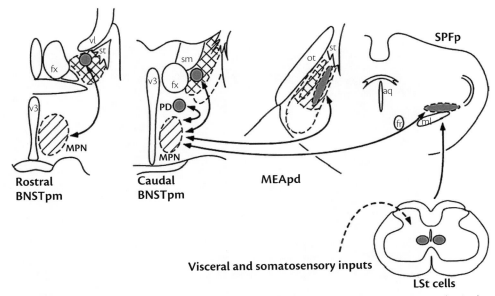

Fig. 10.14 Schematic overview of the distribution of Fos expression following different components of male sexual behavior. Fos induction by anogenital investigation is indicated by diagonal stripes from upper left to lower right; Fos activation by consumatory elements is indicated by diagonal stripes from lower left to upper right; Fos expression specifically induced by ejaculation is depicted in solid gray. Arrows indicate anatomical connections between brain regions. Aq, aqueduct; BNSTpm, posteromedial bed nucleus of the stria terminalis; Fr, fasciculus retroflexus; fx, fornix; LSt, lumbar spinothalamic cells; MEApd, posterodorsal medial amygdala; Ml, medial lemniscus; MPN,medial preoptic nucleus; ot, optic tract; PD, posterodorsal preoptic nucleus; Sm,stria medularis; SPFp, parvocellular subparafascicular thalamic nucleus; St, stria terminalis; v3, third ventricle; vl, lateral ventricle. Reproduced with permission from: L.M. Coolen, Neural Contol of Ejaculation, *Journal of Comparative Neurology* **493**: 39–45, 2005.

in the medial amygdala. Lesions of the medial amygdala result in severe impairment in male copulatory behavior.

The bed nucleus of the stria terminalis (BNST) is also a hormone sensitive, sexually dimorphic area. Lesions of this area also impair copulation in rodents. It appears to be important for preparatory aspects of copulation, including olfactory cues.

The role of the cerebral cortex in sexual function has focused primarily on the medial prefrontal cortex, primarily the prelimbic and infralimbic regions. These project to the BNST, the MPOA, and the subparafascicular nucleus of the thalamus. These anatomical connections indicate a potential role for the cortical control of sexual behavior. However, lesions of the medial prefrontal cortex have produced inconsistent effects on sexual behavior. Further studies are necessary to clarify cortical control of sexual function.

Imaging studies of sexual function in humans

One of the most exciting developments in the neural control of sexual function is the recent use of use of functional imaging of the human brain during sexual arousal and climax. These studies have confirmed some of the results in animal studies and considerably extended them. Unlike animal studies, these experiments can be combined with psychometric analyses and subjective reports. These studies also allow examination of the temporal sequence of activation, which are not possible with Fos studies in animals.

Functional imaging studies have examined brain activation due to visual sexual stimuli (erotic videos) in normal men and women, as well as some patients with sexual dysfunction. In both sexes activation was seen in anterior cingulate, medial prefrontal, orbitofrontal, insular, and occipitotemporal cortices, and the ventral striatum. In men, much greater amygdala and hypothalamic activation was also observed (Fig. 10.15). Previous studies have shown

that men are more sexually aroused by visual sexual stimuli. These imaging findings may represent the neural correlate of the sexual differences. Decreased hypothalamic activation has also been observed in older men who are less aroused by visual sexual stimulation. In men with hypoactive sexual desire or psychogenic erectile dysfunction, orbitofrontal and temporal limbic cortex activity was maintained during visual sexual stimuli. This is consistent with a postulated role of inhibition of motivated behaviors.

Imaging of the human brain during sexual climax has been performed in men and women. In both, the ventral tegmentum, an area associated with reward was strongly activated. There was decreased activity in the amygdala, and in the limbic cortex. A surprising finding was that in both sexes there was a strong activation of the cerebellum by sexual climax in both sexes (Fig. 10.16). Cerebellar involvement in sexual function has not been notable in animal experiments.

Conclusions

There has been considerable recent progress in our understanding of the neural control of sexual function. The peripheral pathways and neurochemical mediators of sexual arousal have been identified in broad terms, although the mediator(s) of vaginal vasocongestion remain undetermined. The central role of the spinal cord in organizing complex sexual responses is now recognized. Further research is needed to determine the neurochemical mediators of several descending pathways. The functional role of several brainstem nuclei projecting to the lumbosacral spinal cord need to be elucidated. This will be a challenging task, since they likely are involved in a multitude of homeostatic functions. Diencephalic and forebrain areas have been identified as important mediators of sexual behavior. There still remain questions with regard to their exact role. The significance of activity patterns seen in brain

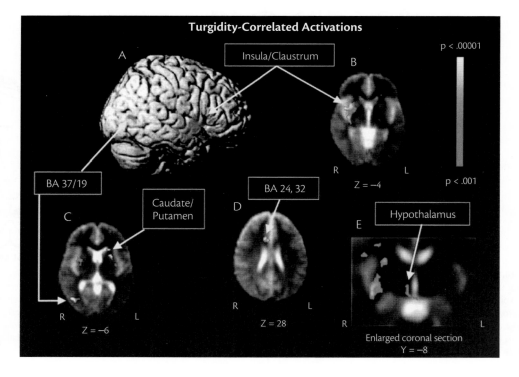

Fig. 10.15 Brain activation correlated with penile erection. The red-yellow color scale indicates regions that exhibit significant correlations with measures of penile turgidity. A) Surface reconstruction depicting projections of activations on the right side of the brain. (B) Axial section depicting the largest brain activation observed in this experiment in the right insula and claustrum. (C) Axial section illustrating activation in left caudate/putamen and right middle temporal/middle occipital gyri. (D) Axial section depicting cingulate gyrus activation. (E) Coronal section illustrating activation in the right hypothalamus. Reproduced with permission from: B.A. Arnow et al., Brain activation and sexual arousal in healthy, heterosexual males, *Brain* **125**, 1014–23, 2002.

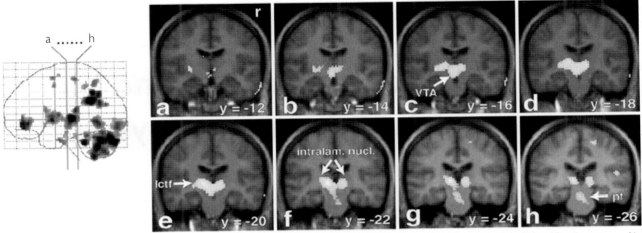

Fig. 10.16 Brain activation during ejaculation in men. A strong activation was seen in the mesodiencephalic transition zone. Increased blood flow is represented in coronal sections (a–h) through the brain. The red lines on the glass brain on the left indicate the orientation and location of the sections. The y value indicates millimeters posterior to the anterior commissure. The activated cluster contains the ventral tegmental area (VTA) (sections a–d). The midline thalamic nuclei are located slightly more caudally (sections d–f). The lateral central tegmental field (lctf; sections c–f) and the zona incerta are located lateral to this area. The activated region extends dorsally into the intralaminar nuclei (intralam. nucl.; sections d–h) and the ventroposterior thalamus. Note also the activation in the medial pontine tegmentum (pt; sections g and h). r, Right side. Reproduced with permission from: G. Holstege et al., Brain Activation during Human Male Ejaculation, *Journal of Neuroscience,* **23**: 9185–93, 2003.

imaging studies, and their temporal patterns require further study. Finally, in all areas, female sexual function requires considerably more research attention.

References

Argiolas, A. and Melis, M. R. (2004). The role of oxytocin and the paraventricular nucleus in the sexual behaviour of male mammals. *Physiol Behav* **83**, 309–17.

Bergman, B., Nilsson, S. and Petersen, I. (1979). The effect on erection and orgasm of cystectomy, prostatectomy and vesiculectomy for cancer of the bladder: A clinical and electromyographic study. *Br J Urol* **51**, 114–20.

Breedlove, S. (1984). Steroid influences on the development and function of a neuromotor system. *Prog Brain Res* **61**, 147–70.

Coolen, L. M. (2005). Neural control of ejaculation. *J Comp Neurol* **493**, 39–45.

Dominguez, J. M., Hull, E. M. (2005). Dopamine, the medial preoptic area, and male sexual behavior. *Physiol Behav* **86**, 356–68.

Hoyle, C. H. V., Stones, R. W., Robson, T., Whitley, K. and Burnstock, G. (1996). Innervation of vasculature and microvasculature of the human vagina by NOS and neuropeptide-containing nerves. *J Anat* **188**, 633–44.

Ignarro, L. J., Bush, P. A., Buga, G. M., Wood, K. S., Fukoto, J. M., and Rajfer, J. (1990). Nitric oxide and cyclic GMP formation upon electrical field stimulation cause relaxation of corpus cavernosum smooth muscle. *Biochem Biophys Res Commun* **170**, 843–50.

Jänig, W. and McLachlan, E. M. (1987). Organization of lumbar spinal outflow to distal colon and pelvic organs. *Physiol Rev* **67**, 1332–404.

Kinsey, A. C., Pomeroy, W. B., Martin, C. E. and Gebhard, P. H. (1953). *Sexual behavior in the human female.* W.B. Saunders Co., Philadelphia.

Kruger, T. H., Hartmann, U. and Schedlowski, M. (2005). Prolactinergic and dopaminergic mechanisms underlying sexual arousal and orgasm in humans. *World J Urol* **23**, 130–8.

Langworthy, O. R. (1965). Innervation of the pelvic organs of the rat. *Invest Urol* **2**, 491–511.

Levin, R. J. (1991). VIP, vagina, clitoral and periurethral glans – An update on human female genital arousal. *Exp Clin Endocrinol* **98**, 61–9.

Lue, T. F. (2000). Erectile dysfunction. *N Engl J Med* **342**, 1802–13.

Marson, L., Cai, R. and Makhanova, N. (2003). Identification of spinal neurons involved in the urethrogenital reflex in the female rat. *J Comp Neurol* **462**, 355–70.

Mason, P. (2005). Ventromedial medulla: Pain modulation and beyond. *J Comp Neurol* **493**, 2–8.

McKenna, K. E., Chung, S. K. and McVary, K. T. (1991). A model for the study of sexual function in anesthetized male and female rats. *Am J Physiol* **261**, R1276–85.

McKenna, K. E. (1999). Central nervous system pathways involved in the control of penile erection. *Ann Rev Sex Res* **10**, 157–83.

Recker, F. and Tscholl, R. (1993). Monitoring of emission as direct intraoperative control for nerve sparing retroperitoneal lymphadenectomy. *J Urol* **150**, 1360–4.

Rosen, R. C. and McKenna, K. E. (2002). PDE-5 inhibition and sexual response: Pharmacological mechanisms and clinical outcomes. *Ann Rev Sex Rev* **13**, 36–88.

Sipski, M., Alexander, C. and Rosen, R. (2001). Sexual arousal and orgasm in women: Effect of spinal cord injury. *Ann Neurol* **44**, 35–44.

Truitt, W. A. and Coolen, L. M. (2002). Identification of a potential ejaculation generator in the spinal cord. *Science,* **297**, 1566–9.

Truitt, W. A., Shipley, M. T., Veening, J. G. and Coolen, L. M. (2003). Activation of a subset of lumbar spinothalamic neurons after copulatory behavior in male but not female rats. *J Neurosci* **23**, 325–31.

CHAPTER 11

Molecular genetics and the autonomic nervous system

Stephen J. Peroutka

Key points

- Molecular genetic advances have advanced significantly the understanding of autonomic nervous system dysfunction.

- Rare genetic variants have been identified that lead to significant developmental abnormalities of the autonomic nervous system.

- More common genetic variants have been identified that explain some of the variation in autonomic activity within the general population.

Introduction

The Human Genome Project and other efforts to sequence the human genome have created vast amounts of information concerning the location and sequence of specific genes. Traditional approaches to understanding the genetic basis of disease have been based on the 'physical mapping' of a single clinical phenotype to a specific region of human DNA and, ultimately, to a specific genetic variant. This method has been very successful for a number of rare, clinically distinct disorders such as Huntington's disease, cystic fibrosis, and breast cancer. This approach has also been increasingly successful, as described below, in the evaluation of autonomic nervous system (ANS) dysfunction.

This chapter is divided into two major sections. The first and largest section reviews genetic mutations that give rise to developmental abnormalities of the ANS that are usually identified at, or shortly after, birth. The second section reviews genetic variants, some of which are fairly common, that alter the function of the ANS in children and adults. In general, common polymorphisms (i.e. those occurring in >1% of the general population) cause variations in autonomic function that are relatively mild. Since the molecular genetic understanding of ANS function continues to grow rapidly, this chapter should be considered a brief overview of a dynamic subject. A much more thorough and continually updated listing of molecular genetic data can be obtained via a search of Online Mendelian Inheritance in Man at the following Internet address:

http://www.ncbi.nlm.nih.gov/entrez/query.fcgi?db
=OMIM&cmd=Limits

Developmental abnormalities of the autonomic nervous system

Multiple specific genetic mutations have been identified that impair the normal development of the ANS (Table 11.1). For example, abnormalities of neural crest development give rise to a number of specific ANS disorders. More specifically, Hirschsprung disease (also known as aganglionic megacolon) is a congenital disorder characterized by absence of enteric ganglia along a variable length of the intestine, leading to functional bowel obstruction and distension shortly after birth. Hirschsprung disease is the most common hereditary cause of intestinal obstruction and it shows considerable variation and complex inheritance. This disorder is multifactorial in its inheritance because it can result from a mutation in any one or more of several genes that play key roles in the development of the ANS from the embryonic neural crest. Coding sequence mutations in the ECE1, EDN3, EDNRB, GDNF, RET, PHOX2B and SOX10 genes are involved in the pathogenesis of Hirschsprung's disease as well as a variety of other autonomic abnormalities. Mutations in these genes can result in dominant, recessive or polygenic patterns of inheritance (Hofstra et al. 1997). Aganglionic megacolon is also observed in some cases of trisomy 21 (Down syndrome). Thus, Hirschsprung disease represents an excellent example of both the complexity, yet definability, of a complex polygenic genetic developmental disorder.

Hirschsprung disease, essential hypertension and endothelin-converting enzyme 1

The endothelins are a family of potent vasoactive peptides the effects of which are mediated via G protein-coupled receptors. Endothelin-converting enzyme-1 (ECE1) is involved in the physiological processing of endothelin-1. A heterozygous C-to-T transition, resulting in the substitution of cysteine for arginine at position 742, in the vicinity of the active site of ECE1 (Valdenaire et al. 1995) was observed in a patient with Hirschsprung's disease, cardiac defects (i.e. ductus arteriosus, small subaortic ventricular septal defect, and small atrial septal defect), craniofacial abnormalities (i.e. cupped ears that were immature and posteriorly rotated and small nose with a high bridge and bulbous tip), other dysmorphic features (tapered fingers with hyperconvex nails, a single left palmar

Table 11.1 Molecular genetic variations affecting autonomic nervous system function

Gene symbol	Gene name	CHR	Polymorphism	Estimated frequency	Autonomic clinical features
ECE1	Endothelin-converting enzyme	1p36.1	ARG742CYS	< 0.0002%	Neural crest developmental abnormalities (e.g. Hirschsprung disease, cardiac defects, essential hypertension)
EDN3	Endothelin-3	20q13.2–13.3	Multiple	< 0.0002%	Neural crest developmental abnormalities (e.g. Hirschsprung disease, Waardenburg–Shah syndrome, central hypoventilation syndrome)
EDNRB	Endothelin receptor type B	13q22	Multiple	< 0.0002%	Neural crest developmental abnormalities (e.g. Hirschsprung disease, Waardenburg–Shah syndrome, ABCD syndrome)
GDNF	Glial derived neurotrophic factor	5p13.1–p12	Multiple	< 0.0002%	Neural crest developmental abnormalities (e.g. Hirschsprung disease)
RET	Rearranged during transfection proto-oncogene (tyrosine kinase receptor for GDNF)	10q11.2	Multiple	< 0.0002%	Neural crest developmental abnormalities (e.g. Hirschsprung disease, central hypoventilation syndrome, multiple endocrine neoplasia syndrome, thyroid carcinoma)
PHOX2B	Paired-like homeobox 2B	4p12	Multiple	< 0.0002%	Neural crest developmental abnormalities (e.g. Hirschsprung disease, neuroblastoma, central hypoventilation syndrome)
SOX10	SRY-Box 10	22q13	Multiple	< 0.0002%	Neural crest developmental abnormalities (e.g. Hirschsprung disease, Waardenburg–Shah syndrome, peripheral demyelinating neuropathy)
SPTLC1	Serine palmitoyltransferase, long chain base subunit 1	9q22.1–q22.3	Multiple	< 0.0002%	Hereditary sensory neuropathy type 1 (HSN1); HSAN1 (sensorimotor axonal neuropathy)
HSN2	HSN2	12p13.33	Multiple	< 0.0002%	HSN2 (large and small axon loss)
IKBKAP	Inhibitor of kappa light polypeptide gene enhancer in B cells, kinase complex-associated protein	9q31	Multiple	< 0.0002%	Hereditary sensory and autonomic neuropathy type 3, HSAN3; familial dysautonomia; Riley–Day syndrome (large and small axon loss)
NTRK1	Neurotrophic tyrosine kinase receptor type 1	1q21–q22	Multiple	< 0.0002%	Congenital insensitivity to pain with anhidrosis (CIPA); also called hereditary sensory and autonomic neuropathy type 4, HSAN4, familial dysautonomia type 2, congenital sensory neuropathy with anhidrosis (C-fibre loss)
NGFB	Nerve growth factor, beta subunit	1p13.1	ARG211TRP	< 0.0002%	Hereditary sensory and autonomic neuropathy type 5, HSAN5 (C-fibre and A-delta fibre loss)
ADRA2B	α_{2b}-adrenergic receptor	2	3 glutamic acid deletion	13% homozygotes	Increased SNS activity
ADRB2	β_2-adrenergic receptor	5q32–q34	THR164ILE	4%	Reduced response to β_2-adrenoceptor agonist; increased mortality from congestive heart failure
DBH	Dopamine-beta-hydroxylase	9q34	Multiple	< 0.0002%	Norepinephrine deficiency secondary to inability to convert endogenous dopamine to norepinephrine
DRD4	Dopamine receptor D4	11p15.5	13-bp deletion	2%	Autonomic hyperactivity
TTR	Transthyretin	18q11.2–q12.1	VAL30MET and multiple others	1.5%	Amyloid polyneuropathy
SLC6A2	Solute carrier family 6 (neurotransmitter transporter, noradrenaline), member 2	16q12.2	ALA457PRO	< 0.0002%	Orthostatic intolerance

crease, contractures at the interphalangeal joint of the thumbs, proximal interphalangeal joints of the fingers bilaterally, and micropenis), and autonomic dysfunction (episodes of severe agitation in association with significant tachycardia, hypertension, and core temperatures as high as 40.5°C, and status epilepticus)

(Hofstra et al. 1999). It has been suggested that the ARG742CYS mutation is responsible for, or at least contributed to, the phenotype of this patient because of an overlap in phenotypic features of between mouse models of this variant and those of the patient (Hofstra et al. 1999). Moreover, the mutation was thought to lead to the phenotype by resulting in reduced levels of endothelin-1 (EDN1) and endothelin-3 (EDN3) (Hofstra et al. 1999). Other mutations of ECE1 have been associated with essential hypertension.

Hirschsprung disease, Waardenburg–Shah syndrome, central hypoventilation syndrome and endothelin-3

The endothelins are a family of potent vasoactive peptides consisting of three isopeptides: EDN1, EDN2 and EDN3. EDN3 exerts a dose-dependent stimulation of proliferation and melanogenesis in neural crest cells. Mice lacking the EDN3 gene display a phenotype similar to that seen in humans with Waardenburg–Hirschsprung syndrome. In humans, at least seven different EDN3 mutations have been found in patients with Hirschsprung disease (McCallion and Chakravarti 2001, Puri and Shinkai 2004). Genetic mutations in the EDN3 gene have also been associated with the Waardenburg–Shah syndrome and the central hypoventilation syndrome (i.e. Ondine's curse).

Hirschsprung disease type 2, Waardenburg–Shah syndrome, ABCD syndrome and endothelin receptor type B

The endothelins mediate their effects via G protein-coupled receptors. Mutations within the endothelin receptor type B (EDNRB) gene are the molecular basis of Hirschsprung disease type 2 (Puffenberger et al. 1994b, Amiel et al. 1996, Kusafuka et al. 1996, Svensson et al. 1998, Auricchio et al. 1999). It has been estimated that EDNRB mutations account for approximately 5% of cases of Hirschsprung disease (Chakravarti 1996). However, penetrance is not 100% for some of the mutations, even in homozygotes with the mutation (Puffenberger et al. 1994a, Duan et al. 2003). These data indicate that the EDNRB gene is an important modifier gene for the development of Hirschsprung disease type 2. Genetic mutations in the EDN3 gene have also been associated with the Waardenburg–Shah syndrome and the ABCD syndrome (albinism, black lock, cell migration disorder).

Hirschsprung disease and glial cell line-derived neurotrophic factor

A causal link between Hirschsprung disease and the glial cell line-derived neurotrophic factor (GDNF) gene was established as a result of an initial observation that Gdnf -/- mice display congenital intestinal aganglionosis and renal agenesis (Moore et al. 1996). A direct screen of 106 unrelated patients with Hirschsprung disease for mutations in GDNF identified one familial GDNF missense mutation (ARG93TRP) in a patient with Hirschsprung disease with a known mutation in the GDNF receptor gene (i.e. RET gene described below) (Angrist et al. 1998). These data suggested that GDNF is a minor contributor to Hirschsprung disease susceptibility and that, in rare instances, GDNF and RET mutations may act in concert to produce the Hirschsprung disease phenotype. Multiple other studies have now confirmed that GDNF mutations alone may be causative in some cases of Hirschsprung disease (Ivanchuk et al. 1996).

Hirschsprung disease, multiple endocrine neoplasia, medullary thyroid carcinoma and rearranged during transfection proto-oncogene

The rearranged during transfection (RET) gene encodes a tyrosine kinase receptor that is activated endogenously by GDNF. Mutations in the RET gene are associated with multiple endocrine neoplasia type IIA, multiple endocrine neoplasia type IIB, medullary thyroid carcinoma and Hirschsprung disease. During embryogenesis, RET and GDNF genes are involved in the migration and differentiation of enteric ganglion cells, sympathetic neurons and melanocytes from the neural crest, thus being critical for normal ANS formation. Mutations in the RET gene exist in 50% of patients with familial Hirschsprung disease (Attie et al. 1994, Edery et al. 1994, Pasini et al. 1996, Gabriel et al. 2002). Penetrance is greater in males than in females, in keeping with the higher frequency of the disorder in males. A large number of mutations exist throughout the gene in the familial cases as well as in approximately 33% of sporadic cases. Specifically, frameshift and missense mutations disrupt or change the structure of the protein.

Hirschsprung disease (short segment), neuroblastoma, central hypoventilation syndrome and paired-like homeobox 2B

The paired-like homeobox 2B gene (PHOX2B) is involved in the early development of the ANS from the neural crest (Pattyn et al. 1999). PHOX2B is one of multiple genes needed for the differentiation and survival of subsets of autonomic neurons. In mice with a targeted deletion of the PHOX2B gene, all autonomic ganglia and the three cranial sensory ganglia (that are part of the autonomic reflex circuits) fail to develop properly and eventually degenerate (Pattyn et al. 1999). In humans, mutations in the PHOX2B gene have been associated with Hirschsprung disease (short segment) (Benailly et al. 2003), both with and without associated and neuroblastoma (Trochet et al. 2004, Mosse et al. 2004), as well as with central hypoventilation syndrome.

Hirschsprung disease, Waardenburg–Shah syndrome and SRY-Box 10

The SRY-Box 10 gene (SOX10) plays a key role in neural crest development. In Waardenburg–Shah syndrome, patients have deafness, pigmentary abnormalities, and Hirschsprung disease, all caused by the failure of embryonic neural crest development. In patients with Waardenburg–Shah syndrome, mutations in the SOX10 gene have been identified (Pingault et al. 1998, Southard-Smith et al. 1999).

Hereditary sensory and autonomic neuropathy type 1 and serine palmitoyltransferase, long-chain base subunit 1

Serine palmitoyltransferase is the key enzyme in sphingolipid biosynthesis. Mutations in the gene can lead to increased activation of the enzyme, causing an increased production of glucosyl ceramide. Ceramide, resulting from catabolism of sphingomyelin, can mediate cell death. Therefore, in theory, increased ceramide synthesis leads directly to neuronal cell death. Multiple mutations within the serine palmitoyltransferase, long-chain base subunit 1 (SPTLC1) gene have been associated with hereditary sensory neuropathy type 1 (HSN1; also called hereditary sensory and autonomic neuropathy type 1 [HSAN1]) (i.e. a dominantly inherited sensorimotor axonal neuropathy) (Bejaoui et al. 2001, Bejaoui et al. 2002).

Hereditary sensory and autonomic neuropathy type 2 and the HSN2 gene

Hereditary sensory neuropathy type 2 (HSN2; also called hereditary sensory and autonomic neuropathy type 2 [HSAN2]), is a rare autosomal recessive disorder that usually begins in childhood and is characterized by an impairment of pain, temperature and touch sensation resulting from the reduction or absence of peripheral sensory neurons. Symptoms often include inflammation of the digits, especially around the nails, usually accompanied by infection of the fingers and on the soles of the feet. A novel gene, designated HSN2, has been identified on chromosome 12p13.33 that co-segregates with the disease (Lafreniere et al. 2004, Riviere et al. 2004). The HSN2 gene encodes a deduced 434-amino acid protein. It has been suggested that the HSN2 protein may play a role in the development and/or maintenance of peripheral sensory neurons or their supporting Schwann cells (Lafreniere et al. 2004). The molecular mechanism by which this gene induces sensory neuronal death remains unknown.

Hereditary sensory and autonomic neuropathy type 3 (also known as familial dysautonomia, Riley–Day syndrome) and inhibitor of kappa light polypeptide gene enhancer in B cells, kinase complex-associated protein

An autosomal recessive clinical syndrome consisting of a congenital lack of tearing, emotional lability, paroxysmal hypertension, increased sweating, cold hands and feet, corneal anaesthesia, erythematous skin blotching, and drooling has been termed the Riley–Day syndrome or hereditary sensory neuropathy type 3 (HSN3; also called hereditary sensory and autonomic neuropathy type 3 [HSAN3]) (Brunt and McKusick 1970). Autonomic dysfunction is the principal symptom, resulting from decreased populations of sensory, sympathetic and parasympathetic neurons. However, the clinical manifestations are variable and may also include absence of fungiform papillae of the tongue, severe scoliosis, and neuropathic joints. The individuals, thus far all Ashkenazi Jewish patients, also have an enhanced response to pressor agents due to a denervation supersensitivity to catecholamines (Bickel et al. 2002). Excretion of both dopamine and noradrenaline metabolites is reduced and plasma dopamine-beta-hydroxylase (DBH) levels are low.

Linkage analysis (Blumenfeld et al. 1993) led to the identification of the inhibitor of kappa light polypeptide gene enhancer in B cells, kinase complex-associated protein (IKBKAP) as the causative gene located on chromosome 9q31–q33 (Slaugenhaupt et al. 2001). IKBKAP is a scaffold protein and a regulator of at least three different kinases involved in proinflammatory signalling. The major haplotype mutation was located at the donor splice site of intron 20. In patients with HSAN3, wildtype IKBKAP transcripts are present, although to varying extents, in all cell lines, blood, and post-mortem tissues (Cuajungco et al. 2003). However, the relative wildtype-to-mutant IKBKAP RNA levels are highest in cultured patient lymphoblasts and lowest in post-mortem central and peripheral nervous tissues. The authors suggested that the relative inefficiency of wildtype IKBKAP mRNA production from the mutant alleles in the nervous system underlies the selective degeneration of sensory and autonomic neurons in HSAN3 (Cuajungco et al. 2003).

Hereditary sensory and autonomic neuropathy type 4 and neurotrophic tyrosine kinase receptor type 1

Neurotrophins and their receptors regulate the development and maintenance of both the central and the peripheral nervous systems. The neurotrophic tyrosine kinase receptor type 1 gene (NTRK1) is located at chromosome 1q32–q41 and is a primary receptor for nerve growth factor (NGF). Defects in the NGF signal transduction pathway leads to a failure to support the survival of sympathetic and primary sensory neurons. In addition, NGF acts as an immunoregulatory cytokine on monocytes.

Hereditary sensory neuropathy type 4 (HSN4; also called hereditary sensory and autonomic neuropathy type 4 [HSAN4]) is an autosomal recessive disorder characterized by the absence of pain sensation often leading to self-mutilation, anhidrosis, recurrent episodic high fever and mental retardation (Indo 2001, Indo 2002). Sweating cannot be elicited by thermal, painful, emotional or chemical stimuli despite the presence of normal sweat glands. The clinical syndrome has also been called congenital insensitivity to pain with anhidrosis (CIPA), familial dysautonomia type 2, and congenital sensory neuropathy with anhidrosis. Patients with HSN4 have a hereditary developmental defect of nerve outgrowth (Verze et al. 2000).

In three unrelated patients with HSN4, different mutations within the NTRK1 gene were identified (Indo et al. 1996). Specifically, a single base C deletion at nucleotide 1726 in exon C causes a frameshift and premature termination of the receptor protein in two individuals with congenital insensitivity to pain. The individuals are homozygous for the mutation. The authors suggested that the clinical symptomatology results from the fact that the NGF–NTRK1 system plays a critical role in the development and function of the peripheral pain and temperature systems (Indo et al. 1996). Over the past decade, approximately 40 specific mutations have been identified in the NTRK1 gene that are involved in the extracellular domain of the receptor that interacts with the binding of NGF as well as in the intracellular signal transduction domain of the receptor (Indo 2001). Many of these mutations have been identified in patients with HSN4.

Hereditary sensory and autonomic neuropathy type 5 and nerve growth factor, beta S subunit

Hereditary sensory and autonomic neuropathy type 5 (HSAN5) is characterized by a loss of deep pain and temperature sensation with a severe reduction of unmyelinated nerve fibres and moderate loss of thin myelinated nerve fibres (Einarsdottir et al. 2004). In contrast to HSAN4, mental abilities and most other neurological functions remain intact. A candidate gene analysis of a large family from Sweden revealed a mutation in the coding region of the nerve growth factor, beta S subunit (NGFB) gene (ARG211TRP) that co-segregated with the disease phenotype (Einarsdottir et al. 2004). Neurotrophins such as NGF regulate the development and maintenance of the central and the peripheral nervous systems, and also play an immunoregulatory role. The authors noted that this NGFB mutation seems to separate the effects of NGF involved in development of central nervous system (CNS) functions from those involved in peripheral pain pathways (Einarsdottir et al. 2004). Indeed, this conclusion is consistent with the observation that NGF plays a key role in the maintenance and regeneration of peripheral sensory neurons (Ramer et al. 2000) but may be less important in the development and maintenance of the CNS.

Functional abnormalities of the autonomic nervous system

Increased sympathetic nervous system activity and the α_{2b}-adrenergic receptor

A polymorphism in the α_{2b}-adrenergic receptor (ADRA2B) gene leading to the deletion of 3 glutamic acids from a glutamic acid repeat element (glu12, amino acids 297 to 309) in the third intracellular loop of the receptor protein has been evaluated (Heinonen et al. 1999). This repeat element had been shown to be important for agonist-dependent alpha-2B-adrenergic receptor desensitization. In subjects homozygous for the short allele compared with subjects with two long alleles, the basal metabolic rate was 6% lower (p = 0.009) than in controls. Since a lower metabolic rate is a risk factor for obesity, the authors concluded that this polymorphism of the ADRA2B subtype could partly explain the variation in basal metabolic rate in an obese population and may therefore contribute to the pathogenesis of obesity (Heinonen et al. 1999).

In addition, the same ADRA2B 3-glutamic acid deletion polymorphism was evaluated in 381 healthy Japanese males using electrocardiogram R-R interval power spectral analysis (Suzuki et al. 2003). In R-R spectral analysis of heart rate variability, homozygous carriers of the short allele (13% of the study group) had significantly greater low frequency and very low frequency than did homozygous carriers of the long allele, as well as a higher sympathetic nervous system index. In general, low frequencies of heart rate variability are associated with both sympathetic nervous system (SNS) and parasympathetic nervous system (PNS) activities and the very low frequencies of heart rate variability reflect thermoregulatory control of SNS activity. Thus, these findings suggested that the ADRA2B deletion polymorphism is associated with increased SNS activity and lower PNS activity in healthy, young males (Suzuki et al. 2003). The authors hypothesized that the increased SNS activity might be secondary to the decreased basal metabolic rate observed by others (Heinonen et al. 1999). Alternatively, the ADRA2B deletion may result in increased SNS activity with a secondary decrease in basal metabolic rate.

Reduced response to β_2-adrenoceptor agonists and the β_2-adrenergic receptor

The Thr164Ile polymorphism of the β_2-adrenoceptor is present in ~4% of the population and is associated with a significant decrease in response to β_2-adrenergic agonists (Brodde et al. 2001, Dishy et al. 2001). Altered adrenergic vascular sensitivity may contribute to the decreased survival observed in patients with congestive heart failure carrying the Ile164 allele. In a study of patients with congestive heart failure, those with the Ile164 polymorphism displayed a striking difference in survival with a relative risk of death or cardiac transplant of 4.81 (p < 0.001) compared with those with the wildtype Thr at this position (Liggett et al. 1998). The 1-year survival for Ile164 patients was 42% compared with 76% for patients with the wildtype β_2-adrenoceptor.

The dose of isoproterenol required to achieve 50% venodilation is significantly higher in individuals with the Ile164 allele than in those without, although the maximal response to isoproterenol does not differ (Dishy et al. 2001). Conversely, the dose of phenylephrine needed to induce 50% venoconstriction is significantly lower in individuals with the Ile164 allele than in those without. Thus, the Thr164Ile polymorphism of the β_2-adrenergic receptor is associated with a five-fold reduction in sensitivity to β_2-receptor agonist-mediated vasodilation while vasoconstrictor sensitivity is increased. The overall effect of the Thr164Ile polymorphism is to shift the balance of adrenergic vascular tone toward vasoconstriction. This suggests a mechanistic explanation for the clinical observation of decreased survival in patients with congestive heart failure heterozygous for the Thr164Ile polymorphism (Dishy et al. 2001).

Norepinephrine deficiency and dopamine-beta-hydroxylase

DBH converts dopamine to norepinephrine in postganglionic sympathetic neurons. The DBH gene is located at chromosome 9q34. Several patients have been analysed with congenital DBH deficiency (Robertson et al. 1986, Robertson et al. 1991, Man in 't Veld et al. 1987a, Mathias et al. 1990). The individuals have noradrenergic denervation and adrenomedullary failure but baroreflex afferents, cholinergic innervation and adrenocortical function are normal. Norepinephrine, epinephrine and their breakdown products are not detectable in plasma, urine and cerebrospinal fluid but dopamine levels are increased significantly. Physiological and pharmacological stimuli of sympathetic nervous system activity cause increases in dopamine but not norepinephrine.

DBH deficient infants have a delay in the opening of the eyes (2 weeks in one case), and ptosis has been observed in almost all DBH-deficient infants. Some of the infants have been reported to be sickly in the neonatal stage and survival is often believed to be unlikely. Hypotension, hypoglycaemia and hypothermia are present early in life. Postural hypotension is exhibited during exercise in childhood and is marked by an increase in heart rate as the blood pressure falls. Syncopal episodes may be misinterpreted as epilepsy in the children, leading to the treatment with anticonvulsants. In general, symptoms worsen during adolescence and severely limit the function of the individual.

Clinical features during adolescence and adulthood include reduced exercise tolerance, skeletal muscle hypotonia, recurrent hypoglycaemia, ptosis of the eyelids, nasal stuffiness, and prolonged or retrograde ejaculation. The severe postural hypotension is attributed to the impairment of sympathetic vasoconstrictor function. Symptoms in DBH deficiency have also been reported to worsen in the morning, after exercise and in warm weather (Mathias et al. 1990). No other neurological or psychiatric abnormalities have been reported.

The symptoms of DBH deficiency respond well from treatment with D-dihydroxyphenylserine (DOPS; also known as Droxidopa) (Biaggioni and Robertson 1987, Man in 't Veld et al. 1987b, Mathias et al. 1990, Thompson et al. 1995). This molecule is converted to norepinephrine by decarboxylation of the terminal carboxyl group. Treatment with DOPS (150–600 mg/day) leads to a reduction in orthostatic hypotension, increased plasma levels of norepinephrine and, in the males, the ability to ejaculate.

Specific mutations within the DBH gene have been identified that appear to be the cause of the enzymatic deficiency (Kim et al. 2002). Specifically, seven novel variants, including four potentially pathogenic mutations in the human DBH gene, were identified from an analysis of two unrelated patients with DBH deficiency and their families. Both patients were found to be compound heterozygotes for variants affecting expression of DBH. Each patient carried one copy of a T—>C transversion in the splice donor site of DBH intron 1, creating a premature stop codon. One patient also had a missense mutation in DBH exon 2 while the other had missense mutations in exons 1 and 6. The authors proposed that deficiency in norepinephrine is an autosomal recessive disorder resulting from heterogeneous molecular lesions with the DBH gene (Kim et al. 2002).

Autonomic hyperactivity and dopamine D4 receptor

The dopamine D4 receptor (DRD4) gene is one of the five known G protein-coupled receptors for which dopamine is the primary neurotransmitter. The gene is located at chromosome 11p15.5 and codes for a receptor protein of 387 amino acids (Van Tol et al. 1991). At least three common polymorphic variants of the gene exist in the human population based as a result of known variations in a 48-base-pair sequence in the third cytoplasmic loop of the receptor (Van Tol et al. 1992).

A 13-base-pair deletion of bases 235–247 in the DRD4 gene has been identified in approximately 2% of the general population (Nothen et al. 1994). The deletion alters the reading frame from amino acid 79 in the receptor and generates a stop codon 20 amino acids downstream, thereby truncating the receptor to an abnormally short 98 amino acids. No major neuropsychiatric disturbances have been observed in heterozygotes with this mutation (Nothen et al. 1994). However, in a single homozygous individual with this mutation, autonomic hyperactivity was observed. Specifically, the 50-year-old (at the time of the study) male reported severe dermatographism and excessive sweating. These symptoms were exacerbated in social gatherings and moderately warm temperatures. The individual denied feeling anxious in these situations but characterized himself as nervous and explosive since early adulthood. He has had severe migrainous headaches since adolescence, successfully treated with a tricyclic antidepressant. He has been obese since adolescence. He had an acoustic neuroma removed at 38 years of age, with a negative family history, and a recurrence removed at 44 years of age. Fluctuations in pulse rate leading to intermittent sinus tachycardia had been treated with beta-blockers since approximately 40 years of age. A consistently reduced body temperature (35.4°C) was documented (Nothen et al. 1994). The authors speculated that at least some of these autonomic disturbances could be attributed directly to the absence of a functional DRD4 receptor (Nothen et al. 1994).

Amyloid polyneuropathy and transthyretin

Transthyretin (TTR) is a prealbumin protein of 127 amino acids and is a primary transport protein for thyroxine and retinol (vitamin A). The protein is a common constituent of neuritic plaques and microangiopathic lesions related to amyloid deposition. More than 70 different mutations associated with amyloid deposition have been identified within the TTR gene located at chromosome 18q11.2–q12.1 (Saraiva 1995, Saraiva 2001). Amyloidogenic mutations in this gene lead to decreased stability of the TTR protein, with the VAL30MET variant (also called the Andrade or Portuguese type) being the most common allelic variant. Most of the mutations result in an amyloid polyneuropathy, which involves small, unmyelinated fibres. The neuropathy disproportionately affects pain and temperature sensation although significant clinical variation exists between the various mutations (Ikeda 2002). Indeed, there is a much larger prevalence of TTR mutations than recognized disease due to the wide variation in phenotypes.

Orthostatic intolerance and solute carrier family 6 (neurotransmitter transporter, noradrenaline), member 2

Orthostatic intolerance (OI) is a clinical syndrome consisting of group of symptoms that can occur after assuming an upright posture.

Although a variety of OI definitions have been used in the medical literature, OI can best be defined as the development of light-headedness or 'dizziness', as well as visual changes and other symptoms, upon arising from the supine position to an upright position. In general, OI can be defined as a standing heart rate increase of at least 30 beats per minute, without orthostatic hypotension. Most patients with a diagnosis of orthostatic intolerance are women of 20–50 years of age (Low et al. 1995). This syndrome has also often been described by a number of other names such as the postural orthostatic tachycardia syndrome (POTS), soldiers' heart, neurocirculatory asthenia and mitral valve prolapse syndrome. It may also play a role in the chronic fatigue syndrome (Schondorf and Freeman 1999).

The reuptake of noradrenaline into sympathetic terminals occurs via a specific Na$^+$-dependent and Cl$^-$-dependent transport system mediated by the solute carrier family 6 (neurotransmitter transporter, noradrenaline), member 2 (SLC6A2) gene. In a patient with orthostatic intolerance, an elevated mean plasma noradrenaline concentration was observed while standing (Shannon et al. 2000). Analysis of the norepinephrine-transporter gene revealed that the proband was heterozygous for a ALA457PRO mutation that resulted in more than a 98% loss of function as compared with that of the wild-type gene. The authors concluded that the impairment of synaptic noradrenaline clearance may result in a syndrome characterized by excessive sympathetic activation in response to physiological stimuli.

Future directions

Molecular genetics allows for a mechanistic analysis of the ANS. Moreover, molecular genetic data offer the potential to provide immediate diagnostic, prognostic and therapeutic guidance. The coupling of molecular genetic diagnoses and rational therapeutic approaches based on these data should continue to have a significant impact on the diagnosis and management of patients with autonomic dysfunction. Hopefully, the molecular insights gained from the genetic analysis of the ANS should significantly decrease the societal morbidity from genetically based autonomic dysfunction.

References

Amiel, J., Attie, T., Jan, D., et al. (1996). Heterozygous endothelin receptor B (EDNRB) mutations in isolated Hirschsprung disease. Hum. Mol. Genet., 5, 355–57.

Angrist, M., Jing, S., Bolk, S., et al. (1998). Human GFRA1: cloning, mapping, genomic structure, and evaluation as a candidate gene for Hirschsprung disease susceptibility. Genomics, 48, 354–62.

Attie, T., Edery, P., Lyonne,t S., Nihoul-Fekete, C. and Munnich, A. (1994). [Identification of mutation of RET proto-oncogene in Hirschsprung disease]. C.R. Seances Soc. Biol. Fil., 188, 499–504.

Auricchio, A., Griseri, P., Carpentieri, M. L., et al. (1999). Double heterozygosity for a RET substitution interfering with splicing and an EDNRB missense mutation in Hirschsprung disease. Am. J Hum. Genet., 64, 1216–21.

Bejaoui, K., Uchida, Y., Yasuda, S., et al. (2002). Hereditary sensory neuropathy type 1 mutations confer dominant negative effects on serine palmitoyltransferase, critical for sphingolipid synthesis. J Clin. Invest, 110, 1301–1308.

Bejaoui, K., Wu, C., Scheffler, M. D., et al. (2001). SPTLC1 is mutated in hereditary sensory neuropathy, type 1. Nat. Genet., 27, 261–62.

Benailly, H. K., Lapierre J. M., Laudier B., et al. (2003). PMX2B, a new candidate gene for Hirschsprung's disease. Clin. Genet., 64, 204–209.

Biaggioni, I. and Robertson, D. (1987). Endogenous restoration of noradrenaline by precursor therapy in dopamine-beta-hydroxylase deficiency. *Lancet*, **2**, 1170–72.

Bickel, A., Axelrod, F. B., Schmelz, M., Marthol, H. and Hilz, M.J. (2002). Dermal microdialysis provides evidence for hypersensitivity to noradrenaline in patients with familial dysautonomia. *J Neurol. Neurosurg. Psychiatry*, **73**, 299–302.

Blumenfeld, A., Slaugenhaupt, S. A., Axelrod, F. B., *et al.*(1993). Localization of the gene for familial dysautonomia on chromosome 9 and definition of DNA markers for genetic diagnosis. *Nat. Genet.*, **4**, 160–64.

Brodde, O. E., Buscher, R., Tellkamp, R., Radke, J., Dhein, S., and Insel, P. A. (2001). Blunted cardiac responses to receptor activation in subjects with Thr164Ile beta(2)-adrenoceptors. *Circulation*, **103**, 1048–50.

Brunt, P. W., and McKusick, V. A. (1970). Familial dysautonomia. A report of genetic and clinical studies, with a review of the literature. *Medicine (Baltimore)*, **49**, 343–74.

Chakravarti, A. (1996). Endothelin receptor-mediated signaling in hirschsprung disease. *Hum. Mol. Genet.*, **5**, 303–307.

Cuajungco, M. P., Leyne, M., Mull, J., *et al.* (2003). Tissue-specific reduction in splicing efficiency of IKBKAP due to the major mutation associated with familial dysautonomia. *Am. J Hum. Genet.*, **72**, 749–58.

Dishy, V., Sofowora, G. G., Xie, H. G., Kim, R. B., Byrne, D. W., Stein, C. M. and Wood, A. J. (2001). The effect of common polymorphisms of the beta2-adrenergic receptor on agonist-mediated vascular desensitization. *N. Engl. J Med.*, **345**, 1030–35.

Duan, X. L., Zhang, X. S. and Li, G. W. (2003). Clinical relationship between EDN-3 gene, EDNRB gene and Hirschsprung's disease. *World J Gastroenterol.*, **9**, 2839–42.

Edery, P., Lyonnet, S., Mulligan, L. M., *et al.* (1994). Mutations of the RET proto-oncogene in Hirschsprung's disease. *Nature*, **367**, 378–80.

Einarsdottir, E., Carlsson, A., Minde, J., *et al.* (2004). A mutation in the nerve growth factor beta gene (NGFB) causes loss of pain perception. *Hum. Mol. Genet.*, **13**, 799–805.

Gabriel, S. B., Salomon, R., Pelet, A., *et al.* (2002). Segregation at three loci explains familial and population risk in Hirschsprung disease. *Nat. Genet.*, **31**, 89–93.

Heinonen, P., Koulu, M., Pesonen, U., *et al.* (1999). Identification of a three-amino acid deletion in the alpha2B-adrenergic receptor that is associated with reduced basal metabolic rate in obese subjects. *J Clin. Endocrinol. Metab*, **84**, 2429–33.

Hofstra, R. M., Osinga, J. and Buys, C. H. (1997). Mutations in Hirschsprung disease: when does a mutation contribute to the phenotype. *Eur. J Hum. Genet.*, **5**, 180–85.

Hofstra, R. M, Valdenaire, O., Arch, E., *et al.* (1999). A loss-of-function mutation in the endothelin-converting enzyme 1 (ECE-1) associated with Hirschsprung disease, cardiac defects, and autonomic dysfunction. *Am. J Hum. Genet.*, **64**, 304–308.

Ikeda, S. (2002). Clinical picture and outcome of transthyretin-related familial amyloid polyneuropathy (FAP) in Japanese patients. *Clin. Chem. Lab Med.*, **40**, 1257–61.

Indo, Y. (2001). Molecular basis of congenital insensitivity to pain with anhidrosis (CIPA): mutations and polymorphisms in TRKA (NTRK1) gene encoding the receptor tyrosine kinase for nerve growth factor. *Hum. Mutat.*, **18**, 462–71.

Indo, Y. (2002). Genetics of congenital insensitivity to pain with anhidrosis (CIPA) or hereditary sensory and autonomic neuropathy type IV. Clinical, biological and molecular aspects of mutations in TRKA(NTRK1) gene encoding the receptor tyrosine kinase for nerve growth factor. *Clin. Auton. Res.*, **12** Suppl 1, I20–32.

Indo, Y., Tsuruta, M., Hayashida, Y., *et al.* (1996). Mutations in the TRKA/NGF receptor gene in patients with congenital insensitivity to pain with anhidrosis. *Nat. Genet.*, **13**, 485–88.

Ivanchuk, S. M., Myers, S. M., Eng, C. and Mulligan, L. M. (1996). De novo mutation of GDNF, ligand for the RET/GDNFR-alpha receptor complex, in Hirschsprung disease. *Hum. Mol. Genet.*, **5**, 2023–26.

Kim, C. H, Zabetian, C. P, Cubells, J. F, *et al.* (2002). Mutations in the dopamine beta-hydroxylase gene are associated with human norepinephrine deficiency. *Am. J Med. Genet.*, **108**, 140–47.

Kusafuka, T., Wang, Y. and Puri, P. (1996). Novel mutations of the endothelin-B receptor gene in isolated patients with Hirschsprung's disease. *Hum. Mol. Genet.*, **5**, 347–49.

Lafreniere, R. G, MacDonald, M. L, Dube, M. P, *et al.* (2004). Identification of a novel gene (HSN2) causing hereditary sensory and autonomic neuropathy type II through the Study of Canadian Genetic Isolates. *Am. J Hum. Genet.*, **74**, 1064–73.

Liggett, S. B., Wagoner, L. E., Craft, L. L., Hornung, R. W., Hoit, B. D., McIntosh, T. C. and Walsh, R. A. (1998). The Ile164 beta2-adrenergic receptor polymorphism adversely affects the outcome of congestive heart failure. *J Clin. Invest*, **102**, 1534–39.

Low, P. A., Opfer-Gehrking, T. L., Textor, S. C., *et al.* (1995). Postural tachycardia syndrome (POTS). *Neurology*, **45**, S19–25.

Man in 't Veld, A. J., Boomsma, F., Moleman, P. and Schalekamp, M. A. (1987a). Congenital dopamine-beta-hydroxylase deficiency. A novel orthostatic syndrome. *Lancet*, **1**, 183–88.

Man in 't Veld, A. J., Boomsma, F., van den Meiracker, A. H., and Schalekamp, M. A. (1987b). Effect of unnatural noradrenaline precursor on sympathetic control and orthostatic hypotension in dopamine-beta-hydroxylase deficiency. *Lancet*, **2**, 1172–75.

Mathias, C. J., Bannister, R. B., Cortelli, P., *et al.* (1990). Clinical, autonomic and therapeutic observations in two siblings with postural hypotension and sympathetic failure due to an inability to synthesize noradrenaline from dopamine because of a deficiency of dopamine beta hydroxylase. *Q J Med.*, **75**, 617–33.

McCallion, A. S. and Chakravarti, A. (2001). EDNRB/EDN3 and Hirschsprung disease type II. *Pigment Cell Res.*, **14**, 161–69.

Moore, M. W., Klein, R. D., Farinas I., *et al.* (1996). Renal and neuronal abnormalities in mice lacking GDNF. *Nature*, **382**, 76–79.

Mosse, Y. P., Laudenslager, M., Khazi, D., Carlisle, A. J., Winter, C. L., Rappaport, E. and Maris, J. M. (2004). Germline PHOX2B mutation in hereditary neuroblastoma. *Am. J Hum. Genet.*, **75**, 727–30.

Nothen, M. M., Cichon, S., Hemmer, S., *et al.* (1994). Human dopamine D4 receptor gene: frequent occurrence of a null allele and observation of homozygosity. *Hum. Mol. Genet.*, **3**, 2207–2212.

Pasini, B., Ceccherini, I. and Romeo, G. (1996). RET mutations in human disease. *Trends Genet.*, **12**, 138–44.

Pattyn, A., Morin, X., Cremer, H., Goridis, C. and Brunet, J. F. (1999). The homeobox gene Phox2b is essential for the development of autonomic neural crest derivatives. *Nature*, **399**, 366–70.

Pingault, V., Bondurand, N., Kuhlbrodt, K., *et al.* (1998). SOX10 mutations in patients with Waardenburg-Hirschsprung disease. *Nat. Genet.*, **18**, 171–73.

Puffenberger, E. G., Hosoda, K., Washington, S. S., Nakao, K., deWit, D., Yanagisawa, M. and Chakravart, A. (1994b). A missense mutation of the endothelin-B receptor gene in multigenic Hirschsprung's disease. *Cell*, **79**, 1257–66.

Puffenberger, E. G., Hosoda, K., Washington, S. S., Nakao, K., deWit, D., Yanagisawa, M. and Chakravart, A. (1994a). A missense mutation of the endothelin-B receptor gene in multigenic Hirschsprung's disease. *Cell*, **79**, 1257–66.

Puri, P. and Shinkai, T. (2004). Pathogenesis of Hirschsprung's disease and its variants: recent progress. *Semin. Pediatr. Surg.*, **13**, 18–24.

Ramer, M. S, Priestley, J.V. and McMahon, S. B. (2000). Functional regeneration of sensory axons into the adult spinal cord. *Nature*, **403**, 312–316.

Riviere, J. B., Verlaan, D. J., Shekarabi, M., *et al.* (2004). A mutation in the HSN2 gene causes sensory neuropathy type II in a Lebanese family. *Ann. Neurol.*, **56**, 572–75.

Robertson, D., Goldberg, M. R., Onrot, J., Hollister, A. S., Wiley, R., Thompson, J. G., Jr. and Robertson, R. M. (1986). Isolated failure of autonomic noradrenergic neurotransmission. Evidence for impaired beta-hydroxylation of dopamine. *N. Engl. J Med.,* **314**, 1494–97.

Robertson, D., Haile, V., Perry, S. E., Robertson, R. M., Phillips, J. A., III and Biaggioni, I. (1991). Dopamine beta-hydroxylase deficiency. A genetic disorder of cardiovascular regulation. *Hypertension,* **18**, 1–8.

Saraiva, M. J. (1995). Transthyretin mutations in health and disease. *Hum. Mutat.,* **5**, 191–96.

Saraiva, M. J. (2001). Transthyretin amyloidosis: a tale of weak interactions. *FEBS Lett.,* **498**, 201–203.

Schondorf, R. and Freeman, R. (1999). The importance of orthostatic intolerance in the chronic fatigue syndrome. *Am. J Med. Sci.,* **317**, 117–23.

Shannon, J. R., Flattem, N. L., Jordan, J., *et al.* (2000). Orthostatic intolerance and tachycardia associated with norepinephrine-transporter deficiency. *N. Engl. J Med.,* **342**, 541–49.

Slaugenhaupt, S. A., Blumenfeld, A., Gill, S. P., *et al.* (2001). Tissue-specific expression of a splicing mutation in the IKBKAP gene causes familial dysautonomia. *Am. J Hum. Genet.,* **68**, 598–605.

Southard-Smith, E. M., Angrist, M., Ellison, J. S., Agarwala, R., Baxevanis, A. D., Chakravarti, A. and Pavan, W. J. (1999). The Sox10(Dom) mouse: modeling the genetic variation of Waardenburg-Shah (WS4) syndrome. *Genome Res.,* **9**, 215–25.

Suzuki, N., Matsunaga, T., Nagasumi, K., *et al.* (2003). Alpha(2B)-adrenergic receptor deletion polymorphism associates with autonomic nervous system activity in young healthy Japanese. *J Clin. Endocrinol. Metab,* **88**, 1184–87.

Svensson, P. J., Anvret, M., Molander, M. L. and Nordenskjold, A. (1998). Phenotypic variation in a family with mutations in two Hirschsprung-related genes (RET and endothelin receptor B). *Hum. Genet.,* **103**, 145–48.

Thompson, J. M., O'Callaghan, C. J., Kingwell, B. A., Lambert, G. W., Jennings, G. L. and Esler, M.D. (1995). Total norepinephrine spillover, muscle sympathetic nerve activity and heart-rate spectral analysis in a patient with dopamine beta-hydroxylase deficiency. *J Auton. Nerv. Syst.,* **55**, 198–206.

Trochet, D., Bourdeaut, F., Janoueix-Lerosey, I., *et al.* (2004). Germline mutations of the paired-like homeobox 2B (PHOX2B) gene in neuroblastoma. *Am. J Hum. Genet.,* **74**, 761–64.

Valdenaire, O., Rohrbacher, E. and Mattei, M. G. (1995). Organization of the gene encoding the human endothelin-converting enzyme (ECE-1). *J Biol. Chem.,* **270**, 29794–98.

Van Tol, H. H., Bunzow, J. R., Guan, H. C., Sunahara, R. K., Seeman, P., Niznik, H. B. and Civelli, O. (1991). Cloning of the gene for a human dopamine D4 receptor with high affinity for the antipsychotic clozapine. *Nature,* **350**, 610–614.

Van Tol, H. H., Wu, C. M., Guan, H. C., *et al.* (1992). Multiple dopamine D4 receptor variants in the human population. *Nature,* **358**, 149–52.

Verze, L., Viglietti-Panzica, C., Plumari, L., Calcagni, M., Stella, M., Schrama, L. H. and Panzica, G. C. (2000). Cutaneous innervation in hereditary sensory and autonomic neuropathy type IV. *Neurology,* **55**, 126–28.

Physiology and Pathophysiology Relevant to Autonomic Failure

CHAPTER 12

Functional neuroimaging of autonomic control

Hugo D. Critchley and Christopher J. Mathias

Background

Behavioural context

Functional neuroimaging increasingly provides insights into the brain's regulation of internal bodily processes, including the generation and representation of individual autonomic responses, the coordinated autonomic control of internal states and the integration of autonomic changes with perceptual, cognitive and somatomotor processes that converge in the adaptive control of behaviour.

The autonomic nervous system represents the principal route for regulation of internal bodily processes at both 'vegetative' autoregulatory level or at the level of dynamic interactions between the organism and environment. The sympathetic and parasympathetic autonomic axes control the baseline balance of 'maintenance' processes by their innervation of every major bodily system. They also mediate rapid bodily arousal reactions that optimize survival-related behaviours in response to environmental challenges. Heuristically, this is achieved as an enhancement of sympathetic activity and withdrawal of parasympathetic activity; facilitating 'fight or flight' motor actions by increasing cardiac output, dilating vessels of the musculature and reducing blood supply to the gut. In contrast, enhanced parasympathetic activity with sympathetic withdrawal promotes recuperative functions; reducing heart rate, lowering blood pressure and slowing gut motility (Cannon 1929). Nevertheless, these are broad generalizations; autonomic function is characterized by goal-orientated organ specificity (Porges 1995, Morrison 2001). Moreover, a subset of autonomic arousal responses have developed into potent social cues that can betray an individual's motivational state (Darwin 1898, Ekman et al. 1983)

The field of autonomic neuroscience has benefited from continued technical advances. Notably, human functional neuroimaging techniques permit brain-wide, non-invasive mapping of changes in cerebral activity during behaviour. Temporal and spatial characteristics of these imaging techniques, particularly functional magnetic resonance imaging (fMRI), hitherto have been typically more sensitive to changes in cortical response. Imaging brainstem and hypothalamic centres poses more problems from a technical standpoint and in relation to experimental design. As a consequence, much of the human imaging autonomic literature relates to cortical correlates of stimulus-evoked shifts in bodily states that accompany behavioural challenges. Thus complementary anatomical and neurophysiological investigations remain essential for dissecting the finer mechanisms of autonomic control. The spatial resolution of functional brain imaging methods is presently suboptimal for visualizing in detail hypothalamic and brainstem control (via spinal or vagal routes) of peripheral neural effectors and mapping in full the subcortical representation of ascending viscerosensory information. Nevertheless, functional brain imaging provides a perspective on the wider brain control of human somatic and visceral processes that extends neuroanatomical understanding of autonomic regulation beyond the brainstem and rudimentary models of limbic functioning. It is anticipated that methodological developments in analytic approaches (e.g. functional connectivity models) and imaging technology (e.g. steady-state free precession pulse sequences in MRI) can provide mechanistic insights into interactions between cortical and subcortical centres that define the central neural substrate supporting adaptive autonomic control.

Anatomical context

Core knowledge regarding central autonomic control has been established from both basic and clinical scientific studies without the aid of human functional brain imaging. Critical to homeostasis is the functional organization of sympathetic and parasympathetic nuclei within hypothalamus, pons and medulla: homeostasis requires feedback control where efferent activity reflects complementary reactions to afferent information. Hence, sympathetic nuclei within hypothalamus and brainstem interact with afferent homeostatic (e.g. thermoregulatory) representations. The combination of modality-specific and organ-specific autonomic processing supported across these medullary, pontine and hypothalamic centres underpins the generation of response patterns evoked differentially across physiological or behavioural challenges (Saper 2002). Their impact is not merely confined to the periphery: notably, within the dorsal pons, such nuclei lie in close proximity to ascending neuromodulator pathways (dopamine, 5-hydroxytryptamine [5-HT], acetylcholine and noradrenaline) implicated in cortical excitation, behavioural arousal and signalling motivational drive. While noradrenergic cell groups within the locus coeruleus and caudal lateral tegmentum influence descending efferent sympathetic drive via spinal projections (Svensson 1987), concurrent activation of noradrenergic (A6 and A4) projections to thalamus and cortex influence central arousal, enhancing attentional alertness and sensory orienting to environmental novelty (Aston-Jones et al. 1991). Control of efferent parasympathetic responses is also dispersed across brainstem centres, including nucleus ambiguus and dorsal motor nucleus of the vagus, Edinger–Westphal nucleus and salivatory nucleus. These interconnect and interact with adjacent sympathetic centres. The motor nucleus of the vagus has a coherent functional relationship with the nucleus of the solitary tract (NTS), which relays and represents visceral information from vagal afferents (e.g. Willette et al. 1984, Blessing 1997, Davidson and Koss 1975, Bennarroch 1997, Chapters 2 and 10).

Both sympathetic and parasympathetic brainstem nuclei are influenced by descending projections from suprathalamic centres. Animal and human experiments emphasize the role of limbic cortices (cingulate, medial temporal, and insula), together with the amygdala, in providing a descending drive to hypothalamus and brainstem for the generation of autonomic responses that accompany emotional behaviour (Kaada 1951, Gelsema et al. 1989, Neafsey 1990, Pool and Ransohoff 1949, Fish et al. 1993, Oppenheimer et al. 1992, Mangina and Buezeron-Mangina 1996, Asahina et al. 2003). However, stimulation or lesions of even 'nonemotional' prefrontal and motor cortices may influence production of autonomic responses in certain contexts (Sequeira et al. 1995, Sequeira and Ba-M'hamed 1999) suggesting a complex relationship between homeostatic control and cognitive and motor processes.

Afferent information from the body is essential for brainstem autonomic centres to maintain homoeostatic control through monitoring the general integrity of the body. This afferent interoceptive information also underpins drive for motivational behaviour. It conveys basic states such as hunger and thirst and sensations of comfort and discomfort. Moreover, where autonomic arousal occurs in anticipation of behavioural responses, feedback of bodily changes reinforces stimulus processing to influence behavioural judgements, implicitly or explicitly (Damasio et al. 1991, Damasio 1994, Bechara et al. 1997). The central representation of these internal motivational signals is hypothesized as the origin of emotional feeling states (James 1894, Lange 1885, Damasio 1994, 1999).

Interoceptive information from bodily organs is conveyed centrally by humoral, spinal and vagal pathways. Central chemoreceptors, including those in the hypothalamus, monitor directly the internal milieu. Studies of afferent neural pathways have highlighted the role of thin fibres conveying information from many sensory receptor subtypes to the spinal cord and along the vagus. It is argued on the basis of neuroanatomical studies (Craig 2002, 2003) that the Lamina 1 spinothalamocortical pathway is especially dedicated to conveying interoceptive information, converging within the diencephalon with afferent information carried by cranial nerves including the vagus nerve. Information is relayed topographically via ventroposterior medial parvicellular (VPpc) thalamic nucleus to insula cortex (Saper 2002, Craig 2003). The stream of interoceptive information then projects onto right anterior insula and orbitofrontal cortices. This representation is further enriched by other motivationally important sensations including metaboreception, pain, itch, temperature and sensual touch (Craig 2003). This neuroanatomical arrangement has been proposed to be evolutionary specialized in primates, bypassing an obligatory pontine (parabrachial) relay (however afferent vagus and spinal information does reach the parabrachial nucleus via collaterals) to enable cortical mapping of salient visceral information (Fig. 12.1).

Neuroimaging techniques as applied to studying autonomic function

Human functional brain imaging techniques share the common aim of capturing the workings of the human brain, and to do so must be sensitive to changes in 'contrast' that reflect differences reflecting changeable brain states. Some techniques map the distribution of blood: Thus, xenon computerized tomography (CT) scanning enables rapid (but anatomically coarse) mapping of brain perfusion and hypoperfusion with X-rays; water ($H_2^{15}O$) positron emission tomography (water PET) uses radiolabelled water to quantify state induced changes in regional cerebral blood flow (rCBF); functional magnetic resonance imaging (fMRI) maps changes in local blood oxygenation level dependent (BOLD) contrast reflecting circumscribed paramagnetic changes consequent

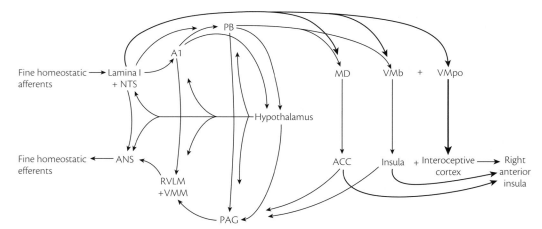

Fig. 12.1 Schematic representation of neuroanatomical pathways in interoception and afferent visceral control. Afferent thin fibres travelling in Lamina 1 of the spinal cord and the vagus nerve convey interoceptive and motivationally salient information to the brain. In primates, a pontine relay is bypassed via an evolutionarily specialized thalamocortical pathway to interoceptive cortices that terminates in right anterior insula (which projects further into orbitofrontal cortex). There is an accessory branch to anterior cingulate cortex. This specialized route is highlighted using a thicker line. A1, catecholaminergic cell group of ventrolateral medulla; ACC, anterior cingulate cortex; ANS, peripheral autonomic nervous system; NTS, nucleus of solitary tract; PAG, periaqueductal grey; PB, parabrachial nucleus; RVLM, rostral ventrolateral medulla; VMM, ventromedial medulla. Thalamic nuclei: MD, mediodorsal; VMb, basal ventromedial; VMpo, parvocellular ventroposterormedial. With permission from *Current Opinion in Neurobiology*, **13**, AD (Bud) Craig, Interoception: the sense of the physiological condition of the body, 500–505, Copyright 2003, with permission from Elsevier.

upon an influx of oxygenated blood in response to local neuronal activity. The spatial and temporal resolution of fMRI, currently the most widely used brain imaging technique, is constrained by the physiology of haemodynamic coupling with neural activity (i.e. the area and time over which arteriolar blood enters a brain region with enhanced activity).

Single photon emission computed tomography (SPECT) and PET both use radioisotopes to track physiological processes. While water PET (described above) maps blood flow across the brain, labelling other molecules can provide more direct insights into metabolic or neuropharmacological processes, for example the uptake of glucose molecules or the occupancy of dopamine receptors in cortex and basal ganglia. The use of radioactive tracers constrains the number of scans that can be acquired (typically twelve 90-second scans in a water PET study) whereas many hundreds of scans can be acquired in fMRI experiments at a frequency of up to one a second. Whatever the technique, ultimately the acquired scans are spatially transformed to correct for movement, co-registered and statistically compared to look for regional changes, which may be further referenced against known anatomy by transforming the statistical images into 'standard' space representing a typical healthy brain.

There are a number of general considerations with respect to cerebral neuroimaging that are significant with respect to autonomic studies. Firstly, not every brain region is imaged with the same degree of clarity in functional experiments. Sensitivity to brainstem changes is limited not only by spatial scale and the small size of adjacent autonomic nuclei but also by:

◆ being at the perimeter of the field of view (when imaging whole brain)

◆ pulsatile movement with both the cardiac and respiratory cycle

◆ the number of tissue interfaces in that region.

In fMRI there are specific types of signal dropout and distortion that differentially affect brain regions. With standard acquisition sequences, caudomedial orbitofrontal cortex (a 'limbic' region) is very susceptible to signal loss and, as with brainstem, may require non-standard approaches to optimize the quality of activation data from that region (Deichmann et al. 2002, 2003, De Pannfilis and Schwarzbaue 2005, Weiskopf et al. 2005) (Fig. 12.2 illustrates the work of Weizkopf and colleagues showing distribution of brain regions requiring special fMRI acquisition approaches to overcome dropout and distortion).

A second general consideration is the constraints of the imaging environment: the patients are typically recumbent and required to maintain a fixed position to limit head movement. The degree to which the scanning environment needs to be free of distraction is typically much greater than required in clinical physiological investigations and invasive procedures are often difficult to implement. In fMRI scanning, a major limiting factor is the degree to which physiological monitoring equipment can be used in the context of a large magnetic field. Electronic equipment may not function, or can represent a physical danger to the subjects or damage the scanner whether by flying into the magnetic field or by induction of electrical currents. Moreover, electrical and radiofrequency (RF) noise generation may interfere significantly with image acquisition. Even 'MRI safe' instrumentation may not be compatible with the acquisition of meaningful fMRI data without local safety testing and quality control of fMRI image acquisition. A number of strategies, including RF filtering and shielding, and the used of fibreoptic signal transduction are frequently implemented for effective subject monitoring in fMRI environments. A compromise has been to replicate the task procedures outside the scanner and index autonomic (or behavioural) responses at a different time to scanning, assuming similar effects occur at the time of scanning. However, this approach lacks the power of simultaneous data acquisition.

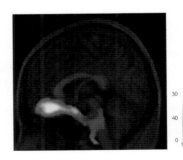

Optimal z-shim gradient moment   Optimal slice tilt

Negative PE polarity

Positive PE polarity

+1.6
+0.6
−0.4
−1.4
−2.4
m Tm ^m II

+30
+15
0
−15
−30
−45
Degree

Gain in BOLD sensitivity if optimal parameters (z-shim moment, slice tilt, phase-encoding polarity) are used.

30
40
0
% BS

Fig. 12.2 Compensatory measures required to optimize functional magnetic resonance imaging (fMRI) signal acquisition from orbitofrontal cortex and brainstem (Weiskopf et al. 2005, Deichmann et al. 2002, 2003). The values are based on group means from five subjects scanned using T2* sensitive echoplanar imaging (EPI) on a Siemens 3T Allegra scanner. The four smaller figures show respectively the optimal slice tilt and z-shim moments for either a positive or negative phase encoding (PE) polarity. The signal (blood oxygenation level dependent [BOLD]) sensitivity gain is determined in comparison with a standard EPI (tilt 0°, z-shim moment = 0, PE positive). See also Plate 1. Reprinted from *Neuroimage* **1**;33(2) Weiskopf N, Hutton C, Josephs O, Deichmann, Optimal EPI parameters for reduction of susceptibility-induced BOLD sensitivity losses: a whole-brain analysis at 3 T and 1.5 T. R., 493–504, Copyright 2006, with permission from Elsevier.

Nevertheless, physiological autonomic recording in an MRI environment is becoming increasingly available, the lag reflecting the rapidity with which psychologists rather than physiologists have embraced the functional imaging techniques.

Special considerations need to be taken with reference to imaging autonomic control. Global (i.e. non-regional) changes in brain perfusion may occur during states of autonomic arousal or as consequences of pharmacological treatments to confound thresholded measurements of regional activity (however SPECT and PET scans are corrected for overall signal). Physiological 'noise' (changes in blood CO_2 or cardiac output [Wise et al. 2004]) is viewed as the major confound in interpreting neurally induced activity changes (Macey et al. 2004, Friston et al. 1995, Triantafyllou et al. 2005). These can be dealt with in part by introducing complex experimental interventions (such as 'CO_2-clamping' the experimental subject to limit respiratory-induced changes in global signal (Evans et al. 2002)) or by further statistical corrections (e.g. measuring changing physiological responses and including them as confounding covariates in analyses). There is, however, always a danger of reduced sensitivity to the process of interest: the phrase 'throwing the baby out with the bathwater' is often used by neuroimagers.

Neuroimaging context

Functional neuroimaging is perhaps the major neuroscientific tool for investigating *in vivo* human brain function. Surprisingly, there have been relatively few functional imaging studies that have examined central autonomic control and representation of visceral bodily responses. Autonomic indices, such as electrodermal activity (EDA), have typically been used in parallel with functional imaging paradigms as objective dependent measures of emotional processing and learning, for example to index the acquisition or expression of fear conditioning (Büchel et al. 1998, Morris et al. 1998).

Nevertheless psychological states, including emotional, cognitive and motor behaviours induce physiological changes in the body that reflect varying degrees of autonomic arousal induced by specific task demands (Fig. 12.3). A full understanding of the neural substrates for psychological processes should perhaps take into account or control for these induced bodily changes. Traditionally studies have been designed to compare an 'active' condition with a resting control state. Often there is an implicit difference in difficulty between the active and control tasks. Thus brain activity evoked during a cognitive or motor task, when compared with an easier control condition, may unintentionally include correlates

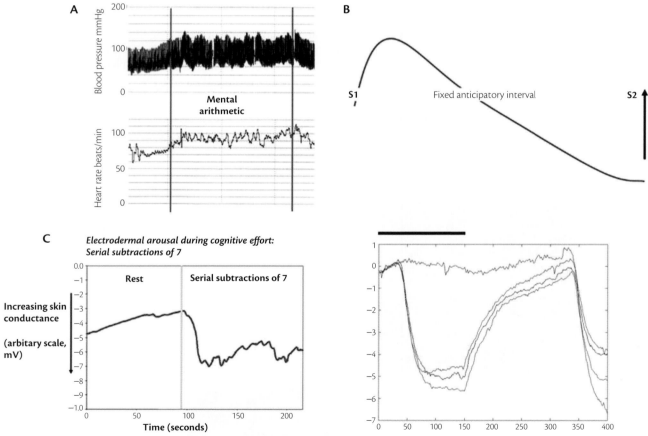

Fig. 12.3 Examples of psychophysiological responses. **A:** Continuous blood pressure and heart rate responses when a subject performs effortful mental arithmetic (serial subtractions of the number seven, out aloud) as a mental stress task. **B:** Schematic of heart rate response when performing a forewarned reaction time task (e.g. Jennings et al. 1990; Frith and Allen 1983) A warning stimulus, S1, may induce a orienting heart rate acceleration (with or without an initial deceleration). Anticipation of a second imperative stimulus, S2, over a predicable time interval induces a marked deceleration in heart rate that recovers once a reaction-time response is made. Such decelerations in daily life occur whenever events are anticipated, (e.g. at traffic lights). **C:** Data of a subject performing serial subtractions of sevens (mental stress task), showing a sustained shift in the skin conductance level and a related increase in phasic (SCR) components of electrodermal activity. Panel A from Critchley HD, Dolan RJ, *et al.* Human cingulate cortex and autonomic control: converging neuroimaging and clinical evidence. *Brain.* 2003, **126**(Pt 10):2139–52, by permission of Oxford University Press.

of effort-induced autonomic arousal. Similar caveats are equally applicable to studies of emotional processing where differential bodily arousal states can be viewed as intrinsic to the concept of emotion (James 1894, Lange 1885, Ekman et al. 1983). It is unsurprising, therefore, that activity in some brain regions have been highlighted as reflecting nonspecific 'task engagement', 'attentional recruitment' or volitional effort: Paus and co-workers (Paus et al. 1998) highlighted the relatively nonspecific engagement of dorsal anterior cingulate cortex during behavioural effort (where stress or effort is crucial, and invariably uncontrolled, variables) and Raichle and co-workers similarly point to activation of ventromedial prefrontal cortex and subgenual cingulate cortices commonly in low-demand control conditions or disengagement with the environment (e.g. Raichle et al. 2001, Raichle and Gusnard 2005).

The developing field of autonomic neuroimaging has the potential to provide a detailed explanation of the functional relationship between brain and body. In so doing, these investigations may inform other disciplines by accounting for regional brain activity currently poorly understood on account of relatively poor psychological specificity.

Changes in the pupillary light reflex reflect attentional and arousal responses to stimuli that are isoluminent with each other, manifest as a blunting of the light reflex amplitude and a more rapid recovery (Critchley et al. 2005c). The stimuli were presented at the time of the black bar.

Studies in healthy individuals

Central cardiovascular control

Efferent cardiovascular responses and reflexes

A first approach to identify central autonomic control centres is to relate peripheral autonomic responses to regional brain activity while individuals perform a range of tasks engendering alteration in cardiovascular state, e.g. increases in heart rate and blood pressure. Such tasks (used clinically as 'autonomic function tests') include the Valsalva manoeuvre (breathing against a closed glottis), isometric handgrip exercise, deep inspiration, mental stress (arithmetic), and cold pressor tests. Autonomic centres may thus be identified by looking for shared features in activity patterns.

Using this approach in a (fMRI) study, King et al. (1999) reported increased activity in anterior and posterior insula, medial prefrontal cortex and ventroposterior thalamus during respiratory, Valsalva and exercise challenges. Similarly, a subsequent study (Harper et al. 2000, using fMRI) described activity increases in ventral and medial prefrontal cortex, anterior cingulate, insula, medial temporal lobe, medial thalamus, cerebellum midbrain and pons during cold pressor challenge and performance of Valsalva manoeuvres. Despite technical limitations, differential responses have also been observed across brainstem sites such periaqueductal grey matter (PAG) and dorsal raphe nucleus and may in fact distinguish respiratory autonomic challenge (maximum inspiration, Valsalva) from isometric exercise (Topolovec et al. 2004).

In one of our early studies of central cardiovascular control (Critchley et al. 2000a), we used positron emission tomography (PET) to examine brain activity during cardiovascular arousal induced by mental arithmetic or physical effort compared to non-effortful control tasks. The rationale was relatively straightforward: regional brain activity during cognitive effort and inner speech (prefrontal and speech-related frontotemporal cortices) would be

largely dissociable from activity associated with sustained physical effort (somatomotor cortices). However, both effortful tasks induced increased heart rate and blood pressure such that activity shared across these conditions would include responses in autonomic centres controlling peripheral cardiovascular arousal (Fig. 12.4). We therefore first tested for activity common to effortful task performance, independent of whether the subject was performing mental arithmetic or isometric exercise, using a conjunction analysis to test for significant commonalities (Price and Friston 1997). This revealed a significant enhancement of activity in right anterior cingulate, dorsal pons and midline cerebellum during effort

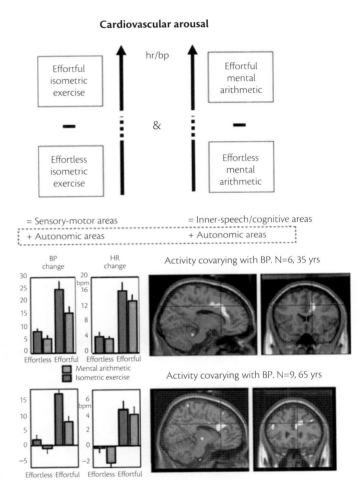

Fig. 12.4 Positron emission tomography (PET) studies of cardiovascular arousal. The upper figure illustrates a PET paradigm where each subject performed three repetitions of four task conditions while undergoing a PET functional scan with simultaneous monitoring of cardiovascular responses. Subjects undertook mental stress and exercise stress tasks to increase heart rate and blood pressure. They also performed corresponding control conditions. By testing for brain activity related to effort or autonomic arousal, independent of task modality (physical or mental) activity can be identified in brain centres mediating autonomic control. The lower figure illustrates data from two studies showing increases in heart rate and blood pressure during effortful task performance with enhanced activity in right dorsal anterior cingulate cortex related blood pressure changes (i.e. sympathetic cardiovascular arousal). Group data from healthy subjects (mean age 35 years and below 65 years) is presented on parasagittal and coronal sections of a normalized template brain scan, showing significant modality-independent correlations of blood pressure and regional cerebral blood flow. Reprinted from *Human Brain Function*, ed Frackowiak et al., Chapter 20, Critchley and Dolan, 397–417, Copyright 2004, with permission from Elsevier.

associated with cardiovascular arousal. To further characterize centres related to autonomic control, brain activity during mental effort and exercise was correlated with direct scan-by-scan measurements of heart rate and blood pressure. We again tested for activity that predicted the magnitude of the cardiovascular response in both cognitive and exercise conditions. Notably, activity in right anterior cingulate, right insula and pons covaried with increases in blood pressure and heart rate independent of task modality (Fig. 12.4). This study provided evidence that cortical regions such as anterior cingulate are important for integrating volitional effort with peripheral states of cardiovascular arousal. The study also suggested a laterality of sympathetic responses to right hemisphere which accords with an earlier proposal based upon stimulation of human insular cortices (Oppenheimer et al. 1992). This relationship between anterior cingulate activity and increases in blood pressure was later confirmed in a replication of this study within an older group) of healthy subjects (mean age 65 years of age; Fig. 12.4) and paralleled by evidence from patients with anterior cingulate cortex lesions and patients with pure autonomic failure.

In an extension of this basic approach of mapping brain activity related to cardiovascular control, we used the better temporal resolution associated with fMRI to determine regions contributing to sympathetic and parasympathetic influences on heart rate (Critchley et al. 2003). We scanned subjects while they performed repetitions of paced motor and cognitive tasks, chosen to induce variability in heart rate across the study session, while simultaneously acquiring electrocardiography (ECG) measures. In the motor tasks, subjects performed isometric handgrip squeezes, either squeezing for 6 seconds then relaxing for 6 seconds or squeezing for 11 seconds and relaxing for 11 seconds repeated over 3-minute blocks. The cognitive tasks took the form of an 'n-back' working memory task, in which subjects monitored serial presentations of letters, responding in the low-demand 'one-back' task to immediate repetitions of stimuli, and in the high-demand '2-back' task to repetitions of letter stimuli separated by an interposing letter. Heart rate variability (HRV) was derived from R-wave intervals of the ECG. Further indices reflecting sympathetic and parasympathetic modulation of heart rate, were derived using power spectral analyses of R-R interbeat intervals. In this procedure, which has become routine in clinical autonomic practice and research, the spectral power of heart rate variability at 'high-frequency' (0.15–0.50 Hz) is closely related to parasympathetic nervous control of the heart, whereas 'low frequency' spectral power (0.05–0.15 Hz) predominantly reflects sympathetic activity.

Changes in heart rate variability (increases or decreases) covaried with activity in anterior/mid cingulate cortex, somatomotor cortex and insulae that partially overlapped with regions activated by the cognitive and physical challenges (Fig. 12.5). Moreover, increases in the low frequency, sympathetic, component of HRV were likewise associated with increased cingulate, somatomotor, and insular activity.

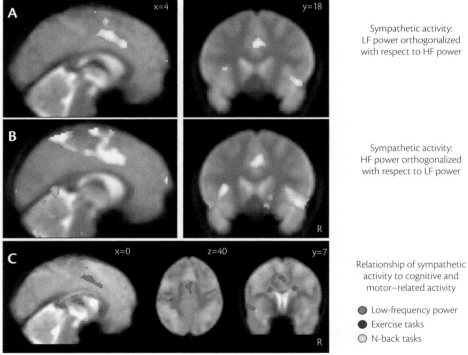

Sympathetic activity:
LF power orthogonalized
with respect to HF power

Sympathetic activity:
HF power orthogonalized
with respect to LF power

Relationship of sympathetic
activity to cognitive and
motor–related activity

◕ Low-frequency power
● Exercise tasks
○ N-back tasks

Fig. 12.5 Functional magnetic resonance imaging (fMRI) study of sympathetic influences on heart rate variability. Subjects were scanned using fMRI performing a cognitive task (n-back) at two levels of difficulty, and two levels of an exercise task, while echocardiography was continuously acquired during scanning. Post hoc analyses enabled extraction of a timeline for sympathetic (low frequency, LF) power in heart rate variability, which could be related to changes in regional brain activity, controlling for the task performance and high frequency (HF, parasympathetic) influences on heart rate. **A** and **B**: The location of brain activity correlated with cardiac sympathetic influences, respectively keeping and losing variance shared with parasympathetic changes. **C**: The activation of dorsal cingulate and insula cortices can be anatomically distinguished from activity related to cognitive work or motor task performance. These group data sets are plotted on sections of a mean functional (echoplanar T2*) image from the group illustrating the anatomical resolution of fMRI and the caudal orbitomedial area of signal loss due to susceptibility artefact. See also Plate 2. Reprinted from Critchley HD et al., Dolan RJ, Human cingulate cortex and autonomic control: converging neuroimaging and clinical evidence. *Brain*. 2003, **126**(Pt 10):2139–52, by permisssion of Oxford University Press.

This contrasts with increases in activity relating purely to parasympathetic components of HRV, observed in anterior temporal lobe (uncal regions bilaterally) and basal ganglia (Lane et al. 2001, Matthews et al. 2004). Some overlap in regions showing covariation with sympathetic and parasympathetic components of HRV was observed in somatomotor and medial parietal lobe cortices. These findings support findings from our earlier studies that indicated that activity within dorsal anterior and mid-cingulate cortex is associated with control of cardiovascular autonomic arousal during volitional behaviour, in particular the activity related to sympathetic autonomic drive to the heart.

A number of other groups have tested for functional brain correlates of heart rate variability to highlight parasympathetic cardiac control centres. In one PET study (Lane et al. 2001), increases in activity of medial prefrontal and insular cortices correlated with heart rate variability as subjects watched emotional films. An extension of this approach, (Lane et al. 2008) found an association between rostral medial prefrontal activity changes and high frequency (parasympathetic) power in heart rate variability, with areas including caudate nucleus and insula and periaqueductal grey matter (PAG) recruited when HRV changes accompany emotional processing. In a much larger group PET study activity within insula, anterior cingulate and parietal cortices was enhanced during mental challenge (working memory) and correlated with increased heart rate, and activity within regions including ventromedial prefrontal cortex and amygdala correlated with heart rate variability measures of parasympathetic cardiac influences (Gianaros et al. 2004). This same group (Gianaros et al. 2005) has since demonstrated linear bilateral correlation of activity within perigenual and mid anterior cingulate cortex with stress-induced increases in blood pressure evoked by performance of a Stroop colour-word interference task.

These studies, coupled with observations in patient groups argue for a contribution of dorsal anterior cingulate cortex to the control of cardiovascular sympathetic responses during behaviour. The engagement of other brain regions appears more contextual. Thus other regions, including insula, ventromedial prefrontal and subgenual cingulate cortices and amygdala, are also implicated in influencing states of cardiovascular arousal. During emotional processing amygdala activation predicts emotion-induced changes in cardiac rate along with dorsal anterior cingulate cortex (Critchley et al. 2005a) and, in fact predicts other autonomic responses (Williams et al. 2001, Phelps et al. 2001). Most strikingly amygdala activity has been shown to predict the direct autonomic modulation of heart muscular response in the context of anxiety (Dalton et al. 2005). Unfortunately simultaneous functional imaging with MRI of heart and brain is not yet possible, so the relationship has to be inferred across separate sessions. The magnitude of cardiac contractility (derived from magnetic resonance imaging of the luminal volume of the heart at end diastole) was modulated by inducing states of heightened anxiety with the threat of electric shock. Repeating the anxiety induction conditions while performing fMRI of the brain showed that activity changes in the amygdala and in prefrontal and insula cortices correlated closely with these cardiac changes (Fig. 12.6). This study importantly paves the way for future use of combined brain and cardiac MRI techniques within the same experiment.

The baroreceptor reflex provides continuous control of arterial pressure, principally in response to orthostatic volumes shifts.

The brainstem sites responsible for this mechanism are well characterized in animals and involve baroreceptor afferents to the nucleus of the solitary tract (NTS) that modulate efferent pressor tone generated and maintained within rostral ventrolateral medulla. Neuroimaging correlates of responses to blood pressure manipulations have been examined in both animal and humans. In anaesthetized cats, decreases in blood pressure (induced by sodium nitroprusside) evoked fMRI signal decreases within the medullary NTS pathway and also cerebellum, pons and right insula (Henderson et al. 2004). The same regions responded to increases in arterial pressure induced by phenylephrine. Interestingly amygdala activity was enhanced by decreases, not increases in blood pressure. In humans, baroreceptor reflex activity (with corresponding increases in heart rate and muscle sympathetic nerve activity) can be induced experimentally using lower body negative pressure. Kimmerly and co-workers (2005) manipulated the baroreflex in an fMRI experiment using lower body negative pressure induced via a sealed pressure chamber. Passive manipulations were repeated over the course of the experiment during fMRI measurement of regional brain activity. Interestingly, induction of baroreflex responses, with corresponding decreases in central venous pressure and elevation of heart rate (blood pressure was maintained) evoked enhanced activity in posterior insula and lateral prefrontal cortex, whereas activity in genual (not dorsal) anterior cingulate cortex, amygdala and anterior insula was observed to decrease suggesting these latter areas suppress, or are suppressed by, sympathoexcitatory tone at rest.

Afferent cardiovascular representation

The above studies have helped identify brain correlates of efferent autonomic drive in healthy controls. However, in presuming that the activity represents central centres for autonomic control, ascribing the activity to efferent or afferent response limbs is not straightforward. However two strategies are available for neuroimaging. First, discrete patients groups may be viewed as 'lesion-deficit' models to examine the functional consequences of failing to generate or feedback a peripheral autonomic cardiovascular response. Second, the widespread observation that attention enhances activity within relevant sensory cortices (e.g. Chawla et al. 1999) provides an alternative means of probing interoceptive cardiovascular representations in healthy controls without confounding induced changes in bodily response.

In a collaborative study, we examined brain activity related to attending to internal, autonomically controlled visceral responses using a biofeedback task (Wiens et al. 2000). The task itself involved playing back to the subject a series of tones, generated by the subject's own heartbeat. A trial consisted of a cue for the subject to attend introspectively to the timing his/her heartbeat. Ten tones were then played after which the subject had to judge if the tones were synchronous with their heartbeat or played back with a half-second delay (which occurred randomly on 50% of trials). In our neuroimaging study (Critchley et al. 2004), we also included an 'exteroceptive' condition to control for nonspecific performance effects in the scanner, in which the subjects were prompted at the start of each trial to attend to the note quality and respond at the end if the one of the sequence of notes subtly changed in pitch. Attending interoceptively enhanced activity in a number of brain regions, including anterior cingulate, somatomotor and anterior and mid insula cortices. Individual differences in interoceptive sensitivity, predicted by feedback theories of emotion to influence

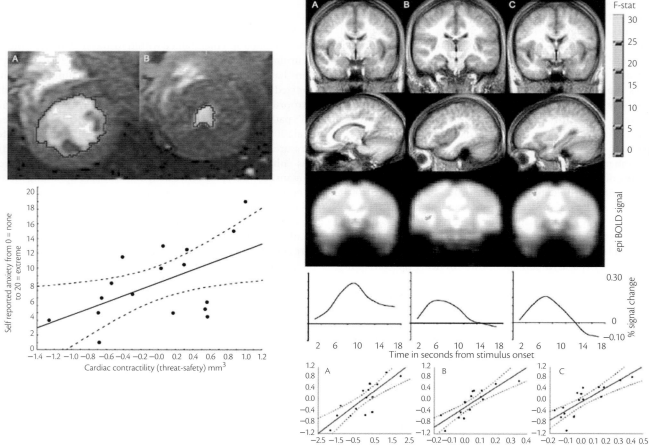

Fig. 12.6 Heart–brain correlations during stress. Correlations between regional brain activity and cardiac end diastolic volume during stress, highlighting a positive relationship between amygdala insula and prefrontal activity and cardiac filling induced autonomically by anticipatory fear. The figure to the left shows cross-sectional magnetic resonance image of the left ventricle at **(A)** maximum diastole and **(B)** maximal systole. The scatter plot beneath relates measured cardiac contractility with self-report measures of anxiety in threat versus safety conditions. The figures to the right illustrate clusters of brain activation during threat in **(A)** amygdala, **(B)** insula and **(C)** prefrontal cortex positively associated with cardiac contractility to the threat of shock. The first two rows display the location and size of the clusters, with the colour of the cluster indexing the size of the effect. The third row is composed of the same clusters superimposed on an averaged EPI BOLD signal indicating adequate signal coverage for each cluster. The fourth row is the averaged haemodynamic response function to the threat condition for each cluster. The last row contains the scatter plots for each cluster with the difference in cardiac contractility (threat minus safety) on the x axis and the difference in percentage signal change (threat minus safety) for each cluster. See also Plate 3. With permission from Dalton KM, Kalin NH, Grist TM, Davidson RJ. 2005. *J Cogn. Neurosci.* MIT Press.

subjective emotional experience, were used to examine brain regions supporting conscious awareness of internal state. Notably, only activity in right anterior insula cortex correlated with interoceptive awareness (performance accuracy on the task). Furthermore, the activity with right anterior insula (and in a parallel structural study, its grey matter volume) predicted general visceral sensitivity and subjective day-to-day emotional experience, at least of anxiety symptoms (Fig. 12.7).

These observations a role for right anterior insula in representing both autonomic cardiovascular symptoms and, more broadly, in representing emotional feeling states associated with visceral arousal. Similar neuroimaging findings are reported in a heartbeat counting task (Pollatos et al. 2004) and the magnitude of a right frontal heartbeat-evoked electroencephalographic potential has been shown to be dependent on interoceptive sensitivity (Pollatos and Schandry 2004). Nevertheless, the link between awareness of cardiovascular responses and emotion may preferentially be expressed in anxiety symptoms and hence may not be generalizable across all emotions. Saper (2002) in reappraising earlier findings

(such as those of Penfield), argues against insula cortex as a (general) emotional integrator. Instead he attributes this function to medial temporal lobe structures, including the amygdala. It is noteworthy that, in the context of threat, processing both amygdala and insula were observed to be sensitive to the presence of changes in autonomic state responses (Critchley et al. 2002b). Anatomically, projections from anterior insula cortex and medial temporal lobe converge within ventromedial prefrontal cortex an area that implicated in both emotional appraisal and autonomic control (Ongur et al. 2003, Price 2005).

Electrodermal arousal

As an index of autonomic arousal, electrodermal activity (EDA) is not confounded by changes in parasympathetic activity, and is used extensively in psychophysical experiments to 'objectively' index attention and emotion (Venables and Christie 1980, Fowles et al. 1981, Boucsein 1992, Ohman and Soares 1993). Functional neuroimaging studies of fear conditioning and subjective affective experience have also used EDA as a dependent measure signifying

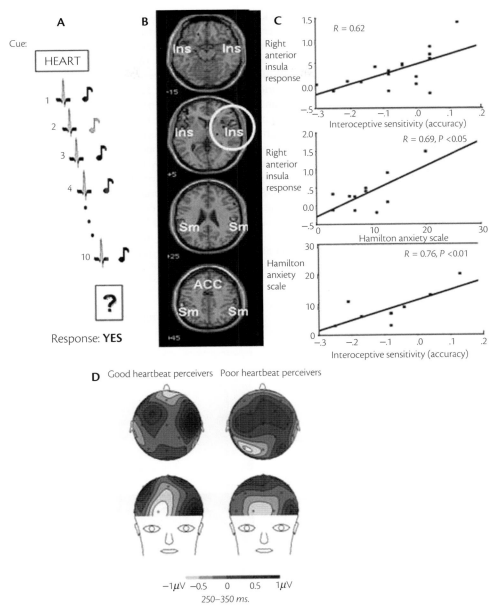

Fig. 12.7 Interoception and feeling states neural activity during interoceptive awareness. Healthy individuals were scanned while they performed a heartbeat detection task (adapted from that used in Wiens et al. 2000) in which they judged the timing of their own heartbeats to auditory tones (triggered by their heartbeats). **A:** Subjects were cued to attend to their heart then a series of 10 tones would be played that were either synchronous with their finger pulse, or delayed by 500 ms. Individuals made the judgement at the end of each trial of 10 beats. In a control condition ('note'), subjects attended only to the quality of the notes, identifying the presence of a subtle change in note pitch in the sequence. **B:** Activity when attending to heartbeat timing was enhanced (relative to the exteroceptive 'note' task) in bilateral insula, bilateral somatomotor and anterior cingulate cortices. **C:** Only activity in right anterior insula correlated with conscious awareness of the timing of heartbeats i.e. interoceptive sensitivity (performance accuracy on the task, relative to the control condition. Across individuals, there were significant correlations between activity of right anterior cortex, interoceptive sensitivity and day-to-day experience of anxiety symptoms, consistent with a proposal that right anterior insula is a substrate for feeling states generated from afferent visceral responses. **D:** Beneath shows a figure from Pollatos and Schandry (2004) showing a right prefrontal brain potential time locked 250–300 ms after the echocardiograph R wave of each heartbeat. With permission from Wiens S, Mezzacappa ES, Katkin ES. (2001). Heartbeat detection and the experience of emotions. *Cognition and Emotion* **14**:417–427, reprinted by permission of the publisher (Taylor and Francis Group, http://informaworld.com). See also Plate 4. Figure D from Pollatos O, Schandry R. 2004. Accuracy of heartbeat perception is reflected in the amplitude of the heartbeat-evoked brain potential. *Psychophsyiology* **41**:476–482, Wiley.

emotional processing (e.g. Morris et al. 1998, Büchel et al. 1998, Lane et al. 1999, Chua et al. 1999). In these experiments, observed activity within amygdala, insula and anterior cingulate have been related to evoked changes in EDA. Similarly amygdala activity predicts the presents of EDA responses to emotive stimuli (Phelps et al. 2001, Williams et al. 2001).

General correlates of EDA activity

The first neuroimaging study to directly explore a general relationship between EDA and regional brain activity was that of Fredrikson et al. (1998). These investigators used PET neuroimaging and continuous electrodermal recording to identify changes in brain activity relating to EDA arousal, while subjects were presented with a variety of orientating and emotive stimuli, including skin shocks and videos of snakes. Stimuli evoking strong EDA responses were associated with modulation of activity in motor cortex, dorsal anterior and posterior cingulate, right insula, right inferior parietal lobe and extrastriate visual cortex. In fact, positive correlations were observed between with EDA and activity in cingulate and motor cortices, and decreased correlations in insula, parietal and visual cortex. This study suggested a distributed neural system governing electrodermal arousal within human brain, and highlighted engagement of anterior cingulate cortex in sympathetic arousal responses. In a similar fMRI experiment, Williams and colleagues (2000) examined processing of visual stimuli during simultaneous EDA monitoring. Stimuli producing EDA responses evoked increased activity (relative to those that did not) in ventromedial prefrontal cortex, anterior cingulate and medial temporal lobe.

In one of our own experiments, we used fMRI (Critchley et al. 2000b) to index brain activity relating to EDA fluctuations evoked naturalistically by performance of a cognitive 'gambling' task. On each trial of this task, subjects saw a pair of playing cards and had to make a two-choice button press decision to win (or lose) money. Visual feedback of overall winnings, and whether the correct response had been made, was given after each response (Elliott et al. 2000) (Fig. 12.8). Activity attributable to these cognitive and sensory aspects of the task were modelled so that EDA related activity could be examined in isolation from confound stimulus-task effects. Subject-specific EDA fluctuations during task performance were used as covariates of interest in two sets of analyses. Firstly, the EDA trace over the course of the experiment was used as a regressor of interest to examine brain activity covarying with this peripheral measure of arousal. Secondly, distinct peaks in the EDA trace were identified. Neural activity occurring approximately 4 seconds before and after these EDA peaks was modelled to highlight and dissociate brain areas associated with generation and feedback re-representation of these discrete EDA responses (Fig. 12.8).

A *Visual presentation during task*

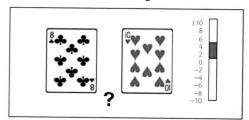

B *Random function determining winnings*

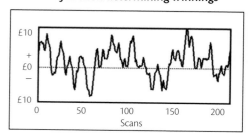

C *EDA in one individual during task*

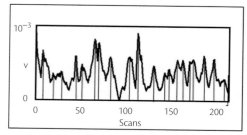

D *Activity covarying with EDA*

Right anterior insula/orbitofrontal cortex

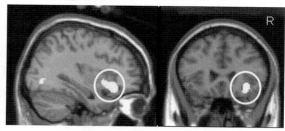

Bilateral ventromedial prefrontal cortex

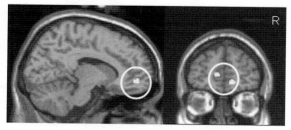

Inferior parietal lobe and extrastriate cortex

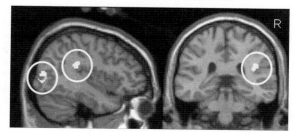

Fig. 12.8 Regional activity relating to electrodermal activity during gambling task performance. **A:** Six subjects were scanned using functional magnetic resonance imaging performing a decision-related gambling task. In individual trials, the subject was presented with pairs of playing cards and was required to respond to one or other in order to win money. Immediate feedback was given (tick/cross replacing the question mark) indicating if the individual had won or lost money, and the level of overall winnings modified accordingly. **B:** Unknown to the subject, feedback (wins/losses) on any particular trial was predetermined by a binomial random walk. **C:** Performing the task produced individualized fluctuations in electrodermal activity (EDA) recorded throughout the task (black line). In a covariance analysis these continuous data were used to examine activity covarying with EDA. Also, peaks in EDA responses were identified (illustrated in red) and used in an event-related analysis. **D:** Brain regions covarying with EDA. Significant group activity is mapped on parasagittal and coronal sections of a template brain and is observed in anterior insula and ventromedial prefrontal cortices, extrastriate visual cortex, and right parietal lobe. See also Plate 5. With permission from Critchley (2000a).

EDA fluctuation over the course of the experiment was associated with increased activity in bilateral ventromedial prefrontal cortex, right insula/orbitofrontal cortex, right inferior parietal cortex and extrastriate visual cortex. Prior to discrete EDA responses there was increased activity within left ventromedial prefrontal cortex, extrastriate cortex and cerebellum, suggesting these regions preferentially contribute to EDA generation. Conversely, following individual EDA responses, there was greater right medial prefrontal cortex suggesting that this region is important for representation of peripheral EDA arousal. These observations suggest a partial segregation, even within ventromedial prefrontal cortex, of regional brain activity supporting generation and representation of EDA.

Patterson and others (2002) also observed activity in ventromedial and orbitofrontal cortices correlating with EDA arousal, in their case during a selection of cognitive tasks. These observation associating ventromedial prefrontal activity with generation and representation of EDA responses during a decision-making task is consistent both with the reported effects of prefrontal lesions on generation of EDA responses (Tranel and Damasio 1994, Bechara et al. 1996, Zahn et al. 1999) and proposed modulation of these areas during motivational decision making by EDA-related arousal (Bechara et al. 1996, 1997, Damasio 1994). The study also showed activity in regions such as inferior parietal lobule and extrastriate visual cortex associated with EDA. These areas are critical to directing visual attention and the imaging findings suggest that sympathetic arousal and attention may share a common neural substrate. However, the study only dealt with the mechanisms by which cognitive or emotional responses are integrated with EDA arousal and notably failed to demonstrate anterior cingulate activity in association with EDA, in contrast to other lesion and neuroimaging observations (Tranel and Damasio 1994, Fredikson et al. 1998, Williams et al. 2000)

Contextual EDA

In a further event-related fMRI study that examined how arousal, indexed by EDA, may influence regional brain activity during anticipation of a rewarding or punishing outcome (Critchley et al. 2001a). A second gambling task was designed, in which the subject had to guess, when presented with one playing card (face value between 1 and 10), if the face value of a successive card would be higher or lower. Correct decisions were associated with financial gain, and wrong decisions with financial loss. These decisions were therefore associated with different but predictable risks that were a function of the face value of the cue card. Although the subjects responded as soon as the saw the first card, the second card (indicating if the subject had won or lost) was presented after a fixed delay period. The question addressed here was how sympathetic arousal (indexed by EDA), and the risk-value of each decision, modulated brain activity during anticipation of outcome. During the anticipatory delay period, anterior cingulate and dorsolateral prefrontal cortex activity varied parametrically with the degree of anticipatory EDA response. Activity in anterior cingulate and insula cortex was influenced by risk, and a conjunction analysis confirmed that anterior cingulate cortex was the sole area modulated by both risk and arousal (Fig. 12.9).

Insights from biofeedback experiments

In a further neuroimaging study we examined the functional neuroanatomy through which conscious 'psychological' processes influence EDA (Critchley et al. 2001b). Although the generation of EDA usually occurs outside of conscious influence, biofeedback relaxation techniques can enable subjects to gain control over autonomic responses. Consequently, prior to PET scanning, we trained subjects to perform a biofeedback relaxation task in which EDA was used as an index of sympathetic arousal, which was continuously presented visually to subjects in the form of a 'thermometer'. As a subject relaxed and decreased the level of EDA arousal, there was a parallel decrease in the column height of the thermometer, eventually reaching the 'bulb' (which served as a fixed end point). During PET scanning, subjects performed repetitions of 4 different tasks:

- the biofeedback relaxation, where they aimed to relax and decrease the column height while receiving accurate EDA-feedback

- attempted relaxation with false feedback and where the display column fluctuated randomly

- no-relaxation with EDA-biofeedback and where subjects attempted to stem any downward drift in their EDA level

- the subjects attempted not to relax while watching a false, randomly fluctuating display; EDA was recorded during all experimental conditions, irrespective of whether or not it contributed to the visual feedback.

The main effect of attempting to relax, and reduce EDA arousal, was associated with increased activity in anterior cingulate, inferior parietal cortex and globus pallidus. Integration of the intention to relax with feedback of subjects EDA level (i.e. the interaction between true versus false EDA-biofeedback and relaxation versus no relaxation), was associated with increased activity in ventromedial prefrontal cortex, anterior cingulate and cerebellar vermis. Finally activity in medial temporal lobe involving the uncus, just anterior to the amygdala, reflected the rate of decrease in EDA-indexed arousal across all experimentally tasks. Together these observations implicate brain regions such as ventromedial prefrontal cortex and anterior cingulate in integration of bodily arousal with cognitive processes (intention to relax). Interestingly, in contrast to studies of sympathetic arousal (Critchley et al. 2000a,b) activity during performance of intentional relaxation tasks was greater in left hemisphere than the right. Also, the observation that activity in the uncus is associated with sympathetic relaxation suggests a mechanism by which relaxation strategies may therapeutically influence brain regions mediating fear and stress responses, such as the adjacent amygdala.

We subsequently developed a similar biofeedback relaxation task for fMRI that utilized the higher spatial and enhanced temporal resolution of this technique. This allowed us to delineate a matrix of regional brain activity relating to volitional decreases in electrodermal activity and examine in more detail the neuroanatomy supporting cognitive influences on autonomic responses (Critchley et al. 2002) We obtained functional magnetic resonance imaging (fMRI) measures in 17 subjects to assess brain activity relating biofeedback relaxation in which a visual index of electrodermal arousal was modulated by accuracy (addition of random 'noise') or sensitivity (by scalar adjustments of feedback). Performance of biofeedback relaxation tasks activated a central autonomic matrix, including insula, cingulate, thalamus, hypothalamus, and brainstem, as well as somatosensory cortex, dorsolateral prefrontal cortex and extrastriate cortical area V5 (Fig. 12.10). 'Noisy' feedback to subjects was associated with increased activity in anterior cingulate, amygdala and V5. Activity within the anterior insula was

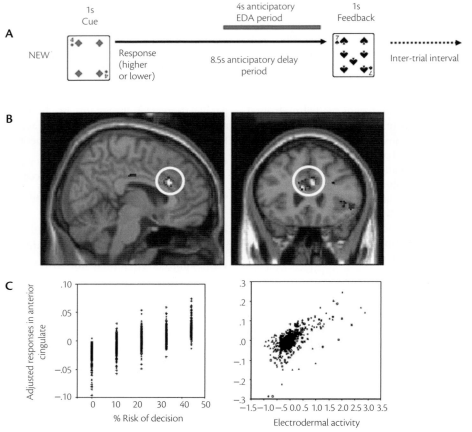

Fig. 12.9 Modulation of delay-period activity by risk and anticipatory electrodermal activity arousal. **A:** Diagram of individual trial. Subjects made a response to a cue card, judging if next (feedback) card would be higher or lower. Activity during the delay period before outcome was examined for modulation by riskiness of decision and by anticipatory electrodermal activity (EDA) response (mean EDA in 4 seconds prior to outcome feedback). **B** and **C:** Activity within anterior cingulate was modulated as function of both risk and EDA. From Critchley et al. 2001a, with permission. Damage to both dorsolateral prefrontal and anterior cingulate cortices has previously been observed to diminish EDA response magnitude (Zahn et al. 1999 Tranel 2000). The neuroimaging findings strongly implicate anterior cingulate cortex in the integration of cognitive processes (e.g. processing risk and expectancy) with EDA and other bodily states of arousal. The role of the dorsolateral prefrontal activation in these studies may reflect a more selective relationship between contextual control of bodily arousal during cognitive processing related to expectation, action, and experience. See also Plate 6. Reprinted from *Neuron*, **29**, Critchley HD, Mathias CJ, Dolan RJ., Neural activity relating to reward anticipation in the human brain, 537–545, Copyright 2001, with permission from Elsevier.

modulated by both accuracy and sensitivity of feedback, and additionally reflected an interaction between these qualities of feedback. Thus, the increased insular response to noise in the feedback signal was further modulated by the perceptual qualities (sensitivity) of the feedback. These findings highlight neural substrates supporting integration of perceptual processing, interoceptive awareness and intentional modulation of bodily states of arousal. In particular, our findings suggest that activity in anterior cingulate mediates the intentional drive to decrease sympathetic activity, whereas insula activity may support *sensory* integration of interoceptive and external information about bodily states, a process likely to be closely related to the experience of interoceptive awareness and 'feeling states'.

The relationship between tonic and phasic components of EDA (respectively, the sympathetic skin conductance response [SCR] and skin conductance level [SCL]) was examined in a study where subjects performed relaxation and arousal biofeedback tasks to respectively decrease and increase electrodermal arousal (Nagai et al. 2004). While transient phasic shifts in electrodermal arousal correlated with fairly widespread activity including regions such as dorsal anterior cingulate cortex, it was noteworthy that decreasing

tonic sympathetic tone (reduced SCL) was associated with increasing activity in subgenual cingulate cortex and adjacent medial orbitofrontal cortex. Not only did this study suggest a functional and behavioural dissociation of EDA arousal 'state' and 'response', inferred from segregation of neural control systems but it also provided a physiological account of the default states of brain activity corresponding to ventromedial prefrontal cortex activity enhancement during control tasks (Raichle et al. 2001) and self-referential processing (Gusnard et al. 2001) where the subject is behaviourally (and autonomically) disengaged from the environment (Fig. 12.11)

Respiratory control

The voluntary and involuntary control of respiration is yoked to reflex control of the heart and cardiovascular system. Respiratory control may in fact represent the major mechanism through which biofeedback may influence autonomic function, despite no direct vagal pathway with electrodermal activity. The muscles of respiration, including the diaphragm are striated and therefore under voluntary control, yet diaphragmatic 'tidal' breathing and other breathing-related reflexes are essentially autonomic processes necessary for homeostatic integrity. Reflexive breathing, regulated

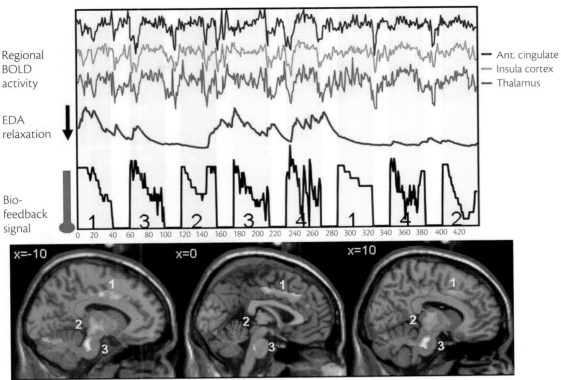

Fig. 12.10 Brain activity during biofeedback relaxation magnetic resonance imaging study. Subjects were scanned while performing biofeedback relaxation tasks, which differed either in the sensitivity or in the accuracy of the feedback signal. Compared with rest, performance of biofeedback tasks was associated with activity in a distributed network of cortical, subcortical and brainstem regions, including many putative autonomic control centres. The upper figure shows the relationship of regional brain activity, measured electrodermal activity (EDA) and the quality of the biofeedback signal during imaging. The figure below shows group activity plotted on a parasagittal section of a template brain illustrating involvement of cingulate, thalamus, hypothalamus pons and cerebellum in biofeedback task performance. The figure to the right illustrates increased activity within anterior cingulate cortex in association with decreasing EDA arousal across the whole experiment. See also Plate 7. Reprinted from *Neuroimage*, **6**, Critchley HD, Melmed RN, Featherstone E, Mathias CJ, Dolan RJ, Volitional control of autonomic arousal: a functional magnetic resonance study, 909–19, Copyright 2002, with permission from Elsevier.

by centres within the brainstem, is observed during anaesthesia and sleep, while skilled volitional respiratory control, ultimately mediated at the level of cortex, underpins the mechanics of speech and related functions such as singing.

Central to reflex control of respiration is the internal monitoring of blood chemistry, reflecting efficiency of gas exchange (Guz, 1975, Banzett et al. 1996). Animal experiments and lesion studies highlight regions of medulla, close to cardiovascular centres, in the control of depth and rhythm of reflexive respiration. Naturally neuroimaging has been applied to assess respiratory control on a system-wide basis, but in this regard precautions must necessarily be taken since the two dependent measures of human functional brain imaging, cerebral blood flow and blood oxygenation level dependent (BOLD) signal are highly sensitive to circulating CO_2 levels. A number of neuroimaging studies have examined brain activity relating to the control of breathing, either in response to respiratory challenges (such as hypoxia or hypercapnia) or respiratory changes occurring during volitional behaviour that directly or indirectly modulate the frequency and depth of breathing. The effects of mild hypoxic challenge healthy subjects (comparable to 3000 metres altitude) (in contrast to ischaemic vascular changes in regions cerebral perfusion) results in a global decline in the fMRI BOLD signal. With respect to the role of CO_2 in respiratory control, PET, Corfield and co-workers (1995) demonstrated using PET widespread increases in brain activity, from brainstem thalamus and limbic system to visual sensory cortices, during states of CO_2-

stimulated breathing. Notably, activity within motor cortices was not enhanced, in contrast to voluntarily-induced hyperventilatory states. Pet studies reliably report and association between dyspnoeic states induced by hypercapnia and activation of particularly of anterior insular cortex (e.g. Banzett et al. 2000, Liotti et al. 2001), consistent with the putative role of anterior insula in translating behaviourally salient internal states into subjective emotional states of discomfort (Critchley et al. 2004).

More recently, fMRI studies have replicated such findings with increased sensitivity: the sophisticated study of Evans et al. (2002) highlighting concurrent activation of dorsal anterior cingulate with (predominantly right) anterior insular cortex during subjective air hunger (Fig. 12.12). Enhanced activity was also apparent in the cerebellar vermis, amygdala and striatum. Furthermore, patients with congenital hypoventilation syndrome, in whom there is impairment of autonomic and respiratory response to hypoxia, demonstrate underactivity across similar cortical, limbic and subcortical regions to that implicated in hypercapnic response (Macey et al. 2005).

PET studies revealed volitional control of respiration, in contrast to changes induced reflexively by chemosensory stimulation, to be associated with activation of typical motor pathways, including motor and cerebellar cortices (Ramsay et al. 1993, Fink et al. 1996). Studies using fMRI extend these observations, highlighting activation of SMA, thalamus and even medullary centres during hyperpnoea in addition to sensorimotor and cerebellar activity (McKay et al. 2003).

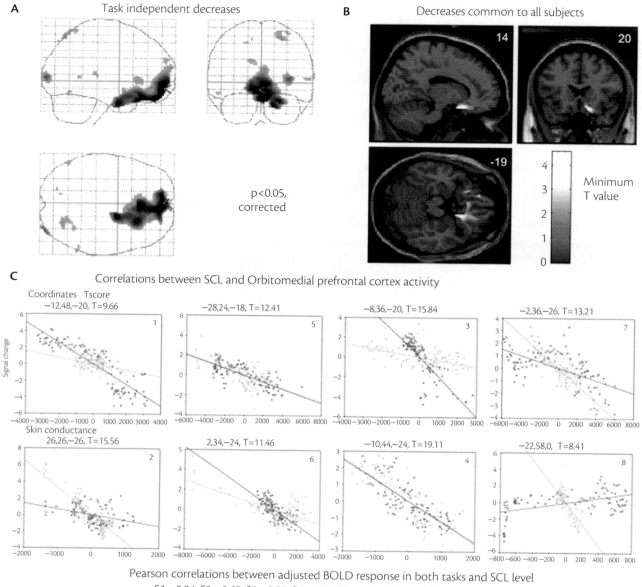

Fig. 12.11 Regional brain activity associated with decreases in skin conductance level. (A) Regional brain activity related to task-independent decreases in skin conductance level (SCL). Decreases in SCL were associated with increased activity in VMPFC and OFC. A conjunction analysis was used to identify regional activity negatively correlating with across both biofeedback relaxation and arousal tasks (*P* < 0.05, corrected). (B) Regional brain activity associated with decreases in tonic skin conductance level common across all subjects (conjunction analysis associated with decreases in skin conductance), presented on a normalized template brain scan (*P* < 0.05, corrected). The scale represents the minimum *t* value shared by all eight subjects contributing to the conjunction analysis. Common brain activity was found in VMPFC and OFC. (C) Plots of individual subjects' data showing correlations between skin conductance and ventromedial and orbitofrontal BOLD activity during biofeedback relaxation (light dots) and arousal tasks (dark dots). Data are plotted for the peak voxels of activity identified in first-level individual subject analyses. Pearson correlations showed significant negative correlation between adjusted VMPFC and OFC BOLD responses and task-independent SCL activity in the eight subjects. See also Plate 8. Copyright from Nagai et al. (2004) with permission from Elsevier.

Autonomic gastrointestinal control

Understanding brain mechanisms influencing the autonomic control of gastrointestinal function have been led predominantly by investigations addressing visceral pain and the understanding of 'functional' disorders such as irritable bowel syndrome (Derbyshire 2003). The emphasis has therefore been on afferent information from the bowel. This work has been led by Qasim Aziz's group in Manchester (Aziz et al. 2000, Hobday et al. 2001) whose focus has been to identify central substrates underlying psychosomatic

conditions such as irritable bowel syndrome. Typically, activation of bowel stretch receptors in the viscera (e.g. lower oesophagus or rectum), with or without associated pain sensation, is associated with enhanced activation of anterior cingulate and insula (Fig. 12.13). The sensitivity of these brain regions to viscerosensory stimulation is underpinned in many studies, many described in this chapter. However, it is noteworthy that the network of brain regions activated in response to visceral challenges overlaps considerably with a general central 'pain matrix', with the possible exception of thalamic activity which perhaps provides the best

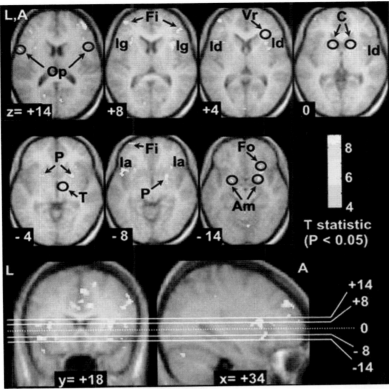
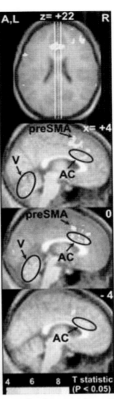

Fig. 12.12 Brain activity related to air hunger. Statistical maps of significant brain activation associated with periods of air hunger for the group (same T statistic map as in Fig. 12.4) superimposed onto the group mean structural image. Selected axial slices are displayed illustrating the effect size of regions of interest: insula, prefrontal cortex, basal ganglia, and amygdala. 'L, A' indicates left anterior. Horizontal slices are depicted on a coronal image and sagittal image. Relevant local maxima are labelled: Am, amygdala; C, caudate; Fi, inferior frontal gyrus; Fo, orbital frontal gyrus; Ia, insula (agranular); Id, insula (dysgranular); Ig, insula (granular); Op, operculum; P, putamen; T, thalamus; Vr, vertical ramus lateral fissure. See also Plate 9. With permission from the American Physiological Society (Evans *et al.* 2002).

indicator of painful sensory experience (Casey,1999). This latter difference highlighted by Derbyshire (2003), contrasts with reports thalamic responses in during visceral gastrointestinal distension in animals, but nevertheless may reflect differential organization of afferent sensory streams within thalamus

Urogenital autonomic control

Bladder sensation and control of voiding

Animal studies have implicated discrete brainstem centres in the control of micturition. These include a pontine micturition centre in the dorsal tegmentum, a ventral pontine storage centre, parabrachial nucleus and PAG. In humans, functional imaging studies have enabled examination of cortical and subcortical correlates of subjective bladder sensation and mechanisms underlying volitional voiding, examined during different degrees of bladder filling. Consistent with the animal evidence, early PET studies identified enhanced dorsal tegmental activity with active voiding. In contrast, a more ventral brainstem region was associated with an inability to void during the scanning procedure (Blok et al. 1997, 1998). The representation of bladder filling appears to be associated with activation in the region of the PAG region and at a cortical level insula and anterior cingulate activity changes, the precise location of the latter varying across studies (Blok et al. 1997, 1998, Athwal et al. 2001, Matsuura et al. 2002) (Fig. 12.14). These observations suggest that bladder sensation is typical of other types of visceral sensation and endorse the notion of common channel supporting visceral response, central autonomic feedback and pain that terminates in

insula and dorsal cingulate (Saper 2002, Craig 2002, Critchley 2003). Nevertheless, there appears to be specificity in responses to bladder stimulation, with concurrent activation of lateral prefrontal cortex suggesting a likely substrate volitional bladder control. Moreover, dysfunctional interactions between these cortical regions (and their influence on pontine centres) are implicated in the pathoaetiology of certain disorders of bladder control and micturition (e.g. Fowler's syndrome: DasGupta et al. 2005, Kavia et al. 2005)

Autonomic correlates of sexual arousal

Neuroimaging as highlighted the patterning of cortical and subcortical brain responses to a number of aspects of sexual bonding and autonomic correlates of sexual arousal and orgasm. In a study of 'romantic love' Bartels and Zeki (2000) showed that viewing a picture of a 'deeply loved' partner (in contrast to pictures of close friends) enhanced middle insula, rostral anterior cingulate activity and striatum, while deactivating amygdala. The activity differences reflected feelings of love and sexual attraction. There have been a number of PET studies of sexual arousal in men: Rauch and co-workers (1999) showed activation of anterior cingulate, anterior temporal cortex and striatum (pallidus) when sexual arousal (in contrast to competitive arousal) was induced using scripts. Similar findings of sexual arousal related cingulate and striatum activation (often with hypothalamus) are also reported in response to erotic pictures or films in PET (Redoute et al. 2000, Beauregard et al. 2001). Hypothalamic activation has also been observed using fMRI in male marmosets aroused by female odours (Ferris et al. 2001).

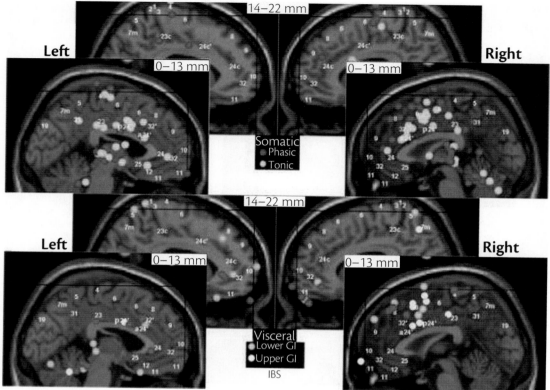

Fig. 12.13 Viscerosensory stimulation. The centre of each reported regional cerebral blood flow increase on the medial surface of the brain during the experience of phasic or tonic somatic pain (top) and during the experience of visceral pain (bottom) in the lower or upper gastrointestinal (GI) tract. Responses to lower GI distension in patients with irritable bowel syndrome are shown in purple. The responses are plotted onto the standard MNI brain provided with SPM99 and the Brodmann's areas shown. The ACC is divided into perigenual (24), anterior midcingulate (a24') and posterior midcingulate (p24'). See also Plate 10. With permission from Derbyshire SW. 2003. Visceral afferent pathways and functional brain imaging. *Scientific World Journal.* **3**:1065–80.

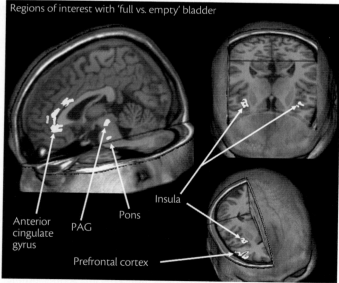

Fig. 12.14 Brain activity related to urinary control. Summary of regions of interest comparing 'full versus empty' bladder conditions based on the coordinates published in five positron emission tomography studies: Athwal et al. 2001, Blok et al. 1997, Blok et al. 1998, Nour et al. 2000, Matsuura et al. 2002. See also Plate 11. With permission from Kavia RB, Dasgupta R, Fowler CJ. 2005. Functional imaging and the central control of the bladder. *J Comp. Neurol.* **493**:27–32, Wiley.

Other PET studies have been less consistent, with effects confined to extrastriate visual regions (Bocher et al. 2001). More widespread cortical and subcortical activation was observed in an early fMRI study of male responses to erotic imagery (Park et al. 2001). Also using fMRI, correlation between brain activity and penile erectile response when viewing erotic films directly highlighted arousal-related activity in striatum, claustrum cingulate insula and hypothalamus (Arnow et al. 2002). In a PET study, sexual penile somatosensory stimulation was associated with insula activation and amygdala deactivation (but surprisingly no hypothalamus) (Georgiadis and Holstege 2005). During male ejaculation enhanced activity is reported in midbrain and striatum (seemingly reflecting a dopaminergic effect) again with amygdala deactivation (Holstege et al. 2003). Neuroimaging studies of sexual arousal in women are largely confined to fMRI investigations. Gender differences are reported in hypothalamus (Karama et al. 2002) and amygdala activation (Hamann et al. 2004). To summarize, while there is increasing neuroanatomical consistency across imaging studies concerning the activity patterns associated with sexual arousal, a mechanistic knowledge remains rather rudimentary. Focusing of functional interactions between regions and specific roles of areas such as hypothalamus and tegmentum in the context of sexual arousal may provide in the future a clinically useful level of detail for understanding the cerebral autonomic mechanisms underlying sexual function and dysfunction.

Pupil responses

Few neuroimaging experiments have explicitly looked at the neural control of pupils, rather pupillometry has occasionally been employed within functional imaging experiments as an objective index of cognitive or emotional processing (Siegle et al. 2003, O'Doherty et al. 2003). Neuroanatomically, the control of pupil diameter in response to luminance changes in mediated via parasympathetic nuclei in the brainstem—the Edinger–Westphal nuclei. Cortical and subcortical descending influences modulate tonic and phasic pupillary responses, reflecting factors such as colour and coherence in visual objects, and the motivational meaning of stimuli (Barbur 2004). Pupil dilatation may have specific social meaning as suggested by cosmetic use of belladonna by 17th century Venetian ladies. Harrison and co-workers (2006) recently examined behaviourally and using neuroimaging the role of pupil size in emotional processing. Subjects viewed faces with neutral, happy, sad and angry facial expressions. The faces also displayed four different sizes of pupils, though none of the subject was explicitly aware of this manipulation. In a behavioural rating of the faces, manipulation of pupil size did not affect ratings of attractiveness of the faces (dismissing a long-standing myth). However, when subjects saw sad faces, there was a clear effect of pupil size on perceived emotional intensity: the smaller the pupil the more intensely sad and negative the face appeared. No such effect was observed with happy, angry or neutral faces. In a functional imaging experiment, subjects only estimated the age of these emotional faces. Nevertheless, perception of small pupils on sad faces modulated activity in amygdala, frontal operculum and superior temporal sulcus (a face-feature processing region). In addition this effect of pupils in the context of sad faces strongly modulated brainstem activity in a region corresponding anatomically to the Edinger–Westphal nuclei. During functional imaging, the pupil size of the subjects was monitored: there was clear correspondence between the pupil response of the observer and the face stimuli only for sad faces, such that perceiving small pupils in the context of sad faces evoked autonomic mimicry (mirroring) in the perceiver, consistent with an emotion-specific automatic empathy response, in this case mediated autonomically via the Edinger–Westphal nuclei (Fig. 12.15). These findings highlight the role of autonomic engagement in action-perception models of emotional exchanges and define the functional anatomy of emotion-related cortical and amygdala influences on this aspect of parasympathetic control.

Patient studies

Abnormalities in efferent autonomic response
Vasovagal syncope and essential hyperhidrosis
There have been few if any neuroimaging studies examining neurocardiogenic (vasovagal) syncope or essential hyperhidrosis from an autonomic 'neurological' perspective. However, insight can be gained from the large number of studies using typical precipitants of these autonomic symptoms: i.e. blood-injury-injection phobia and social stress. There are certain key findings in these experiments, namely hyperexcitability of components of brain regions implicated in both fear and autonomic control system (amygdala, insula, anterior cingulate) during symptom provocation (exposure to blood, blood imagery, anticipation of needle or social challenge) and, in the case of social phobics, in response to negative facial expressions (anger, contempt, disgust)

Cardiovascular patients and stress

Neuroimaging applied to cardiac patients has provided insight into mechanisms underlying the experience and generation of cardiac dysfunction. Changes in brain activity during cardiac ischaemia have been indexed using PET. Rosen and colleagues (1996) showed subcortical changes accompanying electrocardiographic evidence of cardiac ischaemia extending to cortical areas with perception of angina. Later, Soufer and colleagues (1998) also showed cingulate deactivations and shifts in the symmetry of brain activity in patients who develop myocardial ischaemia during mental stress challenge. Further studies (Rosen et al. 2002) highlight the enhancement of right anterior insula activity during patients' experience of cardiac chest pain in cardiac syndrome X.

One of the most important considerations with respect to central autonomic control is the role of the autonomic nervous system in psychosomatic morbidity. Autonomic (and stress hormone) responses to acute and chronic emotional challenges may elicit specific detrimental effects on bodily organs. A florid example of this is stress-induced ventricular arrhythmia and sudden death. Ventricular arrhythmia represents a final pathway before death where the heart cannot pump blood to the brain or body as a result of uncoordinated myocardial activity. The coordinated propagation of excitation over the myocardial surface from the ventricular pacemaker heart is influenced by sympathetic and parasympathetic nerves, predominantly through their effect on the refractory (recovery) period of the cardiac cycle. Electrical recovery is speeded by enhanced sympathetic activity and decreased parasympathetic activity. Different regions of ventricular myocardium are supplied by left and right autonomic nerves hence, if the left/right balance of autonomic input is disrupted this may lead to a proarrhythmic state i.e. some parts of the heart muscle are ready to contract before other parts. This is proposed as a mechanism for sudden death in epilepsy where ictal activity asymmetrically drives efferent cardiac nerves. The smoothness and coherence in cardiac electrical recovery can be measured from the morphology and distribution of T-waves across 12-lead electrocardiography. Inhomogeneity of T-waves suggests a proarrhythmic state. Mental stress shifts the electrical activity of the heart toward this proarrhythmic state, even in healthy people (Taggart et al. 2005) perhaps representing a descending overspill from asymmetrical cortical activity during emotional processing (Lane and Jennings 1996). An afferent efferent loop in cardiac autonomic control exists such that, in health, feedback from the heart regulates the efferent autonomic drive. In patients with ischaemic heart disease, the situation may be further exacerbated by feedback from an abnormal heart. Heart attacks and sudden typically occur during situations of emotional arousal or acute stress. We set out to examine, using PET, changes in regional brain activity during autonomic arousal and stress (mental and exercise pressor tasks) that predict proarrhythmic changes in the electrical activity of the heart (measured from ECG T-waves) in patients with heart disease (Critchley et al. 2005b. The two stress tasks enhanced sympathetic activity to the heart they also evoked proarrhythmic changes on ECG. These correlated with a right-lateralized shift in midbrain activity (in the region of the parabrachial nucleus), representing with a lateralization of activity during stress at the level of an integrative relay controlling efferent sympathetic responses to the heart. Moreover, the right lateralization predicted the extent to which proarrhythmic changes occurred and which patients were at greatest risk (Fig. 12.16). This study has led

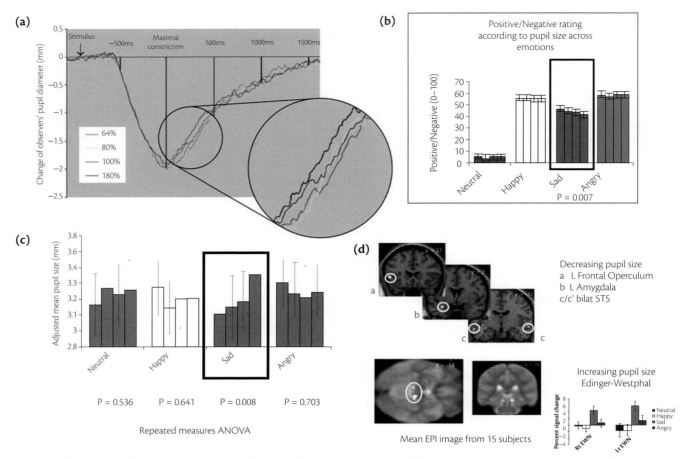

Fig. 12.15 Pupillary contagion during emotional processing. **(a)** Subjects' mean pupil response to a 500 ms stimulus presentation, illustrating the pupillary light response beginning approximately 200 ms after stimulus onset and peaking 200 ms after stimulus offset, followed by a gradual return to baseline. **(b)** Mean ratings for each of the facial expressions according to emotion and pupil size (64% to 180% left to right). 1) Modulus of the positive/negative rating on a 0–100 absolute scale. Small pupils in expressions of sadness are rated as significantly more negative (*—repeated measures ANOVA F (3,30) = 4.340, p = 0.007, Contrasts, 64% vs 100% F (1,30) = 5.481, p = 0.026, 64% vs 180% F (1,30) = 9.311, p = 0.005, 80% vs 180% F (1,30) = 5.377, p = 0.027) than those with larger pupils. **(c)** Subject's mean pupil size in the 500 ms window following maximal pupillary constriction for neutral, happy, sad, and angry facial expressions. Pupil size is plotted in response to observed pupil areas 64%, 80%, 100% and 180% of the original image (from left to right). Observers' own pupil size was significantly smaller when viewing sad faces with small pupils than when viewing those with larger pupils (Repeated measures ANOVA F = 5.04, p = 0.008) with significantly smaller pupil size when viewing sad faces with pupil area 64% (* p = 0.002), 80% (* p = 0.005) and 100% (* p = 0.049) of the original compared with images with pupils 180% of the area of the original image. The horizontal line indicates subjects' mean pupil size across all trials. **(d)** Prefrontal lateral temporal and amygdala brain regions showing a significant correlation with linearly decreasing pupil size in the context of expressions of sadness. All regions shown are significant at the p ≤ 0.001, uncorrected. Midbrain regions showing a significant correlation with linearly increasing pupil size in the context of expressions of sadness. Both regions shown are significant at the p ≤ 0.001 uncorrected. Percent signal change for the right and left brainstem regions plotted against emotional expression. Increasing pupil size effects a significantly greater percentage signal change in sad facial expressions than the other emotional expressions in both brainstem regions shown. See also Plate 12. Harrison N, Singer T, Rotshtein P, Dolan RJ, Critchley HD, Pupil size modulates the empathic experience of sadness. *Social Cognitive and Affective Neuroscience* (SCAN) 2006 **1**, 1–13, by permission of Oxford University Press.

to a number of related investigations of afferent and efferent autonomic mechanisms underlying cardiac vulnerability to stress. Moreover it highlights the usefulness of combining autonomic monitoring with functional brain imaging to address fundamental clinical questions

Spinal cord injury

Patients with high spinal cord injury (SCI) not only lose afferent sensory representation of their peripheral bodily responses transmitted predominantly via the spinal cord, but also the cerebral control of sympathetic autonomic processes is disrupted by interruption of descending spinal signals to the paravertebral sympathetic ganglia. Obviously the extent to which autonomic bodily control is perturbed is critically dependent on the completeness of

the spinal lesion, and it is noteworthy that the American Spinal Injury Association (ASIA) classification of spinal cord injury as yet fails to incorporate autonomic measures. Nevertheless, the integration of brain and body is only partial disrupted, since even in complete high spinal transaction vagal afferent and efferent traffic is intact. Largely on account of logistically difficulties, functional neuroimaging studies of the effects of SCI on regional brain activity have not been extensively undertaken. Nevertheless, the partial lesion-deficit model afforded by SCI can inform both basic neuroscience while providing information directly salient to the clinical understanding and management of SCI patients. In an ambitious study of patients with SCI, Nicotra and co-workers (Nicotra et al. 2005) examined the processing of aversive pain stimuli and emotional learning (in the form of associative fear conditioning)

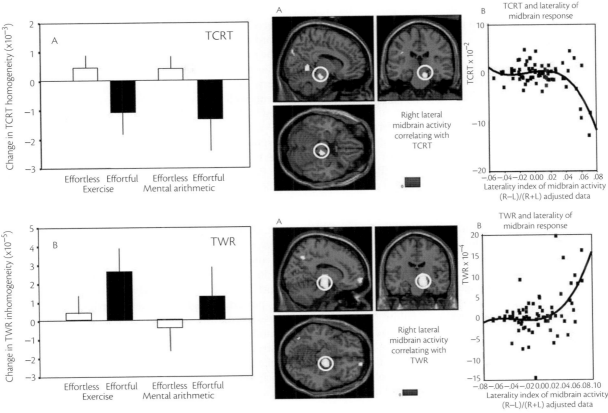

Fig. 12.16 Lateral shift in midbrain activity predicting stress-induced proarrhythmic changes in ECG T-waves (repolarization). Using the same positron emission tomography design illustrated in Fig. 12.4, 10 cardiac patients were scanned with simultaneous 12-lead ECG monitoring. Complementary measures of T-wave changes indicative of proarrhythmic electrical inhomogeneity of myocardial repolarization were derived (decreased TCRT and increased TWR) and shown to be enhanced by cognitive and physical effort (figures to left). The same measures were predicted by right-left right shifts in the activity of the midbrain. The data suggest that a lateralized imbalance in the autonomic drive to the heart, originating in functional imbalance at the level of a midbrain autonomic relay, may predispose to stress-induced arrhythmia and sudden cardiac death. Middle figures illustrate this correlation with midbrain activity across the group, and the effect is plotted for each measure in scatter plots to the right. See also Plate 13. Critchley HD, Taggart P, Sutton PM, Holdright DR, Batchvarov V, Hnatkova K, Malik M, Dolan RJ., Mental stress and sudden cardiac death: asymmetric midbrain activity as a linking mechanism, *Brain*, 2005, **128**:75–85, by permission of Oxford University Press.

reflecting the sensory and autonomic disruption following SCI. Theoretical accounts of emotion have long postulated emotional deficits in SCI patients as a result of their 'disconnection' from their body. Trauma, psychological and physical adjustment to disability and frequently chronic neural pain confound studies of emotion in a patient group in whom depressive symptoms are common. Nevertheless anecdotal evidence suggests a proportion of SCI patients undergo changes emotional and behavioural style that are difficult to attribute only to these adjustments. Nicotra used fMRI and a basic emotional learning paradigm to investigate the expression of emotion-related brain activity consequent upon SCI. During scanning, painful electrical stimuli, delivered above the sensory level of each patient's lesion, were paired with visual presentations of one face stimulus. Not every presentation of this stimulus was paired with the shock, so that unpaired stimuli represented the learned 'threat-of-shock'. A further face stimulus was paired (on half the trials) with equivalent electrical stimulation of the skin below the level of the lesion. Subjects also saw (control) face stimuli that were never paired with electrical shock. There was in fact little evidence that skin stimulation below the lesion level evoked changes in autonomic cardiac or even brain responses in the SCI patients (this contrasts with a study in women with spinal cord transection which reported vagally mediated changes in brain

activity during orgasm [Komisaruk et al. 2004]). However, in both healthy control subjects and SCI patients, painful stimulation above the sensory level of the SCI lesion, evoked both a parasympathetic bradycardic response and brain activation of dorsal anterior cingulate, right insula and medial temporal lobe. However, SCI patients differed from control subjects in the pattern of conditioning-related brain activity. SCI patients showed a relative enhancement of activity within dorsal anterior cingulate, periaqueductal grey matter and superior temporal gyrus (a region implicated in processing salient face stimuli). Conversely SCI patients showed relative attenuation of activity in ventromedial prefrontal and motor cingulate cortices to the threat of painful arm stimulation (Fig. 12.17).

It was also noteworthy that whereas control subjects demonstrated bradycardia in response to the threat of pain, SCI patients also did not. Together these findings provide evidence for differences both in parasympathetic cardiac response and brain activity in SCI patients in response to the threat of pain. The differences in the activity of prefrontal and cingulate cortices and brainstem to emotional threat stimuli represent perhaps an oversensitivity of pain related responses and a failure in integrating external emotional cues with a relative absence of afferent information from the body. It is postulated that these differences account for some of the emotional sequellae of spinal cord damage and perhaps the high incidence of chronic neural pain in patients with SCI.

Autonomic failure

Pure autonomic failure

Pure autonomic failure (PAF) (Bradbury–Eggleston Syndrome) represents a peripheral disorder characterized by peripheral autonomic (sympathetic and parasympathetic) denervation impairing effector responses (Chapter 39, Mathias 2000). Afferent pathways from the viscera are presumed to be intact, accounting for the range of cardiovascular and visceral symptoms experienced by this patient group (Mathias et al. 1999). Patients with PAF present a very interesting model for examining central control of autonomic responses: The absence of centrally generated autonomic responses effectively make PAF a lesion model of afferent integrated bodily changes during a range of volitional cognitive and emotional behaviours i.e. whatever changes and differences are seen the brain must be the consequence of a failure to feedback to the brain the presence of autonomic responses normally generated in health. Early functional imaging studies highlight the intact nature of the basal ganglia and dopamine binding in patients with PAF compared with patients with central autonomic failure (Shy–Drager variant of multiple system atrophy [MSA]) (Brooks et al. 1990, Fulham et al. 1991). Nevertheless, the PAF model is more powerful for studying brain mechanisms underlying autonomic symptoms and the impact of bodily responses on other types of processing, since PAF is confined to the autonomic system and patients with PAF are largely cognitively and emotionally intact in their daily lives (Heims et al. 2004, 2006).

We examined, using PET, regional activity in patients with PAF and matched controls during the performance of cognitive and physical 'stressor' tasks (in fact this replicated a study of young controls described above). By virtue of the diagnosis of PAF, differences in regional brain activity between patients and controls must be consequent to absent feedback of autonomic bodily changes normally accompanying effortful behaviour. We predicted that there would be decreased activity in PAF subjects within brain regions *mapping* autonomic arousal and perhaps increases within regions *generating* autonomic arousal states (from lack of negative feedback). Interestingly across all effortful and effortless task conditions, patients with PAF demonstrated enhanced activity of the dorsal pons compared with controls (Fig 12.18). In the previous study of young healthy controls, activity in this region was observed during performance of effortful pressor tasks associated with increases in cardiovascular arousal. This newer finding in patients with PAF suggests that above and beyond the generation of arousal patterns during effort, the dorsal pontine region is responsible for continuous, autoregulatory efferent control of autonomic responses. In this role pontine activity is governed by afferent feedback and is largely independent of 'higher' cognitive or physical drive. Reduced activity across all tasks was observed in regions including insula and primary somatosensory cortex, consistent with the notion that these areas are primarily involved with the continuous mapping of bodily states (Fig 12.18).

Of particular interest were brain areas that showed context-dependent changes in activity; that is distinct brain areas showed differences between patients with PAF and controls during physical and mental effort (accompanied by autonomic arousal in controls) but not during effortless tasks. In the previous PET study we had observed right anterior cingulate activity covarying with increases in cardiovascular arousal in young controls (mean age, 35 years). In the present study the same effect was observed in older controls (mean age, 65 years) (Fig. 12.4). It was therefore surprising to observe significantly *greater* right anterior cingulate activity in patients with PAF, who generated no cardiovascular arousal, compared with matched healthy controls. Importantly, this observation was in keeping with the notion that anterior cingulate activity is responsible for context-specific autonomic modulation of bodily states to meet behavioural demands (Fig 12.8). Thus, in the patients with PAF, performance of effortful tasks increases the intact efferent drive to modulate bodily arousal but the response is impaired in the periphery. In healthy subjects, these context-specific autonomic responses negatively feedback to regulate efferent sympathetic drive, whereas in patients with PAF there is no such feedback and consequently greater peripheral autonomic drive from anterior cingulate cortex. Not only does this study indicate a basis in functional abnormalities within limbic and paralimbic cortices and brainstem for symptomatology of autonomic failure, but it provides powerful insight into the hierarchical arrangement of brain centres mediating autonomic changes in bodily state to the demands of volitional behaviour. In fact, the study also addressed the structure of first and second-order representations of afferent visceral information with implications for models of emotion and consciousness (Critchley et al. 2001).

In a parallel structural study using MRI, involuntary changes were observed in insula, anterior cingulate and right lateral prefrontal cortices in patients with PAF compared with controls, providing evidence that these regions were somehow affected chronically by long-standing absence of integrated autonomic feedback (Critchley et al. 2001). However, in a study of fear conditioning we were able to use the higher temporal and spatial resolution of fMRI to examine the phasic consequences of absent autonomic responses on brain activity related to the presence and absence of autonomic feedback. In fear conditioning an association is learned between a stimulus and an aversive event such that the stimulus is learned to be a threat. This learning is dependent on the functional integrity of the amygdala. In healthy subjects one can index this learning using autonomic measures of arousal such as skin conductance response or by somatomotor measures such as reaction-time or startle response. In patients with PAF, skin conductance is absent, yet startle responses are intact or exaggerated. Using a fear conditioning paradigm, we showed that the absence of an autonomic response to learned threat stimuli was associated with diminished activity in an amygdala region and, notably in right insula cortex. An extension of the study, in which some of the threat stimuli were presented subliminally (using a method called backward masking) showed that the same region of insula was sensitive to awareness of emotional context and the presence of autonomic arousal, suggesting it to be a site where emotional material is integrated within afferent visceral information. This interpretation is interesting, in that it converges with other evidence (some described above) suggesting right insula to be important for representing emotional feeling states, particularly those arising from autonomic bodily responses. Despite underactivity in this particular experimental context, right anterior cortex is the likely central origin of feelings of discomfort presyncope and fatigue that accompany autonomic failure in daily life.

Ventromedial prefrontal/subgenual cingulate cortex

Motor cingulate/adjacent callosum

Periaqueductal grey

ACC

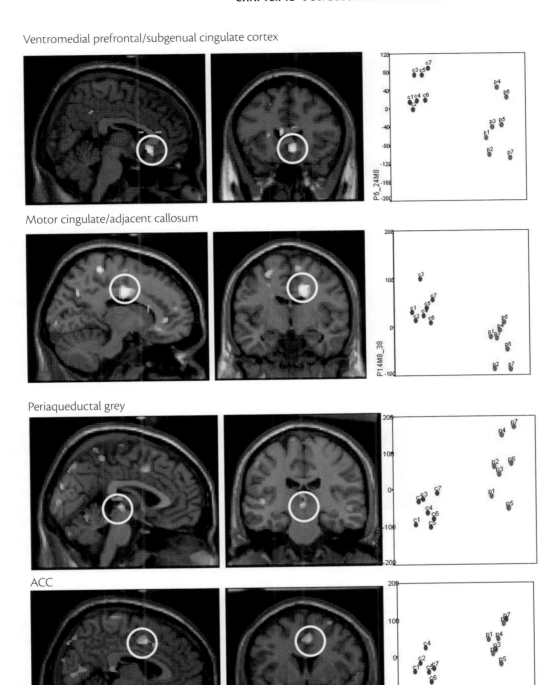

Fig. 12.17 Functional brain activity relating to abnormalities in emotional autonomic responsitivity in patients with high spinal cord transection. Patients with high spinal cord lesions, compared with healthy controls, showed abnormal fear conditioning with heightened activity in pain processing regions, suggesting upregulation of pain systems. When exposed to the threat of pain, they showed attenuated activity within medial orbitofrontal/subgenual cingulate and motor cingulate cortices (top two panels) To the left, the anatomical location of differences in activity is plotted on orthogonal sections of a template brain and to the right responses for threat-related activity is shown for controls (blue) and patients (red). The bottom two panels illustrate enhanced activity in pain reactive regions to the threat of pain in spinal lesioned subjects (i.e. the periaqueductal grey matter and a midcingulate region). These data show an impact on emotional systems of the relative loss of autonomic control and afferent spinal visceral information consequent upon upper thoracic or cervical spinal damage. See also Plate 14. Nicotra A, Critchley HD, Mathias CJ, Dolan RJ, Emotional and autonomic consequences of spinal cord injury explored using functional brain imaging. *Brain*. 2005, **129** (3): 718–728, by permission of Oxford University Press.

(a)

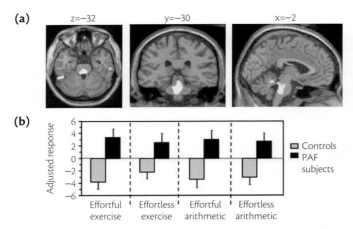

(b)

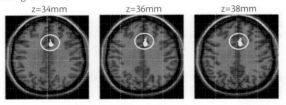

(c) Interaction with effort: Anterior cingulate activity greater in PAF subjects during effortful versus effortless tasks

(d) Interaction with effort: Medial parietal/posterior cingulate activity greater in controls during effortful versus effortless tasks

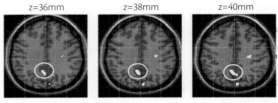

Fig. 12.18 Regional activity differences in patients with pure autonomic failure (PAF). Patients with PAF, a peripheral autonomic denervation, and matched controls were scanned using positron emission tomography during performance of effortful cognitive (mental arithmetic) and physical (isometric exercise) stress tasks and low grade, effortless, control conditions. Consistent with their diagnosis, patients with PAF did not show significant increases in blood pressure or heart rate. **(a)** Independent of task, patients with PAF showed significantly increased blood flow relative to controls in dorsal pons, consistent with increased autoregulatory activity in absence of continuous negative feedback of autonomic responses. The figure plots this group difference in activity on axial coronal and parasagittal sections of a template brain, together with **(b)** bar graphs of the adjusted blood flow responses for the four-task conditions for the patient groups. **(c)** In the absence of autonomic responses during effortful cognitive and physical behaviours, patients with PAF had significantly greater activity than controls in right anterior cingulate (beyond that seen in association with autonomic arousal [see Fig. 12.3B]), suggestive of a context-specific increase in activity in the absence of negative feedback of autonomic arousal. **(d)** In contrast, decreased activity in posterior cingulate/medial parietal cortex was observed in the patients with PAF during effortful behaviour, independent of task modality. The anatomical locations of these second-order differences are illustrated on axial sections of a template brain. See also Plate 15. Reprinted by permission from Macmillan Publishers Ltd: *Nature Neurosci*, Critchley HD, Mathias CJ, Dolan RJ. Copyright (2001).

Multiple system atrophy

As a progressive neurodegenerative condition, imaging studies of patients with multiple system atrophy (MSA) have focused on clinical need for early diagnosis, differentiation form other disorders including Parkinson's disease and characterization of central correlates of pathological mechanisms that may inform future therapy. MSA is associated with a triad of progressive parkinsonian, autonomic and cerebellar symptoms expressed in varying degrees. In MSA with parkinsonism, the prognosis in terms of mortality and treatment responsiveness is worse than in Parkinson's disease (Quinn and Marsden 1993). In the Shy–Drager variant of MSA, autonomic symptoms are prominent. Early autonomic dysfunction (including urogenital and cardiovascular symptoms) may require specifically targeted intervention. Structural changes in the brains of patients with MSA are widespread, with atrophy of putamen and marginal hyperintensity of basal ganglia, and degenerative changes in brainstem, pons, cerebellar peduncles and cerebellum. Other imaging techniques such as magnetic resonance spectroscopy (MRS) may distinguish MSA from Parkinson's disease based on indices of neuronal integrity (NAA/Cr ratios), studies of axonal density and gliosis using magnetic transfer ratios (MTR) may also prove useful in discriminating MSA from other neurodegenerative conditions, as may regional patterns of neurodegeneration measured using voxel based morphometry (VBM) and related techniques (Seppi et al. 2005, Specht et al. 2003, 2005). Similarly, functional imaging studies of MSA have also focused on diagnostic questions. SPECT imaging of dopamine transporter or D2 receptor density suggest a large overlap between striatal changes in MSA with parkinsonism and Parkinson's disease. Nevertheless, using ligands sensitive to midbrain monoamine transporter molecules, a greater degree of differentiation may be achieved, reflecting more diffuse brainstem pathology in MSA (Scherfler et al. 2005) SPECT methods measuring brain perfusion may perhaps offer greater discrimination across diagnostic groups, highlighting reduced brainstem and cerebellar perfusion in MSA compared with Parkinson's disease patients (Cilia et al. 2005). These studies emphasise the relative underdevelopment of functional imaging methods in the clinical arena with respect to progressive neurological disorder. However, the advent of interventions such as deep brain stimulation in the therapeutic management of the conditions such a Parkinson's disease may make advance the usefulness of these techniques for the targeting of specific treatments.

Conclusions

Neuroimaging studies of autonomic control in humans complement and extend data grained in animal experiments emphasizing brainstem and hypothalamic autoregulatory systems. What is particularly added is the ability to observe the system dynamically in the context of behaviour and endorsed by reported subjective experience. Typically autonomic neuroimaging studies emphasize brain processes above the brainstem, particularly in neo- and limbic cortices. As the techniques gain sophistication, the ability to also simultaneously image brainstem responses is increasing (e.g. Harrison et al. 2006). In general, the studies perhaps reveal specialization of cingulate and insula cortex respectively in generating and representing autonomic arousal states during volitional, cognitive and emotional behaviours. Intermediate regions, including orbital and ventromedial prefrontal cortices and basal ganglia, have a more contextual role. In the context of emotional processing, amygdala interactions with insula and cingulate become salient. This summary is heuristic. Regional segregation of 'efferent autonomic drive' even within anterior cingulate is apparent, as might be anticipated given the degree of organ specificity and response patterning in peripheral autonomic control. Further investigations, ideally using multiple autonomic measures, and strengthened by patient studies are required to segregate central axes of autonomic control. No doubt many such investigations are underway.

Functional neuroimaging of autonomic control remains a relatively young and specialized field that is nevertheless providing novel and important insights into physiological processes and clinical conditions. The techniques for integrating acquisition of autonomic data with brain imaging are still developing, and constrained by safety and technical limitations. There is also a degree of philosophical resistance: while many medics and physiologists, particularly those interested in psychosomatic phenomena, have no problem with conceptual integration of brain and body, much of functional neuroimaging is led at present by psychologists who wish the imaging of pure human thought processes to be free from 'physiological noise' or confounding low level interpretations. Only by pursuing these studies can we gain a comprehensive mechanistic understanding of the brain processes governing internal and external behaviours and generate models for understanding and managing pathological disorders and symptom expression arising for autonomically-mediated interaction of brain and body.

References

Arnow, B. A., Desmond, J. E., Banner, L. L., et al. (2002). Brain activation and sexual arousal in healthy, heterosexual males. *Brain* 125, 1014–23.

Asahina, M., Suzuki, A., Mori, M., Kanesaka, T., Hattori, T. (2003). Emotional sweating response in a patient with bilateral amygdala damage. *Int. J Psychophysiol.* 47, 87–93.

Aston-Jones, G., Chiang, C., and Alexinsky, T, (1991). Discharge of noradrenergic locus coeruleus neurons in behaving rats and monkeys suggests a role in vigilance. *Prog. Brain. Res.* 88, 501–20.

Athwal, B. S., Berkley, K. J., Hussain, I., et al. (2001). Brain responses to changes in bladder volume and urge to void in healthy men. *Brain* 124(Pt 2), 369–77.

Aziz, Q., Schnitzler, A., Enck, P. (2000). Functional neuroimaging of visceral sensation. *J Clin. Neurophysiol.* 17(6), 604–12.

Banzett, R. B., Lansing, R. W., Evans, K. C., Shea, S.A. (1996). Stimulus-response characteristics of CO2-induced air hunger in normal subjects. *Respir Physiol.* 103(1),19–31.

Banzett, R. B., Mulnier, H. E., Murphy, K., Rosen, S. D., Wise, R. J., Adams, L. (2000). Breathlessness in humans activates insular cortex. *Neuroreport* 11(10), 2117–20.

Barbur, J. L. (2004) in *The Visual Neurosciences*, L. M. Chalupa, J. S. Werner, Eds. (MIT Press, Cambridge, MA vol. 1, pp. 641–56.

Bartels, A., Zeki, S. (2000). The neural basis of romantic love. *Neuroreport* 11(17), 3829–34.

Beauregard, M., Levesque, J., Bourgouin, P. (2001). Neural correlates of conscious self-regulation of emotion. *J Neurosci.* 21(18), RC165.

Bechara, A., Damasio, H., Tranel, D., Damasio, A. R. (1997). Deciding advantageously before knowing the advantageous strategy. *Science* 275, 1293–5.

Bechara, A., Tranel, D., Damasio, H., Damasio, A. R. (1996). Failure to respond autonomically to anticipated future outcomes following damage to prefrontal cortex. *Cereb. Cortex* 6, 215–25.

Bennarroch, E. E. (1997). Functional anatomy of the central autonomic network. In: Bennarroch, E. E. *Central autonomic network: Functional organization and clinical correlations.* Armonk NY: Futura Publishing Company Inc. 1997, 29–83.

Blessing, W. W. (1997). Inadequate frameworks for understanding bodily homeostasis. *Trends Neurosci.* 20, 235–39.

Blok, B. F., Sturms, L. M., Holstege, G. (1998). Brain activation during micturition in women. *Brain.* 121 (Pt 11), 2033–42.

Blok B. F., Willemsen, A. T., Holstege, G. (1997). A PET study on brain control of micturition in humans. *Brain* 120, 111–21.

Bocher, M., Chisin, R., Parag, Y., et al. (2001). Cerebral activation associated with sexual arousal in response to a pornographic clip: A 15O-H2O PET study in heterosexual men. *Neuroimage* 14, 105–17.

Boucsein, W. (1992). *Electrodermal activity.* New York: Plenum Press.

Brooks, D. J., Salmon, E. P., Mathias, C. J., et al. (1990). The relationship between locomotor disability, autonomic dysfunction, and the integrity of the striatal dopaminergic system in patients with multiple system atrophy, pure autonomic failure, and Parkinson's disease, studied with PET. *Brain* 113:1539–52.

Büchel, C., Morris, J., Dolan, R., Friston, K. (1998). Brain systems mediating aversive conditioning: an event-related fMRI study. *Neuron* 20, 947–57.

Cannon, W.B. (1929). *Bodily Changes in Pain, Hunger, Fear and Rage: An Account of Recent Research into the Function of Emotional Excitement,* 2nd ed. New York: Appleton.

Casey, K.L. (1999). Forebrain mechanisms of nociception and pain: analysis through imaging. *Proc. Natl. Acad. Sci. U S A* 96(14), 7668–74.

Chawla, D., Rees, G., Friston, K. J. (1999). The physiological basis of attentional modulation in extrastriate visual areas. *Nature Neurosci.* 2, 671–76.

Chua P., Krams, M., Toni, I., Passingham, R., Dolan, R. (1999). A functional anatomy of anticipatory anxiety. *Neuroimage* 9, 563–71.

Cilia, R., Marotta, G., Benti, R., Pezzoli, G., Antonini, A. (2005). Brain SPECT imaging in multiple system atrophy. *J Neural. Transm.* 112, 1635–45.

Corfield, D. R., Fink, G. R., Ramsay, S. C., et al. (1995). Evidence for limbic system activation during CO2-stimulated breathing in man. *J Physiol.* 488 (Pt 1), 77–84.

Craig, A.D. (2002). How do you feel? Interoception:the sense of the physiological condition of the body. *Nat. Rev. Neurosci.* 3, 655–66

Craig, A.D. (2003). Interoception: the sense of the physiological condition of the body. *Curr. Opin. Neurobiol.* 13, 500–505

Critchley, H. D., Corfield. D. R., Chandler, M. P., Mathias, C. J., Dolan, R. J. (2000a). Cerebral correlates of autonomic cardiovascular arousal: A functional neuroimaging investigation. *J Physiol. Lond.* 523, 259–70.

Critchley, H. D., Elliot, R., Mathias, C. J., Dolan, R. J. (2000b). Neural activity relating to the generation and representation of galvanic skin conductance response: A functional magnetic imaging study. *J Neurosci.* 20, 3033–40.

Critchley, H. D., Josephs, O., O'Doherty, J., et al. (2003). Human cingulate cortex and autonomic cardiovascular control:Converging neuroimaging and clinical evidence. *Brain* 216, 2139–56.

Critchley, H. D., Mathias, C. J., Dolan, R. J. (2001). Neural correlates of first and second-order representation of bodily states. *Nature Neurosci.* 4, 207–212.

Critchley, H. D., Mathias, C. J., Dolan, R. J. (2001a). Neural activity relating to reward anticipation in the human brain. *Neuron* 29, 537–45.

Critchley, H. D., Mathias, C. J., Dolan, R. J. (2002b). Fear-conditioning in humans: The influence of awareness and arousal on functional neuroanatomy. *Neuron* 33, 653–63.

Critchley, H. D., Melmed, R. N., Featherstone, E., Mathias, C. J., Dolan, R. J. (2001b). Brain activity during biofeedback relaxation: a functional neuroimaging investigation. *Brain* 124, 1003–1012.

Critchley, H. D., Melmed, R. N., Featherstone, E., Mathias, C. J., Dolan, R. J. (2002). Volitional control of autonomic arousal: a functional magnetic resonance study. *Neuroimage.* 6, 909–19.

Critchley, H. D., Wiens, S., Rotshstein, P., Öhman. A., Dolan.R. J. (2004). Neural systems supporting awareness. *Nature Neuroscience* 7,189–95.

Critchley, H. D., Rotshtein, P., Nagai, Y., O'Doherty, J., Mathias, C. J., Dolan, R. J. (2005a). Activity in the human brain predicting differential heart rate responses to emotional facial expressions. *Neuroimage* 24, 751–62.

Critchley, H. D., Taggart, P., Sutton, P. M., Holdright, D. R., Batchvarov, V., Hnatkova, K., Malik, M., Dolan, R. J. (2005b). Mental stress and sudden cardiac death: asymmetric midbrain activity as a linking mechanism. *Brain* **128**, 75–85.

Critchley, H. D., Tang, J., Glaser, D., Butterworth, B., Dolan, R. J. (2005c). Anterior cingulate activity during error and autonomic response. *Neuroimage*, **27**, 885–95.

Dalton, K. M., Kalin, N. H., Grist, T. M., Davidson, R. J. (2005). Neural-cardiac coupling in threat-evoked anxiety. *J Cogn. Neurosci* **17**, 969–80.

Damasio, A. R., Tranel, D., Damasio. H. C. (1991). Somatic markers and the guidance of behavior: Theory and preliminary testing. In: *Frontal lobe function and dysfunction*, edited by H. S. Levin, H. M. Eisenberg, L. B. Benton. New York: Oxford University Press. Chapt 11.

Damasio, A. R. (1994). *Descartes' Error: Emotion, Reason and the Human Brain*. New York: Grosset Putnam.

Damasio, A. R. (1999). *The Feeling of What Happens: Body and Emotion in the Making of Consciousness*. New York: Harcourt Brace.

Darwin, C. (1998). *The expression of the emotions in man and animals*. 3rd edition, edited by P. Ekman. Oxford University Press.

DasGupta, R., Critchley, H. D., Dolan, R. J., Fowler, C.J. (2005). Changes in brain activity following sacral neuromodulation for urinary retention. *J Urol.* **174**(6), 2268–72.

Davison, M. A., Koss, M. C. (1975). Brainstem loci for activation of electrodermal response in the cat. *Am. J Physiol.* **229**, 930–4.

Deichmann, R., Gottfried, J. A., Hutton, C., Turner, R. (2003). Optimized EPI for fMRI studies of the orbitofrontal cortex. *Neuroimage* **19**, 430–41.

Deichmann, R., Josephs, O., Hutton, C., Corfield, D. R., Turner, R. (2002). Compensation of susceptibility-induced BOLD sensitivity losses in echo-planar fMRI imaging. *Neuroimage* **15**, 120–35.

De Panfilis, C., Schwarzbauer, C. (2005). Positive or negative blips? The effect of phase encoding scheme on susceptibility-induced signal losses in EPI. *Neuroimage* **25**, 112–21.

Derbyshire, S. W. (2003). Visceral afferent pathways and functional brain imaging. *ScientificWorldJournal* **3**, 1065–80.

Ekman, P., Levenson, R. W., Friesen, W. V. (1983). Autonomic nervous system activity distinguishes among emotions. *Science* **221**(4616), 1208–10.

Elliott, R., Friston, R. J., Dolan, R. J. (2000). Dissociable responses associated with reward, punishment and risk-taking behaviour. *J. Neurosci.* **20**, 6159–65.

Evans, K. C., Banzett, R. B., Adams, L., McKay, L., Frackowiak, R. S., Corfield, D. R. (2002). BOLD fMRI identifies limbic, paralimbic, and cerebellar activation during air hunger. *J Neurophysiol.* **88**(3), 1500–11.

Ferris, C. F., Snowdon, C. T., King, J. A., *et al.* (2001). Functional imaging of brain activity in conscious monkeys responding to sexually arousing cues. *Neuroreport* **12**, 2231–6.

Fink, G. R., Adams, L., Watson, J. D., *et al.* (1996). Hyperpnoea during and immediately after exercise in man: evidence of motor cortical involvement. *J Physiol* **489**(Pt 3), 663–75.

Fish, D. R., Gloor, P., Quesney, F. L., Olivier, A. (1993). Clinical responses to electrical brain stimulation of temporal and frontal lobes in patients with epilepsy. Pathophysiological implications. *Brain* **116**, 397–414.

Fowles, D.C., Christie, M. J., Edelberg, R., Grings, W. W., Lykken, D. T., Venables, P. H. (1981). Publication recommendations for electrodermal measurements. *Psychophysiology* **18**, 232–39.

Fredrikson, M., Furmark, T., Olsson, M. T., Fischer, H., Andersson, J., Langstrom, B. (1998). Functional neuroanatomical correlates of electrodermal activity: a positron emission tomographic study. *Psychophysiology* **35**, 179–85.

Friston, K. J., Holmes, A. P., Poline, J. B., Grasby, P. J., Williams, S. C., Frackowiak, R. S., Turner, R. (1995). Analysis of fMRI time-series revisited. *Neuroimage* **2**, 45–53.

Frith, C. D. Allen, H. A. (1983). The skin conductance orienting response as an index of attention. *Biol Psychol.* **17**, 27–39.

Fulham, M. J., Dubinsky, R. M., Polinsky, R. J., *et al.* (1991).Computed tomography, magnetic resonance imaging and positron emission tomography with [18F]fluorodeoxyglucose in multiple system atrophy and pure autonomic failure. *Clin Auton Res.* **1**, 27–36.

Gelsema, A. J., Agarwal, S. K., Calaresu, F. R. (1989). Cardiovascular responses and changes in neural activity in the rostral ventrolateral medulla elicited by electrical stimulation of the amygdala of the rat. *J Autonomic Nervous System.* **27**, 91–100.

Georgiadis, J. R., Holstege, G. (2005). Human brain activation during sexual stimulation of the penis. *J Comp Neurol.* **493**, 33–8.

Gianaros, P. J., Van Der Veen, F. M., Jennings, J. R. (2004). Regional cerebral blood flow correlates with heart period and high-frequency heart period variability during working-memory tasks: Implications for the cortical and subcortical regulation of cardiac autonomic activity. *Psychophysiology* **41**(4), 521–30.

Gianaros, P. J., Derbyshire, S. W., May, J. C., Siegle, G. J., Gamalo, M. A., Jennings, J. R. (2005).Anterior cingulate activity correlates with blood pressure during stress. *Psychophysiology* **42**(6), 627–35.

Gusnard, D. A., Akbudak, E., Shulman, G. L., Raichle, M.E. (2001). Medial prefrontal cortex and self-referential mental activity: relation to a default mode of brain function. *Proc Natl Acad Sci U S A* **98**(7), 4259–64. Epub 2001 Mar 20

Guz, A. (1975). Regulation of respiration in man. *Annu Rev Physiol.* **37**, 303–23.

Hamann, S., Herman, R. A., Nolan, C. L., Wallen, K. (2004). Men and women differ in amygdala response to visual sexual stimuli. *Nat Neurosci*, 7411–6.

Harper, R. M., Bandler, R., Spriggs, D., Alger, J. R. (2000). Lateralized and widespread brain activation during transient blood pressure elevation revealed by magnetic resonance imaging. *J Comp. Neurol.* **417**, 195–204.

Harrison, N., Singer, T., Rotshtein, P., Dolan, R. J., Critchley, H. D. (2006). Pupil size modulates the empathic experience of sadnesss. *SCAN* **1**, 1–13.

Heims, H., Critchley, H. D., Mathias, C. J., Cipolotti, L. (2006). Cognitive functioning in orthostatic hypotension due to pure autonomic failure. *Clinical Autonomic Research*

Heims, H. C., Critchley, H. D., Mathias, C. J., Dolan, R. J., Cipolotti, L. (2004). Social and motivational functioning is not critically dependent on autonomic responses: Neuropsychological evidence from patients with pure autonomic failure. *Neuropsychologia*, **42**; 1979–88.

Henderson, L. A., Richard, C. A., Macey, P. M., Runquist, M. L., Yu, P. L., Galons, J. P., Harper, R. M. (2004). Functional magnetic resonance signal changes in neural structures to baroreceptor reflex activation. *J Appl Physiol.* **96**(2), 693–703.

Hobday, D. I., Aziz, Q., Thacker, N., Hollander, I., Jackson, A., Thompson, D. G. (2001). A study of the cortical processing of ano-rectal sensation using functional MRI. *Brain* **124**(Pt 2), 361–8.

Holstege, G., Georgiadis, J. R., Paans, A. M., Meiners, L. C., van der Graaf, F. H., Reinders, A. A. (2003) Brain activation during human male ejaculation. *J Neurosci.* **23**, 9185–93.

James, W. (1894). Physical basis of emotion. *Psychological Review* **1**, 516–29, reprinted in 1994. *Psychological Review* **101**, 205–210.

Jennings, J. R., van der Molen, M. W., Somsen, R. J., Terezis, C. (1990). On the shift from anticipatory heart rate deceleration to acceleratory recovery: revisiting the role of response factors. *Psychophysiology* **27**, 385–95.

Kaada, B. R. (1951). Somato-motor, autonomic and electrocorticographic responses to electrical stimulation of rhinencephalic and other structures in primates, cat and dog. *Acta Physiol Scand* **24**, Suppl. 83, 1–285.

Karama, S., Lecours, A. R., Leroux, J. M., Bourgouin, P., Beaudoin, G., Joubert, S., Beauregard, M. (2002). Areas of brain activation in males and females during viewing of erotic film excerpts. *Hum Brain Mapp*, **16**, 1–13.

Kavia, R. B., DasGupta, R., Fowler, C. J. (2005). Functional imaging and the central control of the bladder. *J Comp Neurol.* **493**, 27–32.

Kimmerly, D. S., O'Leary, D. D., Menon, R. S., Gati, J. S., Shoemaker, J. K. (2005). Cortical regions associated with autonomic cardiovascular regulation during lower body negative pressure in humans. *J Physiol.* **569**(Pt 1), 331–45.

King, A. B., Menon, R. S., Hachinski, V., Cechetto, D. F. (1999). Human forebrain activation by visceral stimuli. *J Comp Neurol* **413**, 572–82.

Komisaruk, B. R., Whipple, B., Crawford, A., Liu, W. C., Kalnin, A., Mosier, K. (2004). Brain activation during vaginocervical self-stimulation and orgasm in women with complete spinal cord injury: fMRI evidence of mediation by the vagus nerves. *Brain Res.* **1024**(1–2), 77–88.

Lane, R. D., Chua, P. M., Dolan, R. J. (1999). Common effects of emotional valence arousal and attention on neural activation during visual processing of pictures. *Neuropsychologia* **37**, 989–97.

Lane, R. D., Jennings, J. R. (1996) Hemispheric asymmetry autonomic asymmetry and the problem of sudden cardiac death. In Davidson, R. J., Hugdahl, K., editors. *Brain Asymmetry*. Massachusetts: The MIT Press; p. 271–304.

Lane, R. D., Reiman, E. M., Ahern, G. L., & Thayer, J. F. (2001). Activity in the medial prefrontal cortex correlates with vagal component of heart rate variability. *Brain and Cognition*, **47**, 97–100.

Lane, R. D., McRae K., Reiman, E. M., Chen K., Ahern, G. L., & Thayer, J. F. (2008). Activity Neural correlates of heart rate variability during emotion. *Neuroimage*, Aug 9. [Epub ahead of print].

Lange, C. G. (1885). The mechanism of the emotions. In editor B. Rand. *The classical psychologist*. Boston:Houghton Mifflin; p.672–85.

Liotti, M., Brannan, S., Egan, G., *et al.* (2001). Brain responses associated with consciousness of breathlessness (air hunger*). Proc Natl Acad Sci U S A* **98**(4), 2035–40.

Macey, P. M., Macey, K. E., Kumar, R., Harper, R. M. (2004). A method for removal of global effects from fMRI time series. *Neuroimage* **22**(1), 360–6.

Macey, P. M., Woo, M. A., Macey, K. E., Keens, T. G., Saeed, M. M., Alger, J. R., Harper, R. M. (2005_. Hypoxia reveals posterior thalamic, cerebellar, midbrain, and limbic deficits in congenital central hypoventilation syndrome. *J Appl Physiol.* **98**(3), 958–69.

Mangina, C. A., Beuzeron-Mangina, J. H. (1996). Direct electrical stimulation of specific human brain structures and bilateral electrodermal activity. *Int J Psychophysiol* **22**, 1–8.

Mathias, C. J., Mallipeddi, R., Bleasdale-Barr, K. (1999). Symptoms associated with orthostatic hypotension in pure autonomic failure and multiple system atrophy. *J Neurol* **246**, 893–98.

Mathias, C. J. (2000). Disorders of the Autonomic Nervous System. in *Neurology in Clinical Practice*. eds. Bradley, W. G., Daroff, R. B., Fenichel, G. M., *et al.* Butterworth-Heinemann, Woburn MA; 2131–65

Matsuura, S., Kakizaki, H., Mitsui, T., Shiga, T., Tamaki, N., Koyanagi, T. (2002). Human brain region response to distention or cold stimulation of the bladder: a positron emission tomography study. *J Urol* **168**(5), 2035–9.

Matthews, S. C., Paulus, M. P., Simmons, A. N., Nelesen, R. A., Dimsdale, J. E. (2004). Functional subdivisions within anterior cingulate cortex and their relationship to autonomic nervous system function. *Neuroimage* **22**(3), 1151–6.

McKay, L. C., Evans, K. C., Frackowiak, R. S., Corfield, D. R. (2003). Neural correlates of voluntary breathing in humans. *J Appl Physiol.* **95**, 1170–8.

Morris, J. S., Ohman, A., Dolan, R. J. (1998). Conscious and unconscious emotional learning in the human amygdala. *Nature* **393**, 467–70.

Morrison, S. F. (2001). Differential control of sympathetic outflow. *Am J Regulatory Integrative Comp Physiol* **281**, R683–98.

Nagai, Y., Critchley, H. D., Featherstone, E., Trimble, M. R., Dolan, R. J. (2004). Activity in ventromedial prefrontal cortex covaries with sympathetic skin conductance level: a physiological account of a 'default mode' of brain function. *Neuroimage* **22**, 243–51.

Neafsey, E. J. (1990). Prefrontal cortical control of the autonomic nervous system: Anatomical and physiological observations. *Prog. Brain. Res.* **85**, 147–65.

Nicotra, A., Critchley, H. D., Mathias, C. J., Dolan, R. J. (2005). Emotional and autonomic consequences of spinal cord injury explored using functional brain imaging. *Brain*. 2005 Dec 5; [Epub ahead of print]

Nour, S., Svarer, C., Kristensen, J. K., Paulson, O. B., Law, I. (2000). Cerebral activation during micturition in normal men. *Brain* **123** (Pt 4), 781–9.

O'Doherty, J. P., Dayan, P., Friston, K., Critchley, H., Dolan, R. J. (2003). Temporal difference models and reward-related learning in the human brain. *Neuron* **38**, 329–37.

Ohman, A., Soares, J. J. (1993). On the automatic nature of phobic fear: conditioned electrodermal responses to masked fear-relevant stimuli. *J Abnorm Psychol* **102**, 121–32.

Ongur, D., Ferry, A. T., Price, J. L. (2003). Architectonic subdivision of the human orbital and medial prefrontal cortex. *J Comp Neurol.* **460**, 425–49.

Oppenheimer, S. M., Cechetto, D. F. (1990). Cardiac chronotropic organization of the rat insular cortex. *Brain Research* **533**, 66–72.

Oppenheimer, S. M., Gelb, A., Girvin, J. P., Hachinski, V. C. (1992). Cardiovascular effects of human insular cortex stimulation. *Neurology* **42**, 1727–32.

Park, K., Seo, J. J., Kang, H. K., Ryu, S. B., Kim, H. J., Jeong, G. W. (2001). A new potential of blood oxygenation level dependent (BOLD) functional MRI for evaluating cerebral centers of penile erection. *Int J Impot Res* **13**, 73–81.

Patterson, J. C. 2nd, Ungerleider, L. G., Bandettini, P. A. (2002). Task-independent functional brain activity correlation with skin conductance changes:an fMRI study. *Neuroimage* **17**, 1797–806.

Paus, T., Koski, L., Caramanos, Z., Westbury, C. (1998). Regional differences in the effects of task difficulty and motor output on blood flow response in the human anterior cingulate cortex: a review of 107 PET activation studies. *Neuroreport* **9**, R37–47.

Phelps, E. A., O'Connor, K. J., Gatenby, J. C., Gore, J. C., Grillon, C., Davis, M. (2001). Activation of the left amygdala to a cognitive representation of fear. *Nat Neurosci.* **4**(4), 437–41.

Pollatos, O., Auer, D. P., Schandry, R., Kaufmann, C. (2004). Autonomic awareness: Neural activity during the perception of cardiovascular stimuli: In *10th Annual Meeting of the Organisation for Human Brain Mapping*; Budapest, Hungary pTU285.

Pollatos, O., Schandry, R. (2004). Accuracy of heartbeat perception is reflected in the amplitude of the heartbeat-evoked brain potential. *Psychophsyiology* **41**, 476–82.

Pollatos, O., Schandry, R., Auer, D. P., Kaufmann, C. (2007). Brain structures mediating cardiovascular arousal and interoceptive awareness. *Brain Res* **1141**, 178–87.

Pool, J. L. and Ransohoff, J. (1949). Autonomic effects on stimulating the rostral portion of the cingulate gyri in man. *J Neurophysiology* **12**, 385–92.

Porges, S. W. (1995). Orienting in a defensive world: Mammalian modification of our evolutionary heritage. A polyvagal theory. *Psychophysiology* 32, 301–18.

Price, C. J., Friston, K. J. (1997) Cognitive conjunction: a new approach to brain activation experiments. *Neuroimage* **5**(4 Pt 1), 261–70.

Price, J. L. (2005). Free will versus survival. *J Comp Neurol* **493**(1), 132–9.

Quinn, N. P., Marsden, C. D. (1993). The motor disorder of multiple system atrophy. *JNNP* **56**, 1239–42.

Raichle, M. E., Gusnard, D. A. (2005). Intrinsic brain activity sets the stage for expression of motivated behavior. *J Comp Neurol* **493**(1), 167–76.

Raichle, M. E., MacLeod, A. M., Snyder, A. Z., Powers, W. J., Gusnard, D. A., Shulman, G. L. (2001). A default mode of brain function. *Proc Natl Acad Sci U S A* **98**(2), 676–82.

Ramsay, S. C., Adams, L., Murphy, K., *et al.* (1993). Regional cerebral blood flow during volitional expiration in man: comparison with volitional inspiration. *J Physiol* **461**, 85–101.

Rauch, S. L., Shin, L. M., Dougherty, D. D., *et al.* (1999). Neural activation during sexual and competitive arousal in healthy men. *Psychiatry Res* **91**, 1–10.

Redoute, J., Stoleru, S., Gregoire, M. C., *et al.* (2000). Brain processing of visual sexual stimuli in human males. *Hum Brain Mapp* **11**(3), 162–77.

Rosen, S. D., Paulesu, E., Nihoyannopoulos, P., *et al.* (1996). Silent ischemia as a central problem: regional brain activation compared in silent and painful myocardial ischemia. *Ann Intern Med* **124**, 939–49.

Rosen, S. D., Paulesu, E., Wise, R. J., Camici, P. G. (2002). Central neural contribution to the perception of chest pain in cardiac syndrome X. *Heart* **87**, 513–19.

Saper, C. B. (2002). The central autonomic nervous system: conscious visceral perception and autonomic pattern generation. *Annu Rev Neurosci.* **25**, 433–69.

Scherfler, C., Seppi, K., Donnemiller, E., *et al.* (2005). Voxel-wise analysis of [123I]beta-CIT SPECT differentiates the Parkinson variant of multiple system atrophy from idiopathic Parkinson's disease. *Brain.* **128**, 1605–12.

Seppi, K., Schocke, M. F., Wenning, G. K., Poewe, W. (2005). How to diagnose MSA early: the role of magnetic resonance imaging. *J Neural Transm* **112**, 1625–34.

Sequeira, H., Ba-M'Hamed, S., Roy, J. C. (1995) Fronto-parietal control of electrodermal activity in the cat. *J Auton Nerv Syst.* **53**, 103–14.

Sequeira, H., Ba-M'hamed, S. (1999). Pyramidal control of heart rate and arterial pressure in cats. *Arch Ital Biol.* **13,** 47–62.

Siegle, G. J., Steinhauer, S. R., Stenger, V. A., Konecky, R., Carter, C. S. (2003). Use of concurrent pupil dilation assessment to inform interpretation and analysis of fMRI data. *Neuroimage* **20**, 114–24.

Soufer, R., Bremner, J. D., Arrighi, J. A., Cohen, I., Zaret, B. L., Burg, M. M., Goldman-Rakic, P. (1998). Cerebral cortical hyperactivation in response to mental stress in patients with coronary artery disease. *Proc Natl Acad Sci U S A* **95**, 6454–9.

Specht, K., Minnerop, M., Abele, M., Reul, J., Wullner, U., Klockgether, T. (2003). In vivo voxel-based morphometry in multiple system atrophy of the cerebellar type. *Arch Neurol* **60**, 1431–5.

Specht, K., Minnerop, M., Muller-Hubenthal, J., Klockgether, T. (2005). Voxel-based analysis of multiple-system atrophy of cerebellar type: complementary results by combining voxel-based morphometry and voxel-based relaxometry. *Neuroimage* **25**, 287–93.

Svensson, T. H. (1987). Peripheral, autonomic regulation of locus coeruleus noradrenergic neurons in brain: putative implications for psychiatry and psychopharmacology. *Psychopharmacology* **92**, 1–7.

Taggart P., Sutton P., Redfern, C., *et al.* (2005). The effect of mental stress on the non-dipolar components of the T wave: modulation by hypnosis. *Psychosom Med* **67**, 376–83.

Topolovec, J. C., Gati, J. S., Menon, R. S., Shoemaker, J. K., Cechetto, D. F. (2004). Human cardiovascular and gustatory brainstem sites observed by functional magnetic resonance imaging. *J Comp Neurol* **471**(4), 446–61.

Tranel, D., Damasio, H. (1994). Neuroanatomical correlates of electrodermal skin conductance responses. *Psychophysiology* **31**, 427–38.

Tranel, D. (2000). Electrodermal activity in cognitive neuroscience: neuroanatomical and neuropsychological correlates. In: *Cognitive neuroscience of emotion*, R. D. Lane, L. Nadel, eds. (New York: Oxford University Press) 192–224.

Triantafyllou, C., Hoge, R. D., Krueger, G., Wiggins, C. J., Potthast, A., Wiggins, G. C., Wald, L. L. (2005). Comparison of physiological noise at 1.5 T, 3 T and 7 T and optimization of fMRI acquisition parameters. *Neuroimage* **26**(1), 243–50.

Venables, P. H., Christie, M. J. (1980). Electrodermal activity. In: *Techniques in psychophysiology*, edited by I. Martin and P. H. Venables. New York: Wiley pp. 3–67.

Weiskopf, N., Hutton, C., Josephs, O., Deichmann, R. (2005). Optimal EPI parameters for BOLD sensitivity dropout reduction: a whole brain map. *Proceedings of ISMRM* **13**. p. 1543.

Weiskopf, N., Hutton, C., Josephs, O., Deichmann, R. (2006). Optimal EPI parameters for reduction of susceptibility-induced BOLD sensitivity losses: a whole-brain analysis at 3 T and 1.5 T. *Neuroimage* **33**(2), 493–504.

Wiens, S. Mezzacappa. E. S., and Katin, E. S. (2000). Heartbeat detection and the experience of emotions. *Cognition Emotion* **14**, 417–27.

Willette, R. N., Punnen, S., Krieger, A. J., Sapru, H. N. (1984). Interdependence of rostral and caudal ventrolateral medullary areas in the control of blood pressure. *Brain Research* **321**, 169–74.

Williams, L. M., Brammer, M. J., Skerrett, D., *et al.* (2000). The neural correlates of orienting: an integration of fMRI and skin conductance orienting. *Neuroreport* **11**, 3011–5

Williams, L. M., Phillips, M. L., Brammer, M. J., *et al.* (2001). Arousal dissociates amygdala and hippocampal fear responses: evidence from simultaneous fMRI and skin conductance recording. *Neuroimage* **14**(5), 1070–9.

Wise, R. G., Ide, K., Poulin, M. J., Tracey, I. (2004) Resting fluctuations in arterial carbon dioxide induce significant low frequency variations in BOLD signal. *Neuroimage* 21,1652–64.

Zahn, T. P., Grafman, J. Tranel. D. (1999). Frontal lobe lesions and electrodermal activity: effects of significance. *Neuropsychologia* **37**, 1227–41.

CHAPTER 13

Autoregulation and autonomic control of the cerebral circulation: implications and pathophysiology

Peter J. Goadsby

Introduction

Autoregulation of the cerebral circulation and autonomic neuronal influences on brain blood flow form an important part of the normal control of cerebral perfusion (Edvinsson and Krause 2002). Although autoregulation of cerebral perfusion has been recognized for many years, neural control or neurogenically mediated changes in cerebral blood flow are a newer concept notwithstanding the observation that nerves exist on the vessels dates to Thomas Willis in 1664. The classic view of the cerebral circulation has been that blood flow and cerebral metabolism are tightly coupled under the influence of substances, such as H^+, adenosine, nitric oxide and K^+, that ensure a rapid and matched supply of blood when required without neural influence (Kuschinsky 1989, Purves 1972). Autoregulation in physiological terms is the very specific phenomenon that brain blood flow remains constant in the face of changing perfusion pressure over a range of pressures. In this chapter currently accepted views of autoregulation and the effects of the neural innervation are set out based largely on data from experimental animals.

The innervation of the cerebral circulation can be divided conveniently into intrinsic and extrinsic systems. The intrinsic systems originate within the central nervous system and, without exiting the brain, innervate cerebral parenchymal vessels (Hartman et al. 1980). They are not strictly autonomic in the classic sense of the word, although as their function is better understood such a distinction may eventually be useful. They have been reviewed well and extensively elsewhere (Goadsby and Edvinsson 2002). The extrinsic systems are those that commence within the central nervous system but exit and have an extra-axial synapse before innervating the cerebral vessels. The autonomic innervation of the cerebral circulation is a subset of these extrinsic nerves (Table 13.1), the sympathetic and parasympathetic nerves. The other component of the extrinsic innervation, the trigeminovascular system, is covered elsewhere in this volume.

Autoregulation

Autoregulation is that property of a vascular bed maintaining a constant blood flow in the face of changes in perfusion pressure. It is not confined to the brain but the discussion in this section relates to the phenomenon as it affects cerebral blood flow (Fig. 13.1). The perfusion pressure for the brain is the difference between the arterial blood pressure and either the venous or cerebrospinal fluid pressure, dependent on which is greater. Autoregulation is achieved by variations in vessel calibre: when perfusion pressure drops there

Table 13.1 Extrinsic cerebrovascular innervation

System	Ganglion	Transmitter
Autonomic innervation		
Parasympathetic	Pterygopalatine[a]	Vasoactive intestinal polypeptide (VIP)
	Otic	Peptide histidine methionine (PHM)[b]
	Carotid miniganglia	Pituitary adenylate cyclase activating peptide (PACAP)
		Helodermin
		Helospectin I and II
		Nitric oxide
Sympathetic	Superior cervical	Noradrenaline
		Neuropeptide Y (NPY)
Sensory innervation		
Trigeminal	Trigeminal	Calcitonin-gene-related peptide (CGRP) Substance P
		Neurokinin A
		Amylin
		Cholecystokinin-8

[a] Sphenopalatine in experimental animals.
[b] Peptide histidine isoleucine (PHI) in experimental animals.

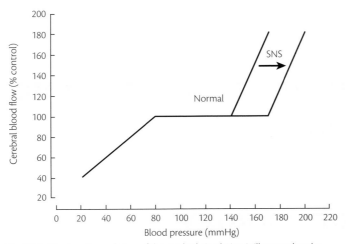

Fig. 13.1 Classic autoregulation of the cerebral circulation is illustrated as the maintenance of cerebral blood flow in the face of change in arterial blood pressure over a range of pressures. It is currently considered that the sympathetic nervous system (SNS) when stimulated acts to extend this range, as indicated by the arrow, thus having an essentially protective effect.

is dilation and flow is maintained, and when perfusion pressure elevates there is vasoconstriction. Experimental data suggest that both small cerebral arterioles and large-calibre vessels contribute to cerebral autoregulation. Autoregulation has a time constant in seconds so that Fig. 13.1 represents the steady-state situation with passive changes being observed during the initial portion of any sudden change in blood pressure. This phenomenon is considered to be a property of vessels and is influenced by the neural innervation, particularly the sympathetic nerves, but locally determined by either myogenic or metabolic mechanisms. The most convincing data explain autoregulation as a myogenic mechanism, such that stretch-dependent vasoconstriction, or vice versa, maintain a constant blood flow. Such a mechanism would be a response to changes in transmural pressure that probably includes an endothelial component and involves calcium entry into endothelial cells during stretch. There is evidence that at lower blood pressures local changes in adenosine may contribute to maintaining cerebral blood flow. It is perhaps of surprise that despite the relatively simple nature of the response and its consistency the precise mechanisms involved in autoregulation remain to be elucidated.

Autonomic neural influences on cerebral autoregulation

Of the currently understood role and effects of the autonomic innervation of the cerebral circulation, the interaction with cerebral autoregulation is by far the best documented. It has been established for some time that stimulation of the sympathetic nerves during hypertension will extend the upper limit of autoregulation. Thus, for a higher blood pressure cerebral blood flow remains constant. It is important that chronic denervation does not alter the limits of autoregulation, so the process is an active one. The clinical implication is that in degenerative nervous system diseases involving the autonomic nervous system, autoregulatory dysfunction is not related to shifts in the normal autoregulatory curve for the cerebral vessels but to disease processes that alter the perfusion pressure. The therapeutic implication is that if perfusion

pressure is maintained, the patient will experience fewer symptoms. It is considered that the shift in the autoregulatory curve seen with sympathetic activation is a protective phenomenon against cerebral damage that can be caused by excessive pressure. Both noradrenaline and neuropeptide Y (NPY) seem to be involved in this protective process. A similar mechanism is thought to be activated to modulate intracranial pressure. Certainly, sympathetic nerve stimulation can alter intracranial pressure. The regulation of venous capacitance and the dense innervation of the choroid plexus by adrenergic nerves is likely to have an important influence upon intracranial pressure and is the subject of ongoing research.

Parasympathetic influences on the cerebral circulation

The parasympathetic innervation of the cerebral circulation represents the most powerful of the neural vasodilator influences upon that bed and its influence cannot be overlooked in any pathophysiological situation. The parasympathetic system is basically vasodilator in nature and is capable of altering brain blood flow independently of the prevailing metabolic demand and perfusion pressure. It is a potential reserve system that is well characterized in experimental animals but still lacks detailed analysis in humans.

Anatomy

The parasympathetic system is that system arising from the superior salivatory nucleus and passing out of the brain in the facial (VIIth cranial) nerve, distributing fibres through the pterygopalatine (sphenopalatine) and otic ganglia and carotid miniganglia to dilate vessels, almost certainly by way of a peptidergic transmitter (Fig. 13.2). The terms pterygopalatine and sphenopalatine imply the same structure, with the former being the correct term in humans because of its relationship to the pterygopalatine fossa. Pharmacologically the system is characterized by the presence of one or more substances, such as acetylcholine, vasoactive intestinal peptide (VIP), and peptide histidine methionine (isoleucine in the rat, thus PHI).

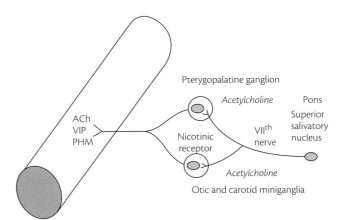

Fig. 13.2 The elements of the parasympathetic innervation of the cerebral circulation. The cell bodies of origin lie in the superior salivatory nucleus of the pons and project from the facial (VIIth) nerve to autonomic ganglia before innervating the vessels.

Origin

Chorobski and Penfield (1932) were the first to describe in detail the anatomy of the facial nerve dilator pathway that runs from the medulla via the greater superficial petrosal to the pial vessels of the cat and monkey. Initially studies examining the parasympathetic innervation of the cerebral vessels defined them as cholinergic. This led to considerable confusion as, although these nerves have cholinergic markers useful for anatomical studies, there was no apparent vasomotor function for the acetylcholine putatively stored in these nerves. It was thus concluded that the nerves had no physiological effect when, in fact, the data, as they were, only demonstrated that acetylcholine plays no immediate role in the effect of activation of parasympathetic nerves. Careful studies using histochemical techniques have shown acetylcholinesterase on the large cerebral vessels. Biochemical and histochemical evidence of choline acetyltransferase (ChAT) activity and the presence of a high-affinity choline uptake system on the vessels have also been useful surrogate markers of the parasympathetic system. Ultrastructural studies have noted a small number of agranular vesicles that store non-adrenergic transmitters. The innervation with cholinergic nerves is regionally variable anterior to posterior and the concentration of nerves along any vessel varies, with the densest innervation being at branching points, particularly in the pial vessels. In the cat and the rat, where detailed studies are available using acetylcholinesterase as a marker, the densest innervation is that of the anterior vessels. Notable variations in ChAT activity are seen between species, with the middle cerebral artery density being less than the basilar in the cat, and other variables such as age being recognized.

The facial/greater superficial petrosal nerve pathway courses to the ipsilateral sphenopalatine and otic ganglia and thence loops back via the ethmoidal nerve to enter the cranial cavity. Ablation of the sphenopalatine ganglion leads to a marked reduction in cholinesterase fibre density in the anterior vessels of the circle of Willis, and it has been shown by direct means that nerves in the posterior circulation innervating the basilar artery also course to the sphenopalatine ganglion. Furthermore, using the transganglionic tracer, pseudorabies virus, it has been established that the central nucleus for these fibres is in the superior salivatory nucleus of the pons.

Transmitters and modulators

The parasympathetic system contains a number of transmitter or neuromodulator substances which are often co-localized in the same neuron. All the substances known to exist in the parasympathetic nerves are vasodilator (Table 13.2) but their precise role and, in particular, relationship to one another remains unclear. Whether these anatomical subgroups with one, two, three, or even four co-localized transmitters have functional correlates remains to be established.

Acetycholine

The cerebral vessels in isolation bind tritiated cholinergic ligands and thus various muscarinic receptors have been shown to exist on them. Acetylcholine dilates most of the cerebral vessels either *in vitro* or *in vivo* by an atropine-sensitive receptor, an effect that is mediated via the release of an endothelium-derived relaxing factor, nitric oxide. Local application of a cholinomimetic (carbachol) into the cerebrospinal fluid causes pial vessel dilatation, which is again antagonized by atropine. Parenteral administration of acetylcholine

Table 13.2 Transmitters of the parasympathetic system

Level	Structure	Transmitter	Antagonist
Brainstem (pons) course	Superior salivatory nucleus	Glutamate	?
	Facial nerve[a]		
Peripheral ganglion	Pterygopalatine Otic Carotid miniganglia	Acetylcholine	Hexamethonium-sensitive nicotinic receptor
End-organ	Cerebral blood vessels	VIP	None available
		PHI	
		Nitric oxide	Nitric oxide synthase inhibitors
		Helospectin-related[b]	

[a] The fibres traverse the facial nerve, passing through but not synapsing in the geniculate ganglion and emerging as the greater superficial petrosal nerve.
[b] Helodermin, Helospectin I and II.
VIP, vasoactive intestinal polypeptide; PHI, peptide histidine isoleucine (methionine);?, unknown.

increases cerebral blood flow, an effect again inhibited by atropine. Curiously, then, it will be seen below that nicotinic antagonists are completely ineffective when tested during parasympathetic stimulation. The role of acetylcholine in these nerves remains unresolved.

Vasoactive intestinal peptide

The characterization of neuropeptides in the 1980s and 1990s led to a substantial re-evaluation of virtually all neuronal systems with respect to transmitter content. Potent vasodilator peptides were characterized, and identified in the parasympathetic nerves of the cranium, particularly VIP and, coexistent with it, peptide histidine methionine (PHM). VIP is a 28-amino-acid basic polypeptide that was first isolated from the porcine duodenum. It belongs to a structural superfamily of peptides along with glucagon, secretin, and gastrin inhibitory peptide. The family is characterized by helodermin/helospectin-like peptides that are distributed in the central nervous system and in endocrine cells, such as the C cells of the thyroid. It has been shown that each of helodermin and the helospectins I and II are vasodilator in the cerebral circulation. There are as yet no data that address the inter-relationship of these transmitters, although they can have added effects.

It has been established clearly that the large cerebral vessels and cortical pial vessels have a rich VIPergic innervation that can be immunohistochemically identified and measured by radioimmunoassay. Indeed, using ultrastructural techniques it can be seen that vasoactive intestinal polypeptide is found in large, dense-core neuronal vesicles in perivascular nerve terminals on the vessels. Two important features characterize this innervation: first, it is predominantly in the anterior segments of the circle of Willis, and, secondly, the fibres may be seen to follow the vessels and penetrate into the parenchyma. However, it has been shown that VIP-immunoreactive nerves that innervate the pial vessels may arise, at least in part, from intracortical neurons. The pattern of innervation of the vessels has further been characterized as having a spiral distribution with respect to the lumen and, importantly, this innervation is seen in human vessels. The origin of the nerves is essentially as it is for the cholinergic system.

Peptide histidine methionine (isoleucine)

The third major marker for the parasympathetic system is PHM. This is cleaved from the same pre-propeptide as VIP and there is at least a 50% sequence homology. PHM and PHI are almost identical, with a difference in two amino acid residues (92, lysine for arginine; 107, methionine for isoleucine), with the latter being the rodent peptide. Immunohistochemical studies have confirmed the existence of PHI(M)-like immunoreactivity on cerebral vessels, and the distribution is essentially parallel to that of VIP. PHI(M) elicits a less potent dose-dependent vasodilatation than VIP *in vitro* and *in vivo*. Microapplication of PHI(M) dilates both arteries and veins *in situ*.

Nitric oxide

The most recent addition to the transmitters or modulators that are involved in parasympathetic cerebrovascular actions is nitric oxide (NO), the physiology of which is dealt with elsewhere in this volume. NO is a short lived, highly reactive molecule, which is capable of dilating cerebral vessels. The effect of blockade of NO production on non-neural responses, such as hypercapnia, remains somewhat controversial in terms of quantity, while its role in parasympathetic responses seems clearer. Blockade of NO synthesis reduces the effect of parasympathetic stimulation in the cerebral circulation (Goadsby et al. 1996). This observation is important because NO can be both deleterious and protective during cerebral ischaemia, thus providing an avenue by which the parasympathetic nervous innervation might mediate protective neurovascular dilatation in the cerebral circulation (Kano et al. 1991).

Physiological effects

Effect of parasympathetic blockade

Given that the cranial parasympathetic outflow to the cerebral vessels via the facial nerve is marked by many neurotransmitters or neuromodulators (acetylcholine, VIP, NO, and PHI(M)), what is the effect of blocking this outflow?

Resting cerebral blood flow and autoregulation

Few experiments have addressed the question of the facial nerve and its role in autoregulation. Sectioning the facial nerve does not alter autoregulation in the cat, while resting cerebral blood flow or glucose utilization are also unaffected.

Hypercapnia and hypoxia

Studies in the baboon, cat, dog, rat, and rabbit all demonstrate no effect of sections of the facial nerve on either hypercapnic or hypoxic vasodilatation. Similarly, Seylaz and colleagues have demonstrated that the main parasympathetic outflow ganglia, the sphenopalatine ganglion, may be ablated without any alteration of hypercapnic vasodilatation.

Stimulation of the parasympathetic nerves

Local nerve stimulation

To further characterize the relationship between anatomically defined parasympathetic nerves and their transmitters, studies have examined carefully the release of the various marker substances of this system *in vitro*. Incubation of cerebral vessels from cat or rabbit with labelled choline chloride, a precursor in the synthesis pathway for acetylcholine, permits measurement of labelled acetylcholine when nerves surrounding the vessels are stimulated. This response may be blocked if calcium is removed from the buffer or tetrodotoxin added, suggesting an active neural process. The method of transmural nerve stimulation has been employed in isolated vessel preparations to examine the possible role of identified putative transmitters. Except in porcine vessels, relaxation is only seen if the vessels are pre-contracted. Transmural nerve stimulation leads to contraction of rabbit, goat, and human pial vessels, in contrast to relaxation in those of the cat, dog, and pig. For the cat and pig it is clear that a non-adrenergic, non-cholinergic dilator mechanism is operating, and available data suggest that the mediator is VIP. Similar studies have also been used to determine the substances that are released when cerebral nerves are stimulated directly *in vitro*. VIP is released when cerebral arterial nerves are stimulated. Indeed, although no antagonist to VIP is available, specific VIP antiserum has been used to inhibit non-cholinergic, non-adrenergic dilator responses in the cranial circulation resulting from both direct and distant nerve stimulation. Finally, an *in vivo* study has demonstrated local cortical release of VIP with facial nerve stimulation. This release is blocked by hexamethonium, demonstrating release of VIP in the context of activation of a classical nicotinic autonomic ganglion in the cerebral circulation.

Effect of direct parasympathetic stimulation on cerebral blood flow

Facial nerve stimulation

Direct stimulation of the facial nerve in humans leads to an increase in total cranial blood flow, as does facial nerve nucleus stimulation in the monkey or stimulation of an area just dorsal to it in the cat. In primates and in cats, stimulation of the nerve with its proximal end intact (that is, attached to the brainstem) reduces cerebral blood flow, while stimulation of the sectioned distal segment will increase it. In the baboon, using the xenon-133 (^{133}Xe) clearance method, it has been shown that facial nerve stimulation increases cerebral blood flow, and a similar effect is seen in the dog, rat, and rabbit. It has been demonstrated in cats, using iodoantipyrine or laser Doppler flowmetry, that such stimulation can increase cerebral blood flow. Clearly, stimulation of the facial nerve increases cerebral blood flow without altering metabolic activity, as reflected by stable glucose utilization and sagittal sinus oxygen content. These responses are meditated through a classical parasympathetic ganglion as they can be blocked by hexamethonium, and probably use vasoactive intestinal polypeptide as the major transmitter of the system.

Sphenopalatine (pterygopalatine) ganglion

Studies of the peripheral ganglion mediating facial nerve vasodilatation have included peripheral reflex (trigeminal ganglion) and central structure (locus coeruleus) stimulation. It is clear that effects mediated by the facial nerve can be blocked by sphenopalatine ganglion removal and that this same response is VIP mediated. Indeed, using at least three different methods of measurement of cerebral blood flow, stimulation of the sphenopalatine ganglion in the cat and rat has been shown to produce strong frequency-dependent cerebral vasodilator responses. Importantly, cerebral glucose utilization and tissue PO_2 are not affected and the response is thus truly neurogenic.

In summary, the cranial parasympathetic pathway to the cerebral vessels arises in the superior salivatory nucleus in the pons; it traverses the facial nerve, joining the greater superficial petrosal nerve to be distributed to the vessels after synapsing chiefly in the sphenopalatine or otic ganglia. A variable small number of fibres in different species (including humans) have this peripheral synapse located in microganglia on the wall of the internal carotid artery, particularly near the carotid siphon. The transmitters contained in this system are acetylcholine, VIP, PHM(I), NO, and helospectin-related peptides. The ganglionic transmission in the periphery is mediated by a classic parasympathetic nicotinic ganglion, while current data would suggest that VIP is the major neuroeffector substance at the nerve–smooth muscle junction. The pathway does not play a role in either hypercapnic or hypoxic vasodilator responses or autoregulatory responses to changes in arterial perfusion pressure. The system can be activated by either direct stimulation or via connections with other important central neural vasoactive nuclei to increase cerebral blood flow independent of cerebral metabolic needs.

Role and clinical implications

Although there have been considerable advances in understanding the basic capabilities and connectivity of the parasympathetic innervation of the cerebral circulation, these data have not indicated a clear physiological role for the system. The nerves are not involved directly in the most basic cerebrovascular responses, such as hypoxic or hypercapnic vasodilatation, nor do they appear to play a role in autoregulation. Their effects are, however, independent of direct metabolic intervention. This latter fact suggests a role in times of threat, such as during ischaemia or in vasospastic conditions, such as subarachnoid haemorrhage (Table 13.3). The parasympathetic system is ideally placed to be engaged to increase cerebral blood flow when ordinary metabolic driving factors are impaired. This protection may, however, be regionally variable since the posterior circulation innervation with VIP is much less than that seen anteriorly. This finding may have implications in situations where predominantly posterior changes are reported, such as migraine. As yet this question has not been adequately addressed. There are, as yet, no studies in human autonomic failure to determine whether there is cranial cerebrovascular parasympathetic dysfunction. The first step will be post-mortem studies to address the anatomical question of whether the nerves are present in usual numbers, while animal physiologists pursue the pathophysiological implications of parasympathetic dysfunction. It may be too narrow a perspective to consider only a vasomotor

function for these nerves as there is evidence that cholinergic mechanisms can alter capillary permeability, including the movement of amino acids. Whatever their function is ultimately revealed to be, it is now clear that the evidence for the existence of the parasympathetic innervation of the cerebral vessels is beyond question.

Sympathetic influences upon the cerebral circulation

The sympathetic innervation of the cerebral circulation was the first to be characterized, with the development of the Falck–Hillarp histofluorescence technique in the early 1960s. The sympathetic innervation of the brain circulation has thus been studied longer and is better understood than that of the parasympathetic system (Fig. 13.3).

Anatomy

The sympathetic nervous innervation of the cerebral circulation arises in the hypothalamus as first-order neurons and projects to the intermediolateral cell column of the spinal cord. Second-order neurons arise from the sympathetic chain and proceed to synapse with third-order neurons in the superior cervical ganglion (Goadsby 2002). The innervation is lateralized and largely respects the midline, with subsequent projection to the cerebral vessels being provided by sympathetic nerves that run rostral with the carotid artery. There is a dense innervation, particularly of more proximal large arteries, which follows vessels out to the pia and along the brain surface but generally only follow penetrating vessels for a short distance into the cerebral parenchyma. The largest part of the adrenergic supply of the intraparenchymal vessels is supplied by the locus coeruleus (Raichle et al. 1975). The sympathetic nerve terminals are often located close to smooth muscle cells in the outer media. The terminals are characterized electron microscopically as small, electron-dense vesicles. The sympathetic innervation of the cerebral vessels accounts for about half the nerves observed in the vessels walls. The innervation is most dense anteriorly, with a relatively sparser supply in the vertebrobasilar territory that is considered to arise largely from the stellate ganglion.

Transmitters and neuromodulators

Noradrenaline

The main transmitter of the sympathetic innervation is the classic autonomic amine transmitter, noradrenaline. Extirpation of the

Table 13.3 Clinical conditions in which parasympathetic activation may be implicated

---

- Stroke
- Subarachnoid hemorrhage
- Migraine (Goadsby et al. 1990)
- Cluster headache (Goadsby and Edvinsson 1994)
- Paroxysmal hemicranias (Goadsby and Lipton 1997)
- Short-lasting unilateral neuralgiform headache attacks with conjunctival injection and tearing (SUNCT) (Goadsby and Lipton, 1997)

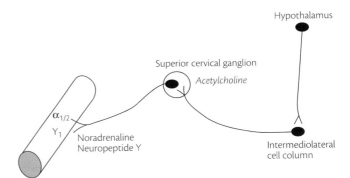

Fig. 13.3 The elements of the sympathetic innervation of the cerebral vessels, including the receptor populations ($\alpha_{1/2}$ and Y_1).

superior cervical ganglion results in a mainly ipsilateral reduction in adrenergic fibres from the vessels. In addition, sympathetic nerve stimulation can cause perivascular release of noradrenaline, while labelled noradrenaline is taken up into the nerves. The effect of noradrenaline release is to constrict the vessels through activation of α-adrenoceptors in the vessels. In humans the predominant receptor subtype is the α_1-adrenoceptor, while in some experimental animals α_2-adrenoceptors can be seen; both mediate vasoconstriction. Of the commonly used experimental species, only the pig cerebral circulation is dominated by dilatory β-adrenoceptors, although all species have dilatory β-adrenoceptors that are unmasked by α-blockade. In humans both β_1- and β_2-adrenoceptors are located on cerebral vessels.

Peptides

In addition to the classic constrictor aminergic transmitter, sympathetic nerves release the vasoconstrictor peptide neuropeptide Y (NPY). NPY is widely distributed in the brain and peripheral nervous system. Fibres that contain NPY form a dense network around cerebral arteries and veins and double stain for noradrenaline (Edvinsson et al. 1983). Retrograde tracing studies have shown NPY-positive fibres that have cell bodies in the superior cervical ganglion, and these fibres are substantially reduced by sympathectomy. Furthermore, NPY co-localizes with dopamine-beta-hydroxylase in cell bodies in the superior cervical ganglion, demonstrating that the peptide exists in cells that synthesize noradrenaline. NPY is potent constrictor of cerebral vessels at the NPY Y_1 receptor. This receptor has been identified on cerebral vessels using polymerase chain reaction (PCR) for the human NPY Y_1 receptor and constriction can be mimicked by the agonist NPY13–36 and blocked by the Y_1 antagonist BIBP.

Physiological effects

Stimulation

Direct stimulation of the cervical sympathetic nerves in experimental animals results in large vessel constriction but no change to small calibre vessels. The effect is more prominent on the cerebral veins and is blocked by α_1-adrenoceptor blockade. Consistent with these data, microapplication of noradrenaline reduces local vessel diameter. The details of this system have been further studied using local transmural nerve stimulation although, because of species variation in nerve supply, the results have not always been consistent.

Physiological roles

The influence of the sympathetic innervation of the cerebral circulation is discussed above under 'Autoregulation' and this is by far its best described effect. There are some data to suggest that hypercapnic vasodilatation is influenced by the sympathetic innervation, such that the response is enhanced, but this requires further study.

Trophic effects

There are excellent data that have established a role for the sympathetic nerves in development, particularly of the muscular layer of the wall of cerebral vessels (Dimitriadou et al. 1988). The trophic effects of the sympathetic nerves deserve further investigation.

Summary

Current understanding of the action of the autonomic innervation of the cerebral circulation is detailed, at least in experimental animals.

The challenge for the next decade is to turn that knowledge into practical applications for patients with disease of the autonomic nervous system. The tools are now available in the form of functional imaging techniques so that we can anticipate advances in pathophysiological understanding in this field.

Acknowledgements

The work of the author reported herein has been supported by the Sandler Family Trust.

References

Chorobski, J., Penfield, W. (1932). Cerebral vasodilator nerves and their pathway from the medulla oblongata. *Arch. Neurol. Psych.* **28**, 1257–89.

Dimitriadou, V., Aubineau, P., Taxi, J., Seylaz, J. (1988). Ultrastructural changes in the cerebral artery wall induced by long-term sympathetic denervation. *Blood Vessels* **25**, 122–43.

Edvinsson, L., Emson, P., McCulloch, J., Tatemoto, K., Uddman, R. (1983). Neuropeptide Y: cerebrovascular innervation and vasomotor effects in the cat. *Neuroscience Letters* **43**, 79–84.

Edvinsson, L., Krause, D. N. (2002). *Cerebral Blood Flow and Metabolism.* Philadelphia: Lippincott Williams & Wilkins.

Goadsby, P. J. (2002). Raeders Syndrome: 'Paratrigeminal' paralysis of oculo-pupillary sympathetic. *Journal of Neurology, Neurosurgery and Psychiatry* **72**, 297–99.

Goadsby, P. J., Edvinsson, L. (1994). Human *in vivo* evidence for trigeminovascular activation in cluster headache. *Brain* **117**, 427–34.

Goadsby, P. J., Edvinsson, L. (2002). Neurovascular control of the cerebral circulation. In: Edvinsson, L. and Krause, D. N., editors. *Cerebral Blood Flow and Metabolism.* Philadelphia: Lippincott Williams & Wilkins, 172–88.

Goadsby, P. J., Edvinsson, L., Ekman, R. (1990) Vasoactive peptide release in the extracerebral circulation of humans during migraine headache. *Ann. Neurol.* **28**, 183–87.

Goadsby, P. J., Lipton, R. B. (1997). A review of paroxysmal hemicranias, SUNCT syndrome and other short-lasting headaches with autonomic features, including new cases. *Brain* **120**, 193–209.

Goadsby, P. J., Uddman, R., Edvinsson, L. (1996). Cerebral vasodilatation in the cat involves nitric oxide from parasympathetic nerves. *Brain Research* **707**, 110–118.

Hartman, B. K., Swanson, L. W., Raichle, M. E., Preskorn, S. H., Clark, H. B. (1980). Central adrenergic regulation of cerebral microvascular permeability and blood flow; anatomic and physiologic evidence. *The Cerebral Microvasculature—Advances in Experimental Medicine and Biology* **131**, 113–26.

Kano, M., Moskowitz, M. A., Yokota, M. (1991). Parasympathetic dennervation of rat pial vessels significantly increases infarction volume following middle cerebral artery occlusion. *J Cereb. Blood. Flow. Metab.* **11**, 628–37.

Kuschinsky, W. (1989). Coupling of blood flow and metabolism in the brain- the classical view. In: Seylaz, J. and Sercombe, R., editors. *Neurotransmission and cerebrovascular function* (vol 2). Amsterdam: Elsevier Science Publishers, 331–42.

Purves, M. J. (1972). *The Physiology of the Cerebral Circulation.* Cambridge: Cambridge University Press.

Raichle, M. E., Hartman, B. K., Eichling, J. O., Sharpe, L. G. (1975). Central noradrenergic regulation of cerebral blood flow and vascular permeability. *Proceedings of the National Academy of Science (USA)* **72**, 3726–30.

CHAPTER 14

Autonomic control of the airways

Peter J. Barnes

Introduction

Autonomic nerves of the airways regulate the calibre of the airways and control airway smooth muscle tone, airway blood flow, and mucus secretion. They may also influence the inflammatory process and play an integral role in host defence.

Overview of airway innervation

Neural control of airway function is more complex than previously appreciated. Many neurotransmitters are now identified and these act on a multitude of autonomic receptors. Three types of airway nerve are recognized (Barnes 1986):

- parasympathetic nerves that release acetylcholine (ACh)
- sympathetic nerves that release noradrenaline
- afferent (sensory nerves), the primary transmitter of which may be glutamate.

In addition to these classic transmitters, multiple neuropeptides have now been localized to airway nerves and may have potent effects on airway function (Barnes et al. 1991). All of these neurotransmitters act on receptors that are expressed on the surface of target cells in the airway. It is increasingly recognized that a single transmitter may act on several subtypes of receptor, which may lead to different cellular effects mediated via different second messenger systems.

Several neural mechanisms are involved in the regulation of airway calibre and abnormalities in neural control may contribute to airway narrowing in disease (Fig. 14.1). Neural mechanisms may be involved in the pathophysiology of airway diseases, such as asthma and chronic obstructive pulmonary disease (COPD), contributing to the symptoms and possibly to the inflammatory response (Barnes 1986). There is a close interrelationship between inflammation and neural responses in the airways, since inflammatory mediators may influence the release of neurotransmitters via activation of sensory nerves leading to reflex effects and via stimulation of prejunctional receptors that influence the release of neurotransmitters (Barnes 1992). In turn, neural mechanisms may influence the nature of the inflammatory response, either reducing inflammation or exaggerating the inflammatory response.

Neural interactions

Complex interactions between various components of the autonomic nervous system are now recognized. Adrenergic nerves may modulate cholinergic neurotransmission in the airways and sensory nerves may influence neurotransmission in parasympathetic ganglia and at postganglionic nerves. This means that changes in the function of one neural pathway may have effects on several other pathways.

Cotransmission

Although it was once the dogma that each nerve has its own unique transmitter it is now apparent that almost every nerve contains multiple transmitters (Fig. 14.2). Thus airway parasympathetic nerves, in which the primary transmitter is ACh, also contain the neuropeptides vasoactive intestinal polypeptide (VIP), peptide histidine isoleucine/methionine (PHI/M), pituitary adenylate cyclase-activating peptide (PACAP), helodermin, galanin and nitric oxide (NO) (Fig. 14.3). These cotransmitters may have either facilitatory or antagonistic effects on target cells, or may influence the release of the primary transmitter via prejunctional receptors. Thus VIP modulates the release of ACh from airway cholinergic nerves. Sympathetic nerves, which release noradrenaline, may also release

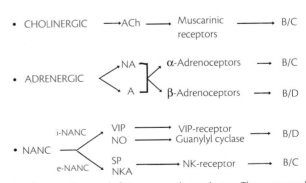

Fig. 14.1 Autonomic control of airway smooth muscle tone. There are neural mechanisms resulting in bronchoconstriction (B/C) and bronchodilatation (B/D). ACh, acetylcholine; NA, noradrenaline; A, adrenaline; VIP, vasoactive intestinal peptide; NO, nitric oxide; i-NANC, inhibitory non-adrenergic non-cholinergic nerves; e-NANC, excitatory non-adrenergic non-cholinergic nerves; NK, neurokinin.

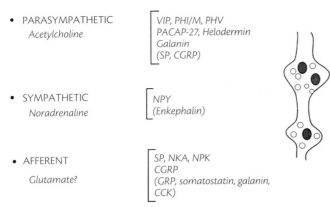

- PARASYMPATHETIC
  Acetylcholine

  [VIP, PHI/M, PHV
  PACAP-27, Helodermin
  Galanin
  (SP, CGRP)]

- SYMPATHETIC
  Noradrenaline

  [NPY
  (Enkephalin)]

- AFFERENT
  Glutamate?

  [SP, NKA, NPK
  CGRP
  (GRP, somatostatin, galanin,
  CCK)]

Fig. 14.2 Cotransmission in airway nerves.

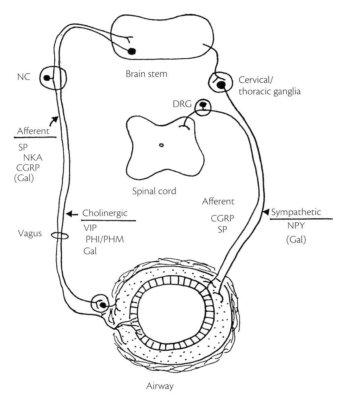

Fig. 14.3 Neurotransmitters and cotransmitters in airway nerves. SP, substance P; NKA, neurokinin A; CGRP, calcitonin-gene-related peptide; Gal, galanin; VIP, vasoactive intestinal peptide; PHI/PHM, peptide histidine isoleucine/methionine; NPY, neuropeptide Y.

neuropeptide Y (NPY) and enkephalins, whereas afferent nerves may contain a variety of peptides, including substance P (SP), neurokinin A (NKA), calcitonin-gene-related peptide (CGRP), galanin, VIP and cholecystokinin.

The physiological role of neurotransmission may be in 'fine-tuning' of neural control. Neuropeptides may be preferentially released by high frequency firing of nerves, and their effects may therefore only become manifest under conditions of excessive nerve stimulation. Neuropeptide neurotransmitters may also act on target cells different from the primary transmitter, resulting in different physiological effects. Thus in airways ACh causes bronchoconstriction, but VIP which is co-released may have its major effect on bronchial vessels, thus increasing blood flow to the airways. In chronic inflammation the role of cotransmitters may be increased by alterations in the expression of their receptors or by increased synthesis of transmitters via increased gene transcription.

Afferent nerves

The sensory innervation of the respiratory tract is mainly carried in the vagus nerve. The neuronal cell bodies are localized to the nodose and jugular ganglia and input to the solitary tract nucleus in the brain stem. A few sensory fibres supplying the lower airways enter the spinal cord in the upper thoracic sympathetic trunks, but their contribution to respiratory reflexes is minor and it is uncertain whether they are represented in humans. There is a tonic discharge of sensory nerves that has a regulatory effect on respiratory function and also triggers powerful protective reflex mechanisms in response to inhaled noxious agents, physical stimuli or certain inflammatory mediators.

Laryngeal innervation

The larynx is richly supplied with sensory nerves that are derived from the superior laryngeal nerve. There are numerous sensory arborizations with the appearance of mechanoreceptors. Electrophysiological studies indicate that many afferents function like rapidly adapting (irritant) receptors in the lower respiratory tract. It is this rich sensory innervation that allows the larynx to function as the first line of defence of the lower airways.

Laryngeal afferents are activated by both hypotonic and hypertonic fluids, although the former are a more potent stimulus. These afferents are particularly sensitive to water and some of these fibres respond primarily to an absence of chloride ions. This sensitivity to low chloride ions appears to be confined to the larynx and upper trachea, and may be important in the coughing response to citrate and bicarbonate aerosols in evoking cough in humans.

Laryngeal afferents are also stimulated by mechanical stimulation and by inhaled particulate matter. There is a wide variety of chemical irritants that stimulate laryngeal afferents, including ammonia, cigarette smoke and CS riot gas. There is a limited sensitivity to capsaicin, which may reflect the paucity of unmyelinated fibres in the larynx. Interestingly, there are also specific cold receptors that appear to be stimulated by l-menthol, and may be involved in reflex responses to cold air, including cough.

Laryngeal reflexes

A major function of laryngeal sensory endings is to trigger defence reflexes in the airways, including bronchoconstriction and mucus secretion, to protect the lower respiratory tract against the harmful effects of inhaled foreign agents. Aspiration of fluids or chemical irritants is associated with ventilatory changes, including cough, inhibition of breathing and swallowing. In immature animals the apnoeic response is predominant, and although evolved to prevent inspiration of fluids into the lungs it has been implicated in cot deaths in human infants. Laryngeal stimulation elicits an increase in tracheal mucus secretion and this effect is due to reflex cholinergic stimulation.

A laryngeal reflex bronchodilatation has also been demonstrated recently in animals and humans, but only becomes apparent when cholinergic reflexes are blocked (Lammers et al. 1992). This appears to be mediated by inhibitory non-adrenergic non-cholinergic (i-NANC) nerves that release NO. It is unlikely that this reflex is important in airway defence as the cholinergic constrictor reflex predominates, but if i-NANC mechanisms become defective, as might occur in chronic inflammation of the airways, then this would lead to exaggerated laryngeal reflex bronchoconstriction.

Lower airway innervation

At least three types of afferent fibre have been identified in the lower airways (Mazzone 2004) (Fig. 14.4). Most of the information on their function has been obtained from studies in anaesthetized animals. It has been difficult to apply electrophysiological techniques to humans, so it is difficult to know how much of the information obtained in anaesthetized animals can be extrapolated to human airways.

Slowly adapting receptors

Myelinated fibres associated with smooth muscle of proximal airways are probably slowly adapting (pulmonary stretch) receptors (SAR), which are involved in reflex control of breathing. Activation of SARs reduces efferent vagal discharge and mediates bronchodilatation. During tracheal constriction the activity of SARs may serve to limit the bronchoconstrictor response. SARs may play a role in the cough reflex, because when these receptors are destroyed by high concentration of SO_2 the cough response to mechanical stimulation is lost.

Rapidly adapting receptors

Myelinated fibres in the epithelium, particularly at the branching points of proximal airways, show rapid adaptation. Rapidly adapting receptors (RAR) account for 10–30% of the myelinated nerve endings in the airways. These endings are sensitive to mechanical stimulation and to mediators such as histamine. The response of RAR to histamine is partly due to mechanical distortion consequent on bronchoconstriction, although if this is prevented by pretreatment with isoprenaline the RAR response is not abolished, indicating a direct stimulatory effect of histamine. It is likely that mechanical distortion of the airway may amplify irritant receptor discharge.

RAR with widespread arborizations are very numerous in the area of the carina, where they have been termed 'cough receptors' as cough can be evoked by even the slightest touch in this region. RAR respond to inhaled cigarette smoke, ozone, serotonin, and prostaglandin $F_{2\alpha}$, although it is possible that these responses are secondary to the mechanical distortion produced by the bronchoconstrictor response to these irritants. Neurophysiological studies using an *in vitro* preparation in guinea pig trachea and bronchi show that most afferent fibres are myelinated and belong to the Aδ-fibre group. Although these fibres are activated by mechanical stimulation and low pH, they are not sensitive to capsaicin, histamine or bradykinin (Fox et al. 1993).

C-Fibres

There is a high density of unmyelinated (C-fibres) in the airways and they greatly outnumber myelinated fibres. In the bronchi C-fibres account for 80–90% of all afferent fibres in cats. C-fibres play an important role in the defence of the lower respiratory tract (Canning 2006). C-fibres contain neuropeptides, including SP, NKA and CGRP, which confer a motor function on these nerves. Bronchial C-fibres are insensitive to lung inflation and deflation, but typically respond to chemical stimulation. *In vivo* studies suggest that bronchial C-fibres in dogs respond to the inflammatory mediators histamine, bradykinin, serotonin, and prostaglandins. They are selectively stimulated by capsaicin given either intravenously or by inhalation and are also stimulated by SO_2 and cigarette smoke. Since these fibres are relatively unaffected by lung mechanics, it is likely that these agents act directly on the unmyelinated endings in the airway epithelium. In the *in vitro* guinea pig trachea preparation C-fibres are stimulated by capsaicin and by bradykinin, but not by histamine, serotonin or prostaglandins (with the possible exception of prostacyclin) (Fox et al. 1993). Both RARs and C-fibres are sensitive to water and hyperosmotic solutions, with RARs showing a greater sensitivity to hypotonic and C-fibres to hypertonic saline. In the *in vitro* guinea pig trachea preparation Aδ-fibres and C-fibres are stimulated by water and by hyperosmolar solutions; a small proportion of Aδ-fibres are also stimulated by low chloride solutions, whereas most C-fibres are.

Pulmonary C-fibres that are activated via the pulmonary circulation appear to have different properties to bronchial C-fibres. Lobeline, which stimulates pulmonary but not bronchial C-fibres, causes cough when perfused through the pulmonary circulation, suggesting that pulmonary C-fibres may be involved in the cough reflex.

Defence reflexes

Afferent nerves play a critical role in defence of the airways. There are powerful protective reflexes evoked by stimulation of afferent nerve endings on the surface of the larynx that serve to limit access of noxious agents to the gas exchanging surface. If this line of defence is breached, there are additional defensive reflexes activated within the lower respiratory tract. These reflexes include changes in the pattern of breathing (rapid shallow breathing or in infants apnoea), constriction of the airways, increased airway secretions, and increased blood flow in the tracheal and bronchial circulations. These responses comprise a coordinated response that limits the access of the noxious agent to the delicate gas exchanging surface of the lung in order to preserve oxygenation.

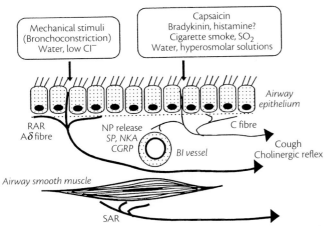

Fig. 14.4 Afferent nerves in airways. Slowly adapting receptors (SAR) are found in airway smooth muscle, whereas rapidly adapting myelinated (RAR) and unmyelinated C-fibres are present in the airway mucosa.

Cough

Cough is an important defence reflex, which may be triggered from either laryngeal or lower airway afferents. It is characterized by violent expiration, which provides the high flow rate needed to expel foreign particles and mucus from the lower respiratory tract. There is still debate about which are the most important afferents for initiation of cough and this may be dependent on the stimulus. Thus RARs are activated by mechanical stimuli (e.g. particulate matter), bronchoconstrictors and hypotonic saline and water, whereas C-fibres are more sensitive to hypertonic solutions, bradykinin, and capsaicin (Carr and Undem 2003). In normal humans inhaled capsaicin is a potent tussive stimulus and this is associated with a transient bronchoconstrictor reflex that is abolished by an anticholinergic drug. It is not certain whether this is due to stimulation of C-fibres in the larynx, but as these are very sparse it is likely that bronchial C-fibres are also involved. Citric acid is commonly used to stimulate coughing in experimental challenges in human subjects; it is likely that it produces cough by a combination of low pH (which stimulates C-fibres) and low chloride (which may stimulate laryngeal and lower airway afferents). Inhaled bradykinin causes coughing and a raw sensation retrosternally, which may be due to stimulation of C-fibres in the lower airways. Bradykinin appears to be a relatively pure stimulant of C fibres (Fox et al. 1993). Prostaglandins E_2 and $F_{2\alpha}$ are potent tussive agents in humans and also sensitize the cough reflex. This may be relevant to airway defences, since noxious agents may stimulate the release of prostaglandins (particularly PGE_2) from airway sensory nerves, and this may lead to enhanced sensitivity of the cough reflex and thus a greater likelihood of expelling the noxious agent if it persists. Bronchoconstriction and increased mucus secretion are often caused by the same stimuli that provoke cough, thereby increasing the efficiency of the cough reflex. C-fibres are activated by capsaicin and acid via vanilloid receptors (TRPV1), for which small molecule inhibitors have now been developed (Jia et al. 2005).

Cholinergic nerves

Cholinergic nerves are the major neural bronchoconstrictor mechanism in human airway, and are the major determinant of airway calibre.

Cholinergic control of airways

Cholinergic nerve fibres arise in the nucleus ambiguus in the brainstem and travel down the vagus nerve and synapse in parasympathetic ganglia, which are located within the airway wall. From these ganglia short postganglionic fibres travel to airway smooth muscle and submucosal glands (Fig. 14.5). In animals, electrical stimulation of the vagus nerve causes release of ACh from cholinergic nerve terminals, with activation of muscarinic cholinergic receptors on smooth muscle and gland cells, which results in bronchoconstriction and mucus secretion. Prior administration of a muscarinic receptor antagonist, such as atropine, prevents vagally induced bronchoconstriction.

Muscarinic receptors

Four subtypes of muscarinic receptor have now been identified by binding studies and pharmacologically in lung (Barnes 1993). The muscarinic receptors that mediate bronchoconstriction in human and animal airways belong to the M3-receptor subtype, whereas

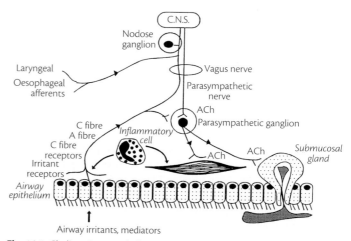

Fig. 14.5 Cholinergic control of airway smooth muscle. Preganglionic and postganglionic parasympathetic nerves release acetylcholine (ACh) and can be activated by airway and extrapulmonary afferent nerves.

mucus secretion appears to be mediated by M1- and M3-receptors. Muscarinic receptor stimulation results in vasodilatation via activation of M3-receptors on endothelial cells that release NO. M1-receptors are also localized to parasympathetic ganglia, where they facilitate the neurotransmission mediated via nicotinic receptors (Fig. 14.6).

Inhibitory muscarinic receptors (autoreceptors) have been demonstrated on cholinergic nerves of airways in animals *in vivo*, and in human bronchi *in vitro* (Barnes 1993). These prejunctional receptors inhibit ACh release and may serve to limit vagal bronchoconstriction. Autoreceptors in human airways belong to the M_2-receptor subtype, whereas those on airway smooth muscle and glands belong to the M_3-receptor subtype. Drugs such as atropine and ipratropium bromide, which block both prejunctional M_2-receptors and postjunctional M_3-receptors on smooth muscle

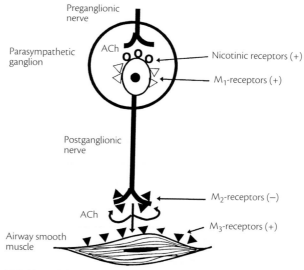

Fig. 14.6 Muscarinic receptor subtypes in airways. M_2-receptors on postganglionic cholinergic nerve terminals inhibit the release of acetylcholine (ACh), thus reducing the stimulation of postjunctional M_3-receptors, which constrict airway smooth muscle.

with equal efficacy, therefore increase ACh release, which may then overcome the postjunctional blockade. This means that such drugs will not be as effective against vagal bronchoconstriction as against cholinergic agonists, and it may be necessary to re-evaluate the contribution of cholinergic nerves when drugs which are selective for the M_3-receptors are developed for clinical use. The presence of muscarinic autoreceptors has been demonstrated in human subjects *in vivo*. A cholinergic agonist, pilocarpine, which selectively activates M_2-receptors, inhibits cholinergic reflex bronchoconstriction induced by sulphur dioxide in normal subjects, but such an inhibitory mechanism does not appear to operate in asthmatic subjects, suggesting that there may be dysfunction of these autoreceptors. Such a defect in muscarinic autoreceptors may then result in exaggerated cholinergic reflexes in asthma, since the normal feedback inhibition of ACh release may be lost. This might also explain the sometimes catastrophic bronchoconstriction that occurs with β-blockers in asthma which, at least in mild asthmatics, appears to be mediated by cholinergic pathways. Antagonism of inhibitory β-receptors on cholinergic nerves would result in increased release of Ach, which could not be switched off in the asthmatic patient (Fig. 14.7). This explains why anticholinergics block β-blocker induced asthma. The mechanisms that lead to dysfunction of prejunctional M_2-receptors in asthmatic airways are not certain, but it is possible that M_2-receptors may be more susceptible to damage by oxidants or other products of the inflammatory response in the airways. Experimental studies have demonstrated that influenza virus infection and eosinophils in guinea pigs may result in a selective loss of M_2-receptors compared with M_3-receptors, resulting in a loss of autoreceptor function and enhanced cholinergic bronchoconstriction.

Cholinergic innervation is greatest in large airways and diminishes peripherally, although in humans muscarinic receptors are localized to airway smooth muscle in all airways (Barnes 2004). In humans, studies that have tried to distinguish large and small

airway effects have shown that cholinergic bronchoconstriction predominantly involves larger airways, whereas β-agonists are equally effective in large and small airways. This relative diminution of cholinergic control in small airways may have important clinical implications, since anticholinergic drugs are likely to be less useful than β-agonists when bronchoconstriction involves small airways.

In animals, there is a certain degree of resting bronchomotor tone caused by tonic parasympathetic activity. This tone can be reversed by atropine, and enhanced by administration of an inhibitor of acetylcholinesterase (which normally rapidly inactivates ACh released from nerve terminals). Normal human subjects also have resting bronchomotor tone, since atropine causes bronchodilatation and inhalation of the acetylcholinesterase inhibitor edrophonium results in bronchoconstriction.

Cholinergic reflexes

A wide variety of stimuli are able to elicit reflex cholinergic bronchoconstriction through activation of sensory receptors in the larynx or lower airways. Activation of cholinergic reflexes may result in bronchoconstriction and an increase in airway mucus secretion through the activation of muscarinic receptors on airway smooth muscle cells and submucosal glands. Cholinergic reflexes may also increase airway blood flow, particularly in proximal airways. Stimulation of the vagus nerve in animals results in vasodilatation in proximal airways that is partially reduced by atropine, suggesting a cholinergic component. The residual component is likely to be due to release of neuropeptides (such as VIP and CGRP) and NO. Cigarette smoke inhalation results in an increase in airway blood flow in pig, through effects of exogenous NO contained in cigarette smoke, but also via release of endogenous NO from airway nerves. Cholinergic reflexes may also increase mucociliary clearance, presumably via an effect of ACh on ciliated epithelial cells.

Several inhaled irritants have been found to activate cholinergic reflexes in human airways, resulting in bronchoconstriction. These include SO_2, metabisulphite and bradykinin. Both water (fog) and hypertonic saline also produce cough and bronchoconstriction in asthmatic patients, although the role of cholinergic reflexes in the bronchoconstrictor responses has not been fully evaluated. The activation of cholinergic reflexes by airway irritants is clearly part of a defensive reflex, since the bronchoconstriction serves to reduce the penetration of the noxious substance and increases the efficiency of the cough mechanism, the increase in mucus secretion and increased mucociliary clearance result in more efficient removal of the irritant and the increase in airway blood flow may serve to bring in inflammatory cells.

Cholinergic reflexes may also be activated from extrapulmonary afferents and these reflexes may also contribute to airway defences. Oesophageal reflux may be associated with bronchoconstriction in asthmatic patients. In some patients this may be due to aspiration of acid into the airways, in other cases acid reflux into the oesophagus activates a reflex cholinergic bronchoconstriction (the 'reflux reflex'). Presumably this reflex evolved to prevent aspiration of stomach contents. There are also reflexes that may be activated by stimulation of sensory receptors in the nose, resulting in bronchoconstriction and laryngeal narrowing. This may serve as an early warning system so that noxious agents inhaled through the nose are prevented from inhalation.

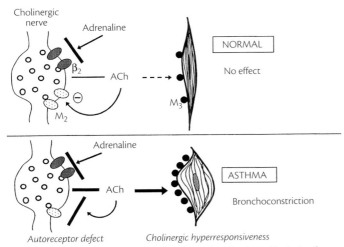

Fig. 14.7 Possible mechanism of beta-blocker induced asthma. Blockade of prejunctional β₂-receptors on cholinergic nerves in normal individuals results in increased release of acetylcholine (ACh), but this is compensated by stimulation of prejunctional muscarinic M₂-receptors to inhibit any increase in ACh. In patients with asthma, prejunctional M₂-receptors are dysfunctional, so that there is a net release of ACh, and ACh also has a greater bronchoconstrictor effect on the airways due to airway hyperresponsiveness.

Extra-neuronal acetylcholine

Recent evidence suggests that ACh may also be released from cells in the airways other than nerves, including epithelial cells, but the role of extraneuronal ACh in human airways is currently uncertain (Wessler and Kirkpatrick 2001). The synthesis of ACh in epithelial cells is increased by inflammatory stimuli, which increase the expression of choline acetyltransferase (ChAT), which synthesizes ACh and this could therefore theoretically contribute to cholinergic effects in airway diseases. Since muscarinic receptors are expressed in airway smooth muscle of small airways, which do not appear to be innervated by cholinergic nerves, this might be important as a mechanism of cholinergic narrowing in peripheral airways that could be relevant in COPD. ChAT is also expressed in inflammatory cells, including macrophages and T-lymphocytes, indicating another source of ACh in inflammatory airway diseases (Wessler and Kirkpatrick 2001). Human T-lymphocytes express ChAT and release ACh on immune activation, but also express muscarinic receptors, so have the ability to respond to ACh.

Cholinergic mechanisms in inflammation

Not only do inflammatory cells have the capacity to synthesize ACh, but they may also respond to ACh through the activation of nicotinic and muscarinic receptors. This suggests the possibility that anticholinergic drugs might have inhibitory effects on inflammatory cells that are activated by neuronal and extra-neuronal release of ACh. A monocyte/macrophage line has been shown to express m_3 and m_5 receptor messenger RNA (mRNA) after treatment with interferon-γ, although it is not certain whether alveolar macrophages have the capacity to respond to ACh. Muscarinic receptors are also expressed on T-lymphocytes but not on neutrophils. T-lymphocytes are activated by ACh via M_1-receptors to release interleukin-2 and thus proliferate (Nomura et al. 2003). ACh stimulates human bronchial epithelial cells to release monocyte and neutrophil chemotactic factors via M_1-receptors

(Koyama et al. 1992). ACh also releases neutrophil chemotactic factors, particularly leukotriene B_4, from bovine alveolar macrophages via M_3-receptors (Sato et al. 1998). Whether anticholinergic drugs have any anti-inflammatory effects is not yet established, but should be further investigated, particularly in cells from patients with COPD.

Neurogenic inflammation

Pain, heat, redness and swelling are the cardinal signs of inflammation. Sensory nerves may be involved in the generation of each of these signs. There is now considerable evidence that sensory nerves participate in inflammatory responses. This 'neurogenic inflammation' is due to the antidromic release of neuropeptides from C-fibres, via an axon reflex. The phenomenon is well documented in several organs, including skin, eye, gastrointestinal tract, and bladder. There is also increasing evidence that neurogenic inflammation occurs in the respiratory tract (Barnes 2001). It may contribute to the inflammatory response in asthma and COPD and may have evolved as an airway defence mechanism.

Activation of airway C-fibres may release several neuropeptides, including tachykinins (SP, NKA) and CGRP. In some population of C-fibres other neuropeptides such as galanin, VIP and NPY are also present. These peptides have potent effects on airway function and may lead to a chronic inflammatory state with narrowing of the airways (Fig. 14.8). This presumably evolved as a mechanism of defence against invading organisms and as a mechanism to repair the airway damaged by noxious agents in the respiratory tract.

Tachykinins

SP and NKA, but not neurokinin B, are localized to sensory nerves in the airways of several species. SP-immunoreactive nerves are abundant in rodent airways, but are sparse in human airways. SP-immunoreactive nerves in the airway are found beneath and

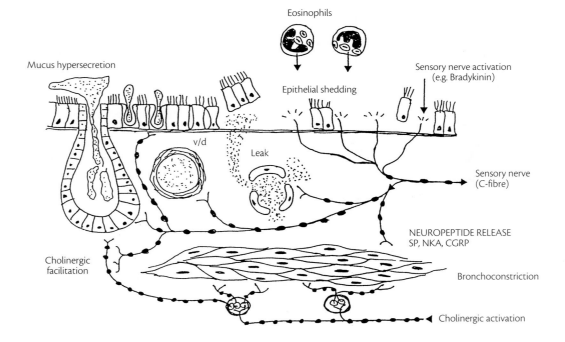

Fig. 14.8 Axon reflex mechanisms. Possible neurogenic inflammation in asthmatic airways via retrograde release of peptides from sensory nerves via an axon reflex. Substance P (SP) causes vasodilatation, plasma exudation and mucus secretion, whereas neurokinin A (NKA) causes bronchoconstriction and enhanced cholinergic reflexes and calcitonin-gene-related peptide (CGRP) vasodilatation.

within the airway epithelium, around blood vessels and, to a lesser extent, within airway smooth muscle. SP-immunoreactive nerves fibres also innervate parasympathetic ganglia, suggesting a sensory input which may modulate ganglionic transmission and so result in ganglionic reflexes. SP in the airways is localized predominantly to capsaicin-sensitive unmyelinated nerves in the airways, but chronic administration of capsaicin only partially depletes the lung of tachykinins, indicating the presence of a population of capsaicin-resistant SP-immunoreactive nerves, as in the gastrointestinal tract. Tachykinins have many different effects on the airways, which are mediated via NK_1-receptors (preferentially activated by SP) and NK_2-receptors (activated by NKA) (Joos et al. 2000). Tachykinins constrict smooth muscle of human airways *in vitro* via NK_2-receptors. The contractile response to NKA is significantly greater in smaller human bronchi than in more proximal airways, indicating that tachykinins may have a more important constrictor effect on more peripheral airways, whereas cholinergic constriction tends to be more pronounced in proximal airways. *In vivo* SP does not cause bronchoconstriction or cough, whereas NKA causes bronchoconstriction in asthmatic subjects. Mechanical removal of airway epithelium potentiates the bronchoconstrictor response to tachykinins, largely because the ectoenzyme neutral endopeptidase (NEP, E.C. 3.4.24.11), which is a key enzyme in the degradation of tachykinins in airways. SP also stimulates mucus secretion from submucosal glands and goblet cells, stimulates plasma extravasation, and increases airway blood flow, effects that are mediated via NK_1-receptors.

Tachykinins are metabolized by NEP, and inhibition of NEP by phosphoramidon or thiorphan markedly potentiates bronchoconstriction and mucus secretion in animal and human airways. The activity of NEP in the airways appears to be an important factor in determining the effects of tachykinins; any factors that inhibit the enzyme or its expression may be associated with increased effects of exogenous or endogenously released tachykinins. Several of the stimuli known to induce bronchoconstrictor responses in asthmatic patients have been found to reduce the activity of airway NEP.

Calcitonin-gene-related peptide

CGRP is co-stored and co-localized with SP in afferent nerves. CGRP is a potent vasodilator, which has long-lasting effects. CGRP is an effective dilator of bronchial vessels *in vitro* and produces a marked and long-lasting increase in airway blood flow in anaesthetized animals. Receptor mapping studies have demonstrated that CGRP receptors are localized predominantly to bronchial vessels rather than to smooth muscle or epithelium in human airways. It is likely that CGRP is the predominant mediator of arterial vasodilatation and increased blood flow in response to sensory nerve stimulation in the bronchi. CGRP is a bronchoconstrictor, largely due to the release of spasmogens, such as endothelin-1. It may also act as an endogenous anti-inflammatory mechanism in the airways (Dakhama et al. 2004).

Neurotrophins

Neurotrophins, such as nerve growth factor (NGF), may be released from inflammatory and structural cells in airways and stimulate the increased synthesis of neuropeptides, such as substance P, in airway sensory nerves, as well as sensitizing nerve endings in the airways (Nockher and Renz 2006). NGF is released from human airway epithelial cells after exposure to inflammatory stimuli (Fox et al. 2001).

Neurotrophins may play an important role in mediating airway hyperresponsiveness (AHR) in asthma and may account for the plasticity of sensory nerves in inflammation, with increased expression of neuropeptides in airway sensory nerves (Myers et al. 2002).

Neurogenic inflammation in human airways

Although there is clear evidence for neurogenic inflammation in rodent airways, it has been difficult to study these mechanisms in human airways. There are few SP-immunoreactive airways in human airways, as discussed above, but there is an apparent increase in patients with asthma, although this has not been confirmed in other studies. The role of neurogenic inflammation in response to inhaled irritants in normal individuals is likely to be minimal or absent. While capsaicin induces bronchoconstriction and plasma exudation in rodents, inhaled capsaicin causes cough and a *transient* bronchoconstriction in humans, suggesting that neuropeptide release does not occur in human airways. Bradykinin is a potent bronchoconstrictor and tussive agent in asthmatic patients which is reduced by a tachykinin antagonist. Since normal subjects fail to constrict to bradykinin, although it induces cough, this provides some evidence that neurogenic inflammation may be enhanced in asthma but is not present under normal conditions. NEP inhibitors potentiate the bronchoconstrictor response to inhaled NKA in normal and asthmatic subjects, but there is no effect on baseline lung function in asthmatic patients, indicating that there is unlikely to be any basal release of tachykinins. It is possible that NEP may become dysfunctional after viral infections or exposure to oxidants and airway irritants such as cigarette smoke, but this has not yet been investigated in humans. Tachykinin antagonists are effective in a variety of animal models of asthma, but there is so far little evidence that they are efficacious in human airway disease.

Bronchodilator nerves

Neural bronchodilator mechanisms exist in airways and there are considerable species differences.

Sympathetic nerves

Sympathetic innervation of human airways is sparse and there is no functional evidence for innervation of airway smooth muscle, in contrast to the sympathetic bronchodilator mechanisms that exist in other species (Fig. 14.9). Sympathetic nerves may regulate bronchial blood flow and to a lesser extent mucus secretion. Sympathetic nerves may also influence airway tone indirectly through a modulatory effect on parasympathetic ganglia; sympathetic nerve profiles have been observed in close proximity to parasympathetic ganglia and postganglionic cholinergic nerve terminals in human airways.

Circulating catecholamines

In the absence of sympathetic nerves, circulating adrenaline may play a role in regulating airway tone. β-adrenergic blockade causes bronchoconstriction in asthmatic patients, but not in normal subjects, implying an increased adrenergic drive in asthma. This might be provided by circulating adrenaline in asthma. However, circulating concentrations of adrenaline (epinephrine), even in acute exacerbations of asthma, are normal. The mechanism whereby beta-blockers may cause bronchoconstriction in asthma is still not

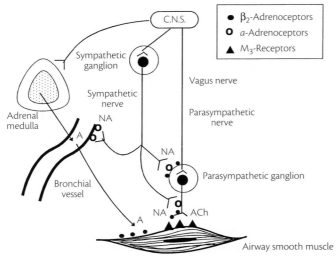

Fig. 14.9 Adrenergic control of airway smooth muscle. Sympathetic nerves release noradrenaline (NA), which may modulate cholinergic nerves at the level of the parasympathetic ganglion or postganglionic nerves, rather than directly at smooth muscle in human airways. Circulating adrenaline (A) is more likely to be important in adrenergic control of airway smooth muscle.

completely understood, but may be due to blockade of prejunctional β_2-receptors on cholinergic nerves in the airways, resulting in increased ACh release in asthma, in which, as discussed above, the normal autoreceptor feedback via prejunctional M_2-receptors may be defective (Fig. 14.7).

i-NANC nerves

There are bronchodilator nerves in human airways that are not blocked by adrenergic blockers and are therefore described as i-NANC. The neurotransmitter for these nerves in some species, including guinea pigs and cats, is VIP and related peptides. The i-NANC bronchodilator response is blocked by α-chymotrypsin, an enzyme that very efficiently degrades VIP and by antibodies to VIP. However, although VIP is present in human airways and VIP is a potent bronchodilator of human airways *in vitro*, there is no evidence that VIP is involved in neurotransmission of i-NANC responses in human airways, and α-chymotrypsin that completely blocks the response to exogenous VIP has no effect on neural bronchodilator responses. It is likely that VIP and related peptides may be more important in neural vasodilatation responses and may result in increased blood flow to bronchoconstricted airways.

The predominant neurotransmitter of human airways is NO. NO synthase inhibitors, such as N^G-L-arginine methyl ester, virtually abolish the i-NANC response (Belvisi et al. 1992). This effect is more marked in proximal airways, consistent with the demonstration that 'nitrergic' innervation is greatest in proximal airways. NO appears to be a cotransmitter with ACh, and NO acts as a 'braking' mechanism for the cholinergic system by acting as a functional antagonist to ACh at airway smooth muscle (Ward et al. 1993). (Fig. 14.10).

Neural control of airways in disease

Autonomic control of airways may be abnormal and contribute to the pathophysiology in several airway diseases.

Asthma

There is compelling evidence that neural mechanisms contribute to the pathophysiology of asthma. It has long been proposed that there is an imbalance in autonomic control in asthma, with a preponderance of bronchoconstrictor mechanisms (muscarinic, α-adrenergic) or a deficit in bronchodilator mechanisms (β-adrenergic). While there is no convincing evidence for a primary defect in autonomic control in asthma, there are several abnormalities that arise as a consequence of the disease.

Activation and sensitization of airway sensory nerves may result in the symptoms of cough and chest tightness that are so unpleasant in asthmatic patients. Cholinergic reflex bronchoconstriction may be important, particularly during exacerbations of asthma, when anticholinergic drugs are relatively effective. The defective function of prejunctional M_2-receptors may contribute to exaggerated reflex bronchoconstriction. Furthermore, loss of neuronally produced NO by the action of superoxide anions, generated from inflammatory cells, may leave the cholinergic neural bronchoconstriction unopposed. Whether neurogenic inflammation is present in asthmatic airways is uncertain, but is favoured by the possible loss of NEP in asthma, by increased synthesis of SP and by increased expression of NK_1-receptors. On the other hand, the clinical response to tachykinin antagonists, which are very effective in animal models of asthma, has been disappointing. Neurotrophins, released from epithelial cells and mast cells, may play an important role in sensitizing sensory nerves of the airways, resulting in airway hyperresponsiveness.

Chronic obstructive pulmonary disease

The airways are structurally narrowed in COPD, which means that the normal vagal cholinergic tone has a relatively greater effect on calibre than in normal airways, purely for geometric reasons. This explains why anticholinergics are as or more effective than inhaled β_2-agonists as bronchodilators in these patients. Neural mechanisms may explain the mucus hypersecretion seen in cigarette smokers, and irritants in cigarette smoke may activate axon reflex mechanisms, resulting in the release tachykinins, which have a potent effect on mucus secretions.

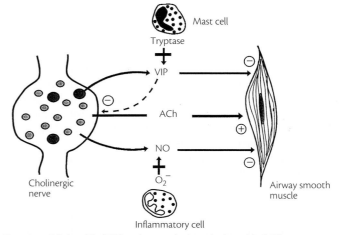

Fig. 14.10 Nitric oxide (NO) and vasoactive intestinal peptide (VIP) may modulate cholinergic neural effects mediated via acetylcholine (ACh). In inflammation NO may be removed by superoxide anions (O_2^-) generated from inflammatory cells and VIP by mast cell tryptase, therefore diminishing their 'braking' effects, resulting in exaggerated cholinergic bronchoconstriction.

References

Barnes, P. J. (1986). Neural control of human airways in health and disease. *Am Rev Respir Dis* **134**, 1289–1314.

Barnes, P. J. (1992). Modulation of neurotransmission in airways. *Physiol Rev* **72**, 699–729.

Barnes, P. J. (1993). Muscarinic receptor subtyes in airways. *Life Sci* **52**, 521–28.

Barnes, P. J. (2001). Neurogenic inflammation in the airways. *Respir Physiol* **125**, 145–54.

Barnes, P. J. (2004). Distribution of receptor targets in the lung. *Proc Am Thorac Soc* **1**, 345–51.

Barnes, P.J., Baraniuk, J., Belvisi, M. G. (1991). Neuropeptides in the respiratory tract. *Am Rev Respir Dis* 144, 1187–98, 391–399.

Belvisi, M. G., Stretton, C. D., Barnes, P. J. (1992). Nitric oxide is the endogenous neurotransmitter of bronchodilator nerves in human airways. *Eur J Pharmacol* **210**, 221–22.

Canning, B. J. (2006). Anatomy and neurophysiology of the cough reflex: ACCP evidence-based clinical practice guidelines. *Chest* **129**, 33S–47S.

Carr, M. J., Undem, B. J. (2003). Bronchopulmonary afferent nerves. *Respirology* **8**, 291–301.

Dakhama, A., Larsen, G. L., Gelfand, E. W. (2004). Calcitonin gene-related peptide: role in airway homeostasis. *Curr Opin Pharmacol* **4**, 215–20.

Fox, A. J., Barnes, P. J., Urban, L., Dray, A. (1993). An in vitro study of the properties of single vagal afferents innervating guinea-pig airways. *J Physiol* **469**, 21–35.

Fox, A. J., Patel, H. J., Barnes, P. J., Belvisi, M. G. (2001). Release of nerve growth factor by human pulmonary epithelial cells: role in airway inflammatory diseases. *Eur J Pharmacol* **424**:, 159–62.

Jia, Y., McLeod, R. L., Hey, J. A. (2005). TRPV1 receptor: a target for the treatment of pain, cough, airway disease and urinary incontinence. *Drug News Perspect* **18**, 165–71.

Joos, G. F., Germonpre, P. R., Pauwels, R. A. (2000). Role of tachykinins in asthma. *Allergy* **55**, 321–37.

Koyama, S., Rennard, S. I., Robbins, R. A. (1992). Acetylcholine stimulates bronchial epithelial cells to release neutrophil and monocyte chemotactic activity. *Am J Physiol* **262**, L466–71.

Lammers, J. W. J., Barnes, P. J., Chung, K. F. (1992). Non-adrenergic, non-cholineergic airway inhibitory nerves. *Eur Respir J* **5**, 239–46.

Mazzone, S. B. (2004). Sensory regulation of the cough reflex. *Pulm Pharmacol Ther* **17**, 361–68.

Myers, A. C., Kajekar, R., Undem, B. J. (2002). Allergic inflammation-induced neuropeptide production in rapidly adapting afferent nerves in guinea pig airways. *Am J Physiol Lung Cell Mol Physiol* **282**, L775–81.

Nockher, W. A., Renz, H. (2006). Neurotrophins and asthma: novel insight into neuroimmune interaction. *J Allergy Clin Immunol* **117**, 67–71.

Nomura, J., Hosoi, T., Okuma, Y., Nomura, Y. (2003). The presence and functions of muscarinic receptors in human T cells: the involvement in IL-2 and IL-2 receptor system. *Life Sci* **72**, 2121–26.

Sato, E., Koyama, S., Okubo, Y., Kubo, K., Sekiguchi, M. (1998). Acetylcholine stimulates alveolar macrophages to release inflammatory cell chemotactic activity. *Am J Physiol* **274**, L970–79.

Ward, J. K., Belvisi, M. G., Fox, A. J., Miura, M., Tadjkarimi, S., Yacoub, M. H., Barnes, P. J. (1993). Modulation of cholinergic neural bronchoconstriction by endogenous nitric oxide and vasoactive intestinal peptide in human airways in vitro. *J Clin Invest* **92**, 736–43.

Wessler, I. K., Kirkpatrick, C. J. (2001). The non-neuronal cholinergic system: an emerging drug target in the airways. *Pulm Pharmacol Ther* **14**, 423–34.

CHAPTER 15

Autonomic function at high altitudes

Mark Drinkhill, Maria Rivera-Ch and
Roger Hainsworth

Key points

- High altitude exposure stresses homeostasis mainly by causing hypobaric hypoxia although the low temperatures can also be a problem.

- Adaptive mechanisms include an increased respiratory drive, erythropoiesis and vascular and enzyme changes.

- Altitude exposure is associated with an increase in sympathetic activity, the extent of which depends on the altitude, the rate of ascent and the time at altitude.

- The mechanisms for the increased sympathetic drive involve chemoreceptor stimulation, altered baroreceptor function, and possibly pulmonary reflexes.

- Chronic mountain sickness occurs in some permanent altitude residents and is characterized by abnormally high haematocrits and packed cell volumes with high blood viscosity and low flows. It is a potentially fatal condition and a serious public health problem in some regions.

- The pathophysiological mechanisms in CMS are unclear but seem to involve a loss of hypoxic ventilatory drive.

- Cardiovascular effects of CMS include impaired cerebrovascular autoregulation and vasomotor reflexes. Orthostatic tolerance, however, is very high, probably due to the large packed cell volumes.

Introduction

Although most human beings live near to sea level, approximately 140 million people live at altitudes over 2500m (WHO, 1996). Populations live at these altitudes in three main regions of the world: the Andes of South America, the highlands of Eastern Africa, and the Himalayas of South-Central Asia (Fig. 15.1).

The main challenges to life at high altitude come from hypobaric hypoxia and the low ambient temperatures. Barometric pressure decreases progressively with increasing height above sea-level and ambient temperature also decreases. The change in temperature is about 1°C for each 150m elevation, so that at an elevation of 4500m temperature is roughly 30°C lower than at sea level. The implication of this is that, even in equatorial regions, temperature in the high mountains, such as Andes or Himalayas does not increase much, if at all, above freezing. The effect of the low temperature

may be offset during clear days by the radiant solar heat although the dangers of radiation at high altitudes should not be forgotten. Night-time temperatures are very low. However, apart from dangers of cold exposure to mountain climbers and trekkers, the main challenge to body homeostasis is from the low barometric pressure and the associated hypoxia.

Up to an altitude of about 2500m (8000ft) most people experience few if any effects of hypoxia, although individuals with mild cardiac or pulmonary disease, insufficient to cause hypoxia at sea-level, could become significantly hypoxic even at these moderate altitudes. Above 3000m some effects of hypoxia are likely to be experienced, and above 4000m adverse effects would be experienced by most unacclimatized visitors. Despite the inhospitable conditions there are many permanent high altitude human habitations. For example in the Peruvian Andes, Cerro de Pasco is a busy mining town of 72,000 inhabitants at 4300m, where much high altitude research has been undertaken. Smaller habitations occur at altitudes up to 5500m.

At 4300m barometric pressure has fallen from the sea level value of 760mmHg to only about 450mmHg. The effect on arterial oxygen tension is proportionately greater because, unlike oxygen tension, water vapour pressure and carbon dioxide tension in the body are not dependent on barometric pressure. Alveolar oxygen tension (PaO_2) can be estimated from the simple version of the alveolar air equation:

$$PaO_2 = (P_{B-W}) \times F_IO_2 - \frac{PaCO_2}{R}$$

Where P_B is barometric pressure, $_W$ is water vapour pressure (47mmHg at body temperature), FiO_2 is fractional concentration of inspired oxygen (0.209), $PaCO_2$ is partial pressure of CO_2 in alveoli, and R is respiratory exchange ratio. At 4300m, assuming no hyperventilation and no acclimatization:

$$PaO_2 = (450 - 47) \times 0.0209 - \frac{40}{0.8} = 34$$

Adaptation to the hypoxia consists of several changes to maximize oxygen availability to tissues.

(i) *Ventilatory responses.* Hypoxia stimulates peripheral chemoreceptors and increases pulmonary ventilation. This decreases alveolar and arterial carbon dioxide tension and consequently

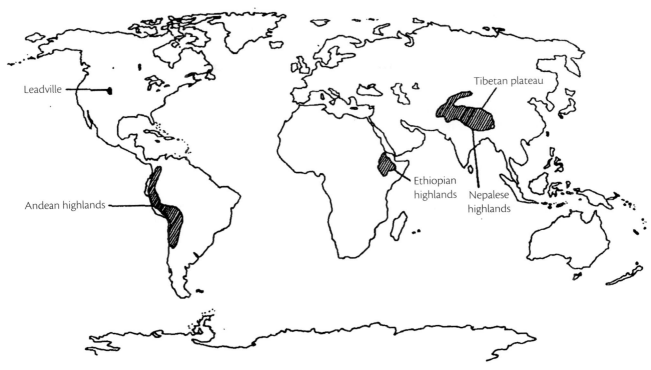

Fig. 15.1 Regions of the world with populations living in excess of 2500m.

oxygen tension increases. This mechanism is of limited effect in the visitor, at least in the initial stages, because the resulting hypocapnia and consequent cerebrospinal fluid alkalaemia decreases central respiratory drive. With adaptation, the ventilatory response is restored, partly by renal bicarbonate excretion, and partly by the active transport of hydrogen ions out of the cerebrospinal fluid thus decreasing the c.s.f. pH and restoring the central drive. The overall effect of this is to reduce $PaCO_2$ in some fully acclimatized residents possibly to as low as 25mmHg. Thus the difference between inspired and alveolar oxygen tensions is reduced (Fig. 15.2).

(ii) *Blood changes.* Hypoxia stimulates the release of erythropoietin and this induces haemopoiesis, and thereby oxygen carrying capacity is increased. This is seen as an increase in blood haemoglobin, haematocrit and packed cell volume. Excessive changes occur in patients with chronic mountain sickness. The other effect is that there is an increase in the amount of 2,3 diphosphoglycerate in the red blood cells. This shifts the haemoglobin-oxygen dissociation curve to the right thereby facilitating the unloading of oxygen to the tissues.

(iii) *Tissue changes.* Delivery and utilization of oxygen are facilitated by an increase in capillary density and an increase in the number of intracellular mitochondria.

Acute mountain sickness

Ideally ascent to high altitude should be gradual with several days spent at increasing heights to allow time for adaptive changes to occur. Too rapid an ascent, and particularly in susceptible subjects, can lead to acute mountain sickness, the severity of which can range from moderate discomfort to life threatening incapacity.

Symptoms include headache, abnormal breathlessness, nausea, appetite loss and sleep disturbances.

The causes of acute mountain sickness are mainly due to the combination of hypoxia and fluid retention. Hypoxia causes vasoconstriction in the pulmonary circulation, partly by a direct effect on the pulmonary vessels and partly through a chemoreceptor-mediated reflex. This, together with fluid retention, results in pulmonary hypertension and oedema. In severe cases, right heart failure may ensue. These effects are exacerbated by increases in pulmonary blood volume or flow as might be caused by physical exercise, or simply by bending forwards which would compress abdominal capacitance vessels.

Cerebral oedema is another serious manifestation. Effects can vary from an unpleasant headache to coma. It results from excessive vasodilatation of the cerebral arteries.

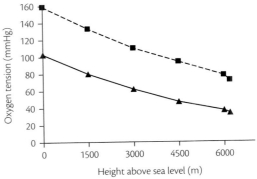

Fig. 15.2 Effects of altitude on inspired oxygen tension ($P_{I}O_2$ ■) and alveolar oxygen tension (Pa_{O_2} ▲). The difference between P_IO_2 and PaO_2 narrows with increasing altitude due to hyperventilation reducing CO_2 tension.

Sleep disturbances arise from the change in the chemical control of breathing. As the individual falls asleep, respiration is depressed. Normally, a small increase in PCO_2 is sufficient to sustain breathing. However, after arrival at altitude control of breathing is changed such that the drive is mainly hypoxic. Sleep causes periodic breathing due to the necessity to increase the hypoxic stimulus.

The only effective treatment for acute mountain sickness, if severe, is immediate descent. It often may be prevented by taking acetazolamide from before ascent until after several days of acclimatization. The drug inhibits carbonic anhydrase and appears to act both as a respiratory stimulant and as a diuretic.

Cardiovascular changes at altitude

Although many studies have been conducted on a variety of subjects, including high altitude natives, lowlanders and acclimatized individuals residing at or transiently exposed to high altitude, integration of the results of the various studies can be difficult due to numerous confounding variables. These include speed of ascent, altitude achieved, duration of stay, the relatively small number of subjects studied and methodological difficulties and differences, such as studies undertaken either in the field or simulated in a hypobaric chamber. Therefore, it is not surprising that many of the findings from these studies are conflicting and difficult to interpret.

The period of initial adaptation, i.e. the first days and weeks following arriving at attitude, is a critical time since it is during this period that acute mountain sickness and/or pulmonary oedema may occur. The processes of adaptation occurring during this initial period may well determine the individual's ability to continue to function normally. Recent studies in animals and man have highlighted the role of the autonomic nervous system in adaptation and in particular the importance of sympathetic activation following high altitude exposure.

An increase in resting heart rate in response to acute hypoxia has been described in several species including man (Kontos et al., 1967). Vogel and Harris (1967) employed simulated exposure to high altitude in man at the equivalent of 600, 3400 and 4600m using a hypobaric chamber. Each chamber elevation was developed over a thirty minute period and was maintained for forty-eight hours. At 3400m resting heart rate was significantly increased at ten hours and by forty hours it had increased by 16% from the resting value at 600m. At 4600m it increased by 34%. Similar findings of an increase in heart rate of 18% have been shown upon ascent to 4300m for periods up to 5 weeks (Vogel, Hansen and Harris 1967). However, this study also demonstrated that the rate of ascent also influenced the magnitude of the heart rate increase. A gradual increase in altitude over a period of two weeks resulted in the resting heart rate increasing by 25% compared with an abrupt ascent which resulted in an increase of only 9%. As subjects acclimatize at altitudes up to about 4500m much of the increase in heart rate is lost and resting heart rates return towards their sea level values.

Acute hypoxia also causes an increase in cardiac output both at rest and for a given level of exercise compared with normoxia. This was demonstrated both at sea level in subjects breathing mixtures of low oxygen (Kontos et al. 1967, Vogel and Harris 1967) and on acute exposure to high altitude (Grollman 1930). The increase in cardiac output at high altitude is due to an increase in heart rate with no consistent change in stroke volume (Vogel & Harris 1967).

As subjects acclimatize to high altitude, cardiac output returns to sea level values although the heart rate can remain high with a fall in stroke volume, possibly resulting from a loss in plasma volume and decreased venous return (Grollman 1930, Reeves et al. 1987).

The effect of hypoxia on the pulmonary circulation is dramatic and results in pulmonary hypertension caused by an increase in pulmonary vascular resistance. The onset has been shown in man to be very rapid, reaching a maximum within 5 minutes (Talbot et al. 2005). Zhao et al. (2001) demonstrated, in human subjects breathing 11% oxygen for 30mins, an increase in mean pulmonary artery pressure of 56%, from 16 to 25mmHg. The effect of hypoxia on the pulmonary circulation is even more pronounced during exercise, as demonstrated in studies carried out on subjects of Operation Everest II (Groves et al. 1987). Resting pulmonary artery pressure increased from 15mmHg at sea level to 34mmHg at 8840m. During near maximal exercise it increased from 33mmHg at sea level to 54mmHg at 8840m. In the short term the mechanism of this pulmonary artery vasoconstriction involves inhibition of O_2 sensitive K^+ channels leading to depolarization of pulmonary artery smooth muscle cells and activation of voltage gated Ca^{2+} channels causing Ca^{2+} influx and vasoconstriction (see Moudgil et al. 2005). This process is immediately reversed by breathing oxygen. However, lowlanders exposed to high altitude for 2–3 weeks develop pulmonary hypertension that is not completely reversed by oxygen breathing (Groves et al. 1987) suggesting vascular remodelling of pulmonary arterioles. This remodelling involves the proliferation of smooth muscle cells and a thickening of the artery wall (Riley 1991).

The autonomic system

Acute hypoxia is a potent activator of the sympathetic nervous system demonstrated by the increase of systemic and regional sympathetic tone (Marshall 1994, Reis et al. 1994). Studies in a number of species including dogs, rats and rabbits showed that breathing low oxygen mixtures stimulated the sympathoadrenal system. Acute hypoxia in spontaneously breathing anaesthetized animals shows increases in sympathetic nerve activity, increased release of catecholamines, regional vasoconstriction and increases in heart rate (Korner et al. 1967, Heistad & Abboud 1980, Rowell & Blackmon 1986). However, the effects of hypoxia on the sympathetic nervous system in spontaneously breathing humans are more difficult to determine and often indirect methods of assessment have been employed.

Catecholamines

Although numerous studies on the effects of hypoxia on catecholamine levels in humans have been published the results have been inconsistent. The inconsistency may reflect the methodology used and differences in the rate of ascent to altitude and differences in the altitudes attained. In man, increased sympathetic activity has classically been assessed through the determination of catecholamine concentrations in urine, venous plasma and arterial plasma. However, the measurement of urinary excretion of catecholamines or their metabolites is non-specific (Rostrup 1998). The sympathetic nervous system is regionally differentiated and determination of plasma noradrenaline concentration gives no indication of regional sympathetic activation, nor does it take account of the rate at which it is being removed from the circulation (Esler 2000).

This means that sympathetic activity may be increased in some regions while being reduced in others. The concentrations of regional venous plasma catecholamines reflect the net effect of both local-release and reuptake as well as the circulating arterial plasma levels.

Mazzeo et al. (1991) studied 7 men at sea level, within 4 hrs and after 21 days at altitude (4300m) and measured arterial plasma noradrenaline and adrenaline concentrations. Acute exposure to altitude decreased noradrenaline by 36% compared to values obtained at sea level but by day 21 it had increased to 52% above sea level values. Arterial plasma adrenaline values were increased by 99% upon acute altitude exposure but declined to only 26% above sea level by day 21. In contrast, in a later study Mazzeo et al. (1998) studied 16 women at sea level and during 12 days of exposure to 4300m. They measured 24hr urinary noradrenaline and adrenaline excretion and measured venous plasma catecholames. Both urinary noradrenaline and adrenaline excretion rose significantly by 44% and 93% respectively after only one day at altitude. Similarly plasma catecholamines were found to be significantly elevated on day 4 at altitude. During the 12 day period noradrenaline continued to increase as assessed both from urinary excretion and in the plasma samples. Adrenaline values however fell back to those recorded at sea level. Rostrup (1998) examined venous plasma catecholamines in 12 men at sea level and on days 2 and 7 at 4200m although 3 days were spent reaching the final altitude. Both plasma noradrenaline and adrenaline fell on day 2 but recovered by day 7.

Results from simulated hypoxia are also conflicting. Johnson et al. (1988) determined urinary catecholamines in eight subjects at a simulated altitude of 4570m for 42h and found that adrenaline increased but noradrenaline was unchanged. Young et al. (1992), however, in Operation Everest II, could not demonstrate any significant change in catecholamines despite exposure to simulated altitudes of 8848m for 40 days. These results taken together, while being confusing, do suggest that in the early stages of exposure to altitude there is an increase mainly in adrenaline, but that later it is noradrenaline that predominates.

The changes in catecholamines are more consistent during exposure to chronic hypoxia. Calbet (2003) measured systemic and skeletal muscle noradenaline and adrenaline spillover in 9 lowlanders after 9 weeks of exposure at 5260m. After 9 weeks plasma arterial noradrenaline and adrenaline concentrations were approximately 4 and 2 fold higher than the sea level values. These values were found to be similar to those patients with compensated chronic heart failure (Azevedo et al. 2000).

The maximal heart rate, i.e. the heart rate at maximal exercise, is reduced at altitude. In Operation Everest II maximal heart rates decreased from 160 at sea level to 118 at 8848m (Reeves et al. 1987). Given the evidence for elevated catecholamines, at altitude at least during chronic exposure, this suggests a down regulation of the β-adrenergic receptors. Studies in animals have shown a number of changes in receptor density in the heart. Voelkel et al. (1981) showed that the density of β-adrenergic receptors in the rat halved following 5 weeks in a hypobaric chamber at a simulated altitude of 4250m. Kacimi et al. (1992) examined β-adrenergic receptor density in rats at 1, 3, 7, 15 and 21 days of exposure to hypobaric hypoxia. Exposure to hypoxia from 1–15 days did not affect β-adrenergic receptor density. However by 21 days there was a 24% reduction. Leon-Velarde et al. (2001) exposed rats to a simulated altitude of 5500m for 21 days and also found a reduction of 24% in β-adrenergic receptor density in both left and right ventricles and an increase in α_1-adrenergic receptor density of 66%, but only in the left ventricle. In contrast Morel et al. (2003) exposed rats to 5500m for 15 days and found no change in α_1-adrenergic receptor density in either left or right ventricle. Density of adenosine receptors has also been shown to be decreased by 46% following 30 day exposure to 5500m simulated altitude in the rat while muscarinic receptor density increased by 49% (Kacimi et al. 1993).

Changes in receptor density have also been reported from studies in man. Richalet et al. (1988) infused intravenous isoprenaline in 9 subjects tested at sea level, after 2 days at 4350m, and after 3 and 21 days at 4800m. The isoprenaline dose required to increase heart rate by 25 beats min^{-1} increased with increasing exposure to altitude and this was attributed to a down regulation of the β-adrenergic receptors. Fischetti et al. (2000) reported a 21% reduction in platelet α_2-adrenergic receptor density after 4 weeks exposure to 5050m. Modifications of the α_2-adrenergic receptor density on platelets may indicate a similar change in the central nervous system (Piletz et al. 1991). In the central nervous system α_2-adrenergic receptors are known to play an important role in cardiovascular regulation (Gavras et al. 2001). Stimulation of these receptors in the ventrolateral medulla has been shown to reduce sympathetic and increase parasympathetic outflow. If a central change in the density of these receptors occurred it may account for the effect of altitude exposure on the autonomic system.

The influence of the parasympathetic system has been assessed in human studies from the effects of muscarinic blockade. Clar et al. (2001) showed that following 8 hours of exposure to hypoxia the sensitivity of heart rate to hypoxia was significantly reduced by muscarinic blockade. Boushel et al. (2001) exposed subjects to an altitude of 5260m for 9 weeks and found that muscarinic blockade increased resting heart rate by 80 beats per minute. This increase in heart rate seen at rest and during exercise to muscarinic blockade suggested to the authors enhanced parasympathetic activity as a mechanism for the reduction in heart rate seen during chronic adaptation to altitude.

Muscle sympathetic nerve activity

Following prolonged altitude exposure heart rate and cardiac output tend to return to sea level values and this suggests a reduction in sympathetic activity. However, as discussed above, the assessment of the role of the sympathetic nervous system to hypoxia has proven difficult to interpret using indirect methods such as urine and plasma catecholamine levels. Microneurography techniques have allowed the direct measurements of muscle sympathetic nerve activity from the peroneal nerve. A number of studies have examined the effects of acute exposure to hypoxic breathing on muscle sympathetic nerve activity and reported an increase in discharge of 6–12 bursts min^{-1} (Duplain et al. 1999, Hansen et al. 2000). Studies of the effects of chronic hypoxia have also shown enhanced sympathetic activity. Hanson et al. (2003) measured peroneal muscle sympathetic nerve activity in 8 subjects at sea level and during exposure to an altitude of 5260m for 4 weeks and found burst frequency to increase from an average of 16 to 48 bursts min^{-1}. Upon returning to sea level, sympathetic activity was still found to be elevated 3 days following descent, at 37 bursts/min.

Heart rate variability

The activity of the cardiac autonomic nerves is often assessed non-invasively using the technique of heart rate variability which is the beat to beat alteration of the R-R intervals. Heart rate variability is known to be heavily influenced by respiratory activity (Brown et al. 1993) and this has largely been ignored in many studies examining hypoxia which itself drives respiration. High frequency components are considered to be associated with cardiac parasympathetic activity whereas the low frequency components are associated with both parasympathetic and sympathetic activity. The ratio of low frequency to high frequency power is said to be an index of the "sympathovagal balance". Kanai et al. (2001) compared heart rate variability in 3 groups of subjects at sea level and 2 hours after arriving at an altitude of 2700m or 3700m. Both high and low frequency bands were decreased at either altitude compared to sea level values although the ratio of the low frequency to high frequency power increased. The increase in the ratio is believed to imply that the sympathetic nervous system is dominant compared to the parasympathetic system at high altitude. Similar results were obtained by Cornolo et al. (2004) who reported that acute exposure to an altitude of 4350m for 1-2 days in 12 subjects reduced power in the high-frequency band but increased the low-frequency power and increased the low to high frequency ratio. From these findings they concluded that acute exposure to hypoxia is associated with decreased parasympathetic and increased sympathetic tone and during acclimatization there is a progressive shift toward still higher sympathetic tone.

Arterial baroreflex

There have been a number of studies in humans of baroreflex control at altitude or simulated altitude but their findings have often been contradictory, reporting an increase, decrease or no change in gain and/or set point of the reflex. Sagawa et al. (1997) exposed seven unacclimatized subjects to a simulated altitude of 4300m and stimulated carotid baroreceptors by applying both positive and negative pressures to a neck chamber. They found baroreceptor response curves to show no change in the set point but there was a 50% reduction in the gain of the carotid baroreflex control of heart rate. Studies by Halliwill & Minson (2002, 2005) in man had subjects breathing room air or 12% oxygen, and induced arterial pressure changes by nitroprusside and phenylephrine. They found

no effect on arterial baroreflex gain of heart rate or sympathetic activity, but in contrast found hypoxia to reset baroreflex control to higher pressures. A number of authors have examined changes in spontaneous baroreflex gain derived from R-R intervals and blood pressure during simulated high altitude and reported a reduction of 35-43% (Sevre et al. 2001, Blaber et al. 2003, Roche et al. 2002). These contradictory findings are likely to be due to differences in the methods used. Hypoxia has a marked effect on ventilation and both frequency and depth of ventilation can affect the baroreflex. In human studies this variable can prove difficult to regulate and therefore makes comparisons between studies impossible.

We recently carried out a study in anaesthetized, artificially ventilated dogs in which we were able to control the relevant variables much better than is possible in conscious humans (Moore et al. 2004a). We compared carotid baroreflex function in dogs living at altitude (4338m) with that in lowland animals and determined vascular responses in a vascularly isolated hind limb (Fig. 15.3). We found that although the gain of the baroreflex was not different between lowland and high altitude animals, the set point was significantly lower in high altitude animals (117±7 versus 90±8mmHg). This difference was reduced by perfusing the carotid sinuses with hyperoxic blood. These results indicate that hypoxia has a direct effect on the carotid baroreflex control of vascular resistance and that it is reset during chronic hypoxia to lower pressures without any significant effect on the gain.

Gastric motility

Gastric motility is regulated through a network of regulatory peptides, hormones and sympathetic and parasympathetic and enteric nervous systems. Yoshimoto et al. (2004) examined the effect of hypobaric hypoxia on gastric motility in conscious rats exposed to a simulated altitude of 5065m, with an ascent time of 8 minutes and 60 minutes exposure. They found significant reductions in the magnitude of frequency and magnitude of gastric contraction wave by 0.5 cycles/min and 65% respectively. Gastric vagotomy abolished the reduction in magnitude of the gastric contraction wave but not the reduction in frequency, suggesting a role for the vagus nerve only in modulating the strength of the contraction wave. These findings may account for nausea, vomiting, and loss of appetite reported at altitude.

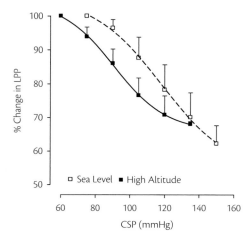
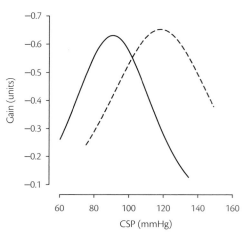

Fig. 15.3 Left. Effect of increasing carotid sinus pressure on isolated limb perfusion pressure (LPP). Carotid baroreflex response curves obtained from sea level --□-- (n = 6) or high altitude ■■■ (n = 8) animals. Right. First differential of the baroreflex response curve to obtain set point and gain. Note that hypoxia results in a reduction in the set point of the baroreflex response curve without affecting its gain.

Mechanism for sympathetic activation at high altitude

The increase in sympathetic activity at altitude is caused by both the direct and indirect effects of the hypoxia. The role of chemoreceptors is reviewed by Marshall (1994). Hypoxia has a direct effect on vascular smooth muscle in the systemic circulation which is to cause it to relax. This would tend to decrease blood pressure resulting in a baroreceptor mediated sympathetic excitation. Alterations in baroreflex function, an increase in "set point" and possibly a decrease in gain, are likely to contribute. An additional mechanism for exciting sympathetic activity may also arise through stimulation of pulmonary arterial baroreceptors. Hypoxia induces pulmonary hypertension (described above) and recent studies in our laboratory in the anaesthetized dog have shown that increasing pulmonary artery pressure significantly increases systemic vascular resistance (McMahon et al. 2000, Moore et al. 2004b). Step increases in pulmonary artery pressure from around 5 to 40 mmHg caused systemic perfusion pressure to increase by an average of 45% (Fig. 15.4). In the same experimental model we have also demonstrated that increases in pulmonary arterial pressure results in an increase in sympathetic efferent nerve activity recorded from the renal nerves (unpublished observations Fig. 15.5).

Autonomic function and chronic mountain sickness

Definition

Chronic mountain sickness (CMS, Monge's disease) is frequently found in long-term residents of high altitudes. It is characterized by excessive polycythemia accompanied by several clinical manifestations, including pulmonary hypertension. It is a major public health problem, especially in Latin America where there are about 30 million people living in the Andean region (Lumbreras and León-Velarde 2003). For a detailed historical account of the CMS see Winslow and Monge-C (1987).

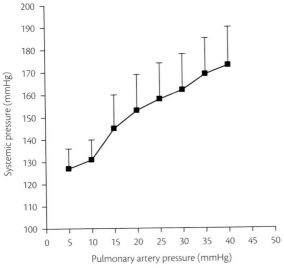

Fig. 15.4 Responses of systemic perfusion pressure to stepwise increases in pulmonary artery pressure (n = 7). Adapted from Moore JP, Hainsworth R and Drinkhill MJ (2004b). Phasic negative intrathoracic pressures enhance the vascular responses to stimulation of pulmonary arterial baroreceptors in closed-chest anaesthetized dogs. *Journal of Physiology*, **555**, 815–824. (c) John Wiley and Sons.

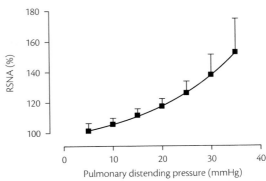

Fig. 15.5 Response of renal sympathetic efferent nerve activity (RSNA) to increasing pulmonary arterial pressure (n = 6, unpublished observations).

Clinical features

Patients with CMS develop excessive polycythemia and an array of clinical features including dyspnoea, palpitations, insomnia, dizziness, headache, confusion, loss of appetite, lack of mental concentration and memory alterations. Patients may also complain of decreased exercise tolerance, bone pain and acral paraesthesias. Occasionally, haemoptysis has been reported. Impairment of mental function, which may be reversed by phlebotomy, was reported in the original description of the syndrome by Monge M (1925). Physical examination reveals cyanosis, due to the combination of polycythemia and low oxygen saturation, and a marked pigmentation of the skin exposed to the sun. Hyperaemia of conjunctivae is characteristic and the retinal vessels are also dilated and engorged. The second cardiac sound is frequently accentuated and there is an increased cardiac size, mainly due to right ventricular hypertrophy. As the condition progresses, overt congestive heart failure becomes evident, characterized by dyspnoea at rest and during mild effort, peripheral oedema, distension of superficial veins, and progressive cardiac dilation. A clinical score was devised in the attempt to assess the severity of the syndrome and to compare CMS cases within and between different countries in the world (León-Velarde et al. 2003).

Pathophysiology of CMS

Extensive comparative physiological research has clearly shown that some species, including humans, are susceptible to CMS whereas other animal species, particularly native animals tolerant to hypoxia, do not develop the condition. The former are considered not to be genetically adapted to high altitude (Monge-C and León-Velarde 1991), whereas native species are (Monge-C and León-Velarde 1991). From this perspective, CMS can be considered as a loss of adaptation or as an inappropriate adaptation to high altitude.

CMS is most likely the result of several influences acting on subjects living at high altitudes. Hypoventilation associated with aging has been proposed as one of the main underlying mechanisms (Sime et al. 1975). Many of the clinical features may be attributed to the excessive polycythemia which leads to hyperviscosity of the blood and consequently impaired blood flow and impaired oxygen delivery to several organs including the brain (Monge-C et al. 1982). There may be a genetic basis for CMS but this is complex to study and, if there is a genetic predisposition it is likely to interact with environmental factors.

Several specific pathophysiological mechanisms have been suggested to explain some of the clinical features of CMS. Vasodilatation in response to CO2 and NO in the region supplied by the middle cerebral artery is defective in Andean natives, both at altitude and in the same subjects at sea level, and this may be implicated in the development of incapacitating migraine. Susceptibility to migraine might depend in part on gene expression with consequent alterations of endothelial function (Appenzeller et al. 2004). Low levels of ATPase found in peripheral nerves were inversely related to symptom scores and CMS scores and may be associated with acral paraesthesias (Appenzeller et al. 2002).

Ventilatory responses

Sime et al. (1975) reported a blunted ventilatory response to hypoxia (VRH) in subjects with CMS. They interpreted this as the basic underlying causative mechanism leading to the condition. The evidence, however, is conflicting. While some studies have found that VRH was lower in subjects with CMS than in healthy high altitude natives (Severinghaus et al. 1966; Vargas and Villena 1993) others have reported a blunted VRH in children and adults without CMS (Sime et al. 1975; Sorensen and Severinghaus 1968; Lahiri et al. 1976).

Several authors have examined the possible role of peripheral chemoreceptors. Bainton et al. (1964) found that high altitude natives have a reduced sensitivity to hypoxia, and suggested that this may lead to CMS. Arias Stella and Valcarcel (1976) found an age-related hyperplasia of carotid body chief cells and they related this with the age-dependent blunted VRH previously suggested as the main cause of CMS (Sime et al. 1975).

Experiments have been carried out to examine the plasticity of chemoreflexes to both long and short term changes in blood gas tensions. Our group at the Universidad Peruana Cayetano Heredia,

in collaboration with investigators from the University of Oxford, studied the plasticity of chemoreflexes in response to longer term alterations in arterial blood gases. In particular, we examined the alterations in the chemoreflexes of chronically hypoxic high-altitude natives. These natives are known to have blunted respiratory responses to hypoxia but there was controversy as to whether this blunting was reversible if they migrated to live at sea level. We found that the natives who had migrated to live at sea level had ventilatory responses to acute hypoxia (few minutes) which had become similar to that of sea-level controls (Gamboa et al. 2003). However, responses to sustained hypoxia (20 min) remained markedly blunted (Gamboa et al. 2003). These results may explain the apparent discrepancy in previous studies. In addition, we demonstrated that healthy high-altitude natives who had been resident at sea level, reacclimatize to high altitude in the same way as sea-level subjects, by increasing their ventilatory sensitivity to hypoxia (Fig. 15.6) (Rivera-Ch et al. 2003). We also showed that, although there was a large overlap in the values for acute HVR from healthy high altitude natives and from subjects with CMS, there was also a strong correlation between haematocrit and end-tidal CO2 pressure which could not be explained only by a reduction in AHVR. These results suggest that the lower levels of ventilation in patients with CMS may arise through mechanisms other than reductions in the peripheral chemoreflex sensitivity to hypoxia. These data do not support the notion that the reduction in the acute HVR plays a major role in the causation of CMS (León-Velarde et al. 2003). Finally, we have demonstrated that, although hypoxia induced a smaller increase in the total ventilatory sensitivity to CO2 in high-altitude subjects than in sea-level subjects, the peripheral chemoreflex sensitivity to CO2 was still no higher in the sea-level subjects under conditions of euoxia (Fatemian et al. 2003). Thus the blunting of the peripheral chemoreflex response in high-altitude natives

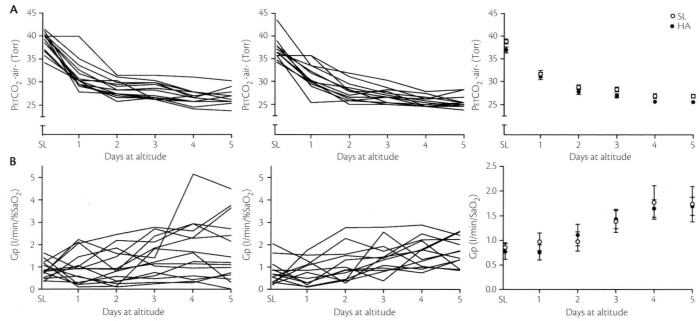

Fig. 15.6 Air-breathing end-tidal PCO_2 (PET_{CO_2}; A) and ventilatory response to acute hypoxia (model parameter of Gp; B) during a 6-day sojourn at high altitude (HA). Left: individual responses for sea-level (SL) natives; center: individual responses for HA natives; right: group responses for SL and HA natives. Group responses are means ± SE. SaO_2, calculated arterial O_2 saturation. Reproduced with permission from Rivera-Ch M, Gamboa A, León-Velarde F, Palacios JA, O'Connor DF and Robbins PA (2003). Hi-altitude natives living at sea level acclimatize to high altitude like sea-level natives. *Journal of Applied Physiology*, **94**, 1263–68. (c) American Physiological Society, 2003.

appeared to be specific for hypoxia, with the response to hypercapnia being either protected or even enhanced. All these findings provide a better understanding of the plasticity of chemoreflexes after lifelong exposure to hypoxia, emphasizing their ability to remodel their properties.

The abnormal polycythemia seen in CMS has been attributed to the diminished ventilatory response to hypoxia. To further explore this area, we determined the respiratory and cardiovascular responses to acute hypoxia, in normal high altitude dwellers and in CMS patients, at high altitude and the day after arrival in Lima. The results showed that at high altitude, with end-tidal PO_2 ($PETO_2$) at 100mmHg, there were no differences between groups in ventilation, blood pressure or heart rate. However, responses to hypoxia (ventilation, blood pressure and heart rate) were smaller in CMS. When the study was repeated at Lima, at $PETO_2$ 100mmHg, ventilation was less in CMS than normals; unlike CMS, normals had greater ventilation during normoxia at Lima than at CP. The hypoxic stimulus, at Lima, again resulted in smaller ventilatory and blood pressure in CMS than in normals. In CMS, ventilatory responses at Lima were even smaller than those at CP.

Cardiovascular responses

Until recently, there had been few studies on the cardiovascular and cerebrovascular control in subjects with CMS. Recently Bernardi et al. (2003) performed a series of studies to assess the baroreflex function and the chemo- and baroreflex interactions in Andean subjects with and without CMS. They found that subjects with CMS showed a reduction in the responses to stimulation of peripheral chemoreflexes. In addition, these subjects also showed a reduction in the baroreflex control of heart rate and blood pressure. The reduction in the arterial baroreflex correlated with an increase in CMS score, and with an increase of haemoglobin levels. Interestingly, upon descent of CMS subjects to sea level, there was an increase in the responses to the arterial baroreflex as well as in minute ventilation, with a parallel drop in CMS score indicative of an improvement of clinical symptoms. The authors interpreted these findings as suggestive of a functional, reversible central depression rather than of the presence of an organic dysautonomia in CMS. They further suggested that the observed baroreflex alteration might be involved in the causation of some of the symptoms of CMS. In another study on subjects with CMS, performed at high altitude, the same authors showed that 1 hour of oxygen administration by a slow breathing pattern or 1 hour of passive oxygen administration were associated with increased oxygen saturation and an increased arterial baroreflex sensitivity (Keyl et al. 2003).

The major mechanism for the control of blood pressure is through regulation of peripheral vascular resistance and most studies have examined only the control of heart rate. We have recently studied the responses of forearm vascular resistance to carotid baroreceptor stimulation in high altitude residents with and without CMS, both at their resident altitude and shortly after descent to sea level. Results showed that in both groups, within a day of exposure to normoxia, the baroreflex was reset to lower pressures but with no apparent change in sensitivity (Moore et al. 2004c).

Blood volumes and orthostatic tolerance. Orthostatic tolerance is a measure of the ability to maintain consciousness and adequate blood pressure during gravitational stress (see Chapter 47). It is known to depend partly on the degree of vasoconstriction and partly on the magnitude of plasma volume. However, the possible influence of packed red cell volume (PCV) is unknown. High altitude residents have high haematocrits but it was not known whether their packed cell volumes were also high or whether their orthostatic tolerance is different from low altitude residents. We therefore determined plasma volume, PCV and orthostatic tolerance in a group of high altitude dwellers, including some with CMS (Claydon et al. 2004). We showed that although high altitude residents have large PCV, their plasma volumes are similar to lowland dwellers. The group with CMS has a particularly large PCV and also has a very high orthostatic tolerance, despite smaller heart rate responses. These results are compatible with the view that PCV is of importance in determining orthostatic tolerance (Claydon et al. 2004). We also showed that the good orthostatic tolerance seen in high altitude dwellers at altitude was also seen at sea level and so it could not have been due to a hypoxia mediated vasoconstriction. There was no difference in orthostatic tolerance between CMS patients, with their exceptionally large blood volumes, and the HA controls. We speculated that this may be because peripheral vascular and cerebrovascular responses (at least at sea level) are impaired in the CMS patients relative to high altitude controls. Thus, the advantage of the large blood volume may be offset by the smaller vascular responses (Claydon et al. 2005).

Cerebrovascular control. Cerebral blood flow is known to be less in CMS patients than in healthy controls and this is attributed to the high viscosity of the blood. The cerebral circulation normally shows an efficient autoregulation whereby changes in cerebral perfusion pressure have minimal effect on flow. Claydon et al. (2005) assessed autoregulation from the correlation between flow and pressure during orthostatic stress, where a significant correlation with a high coefficient indicates poor autoregulation. Results of this study showed that cerebrovascular autoregulation was impaired in CMS patients.

Cerebral blood flow is particularly sensitive to the level of CO2. Roach et al. (2001) have reported an impaired cerebrovascular sensitivity to carbon dioxide in the presence of hypobaric hypoxia in subjects with CMS and this is suggested as another possible link between the autonomic disturbances and the origin of clinical manifestations of CMS.

Norcliffe et al. (2005) determined the cerebrovascular responses to hypoxia and hypercapnia, separately and together, in CMS patients and normal high altitude dwellers. CMS patients did not respond differently to the normals, but in both groups at altitude the sensitivity of the cerebral circulation to hypoxia was less than that in sea level residents. Shortly after descent to sea level, however, sensitivity increased. Sensitivity to hypercapnia during hypoxia decreased after descent.

Concluding remarks

Exposure to high altitude provides a considerable stress on homeostatic mechanisms, the main challenge being the chronic hypoxia. This, in addition to causing a direct stimulation of peripheral chemoreceptors, affects other functions. The adaptation of long-term high altitude residents differs from that of sojourners so that their lives are relatively normal. Adaptation mechanisms, however, may differ in different populations. Interestingly, a significant minority, particularly Andeans, become maladapted and develop chronic mountain sickness characterized by a high haematocrit and the consequences of the high blood viscosity particularly on the brain heart and lungs.

References

Appenzeller, O., Passino, C., Roach, R. *et al.* (2004). Cerebral vasoreactivity in Andeans and headache at sea level. *J Neurol Sci* **219**, 101–6.

Appenzeller, O., Thomas, P. K., Ponsford, S., Gamboa, J. L., Cáceda, R. and Milner, P. (2002). Acral paresthesias in the Andes and neurology at sea level. *Neurology* **59**, 1532–5.

Azevedo, E. R., Newton, G. E., Floras, J. S., and Parker, J. D. (2000). Reducing cardiac filling pressure lowers norepinephrine spillover in patients with chronic heart failure. *Circulation* **101**, 2053–9.

Bainton, C. R., Carcelen, A., and Severinghaus, J. W. (1964). Carotid chemoreceptor insensitivity in Andean natives. *J Physiol* **177**, 30–1.

Bernardi, L., Roach, R. C., Keyl, C. *et al.* (2003). Ventilation, autonomic function, sleep and erythropoietin. Chronic mountain sickness of Andean natives. *Adv Exp Med Biol* **543**, 161–75.

Blaber, A. P., Hartley, T., and Pretorius, P. J. (2003). Effect of acute exposure to 3660 m altitude on orthostatic responses and tolerance. *J Appl Physiol* **95**, 591–601.

Bogaard, H. J., Hopkins, S. R., Yamaya, Y., Niizeki, K., Ziegler, M. G. and Wagner, P. D. (2002). Role of the autonomic nervous system in the reduced maximal cardiac output at altitude. *J Appl Physiol* **93**, 271–91.

Boushel, R., Calbet, J. A., Radegran, G., Sondergaard, H., Wagner, P. D., and Saltin, B. (2001). Parasympathetic neural activity accounts for the lowering of exercise heart rate at high altitude. *Circulation* **104**, 785–91.

Brown TE, Beightol LA, Koh J and Eckberg DL (1993). Important influence of respiration on human R-R interval power spectra is largely ignored. *Journal of Applied Physiology*, **75**, 2310–7.

Calbet, J. A. (2003). Chronic hypoxia increases blood pressure and noradrenaline spillover in healthy humans. *J Physiol* **551**, 379–86.

Clar, C., Dorrington, K. L., Fatemian, M. and Robbins, P. A. (2001). Effects of 8 h of isocapnic hypoxia with and without muscarinic blockade on ventilation and heart rate in humans. *Exp Physiol* **86**, 529–38.

Claydon, V. E., Moore, J. P., Norcliffe, L. J., *et al.* (2003). Cardiac baroreceptor sensitivity in high altitude natives. *Clin Auton Res* **13**, 459.

Claydon, V. E., Norcliffe, L. J., Moore, J. P., *et al.* (2004). Orthostatic tolerance and blood volumes in Andean high altitude dwellers. *Exp Physiol* **89**, 565–71.

Claydon, V. E., Norcliffe, L. J., Moore, J. P., *et al.* (2005). Cardiovascular responses to orthostatic stress in healthy altitude dwellers, and altitude residents with chronic mountain sickness. *Exp Physiol* **90**, 103–10.

Cornolo, J., Mollard, P., Brugniaux, J. V., Robach, P., and Richalet, J. P. (2004). Autonomic control of the cardiovascular system during acclimatization to high altitude: effects of sildenafil. *J Appl Physiol* **97**, 935–40.

Duplain, H., Vollenweider, L., Delabays, A., Nicod, P., Bartsch, P., Scherrer, U. (1999). Augmented sympathetic activation during short-term hypoxia and high-altitude exposure in subjects susceptible to high-altitude pulmonary edema. *Circulation* **99**, 1713–8.

Esler, M. (2000). The sympathetic system and hypertension. *Am J Hypertens* **13**, 99S–105S.

Fatemian, M., Gamboa, A., León-Velarde, F., Rivera-Ch, M., Palacios, J. A., Robbins, P. A. (2003). Ventilatory response to CO2 in high-altitude natives and patients with chronic mountain sickness. *J Appl Physiol* **94**, 1279–87.

Fischetti, F., Fabris, B., Zaccaria, M., *et al.* (2000). Effects of prolonged high-altitude exposure on peripheral adrenergic receptors in young healthy volunteers. *Eur J Appl Physiol* **82**, 439–45.

Gamboa, A., León-Velarde, F., Rivera-Ch, M., *et al.* (2003). Acute and sustained ventilatory responses to hypoxia in high-altitude natives living at sea level. *J Appl Physiol* **94**, 1255–62.

Gavras, I., Manolis, A. J. and Gavras, H. (2001). The alpha2-adrenergic receptors in hypertension and heart failure: experimental and clinical studies. *J Hypertens* **19**, 2115–24.

Grollman, A. (1930). Physiological variations of the cardiac output of man. VII. The effect of high altitude on the cardiac output and its related functions: an account of experiments conducted on the summit of Pikes Peak, Colarado. *Am J Physiol* **93**, 19–40.

Groves, B. M., Reeves, J. T., Sutton, J. R., *et al.* (1987). Operation Everest II: elevated high-altitude pulmonary resistance unresponsive to oxygen. *J Appl Physiol* **63**, 521–30.

Hackett, P. H. and Roach, R. C. (2000). High-altitude medicine. In: Auerbach, P. A. (ed.) *Wilderness Medicine*, pp. 1–37. Mosby, St. Louis.

Hackett, P. H., Rennie, I. D., and Levine, H. D. (1976). The incidence, importance and prophylaxis of acute mountain sickness. *Lancet* **2**, 1149–54.

Halliwill, J. R. and Minson, C. T. (2002). Effect of hypoxia on arterial baroreflex control of heart rate and muscle sympathetic nerve activity in humans. *J Appl Physiol* **93**, 857–64.

Halliwill, J. R. and Minson, C. T. (2005). Cardiovagal regulation during combined hypoxic and orthostatic stress: fainters vs. nonfainters. *J Appl Physiol* **98**, 1050–6.

Hansen, J. and Sander, M. (2003). Sympathetic neural overactivity in healthy humans after prolonged exposure to hypobaric hypoxia. *J Physiol* **546**, 921–9.

Heistad, D. D. and Abboud, F. M. (1980). Circulatory adjustments to hypoxia. *Circulation* **61**, 463–70.

Jefferson, J. A., Escudero, E., Hurtado, M. E. *et al.* (2002). Excessive erythrocytosis, chronic mountain sickness, and serum cobalt levels. *Lancet* **359**, 407–8.

Johnson, T. S., Rock, P. B., Young, J. B., Fulco, C. S. and Trad, L. A. (1988). Hemodynamic and sympathoadrenal responses to altitude in humans: effect of dexamethasone. *Aviat Space Environ Med* **59**, 208–12.

Kacimi, R., Richalet, J. P., Corsin, A., Abousahl, I. and Crozatier, B. (1992). Hypoxia-induced downregulation of beta-adrenergic receptors in rat heart. *J Appl Physiol* **73**, 1377–82.

Kacimi, R., Richalet, J. P. and Crozatier, B. (1993). Hypoxia-induced differential modulation of adenosinergic and muscarinic receptors in rat heart. *J Appl Physiol* **75**, 1123–8.

Kanai, M., Nishihara, F., Shiga, T., Shimada, H. and Saito, S. (2001). Alterations in autonomic nervous control of heart rate among tourists at 2700 and 3700 m above sea level. *Wilderness and Environmental Medicine* **12**, 8–12.

Keyl, C., Schneider, A., Gamboa, A., *et al.* (2003). Autonomic cardiovascular function in high-altitude Andean natives with chronic mountain sickness. *J Appl Physiol* **94**, 213–9.

Kontos, H. A., Levasseur, J. E., Richardson, D. W., Mauck, H. P. Jr, and Patterson J. L. Jr (1967). Comparative circulatory responses to systemic hypoxia in man and in unanesthetized dog. *J Appl Physiol* **23**, 381–6.

Leon-Velarde, F., Bourin, M. C., Germack, R., Mohammadi, K., Crozatier, B. and Richalet, J. P. (2001). Differential alterations in cardiac adrenergic signaling in chronic hypoxia or norepinephrine infusion. *Am J Physiol* **280**, R274–81.

León-Velarde, F., Gamboa, A., Rivera-Ch, M., Palacios, J. A., Robbins, P. A. (2003). Peripheral chemoreflex function in high-altitude natives and patients with chronic mountain sickness. *J Appl Physiol* **94**, 1269–78.

León-Velarde, F., McCullough, R. G., Reeves, J. T., *et al.* (2003). Proposal for scoring severity in chronic mountain sickness (CMS). Background and conclusions of the CMS Working Group. *Adv Exp Med Biol* **543**, 339–54.

Lumbreras, L. G. and León-Velarde, F. (2003). El medio ambiente en los Andes. In: León-Velarde, F. and Monge-C. C. (eds). *El reto fisiológico de vivir en los Andes*. Lima: Instituto Francés de Estudios Andinos, Fondo Editorial de la Universidad Peruana Cayetano Heredia, 29–39.

McMahon, N. C., Drinkhill, M. J., Myers, D. S. and Hainsworth, R. (2000). Reflex responses from the main pulmonary artery and bifurcation in anaesthetised dogs. *Exp Physiol* **85**, 411–20.

Marshall, J. M. (1994). Peripheral chemoreceptors and cardiovascular regulation. *Physiol Rev* **74**, 543–94.

Mazzeo, R. S., Bender, P. R., Brooks, G. A., *et al.* (1991). Arterial catecholamine responses during exercise with acute and chronic high-altitude exposure. *Am J Physiol* **261**, E419–24.

Mazzeo, R. S., Child, A., Butterfield, G. E., *et al.* (1998). Catecholamine response during 12 days of high-altitude exposure (4,300 m) in women. *J Appl Physiol* **84**, 1151–7.

Monge, M. C. (1925). *Sobre un caso de enfermedad de Váquez*. Comunicación presentada a la Academia Nacional de Medicina. Lima, 1–6.

Monge-C. C. and León-Velarde, F. (1991). Physiological adaptation to high altitude: oxygen transport in mammals and birds. *Physiol Rev* **71**, 1135–72.

Monge-C. C. and Whittembury, J. (1982). Chronic mountain sickness and the physiopathology of hypoxemic polycythemia. In: Sutton, J. R., Jones, N. L., Houston, C. S. (eds). *Hypoxia: man at altitude*. New York Thieme-Stratton, pp. 51–6.

Moore, J. P., Rivera-Chira, M., Macarlupu, J. L., *et al.* (2004a). Carotid baroreflex regulation of vascular resistance in lowland and high altitude anaesthetized dogs. *J Physiol* **560**, PC11.

Moore, J. P., Hainsworth, R., and Drinkhill, M. J. (2004b). Phasic negative intrathoracic pressures enhance the vascular responses to stimulation of pulmonary arterial baroreceptors in closed-chest anaesthetized dogs. *J Physiol* **555**, 815–24.

Moore, J. P., Claydon, V. E., Norcliffe, L. J. *et al.* (2004c). Carotid baroreflex regulation of vascular resistance in high altitude Andean natives with CMS. *Clin Auton Res* **14**, 416.

Morel, O. E., Buvry, A., Le Corvoisier, P., *et al.* (2003). Effects of nifedipine-induced pulmonary vasodilatation on cardiac receptors and protein kinase C isoforms in the chronically hypoxic rat. *Pflugers Archiv* **446**, 356–64.

Moudgil, R., Michelakis, E. D., and Archer, S. L. (2005). Hypoxic pulmonary vasoconstriction. *J Appl Physiol* **98**, 390–403.

Norcliffe, L. J., Rivera, M., Palacios, A. J., *et al.* (2003). Cardiovascular and ventilatory reponses to hypoxia in high altitude dwellers. *Clin Auton Res* **13**, 459–60.

Piletz, J. E., Andorn, A. C., Unnerstall, J. R., and Halaris, A. (1991). Binding of [3H]-p-aminoclonidine to alpha 2-adrenoceptor states plus a non-adrenergic site on human platelet plasma membranes. *Biochem Pharmacol* **42**, 569–84.

Reeves, J. T., Groves, B. M., Sutton, J. T., *et al.* (1987). Operation Everest II: preservation of cardiac function at extreme altitude. *J Appl Physiol* **63**, 531–9.

Reis, D. J., Golanov, E. V., Ruggiero, D. A. and Sun, M. K. (1994). Sympatho-excitatory neurons of the rostral ventrolateral medulla are oxygen sensors and essential elements in the tonic and reflex control of the systemic and cerebral circulations. *J Hypertens* **12**, S159–80.

Richalet, J. P., Larmignat, P., Rathat, C., Keromes, A., Baud, P., and Lhoste, F. (1988). Decreased cardiac response to isoproterenol infusion in acute and chronic hypoxia. *J Appl Physiol* **65**, 1957–61.

Riley, D. J. (1991). *Vascular remodelling in the lung: Scientific Foundations* (eds Crstal, R.C., West, J. B.), pp.1189–98. Raven Press, New York.

Rivera-Ch, M., Gamboa, A., León-Velarde, F., Palacios, J. A., O'Connor, D. F., and Robbins, P. A. (2003). Hi-altitude natives living at sea level acclimatize to high altitude like sea-level natives. *J Appl Physiol* **94**, 1263–8.

Roach, R., Passino, C., Bernardi, L., Gamboa, J., Gamboa, A., and Appenzeller, O. (2001). Cerebrovascular reactivity to CO2 at high altitude and sea level in Andean Natives. *Clin Auton Res* **11**, 183.

Roche, F., Reynaud, C., Garet, M., Pichot, V., Costes, F., and Barthelemy, J. C. (2002). Cardiac baroreflex control in humans during and immediately after brief exposure to simulated high altitude. *Clinical Physiology and Functional Imaging* **22**, 301–6.

Rostrup, M. (1998). Catecholamines, hypoxia and high altitude. *Acta Physiol Scand* **162**, 389–99.

Rowell, L. B. and Blackmon, J. R. (1986). Lack of sympathetic vasoconstriction in hypoxemic humans at rest. *Am J Physiol* **251**, H562–70.

Sagawa, S., Torii, R., Nagaya, K., Wada, F., Endo, Y., and Shiraki, K. (1997). Carotid baroreflex control of heart rate during acute exposure to simulated altitudes of 3,800 m and 4,300 m. *Am J Physiol* **273**, R1219–23.

Severinghaus, J. W., Bainton, C. R. and Carcelen, A. (1966). Respiratory insensitivity to hypoxia in chronically hypoxic man. *Resp Physiol* **1**, 308–34.

Sevre, K., Bendz, B., Hanko, E., *et al.* (2001). Reduced autonomic activity during stepwise exposure to high altitude. *Acta Physiol Scand* **173**, 409–17.

Sime, F., Monge-C. C., and Whittembury, J. (1975). Age as a cause of chronic mountain sickness. *Int J Biometeorol* **19**, 93–8.

Singh I, Khanna PK, Srivastava MC, Lal M, Roy SB and Subramanyam CSV (1969). Acute mountain sickness. *New England Journal of Medicine*. **280**, 175–184.

Sutton, J. R., Reeves, J. T., Wagner, P. D. *et al.* (1988). Operation Everest II: Oxygen transport during exercise at extreme simulated altitude. *J Appl Physiol* **64**, 1309–21.

Talbot, N. P., Balanos, G. M., Dorrington, K. L., and Robbins, P. A. (2005). Two temporal components within the human pulmonary vascular response to ⁻2 h of isocapnic hypoxia. *J Appl Physiol* **98**, 1125–39.

Voelkel, N. F., Hegstrand, L., Reeves, J. T., McMurty, I. F., and Molinoff, P. B. (1981). Effects of hypoxia on density of beta-adrenergic receptors. *J Appl Physiol* **50**, 363–6.

Vogel, J. A. and Harris, C. W. (1967). Cardiopulmonary responses of resting man during early exposure to high altitude. *J Appl Physiol* **22**, 1124–8.

Vogel, J. A., Hansen, J. E., and Harris, C. W. (1967) Cardiovascular responses in man during exhaustive work at sea level and high altitude. *J Appl Physiol* **23**, 531–9.

Weil, J. V. (1986). Ventilatory control at high altitude. In: *Handbook of Physiology. The Respiratory System II*. Control of Breathing, Part II, pp.703–27. American Physiological Society.

West, J. B., Boyer, S. J., Graber, D. J., *et al.* (1983). Maximal exercise at extreme altitudes on Mount Everest. *J Appl Physiol* **55**, 688–98.

WHO (1996). *World Health Statistics Annual 1995*. World Health Organization, Geneva.

Winslow, R. M. and Monge, C-C. (1987). *Hypoxia, polycythemia, and chronic mountain sickness*, pp.5–18. The Johns Hopkins University Press, Baltimore.

Yoshimoto, M., Sasaki, M., Naraki, N., Mohri, M. and Miki, K. (2004). Regulation of gastric motility at simulated high altitude in conscious rats. *J Appl Physiol* **97**, 599–604.

Young, P. M., Sutton, J. R., Green, H. J., *et al.* (1992). Operation Everest II: metabolic and hormonal responses to incremental exercise to exhaustion. *J Appl Physiol* **73**, 2574–9.

Zhao, L., Mason, N. A., Morrell, N. W., *et al.* (2001) Sildenafil inhibits hypoxia-induced pulmonary hypertension. *Circulation* **104**, 424–8.

CHAPTER 16

The gut and the autonomic nervous system

Anne E. Bishop and Julia M. Polak

Key points

- The autonomic nervous system of the gut, or the enteric nervous system (ENS), acts to a large degree independently of the rest of the autonomic nervous system.

- The ENS governs gut motility, secretion and absorption.

- It contains a similar number of neurons to that in the spinal cord.

- A dense circuitry of sensory and motor neurons, with interconnecting interneurons, connects the different levels of the gut and coordinates activity along its length.

- ENS neurons lie in two major types of ganglia, the myenteric (Auerbach's) and submucosal (Meissner's) plexuses.

- The range of neurotransmitters in the ENS is similar to that in the CNS.

- Abnormalities of ENS structure and function have been shown to contribute to a number of enteric diseases.

Introduction

Although under the overriding control of the central nervous system (CNS), the gastrointestinal tract is capable of carrying out its functions of food passage, storage, digestion, and absorption after all central connections are severed. Thus, sympathetic denervation has only a transient effect on gut function; denervation of the parasympathetic nervous system usually reduces the tone and degree of peristaltic activity but this is eventually compensated for by increased intrinsic excitability of the enteric plexuses. Afferent pathways relay sensory information on pain, distension, and nausea. The reflex function of the autonomic nervous system of the gut, or the enteric nervous system (ENS), occurs through coordination of sensory neurons, interneurons, and excitatory and inhibitory motor neurons. This autonomy of the gastrointestinal tract has been the subject of much interest and speculation, and terms such as 'minibrain' have been used to describe the gut's intrinsic innervation; some indication of the size and importance of the intramural innervation can be gained from the observation that the number of neurons in the human gut, an estimated 10^8, is similar to that in the spinal cord (Furness and Costa 1987). Far from using only the classic autonomic neurotransmitters, acetylcholine and noradrenaline, the ENS employs a myriad of substances,

including amines, γ-aminobutyric acid (GABA), adenosine triphosphate (ATP), nitric oxide (NO), and a variety of peptides, to relay information. The neuropeptides are probably the most abundant neurotransmitter type in the gut and are found singly or in combinations with other peptides or neuroactive substances.

This chapter describes the composition of the autonomic nervous system of the gut with particular reference to the peptidergic innervation in normal and disease states and during development.

Development

The neurons and glia that make up the ENS are derived from precursor cells in the neural crest (see Heanue and Pachnis 2007 for review). Most enteric neurons and glial cells arise from cells at the vagal level (Le Douarin and Teillet 1973) but some are derived from sacral crest cells (Burns and Le Douarin 1998). The neural crest cells that enter the gut have been termed enteric neural crest-derived cells (ENCCs) and are known to undergo highly active proliferation and migration to form the eventual massive network of neurons and glia in the fully developed gut (Young et al. 2005). Crest cells migrate predominantly in the outer gut mesenchyme and the behaviour of the migrating ENCCs, in terms of their phenotypic changes and their correct location within the myenteric and submucosal plexuses, is subject to a range of physical and chemical (Young et al. 2003). However, little is known about the behaviour of ENCCs at the cellular level largely because the only information has been obtained from fixed samples of gut. Very elegant studies have been carried out using mice and chicks in which ENCCs were labelled with fluorescent markers in order to follow their migration patterns within the embryonic gut (Young et al. 2004, Druckenbrod and Epstein 2005, 2007). Cells were seen to migrate in chains that followed complex and unpredictable trajectories which appeared to depend on their position with respect to the wavefront of the migration. Some of the leading cells and their processes formed a scaffold along which later cells migrate. Migration of ENCCs appears to differ from that of other crest cells in two main ways. Firstly, the scale of migration was found to be greater; the distance they migrate to colonize the entire gastrointestinal tract exceeded that of any other crest cell population. Secondly, in comparison to other environments through which neural crest cells migrate, the gut mesenchyme appears to be relatively uniform. Much of the more recent information that has been obtained regarding the development of the ENS has arisen from genetic studies aimed at uncovering the pathogenesis of congenital aganglionosis or Hirschsprung disease (Heanue and Pachnis 2006, 2007).

General composition

Sympathetic innervation

Preganglionic fibres from T8 to L3 of the spinal cord pass through the sympathetic chains to synapse with postganglionic neurons in the coeliac and superior and inferior mesenteric ganglia. The postganglionic fibres spread from these ganglia to innervate all parts of the gut. The fibres either innervate their effector organ (i.e. muscle layers, blood vessels, or epithelium) directly or synapse with neurons of the main ganglionated (myenteric or submucous) plexuses.

Parasympathetic innervation

The parasympathetic innervation of the gut is either cranial or sacral in origin. Cranial parasympathetic fibres run mostly in the vagus nerves, whereas sacral nerves originate from S2–S4 of the spinal cord and pass through the nervi erigentes to innervate the lower bowel. The fibres synapse in the intramural plexuses and postganglionic fibres radiate to effector organs including other cells in the plexuses.

Intramural plexuses

Most of the fibres that innervate the gut arise from the intramural plexuses. These plexuses form a complex, heterogeneous part of the autonomic nervous system, as was recognized very early in the work of Langley (1898). There are two main ganglionated plexuses—the myenteric (or Auerbach's), which lies between the longitudinal and circular muscle coats, and the submucous (or Meissner's), lying between the circular muscle and the muscularis mucosae. The myenteric plexus contains most of the intrinsic nerve cell bodies of the gut. It can be subdivided into three parts: the primary, secondary, and tertiary plexuses. The primary plexus is composed of the neuronal cells and bundles of fibres running between them (i.e. the core of the plexus). The secondary component is formed by fibres running from ganglia or connecting branches of the primary plexus, which pass to the muscle, whereas the fine fibres that run between the ganglia and branches of the primary plexus are known as the tertiary plexus. The submucous plexus has sometimes been described as having two components, one by the muscularis mucosae, known as Meissner's plexus, and the other against the circular muscle, called Henle's plexus. However, the lack of apparent functional and structural differentiation between the two means that they are unified in most of the relevant literature. The intramural ganglia supply fibres that either synapse with cells in the same or other ganglia, or innervate a range of effector organs in the gut as well as sending afferents to the CNS.

Enteric glia

Although originally assumed to play a solely passive, supportive role in the gut, the enteric glia are now considered to be active in the mediation of gut function by the ENS (Ruhl et al. 2004). Glial cells outnumber neurons by about 4:1 in the ENS (Gabella 1981) and show evidence of morphological and functional heterogeneity (Hanini and Reichenbach 1994). The glia maintain the structural and functional integrity of the enteric neurons (Bush et al. 1998), including through the secretion of GDNF (Hoener et al. 1996, Bar et al. 1997). There is also evidence that the glia are part of the inflammatory response of the gut, interacting with immunocytes and secreting cytokines (Ruhl et al. 2001, Cabarrocas et al. 2003, Tjwa et al. 2003, Ruhl et al. 2004). Enteric glia also appear to help maintain the mucosal epithelial barrier by forming a dense network on the basal side of intestinal mucosa (Steinkamp et al. 2003, Savidge et al. 2003).

Interstitial cells of Cajal

The rhythmical waves of depolarization, known as slow waves, that occur in the gut musculature were long thought to be generated by the smooth muscle cells themselves (Tomita 1981). Eventual study of single gut smooth muscle cells showed that they were incapable of producing slow waves and, furthermore, lacked the necessary ion channels (Farrugia 1999). From this, it was shown that the interstitial cells of Cajal (ICC), that had previously been suggested to act as pacemakers in the gut (Thuneberg 1982), do indeed fulfil this role (Dickens et al. 1999, Hirst and Edwards 2001, Hirst and Ward 2003, Ward et al. 2004, Ward and Sanders 2006). There appears to be two types of ICC; one type forms networks lying in the region of the myenteric plexus (ICC_{MY}) that generate pacemaker potentials, and the other type (ICC_{IM}) is densely innervated and distributed among the smooth muscle cells with which they are tightly electrically coupled (Wang et al. 1999). Abnormalities of these interstitial cells have been described in a number of human gut diseases including oesophageal achalasai, hypertrophic pyloric stenosis, Hirschsprung disease and inflammatory bowel disease (IBD) (Vanderwinder and Rumessen 1999).

Neurochemistry

A number of functionally different neuronal types have been identified in the intramural plexuses of the gut, mainly on the basis of electrophysiology, and attempts have been made to relate the function and morphology of the cells. The work of Dogiel (1899) describing three morphologically and, he hypothesized, functionally distinct types of gut neurons subsequently has been shown by the investigation of morphofunctional correlations to be remarkably prescient. In particular, this has been achieved by injection of dye into cells previously characterized electrophysiologically (for review see Furness and Costa 1987). Table 16.1 summarizes the current knowledge of the neurons of Dogiel's classification, as studied in the guinea pig small intestine. There has been much controversy over the value of Dogiel's work but this classification remains a useful basis for neuronal identification. However, it must be noted that not all gut neurons have been found to fit into the classification.

Chemically mediated neural signalling in the gut is essentially the same as that which occurs in any other part of the nervous system and transmitter release is by Ca^{2+}-triggered exocytosis from storage in axonal vesicles. Neurotransmitters in the gut bind to their specific postsynaptic receptors and elicit synaptic events that are either ionotropic (direct receptor coupling to the ion channel) or metabotropic (indirect effects on ion channel mediated by second messengers). Fast and slow excitatory postsynaptic potentials (EPSPs) and inhibitory postsynaptic potentials (IPSPs) are principal synaptic events in the ENS. A large number of different

Table 16.1 Dogiel's classification[a]

Type	Axons	Dendrites	Function	Electrophysiology[b]	Products[c,d]
I	Project through other ganglia to muscle	4–20; short, end within ganglia	Motor	S	Substance P, dynorphin, NO, enkephalin, VIP GRP, CCK
II	Project to other ganglia	3–10; long	Sensory	AH	Somatostatin, substance P, CCK
III	Termination not traced	2–10; short, end within ganglia	?	S	Somatostatin, VIP, dynorphin, CGRP, NPY, CCK

[a] Dogiel 1899

[b] S, fast excitatory postsynaptic potentials (cholinergic); AH, prolonged after hyperpolarizations.

[c] Furness and Costa 1987; Costa et al. 1992.

[d] NO, nitric oxide; VIP, vasoactive intestinal peptide; GRP, gastrin-releasing peptide (or bombesin); CCK, cholecystokinin; CGRP, calcitonin-gene-related peptide; NPY, neuropeptide Y.

substances have been identified, by pharmacological, physiological, or morphological means, in the autonomic nervous system of the mammalian gut. Not all of these substances have been shown as yet to satisfy all the criteria used to identify neurotransmitters. However, what is clear is that a highly complex, heterogeneous transmitter system exists with subtypes of neurons chemically coded by the presence of a specific substance or combination of substances. Different combinations of the same substances can be found in functionally and morphologically distinct neurons (see Table 16.1, for example). For brevity Table 16.2 provides a list of the main established and candidate transmitters that have been identified in enteric nerves.

Acetylcholine and noradrenaline have long been known to be neurotransmitters in the gut and their excitatory and inhibitory influences on gut function are well described. What has emerged in recent years is the realization that these 'classic' neurotransmitters often coexist with other substances in the gut innervation. For example, in the guinea pig the peptides, cholecystokinin, somatostatin, neuropeptide Y (NPY), and substance P (SP), have been localized to cholinergic neurons, identified by immunostaining of the acetylcholine-synthesizing enzyme choline acetyltransferase (Furness and Costa 1987). Similarly, NPY has been demonstrated in postganglionic sympathetic neurons supplying the stomach and colon of several species (Ekblad et al. 1984, Su et al. 1987).

Although ATP has been put forward as the main transmitter in inhibitory gastrointestinal neurons it seems, at present, that it is more widely accepted as also being present in other types of neurons and acting as some kind of cotransmitter (Burnstock 1981).

Table 16.2 Neurochemicals identified in the innervation of the human gut

- ◆ Acetylcholine (ACh)
- ◆ Adenosine triphosphate (ATP)
- ◆ Dopamine
- ◆ γ-aminobutyric acid (GABA)
- ◆ Haem oxygenase
- ◆ Nitric oxide
- ◆ Noradrenaline
- ◆ Peptides
- ◆ Prostaglandins
- ◆ Serotonin (5-hydroxytryptamine, 5-HT)

Dopamine, a precursor to noradrenaline, has been found in gastrointestinal nerves, but is likely to be related to the sympathetic nerves rather aminobutyric acid. GABA appears to cause differential modulation of gastrointestinal motility by stimulating cholinergic neurons via GABA-A receptors or reducing cholinergic contractions via the GABA-B subtype (Ong and Kerr 1983). The amine has been identified in the myenteric plexus in neurons that seems to innervate other ganglion cells (Jessen et al. 1979).

Serotonin (5-hydroxytryptamine; 5-HT) has long been known to act as a transmitter in the CNS but its presence in gastrointestinal nerves was a matter of debate prior to the advent of specific antibodies to the amine. A major problem with evaluation of serotonin as a neurotransmitter is its relatively high concentration in endocrine cells in all areas of the gastrointestinal mucosa. Serotonin has been localized to the intramural plexuses (Furness and Costa 1987) where it has been suggested to contribute to slow potentials in prolonged after-hyperpolarization neurons. However, the major action of serotonin on the ENS is its role in the transepithelial detection of intraluminal conditions. In this system, serotonin is secreted from specific neuroendocrine cells, known as enterochromaffin cells, that are scattered along the length of the gastrointestinal tract, and activates primary afferent neurons lying in the gut wall (Grider 1994, 2003, Pan et al. 2000, Gershon 2005, Gershon and Tack 2007). Serotoninergic agents have been used to treat irritable bowel syndrome (IBS); for example, ligands acting at the 5-HT$_4$ subtype of receptors, have been used to treat constipation-predominant IBS, although their exact mode of action is not yet fully understood. There are no extracellular enzymes that catabolize serotonin and so responses to the amine are terminated by reuptake. A specific serotonin reuptake transporter (SERT) is present in the plasma membranes of serotonergic neurons but, as the enteric mucosa lacks serotonergic innervation, enterocytes possess SERT and perform the uptake of 5-HT (Wade et al. 1996, Chen et al. 1998, Coates et al. 2004). It is possible that potentiation of the effects of serotonin due to SERT decrease could account for the symptoms of diarrhoea-predominant IBS, while receptor desensitization may cause the form associated with constipation.

NANC innervation: nitric oxide

The major inhibitory innervation of the mammalian gut comes from intrinsic nerves and plays an essential role in most gastrointestinal reflexes. The term non-adrenergic, non-cholinergic (NANC) was coined to describe these nerves as the neurotransmitter/s they contain remained unknown for many years despite extensive investigation. However, now there is a wealth of morphological, physiological, and pharmacological evidence that the inhibitory transmitter in the gut of a variety of species, including man, is NO (Bult et al. 1990, Toda et al. 1990, Sanders and Ward 1992, Stark and Szurszewski 1992, Keef et al. 1993) (Fig. 16.1). This free radical gas is a major regulatory factor in the mammalian body and is produced by a variety of cells in addition to nerves, such as endothelium, epithelium and macrophages (Moncada et al. 1991). NO is unique among neuroactive substances in that it is a gas with no known storage mechanisms and is very labile with a half-life of a few seconds. Instead of interacting with a cell surface receptor, it diffuses across membranes. Once in the cell, it binds to and activates soluble guanylate cyclase, thereby increasing cyclic guanosine monophosphate levels, although it may have other modes of action.

NO is synthesized from the terminal guanidino nitrogen of L-arginine by the enzyme known as NO synthase (NOS) that exists in three main forms: Type I (neuronal) NOS and Type III (endothelial) NOS are expressed constitutively and are calcium and calmodulin dependent, while Type II (inducible) NOS is calcium and calmodulin independent (Moncada et al. 1991). The nature and short half-life of NO preclude its localization in tissues, but the distribution of the Type I enzyme has been studied in several species and it has been found to occur mainly in Type I cells of the Dogiel classification, which fits with a role for NO in the control of motor function in the gut (Costa et al. 1992, Springall et al. 1992, Ward et al. 1992, Young et al. 1992, Desai et al. 1994). Reduced expression of Type I NOS and NO activity has been described in a number of gastrointestinal dysmotility syndromes including oesophageal achalasia (Mearin et al. 1993), Hirschsprung disease (congenital aganglionosis) (Vanderwinden et al. 1993; Bealer et al. 1994, O'Kelly et al. 1994, Larsson et al. 1995, Tomita et al. 1995, Guo et al. 1997) and hypertrophic pyloric stenosis (Vanderwinden et al. 1992, Abel 1996). Interestingly, mice that have had the gene for Type I NOS removed by homologous recombination live and reproduce normally and have no demonstrable abnormality of the CNS (Huang et al. 1993). However, the major pathological feature they do display is gross gastric enlargement with pyloric sphincter hypertrophy.

Neural cell adhesion molecule

A range of cell surface molecules has been studied extensively and shown to contribute to cell-to-cell recognition processes in normal adult and developing tissues. One of the best characterized is neural cell adhesion molecule (NCAM), which mediates the initial interaction between nerve and muscle and acts in subsequent stages of synapse development and stabilization (Reiger et al. 1985) and maintenance of the neuromuscular system (Thiery 1982, Cunningham 1991). Recent study of the human intestine has shown that NCAM expression can be detected on muscle and nerves from 8 weeks of gestation, the earliest stage examined (Romanska et al. 1996a). By 20 weeks of gestation, strong expression was seen on all nerves but only on the muscularis mucosae and the inner edge of the circular muscle. At birth, NCAM was confined to nerves. Thus, muscular expression of NCAM in the human intestine is high during development of the neuromuscular system but tails off once maturation occurs. However, as with skeletal muscle (Cashman et al. 1987, Walsh et al. 1987, 1988), the levels of NCAM seen on the smooth muscle of the intestine can increase in disease conditions such as Hirschsprung disease, where strong expression of NCAM is seen on the muscularis mucosae (Romanska et al. 1993) (Fig. 16.2). The presence of NCAM on muscle in aganglionic bowel is unlikely to be the result of the intractable constipation that occurs as it is not found in bowel taken from individuals

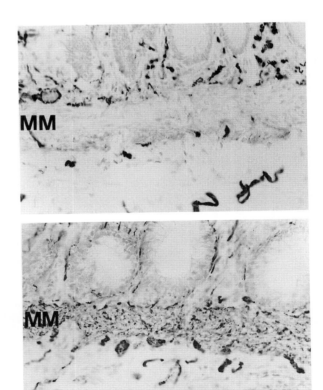

Fig. 16.2 Neural cell adhesion molecule (NCAM) immunostained using the avidin biotin complex method in:

♦ normal large bowel from a neonate—immunoreactivity for NCAM is confined to the nerves (muscularis mucosae [MM])

♦ large bowel from a child with congenital aganglionosis—NCAM is present not only on nerves but also on the MM.

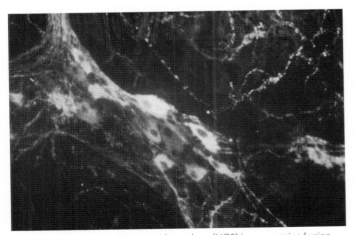

Fig. 16.1 Type I (neuronal) nitric oxide synthase (NOS) immunostained using indirect immunofluorescence in a whole mount preparation of the myenteric plexus of guinea pig stomach and visualized using a confocal laser microscope. The projections of the immunoreactive fibres in three dimensions have been incorporated into a two dimensional image. The NOS-immunoreactive ganglion cells have Type 1 Dogiel morphology.

with idiopathic constipation and normal appearing, ganglionic intestine (Romanska et al. 1996b).

Morphological studies of gut neuropeptides

The most widespread and abundant transmitters in the mammalian gut are the neuropeptides. As yet, not all of them satisfy the classic criteria for neurotransmitters, but they do represent a relatively new discovery in the peripheral nervous system; their numbers are continuously expanding and our understanding of them increasing. The rest of this chapter describes current knowledge of this heterogeneous group of substances, with emphasis on the contribution of morphological investigations.

For brevity, a list of the major peptides currently identifiable in the innervation of the mammalian gut is given in Table 16.3, together with information on their origins and known actions. The information in the table is based on data derived from human and experimental animal (mainly rat and guinea pig) tissues.

Localization of neuropeptides: immunocytochemistry

Most of the literature on the localization of neuropeptides in the gut concerns the application of immunocytochemistry at light or electron microscopical levels. Several immunocytochemical

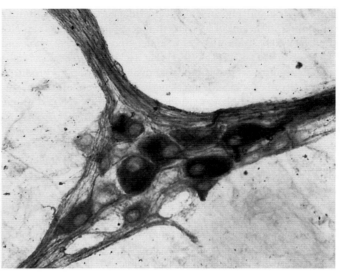

Fig. 16.3 Vasoactive intestinal peptide immunostained using the peroxidase antiperoxidase method in a whole mount preparation of the submucous plexus of the human colon. Both ganglion cells and nerve fibres show dense immunoreactivity.

Table 16.3 Major enteric neuropeptides

Peptides*	Main actions	Main origin(s)
Bombesin (GRP)	Multiple stimulatory effects (e.g. gastrin release)	Local
CGRP	Gastric acid release, muscle constriction	Local and sensory
CCK8	Not known	Local
CRF	Muscle constriction, mucosal permeability	Local
Dynorphin	Opiate effects	Local
Endothelin-1	Vasoconstriction	Local
Galanin	Muscle constriction	Local
Ghrelin	Muscle constriction	Local
Leu-enkephalin	Opiate effects	Local
Met-enkephalin	Opiate effects	Local
Motilin	Muscle constriction	Local
Neuromedin U	Muscle constriction, vasoconstriction	Local
NPY	Vasoconstriction	Local and sympathetic
PACAP	Adenylate cyclase activation	Local
PHM	Muscle relaxation, secretion	Local
Somatostatin	Multiple inhibitory effects e.g. gastric inhibition	Local
Substance P	Vasodilation, muscle constriction	Local and sensory
VIP	Vasodilation, muscle relaxation, secretion	Local

*CGRP, calcitonin-gene-related peptide; CRF, corticotrophin-releasing factor; GRP, gastrin-releasing peptide; CCK, cholecystokinin; NPY, neuropeptide Y; PACAP, pituitary adenylate cyclase-activating peptide; PHM, peptide histidine methionine; VIP, vasoactive intestinal peptide.

techniques exist and those for light microscopy can be divided broadly into transmitted light methods or fluorescent labelling (for review see Polak and Van Noorden 2003). Of the former, the unlabelled antibody enzyme (peroxidase antiperoxidase) or avidin-biotin complex methods are the most widely used. Fluorescence labelling usually employs an indirect method with fluorescein, rhodamine, or some other fluorescent compound coupled to the secondary antibody. The method of choice is often a matter of personal preference but immunostains visible on transmitted light are permanent and therefore more widely used where long-term storage of preparations is required. Immunostains of neuropeptides can be made on tissue sections or on whole mount preparations of intact layers of the gut (e.g. intramural plexuses) (Figs. 16.1 and 16. 3) or muscle layers. Co-localization of neuropeptides is achieved using serial sectioning through ganglion cells or by administering antibodies to separate neuropeptides, labelled with different colours, to the same section. The unravelling of the complexity of the ENS has been aided in recent years by the advent of confocal laser microscopy which allows quantitative, three-dimensional analysis of immunofluorescent tissue preparations (Matsumoto and Kramer 1994) (Fig. 16.1).

Similarly, for electron microscopy a number of methods exist for immunostaining of vesicles containing neuropeptides (and other antigens), the most popular of which are those that employ gold-labelled antibodies. Colloidal gold adsorbs on to the Fc portion of the immunoglobulin molecule and is electron dense. The immunogold staining technique is a straightforward indirect method (De Mey et al. 1981) (Fig. 16.4) and has been adapted to allow immunostaining of multiple antigens in a single tissue section by the use of antibodies labelled with gold particles of different sizes.

Localization of neuropeptide gene expression: *in situ* hybridization

Immunocytochemistry localizes the final products of gut nerves but information on the sites, rates, and control of neuropeptide

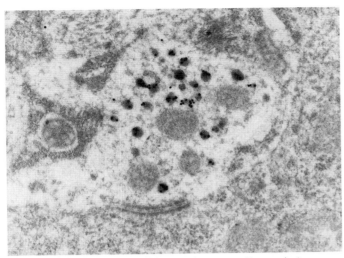

Fig. 16.4 Immunoreactivity for substance P demonstrated in granules in a nerve terminal in guinea pig colon using the indirect immunogold method and visualized using a transmission electron microscope.

gene expression can now be derived from histological preparations using *in situ* hybridization of DNA or RNA species directing neuropeptide synthesis (for review see Polak and McGee 1990). This technique utilizes the capacity of labelled complementary nucleic acid sequences to form stable hybrids with endogenous DNA or mRNA. The complementary sequences, in the form of single-stranded DNA or RNA, double-stranded DNA, or synthetic oligodeoxyribonucleotides, can be labelled with isotopes (e.g. ^{32}P, ^{35}S, ^{3}H) and localized by autoradiography or with substances subsequently localized by immunocytochemistry (e.g. biotin, digoxigenin) (Fig. 16.5).

Neural origins

The nature and projections of neuropeptide-containing gut nerves have been studied extensively in experimental animals. Chemical manipulations in combination with immunocytochemistry can

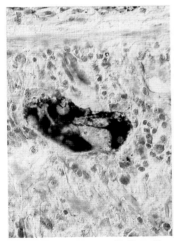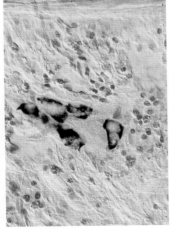

Fig. 16.5 Serial sections of inflamed human colon showing the submucous plexus. In **(a)** the section has been immunostained for vasoactive intestinal polypeptide (VIP) and in **(b)** *in situ* hybridization with a digoxygenin-labelled riboprobe shows the expression of VIP messenger RNA in the same cells.

help to identify particular nerve types containing neuropeptides. For example, immunostaining of NPY in rats treated with 6-hydroxydopamine shows a loss of NPY-immunoreactive fibres from around gut blood vessels, suggesting that these are noradrenergic sympathetic nerves (Su et al. 1987). Similarly, destruction of primary sensory afferents by administration of capsaicin (8-methyl-N-vanillyl-5-nonenamide) removes a proportion of CGRP- and SP-immunoreactive fibres from the rat gut, indicating their sensory nature (Su et al. 1987).

Analysis of the origin and projection fields of neuropeptide-containing innervation of the gut requires further manipulations, in the form of surgical interruption of nerve pathways or retrograde tracing using dyes. Interruption of pathways has been a useful way of establishing nerve origins. To continue with the example of NPY-containing nerves, sympathectomy by removal of the coeliac ganglion and plexus and the superior mesenteric ganglion reduces the population of nerves in the rat gut in a similar way to administration of 6-hydroxydopamine (Su et al. 1987). Lesioning of pathways can also be used to study neural projections within the gut wall. Myotomy, myectomy, and homotopic autotransplants, with immunocytochemical identification of nerve types, have been used successfully to provide detailed information on the projections of neuropeptide-immunoreactive nerves in certain species and the most complete analysis of neuronal circuitry of the mammalian gut has been achieved by application of these methods in the guinea pig small intestine (for review see Furness and Costa 1987, Furness 2000). However, a less invasive method is retrograde tracing of neuronal pathways, which has the major advantage of being applicable in specimens of human gut, thereby yielding information with direct relevance to clinical gastroenterology. Retrograde tracing uses the ability of nerves to transport dyes retrogradely to their perikarya and consists of injection of a suitable chemical (e.g. horseradish peroxidase, radiolabelled amino acids, fluorescent dyes) *in vivo* to the terminal region of interest, which is taken up and labels the cell of origin (for review see Su and Polak 1987). This is then identified by neuropeptide immunocytochemistry. In this way, sympathetic, NPY-immunoreactive nerves supplying, for example, the rat stomach have been shown to arise from perikarya in the coeliac and inferior mesenteric ganglia whereas sensory CGRP-immunoreactive fibres are supplied by bilateral dorsal root ganglia at levels T8–T11 (Su et al. 1987). A refinement of this technology has been to apply it *in vitro* to study human enteric neural pathways. Injection of a fluorescent dye, Fluorogold, into human colon maintained *in vitro*, combined with fluorescein immunofluorescence on whole mount preparations, was used to study the projection field of vasoactive intestinal polypeptide (VIP)-containing nerves in three dimensions (Domoto et al. 1990) and, thus, provide a new means to study human gut neuroanatomy (Fig. 16.6).

Neuropeptides in the developing human gut

Few studies have been made of neuropeptides in human fetal gut. A comprehensive immunocytochemical study of the ontogeny of major neuropeptides in the human oesophagus revealed their appearance in fibres at 11 (VIP, NPY, gastrin-releasing peptide [GRP]), 13 (galanin, SP), 15.5 (somatostatin, met-enkephalin), and 18 weeks (CGRP) (Hitchcock et al. 1992). Some investigation has been made of the way in which the peptide-containing nerves infiltrate the developing human gut. Traditionally, colonization

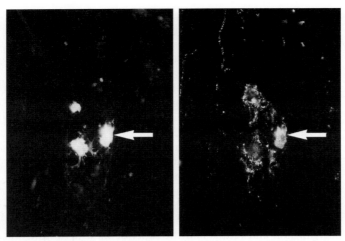

Fig. 16.6 (a) Fluorogold-labelled neurons in a whole mount preparation of the submucous plexus of the human colon after injection of the dye into the submucous layer. **(b)** Vasoactive-intestinal peptide (VIP) immunostained by indirect immunofluorescence in the same specimen. One cell (arrow) is labelled with the dye and also shows immunoreactivity for VIP. Differential visualization of the dye and immunostain in the same cells was achieved by altering the wavelength of observation light.

of the human gut by nerves is considered to occur in a craniocaudal direction, with subsequent passage of neuronal precursors through the muscle to form the major ganglionated plexuses although, in other species, bidirectional migration of neuronal precursors has been detected. Using immunocytochemistry and *in situ* hybridization in combination, the appearance of VIP-containing nerves has been examined in developing human gut (Facer et al. 1992). At the earliest stage examined (8 weeks gestation) nerve cells, demonstrated by immunostaining of the general nerve marker protein gene product 9.5, were found throughout the length of the gut, but not transversely. Ganglion cells were first found in both myenteric and submucous plexuses at 9 weeks gestation. VIP immunoreactivity was seen in fibres from 9 weeks' gestation but could not be found in perikarya until 18 weeks' gestation. With *in situ* hybridization, VIP gene expression in cells was detected much earlier, from 9 weeks' gestation, and its temporal appearance was consistent with craniocaudal, transmural neuronal colonization and/or migration.

Neuropeptides in gastrointestinal diseases

Marked abnormalities of the neuropeptide-containing innervation of the gut have been observed in a number of diseases. In view of the rapid breakdown of most neuropeptides, alterations in circulating levels are rare and most changes have been observed on the basis of morphological investigations sometimes coupled with radioimmunological measurement of peptide concentrations in affected tissues.

Chagas' disease

Severe disturbance of the normal pattern of neuropeptide-containing nerves has been reported in Chagas' disease, an example of acquired aganglionosis. This disease is a common result of long-standing infection with the flagellate protozoan, *Trypanasoma cruzi*. Ganglionitis occurs in the intramural plexuses with subsequent destruction of cells leading to denervation and distension of gut

segments, most commonly manifesting as megaoesophagus and/or megacolon. Comparison with both normal controls and patients with multiple system atrophy (Shy–Drager syndrome) has revealed a reduction in both VIP- and SP-immunoreactive nerves and tissue content of these neuropeptides only in Chagas' disease (Long et al. 1980). Thus the neuropeptides appear to be affected by intrinsic but not extrinsic autonomic neuropathy, indicating that VIP and SP have mainly intrinsic origins in the human bowel. A similar reduction in neuropeptides was found in an equine disease, grass sickness, which is in many ways analogous to human Chagas' disease in being acquired aganglionosis, although the pathogenic agent has yet to be identified (Bishop et al. 1984).

Idiopathic constipation

The pathogenesis of idiopathic, slow-transit constipation has yet to be clearly defined and, at present, colectomy is often used to treat the condition. Some changes in the morphology of intramural neurons have been noted and a recent study has examined the morphology and concentrations of the three major gut neuropeptides, VIP, SP, and NPY, in affected bowel (Milner et al. 1990). It seems that SP- and NPY-containing nerves are not altered in the colon of individuals with severe chronic idiopathic constipation, in comparison with normal control bowel. However, VIP content was reduced in the intramural plexuses of the colon, although no consistent alteration of VIP-immunoreactive nerves was seen on immunocytochemistry.

Hirschsprung disease

Hirschsprung disease, or congenital aganglionosis, is the most common of the congenital gut motility disorders and occurs in sporadic or familial forms. Heterozygous mutations in the *RET* receptor tyrosine kinase, that is expressed in ENCCs during their migration into the gut and persists during later ENS development (Pachnis et al. 1993), account for 15–35% of patients with sporadic Hirschsprung disease and 50% of familial cases (Brooks et al. 2005), whereas non-coding mutations have been suggested to impart susceptibility in other cases of Hirschsprung disease (Brooks et al. 2005, Emison et al. 2005, Griseri et al. 2007). In Hirschsprung disease, the neuronal lesions do not appear to be confined to an absence of intramural ganglion cells. Hypertrophied nerve bundles can be observed, often in the serosa or between the longitudinal and circular muscle layers. In addition, alterations of specific nerve types have been noted including increased adrenergic and cholinesterase-positive nerves and loss of intrinsic serotonin-containing nerves. For the neuropeptides, a mixed pattern of changes are seen in aganglionic bowel. VIP- (and its related molecule, peptide histidine methionine), SP-, met-enkephalin-, somatostatin-, and CGRP-immunoreactive nerves are reduced in aganglionic segments, possibly reflecting their mainly intrinsic origin in the human large bowel (Ehrenpreis and Pernow 1953, Tafuri et al. 1974, Bishop et al. 1981, Hamada et al. 1987). In contrast, fibres containing NPY immunoreactivity show a marked increase in aganglionic bowel, particularly in the circular muscle where few such fibres are normally found (Hamada et al. 1987) (Fig. 16.7). As described earlier, NPY-immunoreactive fibres in the gut have a dual origin from intramural ganglion cells and extrinsic noradrenergic nerves, and the latter innervate mainly the vasculature and myenteric plexus (Ekblad et al. 1984, Su et al. 1987). This change in NPY nerves may thus reflect the reported hyperplasia of aminergic fibres in patients with Hirschsprung disease.

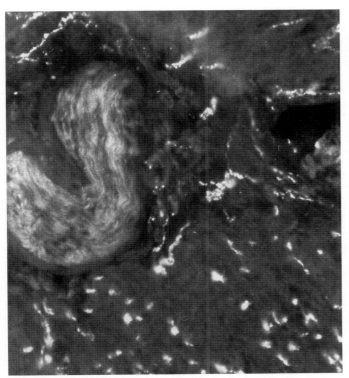

Fig. 16.7 Hyperplastic, numerous neuropeptide Y-immunoreactive fibres demonstrated by indirect immunofluorescence in large bowel from a child with Hirschsprung disease.

Diabetic neuropathy

Specific alterations of peptide-containing nerves are seen in the enteric neuropathy associated with streptozotocin-induced diabetes mellitus in rats. It has been reported that VIP nerve immunoreactivity increases, whereas that of CGRP nerves decreases, while SP- and NPY-immunoreactive nerves remain unchanged (Belai and Burnstock, 1990, Belai et al. 1993).

Inflammatory bowel disease

Neuronal abnormalities have long been known to occur in Crohn's disease (regional enteritis) and take the form of general nerve proliferation, sometimes termed neuromatous hyperplasia (Davis et al. 1955), but their significance remains unknown. Such changes are not characteristic of ulcerative colitis, and it is possible that the transmural inflammatory process that occurs in Crohn's disease stimulates the neural proliferation, as such a stimulus would be absent from all but the most severe cases of ulcerative colitis. No agreement has been reached on the pathology of peptide-containing nerves in IBD and a variety of different findings has been published (for review see Bishop and Polak 1990). The first study reported that VIP-immunoreactive fibres and the tissue content of VIP is increased in Crohn's disease (ileitis and colitis), in comparison with both ulcerative colitis and normal controls (Bishop et al. 1980, O'Morain et al. 1984). No evidence has been obtained that these hyperplastic VIP nerves are functional, but it is tempting to speculate that the peptide's potent stimulation of gut secretion and inhibition of motility may contribute to the symptoms of the disease. In contrast, a separate group of researchers reported a reduction of VIP nerves in Crohn's disease (Sjolund et al. 1983), while

a later study described loss of VIP from the mucosa/submucosa in Crohn's and ulcerative colitis (Koch et al. 1987). More recently, increased immunoreactivity for not only VIP but also NOS was described in Crohn's disease, in nerves and inflammatory cells, leading to the suggestion that neural-immunological interactions occur (Belai et al. 1997) and an increase in VIP-immunoreactive nerves of the submucosa specifically has also been observed in Crohn's disease (Schneider et al. 2001). SP, which is known to be an important mediator in neurogenic inflammation (O'Connor et al. 2004), has been reported to be increased in the rectum and colon of patients with ulcerative colitis and the levels of the neuropeptide correlate with disease activity (Koch et al. 1987).

Corticotrophin releasing factor (CRF) has been found in neuronal cell bodies and fibres of both enteric plexuses in most parts of the gut (Liu et al. 2006). This neuropeptide has been shown to play a pivotal role in mediating the effects of stress on the gut of animal models, some of which may be relevant to stress-induced exacerbation of symptoms in patients with IBD. Peripheral administration of CRF antagonists has been shown to abolish increases in colonic motility and decreases in gastric motility caused by restraint-induced stress. Mucosal permeability also appears to be increased by CRF, because pretreatment with a CRF antagonist reduced the inflammation caused by injection of *C. difficile* toxin into rat terminal ileum (Wlk et al. 2002). It has yet to be seen whether CRF has a similar role in human beings, but there is some preliminary evidence that it does in that CRF levels are increased in mononuclear cells of the lamina propria in colonic biopsies from patients with active ulcerative colitis (Kawahito et al. 1995, Muramatsu et al. 2000).

Conclusion

The intramural plexuses of the mammalian gut have long been known to form a major part of the autonomic nervous system but their importance has only been recognized comparatively recently with the discovery in of their complex neurochemistry and wide range of actions. The application of new techniques for the investigation of nerves allows delineation of the neuroanatomy of the gut and is revealing pathological alterations which may provide the basis for future therapeutic measures.

References

Abel, R. M. (1996). The ontogeny of the peptidergic innervation of the human pylorus, with special reference to understanding the aetiology and pathogenesis of infantile hypertrophic pyloric stenosis. *J. Pediatr. Surg.* **31**, 490–7.

Bar, K. J., Facer, P., Williams, N. S., Tam, P. K., Anand, P. (1997). Glial-derived neurotrophic factor in human adult and fetal intestine and in Hirshcsprung's disease. *Gastroenterol.* **112**, 1381–5.

Bealer, J. F., Natuzzi, E. S., Buscher, C., Ursell, P. C., Flake, A. W., Adzick, N. S. and Harrison, M. R. (1994). NO synthase is deficient in the aganglionic colon of patients with Hirschsprung's disease. *Pediatrics* **93**, 647–51.

Belai, A., Boulos, P. B., Robson, T., Burnstock, G. (1997). Neurochemical coding in the small intestine of patients with Crohn's disease. *Gut* **40**, 767–74.

Belai, A. and Burnstock, G. (1990). Changes in adrenergic and peptidergic nerves in the submucous plexus of streptozotocin-diabetic rat ileum. *Gastroenterology* **98**, 1427–36.

Belai, A., Facer, P., Bishop, A. E., Polak, J. M. and Burnstock, G. (1993). Effect of streptozotocin-diabetes on the level of VIP mRNA in myenteric neurones. *NeuroReport* **4**, 291–94.

Bishop, A. E., Hodson, N. P., Major, J. H., *et al.* (1984). The regulatory peptide system of the large bowel in equine grass sickness. *Experientia* **40**, 801–6.

Bishop, A. E. and Polak, J. M. (1990). Gut endocrine and neural peptides. *Endocrinol. Pathol.* **1**, 4–24.

Bishop, A. E., Polak, J. M., Bryant, M. G., Bloom, S. R. and Hamilton, S. (1980). Abnormalities of vasoactive intestinal polypeptide-containing nerves in Crohn's *disease. Gastroenterology* **79**, 853–60.

Bishop, A. E., Polak, J. M., Lake, B. D., Bryant, M. G. and Bloom, S. R. (1981). Abnormalities of the colonic regulatory peptides in Hirschsprung's disease. *Histopathology* **5**, 679–88.

Brooks, A. S., Oostra, B. A. & Hofstra, R. M. (2005). Studying the genetics of Hirschsprung's disease: unraveling an oligogenic disorder. *Clin. Genet.* **67**, 6–14.

Bult, H., Boeckxstaens G. E., Pelckmans, P. A., Jordaens, F. H., Van Maercke Y. M. and Herman, A. G. (1990). NO as an inhibitory non-adrenergic, non-cholinergic neurotransmitter. *Nature* **345**, 346–47.

Burns, A. J., Le Douarin, N. M. (1998). The sacral neural crest contributes neurons and glia to the post-umbilical gut: spatiotemporal analysis of the development of the ENS. *Development* **125**, 4335–47

Burnstock, G. (1981). Neurotransmitters and trophic factors in the autonomic nervous system. *J. Physiol.* **313**, 1–35.

Bush, T. G., Savidge, T. C., Freeman, *et al.* (1998). Fulminant jejuno-ileitis following ablation of enteric glia in adult transgenic mice. *Cell* **93**, 189–201.

Cabarrocas, J., Savidge, T. C., Liblau, R.S. (2003). Role of enteric glial cells in inflammatory bowel disease. *Glia* **41**, 81–93.

Cashman, N. R., Covault, J., Wollman, R. L. and Sanes, J. R. (1987). Neural cell adhesion molecule in norml, denervated and myopathic human muscle. *Ann. Neurol.* **21**, 481–9.

Chen, J-X., Pan, H., Rothman, T. P., Wade, P. R., Gershon, M. D. (1998). Guinea pig 5-HT transporter: cloning, expression, distribution and function in intestinal sensory reception. *Am. J. Physiol.* **275**, G433–48.

Coates, M. D., Mahoney, C. R., Linden, D. R., *et al.* (2004). Molecular defects in mucosal serotonin content and decreased serotonin reuptake transporter in ulcerative colitis and IBS. *Gastroenterol.* **126**, 1657–64.

Costa, M., Furness, J. B., Pompolo, S., Brookes, S. J. H., Bornstein, J. C., Bredt, D. S. and Snyder, S. H. (1992). Projections and chemical coding of neurons with immunoreactivity for NO synthase in the guinea pig small intestine. *Neurosci. Lett.* 148, 121–25.

Covault, J. and Sanes, J. R. (1985). Neural cell adhesion molecule (NCAM) accumulates in denervated and paralysed skeletal muscle. *Proc. Natl. Acad. Sci.* **82**, 4544–48.

Cunningham, B. A. (1991). Transactions of the ninth annual meeting of The American Gynaecological and Obstetrical Society. *Am. J. Obstet. Gynaecol.* **164**, 939–48.

Davis, D. R., Dockerty, M. B. and Mayo C. W. (1955). The myenteric plexus in regional enteritis: a study of ganglion cells in the ileum in 24 cases. *Surg. Gynaecol. Obstet.* **101**, 208.

De Mey, J., Moeremans, M., Geuens, G., Nuydens, R. and De Brabander, M. (1981). High resolution light and electron microscopic localization of tubulin with the IGS (immunogold staining) method. *Cell Biol. Int. Rep.* **5**, 889–99.

Desai, K. M., Warner, T. D., Bishop, A. E., Moncada, S., Polak, J. M. and Vane, J. R. (1994). NO but not VIP is the main neurotransmitter of vagally-induced relaxation of the guinea pig stomach. *Brit. J. Pharmacol.* **113**, 1197–1202.

Dickens, E. J., Hirst, G. D. S., Tomita, T. (1999). Identification of rhythmically active cells in guinea pig stomach. *J. Physiol. (Lond.)* **514**, 515–31.

Dogiel, A. S. (1899). Ueber den bau der Ganglien in den Gefiechten des Darmes und der Gallenblase des Menschen und der Sdugetiere. *Arch. Anat. Physiol. Leipzig, Anat. Abt.* **130**, 58.

Domoto, T., Bishop, A. E., Oki, M. and Polak, J. M. (1990). An *in vitro* study of the projections of enteric VIP-immunoreactive neurones in the human colon. *Gastroenterology* **98**, 819–27.

Druckenbrod, N. R. & Epstein, M. L. (2005). The pattern of neural crest advance in the cecum and colon. *Dev. Biol.* **287**, 125–33.

Druckenbrod, N. R. & Epstein, M. L. (2007). Behavior of enteric neural crest-derived cells varies with respect to the migratory wavefront. *Dev. Dyn.* **236**, 84–92.

Ehrenpreis, T. and Pernow, B. (1953). On the occurrence of substance P. in the rectosigmoid in Hirschsprung's disease. *Acta Physiol. Scand.* **27**, 380–8

Ekblad, E., Wahlstedt, C., Ekelund, M., Hakanson, R. and Sundler, F. (1984). Neuropeptide Y in the gut and pancreas. Distribution and possible vasomotor function. *Frontiers Horm. Res.* **12**, 85–90.

Emison, E. S., McCallion, A. S., Kashuk, C. S. *et al.* (2005). A common sex-dependent mutation in a RET enhancer underlies Hirschsprung disease risk. *Nature* **434**, 857–63.

Facer, P., Bishop, A.E., Moscoso, G., *et al.* (1992). Vasoactive intestinal peptide gene expression in the developing human gastrointestinal tract. *Gastroenterology* **102**, 47–55.

Farrugia, G. (1999). Ionic conductances in gastrointestinal smooth muscles and interstitial cells of Cajal. *Annu. Rev. Physiol.* **61**, 45–84.

Furness, J. B. and Costa, M. (ed.) (1987). *The ENS.* Churchill Livingstone, Edinburgh.

Furness, J. B. (2000). Types of neurons in the ENS. *J. Auton. Nerv. Syst.* **81**, 87–96.

Gabella, G. (1981). Ultrastructure of the nerve plexuses of the mammalian intestine: the enteric glial cells. *Neurosci.* **6**, 425–36.

Gershon, M. D. (2005). Nerves, reflexes, and the ENS: pathogenesis of the irritable bowel syndrome. *J. Clin. Gastroenterol.* **34**, 189–93.

Gershon, M. D., Tack, J. (2007). The serotonin signaling system: from basic understanding to drug development for functional GI disorders. *Gastroenterol.* **132**, 397–414

Grider, J. R. (1994). CGRP as a transmitter in the sensory pathway mediating peristaltic reflex. *Am. J. Physiol.* **266**, G1139–45.

Grider, J. R. (2003). Neurotransmitters mediating the intestinal peristaltic reflex in the mouse. *J. Pharmacol. Exp. Ther.* **307**, 460–67.

Griseri, P., Lantieri, F., Puppo, F. *et al.* (2007). A common variant located in the 3'UTR of the RET gene is associated with protection from Hirschsprung disease. *Hum. Mutat.* **28**, 168–76.

Guo, R., Nada, O., Suita, S., Taguchi, T. and Masumoto, K. (1997). The distribution and co-localization of NO synthase and vasoactive intestinal polypeptide nerves of the colon with Hirschsprung's disease. *Virchows Arch.* **430**, 53–61.

Hamada, Y., Bishop, A. E., Federici, G., Rivosecchi, M., Talbot, I. C. and Polak, J. M. (1987). Increased neuropeptide Y-immunoreactive innervation of aganglionic bowel in Hirschsprung'.s disease. *Virchow's Arch.* A**411**, 369–77.

Hanani, M., Reichenbach, A. Morphology of horseradish peroxidise (HRP)-injected glial cells in the myenteric plexus of the guinea pig. *Cell Tiss. Res.* **278**, 153–60.

Heanue, T. A., Pachnis, V. (2006). Expression profiling the developing mammalian ENS identifies marker and candidate Hirschsprung disease genes. *Proc Natl. Acad. Sci.* **103**, 6919–24.

Heanue, T. A., Pachnis, V. (2007). ENS development and Hirschsprung's disease: advances in genetic and stem cell studies. *Nat Rev Neurosci.* **8**, 466–79.

Hirst, G. D. S., Edwards, F. R. (2001). Generation of slow waves in the antral region of guinea pig stomach—a stochastic process. *J. Physiol. (Lond.)* **535**, 165–80.

Hirst, G. D. S., Ward, S. M. (2003). Interstitial cells, involvement in rhythmicity and neural control of smooth muscle cells. *J. Physiol. (Lond.)* **550**, 337–46.

Hitchcock, R. J. I., Pemble, M. J., Bishop, A. E., Spitz, L. and Polak, J. M. (1992). The ontogeny and distribution of neuropeptides in the human fetal and infant oesophagus. *Gastroenterology* **102**, 840–8.

Hoehner, J. C., Wester, T., Pahlman, S., Olsen, L. (1996). Localization of neurotrophins and their high affinity receptors during human nteric nervous system development. *Gastroenterol.* **110**, 756–67.

Jessen, K.R., Mirsky, R., Dennison, M.E. and Burnstock, G. (1979). GABA may be a neurotransmitter in the vertebrate peripheral nervous system. *Nature* **281**, 71–4.

Kawahito, Y., Sano, H., Mukai, S., Asai, K., Kimura, S., Yamamura, Y., Kato, H., Chrousos, G.P., Wilder, R.L., Kondo, M. (1995). Corticotropin releasing hormone in colonic mucosa in patients with ulcerative colitis. *Gut* **37**, 544–51.

Keef, K.D., Du, C., Ward, S.M., McGregor, B. and Sanders, K. M. (1993). Enteric inhibitory neural regulation of human colonic circular muscle: role of NO. *Gastroenterology* **105**, 1009–16.

Koch, T. R., Carney, J. A. and Go V. L. W. (1987). Distribution and quantification of gut neuropeptides in normal intestine and inflammatory bowel disease. *Dig. Dis. Sci.* **32**, 369–76.

Langley, J. N. (1898) On the union of cranial autonomic (visceral) fibres with the nerve cells of the superior cervical ganglion. *J. Physiol.* **23**, 240–70.

Larsson, L. T., Shen, Z., Ekblad, E., Sundler, F., Alm, P. and Andersson, K. E. (1995). Lack of neuronal NO synthase in nerve fibres of aganglionic intestine: a clue to Hirschsprung's disease. *J. Pediatr. Gastroenterol. Nutr.* **20**, 49–53.

Le Douarin, N.M., Teillet, M.A. (1973). The migration of neural crest cells to the wall of the digestive tract in avian embryo. *J. Embryol. Exp. Morphol.* **30**, 31–48.

Long, R.G., Bishop, A.E., Barnes, A.J., *et al.* (1980). Neural and hormonal peptides in rectal biopsy specimens from patients with Chagas' disease and chronic autonomic failure. *Lancet* **i**, 559–62.

Matsumoto, B. and Kramer, T. (1994). Theory and applications of confocal microscopy. *Cell Vision* **1**, 190–8.

Mearin, F., Mourelle, M., Guarner, F., Salas, A., Riveros-Moreno, V., Moncada, S. and Malagelada, J. R. (1993). Patients with achalasia lack NO synthase in the gastro-oesophageal junction. *Euro. J. Clin. Invest.* **23**, 724–8.

Milner, P., Crowe, R., Kamm, M. A., Lennard-Jones, J. E. and Burnstock, G. (1990). Vasoactive intestinal polypeptide levels in sigmoid colon in idiopathic constipation and diverticular disease. *Gastroenterology* **99**, 666–75.

Moncada, S., Palmer, R. M. J. and Higgs, E. A. (1991). NO: physiology, pathophysiology and pharmacology. *Pharmacol. Rev.* **43**, 109–42.

Muramatsu Y., Fukushima K., Iino K., *et al.* (2000). Urocortin and corticotropin-releasing factor receptor expression in the human colonic mucosa. *Peptides* **21**, 1799–809.

O'Connor, T., O'Connell, J., O'Brien, D. I. *et al.* (2004). The role of substance P. in inflammatory disease. J. Cell Physiol. **201**, 167–80.

O'Kelly, T. J., Davies, J. R., Tam, P. K., Brading, A. F., Mortensen, N. J. (1994). Abnormalities of NO-producing neurons in Hirschsprung's disease: morphology and implications. *J. Pediatr. Surg.* **29**, 294–9.

O'Morain, C., Bishop, A. E., McGregor, G. P., Levi, A. J., Bloom, S. R., Polak, J. M., and Peters, T. J. (1984). Vasoactive intestinal peptide concentrations and immunocytochemical studies in rectal biopsies from patients with inflammatory bowel disease. *Gut* **25**, 57–61.

Ong, J. and Kerr, D. I. B. (1983). GABAA- and GABAB-receptor-mediated modification of intestinal motility. *Eur. J. Pharmacol.* **86**, 9–17.

Pachnis, V., Mankoo, B., Constantini, F. (1993). Expression of the c-ret proto-oncogene during mouse embryogenesis. *Development* **119**, 1005–1017.

Pan, H., Gershon, M. D. (2000). Activation of intrinsic afferent pathways in submucosal ganglia of the guinea pig small intestine. *J. Neurosci.* **20**, 3295–3309.

Polak, J. M., McGee, J. O'D. (1990). *In situ hybridization.* Oxford University Press, Oxford.

Polak, J. M., Van Noorden, S. (2003). *Introduction to immunocytochemistry* (3rd edn). Bios Scientific Publishers, Oxford.

Rieger, F., Grumet M. and Edelman G. M. (1985) N-CAM at the vertebrate neuromuscular junction. *J. Cell Biol.* **101**, 285–93.

Romanska, H. M., Bishop, A. E., Brereton, R. J., Spitz, L. and Polak, J. M. (1993). Increased expression of muscular neural cell adhesion molecule in congenital aganglionosis. *Gastroenterology* **105**, 1104–1109.

Romanska, H. M., Bishop, A. E., Lee, J. C., Walsh, F. S., Spitz, L. and Polak, J. M. (1996b). Idiopathic constipation is not associated with increased neural cell adhesion molecule expression on intestinal muscle. *Dig. Dis. Sci.* **41**, 1298–302.

Romanska, H. M., Bishop, A. E., Moscoso, G., Walsh, F. S., Spitz, L., Brereton, R. J., and Polak, J. M. (1996a). Neural cell adhesion molecule expression in the nerves and muscle of developing human large bowel. *J. Pediatr. Gastroenter. Nutr.* **22**, 351–8.

Ruhl, A., Franze, S., Collin, S. M., Stremmel, W. (2001). Interleukin 6 expression and regulation in rat enteric glial cells. *Am. J. Physiol.* **280**, G1163–1171.

Ruhl, A., Nasser, Y., Sharkey, K. A. (2004). Enteric glia. *Neurogastroenterol. Moltil.* **16** Suppl. 1, 44–49.

Sanders, K. M. and Ward, S. M. (1992). NO as a mediator of non-adrenergic, non-cholinergic (NANC) neurotransmission. *Am. J. Physiol.* **262**, G379–92.

Savidge, T., Newman, P., Pan, W-H., Hurst, R. (2003). Enteroglia (EGC) are novel cellular regulators of mucosal barrier function in the gastrointestinal tract. *Gastroenterol.* **124**, A27.

Schneider, J., Jehle, E. C., Starlinger, M. J., Neunlist, M., Michel, K., Hoppe, S., Schemann, M. (2001). Neurotransmitter coding of enteric neurones in the submucous plexus is changed in non-inflamed rectum of patients with Crohn's disease. *Neurogastroenterol. Motil.* **13**, 255–64.

Sjolund, K., Schaffalitzky De Muckadell, 0.B., Fahrenkrug, J., Hakanson, R., Peterson, B. G., and Sundler, F. (1983). Peptide-containing nerve fibres in the gut wall in Crohn's disease. *Gut* **24**, 724–33.

Springall, D. R., Suburo, A., Bishop, A. E., Merett, M., Riveros-Moreno, V., Moncada, S. and Polak, J. M. (1992). Distinct localization of NO synthase(s) immunoreactivity in human vasculature and nerves using separate antisera. *Histochem.* **98**, 259–66.

Stark, M. E. and Szurszewski, J. H. (1992). Role of NO in gastrointestinal and hepatic function and disease. *Gastroenterology* **103**, 1928–49.

Steinkamp, M., Geering, I., Seufferlein, T., *et al.* (2003). Glial-derived neurotrophic factor regulates apoptosis in colonic epithelial cells. *Gastroenterol.* **124**, 1748–57.

Su, H. C., Bishop, A. E., Power, R. F., Hamada, Y., and Polak, J. M. (1987). Dual intrinsic and extrinsic origins of CGRP- and NPY-immunoreactive nerves of rat gut and pancreas. *J. Neurosci.* **7**, 2674–87.

Su, H. C. and Polak, J. M. (1987). Combined axonal transport tracing and immunocytochemistry for mapping pathways of peptide-containing nerves in the peripheral nervous system. *Experientia* **43**, 761–7.

Tafuri, W. L., Maria, T. A., Pittella, J. E. and Bogliolo, L. (1974). An electron microscopic study of the Auerbach's plexus and determination of substance P of the colon in Hirschsprung's disease. *Virchow's Arch.* **A362**, 41–50.

Thiery, J. P. (1982). Cell adhesion molecules in early chicken embryogenesis. *Proc. Natl. Acad. Sci.* **79**, 6737–41.

Thuneberg, L. (1982). Interstitial cells of Cajal: intestinal pacemaker cells? *Adv. Anat. Embryol. Cell Biol.* **71**, 1–130.

Tjwa, E. T., Bradley, J. M., Kennan, C. M., Kroese, A. B., Sharkey, K. A. (2003). Interleukin 1β activates specific populations of enteric neuron and enteric glia in the guinea pig ileum and colon. *Am. J. Physiol.* **285**, G1268–1276.

Toda, N., Baba, H. and Okamura, T. (1990). Role of NO in non-adrenergic, non-cholinergic nerve-mediated relaxation in dog duodenal longitudinal muscle strips. *Jap. J. Pharmacol.* **53**, 281–84.

Tomita, T. (1981). Electrical activity (spikes and slow waves) in gastrointestinal smooth muscles. In: Bulbring, E., Brading, A. F., Jones, A. W., Tomita, T., Editors. Smooth muscle: an assessment of current knowledge. Edward Arnold: 1981, pp. 127–56.

Tomita, R., Munakata, K., Kurosu, Y., Tanjoh, K. (1995). A role of NO in Hirschsprung's disease. *J. Pediatr. Surg.* **30**, 437–40.

Vanderwinden, J. M., Rumessen, J. J. (1999). Interstitial cells of Cajal in human gut and gastrointestinal disease. *Microsc. Res. Tech.* **47**, 344–60.

Vanderwinden, J. M., Mailleux, P., Schiffmann, S. N., Vanderhaeghen, J. J. and De Laet, M. H. (1992). NO synthase activity in infantile hypertrophic pyloric stenosis. *New Engl. J. Med.* **327**, 511–5.

Vanderwinden, J. M., De Laet, M. H., Schiffmann, S. N., Mailleux, P., Lowenstein, C. J., Snyder, S. H. and Vanderhaeghen, J. J. (1993). NO synthase distribution in the ENS of Hirschsprung's disease. *Gastroenterology* **105**, 969–73.

Wade, P. R., Chen, J., Jaffe, B., Kassem, I. S., Blakely, R. D., Gershon, M. D. (1996). Localization and function of a 5-HT transporter in crypt epithelia of the gastrointestinal tract. *J. Neurosci.* **16**, 2352–64.

Walsh F. S., Moore, S. and Lake, B. (1987). Cell adhesion molecule NCAM is expressed by denervated myofibres in Werding-Hoffman and Kugelberg-Welander type of spinal muscular atrophies. *J Neurol. Neurosurg. Psychiatry* **50**, 539–42.

Walsh, F. S., Moore, S., and Dickson J. (1988). Expression of membrane antigens in myotonic dystrophy. *J Neurol. Neurosurg. Psychiatry* **51**, 136–8.

Wang, X. Y., Sanders, K. M., Ward, S. M. (1999). Intimate relationship between interstitial cells of Cajal and enteric nerves in the guinea pig small intestine. *Cell Tiss. Res.* **295**, 247–56.

Ward, S. M., Xue, C., Shuttleworth, C. W. R., Bredt, D. S., Snyder, S. H. and Sanders, K. M. (1992). NADPH diaphorase and NO synthase co-localization in enteric neurons of the canine proximal colon. *Am. J. Physiol.* **263**, G277–284.

Ward, S. M., Sanders, K. M., Hirst, G. D. S. (2004). Role of interstitial cells of Cajal in neural control of gastrointestinal smooth muscles. *Neurogastroenterol.* **16** Suppl 1, 112–117.

Ward, S. M. & Sanders, K. M. (2006). Involvement of intramuscular interstitial cells of Cajal in neuroeffector transmission in the gastrointestinal tract. *J. Physiol.* **576**, 675–82.

Wlk, M., Wang, C. C., Venihaki, M., *et al.* (2002). Corticotropin-releasing hormone antagonists possess anti-inflammatory effects in the mouse ileum. *Gastroenterol.* **123**, 505–15.

Young, H. M., Furness, J. B., Shutleworth, C. W. R., Bredt, D. S. and Snyder, S. H. (1992). Co-localization of NO synthase immunoreactivity and NADPH diaphorase staining in neurons of the guinea-pig intestine. *Histochem.* **97**, 375–78.

Young, H. M., Bergner, A. J. and Muller, T. (2003). Acquisition of neuronal and glial markers by neural crest-derived cells in the mouse intestine. *J. Comp. Neurol.* **456**, 1–11.

Young, H. M., Bergner, A. J., Anderson, R. B. Enomoto, H., Milbrandt, J., Newgreen, D. F., Whitington, P. M. (2004). Dynamics of neural crest-derived cell migration in the embryonic mouse gut. *Dev. Biol.* **270**, 455–73.

Young, H. M., Turner, K. N. & Bergner, A. J. (2005). The location and phenotype of proliferating neural-crestderived cells in the developing mouse gut. *Cell Tissue Res.* **320**, 1–9.

CHAPTER 17

Nausea, vomiting, and the autonomic nervous system

Paul L. R. Andrews

Introduction

Nausea (a sensation) and vomiting (a motor event) are among the most common symptoms of disease and are also frequent 'side-effects' of drug therapies (e.g. anticancer chemotherapy) and some treatments (e.g. radiotherapy, postoperative nausea and vomiting). The autonomic nervous system plays a major role in both nausea and vomiting. Visceral afferents, principally in the abdominal vagus, provide one of the most important triggers for their induction. The nucleus tractus solitarius in the brainstem is one of the main nuclei involved in processing visceral afferent information and serves to integrate many of the reflex motor events constituting vomiting. The autonomic motor nuclei in the brainstem (e.g. dorsal motor vagal nucleus, nucleus ambiguus, the presympathetic neurons), thoracolumbar and sacral spinal cord are all involved to varying degrees in generating the physiological events accompanying nausea and the motor components of vomiting. The hypothalamic–pituitary axis is involved in the endocrine changes associated with nausea and 'higher' brain regions are implicated in the emotional (e.g. amygdala) and sensory experiences (insula).

Disorders of the autonomic nervous system also result in nausea and vomiting. For example, brainstem tumours involving the nucleus tractus solitarius cause nausea and vomiting as may disordered gastric motility secondary to damage to the extrinsic or enteric innervation of the upper gut.

Although nausea and vomiting are often encountered in a clinical context, a fact recognized by Hippocrates and other early physicians (Stern et al. 2011), it is important to appreciate that they evolved as components of the body's defensive system, which serves to protect it against accidentally ingested toxins (e.g. viral, bacterial, plant, marine organisms), which may be tasteless or masked by food or even constituents of the food itself (e.g. plant alkaloids and other defensive compounds). This 'biological' role has long been recognized, as elegantly illustrated by the following quotation from Robert Boyle in 1686:

Tis profitable for man that his stomach should nauseate and reject things that have a loathsome taste or smell.

This chapter examines the links between nausea and vomiting and the autonomic nervous system from several aspects: the motor components of nausea and vomiting; the pathways by which they are induced, and the mechanism by which autonomic disorders and drugs used to treat them may induce nausea and vomiting. The chapter concludes with an introduction to the pharmacology of anti-emetics.

Nausea

Nausea (Fig. 17.1) is less well understood than vomiting and yet is considered by patients to be far more of a problem because of its prolonged and debilitating nature. In general nausea is less well treated than is vomiting, to some extent reflecting the relatively poor understanding in contrast to vomiting. For a comprehensive discussion of the physiology of nausea see Stern et al. 2011.

The study of nausea is difficult because it is a subjective sensation relying on the patient to report, describe, and characterize in the light of previous experiences often acquired in childhood. In addition, because it is a subjective sensation it is impossible to study directly in animals, although the behaviour of animals in the pre-expulsion period can be quantified and can be argued to be correlates, equivalents, or surrogates of the sensation (Stern et al. 2011). Nausea is also difficult to identify with certainty in neonates and children before language develops, therefore there is a need to develop biomarkers for use in this population and also in the adult population so that diagnosis does not reply upon self-reporting, and more objective measures of efficacy can be obtained for pharmacological therapies.

Nausea is described variously as 'a feeling that vomiting is about to take place', 'an unpleasant sensation of being about to vomit', 'the imminent desire to vomit', 'a vague discomfort in the epigastric region with 'queasiness' or 'sick-to-the-stomach sensations' (see Stern et al. 2011, Table 1.1, p: 8/9 for 30 'definitions' of nausea from the literature illustrating the difficulty in defining sensory experiences to ensure consistency in clinical trials). In addition to the sensory aspects of nausea, a number of endocrine (e.g. adrenaline [increase], adrenocorticotropic hormone [increase], cortisol [increase in motion sickness but may decrease in patients undergoing chemotherapy], growth hormone [increase], endorphin [increase]), autonomic changes (e.g. sweating), and somatic (e.g. lassitude and weakness) responses occur. One of the problems in identifying the mechanisms by which the sensation is generated is separating which of these changes are a response to the generally stressful nature of nausea and which are a component of the mechanism underlying the genesis of the sensation. It should be noted

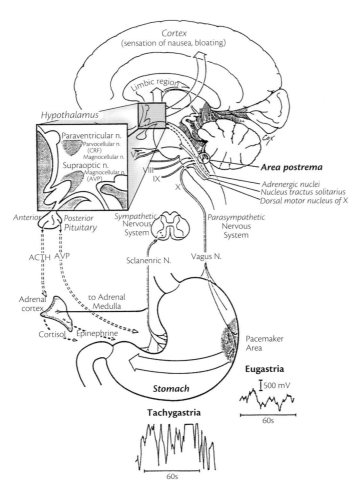

Fig. 17.1 Brain–gut and gut–brain interactions during the shift from eugastria to tachygastria. Vagal and splanchnic nervous systems connect with the central nervous system structures such as the hypothalamus, area postrema, and cortex, areas that are relevant to the perception of visceral sensations such as nausea and bloating. Neural efferent activity from the parasympathetic and sympathetic nervous systems or stress hormones such as epinephrine, cortisol, and vasopressin (AVP), may alter gastric neuromuscular activity, such as the pacesetter potentials. ACTH, adrenocorticotropic hormone; CRF, corticotropin releasing factor. Figure from Koch and Stern 2004, with permission.

that most studies that have investigated the mechanism of nausea have used motion sickness (usually vection/illusory self-motion) as a model and relatively few have studied patients with nausea caused either by their disease or treatment. There are some features of motion sickness such as sensations of light-headedness, disorientation, dizziness and perhaps sopite-syndrome (Muth 2006) that suggest that aspects of motion sickness may differ from nausea induced by other stimuli, but this requires systematic investigation.

It appears that many, if not all, of the autonomic changes that occur in the pre-emetic and peri-emetic period are either components of the 'vomiting motor programme' or are responses to the 'stress' of nausea. Thus, they are not responsible for the genesis of the sensation of nausea and many of them can be induced independently without being accompanied by nausea. It has been reported that all the autonomic signs of motion sickness have been observed in a decorticate person on an airplane (Doig et al. 1953).

Studies, predominantly of motion sickness in man using the vection/illusory self-motion model, have identified two consistent

responses (elevated vasopressin and disturbances in the electrogastrogram [EGG]) that appear to be intimately linked to nausea, although the way in which they are mechanistically linked to the genesis of the sensation is yet to be established.

Vasopressin

An elevation in plasma vasopressin (AVP, antidiuretic hormone) may be expected as a response to the fluid loss expected to occur when vomiting ensues. However, it is difficult to reconcile this function with the very high levels of vasopressin measured in some studies during nausea and vomiting in man and animals as these levels are in excess of those required for antidiuresis. These elevated levels of vasopressin could divert blood away from the gastrointestinal tract argued to reduce absorption of ingested toxins. Experimental studies in man have shown a close temporal correlation between the onset of nausea and the increase in vasopressin levels (Stern et al. 2011) and also with the decline in vasopressin levels and the passing of the sensation. Similar changes in vasopressin but not oxytocin have been seen in animal models (e.g. ferret, dog) in response to emetic stimuli and emphasize the selective nature of the response. Infusions of vasopressin in man can induce nausea and bloating (Caras et al. 1997) and gastric dysrhythmias. Several studies have reported a positive correlation between plasma vasopressin concentration and the intensity of nausea. However, patients with diabetes insipidus incapable of raising vasopressin levels have nausea and vomiting when given apomorphine or oral ipecacuanha (Nussey et al. 1988). It is possible that elevated plasma vasopressin represents the predominant mechanism for genesis of nausea but when it is absent other substances or mechanisms can fulfil a similar role. Plasticity in the emetic reflex has been reported in animals where removal of one pathway may lead to the induction or expression of an additional mechanism (Andrews and Davis 1995). However, the site (central vs. peripheral) at which elevated plasma vasopressin would act to induce the sensation of nausea remains to be identified (Stern et al. 2011).

Overall, plasma vasopressin levels may be a useful biomarker for nausea but until the mechanistic link (if any) is understood should measurements should be used with caution. Developments in vasopressin receptor pharmacology (V_{1a}, V_{1b}, V_2) and antagonists (Ali et al. 2007) will facilitate identification of its role in nausea.

Electrogastrogram rhythm changes

These are abnormalities in the frequency (bradygastria or tachygastria) of the gastric muscle slow wave or pacesetter potential outside the normal range of 2–4 cpm, which is determined by the pacemaker activity of the interstitial cells of Cajal (Owyang and Hasler 2002). The electrical activity of the stomach, the EGG, can be recorded from cutaneous electrodes placed over the stomach (Koch and Stern 2004) and such recordings have been used as a diagnostic aid. Dysrhythmias have been reported in healthy subjects exposed to vection (illusory self-motion), with experimental hyperglycaemia or antral distension, and in patients with symptomatic diabetic and idiopathic gastroparesis, functional dyspepsia, pregnancy sickness, chronic renal failure, visceral neuropathy, after gastric surgery and treatment with anticancer chemotherapy (Koch and Stern 2004). Dysrhythmias (usually tachygastria, 4–9 cpm) evoked by motion sickness have been the most studied and onset a few minutes before nausea is reported. with the degree of change positively correlated with the intensity of nausea. The functional correlate of the dysrhythmias is reduced contractile activity in the gastric antrum and this is consistent with observations that gastric emptying is delayed following exposure to an emetic stimulus. Multiple neuroendocrine mechanisms have been implicated in the genesis of dysrhythmias (Owyang and Hasler 2002) but of most relevance to this chapter are:

- induction of dysrhythmias by vasopressin

- an increase in sympathetic nervous system drive to the stomach associated with a decrease in the vagal drive (Muth 2006, Stern et al. 2011).

For both vasopressin and gastric dysrhythmias, if they are involved in nausea then how could they generate the sensation? The mechanical consequence of gastric dysrhythmias (i.e. antral quiescence) could be detected by visceral afferents projecting to the brainstem and eventually generating the sensation by projection of the signal to higher brain regions. Abdominal vagal afferent activation has been shown to evoke vasopressin secretion so that even if vasopressin secretion was the primary cause of the dysrhythmia, secretion could be enhanced via its effects on the stomach. Systemic vasopressin could also activate the nucleus tractus solitarius via the area postrema. From the nucleus tractus solitarius second order projections have ready access to the higher regions of the brain, with the insular cortex proposed as the visceral sensory area (see Stern et al. 2011, Chapter 4 for detailed discussion of central pathways).

There is a pressing need for functional brain imaging studies (see Van Oudenhove et al. 2007) specifically investigating subjects experiencing nausea. A study using magnetic source imaging with vestibular and ingested ipecac as stimuli implicated the inferior frontal gyrus in the sensation (Miller et al., 1996) and an fMRI study in volunteers experiencing video-induced motion sickness showed activation of the inferior frontal gyrus and the temporal lobe (Ng et al., 2011).

Vomiting

Motor components of the emetic reflex

The motor components of the emetic reflex (Fig. 17.2) can conveniently be divided into three phases. Each will be described together with the pathways that mediate the response.

Pre-expulsion

The phase prior to the onset of retching and vomiting is associated with nausea and responses suggestive of autonomic arousal. While the latter coexist with nausea, perhaps with the exception of the gastric motility changes, there is no evidence that they are directly responsible for genesis of the sensation of nausea and should be regarded as part of the emetic motor programme. Each will be briefly described.

Salivation

Salivation, often accompanied by repetitive swallowing, is a clear prodromal sign of emesis in animals, particularly dogs, and is due to activation of the parasympathetic nerves. However, salivary secretion is reduced during each burst of retching and may be absent between bursts (Furukawa and Okada 1994). In addition, salivation could also be reflexly evoked by oesophageal distension and gastric mucosal stimulation. It has been argued that the increase in alkaline saliva secretion may buffer the acidic nature of the vomitus, which could lead to dental erosion. Hypertrophy of the salivary glands is reported in some patients with bulimia.

In humans, increased salivation is reported to occur prior to emesis, particularly when induced by motion. However, this is based almost exclusively on subjective reports. A study measuring salivary secretion in individuals sick at sea showed that there was a decrease in unstimulated and stimulated salivary flow in 80% of the subjects (Gordon et al. 1989). Eight of the 13 subjects reported an increase in salivation, although in six there was a decrease. This and other studies, which attempt to demonstrate a correlation between salivary secretion and subjective symptoms, highlight the difficulty of extrapolating physiological mechanisms from subjective reports. The subject's perception of increased salivation could be due to a reduction in spontaneous swallowing, perhaps allowing an accumulation of saliva in the mouth. Alternatively, it is possible that there is heightened sensitivity of the oral cavity, which can be considered one of the early lines of defence against ingested toxins. This would appear to make sense teleologically when the warning, protective, and learning roles of nausea are considered.

Tachycardia

An increase in heart rate and blood pressure is often reported prior to the onset of retching and vomiting. However, the magnitude of the tachycardia does not appear to correlate with the severity of symptoms in response to a motion stimulus (Koch 1993). The mechanism is increased sympathetic drive and a reduction in vagal tone. Using illusory self-motion as a nauseogenic stimulus a reciprocal relationship was reported between respiratory sinus arrhythmia and severity of motion sickness symptoms (Gianaros et al. 2003). Once retching and vomiting commence the cardiovascular changes are modulated by the marked oscillations in intrathoracic and intra-abdominal pressure, which modify venous return.

Cutaneous vasoconstriction

Vasoconstriction is presumably due to increased activation of sympathetic adrenergic vasoconstrictor fibres to the skin, and the consequential reduced blood flow gives rise to the characteristic pallid (or even 'green') appearance associated with nausea. However, a role for high concentrations of plasma vasopressin cannot be excluded (see p.206). Regulation of cutaneous blood flow is reviewed by Drummond in Chapter 67.

Sweating

The pathway for sweating is again sympathetic, although involving cholinergic mechanisms (see Goadsby, Chapter 13 and Low and Fealey, Chapter 31). In association with nausea it appears to be particularly prominent on the forehead and may not be present on the palms (Himi et al. 2004). When there is simultaneous activation of the vasoconstrictor and sudomotor fibres 'cold sweating' occurs, a condition associated with mental stress. Both changes are reflected in an increase in skin conductance.

Pupillary dilatation

The pupil is reported to dilate in the prodromal phase, although it has not been formally characterized. Dilation is another indication of a reciprocal change in the balance of sympathetic and parasympathetic activity, with the former predominating. Ambulatory pupilometry may provide useful insights into the time course of the changes in autonomic activity that occur in the prodromal phase.

Peri-expulsion and expulsion

The basic mechanism by which vomiting occurs due to contraction of the diaphragm and abdominal muscles was identified by the

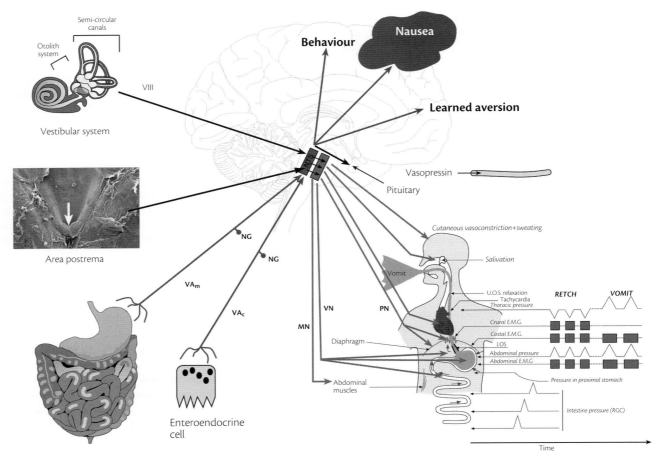

Fig. 17.2 A diagrammatic summary of the main afferent pathways capable of inducing nausea and vomiting converging on the nucleus tractus solitarius (NTS): Vestibular system (semicircular canals and otoliths via cranial nerve VIII and the vestibular nucleus); area postrema and the abdominal vagal afferents (VA_M, vagal afferent mechanoreceptors, VA_C, vagal afferent mucosal chemoreceptors, NG, nodose ganglion). The NTS sends outputs to the major motor nuclei (located in the more ventral parts of the brainstem; motor nuclei such as the ventral respiratory group [VRG], Bötzinger neurons, presympathetic neurons) responsible for the mechanical events of retching and vomiting (e.g. VN, abdominal vagus nerve from dorsal motor vagal nucleus mediating lower oesophageal sphincter [LOS] relaxation, gastric relaxation and giant retrograde contraction of the small intestine; P, phrenic nerve with nuclei in C_3–C_5 driven from VRG; MN, spinal motor neurons), the prodromas of vomiting often associated with nausea (mediated by sympathetic and parasympathetic nerves) and the rostral projections (predominantly via the parabrachial nucleus [PBN]) leading to vasopressin secretion (hypothalamus–posterior pituitary) and the more complex responses requiring cerebral cortical involvement including the genesis of the sensation of nausea itself. UOS, upper oesophageal sphincter; EMG, electromyogram. See text for details. Reproduced from Stern, R.M., Koch, K. and Andrews, P.L.R., *Nausea—Mechanisms and Management*, 2011, with permission from Oxford University Press.

classic studies of Magendie in 1813 who 'replaced' the stomach in a dog with a pig's bladder and demonstrated that the contents of the bladder could be expelled when the animal was given an emetic. More recent studies have revealed many subtle additional features of the process by recording electromyographic activity from a number of skeletal muscles and the gut. The description below is based mainly on studies in dogs (Lang et al. 1993) but the more limited human studies indicate that the mechanism is comparable although is unlikely to be identical in the oesophagus because of the differences in the extent of striated and smooth muscle in the two species. There is a need for studies in humans using more modern techniques, because the key studies describing aspects of the mechanics of vomiting in humans were published over 40 years ago (e.g. Lumsden and Holden 1969)

The main activity occurring during the peri-expulsion period is in the gastrointestinal tract whereas the expulsive phase mainly involves the diaphragm and abdominal muscles.

Gastrointestinal tract

Several specific changes occur in the gut prior to the onset of retching and vomiting, and the major ones are described below. It must be emphasized that these events are not the cause of nausea but are components of the motor response leading to expulsion, with each event having a function.

The initial event appears to be relaxation of the proximal stomach (De Ponti et al. 1990) and while this may occur prior to the onset of emesis to reduce the emptying of an ingested toxin, animal studies have shown that relaxation occurs as a specific component of the emetic reflex. The relaxation allows the stomach to receive the material from the intestine prior to retching and may place the stomach in an anatomically more favourable position for compression by the diaphragm and abdominal muscles. In addition, if the stomach wall is flaccid, the intra-abdominal pressure changes are more likely to be transmitted than if there is a high tone. The mechanism of relaxation is by vagal efferent activation of the intramural non-adrenergic, non-cholinergic inhibitory neurons, using nitric oxide and vasoactive intestinal polypeptide as neurotransmitters. The lower oesophageal sphincter relaxes at this time, again under the influence of the vagus.

When the stomach is relaxed, a single, large amplitude (~1.5 times the amplitude of phase III of the migrating motor complex [MMC]) contraction termed the retrograde giant contraction (RGC) originates in the small intestine and propagates retrogradely to the gastric antrum. The speed of propagation is about 10 cm/s in the dog. This contraction is under vagal control and can be blocked by atropine and hexamethonium but not by phentolamine and propranolol (Lang et al. 1993).

The RGC is proposed to have two functions:

♦ to return any contaminated gastric contents to the stomach for expulsion

♦ to carry alkaline pancreatic and intestinal secretions to the stomach to buffer gastric contents and hence reduce damage to the teeth and oesophagus.

The RGC also carries bile with it, probably accounting for its frequent presence in vomitus, although a reduction in the motility index in the gastric antrum that accompanies nausea will also favour duodenogastric reflux. Studies of the gallbladder and sphincter of Oddi during vomiting have revealed that the gallbladder contracts during retching and the sphincter may undergo transient inhibition, although this usually disappeared before peak contraction of the gallbladder. Thus there appears to be little emptying of the gallbladder during emesis (Qu et al. 1995).

The RGC is a key event in the sequencing of the emetic reflex, as retching does not begin until the RGC has reached the stomach. Other events occurring in the period immediately before retching (in the dog) include tonic contraction of the cricopharyngeus (the upper oesophageal sphincter) and cervical oesophagus (in a longitudinal direction) (Lang et al. 1993). This pulls the abdominal oesophagus and the proximal stomach orad. The net effect is to eliminate the abdominal portion of the oesophagus and to cause funnelling of the stomach—both events will facilitate the expulsion of material. Retching begins shortly after the longitudinal pharyngoesophageal contraction.

Retches occur by synchronous rhythmic contraction of the diaphragm, anterior abdominal muscles, and the external intercostal muscles, leading to an increase in intra-abdominal pressure and a concomitant decrease in intrathoracic pressure, generating a pressure gradient between the stomach and the oesophagus. The lower oesophageal sphincter is relaxed at this time and therefore gastric contents can enter the oesophagus during retching. Between retches the gastric contents return to the stomach and therefore during a burst of retches gastric contents oscillate between the stomach and oesophagus. Retching may be a way of 'testing' whether material is sufficiently liquid to be expelled and, in addition, as the force builds up during a chain of retches it may also increase momentum in the semi-fluid vomitus to facilitate expulsion. The factors that regulate the number of retches in a burst are not known but preclinical studies have implicated gastric volume (low volumes are associated with a greater number of retches prior to a vomit) and end-tidal PCO_2. Also of interest is: what determines when a retch is converted into a vomit? Curiously, although material may reach the cervical oesophagus and the upper

oesophageal sphincter relaxes during each retch, material is not expelled until a vomit is produced.

The vomit is usually a single event at the end of a chain of retches and they are most readily differentiated by the forceful oral expulsion of material, often containing undigested food residue but it may also contain bacteria (e.g. *Helicobacter pylori*) and viruses (e.g. norovirus) and hence is a potential source of infection. The motor events also differ between retching and vomiting in several subtle but critical ways.

♦ The contraction of the diaphragmatic dome muscles and the rectus abdominis is maximal during a vomit.

♦ During a vomit the muscle of the peri-oesophageal (right crus) diaphragm is inhibited, removing another contribution to the pressure barrier between the stomach and the thoracic oesophagus. The crural diaphragm is regulated by the phrenic nerve but the fibres originate from a sub-population of neurons in the phrenic nerve nucleus in the cervical spinal cord (Miller 1990, Pickering and Jones 2002).

♦ During a retch, intra-abdominal pressure undergoes positive oscillations coincident with negative oscillations in the intrathoracic pressure, whereas during a vomit both pressures are positive (Brizzee 1990). The intra-abdominal pressure is greater than 100 mmHg and continence appears to be preserved by increased discharge in the pudendal nerve (Miller et al. 1995).

♦ There is a retrograde contraction of the muscle of the cervical oesophagus and the upper oesophageal sphincter is further opened by contraction of the geniohyoideus muscle during a vomit. This has been observed in dogs (Lang et al. 1993) but requires investigation in humans.

Thus at this stage all barriers to expulsion are removed and the force generated by the compression of the stomach by the diaphragm and abdominal muscles is exerted on the gastric contents to propel them in a single stream up the oesophagus. It should be appreciated that the physical act of vomiting places a considerable physical stress on the body, which may be of particular concern in patients who have recently undergone surgery. In addition, vomiting places a similar burden on the cardiovascular system as does straining at stool.

Post-expulsion

Immediately after the vomit, swallowing usually occurs in animals, often accompanied by profuse licking. Relatively little information is available from humans as studies are usually stopped before emesis is induced and catheters inserted into the gut to monitor activity are expelled or moved by vomiting. One study in which vomiting was recorded showed that about 3 minutes after the vomit a burst of aborally migrating contractions typical of phase III of the migrating motor complex occurred, originating in the duodenum. Also of note was that the increase in skin conductance, which peaked at the time of the onset of the RGC and vomit, took 10–15 minutes to return to pre-emesis levels, suggesting that some of the autonomic changes may be sustained (Thompson and Malagelada 1982).

Three questions are of particular interest regarding this phase.

♦ What determines whether and when the next episode of retching and vomiting will occur?

◆ Why does vomiting produce a sense of relief? Is this due to the removal of a stimulus or is it contributed to by the release of an endogenous opiate?

◆ When and how does the normal pattern of gastrointestinal tract motility resume so that patients with protracted vomiting can resume eating or nutrition can be delivered by nasogastric tube?

Pathways by which the emetic mechanism can be activated

The section below describes the main pathways by which nausea and vomiting can be activated (Fig. 17.2). These pathways provide a framework within which to consider the mechanisms by which the spectrum of clinical conditions and treatments evoke these symptoms.

Visceral afferents

From a purely 'biological' perspective, the abdominal vagal afferents are the most important input by which nausea and vomiting can be triggered. Vagal afferents supply the gastrointestinal tract, possibly as far as the first third of the colon with the information projected predominantly to the nucleus tractus solitarius in the brainstem (Saper 2002, Berthoud et al. 2004, Grundy et al. 2006). Two major types of abdominal vagal afferent have been described.

◆ 'In series' tension receptors signalling distension and contraction of the muscle of the oesophagus, stomach, and small intestine—the physiological role of these afferents is in vago-vagal reflexes and, in particular, those regulating aspects of motility, such as storage of food in the proximal stomach and probably contributing to the initial sensation of comfortable fullness or satiety. These afferents are most likely to be responsible for nausea and vomiting induced by gastric stasis (e.g. diabetic gastroparesis), dysrhythmias, or overdistension, particularly in regions such as the gastric antrum and duodenum, which have little receptive capacity. Vagal mechanoreceptors are also the most likely candidates for mediating the emetic response to intestinal obstruction.

◆ Mucosal afferents monitor features of the luminal environment in the stomach and small intestine, such as shearing of luminal contents against the mucosa and the chemical nature of luminal contents (e.g. osmolarity, pH). They are involved in vago-vagal reflexes regulating the gut but the nature of the sensations they signal is far from clear, although it is likely that they can induce nausea. The emetic response to orally administered hypertonic solutions (e.g. such as may enter the duodenum in dumping syndrome) and copper sulphate is mediated by these afferents. Studies of the mechanism by which cytotoxic drugs (e.g. cisplatin) and radiation induce acute emesis as a side-effect of their antitumour action have provided important insights into a population of these mucosal afferents. (see Fig 17.3, section on 5-HT$_3$ receptor antagonists below; Andrews and Davis 1995).

The gut is also supplied by splanchnic afferents, which signal information about noxious stimuli to the spinal cord and hence the brainstem. Stimulation of the splanchnic afferents does not invoke emesis but nausea is associated with intense pain, and pain can enhance nausea or cause nausea (Desbiens et al. 1997, Drummond and Granston 2004, 2005). There is convergence between vagal and splanchnic afferents in the nucleus tractus solitarius, which could provide a substrate for interactions, with activation of the splanchnic

afferents perhaps lowering the threshold for vagal afferents to induce emesis. In addition, peripherally released mediators from sympathetic efferents can modify visceral afferent sensitivity.

Emesis may also be evoked by vagal afferents from two other sites: the heart and the auditory meatus. In the cat, stimulation of cardiac ventricular vagal afferents induced relaxation of the proximal stomach and vomiting (Abrahamsson and Thoren 1973). These afferents are candidates for inducing the sensation of nausea that may accompany myocardial infarct as well as some of the related circulatory changes. They have also been implicated in the initiation of vaso-vagal syncope. Vomiting may be induced by stimulation of Arnold's nerve (sometimes called The Alderman's nerve) the auricular branch of the vagus supplying part of the pinna and the posterior part of the external auditory meatus.

Vagal and glossopharyngeal afferents are implicated in the induction of nausea and the accompanying EGG changes induced by bitter tasting substances (Peyrot des Gachons et al., 2011).

Area postrema

The role of the area postrema (Figs. 17.2 and 17.3) in emesis is still to some extent controversial although it has long been described as the 'chemoreceptor trigger zone' (CTZ) for emesis (reviewed by Borison 1989, Miller and Leslie 1994). The area postrema is located at the caudal extremity of the fourth ventricle. The presence of fenestrated capillaries means that the blood–brain barrier is incomplete in this and other circumventricular organs (e.g. organum vasculosum laminae terminalis, subfornical organ). Ablation studies (including in humans, Lindstrom and Brizzee 1962) implicated the area postrema in the detection of emetic agents in the bloodstream, a role consistent with its morphological characteristics, and hence led to it being called 'the chemoreceptor trigger zone for emesis'. While ablation of the area postrema can abolish the emetic response to a range of experimental stimuli (e.g. dopamine and opiate receptor agonists), dendrites projecting into the area postrema from the nucleus tractus solitarius (within the blood–brain barrier although there is some evidence of fenestrated capillaries) also provide a substrate at which these agents could act. The role of the area postrema and nucleus tractus solitarius in mediating the emetic response to some drugs (apomorphine, morphine) is not in question and it is likely that peptides or other agents released from the gut mucosa could act here to induce nausea and vomiting, or perhaps sensitize the emetic system to other inputs. However, it should not be assumed that all substances in the circulation use this pathway. Studies of the mechanism by which cytotoxic anticancer drugs and radiation induce nausea and vomiting have implicated abdominal vagal afferents in the acute phase of emesis (reviewed by Andrews and Davis 1995) rather than the area postrema.

The interpretation of the effects of lesions directed at the area postrema is complicated because abdominal vagal afferents project to the area postrema and the subjacent region of the nucleus tractus solitarius. It is inevitable that ablation of the area postrema will cause collateral damage to these afferents. Thus if a systemic emetic agent had a peripheral site of action (e.g. in the gut mucosa) and activated vagal afferents, then a lesion directed at the area postrema could abolish the emetic response leading to the erroneous conclusion that the emetic agent was acting on the area postrema. It is important that the effects of area postrema ablation and abdominal vagotomy are both investigated before drawing conclusions about the site of action of an emetic agent.

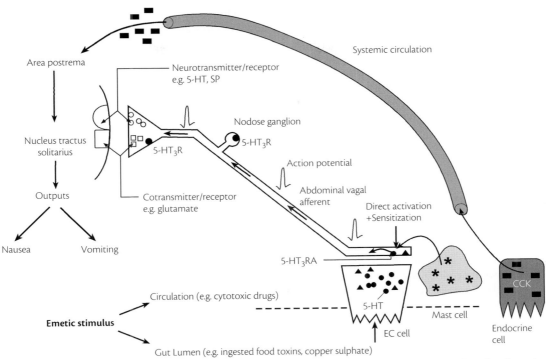

Fig. 17.3 The proposed mechanism by which ingested food toxins and mucosal irritants and systemically administered cytotoxic drugs (e.g. the anticancer agent cisplatin) can drive the nucleus tractus solitarius (NTS) in the dorsal brainstem and hence access pathways responsible for the induction of nausea and vomiting. It is proposed that the enterochromaffin cell (EC) responds to the stimulus by releasing 5-hydroxytryptamine (5-HT, granules) by exocytosis to act locally on 5-HT$_3$ receptors located on the peripheral terminal of the abdominal vagal afferent. 5-HT$_3$ receptors are also found in other locations on the vagal afferent as well as in the NTS, but the peripheral site is considered to be the main one at which 5-HT$_3$ receptor antagonists act against chemotherapy-induced emesis. The 5-HT cannot only stimulate activity in the afferent but can also sensitize the terminal to the action of other locally released agents. Other substances have been implicated, including substance P (SP) from the EC cell, cholecystokinin (CCK) from enteroendocrine cells, and histamine and prostaglandins from mucosal mast cells. In some cases (e.g. CCK), the mucosal released substances enter the systemic circulation and could act via the area postrema. The neurotransmitter(s) used by the abdominal vagal afferent is not known, although glutamate has been implicated and is likely to be a cotransmitter with both 5-HT (5-HT$_3$ receptor) and SP (NK-1 receptor) implicated. However, his has not been studied in detail in species with an emetic reflex. See text for details and references. Reproduced from Stern, R.M., Koch, K. and Andrews, P.L.R., *Nausea—Mechanisms and Management*, 2011, with permission from Oxford University Press.

Vestibular system

The vestibular system is essential for the genesis of motion sickness, which is due to a 'mismatch' between vestibular, visual, and proprioceptive systems (Yates et al. 1998, Golding and Gresty 2005). Care must be taken in distinguishing between vestibular (vertigo) and non-vestibular types of dizziness (Baloh 1993), particularly as nausea and vomiting are common symptoms of the former but not the latter. Non-vestibular dizziness, often described as 'light-headedness', is more likely to be associated with autonomic disorders as it can be induced by diffuse cerebral ischaemia. It is estimated that only 50% of patients complaining of dizziness have vertigo (Baloh 1993). Dizziness and autonomic disorders are reviewed in detail in Chapter 34 by Luxon and Pagarkar, and Yates and Bronstein discuss the vestibular influences on the cardiovascular system in Chapter 8 of this volume.

Disorders affecting vestibular system function and leading to vertigo include benign positional vertigo (due to inner ear disease), Menière's syndrome, viral neurolabyrynthitis, vertebrobasilar insufficiency, and posterior fossa migraine (Baloh 1993).

Higher inputs

The involvement of the higher areas of the brain in triggering the emetic reflex is poorly understood, although the existence of phenomena such as anticipatory emesis to anticancer therapy and vomiting to horrific sights or unpleasant smells, and nausea and vomiting associated with temporal lobe epilepsy illustrate that the cerebral cortex is capable of activating brainstem mechanisms. In view of the growing evidence of the extent of central nervous system damage in 'autonomic' disorders, an understanding of these higher inputs is likely to be of increasing importance in understanding symptoms. In addition, careful investigation of nausea and vomiting in such patients may provide insights into the pathways in humans as may the growing number of studies of brain imaging in patients with migraine where nausea is a common symptom.

The higher regions of the brain have a modulatory effect on the brainstem pathways which are capable of generating the somatic motor responses of retching and vomiting and, as far as has been investigated, the autonomic responses (e.g. proximal gastric relaxation). The level of arousal determines the threshold for activation of the emetic reflex, as indicated by marked suppression of the emetic reflex by general anaesthesia. Emesis is usually preceded by arousal, particularly from sleep, and incomplete arousal (e.g. due to alcohol) increases the chance of aspiration of vomitus. Activation of the cough reflex is also linked to the level of arousal.

Integration of the emetic reflex

The inputs capable of inducing nausea and vomiting converge in the brainstem with the nucleus tractus solitarius being the most likely region involved in the initial processing of the information and co-ordination of outputs. Based primarily upon studies of motion sickness where the stimulus intensity can be readily controlled, the normal sequence appears to be that 'low' intensity stimulation induces nausea (a 'warning') and continued activation at 'higher' intensities induces retching and vomiting. The threshold for the latter must be very carefully regulated to prevent 'accidental' activation by a sudden head movement or a large gastric contraction producing an intense vagal afferent discharge. Studies using electrical stimulation of the vagal afferents suggest that the duration of activation is a factor in addition to the intensity.

At some point in the processing the nausea and vomiting pathways must diverge (Fig. 17.1). The signal for the genesis of the sensation of nausea and the release of vasopressin travels rostrally (cortex, hypothalamus) and the signal for the reflex events of retching and vomiting going to brainstem regions that coordinate the motor outputs. The autonomic motor outflows arise from the dorsal motor vagal nucleus, nucleus ambiguus and the pre-sympathetic nuclei, and these outflows are coordinated by the nucleus tractus solitarius and the reticular formation dorsal to the semi-compact part of nucleus ambiguus termed the 'prodromal sign centre' by Fukuda et al. (2003). The outputs to the diaphragm (phrenic nerve) and to the abdominal muscles arise from the spinal cord and are driven by brainstem neurons in the ventral respiratory group which are themselves driven by central pattern generator neurons located in the reticular formation adjacent to the nucleus ambiguus (Fukuda et al. 2003). Within the motor components the temporal co-ordination is impressive, with retching not beginning until the RGC has reached the stomach.

A knowledge of the central processing is of more than academic interest as an anti-emetic should block both nausea and vomiting. However, unless the drug blocks transmission before the pathways diverge, it is possible that vomiting could be blocked without affecting nausea or *vice versa*.

Nausea, vomiting and disorders of the autonomic nervous system

The preceding sections have provided a framework within which two aspects of autonomic disorders can be discussed. First, how nausea and vomiting may be induced as symptoms of autonomic disorders, such as diabetes mellitus, and, secondly, the mechanism by which pharmacological treatments (e.g. L-3, 4-dihydroxyphenylalanine [L-dopa]) for disorders involving the autonomic nervous system may induce nausea and vomiting.

Nausea and vomiting as symptoms of autonomic disorders

Diabetic gastroparesis

Gastroparesis (Chapters 27 and 53) is common in patients with diabetic autonomic neuropathy and particularly in those who are insulin-dependent. The incidence is not precisely known as it is likely that many patients may have impaired gastric emptying without being symptomatic. The pathophysiological mechanisms leading to the severe retention of gastric contents is unclear, but vagal degeneration has been implicated, although this is not a universal finding (Yoshida et al. 1988). The assessment of the extent of vagal damage is difficult because of the lack of simple tests

of abdominal vagal integrity and function (approximately 90% of the fibres are afferent), the paucity of histological material, and the high proportion of unmyelinated fibres which can only be adequately assessed by electron microscopy.

The incidence of vomiting in patients with diabetic gastroparesis is unclear and may reflect experiences of populations with disease of differing severity, duration, and glycaemic control. In addition, little effort appears to have been made to distinguish nausea from vomiting, although the former is usually of greater concern to patients because of its sustained nature.

In the section on nausea above, the link (not necessarily causal) between nausea and gastric dysrhythmias was noted. Such dysrhythmias have been reported to occur in patients with diabetic gastroparesis. Acute hyperglycaemia in healthy individuals induces gastric dysrhythmias that could be prevented by indomethacin, implicating prostaglandins in the mechanism (Hasler et al. 1995). In addition nitrergic stimulation using an NO donor and the cGMP-PDE$_5$ inhibitor sildenafil was effective in reducing hyperglycaemia-induced tachygastria in healthy volunteers, suggesting that such agents may be of use in treatment of diabetic dysrhythmias (Coleski et al. 2005).

Breaking the cycle of impaired gastric emptying and oscillation in blood glucose levels is therefore of considerable relevance in some of these patients. This is also important because hypoglycaemia can occur with erratic gastric emptying. Studies with the toxin hypoglycin A have shown that hypoglycaemia can rapidly induce vomiting. The mechanism is unclear, although area postrema ablation affected the acute emetic response (Tanaka 1979). One possibility is that the hypoglycaemia induces a release of adrenal catecholamines and these act on the area postrema to induce nausea and vomiting via activation of α-adrenoceptors (mainly α$_2$) that have been implicated in emesis at this site (Hikasa et al. 1991).

An excess glucose or fat load in the small intestine will delay gastric emptying, but if the load in the gut lumen is particularly hypertonic, 'dumping' syndrome may result. The mechanism in part appears to involve release of 5-HT from enterochromaffin cells and activation of abdominal vagal afferents leading to activation of emetic pathways. Lipids in the intestine can modulate the sensations arising from the stomach in response to distension (Feinle et al. 2001). Plasma glucose levels influence gastric emptying, with pronounced hypoglycaemia causing acceleration and hyperglycaemia slowing. A study in normal subjects and patients with insulin-dependent diabetes mellitus showed that emptying of a mixed meal is modulated in both groups by the 'physiological hyperglycaemia' following a meal (Schvarcz et al. 1997).

Treatment of diabetes with metformin can be associated with nausea, vomiting and diarrhoea. These side-effects were not significantly affected by treatment with ondansetron (a 5-HT$_3$ receptor antagonist) although metformin is a biguanide derivative and related biguanides are agonists at 5-HT$_3$ receptors (Hoffmann et al. 2003).

Neurally mediated syncope

Nausea (but usually not vomiting) is a symptom in some patients with vaso-vagal syncope, together with other features, such as light-headedness, dizziness (see also vertigo), blurred vision, weakness, and cognitive impairment. These symptoms may be followed by fainting. Several mechanisms could contribute but these have not been formally investigated.

◆ The sensory disturbances may induce a sensation of illusory self-motion, a very effective experimental nauseogenic stimulus (Koch 1993), producing a vestibulo-visual conflict sufficient to cause mild activation of the motion sickness pathways.

◆ The gradual reduction in cerebral perfusion which eventually leads to fainting may be sufficient to induce a degree of ischaemia-induced firing of neurons in a sensitive site in the emetic pathway, such as the area postrema, the nucleus tractus solitarius, the vestibular system, or inferior frontal gyrus. Of interest is the observation that during experimental centrifugation cerebral hypoperfusion precedes the onset of nausea (Serrador et al. 2005). The regulation of the vertebral circulation is reviewed by Goadsby in Chapter 13 in this volume.

◆ Activation of ventricular cardiac afferents can induce nausea and vomiting in humans and vomiting in cats, and these afferents are thought to be responsible for the occurrence of nausea in myocardial infarct patients (Abrahamsson and Thoren 1973). Activation of these receptors also produces reflex gastric relaxation which could contribute to the genesis of nausea. The ventricular receptors provide a potential mechanism by which reduced ventricular filling could induce nausea. They have been implicated in the genesis of the vaso-vagal syndrome, which Barcroft and Swan (1953) noted shared a likeness to the response to apomorphine, a dopamine D_2-receptor agonist, inducing emesis via a central action (area postrema).

◆ A fall in blood pressure will reduce the activation of the arterial baroreceptors which provide a tonic inhibitory input to the hypothalamic neurons secreting vasopressin. Vasopressin levels will increase, but whether these are sufficient to induce nausea is unclear.

Nausea and the occasional vomiting associated with neurally mediated syncope should be distinguished from posturally evoked vomiting which is associated with posterior fossa lesions.

Disordered dopamine and adrenaline metabolism

Dopamine, adrenaline, and noradrenaline are capable of inducing nausea and vomiting by a direct action on the area postrema and it is likely that they may also act via delaying gastric emptying.

These substances may be secreted in excess by phaeochromocytomas (see Chapter 64, Eisenhofer et al.) in which nausea and vomiting may occur, although they are not major symptoms. While attention correctly focuses on the catecholamines as the most likely cause of nausea and vomiting, neuropeptide Y is also released and may be of significance as it can induce emesis and activate area postrema neurons (Carpenter 1990). Ischaemic enterocolitis is a pathological complication of phaeochromocytoma and vomiting can occur in patients with acute mesenteric ischaemia. The mechanism is not known but is presumably via activation of gut afferents due to ischaemia-induced release of local neuroactive mediators.

A pseudo-phaeochromocytoma has been described in which there were hypertensive episodes, flushing, nausea, epigastric discomfort, and polyuria (Kuchel 1996). Attention was drawn to the importance of measuring sulphated as well as free plasma dopamine, as the former has a half-life 60 times that of dopamine.

Dopamine-beta-hydroxylase deficiency, in which there is a marked increase in plasma dopamine levels, does not appear to induce nausea and vomiting (Chapter 49).

Familial dysautonomia (Riley–Day syndrome)

Vomiting is a feature of the Riley–Day syndrome (Chapter 48), with the episodes being triggered by emotional crises. Although this disorder is characterized by a reduction in noradrenaline synthesis, during the emotional crisis plasma noradrenaline and dopamine levels are markedly elevated and while the vomiting is reported to be correlated with the dopamine levels, both agents are capable of inducing emesis via an action on the area postrema with dopamine D_2, and α_1- and α_2-adrenoceptors implicated. The treatment is aimed at the emotional crisis. Diazepam is used which sedates the patient and thus has an indirect action to alleviate the vomiting, but this does not exclude a direct anti-emetic action.

Alcoholic neuropathy

Although nausea and vomiting are not particularly features of alcoholic neuropathy, chronic alcohol intake blunts the emetic reflex. The evidence emerges from studies of patients with head and neck cancer in which alcohol is implicated in the aetiology. In response to the cytotoxic drug cisplatin (a potent emetogen) such patients have little or no vomiting and less nausea than would be expected (Jones and Cunningham 1993). The mechanism has not been investigated but it could indicate damage to the enterochromaffin–vagal afferent system or the dorsal brainstem complex (area postrema, nucleus tractus solitarius).

Brainstem tumours and related lesions

Nausea and vomiting may be early symptoms of tumours located in or impacting on the fourth ventricle (North and Reilly 1990, Lee et al. 2008). The reason for this is that the tumour itself, or the resulting raised intracranial pressure, or both (i.e. in posterior fossa tumours) compresses the area postrema or, more likely, the subjacent nucleus tractus solitarius, inducing neuronal firing and activation of the emetic pathways, although this has never been demonstrated experimentally. The vagus has a meningeal branch to the dura covering the posterior fossa. It is conceivable that afferents in this branch are implicated in the emesis induced by raised intracranial pressure but this requires experimental investigation. The possibility that neuroactive agents released into the cerebrospinal fluid and acting on the area postrema may contribute should not be excluded.

Vomiting may be induced by postural changes (posturally evoked vomiting, PEV) without the presence of concomitant nystagmus or vertigo, when it is often an indication of a posterior fossa lesion.

Projectile vomiting has been reported in a patient with a solitary metastasis involving the lateral pontine tegmentum and middle cerebellar peduncle without hydrocephalus. In this case it appeared likely that the trigger for emesis was involvement of pathways to or from the 'vomiting centre' (Baker and Bernat 1985). Isolated vomiting not associated with either a rise in intracranial pressure or vertigo was reported in a patient with central nervous system (CNS) lupus who had a unilateral lesion in the dorsal vagal complex (Sawai et al. 2006)

Nausea and vomiting, together with a constellation of other symptoms, are a feature of acute brainstem lesions such as those seen in Wallenberg's syndrome (lateral medullary stroke). In this syndrome there is an ischaemic attack affecting the brainstem. The ischaemic insult may cause neuronal discharge directly by release of excitatory amino acids, by permeabilizing capillaries, or indirectly by producing localized oedema, which may activate the nucleus tractus solitarius by mechanical deformation.

Nausea and vomiting as a side-effect of treatment for autonomic disorders

Bethanecol

The muscarinic receptor agonists carbachol and bethanecol are carbamoyl esters of choline, resistant to the activity of both specific and nonspecific cholinestereases (Broadley 1996). They exert relatively selective effects on the gastrointestinal tract and bladder, with both effects being ascribed to an action on muscarinic M_3-receptors, and they have been used in the treatment of urinary retention and markedly delayed gastric emptying and paralytic ileus. Nausea and vomiting are recognized side-effects of both. The mechanism is unclear as it is the muscarinic M_1 and nicotinic cholinoceptors in the dorsal medulla which are most implicated in emesis. Carbachol does have some nicotinic activity but bethanecol has little or none.

Both agents act by stimulating the muscarinic M_3-receptors located on the smooth muscles. In the gastrointestinal tract other approaches are available, such as using the substituted prokinetic benzamides (e.g. metoclopramide), which have their prokinetic effect by the release of acetylcholine (and other excitatory transmitters) from myenteric neurons via a 5-HT$_4$ agonist effect (Sanger 2009 for review). However, if the myenteric plexus is damaged by autonomic disease then such an approach, although working initially, may not continue to be effective as the disease progresses.

Levodopa and other anti-parkinsonian drugs

Oral levodopa is used in conjunction with a decarboxylase inhibitor (e.g. benserazide, carbidopa) to alleviate the bradykinesia and rigidity of Parkinson's disease. The decarboxylase inhibitor is given to prevent the breakdown of L-dopa to dopamine in the periphery. This is possible as, in contrast to L-dopa, the decarboxylase inhibitors do not cross the blood–brain barrier. It is argued that reducing the conversion of L-dopa to dopamine outside the brain reduces the side-effects of nausea and vomiting. This appears to be supported by clinical experience, with a vomiting frequency of 80% with oral L-dopa in the initial stages of treatment compared to 15% when combined with a decarboxylase inhibitor (Parkes 1986). It is perhaps surprising that the site of the emetic effect of L-dopa is not known with certainty. The most likely site would appear to be the area postrema, which is located outside the blood–brain barrier, as ablation or domperidone abolishes the emetic response to dopamine receptor agonists, such as apomorphine, which is used for 'off' episodes in patients with Parkinson's disease refractory to other treatments. Although decarboxylase inhibitors do not cross the blood–brain barrier they would be expected to act in the area postrema which is outside the blood–brain barrier. However, the possibility of a peripheral (gastrointestinal) effect of L-dopa cannot be excluded even when co-administered with a decarboxylase inhibitor, as there is some peripheral conversion to dopamine and dopamine receptors are present in the gut with activation leading to a delay in gastric emptying. In a few patients who had a vagotomy for pyloric stenosis and who were

subsequently given L-dopa, no 'sickness' was reported (Parkes 1986). This unique anecdotal observation is suggestive of a peripheral contribution and perhaps this accounts for the residual nausea and vomiting in patients treated with L-dopa and decarboxylase inhibitors.

Nausea is a common side-effect of a range of dopamine agonist drugs used to treat Parkinson's disease, including bromocriptine, pergolide, ropinirole and rotigotine (Perez-Lloret and Rascol 2010, Kulisevsky and Pagonabarrag, 2010), and anti-parkinsonian drugs with different mechanisms of action, such as selegiline (monoamine oxidase inhibitor often used in combination with L-dopa) can have nausea and vomiting as a side-effect, consistent with an involvement of catecholamine receptors in the emetic response.

Abnormalities of autonomic function are seen particularly in patients with advanced Parkinson's disease resulting, among other manifestations, in a feeling of early satiety and delayed gastrointestinal motility (Chapter 45) (Kaneoke et al. 1995, Natale et al. 2008), both of which could contribute to the genesis of nausea. Impaired gut motility will also affect the kinetics of L-dopa absorption as shown in a preclinical study (Fernandez et al. 2010).

One intriguing aspect that does require study is the basis of the tolerance to the emetic effects of most anti-parkinsonian drugs, which occurs within 1–6 months (Parkes 1986).

Carbamazepine

Epileptic seizures may occasionally be induced by very low cerebral perfusion due to low blood pressure as a result of autonomic failure. Nausea and vomiting are side-effects of the anti-epileptic drug, carbamazepine, acting via blockade of a population of sodium channels.

Clonidine

Clonidine is an α_2-adrenoceptor agonist, used in the treatment of hypertension. Occasionally nausea is a side-effect of clonidine and is likely to be due to an action on central α_2-receptors in the area postrema or nucleus tractus solitarius. In addition to acting at α_2-adrenoceptors, clonidine may have an action at another binding site, identified as 'imidazoline receptors/binding sites' (Broadley 1996) of which two subtypes are proposed: I_1 and I_2. The I_1 sites preferentially bind clonidine and idazoxan and are located in the brainstem and kidney, whereas the I_2 receptors have a greater affinity for idazoxan over clonidine and are found in kidney, liver, adipocytes, platelets, urethra, pancreatic B cells, adrenal chromaffin cells, and CNS astrocytes (Reis and Regunathan 1996). The possible role of I_1 and I_2 receptors in the genesis of nausea induced by clonidine has not been investigated.

Insulin

Insulin may activate neurons in the area postrema of the dog, and the emesis induced within 1 minute by systemic insulin administration can be abolished by area postrema ablation (Carpenter and Briggs 1986).

Octreotide

Octreotide is a stable analogue of somatostatin used to reduce hormone secretion from tumours, postprandial hypotension, and orthostatic hypotension due to autonomic failure (Chapter 47). Nausea, vomiting, and abdominal cramps are side-effects. The site of the emetic effect has not been investigated and although systemic somatostatin is capable of inducing vomiting in dogs, it failed to activate area postrema neurons when applied directly (Carpenter 1990). This could be taken as a very preliminary indication for a peripheral emetic action but requires direct investigation

Pharmacology of anti-emetics

The 'perfect' anti-emetic agent should be capable of blocking both nausea and vomiting from any cause (Sanger and Andrews 2006). At present such an agent is not available clinically, although several approaches have been identified from preclinical studies. The pharmacology and proposed sites of action of some of the current anti-emetics will be discussed. Until the perfect anti-emetic is available some consideration should be given to the cause of the emesis when deciding which anti-emetic to use. For example, if the cause of the emesis is due to inappropriate activation of vestibular pathways, then an agent acting on appropriate receptors (e.g. histamine$_1$, muscarinic) in the pathway is relevant. There are five main pharmacological classes of anti-emetic.

Dopamine-receptor antagonists

Several compounds (e.g. domperidone, metoclopramide, and phenothiazines such as prochloperazine, chlorpromazine, trifluorperazine) are classed as 'dopamine-receptor antagonists' but this is not necessarily the only pharmacological action they possess or the mechanism by which they exert their anti-emetic effect. The dopamine D_2-receptor subtype acting via inhibition of adenylate cyclase is the one most for which there is the greatest evidence for an involvement in emesis but recently the D_3-receptor has also been implicated. Blockade of dopamine receptors in the dorsal brainstem and in the upper gastrointestinal tract have been implicated in the anti-emetic effects of the antagonists discussed here but the way in which these dopaminergic mechanisms are activated by clinically relevant emetic stimuli are still unclear (Sanger and Andrews 2006).

Domperidone (a benzimidazole derivative) is an antagonist at the dopamine D_2-receptor. Its prokinetic effect, particularly in the stomach and the small intestine, may be the mechanism by which it alleviates nausea and vomiting secondary to delayed gastric emptying (e.g. diabetic gastroparesis). The 'direct' anti-emetic effects of domperidone are still a matter of controversy (Sanger and Andrews 2006). At conventional doses, domperidone penetrates the blood–brain barrier poorly and this explains why extrapyramidal reactions are rare. However, it should not be assumed that poor penetration of the blood–brain barrier means that the drug does have a central effect. The area postrema is outside the blood–brain barrier and this is a site at which D_2-receptor agonists (e.g. apomorphine, L-dopa, lisuride) can induce emesis including via a possible action on receptors of nucleus tractus solitarius dendrites projecting into the area postrema. Of note is that domperidone does not block hiccup or yawning produced by L-dopa (Parkes 1986). Furthermore, sufficient drug may reach a critical site in the emetic pathway (e.g. the nucleus tractus solitarius) to exert an effect if the structure is adjacent to a circumventricular organ (e.g. area postrema).

Metoclopramide is a substituted benzamide and unravelling its pharmacology led directly to the development of 5-HT$_3$-receptor antagonists and 5-HT$_4$-receptor agonists. Metoclopramide is a D_2-receptor antagonist and it was originally thought that this accounted for its anti-emetic and prokinetic effects. However, subsequent studies of the pharmacology revealed that an agonist action at 5-HT$_4$ receptors on myenteric neurons, leading to a release of acetylcholine, makes a major contribution to the prokinetic effects (see Sanger 2009 for references). At usual therapeutic doses the D_2-receptor antagonism and 5-HT$_4$-receptor agonism account for the clinical effects, but at high doses metoclopramide also acts as a 5-HT$_3$-receptor antagonist. It is this latter action which accounts for its improved anti-emetic efficacy against anticancer therapy-induced emesis when given at high doses (Andrews and Sanger 2006).

The phenothiazines, exemplified by prochloperazine, have the most complex pharmacology of the 'dopamine' antagonists with binding at D_2, D_3, H_1 α_1 and muscarinic acetylcholine receptors depending upon the concentration (Andrews and Sanger 2006). Although the anti-emetic effect is most often attributed to dopamine receptor blockade, the presence of histaminic and muscarinic receptors in the motion sickness pathway should not be overlooked. It is possible that by reducing the tonic input to the brainstem from the vestibular system the threshold for activation of the emetic mechanism from other causes is also reduced and this could explain the 'general' anti-emetic effects of prochloperazine. The sedative effects of prochloperazine (and other agents) may also contribute to the anti-emetic effect by reducing arousal.

Muscarinic receptor antagonists

Scopolamine (hyoscine), a plant alkaloid, is perhaps the best known of the non-selective anti-muscarinic agents which are particularly useful in treating emesis involving activation of the labyrinthine system. Studies using more selective agents have implicated M_3/M_5 receptors in the mediation of motion sickness (Golding and Gresty 2005).

Histamine-receptor antagonists

Histamine$_1$-receptor antagonists, such as cinnarizine, cyclizine, meclozine, promethazine, and dimenhydrinate, are particularly useful in the treatment of labyrinthine disorders and motion sickness. The exact site of action is unclear, although H_1 receptors are present in the vestibular-cerebellar pathway and in the nucleus tractus solitarius. The sedative effect of the H_1 antagonists and anti-muscarinic properties (Owyang and Hasler 2002) may also contribute to their anti-emetic effects. The sensitivity to motion sickness is a predictor of sensitivity to other emetic stimuli including pregnancy, chemotherapy and postoperative nausea and vomiting (see Stern et al. 2011). In view of this the vestibular system may be able to modulate the sensitivity of the brainstem emetic mechanism and as a result agents acting against the motion-sickness pathway may have broader spectrum anti-emetic effects than expected.

5-Hydroxytryptamine$_3$ receptor antagonists

Agents in this class include granisetron, ondansetron, tropisetron, dolasetron and palonosetron, and while they are all antagonists at the 5-HT$_3$ receptor, recent studies with palonosetron suggest that it may have positive cooperativity and allosteric binding at the receptor, which may contribute to its superiority demonstrated in clinical trials (Rojas et al. 2008, 2010). In contrast to the 'first generation' 5-HT$_3$ receptor antagonists, palonosetron also has a longer plasma half-life (Navari 2009) The 5-HT$_3$ receptor is a ligand-gated ion channel, non-selectively permeable to small monovalent ions and activation of which leads to depolarization of neurons (Sanger and Andrews 2006). The native receptor involved in emesis is a heteromeric channel consisting of two subunits $5-HT_{3a}$ and $5-HT_{3b}$ and polymorphisms of the latter have been implicated in the determination of the anti-emetic efficacy of $5-HT_3$ receptor antagonists in patients undergoing chemotherapy (Tremblay et al. 2003). The principal locations of $5-HT_3$ receptors relevant to the anti-emetic action are on the peripheral and central terminals of abdominal vagal afferents, neurons in the nucleus tractus solitarius, and probably the 5-HT-containing enterochromaffin cells in the gut mucosa. Activation of $5-HT_3$ receptors has been implicated in the acute phase of the emetic response to radiation and cytotoxic anticancer drugs (e.g. cisplatin, cyclophosphamide) but this does not exclude involvement of other mechanisms such as signalling molecules released from the gut to act on the area postrema (Rudd and Andrews 2005). It is proposed that these stimuli induce emesis via the release of 5-HT (this is proposed to be by generation of free radicals) from the gut mucosal enterochromaffin cells, the 5-HT acts on $5-HT_3$ receptors located on the peripheral terminals of vagal afferents terminating in close proximity to the basal surface of these cells. The activation of the $5-HT_3$ receptors leads to discharge of the vagal afferents which project to the nucleus tractus solitarius and this input together with the sensitization of the afferents to other locally released mediators (e.g. substance P [SP], which is also located in the enterochromaffin cells) constitutes the emetic stimulus. The main site of the anti-emetic effect of the $5-HT_3$ receptors antagonists is considered to be peripheral on the vagal $5-HT_3$ receptors but there may be some contribution from blockade of the receptors in the nucleus tractus solitarius and the proposed autoreceptors on the enterochromaffin cells (Fig. 17.3).

It must be emphasized that the $5-HT_3$-receptor antagonists are not universal anti-emetics. For example, their demonstrated clinical efficacy is limited to emesis induced by radiation and cytotoxic drugs and postoperative emesis. However, they are ineffective against motion and centrally acting emetics such as apomorphine. In addition, they do not block the emetic effect of all experimental stimuli acting via the vagus, suggesting that there are different peripheral transduction mechanisms and that blockade of the $5-HT_3$ receptors in the nucleus tractus solitarius is insufficient to block emesis.

NK-1 receptor antagonists

SP is a member of the mammalian tachykinin family of neuropeptides with neurokinin A (NKA) and B (NKB) being the other main members. These tachykinins are agonists at the three neurokinin receptors (NK-1, NK-2, NK-3), with SP being the most potent ligand at the NK-1 receptors (NK-1 ≥ NKA > NKB). Clinical interest in SP had focused on its role in nociception but the identification of non-peptide, brain penetrant selective antagonists for the NK-1 receptor allowed other potential therapeutic targets to be explored. Preclinical studies in animal models of emesis including the ferret (the species in which the anti-emetic effect of the $5-HT_3$ receptor antagonists was identified) demonstrated that blockade of the NK-1 receptor can markedly reduce or abolish the emetic response to motion and stimuli such as opiates and apomorphine acting at the area postrema and cisplatin and copper sulphate acting via the abdominal vagal afferents. As these agents are effective against both central and peripherally acting stimuli it is proposed that the site of action is at the convergence point of these pathways in the brain stem and although the exact site remains to be identified the blockade appears to be on the pathway(s) leading to activation of the motor outputs rather than on the inputs to the brainstem. Regions of both the nucleus tractus solitarius and the reticular formation adjacent to the semi-compact part of the nucleus ambiguus have been implicated (Andrews and Rudd 2004 for review).

The first NK-1 receptor antagonist (aprepitant), licensed in 2003 for use in chemotherapy, induced nausea and vomiting, but it must be noted that in this setting it is usually used in combination with a $5-HT_3$ receptor antagonist (e.g. ondansetron) and a synthetic corticosteroid (e.g. dexamethasone). Several other NK-1 receptor antagonists are in clinical trials (e.g. casopitant, fosaprepitant, netupitant, SCH619734, vestipitant; Reddy et al. 2006, Navari 2007). The efficacy of aprepitant is most marked in the delayed phase of chemotherapy-induced emesis (Kris et al. 2005). The clinical studies have also revealed that efficacy against vomiting is greater than that against nausea (c.f. $5-HT_3$ receptor antagonists) but the reasons are unclear. The full spectrum of anti-emetic activity is under investigation, but these agents have already been investigated in postoperative nausea and vomiting, with evidence of superiority to 'first generation' $5-HT_3$ receptor antagonists (Apfel et al. 2008, Apfel 2010). As has happened with the $5-HT_3$ receptor antagonists it is likely that they will be used 'off-label' in a number of indications where other agents have failed.

Complementary and non-pharmacological treatments

Ginger is probably the most popular complementary treatment used for treatment of nausea and vomiting. There is limited evidence for efficacy, particularly against nausea, in motion sickness, pregnancy sickness and postoperative nausea and vomiting (Ernst and Pittler 2000, Chaiyakunapruk et al. 2006). A well-controlled study of experimentally induced motion sickness revealed that ingestion of a 1g dried ginger capsule reduced the nausea score, tachygastria and the secretion of vasopressin; however, it was without effect on the nausea score or tachygastria evoked by vasopressin infusion (Lien et al. 2003). These results suggest that the anti-nausea effect of ginger may be secondary to blunting the pituitary secretion of vasopressin and this awaits confirmation in other models of nausea. Pharmacological studies of ginger extract have demonstrated prokinetic effects in the stomach and spasmolytic effects in the intestine, with the former being ascribed to cholinergic activity and the latter to calcium-channel antagonism (Ghayur and Gilani 2005). Constituents of ginger such as [6]-shogaol and [6]-gingerol are able to bind to the $5-HT_3$ receptor, prevent cation influx and contractions of the guinea pig ileum evoked by a selective $5-HT_3$ receptor agonist (Abdel-Aziz et al. 2006). More recent preclinical studies have demonstrated weak antagonist effects of both gingerols and shogaols on $5-HT_3$ and M_3 receptors (Pertz et al. 2011). The latter effect if translated *in vivo* is of interest because M_3 receptors have been implicated in motion sickness. The relationship between these various pharmacological effects and the anti-nausea effects of ginger (if confirmed) requires investigation.

A number of non-pharmacological treatments have been investigated and shown to be beneficial against nausea in various experimental and/or clinical settings, including: acupressure/acupuncture (P6 point) (Stern et al. 2001), controlled/slow deep breathing (Yen Pik Sang et al. 2003), gastric pacing (Lin et al. 2004); high-protein meals with ginger (Levine et al. 2008) and without the addition of ginger (Levine et al. 2004).

Future directions

It is often difficult to identify the precise cause of the nausea and vomiting, and the pathways involved in triggering the response to many emetic stimuli have not been investigated, so a 'universal' anti-emetic would be of considerable clinical use. In animal models, agonists at 5-HT_{1A}, μ-opioid, $GABA_B$, and cannabinoid CB_1 receptor, have such broad-spectrum effects, and additionally the peptide ghrelin has been demonstrated to have an anti-emetic effect in addition to its well-known orexigenic actions (Sanger and Andrews 2006). It is not yet known how these findings will translate to the clinic but this does represent a novel approach and may mimic activation of endogenous pathways capable of inhibiting emesis. Support for this comes from studies in which the threshold for the induction of emesis is reduced by antagonists of opioid and CB_1 receptors (Sanger and Andrews 2006).

Although advances have been made in the pharmacotherapy of vomiting, the treatment of nausea is in general less effective. This is a major challenge as nausea is frequently reported as being of more concern to patients, with protracted nausea having an impact on quality of life and compliance with some treatments. Identification of novel therapies that are effective against nausea represents a major clinical challenge. While the CNS pathways are the most obvious target, until understanding of these pathways in humans is more advanced, the more immediately treatable pathways may be prevention of the rise in plasma vasopressin or blockade of its undesirable effects, and/or correction of gastric dysrhythmias.

References

Abdel-Aziz, H., Windeck, T., Ploch, M. and Verspohl, E.J. (2006). Mode of action of gingerols and shogaols on 5-HT3 receptors: binding studies, cation uptake by receptor channels and contraction of isolated guinea-pig ileum. *Eur.J.Pharmacol.* **530**, 136–43.

Abrahamsson, H. and Thoren, P. (1973). Vomiting and reflex vagal relaxation of the stomach elicited from heart receptors in the cat. *Acta Physiol. Scand.* **88**, 433–9.

Ali, F., Guglin, M., Vaitkevicius, P. and Ghali, J.K. (2007). Therapeuetic potential of vasopressin receptor antagonists. *Drugs*, **67**, 847–58.

Andrews, P. L. R. and Davis, C. J. (1995). The physiology of emesis induced by anti-cancer therapy. In *Serotonin and scientific basis of anti-emetic therapy*, (ed. D. J. M. Reynolds, P. L. R. Andrews, and C. J. Davis), Ch. 2, 25–49. Oxford Clinical Communications, Oxford.

Andrews, P. L. R. and Rudd, J. A. (2004). The Role of Tachykinins and the Tachykinin NK1 Receptor in Nausea and Emesis, In: Holzer, P. (Ed.), pp. 359–440. *Handbook of Experimental Pharmacology*, Tachykinins, Springer.

Apfel, C. C. (2010). Postoperative nausea and vomiting. In R. D. Miller *et al.* (Eds.), *Miller's Anesthesia* (7th ed., pp. 2729–55). New York: Churchill Livingstone Elsevier

Apfel, C. C., Malhotra, A., and Leslie, J. B. (2008). The role of neurokinin-1 receptor antagonists for the management of postoperative nausea and vomiting. *Curr Opinion in Anesth.* **21**, 427–32.

Baker, P. C. H. and Bernat, J. I. (1985). The neuroanatomy of vomiting in man: association of projectile vomiting with a solitary metastasis in the lateral tegmentum of the pons and the middle cerebellar peduncle. *J. Neurol. Psychiat.* **48**, 1165–8.

Baloh, R. W. (1993). Diagnosis and management of vertigo. In *The handbook of nausea and vomiting*, (ed. M. H. Sleisenger), pp. 27–42. Parthenon Publishing Group, New York.

Barcroft, H. and Swan, H. J. C. (1953). *Sympathetic control of human blood vessels.* Edward Arnold, London.

Berthoud, H.R., Blackshaw, L.A., Brookes, S.J. and Grundy, D. (2004). Neuroanatomy of extrinsic afferents supplying the gastrointestinal tract. *Neurogastroenterol. Motil.* **16**, Suppl 1, 28–33.

Borison, H. L. (1989). Area postrema: Chemoreceptor circumventricular organ of the medulla oblongata. *Prog. Neurobiol.* **32**, 351–90.

Borison, H. L. and McCarthy, L. E. (1983). Neuropharmacologic mechanisms of emesis. In *Antiemetics and cancer chemotherapy*, (ed. J. Laszlo), Ch. 2, pp. 6–20. Williams and Wilkins, Baltimore.

Boyle, R. (1996). *A free enquiry into the vulgarly received notion of nature* (E. B. Davis and M. Hunter, Eds.). Cambridge, UK: Cambridge University Press. (Original work published 1686).

Brizzee, K.R. (1990). Mechanics of vomiting: a minireview. *Can. J. Physiol. Pharmacol.* **68**, 221–29.

Broadley, K. J. (1996). *Autonomic pharmacology*, Taylor and Francis, London, UK.

Caras, S. D., Soykan, I., Beverly, V., Lin, Z., and McCallum, R. W. (1997). The effect of intravenous vasopressin on gastric myoelectrical activity in human subjects. *Neurogastroent. Motility* **9**, 151–6.

Carpenter, D. O. (1990). Neural mechanisms of emesis. *Can. J. Physiol. Pharmacol.* **68**, 230–6.

Carpenter, D. O. and Briggs, D. B. (1986). Insulin excites neurons of the area postrema and causes emesis. *Neurosci. Lett.* **68**, 85–9.

Chaiyakunapruk, N., Kitikannakorn, N., Nathisuwan, S., Leeprakobboon, K. and Leelasettagool, C. (2006). The efficacy of ginger for the prevention of postoperative nausea and vomiting: a meta analysis. *Am.J.Obstet. Gynaecol.* **194**, 95–99.

Coleski, R., Gonlachanvit, S., Owyang, C. and Hasler, W.L. (2005). Selective reversal of hyperglycaemia-evoked gastric myoelectric dyscrhythmias by nitregergis stimulation in healthy humans. *J. Pharmacol. Exp.Ther.* **312**, 103–111.

De Ponti, F., Malagelada, J. R., Azpiroz, F., Yaksh, T. L., and Thomforde G. M. (1990). Variations in gastric tone associated with duodenal motor events after activation of central emetic mechanisms in the dog. *J. Gastrointest. Motility*, **2**, 1–11.

Desbiens, N. A., Mueller-Rizner, N., Connors, A. F. and Wenger, N. S. (1997). The relationship of nausea and dyspnea to pain in seriously ill patients. *Pain* **71**, 149–56.

Doig, R.K., Wolf, S. and Wolff, M.S. (1953). Study of gastric function in a 'decorticate' man with a gastric fistula. *Gastroenterology*, **23**, 4–44.

Drummond, P. D. and Granston, A. (2004). Facial pain increases nausea and headache during motion sickness in migraine sufferers. *Brain*, **127**, 526–34.

Drummond, P. D. and Granston, A. (2005). Painful stimulation of the temple induces nausea, headache and extracranial vasodilation in migraine sufferers. *Cephalalgia*, **25**, 16–22.

Ernst, E. and Pittler, M.H. (2000). Efficacy of ginger for nausea and vomiting: a systematic review of randomized clinical trials. *Br.J. Anaesth.* **84**, 367–71.

Feinle, C., Grundy, D. and Fried, M. (2001). Modulation of gastric distension-induced sensations by small intestinal receptors. *Am.J.Physiol Gastrointest Liver Physiol*, **280**, G51–57.

Fernandez, N., Garcia, J.J., Diez, M.J., Sahagun, A.M. and Gonzalez, A. (2010). Effects of slowed gastrointestinal motility on levodopa pharmacokinetics. *Autonom, Neurosc.i: Basic and Clinical*, **156**, 67–72.

Fukuda, H., Koga, T., Furukawa, N., Nakamura, E., Hatano, M. and Yanagihara, M. (2003). The site of the antiemetic action of NK1 receptor antagonists.In *Antiemetic Therapy*. Ed Donnerer, J. Basel, Karger, pp. 33–77.

Furukawa, N. and Okada, H. (1994). Canine salivary secretion from the submaxillary glands before and during retching. *Am. J. Physiol.* **267**, G810–817.

Ghayur, M.N. and Gilani, A.H. (2005). Pharmacological basis for the medicinal use of ginger in gastrointestinal disorders. *Dig.Dis.Sci.* **50**, 1889–97.

Gianaros, P.J., Quigley, K.S., Muth, E.R., Levine, M.E., Vasko, R.C. and Stern, R.M. (2003). Relationship between temporal changes in cardiac parasympathetic activity and motion sickness severity. *Psychophysiology* **40**, 39–44.

Golding, J.F. and Gresty, M.A. (2005). Motion sickness. *Current Opinion in Neurology* **18**, 29–34.

Gordon, C. R., Ben-Aryeh, H., Szargel, R., Attias, J., Rolnick, A., and Laufer, D. (1989). Salivary changes associated with seasickness. *J. Autonom. Nerv. Syst.* **26**, 37–42.

Grundy, D., Al-Chaer, E.D., Aziz, Q., Collins, S.M., Ke, M., Tache, Y. and Wood, J.D. (2006). Fundamentals of neurogastroenterology: basic science. *Gastroenterol.* **130**, 1391–1411.

Grundy, D., Blackshaw, A., and Andrews, P. L. R. (1991). Neural correlates of the gastrointestinal motor changes in emesis. In *Brain gut interactions*, (Ed. Y. Tache and D. Wingate), pp. 325–38. CRC Press, Boca Raton, FL.

Hasler, W. L., Soudah, H. C., Dulai, G., and Owyang, C. (1995). Mediation of hyperglycaemia evoked slow-wave dysrhythmias by endogenous prostaglandins. *Gastroenterol.* **108**, 727–36.

Hikasa, Y., Ogasawara, S., and Takase, K. (1991). Alpha adrenoceptor subtypes involved in the emetic action in dogs. *J. Pharmacol. Exp. Ther.* **261**, 746–54.

Himi, N.,Koga, T., Nakamura, E., Kobashi, M., Yamane, M. and Tsujioka, K. (2004). Differences in autonomic responses between subjects with and without nausea while watching an irregularly oscillating video. *Autonom. Neurosci. :Basic and Clinical* **116**, 46–53.

Hoffmann, I.S., Roa, M., Torrico, F. and Cubeddu, L.X. (2003). Ondansetron and metformin-induced gastrointestinal side effects. *Am J Ther* **10**, 447–51.

Jones, A.L. and Cunninghamn, D. (1993). The clinical care of patients receiving chemotherapy. In: Emesis in Anti-cancer Therapy-Mechanisms and Treatmemt. Eds, P.L.R. Andrews and G.J. Sanger, Chapter 11, p. 229–46. Chapman & Hall, London, UK.

Kaneoke, Y., Koike, Y., Sakurai, N. *et al.* (1995). Gastrointestinal dysfunction in Parkinson's disease detected by electrogastroenterography. *J. Autonom. Nerv. Syst.* **50**, 275–81.

Koch, K. L. (1993). Motion sickness. In *The handbook of nausea and vomiting*, ed. M. H. Sleisenger), pp. 43–60. Parthenon Publishing Group, New York.

Koch, K. L. and Stern, R. (2004). *Handbook of Electrogastrography*, New York, Oxford University Press, Inc.

Kris, M.G., Hesketh, P.J., Herrstedt, J., Rittenberg, C., Einhorn, L.H., Grunberg, S., Koeller, J., Olver, I., Borjeson, S. and Ballatori, E. (2005). Consensus proposals for the prevention of acute and delayed vomiting and nausea following high-risk chemotherapy. *Support. Care Cancer.* **13**, 85–96.

Kuchel, O. (1996). Disorders of dopamine metabolism. In *Primer on the autonomic nervous system*. (Ed. D. Robertson, P. A. Low and R. J. Polinsky) pp. 212–216. Academic Press Inc., San Diego.

Kulisevsky, J. and Pagonabarraga, J. (2010). Tolerability and safety of ropinirole versus other dopamine agonists and levodopa in the treatment of Parkinson's disease: meta-analysis of randomized controlled trials. *Drug Saf.* **33**, 147–61.

Lang, I. M., Sarna, S. K., and Dodds, W. J. (1993). Pharyngeal, esophageal, and proximal gastric responses associated with vomiting. *Am. J. Physiol.* **265**, G963–972.

Lee, J.W., Bromfield, E. and Kesari, S. (2008). Emesis responsive to levetiracetam. *J.Neurol. Neurosurg. Psychiatry*, **79**, 847–49.

Levine, M.E., Gillis, M.G., Koch, S.Y., Voss, A.C., Stern, R.M. and Koch, K.L. (2008). Protein and ginger for the treatment of chemotherapy-induced delayed nausea. *Journal of Alternative and Complimentary Medicine*, **14**, 545–51.

Levine, M.E., Muth, E.R., Williamson, M.J. and Stern, R.M. (2004). Protein-predominant meals inhibit the development of gastric tachyarrythmia, nausea and the symptoms of motion sickness. *Aliment. Pharmacol. Ther.* **19**, 583–90.

Lien, H-C., Sun, W.M., Chen, Y-H., Kim, H., Hasler, W. and Owyang, C. (2003). Effects of ginger on motion sickness and gastric slow-wave dysrhythmias induced by circular vection. *Am.J.Physiol. Gastrointest. Liver Physiol.* **284**, G481–89.

Lin, Z., Forster, J., Sarosiek, I. and McCallum, R.W. (2004). Effect of high-frequency gastric electrical stimulation on gastric myoelectric activity in gastroparetic patients. *Neurogastroeneterol. Motil.* **16**, 205–212.

Lindstrom, P.A., and Brizzee, K.R. (1962). Relief of intractable vomiting from surgical lesions in the area postrema. *J.Neurosurg.*, 19, 228–36.

Lumsden, K. and Holden, W. S. (1969). The act of vomiting in man. *Gut,* **10**, 173–79.

Miller, A.D. (1990). Respiratory muscle control during vomiting. *Can. J. Physiol. Pharmacology.* **68**, 237–41.

Miller, A. D., Nonaka, S., Siniaia, M. S., & Jakus, J. (1995). Multifunctional ventral respiratory group: Bulbospinal expiratory neurons play a role in pudendal discharge during vomiting. *J Auton Nerv Syst,* **54**, 253–60.

Miller, A. D., Rowley, H. A., Roberts, T. P. L., and Kucharczyk, J. (1996). Human cortical activity during vestibular- and drug-induced nausea detected using MSI. *Ann. New York Acad. Sci.* **781**, 670–2.

Miller, A. D., and Leslie, R. A. (1994). The area postrema and vomiting. *Frontiers in Neuroendocrin.* **15**, 1–20.

Muth, E. (2006). Motion and space sickness: Intestinal and autonomic correlates. *Autonomic Neuroscience: Basic and Clinical,* **129**, 58–66

Natale, G., Pasquali, L., Ruggieri, S., Paparelli, A. and Fornai, F. (2008). Parkinson's disease and the gut: a well known clinical association in need of an effective cure and explanation. *Neurogastroenterol Motil,* **20**, 741–49.

Navari, R.M. (2007). Fosaprepitant (MK-0517): a neurokinin –1 receptor antagonist for the prevention of chemotherapy-induced nausea and vomiting. *Expert Opin Investigational Drugs,* **16**, 1977–85.

Navari, R.M. (2009). Palonosteron: a second generation 5-hydroxytryptamine 3 receptor antagonist. *Expert Opin Drug Metab Toxicol,* **5**, 1577–86.

Ng, K.S., Chua, Y.C., Ban, V.F. *et al.* (2011). Identifying human biomarkers of nausea for refining animal studies on emesis. *Gastroenterology* **140**, Supplement, S-368.

North, B., and Reilly, P. (1990). *Raised intracranial pressure. A clinical guide.* Heinemann Medical Books, pp. 30–1. Heinemann, New York.

Nussey, S. S., Hawthorn, J., Page, S. R., Ang, V. T. Y., and design and pharmacology of nove. (1988). Responses of plasma oxytocin and arginine vasopressin to nausea induced by apomorphine and ipecacuanha. *Clin. Endocrinol.* **28**, 297–304.

Owyang, C. and Hasler, W.L. (2002). Physiology and pathophysiology of the interstitial cells of Cajal: From bench to bedside:VI. Pathogenesis and therapeutic approaches to human gastric dysrythmias. *Am.J.Physiol. Gastrointest. Liver Physiol* **283**, 8–15.

Parkes, J. D. (1986). A neurologist's view of nausea and vomiting. Introduction: vomiting is common in neurological disorders. In *Nausea and vomiting: mechanism and treatment*, (Eds. C. J. Davis, G. V. Lake-Bakaar, and D. G. Grahame-Smith), pp. 160–6. Springer-Verlag, Berlin.

Perez-Lloret, S. and Rascol, O. (2010). Dopamine receptor agonists for the treatment of early or advanced Parkinson's disease. *CNS Drugs* **24**, 941–68.

Pertz, H.H., Lehmann, J., Roth-Ehrang, R. and Elz, S. (2011). Effects of ginger constituents on the gastrointestinal tract: Role of cholinergic M3 and Serotonergic 5-HT3 and 5-HT4 receptors. *Planta Med*, Feb 8th epub ahead of print.

Peyrot des Gachons, C., Beauchamp, G.K., Stern, R.M., Koch, K.L. and Breslin, P.A.S. (2011). Bitter taste induces nausea. *Curr. Biol.,* **21**, R247–248.

Pickering, M. and Jones, J.F. (2002). The diaphragm: two physiological muscles in one. *J. Anat.* **201**, 305–312.

Qu, R., Furukawa, N., and Fukuda, H. (1995). Changes in extrahepatic biliary motilities with emesis in dogs. *J. Autonom. Nerv. Syst* **56**, 87–96.

Reddy, G.K., Gralla, R.J. and Hesketh, P.J. (2006). Novel neurokinin-1 antagonists as antiemetics for the treatment of chemotherapy-induced emesis. *Support Cancer Ther* **3**, 140–42.

Reis, D. J. and Regunathan, S. (1996). Imidazoline receptors and their native ligands. In *Primer on the Autonomic Nervous System* (ed. D. Robertson, P. A. Low and R. J. Polinsky) pp. 107–8. Academic Press Inc., San Diego.

Rojas, C., Stathis, M., Thomas, A.G., Massuda, E.B., Alt, J., Zhang, J., Rubenstein, E., Sebastiani, S. and Cantoreggi, S., Snyder, S.H., Slusher, B. (2008). Palonosetron exhibits unique molecular interactions with the 5- HT_3 receptor. *Anesth Anlag* **107**, 469–78.

Rudd, J.R. and Andrews, P.L.R. (2005). Mechanisms of acute, delayed and anticipatory emesis induced by anticancer therapies. In: Hesketh, P.J, pp. 15–65. (Ed), *Management and Treatment of Nausea and Vomiting in Cancer and Cancer Treatment*. Jones and Bartlett, Sudbury, MA.

Sanger, G.J. (2009). Translating 5-HT receptor pharmacology. *Neurogastroenterol Motil* **21**, 1235–38.

Sanger, G.J. and Andrews, P.L.R. (2006). Treatment of nausea and vomiting: Where are the gaps in our knowledge? *Autonomic Neuroscience: Basic and Clinical* **129**, 3–16.

Saper, C. B. (2002). The central autonomic nervous system: Conscious visceral perception and autonomic pattern generation. *Ann Rev Neurosci*, **25**, 433–69.

Sawai, S., Sakakibara, R., Kanai, K., Kawaguchi, N., Uchiyama, T., Yamamoto, T., Ito, T., Liu, Z. and Hattori, T. (2006). Isolated vomiting due to a unilateral dorsal vagal complex lesion. *Eur.J.Neurol.* **56**, 246–48.

Schvarcz, E., Palmer, M., Aman, J., Horowitz, M., Stridsberg, M., and Berne, C. (1997). Physiological hyperglycemia slows gastric emptying in normal subjects and patients with insulin-dependent diabetes mellitus. *Gastroenterology* **113**, 60–6.

Serrador, J.M., Schlegel, T.T., Balck, F.O. and Wood, S.J. (2005). Cerebral hypoperfusion precedes nausea during centrifugation. *Aviat. Space Environ. Med.* **76**, 91–96

Stern, R.M., Jokerst, M.D., Muth, E.R. and Hollis, C. (2001). Acupressure relieves the symptoms of motion sickness and reduces abnormal gastric activity. *Altern. Ther. Health Med.* **7**, 91–94.

Stern, R.M., Koch, K. and Andrews, P.L.R. (2011). *Nausea-Mechanisms and Management*. Oxford University Press.

Tanaka, K. (1979). Jamaican vomiting sickness. In *Handbook of clinical neurology*, (ed. P. J. Vinken and G. W. Bruyn), Vol. 37, Chapter 17, pp. 511–39. North Holland Publishing Company, Amsterdam.

Thompson, D. G. and Malagelada, J. R. (1982). Vomiting and the small intestine. *Dig. Dis. Sci.* **27**, 1121–5.

Tremblay, P-B., Kaiser, R., Sezer, O., Rosler, N., Schelenz, C., Possinger, K., Roots, I. and Brockmoller, J., (2003). Variations in the 5-hydroxytryptamine type 3B receptor gene as predictors of the efficacy of antiemetic treatment in cancer patients. *J. Clin. Oncol.* **21**, 2147–55.

Van Oudernhove, L., Coen, S.J. and Aziz, Q. (2007). Functional brain imaging of gastrointestinal sensation in health and disease. *World J. Gastroenterol.* **13**, 3438–45.

Yates, B.J., Miller, A.D. and Lucot, J.B. (1998). Physiological basis and pharmacology of motion sickness. *Brain Res. Bull.*, **47**, 395–406.

Yen Pik Sang, F.D., Golding, J.F. and Gresty, M.A. (2003). Suppression of sickness by controlled breathing during mildly nauseogenic motion. *Avait.Space Environ.Med.* **74**, 998–1002.

Yoshida, M. M., Schuffler, M. D. and Sumi, S. M. (1988). There are no morphologic abnormalities of the gastric wall or abdominal vagus in patients with diabetic gastroparesis. *Gastroenterology* **94**, 907–14.

CHAPTER 18

The influence of the autonomic nervous system on metabolic function

Ian A. Macdonald

Key points

◆ The sympathoadrenal system has direct effects on carbohydrate and fat metabolism, leading to mobilization of fuel stores.

◆ Indirect effects of the sympathoadrenal system on metabolism are mediated via alterations in insulin release from the pancreas and interactions with thyroid function.

◆ The sympathoadrenal system has direct stimulatory effects on resting energy expenditure, which may be involved in responses to over and underfeeding.

◆ Nutritional status can affect sympathoadrenal activity and increased sympathetic activity may contribute to hypertension in obesity.

Introduction

The autonomic innervation of peripheral tissues is important in the regulation of metabolism, but there is also a key role for catecholamines released from the adrenal medulla. This chapter will deal with the influences of both autonomic (mainly sympathetic) postganglionic nerves and plasma catecholamines on metabolism. These effects can occur either through direct actions of catecholamines within metabolically active tissue, or as a consequence of alterations in the major hormones that regulate metabolism. There is now substantial evidence that changes in metabolic or nutritional status can affect the autonomic nervous system (in particular the sympathoadrenal component), and these effects will be considered. Afferent components of the autonomic nervous control of metabolism are now recognized to include signals from peripheral tissues, such as the liver and adipose tissue. For example, afferent neural connections between the liver/hepatic portal vein region and the brain affect glucose metabolism, whilst cytokine/endocrine signals from adipose tissue (e.g. leptin) affect the hypothalamic control of energy metabolism and also possibly affect blood pressure. The mechanisms by which diabetes mellitus has profound effects on the autonomic and sensory nervous system are not fully understood. However, it is well established that the pathological consequences of this neuropathy for sympathetic function are extremely serious with regard to the postural control of blood pressure and the regulation of sweating. The implications of such diabetic neuropathy on the control of metabolism will be described.

Control of metabolism

There are numerous intracellular biochemical processes that may be under sympathoadrenal regulation. This chapter will focus on the metabolism of two of the dietary macronutrients (carbohydrate and fat), concentrating on effects that have been established through *in vivo* studies (mainly in humans). Consideration will also be given to overall energy metabolism—assessing the effects of the sympathoadrenal system on resting energy expenditure (thermogenesis). Detailed reviews include those by Young and Landsberg (1977), Macdonald et al. (1985), Webber and Macdonald (1993), Nonogaki (2000), and Snitker et al. (2000).

Direct sympathoadrenal control of metabolism

Carbohydrate metabolism

The maintenance of an adequate supply of glucose to neural tissue is a fundamental component of homeostasis (Fig. 18.1). The carbohydrate component of food is stored in the liver and skeletal muscle as glycogen, under the influence of insulin released from the β-cells of the islets of Langerhans in the pancreas. During the intervals between meals, or in periods of prolonged starvation, the stored liver glycogen is used to produce free glucose, which maintains an adequate blood glucose concentration, thus sustaining neural function. During short periods of starvation (less than 24 hours), blood glucose is maintained mainly by the breakdown of the liver glycogen store (the process of glycogenolysis), and partly by the synthesis of glucose (gluconeogenesis) in the liver. This hepatic glycogenolysis is regulated in part by glucagon released from the α-cells of the pancreatic islets, but it is now clear that adrenaline stimulation of glycogenolysis is also important.

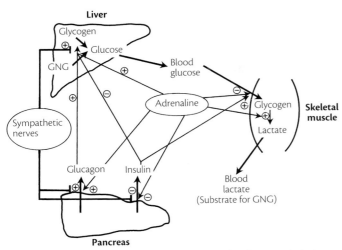

Fig. 18.1 Effects of sympathetic nerves and plasma adrenaline on carbohydrate metabolism. Both direct effects on liver and muscle metabolism and indirect effects via alterations in insulin and glucagon release are illustrated. GNG, gluconeogenesis; +, stimulated; −, inhibited.

In humans, adrenaline stimulates glycogenolysis mainly via activation of β-adrenoceptors, but this is of minor importance during short periods of fasting. A small component of hepatic glycogenolysis after an overnight fast is due to stimulation of α-adrenoceptors, probably through the sympathetic innervation of the liver. After more prolonged fasting (i.e. several days), adrenaline contributes to the maintenance of glucose homeostasis but glucagon is still of primary importance (Boyle et al. 1989).

The liver glycogen store is depleted after 2 days of starvation, and the synthesis of glucose (gluconeogenesis) from precursors such as lactate, alanine, and glycerol becomes of major importance. This gluconeogenesis occurs mainly in the liver (although the kidneys do contribute) and is stimulated by glucagon and adrenaline. In addition to a direct effect on hepatic gluconeogenesis, adrenaline is one of the main stimuli for increasing muscle glycogenolysis in the resting state. By contrast to the liver, muscle glycogen cannot be broken down to free glucose, but instead lactate is produced and passes into the blood. This lactate is a substrate for hepatic gluconeogenesis and thus muscle glycogen can indirectly contribute to the maintenance of blood glucose (the Cori cycle).

The liver has a sympathetic innervation that has been studied extensively by Lautt (1980). Stimulation of the hepatic sympathetic supply leads to increased glycogenolysis and glucose release. There is no direct evidence that these nerves are involved in the regulation of carbohydrate metabolism under normal conditions. For example, applications of local anaesthetic to the coeliac ganglion (preventing sympathetic activation of the liver) has no effect on the increase in release of glucose from the liver during exercise (Kjaer et al. 1993). Denervation of the liver, such as with transplantation, does not produce any gross abnormalities of carbohydrate metabolism, with transplant recipients having the same hepatic glucose production responses to exercise to those seen in healthy individuals (Kjaer et al. 1995). However, with liver transplantation it would be rather difficult to identify more subtle alterations, given the previous metabolic disease and post-transplant immunosuppression. It is more likely that hepatic sympathetic nerves are of importance in severe hypoglycaemia or when the other mechanisms are defective.

It is well recognized that the sympathetic innervation of skeletal muscle has a major influence on resting blood flow in muscle. There is also some evidence from animal studies that stimulation of the sympathetic innervation of resting skeletal muscle increases glucose uptake into the muscle (reviewed by Nonogaki 2000), but there is no direct evidence of similar effects in humans.

Fat metabolism

The major direct metabolic effects of the sympathoadrenal system are in the control of fat metabolism (Fig. 18.2). The storage of fatty acids as triacylglycerols in adipose tissue is regulated by insulin, which stimulates the storage process and inhibits the breakdown of triacylglycerol to non-esterified fatty acids (NEFA or FFA). This breakdown process (lipolysis) increases if plasma insulin levels fall, but the major stimulation is achieved by several hormones, including adrenaline, and by the sympathetic innervation of the adipose tissue. With short periods of starvation (up to 20 hours), there appears to be little involvement of sympathoadrenal stimulation of lipolysis, with the fall in plasma insulin and rise in plasma cortisol being the likely stimuli for an increase in NEFA release from adipose tissue (Samra et al. 1996). More prolonged starvation, and a variety of other stressors, leads to increased lipolysis via sympathoadrenal stimulation. The sympathoadrenal stimulation of lipolysis occurs via β-adrenoceptor-mediated processes. By contrast, the stimulation of α-adrenoceptors in adipose tissue inhibits lipolysis. This may prevent the occurrence of excessive rates of lipolysis during periods of starvation, as there is evidence that such a state is accompanied by a fall in β-adrenoceptor density and a rise in α-adrenoceptor density in adipose tissue.

The sympathetic innervation of white adipose tissue mainly supplies the vasculature, but in some depots there is a direct innervation of the adipose tissue cells. There is histological evidence that neurotransmitters released from the sympathetic nerves may also stimulate non-innervated adipose tissue cells, thus providing a key role for the sympathetic nervous system in the regulation of adipose tissue blood flow and metabolism (Fredholm 1985). There is some evidence from animal studies of a parasympathetic innervation of adipose tissue (Kreier et al. 2002) which may be involved in regulating the storage of fat in the adipose tissue independently of the normal insulin mediated effects.

During conditions such as orthostasis, there are transient reductions in human adipose tissue blood flow, mediated by sympathetic

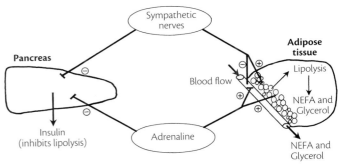

Fig. 18.2 Effects of sympathetic nerves and plasma adrenaline on fat metabolism. Both direct effects on adipose tissue blood flow and metabolism and indirect effects through inhibition of insulin release are illustrated. NEFA, non-esterified fatty acids; +, stimulated; −, inhibited.

nervous innervation of vascular smooth muscle. However, these blood vessels also contain β-adrenoceptors which mediate vasodilatation in response to an increase in plasma adrenaline, or possibly due to diffusion of noradrenaline from the sympathetic neuroeffector junctions. Thus, prolonged sympathetic nervous stimulation to white adipose tissue is accompanied by a type of vasoconstrictor escape, while a rise in plasma adrenaline levels products active vasodilatation (Hjemdahl and Linde 1983). Furthermore, the stimulation of lipolysis by the sympathetic nerves, or plasma adrenaline, leads to a rise in adipose tissue blood flow through metabolic effects—facilitating the transport of fatty acids to other tissues in the body (reviewed by Frayn and Macdonald 1996).

Brown adipose tissue has a more dense vascular supply and innervation than white adipose tissue. Furthermore, many more brown adipose tissue cells are sympathetically innervated directly. The vascular innervation appears to be predominantly vasodilator, with the released noradrenaline acting on β-adrenoceptors. The stimulation of lipolysis in brown adipose tissue is accompanied by a marked increase in the oxygen consumption of the tissue (brown adipose tissue thermogenesis). This metabolic event is mediated by β-adrenoceptors that appear to be somewhat atypical, and have been designated β₃ (Arch et al. 1984). In humans, brown adipose tissue is important as a site of thermogenesis in the newborn, but is of limited significance in the adult.

Studies in animals of sympathetic activation of skeletal muscle have demonstrated an activation of muscle lipoprotein lipase (LPL). This activation of LPL would facilitate the breakdown of plasma triacylglycerol and enable the FFA thus liberated to be taken up by the muscle fibres and either used as a fuel for oxidation or stored as triacylglycerol. It is not known whether such effects also occur in humans, but there is some evidence that sympathetic activation can activate fat breakdown in skeletal muscle. The latter is based on the observation that sympathetic activation produced by lower body negative pressure (LBNP) was accompanied by an increase in extracellular glycerol concentration (an index of increased intramuscular lipolysis) in forearm muscle (Henry et al. 1998). However, a subsequent study failed to confirm this observation (Navegantes et al. 2003) and so it remains unclear whether the sympathetic innervation of skeletal muscle in humans has direct metabolic effects.

Indirect autonomic effects on metabolism

The main indirect effect on metabolism is through the modulation of insulin and glucagon release from the pancreas. Stimulation of the sympathetic innervation of the β-cell leads to α-adrenoceptor mediated inhibition of insulin release. Evidence from *in vitro* studies suggests plasma catecholamines inhibit insulin release through activation of α₂-adrenoceptors, but is not known whether these also mediate the sympathetic nervous effects. The pancreatic β-cells also contain β₂-adrenoceptors, although it is uncommon for these to be stimulated by plasma adrenaline under physiological conditions—the stimulation of α-adrenoceptors seems to predominate. However, β₂-adrenoceptor agonists such as salbutamol will stimulate insulin release.

An important physiological role of the autonomic nervous system in the control of insulin release is the stimulatory effect of the vagus supply to the pancreas. Stimulation of the parasympathetic innervation of the β-cells leads to insulin release, and is an important component of the cephalic and gastric phases of feeding. Thus, the sight, smell, and taste of food, and its presence in the stomach, will elicit an insulin secretory response, which primes the liver to maximize glucose retention when the food is absorbed. Once nutrient absorption occurs, further insulin release is due to direct effects of glucose and amino acids (and of gastrointestinal hormones) on the β-cells. Stimulation of the parasympathetic nerve supply to the pancreas also gives rise to the secretion of the hormone pancreatic polypeptide. The functions of this hormone are unclear, but its release in response to a variety of stimuli (including food and hypoglycaemia) provides a marker of pancreatic vagal function.

The pancreatic α-cells are stimulated by both their sympathetic innervation and by plasma catecholamines. Glucagon release results from activation of β-adrenoceptors, although such release has not been demonstrated in all studies of the effects of the infusion of adrenaline.

One of the consequences of pancreatic transplantation is to produce a denervated pancreas. However, this cannot readily be used to judge the overall importance of the innervation, as the transplant recipients are patients with insulin-dependent diabetes mellitus (IDDM) who also have severe diabetic complications such as endstage renal failure. Such pancreatic transplantation is judged to be successful if the patient no longer needs to inject insulin (although this is only achieved with continued immunosuppression). The transplanted pancreas is capable of controlling postprandial blood glucose satisfactorily, and releases glucagon in response to hypoglycaemia. However, it is not known whether the effectiveness of the pancreas in regulating metabolism is compromised by its lack of autonomic innervation.

One of the most important indirect effects of the sympathoadrenal system on metabolism is to reduce the sensitivity of the peripheral tissues to insulin. Thus, under conditions of sympathetic activation or increased adrenal medullary secretion (such as in trauma or after a myocardial infarction) there is a reduction in the effectiveness of insulin to stimulate glucose uptake and utilization in adipose tissue and skeletal muscle. These peripheral effects of the catecholamines seem to be mediated through activation of β₂-adrenoceptors and thus are also produced by drugs such as salbutamol, ritodrine, and terbutaline. Such drugs are commonly used to prevent premature labour. If used in pregnant women with IDDM, these drugs lead to a marked increased in the insulin requirements for achieving adequate control of blood glucose. The latter is of major importance in preventing the occurrence of macrosomia in the fetus. Large doses of these β₂-agonists can stimulate adipose tissue lipolysis and pancreatic glucagon secretion, leading to increased ketone production which may develop into diabetic ketoacidosis. In such conditions of possible premature labour, steroids are sometimes given intravenously to the woman to stimulate the fetal lung maturation process, and in patients with IDDM these high doses of steroids will increase the likelihood of occurrence of diabetic ketoacidosis.

In summary, physiologically the predominant effects of the sympathoadrenal system are to raise blood glucose concentration through direct effects on glycogenolysis and gluconeogenesis and indirectly through reducing insulin release, decreasing insulin sensitivity, and possibly stimulating glucagon release. Of equal, if not greater, importance is the effect of the sympathoadrenal system on the regulation of lipolysis. The sympathetic innervation to adipose tissue and plasma catecholamines both stimulate lipolysis, an effect that is enhanced if there is also a catecholamine-mediated suppression of insulin release. The parasympathetic innervation of the pancreatic β-cell can stimulate insulin release, and is of importance in the early stages of food ingestion.

Thermogenesis

Given the profound effects of the catecholamines on metabolism described above, it would be surprising if there was not also an effect on energy metabolism. It was demonstrated over 60 years ago that the infusion of adrenaline into humans (in amounts that we now know produce plasma adrenaline levels in the physiological range) caused an increase in whole-body energy metabolism, as well as stimulating heart rate and respiration. This effect is now known as adrenaline (catecholamine)-induced thermogenesis (the stimulation of energy metabolism above resting, baseline levels) and does not involve an increase in physical activity, although adrenaline will, of course, increase skeletal muscle tremor. The existence of this catecholamine-induced thermogenesis has been confirmed many times, and may be of physiological importance in the control of energy balance and of body temperature.

The infusion of noradrenaline also stimulates thermogenesis, mainly through an increase in lipolysis and oxidation of free fatty acids (as is the case with adrenaline), although the amounts that have to be used are somewhat larger than for adrenaline. In fact, the plasma adrenaline threshold for increasing thermogenesis is toward the lower end of the physiological range. Higher plasma levels of noradrenaline are needed to stimulate thermogenesis, indicating that under physiological conditions, it is more likely that direct stimulation of thermogenesis by noradrenaline occurs due to activation of the sympathetic nerves rather than through an effect of plasma noradrenaline.

When the human neonate is exposed to a cool environment, its total heat production increases (cold-induced thermogenesis) to maintain body temperature. It seems most probable that this cold-induced thermogenesis is mediated through the sympathetic nervous system activating thermogenesis in brown adipose tissue—as also seen in cold-adapted rodents and hibernating mammals. Thus, catecholamine-induced thermogenesis is of major importance in neonatal thermoregulation. Studies in adult humans also indicate that cold-induced thermogenesis occurs in the absence of muscle contraction (Jessen et al. 1990) and it has been suggested that this is also stimulated by catecholamines. However, the normal human adult has insufficient brown adipose tissue to contribute significantly to heat production in the cold, and it seems more probable that the splanchnic region and skeletal muscle are the major sites of such thermogenesis. Nevertheless, such non-shivering thermogenesis would be of minor importance in the regulation of body temperature in most situations.

There is an increasing volume of evidence that sympathoadrenal effects on thermogenesis may be of importance in the overall regulation of energy metabolism. It has been apparent for many years that experimental animals (e.g. rats, pigs), and in some cases humans, can regulate overall thermogenesis to maintain energy balance over a wide range of energy intake. Studies in the rat by Rothwell and Stock (1981) indicated that the consumption of excessive amounts of a varied, palatable diet did not produce the expected degree of weight gain, because of a profound increase in energy expenditure. This increased energy expenditure was not due to physical activity, but was a result of increased sympathetic nervous stimulation of brown adipose tissue and of an increased mass of this tissue. Attempts to make similar observations in adult humans foundered because of the small amounts of this tissue. However, there have now been several demonstrations of marked sympathoadrenal effects on overall energy metabolism.

The first of these demonstrations relates to the effects of insulin and glucose in normal humans. If one raises plasma insulin levels by exogenous infusion, but then infuses glucose to maintain a constant blood glucose, the amount of glucose infused matches the glucose taken up by the tissues and is a measure of the sensitivity of the individual to insulin (the glucose clamp method). In healthy subjects, the glucose taken up by the tissues is either oxidized, or stored as glycogen. Acheson and colleagues demonstrated that this combined infusion of insulin and glucose stimulated thermogenesis (increasing resting energy expenditure by 10–20%), and that the observed increase was substantially greater than the expected increase required to provide the necessary energy for the amount of glycogen being synthesized. The demonstration that this extra energy expenditure could be suppressed by administration of a β-adrenoceptor antagonist led to the proposition that part of the observed glucose-induced thermogenesis was due to sympathoadrenal activation (Acheson 1988). However, it should be noted that this effect is most noticeable at high insulin concentrations, which exceed those seen with normal dietary carbohydrate intakes.

Further support for a link between glucose metabolism, the sympathoadrenal system and thermogenesis comes from the studies of Astrup and colleagues. They demonstrated an increase in thermogenesis in resting skeletal muscle, approximately 4 hours after ingestion of a glucose load, coincident with an increase in plasma adrenaline levels. Subsequent studies by this group showed that the ingestion of a mixed meal has a similar effect and that in both cases this delayed stimulation of thermogenesis can be prevented by β-adrenoceptor blockade (Astrup et al. 1990). In the same review, these authors provided a useful analysis of previous studies which indicated that β-blockade only reduced meal-induced thermogenesis in the later stages and when there was a high carbohydrate content of the ingested food.

Work by Schwarz and colleagues has shown a positive correlation between the increase in thermogenesis seen after consuming a mixed meal and the stimulation of the sympathetic nervous system (assessed by measuring plasma noradrenaline turnover). Furthermore, the administration of clonidine, to suppress central sympathetic outflow, reduced both the sympathetic stimulation and the thermogenic response to the meals (Schwarz et al. 1988). There is evidence that the thermogenic response to meals decreases with ageing, and that it is higher in individuals of all ages who are physically active compared to those who are sedentary (reviewed by Seals and Bell 2004). However, the overall level of sympathetic activation (assessed by either microneurography or plasma catecholamines) does not appear to be related to these age or physical activity related differences in thermogenic response.

In summary, the sympathoadrenal system can stimulate thermogenesis, and there are a number of physiological conditions in which this effect may operate. The final part of this chapter will consider whether disorders of such effects are involved in the aetiology of obesity, or in disturbances of thermoregulation.

Metabolic and nutritional effects on the sympathoadrenal system

In addition to the sympathoadrenal system being important in the regulation of metabolism, it is apparent that alterations in metabolic or nutritional status can affect the activity of the sympathoadrenal system. Some of these effects would be entirely predictable on the basis of the regulation of metabolism discussed above. The best example of this is the effect of an acute reduction in blood glucose concentration producing hypoglycaemia, which leads to adrenaline release from the adrenal medulla and altered sympathetic nervous system activity. However, there are a variety of other metabolic and nutritional effects on the sympathoadrenal system which are considered below.

Dietary effects on the sympathetic nervous system: animal studies

The possibility that the amount and composition of the diet may affect the sympathetic nervous system has been addressed by the studies of Landsberg, Young, and colleagues (Landsberg and Young 1985). They assessed the activity of the sympathetic nervous system by measuring the rate of turnover of the neurotransmitter noradrenaline in specific organs and tissues of rats and mice. These studies have shown that starvation suppresses and overfeeding enhances sympathetic activity, with an increased dietary carbohydrate content being a particularly potent stimulus. This effect of carbohydrate to stimulate the sympathetic nervous system appears to involve an action of insulin in the hypothalamus. This has led to a series of studies on the effects of insulin on the sympathetic nervous system in humans which will be discussed below.

There are impressive correlations between increased noradrenaline turnover and thermogenesis in brown adipose tissue during both excess dietary intake and cold adaptation in rodents. Thus, it would appear that there is an important functional role for diet-induced changes in sympathetic activity. This is supported by the demonstration that a reduced energy intake leads to a fall in sympathetic activity and in blood pressure in spontaneously hypertensive rats.

Human studies

Assessing the activity of the sympathetic nervous system in humans is restricted to intraneural recordings in superficial nerves, measuring plasma noradrenaline turnover (Esler et al. 1990) or measuring plasma or urinary catecholamine concentrations. Each of these techniques has some limitations, and caution must be exercised when interpreting any results obtained, especially if there are no associated functional measurements. Alterations in dietary intake in humans are accompanied by changes in sympathetic activity (assessed by plasma noradrenaline turnover and plasma and urinary levels) that are qualitatively similar to the effects seen in animals. A reduced energy intake is accompanied by evidence of reduced sympathetic activity and decreased supine blood pressure, with increased energy intake being associated with opposite changes. Horowitz et al. (1999) observed that short-term fasting reduced plasma noradrenaline turnover in non-obese, but not in obese, women, and it is now clear that altered sympathoadrenal function may play a role in the development of obesity or its comorbidities (Snitker et al. 2000).

Metabolic effects on the sympathoadrenal system

Hypoglycaemia

The most potent metabolic disturbances affecting the sympathoadrenal system relate to alterations in glucose metabolism, or in plasma insulin concentrations. In healthy adult humans an overnight fast produces blood glucose concentrations of 4–5 mmol/litre. Acute reduction of blood glucose to approximately 3.5 mmol/litre (with insulin) is followed within 10 minutes by the secretion of adrenaline from the adrenal medulla. More severe hypoglycaemia is associated with progressively increasing adrenaline responses (Fig. 18.3). This release of adrenaline at a relatively high blood glucose level is part of the early endocrine response that opposes the effect of insulin and occurs before any detectable impairment in cerebral function caused by the fall in blood glucose.

More profound hypoglycaemia (blood glucose 2–3 mmol/litre) is accompanied by an increase in plasma noradrenaline concentrations, the rate of appearance of noradrenaline in plasma, and by an increase in muscle and skin nerve sympathetic activity (measured by microneurography) (reviewed by Heller and Macdonald 1991). The effect on muscle sympathetic activity is interesting as this appears to be occurring in vasoconstrictor fibres, yet muscle vasodilatation occurs in hypoglycaemia. The latter is not due to the

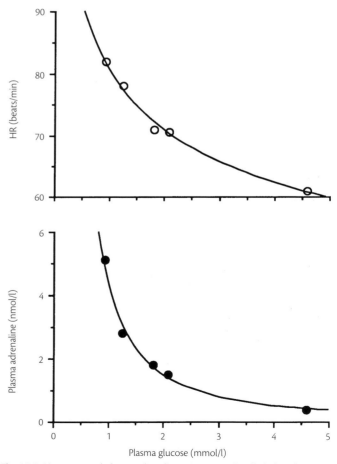

Fig. 18.3 Heart rate and plasma adrenaline responses to insulin-induced hypoglycaemia. In both cases there is a curvilinear relationship with more profound hypoglycaemia having a progressively greater effect.

effects of insulin as it occurs when hypoglycaemia is induced with relatively low plasma insulin levels (below 120 mU/litre) whereas the effect of insulin to produce vasodilatation in skeletal muscle does not occur until insulin levels exceed 140 mU/litre. It is far more likely that the muscle vasodilatation in hypoglycaemia is due to the increased plasma adrenaline levels as it can be prevented by β-adrenoceptor antagonism. The muscle blood flow response to hypoglycaemia illustrates the need to assess sympathetically mediated function as well as sympathetic nervous system activity.

Such hypoglycaemia occurs most commonly in patients with IDDM. When these patients first develop diabetes, their responses to hypoglycaemia are the same as in non-diabetic subjects. However, within 5 years of the onset of IDDM, most patients lose the ability to release glucagon in response to hypoglycaemia (although not in response to other stimuli). Such patients are then dependent on an adequate adrenaline response and on the disappearance of the injected insulin, for blood glucose recovery after hypoglycaemia (unless they eat). When such diabetic patients develop autonomic neuropathy of such a severity that they fail to release adrenaline from the adrenal medulla, they will then be at risk of developing prolonged, severe hypoglycaemia if their insulin dose and food intake are poorly matched.

The symptomatic responses and physiological disturbances that occur with hypoglycaemia are reduced when patients experience regular episodes of low blood glucose. This phenomenon is not well understood, but an episode of hypoglycaemia on one day reduces the adrenomedullary response to the same degree of hypoglycaemia the next day. This reduced response does not appear to be due to an adrenal medullary defect, as the plasma adrenaline response to postural change or to mental arithmetic is unaffected by antecedent hypoglycaemia (Robinson et al. 1995). However, other recent studies have suggested that the adrenaline and sympathetic nervous system responses to hypoglycaemia may be reduced by moderate intensity exercise in the previous 24 hours (Sandoval et al. 2004). This suggests that activation of the sympathoadrenal system may reduce responses to subsequent stimulation, and the functional consequences of this will need to be determined in the future.

Hyperglycaemia and insulin

A rise in blood glucose concentration is often accompanied by an increase in plasma noradrenaline, heart rate, and blood pressure consistent with stimulation of the sympathetic nervous system. This is confirmed by the demonstration of increased muscle sympathetic nerve activity after glucose ingestion (Berne et al. 1989). The effect of glucose can be explained at least partly by an action of insulin on the sympathetic nervous system. The technique of insulin and glucose infusion (glucose clamping) described above leads to a rise in plasma noradrenaline, heart rate, and systolic blood pressure in normal humans. Studies with microneurography have shown increased muscle sympathetic (vasoconstrictor) nerve activity, but again it is interesting to note that forearm (predominantly muscle) blood flow increases in these circumstances (Scott et al. 1988a). This raises the possibility that insulin may have direct effects on the vascular smooth muscle (or the sympathetic nerve terminals) to produce vasodilatation which leads to reflex activation of the sympathetic nervous system.

A disturbance of the balance between vasodilator effects of insulin and sympathetic nervous system activation may contribute to the falls in blood pressure seen after high carbohydrate meals in the elderly. The normal muscle vasoconstrictor responses to high-fat meals are converted into vasodilator responses (with a fall in blood pressure) by the infusion of insulin to produce plasma concentrations similar to those seen after carbohydrate-rich meals (Kearney et al. 1998).

Changes in sympathoadrenally regulated processes during metabolic/nutritional disturbances

Acute (48-hour) starvation in healthy humans is accompanied by functional changes consistent with altered sympathoadrenal activity. The regulation of body temperature during cold exposure is impaired with an inadequate increase in thermogenesis and reduction in limb blood flow contributing to a fall in core temperature (Macdonald et al. 1984). In addition, there is no increase in thermogenesis during insulin and glucose infusion in starvation. As the latter response is normally mediated by the sympathetic nervous system, this is consistent with reduced sympathetic activity in starvation. Further evidence of functional impairment of sympathetic control during starvation is provided by the falls in arterial blood pressure on standing seen after 48 hours' starvation in young men with normal orthostatic responses in the fed state (Bennett et al. 1984). These functional impairments seen in acute starvation are not due to the inability to respond to catecholamines, as the cardiac and thermogenic responses to infused adrenaline are actually enhanced after 48 hours' starvation.

These demonstrations of functional impairments consistent with reduced sympathetic activity are not restricted to acute starvation. Severe weight loss in human babies (due to inadequate food intake) and adults (with Crohn's disease, coeliac disease, or postoperative fistulas) is accompanied by impaired thermoregulation, particularly with reduced or absent thermogenic responses, which is reversed by weight gain. Impaired thermoregulation also occurs in anorexia nervosa, although it is not clear whether these changes are also reversible. It seems most unlikely that weight loss in anorexia nervosa is contributed to by enhanced thermogenic responses to food or to catecholamines, which would increase overall energy expenditure, producing the opposite effect to that which may occur in obesity. However, the weight loss associated with chronic respiratory disease is accompanied by increases in resting energy expenditure and urinary catecholamine excretion, providing further evidence of an effect of the sympathoadrenal system on energy metabolism.

Many studies have also shown poor orthostatic tolerance during chronic undernutrition, although this may of course be due to disturbances of fluid and electrolyte balance rather than to nutritional effects on the sympathetic nervous system.

Obesity

The role of the sympathoadrenal system in controlling substrate mobilization and thermogenesis, and the links between nutritional factors and the sympathetic nervous system, have led to the proposition that reduced sympathetic activity contributes to the development or maintenance of obesity. It is now clear that in several animal models of obesity reduced sympathetic nervous stimulation of thermogenesis is a contributory factor to the development of the obese state. The genetically obese *ob/ob* mouse cannot produce the peptide leptin in its adipose tissue, and becomes obese through excessive eating and low rates of thermogenesis. Administration of leptin to these animals lowers food intake and increases sympathetic nervous stimulation of brown adipose tissue thermogenesis, causing the animals to lose weight. This observation led to great interest in the possibility that a defect in the production of leptin may contribute to the production of leptin in obese humans. However, with the exception of a few, rare, cases of deficiencies of leptin production or defects in the hypothalamic leptin receptor, it is clear that obese humans have markedly elevated plasma leptin concentrations, which are in direct proportion to their level of body fatness.

Leptin release from adipose tissue provides a feedback signal to the hypothalamus on the state of the body's energy reserves. In animals such as rats and mice, this can lead to activation of the sympathetic nervous system, increasing resting energy expenditure, and also reduce energy intake. Whilst it is clear that in obese humans the high leptin concentrations are not very effective at affecting feeding behaviour, if leptin is administered to leptin deficient humans it does reduce food intake. Thus, the same feedback pathways linking adipose tissue, the hypothalamus and the sympathetic nervous system are also likely to operate in humans. This has led to interest in the possibility that increased plasma leptin levels in obese humans might lead to increased sympathetic activation, which may in turn contribute to the hypertension often seen in obesity. Esler's group have demonstrated a positive relationship between plasma leptin and renal sympathetic activity (Eikelis et al. 2003) that could contribute to the development of hypertension in the obese.

It has been suggested from a number of animal studies that leptin release from adipose tissue may be under inhibitory feedback control by the sympathetic innervation of the tissue. Such feedback control may also occur in humans, although there is no direct evidence to support this possibility. Plasma leptin concentration in humans is affected by short-term (over 2–3 days) changes in energy balance, with underfeeding lowering the levels and overfeeding increasing them. As such changes in energy balance also affect the sympathetic nervous system, it remains possible that a feedback control loop between the sympathetic nervous system and leptin release from adipose tissue does operate in man. However, this does not seem to be of clinical importance as a variety of conditions in which sympathetic activity is known to be altered (e.g. autonomic failure, essential hypertension) are not associated with abnormal levels of plasma leptin (Eikelis et al. 2003).

In obese humans, some investigators have shown reduced catecholamine-induced thermogenesis, and others have observed altered plasma catecholamine kinetics. However, there have been many conflicting reports, and it seems most probable that human obesity is not due to a single metabolic defect, but has varied aetiologies. However, there is no doubt that if an individual fails to respond to increased carbohydrate intake by activating thermogenesis (possibly through the sympathetic nervous system) then he or she will have a greater tendency to develop obesity than someone who does increase thermogenesis. This is illustrated by studies on Pima Indians and other groups with a high susceptibility to develop obesity, where altered metabolism and low sympathetic activity are risk factors for subsequent weight gain (Astrup and Macdonald 1998).

There have now been several studies of already obese patients that revealed minor impairments of autonomic function associated with obesity (Peterson et al. 1988). Most of these changes were in the parasympathetic nervous system (analogous to the early

stages of autonomic neuropathy in diabetes mellitus). There is also evidence of abnormal regulation of platelet α-adrenoceptors in obesity, although there is little disturbance of β-adrenoceptor sensitivity unless such patients are underfed (Berlin et al. 1990).

It has become clear over the past few years that undernutrition during fetal and early postnatal life increases the risks of developing obesity, cardiovascular disease and diabetes in adult life. A recent study by Weitz et al. (2003) showed that altered sympathetic nervous system activity may contribute to the development of obesity in people of low birth weight. Young adult subjects with a low birth weight had a lower resting sympathetic nervous system activity than matched subjects with a normal birth weight. This raises the possibility that nutritional disturbances in early life may have a long-term influence on the sympathetic nervous system and affect the control of metabolism.

Sympathoadrenal dysfunction

The main consequences of sympathoadrenal dysfunction are considered in other sections of this book, but it is worth noting here that patients with autonomic failure are frequently insulin resistant and can have impaired glucose tolerance. However, this is likely to result mainly from their low levels of physical activity, and possibly reduced carbohydrate intake, rather than from defects in the autonomic nervous system. The other two clinical situations in which one might expect altered control of metabolism are in adrenal insufficiency (either Addison's disease or post-adrenalectomy) or in diabetic autonomic neuropathy.

Addison's disease is characterized by adrenocortical degeneration and loss of corticosteroids, but the adrenal medulla is usually preserved. However, the enzyme phenylethanolamine-N-methyltransferase (PNMT), involved in the conversion of noradrenaline to adrenaline, is only produced in the presence of cortisol. Thus, in untreated Addison's disease there would be a deficiency of adrenaline that would contribute to the problems of hypoglycaemia and intolerance of other stresses that characterize this condition. Once the patients are given glucocorticoid replacement therapy there should be normal production of adrenaline, provided the adrenal medulla is preserved.

There is little evidence of impaired thermoregulation or other aspects of metabolism in adrenalectomized patients, although there have been few studies of such patients using the more sensitive methods now available. The fact that adrenalectomy does not produce serious metabolic disturbances (provided that corticosteroid replacement therapy is adequate) is not too surprising as the sympathetic innervation of blood vessels (to regulate heat loss in thermoregulation) and of the metabolically active tissues and endocrine glands, are probably more important than the effects of circulating adrenaline. The major exception is the prevention of hypoglycaemia during exercise, starvation, or in the presence of excess insulin. The primary factor acting to raise blood glucose under these conditions is glucagon, with adrenaline providing a secondary role. Obviously, the absence of a glucagon response in an adrenalectomized patient would then lead to serious problems in the defence of blood glucose concentration. Such an occurrence is likely to be rare, as (apart from the failure to release glucagon in IDDM as mentioned above) the only circumstances likely to affect glucagon release are the infusion of somatostatin or its analogues, and of course, pancreatectomy.

The problems of impaired responses to hypoglycaemia in diabetic autonomic neuropathy were considered above. However, diabetic autonomic neuropathy has other implications for metabolism, as these patients have impaired thermoregulatory responses to cold exposure. Such patients have less vasoconstriction in the feet and legs when exposed to the cold, and are more likely to shiver than diabetic patients without such complications. Furthermore, the rate of resting energy expenditure under thermoneutral conditions of the neuropathic patients who shivered was higher than in non-neuropathic patients who did not shiver when cooled (Scott et al. 1988b). This indicates that inadequate control of the peripheral circulation through impaired sympathetic function is likely to lead to increased heat loss, which requires an elevated resting metabolic rate to maintain thermal balance.

Conclusion

The parasympathetic nervous system has a minor role in the regulation of metabolism, via effects on insulin release. Impaired parasympathetic activity is seen in obesity, but the effects are not as marked as in diabetes. By contrast, the sympathoadrenal system is an important regulator of metabolism, and an essential feature of homeostasis is the activation of the sympathoadrenal system when tissue fuel supplies are compromised (e.g. the adrenaline response to hypoglycaemia). However, there does appear to be a more fundamental link between nutritional status and the sympathetic nervous system which may have important implications for the development/maintenance of obesity and may also contribute to the increased cardiovascular disease seen in obese individuals.

References

Acheson, K. J. (1988). Nutrient induced thermogenesis. In *Clinical progress in nutrition research*, (ed. A. Sitges-Serra, A. Sitges-Creus, and S. Schwartz-Riera), pp. 255–64. Karger, Basel.

Arch, J. R. S., Ainsworth, A. T., and Cawthorne, M. A. (1984). Atypical β-adrenoceptor on brown adipocytes as target for antiobesity drugs. *Nature* 309, 163–5.

Astrup, A., Christensen, N. J., Simonsen, L., and Bulow, J. (1990). Effects of nutrient intake on sympathoadrenal activity and thermogenic mechanisms. *J. Neurosci. Methods* 34, 187–92.

Astrup, A. and Macdonald, I. A. (1998). Sympathoadrenal system and metabolism. In *Handbook of obesity*, (ed. G. A. Bray, C. Bouchard, and W. P. T. James), pp. 491–511. Marcel Dekker, New York.

Bennett, T., Macdonald, I. A., and Sainsbury, R. (1984). The influence of starvation on the cardiovascular responses to lower body subatmospheric pressure or to standing in man. *Clin. Sci.* 66, 141–6.

Berlin, I., Berlan, M., Crespo-Laumonier, B. *et al.* (1990). Alterations in β-adrenergic sensitivity and platelet α₂-adrenoceptors in obese women: effect of exercise and calorie restriction. *Clin. Sci.* 78, 81–7.

Berne, C., Fagius, J., and Niklasson, F. (1989). Sympathetic response to oral carbohydrate administration. Evidence from micro-electrode recordings. *J. Clin. Invest.* 84, 1043–9.

Boyle, P. J., Shah, S. D., and Cryer, P. E. (1989). Insulin, glucagon and catecholamines in prevention of hypoglycemia during fasting. *Am. J. Physiol.* 256, E651–61.

Eikelis, N., Schlaich, M., Aggarwal, A., Kaye, D. and Esler, M. (2003). Interactions between leptin and the human sympathetic nervous system. *Hypertension,* 41, 1072–79.

Esler, M. Jennings, G., Meredith, I., Horne, M., and Eisenhofer, G. (1990). Overflow of catecholamine neurotransmitter to the circulation: source, fate and function. *Physiol. Rev.,* 70, 963–85.

Frayn, K. N. and Macdonald I. A. (1996). Adipose tissue circulation. In *Nervous control of blood vessels*, (ed. T. Bennett and S. M. Gardiner), pp. 505–39. Hardwood Academic Publishers, UK.

Fredholm, B. B. (1985). Nervous control of circulation and metabolism in white adipose tissue. In *New perspectives in adipose tissue: structure, function and development*, (ed. A. Cryer and R. L. R. Van), pp. 45–64. Butterworths, London.

Heller, S. R. and Macdonald, I. A. (1991). Physiological disturbances in hypoglycaemia: effect on subjective awareness. *Clin. Sci.* 81, 1–9.

Henry, S., Trueb, L., Sartori, C., Scherrer, U., Jequier, E. and Tappy, L. (1998) Effects of sympathetic activation by a lower body negative pressure on glucose and lipid metabolism. *Clinical Physiology,* 18, 562–69.

Hjemdahl, P. and Linde, B. (1983). Influence of circulating NE and Epi on adipose tissue vascular resistance and lipolysis in humans. *Am. J. Physiol.* 245, H447–52.

Horowitz, J.F., Coppack, S.W., Paramore, D., Cryer, P.E., Zhao, G. and Klein, S. (1999). Effect of short-term fasting on lipid kinetics in lean and obese women. *Am J Physiol,* 276, E278–84.

Jessen, K., Rabol, A., and Winkles, K. (1990). Total body and splanchnic thermogenesis in curarized man during a short exposure to cold. *Acta Anaesth. Scand.* 24, 339–44.

Kearney, M. T., Cowley, A. J., Evans, A., Stubbs, T. A., and Macdonald, I. A. (1998). Insulin's depressor action on skeletal muscle vasculative: a novel mechanism for postprandial hypotension in the elderly. *J. Am. Coll. Cardiol.* 31, 209–16.

Kjaer, M., Engfred, K., Fernandes, A., Secher, N. H., and Galbo, H. (1993). Regulation of hepatic glucose production during exercise in humans: role of sympathoadrenergic activity. *Am. J. Physiol.* 265, E275–83.

Kjaer, M., Keiding, S., Engfred, K. *et al.* (1995). Glucose homeostasis during exercise in humans with a liver or kidney transplant. *Am. J. Physiol.* 268, E636–44.

Kreier, F., Fliers, E., Voshol, P.J., Havekes, L.M., Kalsbeek, A., van Heijningen, C.L., Mettenleiter, T.C., Romijn, J.A., Sauerwein, H.P. and Buijs, R.M. (2002). Selective parasympathetic innervation of subcutaneous and intra-abdominal fat—functional implications. *J. Clin. Invest.* 110, 1235–37.

Landsberg, L. and Young, J. B. (1985). The influence of diet on the sympathetic nervous system. In *Neuroendocrine perspectives*, (ed. E. E. Muller, R. M. McLeod and L. A. Frohman), pp. 191–218. Elsevier, Amsterdam.

Lautt, W. W. (1980). Hepatic nerves. A review of their functions and effects. *Can. J. Physiol. Pharmacol.* 58, 105–23.

Macdonald, I. A., Bennett, T., and Fellows, I. W. (1985). Catecholamines and the control of metabolism in man. *Clin. Sci.* 68, 613–19.

Macdonald, I. A., Bennett, T., and Sainsbury, R. (1984). The effect of a 48 h fast on the thermoregulatory responses to graded cooling in man. *Clin. Sci.* 67, 445–52.

Navegantes, L.C., Sjostrand, M., Gudbjornsdottir, S., Strindberg, L., Elam, M. and Lonnroth, P. (2003). Regulation and counterregulation of lipolysis in vivo: different roles of sympathetic activation and insulin. *J. Clin. Endocrinol. Metab* 88, 5515–20.

Nonogaki, K. (2000). New insights into sympathetic regulation of glucose and fat metabolism. *Diabetologia.* 43, 533–49.

Peterson, H. R., Rothschild, M., Winberg, C. R., Fell, R. D., McLeish, K. R., and Pfeiffer, M. A. (1988). Body fat and the activity of the autonomic nervous system. *New Engl. J. Med.* 318, 1077–83.

Robinson, A. M., Parkin, H. M., Macdonald, I. A., and Tattersall, R. B. (1995). Antecedent hypoglycaemia in non-diabetic subjects reduces the adrenaline response for 6 days but does not affect the catecholamine response to other stimuli. *Clin. Sci.* 89, 359–66.

Rothwell, N. J. and Stock, M. J. (1981). Regulation of energy balance. *Ann. Rev. Nutr.* 1, 235–56.

Samra, J. S., Clark, M. L., Humphreys, S. M., Macdonald, I. A., Matthews, D. R., and Frayn, K. N. (1996). Effects of morning rise in cortisol concentration on regulation of lipolysis in subcutaneous adipose tissue. *Am. J. Physiol.* **271**, E996–E1002.

Sandoval, D.A., Guy, D.L., Richardson, M.A., Ertl, A.C. and Davis, S.N. Effects of low and moderate antecedent exercise on counterregulatory responses to subsequent hypoglycemia in type 1 diabetes. *Diabetes*, **53**, 1798–1806.

Schwartz, R. W., Jaeger, L. F., and Veith, R. C. (1988). Effect of clonidine on the thermic effect of feeding in humans. *Am. J. Physiol.* **254**, R90–94.

Scott, A. R., Bennett, T., and Macdonald, I. A. (1988*a*). Effects of hyperinsulinaemia on the cardiovascular responses to graded hypovolaemia in normal and diabetic subjects. *Clin. Sci.* **75**, 85–92.

Scott, A. R., Macdonald, I. A., Bennett, T., and Tattersall, R. B. (1988*b*). Abnormal thermoregulation in diabetic autonomic neuropathy. *Diabetes* **37**, 961–8.

Seals, D.R. amd Bell, C. Chronic sympathetic activation: consequence and cause of age-associated obesity? *Diabetes*, **53**, 276–84.

Snitker, S., Macdonald, I., Ravussin, E. and Astrup, A. The sympathetic nervous system and obesity: role in aetiology and treatment. *Obesity Reviews*, **1**, 5–15.

Webber, J. and Macdonald, I. A. (1993). Metabolic actions of catecholamines in man. *Baillière's Clin. Endocrinol. Metab.* **7**, 393–413.

Weitz, G., Deckert, P., Heindl, S., Struck, J., Perras, B. and Dodt, C. (2003). Evidence for lower sympathetic nerve activity in young adults with low birth weight. *J Hypertens.* **21**, 943–50.

Young, J. B. and Landsberg, L. (1977). Catecholamines and intermediary metabolism. *Clin. Endocrinol. Metab.* **6**, 599–631.

CHAPTER 19

The kidney and the sympathetic nervous system

Edward J. Johns

Introduction

Cardiovascular homeostasis requires a balance to exist between the volume of blood in the vascular system, the ability of the heart to pump effectively and the functioning of the kidney to ensure that the degree of fluid reabsorption and loss in the urine is appropriate. This cardiovascular–renal axis is fundamental to homeostasis and should one component be defective, then cardiovascular disease becomes evident. The primary role of the kidney is to ensure that extracellular fluid volume is maintained at a level that is required for cardiovascular homeostasis. A secondary underlying dynamic regulatory mechanism is renal renin release and the production of angiotensin II, which also determines vascular tone as well as the secretion of aldosterone. Regulation of these functions are achieved to a large degree by the autonomic nervous system and the renal innervation, which enables the kidney to efficiently and effectively retain or excrete fluid as well as secrete renin in the face of a varying intake and loss of sodium and water as occurs during normal everyday activities.

Almost a quarter of cardiac output passes though the two kidneys and of this 20% is filtered, representing a volume of some 180 litres per day. As the fluid passes along the nephron, some 98–99% is absorbed, while there is secretion of various metabolites into the tubule to enable their elimination from the body. The processing of the fluid varies greatly along the different nephron segments. At the proximal tubule some 67% of the sodium and water is reabsorbed isosmotically across the high permeability epithelial. The loop of Henle dips deeply into the medulla and papilla, but the ascending limb is impermeable to water yet sodium is reabsorbed via the sodium/potassium/two chloride transporter, which is the fundamental mechanism allowing generation of the medullary concentration gradients, and at this stage a further 25% of the fluid is reabsorbed. The distal tubule and collecting duct are low permeability epithelia and are relatively impermeable but can be made selectively permeable to water, under the influence of anti-diuretic hormone, while aldosterone acts on the principal cells to stimulate sodium reabsorption and together this amounts to some 8% of the filtered load (Boron and Boulepaep 2003). The hormonal control of fluid balance is a relatively slow regulation, but the renal sympathetic nerves exert a more rapid and dynamic control of fluid output.

Renal sympathetic nerves

The kidney has a very dense innervation comprising postganglionic sympathetic fibres that arise from spinal segments ranging from T11 to L3. Sympathetic preganglionic fibres arise from the rostral ventrolateral medulla, paraventricular nucleus, to a lesser degree from the raphe nuclei and A5 region, and project to the intermediolateral areas of the spinal cord. These fibres then track from the spinal segments to the prevertebral, aortico-renal and splanchnic ganglia, to the paravertebral coeliac and mesenteric ganglia, and it is from these ganglia that the postganglionic fibres arise and traverse along the renal artery and vein to enter the kidney at the hilus (Fig. 19.1).

On entering the kidney, the nerves divide into smaller bundles and generally course alongside the blood vessels as they branch into interlobar, arcuate, interlobular, and then afferent and efferent arterioles. At this level, they divide further and pass into close proximity to the different tubular elements of the nephron.

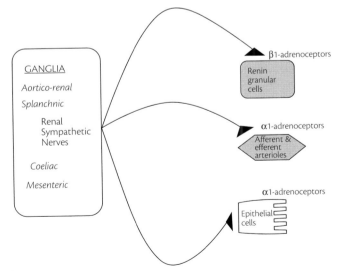

Fig. 19.1

Generally, the primary innervation lies within the cortex and outer medulla with much less being present at the inner medulla and virtually none in the papilla. The nerves are typical of sympathetic fibres, having varicosities on their axons as they trail through the tissue. The density of the neuroeffector junctions vary along both the vasculature and nephrons, being greatest at the afferent and efferent arterioles, with fewer being present on the remainder of the vasculature. Along the nephron, the highest density is found at the ascending thick ascending limb of the loop of Henle and is lower along the distal and proximal tubules (Barajas et al. 1992, Barajas et al. 1984).

Physiology of the renal nerves

Noradrenaline is contained within dense cored vesicles present in the varicosities of the sympathetic fibre. As an action potential passes along the fibre, it is depolarized and exocytosis releases the transmitter into the neuroeffector junction where it diffuses to the postsynaptic adrenoceptors present on the plasma membrane of the target cells.

Renal vasculature

The frequency of action potentials travelling along the nerve fibre recruits different functionalities. From the early reports, it became evident that high rates of electrical stimulation of the renal nerves caused marked reductions in renal blood flow and glomerular filtration rate. This was due to their vasoconstrictor action at the major resistance vessels, the afferent and efferent arterioles and, to a lesser degree, at the interlobular arteries (Coote et al. 1972). It is important to emphasize that there can be a degree of activation of the renal sympathetic nerves, which can cause modest decreases in renal blood flow of up to some 20%, without changing glomerular filtration rate (Johns et al. 1976, Handa and Johns 1985). This is due to a differential impact of the renal sympathetic nerves at the afferent and efferent arterioles whereby tone increases to a relatively greater extent at the efferent arteriole with the result that glomerular filtration pressure remains unchanged.

More recently attention has focussed on potential differences in the neural control of blood flow through the cortical and medullary regions of the kidney. Direct electrical stimulation of the renal sympathetic nerves can cause frequency related reductions in blood flow through the cortex to a large degree paralleling total renal blood flow, but, by contrast, the medulla appears much less influenced by changes in renal sympathetic nerve activity (Eppel et al. 2004, Walkowska et al. 2005). The reasons for this insensitivity of the medulla to neural control are unclear, but may be dependent on the relative lack of innervation or the interplay of complex autocrine/paracrine factors, such as angiotensin II, arachidonic acid metabolites, nitric oxide and superoxide anions acting to offset the vasoconstrictor actions of the renal nerves (Evans et al. 2004, La Grange et al. 1973).

Tubular actions

Early studies in the dog by LaGrange and co-workers (La Grange et al. 1973, Bello-Reuss et al. 1975) demonstrated that there was a low level of electrical stimulation of the renal sympathetic nerves at which there was no change in renal blood flow or glomerular filtration but a marked 30–40% reduction in urinary sodium excretion. The later reports of Gottschalk and co-workers (Bello-Reuss et al. 1975), using micropuncture approaches, clearly demonstrated that

the nerves acted primarily on proximal tubular fluid reabsorption; thus proximal tubular fluid decreased when the renal nerves were sectioned, but was increased when the renal sympathetic nerves were stimulated at low levels which did not change renal haemodynamics. Further, it was reported (DiBona and Sawin 1982) that electrical renal sympathetic nerve stimulation could also increase sodium, but not water, reabsorption at the thick limb of the ascending loop of Henle.

Sodium reabsorption across the proximal tubular epithelial cells is dependent upon the two main transporters, the sodium/potassium/ATPase at the basolateral membrane, and the apical sodium/hydrogen exchanger (NHE). This latter exchanger is present in a number of isoforms but it is isoform 3, NHE3, which is recognized as the entity that can be subjected to regulation by adrenergic stimuli (Liu and Gesek 2001, Liu et al. 1997). It would appear that the NHE3 protein is incorporated into the plasma membrane where it is active but is also present in sub-endosomal layers where the transporter is likely to be an inactive state (McDonough et al. 2003). The mechanisms regulating the amount of the sub-endosomal versus membrane incorporated NHE3 are not clearly defined but reflex activation of the renal sympathetic nerves, accompanied by a rise in blood pressure, has been demonstrated to increase NHE3 in the apical membrane (Ye et al. 2002).

Renin release

Renin is contained in granular cells which are phenotypically smooth muscle cells but have become modified to generate renin. These granular cells are typically found along that part of the afferent arteriole just before it enters the glomerulus. The number of granular cells within the afferent arteriole changes in response to physiological demands, for example the number increases when subjected to a low dietary sodium intake or a reduced blood pressure. Because the granular cells are interdigitated with the afferent arteriolar smooth muscle cells, they will also have neuroeffector junctions with the renal sympathetic nerves. Initial studies demonstrated that there was a rapid large release of renin into the circulation when the renal sympathetic nerves were electrically activated (Coote et al. 1972). Frequently, these investigations were compromised by the difficulty that the level of renal nerve stimulation also caused concomitant reductions in renal blood flow and it was not clear whether the neurally mediated stimulation of renin secretion was due to a direct action of the nerves at the renin-containing granular cells or indirectly via changes in renal blood flow. The situation was clarified by Kopp and co-workers (Kopp et al. 1980) who demonstrated in the dog, that low level renal nerve stimulation could increase renin secretion in the absence of changes in renal haemodynamics. These observations, together with those of others (Osborn et al. 1981), gave credence to the concept that the renal nerves could directly cause renin secretion, which was independent of neural changes in renal blood flow or glomerular filtration rate.

Summary

The body of evidence arising from the studies investigating the renal functional responses when the renal sympathetic nerves are electrically stimulated give rise to a number of important points.

◆ At the lowest levels of renal nerve activation there are no changes in fluid output and renal haemodynamics, but there is a direct nerve-mediated increase in renin secretion.

- At higher rates of renal nerve stimulation there will be a greater increase in renin secretion rate but this is then associated with a decrease in fluid output, representing an increase in tubular sodium and water reabsorption, but again occurring in the absence of changes in either renal blood flow or glomerular filtration rate. In this range, the increase in fluid reabsorption reflects a direct action of the neurotransmitter on the tubular epithelial cells of the proximal tubule and thick limb of the ascending loop of Henle.

- At a relatively high rate of renal sympathetic nerve stimulation, there will be a renal nerve induced constriction of afferent and efferent arterioles which will decrease renal haemodynamics in a frequency related manner, initially as a fall in renal blood flow and then, at higher levels, as reductions in both renal blood flow and glomerular filtration rate.

Together these studies demonstrate that there is a progressive and cumulative recruitment of functionalities as the level of renal sympathetic nerve activity increases (Fig. 19.1). The important concept highlighted by these observations is that there is a degree of sympathetic outflow to the kidney that can have a major impact on renin secretion and fluid reabsorption and, over the longer term, plasma angiotensin II and extracellular fluid volume can significantly determine the level at which blood pressure is set. It is likely that in normal everyday activity, standing, lying, digesting and drinking, it is this low level of renal sympathetic activity that is important in ensuring fluid homeostasis is maintained. By contrast, the high levels of renal sympathetic nerve activation required to reduce renal blood flow and glomerular filtration rate will only come into play when more urgent and demanding regulation by the sympathetic nervous system is required, for example, when cardiac output has to be redirected as occurs during exercise and in 'fight and flight' scenarios. However, it is important to point out that this level of sympathoexcitation is generally short lived and unlikely to have a long-lasting influence on cardiovascular homeostasis.

Pharmacology of the renal nerves

Recent molecular biological and cloning studies have revealed that adrenoceptors can be expressed as different subtypes of α_1-adrenoceptors (α_{1A}, α_{1B} and α_{1D}), of α_2-adrenoceptors (α_{2A}, α_{2B} and α_{2C}) and β-adrenoceptors (β_1, β_2- and β_3) and that they all couple to G-proteins that initiate signalling cascades necessary to elicit the cellular response to the catecholamines (Summers et al. 2004). A variety of these subtypes of adrenoceptors exist within the kidney and each mediates adrenergic control of a particular functionality.

Initial studies demonstrated that renal nerve induced reductions in renal blood flow were blocked by α-adrenoceptor antagonists such as phentolamine and prazosin (Johns 1991), indicating that at the renal vasculature α_1-adrenoceptors were involved, which in later studies were shown to be primarily of the α_{1A}-adrenoceptor subtype (Sattar and Johns 1994). Investigations into the neural regulation of fluid reabsorption found that the antinatriuresis caused by low level renal nerve stimulation could be blocked by prazosin but not yohimbine, compatible with α_1-adrenoceptors present at the epithelial cells (Johns and Manitius 1986) and later reports (Sattar and Johns 1994) provided evidence indicating that α_{1A}-adrenoceptors were the primary receptor subtype involved. Investigations into the renal nerve-induced increase in renin secretion found it to be blocked by β-adrenoceptor antagonists such as

propranolol (Kopp et al. 1980). Thereafter, attention was focused on determining which subtype was involved and reports in the dog (Osborn et al. 1981) and cat (Johns 1981) demonstrated that neurally induced renin release could be prevented following the administration of selective β_1-adrenoceptor but not β_2-adrenoceptor antagonists indicating that β_1-adrenoceptors were the functionally important subtype.

Thus, the renal sympathetic nerves exert their control over different aspects of kidney function by activating different adrenoceptor subtypes (Fig. 19.1). This means that in disease states in which autonomic outflow may be elevated, administration of different adrenergic blocking drugs may have different effects on kidney function. For example, while administration of β-blockers to hypertensive patients will prevent neurally induced renin release, and thereby remove one important contributor to the chronically elevated blood pressure, the neural drive to retain sodium, via an action of the nerves at the tubular epithelial cells, will remain unchecked. On the other hand, administration of α-adrenergic blockers, such as prazosin, may prevent renal nerve mediated sodium retention, but neurally induced renin secretion will not be affected and, indeed, may be enhanced.

Reflex neural regulation of the kidney

Examination of a multifibre recording of renal sympathetic nerve activity reveals a complex electrical signal that is characterized by a bursting pattern the magnitude of which may be influenced by the alertness of the individual, it has a cardiac entrainment and also demonstrates a respiratory rhythm. The actual level of activity within the renal sympathetic nerves is determined by the central integration of sensory information arising from different areas of the body and this will change over time dependent upon normal everyday demands and behavioural states, such as feeding, exercise or sleeping. A number of sensory systems contribute afferent information into the central nervous system and their importance and significance may undergo major changes in pathophysiological states (Fig. 19.2).

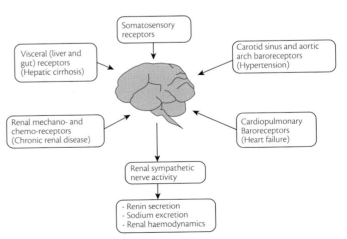

Fig. 19.2

Cardiovascular baroreceptor

Carotid sinus and aortic arch baroreceptors

It is now generally recognized that sensory mechanoreceptors within the carotid sinuses and aortic arch are depolarized as the vessel walls are stretched as a consequence of increased blood pressure, and result in a reflex decrease in sympathetic outflow, including that to the kidney. The receptors transmit information related to blood pressure in two ways; firstly, as an increase or decrease in mean pressure; and secondly, on a beat by beat basis, that is, varying over the cardiac cycle. Thus, within the renal sympathetic nerve signal, there is a bursting activity entrained with heart rate, increasing during diastole and decreasing during systole, although this latter pattern is more evident in anaesthetized preparations (Zhang and Johns 1997, Huang et al. 2006). However, if the integrated signal from the multifibre recording is measured, as blood pressure is increased or lowered by the acute administration of vasoactive drugs, then there is a reciprocal decrease or increase in renal sympathetic nerve activity which allows a baroreceptor gain curve to be produced (Huang et al. 2006). The slope, or sensitivity, of this relationship can be raised or lowered by other sensory inputs to the central nervous system and it would seem that this baroreceptor regulation of renal sympathetic nerve activity is one of the most important (Johns 2005, Johns 2002).

There are a number of functional consequences to the baroreceptor regulation of renal sympathetic nerve activity. Early reports in the dog demonstrated that reduction in carotid sinus pressure, induced either mechanically or as a consequence to head-up tilt, increased renal sympathetic nerve activity, raised renin secretion rate and resulted in a renal nerve-dependent antinatriuresis and antidiuresis with no measurable alteration in renal haemodynamics (DiBona and Kopp 1997, Johns, 2005, Johns, 2002). The significance of these observations is that in response to normal physiological activity of the individual, the baroreflex control of blood pressure will impinge on kidney function, but primarily in relation to the secretion of renin and the regulation of fluid balance rather than regulation of renal vascular resistance and renal haemodynamics. Valuable insight into the way the baroreceptor control of renal sympathetic outflow has been revealed by studies in the conscious rat by (Miki and Yoshimoto 2005) who reported that baroreflex gain control moved to a higher pressure with greater sensitivity during raised physical activity such as grooming, but was decreased with less sensitivity during the sleep state.

Low pressure baroreceptors

Mechanoreceptors are also present in the walls of the vessels in the cardiopulmonary areas of the circulation. These sites, which comprise the atria and the great veins (superior and inferior venae cavae, and pulmonary vein) are low pressure areas and the degree of stretch in the vessel walls is determined by the volume or blood contained within them rather than pressure per se. There is a body of information demonstrating that mechanical balloon inflation of the left atria causes a reflex inhibition of renal sympathetic nerve activity and a renal nerve-dependent increase in sodium and water excretion (DiBona & Kopp 1997). Moreover, earlier reports (Miki et al. 1989, Miki et al. 2002) demonstrated in conscious dogs that the renal sympathoinhibition and natriuretic responses to a period of head-out total body water immersion (to shift fluid to central compartments) was prevented following chronic cardiac denervation. Further supportive evidence for this reflex has been obtained in both the conscious and anaesthetized rat preparations (DiBona & Kopp 1997) where an acute saline volume load resulted in a marked reduction in renal sympathetic nerve activity.

Somatosensory receptors

The somatosensory system is richly endowed with both mechanoreceptors, residing in the muscle tendons and joints, chemoreceptors within skeletal muscle tissue (metaboreceptors) while in the skin there are nociceptors and thermoreceptors. Electrical stimulation of the sciatic nerve, containing all these sensory nerve fibres, in the anaesthetized dog (Thames and Abboud 1979) was found to reduce total renal blood flow which was dependent on an intact renal innervation. Those initial studies were extended in the anaesthetized rat, using electrical stimulation of the brachial nerves, application of noxious substances, either subcutaneously or via inhalation to stimulate somatosensory receptors (Davis and Johns 1991, Huang and Johns 1998, Zhang and Johns 1997). These experimental manoeuvres were found to cause modest rises in blood pressure, transient increases in renal sympathetic nerve activity and a renal nerve-dependent antinatriuresis and antidiuresis, but in the absence of any meaningful change in renal haemodynamics (Johns 2005, Johns 2002). In a more selective fashion (DiBona 2000) demonstrated that a thermal challenge to the tail of the anaesthetized rat resulted in a marked sympathoexcitation in some, but not all, single renal sympathetic nerve fibres.

Visceral receptors

There are chemoreceptors and mechanoreceptors contained within different visceral organs that have a significant input into the central nervous system and can contribute to autonomic control. The gut would appear to be an important site of sensory information as studies using the anaesthetized rat (Weaver et al. 1987) found that exposure of the small intestine to externally applied bradykinin to depolarize sensory nerve endings led to an increase in blood pressure and a concomitant rise in renal sympathetic nerve activity associated with a renal nerve-dependent antinatriuresis and antidiuresis.

The situation with regard to the liver is more complex but there is a growing awareness that chemoreceptors and mechanoreceptors are present within this region that provide important afferent information. Hevener and colleagues (2000) have demonstrated that a lowered plasma glucose in the hepatic portal vein, but not hepatic artery, leads to a marked secretion of adrenaline, which was blocked following deafferentation of the hepatic portal vein. These observations indicate a sympathoactivation of the adrenal which may include the renal sympathetic nerves. By contrast Ishiki et al. (1991) and Morita et al. (1991) demonstrated that perfusion of a hypertonic saline solution into the hepatic portal vein caused a reduction in renal sympathetic nerve activity and associated diuretic and natriuretic responses. These findings would form the basis of a reflex where an intake of sodium in the diet when absorbed by the gut, would initially traverse the hepatic portal vein where an increase in osmolarity would be detected leading to a reflex decrease in renal sympathetic nerve activity and a homeostatic loss of sodium from the kidney.

Interestingly, there have been a series of reports suggesting that there are pressure (mechano-) receptors present in the splenic circulation that can influence autonomic control. In the anaesthetized rat, when splenic venous pressure was increased, splenic afferent nerve activity rose while blood pressure and renal blood flow decreased (Hamza and Kaufman 2004, Moncrief and Kaufman 2006). This group went on to show that the reduced renal blood flow was a renal nerve-dependent event as it was blunted by prior renal denervation. Moreover, they found that this splenorenal reflex was mediated by increases in pressure within, but not blood flow through, the splenic vein. Clearly, venous pressure within the spleen area will cause a reflex increase in renal sympathetic nerve activity and this could well contribute to the increase in the neural control of the kidney in portal hypertension and liver disease.

Renal receptors

Sensory nerves have been described within the kidney itself and these comprise the afferent limb of the renorenal reflex. They are found in greatest density in the pelvic wall where they probably act as mechanoreceptors, transducing stretch caused by either pressure within the renal interstitium or renal hilus, or chemoreceptors sensing the urinary composition in the pelvis. The afferent nerve fibres project to their cell bodies located in the ipsilateral dorsal root ganglia, from T6 to L4 and thereafter to the ipsilateral dorsal horn of the spinal cord.

On raising pelvic hydrostatic pressure, from approximately 3 mmHg to 20 mmHg, renal afferent nerve activity increased roughly in proportion to the change in pressure and is considered a response of the mechanoreceptors. The chemoreceptors appear more diverse as they can be activated by renal ischaemia, but other chemoreceptors can be activated by pelvic perfusions of hypertonic sodium chloride solutions. The mechanoreceptor and chemoreceptor challenges used experimentally fall within the physiological range of pressures and concentrations normally found within the pelvis (DiBona and Kopp 1997).

Acute surgical denervation of one kidney in the anaesthetized rat results in a denervation diuresis and natriuresis in that kidney, but at the contralateral kidney, there is an increase in efferent renal sympathetic nerve traffic and an antidiuresis and antinatriuresis. Conversely, stimulation of mechanoreceptors by increasing pelvic pressure in the ipsilateral kidney, results in a renal sympathetic nerve-dependent diuresis and natriuresis at the contralateral kidney. Taken at a simplified level, this means that the renorenal reflex functions to ensure that should there be excessive loss of fluid from one kidney, there is a prompt neurally mediated compensatory excretory response in the contralateral kidney. Interestingly in the dog, and to some extent the cat, the reflex functions in a somewhat different way in that increasing renal pelvic pressure increases the ipsilateral efferent nerve activity which causes a reflex sympathoexcitation in the contralateral kidney and renal nerve-mediated reductions in renal blood flow and sodium excretion. The meaning of the inhibitory renorenal reflex in the rat as against the excitatory renorenal reflex in the dog is unclear (DiBona and Kopp 1997)

The transduction mechanism at the sensory nerve terminals leading to a depolarization has now been defined in some detail. The increase in renal pelvic pressure results in bradykinin production which activates protein kinase C (PKC) to stimulate cyclooxygenase-2 (COX-2) to generate prostaglandin E2 (PGE2). This signalling cascade stimulates adenylyl cyclase to generate cyclic adenosine monophosphate (cAMP), which, via protein kinase A (PKA), generates substance P and initiates depolarization of the sensory nerve terminal. The effectiveness of the pathway has been found to be modulated by angiotensin II (Kopp et al. 2006).

Pathophysiological states

There is a growing realization that in many pathophysiological states where there are derangements of the cardiovascular system, there is an inappropriate response in the autonomic nervous system. In many instances a deranged sympathetic drive is caused by the disease process eliciting aberrant sensory signals from the tissue itself, which then becomes the initiator of the pathophysiological state (Fig. 19.2).

Hypertension

Many early investigations were directed towards determining whether the renal sympathetic nerves had a potential role in the genesis and maintenance of hypertension. To this end, animal models of hypertension were used, for example, the spontaneously hypertensive rat (SHR) as a model of genetic or essential hypertension, the Goldblatt (2K1C, IKIC) hypertensive rat model of renovascular hypertension and the DOCA-salt (deoxycorticosterone acetate) representing a volume expansion model of hypertension. The initial studies demonstrated that in the SHR, renal denervation at the pre-hypertensive stage either prevented or markedly reduced the rate at which blood pressure rose into the hypertensive phase. Interestingly, a similar effect of renal denervation was reported in both the Goldblatt and DOCA-salt hypertensive rate models (DiBona and Kopp 1997). Moreover, definitive studies using single renal sympathetic nerve fibre recordings found the rate of action potential firing was approximately doubled in the SHR compared with the normotensive control rats (Lundin et al. 1984).

The question arises as to whether a similar renal sympathoexcitation occurs in essential hypertension which comprises the largest proportion of hypertensive patients. One option has been to undertake recordings from peripheral sympathetic nerves by inserting recording electrodes into the peroneal nerve and this has provided convincing evidence that in the younger essential hypertensive patients, the bursting pattern of muscle sympathetic nerve activity is much higher than in normal subjects (Esler and Kaye 2000). An alternative approach has been to utilize the noradrenaline 'spillover' technique whereby sampling regional venous blood and comparing noradrenaline concentrations in arterial blood, neurotransmitter release from organs such as the kidney and heart can be measured. In studies using this technique, it is clear that there is a marked elevation in neurotransmitter release from the kidneys of hypertensive patients (Esler et al. 2003).

Together these studies support the view that hypertension, and certainly that arising from a genetic source, occurs with an elevated renal sympathetic nerve activity that would impact on kidney function. Indeed, under these conditions there would be an inappropriately raised renin secretion from the kidney together with fluid retention and these two factors would exacerbate the hypertensive state creating a spiral of increasing stress on the cardiovascular system.

Heart failure

Heart failure is a state where there is an inability of the heart to pump blood around the body sufficient to meet metabolic demands. It occurs when there is atherosclerosis causing narrowing or even blocking of the coronary arteries and impairing perfusion of parts of the myocardium thereby preventing the remainder from providing sufficient cardiac output. Congestive heart failure occurs most frequently following a period of hypertension with a chronically raised afterload on the heart, which eventually begins to fail. There are experimental studies in animal models of heart failure (Zucker et al. 2004) in which renal sympathetic nerve activity has been measured directly, and in human cardiac failure, using noradrenaline spillover (Esler et al. 2003), indicating that there is an activation of the sympathetic nervous system, primarily to drive the failing heart to ensure adequate output, but also inappropriately to the kidney causing it to retain fluid.

A further important point arising from these observations is that not only is basal renal sympathetic nerve activity elevated, but there is also a deficit in the reflex modulation of sympathetic outflow. Thus, the sensitivity the baroreflex gain curves for renal sympathetic nerve activity was depressed while the renal sympathoinhibition in response to an acute saline volume load was lost (Zucker et al. 2004) in the experimental models of heart failure. Interestingly, these deficits in autonomic regulation also become apparent in situations of cardiac hypertrophy, a state likely to precede the development of an overt compromise in cardiac output. Using two models of cardiac hypertrophy, induced with either thyroxine or treatment with a caffeine/isoprenaline mixture, there was a depressed regulation of sympathetic outflow to the kidney in response to activation of both the high and low pressure baroreceptors (Flanagan et al. 2008). All these observations point to the fact that the kidney is subjected to a raised sympathetic outflow in two ways—as an increased basal level of nerve traffic, and as a consequence of an inability to reflexly modulate nerve activity. Either way, the functional consequences are that the kidney would be unable to dynamically and rapidly respond to varying sodium and water intake as occurs in normal everyday activity, there would be inappropriate fluid retention, which would exacerbate the load on the heart and contribute to the progression of the disease.

Cirrhosis

Hepatic cirrhosis is associated with oedema, which is caused by increased fluid reabsorption by the kidney. As indicated above, sensory receptors are present in the liver and spleen which, when activated, can elicit a renal sympathoexcitation. The animal model most widely used is the rat in which the common bile duct is ligated and over several weeks a state of cirrhosis becomes apparent. There is a blunted ability to excrete a sodium load in this model but if the animals are subjected to a prior renal denervation, a greater proportion of the load is excreted. Moreover the renal sympathoinhibition that occurs in response to a saline load is markedly attenuated (DiBona and Kopp 1997). It would seem that in patients with cirrhosis there is a heightened neural control of kidney as administration of α-adrenoceptor antagonists, or bilateral lumbar spinal anaesthetic block results in diuretic and natriuretic responses, consistent with withdrawal of renal sympathetic tone. Taken together, these findings point to a raised sympathetic output in hepatic cirrhosis and the underlying causes are likely to be due to an inappropriate stimulation of afferent receptors within the hepatic and splenic areas of the body.

Renal failure

There is a strong association between hypertension and chronic renal disease and, in fact, renal diseases are the most common cause of secondary hypertension (Campese et al. 2006). The mechanisms underlying the origin of the hypertension is unclear, but there have been a number of experimental and clinical studies that have implicated the sympathetic nervous system. As indicated above, there are sensory receptors within the kidney which, when challenged with physiological stimuli, can increase or decrease sympathetic nerve activity as part of the renorenal reflex. There have been a number of reports using a rat model of renal injury, induced by injecting small amounts of phenol into the lower pole of the kidney (Ye et al. 2002), which have shown the manoeuvre to elicit an immediate and sustained increase in blood pressure, plasma noradrenaline and contralateral renal sympathetic nerve activity. The consensus is that this inappropriate and excessive stimulation of the sensory receptors within the kidney elicits raised sympathetic drive contributing to a state of hypertension. A key study by Hausberg et al. (2002) gave some insight into the situation in man. They observed that the rate of bursting activity in muscle sympathetic nerves was some three times higher in renal transplant patients who retained their diseased kidneys, compared with normal subjects. Moreover if during transplant surgery the diseased kidney was removed, the rate of bursting activity could not be distinguished from that in control subjects. What these findings reveal is that within the diseased kidney the tissue degeneration causes an excessive stimulation of the sensory nerves, which reflexly elevates sympathetic nervous activity, increases peripheral vascular resistance and ultimately blood pressure.

Summary

The renal sympathetic nerves exert an important regulatory influence over the secretory, excretory and haemodynamic functions of the kidney, all of which serve to ensure cardiovascular homeostasis. The autonomic nervous system receives sensory information from all body systems, cardiovascular, somatosensory and visceral, and integrates the information to ensure that sympathetic outflow to all organs, including the kidney, results in compensatory functional adjustments. Frequently in pathophysiological states, excessive sensory information can pass to the central nervous system, with the result that there can be inappropriate sympathetic outflow to the kidney with functional responses that exacerbate the disease process. This scenario can place the kidney at a key position in the therapeutic and management considerations of the disease process.

References

Barajas, L., Liu, L. & Powers, K. (1992).Anatomy of the renal innervation: intrarenal aspects and ganglia of origin. *Can J Physiol Pharmacol*, **70**, 735–49.

Barajas, L., Powers, K. & Wang, P. (1984). Innervation of the renal cortical tubules: a quantitative study. *Am J Physiol*, **247**, F50–60.

Bello-Reuss, E., Colindres, R. E., Pastoriza-Munoz, E., Mueller, R. A. & Gottschalk, C. W. (1975). Effects of acute unilateral renal denervation in the rat. *J Clin Invest*, **56**, 208–17.

Boron, W. F. & Boulepaep, E. L. (2003). *Medical Physiology: a cellular and molecular approach*, Philadelphia, Saunders.

Campese, V. M., Mitra, N. & Sandee, D. (2006). Hypertension in renal parenchymal disease: why is it so resistant to treatment? *Kidney Int*, **69**, 967–73.

Coote, J. H., Johns, E. J., Macleod, V. H. & Singer, B. (1972). Effect of renal nerve stimulation, renal blood flow and adrenergic blockade on plasma renin activity in the cat. *J Physiol*, **226**, 15–36.

Davis, G. & Johns, E. J. (1991). Effect of somatic nerve stimulation on the kidney in intact, vagotomized and carotid sinus-denervated rats. *J Physiol*, **432**, 573–84.

DiBona, G. F. (2000). Neural control of the kidney: functionally specific renal sympathetic nerve fibers. *Am J Physiol Regul Integr Comp Physiol*, **279**, R1517–24.

DiBona, G. F. & Kopp, U. C. (1997). Neural control of renal function. *Physiol Rev*, **77**, 75–197.

DiBona, G. F. & Sawin, L. L. (1982). Effect of renal nerve stimulation on NaCl and H2O transport in Henle's loop of the rat. *Am J Physiol*, **243**, F576–80.

Eppel, G. A., Malpas, S. C., Denton, K. M. & Evans, R. G. (2004). Neural control of renal medullary perfusion. *Clin Exp Pharmacol Physiol*, **31**, 387–96.

Esler, M. & Kaye, D. (2000). Sympathetic nervous system activation in essential hypertension, cardiac failure and psychosomatic heart disease. *J Cardiovasc Pharmacol*, **35**, S1–7.

Esler, M., Lambert, G., Brunner-La Rocca, H. P., Vaddadi, G. & Kaye, D. (2003). Sympathetic nerve activity and neurotransmitter release in humans: translation from pathophysiology into clinical practice. *Acta Physiol Scand*, **177**, 275–84.

Evans, R. G., Eppel, G. A., Anderson, W. P. & Denton, K. M. (2004). Mechanisms underlying the differential control of blood flow in the renal medulla and cortex. *J Hypertens*, **22**, 1439–51.

Flanagan, E. T., Buckley, M. M., Aherne, C. M., Lainis, F., Sattar, M. & Johns, E. J. (2008). Impact of cardiac hypertrophy on arterial and cardiopulmonary baroreflex control of renal sympathetic nerve activity in anaesthetized rats. *Exp Physiol*, **93**, 1058–64.

Hamza, S. M. & Kaufman, S. (2004). Splenorenal reflex modulates renal blood flow in the rat. *J Physiol*, **558**, 277–82.

Handa, R. K. & Johns, E. J. (1985). Interaction of the renin-angiotensin system and the renal nerves in the regulation of rat kidney function. *J Physiol*, **369**, 311–21.

Hausberg, M., Kosch, M., Harmelink, P., Barenbrock, M., Hohage, H., Kisters, K., Dietl, K. H. & Rahn, K. H. (2002). Sympathetic nerve activity in end-stage renal disease. *Circulation*, **106**, 1974–9.

Hevener, A. L., Bergman, R. N. & Donovan, C. M. (2000). Portal vein afferents are critical for the sympathoadrenal response to hypoglycemia. *Diabetes*, **49**, 8–12.

Huang, C. & Johns, E. J. (1998). Role of ANG II in mediating somatosensory-induced renal nerve-dependent antinatriuresis in the rat. *Am J Physiol*, **275**, R194–202.

Huang, C., Yoshimoto, M., Miki, K. & Johns, E. J. (2006). The contribution of brain angiotensin II to the baroreflex regulation of renal sympathetic nerve activity in conscious normotensive and hypertensive rats. *J Physiol*, **574**, 597–604.

Ishiki, K., Morita, H. & Hosomi, H. (1991). Reflex control of renal nerve activity originating from the osmoreceptors in the hepato-portal region. *J Auton Nerv Syst*, **36**, 139–48.

Johns, E. J. (1981). An investigation into the type of beta-adrenoceptor mediating sympathetically activated renin release in the cat. *Br J Pharmacol*, **73**, 749–54.

Johns, E. J. (1991). The physiology and pharmacology of the renal nerves. *Pol Arch Med Wewn*, **85**, 141–9.

Johns, E. J. (2002) The autonomic nervous system and pressure-natriuresis in cardiovascular-renal interactions in response to salt. *Clin Auton Res*, **12**, 256–63.

Johns, E. J. (2005). Angiotensin II in the brain and the autonomic control of the kidney. *Exp Physiol*, **90**, 163–8.

Johns, E. J. & Manitius, J. (1986). An investigation into the alpha-adrenoceptor mediating renal nerve-induced calcium reabsorption by the rat kidney. *Br J Pharmacol*, **89**, 91–7.

Johns, E. J., Lewis, B. A. & Singer, B. (1976). The sodium-retaining effect of renal nerve activity in the cat: role of angiotensin formation. *Clin Sci Mol Med*, **51**, 93–102.

Kopp, U., Aurell, M., Nilsson, I. M. & Ablad, B. (1980). The role of beta-1-adrenoceptors in the renin release response to graded renal sympathetic nerve stimulation. *Pflugers Arch*, **387**, 107–13.

Kopp, U. C., Cicha, M. Z. & Smith, L. A. (2006). Differential effects of endothelin on the activation of renal mechanosensory nerves: stimulatory in high sodium diet and inhibitory in low sodium diet. *Am J Physiol Regul Integr Comp Physiol*.

La Grange, R. G., Sloop, C. H. & Schmid, H. E. (1973). Selective stimulation of renal nerves in the anesthetized dog. Effect on renin release during controlled changes in renal hemodynamics. *Circ Res*, **33**, 704–12.

Liu, F. & Gesek, F. A. (2001). alpha(1)-Adrenergic receptors activate NHE1 and NHE3 through distinct signaling pathways in epithelial cells. *Am J Physiol Renal Physiol*, **280**, F415–25.

Liu, F., Nesbitt, T., Drezner, M. K., Friedman, P. A. & Gesek, F. A. (1997). Proximal nephron Na +/H + exchange is regulated by alpha 1A- and alpha 1B-adrenergic receptor subtypes. *Mol Pharmacol*, **52**, 1010–8.

Lundin, S., Rickstein, S. E. & Thoren, P. (1984). Renal sympathetic activity in spontaneously hypertensive rats and normotensive controls, as studied by three different methods. *Acta Physiol Scand*, **120**, 265–72.

McDonough, A. A., Leong, P. K. & Yang, L. E. (2003). Mechanisms of pressure natriuresis: how blood pressure regulates renal sodium transport. *Ann N Y Acad Sci*, **986**, 669–77.

Miki, K. & Yoshimoto, M. (2005). Differential effects of behaviour on sympathetic outflow during sleep and exercise. *Exp Physiol*, **90**, 155–8.

Miki, K., Hayashida, Y. & Shiraki, K. (2002). Role of cardiac-renal neural reflex in regulating sodium excretion during water immersion in conscious dogs. *J Physiol*, **545**, 305–12.

Miki, K., Hayashida, Y., Sagawa, S. & Shiraki, K. (1989). Renal sympathetic nerve activity and natriuresis during water immersion in conscious dogs. *Am J Physiol*, **256**, R299–305.

Moncrief, K. & Kaufman, S. (2006). Splenic baroreceptors control splenic afferent nerve activity. *Am J Physiol Regul Integr Comp Physiol*, **290**, R352–6.

Morita, H., Ishiki, K. & Hosomi I, H. (1991). Effects of hepatic NaCl receptor stimulation on renal nerve activity in conscious rabbits. *Neurosci Lett*, **123**, 1–3.

Osborn, J. L., Dibona, G. F. & Thames, M. D. (1981). Beta-1 receptor mediation of renin secretion elicited by low-frequency renal nerve stimulation. *J Pharmacol Exp Ther*, **216**, 265–9.

Sattar, M. A. & Johns, E. J. (1994). Evidence for an alpha 1-adrenoceptor subtype mediating adrenergic vasoconstriction in Wistar normotensive and stroke-prone spontaneously hypertensive rat kidney. *J Cardiovasc Pharmacol*, **23**, 232–9.

Summers, R. J., Broxton, N., Hutchinson, D. S. & Evans, B. A. (2004). The Janus faces of adrenoceptors: factors controlling the coupling of adrenoceptors to multiple signal transduction pathways. *Clin Exp Pharmacol Physiol*, **31**, 822–7.

Thames S, M. D. & Abboud, F. M. (1979). Interaction of somatic and cardiopulmonary receptors in control of renal circulation. *Am J Physiol*, **237**, H560–5.

Walkowska, A., Badzynska, B., Kompanowska-Jezierska, E., Johns, E. J. & Sadowski, J. (2005). Effects of renal nerve stimulation on intrarenal blood flow in rats with intact or inactivated NO synthases. *Acta Physiol Scand*, **183**, 99–105.

Weaver R, L. C., Genovesi, S., Stella, A. & Zanchetti, A. (1987). Neural, hemodynamic, and renal responses to stimulation of intestinal receptors. *Am J Physiol*, **253**, H1167–76.

Ye, S., Zhong, H., Yanamadala, V. & Campese, V. M. (2002). Renal injury caused by intrarenal injection of phenol increases afferent and efferent renal sympathetic nerve activity. *Am J Hypertens*, **15**, 717–24.

Zhang, T. & Johns, E. J. (1997). Somatosensory influences on renal sympathetic nerve activity in anesthetized Wistar and hypertensive rats. *Am J Physiol*, **272**, R982–90.

Zucker, I. H., Schultz, H. D., Li, Y. F., Wang, Y., Wang, W. & Patel, K. P. (2004). The origin of sympathetic outflow in heart failure: the roles of angiotensin II and nitric oxide. *Prog Biophys Mol Biol*, **84**, 217–32.

CHAPTER 20

Pain and the sympathetic nervous system: pathophysiological mechanisms

Wilfrid Jänig

Introduction

The relationship between the autonomic nervous system and the nociceptive system has many facets that are interesting from the biological, pathobiological, and clinical point of view. I will discuss this field in a broad context and focus mainly on the sympathetic nervous system. The peripheral sympathetic noradrenergic neuron may have, in addition to its conventional function, transmitting signals generated in the brain to peripheral target cells, quite different functions that are directly or indirectly related to protection of body tissues (i.e. related to pain, hyperalgesia and inflammation). Some of these functions have not been studied as extensively as the function to regulate autonomic target cells (Chapter 1) (Jänig 2006). The parasympathetic nervous system is not involved in the generation of pain, yet may also be important in protection of body tissues (e.g. the gastrointestinal tract). Vagal afferents are involved in integrative aspects of pain, hyperalgesia and inflammation. This is discussed elsewhere (Jänig 2005, 2009a, Jänig and Levine 2006).

Table 20.1 lists different functions of the sympathetic nervous system related to pain and protection of body tissues in biological and pathobiological conditions. It shows that peripheral as well as central mechanisms have to be considered and that, in addition to the sympathetic nervous system, neuroendocrine systems and the immune system are involved. Often biology and pathobiology are not clearly separated.

Three aspects of the topic *sympathetic nervous system and pain* should be distinguished (Table 20.1):

1 Reactions of the sympathetic nervous system in pain—addresses the autonomic reactions during pain and includes reflexes to noxious stimulation and adaptive reactions (behaviour) during pain.

2 Mechanisms underlying coupling (cross-talk) from sympathetic (noradrenergic) neurons to afferent neurons in the generation of pain involving (a) excitation of the sympathetic postganglionic neurons and release of noradrenaline, (b) the sympathetic postganglionic fibres and inflammatory mediators (such as prostanoids, nerve growth factor or cytokines), or (c) the sympathoadrenal system.

3 Based on observations made on patients and in animal experimentation, it is likely that activity in sympathetic noradrenergic neurons or in the sympathoadrenal system, both generated in the brain, contributes directly or indirectly to pain. This central aspect includes the various forms of sympathetic-afferent coupling (see part 2). It additionally involves the immune system and the hypothalamo-pituitary-adrenal system. These central mechanisms appear to be important to understand the mechanisms of chronic pain and inflammation (e.g. in rheumatic diseases, fibromyalgia or complex regional pain syndrome [Chapter 69]).

The reasoning in this chapter is based on clinical observations made on patients with pain and hyperalgesia (in particular patients with complex regional pain syndrome [CRPS]; Chapter 69), on experimental investigations of these patients, and on animal experiments using *in vivo* and *in vitro* models (parts 1 and 2 in Table 20.1). The role of the sympathetic nervous system and its transmitters in acute inflammation and pain (e.g. bradykinin-induced synovial plasma extravasation) or chronic inflammation (such as rheumatoid arthritis) and its interaction with the peptidergic afferent innervation as well as the hypothalamo-pituitary-adrenal system will not be discussed. We are just at the beginning of the experimental investigation of these control mechanisms (part 3 in Table 20.1) (Straub and Härle 2005, Jänig and Levine 2006).

Reactions of the sympathetic nervous system in pain

Any acute and chronic tissue injury affects the sympathetic nervous system. Neurons of sympathetic systems exhibit generalized and specific reactions to these stimuli. The generalized reactions probably only occur in certain types of sympathetic system (e.g. muscle

Table 20.1 Sympathetic nervous system and pain

(1) Reactions of the sympathetic nervous system in pain
◆ Protective spinal and supraspinal reflexes
◆ Fight, flight and quiescence organized at the level of the periaqueductal gray
◆ Sympathetically mediated changes in refereed hyperalgesic zones during visceral and deep somatic pain
(2) Role of the sympathetic nervous system in the generation of pain
(Sympathetic-afferent coupling in the periphery)
◆ Coupling after nerve lesion (noradrenaline, α-adrenoceptors)
◆ Coupling via the micromilieu of the nociceptor and the vascular bed
◆ Sensitization of nociceptors mediated by sympathetic terminals independent of excitation and release of noradrenaline
◆ Sensitization of nociceptors initiated by cytokines or nerve growth factor and mediated by sympathetic terminals
◆ Sensitization of nociceptors by adrenalin released by the sympathoadrenal system
(3) Sympathetic nervous system and central mechanisms
(Control of inflammation and hyperalgesia by sympathetic and neuroendocrine mechanisms)
◆ Complex regional pain syndrome and sympathetic nervous system
◆ Immune system and sympathetic nervous system
◆ Rheumatic diseases and sympathetic nervous system
◆ Persistent generalizing pain syndromes (e.g. fibromyalgia, irritable bowel syndrome) and sympathetic nervous system

vasoconstrictor, visceral vasoconstrictor, sudomotor neurons or sympathetic cardiomotor neurons) but are weak or absent in other systems (e.g. sympathetic systems to pelvic organs). They are organized in spinal cord, brainstem (medulla oblongata, mesencephalon) and hypothalamus and are probably best understood as components of the different patterns of defence behaviour, such as 'confrontational defence', 'flight' and 'quiescence'. Confrontational defence and flight are typical of an active defence strategy when animals encounter threatening stimuli that are potentially injurious for the body, confrontational defence leading potentially to fight and flight to forward avoidance. Both patterns are represented in the lateral and dorsolateral periaqueductal grey of the mesencephalon, activated from the body surface or cortex, and associated with endogenous non-opioid analgesia, hypertension, and tachycardia. Quiescence is similar to the natural reactions of mammals during *serious injury* and *chronic pain* occurring particularly in the deep and visceral tissues. It is represented in the ventrolateral periaqueductal grey, activated from the deep tissues and consists of hyporeactivity, hypotension, bradycardia and an endogenous opioid sensitive analgesia. These stereotyped pre-programmed elementary behaviours and their association with the endogenous control of analgesia enable the organism to cope with dangerous situations that are always accompanied by pain or impending pain. The dorsolateral, lateral and ventrolateral columns of the periaqueductal grey have distinct reciprocal connections with the autonomic centres in the lower brainstem and hypothalamus that differentially regulate the activity in neurons of the sympathetic pathways. Furthermore, they are under differential control of the

medial and orbital prefrontal cortex (Keay and Bandler 2004, see Jänig 2006, 2009a).

There also exist more localized and distinct reactions of the sympathetic nervous system to noxious stimuli that are organized within the spinal cord and trigeminal nucleus and in the periphery (i.e. somatosympathetic, viscerosympathetic and viscerovisceral reflexes). For example cutaneous vasoconstrictor neurons exhibit distinct inhibitory reflexes to noxious stimuli of territories innervated by these neurons (Jänig 2006).

The hypothalamo-mesencephalic and the spinal level of integration are presumably protective under normal biological conditions. Activation of these integrative mechanisms leads to an activation of the hypothalamo-pituitary-adrenocortical system too. Spinal nociceptive reflexes are also at the base of pain, changes of blood flow and sweating, trophic changes of tissue and oedema in referred somatic zones during chronic injuries in visceral and deep somatic tissues. Most of these changes in the referred zones involve the sympathetic nervous system.

Role of the sympathetic nervous system in the generation of pain

Under physiological conditions there exists almost no influence of activity in sympathetic neurons on sensory neurons projecting to skin and deep somatic tissues in mammals. The effects that have been measured under experimental conditions on receptors with myelinated and unmyelinated axons are weak and can in part be explained by changes of the effector organs (erector pili muscles, blood vessels) induced by the activation of sympathetic neurons. These rather negative results do not rule out that noradrenaline or co-localized substances released by the postganglionic terminals have secondary long-term effects on the excitability of sensory receptors although we have no experimental evidence for this (Jänig 2009a).

Pain being dependent on activity in sympathetic neurons is called *sympathetically maintained pain* (SMP). SMP is a symptom and includes generically spontaneous pain and pain evoked by mechanical or thermal stimuli. It may be present in the complex regional pain syndrome (CRPS) type I and type II and in other pain syndromes. The idea about the involvement of the (efferent) sympathetic nervous system in pain is based on various clinical observations which have been documented in the literature since tens of years. These experiments demonstrate that:

◆ activation of sympathetic postganglionic neurons can produce pain

◆ blockade of sympathetic activity can relieve the pain

◆ noradrenaline injected intracutaneously is able to rekindle the pain

◆ α-adrenoceptor blockers or guanethidine (which depletes noradrenaline from its stores) can relieve the pain (Chapter 69) (Jänig 2009a).

The interpretation of these data is: Nociceptors are excited and possibly sensitized by noradrenaline released by the sympathetic fibres. Either the nociceptors have expressed adrenoceptors and/or the excitatory effect is generated indirectly (e.g. via changes in blood flow or via cells releasing inflammatory mediators). Sympathetically maintained activity in nociceptive neurons may

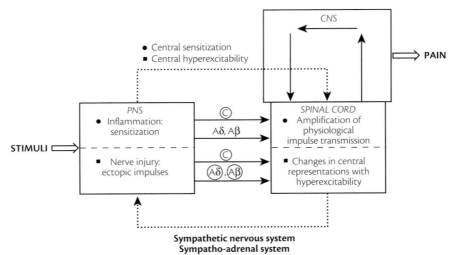

Fig. 20.1 Concept of generation of peripheral and central hyperexcitability during inflammatory pain and neuropathic pain. The upper interrupted arrow indicates that the central changes are generated (and possibly maintained): (a) by persistent activation of nociceptors with C-fibres (e.g. during chronic inflammation) called here 'central sensitization' or (b) after trauma with nerve lesion by ectopic activity and other changes in lesioned afferent neurons called here 'central hyperexcitability'. The lower interrupted arrow indicates the efferent feedback via the sympathetic nervous system or the sympathoadrenal system to the primary afferent neurons. Primary afferent nociceptive neurons (in particular those with C-fibres, encircled) are sensitized during inflammation. The biochemical and physiological changes occurring in these neurons during sensitization (and therefore also the central sensitization) are principally reversible. After nerve injury *all* lesioned primary afferent neurons (unmyelinated as well as myelinated ones, encircled) undergo biochemical, physiological and morphological changes, which become irreversible with time. These peripheral changes entail changes of the central representations (of the somatosensory system) which become irreversible (and therefore also the central hyperexcitability) if no regeneration of primary afferent neurons to their target tissue occurs. The central changes, induced by persistent activity in sensitized afferent nociceptive neurons or injured afferent neurons, are also reflected in the activity of the efferent feedback systems. The transmission of nociceptive impulses is under multiple excitatory and inhibitory controls of supraspinal centres (see central nervous system [CNS] loop). This supraspinal control changes too under pathophysiological conditions. Aβ, Aδ, afferent neurons with large diameter or small diameter myelinated axons; C, afferent neurons with unmyelinated axons; PNS, peripheral nervous system.

generate and maintain a state of central sensitization/hyperexcitability leading to spontaneous pain and secondary evoked pain (mechanical and possibly cold allodynia) (Fig. 20.1).

Coupling between sympathetic postganglionic neurons and primary afferent neurons following nerve trauma

Under pathophysiological conditions, which develop after peripheral nerve injury, sympathetic noradrenergic neurons may influence afferent neurons in several ways. This is illustrated schematically in Fig. 20.2. Various types of experiments on animal models with nerve injury have shown that the coupling may occur at, or close to, the lesion site, as well as remote from the lesion site.

Coupling between lesioned postganglionic and afferent nerve terminals

Coupling may occur between sympathetic fibres and afferent terminals in a neuroma, following nerve transection or ligation. Some myelinated as well as unmyelinated nerve fibres in the neuroma can be excited following electrical stimulation of the sympathetic supply or by noradrenaline or adrenaline injected systemically. The coupling has been observed in young neuromas but less so in old ones weeks and months after nerve lesion. This is compatible with clinical experience showing that neuroma pain is usually not dependent on sympathetic activity. It is also compatible with histological observations showing that catecholamine-containing axon profiles are rare within the neuroma and for several centimetres proximal to it, many weeks after cutting and ligating the nerve. Thus, this coupling is chemical and occurs via noradrenaline acting on α-adrenoceptors, although other mediator substances may also be involved. Ephaptic coupling between sympathetic fibres

and afferent fibres has so far not been observed in a neuroma (Blumberg and Jänig 1982, Jänig and Koltzenburg 1991, Jänig 2009a).

The situation is different when afferent and sympathetic fibres are allowed to regenerate to the target tissue. This has been shown experimentally for the chronic situation more than a year after cross-union of nerves (proximal stump of the sural or superficial peroneal nerve to the distal stump of the tibial nerve, in the cat) and after reinnervation of appropriate and inappropriate target tissues. Now unmyelinated afferent fibres may be vigorously excited by electrical low-frequency stimulation of the sympathetic supply (Häbler et al. 1987). Also this excitation is adrenoceptor-mediated (Fig. 20.3). It can be mimicked by adrenaline or noradrenaline and blocked by α-adrenoceptor blockers.

Coupling between intact postganglionic and afferent nerve terminals following partial nerve lesion

Intact C-fibre polymodal nociceptors in skin may develop sensitivity to catecholamines following partial nerve injury. Sympathetic nerve stimulation and noradrenaline may excite the polymodal nociceptors or sensitize them for heat stimuli. The activation and sensitization is already seen 4–10 days after partial nerve lesion and is maintained for at least 150 days. This sympathetic–afferent coupling apparently involves the non-lesioned polymodal nociceptive afferent axons that still projected through the lesion site, and non-lesioned postganglionic axons. It is assumed that the unlesioned unmyelinated afferents develop some sort of hyperreactivity to catecholamines following degeneration of the sympathetic postganglionic axons. Expression of adrenoceptors in afferent fibres may be triggered by collateral sprouting of both afferent fibres and postganglionic fibres in the target tissue (Sato and Perl 1991).

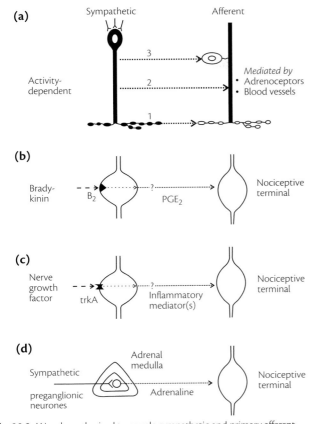

Fig. 20.2 Ways hypothesized to couple sympathetic and primary afferent neurons following peripheral nerve lesion **(a)** or during inflammation **(b to d)**. **(a)** These types of coupling depend on activity in the sympathetic neurons and on the expression of functional adrenoceptors by the afferent neurons or is mediated indirectly (e.g. via blood vessels [blood flow] or inflammatory cells). It can occur in the periphery (1), in the dorsal root ganglion (3) or possibly also in the lesioned nerve (2). **(b)** The inflammatory mediator bradykinin acts at B_2 receptors in the membrane of the sympathetic varicosities or in cells upstream of these varicosities, inducing release of prostaglandin E_2 (PGE_2) and sensitization of nociceptors. This way of coupling is probably not dependent on activity in the sympathetic neurons. **(c)** Nerve growth factor released during an experimental inflammation reacts with the high-affinity receptor for trkA in the membrane of the sympathetic varicosities, inducing release of an inflammatory mediator or inflammatory mediators and sensitization of nociceptors. This effect is probably not dependent on activity in the sympathetic neurons. **(d)** Activation of the adrenal medulla by sympathetic preganglionic neurons leads to release of adrenaline which generates sensitization of nociceptors. The ? in **b** and **c** indicates that PGE_2 or other inflammatory mediators may be released by cells other than the sympathetic varicosities. Modified from Jänig and Häbler 2000, with permission.

However, this sympathetic-afferent coupling leading to activation and sensitization of nociceptors required sympathetic stimulation at high non-physiological frequencies.

Coupling in the dorsal root ganglion and collateral sprouting following peripheral nerve lesion

A possibility of chemical sympathetic–afferent coupling following peripheral nerve lesion (e.g. cutting and ligating the sciatic nerve in rats) may occur a long way proximally to the injury site, such as in the proximal part of the nerve or in the dorsal root ganglion (DRG; 3 in Fig. 20.2a). Sympathetic postganglionic fibres reach the spinal nerves via grey rami. Most of these fibres project distally to peripheral target cells, others project proximally (e.g. to the DRG) and are

normally found along blood vessels. This situation changes after an experimental nerve lesion (e.g. transection and ligation of the sciatic nerve). Now many perivascular fine catecholamine-containing axons of the unlesioned proximally projecting neurons start to penetrate the DRGs which contain somata with lesioned axons. The extent of this novel *collateral* sprouting increases with time after the nerve lesion. Several weeks after the nerve lesion some somata are partially or almost completely surrounded by varicose catecholaminergic terminals; the frequency of these catecholamine-fluorescent structures increases for more than 70 days after the nerve lesion. The noradrenergic axons sprout preferentially in DRGs which contain somata of lesioned neurons, and here preferentially to large-diameter neurons which are lesioned (McLachlan et al. 1993).

Neurophysiological experiments on rats with the same nerve lesion show that afferent neurons projecting in the lesioned nerve can be affected via the DRG by sympathetic stimulation and by catecholamines. Afferent neurons with myelinated fibres are mainly involved; they are preferentially excited in the first weeks after lesion and predominantly inhibited in their activity at later times when the catecholaminergic sprouting in the DRG is more prominent (McLachlan et al. 1993, Michaelis et al. 1996). This coupling probably occurs only to muscle afferent neurons with Aδ-fibres (Michaelis et al. 2000). Furthermore, activation of afferent neurons requires stimulation of the sympathetic neurons at high non-physiological frequencies. Finally the afferent neurons in the dorsal root ganglion may be activated indirectly by decrease of blood flow and not directly via adrenoceptors in the dorsal root ganglion cells (Häbler et al. 2000).

The mechanism leading to the collateral sprouting in the DRG is possibly related to some trophic signal generated by afferent cells with lesioned axons in the DRG or their surrounding Schwann cells. Whether these aberrant pathological connections account for spontaneous pain and allodynia in some patients after peripheral nerve lesions awaits further investigations (for discussion see Jänig et al. 1996, Jänig 2009).

Adrenoceptors involved in chemical sympathetic–afferent coupling following nerve lesion

Excitation and depression of lesioned primary afferent neurons (in the DRG at their lesioned terminals in the neuroma), or of unlesioned collaterally sprouting primary afferents generated by activation of the sympathetic innervation, is mimicked by systemic injection of noradrenaline or adrenaline and blocked by phentolamine application. Thus, both excitation and depression are suggested to be mediated by α-adrenoceptors. The cellular mechanisms underlying the increased sensitivity are unknown. Novel expression or up-regulation of adrenoceptors occurs; alternatively, normally present adrenoceptors that are not functional become uncovered and effective during the response to damage. The subtype of α-adrenoceptor being involved in the sympathetic–afferent coupling in the different rat models is predominantly α_2. Knowledge about the subtypes of adrenoceptor following nerve trauma may turn out to be useful in the design of more specific treatment modalities for neuropathic pain conditions involving sympathetic efferent activity (Jänig et al. 1996; Jänig and Häbler 2000).

Synopsis

Peripheral trauma with nerve injury may lead to sensitization and activation of nociceptive and activation of other primary afferent

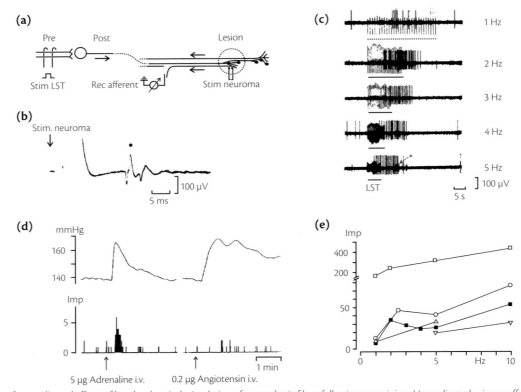

Fig. 20.3 Excitation of unmyelinated afferent fibres by electrical stimulation of sympathetic fibres following nerve injury. Unmyelinated primary afferents were recorded in cats 11–20 months following a nerve lesion. The central cut stump of a cutaneous nerve innervating hairy skin (sural or superficial peroneal nerve) had been adapted to the distal stump of a transected mixed nerve (tibial nerve). This preparation was designed to mimic the consequences of a mixed nerve lesion. There was a 'neuroma-in-continuity' at the site of the lesion and cutaneous nerve fibres had regenerated into skin or deep somatic tissue supplied by the mixed nerve. **(a)** Experimental set-up. pre, preganglionic; post, postganglionic; LST, lumbar sympathetic trunk. **(b)** The afferent fibres were identified as unmyelinated by electrical stimulation of the neuroma with single impulses. The signal indicated by the dot was the same as in **c**; the afferent fibre conducted at 1.3 m/s. **(c)** Record from a single unmyelinated afferent unit. Supramaximal stimulation of the LST with trains of 30 pulses at 1–5 Hz (stimulation artefacts indicated by bars and dots in upper record). Note that the afferent unit had some low rate of ongoing activity (impulses before the trains at 1 and 4 Hz) and that a second unit was recruited at 5 Hz (marked by *). **(d)** Adrenaline (5μg injected intravenously) activated the fibre. Angiotensin (0.2μg injected intravenously) generated a large increase of blood pressure (MAP, mean arterial blood pressure) but did not activate the afferent fibre. **(e)** Stimulus response curves for the single unit (■) and four filaments containing 2–3 (O, ∇, Δ) or more than 5 (□) afferent units. Ordinate scale is the total number of impulses exceeding ongoing activity in response to variable stimulation frequency of the LST. Reprinted from *Neurosci. Lett.*, **82**, Häbler, H.-J., Jänig, W., and Koltzenburg, M., Activation of unmyelinated afferents in chronically lesioned nerves by adrenaline and excitation of sympathetic efferents in the cat, 35–40, Copyright (1987), with permission from Elsevier.

neurons. These processes depend on and are maintained by the sympathetic nervous system. Several ways of coupling between sympathetic postganglionic neurons and primary afferent neurons are possible and have been worked out experimentally on animal models with controlled nerve lesions, showing that there may be intimate relationships between sympathetic neurons and afferent neurons under pathophysiological conditions (Fig. 20.4):

◆ The sympathetic postganglionic neuron may develop chemically mediated 'cross-talk' to primary afferent neurons. Whether this occurs probably depends on the time after nerve lesion as well as on the type of nerve lesion (partial, complete).

◆ Following peripheral nerve lesion, remote collateral sprouting of unlesioned postganglionic fibres occurs in the dorsal root ganglion, preferentially toward the large-diameter cells. Collateral sprouting of unlesioned postganglionic fibres may also occur in the peripheral target tissue (in particular after partial nerve lesion). The signal(s) initiating this sprouting probably derive from primary afferent neurons and/or Schwann cells and may be neurotrophic substances.

◆ This interaction is mediated by noradrenaline, but additional mediator substances cannot be excluded.

◆ Primary afferent neurons express functional adrenoceptors. The type of adrenoceptor involved is preferentially α_2 in the animal models. Signal(s) that initiate the functional expression of adrenoceptors may be related to a decrease of density of noradrenergic innervation (i.e. relative or complete denervation), to activity in the sympathetic neurons, or to neurotrophic signals that derive from the Schwann cells or other cells.

◆ Plastic changes of primary afferent and sympathetic postganglionic neurons following peripheral trauma with nerve lesion may explain some of the clinical sensory phenomena in patients with sympathetically maintained pain (SMP) (e.g. in CRPS type II). It does not explain SMP in patients without nerve lesion (e.g. CRPS type I) (Chapter 69).

Indirect coupling between noradrenergic nerve terminals and nociceptors in the periphery

Nociceptive afferents are embedded in a complex micromilieu (Fig. 20.5). The state of this micromilieu surrounding the receptive terminals depends on mediator substances that are released during

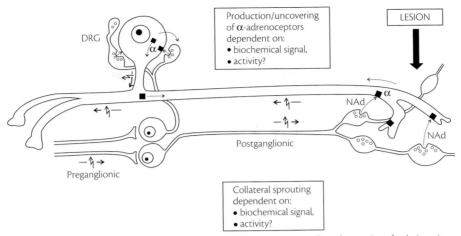

Fig. 20.4 Relation between afferent neurons and sympathetic neurons following peripheral nerve lesion. Collateral sprouting of unlesioned sympathetic neurons in the dorsal root ganglion (DRG) and in the peripheral target tissue. Synthesis or up-regulation of functional adrenoceptors (preferentially α-adrenoceptors) by afferent neurons after nerve lesion. It is unclear in which way these processes are related to the biochemical signals (e.g. neurotrophins) synthesized by neurons, Schwann cells, and other cells in the DRG or in the periphery and the expression of their receptors. In which way are these processes dependent on activity in the afferent neurons, on the presence/absence of postganglionic noradrenergic neurons or on the activity in the postganglionic neurons? NAd, noradrenaline. Reprinted from *Prog. in Brain Res.*, **113**, Jänig, W., Levine, J. D., and Michaelis, M., Interaction of sympathetic and primary afferent neurons following nerve injury and tissue trauma, 161–84, Copyright 1996 with permission from Elsevier.

inflammatory processes following trauma from non-neural cells such as mast cells, polymorphonuclear leucocytes, macrophages, fibroblasts, endothelial cells, and other cells. The microcirculation is under neural control of sympathetic vasoconstrictor neurons. Moreover, activation of subgroups of nociceptive primary afferents (in human skin mechanoinsensitive C-fibre afferents; see Schmelz et al. (2000) in Jänig (2006)) not only causes orthodromic impulse traffic but also *arteriolar (precapillary) vasodilation* and (in some tissues) *venular plasma extravasation* by release of neuropeptides from the receptive terminals (e.g. substance P and calcitonin-gene-related peptide [CGRP]). Both afferent-induced changes are called neurogenic inflammation. Thus, there are possibilities for indirect coupling between sympathetic and afferent nerve terminals (Fig. 20.5): first, vascular perfusion of the micromilieu surrounding the nociceptors after nerve trauma may change as consequence of denervation and reinnervation by postganglionic vasoconstrictor neurons and afferent nociceptive neurons and the development of hyperreactivity of blood vessels (Jobling et al. 1992, Koltzenburg et al. 1995); second, nociceptors may be sensitized by inflammatory mediators such as prostaglandins and interleukins, the release of which from non-neuronal cells of the micromilieu may be mediated by noradrenergic nerve terminals.

Changes of neurovascular transmission and development of hyperreactivity of blood vessels

Neural control of blood vessels can change dramatically after trauma with nerve lesion, but possibly also after trauma without lesion of nerves (Koltzenburg et al. 1995):

◆ Cutaneous blood vessels that are reinnervated after a nerve lesion might exhibit stronger than normal vasoconstriction to impulses in sympathetic neurons.

◆ The sympathetically reinnervated cutaneous blood vessels may show stronger than normal vasoconstrictions to systemic catecholamines and appear to be hyperreactive.

◆ The blood vessels may exhibit changes in vasodilation to antidromic activation of reinnervated unmyelinated afferents.

The reinnervated blood vessels may therefore be under stronger than normal vasoconstrictor influence, probably due to a decreased reuptake of noradrenaline released by the postganglionic vasoconstrictor axons, which can no longer be counteracted by an afferent-mediated vasodilation. *In vitro* investigation of the rat tail artery has shown that the functional recovery of neurovascular transmission may remain permanently disturbed after a nerve lesion (Jobling et al. 1992).

The altered neural and non-neural control of blood vessels will contribute to abnormal regulation of microcirculation following trauma due to nerve injury. These changes can contribute to the abnormal regulation of blood flow through skin and deep somatic tissues and possibly to the trophic changes (including the oedema) both present in patients with CRPS (Chapter 69). They may furthermore be a permissive factor in the generation of afferent nociceptive impulse activity and therefore in the sensitization of nociceptors and in the generation of pain.

Finally, it is commonly believed that skin temperature changes during painful disorders following trauma with or without nerve injury (e.g. in CRPS I or II) reflect changes of activity in cutaneous vasoconstrictor neurons. Thus, cold skin may then be associated with a high level and warm skin with a low level of activity in these neurons. This is probably a misconception, and there is no proof that the relation between skin temperature and activity in sympathetic neurons holds under these pathophysiological conditions. Therefore, it is also not correct to conclude, *only* on the basis of cold feet or hands of these patients, that there is a 'high sympathetic tone' or 'hyper-sympathetic' activity (Chapter 69).

Sensitization of nociceptors mediated by sympathetic fibres or by adrenaline released by the adrenal medulla

Based on experimental studies of standardized behaviour in rats it has been shown that sensitization of nociceptors for mechanical and heat stimuli may be mediated by sympathetic nerve fibres independent of impulse activity and noradrenaline release or by adrenaline released from the adrenal medulla (Fig. 20.2b-d). These ways

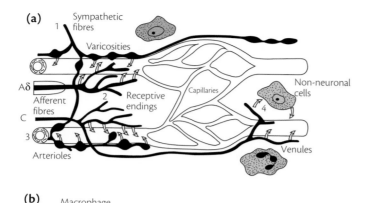

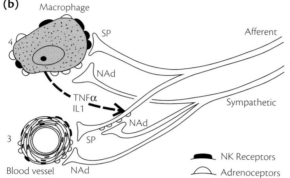

Fig. 20.5 (a) The micromilieu of nociceptors. The microenvironment of primary afferents is thought to affect the properties of the receptive endings of myelinated (A) and unmyelinated (C) afferent fibres. This has been particularly documented for inflammatory processes, but pathological changes in the direct surroundings of primary afferents may contribute to pain states. The vascular bed consists of arterioles (directly innervated by sympathetic and afferent peptidergic fibres), capillaries (not innervated and not influenced by nerve fibres) and venules (not directly innervated but influenced by nerve fibres). The micromilieu depends on several interacting components: Activity in postganglionic noradrenergic fibres (*1*) supplying blood vessels (*3*) causes release of noradrenaline (NAd) and possibly other substances and vasoconstriction. Excitation of primary afferents (Aδ- and C-fibres) (*2*) causes vasodilation in precapillary arterioles and plasma extravasation in postcapillary venules (C-fibres only) by the release of calcitonin-gene-related peptide (CGRP; only vasodilation) and substance P (SP). Some of these effects may be mediated by non-neuronal cells such as mast cells and macrophages (*4*). Other factors that affect the control of the microcirculation are the myogenic properties of arterioles (*3*) and more global environmental influences such as a change of the temperature and the metabolic state of the tissue. With permission from Jänig, W. and Koltzenburg, M. (1991). What is the interaction between the sympathetic terminal and the primary afferent fibre? In *Towards a new pharmacotherapy of pain*, (ed. A. I. Basbaum and J. M. Besson), Wiley. **(b)** Hypothetical relation between sympathetic noradrenergic nerve fibres (*1*), peptidergic afferent nerve fibres (*2*), blood vessels (*3*) and macrophages (*4*). The activated and sensitized afferent nerve fibres activate macrophages possibly via substance P release. The immune cells start to release cytokines, such as tumour necrosis factor α (TNF-α) and interleukin 1 (IL-1) which further activate afferent fibres. Substance P released from the afferent nerve fibres reacts with neurokinin 1 (NK-1) receptors in the blood vessels (causing neurogenic inflammation). The sympathetic nerve fibres are hypothesized to interact with this system on three levels: (*1*) via adrenoceptors (mainly α) on the blood vessels (vasoconstriction); (*2*) via adrenoceptors (mainly β) on macrophages (further release of cytokines), and (*3*) via adrenoceptors (mainly α) on afferents (further sensitization of these fibres). Modified from *The Lancet Neurology*, **2**, Jänig and Baron, Complex regional pain syndrome: mystery explained? 687–697, Copyright (2003), with permission from Elsevier.

of coupling between sympathetic postganglionic neurons and primary afferent neurons have no clinical correlate on humans yet. However, they indicate that the sympathetic nervous system may be involved in the generation of pain in an unprecedented way.

Sensitization of nociceptors mediated by sympathetic terminals independent of excitation and release of noradrenaline

Withdrawal threshold to stimulation of the rat hind paw with a linearly increasing mechanical stimulus applied to the dorsum of the paw decreases dose-dependently after intradermal injection of the inflammatory mediator bradykinin (an octapeptide cleaved from plasma α_2-globulins, by kallikreins circulating in the plasma) (Fig. 20.2b; Fig. 20.6). Following a single injection of bradykinin this decrease lasts for more than one hour for mechanical stimulation. This type of mechanical hyperalgesic behaviour is mediated by the B_2 bradykinin-receptor and is not present when bradykinin is injected subcutaneously (Jänig et al. 2000). Bradykinin-induced hyperalgesic behaviour is blocked by the cyclo-oxygenase inhibitor indomethacin and therefore mediated by a prostaglandin (probably PGE_2) that sensitizes nociceptors for mechanical stimulation (Fig. 20.6). However, in vagotomized rats in which the bradykinin-induced mechanical hyperalgesia is significantly enhanced indomethacin has almost no effect on bradykinin-induced hyperalgesia. This failure is not related to a switch from B2- to B1-receptor subtype because the selective B1-receptor agonist des-Arg9-BK fails to produce hyperalgesia in

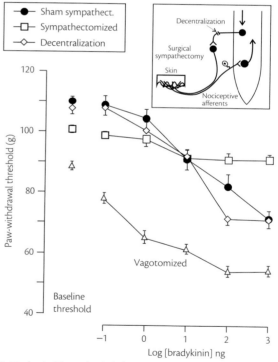

Fig. 20.6 Mechanical hyperalgesic behaviour and sympathetic innervation. Bradykinin-induced hyperalgesia (decrease of paw-withdrawal threshold) in sham sympathectomized rats (●; n = 6 hindpaws) and in sympathectomized rats (□; n = 12 hindpaws) and in rats with decentralized lumbar sympathetic chains (preganglionic axons in lumbar sympathetic chain interrupted 8 days before, ◊; n = 10 hindpaws) (right inset). Bradykinin was injected intracutaneously at the site of stimulation and at the dose indicated (abscissa scale) in volumes of 2.5 μL. Both sham sympathectomy and sympathetic decentralization groups were significantly different from the sympathectomy group. After vagotomy paw-thresholds (baseline and after bradykinin) significantly decrease (Δ; 16 hindpaws). This is the control for the experiment in Fig. 20.8. With permission from Khasar, S.G., Miao, F.J.-P., Jänig, W., and Levine, J.D. (1998a). *Eur. J. Neurosci.* Wiley.

vagotomized rats (Khasar et al. 1998a). This shows that bradykinin-induced hyperalgesia may not be mediated by prostanoids in vagotomized rats. This interesting finding needs to be followed experimentally.

The decrease in paw-withdrawal threshold provided by bradykinin is significantly reduced after surgical sympathectomy. This shows that the sympathetic innervation of the skin is involved in the sensitization of nociceptors for mechanical stimulation. Interestingly, decentralization of the lumbar paravertebral sympathetic ganglia (denervating the postganglionic neurons by cutting the preganglionic sympathetic axons) does not abolish the bradykinin-induced mechanical hyperalgesic behaviour (Fig. 20.6). This indicates that the sensitizing effect of bradykinin is not dependent on activity in the sympathetic neurons innervating skin and therefore not on release of noradrenaline (Khasar et al. 1998a, Jänig and Häbler 2000). It is believed that bradykinin stimulates the release of prostaglandin from the sympathetic terminals. However this release could also occur from other cells in association with the sympathetic terminals in the skin (Fig. 20.2b).

Mechanical hyperalgesic behaviour generated by intracutaneous injection of the inflammatory mediator bradykinin and its dependence on the sympathetic innervation of the skin is an interesting phenomenon. However, the conventional explanation that this mechanical hyperalgesia is due to prostanoids sensitizing nociceptors since indomethacin prevents it appears to be too simple. The reasons are:

- the finding that sympathetic fibres mediate this hyperalgesia independent of neural activity and release of noradrenaline

- indomethacin does not block this behaviour under certain conditions (e.g. when the adrenal medullae are activated after vagotomy)

- in humans sensitization of cutaneous nociceptors by bradykinin to mechanical stimulation is weak or absent.

Thus, this phenomenon has to be reinvestigated using a rigorous experimental approach (see Jänig 2009a).

Sensitization of nociceptors initiated by cytokines or nerve growth factor possibly mediated by sympathetic terminals

Nerve growth factor

Systemic injection of nerve growth factor (NGF) is followed by a transient thermal and mechanical hyperalgesia in rats (Lewin et al. 1993, 1994) and humans (Petty et al. 1994). During experimental inflammation (evoked by Freund's adjuvant in the rat hindpaw) NGF increases in the inflamed tissue paralleled by the development of thermal and mechanical hyperalgesia. Both are prevented by anti-NGF antibodies (Lewin et al. 1994). The mechanisms responsible are sensitization of nociceptors via high-affinity NGF-receptors (trkA receptors) and an induction of increased synthesis of CGRP and substance P in the afferent cell bodies by NGF taken up by the afferent terminals and transported to the cell bodies. The NGF-induced sensitization of nociceptors also seems to be mediated indirectly by the sympathetic postganglionic terminals. Heat and mechanical hyperalgesic behaviour generated by local injection of NGF into the skin is prevented or significantly reduced after chemical or surgical sympathectomy (Woolf et al. 1996). These experiments suggest that NGF released during inflammation

by inflammatory cells acts on the sympathetic terminals via high-affinity trkA receptors inducing the release of inflammatory mediators and subsequently sensitization of nociceptors for mechanical or heat stimuli (Fig. 20.2c) (McMahon 1996, Woolf 1996, Jänig and Häbler 2000). It is unclear whether this sensitization of nociceptors mediated by terminal sympathetic nerve fibres is:

- dependent on activity in the sympathetic neurons, release of noradrenaline and adrenoceptors expressed in the nociceptive afferent neurons

- independent of activity and release of noradrenaline.

Proinflammatory cytokines

Based on behavioural experiments conducted on rats (studying mechanical or heat hyperalgesia) it has been shown, that tissue injury, injection of the bacterial cell wall endotoxin lipopolysaccharide or injection of carrageenan (a plant polysaccharide), stimulates tissue inflammation and leads to sensitization of nociceptors. Systematic pharmacological interventions using blockers or inhibitors of the various mediators demonstrate that the proinflammatory cytokines, tumour necrosis factor α (TNF-α), interleukin (IL)-1, IL-6, and IL-8 may be involved in this process of sensitization and therefore in the generation of hyperalgesia (Cunha et al. 2007, Woolf et al. 1996, Verri et al. 2006). Pathogenic stimuli lead to activation of resident cells and release of the inflammatory mediator bradykinin and other mediators. The inflammatory mediators and the pathogenic stimuli themselves activate macrophages, monocytes and other immune-related cells. These cells release TNF-α, which is believed to generate sensitization of nociceptor by two possible pathways (Fig. 20.7):

- It induces production of IL-6 and IL-1β by immune cells, whereby IL-6 enhances the production of IL-1β. These interleukins stimulate cyclo-oxygenase 2 (COX 2) and the production of prostaglandins (PGE$_2$, PGI$_2$) which in turn react with the nociceptive terminal via E-type prostaglandin receptors.

- It induces the release of IL-8 from endothelial cells and macrophages. IL-8 reacts with the sympathetic terminals that are supposed to mediate sensitization of nociceptive afferent terminals by release of noradrenaline to act via β_2-adrenoceptors.

These two peripheral pathways by which nociceptive afferents can be sensitized involving cytokines are under inhibitory control of circulating glucocorticoids (indicated by asterisks in Fig. 20.7) and of other, anti-inflammatory, interleukins (e.g. IL-4 and IL-10 indicated by # in Fig. 20.7).

It is important to emphasized that the mechanisms, involving NGF, proinflammatory cytokines and noradrenergic sympathetic postganglionic fibres in the sensitization of nociceptive afferents, have been deduced on the basis of behavioural and pharmacological experiments. Proof of such interaction by directly assessing the activity of nociceptors with electrophysiological techniques and of the effect of noradrenergic nerve fibres on the afferent nerve fibres are lacking. These experiments have to be done.

Sympathoadrenal system and nociceptor sensitization

In rats, activation of the sympathoadrenal system (adrenal medulla; e.g. by release of central neurons, connected to preganglionic neurons that innervate the adrenal medulla, from vagal inhibition),

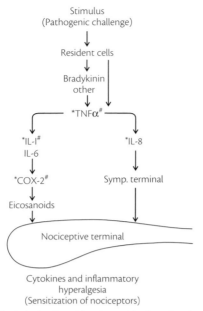

Fig. 20.7 Hypothetical role of cytokines in sensitization of nociceptors during inflammation and the underlying putative mechanisms leading to hyperalgesia. Pathogenic stimuli activate resident cells and lead to release of inflammatory mediators (such as bradykinin). Pro-inflammatory cytokines are synthesized and released by macrophages and other immune or immune-related cells. Nociceptors are postulated to be sensitized by two pathways involving the cytokines: *(1)* Tumour necrosis factor α (TNF-α) induces synthesis and release of interleukin 1 (IL-1) and IL-6 which, in turn, induce the release of eicosanoids (prostaglandin E_2 and I_2 [PGE_2, PGI_2]) by activating cyclo-oxygenase-2 (COX-2). *(2)* TNF-α induces synthesis and release of IL-8. IL-8 activates sympathetic terminals that sensitize nociceptors via β_2-adrenoceptors. Glucocorticoids inhibit the synthesis of the cytokines and the activation of COX-2 (indicated by asterisks). Anti-inflammatory cytokines (such as IL-4 and IL-10) that are also synthesized and released by immune cells inhibit the synthesis and release of pro-inflammatory cytokines (indicated by #). This scheme is fully dependent on behavioural experiments and pharmacological interventions. The different steps will need to be verified experimentally using neurophysiological experiments. After Verri et al. 2006, with permission.

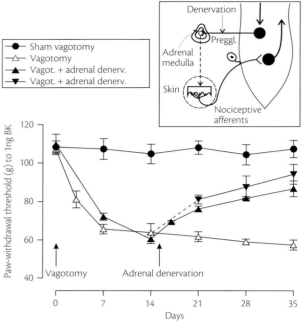

Fig. 20.8 Long-term enhancement of bradykinin-induced behavioural mechanical hyperalgesia after vagotomy and its attenuation after denervation of the adrenal medullae (AM). Vagotomy activates the adrenal medullae, probably by removal of central inhibition. Paw-withdrawal threshold in response to intradermal injection of 1 ng bradykinin (BK) in rats before and 3–35 days after vagotomy (Δ, n = 6), before and 7–35 days after sham-vagotomy ($\bullet$, n = 8; control) and in rats that are first vagotomized and whose AM are denervated 14 days after vagotomy (see inset upper right) and measurements taken up to 35 days after initial surgery. The latter group of animals consists of two subgroups: rats which are tested after vagotomy and after additional denervation of the AM ($\blacktriangle$, n = 6) and rats which are only tested after additional denervation of the AM ($\blacktriangledown$, n = 4). Intradermal injection of 1 ng bradykinin does not significantly decrease paw-withdrawal threshold to mechanical stimulation in control rats (Fig. 20.6). Ordinate scale is threshold in grams. Data of the sham-vagotomy and the vagotomy group of rats are significantly different ≥7 days after vagotomy (p < 0.01). Data of vagotomized rats with denervated AM and rats that are only vagotomized are significantly different on days 28 and 35 (p < 0.01). Data between sham-vagotomized rats and vagotomized rats in which the AM are denervated are not significantly different on days 28 and 35. Ordinate scale, change of baseline threshold and threshold to intracutaneous bradykinin together. With permission from Khasar, S.G., Miao, F.J.-P., Jänig, W., and Levine, J.D. (1998b). Society for Neuroscience.

but not of the sympathoneural system, generates mechanical hyperalgesia and enhances bradykinin-induced mechanical hyperalgesia (decrease of paw-withdrawal threshold to mechanical stimulation of the skin, compare $\bullet$ with Δ in Fig. 20.6). Both develop slowly over 7–14 days following activation of the adrenal medullae (induced by vagotomy) and are maintained over 5 weeks tested (Δ in Fig. 20.8). They are reversed slowly after denervation of the adrenal medullae ($\blacktriangle$,$\blacktriangledown$ in Fig. 20.8) (Khasar et al. 1998a,b). Application of adrenaline through a minipump over 3–14 days slowly enhances the development of mechanical hyperalgesia. Furthermore, continuous application of a β_2-adrenoceptor blocker over 7–14 days by way of a minipump prevents the enhancement of bradykinin-induced hyperalgesic behaviour generated by activation of the adrenal medullae (Khasar et al. 2003).

The results of this experiment are interpreted in the following way: Adrenaline released by persistent activation of the adrenal medullae sensitizes cutaneous nociceptors for mechanical stimuli. This sensitization of nociceptors and its reversal are slow and take days to develop. The slow time course implies that the nociceptor sensitization cannot acutely be blocked by an adrenoceptor antagonist given intracutaneously. Adrenaline probably does not

act directly on the cutaneous nociceptors but on cells in the micro-environment of the nociceptors inducing slow changes, which result in nociceptor sensitization. Candidate cells may be mast cells, macrophages or keratinocytes which then release substances that generate sensitization (Jänig and Häbler 2000, Jänig et al. 2000, Khasar et al. 1998b). The change of sensitivity of a population of nociceptors generated by adrenaline released by the adrenal medullae, which is regulated by the brain, would be a novel mechanism of sensitization. This novel mechanism would be different from mechanisms that lead to activation and/or sensitization of nociceptors by sympathetic-afferent coupling as discussed above (Fig. 20.2d).

This novel mechanism of pain and hyperalgesia involving the sympathoadrenal system may operate in ill-defined chronic pain syndromes such as irritable bowel syndrome, functional dyspepsia, fibromyalgia, chronic fatigue syndrome, etc. (see Mayer and Bushnell 2009). The conclusions on long-term sensitization of nociceptors for mechanical stimulation by adrenaline are indirect and fully rest on behavioural experiments. Neurophysiological experiments *in vivo* on primary afferent nociceptive neurons are required to test whether all or only a subpopulation of nociceptors are sensitized.

Conclusion

In healthy individuals, tissue-damaging stimuli in the periphery are encoded by nociceptive afferent neurons. The nociceptive impulse activity is transformed in the spinal cord and faithfully transmitted to the thalamocortical system and to other supraspinal brain centres, leading to pain perception, appropriate control of the spinal transmission of nociceptive information, and appropriate somatomotor, autonomic, and endocrine reactions. This concerted action of the central nervous system may become disturbed under pathological conditions such as CRPS and related pain states (Chapter 69). Peripheral injury (trauma with and without obvious nerve injuries; chronic inflammation) leads to nociceptor sensitization or ectopically generated afferent impulse traffic to the central nervous system. The peripheral changes entail changes of central neurons (globally described here as 'central sensitization' or 'central hyperexcitability'), resulting in distorted sensations and distorted autonomic, somatomotor, and endocrine reactions.

The sympathetic outflow to the affected peripheral part of the body may be actively involved in the generation of pain and associated processes by way of a positive feedback loop. Stimuli which normally are non-painful may now elicit painful reactions that are dependent on an intact sympathetic innervation. Several pathophysiological mechanisms may be involved in this process:

- abnormal coupling of noradrenergic postganglionic fibres to primary afferent neurons

- alterations of the micromilieu of afferent receptors by changes of neurovascular transmission and by development of hyperreactivity of blood vessel

- alterations of the micromilieu of nociceptors by interference of noradrenergic fibres with non-neural inflammatory and immune-competent cells

- changes of the impulse pattern in neurons of the sympathetic outflow, possibly as a consequence of the central changes (Chapter 69).

Novel ways of involvement of sympathetic postganglionic neurons in the sensitization of nociceptors and subsequent generation of pain and hyperalgesia have only been studied in animal behavioural models. Terminals of sympathetic neurons may mediate sensitization of nociceptors involving nerve growth factor, cytokines or bradykinin. This function of the sympathetic fibre may be independent of its excitability and release of noradrenaline. Finally adrenaline released by the adrenal medulla sensitizes nociceptors for mechanical stimulation. This sensitizing effect takes 1–2 weeks to develop.

The complexity of the somatosensory and autonomic abnormalities observed in patients with chronic pain that may be, in some way or another, associated with the sympathetic nervous system, indicates that several pathobiological processes operate in parallel, on the sensory as well as on the efferent site, and that the actual clinical phenomenology may be dependent on the predominance of one type of pathological mechanism (Chapter 69).

Acknowledgement

This work was supported by the Deutsche Forschungsgemeinschaft.

References

Blumberg, H. and Jänig, W. (1982). Activation of fibers via experimentally produced stump neuromas of skin nerves:ephaptic transmission or retrograde sprouting? *Exp. Neurol.* **76**, 462–82.

Cunha, T. M., Verri, W. A. Jr., Poole, S., Parada, C. A., Cunha, F. Q., and Ferreira, S. H. (2007). Pain facilitation of proinflammatory cytokine actions at peripheral nerve terminals. In *Immune and glial regulation of pain* (ed. J.A. DeLeo, L.S. Sorkin and L.R. Watkins), pp. 67–83. IASP Press, Seattle.

Häbler, H.-J., Eschenfelder, S., Liu, X.-G., and Jänig, W. (2000). Sympathetic-sensory coupling after L5 spinal nerve lesion in the rat and its relation to changes in dorsal root ganglion blood flow. *Pain* **87**, 335–45.

Häbler, H.-J., Jänig, W., and Koltzenburg, M. (1987). Activation of unmyelinated afferents in chronically lesioned nerves by adrenaline and excitation of sympathetic efferents in the cat. *Neurosci. Lett.* **82**, 35–40.

Jobling, P., McLachlan, E. M., Jänig, W., and Anderson, C. R. (1992). Electrophysiological responses in the rat tail artery during reinnervation following lesions of the sympathetic supply. *J. Physiol. London* **454**, 107–28.

Jänig, W. (2005). Vagal afferents and visceral pain. In *Advances in vagal afferent neurobiology* (ed. B. Undem and D. Weinreich D), pp. 461—89. CRC Press, Boca Raton.

Jänig, W. (2006). *The integrative action of the autonomic nervous system. Neurobiology of homeostasis.* Cambridge University Press, Cambridge, New York.

Jänig, W. (2009b). Autonomic nervous system and pain. In *Science of pain* (ed. E.A. Mayer and M.C. Bushnell), pp. 265–300. IASP Press, Seattle.

Jänig, W. (2009a). Autonomic nervous system dysfunction. In *Science of pain* (ed. A.I. Basbaum and M.C. Bushnell), pp. 193–225. Academic Press, San Diego.

Jänig, W., Khasar, S. G., Levine, J. D., and Miao, F. J.-P. (2000). The role of vagal visceral afferents in the control of nociception. *Prog. Brain Res.* **122**, 273–87.

Jänig, W., Levine, J. D., and Michaelis, M. (1996). Interaction of sympathetic and primary afferent neurons following nerve injury and tissue trauma. *Prog. in Brain Res.* **112**, 161–84.

Jänig, W. and Häbler, H. J. (2000). Sympathetic nervous system: contribution to chronic pain. *Prog. Brain. Res.* **129**, 451–68.

Jänig, W. and Koltzenburg, M. (1991). What is the interaction between the sympathetic terminal and the primary afferent fibre? In *Towards a new pharmacotherapy of pain,* (ed. A. I. Basbaum and J. M. Besson), Dahlem Workshop Reports, pp. 331–52. John Wiley & Sons, Chichester.

Jänig, W. and Levine, J. D. (2012). Autonomic-endocrine-immune responses in acute and chronic pain. In *Wall and Melzack´s textbook of pain* (6th edn.)(ed. S.B. McMahon and M. Koltzenburg). Elsevier Churchill Livingstone, Edinburgh.

Keay, K. A. and Bandler, R. (2004). Periaqueductal gray. In *The rat nervous system,* (3rd edn.)(ed. G. Paxinos), pp. 243–57. Academic Press, San Diego.

Khasar, S. G., Green, P. G., Miao, F.-J. P., and Levine, J. D. (2003). Vagal modulation of nociception is mediated by adrenomedullary epinephrine in the rat. *Eur. J. Neurosci.* **17**, 909–15.

Khasar, S. G., Miao, F. J.-P., Jänig, W., and Levine, J. D. (1998b). Vagotomy-induced enhancement of mechanical hyperalgesia in the rat is sympathoadrenal-mediated. *J. Neurosci.* **18**, 3043–9.

Khasar, S. G., Miao, F. J.-P., Jänig, W., and Levine, J. D. (1998a). Modulation of bradykinin-induced mechanical hyperalgesia in the rat by activity in abdominal vagal afferents. *Eur. J. Neurosci.* **10**, 435–44.

Koltzenburg, M., Häbler, H.-J., and Jänig, W. (1995). Functional reinnervation of the vasculature of the adult cat paw by axons originally innervating vessels in hairy skin. *Neuroscience* **67**, 245–52.

Lewin, G. R., Ritter, A. M., and Mendell, L. M. (1993). Nerve growth factor-induced hyperalgesia in the neonatal and adult rat. *J. Neurosci.* 1993; **13**, 2136–48.

Lewin, G. R., Rueff, A., and Mendell, L. M. (1994). Peripheral and central mechanisms of NGF-induced hyperalgesia. *Eur J Neurosci* **6**, 1903–12.

Mayer, E. A. and Bushnell, M. C. (eds.)(2009). Functional pain syndromes: presentation and pathophysiology. IASP Press, Seattle.

McLachlan, E. M., Jänig, W., Devor, M., and Michaelis, M. (1993). Peripheral nerve injury triggers noradrenergic sprouting within dorsal root ganglia. *Nature* **363**, 543–6.

McMahon, S. B. (1996). NGF as a mediator of inflammatory pain. *Philos. Trans. R. Soc. Lond B Biol. Sci.* **351**, 431–40.

Michaelis, M., Devor, M., and Jänig, W. (1996). Sympathetic modulation of activity in rat dorsal root ganglion neurons changes over time following peripheral nerve injury. *J. Neurophysiol.* **76**, 753–63.

Michaelis, M., Liu, X.-G., and Jänig, W. (2000). Peripheral nerve lesion induces ongoing discharges originating from dorsal root ganglia in axotomized and unlesioned muscle afferents. *J. Neurosci.* **20**, 2742–48.

Petty, B. G., Cornblath, D. R., Adornato, B. T., *et al.* (1994). The effect of systemically administered recombinant human nerve growth factor in healthy human subjects. *Ann. Neurol.* **36**, 244–6.

Sato, J. and Perl, E. R. (1991). Adrenergic excitation of cutaneous pain receptors induced by peripheral nerve injury. *Science* **251**, 1608–10.

Straub, R. H. and Härle, P. (2005). Sympathetic transmitters in joint inflammation. *Rheum. Dis. Clin. North Am.* **31**, 43–59.

Verri, W. A. Jr., Cunha, T. M., Parada, C. A., Poole, S., Cunha, F. Q., Ferreira, S. H. (2006). Hypernociceptive role of cytokines and chemokines: targets for analgesic drug development? *Pharmacol. Ther.* **112**, 116–38.

Woolf, C. J. (1996). Phenotypic modification of primary sensory neurons: the role of nerve growth factor in the production of persistent pain. *Phil. Trans. R. Soc. Lond B* **351**, 441–8.

Woolf, C. J., Ma, Q.-P., Allchorne, A., and Poole, S. (1996). Peripheral cell types contributing to the hyperalgesic action of nerve growth factor in inflammation. *J. Neurosci.* **16**, 2716–23.

CHAPTER 21

Temperature regulation and the autonomic nervous system

Kenneth J. Collins

Key points

- Destabilization of thermal control can arise from failure of central or peripheral components of the autonomic nervous system, resulting in syndromes of poikilothermia, hypothermia or hyperthermia.

- Core temperature is the predominant factor in the regulation of autonomic effector responses while both core and skin temperatures contribute equally in behavioural responses that are aimed at achieving thermal comfort.

- The coexistence of numerous neuropeptides in the thermoregulatory autonomic transmitter system suggests a sequence of relationships in the neuronal hierarchy controlling body temperature.

- Recent enquiry has focused on the central nervous co-ordination of thermal and non-thermal pathways; heat stress appears to modify baroreflex control of muscle sympathetic nerve activity and an orthostatic challenge may decrease skin blood flow in heat-stressed individuals.

- More attention has been directed to vagal afferent pathways in the thermoregulatory network that are involved in modulation of energy balance.

- Investigations into the nature of the sympathetic vasodilator nerves in the skin have highlighted the important role of vasoactive peptides, particularly vasoactive intestinal peptide, released from activated sympathetic sudomotor nerves.

- Central modulation of vasoconstrictor and vasodilator activities can be demonstrated and analysed by spectral characteristics of skin sympathetic nerves during heating and cooling.

- A pattern of regional sympathetic differentiation during the cold response phase in fever has been established, which differs from the sympathetic response to cold exposure.

Introduction

The stability of body temperature in humans and other homeostatic mammals requires active defence of set levels of temperature. The means by which homeostatic set levels could be generated by basic neuronal connections between sensors and correction effectors is mostly understood for many systems including thermoregulation. The nature of the set level determinant, however, remains largely ill-defined or undefined in most biological systems, except in one area—that of thermoregulation, which has received considerable theoretical consideration. The autonomic nervous system plays a crucial role in the integrative processes of thermoregulation, in its central nervous organization, in behavioural and metabolic responses, and in the peripheral effector mechanisms. Failure of any part of this system can bring about destabilization of thermal control, which is a feature of many of the important clinical syndromes involving autonomic dysfunction.

Central nervous control

The POAH region (preoptic area, anterior hypothalamus and septum) is a predominant site for integration of central and peripheral information and for control of thermoregulatory effector responses through the autonomic nervous system. Swaab (2004) has reviewed a number of case histories focusing on hypothalamic pathology in disorders of temperature regulation. Hypothermia, hyperthermia or poikilothermia may occur when the POAH area is damaged by infarction, subarachnoid haemorrhage, trauma or surgery. The literature suggests that large lesions in the posterior hypothalamus may impair heat production. Various converging excitatory and inhibitory influences on the control centres markedly change the relationship between activities of core temperature sensors and thermoregulatory responses, thereby temporarily altering the temperature thresholds of effector mechanisms. Hypothalamic thermoregulatory processing can be affected by higher cerebral activities such as in sleep or mental stress. In the schematic representation of human temperature regulation shown in Fig. 21.1, the heat loss effectors (HLE) and heat production effectors (HPE) function partly for behavioural thermocorrection (involving movement of the whole organism relative to the environment) and partly for autonomic thermocorrection (involving activities only of specialized cells and organs). At the hypothalamic interface, various techniques of examining central events in thermoregulation—disturbance/response analysis, effects of temperature upon central neuronal activities, and the effects of central synaptic interference—have led, quite independently, to the notion of reciprocal crossing inhibition in the central pathways.

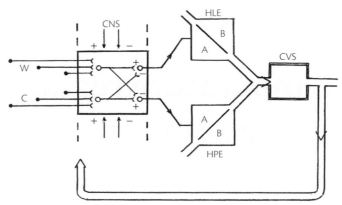

Fig. 21.1 A representation of the mammalian thermoregulatory system. Warm (W) and cold (C) thermosensors are located in the skin, in deep body tissues, and in the hypothalamus. The efferent pathways from the CNS control the activities of behavioural (B) and autonomic (A) heat loss effectors (HLE) and heat production effectors (HPE). The cardiovascular system (CVS) functions as a thermal mixer, the temperature of arterial blood acting as a thermal feedback to the thermosensors. Reprinted from *Journal of Thermal Biology*, **23**, Bligh J, Mammalian homeothermy: an integrative thesis, 143–258, Copyright 1998, with permission from Elsevier.

Many of the POAH neurons are sensitive to change in temperature, but most are temperature insensitive (Boulant 1998) (Fig 21.2). The possible set point role for separate interactions of temperature insensitive neurons with pathways from warm and cold sensors has been discussed by Bligh (1998). The proposition is that the basic set level determination is the consequence of interplay between two species of hypothalamic neurons, one strongly temperature sensitive and the other only weakly or totally unresponsive, and the influence of their activities upon opposing thermocorrective effectors. It has been postulated that there must be some as yet undefined differential gating in the various final pathways that control heat production or loss processes by the central nervous system (CNS). While it is recognized that the POAH region of the brain plays a major role in the integration of nervous pathways, temperature regulation has been shown to involve a hierarchical neuronal network extending from the cerebral cortex, hypothalamus and limbic system to the lower brainstem, reticular formation, spinal cord and sympathetic pathways. The theory built around the dominance of hypothalamic thermosensitivity, however, remains presumptive rather than proven (Romanovsky 2007). There are, for example, circumstances when the influence of extrahypothalamic and indeed extra-central thermosensitivity could be the dominant influence on the activities of thermocorrection effectors, and therefore on body temperature.

Central synaptic studies

Studies of mammalian thermoregulation based on specific chemical interference with synaptic events followed the discovery that the hypothalamus contains relatively large concentrations of noradrenaline (NA) and 5-hydroxytryptamine (5-HT). It was proposed that the intrahypothalamic release of these two monoamines controlled normal thermoregulation. The technique of introducing substances into the brain side of the blood–brain barrier, pioneered by W. Feldberg in the 1960s, revealed that there were accompanying changes in body temperature. Intraventricular injections of 5-HT in cats and primates caused peripheral vasoconstriction, shivering, and huddling, leading to a raised body temperature. In contrast, NA activated processes led to a fall in body temperature. It is difficult to accept the suggestion made at the

time that the differential release of two endogenous monoamines could be the set point determinant (Bligh 1998). Their roles are more likely that of synaptic transmitters, the release of which are caused by afferent events. Microinjection experiments show that cholinoceptive sites are widely scattered between the levels of the optic chiasma and mammillary bodies, in contrast to the more restricted sites in the POAH for NA and 5-HT.

A great number of known and putative transmitter substances have now been shown to have effects upon thermoregulation in central synaptic interference studies. However, opposite effects on thermoregulatory responses with the same transmitter substance have been shown in different mammalian species. Apart from prostaglandin E, which plays a crucial role in the genesis of fevers, no putative neurotransmitter or mediator has had the same effect in all mammals tested. As a systemic mediator, nitric oxide (NO) has been shown to facilitate thermolytic mechanisms, mainly due to its circulatory action. It does not seem to affect most thermoregulatory effectors in a manner sufficient to be attributable to a specific messenger function in control of body temperature. At the central level, however, there seems to exist a consistent inverse relationship between body temperature and systemic NO action in fever (Schmid et al. 1998).

A number of hypothalamic neuropeptides have also been identified that are of importance in normal central thermoregulatory control. For many of these peptides, the information available is insufficient to establish their role (e.g. cholecystokinin, luteinizing hormone-releasing factor, neurotensin), but for some (e.g. glucocorticoids, α-melanocyte-stimulating hormone, arginine vasopressin) there is good evidence that they may participate as thermolytic substances acting within the brain to reduce fever (Kluger et al. 1998). Endogenous opioids such as β-endorphin and met-enkephalin appear to participate in changes in body temperature evoked by stress. The coexistence of so many peptides that alter temperature suggests that there must be a sequence of relationships between peptides and temperature in specific brain tissues, with some specifically involved in hypothalamic pathways and others more important for autonomic effector functions influencing temperature.

Sympathetic pre-motor neurons play a crucial role mediating efferent signals from higher autonomic centres directly to

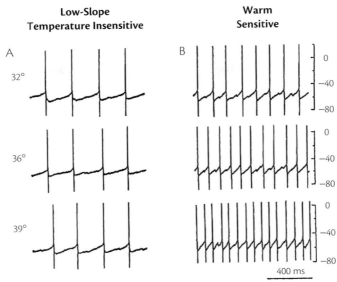

Fig. 21.2 Effect of temperature on the firing rate and interspike interval of two types of POAH (preoptic area, anterior hypothalamus and septum) neurons: **(A)** temperature insensitive neurons and **(B)** warm sensitive neurons. Warming increases the firing rate only in the warm-sensitive neurons and decreases action potential amplitude in both types of neuron. Reprinted from *Brain Function in Hot Environments*, HS Sharma and G Westman eds., Cellular mechanisms of temperature sensitivity in hypothalamic neurons, Boulant JA pp. 3–8 Copyright 1998, with permission from Elsevier.

sympathetic preganglionic neurons in the intermediolateral cell columns of the spinal cord. Excitatory pre-motor sympathetic neurons controlling thermoregulatory structures have been identified with expression of vesicular glutamate transporter (VGLUT)3 whereas those for cardiovascular control are characterized with (VGLUT)2 expression (Nakamura et al. 2005).

Non-thermal/thermal central interactions

The model of the central pathways in Fig. 21.1 is not presented as if it were an isolated and independently operating function for thermoregulation. There are many non-thermal convergent influences derived from the activities of other pathways through the CNS (Mekjavic and Eiken 2006). For example, POAH neurons send axons to and receive projections from the ventromedial and lateral hypothalamus, pathways that affect feeding behaviour. Hypothalamic control of thermoregulatory responses is considerably influenced by other biological responses, such as changes in fluid and electrolyte balance, hypercapnia etc. Heat stress appears to modify the human baroreflex control of muscle sympathetic nerve activity (MSNA) independently of heat-induced hypovolaemia in humans and it is suggested that this stems from central neural interactions between thermoregulatory and baroreflex systems (Kamiya et al. 2003). The effects of baroreceptor loading/unloading on sweating and skin blood flow are less clear. Skin sympathetic nerve activity (SSNA) and sweat rate do not appear to be modulated by arterial baroreflexes in normothermic or moderately heated individuals (Wilson et al. 2001). However, in heat-stressed individuals, there is evidence that the cutaneous vasoconstrictor system is engaged, and is capable of decreasing skin blood flow during an orthostatic challenge (Shibasaki et al. 2006). Integration of thermal and non-thermal regulatory functions is involved in selective brain cooling (Caputa 2004), which allows the brain to remain cooler than the rest of the body. This type of cooling in homeotherms is achieved by the pre-cooling of blood destined for the brain with cool venous blood returning from the nose and head skin, and by cooling the brain directly by venous blood. Common to both is a reduced sympathetic nerve activity, which leads simultaneously to dilatation of the angular oculi veins supplying the intracranial heat exchangers and constriction of the facial veins supplying the heart. Selective brain cooling is shown to be enhanced during heat exposure, exercise and NREM sleep, and is absent in cold conditions.

Behavioural thermoregulation

Behavioural responses (e.g. postural changes in heat or cold), are of primary importance in thermoregulation. The frontal cortex participates through its connections with the ipsilateral POAH (Nagashima et al. 2000). Dysfunction of the cortical or POAH structures or loss of peripheral thermosensitivity can jeopardize inherent learned behavioural thermoregulation (see section on poikilothermia). One effect of behavioural responses is to modify the relationship between the organism and its environment, thereby altering the need for autonomic thermoregulation. The autonomic reactions are principally directed at achieving a virtual constant core temperature. Thermoregulatory behaviour, on the other hand, appears to be aimed at maintaining skin temperature at a level of thermal comfort. Achieving thermal comfort is therefore a primary stimulus for behavioural thermoregulation. Investigations have been made by independently altering core temperature and skin temperature while measuring thermal comfort and autonomic responses (Frank et al. 1999). It is suggested that core temperature and skin temperature contribute equally to thermal comfort, while core temperature predominates in the regulation of autonomic effector and metabolic responses.

Autonomic effector systems

The main sympathetic efferent pathways controlling the effector systems in human thermoregulation are those for heat gain (metabolic) and those for heat loss (vasomotor and sudomotor). Attention has been paid recently to the afferent side of the thermoregulatory network through the vagus nerve conveying signals for peripheral infection responsible for the induction of fever, as well as for the transfer of nutritional and/or metabolic signals to the brain.

Thermogenesis

Homeotherms have five major physiological defences against cold, behavioural responses, cutaneous vasoconstriction, piloerection, metabolic thermogenesis and shivering. Heat production by shivering is controlled through somatic innervation to skeletal muscles with a primary motor centre in the dorsomedial region of the posterior hypothalamus and is not a peripheral autonomic function. Metabolic thermogenesis in cold conditions is, however, a function of sympathetic nervous regulation through the control of non-shivering thermogenesis (NST).

An important source of NST is brown adipose tissue, a specialized tissue innervated by adrenergic nerves and easily identifiable in cold-acclimatized animals and young mammals including human neonates. In brown adipose tissue there is a dense sympathetic innervation. Noradrenaline activates G-protein-coupled β-adrenergic receptors, thus initiating a cascade of metabolic events culminating in the activation of uncoupling protein 1 (UCP1). In recent years, several new members of the mitochondrial carrier protein family have been identified. All appear to possess uncoupling properties in genetically modified systems, with two of them, UCP2 and UCP3 (homologues of UCP1), being expressed in adipose tissue and skeletal muscle, which are recognized as important sites for variations in thermogenesis (Dulloo and Samec 2001). The expression of UCP1 is strongly induced by cold exposure and is modulated by diet and metabolic hormones such as leptin and glucocorticoids (Sell et al. 2004).

NST may also be produced in the adult human by the calorigenic action of catecholamines and other hormones acting on muscles and other tissues. In subjects exposed to air at 12°C for 8 hours daily, electromyographic activity resulting from shivering, together with increased oxygen consumption, both decline with successive exposures. Oxygen consumption, however, declines less than muscle activity, and this has been interpreted as evidence for the development of NST in adults. Outdoor workers such as lumberjacks are reported to develop deposits of brown adipose tissue, while indoor workers of the same age do not. The inference is that those who spend much time exposed to cold can develop brown adipose tissue as a cold defence mechanism in addition to catecholamine NST in other tissues. Thyroxine may play a part as an endogenous transmitter (mediator) for NST. Evidence is lacking, however, that thyroid stimulation is a prerequisite for the development of cold adaptation, for in humans there is no consistent thyroid-stimulating hormone response to acute cooling. Thyroid hormone may increase adrenergic stimulation, however, in part by increasing the number of β-receptors. Patients with pathological elevations of calorigenic hormones as in thyrotoxicosis and phaeochromocytoma often have an associated hyperthermia and in a severe thyroid crisis the body temperature can rise quite rapidly to levels observed in heat stroke.

As mentioned above, the vagus nerve may influence thermoregulation by modulation of energy balance: its afferent fibres convey signals on feeding states resulting in depression or stimulation of metabolic processes. Vagally transmitted neural signals associated with hunger, stimuli from the gut and hepatoportal region, and decline in blood glucose, alter rates of discharge of vagal afferents and the activity of the nucleus of the solitary tract. The biological role of these vagal afferent functions is seen not as directly related to the regulation of body temperature but rather to the regulation of energy balance and the body's energy content (Székely 2000).

Vasomotor control of sensible heat transfer

The flow of energy by convection, conduction, and radiation at the skin interface that can be sensed and measured as heat is referred to as sensible heat transfer. It is largely a function of the autonomic control of vasomotor responses in the skin. The largest group of sympathetic neurons supplying the skin is the noradrenergic vasoconstrictor fibres. At rest in normal ambient temperatures, spontaneous cutaneous sympathetic activity consisting of bursts of impulses have been recorded intraneurally in peripheral nerves, which appear to represent centrally entrained bursts of vasoconstrictor activity. Cold-induced vasoconstriction in skin blood vessels is mediated at least in part by increased activity of vascular smooth muscle α_2-adrenoceptors (Bailey et al. 2004). Investigations of the α_1- and α_2-adrenoceptors involved in the contraction of deep and superficial cutaneous vessels in the limbs have shown that superficial vessels constrict more strongly to noradrenaline than deep vessels when cooled. These differences may relate to the differences in the adrenoceptors and to the local modulation of NO. It is possible that the different responsiveness of superficial and deep cutaneous vessels could allow limbs to dissipate more heat when warm and conserve heat when cool (Roberts et al. 2002).

In extremities such as the hands and feet, blood vessels in the skin are normally subjected to high levels of vasoconstrictor tone that is released when core temperature rises. In the forearm, vasodilatation is mediated by vasodilator nerves associated with sweating which is greater than can be explained by complete release of the vasoconstrictor tone. Active vasodilatation in human skin depends on functional cholinergic fibres but appears mainly to be synchronized with the occurrence of sweating; sympathetic bursts of activity followed by a vasodilator response without sweat expulsion have not been observed. The active vasodilatation is therefore thought to be elicited by sympathetic cholinergic sudomotor nerves.

The spectral power and its distribution in skin sympathetic nerve activity is a useful index for quantitative description. Thus it is found that whole body heating and cooling significantly increase integrated spectral power, the greatest increase occurring in the very high frequency region during heating but not during cooling. The spectral distribution of skin sympathetic nerve activity during heat stress is different from that during normothermia and cooling, which may reflect differences in central modulation of sudomotor/vasodilator effects relative to vasoconstrictor neural activities (Fig. 21.3) (Cui et al. 2006).

Varicosities in cholinergic nerves surrounding sweat glands show strongly immunohistochemically stained antibodies against vasoactive intestinal peptide (VIP). Intradermal microdialysis of VIP has been investigated in discrete areas of the skin in the presence of different levels of the VIP receptor antagonist, VIP (10–28)

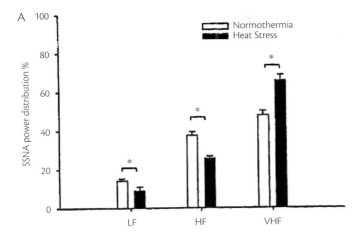

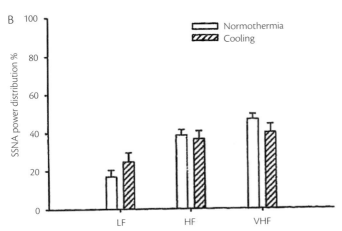

Fig. 21.3 Distribution of skin sympathetic nerve activity (SSNA) spectral power during: **(A)** normothermia and heat stress in human subjects (n = 17) and **(B)** normothermia and cooling (n = 7). Values are means ± SE. Spectral power in low frequency (LF), high frequency (HF) and very high frequency (VHF) regions is expressed as a percentage of total power in each thermal condition. (* significantly different from normothermia, p < 0 05). With permission from The American Physiological Society (Cui et al. 2006).

(Bennett et al. 2003). At the control site, VIP caused a vasodilatation typical of heat stress, and this was attenuated by VIP (10–28). NO may also contribute to the vasodilator response, but does not appear to be the prime agent (Shastry et al. 2000). At least part of the vasoconstrictor response to local skin cooling appears to involve an inhibitory effect on nitric oxide synthase (NOS) activity (Hodges et al. 2006).

Sudomotor control of insensible heat loss

Heat loss through sweating involves evaporative latent heat and is described as insensible heat transfer because it cannot be sensed instrumentally. Sudomotor nerves surrounding the eccrine sweat glands are composed of non-myelinated class C fibres that react strongly in tests for cholinesterase. The predominantly cholinergic sympathetic neurons are accompanied by a few adrenergic terminals. Cytological studies of the glands show that in the early stages of development sudomotor nerves appear to be adrenergic. During development, however, noradrenergic neurons lose their store of endogenous catecholamines, but not their capacity for uptake and

storage. It is proposed that this constitutes evidence of neurotransmitter plasticity as sudomotor neurons appear to undergo transition from noradrenergic to cholinergic function during development *in vivo*, similar to that described in cell cultures.

An overview of the effects and correlates of ageing in the autonomic nervous system (Cowen and Santer 2002) include some of the most striking features of plasticity and neurotrophic actions in the sudomotor system. Immunohistochemical studies demonstrate marked regression of secretory coil morphology with age accompanied by a significant decrease in the number of immunoreactive nerve varicosities and nerve bundles. Only traces of normally strongly acetylcholinesterase-positive sudomotor nerve fibres have been found in elderly people, together with diminished content of VIP and calcitonin-gene-related peptide (CGRP)-like immunoreactivity. VIP, CGRP, atrial natriuretic peptide (ANP) and substance P (SP) have all been identified as possible cotransmitters.

Some of the more important primary autonomic disorders, central nervous disorders and peripheral neuropathies associated with anhidrosis and thermoregulatory failure have been classified by Fealey (2000). Acquired idiopathic generalized anhidrosis represents a heterogeneous clinical syndrome that includes sudomotor neuropathy and failure of the sweat glands. Sudomotor function testing reveals a complete absence of thermoregulatory sweating. Pilocarpine did not induce sweating, microneurography showed that bursts of skin sympathetic nerve activity were not decreased, and skin biopsy showed no abnormalities in the sweat glands (Nakazato et al. 2004). These findings suggest lesions on the postsynaptic side of the of the neuroglandular junctions, the lesion being located in the muscarinic cholinergic receptors. Sweating dysfunction has also been investigated in cases of familial dysautonomia (Hilz et al. 2004). The average density of epidermal nerve fibres is greatly diminished with severe loss from the subepidermal neural plexus and deep dermis. The few sweat glands present had reduced innervation density. SP and CGRP were virtually absent, but VIP immunoreactive nerves were present in the subepidermal plexus. Decreased SP and CGRP in sudomotor endings suggest that in familial disautonomia, gene mutation causes secondary neurotransmitter depletions.

Autonomic nervous system in disorders of thermoregulation

Central autonomic failure, preganglionic and postganglionic neuronal degeneration, and peripheral neuropathies are frequently associated with thermoregulatory dysregulation. Thermoregulatory tests are described in Chapter 22, and it should be emphasized that it is crucial to determine whether the primary cause of autonomic dysfunction could result from failure of the target organ. In clinical practice it is also important to establish whether an abnormal autonomic response might be based on the effects of any of a wide range of drugs that enhance or interfere with autonomic nervous function. Disorders of thermoregulation that help to characterize autonomic involvement often destabilize the control of core temperature and result in syndromes of poikilothermia, hypothermia or hyperthermia.

Poikilothermia

Poikilothermia, the lack of regulated constancy of body temperature, may be diagnosed by abnormal fluctuation in core temperature of more than 2°C caused by small changes in ambient temperature. The condition usually relates to disturbances in central thermoregulatory control even under normal temperature conditions. Although there appears to be a heterogeneity of brain lesions responsible for the condition, it is claimed that poikilothermia in humans is caused principally by lesions in the posterior hypothalamus or midbrain. It is known, however, that paraplegics and tetraplegics may suffer from a condition of partial poikilothermia. They show a lower core temperature in the cold and higher core temperature in the heat when compared with physically non-disabled. The partial failure to maintain a constant core temperature independent of fluctuations in ambient temperature appears to be due to a lack of effector control. Patients with acquired poikilothermia studied by MacKenzie et al. (1996) did not have generalized autonomic failure and the poikilothermia was attributed predominantly to disorders of the central thermoregulatory pathways. Relative poikilothermia, usually in the absence of acquired

hypothalamic disease, is frequently encountered in the newborn and also in old age when elderly people fail to respond adequately to thermal stress.

Hypothermia

Hypothermia, defined by the Royal College of Physicians in 1966 as a deep body temperature below 35°C, most commonly arises as a result of accidental and excessive exposure to cold. Dysfunction or failure of central or peripheral autonomic control is one of many settings associated with primary hypothermia due to impairment of the thermoregulatory system. Many clinical conditions can lead to cold intolerance when low body temperature results from secondary causes such as endocrine, neural, and cardiovascular disease or commonly to the effects of drugs. Ageing is often associated with hypothermia and autonomic dysfunction (Collins 2006). Skin sympathoexcitatory responses to cooling are attenuated in

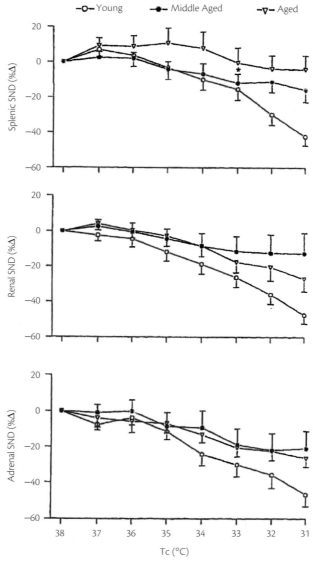

Fig. 21.4 Percentage change in splenic, renal and adrenal sympathetic nerve discharge (SND) during progressive hypothermia (core temperature T c reduced to 31°C) in young, middle-aged and elderly rats (means ± SD). With permission from The American Physiological Society (Helwig et al. 2006).

elderly people compared with young people. Ageing also appears to alter visceral sympathetic nerve responses to acute hypothermia (Helwig et al. 2006) (Fig. 21.4).

Acute central nervous dysfunction with hypothalamic involvement and with transient hypothermia has been described. Agenesis of the corpus callosum, a developmental anomaly causing epilepsy and mental retardation, is often associated with periodic hypothermia (Shapiro's syndrome) through central nervous abnormalities affecting central thermoregulatory control (Tambasco et al. 2005). Hypothermia after acute blood loss has been regarded as an adaptive response that enables the organism to adapt to hypoxic conditions by decreasing cellular metabolism. The hypothermic response appears to involve a centrally mediated component with a high incidence of baroreceptor input to POAH thermosensitive neurons (Hori and Katafuchi 1998).

Hyperthermia

The condition of a thermoregulator whose core temperature is above its set range of temperatures for its normal active state is described as hyperthermia. From the point of view of temperature regulation, hyperthermia exists when heat defence processes such as skin vasodilatation and sweating are working near the limit of their capacity. Central nervous dysfunction leading to hyperthermia originates from many of the lesions also reported for hypothermia and depends on the exact site of the lesion in the thermoregulatory neuraxis. Similarly many of the drugs capable of

inducing hypothermia such as alcohol, antidepressants, psychotropics, and anaesthetics may also induce hyperthermia, depending on the dose and prevailing temperature conditions. Heatstroke is characterized by a core temperature of 4°C or more, accompanied by central nervous disturbances leading to convulsions and coma, and usually anhidrosis (Collins 2003). There are prodromal features of mental confusion and hyperthermia. Anhidrosis is not pathognomic of heat stroke, but autopsy studies reveal oedema of the brain and meninges, and degenerative changes in neurons and petechiae that are common in the walls of the third and fourth ventricles. Neuroleptic malignant syndrome is a rare but potentially lethal complication of medication with neuroleptic agents such as phenothiazines and butyrophenones, particularly in combination with lithium. Symptoms usually progress rapidly over 1–3 days and include hyperthermia, rigidity and tremor, impaired consciousness, and autonomic dysfunction resulting in tachycardia, sweating and labile blood pressure. There is evidence to support the hypothesis that dysregulated sympathetic nervous system hyperactivity is responsible for most of the features of the syndrome (Gurrera 1999). Malignant hyperthermia is a rare hereditary disorder that presents during anaesthesia, especially with halothane and the use of succinylcholine. Skeletal muscle rigidity leading to hyperthermia appears to be due to a sudden rise in the concentration of calcium in muscle cytoplasm. Autonomic cardiovascular disturbances occur including ventricular arrhythmia, tachycardia, sweating, and falling blood pressure, and these may herald a hyperthermic crisis.

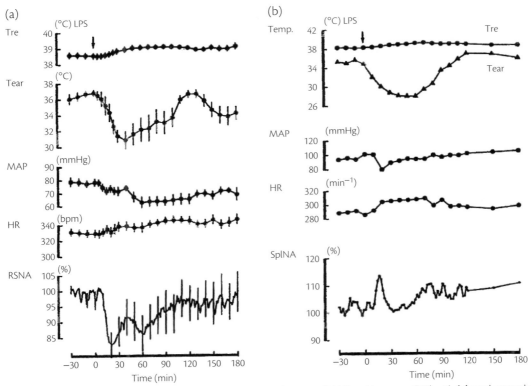

Fig. 21.5 Time course of rectal temperature (Tre), ear temperature (T ear), mean arterial pressure (MAP) and heart rate (HR) with **(a)** renal sympathetic nerve activity (RSNA) and **(b)** splanchnic nerve activity (SplNA) after intravenous injection of lipopolysaccharide (LPS) in rabbits (means ± SE). Reprinted from *Brain Function in Hot Environments*, HS Sharma and G Westman eds., Regional differentiation of sympathetic afferents during fever, Iriki M and Saigusa T, pp. 477–97 Copyright 1998, with permission from Elsevier.

Fever

Fever is not itself a pathological condition, but a physiological response to a foreign substance, usually a microbial endotoxin. It is defined as a state of elevated core temperature which is often, but not necessarily, part of the defensive response to the invasion of pathogens. In contrast to hyperthermia, fever, at least in the phase of rising core temperature, causes activation of cold defence responses such as vasoconstriction and shivering that raise the core temperature to a new level at which thermal neutrality is achieved. The core temperature is then actively defended at the febrile level by intact autonomic and behavioural mechanisms. As the fever abates, regulatory processes appear that are opposed to excess warming and as a result the core temperature falls to normal level again. There is evidence to suggest that a vagal afferent input from abdominally located sensors is part of the pathway through which microbial endotoxins give rise to fever (Romanovsky et al. 1997).

Autonomic failure, either centrally or in the periphery, could presumably alter the febrile response and compromise the physiological defence systems. The elderly, a group in whom there is strong evidence of incipient autonomic dysfunction (Collins 2006), show a blunted or absent fever response to infection in a significant proportion of patients with bacteraemia. Experimental evidence from animal studies also suggests age-related impairments in the fever reaction induced by endogenous pyrogens.

There is a pattern of regional sympathetic differentiation during fever that differs from the sympathetic response during cold exposure (Iriki and Saigusa 1998) (Fig. 21.5). Fever was studied in rabbits by administering lipopolysaccharide as a pyrogenic substance. Within 10–20 minutes rectal temperature started to rise and ear skin temperature decreased indicating enhanced vasoconstriction due to increased skin sympathetic nerve activity (SkSNA). Directly recorded renal sympathetic nerve activity (RSNA), however, was reduced. Since mean arterial pressure (MAP) decreased, it is unlikely that this inhibition was reflexly induced. At the same time, splanchnic sympathetic nerve activity (SplSNA) was augmented rather than inhibited. The response occurred before MAP decreased, and again was probably not generated reflexly although it may have been modified by the change in baroreceptor input. Unlike the febrile response, SplSNA decreased rather than increased (and also RSNA decreased) when a cold defence response was induced by spinal cord cooling. These responses indicate that the pattern of regional sympathetic differentiation during fever is different from that during cold exposure. Other studies of the manner in which pyrogenic cytokines exert their influence on the brain side of the blood–brain barrier (Blatteis 2006), give evidence that a vagal afferent input from hepatic sensors projecting to the POAH is part of the pathway through which microbial endotoxins give rise to fever.

References

Bailey, S. R., Eid, A. H., Mitra, S. and Flavahan, N. A. (2004). Rho/kinase mediates cold-induced constriction of cutaneous arteries: role of (alpha) 2C-adrenoceptor translocation. *Circulation Research* **94**, 1367–74.

Bennett, L. A. T., Johnson, J. M., Stephens, D. P., Saad, A. R. and Kellogg, D. L. (2003). Evidence for a role for vasoactive intestinal peptide in active vasodilatation in cutaneous vasculature of humans. *J Physiol.* **552**, 223–32.

Blatteis, C. M. (2006). Endotoxic fever. New concept of its regulation suggests new approaches to its management. *Pharmacology and Therapeutics*, **111**, 194–223.

Bligh, J. (1998). Mammalian homeothermy: an integrative thesis. *Journal of Thermal Biology* **23**, 143–258.

Boulant, J. A. (1998). Cellular mechanisms of temperature sensitivity in hypothalamic neurons. In H.S. Sharma and J. Westman, eds. *Progress in Brain Research 115, Brain Function in Hot Environments*, pp. 3–8. Elsevier, Amsterdam.

Caputa, M. (2004). Selective brain cooling: a multiple regulatory mechanism. *Journal of Thermal Biology* **29**, 691–702.

Collins K. J. (2003). Heat stress and associated disorders. In G.C. Cook and A.I. Zubin, eds. *Manson's Tropical Diseases, 21st Edition*, pp. 545—54. Saunders, Elsevier, Amsterdam.

Collins, K. J. (2006). Abnormalities of the autonomic nervous system. In M. S. J. Pathy, A. J. Sinclair and J. E. Morley, eds. *Principles and Practice of Geriatric Medicine, 4th Edition, Volume 1*, pp. 969—80. John Wiley & Sons Ltd, Chichester.

Cowen, T. and Santer, R. M. (2002). Ageing in the autonomic nervous system: processes and mechanisms. *Autonomic Neurosciences: Basic and Clinical* **96**, 1—83.

Cui, J., Sathishkumar, M., Wilson, T. E., Shibasaki, M., Davis, S. L. and Crandall, C. G. (2006). Spectral characteristics of skin sympathetic nerve activity in heat-stressed humans. *Am. J Physiol. Heart Circ. Physiol.* **290**, H1601–9.

Dulloo, A. G. and Samec, S. (2001). Uncoupling proteins: their roles in adaptive thermogenesis and substrate metabolism reconsidered. *British Journal of Nutrition* **86**, 123–39.

Fealey, R. D. (2000). Thermoregulatory failure. In O. Appenzeller, ed. *Handbook of Clinical Neurology*, 75, *The Autonomic Nervous System. Part II. Dysfunctions*. pp. 53—83. Elsevier Science BV, Amsterdam.

Frank, S. M., Raja, S. N., Bulcao, C. F. and Goldstein, D. S. (1999). Relative contribution of core and cutaneous temperatures to thermal comfort and autonomic responses in humans. *J Appl. Physiol.*, **86**, 1588–93.

Gurrera, R. J. (1999). Sympathoadrenal hyperactivity and the etiology of neuroleptic malignant syndrome. *Am. J Psych.* **156**, 169–80.

Helwig, B. G., Parimi, S., Ganta, C. K., Cober, R., Fels, R. J. and Kenney, M. J. (2006). Aging alters regulation of visceral sympathetic nerve responses to acute hypothermia. *American Journal of Physiology. Regulation, Integration and Comparative Physiology* **291**, R573–9.

Hilz, M. J., Axelrod, F. B., Bickel, A., Stemper, B., Brys, M., Wendelschafer-Crab, G. and Kennedy, W. R. (2004). Assessing function and pathology in familial dysautonomia: assessment of temperature perception, sweating and cutaneous innervation. *Brain*, **127**, 2090–8.

Hodges, G. J., Zhao, K., Kosiba, W. A. and Johnson, J. M. (2006). The involvement of nitric oxide in the cutaneous vasoconstrictor response to local cooling in humans. *J Physiol.*, **574**, 849–57.

Hori, T. and Katafuchi, T. (1998). Cell biology and the functions of thermosensitive neurons in the brain. In H. S. Sharma and G. Westman, eds. *Progress in Brain Research 115, Brain Function in Hot Environments*, pp.9–23, Elsevier, Amsterdam.

Iriki, M. and Saigusa, T. (1998). Regional differentiation of sympathetic afferents during fever. In H. S. Sharma and G. Westman, eds. *Progress in Brain Research 115, Brain Function in Hot Environments*, pp. 477–97, Elsevier, Amsterdam.

Kamiya, A., Michikami, D., Hayano, J. and Sunagawa, K. (2003). Heat stress modifies human baroreflex function independently of heat-induced hypovolemia. *Jpn. J Physiol.* **53**, 49–62.

Kluger, M. J., Kozak, W., Leon, L. R., Soszynski, D. and Conn, C. A. (1998). Fever and antipyresis. In H. S. Sharma and G. Westman, eds. *Progress in Brain Research 115, Brain Function in Hot Environments*, pp. 465–75, Elsevier, Amsterdam.

MacKenzie, M. A., Wollersheim, H. C., Lenders, J. W., Hermus, A. R. and Thien, T. (1996). Skin blood flow and autonomic reactivity in human poikilothermia. *Clin. Aut. Res,* **6**, 91–7.

Mekjavic, I. B. and Eiken, O. (2006). Contribution of thermal and nonthermal factors to the regulation of body temperature in humans. *J Appl. Physiol.,* **100**, 2065–72.

Nagashima, K., Nakai, S., Tanaka, M. and Kanosue,K. (2000). Neuronal circuitries involved in thermoregulation. *Autonomic Neuroscience: Basic and Clinical* **85**, 18–25.

Nakamura, K., Matsumura, K., Kobayashi, S. and Kaneko, T. (2005). Sympathetic premotor neurons mediating thermoregulatory functions. *Neurosci. Res.* **51**, 1–8.

Nakazato, Y., Tamura, N., Ohkuma, A., Yoshimaru, K. and Shimazu, K. (2004). Idiopathic pure sudomotor failure: anhidrosis due to deficits in cholinergic transmission. *Neurology* **63**, 1476—80.

Roberts, M., Rivers, T., Oliveria, S., Texeira, P. and Raman, E. (2002). Adrenoceptor and local modulator control of cutaneous blood flow in thermal stress. *Comparative Biochemistry and Physiology. A molecular and integrative physiology* **131**, 485–96.

Romanovsky, A. A. (2007). Thermoregulation: some concepts have changed. Functional architecture of the thermoregulatory system. *American Journal of Physiology. Regulatory, integrative and comparative physiology.* **292**, 37–46.

Romanovsky, A. A., Simons, C. J., Székely, M. and Kulchitsky, V. A. (1997). Febrile irresponsiveness of vagotomised rats to a pyrogenic signal: non-sensing brain or non-heating body. *Proceedings of the New York Academy of Sciences,* **813**, 437–44.

Schmid, H. A., Riedel, W. and Simon, E. (1998). Role of nitric oxide in temperature regulation. In H. S. Sharma and J. Westman, eds. *Progress in Brain Research 115, Brain function in hot environments,* pp. 87—110. Elsevier, Amsterdam.

Sell, H., Deshaies, Y. and Richard, D. (2004). The brown adipocyte: update on its metabolic role. *Int. J Biochem. Cell. Biol.* **36**, 2098—104.

Shastry, S., Minson, C. T., Wilson, S. A., Dietz, N. M. and Joyner, M. J. (2000). The effect of atropine and L—NAME on cutaneous blood flow during body heating in humans. *J Appl. Physiol.* **88**, 467–72.

Shibasaki, M., Davis, S. L., Cui, J., Low, D. A., Keller, D. M., Durand, S. and Crandall, C. G. (2006). Neurally mediated vasoconstriction is capable of decreasing skin blood flow during orthostasis in the heat-stressed human. *J Physiol.,* **575**, 953–9.

Swaab, D. F. (2004). Autonomic disorders. Temperature regulation and disturbed thermoregulation. In *Handbook of Clinical Neurology* **80**, 355—60.

Székely, M. (2000). The vagus nerve in thermoregulation and energy metabolism. *Autonomic Neuroscience,* **85**, 26–38.

Tambasco, N., Corea, F. and Bocola, V. (2005). Subtotal corpus callosum agenesis with recurrent hyperhidrosis-hypothermia (Shapiro syndrome). *Neurology* **65**, 124.

Wilson, T. E., Cui, J. and Crandall, C. G. (2001). Absence of arterial baroreflex modulation of skin sympathetic activity and sweat rate during whole-body heating in humans. *J Physiol.* **536**, 615–23.

PART III

Clinical Autonomic Testing

CHAPTER 22

Investigation of autonomic disorders

Christopher J. Mathias, David A. Low,
Valeria Iodice and Roger Bannister

Introduction

In a patient with a suspected autonomic disorder the major aims of investigation are:

1 to determine whether autonomic function is normal or abnormal

2 to assess the degree of dysfunction, in determining the site of the lesion

3 to ascertain whether the abnormality is of primary or secondary to recognized disorders, as the prognosis and management will depend on the diagnostic category.

4 to obtain information on the underlying pathophysiological processes, and effect of stimuli in daily life on autonomic responses as the former are of importance in development of novel treatment, and the latter for ensuring holistic management especially in generalized autonomic disorders.

In this chapter an overview of the ways to investigate the autonomic nervous system is provided (Table 22.1). A range of systems is covered, with an emphasis on the cardiovascular system, where there have been numerous advances, especially in non-invasive measurement and in recognizing the role of compensatory systems, including various hormones. It should be emphasized that assessment of autonomic function depends not only on reflex arcs and on efferent nerve activity but also on end-organ responsiveness, where factors that include the metabolic clearance and disposition of transmitters, postsynaptic receptors, and second messenger systems influence the final response. Therefore each test, and the information from it, should be considered in relation to the whole clinical picture, and closely linked with factors in daily life where relevant. The information from investigations is needed not only for diagnosis but also for evaluation of therapy and assessment of its benefits.

In certain autonomic disorders specific 'non-autonomic' investigations may be needed. An example is in Horner's syndrome where further investigation in identifying the cause is of greater importance than the assessment of the autonomic deficit. The tests may include a computed tomography (CT) or magnetic resonance imaging (MRI) scan to exclude midbrain or medullary infarction, a CT scan of the thorax along with bronchoscopy to exclude Pancoast's syndrome (a malignancy in the apex of the lung), or carotid angiography to exclude dissection of the internal carotid artery.

Interpretation of test results

No single test can provide a global assessment of autonomic function. Even if directed towards a single system, testing usually involves a variety of procedures. Those used as 'screening' or 'standard' tests in our Autonomic Units in London are listed in Appendix I. These are directed predominantly towards cardiovascular autonomic function. This is of particular value as postural hypotension is often a cardinal feature, especially in patients with a generalized autonomic disorder and syncope for the presentation in intermittent disorders. The detection and evaluation of postural hypotension is important because it may be an early sign of sympathetic vasoconstrictor failure; many also have impaired heart rate responses to various stimuli because of cardiac parasympathetic failure. This is often the reverse of what is observed in the intermittent disorders. If the responses to cardiovascular reflex testing are within expected limits, this information, in conjunction with the rest of the clinical picture, is often helpful in excluding the primary autonomic failure syndromes and indicates that other explanations for the features should be sought. If the responses are abnormal and suggest autonomic failure, they reinforce the case for further evaluation. The majority of screening tests are directed towards the determination of autonomic impairment. However, autonomic overactivity is of importance in certain disorders and contributes to morbidity or even mortality. Examples are increased cardiac vagal activity in autonomic mediated syncope (Chapters 55 and 56), and paroxysmal hypertension as part of autonomic dysreflexia in high spinal cord injuries (Chapter 66); specific testing is needed if such disorders are suspected.

The need for 'normal' and ideally 'control' values, and their relevance, warrants discussion. Although the principles of autonomic testing, and the interpretation of the results should be universally applied, the precise levels and ranges of responses to various stimuli depend upon a large number of factors. Some of these include the specific laboratory conditions during testing (such as the room temperature), the nature and specification of testing equipment used, the sophistication of the recording equipment and computer

Table 22.1 Outline of investigations in autonomic failure

Cardiovascular	Head-up tilt (60°)*; Standing*; Valsalva manoeuvre*
	Pressor stimuli—isometric exercise*, cutaneous cold*, mental arithmetic*
	Heart rate responses—deep breathing*, hyperventilation*, standing*, head-up tilt*
	Liquid meal challenge
	Exercise testing
	Carotid sinus massage, head and neck movements
	24-hour ambulatory blood pressure and heart rate monitoring
Biochemical	Plasma noradrenaline, adrenaline, dopamine—supine and head-up tilt or standing; urinary catecholamines; plasma renin activity and aldosterone
Pharmacological	Noradrenaline—α-adrenoceptors, vascular
	Isoprenaline—β-adrenoceptors, vascular and cardiac
	Tyramine—pressor and noradrenaline response
	Edrophonium—noradrenaline response
	Atropine—parasympathetic cardiac blockade
	Clonidine—stimulation or suppression test
Sudomotor	Central regulation—thermoregulatory sweat test
	Sweat gland response—intradermal acetylcholine, quantitative sudomotor axon reflex test (QSART), localized sweat test
	Sympathetic skin response, sympathetic vasomotor response
Gastrointestinal	Barium studies, videocinefluoroscopy, endoscopy, gastric emptying studies
Renal function and urinary tract	Day and night urine volumes and sodium/potassium excretion
	Urodynamic studies, intravenous urography, ultrasound examination, sphincter electromyography
Sexual function	Penile plethysmography
	Intracavernosal papaverine
Respiratory	Laryngoscopy
	Sleep studies to assess apnoea/oxygen desaturation
Eye	Schirmer's test
	Pupillary function—pharmacological and physiological

* Indicate autonomic screening tests used in our London Units.

facilities, the protocol followed, and equally important the quality of staff, who should be trained to conscientiously, consistently and rigorously follow testing schedules. To obtain normal values, the basic requirements are age, gender, body weight, and control of food intake, including, in certain investigations, the avoidance of laboratory personnel as their responses may reflect the effects of habituation. To obtain true 'control' values many other factors may need to be matched, and some of these include drug therapy (which can affect either autonomic nerve activity or function of the target organ from which measurements often are derived), the level of physical fitness, smoking, alcohol intake, and previous medical disorders (such as a myocardial infarction) that may influence

the results. In clinical practice, therefore, information from testing if matched against normal values alone may be of limited value, and may even be misleading if not considered along with the overall clinical picture and in relation to the individual case. However, each laboratory, needs to have a range of values, preferably within different age bands (Appendix I).

Cardiovascular autonomic tests lend themselves to objective rather than descriptive assessment that may not be applied as readily to the testing of other areas affected in autonomic disorders. An example is the videocinefluoroscopic examination of dysphagia, which may provide a clear indication of dysfunction and the risk of aspiration. It is less easy to quantify precisely and therefore interpret if used in longitudinal studies to assess progression of disease, or to determine the responses to therapy. The natural history of certain autonomic disorders also is important when evaluating the responses to intervention. For instance, pancreatic transplantation in diabetic autonomic neuropathy and hepatic transplantation in familial amyloid polyneuropathy prevent further neurological and autonomic damage, but testing may not show improvement; however, this in itself is a positive response, as relentless progression would occur without such intervention.

Cardiovascular testing

The prime concern of the cardiovascular system is tissue perfusion, with blood pressure and blood flow therefore of critical importance. These are influenced by a number of factors, with beat-to-beat control of blood pressure dependent upon the autonomic nervous system and, in particular, the sympathetic efferent pathways. In addition, a number of secondary mechanisms, involving systemically acting hormones, such as angiotensin II and aldosterone, and locally acting substances, such as the prostaglandins, nitric oxide, and endothelin, play a role. These substances may act directly or indirectly on the heart and vasculature, and may control or influence the intravascular and extravascular fluid compartments, each of which may modify the level of blood pressure and thus tissue perfusion. A schematic diagram of the main neurological pathways involved in the regulation of blood pressure is provided in Fig. 22.1. There are cortical, limbic, anterior and posterior hypothalamic, and medullary centres, where the input from a range of afferents can be integrated. The major cardiovascular afferents are those from the carotid sinus, the aortic arch, and the cardiopulmonary region. A range of other afferents (from skeletal muscle, skin, and viscera) also contribute, as is observed in patients with cervical or high thoracic spinal cord transection (in whom the spinal and peripheral autonomic pathways are devoid of cerebral control), in whom stimulation of such afferents may induce autonomic dysreflexia (Chapter 66). Normally from the cerebral centres, the output is co-ordinated through the vagus and the sympathetic nervous system to the heart and blood vessels. Investigative approaches in animals (Chapter 2) indicate that the major baroreceptor afferents pass to the nucleus tractus solitarius, that the vagal output is through the nucleus ambiguus, and that the sympathetic output is through the reticular paramedian nucleus.

Lesions resulting in autonomic dysfunction may involve the afferent pathways, the central connections, the efferent pathways, the target organs, or a combination of these, depending upon the disorder. Impairment of cardiovascular reflex activity usually results in abnormalities of blood pressure control, although

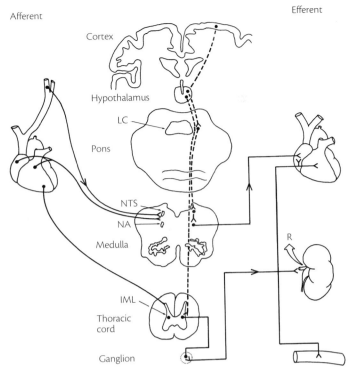

Afferent

Cortex

Hypothalamus

LC

Pons

NTS

NA

Medulla

R

IML

Thoracic cord

Ganglion

Efferent

Fig. 22.1 Diagram of cardiovascular control mechanism. LC, locus ceruleus; NA, nucleus ambiguus; NTS, nucleus tractus solitarius; IML, intermediolateral column; R, renin. Reprinted from *The Lancet*, **ii**, Bannister, R., Chronic autonomic failure with postural hypotension, 404–6, Copyright 1979, with permission from Elsevier.

hormones that influence blood vessels, intravascular volume and the kidneys may help to buffer these abnormalities. These aspects need to be borne in mind when we consider the range of tests to assess cardiovascular aspects of autonomic function, to determine the site or sites of lesions, and to ascertain hormonal factors which may be contributing to, or may be utilized for, the benefit of the patient.

The responses to postural change (head-up tilt and standing), pressor tests, the Valsalva manoeuvre, deep breathing, and hyperventilation form the core of screening tests in most laboratories, as in our two London Autonomic Units. These are described below, together with the results obtained from subjects without autonomic abnormalities that provide 'expected' results in different age bands (see Appendix I). When non-invasive techniques are used with standard laboratory precautions, these screening tests are safe, as in the experience of our units (starting in 1975 and with now over 3000 investigations per year), and that of other major centres. During certain tests (such as isometric hand grip) cardiac dysrhythmias may be more likely to occur in patients with cardiac disease, as after a myocardial infarction; however an electrocardiograph (ECG) analysis of 925 consecutive patients indicated rhythm disturbances during testing in only nine subjects, in whom these resolved without intervention (Piha and Voipio-Pulkki 1993). Although the risk is minimal, continuous ECG monitoring and resuscitation facilities should be available. Depending upon the questions raised, investigations additional to the screening tests may be needed, such as evaluating the responses to food ingestion and exercise. The limitations and risks of these investigations are individually listed where relevant.

Head-up postural challenge

Postural (orthostatic) hypotension is a cardinal manifestation of autonomic failure and therefore the cardiovascular responses to head-up postural change are particularly important (Fig. 22.2). It is defined as a fall of more than 20 mmHg systolic blood pressure and/or a fall in diastolic blood pressure of at least 10 mmHg within 3 minutes on standing/head up tilting (to 60°) (Consensus Statement 1996, Lahrmann et al. 2006). In some patients with Parkinson's disease (PD) a postural fall in blood pressure has been demonstrated even 3 minutes after being upright (Jamnadas-Kohda et al. 2009). Postural hypotension results in a number of symptoms (Table 22.2), characteristically associated with head-up postural change and relieved by sitting or lying flat. In some there may be few symptoms, despite postural hypotension (Fig. 22.3), presumably because of improved cerebral autoregulation (Brooks et al. 1989). In the presence of relevant symptoms, a fall of less than 20 mmHg systolic blood pressure also may be of importance and will warrant further investigation. The presence of vascular disease may enhance susceptibility to cerebral ischaemia, as in patients with carotid artery stenosis (Fig. 22.4).

In the clinic, brachial artery blood pressure usually is measured non-invasively using a standard mercury or aneroid sphygmomanometer. Semi-automated machines, that utilize the auscultatory or oscillometric method to measure systolic and diastolic blood pressure in addition to deriving heart rate, are of value in the laboratory. A considerable advance has been the non-invasive technique to measure finger arterial blood pressure, using a sophisticated system (Finometer; Chapter 23) which provides beat-to-beat pressure and estimations of cardiac output, stroke volume and derived peripheral vascular resistance. This obviates the need for invasive intra-arterial (radial or brachial artery) catheterization, which previously was the only reliable means of obtaining continuous blood pressure measurements. The Finometer provides a reliable measure of change in blood pressure, especially when there are rapid responses, as during the Valsalva manoeuvre (Fig. 22.5).

Basal measurements need to be performed with the subject lying supine in a quiet room and as comfortable as possible. An adequate number of readings, over at least a 5–10-minute interval, may be needed to determine the stability (or lability), of supine blood pressure. Recumbent (supine) hypertension may occur in patients with autonomic failure for reasons that include impaired baroreceptor control, supersensitivity of denervated blood vessels to even small amounts of neurotransmitters or to pressor drug treatment, and fluid shifts from the periphery into the central compartment when changing posture. In our laboratories, blood pressure recordings are performed with the Finometer or Portapres and also with automated machines using brachial blood pressure measurement. The latter allows comparison with conventional clinic blood pressure recordings as factors such as cold fingers, especially in those with Raynaud's phenomenon, may impair monitoring. Most intermittent non-invasive blood pressure measurements take around a minute, and as they involve cuff inflation above systolic blood pressure they should not be repeated too frequently. Postural change can be induced using a manual or electrically operated tilt table (to 60°), or by making the subject initially sit and then stand, or stand. A tilt table is advantageous, especially in subjects who have neurological disabilities, severe postural hypotension, or both, as it also enables rapid return to the horizontal if symptoms occur. Measurements of brachial blood pressure and heart rate during

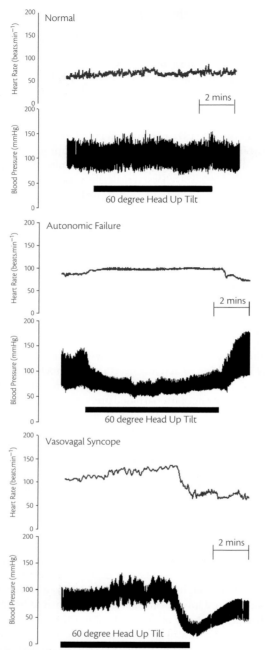

Fig. 22.2 Blood pressure and heart rate before, during and after head-up tilt in a normal subject (uppermost panel), an autonomic mediated patient with pure autonomic failure (middle panel), and a patient with vasovagal syncope (lowermost panel). In the normal subject, there is no fall in blood pressure during head-up tilt, unlike the patient with autonomic failure in whom blood pressure falls promptly and remains low with a blood pressure overshoot on return to the horizontal. In the patient with autonomic failure, there is only a minimal change in heart rate despite the marked blood pressure fall. In the patient with vasovagal syncope, there was initially no fall in blood pressure during head-up tilt; in the latter part of tilt, as indicated in the record, blood pressure initially rose and then markedly fell, to extremely low levels, so that the patient had to be returned to the horizontal. Heart rate also fell.

Table 22.2 Some of the symptoms resulting from postural (orthostatic) hypotension and impaired perfusion of various organs

Cerebral hypoperfusion
◆ Dizziness
◆ Visual disturbances
o Blurred—tunnel
◆ Scotoma
o Greying out—blacking out
o Colour defects
◆ Loss of consciousness
◆ Impaired cognition
Muscle hypoperfusion
◆ Paracervical and suboccipital ('coathanger') ache
◆ Lower back/buttock ache
Renal hypoperfusion
◆ Oliguria
Non-specific
◆ Weakness, lethargy, fatigue
◆ Falls

With permission from Mathias, C. J. (1995a) Orthostatic hypotension – causes, mechanisms and influencing factors. *Neurology* **45**, (Suppl. 5), s6–s11..

head-up tilt ideally should be made every 2 minutes, preferably for a period of 10 minutes, as this also enables blood collection for measurements of catecholamines and other vasoactive hormones released during postural change. It is important with Finometer/Portapres recordings that the hand is at heart level; this is more reliably and comfortably maintained with an adjustable sling, especially during manoeuvres that cause arm movement. An automated arm-heart height correction system is incorporated in the latest models.

In normal subjects, head-up tilt or standing results in minimal changes in blood pressure. In autonomic disorders, however, the pressure often falls. The degree and rapidity of fall and extent of recovery can vary considerably even within the same individual. The blood pressure may fall rapidly and progressively in severe autonomic failure (Figs 22.2 and 22.6a); this may not occur in other patients, especially those with incomplete autonomic failure, as the rate and degree of fall also depends on the ability to recruit non-neurogenic mechanisms that help maintain blood pressure. Thus in patients with high thoracic or cervical spinal cord transaction, especially those who have been rehabilitated, initially there is a rapid fall in blood pressure because of their inability to activate sympathetic vasoconstrictor pathways in response to postural change; this is followed by partial recovery of blood pressure (Fig. 22.6b) (Chapter 66). The recovery results from activation of spinal sympathetic reflexes or humoral compensatory mechanisms, which include the renin–angiotensin–aldosterone system. In patients with autonomic failure who have an immediate and profound fall in blood pressure on postural change it may be difficult, if not impossible, to make accurate measurements using non-invasive techniques other than with the Finometer. Varying the degree of head-up tilt may help.

There is normally a small to moderate rise in heart rate during postural change. In the presence of a substantial fall in blood pressure, a lack of change in heart rate is indicative of a baroreflex abnormality, as occurs when there is an afferent baroreceptor lesion or when

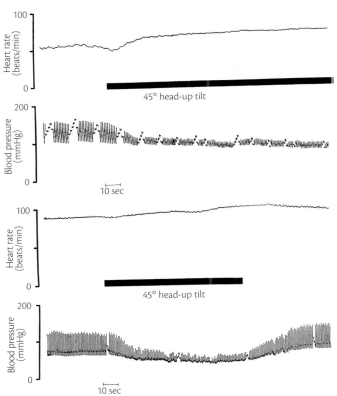

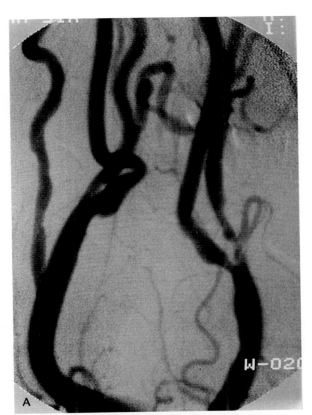

Fig. 22.3 Blood pressure and heart rate, measured by the Finometer, in two patients with autonomic failure. In the patient in the upper panel blood pressure falls to low levels, with the patient maintaining head-up tilt for over 20 minutes with virtually no symptoms. This patient had autonomic failure for many years and could tolerate such levels of blood pressure, presumably because of the improved cerebrovascular autoregulation. This is in contrast to the patient in the lower panel, who had to be put back to the horizontal after a short period of head-up tilt; she recently had developed severe postural hypotension after surgery. With permission from Mathias, C.J. (1996a). Disorders affecting autonomic function in Parkinsonian patients. In Parkinson's disease, (ed. L. Battistin, G. Scarlato, T. Caraceni, and S. Ruggieri), *Advances in Neurology*, **69**, pp. 383–91. Lippincott-Raven Press, New York.

there is both sympathetic and parasympathetic failure, as often occurs in primary autonomic failure. In tetraplegic patients, there is a rise in heart rate in response to the fall in blood pressure, because the vagal and glossopharyngeal afferent and the vagal efferent pathways are intact (Fig. 22.6b). The heart rate, however, does not usually rise above 110 beats/minute, which is similar to levels observed after atropine administration and vagal blockade; further elevation of heart rate probably is dependent on adrenomedullary stimulation and elevation of plasma adrenaline levels, which does not occur in such patients. This adrenal component probably accounts for the greater tachycardia observed in subjects with an intact sympathetic nervous system when they have a low blood pressure, as may occur in haemorrhagic shock.

The degree of postural hypotension is dependent upon a large number of factors (Table 22.3). In primary autonomic failure, postural hypotension is often greater in the morning because of nocturnal diuresis, after food ingestion because of splanchnic vasodilatation, after exercise because of skeletal muscle vasodilatation, and in hot weather because of cutaneous vasodilatation. Vasodilatation induced by drugs, including those normally not considered to have significant cardiovascular effects, may cause

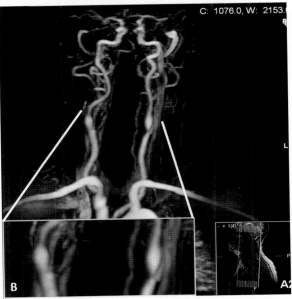

Fig. 22.4 A. Intravenous digital subtraction angiogram of the cerebral vessels in a patient with hypertension and widespread atherosclerosis, indicating left carotid artery stenosis. She had symptoms that initially were considered to be transient ischaemic attacks resulting from thromboembolism. The history, however, indicated symptoms closely associated with postural change. She had a postural fall in systolic blood pressure of only 10 mmHg, which presumably was sufficient to induce symptoms of cerebral ischaemia because of cerebrovascular disease. A reduction in antihypertensive therapy abolished the small postural fall in blood pressure and also her symptoms. This figure was published in Autonomic disorders, Mathias, C. J. in *Textbook of neurology* (ed. J. Bogousslavsky and M. Fisher), pp. 519–45, Copyright Elsevier (1998). B. Non-invasive assessment of the brain and carotid arteries with magnetic resonance angiography in a 68 yr old male patient indicating bilateral carotid artery stenosis with ~50% narrowing of both proximal internal carotid arteries. The patient had experienced 2 episodes of syncope.

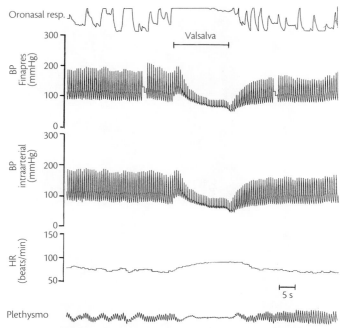

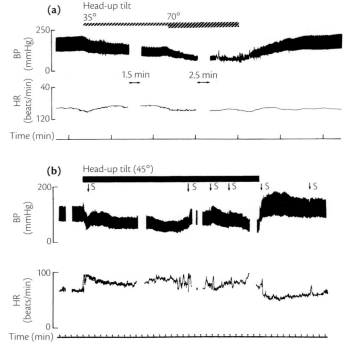

Fig. 22.5 Changes in non-invasive finger blood pressure (BP, Finometer) compared with intra-arterial blood pressure (BP) in a patient with autonomic impairment, before, during, and after a Valsalva manoeuvre. Respiratory rate (oronasal resp.), heart rate (HR), and plethysmograph (Plethysmo) are also continuously recorded; the Finometer recording appears identical to the intra-arterial trace; the breaks indicate an internal calibration signal. Reprinted from *Clinical Neurophysiology* (ed. J. Osselston with C. Binnie, R. Looper, C. Fowler, F. Maguire and P. Prior). Mathias, C. J., 'Assessment of autonomic function.' Heinemann, Butterworth, London. pp. 218–32 © 1995, with permission from Elsevier.

Fig. 22.6 (a) Continuous intra-arterial recording of blood pressure (BP) and heart rate (HR) in a patient with postural hypotension and the Holmes–Adie syndrome. Both systolic and diastolic blood pressure fall progressively during head-up tilt, with no recovery. There are minimal changes in heart rate. There was no change in plasma noradrenaline levels following tilt. Other investigations indicated that the lesion was likely to be on the afferent side of the baroreflex arc. (From Mathias 1987.) **(b)** Blood pressure (BP) and heart rate (HR) in a tetraplegic patient before, during and after head-up tilt to 45°. Blood pressure falls promptly with partial recovery, which in this case is linked to skeletal muscle spasms (S), inducing spinal sympathetic activity. Some of the later oscillations are probably due to the rise in plasma renin, measured where there are interruptions in the intra-arterial record. In the later phases, muscle spasms occur more frequently and further elevate blood pressure. On return to the horizontal, blood pressure rises rapidly above the previous basal level and slowly returns to supine levels. Heart rate tends to move in the opposite direction. There is a transient increase in heart rate during muscle spasms. With permission from Mathias, C. J. and Frankel, H. L. (1988). Cardiovascular control in spinal man. *Ann. Rev. Physiol.* **50**, 577–92.

substantial changes in blood pressure when there is a baroreflex deficit (Fig. 22.7). It is also necessary to consider non-neurogenic causes of postural hypotension (Table 22.2) as these may enhance hypotension considerably in autonomic failure.

A further advance in the assessment of cardiovascular autonomic abnormalities has been the development of 24-hour non-invasive ambulatory blood pressure and heart rate readings, that are of value both in the investigation and also in the evaluation of cardio-vascular autonomic abnormalities (Fig. 22.8a,b,c). In normal subjects, blood pressure is usually higher in the day and lower when the subject is asleep at night. This circadian fall usually does not occur in autonomic failure. The technique also allows, with suita-ble protocols, recordings at different times of the day of responses to stimuli that include postural change, food ingestion, and exercise, each of which can lower blood pressure in autonomic failure. A par-ticular advantage is that the effects of treatment on postural hypoten-sion (Alam et al. 1995), and on hypotension induced by stimuli in daily life, can be assessed in the home situation. These techniques are of value when paroxysmal hypertension also occurs, as in tetraple-gia (Chapter 66) or when episodes of excessive tachycardia occur, as in the Postural Tachycardia Syndrome (PoTS; Fig. 22.8c).

There are methods of quantifying the heart rate changes during standing, one of which is the '30–15 ratio'. Normally, on standing the rise in heart rate is greatest by the fifteenth beat, followed by slowing which is maximal at the thirtieth beat. The ratio of the longest P–R interval of the thirtieth to the shortest interval on the fifteenth beat should normally be over one. In the absence of change in heart rate on standing it is 1.0 or less than 1.0. It thus provides

Table 22.3 Factors influencing postural (orthostatic) hypotension

---

◆ Speed of positional change

◆ Time of day (worse in the morning)

◆ Prolonged recumbency

◆ Warm environment (hot weather, central heating, hot bath)

◆ Raising intrathoracic pressure—micturition, defaecation or coughing

◆ Food and alcohol ingestion

◆ Physical exertion

◆ Manoeuvres and positions (bending forward, abdominal compression, leg crossing, squatting, activating calf muscle pump)*

◆ Drugs with vasoactive properties (including dopaminergic agents)

---

* These manoeuvres usually reduce the postural fall in blood pressure, unlike the others.
Adapted from Mathias 1995a.

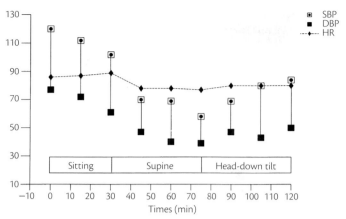

Fig. 22.7 Systolic and diastolic blood pressure in a patient considered to have Parkinson's disease before and after a standard levodopa challenge (250 mg of L-dopa along with 25 mg carbidopa). The patient was initially seated but blood pressure fell and was so low that he needed to be laid supine and horizontal, and then head down. On further investigation, the final diagnosis in this patient was autonomic failure and the parkinsonian form of multiple system atrophy. From Mathias 1999.

Table 22.4 Non-neurogenic causes of postural hypotension

Low intravascular volume	
Blood/plasma loss	Haemorrhage, burns, haemodialysis
Fluid/electrolyte	Inadequate intake—anorexia nervosa
	Fluid loss—vomiting, diarrhoea, losses from ileostomy
	Renal/endocrine—salt-losing nephropathy, adrenal insufficiency (Addison's disease), diabetes insipidus, diuretics
Vasodilatation	
	Drugs
	Glyceryl trinitrate, alcohol
	Heat, pyrexia
	Hyperbradykinism
	Systemic mastocytosis
	Extensive varicose veins
Cardiac impairment	
Myocardial	Myocarditis
Impaired ventricular filling	Atrial myxoma, constrictive pericarditis
Impaired output	Aortic stenosis

a numerical assessment that may be of value in longitudinal or interventional studies; whether it contributes further to assessing or understanding autonomic deficits is debatable. There clearly are difficulties in those who cannot readily stand.

The responses in patients with intermittent autonomic dysfunction, and who do not have detectable autonomic impairment but are prone to fainting or presyncopal symptoms, can differ substantially from patients with autonomic failure. In autonomic mediated syncope (AMS), due to vasovagal syncope or emotional fainting (Chapters 55 and 56), there may be a family history of syncope, especially when the onset is below 20 years of age (Mathias et al. 1998). In these patients, detailed autonomic testing usually

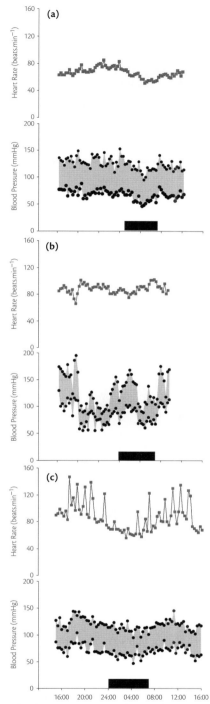

Fig. 22.8 Twenty-four hour non-invasive ambulatory blood pressure profiles showing systolic and diastolic blood pressure and heart rate at intervals through the day and night. (a) The changes in a normal subject with no postural fall in blood pressure; there was a fall in blood pressure at night whilst asleep, with a rise in blood pressure on wakening. (b) Marked fluctuations in blood pressure in a patient with autonomic failure. The marked falls in blood pressure are usually the result of postural changes, either sitting or standing. Supine blood pressure, particularly at night, is elevated. There is reversal of the diurnal changes in blood pressure. There are relatively small changes in heart rate, considering the marked changes in blood pressure. (c) Marked fluctuations in heart rate in a patient with Postural Tachycardia Syndrome. The elevations in heart rate are usually related to periods of being upright and/or during/just after various daily activities, e.g., food, physical activity. Black bars indicates periods of sleep.

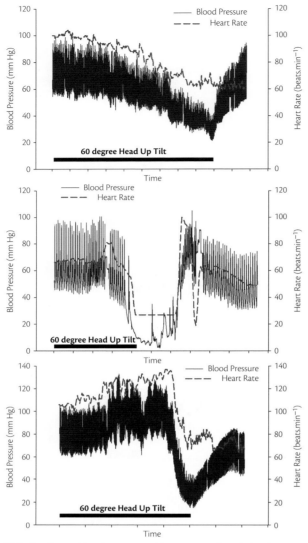

Fig. 22.9 Continuous blood pressure and heart rate tracings during the predominantly vasodepressor (A), cardio-inhibitory (B) and mixed (cardio-inhibitory and vasodepressor, C) forms of autonomic mediated syncope during 60 degree head up tilt tests. From Mathias and Galizia (2010).

reveals no abnormalities, but they may faint during postural change (Fig. 22.2 and 22.9), sometimes when prolonged, or when exposed to a variety of stimuli, including the sight or mere mention of a venipuncture needle. Continuous blood pressure and heart rate monitoring is necessary in such cases. Additional physiological and pharmacological stimuli have been used to induce an episode, including simultaneous lower-body negative pressure, and drugs such as isoprenaline and glyceryl trinitrate. It is debatable whether such stimuli provide information of value, especially as they may induce syncope in normal subjects without a previous history of fainting; moreover, some carry a potential risk. In patients with vasovagal syncope, the blood pressure is often maintained initially during head-up tilt, but then falls and this may be the result of a provoking stimulus, such as venipuncture. The fall in blood pressure may be preceded by a fall in heart rate. The fall in blood pressure typically (but not always) results from withdrawal of sympathetic

nervous activity to blood vessels, while the fall in heart rate is due to increased cardiac parasympathetic activity (Chapter 23). The mixed form (vasodepressor and cardioinhibitory) is more common. There is a vasodepressor form with mainly a fall in blood pressure, while in the cardioinhibitory form asystole occurs (see Fig. 22.9). The latter may warrant a cardiac demand pacemaker. In the mixed form it may be difficult to determine whether vasodepression or cardioinhibition predominates, as this has therapeutic implications. Repeat testing with intravenous atropine that causes vagal blockade often helps with diagnosis (Fig. 22.10). In the predominantly vasodepressor form the blood pressure continues to fall despite the heart rate being maintained thus indicating that a cardiac pacemaker will not be of benefit. If atropine prevents an episode, however, there may be difficulties with interpretation, as the unpredictable nature of the provoking stimulus needs to be considered. The history then becomes important, especially if syncope occur with little or no warning and results in injury.

In carotid sinus hypersensitivity, the ideal provoking stimulus is carotid massage. There are potential risks, however, even though small, and our practice, especially as the diagnosis is being considered in older subjects, is to image the carotid vessels, either with Doppler scanning or magnetic resonance angiography (MRA) of the extracranial vessels (see Fig. 22.4). In those with carotid impairment, in whom massage is considered unsafe, movements of the

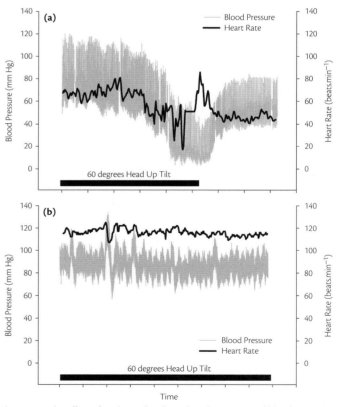

Fig. 22.10 The effect of 60 degree head up tilt on heart rate and blood pressure in a patient with autonomic mediated syncope before (upper panel) and after (lower panel) 1 mg of atropine intravenously. The bradycardia and hypotension were prevented by atropine and syncope did not occur indicating that cardioinhibition predominates in the patient's syncopal events and that a cardiac demand pacemaker is warranted.

head and neck, to mimic provoking stimuli in daily life can be tried. In situational syncope, one can attempt to replicate the stimulus thought to cause syncope, although this may be difficult.

A further group of patients with symptoms on postural change but in whom an autonomic deficit cannot be clearly defined are those who have a pronounced tachycardia during postural change, while blood pressure is maintained. They have the postural tachycardia syndrome (PoTS) defined as a marked rise in heart rate while upright, of 30 bpm within 10 minutes of head-up tilt or standing, or a heart rate of over 120 bpm, but without orthostatic hypotension (see Fig. 22.11) (Schondorf and Low 1993, Freeman et al. 2011; Mathias et al. 2012). It mainly affects young individuals, predominantly female, of 15–40 years of age. Many have symptoms of postural intolerance despite a lack of postural hypotension. Pooling in the dependent limbs, causing cutaneous blotchiness or purplish discoloration may also be evident. The marked chronotropic cardiac response occurs for reasons that may be unclear, and include a compensatory response to inappropriate vasodilatation occurring either in the periphery (in the lower limbs when upright) or in major vascular regions (such as the splanchnic, skeletal muscle or cutaneous beds); activation of cardiac β-adrenergic receptors resulting from increased circulating adrenaline and/or increased central discharge due to an anxiety state; or a reduction in cardiac vagal activity. The onset of the syndrome may be linked to infection, trauma, surgery or stress. The mechanisms causing PoTS vary and include regional autonomic denervation, usually in the lower limbs, hyperadrenergic activity, either neurally

or humorally caused, hypovolaemia linked to changes in the level or responsiveness to hormones (such as the renin–angiotensin–aldosterone system) or in the renal control of fluid secretion, local vascular abnormalities (e.g. cerebral, splanchnic or dependent limbs), physical deconditioning and/or reduced cardiac size, and genetic predisposition due to mutations (Mathias et al. 2012). Patients with PoTS have a variety of associated disorders and conditions, and this is likely to account for the numerous proposed pathophysiological mechanisms, which differs in individuals. The most common association in our Units is with the joint hypermobility syndrome/Ehlers Danlos III (see Fig.22.12).

The Valsalva manoeuvre

The changes in blood pressure and heart rate during the Valsalva manoeuvre, when intrathoracic pressure ideally is raised to 40 mmHg, provide a further assessment of the baroreflex pathways. To perform this, the subject blows with an open glottis into a disposable syringe connected to the mercury column of a sphygmomanometer and maintains a forced expiratory pressure of up to 40 mmHg for 10 seconds. This may be difficult in some subjects, in whom levels between 20 mmHg and 40 mmHg often suffice to induce the necessary changes. The performance of the manoeuvre as well as the blood pressure and heart rate responses can be broken down into distinct phases for further analyses. Normally, with the rise in intrathoracic pressure the venous return falls along with blood pressure (Fig. 22.13). On releasing intrathoracic pressure there is a blood pressure overshoot because of persistence of

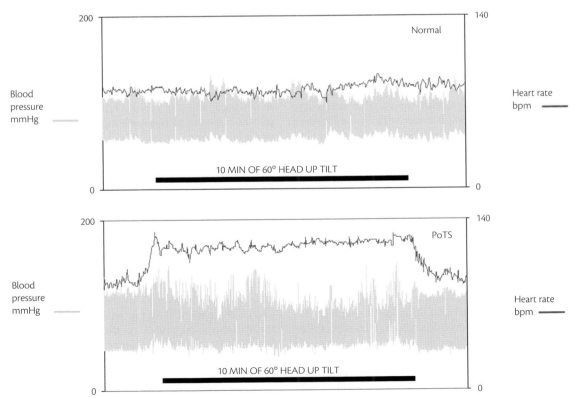

Fig. 22.11 Blood pressure and heart rate profiles obtained while supine and during head-up tilt. (a) Profile of a healthy individual. (b) Profile from a patient with PoTS. Excessive tachycardia is observed after the onset of head-up tilt in the patient with PoTS. From Mathias et al. (2012)..

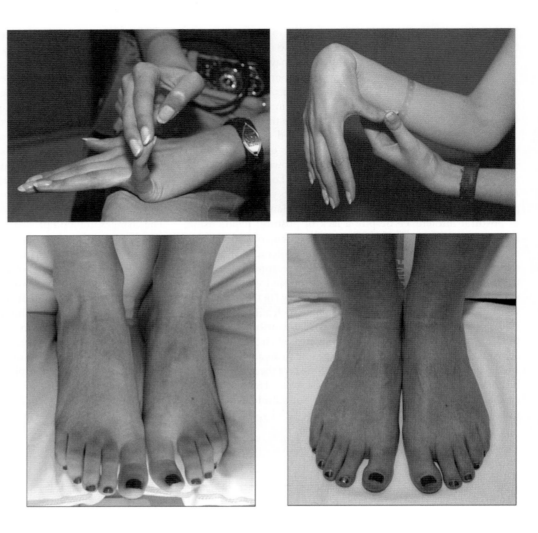

Fig. 22.12 Clinical signs of PoTS. Joint hypermobility in a patient with PoTS and Ehlers-Danlos syndrome type III (also known as EDS hypermobility type). From Mathias et al. (2012).

sympathetic activity. Baroreflex activation then results in a secondary fall in heart rate to below basal levels.

In sympathetic vasoconstrictor failure, the Valsalva manoeuvre results in a continuous fall in blood pressure with no stabilization; following release there is no blood pressure overshoot and thus there is no compensatory bradycardia. If the afferent and vagal efferent components of the baroreflex pathways are intact, as in tetraplegics and some patients with autonomic failure, heart rate rises while the blood pressure falls. There is also a sympathetic component to this response, because in normal subjects the rise in heart rate is blunted following administration of the β-adrenoceptor blocker propranolol. In diabetics with a proliferative retinopathy, some feel that there may be a risk of intraocular haemorrhage, because of the pressure transients.

It often is not possible, without a Finometer, to obtain beat-to-beat blood pressure during the Valsalva manoeuvre; the continuous measurement of heart rate with an electrocardiograph (ECG) often suffices in obtaining relevant information. However, spurious abnormal responses may occur if the cheek muscles are used to produce an apparent but false rise in intrathoracic pressure. Beat-to-beat blood pressure monitoring, as with the Finometer (Fig. 22.5), is of particular value in this situation, as it will identify a lack of fall in blood pressure, indicating that intrathoracic pressure was not elevated adequately.

There are various measurements and derived ratios of heart rate during the different phases of the Valsalva manoeuvre. A commonly used ratio (the Valsalva ratio), relates to the changes in heart rate in response to the variations in blood pressure. Normally, when intrathoracic pressure is elevated (phase II), the blood pressure falls and heart rate rises, while in the first 30 seconds after release of intrathoracic pressure (phase IV), the heart rate should fall in response to the rise in blood pressure. The Valsalva ratio is the derivative of the maximum rise and fall in these two phases (phase II/phase IV) and should normally be over 1, it is 1 or less in the presence of autonomic failure. In our laboratories in London we attempt to obtain a Valsalva in the supine position while maintaining intrathoracic pressure at 40 mmHg, but this may not be achieved for reasons that include the patient's co-operation and strength, especially if there is impairment of muscles (diaphragm, intercostal, and accessory) involved in respiratory effort. The position of the patient (lying or sitting), and the time of day when the Valsalva manoeuvre is performed, are also factors that may influence the response (Chapter 23). The responses also need to be considered in relation to factors known to affect heart rate, such as drug therapy and the myocardial state. We record the responses to three well-performed Valsalva manoeuvres as this verifies an abnormal response, if present. It is debatable if averaging the results from three manoeuvres provides any further

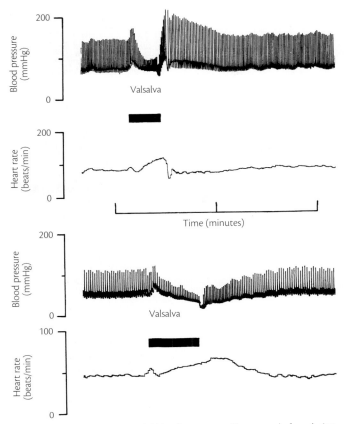

Fig. 22.13 Changes in intra-arterial blood pressure and heart rate before, during, and after the Valsalva manoeuvre, when intrathoracic pressure was raised to 40 mmHg in a normal subject (upper trace) and in a patient with autonomic failure (lower trace). In the normal subject, release of intrathoracic pressure was accompanied by an increase in blood pressure and a reduction in heart rate below basal levels. In the patient, there was a gradual increase in blood pressure implying impairment of sympathetic vasoconstrictor pathways. The heart rate scale varies in the two subjects.

cold there is activation of peripheral receptors, although there is an important cerebral component, especially with the former. Other stimuli, such as sudden noise or mental arithmetic, are dependent predominantly on cerebral stimulation.

Isometric exercise is performed by using either a dynamometer or a partially inflated sphygmomanometer cuff, and sustaining handgrip for 3 minutes, usually at a third of the maximum voluntary contraction pressure. The cold pressor (cutaneous cold) test consists of immersing the hand for up to 2 minutes in ice slush, usually just below 4°C. Cortical arousal is performed by sudden noise, mental arithmetic (subtraction or addition of 7 or 17), or a variety of more complex tasks. These stimuli normally elevate blood pressure and heart rate (Fig. 22.14a, b). In patients with central or efferent sympathetic lesions, the response to these stimuli is impaired or absent.

In tetraplegic patients with complete cervical spinal cord lesions, mental arithmetic and stimuli above the cutaneous level of the lesion (such as with an ice pack) do not raise blood pressure, in contrast to stimuli below the lesion, which activate spinal sympathetic reflexes (independently of the brain) and cause a rise in pressure, often accompanied by a fall in heart rate because of a baroreflex induced increase in vagal activity. Stimuli capable of such effects include cutaneous cold or other noxious, and even non-noxious, cutaneous stimuli (including pin-prick), activation of abdominal or pelvic visceral reflexes by urinary bladder or large bowel contraction, and skeletal muscle spasms (Fig. 22.14c) (Chapter 66). This elevation in blood pressure, along with a range of other cardiovascular changes, is an important component of the syndrome of autonomic dysreflexia and may be mistaken for a hypertensive crisis as in patients with a phaeochromocytoma, when there is excessive secretion of catecholamines from the tumour. Exaggerated pressor responses may occur in patients with partial or complete afferent baroreceptor impairment.

Responses to isometric exercise, cutaneous cold, and mental arithmetic can be obtained within a short period of time, and often provide valuable information in a wide range of disorders. The most useful responses probably are those induced by isometric exercise and cutaneous cold. Factors independent of the autonomic nervous system may affect the responses; thus disordered muscle function may influence the pressor response during isometric exercise and the presence of a sensory deficit may limit the response to cutaneous cold. The sensitivity, specificity, and reproducibility of these tests have been studied. The results obtained during isometric exercise with handgrip compare favourably with tilt-table tests (Khurana and Setty 1996). With the cold pressor test, systolic blood pressure was the more reliable measurement; reproducibility however, was lower when testing was repeated over the same day, or over three consecutive days, presumably because of habituation or anticipation (Fasano et al. 1996). The responses to mental arithmetic can vary; these may be reduced when the stimulus is too trivial as in those who are highly numerate, or when they cannot be performed adequately as in those with dementia. There is a variety of mental stress tests, many computerized both for execution and evaluation, that have been used successfully for research purposes (Mounier-Vehier et al. 1995). Interpretation of the results of pressor tests, therefore, should be linked with the clinical characteristics and diagnosis of each patient, and related to the information that needs to be derived from such testing.

information; it may even be misleading in a subject with normal autonomic function who, for a variety of reasons, may be unable to adequately perform the Valsalva repeatedly. It may be that the best 'normal' response should be considered for the ratio in such subjects.

Analysis of the continuous blood pressure and heart rate record during the Valsalva often provides valuable information on the baroreflex. A rise in heart rate in response to the rise in intrathoracic pressure, when the blood pressure falls, suggests that the afferent and vagal efferent pathways are operative. Recovery of the blood pressure while intrathoracic pressure is maintained often occurs in normal subjects, but not in those with sympathetic vasoconstrictor failure, when blood pressure usually falls inexorably; with release of intrathoracic pressure in such patients there is only a slow return to the baseline without the overshoot, consistent with the lack of sympathetic vasoconstrictor function. These form the characteristic blood pressure features of a 'blocked' Valsalva manoeuvre (Fig. 22.13).

Pressor stimuli

These raise blood pressure by stimulating sympathetic efferent pathways in a variety of ways. With isometric exercise or cutaneous

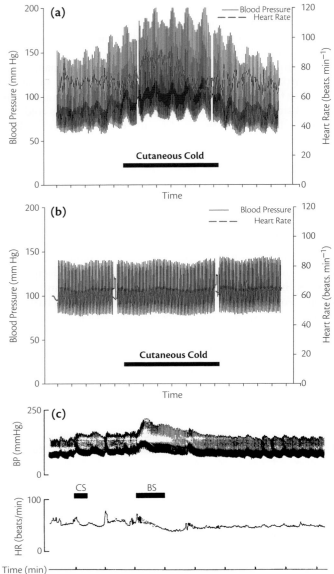

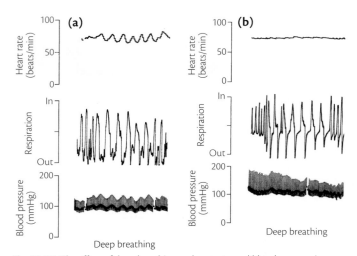

Fig. 22.15 The effect of deep breathing on heart rate and blood pressure in **(a)** a normal subject and **(b)** a patient with autonomic failure. There is no sinus arrhythmia in the patient, despite a fall in blood pressure. Respiratory changes are indicated in the middle panel.

Fig. 22.14 Blood pressure (BP) and heart rate (HR) responses to cutaneous cold (hand up to wrist in ice slush) **(a)** in a normal subject and **(b)** in a patient with autonomic failure. The time scale is similar in **(a)** and **(b)**. In the patient there is no rise in BP. Non-invasive recordings were made with the Finometer. **(c)** Intra-arterial BP and HR in a chronic tetraplegic before, during and after cutaneous stimulation (CS) and bladder stimulation (BS) 6 months after injury when reflex isolated spinal cord activity had returned. Cutaneous stimulation is performed by the application of ice over the chest below the level of the lesion, and urinary bladder stimulation is by suprapubic percussion of the anterior abdominal wall. There is a rise in BP with both stimuli, this being greater with bladder stimulation. From Mathias et al. 1979, with permission.

Heart rate responses to respiratory change

Changes in respiration result in rapid responses in heart rate and often provide a guide to the activity of the cardiac vagi. These results can be used in conjunction with the heart rate response to head-up tilt, standing, and the Valsalva manoeuvre. Normally with inspiration there is a rise, and with expiration a fall, in heart rate; this is the basis of sinus arrhythmia (Fig. 22.15). A considerable number of variations are available to exploit and standardize

this objectively. A single deep breath, a short period of quiet breathing, or a fixed rate of 6 breaths/minute has been used; each is claimed to be a better discriminator. Hyperventilation is probably a stronger stimulus to vagal withdrawal and causes a rise in heart rate. However, it may also lower blood-pressure and this could influence heart rate; the precise mechanisms for the fall in pressure with hyperventilation are unclear. Heart rate responses to respiratory manoeuvres diminish with age, and this is an important factor in interpretation of results (Appendix I).

In autonomic neuropathy complicating diabetes mellitus and alcoholism, cardiac vagal lesions may occur prior to sympathetic impairment, and the heart rate responses to these tests may be abnormal before postural hypotension ensues. Although this provides evidence of an autonomic neuropathy, this should not be equated with a generalized or sympathetic deficit, or both.

Food challenge

Food lowers supine blood pressure in a large number of patients with primary autonomic failure (Chapter 28). In these patients, postprandial hypotension is linked to the release of vasodilatatory gut peptides and splanchnic vasodilatation, which is not accompanied by compensatory changes in cardiac output and skeletal muscle resistance vessels, as occur in normal subjects in whom blood pressure does not fall after food ingestion. In addition to the fall in supine blood pressure, food is now recognized as unmasking or aggravating postural hypotension in autonomic failure, as well as tachycardia in PoTS (see Fig. 22.16). The responses to food ingestion are thus of value in the assessment of postprandial hypotension, and in determining whether drugs (such as octreotide) reduce the blood pressure fall. This can be measured objectively by assessing the responses to head-up tilt ideally after an overnight fast, before and 45 minutes after food ingestion. For practical reasons, ingestion of liquids is preferable. Glucose can be used but the solution provides a caloric load of high osmolality, which may be a problem, especially in diabetics. A clinically relevant and probably more physiological alternative is a balanced liquid meal using commercially available Complan (containing various food

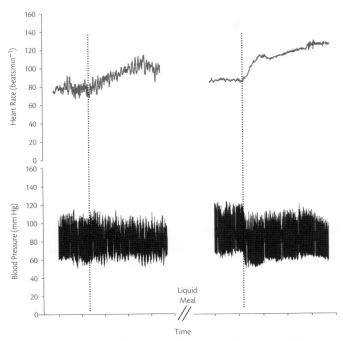

Fig. 22.16 Changes in blood pressure and heart rate while supine and during head-up tilt, before and after ingestion of a balanced liquid meal in a patient with PoTS. A greater rise in heart rate is observed on head-up tilt after ingestion of the meal, compared with heart rate during head-up tilt before the meal. From Mathias et al. (2012).

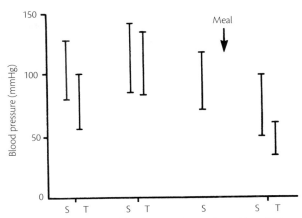

Fig. 22.17 Systolic and diastolic blood pressure in a patient with multiple system atrophy, while supine (S) and after 45° head-up tilt (T) on three occasions. On the first, food intake was not controlled and the patient had eaten earlier. On the second the patient had not eaten and the postural blood pressure fall was negligible. The patient then had a liquid meal. Following food challenge supine blood pressure fell and on the third occasion of tilt there was a considerably greater fall in blood pressure. These observations emphasize the importance of food intake on postural hypotension. From Mathias et al. 1991b.

components) with added glucose, either in a milk or soya-bean base, made up to 300 ml with a caloric load of 330 Kcal (Mathias et al. 1991b). This can be prepared easily and ingested readily via a straw while lying flat, so that the effects of food ingestion also can be obtained independently of postural change. A fall of more than 20 mmHg systolic while supine clearly is abnormal; comparison of blood pressure during head-up tilt preprandially and postprandially enables determination of whether there is enhancement or unmasking of postural hypotension by food. This can be of importance as there are patients who, when fasted, have modest postural hypotension, which is considerably exaggerated by food ingestion (Fig. 22.17).

Exercise testing

It is recognized increasingly that exercise, even in the supine position, lowers blood pressure in patients with autonomic failure (Smith et al. 1995; Chapter 30). In these patients the hypotension induced by exercise is accompanied by a rise in cardiac output similar to that in normal subjects, but there is a coincidental marked fall in systemic vascular resistance (Low et al. 2012). The latter is probably the result of vasodilatation in exercising skeletal muscle, without the compensatory responses elsewhere of increased sympathetic nerve traffic and sympathoadrenal activation which occur normally (Puvi-Rajasingham et al. 1997). Separating the responses of exercise from posture and gravity is important, and a technique has been devised so that increasing workloads (from 25 watts to 75 watts) on a bicycle ergometer can be performed while horizontal (Fig. 22.19). The responses to supine exercise therefore can be assessed, in addition to responses to either head-up

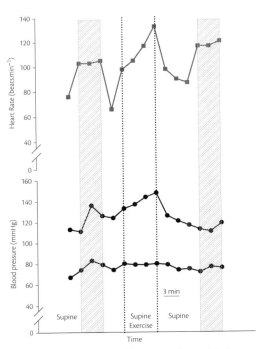

Fig. 22.18 Changes in blood pressure and heart rate observed during standing, as well as before and after graded supine cycling exercise in a patient with PoTS. The patient's blood pressure (top line, systolic blood pressure; bottom line, diastolic blood pressure) and heart rate responses to exercise are preserved, but while standing after exercise (even 10–15 min later) the heart rate remains elevated and above the rate measured before exercise. From Mathias et al. (2012).

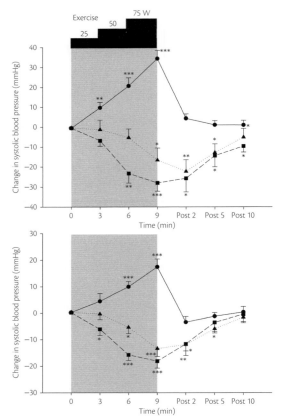

Fig. 22.19 Change in systolic (upper panel) and diastolic (lower panel) blood pressure during 9 minutes of incremental supine exercise on a bicycle at 25, 50, and 75 watts, with supine measurements continued post exercise at 2, 5, and 10 minutes. Blood pressure rises in normal subjects (●--●), and rapidly falls back towards normal on cessation of exercise. In patients with multiple system atrophy (MSA; ▲—▲) and pure autonomic failure (PAF; ■—■), there is a work-related fall in blood pressure that is at its lowest towards the end of the exercise period; post-exercise, blood pressure slowly recovers and even 10 minutes later has not entirely returned to normal. From Smith et al. 1995, with permission.

tilt or standing, before and after exercise. In normal subjects exercise raises blood pressure; in primary autonomic failure usually there is a fall during the period of exercise. In some, however, the pressure does not fall (or rise) during exercise, but falls immediately on ceasing exercise; this is presumably due to peripheral vasodilatation and pooling not opposed by the calf muscle pump (Fig. 22.20). In autonomic failure, there is often an aggravation of postural hypotension post-exercise (Fig. 22.21), which is likely to be of importance in daily life. In patients who also have suspected ischaemic heart disease it may be best to limit or avoid even the mild degree of exercise that these patients are subjected to during this test.

The responses to exercise vary in the different autonomic disorders, with a greater fall in blood pressure in pure autonomic failure (PAF) than in multiple system atrophy (MSA) (Smith et al. 1995). Furthermore, differences may occur even with the various forms of MSA; in the parkinsonian form, there is a smaller fall in blood pressure while supine when compared with the cerebellar form, although the enhancement of postural hypotension post-exercise is similar in the two groups (Smith and Mathias 1996). The reasons are unclear. It may be that there is more extensive autonomic

impairment in the cerebellar form as the lesions are more caudal, and in closer proximity and more likely to impair central autonomic mechanisms. In patients with an isolated peripheral autonomic disorder (dopamine-beta-hydroxylase deficiency), there is neither a rise nor a fall in blood pressure during exercise while supine, but there is a considerable worsening of postural hypotension post-exercise (Fig. 22.21). The reasons for the lack of blood pressure fall while supine are probably similar to those that prevent supine postprandial hypotension in these patients (Chapter 28).

Exercise testing is of particular importance in patients with POTS who usually have exercise intolerance, sometimes associated with fatigue. Excessive tachycardia may occur during even modest exertion and post-exercise tachycardia may persist (see Fig. 22.18).

Carotid sinus massage

This should be performed if the history suggests that syncope is caused by movements of the neck or pressure over the carotid sinus by a collar or tie, especially in the presence of apparently normal cardiovascular autonomic function. Carotid sinus hypersensitivity is recognized increasingly in the elderly as a potential cause of unexplained falls (McIntosh et al. 1993), and needs to be sought actively in this group. The ideal provoking stimulus is carotid massage. However there are potential risks, however small and in our practice the policy is to image the carotid vessels, either with Doppler scanning or MR angiogram (see Fig. 22.4). In those with carotid impairment, in whom massage is considered unsafe, movements of the head and neck to mimic provoking stimuli in daily life can be tried while supine and tilted.

The European Society of Cardiology guidelines on syncope suggest considering the diagnosis of carotid sinus hypersensitivity in patients over 40 years of age in whom the cause of syncope is unclear, despite testing (Moya et al. 2009). In our series, 50 years appeared a more relevant age (Humm and Mathias 2010). In younger patients, syncope provoked by carotid massage may not necessarily indicate carotid sinus hypersensitivity as the stimulus may mimic one of many stimuli capable of inducing such a response (Humm and Mathias 2010). Carotid sinus massage may provoke asystole and cardiac dysrhythmias, so it is essential that adequate resuscitation measures are available readily in the event of cardiovascular collapse. Continuous monitoring of heart rate, the ECG (on an oscilloscope, preferably with a printing facility), and blood pressure, ideally with a non-invasive beat-to-beat machine such as the Finometer, is needed. Only one carotid sinus should be stimulated each time, using gentle pressure that compresses the carotid bulb against the transverse processes of the upper cervical vertebrae. There are normally minor changes in heart rate and blood pressure. In carotid sinus hypersensitivity, severe bradycardia and hypotension may occur (Fig. 22.22). The former may precede the hypotension, and in the cardioinhibitory form may be prevented by atropine or a demand cardiac pacemaker. There is a less common vasodepressor form, where hypotension occurs without bradycardia; this appears to be due to withdrawal of sympathetic nerve activity (Chapter 24). Many fall into the mixed form, with a fall in both heart rate and blood pressure. Therapeutic approaches in the vasodepressor and mixed forms include unilateral or bilateral carotid sinus denervation. Predicting the outcome can be difficult and testing may need to be repeated after intravenous atropine.

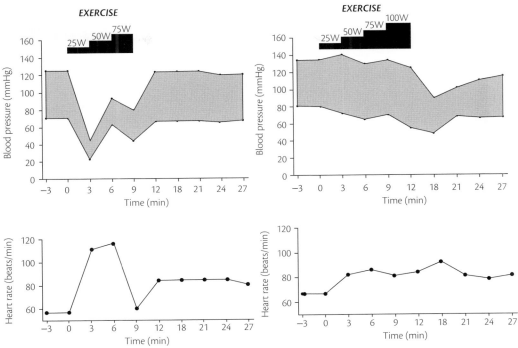

Fig. 22.20 Systolic and diastolic blood pressure (top) and heart rate (lower panel) in two patients with primary autonomic failure, before, during, and after bicycle exercise performed with the patients in the supine position at different workloads, ranging from 25 watts to 100 watts. In the patient on the left there is a marked fall in blood pressure on initiating exercise; she had to crawl upstairs because of severe exercise-induced hypotension. In the patient on the right, there are minor changes in blood pressure during exercise, but a marked decrease soon after stopping exercise. This patient was usually asymptomatic while walking, but developed postural symptoms when he stopped walking and stood still. It is likely that the decrease in blood pressure post-exercise was due to vasodilatation in exercising skeletal muscle, not opposed by the calf muscle pump. From Mathias and Williams 1994, with permission.

Other measures of assessing baroreceptor reflex function

A variety of techniques ranging from lower-body suction to stimulation of carotid sinus afferents by a neck chamber have been utilized. Negative pressure to the lower half of the body can be exerted by having the subject in a box or capsule extending up to the midthoracic region, with an airtight seal allowing suction, usually by a vacuum cleaner, which unloads and thus stimulates cardiopulmonary and aortic baroreceptor afferents. In normal subjects this should increase sympathetic neural activity, with constriction of resistance vessels, a rise in heart rate, and maintenance of blood pressure. This does not occur in sympathetic vasoconstrictor failure, when blood pressure rapidly falls (Fig. 22.23). In autonomically mediated syncope the combination of lower-body negative pressure along with head-up tilt has been used to provoke syncope (El-Badawi et al. 1994).

A specially designed cervical collar enables assessment of carotid sinus afferents, which may be either inhibited or stimulated by localized elevation or lowering of pressure. The relationship between heart rate and blood pressure helps to construct indices of baroreflex sensitivity. Pharmacological approaches using pressor agents (phenylephrine) or vasodilators (glyceryl trinitrate, nitroprusside), given either as a bolus injection, or sublingually, to transiently raise or lower blood pressure respectively, have also been used. The use of physiological and pharmacological approaches have particular value in the research setting and provide considerable information when combined with haemodynamic measurements in different regions.

Cardiac and regional haemodynamic measurements

Non-invasive techniques are now used widely to measure cardiac and regional haemodynamics. Their main value has been in clinical research laboratories, although the information derived in various disorders increasingly has been utilized in diagnosis and management. The measurements include various aspects of cardiac function (such as stroke volume and cardiac output), and blood flow to skin, skeletal muscle, the splanchnic region, and the brain. Some techniques, such as those for cardiac function and skeletal muscle blood flow, are widely available (Smith et al. 1995). Technological advances have contributed substantially to measurements in other regions. In the splanchnic region, measurement of superior mesenteric artery blood flow can be measured accurately and reproducibly and has enhanced our understanding of the role of the splanchnic circulation in various disorders (Chaudhuri et al. 1991) (Chapter 28). Cutaneous blood flow can be measured continuously using laser Doppler flowmetry that has been used in various disease states (Abbott 1993, Faes et al. 1993). Blood velocity in the middle cerebral artery can be measured using Doppler sonography, which has provided useful information in patients with autonomic failure (Brooks et al. 1989, Lagi et al. 1994) and in autonomic mediated syncope (Diehl et al. 1996) (Fig. 22.24). Near infrared spectroscopy (Elwell et al. 1994), positron emission tomography scanning (Dolan et al. 1997), and functional magnetic resonance imaging provide further information on cerebral blood flow changes, especially in localized regions of the brain (Morris et al. 1996).

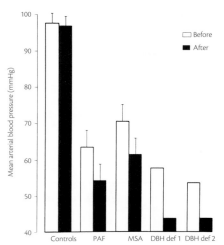

Fig. 22.21 Mean arterial blood pressure during head-up tilt before (open histograms) and 10 minutes after supine exercise (filled histograms) in normal subjects (controls), patients with pure autonomic failure (PAF), multiple system atrophy (MSA), and in two siblings (a brother and sister) with dopamine-beta-hydroxylase (DBH) deficiency. Blood pressure on standing does not change in the controls, either before or after exercise, unlike the autonomic failure groups in whom standing blood pressure after exercise is considerably lower in PAF and MSA, with a substantial accentuation of postural hypotension in the two patients with DBH deficiency. From Smith and Mathias 1995, with permission.

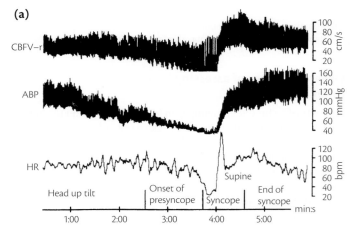

Fig. 22.23 The effect of lower-body negative suction on arterial blood pressure, forearm vascular resistance, and forearm blood flow in a normal subject (upper panel, and in a patient with autonomic failure (lower panel). This rise in forearm vascular resistance in the normal subject during suction is not seen in the patient, in whom there is a substantial fall in blood pressure. From Bannister et al. 1967, with permission.

Spectral analytical techniques to study short-term and long-term cardiovascular changes

These are being utilized increasingly, although largely in a research setting (details in Chapter 24). Beat-to-beat arterial blood pressure and either cerebral blood velocity or heart rate data can be subjected to power spectral transfer function analyses (e.g. estimates of gain, phase and coherence between the two variables) in order to examine cerebrovascular (e.g. cerebral autoregulation) and cardiac baroreflex function (e.g. the 'alpha index'), respectively (Parati et al. 2000). Baroreflex function can also indexed by the calculation of baroreflex sensitivity using the sequence technique, which focuses on the baroreflex (heart rate) response to systolic blood pressure transients (Persson et al. 2001). Furthermore, power

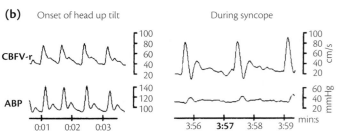

Fig. 22.24 Continuous measurements of right middle cerebral blood velocity (CBV-r), arterial blood pressure (ABP) and heart rate (HR) in a patient before, during, and after tilt-induced neurally mediated (vasovagal) syncope **(a)**. There is a marked fall in ABP that precedes the fall in HR. **(b)**. In the left panel, cerebral blood velocity during head-up tilt before the fall in blood pressure shows a relatively low pulsatility, unlike the arterial blood pressure wave, while this is interchanged during syncope. The findings favour cerebral vasoconstriction during neurally mediated syncope with milder proximal and stronger peripheral vasoconstriction in the cerebral vessels. From Diehl et al. 1996, with permission.

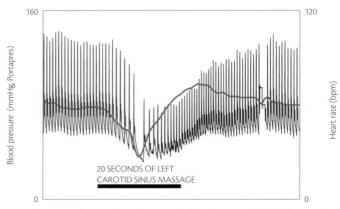

Fig. 22.22 Heart rate and blood pressure before, during, and after left carotid sinus massage in a patient with syncopal episodes. There is a fall in both heart rate and blood pressure during carotid sinus massage, typical of the mixed (cardioinhibitory and vasodepressor) form of this disorder.

spectral analyses of heart rate (e.g. low and high frequencies) can supposedly provide indirect indexes of sympathetic and parasympathetic tone (Chapter 24) or baroreflex function (Rahman et al. 2011). The use of such techniques to study heart rate changes as a measure of cardiac autonomic function during sleep has been of value, especially in certain neuropsychiatric disorders (Ferini-Strambi and Smirne 1997); in narcolepsy there are changes related to impairment of the sleep–awake cycle while in panic disorders sympathetic overactivity occurs only in the day and not at night, thus excluding an intrinsic defect in autonomic regulation.

Electrophysiological assessment of sympathetic activity

Intraneural recordings of sympathetic activity

Skin and muscle sympathetic nerve activity can be recorded using tungsten microelectrodes inserted into a cutaneous nerve in the arm or leg (Chapter 25). Skin sympathetic activity is affected by thermal stimuli and contains neural signals of sudomotor, vasoconstrictor and vasodilator origin (activity can therefore increase with both cold and heat), in contrast to muscle sympathetic activity which responds to manoeuvres activating baroreceptors and is time-locked to blood pressure changes within the cardiac cycle.

Microneurographic techniques have confirmed and advanced our understanding of a considerable number of physiological and pathophysiological processes. However, there are limitations to this technique. Measurements can only be made in a restricted region and although there is a surprisingly good correlation with plasma noradrenaline levels, it may not provide specific answers when stimuli cause differential regional sympathetic responses. More importantly, the procedure is dependent upon considerable skill and, although safe, is an invasive one. It is likely to be unreliable or of no value when sympathoneuronal activity is low or absent, as in autonomic failure.

Sympathetic skin response

Electrical potentials can be recorded from electrodes on the foot and hand using standard electromyographic equipment, before and after stimuli which increase sympathetic cholinergic activity to sweat glands. A variety of these stimuli activate sweat glands, produce of sweat, and change skin resistance, hence the use of the terms sympathetic skin response (SSR), electrodermal activity, and galvanic skin response (Fig. 22.25a). The SSR can be induced by stimuli that are physiological (inspiratory gasp, loud noise, or touch) or electrical (median nerve stimulation) or magnetic (transcranial or neck stimulation). The response is usually absent in axonal neuropathies, but is present in demyelinating disorders (Shahani et al. 1984); this was the original basis of the test which was later adapted as a means of determining sympathetic cholinergic function.

There have been numerous reports on the SSR in a variety of disorders (Arunodaya and Taly 1995), but limited observations on influencing factors and few studies in adequate numbers of clearly defined autonomic disorders. This is compounded by the variability of responses when latency and amplitude are incorporated into calculations. This results in poor sensitivity and specificity, as has been observed previously with polygraph recordings used as a 'lie detector', when the response was measured along with blood

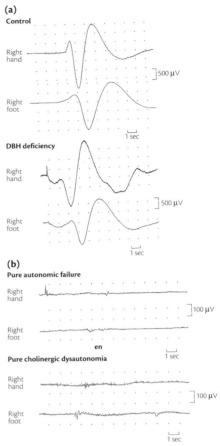

Fig. 22.25 (a) The sympathetic skin response (in microvolts) from the right hand and right foot of a normal subject (control) and a patient with dopamine-beta-hydroxylase (DBH) deficiency. **(b)** The sympathetic skin response could not be recorded in two patients, one with pure autonomic failure (PAF) and the other with pure cholinergic dysautonomia. From Magnifico et al. 1998, with permission.

pressure, heart rate, and respiration rate (Brett et al. 1986). This problem may be avoided by using responses that are either consistently present or absent. When this approach is used the SSR has been reproducibly elicited in normal subjects and patients with dopamine-beta-hydroxylase (DBH) deficiency (with preserved cholinergic function) and is absent in patients with pure autonomic failure and pure cholinergic dysautonomia (Fig. 22.23a, b) (Magnifico et al. 1998). Thus, the SSR may be helpful in patients with peripheral autonomic lesions.

The SSR has the advantage of being a non-invasive test that can be applied readily in most laboratories. However, its value needs further assessment, especially in patients with different types of central autonomic disorders. In MSA with confirmed sympathetic adrenergic failure, up to a third with either the parkinsonian or cerebellar forms had a definite SSR (Fig. 22.26), making it unlikely that it would be a valuable discriminatory test in separating MSA from idiopathic PD (without autonomic failure) (Asahina et al. 2012), especially in the early stages (Magnifico et al. 1997). This is of relevance to observations where the SSR was present, although with a diminished amplitude, in patients who were treated successfully for palmar hyperhidrosis by endoscopic thoracic sympathectomy (Magnifico et al. 1996).

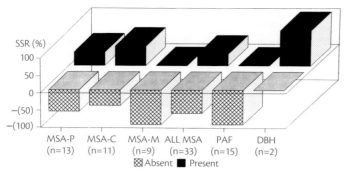

Fig. 22.26 Presence or absence of the sympathetic skin response (SSR) in 33 patients with MSA, 15 patients with pure autonomic failure (PAF), and two siblings with dopamine-beta-hydroxylase (DBH) deficiency. The SSR (as occurs in normal subjects) was present in the two DBH-deficiency patients who had adrenergic failure but preserved cholinergic function; it was absent in all PAF patients with a peripheral sympathetic lesion. A proportion of patients (up to 30%) with the parkinsonian (MSA-P) and cerebellar (MSA-C) forms had preservation of the SSR, despite postural hypotension and definite sympathetic adrenergic failure. Data from Magnifico et al. 1997, with permission.

Similar to the SSR, sympathetic adrenergic pathways can also be evaluated noninvasively using laser Doppler flowmetry by recording the extent of vasoconstriction in the cutaneous circulation (skin vasomotor reflex [SkVR]) (Nicotra et al. 2005). The effects of different stimuli such as inspiratory gasp, mental arithmetic or touch that increase sympathetic activity (SkVR) can be quantified in the hands and feet and also the trunk, as in spinal injury patients. The SkVR responses are generally preserved in MSA but typically reduced in PAF, reflecting extensive postganglionic sympathetic denervation in this group (Young et al. 2006, Asahina et al. 2009).

Biochemical and hormonal

Catecholamines and their metabolites

Noradrenaline is the major neurotransmitter at sympathetic nerve endings, while adrenaline and noradrenaline are both released from the adrenal medulla. Stimuli, such as head-up tilt, that result in sympathoneural activation, elevate levels of noradrenaline in plasma. In sympathetic failure there is no rise in plasma noradrenaline levels and thus the combination of measurement of basal levels along with the response to head-up tilt or standing is necessary (Fig. 22.27). The concentration of noradrenaline in plasma, however, is the net result of a number of processes, involving secretion, neuronal uptake, intraneuronal and extraneuronal metabolism, and clearance. The measurement of metabolites of catecholamines, such as dihydroxyphenylglycol (DHPG), dihydroxyphenylacetic acid (DOPAC) and normetanephrine (NMN), can also be informative. As arterial measurements usually are not made, changes in a venous bed may reflect regional characteristics, which may not be applicable globally.

The basal supine plasma level itself may help in pointing to the possible diagnosis. In PAF, noradrenaline levels, as well as DHPG, and NMN levels (Goldstein et al. 1989), are often low because these patients are likely to have more complete distal lesions, while in MSA, with more central lesions, levels are often within the normal range (Fig. 22.25). Patients with PD who have autonomic failure

also have lower noradrenaline levels than patients without autonomic failure (Senard et al. 1990, Goldstein et al. 2003). It should be noted that basal levels in tetraplegics with a definite preganglionic lesion are about 35% of normal (Chapter 66). Extremely low or virtually undetectable levels of plasma noradrenaline and adrenaline occur in patients with deficiency of the enzyme DBH (Chapter 49). The characteristic difference from other groups with low levels, such as PAF, is that plasma dopamine levels uniquely are elevated (Fig. 22.25). The diagnosis can be confirmed by the absence of DBH in both plasma and tissue. Levels of plasma adrenaline normally often are just at the detection limit of most assays, and basal levels alone do not usually provide useful information. In normal subjects, hypoglycaemia and exercise predominantly raise plasma adrenaline levels; this does not occur in autonomic failure. An excess of plasma noradrenaline and adrenaline may suggest a phaeochromocytoma; such patients characteristically have paroxysms of hypertension, headache and sweating but also may suffer from postural hypotension, because of a low plasma volume and subsensitivity of α-adrenoceptors.

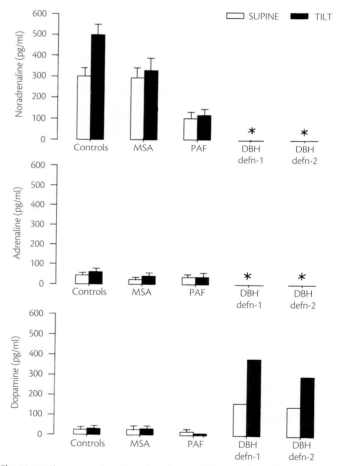

Fig. 22.27 Plasma noradrenaline, adrenaline, and dopamine levels (measured by high pressure liquid chromatography) in normal subjects (controls), patients with multiple system atrophy (MSA), pure autonomic failure (PAF), and two individual patients with dopamine-beta-hydroxylase deficiency (DBH def) while supine and after head-up tilt to 45° for 10 minutes. The asterisk indicates levels below the detection limits for the assay, which are less than 5 pg/ml for noradrenaline and adrenaline and less than 20 pg/ml for dopamine. Bars indicate ± SEM.

Measurements of catecholamines and their metabolites in urine have certain advantages, as they provide a measure of secretion over a longer period, which may be of value in phaeochromocytoma where there may be intermittent secretion. They also may help in the diagnosis of rarer forms of autonomic failure and the monitoring of their treatment. In DBH deficiency, urinary dopamine metabolites are normal or elevated, while those of noradrenaline and adrenaline are almost undetectable; with adequate treatment with DL- or L-threo-dihydroxyphenylserine, noradrenaline metabolites increase (Chapter 49). A number of other urinary metabolites provide indices of central or peripheral catecholamine metabolism.

Techniques such as total-body and regional noradrenaline spillover have provided valuable information on sympathetic activation in the body, heart, and vascular regions (such as the splanchnic and renal circulations), and in the brain (Esler et al. 1993, Lambert et al. 1997). Patients with PD and PAF have low cardiac norepinephrine spillover their reductions in cardiac sympathetic innervation (Goldstein et al. 1997, 2000). The use of radioactive substances and cannulation of arteries and major veins, however, restrict their use to highly specialized research laboratories.

There also are non-invasive approaches to assess regional sympathetic innervation and function. Imaging techniques have been developed to determine cardiac sympathetic innervation using myocardial scintigraphy of the physiological analogue of noradrenaline, [^{123}I]meta-iodobenzyl guanidine (MIBG), that is taken up into sympathetic nerve terminals and can be measured by single photon emission computed tomography (SPECT). Alternatively, 6-[^{18}F]fluorodopamine can be used to visualize sympathetic innervation of cardiac tissue using positron emission tomographic (PET) scanning (Goldstein et al. 1997ab). In MSA, consistent with a preganglionic lesion, noradrenaline transport is preserved, as in normal subjects (Braune et al. 1999), with some exceptions (Raffel et al. 2006). There is impaired uptake in both PD and PAF, suggesting cardiac sympathetic denervation (Goldstein et al. 2000, Sharabi et al. 2008). Impaired uptake has also been shown to occur in some patients with PD prior to the presentation of clinical features suggesting autonomic failure and the motor stages of PD (Goldstein et al. 2007, Haensch et al. 2009). Decreased noradrenergic innervation has also been shown in the renal cortex (Tipre and Goldstein 2005) in PD with autonomic failure (PD + AF) and PAF and in the thyroid (Matsui et al. 2005) in PD + AF. MIBG scanning also successfully images adrenal and extra-adrenal phaeochromocytoma.

Renin–angiotensin–aldosterone system

This system has a major influence on blood pressure. Renin is released from the juxtaglomerular cells of the renal afferent arterioles and, by a series of steps, results in the formation of the active pressor agent, angiotensin II, which has multiple actions on blood vessels, sympathetic nerves, the brain, and also on the adrenal cortex (to cause secretion of aldosterone). In adrenocortical deficiency (such as Addison's disease), postural hypotension may occur, and there is a compensatory and marked elevation in renin and angiotensin II levels while plasma aldosterone levels are extremely low. In such patients plasma cortisol levels do not rise after administration of adrenocorticotrophic hormone.

In autonomic disorders, the renin response to head-up tilt or standing may be of relevance to the use of head-up tilt at night to reduce postural hypotension (Chapter 47). In some patients with primary autonomic failure the renin response is impaired, especially when related to their marked hypotension during head-up tilt (Bannister et al. 1979). In others, however, there may be an exaggerated rise (Mathias et al. 1977), as is also observed in tetraplegic patients (Chapter 66). If renin measurements are made, care should be taken to obtain an adequate basal level, keeping in mind the long half-life of renin. A 10-minute period of tilt may suffice to demonstrate an exaggerated response (Fig. 22.28), although a longer period is preferable, especially if plasma aldosterone is also being measured. A variety of influences, including salt intake and drugs, such as fludrocortisone, can modify renin release.

Antidiuretic hormone (vasopressin)

In normal subjects, there is a rise in plasma vasopressin levels with head-up tilt and with hyperosmotic stimuli. Vasopressin levels have been used to assess the integrity of the afferent and central autonomic pathways. In afferent lesions vasopressin levels do not rise with head-up tilt, unlike patients with central lesions of the baroreceptor pathways, in whom there is no response; in both however, there is a preserved response to an osmotic stimulus, confirming integrity of the relevant hypothalamic nuclei and their posterior pituitary connections. In PAF, vasopressin levels rise with head-up tilt, unlike in MSA (Kaufmann et al. 1992). In patients with cervical spinal-cord injuries there is an exaggerated rise in vasopressin levels with head-up tilt (Chapter 66).

Pharmacological

Information on the integrity of autonomic pathways, the number and sensitivity of receptors on target organs, and on functional components of the autonomic nervous system may be obtained by using drugs that are either agonists or antagonists. When combined with relevant hormonal responses they provide further

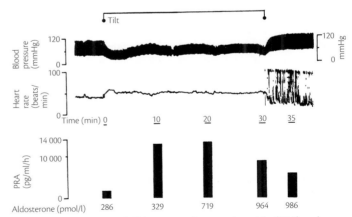

Fig. 22.28 Blood pressure (BP), heart rate, plasma renin activity (PRA), and plasma aldosterone levels in a patient with autonomic failure before, during and after head-up tilt to 45° for 30 minutes. There was an immediate fall in both systolic and diastolic BP which gradually recovered. There was a small elevation in BP over previous basal levels on return to the horizontal. Heart rate rose when BP fell, but the response was modest. Following return to the horizontal, bigeminal rhythm occurred, accounting for the abnormal trace. Levels of plasma renin activity rose markedly during head-up tilt, reaching the levels often seen in severely hypertensive patients with renal artery stenosis. Plasma aldosterone levels rose later. From Bannister et al. 1986, with permission.

information on central and peripheral autonomic pathways and on autonomic receptors. It is important, especially in patients with suspected autonomic disorders who may have abnormal responses, that drugs to reverse their effects are available along with resuscitation facilities.

Drugs acting on the sympathetic nervous system

Noradrenaline

Noradrenaline is the major neurotransmitter at sympathetic nerve endings and predominantly stimulates α-adrenoceptors, with some effects on β-adrenoceptors. Pressor sensitivity to noradrenaline can be tested by intravenous infusion, beginning with a low dose (in case of supersensitivity) followed by increments every 5–10 minutes, with careful monitoring of blood pressure, heart rate, and the ECG. Construction of a dose–response curve will indicate whether there is an enhanced pressor response, when compared to normal responses. In more distal sympathetic lesions, as in PAF, the dose–response curve is shifted considerably to the left, and there is also a greater slope, indicating that these patients have a greater degree of pressor supersensitivity than MSA patients (Fig. 22.29). The mechanisms responsible for pressor supersensitivity appear to be multiple. Indirect evidence from studies of α_2-adrenoceptors on platelets suggest that there is up-regulation of adrenoceptors, probably because of the low levels of plasma noradrenaline. This may account for the difference in slope. The shift to the left that occurs in both PAF and MSA suggests that impairment of the baroreceptor reflex and the inability to compensate in different vascular beds (as also occurs in tetraplegic patients), may be major factors. Finally, clearance of noradrenaline is likely to be affected, depending upon both the site and the degree of sympathetic nerve impairment. The reverse, an impaired pressor response to noradrenaline and other vasopressor agents, may occur in systemic amyloidosis because of infiltration of blood vessels by amyloid tissue.

Assessment of sensitivity to noradrenaline or other adrenoceptor agonists (such as phenylephrine), is of value in providing evidence of sensitivity of blood vessels and the possible response to sympathomimetic treatment. As with other pharmacological tests, these should be performed in laboratories familiar with the techniques. Because of pressor supersensitivity, testing in patients with suspected autonomic disorders should begin cautiously, using doses of a fifth or less than usual. Supine hypertension may occur in patients with autonomic failure and the clinical investigator will need to decide which level of blood pressure can be reached safely in individual patients. One should be on guard for cardiac dysrhythmias. The ready availability of suitable drugs and resuscitation measures in an emergency is a necessity. Rapid relief of severe hypertension may be obtained by placing patients in the head-up position.

Tyramine

Tyramine releases noradrenaline from both the granules and the cytosol within the sympathetic nerve terminal. A lack of rise in blood pressure and in plasma noradrenaline or DHPG levels is indicative of absent noradrenaline stores and is characteristic of widespread postganglionic denervation or noradrenaline depletion, as in PAF and PD + AF (Sharabi et al. 2008) and DBH deficiency (Chapter 49). In incomplete lesions, however, release of even subnormal amounts of noradrenaline may cause a substantial

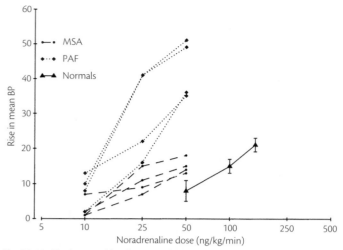

Fig. 22.29 Rise in mean blood pressure (BP) in four patients with pure autonomic failure (PAF), four patients with multiple system atrophy (MSA), and normal subjects (± SEM) during graded intravenous infusions of noradrenaline. Both groups of patients with autonomic failure had increased sensitivity to infused noradrenaline. In the PAF patients there appears to be a considerably greater response.

pressor response because of super-sensitivity; this impairs interpretation of tyramine-induced responses.

Yohimbine

Yohimbine is an α_2-adrenoreceptor antagonist that blocks α-receptors on sympathetic nerve terminals and increases sympathetic nerve activity and thereby noradrenaline. The pressor response to yohimbine can therefore be related to the ability of the sympathetic nerves to activated and thus to release noradrenaline. PAF and PD + AF have small plasma noradrenaline responses to yohimbine (Sharabi et al. 2008) that may be lower than those in MSA. The pressor response is however much lower in PD + AF and PAF compared with MSA with the increase directly related to the baseline noradrenaline levels (Sharabi et al. 2006). Yohimbine challenge testing may show excessive noradrenaline release in patients with anxiety or panic disorder (Goldstein 2010).

Isoprenaline

Isoprenaline is a β-adrenoceptor agonist which acts on both the β_1 and β_2 subtypes. The β_1 subtype is concerned predominantly with raising heart rate, and the β_2 subtype with vasodilatation and bronchodilatation. Isoprenaline can be given either as a bolus or as an intravenous infusion and its effects on heart rate and blood-pressure provide an indication of β-adrenoceptor responsiveness. In patients with autonomic failure and in tetraplegics, bolus intravenous injections cause an exaggerated but transient fall in both systolic and diastolic blood pressure (Fig. 22.30).

Similar changes occur with intravenous infusion of isoprenaline (Fig. 22.31). This may result from β_2-adrenoceptor supersensitivity, and from unopposed β_2-adrenoceptor-induced vasodilatation because of the baroreceptor deficit. PAF and PD + AF patients have virtually absent noradrenaline responses to Isoprenaline (Sharabi et al. 2008). Chronotropic supersensitivity to isoprenaline does not occur in autonomic failure with vagal denervation (Fig. 22.32), despite indirect *in vitro* evidence from lymphocyte studies that suggest an increase in β-adrenoceptor numbers. In tetraplegic

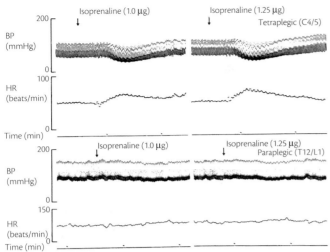

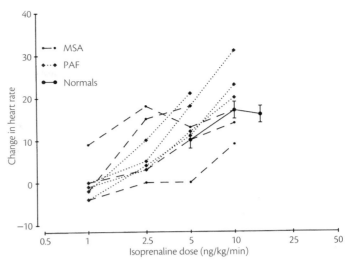

Fig. 22.30 Blood pressure (BP) and heart rate (HR) in a tetraplegic patient (upper panel) and a paraplegic patient with an almost intact sympathetic nervous system (lower panel) in response to bolus injections of isoprenaline. In the tetraplegic patient, there is a clear fall in blood pressure after isoprenaline. This probably results from β$_2$-adrenoceptor-mediated vasodilatation. There is a rise in heart rate before the blood pressure falls and this is likely to be β$_1$-adrenoceptor-mediated effect, which is then enhanced by the fall in blood pressure. In the paraplegic patient, there are considerably smaller changes. From Mathias and Frankel 1986, with permission.

Fig. 22.32 Change in heart rate in response to incremental infusion of isoprenaline in four patients with pure autonomic failure (PAF) and in four patients with multiple system atrophy (MSA). The response in normal subjects (± SEM) is indicated. Despite a fall in blood pressure in most patients with autonomic failure, only a few had a greater increase in sensitivity. Chronotropic β-adrenergic supersensitivity does not appear, therefore, to be as marked as pressor sensitivity in autonomic failure patients.

patients, the fall in blood pressure in the presence of the preserved afferent baroreceptor and efferent vagal pathways may result in a greater rise in heart rate, which is not necessarily attributable to β-adrenoceptor supersensitivity.

Clonidine

Clonidine is an α2-adrenoceptor agonist which has a number of effects, including a predominant cerebral action in reducing

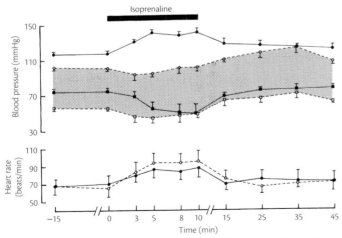

Fig. 22.31 Blood pressure and heart rate in five tetraplegic patients (open circles and squares and broken line) and five control subjects (full circles and squares and continuous line) before, during, and after intravenous infusion of isoprenaline (0.01 μg/min/kg). The shaded area indicates blood pressure in the tetraplegic patients; bars indicate ± SEM. In the tetraplegics, there is a fall in both systolic and diastolic blood pressure. From Mathias et al. 1981, with permission.

sympathetic neural activity and thus lowering blood pressure. In normal subjects after clonidine, plasma noradrenaline levels fall and serum growth hormone levels rise. The latter is dependent upon intact central autonomic pathways. Clonidine can be given intravenously (2 μg/kg body weight over 10 minutes to avoid a transient pressor effect), with observations for a period of 75–90 minutes after administration. Its side-effects include dryness of mouth and sedation. After an hour following intravenous infusion most subjects are awake, although drowsy.

The uses of clonidine include:

- Determining residual sympathetic nervous activity and its contribution to the maintenance of blood pressure. In patients with PAF there is usually an initial rise followed by a fall in blood pressure (because of supersensitivity) with a small fall or no further reduction in the low levels of plasma noradrenaline, unlike normal subjects in whom both blood pressure and plasma noradrenaline levels fall (Thomaides et al. 1992). In patients with MSA or with incomplete autonomic lesions, there is usually a fall in supine blood pressure and plasma noradrenaline levels and to a greater extent than in PAF (Young et al. 2006). Similar changes to those in PAF are observed in DBH deficiency (Chapter 49). In tetraplegics there is a transient pressor response with intravenous clonidine; after oral clonidine, blood pressure is unchanged (Chapter 66).

- Distinguishing phaeochromocytoma patients with autonomous noradrenaline secretion from patients with essential hypertension and labile hypertension who have elevated basal noradrenaline levels—in phaeochromocytoma, plasma noradrenaline levels remain elevated, unlike normal subjects or essential hypertensive patients in whom levels fall after clonidine (Fig. 22.33).

- Measuring the growth hormone response as a neuroendocrine marker of integrity of the central adrenergic system—in normal

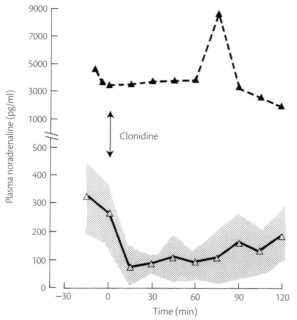

Fig. 22.33 Plasma noradrenaline levels in a patient with a phaeochromocytoma (▲– –▲) and in a group of patients with essential hypertension (Δ––Δ) before and after intravenous clonidine, indicated by an arrow (2 μg/kg over 10 minutes). Plasma noradrenaline levels fall rapidly in the essential hypertensives after clonidine and remain low over the period of observation. The stippled area indicates the ± SEM. Plasma noradrenaline levels are considerably higher in the phaeochromocytoma patient and are not affected by clonidine.

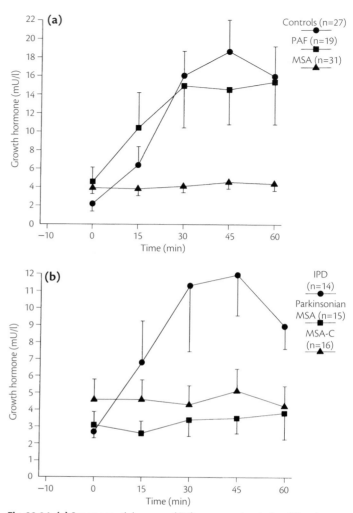

Fig. 22.34 **(a)** Serum growth hormone (GH) concentrations before (0) and at 15-minute intervals for 60 minutes after clonidine (2 μg/kg/min) in normal subjects (controls) and in patients with pure autonomic failure (PAF) and multiple system atrophy (MSA). GH concentrations rise in controls and in patients with PAF with a peripheral lesion; there is no rise in patients with MSA with a central lesion. (From Kimber et al. 1997.) **(b)** Indicates lack of serum GH response to clonidine in MSA (the cerebellar form; MSA-C and the parkinsonian form) in contrast to patients with idiopathic Parkinson's disease with no autonomic deficit IPD), in whom there is a significant rise in GH levels. From Kimber et al. 1997, with permission.

subjects, serum growth hormone levels rise substantially within 15 minutes after clonidine. There is a similar rise in growth hormone levels in patients with PAF in whom the lesions are peripheral, unlike those with MSA in whom there is no rise (Thomaides et al. 1992). These results have been confirmed in larger numbers of PAF and MSA patients, and include MSA with either the parkinsonian or cerebellar form (Fig. 22.34a) (Kimber et al. 1997). More important, in patients with PD, there is a rise in serum growth hormone levels after clonidine (Fig. 22.34b), indicating that in addition to being a useful means of distinguishing central from peripheral autonomic failure, the clonidine–growth hormone test may distinguish MSA from PD (Iodice et al. 2011). In MSA patients who have an absent or impaired growth hormone response to clonidine, the oral administration of the growth hormone secretagogue, L-dopa, raises levels of plasma growth hormone releasing factor (GHRF) and growth hormone, thus indicating the integrity of hypothalamic GHRF-secreting neurones and confirming responsiveness of the anterior pituitary cells. Furthermore, this favours a specific α2-adrenoceptor–hypothalamic deficit in MSA. The clonidine–growth hormone test therefore, may help further in the evaluation of central neurotransmitter abnormalities, in addition to its potential diagnostic capabilities.

Drugs acting on the cholinergic system

Edrophonium

This is a short-acting cholinesterase inhibitor which may help differentiate pre- from postganglionic sympathetic lesions by

stimulating nicotinic receptors within paravertebral ganglia (Gemmill et al. 1988). In PAF with distal lesions edrophonium has no effects, and there is no change in plasma noradrenaline levels. In MSA, where it is presumed there is an intact postganglionic system, there is a rise in noradrenaline levels. The limitations and value of edrophonium testing in different autonomic disorders remain to be evaluated.

Atropine

Postsynaptic parasympathetic and sympathetic cholinergic receptors are of the muscarinic subtype and are effectively blocked by atropine sulphate. It can be used to determine the degree of cardiac vagal (cholinergic) involvement. In normal subjects bolus intravenous doses of 5 μg/kg body weight at 2-minute intervals raise heart rate. Doses up to a total of 1800 μg are usually sufficient to assess responsiveness and construct a dose–response curve (Fig. 22.35). Further atropine should not be given if the heart rate rises above about 110 bpm, or if there is evidence of an abnormal cardiac rhythm. After atropine, side-effects are usually mild, but may be troublesome. Dilatation of the pupils and blurring of vision, because of its cycloplegic effects, may occur. It may impair detrusor muscle activity and the urinary bladder should be emptied before the test. A dry mouth is common and may last for an hour. Subjects should be cautioned not to drink fluids in excess.

In the majority of patients with PAF and MSA, there is vagal impairment with a flat dose–response curve. This is consistent with neuropathological observations on the vagus that indicate lesions either in the dorsal vagal nuclei within the brainstem or more peripherally.

Thermoregulatory and sweat testing

The regulation of body temperature is dependent upon a number of factors that influence heat generation and disposal. Heat disposal depends upon the sudomotor system and the ability of the cutaneous circulation to respond appropriately. Thermoregulatory sweating is tested by raising the core temperature by 1°C, using a variety of methods, such as, a hot room (e.g. a heat chamber) and space blankets. Normally, sweating occurs through stimulation of eccrine sweat glands which are widely distributed over the body. This can be aided by pretreatment with a diaphoretic, paracetamol (0.5 or 1 g orally). The detection of sweat production can be enhanced by using indicator dyes such as quinizarine red, ponso red or alizarin red; when sprinkled on the skin they turn from pale pink to bright red on exposure to moisture. In patients with PAF and MSA thermoregulatory sweating is often impaired. In DBH deficiency, however, sweating is preserved and provides an important clue to the diagnosis (Chapter 49). Other tests of sweat gland function are described in Chapter 31.

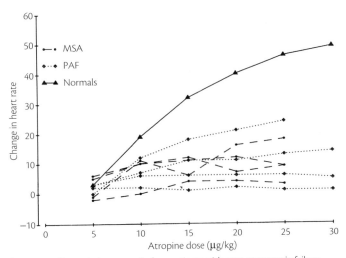

Fig. 22.35 Change in heart rate in four patients with pure autonomic failure (PAF) and four patients with multiple system atrophy (MSA) in response to atropine. In most patients, there is minimal change in heart rate unlike the change expected in normal subjects. Cardiac vagal impairment seems to occur equally in both groups of patients.

The indicator dyes can be used to determine local abnormalities of sudomotor function as in the patchy denervation caused by leprosy (Karat et al. 1969). When applied over the skin and covered by a transparent tape, especially with the subject in a warm room, a colour change occurs in normal but not denervated areas; this may provide a rapid and semi-quantitative assessment applicable to multiple sites if needed, as has been demonstrated in PAF and MSA patients (Riedel and Mathias 1997). Other approaches include the acetylcholine sweatspot test (Ryder et al. 1988). Local disorders of sweating may need special methods of study. In gustatory sweating (Frey's syndrome), severe and socially embarrassing sweating may occur after ingestion of spicy or acidic foods and those containing tyramine. Challenge with food, together with the use of the indicator dye over the head, neck, and trunk, helps determine the area of distribution.

In patients who cannot control their cutaneous circulation, hypothermia may occur in temperate or cold climates, especially in tetraplegics who are unable to shiver (Chapter 66). The reverse, hyperpyrexia, may occur in extremely hot weather, especially when sweating is also impaired. In such patients it is important that core temperature (for example, using a rectal or sublingual thermometer) is measured. If hypothermia is suspected, a low-reading thermometer should be used. In patients with MSA and PAF there is a lack of circadian variation in body temperature, which either does not fall at night, or only minimally in MSA with autonomic failure, unlike in normal subjects (Pierangeli et al. 1997). Details of thermoregulation and its investigation are in Chapter 21.

Gastrointestinal system

The gastrointestinal system is often involved in autonomic disorders. Investigations will depend upon the specific problem.

Oropharyngeal dysphagia may occur, especially in the later states of MSA. Although often asymptomatic, it is of clinical importance as it may result in tracheal aspiration, especially in the presence of laryngeal abductor cord paresis. Videocinefluoroscopic examination is a valuable means of assessing swallowing disturbances (Fig. 22.36) (Mathias 1996). The upper gastrointestinal tract may be assessed using a barium swallow and follow-through. In localized oesophageal involvement (as in Chagas' disease) a barium swallow alone may help. Studies of pressure changes, especially in the oesophagogastric sphincter region may show a different value. If gastroscopy is utilized, an advantage is biopsy of tissue, thus enabling diagnosis of conditions such as systemic amyloidosis. Assessment of gastric motility may be of importance (Chapter 27). In some disorders, rapid gastric emptying is a problem, while in others, such as diabetes, gastroparesis may be particularly troublesome (Chapter 53).

Constipation is a common complaint in autonomic failure. Occasionally other coincidental disorders, such as neoplasia in the elderly, need to be considered. A barium enema or colonoscopy may be helpful. A rectal biopsy and staining with Congo red may provide a definitive diagnosis in amyloidosis.

Renal and urinary bladder function

Nocturnal polyuria is common in autonomic disorders, and in autonomic failure may result in overnight weight loss of over a kilogram with a reduction in extracellular fluid volume; this

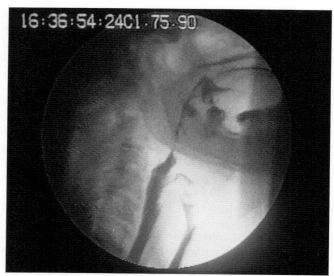

Fig. 22.36 Still from a videocinefluoroscopic examination in a subject with oropharyngeal dysphagia, showing contrast medium in the larynx, with the potential to lead to tracheal aspiration. From Mathias 1996c, with permission.

appears to aggravate postural hypotension in the morning. This can be assessed by 12-hourly evaluations (day and night) of urine volume and, if possible, of sodium and potassium secretion (Mathias et al. 1986). If there is urinary bladder or sphincter involvement, nocturnal polyuria may cause even greater difficulties because of the frequency of micturition, and at times incontinence. The assessments are helpful in predicting the value of the antidiuretic agent, desmopressin, which may be used intranasally or in an oral form at night to reduce nocturnal polyuria (Chapter 47).

Urodynamic measurements provide information on the nature of bladder dysfunction, such as detrusor areflexia or hyper-reflexia. Urethral sphincter electromyography shows a distinct pattern in patients with MSA, and may help distinguish them from those with PD (Chapter 37). Urinary infections and calculi may complicate bladder dysfunction, and suitable investigations, including intravenous urography and ultrasound examination, may be needed.

Sexual function

Impotence in the male is usual in autonomic failure. Organic erectile failure can be difficult to distinguish from psychogenic impotence, though nocturnal erections do not occur in the former. Penile plethysmography may help. Intracorporeal injection of papavarine causes an erection in both groups and therefore is not a means of differentiating between the two (Chapter 37). In situations such as diabetes mellitus, vascular factors also may contribute. In DBH deficiency erection is preserved but there is delayed ejaculation, which can be improved by the drug dihydroxyphenylserine (DOPS), which replenishes noradrenaline levels (Chapter 49).

Respiratory system

Stridor, particularly at night, may occur in the later stages in MSA because of paralysis of abductor muscles of the vocal cord (Chapter 33). This can be detected by laryngoscopy. Brainstem dysfunction causing periods of apnoea may further contribute to hypoxia and complicate the problem. Blood gas monitoring during sleep may be necessary to determine whether significant oxygen desaturation occurs. These investigations are of relevance to management, including the decision on proceeding to a tracheostomy (Harcourt et al. 1996).

The eye

Lacrimal secretion may be diminished as a result of direct involvement of the gland, as in Sjögren's syndrome. Lacrimal secretion can be tested by using a special absorbent paper, which forms the basis of Schirmer's test. Diminished secretion or alacrima may result in corneal abrasions which may need to be assessed using either fluorescein or Bengal red dyes, and a slit lamp.

Intraocular pressure may be reduced in sympathetic lesions, as in Horner's syndrome, but has minimal clinical significance when compared with the elevation of intraocular pressure that may occur with anticholinergic drugs, especially in patients who are prone to glaucoma. Intraocular pressure may be dependent on systemic blood pressure, as has been demonstrated in patients with PAF and MSA (Dumskyj et al. 1997). In these patients, intraocular pressure was lower when blood pressure was reduced during head-up tilt and rose when blood pressure was elevated by returning them to the horizontal and during head-down tilt. This may have implications in the consideration and assessment of glaucoma in such patients.

The pupil is involved in a number of autonomic disorders and can be assessed using either pharmacological approaches (sympathomimetics and cholinomimetics and testing for supersensitivity) or specialized physiological function tests (Chapter 36).

Olfactory function

Anosmia can be present in autonomic failure and may be a means of determining the underlying pathology. The presence of alpha-synuclein in the olfactory bulb is one of the earliest pathologic findings in PD (Braak et al. 2004). Olfactory function can be assessed using the University of Pennsylvania Smell Identification Test (UPSIT) or the 'Sniffin Sticks' smell test. A variety of odours are presented to the patient and one of four options must be chosen with an allotted time for each one. When compared with healthy control individuals, olfactory function is lower in MSA, PAF and PD (Wenning et al. 1995, Muller et al. 2002, Silveira-Moriyama et al. 2009) with the lowest scores reported in PD (Muller et al. 2002, Silveira-Moriyama et al. 2009), or in both PD and PAF presumed to be due to Lewy bodies in both these disorders (Goldstein and Sewell 2009). In PD, anosmia is associated with baroreflex failure and cardiac and organ-selective extracardiac noradrenergic denervation, independently of parkinsonism or striatal dopaminergic denervation (Goldstein et al. 2010) and can pre-date motor symptoms in PD (Ponsen et al. 2004).

Miscellaneous investigations

In this section a range of investigations which may be of value in the assessment of patients with autonomic disorders are described briefly. Some of these investigations are concerned directly with diagnosis, others with elimination of disorders that may mimic autonomic failure, and in addition there are those that provide valuable information in understanding the pathophysiological basis of certain autonomic disorders.

Neurophysiological tests

Electroencephalography may be needed as the distinction between syncope (due to autonomic impairment) and epilepsy can be difficult (Lempert 1996). Occasionally, epileptic seizures may be induced because of an extremely low cerebral perfusion pressure. A variety of transient motor abnormalities, including myoclonic jerks, have been recorded in normal subjects in whom syncope was induced (Lempert et al. 1994).

Auditory evoked responses are of value in separating patients with cerebral lesions as in MSA, from those with more distal lesions as in PAF (Chapter 39). A variety of peripheral electrophysiological studies are of value to determine the specific type of neuropathy, or its absence. Thermal threshold testing is a sensitive means of determining unmyelinated fibre involvement. The absence of the 'H' reflex is characteristic of patients with the Holmes–Adie syndrome, where there is a myotonic pupil and absent tendon reflexes.

Neuro-otological studies

Dizziness is a common symptom in both neuro-otological and autonomic disorders (Chapter 8). In most patients the history and clinical examination separates one from the other, although in some this may not be so. Neuro-otological investigations are of particular value in excluding or confirming primary or coincidental vestibular dysfunction when suspected.

Cardiac investigations

There are a number of cardiac causes of syncope, the most dramatic probably being Stokes–Adams attacks (Chapter 57). In the young the long Q–T syndrome needs to be excluded, while in the elderly cardiac dysrhythmias are common and the use of a 24-hour tape with computerized analysis of cardiac rhythm may be necessary. In rare cases, postural hypotension may be the result of an atrial myxoma and two-dimensional echocardiography is the ideal non-invasive means of making or excluding this diagnosis.

Biopsies

Tissue can be subjected to light microscopy, electron microscopy, and a range of immunohistochemical studies. In amyloidosis, biopsy of the kidney or a sural nerve may provide the diagnosis when tissues are stained with Congo red. Sural nerve biopsies provide valuable information on the nerve fibres and on both degenerative and regenerative peripheral neural processes (Chapter 51). Muscle biopsies in autonomic failure are described in Chapter 39. Skin biopsies have proved to be of value in patients with DBH deficiency, as they have confirmed the integrity of perivascular sympathetic nerves and demonstrated the normal distribution of a range of neuropeptides, some associated with sympathetic nerves (such as neuropeptide Y) and others with parasympathetic nerves (such as vasoactive intestinal peptide) (Chapter 49). In these patients, there is lack of immunoreactivity to DBH in skin tissue containing sympathetic nerves that further confirms the diagnosis. Immunoreactivity to DBH, tyrosine hydroxylase, and the sensory neuropeptides, substance P and CGRP, could not be detected in a skin biopsy in a patient with autonomic and sensory neuropeptide deficiency resulting from a presumed nerve growth factor deficiency (Chapter 49). Based on morphological analyses of skin biopsies, autonomic and somatic innervation has been reported to be impaired in individual case reports of patients with

PD (Donadio et al. 2005, Nolano et al. 2008). PD patients have a significant increase in tactile and thermal thresholds, a significant reduction in mechanical pain perception and loss of epidermal nerve fibres and Meissner corpuscles (Doandio et al. 2005, Nolano et al. 2008). Reduced autonomic innervation of the blood vessels, sweat glands and the erector pili muscles is not restricted to severe cases and may precede the onset of autonomic symptoms in PD at early stages of the disease (Dabby et al. 2006).

Intradermal histamine test

The use of the intradermal histamine test to assess the Lewis response may be of value in certain disorders, especially if correlation with the composition of skin tissue is possible. An abnormal skin histamine response is a characteristic feature of patients with familial dysautonomia (Riley–Day syndrome; Chapter 48); in a patient with diminished sensory neuropeptides (Chapter 51), there was a diminished histamine response consistent with low or absent sensory neuropeptide levels in skin.

Neuroimaging

A range of non-invasive technological advances now enables assessment of cerebral and spinal morphology. A CT scan is often of value but there are considerable advantages in performing an MRI scan (Schrag et al. 1998), especially when determining abnormalities within the basal ganglia, brainstem, and spinal cord. Changes in the basal ganglia and brainstem, including posterior putaminal hypointensity, hyperintense lateral putaminal rim, hot cross bun sign, and middle cerebellar peduncle hyperintensities occur in MSA (see Figure; Gilman et al. 2008). In addition, positron emission tomography (PET) or single photon emission computed tomography (SPECT) scans can provide details of the formation, distribution, and receptor configuration of neuro-transmitters within the central nervous system. Imaging the dopamine active transporter (DAT) provides a measure of dopamine terminal function and can detect striatal dopamine deficiency in idiopathic PD and atypical neurodegenerative parkinsonian disorders such as MSA (see Figure; Brooks, 2011). The value of PET and SPECT scans in separating MSA from PAF, and in the evaluation of neuro-chemical abnormalities, is discussed in Chapters 39 and 40.

Genetic analyses

Recent developments in genetic analyses have increased the understanding of the pathophysiology and hereditary components of autonomic disorders. Genome wide association studies have shown that single nucleotide polymorphism at the alpha-synuclein gene locus are significantly associated with an increased risk for the development of MSA (Scholz et al. 2009) with the strongest association in the cerebellar subtype of MSA (Al-Chalabi et al. 2009). Similarly, in a series of familial PD + AF cases, mutation of the gene encoding alpha-synuclein; whole-gene triplication, was reported (Singleton et al. 2004). Genetic analyses may also be important in cases of suspected familial amyloid polyneuropathy where autonomic dysfunction can occur (Reilly and Staunton, 1996).

Conclusions

The autonomic nervous system innervates every organ and in the generalized autonomic disorders there may be impaired function of virtually every organ in the body. As indicated in this chapter, there is a wide range of investigative approaches and, depending upon the clinical questions raised, specific tests will need to be performed. Further details of certain tests can be found in relevant chapters.

Advances in investigation and diagnosis of various autonomic disorders, and recognition of their complications in various diseases, have resulted in autonomic laboratories now fulfilling an important clinical service role, as distinct from the past where these activities were incorporated, sometimes loosely, into research units. A basic requirement of such laboratories should be the provision of screening autonomic function tests, the capacity to perform additional investigations (such as food challenge, exercise, carotid sinus massage and sudomotor/thermoregulatory tests), and in conjunction with other specialties (such as with gastroenterology, cardiology and endocrinology, as examples) if needed, the ability to advise on, and direct, the evaluation and management of suspected autonomic disorders. Such activities are probably best incorporated into a regional neuroscience or cardiovascular unit or, as in our case, national referral units. The setting up of an autonomic laboratory will depend upon the acquisition of appropriate equipment, which is likely to vary because of dependence on a large number of factors ranging from finance to access for servicing and maintenance of equipment. A crucial factor however, is the training of the physicians directing the unit, and the technical staff performing the investigations. The increasing complexity of autonomic testing, and more importantly its interpretation, now demands that a trainee spends an adequate period in an established autonomic unit, which ideally deals with an extensive range of disorders and has wide expertise on many fronts. The formalized training of technical staff may also need to be considered. This would be similar to medical and paramedical training programmes in neurophysiological, cardiovascular, and cardiology laboratories. A recognized period of training, with accreditation when completed, may become a necessary requirement as autonomic investigation increasingly becomes an integral part of clinical practice in the diagnosis and management of a wide variety of neurological and other medical disorders. Furthermore, interpretation of autonomic testing may be of crucial importance in litigation, especially involving the effects of drugs and toxins.

It is re-emphasized that results obtained from the investigation of autonomic disorders need to be interpreted in conjunction with the clinical state and confounding variables that relate not only to the autonomic nervous system but also to organs they supply, as most tests are dependent upon target organ function. The complexities in many of the systems involved also make it more appropriate that responses to testing are described individually, to have a measure of both the defect and the associated dysfunction, rather than having them incorporated as part of a scoring system. Some of these scoring systems (Low 1993) combine the results of adrenergic, cardiovagal, and sudomotor testing, and although they provide a numerical figure, this often does not aid understanding of the specific attendant abnormalities, or recognition of functional deficits. However, in certain situations as in a research setting, they may be of value.

Finally, it cannot be stressed too strongly that autonomic investigation has to be determined selectively, ideally by a clinician, and preferably by one with a background in integrative physiology, who will take account of various factors, which should also include time,

patient tolerance, and cost. This is because after the initial screening tests, subsequent investigations are often not routine and must be designed to answer specific questions. It is intended that this chapter, by providing an overview of the investigation of those autonomic abnormalities that cause morbidity and contribute to mortality, will help in early diagnosis and comprehensive assessment, each of which is important for prognosis and for appropriate management.

References

Abbott, N. G., Beck, J. S. Wilson, S. B., and Khan, F. (1993). Vasomotor reflexes in the fingertip skin of patients with Type 1 diabetes mellitus and leprosy. *Clin. Auton. Res.* **3**, 189–93.

Alam, M., Smith, G. D. P., Bleasdale-Barr, K., Pavitt, D. V., and Mathias, C. J. (1995). Effects of the peptide release inhibitor, Octreotide, on daytime hypotension and on nocturnal hypertension in primary autonomic failure. *J. Hypertension* **13**, 1664–9.

Al-Chalabi, A., Dürr, A., Wood, N. W., *et al.*; NNIPPS Genetic Study Group. (2009). Genetic variants of the alpha-synuclein gene SNCA are associated with multiple system atrophy. *PLoS One.* **4**, e7114.

Arunodaya, G. R. and Taly, A. B. (1995). Sympathetic skin response: a decade later. *J. Neurol. Sci.* **129**, 81–9.

Asahina, M., Akaogi, Y., Yamanaka, Y., Koyama, Y. and Hattori, T. (2009). Differences in skin sympathetic involvements between two chronic autonomic disorders: multiple system atrophy and pure autonomic failure. *Parkinsonism Relat. Disord.* **15**, 347–50.

Asahina, M., Vichayanrat, E., Low, D. A., Iodice, V. and Mathias, C. J. (2012). Autonomic dysfunction in parkinsonian disorders: assessment and pathophysiology. *J. Neurol. Neurosurg. Psychiatry.* [Epub ahead of print].

Bannister, R. (1979). Chronic autonomic failure with postural hypotension. *Lancet* **ii**, 404–6.

Bannister, R., Ardill, L., and Fentem, P. (1967). Defective autonomic control of blood vessels in idiopathic orthostatic hypotension. *Brain* **90**, 725–46.

Bannister, R., Davies, I. B., Holly, E., Rosenthal, T., and Sever, P. S. (1979). Defective cardiovascular reflexes and supersensitivity to sympathomimetic drugs in autonomic failure. *Brain* **102**, 163–76.

Bannister, R., da Costa, D. F., Hendry, W. G., Jacobs, J., and Mathias, C. J. (1986). Atrial demand pacing to protect against vagal overactivity in sympathetic autonomic neuropathy. *Brain* **109**, 345–56.

Braak, H., Ghebremedhin, E., Rub, U., Bratzke, H. and Del Tredici, K. (2004). Stages in the development of Parkinson's disease-related pathology, *Cell Tissue Res* **318**, 121–34.

Braune, S., Reinhardt, M., Schnitzer, R., Riedel, A. and Lucking, C. H. (1999). Cardiac uptake of [123I]MIBG separates Parkinson's disease from multiple system atrophy. *Neurology*, **53**, 1020–25.

Brett, A. S., Phillips, M., and Beary, J. F. (1986). Predictive power of the polygraph: Can the 'lie detector' really detect liars? *Lancet* **i**, 544–7.

Brooks, D. J. (2011). Imaging dopamine transporters in Parkinson's disease. *Biomark Med.* **4**, 651–60.

Brooks, D. J., Redmond, S., Mathias, C. J., Bannister, R., and Symon, L. (1989). The effect of orthostatic hypotension on cerebral blood flow and middle cerebral artery velocity in autonomic failure, with observations on the action of ephedrine. *J. Neurol. Neurosurg. Psychiat.* **52**, 962–6.

Chaudhuri, K. R., Thomaides, T., Hernandez, P., Alam, M., and Mathias, C. J. (1991). Non-invasive quantification of superior mesenteric artery blood flow during sympathoneural activation in normal subjects. *Clin. Auton. Res.* **1**, 37–42.

Consensus statement (1996). Consensus statement on the definition of orthostatic hypotension, pure autonomic failure and multiple system atrophy. *Clin. Auton. Res.* **6**, 125–6.

Dabby, R., Djaldetti, R., Shahmurov, M. *et al.* (2006). Skin biopsy for assessment of autonomic denervation in Parkinson's disease. *J Neural. Transm.* **113**(9), 1169–76.

Diehl, R. R., Linden, D., Chalkiadaki, A., Ringelstein, E. B., and Berlit, P. (1996). Transcranial doppler during neurocardiogenic syncope. *Clin. Auto. Res.* **6**, 71–4.

Dolan, R. J., Fink, G. R., Rolls, E. *et al.* (1997). How the brain learns to see objects and faces in an impoverished context. *Nature* **389**, 596–9.

Donadio, V., Montagna, P., Nolano, M., *et al.* (2005). Generalised anhidrosis: different lesion sites demonstrated by microneurography and skin biopsy. *J Neurol. Neurosurg. Psychiatry* **76**, 588–91.

Dumskyj, M. J., Mathias, C. J., Dore, C. J., Bleasdale-Barr, K., and Kohner, E. M. (1998). Intraocular pressure, blood pressure and body position in normal human subjects and patients with autonomic failure. *Clin. Auton. Res.* **8**, 9.

El-Badawi, K. M. and Hainsworth, R. (1994). Combined head-up tilt and lower body suction: a test of orthostatic tolerance. *Clin. Auton. Res.* **4**, 41–7.

Elwell, C. E., Cope, M., Edwards, A. D., Wyatt, J. S., Delpy, D. T., and Reynolds, E. O. (1994). Quantification of adult cerebral hemodynamics by near-infrared spectroscopy. *J. Appl. Physiol.* **77**, 2753–60

Esler, M. (1993). Clinical application of noradrenaline spillover methodology: delineation of regional human sympathetic nervous responses. *Pharmacol. Toxicol.* **75**, 243–53.

Faes, T. J. C., Wagemans, M. F. M., Cillekens, J. M., Scheffer, G.-J., Karemaker, J. M., and Bertelsmann, F. W. (1993). The validity and reproducibility of the skin vasomotor test—studies in normal subjects, after spinal anaesthesia, and in diabetes mellitus. *Clin. Auton. Res.* **3**, 319–24.

Fasano, M. L., Sand, T., Brubakk, A. O., Kurszewski, P., Bordini, C., and Sjaastad, O. (1996). Reproducibility of the cold pressor test: studies in normal subjects. *Clin. Auton. Res.* **6**, 249–53.

Ferini-Strambi, L. and Smirne, S. (1997). Cardiac autonomic function during sleep in several neuropsychiatric disorders. *J. Neurol.* **244**, S29–36.

Freeman, R. *et al.* (2011). Consensus statement on the definition of orthostatic hypotension, neurally mediated syncope and the postural tachycardia syndrome. *Auton Neurosci.*

Gemmill, J. D., Venables, G. S., and Ewing, D. J. (1988). Noradrenaline response to edrophonium in primary autonomic failure: distinction between central and peripheral damage. *Lancet* **i**, 1018–21.

Gilman, S., Wenning, G. K., Low, P. A., *et al.* (2008). Second consensus statement on the diagnosis of multiple system atrophy. *Neurology.* **71**, 670–76.

Goldstein, D. S. (2004). Association between cardiac denervation and parkinsonism caused by alpha-synuclein gene triplication. *Brain.* **127**, 768–72.

Goldstein, D. S. (2010). Catecholamines 101. *Clin Auton Res.* **20**, 331–52.

Goldstein, D. S., Holmes, C., Stuhlmuller, J. E., Lenders, J. W. M., and Kopin I. J. (1997a). 6-[^{18}F] Fluorodopamine positron emission tomographic scanning in the assessment of cardiac sympathoneural function—studies in normal humans. *Clin. Auton. Res.* **7**, 17–29.

Goldstein, D. S., Holmes, C., Cannon, R. O. III, Eisenhofer, G., and Kopin, I. J. (1997b). Sympathetic cardioneuropathy in dysautonomias. *New Engl. J. Med.* **336**, 696–702

Goldstein, D. S., Polinsky, R. J., Garty, M., *et al.* (1989). Patterns of plasma levels of catechols in neurogenic orthostatic hypotension. *Ann Neurol.* **26**, 558–63.

Goldstein, D. S., Holmes, C., Sharabi, Y., Brentzel, S. and Eisenhofer, G. (2003). Plasma levels of catechols and metanephrines in neurogenic orthostatic hypotension. *Neurology* **60**, 1327–32.

Goldstein, D. S., Holmes, C., Cannon, R. O. 3rd, Eisenhofer, G. and Kopin, I. J. (1997). Sympathetic cardioneuropathy in dysautonomias. *N Engl J Med.* **336**, 696–702.

Goldstein, D. S., Holmes, C., Li, S. T., Bruce, S., Metman, L. V. and Cannon, R. O. 3rd. (2000). Cardiac sympathetic denervation in Parkinson disease. *Ann. Intern. Med.* **133**, 338–47.

Goldstein, D. S. and Sewell, L. (2009). Olfactory dysfunction in pure autonomic failure: Implications for the pathogenesis of Lewy body diseases. *Parkinsonism Relat Disord.* **15**, 516–20.

Goldstein, D. S., Sewell, L. and Holmes, C. (2010). Association of anosmia with autonomic failure in Parkinson disease. *Neurology,* **74**, 245–51.

Goldstein, D. S., Holmes, C., Li, S. T., Bruce, S., Metman, L. V. and Cannon, R. O., 3rd. (2000). Cardiac sympathetic denervation in Parkinson disease. *Ann. Intern. Med.* **133**, 338–47.

Goldstein, D. S., Sharabi, Y., Karp, B. I., *et al.* (2007). Cardiac sympathetic denervation preceding motor signs in Parkinson disease. *Clin Auton Res.* **17**, 118–21.

Harcourt, J., Spraggs, P., Mathias, C. J., and Brookes, G. (1996). Sleep-related breathing disorders in the Shy-Drager syndrome. Observations on investigation and management. *Eur. J. Neurol.* **3**, 186–90

Haensch, C. A., Lerch, H., Jorg, J. and Isenmann, S. (2009). Cardiac denervation occurs independent of orthostatic hypotension and impaired heart rate variability in Parkinson's disease. *Parkinsonism Relat. Disord.* **15**, 134–37.

Humm, A. M. and Mathias, C. J. (2010). Abnormal cardiovascular responses to carotid sinus massage also occur in vasovagal syncope—implications for diagnosis and treatment. *Eur. J Neurol.* **17**, 1061–67.

Hutchinson, E. C. and Stock, J. P. P. (1960). Carotid sinus syndrome. *Lancet* **ii**, 445–9.

Iodice, V., Low, D. A., Vichayanrat, E. and Mathias, C. J. (2011). Cardiovascular autonomic dysfunction in MSA and Parkinson's disease: similarities and differences. *J Neurol. Sci.* **310**, 133–8.

Jamnadas-Khoda, J., Koshy, S., Mathias, C. J., Muthane, U. B., Ragothaman, M. and Dodaballapur, S. K. (2009). Are current recommendations to diagnose orthostatic hypotension in Parkinson's disease satisfactory? *Mov Disord.* **15**, 1747–451.

Karat, A. B. A., Karat, S., and Pallis, C. (1969). Sweating under cellulose tape. A test of autonomic function. *Lancet* **i**, 651–2

Kaufmann, H., Oribe, E., Miller, M., Knott, P., Wiltshire-Clement, M., and Yahr, M. (1992). Hypotension induced vasopressin release distinguishes between PAF and MSA with autonomic failure. *Neurology* **42**, 590–3.

Khurana, R. K. (1995). Orthostatic intolerance and orthostatic tachycardia: a heterogeneous disorder. *Clin. Auton. Res.* **5**, 12–18.

Khurana, R. K. and Setty, A. (1996). The value of the isometric hand-grip test—studies in various autonomic disorders. *Clin. Auton. Res.* **6**, 211–18.

Kimber, J. R., Watson, L., and Mathias, C. J. (1997). Distinction of idiopathic Parkinson's disease from multiple system atrophy by stimulation of growth hormone release with clonidine. *Lancet* **349**, 1877–81.

Lagi, A., Bacalli, S., Cencetti, S., Paggetti, C., and Colzi, L. (1994). Cerebral autoregulation in orthostatic hypotension: a transcranial doppler study. *Stroke* **25**, 1771–75.

Lahrmann, H., Cortelli, P., Hilz, M., Mathias, C. J., Struhal, W., Tassinari, M. (2006). EFNS guidelines on the diagnosis and management of orthostatic hypotension. *Eur. J Neurol.* **13**, 930–36.

Lambert, G. W., Thompson, J. M., Turner, A. G. *et al.* (1997). Cerebral noradrenaline spillover and its relation to muscle sympathetic nervous activity in healthy human subjects. *J. Autonom. Nerv. Syst.* **64**, 57–64.

Lempert, T. (1996). Recognizing syncope: pitfalls and surprises. *J. R. Soc. Med.* **89**, 372–5.

Lempert, T., Bauer, M., and Schmidt, D. (1994). Syncope: a videometric analysis of 56 episodes of transient cerebral hypoxia. *Ann. Neurol.* **36**, 233–7.

Low, D. A., da Nóbrega, A. C., and Mathias, C. J. (2012). Exercise-induced hypotension in autonomic disorders. *Auton. Neurosci.* **171**(1–2), 66–78.

Low, P. A. (1993). Composite autonomic scoring scale for laboratory quantification of generalized autonomic failure. *Mayo Clin. Proc.* **68**, 748–52.

McIntosh, S. J., Lawson, J., and Kenny, R. A. (1993). Clinical characteristics of vasodepressor, cardioinhibitory and mixed carotid sinus syndrome in the elderly. *Am. J. Med.* **95**, 203–8.

Magnifico, F., Misra, V. P., Murray, N. M. F., and Mathias. C. J. (1996). The sympathetic skin response following successful upper limb sympathectomy in primary hyperhidrosis. *Clin. Auton. Res.* **6**, 289.

Magnifico, F., Misra, V. P., Murray, N. M. F., and Mathias, C. J. (1997). The laboratory detection of autonomic dysfunction in multiple system atrophy—the role of the sympathetic skin response. *Neurology* **48**(suppl), A190.

Magnifico, F., Misra, V. P., Murray, N. M. F., and Mathias, C. J. (1998). The sympathetic skin response in peripheral autonomic failure—evaluation in pure autonomic failure, pure cholinergic dysautonomia and dopamine beta-hydroxylase deficiency. *Clin. Auton. Res.*, **8**, 133–8.

Mathias, C. J. (1987). Autonomic dysfunction. *Br. J. Hosp. Med.* **38**, 238–43.

Mathias, C. J. (1995*a*). Orthostatic hypotension—causes, mechanisms and influencing factors. *Neurology* **45**, (Suppl. 5), s6–s11.

Mathias, C. J. (1995*b*). Assessment of autonomic function. In *Clinical Neurophysiology*, (ed. J. Osseslton with C. Binnie, R. Looper, C. Fowler, F. Maguire and P. Prior). Heinemann, Butterworth, London. pp. 218–32.

Mathias, C. J. (1996*a*). Disorders affecting autonomic function in Parkinsonian patients. In *Parkinson's disease*, (ed. L. Battistin, G. Scarlato, T. Caraceni, and S. Ruggieri), Advances in Neurology, **69**, pp. 383–91. Lippincott-Raven Press, New York.

Mathias, C. J. (1996*b*). Disorders of the autonomic nervous system in childhood. In *Principles of child neurology*, (ed. B. Berg), pp. 413–36. McGraw-Hill, New York.

Mathias, C. J. (1996*c*). Gastrointestinal dysfunction in multiple system atrophy. *Semin. Neurol.* **16**, 251–8.

Mathias, C. J. (1997). Pharmacological manipulation of human gastrointestinal blood flow. *Fund. Clin. Pharmacol.* **11**, 29–34.

Mathias, C. J. (1998). Autonomic disorders. In *Textbook of neurology*, (ed. J. Bogousslavsky and M. Fisher). Chap. 35, pp. 519–45. Butterworth Heinemann, Massachusetts.

Mathias, C. J. (1999). Autonomic dysfunction and the elderly. In *Oxford textbook of geriatric medicine*, (2nd edn), (ed. J. Grimley-Evans). Oxford University Press, Oxford, in press.

Mathias, C. J. and Frankel, H. L. (1986). The neurological and hormonal control of blood vessels and heart in spinal man. *J. Autonom. Nerv. Syst.* (suppl.), 457–64.

Mathias, C. J. and Frankel, H. L. (1988). Cardiovascular control in spinal man. *Ann. Rev. Physiol.* **50**, 577–92.

Mathias, C. J. and Galizia, G. (2010). Orthostatic hypotension and orthostatic intolerance. In: *Endocrinology; adult and pediatric.* 6th ed. Eds. Jameson J. L. and De Groot L. J. Elsevier: 2063–83.

Mathias, C. J. and Williams, A. C. (1994). The Shy Drager syndrome (and multiple system atrophy). In *Neurodegenerative diseases*, (1st edn), (ed. Donald B. Calne), Chap. 43, pp. 743–68. WB Saunders, Philadelphia, Pennsylvania, USA.

Mathias, C. J., Matthews, W. B., and Spalding, J. M. K. S. (1977). Postural changes in plasma renin activity and responses to vasoactive drugs in a case of Shy–Drager syndrome. *J. Neurol. Neurosurg. Psychiat.* **40**, 138–43.

Mathias, C. J., Christensen, N. J., Frankel, H. L., and Spalding, J. M. K. (1979). Cardiovascular control in recently injured tetraplegics in spinal shock. *Q. J. Med. New Series* **48**, 273–87.

Mathias, C. J., Frankel, H. L., Davies, I. B., James, V. H. T., and Peart, W. S. (1981). Renin and aldosterone release during sympathetic stimulation in tetraplegia. *Clin. Sci.* **60**, 399–604.

Mathias, C. J., Fosbraey, P., da Costa, D. F., Thornley, A., and Bannister, R. (1986). Desmopressin reduces nocturnal polyuria, reverses overnight weight loss and improves morning postural hypotension in autonomic failure. *BMJ* **293**, 353–4.

Mathias, C. J., Armstrong, E., Browse, N., Chaudhuri, K. R., Enevoldson, P., and Ross-Russell, R. W. (1991*a*). Value of non-invasive continuous blood pressure monitoring in the detection of carotid sinus hypersensitivity. *Clin. Auton. Res.* **1**, 157–9.

Mathias, C. J., Holly, E. R., Armstrong, E., Shareef, M., and Bannister, R. (1991*b*). The influence of food and postural hypotension in three groups of chronic autonomic failure; clinical and therapeutic implications. *J. Neurol. Neurosurg. Psychiat.* **54**, 726–30.

Mathias, C. J., Deguchi, K., Bleasdale-Barr, K., and Kimber, J. (1998). Frequency of family history in vasovagal syncope. *Lancet* **352**, 33–4.

Mathias, C. J., Low, D. A., Iodice, V., Owens, A. P., Kirbiš, M., and Grahame, R. (2012). The Postural Tachycardia Syndrome (PoTS) – Current experiences and concepts. *Nat. Neurol. Rev.* **8**, 22–34.

Matsui, H., Udaka, F., Oda, M., *et al.* (2005). Metaiodobenzylguanidine (MIBG) uptake in Parkinson's disease also decreases at thyroid. *Ann. Nucl. Med.* 19, 225–29.

Morris, J. S., Frith, C. D., Perrett, D. I. *et al.* (1996). A differential neural response in the human amygdala to fearful and happy facial expressions. *Nature* **383**, 812–15.

Mounier-Vehier, C., Girard, A., Consoli, S., Laude, D., Vacheron, A., and Elghozi, J. L. (1995). Cardiovascular reactivity to a new mental stress test: the maze test. *Clin. Auton. Res.* **5**, 145–50.

Moya, A., Sutton, R., Ammirati, F., *et al.* (2009). Guidelines for the diagnosis and management of syncope (version 2009). *Eur. Heart J.* **30**, 2631–71.

Muller, A. Mungersdorf, M. Reichmann, H. Strehle, G. and Hummel, T. (2002). Olfactory function in Parkinsonian syndromes, *J Clin. Neurosci*, **9**, 521–24.

Nicotra, A., Young, T. M., Asahina, M. and Mathias, C. J. (2005). The effect of different physiological stimuli on skin vasomotor reflexes above and below the lesion in human chronic spinal cord injury. *Neurorehabil Neural Repair.* **19**, 325–31.

Nolano, M., Provitera, V., Estraneo, A., *et al.* (2008). Sensory deficit in Parkinson's disease: evidence of a cutaneous denervation. *Brain*, **131** (Pt 7), 1903–1911.

Parati, G., Di Rienzo, M., and Mancia, G. (2000). How to measure baroreflex sensitivity: from the cardiovascular laboratory to daily life. *J Hypertension* **18**, 7–19.

Persson, P. B., DiRienzo, M., Castiglioni, P., *et al.* (2001). Time versus frequency domain techniques for assessing baroreflex sensitivity. *J Hypertension* **19**, 1699–1705.

Pierangeli, G., Cortelli, P., Provini, F., Plazzi, G., and Lugaresi, E. (1997). Circadian rhythm of body core temperature in neurodegenerative diseases. In *Somatic and autonomic regulation in sleep: physiological and clinical aspects*, pp. 55–71, (ed. E. Lugaresi and P. L. Parmeggiani). Springer-Verlag, Italia, Milano.

Piha, S. J. and Voipio-Pullki, L. M. (1993). Cardiac dysrhythmias during cardiovascular autonomic reflex tests. *Clin. Auton. Res.* **3**, 183–7.

Ponsen, M. M., Stoffers, D., Booij, J., van Eck-Smit, B. L., Wolters, E. and Berendse, H. W. (2004). Idiopathic hyposmia as a preclinical sign of Parkinson's disease. *Ann. Neurol.*, **56**, 173–81.

Puvi-Rajasingham, S., Smith, G. D. P., Akinola, A., and Mathias, C. J. (1997). Abnormal regional blood flow responses during and after exercise in human sympathetic denervation. *J. Physiol.* **505**, 481–9.

Puvi-Rajasingham, S., Smith, G. D. P., Akinola, A., and Mathias, C. J. (1998). Hypotensive and regional haemodynamic effects of exercise, fasted and after food, in human sympathetic denervation. *Clin. Sci.* 94, 49–55.

Raffel, D. M., Koeppe, R. A., Little, R., Wang, C. N., Liu, S., Junck, L., Heumann, M., and Gilman, S. (2006). PET measurement of cardiac and nigrostriatal denervation in Parkinsonian syndromes. *J Nucl. Med.* **47**, 1769–77.

Rahman, F., Pechnik, S., Gross, D., Sewell, L. and Goldstein, D. S. (2011). Low frequency power of heart rate variability reflects baroreflex function, not cardiac sympathetic innervation. *Clin. Auton. Res.*, **21**, 133–41.

Reilly, M. M., and Staunton, H. (1996). Peripheral nerve amyloidosis. *Brain Pathol.* **6**, 163–77.

Riedel, A. and Mathias, C. J. (1997). A rapid response sweat test with potential clinical applications—studies in normal subjects, pure autonomic failure and multiple system atrophy. *Clin. Auton. Res.* **7**, 208.

Ryder, R. E. J., Johnson, K., Owens, D. R., Marshall, R., Ryder, A. P. P., and Hayes, T. M. (1988). Acetylcholine sweatspot test for autonomic denervation. *Lancet* **ii**, 1303–5.

Scholz, S. W., Houlden, H., Schulte, C., *et al.* (2009). SNCA variants are associated with increased risk for multiple system atrophy. *Ann. Neurol.* **65**, 610–614.

Schondorf, R. and Low, P.A. (1993). Idiopathic postural orthostatic tachycardia syndrome: an attenuated form of acute pandysautonomia? *Neurology.* **43**, 132–37.

Schrag, A., Kingsley, D., Phatouros, C. *et al.* (1998). Clinical usefulness of magnetic resonance imaging in multiple system atrophy. *J. Neuroc. Neurosurg. Psychiat.* **65**, 65–71.

Senard J. M., Valet P., Durrieu G., *et al.* (1990). Adrenergic supersensitivity in parkinsonians with orthostatic hypotension. *Eur. J Clin. Invest.* **20**, 613–619.

Shahani, B. T., Halpern, J. J., Boulu, P., and Cohen, J. (1984). Sympathetic skin response-a method of assessing unmyelinated axon dysfunction in peripheral neuropathies. *J. Neurol. Neurosurg. Psychiat.* **47**, 536–42.

Sharabi, Y., Eldadah, B., Li, S. T., Dendi, R., Pechnik, S., Holmes, C., and Goldstein, D. S. (2006). Neuropharmacologic distinction of neurogenic orthostatic hypotension syndromes. *Clin. Neuropharmacol.* **29**, 97–105.

Sharabi, Y., Imrich, R., Holmes, C., Pechnik, S. and Goldstein, D. S. (2008). Generalized and neurotransmitter-selective noradrenergic denervation in Parkinson's disease with orthostatic hypotension. *Mov. Disord.* **23**, 1725–32.

Singleton A., Gwinn-Hardy K., Sharabi Y., *et al.* (1995). Postural hypotension enhanced by exercise in patients with chronic autonomic failure. *Q. J. Med.* **88**, 251–6.

Smith, G. D. P. and Mathias, C. J. (1996). Differences in the cardiovascular responses to supine exercise and to standing post-exercise in two clinical subgroups of the Shy–Drager syndrome (multiple system atrophy). *J. Neurol. Neurosurg. Psychiat.* **61**, 297–303.

Smith, G. D. P., Watson, L. P., Pavitt, D. V., and Mathias, C.J. (1995). Abnormal cardiovascular and catecholamine responses to supine exercise in human subjects with sympathetic dysfunction. *J. Physiol. (London)* **484**, 255–65.

Silveira-Moriyama, L., Mathias, C., Mason, L., Best, C., Quinn, N. P. and Lees, A. J. (2009). Hyposmia in pure autonomic failure. *Neurology* **72**, 1677–81.

Thomaides, T., Chaudhuri, K. R., Maule, S., Watson, L., Marsden, C.D., and Mathias, C. J. (1992). The growth hormone response to clonidine in central and peripheral primary autonomic failure. *Lancet* **340**, 263–6.

Tipre, D. N. and Goldstein, D. S. (2005). Cardiac and extracardiac sympathetic denervation in Parkinson's disease with orthostatic hypotension and in pure autonomic failure. *J Nucl Med.* **46**, 1775–81.

Wenning, G. K., Shephard, B., Hawkes, C., Petruckevitch, A., Lees, A. and Quinn, N. (1995). Olfactory function in atypical parkinsonian syndromes. *Acta Neurol Scand* **91**, 247–50.

Young, T. M., Asahina, M., Nicotra, A. and Mathias, C. J. (2006). Skin vasomotor reflex responses in two contrasting groups of autonomic failure: multiple system atrophy and pure autonomic failure. *J Neurol.* **253**, 846–50.

Young, T. M., Asahina, M., Watson, L. and Mathias, C. J. (2006). Hemodynamic effects of clonidine in two contrasting models of autonomic failure: multiple system atrophy and pure autonomic failure. *Mov Disord.* **21**, 609–615.

Appendix

Data from standard autonomic function tests in 122 subjects who are grouped in different age bands. None of the subjects had autonomic failure or were on drugs that could have interfered with the responses. All measurements were made with an automated sphygmomanometer. Mean change in systolic or diastolic blood pressure (SBP and DBP respectively) or in heart rate (HR), with the standard error of the mean are provided. The figures below these are the 95% confidence intervals, with both lower and upper values.

There is no age relationship of blood pressure responses to standing and head-up tilt. With isometric exercise and cutaneous cold, with increasing age there is a rise in SBP but not DBP and heart rate. The responses to mental arithmetic are not age related. The heart rate responses to the Valsalva manoeuvre (as the Valsalva ratio), and to deep breathing and hyperventilation, show an age dependency.

These values are not a definitive source of normal data, for reasons outlined in the text. The data were collected from our two London Autonomic Units (at the National and St Mary's Hospitals), and compiled by A. Akinola, K. Bleasdale-Barr, L. Everall and C. J. Mathias.

Age groups (years)	20–29	30–39	40–49	50–59	60–69	≥70
Standing						
2 minutes						
Δ SBP	3 ± 2	−1 ± 3	−2 ± 2	2 ± 3	2 ± 3	7 ± 3
	(−1 to 7)	(−7 to 6)	(−6 to 3)	(−1 to 5)	(−1 to 5)	(4 to 10)
Δ DBP	6 ± 3	5 ± 3	6 ± 2	5 ± 3	3 ± 1	5 ± 2
	(0 to 12)	(−1 to 11)	(1 to 11)	(−1 to 11)	(0 to 6)	(1 to 9)
Δ HR	15 ± 3	10 ± 3	11 ± 2	8 ± 2	8 ± 2	7 ± 1
	(9 to 21)	(4 to 16)	(8 to 15)	(4 to 12)	(4 to 12)	(5 to 9)
5 minutes						
Δ SBP	1 ± 3	0 ± 2	−1 ± 2	1 ± 2	4 ± 2	5 ± 3
	(−4 to 6)	(−3 to 4)	(−5 to 3)	(−1 to 3)	(2 to 6)	(2 to 8)
Δ DBP	4 ± 3	4 ± 2	5 ± 2	5 ± 2	6 ± 1	4 ± 2
	(−2 to 10)	(0 to 8)	(1 to 9)	(1 to 9)	(4 to 8)	(0 to 8)
Δ HR	14 ± 3	11 ± 2	11 ± 2	8 ± 2	9 ± 1	9 ± 1
	(8 to 20)	(7 to 15)	(7 to 14)	(4 to 12)	(7 to 11)	(7 to 11)
Head-up tilt						
2 minutes						
Δ SBP	−1 ± 3	3 ± 3	−3 ± 2	−2 ± 4	−8 ± 2	−7 ± 2
	(−7 to 9)	(0 to 9)	(−7 to 1)	(−10 to 2)	(−12 to −4)	(−11 to −3)
Δ DBP	4 ± 3	7 ± 2	2 ± 1	0 ± 2	3 ± 1	2 ± 3
	(−2 to 10)	(3 to 11)	(0 to 4)	(−4 to 4)	(0 to 6)	(−4 to 8)
Δ HR	8 ± 3	8 ± 3	7 ± 2	3 ± 5	2 ± 2	1 ± 2
	(2 to 14)	(2 to 14)	(3 to 11)	(−7 to 13)	(−2 to 6)	(−3 to 5)
5 minutes						
Δ SBP	−4 ± 3	7 ± 2	−2 ± 2	0 ± 4	−5 ± 3	3 ± 4
	(−10 to 2)	(3 to 11)	(−6 to 2)	(−8 to 8)	(−11 to 1)	(−5 to 11)
Δ DBP	0 ± 4	5 ± 2	3 ± 1	3 ± 2	1 ± 2	1 ± 2
	(−8 to 8)	(1 to 9)	(1 to 5)	(−1 to 7)	(−3 to 5)	(−3 to 5)
Δ HR	10 ± 4	7 ± 2	5 ± 1	4 ± 3	3 ± 1	4 ± 2
	(2 to 18)	(3 to 11)	(3 to 7)	(−2 to 10)	(1 to 5)	(0 to 8)

(Contd.)

Age groups (years)	20–29	30–39	40–49	50–59	60–69	≥70
Isometric exercise						
Δ SBP	15 ± 3	13 ± 2	15 ± 3	19 ± 3	17 ± 3	2 ± 4
	(9 to 21)	(9 to 17)	(9 to 21)	(13 to 25)	(11 to 23)	(14 to 30)
Δ DBP	13 ± 2	11 ± 2	12 ± 2	11 ± 3	11 ± 2	11 ± 1
	(9 to 17)	(7 to 15)	(8 to 14)	(5 to 17)	(7 to 15)	(9 to 13)
Δ HR	7 ± 1	7 ± 2	9 ± 2	7 ± 2	4 ± 1	6 ± 1
	(5 to 9)	(3 to 11)	(5 to 13)	(3 to 11)	(2 to 6)	(4 to 8)
Cutaneous cold						
Δ SBP	9 ± 1	9 ± 2	12 ± 3	16 ± 3	15 ± 2	21 ± 3
	(7 to 11)	(5 to 13)	(6 to 18)	(10 to 22)	(11 to 19)	(15 to 27)
Δ DBP	10 ± 2	12 ± 3	10 ± 2	8 ± 4	10 ± 2	12 ± 4
	(6 to 13)	(7 to 17)	(6 to 14)	(5 to 12)	(7 to 13)	(5 to 19)
Δ HR	0 ± 1	3 ± 2	3 ± 2	3 ± 2	1 ± 1	5 ± 1
	(−2 to 2)	(−1 to 7)	(−1 to 7)	(−1 to 7)	(−2 to 3)	(3 to 7)
Mental arithmetic						
Δ SBP	17 ± 4	10 ± 2	12 ± 3	19 ± 3	13 ± 3	13 ± 4
	(10 to 24)	(5 to 15)	(7 to 17)	(16 to 21)	(7 to 19)	(6 to 20)
Δ DBP	12 ± 2	5 ± 3	8 ± 2	6 ± 2	9 ± 2	8 ± 2
	(9 to 15)	(0 to 11)	(5 to 11)	(2 to 10)	(5 to 13)	(3 to 13)
Δ HR	7 ± 3	5 ± 2	8 ± 2	8 ± 2	8 ± 2	5 ± 1
	(2 to 12)	(1 to 9)	(5 to 11)	(6 to 10)	(5 to 11)	(3 to 7)
Valsalva ratio	1.84 ± 0.12	1.81 ± 0.1	1.76 ± 0.06	1.72 ± 0.11	1.62 ± 0.06	1.33 ± 0.06
	(1.6 to 2.08)	(1.6 to 2.02)	(1.67 to 1.92)	(1.50 to 1.94)	(1.50 to 1.74)	(1.21 to 1.45)
Deep breathing						
Δ HR	20 ± 2	19 ± 3	15 ± 2	17 ± 2	12 ± 1	9 ± 1
	16 to 24	13 to 24	11 to 19	15 to 19	11 to 13	(8 to 10)
Hyperventilation						
Δ HR	21 ± 3	21 ± 3	16 ± 2	18 ± 3	11 ± 1	7 ± 1
	(15 to 27)	(15 to 26)	(12 to 21)	(15 to 21)	(10 to 12)	(6 to 8)

CHAPTER 23

Measurement of heart rate and blood pressure to evaluate disturbances in neurocardiovascular control

Wouter Wieling and John M. Karemaker

Introduction

The basis of testing any control system is to induce a disturbance and observe the system's response. In the case of the cardiovascular system quick correction of the disturbance is dependent on reflexes, of which the arterial baroreflex is the most important one. This reflex acts in response to blood pressure changes by changing heart rate, cardiac performance, and vasoconstrictor tone. To correctly evaluate the control system's performance, therefore, the physician requires measurement techniques for blood pressure and heart rate to a degree of precision that is adapted to the characteristics of the response under investigation. This implies that for some clinical measurements arm cuff readings combined with pulse counting may be sufficient, for other measurements a continuous beat-by-beat account of blood pressure and heart rate is required.

In this chapter we will explain, first, the use of non-invasive continuous (finger-) blood pressure by the Finapres technique. Next, we give a short account of the role of the arterial baroreflex in the complex of cardiovascular control mechanisms and we explain the difficulties inherent in quantification of its function. The remainder of the chapter is devoted to a systematic account of cardiovascular reflex tests that are commonly used to evaluate specific aspects of baroreflex function. Additionally, a number of reflex tests are discussed that bypass the baroreflex system while still exciting its efferents. Such tests are useful to ascertain the integrity of these pathways when the baroreflex afferents are involved in a disease process.

Non-invasive monitoring of arterial pressure—the Finapres technique

Counting the pulse and carefully measuring blood pressure with a sphygmomanometer suffices for the routine clinical assessment of patients in the office or at the bedside. Multiple blood pressure readings supine and after standing provide a fair assessment of the typical blood pressure response for an individual. For the evaluation of a patient with disturbances in cardiovascular control mechanisms conventional sphygmomanometry has a major disadvantage: the investigator is not informed about the beat-to-beat fluctuations in arterial pressure. Sphygmomanometry, therefore, is not suitable for evaluation of conditions with sudden transient changes in the circulation. Intra-arterial measurements are not routinely used in cardiovascular laboratories in view of the potential complications. In addition, intravascular instrumentation has the inherent disadvantage of affecting autonomic tone. In this context, the Finapres or volume clamp method with its ability to measure the arterial pressure in the finger non-invasively and continuously, has been an important step forward in the evaluation of autonomic cardiovascular control. The principle of the measurement of finger arterial pressure and its usefulness to assess rapid changes in arterial blood pressure has been described in detail elsewhere (Imholz et al. 1998) and will not be addressed here further.

Measurement of finger arterial pressure is almost always possible. Conditions that provoke severe peripheral arterial contraction and, consequently, low arterial flow to the hand are the major limitations. Warming of the hand will improve measurements. When using Finapres, it is essential that a proper size cuff is snugly applied to the middle or ring finger and, to avoid hydrostatic pressure effects, the finger cuff must be kept at heart level. This can quite simply be accomplished by placing a skin electrode as a reference at a point in the mid-axillary line at heart level (the 4th intercostal space at the sternum). The subject holds the cuffed finger at this place at all times (Fig. 23.1). The measured hand is further supported by a sling. Alternatively, the pressure measurement at the finger can be corrected for hydrostatic effects by pressure measurement in a liquid-filled tube, one end at finger level, the other end at heart level. Such a height correction device is part of some Finapres-based instruments, and is obviously very useful in ambulatory measurements where the hand cannot be held at heart level at all times. However, this device can also induce noise in the recording (movement artefacts) and can be an extra source of equipment failure. It is, therefore, to be applied with caution.

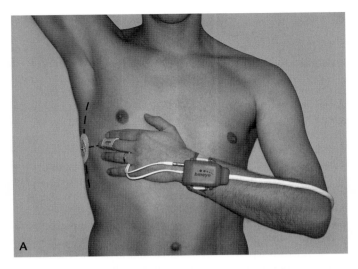

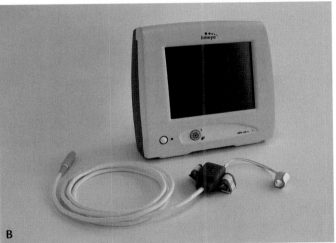

Fig. 23.1 **A**: Basic components of the BMEYE ABM-100 monitor. An inflatable finger sensor is connected to the small wrist box, which is connected via a 5 m long cable to the portable touch screen monitor. **B**: To avoid hydrostatic pressure effects, the finger is held at heart level.

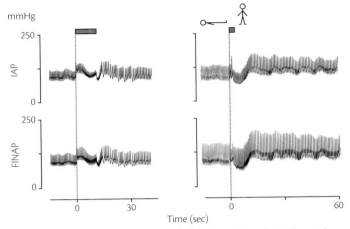

Fig. 23.2 Original recordings of intrabrachial (IAP) and finger (FINAP) arterial blood pressure responses induced by Valsalva manoeuvre (left panel) and standing up (right panel). Duration of Valsalva strain and time needed to stand up are indicated. Note similarity between the IAP and FINAP tracings.

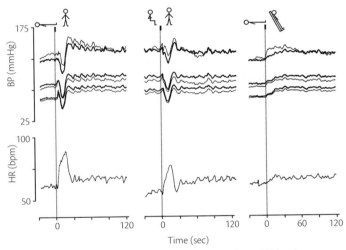

Fig. 23.3 Average intrabrachial (IAP) and finger (FINAP) arterial blood pressure and heart rate responses in 11 healthy adult subjects aged 22–40 years to three orthostatic manoeuvres. Bold trace = IAP, thin trace = FINAP. From Imholz et al. 1998, with permission.

Finapres recordings are similar in appearance to intra-arterial blood pressure recordings (Fig. 23.2), but the measurements are not identical. It has long been known that propagation of the pressure wave towards the periphery changes the pulse wave form, and consequently finger blood pressure values differ from values obtained more proximally. The physiological brachial to finger pressure gradient causes mean and diastolic pressures to be lower in the finger compared to brachial pressure; amplification of the pulse wave, especially in young subjects, may result in higher finger systolic pressure values (Imholz et al. 1998).

When results are averaged for a group of subjects, the differences between intra-arterial and finger pressures are small, for systolic and diastolic pressure usually less than 5 mmHg (Fig. 23.3). However, the standard deviation of these differences is not small and Finapres readings, therefore, do not guarantee a reliable estimate of actual intrabrachial pressure levels in the individual patient. We still recommend a sphygmomanometric reading for this.

In practice, the clinician must interpret a blood pressure response in an individual patient; a reliable estimate of the *changes* in blood pressure is therefore of crucial importance. Finapres is an excellent device in this respect; changes in mean and diastolic pressure during steady state conditions and during manoeuvres such as Valsalva and hypotensive orthostatic stress are reliably measured (Jellema et al. 1996, Imholz et al. 1998). The finger to brachial differences within one subject are relatively stable; the 95% individual limits of agreement of the standard deviation are 0–4 mmHg. Finger systolic pressures are more variable, but on the whole the performance of Finapres allows it to be used to evaluate autonomic cardiovascular control even in patients over 70 years of age.

Solutions to the drawbacks of peripheral finger blood pressure measurements have been described. Reconstruction of brachial artery pressure waves from finger measurements by correction for pulse wave distortion and individual pressures gradients has been found feasible and reliable (Bos et al. 1996, Gizdulich et al. 1997, Guelen et al. 2003).

Monitoring of finger arterial pressure enables one to study the dynamics of circulatory responses in detail. Components of blood pressure and heart rate variability can be studied by techniques such as spectral analysis and sequence analysis, which attempt to dynamically assess baroreflex function (Chapter 24). The ambulatory version of Finapres, the Portapres™ device, enables the study of circulatory responses during 24 hours under everyday circumstances (Imholz et al. 1993). Finapres and Portapres even have made it into space as key instruments in complex experimental human physiology settings (Eckberg 2003).

Once a continuous arterial pulse wave is available, more than just beat-by-beat values for systolic and diastolic pressure can be obtained. A further refinement of pulse wave analysis is the calculation of beat-to-beat changes in stroke volume. This technique has originally been designed for aortic pressure waves, but may be applied to peripheral pressure waves like those obtained by Finapres as well (Stok et al. 1993, Wesseling et al. 1993, van Lieshout and Wesseling 2001). This enables the clinician to evaluate the haemodynamics underlying observed changes in blood pressure in terms of cardiac output and total peripheral resistance. This has opened new avenues of investigation in the laboratory like the evaluation of the hemodynamic mechanisms underlying til-table induced syncope (Wieling et al. 1992, De Jong et al. 1995, De Jong et al. 1997a, Gisolf et al 2004). The technology can also be applied to pressure signals that have been obtained under ambulatory conditions (Veerman et al. 1995, Omboni et al. 2001).

Cardiovascular control and the arterial baroreflex

The control mechanisms involved in circulatory homeostasis include the following major subsets of pressure buffering systems (in acting order from fast (seconds to minutes) to slow (onset hours to days): the neurocardiovascular or neural system, the humorocardiovascular or humoral system, the capillary-fluid-shift system, and the renal-body-fluid control system. The renal-body-fluid system acts as a slow long-term blood pressure integral controller, with the humoral and, especially the neural control system serving as fast fine-tuning feedback mechanisms (reflexes) to match the needs of the body more closely. In the following we will focus exclusively on the neural reflex adjustments (Cowley et al. 1992).

Among the many reflexes that act upon the cardiovascular system, the arterial baroreceptor reflex is the most relevant reflex in autonomic function testing; it is the key regulatory mechanism for short-term control of systemic blood pressure (Eckberg and Sleight 1992, Wieling and Wesseling 1993, Timmers et al. 2003). We will restrict the following discussion to the arterial baroreflex for the sake of brevity, although we are aware that this neglects other neural mechanisms impinging on the cardiovascular system.

Arterial baroreceptors are stretch receptors located in the blood vessel walls of the carotid sinuses and aortic arch, which mainly react to increases in arterial pressure at each arterial pulse wave. The afferents from the carotid sinus areas form, together with the chemoreceptor afferents from the carotid bodies, the (bilateral) carotid sinus nerves, which join the glossopharyngeal nerves on their way to the brain stem. Afferents from the aortic baroreceptors join the vagus nerves inside the thorax. The baroreceptor afferents, both from the carotid sinuses and the aortic arch, have their first synapse in the nucleus tractus solitarii in the brainstem. After this synapse the central 'wiring diagram' very quickly becomes

extremely complex, since even the most simple cardiovascular reflexes are known to have a large degree of central integration.

To regulate beat-to-beat blood pressure the autonomic nervous system has three levers to operate: the heart (heart rate, inotropy), venous supply, and systemic vascular resistance. The efferent limbs of the autonomic nervous system consist of sympathetic and parasympathetic fibres to the heart as well as sympathetic fibres to the smooth muscles in the peripheral blood vessels (Fig. 23.4).

The arterial baroreceptors excite the cardiac vagal centres and, at the same time, inhibit sympathetic outflow from the vasomotor centres in the brainstem. A decrease in arterial pressure and thereby in vascular stretch diminishes vagal excitation and sympathetic inhibition with a resultant decrease in vagal outflow to the heart and increase in sympathetic outflow causing increases in heart rate, cardiac contractility and vasomotor tone, all geared towards blood pressure restoration. Conversely, augmented arterial pressure increases baroreceptor discharge and results in neural reflex adjustments that oppose the blood pressure rise. These adjustments are rapidly acting. Modulation of vagus nerve activity allows changes in heart rate even within the ongoing heart beat or the next beat

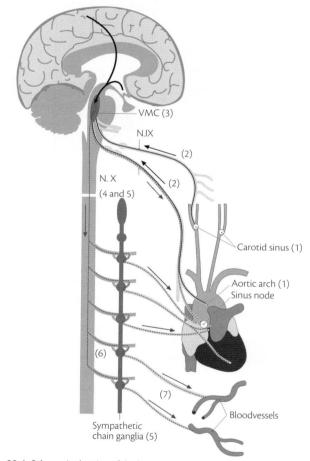

Fig. 23.4 Schematic drawing of the baroreceptor afferent and autonomic efferent pathways of the baroreflex arc. VMC indicates vasomotor centres in brainstem. Possible mechanisms of failure of cardiovascular control are indicated. 1, lesion of carotid sinus/aortic baroreceptors; 2, lesion in afferent carotid and/or aortic afferents; 3, lower brainstem lesion; 4, spinal cord transection; 5, lesion in intermediolateral columns; 6, preganglionic/ganglionic lesion; 7, postganglionic lesion.

after a changed pulse pressure. Sympathetically mediated changes in heart rate, cardiac contractility and arteriolar vasomotor tone need 2–3 seconds to begin.

Quantification of baroreflex function

Theoretically, direct evaluation of baroreflex effectiveness in the intact human is not possible. In order to do so, one would have to vascularly isolate the baroreceptor afferent areas and impose stable blood pressures to them while observing the induced level of blood pressure and heart rate in the remaining part of the vascular tree. Such experiments have been performed in acute animal studies under general anaesthesia. Since then we know 'Koch's blood pressure characteristic curves' (Koch 1931), which relate blood pressure in the isolated receptor areas to effective blood pressure or heart rate. In the intact organism we are in the 'closed loop situation': when blood pressure changes, activation of the baroreflex will tend to annihilate this change. Therefore, input to the arterial baroreflex system, the blood pressure change, cannot be quantified separately from the output of the same system, the new level of blood pressure.

One way around this predicament is to impose a very fast blood pressure change and observe the ensuing vagal change in heart rate. Since the vagal effects are much faster than the sympathetically induced effects on heart and vessels, we may consider the relation between the change in blood pressure and heart rate, with some restrictions, without having to take the closed loop into account. This way of measuring baroreflex sensitivity (BRS) is exploited in a common test as the phenylephrine test. Here a bolus injection of the vasoactive drug induces a rapid blood pressure rise, which provokes a vagally mediated heart rate drop via the baroreflex. BRS is commonly quantified as the quotient of induced change in pulse interval over the causing change in (systolic) blood pressure, thus yielding a measure in ms/mm Hg. Normal values for baroreflex sensitivity range from 15 ms/mm Hg to 50 ms/mm Hg for young adult subjects (Eckberg and Sleight 1992).

We must be aware that this measure of baroreflex quality is restricted to the blood pressure to heart rate arm of the reflex. Important though this may be, it is not essential for blood pressure control in normal daily life: heart transplant patients do not have this reflex, since their hearts are essentially denervated, but they still maintain a normal blood pressure, even when quickly standing up (Wieling and Wesseling 1993). Obviously, a good control of vascular resistance is much more important for the cardiovascular system, but this cannot be quantified as easily as the vagal arm by BRS due to the closed loop problem.

Direct information on activity of sympathetic nerves in humans can be obtained by transcutaneous microneurographic recordings of superficial peripheral nerves in the limbs. By careful positioning of the electrode and selection of nerve fascicles the experienced microneurographer can select activity of postganglionic fibres to skeletal muscle or to the skin. The former is mostly related to blood pressure control, the latter to emotion and thermoregulation. The muscular sympathetic nerve activity (MSNA) signals have taught us a great deal on the nature of baroreflex modulated sympathetic outflow. The nerves are active in bursts; each burst probably requires baroreceptor activity to be at a sufficiently low level to start (i.e. in the diastolic portion of the blood pressure pulse). This burst increases in intensity until it is shut off by the baroreceptor afferent burst induced by the next pulse wave. Sympathetic bursts do not occur in all heart beats; the average number of bursts per 100 beats is an accepted measure to quantify the activity. This may be increased by blood pressure lowering interventions as lower body negative pressure (LBNP) or nitroprusside infusion or decreased by blood pressure increasing infusions like phenylephrine. There is no clear-cut relation between the prevalence of high or low blood pressure and MSNA activity. Recent studies have shown that subjects with higher cardiac output at rest tend to have lower sympathetic nerve activity (Charkoudian et al. 2005). The number of bursts per 100 beats seems to be some individually determined parameter, which is highly reproducible even over periods of years (Fagius and Wallin 1993). For more details on microneurography of sympathetic efferents the reader is referred to Chapter 25.

A more global measure of sympathetic activity may be obtained by measuring the amount of noradrenaline that appears in the bloodstream as a result of neurotransmitter spill-over. Unfortunately one cannot simply take a venous sample and measure catecholamine levels. Each organ has a specific rate of extraction of noradrenaline from the arterial blood and another rate of excretion to the venous blood due to its own sympathetic activity and the reuptake of transmitter by its sympathetic nerve endings. Therefore, one should either obtain arterial samples (where the lung will have exerted its own process of extraction and excretion on the mixed venous blood that enters the heart), or one should go for organ-specific rates by radiotracer methodology involving elaborate catheterization and infusion schemes. For more details the reader is referred to Chapter 26.

Alternatives to the baroreflex sensitivity measurement are offered by computer-oriented techniques applied to continuous recordings of arterial blood pressure and heart rate. For more details on computer analysis of heart rate and blood pressure variability the readers are referred to Chapter 24.

The following paragraphs will detail a set of more or less classical non-invasive methods of arterial baroreflex pathway testing based on analysis of blood pressure and heart rate responses to a variety of physiological stresses. These stresses are easy to apply and provide valuable information about the presence or absence of functional disturbances in baroreflex control of systemic pressure.

For these tests more or less well-established lower limits of normal values per age-group are known. In as far as heart rate responses are important for the test outcome, the reflex tests suffer much less by cardiac rhythm disturbances than spectral analysis techniques tend to do. On the other hand, most tests require some form of patient cooperation, which may be difficult to obtain in elderly, physically or mentally disabled patients. In the latter cases spectral measures, where patient compliance is much less an issue, can have certain advantages.

In general these laboratory stress tests are models for what patients do in their everyday life. As such, the provoked changes in autonomic nervous outflow mimic the various stresses that people impose on themselves willingly during the day. The observable 24-hour variability in blood pressure and heart rate mirrors the underlying efferent autonomic variability (Ewing et al. 1991, Roach et al. 1999) (Chapter 24).

Cardiovascular reflex tests
Procedures and analysis of data

In early studies we used the combination of continuous heart rate monitoring and conventional sphygmomanometry to define normal and abnormal circulatory responses. Presently, in our laboratory continuous blood pressure recording by Finapres is used instead of sphygmomanometry. In the following both methods will be discussed. Various companies now offer the products for the Finapres technique or volume-clamp technique, as invented by Jan Peňaz and further developed by Karel Wesseling. It is beyond the scope of this chapter to give advice on which one to choose. We have had experience with Finapres in experimental and clinical settings from its very beginning and with various successors, as the Portapres and Finometer.

Standardization is a key factor in the assessment of cardiovascular reflex control. Ambient conditions like time of day and room temperature, breathing pattern and body posture during the test, and the preceding period of supine rest should all be considered. In our laboratory studies are performed in the morning in a quiet room at a pleasant ambient temperature (21–23°C) at least 1 hour after breakfast. Subjects abstain from coffee and cigarettes from the previous evening. Medications known to influence the cardiovascular system are not allowed from 48 hours prior to testing. Subjects are informed about the procedures involved and instructed to empty their bladder prior to the start of testing. The actual protocol is begun after a test run to train the subject to perform the test manoeuvres correctly.

Our common order of tests is a forced breathing test in supine position, followed by a standing up test from supine and a Valsalva manoeuvre in sitting position (Table 23.1). This 'classic series' may be followed by long-duration orthostatic stress testing using a tilt table. The latter is performed on special indication after previous testing. We want to have the classic tests performed first, since long-duration tilt (in particular if it leads to fainting) may have prolonged effects on cardiovascular control due to neurohormonal changes. Compared with the test times in the classic battery (Table 23.1) longer supine resting periods (at least 20 minutes) are advised for the assessment of disturbances in humoral control. This issue will not be elaborated further in this chapter.

To keep track of the procedure we use a strip chart recorder at low speed (50 mm/minute) or its computer-based equivalent. Beat-by-beat heart rate from the Finapres arterial pulse pressure interval is represented as a separate tracing. Arm cuff blood pressure is measured supine and in the upright position with the arm relaxed at the side when sphygmomanometry is used. When using Finapres the cuffed finger is kept at heart level, to avoid hydrostatic pressure influences (Fig. 23.1). Just prior to the procedure Finapres'

Table 23.1 Order of observations in standard cardiovascular reflex testing

- Supine instrumentation
- Instruction of manoeuvres
- 5 minutes supine rest
- 1 minute forced breathing test
- 2–3 minutes supine rest
- Standing up
- 5 minutes free standing
- 2–3 minutes sitting
- Valsalva's manoeuvre (sitting)

Physiocal or Servo-selfadjust option is switched off to ascertain a continuous recording during the transient phases of the manoeuvres.

Calculations are made from the original tracings. Control values for heart rate are obtained by averaging a 10 s period prior to the manoeuvres. In case of marked fluctuations in heart rate a 10–30-second period prior to the manoeuvres should be used. Changes in heart rate from control values induced by forced breathing, standing and Valsalva manoeuvre are computed. Control sphygmomanometer blood pressure values are obtained by averaging three measurements. Control values for finger arterial pressure are computed by averaging a 10–30-second period prior to the manoeuvres. Changes in blood pressure from control values induced by the three test manoeuvres are computed.

Overall baroreflex integrity

Overall integrity of the baroreflex arc can be assessed by analysing continuous heart rate and blood pressure responses to orthostasis and Valsalva straining. These manoeuvres impede venous return and reduce cardiac output, thus taxing arterial baroreflex regulatory mechanisms aimed at the stabilization of systemic blood pressure.

Orthostatic stress testing using standing

It is useful to divide the short-term circulatory response to the upright posture into an initial phase (first 30 seconds) with marked changes in heart rate and blood pressure and an early phase of stabilization (after 1–2 minutes standing) (Fig. 23.5A). Prolonged standing is defined as at least 5 minutes upright.

Initial heart rate and blood pressure responses to standing

After a total of 5 minutes of preceding rest, subjects are instructed to move from supine to standing in about 3 seconds, if necessary with assistance (Table 23.1). They stand for at least 2 minutes without support. Standing up in healthy adult subjects induces characteristic changes in heart rate (Fig. 23.5A). The heart rate increases abruptly towards a primary peak around 3 seconds, increases further to a secondary peak around 12 seconds, declines to a relative bradycardia around 20 seconds, and then gradually rises again. The primary (3-second) heart rate peak is vagally mediated and may be attributed to an exercise reflex that operates when voluntary muscle contractions are performed. The more gradual secondary heart rate rise, starting around 5 seconds after stand up, is mainly due to further reflex inhibition of cardiac vagal tone and increased sympathetic outflow to the sinus node and can be attributed to diminished activation of arterial baroreceptors by the fall in arterial pressure. The subsequent decrease in heart rate is associated with the recovery of arterial pressure and is again mediated through the arterial baroreflex by an increase in vagal outflow to the sinus node (Fig. 23.5A) (Borst et al. 1982, Sprangers et al. 1991).

For quantification of the initial heart rate response to standing the secondary heart rate peak is generally used. The highest heart rate in the first 15 seconds from the onset of standing is determined and expressed as the increase from baseline (ΔHRmax, 1 in Fig. 23.5A). This approach also allows a quantification of the response in patients who only show a more gradual heart rate increase, but without a relative bradycardia and consequently without a clear secondary peak. Ewing expressed the relative bradycardia originally as the ratio between the thirtieth and fifteenth R–R interval after the onset of standing. Indeed, on average, the maximal heart rate increase is reached at around the fifteenth beat and the relative bradycardia at around beat 30. However, since there are considerable differences

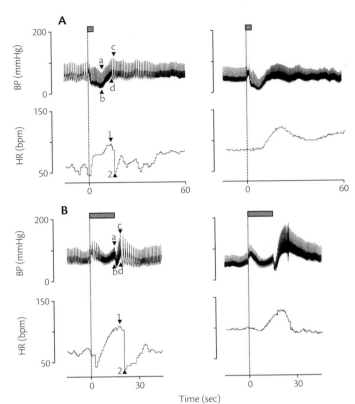

Fig. 23.5 Original tracings in a 33-year-old male subject of blood pressure and heart rate responses induced by **A:** (upper panels) standing and **B:** (lower panels) Valsalva manoeuvre. Pharmacological blockade with atropine (right-hand panels) abolished the large vagally mediated transient heart rate changes, a sluggish sympathetically mediated heart rate increase remains. The arrows indicate the timing of characteristic response extremes of interest. For standing: a, systolic pressure and b, diastolic pressure trough; c, systolic pressure and d, diastolic pressure overshoot; 1, initial peak heart rate increase (HRmax); 2, relative bradycardia (HRmin). For Valsalva manoeuvre: a, systolic and b, diastolic pressure at the end of straining; c, systolic and d, diastolic pressure overshoot; 1, initial peak heart-rate increase (HRmax); 2, bradycardia (HRmin).

Table 23.2 Assessment of initial heart rate (HR) response following 5–10-minute resting period and assessment of early steady-state heart rate response

Age (years)	Initial heart rate response		Early steady state
	ΔHRmax* (beats/minute)	HRmax/HRmin♦	ΔHR 2 minutes▲ (beats/minute)
10–14	< 20	< 1.20	> 35
15–19	19	1.18	> 34
20–24	19	1.17	> 33
25–29	18	1.15	> 32
30–34	17	1.13	> 31
35–39	16	1.11	> 30
40–44	16	1.09	> 29
45–49	15	1.08	> 28
50–54	14	1.06	> 27
55–59	13	1.04	> 26
60–64	13	1.02	> 25
65–69	12	1.01	> 24
70–74	12	1.00	> 23
75–80	11	-	> 22

* Abnormally low scores for ΔHRmax are defined as scores below $P_{0.025}$.

♦ Abnormally low values for relative bradycardia are numerically expressed as HRmax/HRmin ratio.

▲ Heart rate increases above $P_{0.975}$ of early steady-state values (after 2 minutes standing) are defined as excessive increase in heart rate.

between individuals, measurement of the 30/15 ratio at exactly beats 15 and 30 may underestimate the true RRmax/RRmin ratio. It is now generally recommended to use the highest and lowest heart rate in the first 30 seconds from the onset of standing (1 and 2 in Fig. 23.5A) to quantify the relative bradycardia (HRmax/HRmin ratio) (Wieling et al. 1997). The magnitude of ΔHRmax and the HRmax/HRmin ratio decreases with age. Another factor that has a large influence on the initial circulatory response is the duration of the period of supine rest prior to standing (Ten Harkel et al. 1990). The magnitude of ΔHRmax after 20 minutes rest exceeds the value after 1 minute rest by about 30%. Our reference values (Table 23.2) are therefore only valid for resting periods between 5 and 10 minutes. The influence of the level of resting heart rate on the magnitude of test scores is small compared with the effect of age and supine rest both in healthy subjects and in patients.

The test range for ΔHRmax is sufficient also in the elderly and its long-term within-subject repeatability is high. Thus ΔHRmax is a good test to assess instantaneous heart rate control. In contrast, the test range for the HRmax/HRmin ratio does not allow distinguishing between normal and abnormal heart rate control in subjects over 65 years of age (Table 23.2) (Piha 1993).

Using Finapres, the magnitude of the initial blood pressure response can be quantified by determining the systolic and diastolic blood pressure trough (a and b in Fig. 23.5A) and the subsequent systolic and diastolic blood pressure overshoot (c and d in Fig. 23.5A). In patients in whom a recovery of blood pressure is not observed, the value at 10 seconds after the onset of standing up is taken to indicate the trough and the value at 20 seconds to indicate the (absence of an) overshoot. The ratio of the change in pulse interval to mean arterial pressure (ms/mmHg) at the moment of the blood pressure trough (1 and a, b in Fig. 23.5A) has been used to compute an estimate of the sensitivity of the arterial baroreflex. This estimate decreases linearly with age.

Reference values for the magnitude of the initial blood pressure trough have not yet been established. Based on preliminary experience we consider an initial fall of more than 40 mm Hg in systolic pressure and/or more than 25 mm Hg in diastolic pressure as abnormally large (Wieling et al. 1992, Tanaka et al. 1994, Wieling et al. 2006). The initial fall in blood pressure does not increase with age (Fig. 23.6). An initial overshoot of systolic and or diastolic pressure is generally observed in healthy adult subjects. Its absence has been suggested as an indicator of sympathetic vasomotor dysfunction (Lindqvist et al. 1997).

Heart rate and blood pressure adjustments in the early phase of stabilization (1–2 minutes standing) and during prolonged standing (5–10 minutes standing)

The circulatory response in the early phase of stabilization is commonly used in the evaluation of neural circulatory control. This can be established by sphygmomanometer blood pressure readings

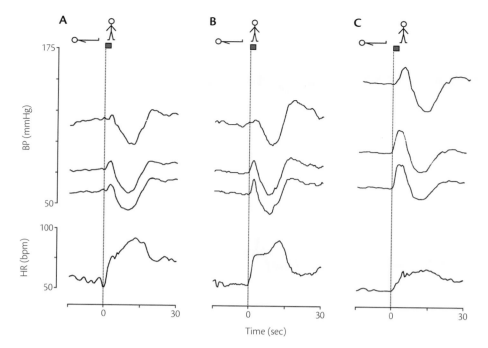

Fig. 23.6 Average systolic, mean and diastolic blood pressure and heart rate responses upon standing in **A:** ten 10–14-year old boys, **B:** ten 20–40-year old adult subjects and **C:** twenty over 70-year-old male subjects. Data kindly provided by Ten Harkel et al. 1998, Imholz et al. 1998 and Dambrink et al. 1991.

or by averaging 10-second periods of heart rate and finger blood pressure centred at 1 minute (3 and e, f in Fig. 23.5A) and 2 minutes after the change of posture. When there are marked fluctuations in heart rate and blood pressure a 30 s period of the Finapres recording should be averaged. Sphygmomanometric readings are erratic under these conditions. To quantify the circulatory response during prolonged standing, heart rate and blood pressure are taken at 5 minutes and 10 minutes after the onset of standing.

The normal adjustments in the early phase of stabilization are an increase in diastolic pressure by about 10 mm Hg, with little or no change in systolic pressure, and an increase in heart rate of about 10 beats/minute. During prolonged standing only minor further changes in heart rate and blood pressure are observed in this phase in healthy adult subjects and in the vast majority of patients with abnormal orthostatic responses (Atkins et al. 1991, Gehrking et al. 2005). Nevertheless, measurements should be continued for 10 minutes if there is a strong clinical suspicion of orthostatic hypotension without the earlier finding of a drop in blood pressure (Streeten et al. 1992, Gibbons and Freeman 2006). Sympathetic vasomotor control continues to play the central role in the maintenance of arterial pressure during prolonged standing (Joyner et al. 1990, Fu et al. 2006). During prolonged standing activation of the humoral system becomes more important, particularly in combating imminent arterial hypotension in the volume-depleted state (Cowley et al. 1992).

The heart rate increase after 1–2 minutes standing depends mainly on vagal withdrawal; an excessive increase (postural tachycardia) indicates functionally intact neurocardiovascular control and a strong adrenergic drive to the sinus node. Although the diagnostic criteria for what will be called postural tachycardia may differ between laboratories, all seem to agree that a sustained heart rate increase of more than 30 bpm within the first 10 minutes of orthostatic stress irrespective of age is abnormal (Low et al. 1995, Jacob 2000, Bonyhay 2004). However, it is well recognized that the postural increase in heart rate decreases with age (Taylor 1992,

Wieling 1992, Low et al. 1997), the decline amounting to about 2 bpm per decade (Table 23.2). The use of one single normative value of 30 bpm for all age groups will thus reduce the diagnostic discrimination of this test and may result in a false-positive test result in younger patients and a false-negative result in older patients.

A decrease in arterial pressure in the upright position can involve both systolic and diastolic pressures at the same time or it may be restricted to systolic pressure only. A fall of systolic pressure only is most likely caused by a non-neurogenic disturbance such as central hypovolaemia. Orthostatic hypotension due to autonomic failure involves both systolic and diastolic pressures. Ageing per se has little effect on sympathetic-circulatory regulation of arterial pressure during orthostasis; in upright, well-hydrated, normotensive elderly subjects arterial pressure is maintained just as well as in young adult subjects (Taylor et al. 1992). A persistent fall of more than 20 mmHg in systolic pressure after 1–2 minutes standing and/or in diastolic pressure of more than 5–10 mmHg is considered abnormal. Patients with a high supine systolic pressure tend to have a larger fall in pressure (Van Dijk et al. 1994).

Orthostatic stress testing using head-up tilting

The initial circulatory response upon a passive change of posture distinctly differs from the response on standing. A 70° head-up tilt results in a gradual rise in diastolic pressure, little change in systolic pressure and a gradual initial heart rate rise with little or no overshoot (Fig. 23.7). The different initial responses can be attributed to the effects of contraction of leg and abdominal muscles on the circulation during standing up; the underlying mechanisms have been addressed elsewhere (Borst et al. 1982, Sprangers et al. 1991, Wieling and Krediet 2006). A 70° angle of tilt may be considered to induce an almost identical hydrostatic effect as a 90° head-up tilt since sin 70° = 0.94 and sin 90° = 1.00. Even with tilt times between 2 seconds and 5 seconds, the speed of the manoeuvre has little or no influence on the initial orthostatic response to upright tilting (for review see Wieling and Wesseling 1993).

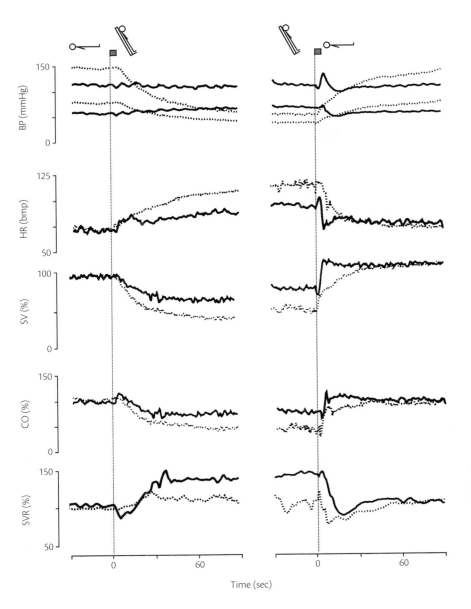

Fig. 23.7 Blood pressure (BP), heart rate (HR), stroke volume (SV), cardiac output (CO) and systemic vascular resistance (SVR) responses to head-up tilt (left panel) and tilt-back (right panel) in six patients with orthostatic hypotension due to autonomic failure (dotted line) and six healthy control (continuous line). From Wieling et al. 1998, with permission.

The initial heart rate response induced by a 70° head-up tilt does not differentiate between patients with mild vagal impairment and those with normal heart rate control; this is in contrast to the response induced by active standing up. Active standing is, therefore, more suitable to assess orthostatic neural control in the initial phase. The circulatory adjustments during quiet standing and passive head-up tilting in the early phase of stabilization (after 1–2 minutes upright) and during prolonged orthostatic stress (5–10 minutes upright) are similar (Low 1997). Both procedures seem appropriate in the clinical evaluation of neural circulatory control in these phases. In subjects with neurological disabilities head-up tilting is preferred since it gives the experimenter better control and allows rapid return to the supine posture in case of impending syncope in the head-up posture. Long-duration head-up tilting (20–45 minutes upright) with or without pharmacological stimulation has been used worldwide to assess a tendency for vasovagal syncope in patients with unexplained syncope (Brignole et al. 2004). However, recent studies with implantable loop recorders

have shown that tilt-table testing is not a reliable test to identify syncopal events in real life in subjects over 50 years of age (Brignole et al. 2006). Our present application of tilt-table testing focuses on teaching the patient to recognize premonitory symptoms and to use physical countermanoeuvres (Krediet et al. 2002, Wieling et al. 2004).

Haemodynamic responses induced by tilt back to supine position

The gradual initial (first 30 seconds) circulatory adjustments to tilt-up in healthy subjects contrast with the pronounced abrupt initial circulatory changes on tilt-back (Fig. 23.8) (Wieling et al. 1998, Toska et al. 2002, van Heusden 2006). Mechanical factors underlie these strikingly different dynamic initial adjustments. After head-up tilt, left ventricular stroke volume is maintained during the first 4–6 s and cardiac output may even increase. This time delay can be attributed to the amount of blood available in the heart and the pulmonary vessels. Stroke volume and cardiac

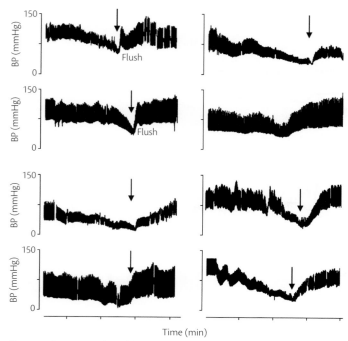

Fig. 23.8 Continuous finger blood pressure recordings during tilt-induced faints. Arrows indicate tilt to horizontal. Pronounced flushing was observed in the patients in the upper left panels. The presence of facial flushing was associated with a rapid return to physiological blood pressure levels suggesting that the faints in these two patients were cardiac output mediated. With permission from Wieling, Krediet, Wilde, *Journal of Cardiovascular Electrophysiology*, Wiley.

output then decrease steadily during the next 30 s to a stable level about 25% below pre-tilt values.

About 2–3 seconds after the onset of tilt-back left ventricular stroke volume increases rapidly to its pre-tilt value in less than 10 seconds. The time delay of 2–3 seconds may be explained by the right-to-left ventricular transit time of blood. The rather abrupt circulatory changes induced by tilt-back compared to the gradual changes on tilt-up appear to indicate that the venous pooling of blood during head-up tilt takes place more gradually than the transfer of stagnant venous blood back to the heart on release of orthostatic stress. Probably this is due to the slow filling of the dependent veins via the (high) resistance of the microvasculature, as opposed to their sudden emptying against almost no resistance on tilt-back

In patients who lack neural circulatory reflex adjustments, gradual blood pressure decreases to head-up tilt and gradual increases to tilt back are observed (Wieling et al. 1998). In patients with a vasovagal reaction during tilt-table testing a similar gradual recovery has been described (de Jong et al. 1997a). However, in some subjects with a vasovagal reaction the recovery of blood pressure is steep and a flush can be observerd (Wieling et al. 2006).

Valsalva manoeuvre

Valsalva manoeuvre as used in the cardiovascular laboratory is an abrupt voluntary elevation of intrathoracic and intra-abdominal pressure by straining. It is provoked by blowing through a mouthpiece in a closed system where pressure is measured (e.g. a blood pressure meter). The patient maintains a prescribed airway pressure and to force an open connection between mouth and airways

a small leak in the tubing (e.g. via a fine-bore hypodermic needle) is advised. After a brief period of increased peripheral arterial pressure, the blood pumped out is not adequately replenished due to the pressure-induced hindrance of inflow of blood to the trunk; this results in a temporary fall in blood volume in the central vessels. A serious fall in arterial pressure is prevented by reflex vasoconstriction (Sandroni et al. 1991, Smith et al. 1996). Typical responses are shown in Figure 5B. Valsalva manoeuvre is performed preferably while sitting, because the circulatory effects are larger in that position compared to the changes observed in the supine position Fig. 23.9) (Ten Harkel et al. 1990).

An expiratory pressure of 40 mmHg is maintained for 15 seconds. Care is taken to prevent deep breathing prior to and directly following release of the strain, since this influences test scores considerably. If straining produces marked falls in blood pressures the manoeuvre should be performed supine. Some elderly patients, especially those with neurological disorders and most very young subjects, in our experience cannot carry out the procedure adequately (De Jong et al. 1997b). Valsalva straining should be avoided in patients with proliferative retinopathy.

Valsalva's manoeuvre elicits typical changes in heart rate in young adult subjects (Fig. 23.5B). An immediate heart rate decrease during the rise in systolic and diastolic pressure at the onset of straining is usually observed. It is followed by an increase in heart rate during and directly after release of intrathoracic pressure and a subsequent bradycardia.

The heart rate increase during and directly after release of the strain (peak 1 in Fig. 23.5B) is mediated by withdrawal of vagal tone and increased sympathetic outflow to the sinus node due to the fall in blood pressure. The bradycardia (2 in Fig. 23.5B) is the result of a vagal reflex, which depends on a blood pressure overshoot relative to control blood pressure. The magnitude of the heart rate responses induced by Valsalva manoeuvre decreases with age (Table 23.3).

In quantifying the heart rate increase induced by Valsalva manoeuvre the maximum heart rate is determined and expressed as the difference from baseline (ΔHRmax, peak 1 in Fig. 23.5B). The ratio between highest and lowest heart rate directly after release of the strain (1 and 2 in Fig. 23.5B) is generally used to quantify the relative bradycardia (HRmax/HRmin ratio or Valsalva ratio). The test range for the Valsalva ratio does not allow distinguishing between normal and abnormal heart rate control in subjects older than 65 years of age (Table 23.3) (Piha 1993). Long-term reproducibility of the Valsalva ratio in adult subjects it is high.

Using Finapres the magnitude of the blood pressure response can be quantified by determining the systolic and diastolic blood-pressure at the end of straining (a and b in Fig. 23.5B) and the subsequent systolic and diastolic blood pressure overshoot after release of Valsalva straining (c and d in Fig. 23.6B) relative to control levels of blood pressure. An overshoot of systolic and or diastolic pressure is generally observed in healthy adult subjects. These pressure elevations provide acceptable estimates of preceding sympathetic nerve responses and the integrity of arterial baroreceptor sympathetic vasomotor control mechanisms (Smith et al. 1996). In patients without a blood-pressure overshoot the highest blood pressure in the first 15 seconds after release of the strain is taken.

It has been suggested that the absence of a partial recovery of arterial pressure during straining is an index of impairment of sympathetic vasomotor function that occurs earlier than the lack

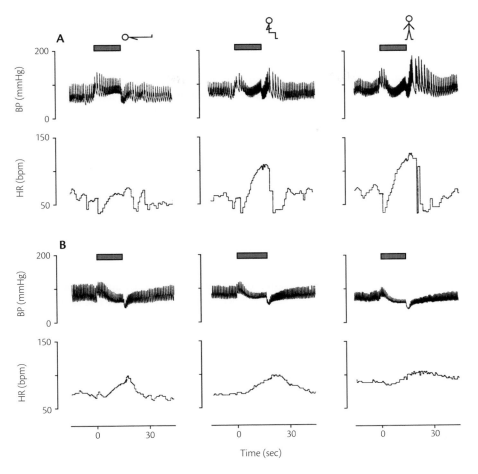

Fig. 23.9 Influence of posture on Valsalva's manoeuvre in **A:** a healthy 33-year-old subject and **B:** a 43-year-old patient with autonomic failure. Note marked influences of posture on the blood pressure responses in both subjects. The square wave response observed in the healthy adult subject in supine position is a normal finding. Ten Harkel et al., *J Appl Physiol* (1990), Am Physiol Soc, used with permission.

Table 23.3 Assessment of heart rate responses induced by forced breathing and the Valsalva manoeuvre

Age (years)	I-E difference* (beats/minute)	Valsalva ratio♦
10–14	< 17	< 1.53
15–19	< 16	< 1.48
20–24	< 15	< 1.43
25–29	< 14	< 1.38
30–34	< 13	< 1.33
35–39	< 12	< 1.28
40–44	< 11	< 1.24
45–49	< 11	< 1.20
50–55	< 10	< 1.16
55–60	< 9	< 1.12
60–65	< 9	< 1.08
65–70	< 8	< 1.04
70–75	< 7	< 1.00
75–80	< 7	-

* Abnormally low scores for I⁻-E difference are defined as scores below $P_{0.025}$.
♦ Abnormally low values for heart rate changes induced by the Valsalva manoeuvre are expressed as the Valsalva ratio.

of overshoot of arterial pressure above baseline values (Sandroni et al. 1991). For older subjects, no data are available on this topic. Blood pressure recovery time after release of the strain is a valuable index of adrenergic failure (Vogel et al. 2005). Baroreflex sensitivity on heart rate can be estimated by measuring the change in inter-beat interval per unit change in systolic blood pressure (ms/mmHg) during the overshoot of blood pressure after the straining (Palmero et al. 1981). This estimate, again, decreases with age.

Afferent arterial baroreflex pathways

If failure of the baroreflex arc is demonstrated by orthostatic stress or Valsalva straining, the question is whether the lesion on the arterial baroreflex arc is on the afferent, central or efferent side. Afferent and central lesions cannot be assessed directly in patients. The common approach is to evaluate efferent sympathetic and parasympathetic pathways. If these are normal the lesion is supposed to be on the afferent or central site of the arterial baroreflex arc.

Efferent sympathetic pathways

Placing one hand in ice water (*cold pressor test*), mental stress and isometric exercise such as sustained handgrip, result in increased systemic blood pressure. The afferent pathways involved in these stresses (pain, central command, muscle receptors) are distinct from the afferent pathways of the arterial baroreflex. In subjects with evidence of disturbances in control of systemic blood pressure during orthostatic stress or Valsalva straining, a rise in blood pressure

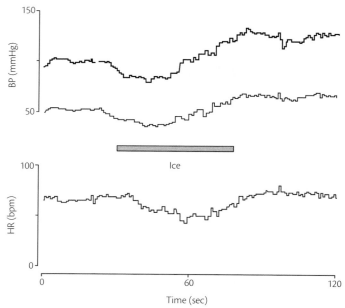

Fig. 23.10 Cold face test in a 51-year-old patient with afferent baroreflex failure. Upper panel shows excessive (> 30 mm Hg) blood pressure elevation. Lower panel demonstrates initial decline in heart rate. With kind permission from Springer Science+Business Media: *Clin Autonom Res*, Baroreflex failure following radiation therapy for nasopharyngeal carcinoma, **9**, 1999, 317–324, Timmers, H.J.L.M., Karemaker, J.M., Lenders J.W.M, and Wieling, W.

in response to these stresses suggests that efferent sympathetic pathways are functioning. The influence of age on the blood pressure responses to such acute stresses is not agreed upon; hyperreactivity and hyporeactivity have been reported. Evidence suggests that application of the above mentioned stressors evokes similar absolute increases in sympathetic neural activity and arterial pressure in healthy young and elderly subjects (Ng et al. 1994).

The arterial blood pressure response to the cold pressor test is in our experience a useful index of sympathetic outflow to systemic blood vessels. Sustained handgrip has consistently been found of limited sensitivity and specificity in the assessment of efferent sympathetic activity (Piha 1993, Ziegler et al. 1992). The cold pressor test is easily applied even in older subjects. The test is performed in the semi-recumbent position. Responses are measured before and during immersion of one hand in ice water for 2 minutes. The changes in blood pressure during the last 10 seconds of the test are compared to baseline values. A blood pressure rise of 10–15 mmHg in systolic pressure and of 10 mmHg in diastolic pressure is considered to be a normal response and an increase of more than 20 mm Hg in systolic pressure *and* 15 mmHg in diastolic pressure as excessive. Pronounced hyperactivity is found in patients with afferent baroreflex lesions (Fig. 23.10) (Timmers et al. 1999, Smit et al. 2002, Timmers et al. 2003). Hyperreactivity is also a frequent finding in hypertensive subjects. Little or no increase in arterial pressure is supposed to indicate failure of efferent sympathetic vasomotor pathways, but some normal subjects may also have little or no response.

Efferent cardiac vagal control

The instantaneous heart rate responses elicited by changes in arterial pressure induced by stand up and Valsalva straining (Fig. 23.5A and 23.5B) are used as measures of the arterial baroreflex effectiveness

on heart rate as discussed above. For a selective evaluation of efferent cardiac vagal pathways it is useful to apply manoeuvres that elicit non-baroreflex mediated changes in vagal outflow to the heart. Stimulation of vagal outflow can be evoked by apnoeic face immersion (diving reflex), the cold face test (Fig. 23.10) or eye-ball pressure (oculovagal reflex). An instantaneous heart rate decrease induced by these manoeuvres indicates intact efferent cardiac vagal pathways (Khurana & Wu 2006). Since heart rate responsiveness decreases at older age the responses to these manoeuvres do not allow distinguishing between normal and diminished efferent cardiac vagal control in the elderly.

Cardiac vagal stimulation and inhibition can be tested by the forced breathing manoeuvre. The afferent pathways and central mechanisms underlying the heart response to this test are complex and the mechanisms involved remain uncertain. There is, however, general agreement that the efferent path is predominantly the parasympathetic supply to the heart by the vagus nerve and the magnitude of the oscillations in heart rate are used as estimate of efferent neural traffic of the vagus nerve to the heart in man. Compliance to the test is easy, the test range is sufficient (also in the elderly, see Table 23.3) and long-term reproducibility is good.

The forced breathing test is performed supine, since vagal effects are then most pronounced. After 5 minutes' rest the subject is instructed to perform six consecutive maximal inspiration and expiration cycles at a rate of 6 breaths/minute. To quantify the test score the difference between maximal and minimal heart rate for each of the six cycles is determined and averaged to obtain the inspiratory-expiratory (I-E) difference in beats per minute. The magnitude of the I-E difference is age-related (Fig. 23.11) (Wieling et al. 1982, Low 1997). The norm values of these two data sets are remarkably similar

The influence of the level of resting heart rate on the I-E difference is small compared to the effect of age. Thus, a correction for resting heart rate is not important in the measurement of the I-E difference. However, to observe modulations in vagally mediated changes in heart rate some vagal tone should be present to be modulated. This test, therefore, cannot be interpreted when the resting heart rate is

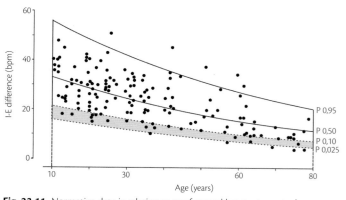

Fig. 23.11 Normative data in relation to age for vagal heart rate control quantified by the heart variations during maximal inspiration and expiration cycles at a rate of 6 breaths/minute (I-E difference). The regression line ($P_{0.50}$) and confidence limits were calculated from log-transformed values. The shaded area indicates values between the lower 2.5th and 10th percentile, which we have defined as borderline. The values below this range are considered abnormally small, values above it are considered normal. Data from Wieling et al. 1982 and Dambrink et al. 1991a.

high (>100 bpm). This principle applies to all tests aiming to assess cardiac vagal tone.

Test battery: clinical interpretation of one or more abnormal test results

We are in favour of using a combination of tests in the evaluation of patients suspected of suffering from autonomic disturbances. We feel that a (patho)physiological interpretation of test results is more important in the evaluation of individual patients than simply to add test scores as was done in the now almost classic 'Ewing-protocol'. Here outcomes of various tests were scored as normal, borderline or pathological, points were awarded per score and all scores added to find a final label (Ewing 1985). If the Ewing battery is used to assess cardiovascular nerve damage age-adjusted reference values should be used (Tables 23.2 and 23.3) (Wieling et al. 1982, Low et al. 1997, Freeman 2006).

The clinical relevance of the search for highly sensitive estimates of alterations in short-term cardiovascular control, be it cardiovagal (Weston et al. 1996) or adrenergic (Low et al. 1996, Lindqvist 1997), needs to be reconsidered. A sensitive test to screen patients for an abnormality is only indicated if efficacious treatments for the primary disease exist and/or efficacious preventive manoeuvres for its sequelae. Early detection of subclinical autonomic dysfunction has been suggested to be important for risk stratification and subsequent management in patients with cardiovascular disease. However, at this moment there is neither efficacious treatment for autonomic dysfunction nor for the associated increase in sudden death. Large-scale screening for impairment of short-term cardiovascular control is, therefore, not yet indicated, except maybe for research purposes (Wieling et al. 1997). In addition, it is important to realize that cardiovascular reflex tests are more difficult to interpret than for example nerve conduction measurements, since both autonomic nerve function and cardiovascular haemodynamics are involved. Moreover, medication and unstable clinical conditions can greatly influence test scores. In daily practice, therefore, it is of far more importance to work towards a definite (patho)physiological diagnosis than to aim for detection of subtle abnormalities.

We use the I-E difference induced by forced breathing as a sensitive measure to assess vagal heart rate control. We have found the combination of abnormally low test scores for both the I-E difference and for ΔHRmax upon standing well suited to identify definite cardiac vagal neuropathy in individual patients (Wieling et al. 1982). HRmax/HRmin ratios induced by standing and the Valsalva heart rate ratios are in our experience in these conditions abnormally low as well.

Spectrum of normal and abnormal orthostatic responses

Five main types of responses are clinically important in the evaluation of complaints of orthostatic dizziness (Table 23.4). The first three are common and transient and are found in subjects with intact circulatory reflexes. The last two are rare and characterized by a significant and persistent fall in blood pressure in the upright position due to autonomic failure.

A careful evaluation of the patient's history and the conventional measurement of blood pressure (sphygmomanometer) and heart rate (pulse counting) supine and after 1–2 minutes standing are simple procedures to evaluate complaints of orthostatic dizziness in general practice. Based on the heart rate and blood pressure responses in the early phase of stabilization a distinction can be made into:

♦ normal orthostatic heart rate and blood pressure control

♦ normal orthostatic blood pressure control in combination with postural tachycardia

♦ orthostatic hypotension with or without postural tachycardia (Table 23.4).

Below we will show that, although continuous measurement of arterial blood pressure is no prerequisite for a classification of patients, analysis of both heart rate and blood pressure changes contributes to a more fundamental understanding of the pathophysiological mechanisms involved.

Initial orthostatic light-headedness on standing in healthy subjects

A normal initial heart rate response including an immediate heart rate increase, a large secondary heart rate peak, and a marked subsequent bradycardia (1 and 2 in Fig. 23.5A) is an important clinical finding. For reasons explained above it indicates, intact afferent, central, and efferent cardiac vagal and sympathetic vasomotor pathways.

Table 23.4 Classification of patients according to their response to standing

Response	Early steady-state blood pressure	Initial heart rate response	Early steady-state	Heart rate response
Normal	Systolic	=	Biphasic	↑
	Diastolic	↑		
Hyperadrenergic	Systolic	↓	Large ΔHRmax	↑↑
	Diastolic	↑↑	– little or no relative brachycardia	
Vasovagal	Systolic	N	Normal or	↓
	Diastolic	N	hyperadrenergic	
Hypoadrenergic	Systolic	↓	Large ΔHRmax	↑↑
(vagus intact)	Diastolic	↓	– no relative bradycardia	
Hypoadrenergic	Systolic	↓	Absent	=
(with cardiac denervation)	Diastolic	↓		

Nevertheless, it should be realized that subjects with intact autonomic cardiovascular control can still have complaints of light-headedness shortly after standing up. In fact most people have experience with a brief feeling of dizziness 5–10 seconds after standing up rapidly, especially after prolonged supine rest. Such common spells of dizziness are characterized by their time of onset and short duration and appear to be more common in young subjects. In teenagers with severe complaints of orthostatic light-headedness immediately at standing up an extraordinary large initial blood pressure drop and sluggish recovery has been observed (see Chapter 60) (Dambrink et al. 1991, Tanaka et al. 1994, Wieling and Krediet 2006). For more details on initial orthostatic hypotension the reader is referred to Chapter 60.

Hyperadrenergic orthostatic response

An excessive heart rate increment (see Table 23.2) after 1–2 minutes of standing can be considered as a compensatory response to a variety of conditions; an abnormal degree of central hypovolaemia and a strong adrenergic drive in the upright posture are common to these conditions (Low et al. 1995). After spaceflight and prolonged bed rest excessive postural heart rate increases are common in otherwise healthy subjects (Baisch 1992, Levine et al. 2002, Fu et al. 2005, Gisolf et al. 2005).

Classically, such a response consists of an immediate heart rate increase and a large secondary peak with little or no subsequent relative bradycardia, resulting in an excessive increase in heart rate in the upright position, together with a fall in systolic pressure and a marked increase in diastolic pressure. A marked increase in both systolic and diastolic pressure has also been described. Augmented responses to Valsalva manoeuvre in these conditions confirms functionally intact arterial baroreflex pathways (Muenter Swift et al. 2005). This augmented response to Valsalva manoeuvre can be observed in normal subjects when thoracic blood volume is decreased by performing the manoeuvre in sitting or standing position (Fig. 23.9).

Vasovagal orthostatic response

Typical for a vasovagal response is a temporary phase of tachycardia in the upright position, which changes into a decrease in heart rate and a fall in blood pressure due to reflex vagal facilitation and adrenergic inhibition, respectively (see Chapter 60) (Van Lieshout et al. 1991a). Using pulse wave analysis the variability of haemodynamic responses leading up to a vasovagal faint can be analysed. The variability in haemodynamic profiles between young subjects is marked (Fig. 23.12). An impaired ability to generate or to maintain vasomotor tone and vagal bradycardia seems to be the key factor in vasovagal fainting in younger subjects during orthostatic stress (Ten Harkel et al. 1993, De Jong et al. 1995, Tanaka et al. 1997). In elderly subjects decreases in cardiac output underlie vasovagal syncope during orthostatic stress testing. Vagal bradycardia is far less pronounced.

Hypoadrenergic orthostatic response with intact heart rate control

In patients with sympathetic vasomotor lesions but intact vagal heart rate control, an immediate large heart rate increase without a relative bradycardia is observed (Van Lieshout et al. 1989). This is accompanied by a progressive fall of both systolic and diastolic blood pressures (Fig. 23.13A). This response can be attributed to

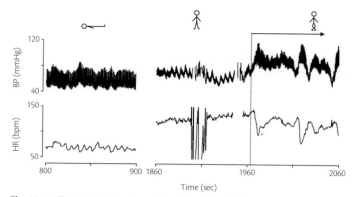

Fig. 23.12 Ten-minute stand test 5 days after spaceflight in a cosmonaut. Note marked postural tachycardia and blood pressure instability with decreased pulse pressure. Leg crossing and muscle tensing at the end of the stand test rapidly restored the reduced pulse pressure and decreased heart rate. With permission from The American Physiological Society (Gisolf et al. 2005).

baroreceptor sensing of an absence of recovery of blood pressure due to the defective vasoconstrictor mechanisms (compare Fig. 23.5A with Fig. 23.13A). Hypoadrenergic orthostatic hypotension, combined with a marked postural tachycardia can be found

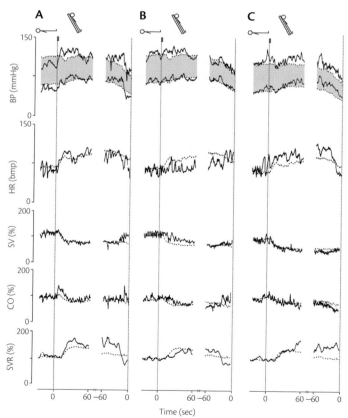

Fig. 23.13 Typical individual responses of a vasovagal response **(A)**, a vasodepressor response **(B)**, and a vagal response **(C)**. The dotted lines represent the group averages of 29 near-fainting subjects of 6–16 years of age. Supine control, the first 60s of the head-up tilt and the last 60s prior to tilt-back are presented. SBP, systolic blood pressure; DBP, diastolic blood pressure; HR, heart rate; SV, stroke volume; CO, cardiac output; SVR, systemic vascular resistance. Reproduced with permission, from De Jong-de Vos van Steenwijk, C.C.E., Wieling, W., Harms, M.P.M. and Wesseling, K.H., (1997), *Clinical Science*, **93**, 205–211, © the Biochemical Society.

in some patients with dysautonomia, in tetraplegic patients, and after extensive sympathectomy.

The blood pressure response induced by Valsalva manoeuvre in these patients indicates loss of sympathetic vasomotor control. If the heart rate response is considered without the simultaneous blood pressure recording, the registration can be misleading, since a normal reflex bradycardia and high Valsalva ratios can be observed in some of these patients (Fig. 23.13A). The rare combination of a hypoadrenergic orthostatic response with intact vagal heart rate control (Fig. 23.13A) may be interpreted as the mirror image of the common pattern of autonomic circulatory denervation (as observed in patients with diabetes mellitus), where impaired vagal heart rate control precedes overt sympathetic damage (i.e. orthostatic hypotension) (Fig. 23.13B).

Hypoadrenergic hypostatic response with impairment of vagal and sympathetic innervation of the heart

In subjects with a normal resting heart rate, a delayed and sluggish primary heart rate response upon standing indicates that vagal heart rate control is absent (Fig. 23.5A and B). The heart rate increase in these patients represents the remaining sympathetic response mentioned before. Thus, a delayed onset of cardioacceleration and a substantial heart rate increase afterwards suggest cardiac vagal denervation with intact sympathetic heart rate control. A small heart rate increase after prolonged standing in patients with orthostatic hypotension should be interpreted as a sign of impaired sympathetic heart rate control. Valsalva manoeuvre will confirm the abnormality. Complete denervation of the heart can be found in patients with a cardiac transplant. The blood pressure adjustment to orthostatic stress shows that when vasomotor innervation is intact, orthostatic blood pressure control remains undisturbed in spite of complete cardiac denervation (Fig. 23.13C) (Wieling and Wesseling 1993). A square wave response is induced by Valsalva manoeuvre. Obviously, the marked blood pressure changes induced by standing and Valsalva manoeuvre will not be noticed in this patient if continuous monitoring is not available.

Square wave response during Valsalva straining

A square wave response during Valsalva straining occurs in subjects with congestive heart failure, but also during a supine Valsalva manoeuvre in some normal subjects (Ten Harkel et al. 1990). In the latter the square wave response changes to 'normal' in the sitting and the standing position (Fig 23.9). These observations suggest that the blood pressure responses during Valsalva straining can be used to monitor changes in central blood volume. The diurnal and postural effects on blood pressure during Valsalva straining in a patient with autonomic failure are another example of this concept (Fig. 23.14) (Van Lieshout et al. 1991b).

Conclusion

An active stand test provides much insight about human neurocardiovascular control; both instantaneous and sustained orthostatic circulatory responses can be assessed. ΔHRmax is a good test to assess instantaneous heart rate control in the elderly, but the HRmax/HRmin ratio is *probably* not. The combination of sphygmomanometric blood pressure readings in the supine position and after 1–2 minutes standing, and monitoring of the instantaneous heart rate response on standing, provides sufficient information

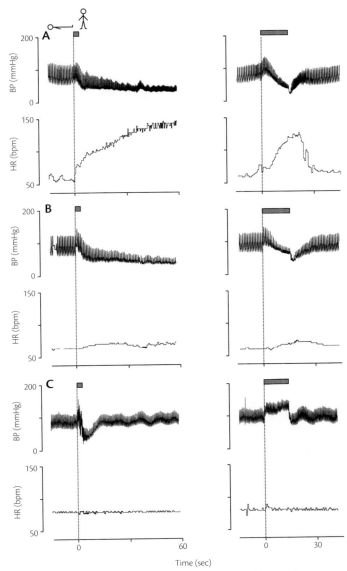

Fig. 23.14 Blood pressure and heart rate responses induced by standing (short bar) and Valsalva's manoeuvre (long bar). **A:** orthostatic hypotension (hypoadrenergic) with intact heart rate control in a 23-year-old female patient. **B:** a 69-year-old male patient with orthostatic hypotension (hypoadrenergic) with impairment of vagal and sympathetic cardiac control (Valsalva manoeuvre is performed supine). **C:** total cardiac denervation with intact vasomotor control in a 38-year-old fit patient with a cardiac transplant.

for a classification of normal and abnormal orthostatic circulatory responses. However, for a full physiological evaluation of an abnormal heart rate response it is necessary to monitor the concomitant blood pressure responses continuously using Finapres.

In contrast to the orthostatic stress test, Valsalva manoeuvre only assesses instantaneous circulatory responses. The advantage of Valsalva manoeuvre is that both the capacities for cardioacceleration and cardiodeceleration are tested. Lack of reference values for blood pressure indices of the manoeuvre in elderly subjects and problems in the correct execution make the procedure less suitable for the assessment of cardiovascular control than orthostatic stress testing.

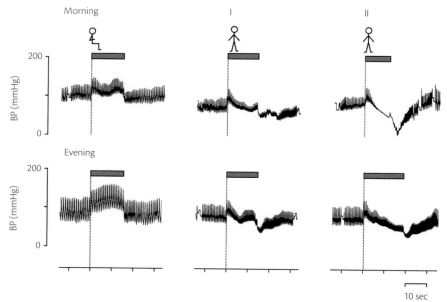

Fig. 23.15 Diurnal and postural effects on the blood pressure response to Valsalva manoeuvre in a 23-year-old female patient with autonomic failure. The manoeuvre was performed in the sitting position, after 10 minutes of standing upright (Standing I) and was repeated after a further 2 minutes in the upright position (Standing II). Bars indicate the duration of the straining period. Note the higher sitting and standing mean blood pressure in the evening and the square wave response during Valsalva's manoeuvre in the sitting position in the evening. With permission from *Neth. J. Med*, Van Lieshout et al. (1991b).

References

Atkins, D., Hanusa, B., Sefcik, T., and Kapoor, W. (1991). Syncope and orthostatic hypotension. *Am. J Med.*, **91**, 179–85

Baisch, F., Beck, L., Karemaker, J. M., Arbeille, P., Gaffney, F. A., and Blomquist, G. (1992). Head-down tilt bedrest. HDT'88- an international collaborative eeffort in integrated systems physiology. *Acta. Physiol. Scand. Suppl.* **604**, 1–12.

Bonyhay, I., Freeman, R.(2004). Sympathetic nerve activity in response to orthostatic stress in the postural tachycardia syndrome. *Circulation* **110**, 3193–98.

Borst, C., Wieling, W., Van Brederode, J.F.M., Hond, A., De Rijk, L.G., and Dunning, A.J. (1982). Mechanisms of initial heart rate response to postural change. *Am. J Physiol.*, **243** (Heart Circ Physiol 12), H676–81.

Bos, W.J., Van Goudoever, J., Van Montfrans, G.A., Van den Meiracker, A.J. and Wesseling, K.H. (1996). Reconstruction of brachial artery pressure from non-invasive finger pressure measurements. *Circulation*, **94**, 1870–75.

Brignole, M., Alboni, P., Benditt, D. G., *et al.*(2004). Guidelines on management (diagnosis and treatment) of syncope-update 2004. Executive Summary. *European Heart J*, **25**, 2054–72.

Brignole, M., Sutton, R., Menozzi, C., *et al.* (2006). ISSUE 2-group. Lack of correlation between the responses to tilt testing and adenosine triphosphate test and the mechanism of spontaneous neurally mediated syncope. *Eur Heart J*, **27**, 2232–39

Charkoudian, N., Joyner, M. J., Johnson, C. P., Eisenach, J. H., Dietz, N. M., Wallin, B. G. (2005). Balance between cardiac output and sympathetic activity in resting humans: role in arterial pressure regulation. *J Physiol.*, **568**, 315–21.

Cowley, A. W. Long-term control of arterial pressure (1992). *Physiol Rev*, **72**, 231–78.

Dambrink, J. H. A., Imholz, B. P. M., Karemaker, J. M. and Wieling, W. (1991b). Postural and transient hypotension in two healthy teenagers. *Clin Aut Res*, **1**, 281–87.

De Jong-de Vos van Steenwijk, C. C. E., Imholz, B. P. M., Wesseling, K. H., and Wieling, W. (1997b). The Valsalva manoeuvre as a cardiovascular reflex test in healthy children and teenagers. *Clin Auton. Res*, **7**, 167–71.

De Jong-de Vos van Steenwijk, C. C. E., Wieling, W., Harms, M. P. M. and Wesseling, K. H. (1997a). Variability of near-fainting responses in healthy 6–16 year old subjects. *Clin. Sci.*, **93**, 205–11.

De Jong-de Vos van Steenwijk, C. C. E., Wieling, W., Johannes, J. M., Harms, M. P. M., Kuis, W. and Wesseling K. H. (1995). Incidence and hemodynamics of near-fainting in healthy 6–16 year old subjects. *J Am. Col. Cardiol.*, **25**, 1615–21

Eckberg, D. L. Bursting into space: alterations of sympathetic control by space travel. (2003). *Acta Physiol Scand*, **177**, 299–311.

Eckberg, D. L. and Sleight, P. (1992). *Human baroreflexes in health and disease*. Oxford University Press, Oxford.

Ewing, D. J., Martyn, C. N., Young, R. J., and Clarke, B. F. (1985). The value of cardiovascular autonomic function tests: 10 year experience in diabetes. *Diabetes Care*, **8**, 491–98.

Ewing, D. J., Neilson, J. M. M., Shapiro, C. M., Stewart, J. A., Reid, W. (1991). Twenty four hour heart rate variability: effects of posture, sleep, and time of day in healthy controls and comparison with bedside tests of autonomic function in diabetic patients. *Br Heart J*, **65**, 239–44.

Fagius, J. and Wallin, B. G. (1993). Long-term variability and reproducibility of resting human muscle nerve sympathetic activity at rest, as reassessed after a decade. *Clin. Auton. Res.* **3**, 201–205.

Freeman, R. Assessment of cardiovascular autonomic function.(2006). *Clin Physiol*, **117**, 716–30.

Fu, Q., Shook, R.P., Okazaki, K., *et al.* (2006). Vasomotor sympathetic neural control is maintained during sustained upright posture in humans. *J Physiol.*, in press

Fu, Q., Witkowski, S., Okazaki, K., and Levine, B.D. (2005). Effects of gender and hypovolemia on sympathetic neural responses to orthostatic stress. *Am. J Physiol. Regul. Integr. Comp. Physiol.*, R109–116.

Gehrking, J. A., Hines, S. M., Benrus-Larsen, L. M., Opher-Gehrking, T. L. and Low, P. A. (2005). What is the minimum duration of a head-up tilt necessary to detect orthostatic hypotension? *Clin. Autonom. Res.*, **15**, 71–75.

Gibbons, C. H., and Freeman, R. (2006). Delayed orthostatic hypotension. *Neurology*, **67**, 28–32.

Gisolf, J., Imink, R. V., van Lieshout, J. J., Stok, W. J., Karemaker, J. M. (2005). Orthostatic blood pressure control before and after space flight determinded by time domain baroreflex method. *J Appl. Physiol.* **98**,1682–90.

Gisolf, J., Westerhof, B. E., Van Dijk, N., Wesseling, K. H., Wieling, W., and Karemaker, J. M. (2004). Sublingual nitroglycerin used in routine tilt testing provokes a cardiac output mediated vasovagal response. *J Am. Coll. Cardiol.*, **44**, 588–93.

Gizdulich, P., Prentza. A. and Wesseling, K. H. (1997). Models of brachial to finger pulse wave distorsion and pressure decrement. *Cardiovasc Res*, **33**, 698–705.

Guelen, I., Westerhof, B. E., Van Der Sar, G. L., Van Montfrans, G. A., Kiemeneij, F., Wesseling, K. H., Bos, W. J. (2003). Finometer, finger pressure measurements with the possibility to reconstruct brachial pressure. *Blood Press. Monit.*, **8**, 27–30.

Imholz, B. P. M., Langewouters, G. J., Van Montfrans, G. A., *et al.* (1993). Feasibility of ambulatory, continuous 24-hour finger arterial pressure recording. *Hypertension*, **21**, 65–73.

Imholz, B. P. M., Wieling, W., Van Montfrans, G. A., Wesseling, K. H. (1998). Fifteen years experience with finger artrial pressure monitoring: assessment of the technology. *Cardiovasc. Res.*, **38**, 605–16

Jacob, G., Costa, F., Shannon, J. R., *et al.*, (2000). The neuropahic postural tachycardia syndrome. *N Engl. J Med.* **343**, 1008–14

Jellema, W. T., Imholz, B. P. M., Van Goedoever, J., Wesseling, K. H. and Van Lieshout, J. J. (1996). Finger arterial versus intrabrachial pressure and continuous cardiac output during head-up tilt testing in healthy subjects. *Clin. Sci.*, **91**, 193–200.

Joyner, M. J. (1990). Sustained increases in sympathetic outflow during prolonged lower body negative pressure in humans. *J Appl. Physiol.* **68**, 1004–09.

Khurana, R.K., and Wu, R. (2006). The cold face test: A non-baroreflex mediated test of cardiac vagal function. *Clin. Autonom. Res.*, **16**, 202–07.

Koch, E. (1931). *Die reflektorische Selbssteuerung des Kreislaufes.* Steinkopff Verlag, Dresden.

Krediet, C. T. P., Van Dijk, N., Linzer, M., Van Lieshout, J. J., Wieling, W. (2002). Management of vasovagal syncope: controlling or aborting faints by the combination of legcrossing and muscle tensing. *Circulation*, **106**, 1684–89.

Levine, B. D., Pawelczyk, J. A., Ertl, A. C., *et al.* (2002). Human sympathetic neural and hemodynamic responses to tilt following spaceflight. *J. Physiol.* **538**(1), 331–40.

Lindqvist, A., Torffvit, O., Rittner, R., Agardh, C. D. and Pahlm, O. (1997). Artery blood pressure oscillation after active standing up: an indicator of sympathetic function in diabetic patients. *Clin. Physiol.*, **17**, 159–69.

Low, P. A. (1996). Clinical autonomic testing report of the therapeutics and technology assessment subcommittee of the American Academy of Neurology. *Neurology*, **46**, 873–80.

Low, P. A., Denq, J. C., Opfer-Gehrking, T. L., Dyck P. J., O'Brien P. C., Slezak J. M. (1997). Effect of age and gender on sudomotor and cardiovagal function and blood pressure response to tilt in normal subjects. *Muscle Nerve* **20**, 1561–68.

Low, P. A., Opfer-Gehrking, T. L., Textor, S. C., *et al.* (1995). Postural Tachycardia Syndrome. *Neurology*, **45**, S19–25.

Muenter Swift, N., Charkoudian, N., Dotson, R.M., Suarez, G.A., Low, P.A. (2005). Baroreflex control of muscle sympathetic nerve activity in postural orthostatic tachycardia syndrome. *Am. J Physiol. Heart Circ. Physiol.* **289**, H1226–33.

Ng, A. V., Callister, R., Johnson, D. G. and Seals, D. R. (1994). Sympathetic neural reactivity to stress does not increase with age in healthy humans. *Am. J Physiol.*, **267**, H344–53.

Omboni, S., Smit, A. A. J. Van, Lieshout, J. J., Settels, J. J., Langewouters, G. J., and Wieling, W. (2001). Mechanisms underlying the impairment in orthostic tolerance after nocturnal recumbancy in patients with autonomic failure. *Clin. Sci.*, **101**, 609–18.

Palmero, H. A., Caeiro, T.F., Iosa, D.J. and Bas, J. (1981). Baroreceptor reflex sensitivity index derived from Phase 4 of the Valsalva maneuver. *Hypertension*, **3**, II-134–7.

Piha, S. J. (1993). Age-related diminution of the cardiovascular autonomic responses: diagnostic problems in the elderly. *Clin. Physiol.*, **13**, 507–17.

Roach, D., Malik, P., Koshman, L. K. and Sheldon, R. (1999). Origins of Heart Rate Variability. Inducibility and Prevalence of a Discrete, Tachycardic Event. *Circulation*, **99**, 3279–85.

Sandroni, P., Benarroch, E. E. and Low, P. A. (1991). Pharmacologic dissection of components of the Valsalva maneuver in adrenergic failure. *J Appl. Physiol.*, **71**, 1563–67.

Smit, A. A. J., Timmers, H. J. L. M., Wieling, W., *et al.* (2002). Long-Term effects of carotid sinus denervation on arterial pressure in humans. *Circulation*, **105**,1329–35.

Smith, M. L., Beightol, L. A., Fritsch-Yelle, J. M., Ellenbogen, K. A., Porter, T. R. and Eckberg, D. L. (1996). Valsalva's maneuver revisited—A quantitative method yielding insights into human autonomic comtrol. *Am. J Physiol.*, **271**, 1240–49.

Sprangers, R. L. H., Wesseling, K. H., Imholz, A. L. T., Imholz, B. P. M. and Wieling, W. (1991). The initial blood pressure fall upon stand up and onset to exercise explained by changes in total peripheral resistance. *J Appl. Physiol.*, **70**, 523–30.

Stok, W. J., Baisch, F., Hillebrecht, A., Schulz, H., Meyer, M. and Karemaker, J. M. (1993). Noninvasive cardiac output measurement by arterial pulse analysis compared with inert gas rebreathing. *J Appl. Physiol.*, **74**, 2687–93.

Streeten, D. H. P. and Anderson, G. H. (1992). Delayed orthostatic tolerance. *Arch. Intern. Med.*, **152**, 1066–72.

Tanaka, H., Thulesius, O., Yamaguchi, H. and Mino, M. (1994). Circulatory responses in children with unexplained syncope evaluated by continuous non-invasive finger blood pressure monitoring. *Acta Paediatr*, **83**, 754–61.

Tanaka, H., Yamaguchi, H., Tamai, H., Mino, M., Konishi, K. and Thulesius, O. (1997). Haemodynamic changes during vasodepressor syncope in children and autonomic function. *Clin. Physiol.*, **17**, 121–33.

Taylor, J. A., Hand, G. A., Johnson, D. G. and Seals, D. R. (1992). Sympathoadrenal-circulatory regulation of arterial pressure during orthostatic stress in young and older men. *Am. J Physiol.*, **263**, R1147–55.

Ten Harkel, A. D. J., Van Lieshout, J. J., Van Lieshout, E. J. and Wieling, W. (1990). Assessment of cardiovascular reflexes: influence of posture and period of preceding rest. *J Appl. Physiol.*, **68**, 147–53.

Ten Harkel, A. D., van Lieshout, J. J., Karemaker, J. M. and Wieling, W. (1993). Differences in circulatory control in normal subjects who faint and who do not faint during orthostatic stress. *Clin. Auton. Res.* **3**, 117–24.

Timmers, H. J. L. M., Karemaker, J. M., Lenders J. W. M., and Wieling, W. (1999). Baroreflex failure following radiation therapy for nasopharyngeal carcinoma. *Clin. Autonom. Res.*, **9**, 317–24.

Timmers, H. J. L. M., Wieling, W., Karemaker, J. M., and Lenders J. W. M. (2003). Denervation of carotid baro- and chemoreceptors in humans. *J Physiol.*, **553**, 3–11.

Toska, K., and Walloe, L. (2002). Dynamic time course of hemodynamic responses after passive head-up tilt and tilt back to supine position. *J Appl. Physiol.*, **92**, 1671–76.

Van Dijk, J. G., Tjon-A-Tsien, A. M. L., Kamzoul, B. A., Kramer, C. G. S. and Lemkes, H. H. P. J. (1994). Effects of supine blood pressure on interpretation of standing up test in 500 patients with diabetes mellitus. *J Autonom. Nerv. System*, **47**, 23–31.

Van Heusden, K., Gisolf, J., Stok, W. J., Dijkstra, S., and Karemaker, J. M. (2006). Mathematical modelling of gravitational effects on the circulation: importance of the time course of venous pooling and blood volume changes in the lung. *Am. J Physiol. Heart Circ. Physiol.*, **291**, H2152–65

Van Lieshout, J. J., Wieling, W., Karemaker, J. M. and Eckberg, D. L. (1991a). The vasovagal response. *Clin. Sci.*, **81**, 575–86.

Van Lieshout, J. J., Wieling, W., Wesseling, K. H. and Karemaker, J. M. (1989). Pitfalls in the assessment of cardiovascular reflexes in patients with sympathetic failure but intact vagal control. *Clin. Sci.*, **76**, 523–28.

Van Lieshout, J. J., and Wesseling K. H. (2001). Continuous cardiac output by pulse contour analysis? *Br. J Anaesth.*, **86**, 467–69.

Van Lieshout, J. J., ten Harkel, A. D., van Leeuwen, A. M. and Wieling, W. (1991b) Contrasting effects of acute and chronic volume expansion on orthostatic blood pressure control in a patient with autonomic circulatory failure. *Neth. J. Med.* **39**, 72–83.

Veerman, D. P., Imholz, B. P. M., Wieling, W., Wesseling, K. H. and Van Montfrans, G. A. (1995). Circadian profile of systemic hemodynamics. *Hypertension*, **26**, 55–59.

Vogel, E. R., Sandroni, P., Low, P. A.(2005). Blood pressure recovery from Valsalva maneuver in patients with autonomic failure. *Neurology*, **65**, 1533–37.

Wesseling, K. H., Jansen, J. R. C., Settels, J. J. and Schreuder, J. J. (1993). Computation of aortic flow from pressure in humans using a nonlinear, three-element model. *J Appl. Physiol.*, **74**, 2566–73.

Weston, P. J., James, M. A., Panerai, R., McNally, P. G., Potter, J. F., Thurston, H. and Swales, J. D. (1996). Abnormal baroreceptor-cardiac reflex sensitivity is not detected by conventional tests of autonomic function in patients with insulin-dependent diabetes mellitus. *Clin. Sci.*, **91**, 59–64.

Wieling, W., Colman, N., Krediet, C. T., and Freeman, R. (2004). Nonpharmacological treatment of reflex syncope. *Clin. Autonom. Res.*, **Suppl 1**, 62–70.

Wieling, W., Krediet, C. P. T, and Wilde, A. A.. (2006). Flush after syncope: not always an arrhythmia. *J Cardiovasc. Electrophysiol.* **17**, 804–805.

Wieling, W., Krediet, C. T. P., Van Dijk, N., Linzer, M. and Tschakovsky, M. (2007). Initial orthostatic hypotension: review of a forgotten condition. *Clin. Sci.*, **112**, 157–65.

Wieling, W., Smit, A. A. J. and Karemaker, J. M. (1997). Autonomic dysfunction in diabetic patients. *Neuroscience Reseserch Communications*, **21**, 67–74.

Wieling, W., Ten Harkel, A. D. J., Van Lieshout, J. J. (1991). Spectrum of orthostatic disorders: classification based on an analysis of the short-term circulatory response upon standing. *Clin. Sci.*, **81**, 241–48.

Wieling, W., Van Brederode, J. F. M., De Rijk, L. G., Borst, C. and Dunning, A. J. (1982). Reflex control of heart rate in normal subjects in relation to age; a data base for cardiac vagal neuropathy. *Diabetologia*, **22**, 163–66.

Wieling, W., Van Lieshout, J. J., Ten Harkel, A. D. (1998). Dynamics of circulatory adjustments to head-up tilt and tilt back in healthy and sympathetically denervated subjects. *Clin. Sci.* **94**, 347–52.

Wieling, W., Veerman, D. P., Dambrink, J. H. A. and Imholz, B. P. M. (1992). Disparities in circulatory adjustment to standing between young and elderly subjects explained by pulse contour analysis. *Clin. Sci.*, **83**, 149–55.

Wieling, W. and Wesseling, K. H. (1993). Importance of reflexes in the circulatory adjustments to postural change. In: *Cardiovascular reflex control in health and disease.* (ed. R. Hainsworth and A.L. Mark), pp. 35–65. WB Saunders Company, London.

Ziegler, D., Laux, G., Dannehl, K., Spüler, M., Mühlen, H., Mayer, P. and Gries, F. A. (1992). Assessment of cardiovascular autonomic function: age-related normal ranges and reproducibility of spectral analysis, vector analysis, and standard tests of heart rate variation and blood pressure responses. *Diab. Med.*, **9**, 166–75.

CHAPTER 24

Computer analysis of blood pressure and heart rate variability in subjects with normal and abnormal autonomic cardiovascular control

G. Parati, M. Di Rienzo, P. Castiglioni and G. Mancia

Introduction

Autonomic cardiovascular regulation in humans is usually investigated by measurement of blood pressure and/or heart rate responses to laboratory stimuli, which interfere in different ways with the central and reflex control of circulation. Although providing important information on autonomic cardiovascular control in health and disease, this approach is affected by several limitations. Some of these can be overcome by analysis of spontaneous fluctuations in cardiovascular signals, which appear to offer, in several instances, a deeper insight into normal and deranged mechanisms of autonomic cardiovascular control. The aim of this chapter is to describe basic features of spontaneous blood pressure and heart rate variability, and to discuss the possible diagnostic value of the data obtained in patients with autonomic dysfunction.

Laboratory methods for the assessment of autonomic cardiovascular regulation

Typical examples of laboratory methods used to investigate autonomic cardiovascular control are:

- the assessment of the reflex changes in R-R interval induced by blood pressure changes that follow intravenous injection or infusion of vasopressor and vasodepressor drugs and thus the increase and decrease in the activity of arterial baroreceptors, respectively (Mancia and Mark 1983)

- the reflex blood pressure and heart rate responses to changes in carotid baroreceptor activity obtained through the application of either positive or negative pneumatic pressures within a neck-chamber device (Ludbrook et al. 1977)

- the cardiovascular responses to mental or physical stressors (Parati et al. 1988b)

- the reflex cardiovascular changes that accompany application of negative pneumatic pressure within a lower-body chamber and thus the unloading of volume cardiac receptors (Mancia et al. 1988); and

- the cardiovascular responses to changes in respiratory activity or posture (Chapters 22 and 23).

This enables important knowledge to be obtained on autonomic cardiovascular regulation, together with assessment of whether this regulation is altered in a number of diseases, including primary and secondary autonomic failure. There are limitations with this approach, however, because:

- some of the stimuli delivered to the cardiovascular system may interfere with the autonomic mechanisms under evaluation

- the assessment of neural cardiovascular control is usually in a stressful laboratory environment

- the reproducibility of the haemodynamic responses is low (Parati et al. 1985)

- responses are usually measured as average stimulus-induced stepwise changes, thus disregarding information on the dynamic features of neural cardiovascular modulation.

Spontaneous blood pressure and heart rate variability: historical and methodological aspects

Blood pressure, although continuously perturbed by external stimuli, invariably displays a tendency to return to a reference level. This suggests that attention has to be paid not only to the average blood pressure value but also to the fluctuations of blood pressure around its average level. These fluctuations appear therefore to be not an undesirable noise but phenomena that need to be understood in order to determine how cardiovascular regulation normally operates and whether a derangement has occurred (Parati et al. 1995c).

Important findings in this direction, were obtained in the 1960s with the introduction of a technique for continuous intra-arterial blood pressure monitoring in ambulant individuals, which provided unequivocal evidence that blood pressure fluctuates continuously and markedly in normal individuals (Mancia et al. 1983; Mancia et al. 1997b), that heart rate behaves in a similar fashion, and that the degree of these fluctuations vary in different clinical conditions. For example, when blood pressure variability was quantified by the standard deviation of its average 24-hour value, blood pressure fluctuations were greater in hypertensive subjects compared with normotensive subjects, and in the elderly compared with young individuals. Conversely, when similarly quantified as the standard deviation of their average value, heart rate fluctuations were reduced in diseases such as diabetes mellitus, congestive heart failure, myocardial infarction, and autonomic failure.

Statistical indexes

These findings suggested that also other indexes of variability, more complex than the 24-hour standard deviation, could be used to study specific aspects of the autonomic control (Task Force of the European Society of Cardiology and the North American Society of Pacing and Electrophysiology 1996). For instance, the overall standard deviation over the 24 hours can be split into a short-term component, obtained as the mean of the standard deviations of contiguous 5-minute segments covering the entire recording, and into a long-term component, computed as the standard deviation of the averages in all 5-minute segments of the entire recording. Indexes derived from the series of normal-to-normal (NN) heart intervals (that is, all intervals between adjacent QRS complexes resulting from sinus node depolarization) are: the square root of the mean squared differences of successive NN intervals (RMSSD); the number of interval differences of successive NN intervals greater than 50 ms (NN50); and the proportion derived by dividing NN50 by the total number of NN intervals (pNN50). RMSSD, NN50 and pNN50 mainly reflect the fastest components of heart rate variability, which are largely due to the vagal control.

Frequency domain analysis

Statistical indexes, although providing a comprehensive description of the signal dispersion around the mean, offer no information on the patterns that characterize the variability of the signal under study over a period of time (deBoer et al. 1987, Mancia et al. 1997b). This has led to the development of other methods for quantification of cardiovascular signal variability, among which spectral analysis has been used widely (Kamath and Fallen 1993). This approach allows the overall variance to be split into its frequency

components (Fig. 24.1). Attention has been largely focused on the spectral peaks that correspond to regular oscillations with frequency greater than 0.025 Hz (i.e. relatively fast oscillations with period shorter than 30 s), which appear to reflect sympathetic and parasympathetic modulation of the heart and vascular tone. This offers a method for quantifying the autonomic cardiovascular modulation either under controlled laboratory conditions, or during daily life activities when a segment of stationary signal can be identified.

The more popular spectral methods for the analysis of cardiovascular signals are the fast Fourier transform (FFT) and the autoregressive modelling (AR) methods (Parati et al. 1995c). The FFT spectrum is derived by transforming all signal data into the frequency domain, regardless of whether their frequency components appear as spectral peaks (reflecting regular oscillations) or as irregular fluctuations, which do not result in clearly identifiable peaks in the spectrum (Fig. 24.1). In contrast, with the AR approach the raw data are used to identify the best-fitting model from which the final spectrum, consisting of the 'direct current' (d.c.) component and a variable number of peaks, is derived.

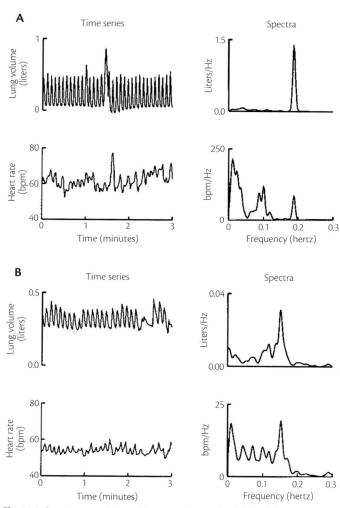

Fig. 24.1 Respiratory activity and heart rate time series (left) and their spectra (right) from one subject with 'peaky' **(A)** and one with 'broad-band' **(B)** heart rate spectrum. With permission from Parati G, Saul JP, Di Rienzo M, and Mancia G, Spectral analysis of blood pressure and heart rate variability in evaluating cardiovascular regulation. A critical appraisal, *Hypertension*, **25**(6):1276–1286. (1995c).

These methods yield similar results when FFT is used with some degree of smoothing and the AR method is applied with a sufficiently high model order (Fig. 24.2). Yet, specific differences between the FFT and AR algorithms make the choice of one of the two approaches preferable in some studies. For instances, the AR method provides spectral estimates with higher frequency resolution, making this method preferable for estimating relatively fast oscillations when only short segments of data are available. Moreover, it is easier to identify power and central frequency of spectral peaks with the AR approach. With the FFT method, attention can be also directed to the slower components of variability and the ability of this method to include the whole blood pressure or heart rate recording in a single spectrum has allowed assessment of spectral components over a broad range of frequencies, from the lowest to the highest (Fig. 24.3). This broad-band approach indicates that 24-hour blood pressure and heart rate spectra are characterized by a $1/f$ trend (i.e. that the power of fluctuations decreases hyperbolically with the frequency), which implies that the total blood pressure and heart rate power depends more on lower than on higher frequencies. The $1/f$ spectral trend also undergoes marked changes following surgical or pharmacological interventions interfering with autonomic cardiovascular influences (Fig. 24.4) and varies in different diseases and conditions, thus

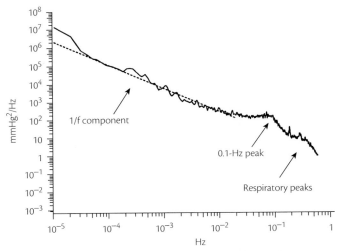

Fig. 24.3 Broad-band spectrum of systolic blood pressure from 24-hour ambulatory intra-arterial recording. Spectral components with frequencies ranging from 0.5 to 2×10^{-5} Hz (i.e. with period between 2 seconds and 12 hours) are considered. The dashed line is the $1/f$ trend modelling the spectrum in a very-low frequency region. From Di Rienzo et al. 1995, with permission from IOS Press.

offering an additional means by which to assess normal and deranged autonomic mechanisms (Fig. 24.5).

Regardless of the method, there are concerns about specificity and reproducibility of the information provided by spectral analysis. The specificity of the low-frequency (LF, around 0.1 Hz) and high-frequency (HF, the respiratory frequency) powers of heart rate as markers of sympathetic and vagal cardiac tone, respectively, is debated, particularly when signal variability is reduced (Daffonchio et al. 1991, Kingwell et al. 1995). Controversial is also the interpretation of LF powers of blood pressure as markers of sympathetic vasomotor tone. Discordant evidence also exists as to the reproducibility of these and other spectral indices (Freed et al. 1994, Parati et al. 1995c). Autonomic cardiovascular modulation is characterized by a high degree of non-linearity in the relationship between external inputs and cardiovascular response; this may impair the use of spectral analysis to assess autonomic cardiovascular control. This issue, exemplified for baroreflex control of R-R interval in Fig. 24.6 (Parati et al. 1995c), is largely ignored as the generally accepted, but incorrect, assumption is that cardiovascular responses are approximately linear. Additional methodological problems are:

- the need of signal stationarity for the correct interpretation of the spectra

- that there has to be an appropriate degree of spontaneous fluctuations to avoid the risk of having no input data in the frequency range of interest

- that frequency domain techniques may better quantify changes in autonomic cardiovascular modulation than mean neural autonomic activity.

As an example, Fig. 24.7 (Parati et al. 1995c) shows how a marked increase in parasympathetic cardiac drive was associated with a reduction, rather than an increase, in heart rate variability.

Time-frequency distributions

The interpretation of classic Fourier analysis is problematic when the signal is non-stationary and the frequency content changes

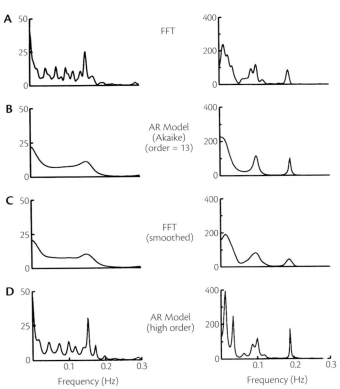

Fig. 24.2 Spectra of the same data as in Fig. 24.1, obtained by different analysis methods. **A:** by unsmoothed fast Fourier transform (FFT) algorithm; **B:** by an autoregressive (AR) model, the order of which (= 13) was determined by the Akaike criterium; **C:** by FFT algorithm smoothed with a Gaussian window (note that it appears very similar to the AR spectrum with model order = 13 in panel **B**; **D:** by an AR model with a high order (= 30) (note that it appears like the unsmoothed FFT spectrum in panel **A**. With permission from Parati G, Saul JP, Di Rienzo M, and Mancia G, Spectral analysis of blood pressure and heart rate variability in evaluating cardiovascular regulation. A critical appraisal, *Hypertension*, **25**(6):1276–1286. (1995c).

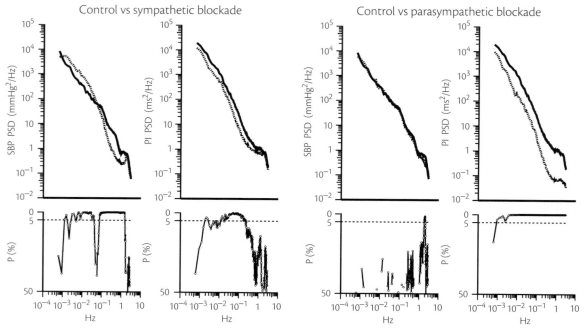

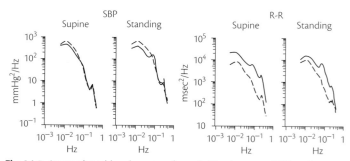

Fig. 24.4 Broad-band power spectral densities (PSD) of systolic blood pressure (SBP), and pulse interval (PI, the reciprocal of heart rate), from 90' recordings in control rats (N = 16, thick line), and in rats after (dashed lines) chemical sympathectomy (N = 13, left panels) or parasympathetic blockade (N = 10, right panels). Lower panels show the significance P of the differences between control and each autonomic blockade, for each spectral line (5% significance is shown by a dotted horizontal line); differences at a given frequency are significant if the corresponding P value falls above the dotted line. Note that the parasympathetic blockade decreases all the PI spectral components, affecting the '1/f' spectral trend and both the LF and HF bands (which in rats are defined between 0.15 Hz and 0.8 Hz and between 0.8 Hz and 2.5 Hz), while it does not practically affect the SBP spectrum; and that sympathetic blockade decreases the PI power mainly in the LF band, and has complex effects on the SBP spectrum, decreasing the power at low frequencies and increasing it at very-low frequencies. Adapted from Castiglioni et al. 1993, with permission (© 1993 IEEE).

over time. In fact, the power spectrum cannot indicate when specific spectral components occur, or how they change in intensity and frequency. Thus, when the signal is characterized by a time-varying spectrum, it is preferable to decompose the signal power by a joint function of time and frequency. The type of time-frequency distribution which better represents a non-stationary signal depends on how fast are the changes of the frequency content. When they are relatively slow, the standard method is the Spectrogram (i.e. the calculation of the Fourier spectrum over a short-time running window). Alternatively, spectral methods based on adaptive AR models are also used (Mainardi et al. 1997). In both these cases it is assumed that locally the signal is approximately stationary. Spectrograms allow to dynamically quantify the profiles of relatively slow-changing spectral powers over long-term periods, thus providing an indirect measure of changes in the autonomic cardiovascular regulation associated, for instance, to different daily life activities during the 24 hours (Fig. 24.8), or to different sleep stages during night. Spectrograms of blood pressure and heart rate series have been also used for the diagnosis of brain death, quantifying the dramatic changes in spectral powers following the loss of the baroreflex brainstem nuclei (Fig. 24.9). When the spectral characteristics change more rapidly, a higher resolution in time and frequency is needed, and methods like the Wigner–Ville distribution or the Choi–Williams distribution are preferred (Cohen 1989). The Wigner–Ville distribution represents the fraction of the power of a non-stationary signal at the frequency *f* and at the time instant *t*. This distribution satisfies the marginal conditions (i.e. the integral over *f* at time *t* gives the instantaneous power, and the integral over *t* at each frequency *f* gives the power spectrum). Thus the Wigner–Ville corresponds to the intuitive idea of

a time-varying spectrum. Unfortunately, interference terms due to undesired interactions between different signal components may be present, and this distribution may not be zero during time periods where the signal is absent or in frequency bands where spectral components are not expected. Interference terms can be in part suppressed by smoothing in time and frequency, or by computing the Choi–Williams distribution (a mathematical variant of the Wigner–Ville) at the cost, however, of a loss of time and frequency resolution.

Wigner–Ville and Choi–Williams distributions have been used to quantify fast spectral changes, like those associated with controlled breathing (Novak et al. 1993), postural changes (Chan et al. 2001), or autonomic tests (Pola et al. 1996).

Fig. 24.5 Average broad-band spectra of systolic blood pressure (SBP) and R–R interval for the supine and standing positions in adult (N = 28, continuous line) and very elderly (N = 20, dashed line) individuals. With permission from Parati G, Frattola A, Di Rienzo M, Castiglioni P, and Mancia G, Broadband spectral analysis of blood pressure and heart rate variability in very elderly subjects, *Hypertension*, **30**(4):803–808 (1997b).

Static (Steady state) gain

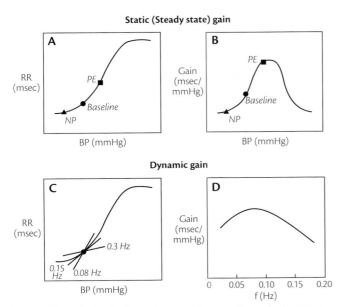

Dynamic gain

Fig. 24.6 Schematic drawing illustrating several features of baroreflex heart rate control. **A:** Sigmoid curve describing the relationship between changes in the input (blood pressure, BP) and reflex changes in the output (R–R interval [RR]). As BP increases, R-R interval increases, approximating a sigmoidal relationship with threshold and saturation values at either end of the curve. The gain of the heart rate baroflex is defined as the slope at any given point on the response curve. Administration of vasoactive agents (nitroprusside, NP, or phenylephrine, PE) induces changes in mean arterial pressure, moving the normal baroreflex operating point (baseline) into a different operating range. This may lead potentially to different gains. **B:** Plot of the baroreceptor heart rate gain as a function of BP. As the baroreflex stimulus-response curve is sigmoidal, maximal gain is observed in the linear portion of the curve, occurring at intermediate BP levels. At more extreme BP values, steady-state gain is diminished. **C:** Dynamic or beat-to-beat baroreflex gain as measured by the autoregressive moving average (ARMA), the spectral and the sequence techniques at the mean operating point in a may be higher or lower than the 'steady-state' gain, depending on the characteristics of the BP signal. **D:** In particular, the dynamic gain may depend on the frequency content of the input signal. In this example the maximal gain is found to occur around 0.10 Hz, with a decreased gain at both ends of the frequency range, suggesting band-pass characteristics. With permission from Parati G, Saul JP, Di Rienzo M, and Mancia G, Spectral analysis of blood pressure and heart rate variability in evaluating cardiovascular regulation. A critical appraisal, *Hypertension*, **25**(6):1276–1286, (1995c).

Non-linear and complexity based methods

In the past decade evidence has been provided that cardiovascular time series may display not only a random stochastic behaviour, quantifiable by spectral methods, but also complex nonlinear dynamics, including deterministic chaos (Poon and Merrill 1997). So far, several methods have been proposed for the analysis of cardiovascular complexity and nonlinear dynamics. Among these methods, the assessment of self-similarity has received particular attention. This is due to fact that fractal-like anatomical structures in the heart and vasculature, and complex interactions among vascular beds, suggest that the cardiovascular signals may be generated by fractal (i.e. self-similar) processes, which lack a characteristic scale of time. Self-similarity means that a plot of the signal versus time behaves like a fractal object, showing statistically similar characteristics after a proper scaling transformation of the horizontal and vertical axes. More precisely, a signal $x(t)$ is defined 'self affine' if it has the same statistical properties of the signal $a^{-H}x(at)$, for any a greater than zero, and it is defined 'self similar' if the previous relation holds for $H = 1$. Thus evaluating the

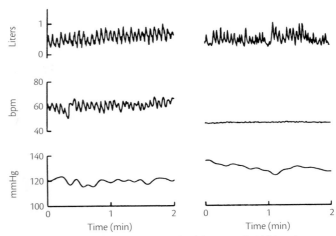

Fig. 24.7 Time series of respiratory volume (top), heart rate (middle), and mean blood pressure (bottom) in one subject under control conditions (left) and during intravenous infusion of phenylephrine (right), which determined an increase in blood pressure and a reflex bradycardia. Note that at the time of maximal reflex cardiac vagal stimulation under phenylephrine infusion, respiratory sinus arrhythmia disappeared. With permission from Parati G, Saul JP, Di Rienzo M, and Mancia G, Spectral analysis of blood pressure and heart rate variability in evaluating cardiovascular regulation. A critical appraisal, *Hypertension*, **25**(6):1276–1286, (1995c).

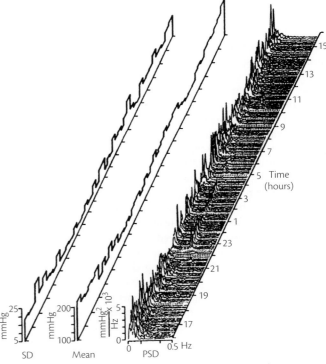

Fig. 24.8 Example of 24-hour spectrogram (PSD) of systolic blood pressure computed over consecutive segments of 256 beats. Mean and standard deviation (SD) in each half-hour is also shown. With permission from Parati G, Castiglioni P, Di Rienzo M, Omboni S, Pedotti A, and Mancia G, Sequential spectral analysis of 24-hour blood pressure and pulse interval in humans, *Hypertension*, **16**(4):414–421, (1990).

self-similarity of a time series implies the estimation of its scaling exponent H. The index H, which is also called Hurst exponent, is related to the slope of the spectrum plotted in a log-log scale (the 1/f spectral trend previously described in Fig. 24.4) and to the

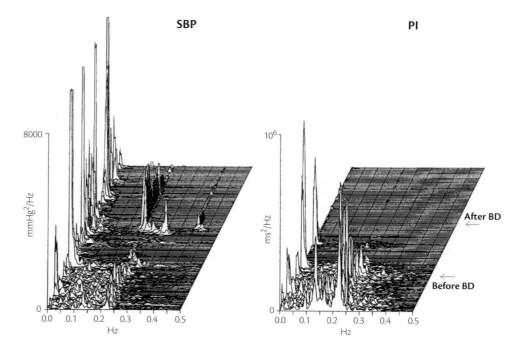

Fig. 24.9 Spectrogram of systolic blood pressure (SBP) and pulse interval (PI) in a patient before and after brain death (BD), showing the changes induced by the loss of brainstem nuclei related to the autonomic control of circulation. Reproduced from *J Neurol Neurosurg Psychiatry*, Conci F, Di Rienzo M, and Castiglioni P, **71**, 621–631, 2001 with permission from BMJ Publishing Group Ltd.

fractal dimension of the time-series (Schepers et al. 1992). It has been shown that *H* may be influenced by autonomic activations and may change with changes of posture (Fischer et al. 2003), with age, and during chronic heart failure (Goldberger et al. 2002). Comparing normal controls and paraplegic subjects with low-level and high-level spinal cord lesions, it has been shown that *H* can discriminate alterations in the autonomic control better than traditional spectral methods do (Merati et al. 2006). More recently, different authors have independently extended this approach in order to provide a more detailed description of the fractal structure of cardiovascular signals. These authors suggested to estimate a whole spectrum of scale exponents, *H(n)*, as a function of the time scale *n* (Castiglioni et al. 2009; Bojorges-Valdez et al. 2007). The estimation of a whole scaling pattern *H(n)* appears to provide a more accurate picture of the effects of autonomic activations. In particular, *H(n)* has been estimated to fully describe the effects on the fractal dynamics of heart rate and blood pressure of autonomic activations physiologically induced by changing posture or by physical exercise, or of long-term autonomic alterations, as those associated with ageing or with a prolonged exposure to high-altitude hypobaric hypoxia (Castiglioni et al. 2009; Di Rienzo et al. 2010).

Another popular 'complexity based' method used for the analysis of blood pressure and heart rate is a measure of signal 'regularity' called entropy (Richman and Moorman 2000). Signal entropy is mathematically defined as the negative logarithm of the probability that two data segments which are similar for a given number of samples remain similar also adding a new sample. In practice, if the signal is very regular and therefore predictable, then it is high the probability that two similar segments remain similar when their length increases: in this case, the high probability produces a low value of entropy. By contrast, if adding a new sample the quantity of generated new information is high, it is unlikely that similar segments remain similar when the length increases, and the resulting entropy is high. It has been shown that ageing and some specific diseases can decrease entropy increasing the overall regularity of cardiovascular signals (Pincus and Goldberger 1994; Voss et al. 1996).

The methods so far described are aimed at quantifying blood pressure and heart rate dynamics separately. However, since the autonomic control of circulation affects simultaneously blood pressure and heart rate, also methods aimed at assessing the coupling between these two signals are of paramount importance in the evaluation of the autonomic cardiovascular control from the spontaneous variability.

Coherence analysis

To understand how the coherence function $k(f)$ quantifies the coupling between two signals, it is useful to recall how the link between two datasets, let us say X and Y, is quantified by r^2, the square of the linear correlation coefficient. The r^2 coefficient is the ratio between the cross-variance of X and Y, σ^2_{XY}, and the product of the standard deviations, σ_{XX} and σ_{YY}: thus r^2 may range between 1 (perfect linear correlation between X and Y) and 0 (when X and Y are completely uncorrelated). Since the coupling between blood pressure and heart rate depends on the frequency of the oscillation, it is useful to calculate r^2 as a function of the frequency *f*. This is possible by evaluating the modulus of the squared coherence function, $|k^2(f)|$. The mathematical definition of $|k^2(f)|$ is formally the same as r^2, being the ratio between the cros-spectrum modulus, $|G^2_{XY}(f)|$, and the product of the square root of the two spectra, $G_{XX}(f)$ and $G_{YY}(f)$. Similarly to r^2, also $|k^2(f)|$ may range between 1 (perfect linear correlation between X and Y at frequency *f*) and 0 (completely uncorrelated signals at frequency *f*). Typically, the squared coherence between systolic blood pressure and R-R interval shows two peaks, at the respiratory frequency and around 0.1 Hz, indicating that respiratory oscillations and LF powers are linearly correlated (Fig. 24.10). By contrast, coherence is remarkably low at lower frequencies, suggesting that oscillations of longer periods are uncoupled, or nonlinearly coupled (de Boer et al. 1985a; de Boer et al. 1985b). It has been shown that the shape of the coherence function strongly depends on the baroreflex, being the coherence spectrum dramatically altered by the opening of the baroreflex loop (Di Rienzo et al. 1996).

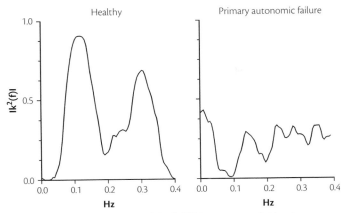

Fig. 24.10 Squared coherence modulus $|k(f)^2|$ between systolic blood pressure and R-R interval in a healthy subject and in a patient with primary autonomic failure at rest from 2-minutes recordings. Values close to zero in the very-low frequency band and two peaks, at 0.1 Hz and at the respiratory frequency, characterize coherence of healthy subjects.

Z-analysis

A different approach for evaluating the coupling between two time series is based on the assessment of the probability to observe specific couples values (Ducher et al. 1994). The method determines the association between two probabilistic events, X and Y, calculating a statistical link coefficient, Z(X,Y). The Z coefficient ranges between −1, when X and Y are mutually exclusive events, and +1, when X is included within Y, and is equal to 0 when X and Y are independent. Intermediate values between −1 and 0 quantify the partial exclusion of Y by X, while values between 0 and +1 quantify the partial dependence of Y on X. Z is estimated by counting the number of times that the X and Y events occurred, n_X and n_Y, and the number of times that they occurred simultaneously, n_{XY}, in a total of N observations. If $(n_{XY}/n_X - n_Y) > 0$, then Z(X,Y) = $(n_{XY}/n_X - n_Y /N) /(1 - n_Y /N)$, otherwise Z(X,Y) = $(n_{XY}/n_X - n_Y /N) /(n_Y /N)$. To quantify the statistical link between two cardiovascular series, let's say systolic blood pressure and heart rate, the X and Y events are the occurrence of systolic blood pressure and heart-rate values within specific amplitude intervals. By choosing Q intervals for systolic blood pressure and M for heart rate, Z(X,Y) is defined over a grid of QxM couples of (X,Y) events. An example is

shown in Fig. 24.11, where a matrix of Z(X, Y) estimates is obtained from 24-hour monitoring of systolic blood pressure and R-R interval data. Similar grids have been used to separately quantify the links between blood pressure and heart rate time series due to direct central controls from those due to the baroreflex control of blood pressure (Cerutti et al. 1995).

Models

An alternative way to assess the relationship between two or more cardiovascular signals is to identify mathematical models whose outputs fit the observed data. Some multivariate models are based on the evaluation of the gain and phase relationship between respiration and either blood pressure or heart rate changes by transfer function analysis (Saul et al. 1991), the relationship between specific components of blood pressure and pulse interval fluctuations in the time or frequency domain to obtain a dynamic assessment of 'spontaneous' baroreflex sensitivity, and the relationship between blood pressure and pulse interval in a closed-loop fashion by either autoregressive moving average techniques (ARMA models) (Patton et al. 1996) or, more simply, through Fourier-based transfer function techniques (Parati et al. 1995a). In a number of instances these approaches have also been employed in the analysis of longer-term blood pressure or heart rate recordings in ambulant subjects, which has allowed study of autonomic cardiovascular influences out of an artificial laboratory setting and under the conditions of daily life.

Insights into neural cardiovascular regulation from blood pressure and heart rate variability analysis

Between-subject differences in blood pressure or heart rate variability can be related to differences in the neural influences responsible for cardiovascular regulation. These factors include both central and reflex influences, with the arterial baroreflex playing a fundamental role (Mancia et al. 1997b). Examples of central influences are hypotension and bradycardia due to the transition from wakefulness to sleep (Mancia et al. 1983, Mancia et al. 1997b), the pressor and tachycardic responses to physical exercise, to unusual emotional stresses, such as gambling or medical visits, or even to common

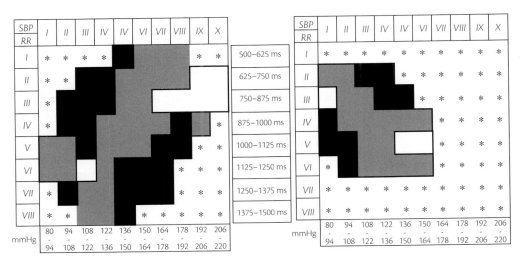

Fig. 24.11 Z values between systolic blood pressure (SBP) and R-R interval (RR) derived from 24-hour recordings in a young healthy subject (left) and in a patient with primary autonomic failure (right). First row and first column define 10 SBP classes from 80 mmHg (class I) to 220 mmHg (class X), and 8 RR classes, from 500 ms (class I) to 1500 ms (class VIII). Z has not been computed for cells with less than 10 couples of SBP and RR values, shown by *. Black, grey and white backgrounds indicate cells of exclusion (Z≤−0.2), independence (−0.2<Z<0.2) and bond (Z≥0.2) respectively.

situations, such as talking (Parati et al. 1992a). These cannot, however, be used easily to quantify whether autonomic cardiovascular influences are normal, reduced, or enhanced because the behavioural challenges are difficult to standardize between individuals.

Different conclusions can be reached for the arterial baroreflex, however. Evidence is available that this reflex exerts an important buffering action on spontaneous blood pressure variability in conscious animals (Cowley, Jr et al. 1973, Di Rienzo et al. 1991, Ramirez et al. 1985) with its inactivation by section of the carotid sinus and aortic nerves, followed by a striking increase in the magnitude of blood pressure fluctuations. Increased variability in blood pressure following anaesthesia or section of the carotid sinus nerves occurs in human subjects undergoing neck surgery (Mancia et al. 1997b). The buffering effect of the arterial baroreflex on blood pressure variability in humans is also demonstrated by the finding that baroreflex sensitivity is inversely related to the 24-hour blood pressure standard deviation (Mancia et al. 1986).

Baroreflex sensitivity also enhances heart rate variability. Sinoaortic denervated animals display reduced heart rate fluctuations (Ramirez et al. 1985). Between-subject differences in heart rate variability are related to differences in their baroreflex sensitivity as assessed by traditional methods (Mancia et al. 1986). Also, changes in baroreflex sensitivity over 24 hours are inversely related to changes in blood pressure variability but directly related to changes in heart rate variability. Thus the stabilizing effect of the baroreflex on blood pressure may be exerted through the ability of baroreceptors to modulate neural cardiac drive in a way that compensates, through changes in cardiac output, for the blood pressure changes. This is further supported by studies in the rat where an atropine-induced reduction in heart rate variability is accompanied by an increase in blood pressure variability (Mancia et al. 1997b). However, in other animals and in humans this is not the only stabilizing blood pressure mechanism, because blood pressure variability is not increased by reducing heart rate variability through atropine (Fig. 24.12) or by abolishing heart rate variations through cardiac pacing (Mancia et al. 1997b), indicating that the stabilizing effect on blood pressure is also accounted for by vascular influences of the baroreflex.

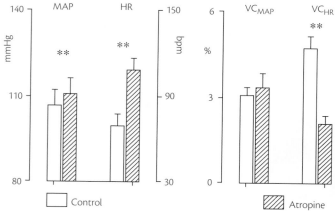

Fig. 24.12 Mean arterial pressure (MAP), heart rate (HR) and their coefficients of variation (VC, i.e. (SD/average value) x 100) in control condition and during intravenous bolus injection of atropine in 10 subjects (mean + SEM). Recordings before and under atropine administration were both carried out over 1 hour. With permission from Parati G, Pomidossi G, Casadei R et al, Role of heart rate variability in the production of blood pressure variability in man, *J Hypertens*, **5**(5):557–560.

Studies in animals and humans (Mancia et al. 1997b, Parati et al. 1995c, Saul et al. 1991) allowed the following additional conclusions. Heart rate fluctuations at frequencies above 0.15 Hz (i.e. in the HF or respiratory band) are due primarily to modulation of sinus node activity by changing vagal cardiac influences, associated with the respiratory cycle, although mechanical modulation of sinus rate by atrial stretch also seems to be involved to some degree (Bernardi et al. 1989). These fluctuations, therefore, can be considered as a relatively satisfactory parasympathetic marker. On the other hand, HF blood pressure fluctuations are caused by the mechanical effects of respiration and no direct vagal modulation of vasomotor tone is involved (Mancia et al. 1997b). Heart rate fluctuations between 0.025 and 0.15 Hz (i.e. in the LF band) are mediated by both sympathetic and parasympathetic influences and, to a minor degree, also by non-neural influences; thus, they cannot be regarded invariably as purely sympathetic markers (Mancia et al. 1997b). For this reason, in the attempt to obtain an index less influenced by the parasympathetic activity, often the LF power is expressed in normalized units after dividing it by the sum of the LF and HF powers, or the LF/HF powers ratio is computed as a measure of the sympathovagal balance (Task Force of the European Society of Cardiology and the North American Society of Pacing and Electrophysiology 1996). The specificity of these fluctuations as indices of sympathetic cardiac modulation can be enhanced in conditions where the sympathetic system is activated (Saul et al. 1990). When blood pressure is considered, spectral powers below 0.15 Hz predominantly reflect fluctuations in vasomotor tone and systemic vascular resistance. At frequencies between 0.04 and 0.025 Hz, this vascular modulation may depend on the renin–angiotensin system, endothelial factors, and local influences related to thermoregulation (Mancia et al. 1997b), although conclusive evidence is not available. In contrast, at frequencies between 0.04 and 0.15 Hz blood pressure fluctuations have repeatedly been interpreted as a marker of sympathetic vasomotor tone (Malliani et al. 1991, Mancia et al. 1993, Mancia et al. 1997b) although this is not invariably so in both animals and man when correlated with other measures of sympathetic activity (Parati et al. 1995c); furthermore, they persist even after substantial removal of sympathetic vascular influences by surgical and/or pharmacological sympathectomy (Mancia et al. 1993).

In conclusion, while spectral analysis of blood pressure and heart rate variability provides substantial information, the interpretation of blood pressure and heart rate spectra as quantitative markers of autonomic cardiovascular influences is still controversial, particularly when signals are recorded in the absence of standardized conditions and without simultaneous recording of respiratory activity (Bernardi et al. 1989, Mancia et al. 1993, Saul et al. 1991).

Broad-band spectral analysis of slower blood pressure and heart rate fluctuations (i.e. below 0.025 Hz) has raised interest because it offers further insights into cardiovascular control mechanisms (Parati et al. 1997b, Di Rienzo et al. 2009). Examples are the spectral alterations observed in rats or cats after baroreceptor denervation by sinoaortic nerve section (Cerutti et al. 1991, Di Rienzo et al. 1996, Parati et al. 1995a). Baroreceptor denervation changed all the spectral components of blood pressure and heart rate, indicating that the baroreflex is responsible for the genesis of a very broad band of spectral frequencies. After denervation in conscious cats, heart rate powers were reduced at all frequencies while blood pressure powers showed more complex changes (Fig. 24.13).

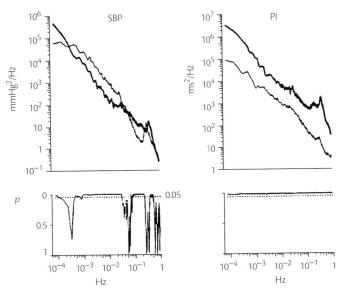

Fig. 24.13 Broad-band spectra of systolic blood pressure (SBP) and pulse interval (PI, reciprocal of heart rate), in intact condition (thick line) and 7 days after surgical baroreceptor deafferentation (thin line) in eight cats. Lower traces show the probability p of the null hypothesis for the differences between conditions. Power differences are statistically significant when p is above the 0.05 level, shown by a dotted line. With kind permission from Springer Science+Business Media: *Med Biol Eng Comput*, Effects of sino-aortic denervation on spectral characteristics of blood pressure and pulse interval variability: a wide-band approach, **34**, 1996, 133–141, Di Rienzo M, Castiglioni P, Parati G, Mancia G, and Pedotti A.

These included a reduction in the LF band and an increase of slower spectral components, which were responsible of changes in the 1/f spectral trend. However, the lowest frequencies analyzed (with period up to 1.5 hours) were significantly reduced after denervation. The arterial baroreflex thus plays different roles depending on the frequency of blood pressure fluctuations; it has a negligible effect on respiratory blood pressure fluctuations; it buffers fluctuations at frequencies lower than 0.1 Hz, and it exerts a pro-oscillatory role on fluctuations around 0.1 Hz and at very low frequencies. This paradoxical pro-oscillatory role of the baroreflex is in agreement with the hypothesis that the spectral peak observed at 0.1 Hz is at least in part due to resonance in the baroreflex loop, and that long term modulations of the baroreflex gain are responsible for very-low frequency blood pressure fluctuations (Wesseling and Settels 1985).

Dynamic assessment of baroreflex sensitivity through analysis of blood pressure and heart rate variability

Because the arterial baroreflex is involved in a major way in the modulation of both spontaneous blood pressure and heart rate variability, joint analysis of these phenomena has been proposed to obtain information on baroreflex function in daily life (Parati et al. 1992b). This can be achieved by different methods of analysis (Laude et al. 2004), both in the time and in the frequency domain, the more popular being 'the sequences technique' and 'the spectral method' (Parati et al. 2000, Parati 2005).

Sequences technique

By a time-domain analysis of continuous blood pressure recordings, this technique identifies sequences of three or more contiguous heart beats in which a progressive increase in systolic blood pressure (called SBP increasing ramp) is followed, with a delay of zero, one or two beats, by a progressive increase of heart interval quantified by the pulse interval PI (this pattern is called hypertension/bradycardia sequence: + PI/+ SBP); or in which an SBP decreasing ramp is similarly followed by progressive reduction in pulse interval (hypotension/tachycardia sequence: –PI/–SBP). As with the laboratory technique based on injection of vasoactive drugs, the slope of the regression line between changes in SBP and subsequent changes in PI is taken as a measure of the sensitivity of baroreflex control of the heart (Bertinieri et al. 1988, Di Rienzo et al. 1985, Parati et al. 1988a, Parati et al. 1995a). Other useful indexes for describing the baroreflex function provided by this method are the number of sequences occurring in a given time period, and the baroreflex effectiveness index (Di Rienzo et al. 2001), defined as the ratio between the number of sequences and the total number of SBP ramps. The effectiveness index is a measure of the capability of the baroreflex to activate 'buffering' heart rate sequences. Application of this technique in animals and humans has led to various conclusions. In cats, these sequences disappear following surgical baroreceptor denervation, demonstrating their dependence on the arterial baroreflex (Bertinieri et al. 1988, Parati et al. 1995a). In normotensive subjects the slope of the hundreds of sequences seen over 24 hours changes over time and displays a clear day–night difference, with a marked increase in slope (i.e. in baroreflex sensitivity) from wakefulness to sleep. In hypertensive patients (Fig. 24.14) (Parati et al. 1988a, Parati et al. 1994) and in the elderly (Fig. 24.15) (Parati et al. 1995b) number and slope of sequences are reduced, with an altered day–night modulation. Also patients suffering from obstructive sleep apnoea syndrome present an important impairment of the sensitivity of the 'spontaneous' cardiac baroreflex at night as assessed by the sequence technique (Parati et al. 1997a), which can be in part restored by acute or chronic treatment with continuous positive airway pressure (Bonsignore et al. 2002, Bonsignore et al. 2006).

Spectral method

Spontaneous baroreflex sensitivity can be assessed in the frequency domain by computing the modulus of the cross-spectrum (Robbe et al. 1987) or the squared ratio (Pagani et al. 1988, Parati et al. 1995a, Parati et al. 1992b) between blood pressure and heart rate powers in the frequency regions where these powers are coherent (Fig. 24.10) (e.g. around 0.1 Hz). As in the case for the sequence slope, this index of baroreflex sensitivity (often termed alpha coefficient), displays a clear 24-hour modulation in normotensive individuals, with a marked increase during night sleep, its magnitude and day–night modulation being markedly reduced in hypertensives and in the elderly with patterns similar to those seen with the sequence technique (Parati et al. 1995a, Parati et al. 1992b, Parati et al. 1995b). Blood pressure and heart rate powers are usually also coherent around the respiratory frequency (about 0.25 Hz), but at variance from the 0.1 Hz coherence, this coherence partially survives sinoaortic denervation (Di Rienzo et al. 1996). Thus, in certain conditions, the high-frequency coherence is accounted for substantially non-baroreceptor mechanisms, making questionable the use of the alpha coefficient in this band. As for the sequence

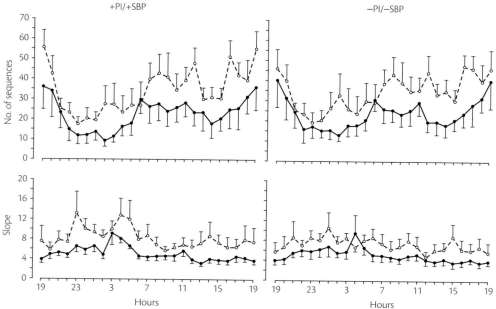

Fig. 24.14 Number and slope of +PI/+SBP and −PI/−SBP sequences during each hour of a 24-hour intra-arterial ambulatory blood pressure recording (means ± SE) for 10 normotensive (o) and 10 hypertensive (●) subjects. With permission from Parati G, Di Rienzo M, Bertinieri G et al, Evaluation of the baroreceptor-heart rate reflex by 24-hour intra-arterial blood pressure monitoring in humans, *Hypertension*, **12**(2):214–222.

technique, also the spectral method has been validated by data collected in animals before and after surgical baroreceptor denervation (Mancia et al. 1999).

Analysis of 'spontaneous' baroreflex sensitivity by time- and frequency-domain methods allows assessing the baroreflex control without interfering importantly with the subject's activities. This is possible because spontaneous methods do not require the use of relatively complex procedure for applying external perturbations to the cardiovascular system, like the stimuli provided by injections of vasoactive drugs or by pneumatic suctions with neck chambers.

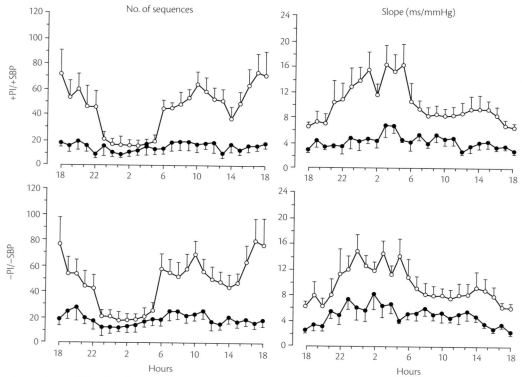

Fig. 24.15 Number and regression coefficients (or slope) of +PI/+SBP and −PI/−SBP sequences in a group of eight young and eight elderly (o) subjects: average ± SE for each hour of 24-hour ambulatory intra-arterial blood pressure recordings. Parati et al., *Am J Physiol*, (1995), Am Physiol Soc, used with permission.

This makes it feasible the assessment of the cardiac baroreflex even in extreme conditions, where classic laboratory methods are difficult to use or may interfere importantly with the measure. For instance, it has been possible to assess the baroreflex sensitivity even in astronauts during a 16-day space shuttle flight by applying the sequence technique and the spectral 'alpha' method (Di Rienzo et al. 2008). This allowed describing the process of adaptation of the cardiovascular control during prolonged exposure to microgravity.

Assessment of the spontaneous baroreflex sensitivity has been also shown to be able to identify early autonomic abnormalities.

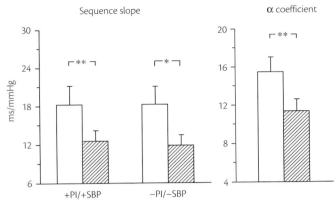

Fig. 24.17 Slope of sequences and alpha (α) coefficient in 10 subjects (average ± SE) during 1-hour non-smoking period (open bars) and during 1-hour period smoking one cigarette every 15 minutes (hatched bars): *p < 0.05; **p < 0.01. Mancia et al., *Am J Physiol* (1997), Am Physiol Soc, used with permission.

In diabetic patients with normal autonomic function, based on deep breathing and heart rate and blood pressure changes from lying to standing, the sequence and spectral methods showed evidences of reduced baroreflex modulation of the heart (Fig. 24.16) (Frattola et al. 1997). This was found also in smokers, where these methods identified baroreflex impairment (Fig. 24.17) which escaped recognition when traditional baroreflex evaluation by laboratory stimuli, such as the neck chamber, was employed (Mancia et al. 1997a).

More recently, in the diagnostic assessment of young individuals with syncopal episodes of suspected 'vasovagal' origin, assessment of spontaneous baroreflex sensitivity by the sequence method was found able to identify those with a positive response to tilt-table testing (Fig. 24.18) (Pitzalis et al. 2003). Moreover, spectral and sequence analysis of blood pressure and heart rate variability suggested that alterations of autonomic cardiac modulation and baroreflex sensitivity during sleep may play a role in determining the phenomenon of excessive daytime sleepiness (EDS), which may dramatically affect patients with sleep related breathing disorders. In fact, patients with EDS showed significantly lower nocturnal baroreflex sensitivity and low-to-high frequency powers ratio of heart rate compared to a control group without EDS but with

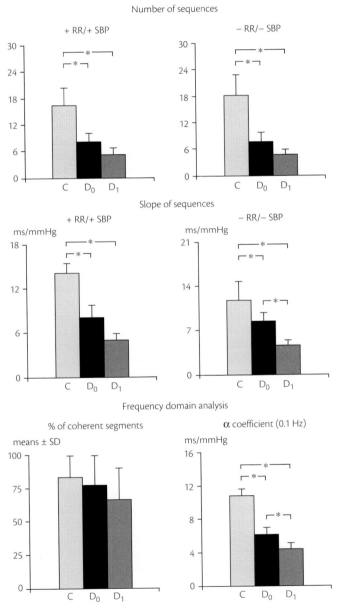

Fig. 24.16 Time-domain and frequency-domain estimates of the spontaneous baroreceptor–heart rate reflex in control subjects (C) and in diabetic patients with no or with autonomic dysfunction at classic laboratory tests (D_0 and D_1, respectively), *p < 0.05. With kind permission from Springer Science+Business Media: *Diabetologia*, Time and frequency domain estimates of spontaneous baroreflex sensitivity provide early detection of autonomic dysfunction in diabetes mellitus, **40**, 1997, 1470–1475, Frattola A, Parati G, Gamba P et al.

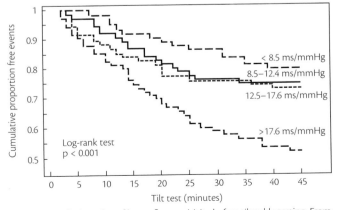

Fig. 24.18 Predictive value of baroreflex sensitivity before tilt-table testing. From Pitzalis et al. 2003, with permission.

the same degree of sleep related breathing disorders (Lombardi et al. 2008).

These observations support the conclusion that joint computer analysis of blood pressure and heart rate variability provide a sensitive method of quantifying the efficiency of the baroreceptor–heart rate reflex in conditions of daily life. This approach avoids the limited number of measurements, the artificial external stimuli, and the abnormal environmental conditions typical of laboratory methods, which may influence neural control of the circulation.

Intra-arterial and non-invasive blood pressure monitoring in the assessment of autonomic cardiovascular regulation in daily life

Analysis of blood pressure variability requires beat-to-beat time series of good quality, that previously have been possible only by intra-arterial recordings. The recent development of non-invasive devices based on finger plethysmography or on applanation tonometry has offered a non-invasive alternative to the intra-arterial approach (Chapter 22). In particular, devices for the continuous measurement of blood pressure at the finger artery are now widely used, and their use for the assessment of blood pressure and heart rate variability has been tested in a number of studies. Finger pressure recordings provide reliable blood pressure values not only at rest but also during laboratory tests inducing pressor or depressor responses (Parati et al. 1989). They also offers a reliable quantification of the standard deviation of mean arterial pressure (although less so for systolic blood pressure), thereby also being suitable for an estimate of overall blood pressure variability. Studies have also focused on whether this approach is adequate for more complex time- and frequency-domain analysis of blood pressure variability. In 14 untreated mild or moderate essential hypertensive patients, spectral analysis was performed on finger (Finapres, TNO) and intra-arterial blood pressure recordings simultaneously obtained for 30 minutes at rest while supine. The standard deviations of the average blood pressures of the whole recording period were slightly higher when assessed by finger than by intra-arterial recordings, the difference being statistically significant for systolic blood pressure only. Spectral powers of heart rate were similar for finger and intra-arterial recordings at all frequencies; this being the case also for spectral powers of mean and diastolic blood pressure. However, low and very-low frequency powers of systolic blood pressure were overestimated by finger blood pressure (Omboni et al. 1993). Despite this, the coherence between intra-arterial and finger blood pressures was greater than 0.5 at all frequencies, and was highest at approximately 0.1 Hz (Omboni et al. 1993). Based on these data, analysis of finger blood pressure recordings should, in general, be accepted in estimating blood pressure variability, even on the background of the reported overestimation of systolic blood pressure powers. This is because such an overestimation represents a nearly constant offset, which can be accounted for by use of correction factors, and the occurrence of a high coherence between finger blood pressure and intra-arterial powers in the frequency regions where the analysis of blood pressure variability is of clinical interest. When finger blood pressure recordings are used to assess spontaneous baroreflex sensitivity noninvasively through the sequence technique, the number of sequences and their slope can be superimposed onto the data derived from analysis of intra-arterial recordings (Omboni et al. 1993).

Similar analyses were carried out on non-invasive and intra-arterial 24-hour ambulatory blood pressure recordings obtained simultaneously through Portapres, the portable version of the Finapres device (Imholz et al. 1993), and Oxford recorder. Results confirmed the data obtained in resting conditions, i.e. that heart rate, diastolic and mean blood pressure powers are similar when derived from finger and intra-arterial signals, while systolic blood pressure powers, in particular very low frequency (with periods up to few hours) and LF powers, are overestimated by finger blood pressure recordings (Castiglioni et al. 1999). The overestimation appears to be relatively constant with time and does not prevent reliable tracking of changes in blood-pressure variability in different clinical and experimental conditions (Omboni et al. 1998).

Data from patients with autonomic failure

In patients with orthostatic hypotension due to primary or secondary autonomic failure the combined use of beat-to-beat finger blood pressure monitoring and computerized assessment of baroreflex sensitivity helps in the determination of the autonomic dysfunction (Omboni et al. 1995). This can be done in the laboratory, during controlled conditions and standardized activities, and over 24 hours, during the dynamic conditions of daily life, using the Portapres device (Chapter 22).

An example of the usefulness of finger blood pressure monitoring in evaluating autonomic failure is provided in Fig. 24.19, which shows beat-to-beat finger blood pressure and heart rate in a young normal subject and in a patient with orthostatic hypotension. The patient had a marked fall in blood pressure, with presyncopal symptoms, and a small heart rate change during standing, in contrast with the young subject who maintained his blood pressure with a normal heart rate increase during standing. Autonomic tests (Valsalva manoeuvre, forced respiratory sinus arrhythmia, and hand-grip exercise) confirmed that the patient had cardiac vagal and sympathetic vasomotor denervation. Use of spectral analysis and sequence analysis indicated minimal baroreflex sensitivity in the patient compared with the normal subject not only during supine rest (1 ms/mmHg vs 15 ms/mmHg) but also during active standing (1 ms/mmHg vs 14 ms/mmHg). The percentage of coherent segments between blood pressure and heart rate was similarly reduced in a striking fashion (i.e. it was 7% in supine and 4% in standing position in the patient, compared with 86% and 79% respectively in the normal subject). Sequence analysis showed very few sequences in the dysautonomic patient (none in supine position and two during standing) compared with the normal subject (3 in supine position and 19 during standing). Thus, although an alteration of neural cardiovascular control was evident using traditional tests, this was complemented by the computerized assessment of baroreflex sensitivity that quantified the striking impairment of 'spontaneous' reflex cardiac control.

The usefulness of computer analysis of blood pressure and heart rate variability in assessing autonomic dysfunction is further emphasized by the data obtained in 10 patients with orthostatic hypotension due to pure autonomic failure, in whom 24-hour beat-to-beat finger blood pressure recordings were performed by Portapres. As previously observed by intra-arterial recordings (Tulen et al. 1991), their 24-hour blood pressure variability is greater, while pulse interval variability is less, when compared with normal subjects (Omboni et al. 1996). Night sleep was associated

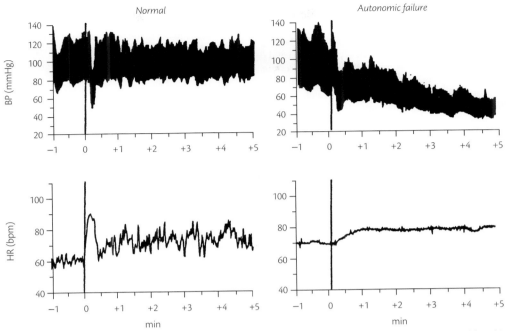

Fig. 24.19 Blood pressure (upper panels) and heart rate (lower panels) tracing obtained by Finapres in a young normal subject (left panels) and in a patient with autonomic failure (right panels) during supine rest and active standing.

either with a small blood pressure reduction, no blood pressure reduction, or in some instances even a reversal of the circadian blood pressure profile. In patients with autonomic failure, the sensitivity of the baroreflex, as assessed by the sequence slope and the alpha coefficient, was strikingly lower than in control subjects throughout the 24 hours, with a loss of its day–night modulation. The percentage of segments with a high coherence was smaller in patients with autonomic failure than in control subjects, indicating a reduced ability of the baroreflex to couple pulse interval with systolic blood pressure changes. An example of these alterations in a representative patient as compared to a healthy control, is provided (Fig. 24.20).

Conclusion

The data reviewed suggest that analysis of blood pressure and heart rate variability provides insight into cardiovascular regulation that cannot be obtained by traditional analysis of stepwise changes in mean blood pressure and heart rate, when induced by external stimuli. Furthermore, these approaches can be used in daily life and with techniques that allow non-invasive beat-to-beat blood pressure recordings. However, cautious interpretation of result is needed, especially for clinical application, and particularly when dealing with fluctuations in a single cardiovascular signal obtained in uncontrolled conditions, when no information on respiratory activity is available. Multivariate analysis techniques, such as the joint quantification of blood pressure and heart rate fluctuations, may provide more reliable information. Studies in autonomic failure suggest that these methods may be complementary to, and sometimes even more sensitive and specific than, traditional laboratory tests. However, the clinical impact of these methods in the diagnostic and prognostic evaluation of patients with autonomic failure needs to be tested in longitudinal controlled studies.

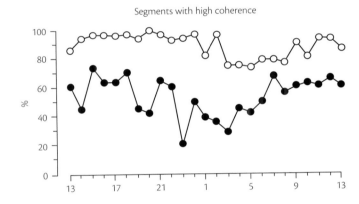

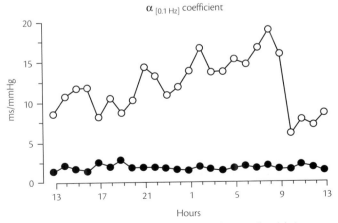

Fig. 24.20 Frequency of segments with high coherence (top panel) and their corresponding alpha (α) coefficient values (bottom panel) in one young healthy subject (o) and in one patient with pure autonomic failure (●). Data are shown as hourly average values. With kind permission from Springer Science+Business Media: *Clin Auton Res*, Blood pressure and heart rate variability in autonomic disorders: a critical review. **6**, 1996, 171–182, Omboni S, Parati G, Di Rienzo M, Wieling W, and Mancia G..

References

Bernardi, L., Keller, F., Sanders, M. *et al.* (1989). Respiratory sinus arrhythmia in the denervated human heart. *J Appl. Physiol.*, **67**, 1447–55.

Bertinieri, G., Di Rienzo, M., Cavallazzi, A., Ferrari, A. U., Pedotti, A., and Mancia, G. (1988). Evaluation of baroreceptor reflex by blood pressure monitoring in unanesthetized cats. *Am. J Physiol.*, **254**, H377–83.

Bojorges-Valdez, E. R., Echeverría, J. C., Valdés-Cristerna, R., and Peña, M. A. (2007). Scaling patterns of heart rate variability data. *Physiol. Meas.*, **28**, 721–30.

Bonsignore, M. R., Parati, G., Insalaco, G., *et al.* (2002). CPAP treatment improves baroreflex control of heart rate during sleep in severe OSAS. *Am. J Respir. Crit. Care Med.*, **166**, 279–86.

Bonsignore, M. R., Parati, G., Insalaco, G. *et al.* (2006). Baroreflex control of heart rate during sleep in severe obstructive sleep apnoea: effects of acute CPAP. *Eur. Respir. J.* **27**, 128–35.

Castiglioni, P., Daffonchio, A., Ferrari, A. U., Mancia, G., Pedotti, A., and Di Rienzo, M. (1993). Blood pressure and heart rate variability in conscious rats before and after autonomic blockade: evaluation by wide band spectral analysis. *Proc. Computers in Cardiology* 1993, 487–90.

Castiglioni P., Parati G., Omboni S. *et al.* (1999). Broad-band spectral analysis of 24 h continuous finger blood pressure: comparison with intra-arterial recordings. *Clin. Sci. (Lond)*, **97**, 129–39.

Castiglioni, P., Parati, G., Civijian, A., Quintin, L., and Di Rienzo, M. (2009). Local scale exponents of blood pressure and heart rate variability by detrended fluctuation analysis: effects of posture, exercise, and aging. *IEEE Trans. Biomed. Eng.*, **56**(3), 675–84.

Cerutti, C., Ducher, M., Lantelme, P., Gustin, M. P., and Paultre, C. (1995). Assessment of spontaneous baroreflex sensitivity in rats a new method using the concept of statistical dependence. *Am. J Physiol.*, **268**, R382–88.

Cerutti, C., Gustin, M. P., Paultre, C. Z. *et al.* (1991). Autonomic nervous system and cardiovascular variability in rats: a spectral analysis approach. *Am. J Physiol.*, **261**, H1292–99.

Chan, H. L., Huang, H. H., and Lin, J. L. (2001). Time-Frequency analysis of heart rate variability during transient segments. *Ann. Biomed. Eng.*, **29**, 983–96.

Cohen, L. (1989). Time-frequency distributions -a review. *Proceedings of the IEEE*, **77**, 941–81.

Conci, F., Di Rienzo, M., and Castiglioni P. (2001). Blood pressure and heart rate variability and baroreflex sensitivity before and after brain death. *J Neurol. Neurosurg. Psychiatry*, **71**, 621–31.

Cowley, A. W., Jr., Liard, J. F., and Guyton, A. C. (1973). Role of baroreceptor reflex in daily control of arterial blood pressure and other variables in dogs. *Circ. Res.*, **32**, 564–76.

Daffonchio, A., Franzelli, C., Di Rienzo, M. *et al.* (1991). Effect of sympathectomy on blood pressure variability in the conscious rat. *J Hypertens. Suppl.*, **9**, S70–71.

de Boer, R. W., Karemaker, J. M., and Strackee, J. (1985a). Relationships between short-term blood-pressure fluctuations and heart-rate variability in resting subjects. I: A spectral analysis approach. *Med. Biol. Eng. Comput.*, **23**, 352–58.

de Boer, R. W., Karemaker, J. M., and Strackee, J. (1985b). Relationships between short-term blood-pressure fluctuations and heart-rate variability in resting subjects. II: A simple model. *Med. Biol. Eng. Comput.*, **23**, 359–64.

de Boer, R. W., Karemaker, J. M., and Strackee, J. (1987). Hemodynamic fluctuations and baroreflex sensitivity in humans: a beat-to-beat model. *Am. J Physiol.*, **253**, H680–89.

Di Rienzo, M., Bertinieri, G., Mancia, G., and Pedotti, A. (1985). A new method for evaluating the baroreflex role by a joint pattern analysis of pulse interval and systolic blood pressure series. *Med. Biol. Eng. Comput.*, **23** Suppl.1, 313–14.

Di Rienzo, M., Castiglioni, P., Iellamo, F. *et al.* (2008). Dynamic adaptation of cardiac baroreflex sensitivity to prolonged exposure to microgravity: data from a 16-day spaceflight. *J Appl. Physiol.*, **105**, 1569–75.

Di Rienzo, M., Castiglioni, P., Parati, G., Mancia, G. and Pedotti, A. (1995). The wide-band spectral analysis: a new insight into long term modulation of blood pressure, heart rate and baroreflex sensitivity. In Di Rienzo, M., Mancia, G., Parati, G., Pedotti, A., and Zanchetti, A. ed. *Computer Analysis of Cardiovascular Signals*, pp. 67–74. IOS Press, Amsterdam.

Di Rienzo, M., Castiglioni, P., Parati, G., Mancia, G., and Pedotti, A. (1996). Effects of sino-aortic denervation on spectral characteristics of blood pressure and pulse interval variability: a wide-band approach. *Med. Biol. Eng. Comput.*, **34**, 133–41.

Di Rienzo, M., Castiglioni, P., Rizzo, F., *et al.* (2010). Linear and Fractal Heart Rate Dynamics during Sleep at High Altitude. *Methods Inf. Med.*, **49**: (in press)

Di Rienzo, M., Parati, G., Castiglioni, P. *et al.* (1991). Role of sinoaortic afferents in modulating BP and pulse-interval spectral characteristics in unanesthetized cats. *Am. J Physiol.*, **261**, H1811–H1818.

Di Rienzo, M., Parati, G., Castiglioni, P., Tordi, R., Mancia, G., and Pedotti, A. (2001). Baroreflex effectiveness index: an additional measure of baroreflex control of heart rate in daily life. *Am. J Physiol. Regul. Integr. Comp. Physiol.*, **280**, R744–51.

Di Rienzo, M., Parati, G., Radaelli, A., and Castiglioni, P. (2009) Baroreflex contribution to blood pressure and heart rate oscillations: time scales, time-variant characteristics and nonlinearities. *Philos. Transact. A. Math. Phys. Eng. Sci.*, **13**, 1301–18.

Ducher, M., Cerutti, C., Gustin, M. P., and Paultre, C. Z. (1994). Statistical relationships between systolic blood pressure and heart rate and their functional significance in conscious rats. *Med. Biol. Eng. Comput.*, **32**, 649–55.

Fischer, R., Akay, M., Castiglioni P., and Di Rienzo, M. (2003). Multi- and monofractal indices of short-term heart rate variability. *Med. Biol. Eng. Comput.*, **41**, 543–49.

Frattola, A., Parati, G., Gamba, P. *et al.* (1997). Time and frequency domain estimates of spontaneous baroreflex sensitivity provide early detection of autonomic dysfunction in diabetes mellitus. *Diabetologia*, **40**, 1470–75.

Freed, L. A., Stein, K. M., Gordon, M., Urban, M., and Kligfield, P. (1994). Reproducibility of power spectral measures of heart rate variability obtained from short-term sampling periods. *Am. J Cardiol.*, **74**, 972–73.

Goldberger, A. L., Amaral, L. A., Hausdorff, J. M., Ivanov, P. C., Peng, C. K., and Stanley, H. E. (2002). Fractal dynamics in physiology: alterations with disease and aging. *Proc. Natl. Acad. Sci. U S A*, **99** Suppl 1, 2466–72.

Imholz, B. P., Langewouters, G. J., van Montfrans, G. A. *et al.* (1993). Feasibility of ambulatory, continuous 24-hour finger arterial pressure recording. *Hypertension*, **21**, 65–73.

Kamath, M. V. and Fallen, E. L. (1993). Power spectral analysis of heart rate variability: a noninvasive signature of cardiac autonomic function. *Crit. Rev. Biomed. Eng.*, **21**, 245–311.

Kingwell, B. A.,Thompson, J. M., McPerson, G. A., Kaye, D. and Jennings, G. L. (1995). Comparison of heart rate spectral analysis with cardiac noradrenaline spillover and muscle sympathetic nerve activity in human subjects. In Di Rienzo, M., Mancia, G., Parati, G., Pedotti, A., and Zanchetti, A. ed. *Computer Analysis of Cardiovascular Signals*, pp. 167–76. IOS Press, Amsterdam.

Laude, D., Elghozi, J. L., Girard, A. *et al.* (2004) Comparison of various techniques used to estimate spontaneous baroreflex sensitivity (the EuroBaVar study). *Am. J Physiol. Regul. Integr. Comp. Physiol.*, **286**, R226–31

Lombardi, C., Parati, G., Cortelli, P. *et al.* (2008). Daytime sleepiness and neural cardiac modulation in sleep-related breathing disorders. *J Sleep Res.*, **17**, 263–70.

Ludbrook, J., Mancia, G., Ferrari, A., and Zanchetti, A. (1977). The variable-pressure neck-chamber method for studying the carotid baroreflex in man. *Clin. Sci. Mol. Med.*, **53**, 165–71.

Mainardi, L. T., Bianchi, A. M., Furlan, R. *et al.* (1997). Multivariate time-variant identification of cardiovascular variability signals: a beat-to-beat spectral parameter estimation in vasovagal syncope. *IEEE Trans. Biomed. Eng.*, **44**, 978–89.

Malliani, A., Pagani, M., Lombardi, F., and Cerutti, S. (1991). Cardiovascular neural regulation explored in the frequency domain. *Circulation*, **84**, 482–92.

Mancia, G., Ferrari, A., Gregorini, L. *et al.* (1983). Blood pressure and heart rate variabilities in normotensive and hypertensive human beings. *Circ. Res.*, **53**, 96–104.

Mancia, G., Grassi, G., and Giannattasio, C. (1988). Cardiopulmonary receptor reflex in hypertension. *Am. J Hypertens.*, **1**, 249–55.

Mancia, G., Grassi, G., Parati, G., and Daffonchio, A. (1993). Evaluating sympathetic activity in human hypertension. *J Hypertens. Suppl.*, **11**, S13–S19.

Mancia, G., Groppelli, A., Di Rienzo, M., Castiglioni P., and Parati, G. (1997a). Smoking impairs baroreflex sensitivity in humans. *Am. J Physiol.*, **273**, H1555–60.

Mancia, G. and Mark, A. L. (1983). Arterial baroreflexes in humans. In Shepherd, J. T. and Abbout, F. M. ed. *Handbook of physiology, Sect 2, The cardiovascular system IV, Peripheral circulation and organ blood flow*, pp. 755–94. American Physiological Society, Bethesda, MD.

Mancia, G., Parati, G., Castiglioni, P., and Di Rienzo, M. (1999). Effect of sinoaortic denervation on frequency-domain estimates of baroreflex sensitivity in conscious cats. *Am. J Physiol.*, **276**, H1987–93.

Mancia G.,Parati, G., Di Rienzo, M. and Zanchetti, A. (1997b). Blood pressure variability. In Zanchetti, A. and Mancia, G. ed. *Handbook of hypertension*, pp. 117–69. Elsevier Science, Amsterdam.

Mancia, G., Parati, G., Pomidossi, G., Casadei, R., Di Rienzo, M., and Zanchetti, A. (1986). Arterial baroreflexes and blood pressure and heart rate variabilities in humans. *Hypertension*, 8, 147–53.

Merati, G., Di Rienzo, M., Parati,G., Veicsteinas, A., and Castiglioni, P. (2006). Assessment of the autonomic control of heart rate variability in healthy and spinal-cord injured subjects: contribution of different complexity-based estimators. *IEEE Trans. Biomed. Eng.*, **53**(1), 43–52.

Novak, V., Novak, P., de Champlain, J., Le Blanc, AR., Martin, R., and Nadeau, R. (1993). Influence of respiration on heart rate and blood pressure fluctuations. *J Appl. Physiol.*, **74**, 617–26.

Omboni, S., Parati, G., Castiglioni, P. *et al.* (1998). Estimation of blood pressure variability from 24-hour ambulatory finger blood pressure. *Hypertension*, **32**, 52–58.

Omboni, S., Parati, G., Di Rienzo, M., Wieling, W., and Mancia, G. (1996). Blood pressure and heart rate variability in autonomic disorders: a critical review. *Clin. Auton. Res.*, **6**, 171–82.

Omboni, S., Parati, G., Frattola, A. *et al.* (1993). Spectral and sequence analysis of finger blood pressure variability. Comparison with analysis of intra-arterial recordings. *Hypertension*, **22**, 26–33.

Omboni, S., Smit, A. A., and Wieling, W. (1995). Twenty four hour continuous non-invasive finger blood pressure monitoring: a novel approach to the evaluation of treatment in patients with autonomic failure. *Br. Heart J*, **73**, 290–92.

Pagani, M., Somers, V., Furlan, R. *et al.* (1988). Changes in autonomic regulation induced by physical training in mild hypertension. *Hypertension*, **12**, 600–610.

Parati, G. (2005). Arterial baroreflex control of heart rate: determining factors and methods to assess its spontaneous modulation. *J Physiol.*, **565**, 706–707.

Parati, G., Casadei, R., Groppelli, A., Di Rienzo, M., and Mancia, G. (1989). Comparison of finger and intra-arterial blood pressure monitoring at rest and during laboratory testing. *Hypertension*, **13**, 647–55.

Parati, G., Castiglioni, P., Di Rienzo, M., Omboni, S., Pedotti, A., and Mancia, G. (1990). Sequential spectral analysis of 24-hour blood pressure and pulse interval in humans. *Hypertension*, **16**, 414–21.

Parati, G., Di Rienzo, M., Bertinieri, G. *et al.* (1988a). Evaluation of the baroreceptor-heart rate reflex by 24-hour intra-arterial blood pressure monitoring in humans. *Hypertension*, **12**, 214–22.

Parati, G., Di Rienzo, M., Bonsignore, M. R., *et al.* (1997a) Autonomic cardiac regulation in obstructive sleep apnea syndrome : evidence from spontaneous baroreflex analysis during sleep. *J Hypertens.*, **15**, 1621–26

Parati, G., Di Rienzo, M., Castiglioni, P., Frattola, A., Omboni, S., Pedotti, A. and Mancia, G. (1995a). Daily life baroreflex modulation: new perspectives from computer analysis of cardiovascular signals. In Di Rienzo, M., Mancia, G., Parati, G., Pedotti, A., and Zanchetti, A. ed. *Computer Analysis of Cardiovascular Signals*, pp. 209–218. IOS Press, Amsterdam.

Parati, G., Di Rienzo, M., and Mancia, G. (2000). How to measure baroreflex sensitivity: from the cardiovascular laboratory to daily life. *J Hypertens.*, **18**, 7–19.

Parati, G., Frattola, A., Di Rienzo, M., Castiglioni, P., and Mancia, G. (1997b). Broadband spectral analysis of blood pressure and heart rate variability in very elderly subjects. *Hypertension*, **30**, 803–808.

Parati, G., Frattola, A., Di Rienzo, M., Castiglioni, P., Pedotti, A., and Mancia, G. (1995b). Effects of aging on 24-h dynamic baroreceptor control of heart rate in ambulant subjects. *Am. J Physiol.*, **268**, H1606–H1612.

Parati, G., Mutti, E., Frattola, A., Castiglioni, P., Di Rienzo, M., and Mancia, G. (1994). Beta-adrenergic blocking treatment and 24-hour baroreflex sensitivity in essential hypertensive patients. *Hypertension*, **23**, 992–96.

Parati, G., Mutti, E., Omboni, S. and Mancia, G. (1992a). How to deal with blood pressure variability. In Brunner, H. and Waeber, B. ed. *Ambulatory blood pressure recording*, pp. 71–99. Raven Press, New York.

Parati, G., Omboni, S., Frattola, A., Di Rienzo, M. and Zanchetti, A. (1992b). Dynamic evaluation of the baroreflex in ambulant subjects. In Di Rienzo, M., Mancia, G., Parati, G., Pedotti, A., and Zanchetti, A. ed. *Blood Pressure and Heart rate Variability*, pp. 123–37. IOS Press, Amsterdam.

Parati, G., Pomidossi, G., Casadei, R. *et al.* (1987). Role of heart rate variability in the production of blood pressure variability in man. *J Hypertens.*, **5**, 557–60.

Parati, G., Pomidossi, G., Casadei, R. *et al.* (1988b). Comparison of the cardiovascular effects of different laboratory stressors and their relationship with blood pressure variability. *J Hypertens.*, **6**, 481–88.

Parati, G., Pomidossi, G., Ramirez, A., Cesana, B., and Mancia, G. (1985). Variability of the haemodynamic responses to laboratory tests employed in assessment of neural cardiovascular regulation in man. *Clin. Sci. (Lond)*, **69**, 533–40.

Parati, G., Saul, J. P., Di Rienzo, M., and Mancia, G. (1995c). Spectral analysis of blood pressure and heart rate variability in evaluating cardiovascular regulation. A critical appraisal. *Hypertension*, **25**, 1276–86.

Patton, D. J., Triedman, J. K., Perrott, M. H., Vidian, A. A., and Saul, J. P. (1996). Baroreflex gain: characterization using autoregressive moving average analysis. *Am. J Physiol.*, **270**, H1240–49.

Pincus, S. M. and Goldberger, A. L. (1994). Physiological time-series analysis: what does regularity quantify? *Am. J Physiol.*, **266**, H1643–56.

Pitzalis, M., Parati, G., Massari, F. *et al.* (2003). Enhanced reflex response to baroreceptor deactivation in subjects with tilt-induced syncope. *J Am. Coll. Cardiol.*, **41**, 1167–73.

Pola, S., Macerata, A., Emdin, M., and Marchesi, C. (1996). Estimation of the power spectral density in nonstationary cardiovascular time series: assessing the role of the time-frequency representations (TFR). *IEEE Trans. Biomed. Eng.*, **43**, 46–59.

Poon, C. S. and Merrill, C. K. (1997). Decrease of cardiac chaos in congestive heart failure. *Nature*, **389**, 492–95.

Ramirez, A. J., Bertinieri, G., Belli, L. *et al.* (1985). Reflex control of blood pressure and heart rate by arterial baroreceptors and by cardiopulmonary receptors in the unanaesthetized cat. *J Hypertens.*, **3**, 327–35.

Richman, J. S. and Moorman, J. R. (2000). Physiological time-series analysis using approximate entropy and sample entropy. *Am. J Physiol. Heart Circ. Physiol.*, **278**, H2039–49.

Robbe, H. W., Mulder, L. J., Ruddel, H., Langewitz, W. A., Veldman, J. B., and Mulder, G. (1987). Assessment of baroreceptor reflex sensitivity by means of spectral analysis. *Hypertension*, **10**, 538–43.

Saul, J. P., Berger, R. D., Albrecht, P., Stein, S. P., Chen, M. H., and Cohen, R. J. (1991). Transfer function analysis of the circulation: unique insights into cardiovascular regulation. *Am. J Physiol.*, **261**, H1231–45.

Saul, J. P., Rea, R. F., Eckberg, D. L., Berger, R. D., and Cohen, R. J. (1990). Heart rate and muscle sympathetic nerve variability during reflex changes of autonomic activity. *Am. J Physiol.*, **258**, H713–21.

Schepers, H. E., van Beek, J. H. G. M., and Bassingthwaighte, J. B. (1992). Four methods to estimate the fractal dimension from self-affine signals. *IEEE Eng. Med. Biol. Mag.*, **11**, 57–64.

Task Force of the European Society of Cardiology and the North American Society of Pacing and Electrophysiology (1996). Heart rate variability: standards of measurement, physiological interpretation and clinical use. *Circulation*, **93**, 1043–65.

Tulen, J. H., Man in 't Veld, A. J., van Steenis, H. G., and Mechelse, K. (1991). Sleep patterns and blood pressure variability in patients with pure autonomic failure. *Clin. Auton. Res.*, **1**, 309–315.

Voss, A., Kurths, J., Kleiner, H. J. *et al.* (1996). The application of methods of non-linear dynamics for the improved and predictive recognition of patients threatened by sudden cardiac death. *Cardiovasc. Res.*, **31**, 419–33.

Wesseling, K. H. and Settels, J. J. (1985). Baromodulation explains short-term blood pressure variability. In Orlebeke, T. F., Mulder, G., and van Dooechen, J. J. P. ed. *Psychophysiology of cardiovascular control. Models, methods and data*, pp. 69–97. Plenum, New York.

CHAPTER 25

Intraneural recordings of normal and abnormal sympathetic activity in humans

B. Gunnar Wallin

Introduction

Sympathetic neural activity is difficult to evaluate in humans. Clinically, it is common to record sympathetic effector activities, such as heart rate, blood flow, or sweat production, and use the results to draw conclusions about the neural drive. Unfortunately, such data are difficult to interpret because effector organs react slowly to variations in sympathetic neural drive and because they may respond also to hormonal, local chemical stimuli, and mechanical stimuli. In addition, resting sympathetic activity cannot be evaluated by these indirect approaches. By using percutaneous microelectrodes to record action potentials from postganglionic sympathetic axons in human peripheral nerves (microneurography), many of these difficulties can be circumvented. The method, which was developed in the 1960s (Vallbo et al. 2004), provides direct information about sympathetic impulse traffic to skin and muscle at rest and during manoeuvres (visceral sympathetic activity and parasympathetic activity are still inaccessible). The technique is not used for routine diagnostic work but is well suited for the study of physiology and pathophysiology.

This chapter will describe technique, methods of analysis, basal characteristics of normal sympathetic activity and examples of different types of applications. Microneurography has been used for a large number of studies both in healthy subjects and patients with various diseases. Most of these will not be described or referred to here but information may be found in other chapters dealing with the specific areas of interest. Early references may be found in Vallbo et al. (1979), Wallin (1994), Mitchell and Victor (1996), Mano (1999), Mano et al. (2006), Wallin and Charkoudian (2007).

Methods

Equipment

Most microneurographic recordings are made with monopolar tungsten microelectrodes with tip diameters of a few micrometres, but a concentric electrode type has also been described. Electrode impedances range from 50 kΩ to several MΩ; single fibre recordings require electrodes with smaller uninsulated tips and higher impedance. The neurogram is amplified (gain 50–100 k), first in a preamplifier/

impedance converter positioned close to the recording site, and then in a main amplifier. To quantify multiunit activity the raw neurogram is full wave rectified and passed through a leaky integrator with a time constant of 0.1 s. Audio-monitoring, after noise reduction achieved by filters and a discriminator, facilitates the location and recording of an optimal neural signal. For technical details, see Vallbo et al. (1979), Gandevia and Hales (1997).

Procedure

Human peripheral nerves contain several fascicles, each of which is surrounded by a connective tissue barrier, the perineurium (Fig. 25.1). Action potentials can be recorded only with the electrode tip inside a fascicle and then there is no cross-talk between fascicles.

The recording electrode is inserted manually through the skin into an underlying nerve and a reference electrode is placed subcutaneously, 1–2 cm away. Usually, recordings are made in large extremity nerves, such as the peroneal, tibial or median nerves, but small cutaneous nerves in arm, leg, face, and mouth have also been used. In most cases the neurogram contains impulses from many sympathetic fibres (multiunit activity), but impulse traffic in single fibres may be recorded (single unit activity) (Fig. 25.1). The microelectrode can also be used for evoking action potentials by intraneural electrical stimulation.

To find a sympathetic recording site, the following three-step procedure is usually followed.

1. The nerve is located by the paraesthesiae/muscle twitches evoked by electrical stimulation, first percutaneously and then through the microelectrode after it has been inserted through the skin. Some superficially located nerves may also be impaled without stimulation through the microelectrode.

2. When impaled by the electrode tip, a nerve fascicle is identified by the type of mechanoreceptor stimulus within the innervation zone that evokes afferent activity: muscle stretch and light touch evoke responses in muscle and skin fascicles, respectively.

3. Since sympathetic nerve fibres are not diffusely distributed in the fascicle but lie in bundles inside Schwann cells, repeated intrafascicular electrode adjustments may be necessary before a sympathetic recording site is found.

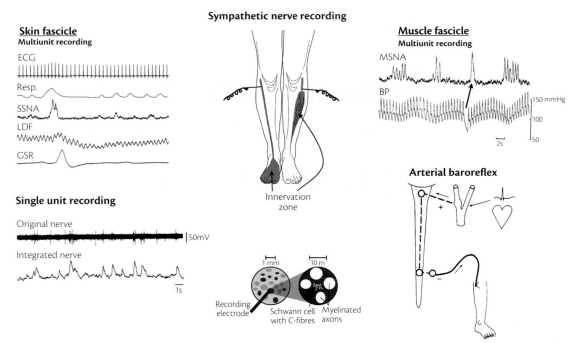

Fig. 25.1 Schematic figure of microneurographic recordings from the peroneal nerves at the fibular heads (*upper middle panel*). The nerve contains skin and muscle fascicles and in both types of fascicles sympathetic fibres are located in bundles inside Schwann cells and surrounded by myelinated axons (*lower middle panel*). *Upper left panel* shows integrated record from multiunit recording from right leg, records of laser Doppler flow (LDF) and skin resistance variations (GSR) from innervation zone in the foot (reduction of resistance upwards); note strong burst evoked by deep inspiration. *Lower left panel* shows original and integrated neural records from cutaneous single unit recording. Note that the single unit can be identified only in the original neurogram (bandpass 0.3—5 kHz). *Upper right panel* illustrates multiunit recording of spontaneous muscular sympathetic nerve activity (MSNA) and intra-arterial blood pressure (innervation zone in left anterior tibial muscle). Arrow indicates the latency in the arterial baroreflex arc which is indicated schematically in *lower right panel*. Note cardiac rhythmicity and inverse relationship between neurogram and blood pressure records. Upper right, lower left and lower middle panels reproduced with permission from Robertsson, Copyright Elsevier 1996.

The procedure involved in microneurography is challenging and requires training. Furthermore, once a good recording site is found, subjects have to be relaxed and lie still, otherwise the electrode may move and the site may be lost.

Identification of sympathetic activity

Sympathetic fibres discharge spontaneously in synchronized bursts, which occur in characteristic temporal patterns (Fig. 25.1). The patterns differ between skin and muscle nerve fascicles, as discussed below. In skin nerves there is a mixture of vasoconstrictor, sudomotor, and vasodilator fibres, all primarily involved in temperature regulation, and some of them probably also in metabolic regulation. Muscle nerves seem to contain only vasoconstrictor fibres, the main function of which is to participate in blood pressure regulation.

In muscle nerves the sympathetic bursts display a prominent cardiac rhythmicity and an inverse relationship to transient blood pressure variations. This is not the case in skin nerves, where the sympathetic bursts have more variable duration and shape. In addition, some manoeuvres lead to marked increases of skin sympathetic nerve activity (SSNA) but not of muscle sympathetic nerve activity (MSNA) (e.g. changes of ambient temperature or arousal), whereas others increase MSNA but not SSNA (e.g. a prolonged apnoea or a Valsalva manoeuvre). For evidence of the sympathetic nature of the recorded impulses, see Vallbo et al. (1979). The differences in temporal pattern and in responses to simple manoeuvres between the two types of activity are so typical that they allow reliable identification of SSNA and MSNA.

Discomfort

During the search for a sympathetic recording site, subjects may experience minor discomfort, but they feel nothing during the recording. In most cases there are no after-effects, but around 10% of the subjects may feel skin paraesthesia or mild muscle tenderness for a few days after the recording (Eckberg et al. 1989). The incidence of symptoms increases if the search procedure exceeds 45 minutes.

Analysis

For analysis, *multiunit* bursts of sympathetic impulses in the integrated neurogram are detected, either visually or by computer. These bursts represent the collective action potentials of several sympathetic fibres. In a given electrode site, the strength of multiunit activity is quantified as the number of bursts multiplied by their mean amplitude or area (total activity). Total activity is well suited to quantify effects of manoeuvres. However, since burst amplitude/area depends on the electrode site, only the number of bursts (burst incidence = bursts/100 heart beats, or burst frequency = bursts/minute) can be used for comparisons between individuals. Recently it has been shown that wavelet analysis can be used to extract single units from multiunit records (Steinback et al. 2010).

Single unit analysis requires fibre identification and evidence that all accepted action potentials ('spikes') derive from the same fibre.

◆ To aid fibre identification in skin nerves, a thermally induced bias of the activity during recordings should be used.

◆ In skin nerve recordings, spike triggered averaging of effector responses should be used, whenever possible.

◆ To make sure all impulses derive from one fibre, spike amplitude is important but, since signal-to-noise ratio often is low, considerable spike amplitude variability may be induced by the noise.

Therefore, identification of single unit activity solely by triggering based on a certain spike amplitude is inadequate: spikes may be missed, or alternatively spikes from other axons may be included. For this reason, computer assisted inspection of wave form and amplitude, combined with spike superimposition is necessary before a population of spikes can be attributed to a single axon (Fig. 25.2). Single unit activity can be quantified in terms of mean frequency, instantaneous frequency (based on the interval between two successive spikes) and spikes per cardiac interval. In general, mean frequencies are low and rarely exceed 1 Hz even when multiunit activity is intense.

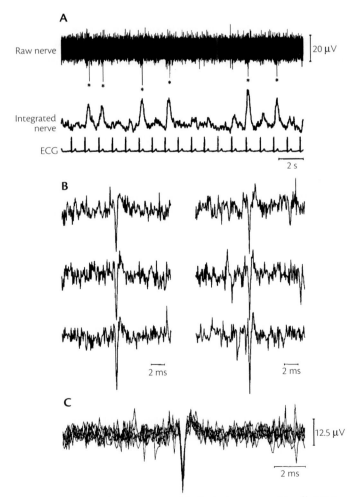

Fig. 25.2 Recording of spontaneous activity in single vasoconstrictor fibre in a muscle nerve fascicle in the peroneal nerve (**A**). Note, that when the fibre is active (*) there is only one spike per sympathetic burst. Rastered (**B**) and superimposed (**C**) action potentials provide evidence that the spikes originate from one axon. With permission from Macefield GV, Vallbo AB and Wallin BG (1994). The discharge behaviour of single vasoconstrictor motoneurones in human muscle nerves. *Journal of Physiology (Lond)*, **481**, 799–809, Wiley.

Areas of application of sympathetic microneurography

Sympathetic microneurography has proved to be of value in a number of research areas (Table 25.1). A disappointment is, however, that the technique has not become useful in clinical diagnostic work. In part this is because the differences between individuals in the strength of resting activity are so wide that it is impossible to define a normal upper limit, above which the strength is pathological.

Physiology

Functional organization of sympathetic outflow

Simultaneous recordings in different nerves—at one time sympathetic reactions were thought to occur in parallel in nerves to all tissues in the body. This view of a diffusely acting system led to the term 'sympathetic tone' to describe the strength of a presumed global level of sympathetic activity. This concept is no longer tenable: simultaneous double recordings reveal clear differences in the control of sympathetic traffic between of skin and muscle nerve sympathetic activity (Fig. 25.5A). On the other hand, *at rest* there is a remarkable parallelism between sympathetic traffic in two muscle nerves (and between some skin nerves) in arm and leg (Fig. 25.3). In spite of this, when comparing burst amplitude distributions between arm and leg neurograms, systematic differences have been found, suggesting that even within the same type of tissue there may be differences in neural control between different territories.

Simultaneous recordings of muscle sympathetic nerve activity (MSNA) and noradrenaline spillover suggest that at rest, there is a parallelism between the strengths of sympathetic outflows to muscle, kidney and the heart (Wallin et al. 1996).

Taken together the findings show that there are different populations of sympathetic neurons, which are controlled separately and, depending on the functional demand, may or may not be coactivated.

Recordings of MSNA during functional magnetic resonance imaging (fMRI) of the brain—Activation of a circumscribed population of nerve cells in the brain leads to a local increase of blood flow (a BOLD effect), which can be detected by fMRI. Recently Macefield and Hendersson (2010) managed to record MSNA during fMRI and correlated the occurrence of sympathetic bursts to BOLD effects in medulla oblongata. In the future, this ground-breaking combination of technologies is likely to provide marked advances in our understanding of central nervous sympathetic function.

Table 25.1 Sympathetic microneurography is useful for studying

◆ Physiology
· Functional organization
· Resting activity
· Reflex effects
· Mental stress
· Relationship of nerve traffic to neurotransmitter release
· Neuro-effector relationship
· Neuro-hormonal interaction
◆ Pathophysiology
◆ Clinical procedures

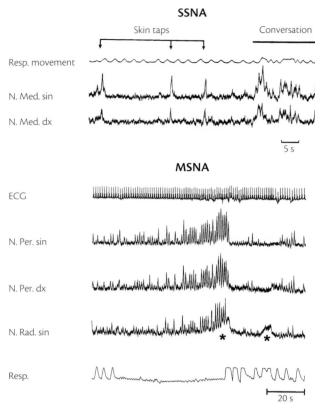

Fig. 25.3 Simultaneous recordings of skin sympathetic nerve activity (SSNA) (upper) in two and muscular sympathetic nerve activity (MSNA) (lower) in three extremity nerves. Note the similarity between the integrated records. In the recording of spontaneous MSNA from the left radial nerve the baseline deflections marked with * are due to artefacts evoked by muscle tension. SSNA records taken from Lidberg L and Wallin BG (1981), *Psychophysiology*, **18**, 268–70, with permission from Wiley.

Resting activity

Microneurography is the only technique that provides detailed information on the character and strength of *resting* sympathetic nerve traffic in humans. Such data can be obtained in both awake and asleep subjects

Multiunit activity—in SSNA burst durations may vary markedly, in addition baroreflex influence is weak or absent, which explains why cardiac rhythmicity is difficult to detect in the multiunit neurogram. In contrast, the strength of resting SSNA is very sensitive to both the thermal and the emotional state of the subject. At thermoneutrality there is little or no sympathetic traffic; in cold subjects there are spontaneously occurring sympathetic bursts dominated by vasoconstrictor impulses, and in warm relaxed subjects, who are sweating, the bursts contain predominantly sudomotor and vasodilator impulses. Emotional stress, on the other hand, coactivates vasoconstrictor and sudomotor impulses and may lead to cold sweat. The sensitivity to stress and temperature, as well as the difficulty of separating different types of impulses in the neurogram, make meaningful quantification of resting multiunit SSNA difficult to achieve.

MSNA is strongly modulated by the arterial baroreflex. This is evidenced by the fact that the bursts display cardiac rhythmicity and occur during transient reductions of blood pressure. Additionally, electrical stimulation of the carotid sinus nerves inhibits the bursts, and their cardiac rhythmicity is eliminated by temporary baroreceptor deafferentation (Fagius et al. 1985).

Baroreflex control within each cardiac cycle implies that bursts of activity correspond to arterial pressure reductions during diastole, and pauses between successive bursts are due to inhibition by increased pressure during systole. In the peroneal nerve the baroreflex latency between the R-wave of the ECG and the start of the neural inhibition is approximately 1.3 seconds.

The number of bursts at rest is similar in arm and leg nerves and remarkably constant in repeated recordings at intervals of up to 12 years (Fagius and Wallin 1993). There are, however, large differences between individuals; in healthy subjects the range may be from only a few to over 90 bursts/100 heart beats (Fig. 25.4). In studies of resting activity food intake is a potential confounder, since it causes an increase of MSNA, which lasts more than 90 minutes. Thus, there should be no food intake later than 2–3 hours before a microneurographic recording.

The parallelism between MSNA recorded from different nerves, together with the reproducibility over time, have two important consequences:

◆ A single recording in a randomly chosen muscle nerve fascicle provides representative information on the strength of the subject's sympathetic nerve activity, thereby making it possible to compare resting activity between individuals in health and disease.

◆ Repeated recordings provide longitudinal information of resting activity, allowing assessment of its changes with age, physical training, drug therapy or other interventions.

The differences between individuals in resting multiunit MSNA are probably of genetic origin (Wallin et al. 1993); no difference has been found between black and white subjects. Young women have fewer bursts than do young men. The number of bursts increases with age (about 1 burst/min/year) and body weight. Plasma insulin-like growth factor-1 (IGF-1) levels are inversely related to resting MSNA but the functional significance of this finding is unclear. Recently, resting burst incidence was also found to be related to respiratory rate: males with higher respiratory rates have more sympathetic bursts than subjects with lower respiratory rates (Narkiewicz et al. 2006). In young women, on the other hand, this relationship is not present (Wallin et al. 2010).

There is no relationship between resting levels of MSNA and arterial blood pressure in young men and women, which may seem surprising in view of the differences between individuals in vasoconstrictor activity. In young men, part of the explanation is that the effects of the sympathetic activity on blood pressure are counteracted by a reciprocal relationship between MSNA and cardiac output (Charkoudian et al. 2005). In addition, noradrenergic receptor sensitivity has been found to be down-regulated in proportion to the level of resting MSNA (Charkoudian et al. 2006). Interestingly, the inverse relationship between MSNA and cardiac output is not present in older men and young women (Hart et al. 2009a and 2009b).

During sleep the strength of resting multiunit sympathetic activity is successively reduced with increasing depth of non-rapid eye movement (REM) sleep but increases during REM sleep. Findings are qualitatively similar in skin and muscle nerves.

Single unit activity—at rest mean firing frequencies in single sympathetic neurons range around 0.5 Hz or less and are similar in muscle vasoconstrictor, skin vasoconstrictor, and sudomotor neurons (Macefield et al. 2002). Each neuron discharges very irregularly and usually only one spike per cardiac interval. Sometimes, however, two or more spikes may occur with short intervals, the consequence being that maximum instantaneous firing frequency

Muscle sympathetic nerve activity at rest

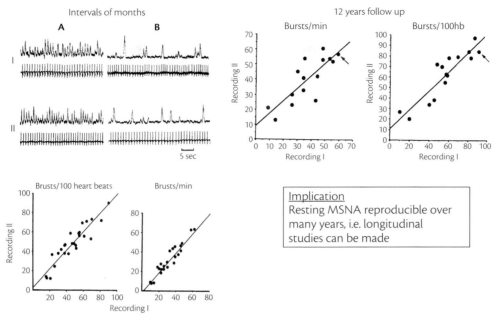

Fig. 25.4 Similarity of muscular sympathetic nerve activity (MSNA) in repeated recordings in the same subjects. Peroneal mean voltage neurograms and ECG from two subjects; interval between recordings 2 months **(A)** and 3 weeks **(B)**, respectively (upper left panel). Correlation between the number of sympathetic bursts in repeated recordings of MSNA in healthy subjects made with intervals of weeks or months (lower left diagrams) and mean interval of 12 years (right diagrams). Note the marked differences between individuals in number of bursts. Upper left panel taken with permission from Sundlöf G and Wallin BG (1977). The variability of muscle nerve sympathetic activity in resting recumbent man. *Journal of Physiology*, Wiley, and bottom left and top right diagrams with kind permission from Springer Science + Business Media: Clinical Autonomic Research, Long-term variability and reproducibility of resting human muscle nerve sympathetic activity at rest, as reassessed after a decade, **3**, 1993, 201–5, Fagius J and Wallin BG.

may exceed 100 Hz. Subjects with high multiunit burst incidence in MSNA at rest do not have higher mean firing frequencies in single fibres than subjects with low burst incidence. Thus, the higher burst incidence must be due to a higher number of active fibres.

Single unit firing frequencies are also low during manoeuvres. Thus, during a prolonged apnoea (which leads to a marked increase of multiunit MSNA) mean firing frequency in 9 single fibres increased to around 1 Hz. This was due to increases of both probability of firing and probability of multiple firing.

Reflex effects

A variety of manoeuvres or stimuli evoke sympathetic reflex effects (Table 25.2) and microneurographic recordings have been an important tool in many studies dealing with the underlying mechanisms.

For example, many studies have been published on the reflex effects associated with different forms of exercise (Mitchell and Victor 1996). Several receptor populations induce reflex effects both in SSNA and MSNA but the strength of the influence may vary markedly between the two sympathetic subdivisions. This is illustrated by the respective effects of arterial baroreflexes and thermoregulatory reflexes.

Arterial baroreflex effects—the arterial baroreflex has pronounced effects on MSNA but little or no effects on SSNA. Baroreflexes are essential for circulatory control during maintenance of upright postures. Recently, many studies have investigated how baroreflex mechanisms are influenced by prolonged bed rest, head-down tilt and microgravity; microneurographic recordings have even been performed in space (Ertl et al. 2002).

Different approaches have been devised to test the arterial baroreflex influence on MSNA in terms of set point and sensitivity, but no

systematic comparison has been made among methods within the same group of subjects. The most common method to determine baroreflex sensitivity is to use vasoactive drugs to alter blood pressure, and then record the associated changes of MSNA (Ebert and Cowley 1992). This technique aims at eliciting relatively large baroreflex responses by inducing rapid, transient changes in arterial pressure (approximately 15–20 mmHg); thus, by definition, it is not a steady state method. The drugs may also alter the distensibility of

Table 25.2 Effects of receptor stimulation and simple manoeuvres on sympathetic nerve traffic studied by microneurography

SSNA	MSNA
◆ Temperature receptors (in CNS and skin)	◆ Arterial baroreceptors
◆ Arousal and stress	◆ Cardiopulmonary stretch receptors
◆ Respiration	◆ Systemic chemoreceptors
◆ Cardiopulmonary receptors	◆ Intramuscular metaboreceptors
◆ Sleep	◆ Respiration/apnoea
◆ Pain	◆ Vestibular receptors
	◆ Laryngeal mechanoreceptors
	◆ Stretch receptors in the urinary bladder
	◆ Temperature receptors (in CNS and skin)
	◆ Arousal and stress
	◆ Sleep
	◆ Pain

the walls of the vessels harbouring the baroreceptors, which complicates the interpretation. The method has not been used to study differences between individuals in baroreflex control.

Another approach is to use records obtained at rest to construct so-called threshold variability diagrams, which relate the percentage occurrence of bursts to the diastolic blood pressure (Kienbaum et al. 2001). The resulting regression line provides reproducible information about the blood pressure thresholds for the occurrence of a sympathetic burst; a convenient measure is the pressure at which 50% of cardiac cycles have bursts. The slope of the regression represents the variability of the threshold in individual subjects and has also been found to provide a measure of baroreflex sensitivity (Hart et al. 2010).

Thermoregulatory reflexes—sympathetic nerve activity may be influenced by thermal stimulation of the skin and by activation of hypothalamic temperature receptors. The effects are differentiated: the influence on SSNA is marked whereas effects on MSNA are much less prominent. Body cooling selectively increases outflow of cutaneous vasoconstrictor impulses, and moderate warming decreases the strength of this activity to a minimum. When body warming leads to sweating, SSNA increases due to activation of sudomotor and vasodilator impulses (Vallbo et al. 1979, Sugenoya et al. 1998). Thus, changes of environmental temperature may activate, relatively selectively, either the vasoconstrictor or the sudomotor and vasodilator neural systems. However, since effects of body warming or cooling on body core temperature occur after long delays the interaction between reflex effects on SSNA evoked from the skin and from central temperature receptors is complex (Iwase et al. 2002). There is also evidence of a moderate MSNA increase during both body cooling (Fagius and Kay 1991) and body warming (Niimi et al. 1997) but the underlying mechanisms are unclear.

Mental stress

Microneurography is useful for studying effects induced by emotional reactions; however, since subjects often tense or move in such situations, there is a risk for changes of the electrode site or contamination of the neurogram by EMG or movement artefacts. The sympathetic reactions are complex.

In SSNA any sensory stimulus causing arousal regularly evokes a single burst (Fig. 25.5A) after a latency of 0.5–1.0 seconds, (depending on the recording site and the subject's height), whereas mental stress (e.g. induced by mental arithmetic) leads to a more long-lasting increase of sympathetic activity. The increase of activity is due to activation of both sudomotor and vasoconstrictor impulses. Arousal-induced changes of electrodermal activity (skin resistance or potential) have been used as indirect measures of the strength of SSNA. However, such data have to be interpreted with great caution; there is no simple quantitative relationship between the number of sudomotor impulses and the size of the electrodermal response (Kunimoto et al. 1992).

In awake subjects an arousal stimulus inhibits one or two sympathetic bursts in MSNA. The degree of inhibition varies among individuals but, in a given individual, it is reproducible over several months (Donadio et al. 2002). In contrast, during stage 2 sleep a K-complex (considered an indicator of arousal) is associated with the opposite response (i.e. a distinct burst in MSNA). An arousal stimulus after acute baroreceptor deafferentation also evokes a burst in MSNA (Fig. 25.5A).

A period of mental arithmetic causes some reduction of MSNA over the first 30–60 seconds, but then there is an increase, the strength of which is influenced by task difficulty and the subject's emotional state (Callister et al. 1992). Intravenous infusion of adrenaline has been found to increase MSNA and therefore, if the stress leads to an increased plasma adrenaline concentration, this may also contribute to the increase of sympathetic traffic.

The relationship between sympathetic activity and neurotransmitter release

Noradrenaline is the principal postganglionic sympathetic transmitter, and simultaneous recordings of sympathetic nerve traffic and measurements of regional *noradrenaline spillover* may provide valuable information. As an example, there is a significant correlation between resting levels of MSNA and noradrenaline spillover to jugular venous blood, suggesting a coupling between brainstem and peripheral noradrenergic activity (Lambert et al. 1997). In patients with cardiac failure both MSNA and jugular noradrenaline spillover are significantly increased (Lambert et al. 1995).

At one time the *concentration of noradrenaline* in forearm venous plasma was thought to be a useful index of sympathetic nerve traffic. However, since the plasma concentration depends on both spillover to the blood, and clearance from the blood, of noradrenaline, as well as on local blood flow, the noradrenaline concentration is not a reliable measure of sympathetic activity. This is illustrated by the finding that the increase of MSNA during systemic hypoxia is associated with unchanged plasma concentration of noradrenaline, which occurs because of an increased plasma clearance of noradrenaline.

Nevertheless, *at rest* there is a positive linear correlation between the sympathetic burst incidence of MSNA and the plasma concentration of noradrenaline. Similar correlations have also been found in pathological conditions, such as hypertension, cardiac failure, and liver cirrhosis with ascites. The relationships probably arise because:

- skeletal muscle is a large tissue, responsible for 10–20% of total spillover

- the contribution of noradrenaline from muscle is disproportionately high in forearm venous blood

- at rest, the strength of MSNA is correlated with noradrenaline spillover in other tissues, such as the heart and the kidney.

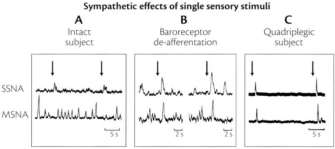

Sympathetic effects of single sensory stimuli

A	B	C
Intact subject	Baroreceptor de-afferentation	Quadriplegic subject

SSNA

MSNA

Fig. 25.5 Effects of single sensory stimuli (arrow) on skin sympathetic nerve activity (SSNA) and muscular sympathetic nerve activity (MSNA) recorded simultaneously in the two peroneal nerves in intact subject **(A)**, after temporary barorecptor deafferentation **(B)** and in quadriplegic subject with complete cervical spinal cord lesion **(C)**. Note that in the intact subject no burst is evoked in MSNA by the stimuli. Panels taken from Stjernberg et al. (1986) (A) and Fagius et al. (1985) (B), with permission. Data in C from Stjernberg et al. (1986).

Neuroeffector relationships

Microneurographic studies usually involve *recordings* of sympathetic nerve traffic. In skin nerves it is also possible, however, to use the electrode to *induce* nerve activity by intraneural electrical stimulation with the purpose of studying neuroeffector mechanisms. Corresponding studies have not been made in muscle nerves, since each stimulus would evoke a strong muscle contraction.

A drawback of this method is that the interpretation of the results is complicated by the fact that electrical stimuli activate several types of nerve fibres. This is most noticeable when studying vascular effector responses, which may result from stimulation of sympathetic efferents as well as afferent unmyelinated fibres. However, by using carefully graded stimuli and local anaesthetic blocks of the nerve, proximal and distal to the stimulation site, evidence was obtained for several vasodilating mechanisms in human skin (Blumberg and Wallin 1987).

Data on sudomotor function obtained with intraneural electrical stimulation is easier to interpret. By stimulating the median nerve at the wrist (after application of local anaesthetic block of the axillary plexus) the relationship between stimulation frequency and skin resistance changes in the hand (a measure of sweat production) was found to be highly nonlinear and depend on the strength of previous activity. The findings show that the amplitude of a skin resistance change is a useful index of sympathetic sudomotor activity only if background sympathetic activity remains constant (i.e. that thermal conditions are constant and that all forms of stress are minimized).

Intraneural electrical stimulation of the lateral femoral cutaneous nerve has been used to study a possible sympathetic contribution to metabolic control of subcutaneous adipose tissue in the thigh (Dodt et al. 1999). A difficulty with this approach is to exclude reflex effects: for practical reasons it is impossible to apply local anaesthetic block of the nerve proximal to the stimulation site.

Neurohormonal interaction

Several microneurographic studies have shown hormonal effects on sympathetic nerve traffic (Table 25.3).

Thus, *insulin*-induced effects on glucose metabolism have been found to be associated with marked changes of MSNA and SSNA. Insulin-induced hypoglycaemia or infusion of 2-deoxy-D-glucose increase MSNA and sudomotor activity in SSNA but inhibit vasoconstrictor activity in SSNA. The underlying mechanisms are complex, but central nervous effects may be important (Munzel et al. 1995).

A central nervous mechanism has been implied for the transient increase of MSNA following subcutaneous injections of *thyrotrophin*-releasing hormone. MSNA correlates negatively with serum levels of free *triiodothyronine and thyroxine*, and positively with thyroid-stimulating hormone. Taken together, the findings suggest an inverse relationship between thyroid function and sympathetic nerve activity.

Table 25.3 Hormonal effects on sympathetic nerve traffic studied by microneurography

Insulin	Cortisone
Glucagon	Growth hormone
Thyroid hormones	Oestrogen
Vasopressin	ANF

Pathophysiology

Theoretically, diseases may result in pathological sympathetic activity which could be detected by microneurography. Unfortunately, the differences between individuals in muscle sympathetic bursts at rest are so wide that it is impossible to define a normal upper limit of burst incidence, above which the strength of resting activity is pathological. Several obstacles prevent the definition of a normal range of resting activity also in skin nerves. In addition, it is sometimes impossible in normal subjects to find a recording site with acceptable signal-to-noise ratio (i.e. failure to find a sympathetic site in an individual patient has no diagnostic significance). The consequence of these limitations is that microneurography is useful mainly for comparing the strength of activity among groups of subjects, but not as a diagnostic tool in individual patients.

In *groups of patients* the technique has proved useful in detecting abnormalities of MSNA both at rest and in response to manoeuvres. Because of the wide differences between individuals it is important to use sufficiently large sample sizes when comparing MSNA between groups (preferably 15–20 subjects in each group). The strength of SSNA is more difficult to assess in a meaningful way: several types of impulses contribute to the multiunit neurogram and, in addition, the sensitivity to thermal changes and emotions make it difficult to define reproducible basal conditions.

Virtually all sympathetic tests aim at measuring reflex response(s) evoked by a more or less well-defined stimulus. It is important to realize that a pathological response can originate anywhere in a reflex arc (i.e. both in neural structures and in the effectors), and microneurography can identify only neural dysfunction proximal to the recording site. A *qualitative* abnormality may occur if a reflex effect is evoked from a stimulus that normally is ineffective, or if a normally excitatory response is turned into an inhibitory one (or vice versa). Such abnormalities are rare. One example is that in patients with spinal cord injury, a strong cutaneous stimulus below the lesion evokes a neural discharge in MSNA below the lesion (Fig. 25.5C) (Stjernberg et al. 1986). In contrast, similar stimuli to intact subjects inhibit one or two sympathetic discharges.

Quantitative abnormalities of multiunit activity have been demonstrated in many diseases (Table 25.4). For example, increases of MSNA at rest have been found in cardiac failure and in several forms of hypertension; an example of the opposite finding (a decrease of resting MSNA) has been reported in patients with recurrent syncope. The interpretation of abnormal findings is often difficult and depends on whether the involved reflexes are excitatory or inhibitory, and whether the lesion is located in the afferent or efferent limb of the reflex arc. Acute total inhibition of MSNA, reduction of blood pressure and syncope may occur as a consequence of a pathological increase of activity in the *afferent* limb of (the inhibitory) arterial baroreflex. Conversely, a lesion resulting in reduced afferent activity in the baroreflex arc is associated with increases of MSNA, heart rate and blood pressure.

In type 2 diabetes there is an increase of resting multiunit MSNA (Huggett et al. 2003). On the other hand, in diabetic polyneuropathy involving lesions in the *efferent* limb of the reflex arc may lead to impaired or failed conduction in postganglionic sympathetic fibres, the net result of which may be weak reflex responses and ultimately no detectable sympathetic activity. Thus, the interpretation of microneurographic findings in diabetic patients is difficult.

Table 25.4 Diseases studied with microneurography

Cardiovascular	Neurological
Cardiac arrhythmia	ALS
Cardiac failure	Cerebellar degeneration
Dopamine-beta-hydroxylase deficiency	Cervical spondylosis
Essential hypertension	Cluster headache
Hypersensitive carotid sinus syndrome	Generalized anhidrosis
Ischaemic heart disease/cardiac infarction	Hemianhidrosis
Orthostatic hypotension	Guillain-Barré syndrome
Renal hypertension	Migraine
Syncope	Palmo-plantar hyperhidrosis
Hormonal	Panic attacks
Hyperaldosteronism	Parkinsonism
Hypopituitary growth hormone deficiency	Polyneuropathy
Thyroid diseases	**Miscellaneous**
	Fabry´s disease
	Fibromyalgia
	Liver cirrhosis with ascites
	McArdle's disease
	Pre-eclampsia
	Trombangitis obliterans

Single fibre recordings have shown increases of firing frequencies both in lean and obese hypertensive patients (Lambert et al. 2007), and in patients with cardiac failure (Macefield et al. 1999, Murai et al. 2009).

Clinical procedures

With microneurography the main technical difficulties are related to the subject moving or tensing the extremity recorded from, or to interference from other types of equipment. In spite of this the method has proved to be robust enough to permit recordings during complex clinical procedures performed in less than optimal environments. For example, studies have been performed during induction and maintenance of general or regional anaesthesia, during operative procedures and during transluminal angioplasty.

Acknowledgement

Supported by the Swedish Medical Research Council, Grant No 12170

References

Blumberg, H. and Wallin, B. G. (1987). Direct evidence of neurally mediated vasodilatation in hairy skin of the human foot. *Journal of Physiology (Lond)*, **382**, 105–21.

Callister, R., Suwarno, N. O. and Seals, D. R. (1992). Sympathetic activity is influenced by task difficulty and stress perception during mental challenge in humans. *Journal of Physiology (Lond)*, **454**, 373–87.

Charkoudian, N., Joyner, M. J., Johnson, C. P., Eisenach, J. H., Dietz, N. M. and Wallin, B. G. (2005). Balance between cardiac output and sympathetic nerve activity in resting humans: role in arterial pressure regulation. *Journal of Physiology (Lond)*, **568**, 315–21.

Charkoudian, N., Joyner, M. J., Sokolnicki, L. A., Johnson, C. P., Eisenach, J. H., Dietz, N. M., Curry, T. B. and Wallin, B. G. (2006). Vascular adrenergic responsiveness is inversely related to tonic activity of sympathetic vasoconstrictor nerves in humans. *Journal of Physiology (Lond)*, **572**, 821–27.

Dodt, C., Lönnroth, P., Fehm, H. L. and Elam, M. (1999). Intraneural stimulation elicits an increase in subcutaneous interstitial glycerol levels in humans. *Journal of Physiology (Lond)*, **521**, 545–52.

Donadio, V., Karlsson, T., Elam, M. and Wallin, B. G. (2002). Interindividual differences in sympathetic and effector responses to arousal in humans. *Journal of Physiology (Lond)*, **544**, 293–302.

Ebert, T. J. and Cowley, A. W. (1992). Baroreflex modulation of sympathetic outflow during physiological increases of vasopressin in humans. *Am. J Physiol.*, **262**, H1372–8.

Eckberg, D. L., Wallin, B. G., Fagius, J., Lundberg, L. and Torebjörk, H. E. (1989). Prospective study of symptoms after human microneurography. *Acta Physiologica Scandinavica*, **137**, 567–9.

Ertl, A. C., Diedrich, A., Biaggioni, I. *et al.* (2002). Human muscle sympathetic nerve activity and plasma noradrenaline kinetics in space. *Journal of Physiology (Lond)*, **538**, 321–9.

Fagius, J., Wallin, B. G., Sundlöf, G., Nerhed, C. and Englesson, S. (1985). Sympathetic outflow in man after anaesthesia of glossopharyngeal and vagus nerves. *Brain*, **108**, 423–38.

Fagius, J. and Kay, R. (1991). Low ambient temperature increases baroreflex-governed sympathetic outflow to muscle vessels in humans. *Acta Physiologica Scandinavica*, **142**, 201–9.

Fagius, J. and Wallin, B. G. (1993). Long-term variability and reproducibility of resting human muscle nerve sympathetic activity at rest, as reassessed after a decade. *Clinical Autonomic Research*, **3**, 201–5.

Gandevia, S. C. and Hales, J. P. (1997). The methodology and scope of human microneurography. *Journal of Neuroscience Methods*, **74**, 123–36.

Hart, E. C., Charkoudian, N., Wallin, B. G., Curry, T. B., Eisenach, J. H. and Joyner, M. J. (2009a). Sex differences in neural-hemodynamic balance: implications for human blood pressure regulation. *Hypertension*, **53**, 571–6.

Hart, E. C., Joyner, M. J., Wallin, B. G., Johnson, C. P., Curry, T. B., Eisenach, J. H., and Charkoudian, N. (2009b). Age-related differences in sympathetic-hemodynamic balance in men. *Hypertension*, **54**, 127–33.

Hart, E. C., Joyner, M. J., Wallin, B. G., Karlsson, T., Curry, T. B. and Charkoudian, N. (2010). Baroreflex control of muscle sympathetic nerve activity: a nonpharmacological measure of baroreflex sensitivity. *Am. J. Physiol. (Heart and Circulatory Physiology)*, **298**, H816–22.

Huggett, R. J., Scott, E. M., Gilbey, S. G., Stoker, J. B., Mackintosh, A. F. and Mary, D. A. (2003). Impact of type 2 diabetes mellitus on sympathetic neural mechanisms in hypertension. *Circulation*, **108**, 3097–101.

Iwase, S., Cui, J., Wallin, B. G. and Mano, T. (2002). Effects of increased ambient temperature on skin sympathetic activity and core temperature in humans. *Neuroscience Letters*, **327**, 37–40.

Kienbaum, P., Karlsson, T., Sverrisdottir, Y. B., Elam, M. and Wallin, B. G. (2001). Two sites for modulation of human sympathetic activity by arterial baroreceptors? *Journal of Physiology (Lond)*, **531**, 861–9.

Kunimoto, M., Kirnö, K., Elam, M., Karlsson, T. and Wallin, B. G. (1992). Non-linearity of skin resistance response to intraneural electrical stimulation of sudomotor nerves. *Acta Physiologica Scandinavica*, **146**, 385–92.

Lambert, E., Straznicky, N., Schlaich, M. *et al.* (2007). Differing pattern of sympathoexcitation in normal-weight and obesity-related hypertension. *Hypertension*, **50**, 862–8.

Lambert, G. W., Kaye, D. M., Lefkovits, J. *et al.* (1995). Increased central nervous system monoamine neurotransmitter turnover and its association with sympathetic nervous activity in treated heart failure patients. *Circulation*, **92**, 1813–8.

Lambert, G. W., Thompson, J. M., Turner, A. G. *et al.* (1997). Cerebral noradrenaline spillover and its relation to muscle sympathetic nervous activity in healthy human subjects. *J Auton. Nerv. Syst.*, **64**, 57–64.

Lidberg, L. and Wallin, B. G. (1981). Sympathetic skin nerve discharges in relation to amplitude of skin resistance responses. *Psychophysiology*, **18**, 268–70.

Macefield, G. V., Vallbo, Å. B. and Wallin, B. G. (1994). The discharge behaviour of single vasoconstrictor motoneurones in human muscle nerves. *Journal of Physiology (Lond)*, **481**, 799–809.

Macefield, V. G., Rundqvist, B., Sverrisdottir, Y. B., Wallin, B. G. and Elam, M. (1999). Firing properties of single muscle vasoconstrictor neurons in the sympathoexcitation associated with congestive heart failure. *Circulation,* **100**, 1708–13.

Macefield, V. G., Elam, M. and Wallin, B. G. (2002). Firing properties of single postganglionic sympathetic neurones. *Autonomic Neuroscience*, **95**, 146–59.

Macefield, V. G. and Henderson, L. A. (2010). Real-time imaging of the medullary circuitry involved in the generation of spontaneous muscle sympathetic nerve activity in awake subjects. *Human Brain Mapping*, **31**, 539–49

Mano, T. (1999). Muscular and cutaneous sympathetic nerve activity. In: Appenzeller O, ed. *Handbook of Clinical Neurology* Vol 74: The Autonomic Nervous System. Part I. Normal function. Chapter 20, pp. 261–5. Elsevier BV.

Mano, T., Iwase, S., Toma, S. (2006). Microneurography as a tool in clinical neurophysiology to investigate peripheral neural traffic in humans. *Clinical Neurophysiology*, **117**, 2357–84.

Mitchell, J. H. and Victor, R. G. (1996). Neural control of the cardiovascular system: insights from muscle sympathetic nerve recordings in humans. *Medical Sciences in Sports and Exercise*, **28**, S60–9.

Munzel, M. S., Anderson, E. A., Johnson, A. K. and Mark, A. L. (1995). Mechanisms of insulin action of sympathetic nerve activity. *Clin. Exp. Hypertens.*, **17**, (1 and 2), 39–50.

Murai, H., Takamura, M., Maruyama, M. *et al.* (2009). Altered firing pattern of single-unit muscle sympathetic nerve activity during handgrip exercise in chronic heart failure. *Journal of Physiology (Lond)*, **587**, 2613–22.

Narkiewicz, K., van de Borne, P., Montano, N., Hering, D., Kara, T., Somers, V. K. (2006). Sympathetic neural outflow and chemoreflex sensitivity are related to spontaneous breathing rate in normal men. *Hypertension*, **47**, 51–5.

Niimi, Y., Matsukawa, T., Sugiyama, Y. *et al.* (1997). Effect of heat stress on muscle sympathetic nerve activity in humans. *J Auton. Nerv. Syst.*, **63**, 61–7.

Salmanpour, A., Brown, L. J., Shoemaker, J. K. (2008) Detection and classification of raw action potential patterns in human Muscle Sympathetic Nerve Activity. *Conf Proc IEEE Eng Med Biol Soc 2008*, 2928–31

Stjernberg, L., Blumberg, H. and Wallin, B. G. (1986). Sympathetic activity in man after spinal cord injury. Outflow to muscle below the lesion. *Brain*, **109**, 695–715.

Sugenoya, J., Iwase, S., Mano, T. *et al.* (1998). Vasodilator component in sympathetic nerve activity destined for the skin of the dorsal foot of mildly heated humans. *Journal of Physiology (Lond)*, **507**, 603–10.

Sundlöf, G. and Wallin, B. G. (1977). The variability of muscle nerve sympathetic activity in resting recumbent man. *Journal of Physiology (Lond)*, **272**, 383–97.

Vallbo, Å. B., Hagbarth, K-E., Torebjörk, H. E. and Wallin, B. G. (1979). Somatosensory, proprioceptive and sympathetic activity in human peripheral nerves. *Physiological Reviews*, **59**, 919–57.

Vallbo, Å. B., Hagbarth, K-E. and Wallin, B. G. (2004). Microneurography: how the technique developed and its role for the investigation of the sympathetic nervous system. *Journal of Applied Physiology*, **96**, 1262–9.

Wallin, B. G. (1994). Assessment of sympathetic mechanisms from recordings of postganglionic efferent nerve traffic. In: Hainsworth R, Mark AL, eds. *Cardiovascular reflex control in health and disease*, pp. 65–93. Saunders, London.

Wallin, B. G., Hart, E. C., Wehrwein, E. A., Charkoudian, N. and Joyner, M. J. (2010). Relationship between breathing and cardiovascular function at rest: Sex related differences. *Acta Physiologica* E-publ 25 March.

Wallin, B. G., Kunimoto, M. and Sellgren, J. (1993). Possible genetic influence on the strength of human muscle nerve sympathetic activity at rest. *Hypertension*, **22**, 282–4.

Wallin, B. G., Thompson, J. M., Jennings, G. L. and Esler, M. D. (1996). Renal noradrenaline spillover correlates with muscle sympathetic activity in humans. *Journal of Physiology (Lond)*, **491**, 881–7.

Wallin, B. G. and Charkoudian, N. (2007) Sympathetic neural control of integrated cardiovascular function: insights from measurement of human sympathetic nerve activity. *Muscle & Nerve*, **36**, 595–614.

CHAPTER 26

Biochemical investigation of autonomic function— measurement of catecholamines and metabolites, and the use of spillover and allied techniques to determine regional sympathetic activation

Murray Esler and Gavin Lambert

Biochemical investigation of autonomic function: 'False starts'

Efforts to chemically quantify sympathetic nervous system activity have a long history (Esler et al. 1990). Over the past 50 years a truly extraordinary range of chemical measurements relating to individual aspects of the biology of sympathetic nerves have been utilized as measures of sympathetic nervous system activity in clinical and experimental studies. Here is a list of these diverse (and in many cases, failed) indices:

◆ tissue activity of enzymes involved in noradrenaline synthesis, in particular tyrosine hydroxylase DeQuattro et al. 1975), the rate-limiting enzyme, which provides a valid marker for noradrenaline synthesis rate

◆ plasma concentration of another enzyme, dopamine-beta-hydroxylase (DBH), involved in noradrenaline synthesis (Weinshilboum et al. 1973)

◆ concentration of noradrenaline in tissues, plasma (Engelman et al. 1968), and in blood platelets after uptake from plasma (Zweifler and Julius 1982) and excretion in urine (von Euler et al. 1954)

◆ concentration of metabolites of noradrenaline in urine and plasma (Eisenhofer et al. 1988)

◆ plasma concentration of the sympathetic cotransmitter, neuropeptide Y (NPY) (Morris et al. 1986)

◆ plasma concentration of other sympathetic vesicle constituents, including chromogranin A (O'Connor and Bernstein 1984).

It is clear, from the use of so many neurochemical indicators of sympathetic nervous activity, that none is entirely satisfactory, while some are quite misleading. The tissue content of noradrenaline provides little direct information about rates of synthesis and release of the neurotransmitter. In heart failure, for example, sympathetic nerve firing rates and noradrenaline release are elevated (Hasking et al. 1986, Grassi et al. 1998), but the concentration of noradrenaline in the heart is reduced (Chidsey and Braunwald 1966). The generation of noradrenaline metabolites is not always closely related to rates of sympathetic nerve firing and transmitter release. Most dihydroxyphenylglycol (DHPG) is derived from the intraneuronal metabolism of noradrenaline leaking from vesicles, and not from released transmitter (Eisenhofer et al. 1996).

The concentration in plasma of DBH was proposed, almost unaccountably given that it is not the rate- limiting enzyme in noradrenaline synthesis, as an index of sympathetic nervous activity but has been discredited. In addition to the flaw in logic, it is now known that the enzyme plasma concentration is determined primarily by genetic factors unrelated to nerve firing rates. More reliable as a measure of sympathetic activity is the concentration in plasma of the sympathetic vesicle constituent, chromogranin A (O'Connor and Bernstein 1984), which is released to plasma during discharge of vesicles in neurotransmission. Given that the sympathetic cotransmitter NPY, unlike noradrenaline, is not subject to neuronal reuptake after release, it was thought that the plasma concentration of NPY might provide a better index of overall sympathetic nervous activity than noradrenaline. This is not the case, however, as most NPY is derived from a single site, the sympathetic nerves of the gut, entering systemic venous plasma via the hepatic vein (Morris et al. 1997).

Plasma noradrenaline, and noradrenaline precursors and metabolites

Following von Euler's characterization of the sympathetic neurotransmitter as noradrenaline (von Euler 1946), and the demonstration that the washout of noradrenaline from an organ was proportional to the rate of electrical stimulation of its sympathetic nerves (Brown and Gillespie 1957), the potential value of noradrenaline release rate measurements as an index of sympathetic nerve firing was seen early. This relationship provided the foundation for the use of noradrenaline measurements, initially in urine, as an index of sympathetic nervous system activity in humans. In a large-scale clinical study involving 500 patients with hypertension, von Euler and colleagues (von Euler et al. 1954) were the first to apply neurochemical measurements of transmitter release, based on urinary noradrenaline excretion rates, in clinical research. Nothing comparable is possible for the parasympathetic nervous system, because the half-time of the parasympathetic neurotransmitter, acetylcholine, in plasma is so short, due to the speedy action of acetylcholine esterases.

Noradrenaline plasma measurements

The development of a sensitive and specific isotope-derivative method for the assay of noradrenaline in plasma, by Engelman and colleagues (Engelman et al. 1968), represented an important technical refinement of the biochemical approach. Prior to this, purported plasma noradrenaline assays were grossly nonspecific and inaccurate, registering values up to 10-fold higher than really was the case. Development of the methodology was quickly followed by its enthusiastic application to clinical research. Plasma noradrenaline measurements do provide a useful guide to sympathetic nervous system function (Robertson et al. 1979), but have substantial limitations.

Perhaps the principal one is that this, and in fact any other global index of sympathetic nervous function, provides no information on the regional patterning of sympathetic nervous outflow. This runs contrary to the functional organization of the sympathetic nervous system, which shows regional differentiation (Esler et al. 1990). A second deficiency of plasma noradrenaline measurements when used as an index of sympathetic nervous activity is the dependence of noradrenaline plasma concentrations on rates of removal of the neurotransmitter from plasma, not just sympathetic tone and noradrenaline release (Esler et al. 1990). An example is provided by the demonstration that a time-honoured clinical test for detecting sympathetic nervous failure in the setting of postural hypotension, measurement of the plasma noradrenaline response to upright posture, is confounded by a large, posture-dependent fall in noradrenaline plasma clearance in the autonomic

insufficiency patients. This elevates their plasma noradrenaline concentration during the postural test (Meredith et al. 1992).

Plasma concentration of the noradrenaline precursor, DOPA: an index of noradrenaline synthesis?

Overflow of the noradrenaline precursor, DOPA (dihydroxyphenylalanine), to plasma gives additional information concerning noradrenaline synthesis, complementing measurements of noradrenaline release (Eisenhofer et al. 1991a). The rate-limiting step in the synthesis of noradrenaline is the hydroxylation of tyrosine to DOPA by tyrosine hydroxylase (Nagatsu et al. 1964). Spontaneous efflux of some of the synthesized DOPA to plasma occurs, creating positive venoarterial plasma DOPA concentration gradients across most organs (Eisenhofer et al. 1991a, Goldstein et al. 1987). Release of DOPA from the heart is near zero when cardiac sympathetic nerves are lost after cardiac transplantation (Kaye et al. 1993), and with the sympathetic nerve degeneration of pure autonomic failure (Meredith et al. 1991b). Based on these observations, and additionally, because in a range of circumstances sympathetic nervous stimulation increases regional overflow of DOPA to plasma, DOPA overflow has been advocated, with justification, as an index of regional noradrenaline synthesis rates (Eisenhofer et al. 1991a, Goldstein et al. 1987).

Plasma concentration of noradrenaline metabolites: DHPG, MHPG and normetanephrine

Noradrenaline metabolites are measurable in plasma. Dihydroxyphenylglycol (DHPG) is mainly formed intraneuronally, via the action of monoamine oxidase on noradrenaline derived from two sources—from transmitter leaking from storage vesicles and from recaptured noradrenaline returned to the sympathetic neuron via active neuronal reuptake (Eisenhofer et al. 1996). Although DHPG overflow from individual organs such as the heart increases with increases in sympathetic nerve firing rates, resulting from increases in noradrenaline synthesis and reuptake after release (Eisenhofer et al. 1991b), the plasma concentration of DHPG is an insensitive measure of sympathetic nervous activity. The same applies for its methylated product, 3-methoxy-4-hydroxyphenylglycol (MHPG), which primarily derives from noradrenaline released from sympathetic nerves (Lambert et al. 1995), and not as was once thought largely from the brain. The latter misconception at one time leading to invalid claims that plasma and urine MHPG measurements could be used to quantify brain noradrenaline turnover. Plasma normetanephrine measurements are primarily used in the diagnosis of phaeochromocytoma, not in assessing sympathetic nervous function.

Whole-body noradrenaline spillover

Given that plasma noradrenaline measurements provide a rather ambiguous guide to sympathetic nervous activity, kinetics techniques for estimating the rate of release of noradrenaline to plasma have been developed (Esler et al. 1990, Esler et al. 1979). The central feature of these methods is determination of the metabolic clearance rate of noradrenaline in plasma, using an isotope dilution technique, with intravenous infusion of tritiated noradrenaline:

$$\text{NA plasma clearance plasma} = \frac{[3H] \text{ NA infusion rate}}{\text{plasma } [3H] \text{ NA conc}}.$$

$$\text{Whole-body NA spillover} = \text{plasma NA conc.} \times \text{NA plasma clearance}$$

Rather than the rate of release of noradrenaline from sympathetic nerves, the noradrenaline 'spillover rate' represents the rate at which released noradrenaline enters plasma. In humans this appears to be approximately 5–20% only of the release rate (Eisenhofer et al. 1996).

The noradrenaline spillover measurement has the advantage over plasma concentration measurements of avoiding the confounding influence of noradrenaline plasma clearance. In many contexts the concentration of noradrenaline in plasma is distorted by altered plasma noradrenaline clearance, rendering the plasma concentration unreliable as a measure of sympathetic nervous activity. Examples are the elevation of plasma concentration of noradrenaline, beyond that expected from existing rates of noradrenaline release, with lowered noradrenaline plasma clearance during upright posture and in cardiac failure (where in both reduced organ blood flow lowers noradrenaline extraction from plasma) (Esler et al. 1990, Hasking et al. 1986, Meredith et al. 1992), and with pure autonomic failure and administration of tricyclic antidepressants (where loss of sympathetic nerves or pharmacological blockade of noradrenaline transporter sites reduces neuronal noradrenaline reuptake from plasma) (Meredith et al. 1991b, Esler et al. 1991b).

There is one additional important point. All global measures of sympathetic function, including this one, do not register the fact that the sympathetic nervous system shows regional differentiation. This technical deficiency is avoided with the use of organ-specific measurements of noradrenaline release.

Neurochemical investigation of regional sympathetic function

Organ-specific noradrenaline spillover

The various elements in the neural control of the circulation have each provided a basis for the development of tests of regional sympathetic nervous system function in humans.

- Sympathetic nerve firing rates in subcutaneous postganglionic sympathetic efferents can be measured with multiunit or single fibre electrophysiological recordings (clinical microneurography) (Hagbarth and Vallbo 1968).

- Pharmacological autonomic blockade can be used to quantify, by subtraction, the prevailing levels of neurally sustained cardiovascular tone.

- Analysis of spontaneous, superimposed circulatory rhythms, including power spectral analysis of heart rate and blood pressure variability (Akselrod et al. 1985) is widely used, despite evident deficiencies (Eckberg 1997, Kingwell et al. 1994, Grassi and Esler 1999) to non-invasively study autonomic neurocirculatory control.

- Sympathetic nerve transmitter release can be studied using radiotracer-derived measures of organ-specific noradrenaline spillover to plasma (Esler et al. 1990, Esler et al. 1984).

These tests are complementary, rather than competing methodologies, and measure different aspects of sympathetic nervous function, although clinical microneurography and noradrenaline spillover measurements have greater specificity than the other two methods, which are indirect.

The regional noradrenaline spillover technique is the 'gold standard' methodology for investigation of sympathetic nervous function in internal organs, such as the heart and kidneys, which are out of reach of clinical microneurography. The sympathetic nerve firing rate of an organ and the rate of spillover of noradrenaline into its venous effluent usually correlate closely (Brown and Gillespie 1957, Bradley and Hjemdahl 1984). During constant rate infusion of radiolabelled noradrenaline, the regional rate of spillover of noradrenaline to plasma can be determined by isotope dilution (Esler et al. 1990, Eisenhofer et al. 1996, Esler et al. 1984, Esler et al. 1982) (Figure 26.1):

$$\text{Regional noradrenaline spillover} = [(C_V - C_A) + (C_A.E)].PF$$

where C_V and C_A are the plasma concentration of noradrenaline in regional venous and arterial plasma, E is the fractional extraction of tritiated noradrenaline and PF is the organ plasma flow. Use of the radiotracer is necessary, because flux of noradrenaline is in two directions. 'Noradrenaline spillover' signifies the outward flux of noradrenaline. In essence, the '$C_A.E$' term in the equation adjusts the organ venous outflow plasma concentration to what it would have been if there had been no noradrenaline uptake from plasma, thereby allowing the Fick Principle to be applied, to calculate noradrenaline spillover.

It should be emphasized that noradrenaline spillover is measured, and from this noradrenaline release (and sympathetic activity) is inferred. A variety of other factors, however, influence the rate at which noradrenaline released into the interstitial space diffuses into plasma. Released noradrenaline is subject to several possible fates: reuptake into sympathetic nerves, O-methylation after uptake into extraneuronal cells, or diffusion into plasma. The rate of overflow of noradrenaline is determined not only by the rate of

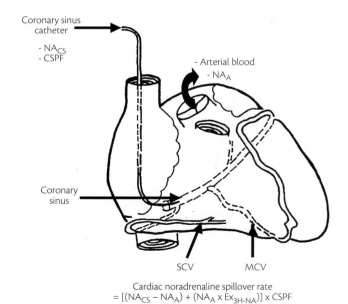

Cardiac noradrenaline spillover rate
= [(NA$_{CS}$ − NA$_A$) + (NA$_A$ × Ex$_{3H-NA}$)] × CSPF

Fig. 26.1 Measurement by isotope dilution of regional noradrenaline spillover to plasma, in the heart (Esler et al. 1984). Measured are the venoarterial plasma noradrenaline concentration gradient across the heart, with coronary sinus venous sampling (NA$_{CS}$-NA$_{ART}$), the transcardiac fractional extraction from plasma of infused tritiated noradrenaline (EX$_{3HNA}$), and the coronary sinus plasma flow (CSPF) measured by thermodilution. MCV, middle cardiac vein; SCV, small cardiac vein.

noradrenaline release (and hence sympathetic nerve firing and nerve density) but also by the activity of the competing disposition mechanisms of uptake, metabolism, and diffusional flow to the circulation, the latter being influenced by factors such as regional blood flow (Chang et al. 1987) and the exchange conductivity of the capillary bed (Cousineau et al. 1984).

Tissue noradrenaline microdialysis

Given that only a small percentage of noradrenaline released from sympathetic nerves spills over into the circulation a substantial synaptic cleft interstitial-extracellular-plasma noradrenaline concentration gradient exists (Khan et al. 2002). While *in vivo* microdialysis provides a measure of noradrenaline in the extracellular fluid a number of limitations have hampered the technique's widespread utility as an index of noradrenaline release. The methodology might be particularly suitable for adipose tissue, where accessing the draining vein for noradrenaline spillover determination can be challenging.

As for noradrenaline spillover measurements, organ blood flow influences the microdialysis noradrenaline measurement, high rates of regional blood flow tending to wash out the neurotransmitter from tissue, and to lower the interstitial value. A second problem is technical; noradrenaline concentrations in the dialysis effluent are typically low, and may be less than the lower limit of sensitivity of the noradrenaline assay. To rectify this multiple dialysis probes may be inserted and effluent pooled, collection times may be increased or microanalytical approaches may be employed. A third difficulty concerns the need to convert the 'effluent concentration' to the true interstitial noradrenaline concentration, which necessitates the use of a locally infused marker chemical.

Despite these challenges, parallel increases in interstitial noradrenaline, plasma noradrenaline concentrations and muscle sympathetic nerve activity in response to sympathetic activation have been demonstrated (Khan et al. 2002).

Sympathetic nerve proteins

One limitation of neurochemical analysis of the sympathetic nervous system is the lack of ready availability of sympathetic nerve tissue, which might allow analysis of the proteins involved in sympathetic neurotransmission. This can be overcome with the biopsy of small subcutaneous hand or forearm veins, which is both aesthetically and ethically acceptable.

Veins are sufficiently densely innervated to provide an adequate source of neural proteins for investigation of such things as the enzymes involved in catecholamine synthesis, abundance of the noradrenaline transporter, and presence of the sympathetic nerve receptors mediating neurotrophic support by nerve growth factor, which is produced in the vein wall (Fig. 26.2). Analysis of messenger RNA (mRNA) is usually not possible, as given the distance between the cell nuclei in the sympathetic ganglia and the peripheral sampling site in the arm or hand, mRNA levels are very low or undetectable.

An example of the application of this methodology is in the investigation of sympathetic nerve biology in patients with essential hypertension, which is often 'neurogenic', the blood pressure elevation being initiated and sustained by sympathetic nervous activation (Esler 2004). Western blot analysis displays lowered content of the neuronal noradrenaline transporter (Fig. 26.2). Patients with essential hypertension commonly display a phenotype

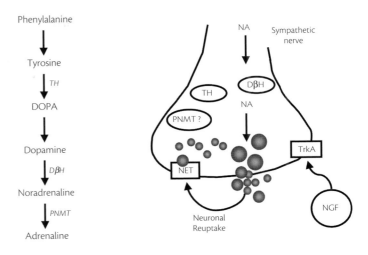

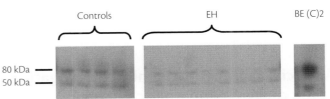

Fig. 26.2 Top panel: Schematic diagram of the sympathetic nerve proteins involved in noradrenaline and adrenaline synthesis, in noradrenaline neuronal reuptake, and in sympathetic nerve neurotrophic support by nerve growth factor. Adrenaline synthesis in sympathetic nerves only occurs with chronic mental stress. TH, tyrosine hydroxylase; DBH, dopamine-beta hydroxylase; PNMT, phenylethanolamine methyltransferase; NA, noradrenaline; NET, noradrenaline transporter; NGF, nerve growth factor; TrkA, NGF receptor. **Lower panel:** Western blot analysis of noradrenaline transporter (NET) protein in hand vein biopsies. The protein is contained only in sympathetic nerves in the biopsy. Data are shown for untreated patients with essential hypertension (EH) and healthy people, with a human neuroblastoma cell line, BE(C)2, serving as the positive control. NET protein abundance was reduced in the patients with hypertension.

of impairment of neuronal noradrenaline reuptake (Esler et al. 1981), which through augmenting the sympathetic neural signal, would be expected to contribute to the blood pressure elevation. The lower NET protein levels appear to explain this.

Differentiation (regionalization) of sympathetic outflows

Sympathetic nervous system responses typically show regional differentiation, with non-uniform engagement of the sympathetic outflows to different organs. The regional patterning of human sympathetic nervous system responses has now been extensively studied, in a variety of clinical contexts (Table 26.1) (Esler et al. 1990, Grassi and Esler 1999). Regional noradrenaline measurements have been used to quantify the distribution and degree of differentiated sympathetic nervous responses accompanying aerobic and isometric exercise, syncope from a vasovagal reaction, dietary sodium restriction and laboratory mental stress, and to study drug effects (Esler et al. 1990, Grassi and Esler 1999).

Simultaneous determination of regional rates of noradrenaline release to plasma from a battery of organs has been used to delineate the patterns of sympathetic nervous activation in disease states,

Table 26.1 Differentiation (regionalization) of human sympathetic responses

	Sympathetic nerve traffic		Noradrenaline spillover		Adrenal
	Muscle	Skin	Heart	Kidneys	Medulla
Physiological responses					
◆ Ageing	↑	0	↑	0	↓
◆ Mental stress	↓	↑	↑	↑	↑
◆ Aerobic exercise	↑	?↓	↑	↑	↑
◆ Low salt diet	↑	?	0	↑	0
◆ Vasovagal syncope	↓	?	↓	↓	↑
Diseases					
◆ Cardiac failure	↑	0	↑	↑	?↑
◆ Essential hypertension	↑	0	↑	↑	0
◆ Hepatic cirrhosis	↑	?	↑	↑	0

Human sympathetic nervous responses, in health and disease are organ-specific (differentiated), rather than global. Sympathetic nervous and adrenal medullary responses are often incongruent (Esler et al. 1990).

such as essential hypertension, cardiac failure, panic disorder, ventricular arrhythmias and hepatic cirrhosis (Table 26.1).

A special case: neurochemical investigation of the cardiac sympathetic nerves

For the sympathetic nerves of the heart, application of neurochemical methodology has had a major impact on the practice of medicine. The cardiac sympathetic nerves are markedly and preferentially stimulated in severe heart failure, so that noradrenaline spillover from the heart is elevated 4–20 fold (Hasking et al. 1986). It was the demonstration of the precise pathophysiology of the cardiac sympathetic nerves in heart failure patients (Hasking et al. 1986, Esler et al. 1997) which provided the logical justification for the testing of β-adrenergic blocking drugs (Packer et al. 1996), which are now successfully used as part of standard heart failure care.

The measurement techniques for quantifying cardiac sympathetic activity are complex, and primarily confined to research applications such as this. The 'gold standard' technique, giving a reliable neurochemical measure of cardiac sympathetic activity, involves the measurement of the rate of overflow of noradrenaline from the heart, the 'noradrenaline spillover rate' (Esler et al. 1990). Imaging methodologies, several of which are available, are also useful, and less invasive, although involving radio-ligand radiation exposure. Most widely used is the meta-iodobenzyl guanidine (MIBG) scan (Wieland et al. 1980, Kline et al. 1981). MIBG is a substrate for the noradrenaline transporter, and taken up into the sympathetic nerves of the heart. MIBG scanning demonstrates very well the anatomy of cardiac sympathetic innervation. Simpler methods for estimating cardiac sympathetic nervous activity are of lower validity. Heart rate is importantly influenced by vagal tone, so its value is limited. Heart rate spectral analysis methods continue to be widely used, but are flawed as measures of cardiac sympathetic tone, and have been discredited (Eckberg 1997, Kingwell et al. 1994, Grassi and Esler 1999).

Activation of the cardiac sympathetic outflow

Activation of the sympathetic outflow to the heart, demonstrable by measurement of cardiac noradrenaline spillover, can be a prime mechanism of physiological response, perhaps most notably in the cardiac output increase with exercise, where noradrenaline spillover can increase 4–20 fold (Esler et al. 1990). As described, an increase in cardiac sympathetic activity of similar magnitude also characterises heart failure, contributing to complications and death (Hasking et al. 1986).

Cardiac sympathetic nerve inhibition

The common faint ('vasovagal syncope') has been thought to be characterized by abrupt, almost total, but reversible sympathetic nervous inhibition. Noradrenaline spillover from the heart falls to near-zero (Esler et al. 1990), contributing to the bradycardia, as does the associated increase in vagal tone when fainting is caused by the discomfort accompanying cardiac catheterization. A recent report, however, demonstrates unequivocally that sympathetic nerve firing measured by microneurography is usually preserved in fainting occurring during head-up tilting (Vaddadi et al. 2010), suggesting that sudden unexplained vasodilation causes the faint.

Measurement of regional sympathetic nerve cotransmission

With regional venous sampling it is possible to test for organ-specific release of the sympathetic cotransmitters neuropeptide Y (Tidgren and Hjemdahl 1989, Kahan et al. 1992) and adrenaline (Esler et al. 1991a). In contrast to release of the major sympathetic neurotransmitter, cotransmitter release is detected only with some difficulty. Net overflow of NPY to plasma has been reported across the forearm (Kahan et al. 1992) and the human kidney (Tidgren and Hjemdahl 1989) under resting conditions. Overflow of NPY from the heart is not evident at rest in healthy subjects, but becomes readily apparent with high rates of cardiac sympathetic nerve firing, such as accompanying aerobic exercise (supine cycling) and in patients with cardiac failure (Morris et al. 1997).

Adrenaline exists in peripheral tissues, where it appears to be largely derived from hormone circulating in plasma, not synthesis *in situ*. To detect outward flux of adrenaline to plasma, indicative of release of adrenaline from neuronal stores, in the face of the net extraction of plasma adrenaline which occurs across all organs except the adrenal medulla, radiotracer methodology is needed (Esler et al. 1991a).

Regional neuronal release of adrenaline in young healthy human subjects is not evident at rest, and can be demonstrated only under special circumstances, such as from the heart with the stimulation of the cardiac sympathetic outflow accompanying aerobic exercise. Adrenaline cotransmission in sympathetic nerves is also present in patients with panic disorder (Wilkinson et al. 1998). Whether this derives from the uptake of adrenaline from plasma during adrenaline surges accompanying panic attacks, or from *in situ* synthesis by phenylethanolamine-N-methyltransferase (PNMT) is uncertain. PNMT, which catalyzes the conversion of noradrenaline to adrenaline, is induced in sympathetic nerves in experimental animals subjected to chronic mental stress (Micutkova et al. 2004).

Quantification of noradrenaline synthesis and release rates in humans

The terms noradrenaline release, spillover, and turnover are often used interchangeably, but actually refer to distinct processes. In order to maintain neuronal stores of noradrenaline, under steady state conditions the rate of noradrenaline synthesis (Fig. 26.3) must equal the rate of noradrenaline turnover, where turnover specifically denotes the depletion of previously synthesized stores of noradrenaline. Hence, in the heart, cardiac noradrenaline turnover may be estimated from the sum of differences in rates at which noradrenaline and its metabolites enter and leave the coronary circulation (Fig. 26.3).

The enzymes typically involved in noradrenaline metabolism are monoamine oxidase (MAO) and catechol-*O*-methyltransferase (COMT). DHPG is produced by intraneuronal deamination (via MAO) of noradrenaline after either leakage of transmitter into the axoplasm from storage vesicles or reuptake of transmitter after exocytotic release (Fig. 26.3); the contribution of the latter process is reflected by the decrease in DHPG production after neuronal uptake blockade. Given the minor reduction in overflow of endogenous DHPG from the heart at rest after pharmacological reuptake-blockade with desipramine, little of the DHPG produced by the heart is from recaptured noradrenaline.

Thus, the major determinant of DHPG production and noradrenaline turnover in the human heart at rest is leakage of transmitter from vesicles (Eisenhofer et al. 1996). Consistent and substantial arterial-venous increments in plasma DHPG across the coronary circulation (Eisenhofer et al. 1992a) and the far greater cardiac spillover of DHPG than of noradrenaline and of MHPG (Eisenhofer et al. 1996, Lambert et al. 1995) illustrate the importance of local deamination as a major determinant of noradrenaline turnover. The combined cardiac spillover of noradrenaline and its deaminated metabolites, most notably DHPG, better reflects local transmitter turnover than does cardiac noradrenaline spillover alone.

The initial rate-limiting step in catecholamine synthesis involves the enzymatic conversion of the amino acid tyrosine to DOPA via the action of tyrosine hydroxylase (Nagatsu et al. 1964) (Fig. 26.2). Subsequently, DOPA is decarboxylated, by the action of aromatic amino acid decarboxylase, to form dopamine, which, in turn, is

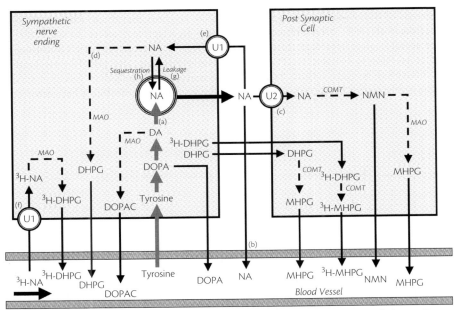

Fig. 26.3 Schematic representation of the disposition of noradrenaline in sympathetic nerve endings and postsynaptic cells (e.g. cardiac myocyte) and overflow into the circulation at rest and during a steady state infusion of a tracer dose of tritiated noradrenaline (^{3}H-NA). At steady state the rate of noradrenaline synthesis (a), by definition, must equal the rate of noradrenaline turnover; where, turnover is equal to the sum of the rates of: spillover of noradrenaline to plasma (b), extraneuronal uptake and subsequent metabolism of noradrenaline (c) and, intraneuronal metabolism of noradrenaline (d). The availability of noradrenaline for intraneuronal metabolism is dependent on the balance between the entry of noradrenaline into the axoplasm via the processes of reuptake (e) and leakage (g) and removal from the axoplasm by vesicular sequestration. Circulating ^{3}H-NA may be extracted from plasma via the process of uptake 1 (U1) and metabolized intraneuronally (f) or extraneuronally. The synthesis of noradrenaline from tyrosine is indicated in grey, catabolic pathways are indicated by dotted arrows. Figure adapted from Eisenhofer and colleagues (Eisenhofer et al. 1996, Eisenhofer et al. 1992a). DOPA, dihydroxyphenylalanine; DA, dopamine; NA, noradrenaline; DHPG, dihydroxyphenylglycol; DOPAC, dihydroxyphenylacetic acid; MHPG, 3-methoxy-4-hydroxyphenylglycol; NMN, normetanephrine; U1, uptake 1; U2, uptake 2; MAO, monoamine oxidase; COMT, catechol-O-methyltransferase; ^{3}H, tritium.

converted to noradrenaline by side-chain hydroxylation through the action of DBH. Use of DOPA overflow from the heart as an index of tyrosine hydroxylase activity is based on considerable experimental evidence (Eisenhofer et al. 1991a, Eisenhofer et al. 1992b). Lack of cardiac DOPA production in the hearts of patients with pure autonomic failure (Meredith et al. 1991b) in whom there was biochemical evidence of almost complete postganglionic sympathetic denervation, or in patients after cardiac transplantation (Kaye et al. 1993, Rundquist et al. 1993) indicates that sympathetic nerves are the source of the DOPA produced by the heart. Positive relationships between cardiac noradrenaline turnover and cardiac DOPA overflow to plasma and parallel changes in fold increases in cardiac DOPA overflow and noradrenaline turnover during sympathetic activation (Eisenhofer et al. 1996, Eisenhofer et al. 1991a) support the use of DOPA overflow to plasma from the heart as an index of cardiac tyrosine hydroxylase activity.

Measurement of neuronal noradrenaline reuptake

Reuptake of noradrenaline into sympathetic nerves after its release terminates the neural signal. A fault in transmitter inactivation may augment the effects of sympathetic nerve traffic. In the heart approximately 95% of released noradrenaline is recaptured into sympathetic nerves (Goldstein et al. 1988a, Goldstein et al. 1988b), so the heart is more sensitive than all other organs to impairments in transmitter reuptake (Rumantir et al. 2000, Shannon et al. 2000). Indeed, an abnormality in neuronal noradrenaline reuptake could sensitise the heart to sympathetic activation. The most precise measurement of human sympathetic nerve reuptake of noradrenaline can be achieved with analysis of tracer noradrenaline kinetics in the heart (Esler et al. 1979, Esler et al. 1984). Measurement of the extraction of infused tritiated noradrenaline in passage through the heart, and its intraneuronal conversion to tritiated DHPG allows direct quantification of neuronal noradrenaline reuptake (Fig. 26.3). In healthy young subjects the extraction of tritium

labelled noradrenaline in passage through the heart is typically in the order of 80% and is reduced with aging (Esler et al. 2002a) in patients with pure autonomic failure (Meredith et al. 1991b) and following uptake-1 blockade with desipramine (Esler et al. 1991a) (Fig. 26.4). Phenotypic evidence of a defect in noradrenaline transporter function has also been documented in patients with essential hypertension, congestive heart failure and renal artery stenosis (Eisenhofer et al. 1996, Schlaich et al. 2004, Petersson et al. 2002) (Fig. 26.4). Interestingly, given the historical importance of tricyclic antidepressant medications in theories underpinning the development of affective disorders (Schildkraut 1965), we also observe a reduction in tritiated noradrenaline extraction by the heart in patients with depression and in subjects with panic disorder (Fig. 26.4).

The mechanism(s) responsible for the defect in noradrenaline reuptake observed in different patient groups has not been unequivocally elucidated. In pure autonomic failure the defect in uptake is undoubtedly due to the absence of functional sympathetic nerves, perhaps as a result of diminished or absent neurotrophic support by nerve growth factor (Kaye et al. 2000). In conditions of high cardiac sympathetic tone, such as heart failure, essential hypertension or renal artery stenosis, activation of the cardiac sympathetic outflow may lead to the development of left ventricular hypertrophy (Schlaich et al. 2003) with subsequent increased synaptic cleft width and reduced efficiency of tritiated noradrenaline extraction. While it remains unknown as to whether elevated rates of sympathetic nerve firing per se exert a regulatory influence on noradrenaline transporter function, the observation that exposure of isolated cardiomyocytes to noradrenaline results in a down-regulation of nerve growth factor (NGF) gene expression, suggests that myocardial NGF down-regulation may represent an adaptive response to sympathetic overactivity (Kaye et al. 2000). In neuropsychiatric conditions, such as depression and panic disorder, the possible mechanisms underlying defective noradrenaline transporter function are difficult to reconcile. Given the significant comorbidity between depression and panic disorder

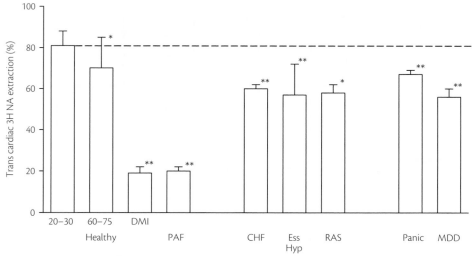

Fig. 26.4 Extraction of tritium labelled noradrenaline (^{3}H NA) by the heart in healthy (Esler et al. 2002b), younger (20–30 years old) and older (60–75 years old) subjects at rest and following desipramine (DMI) infusion (Esler et al. 1991b, Schlaich et al. 2004) and in patients with pure autonomic failure (PAF) (Meredith et al. 1991b), congestive heart failure (CHF) (Eisenhofer et al. 1996, Meredith et al. 1993), essential hypertension (Ess Hyp), renal artery stenosis (RAS) (Petersson et al. 2002), panic disorder (Panic) and major depressive disorder (MDD). Values shown are mean + SEM, * p < 0.05, ** p < 0.01

it is conceivable that a similar mechanism is operative in both conditions. Of note, functionally relevant polymorphisms in the noradrenaline transporter gene have been described (Runkel et al. 2000); moreover, there exists a growing body of evidence implicating epigenetic modification of DNA causing gene silencing (El-Osta 2004). In humans, this modification occurs only on cytosines that precede a guanosine (CpG dinucleotide) in the DNA sequence. The noradrenaline transporter gene promoter is rich in CpG islands and may be a target for DNA methylation.

Measurement of tissue noradrenaline stores by isotope dilution

The content of noradrenaline stored in the heart may be estimated, using radioisotope methodology, from the specific activity of ^{3}H-DHPG produced by the heart during an intravenous infusion of tritiated noradrenaline as a surrogate measure of sympathetic innervation of the heart (Eisenhofer et al. 1996, Eisenhofer et al. 1991b). The ratio of [^{3}H]DHPG to DHPG overflowing into coronary sinus plasma varies inversely with the amount of stored noradrenaline diluting the sequestered ^{3}H-noradrenaline. The linear time-dependent increase in [^{3}H]DHPG specific activity reflects the increase in the specific activity of ^{3}H-noradrenaline in vesicular stores secondary to accumulation of infused ^{3}H-noradrenaline. The rate of increase varies directly with the rate of entry of ^{3}H-noradrenaline into vesicular stores and inversely with the amount of endogenous noradrenaline available to dilute the sequestered ^{3}H-noradrenaline.

The amount of noradrenaline in vesicular stores may therefore be estimated by dividing the rate of vesicular sequestration of ^{3}H-noradrenaline by the rate of increase in specific activity of ^{3}H-DHPG. Using this methodology, Eisenhofer and colleagues demonstrated that the decreased noradrenaline store size in the failing heart occurs as a consequence of chronically increased noradrenaline turnover and reduced efficiency of noradrenaline reuptake and storage (Eisenhofer et al. 1996).

Sympathetic denervation

While the heart receives a rich outflow of postganglionic sympathetic fibres, distributed to all tissue types, including cardiac myocytes, conducting tissue and the vasculature, the cardiac sympathetic nerves are not essential for life. Their loss due to unexplained degeneration, in pure autonomic failure, or when they are cut surgically during cardiac transplantation, does impair exercise responses but causes surprisingly limited disability. Similarly, the selective sympathetic denervation of the donor heart in patients having cardiac transplantation is not sufficient to cause postural hypotension. This contrasts with patients who have pure autonomic failure, where the loss of sympathetic nerves is generalized, and not confined to the heart, extending to the capacitance and resistance components of the circulation. The cardiac sympathetic nerves are not important in postural circulatory homeostasis, but their loss does impair exercise responses.

A particular application of DOPA and DHPG overflow measurements has been in the study of denervation and reinnervation of the human heart, where these and other neurochemical measures of sympathetic neuronal integrity have been applied in the clinical setting of autonomic insufficiency syndromes and cardiac transplantation (Kaye et al. 1993, Meredith et al. 1991b, Rundquist et al. 1993), and in cardiac failure, where cardiac sympathetic denervation had been surmised (Meredith et al. 1993). In patients with recent orthotopic transplantation of the heart, as expected the overflow of DOPA, noradrenaline and DHPG from the heart are near zero (Kaye et al. 1993). Similarly, the extraction of tritiated noradrenaline from plasma in passage through the heart, during infusion of the tracer, is identical to the extraction occurring in healthy human subjects after pharmacological blockade of neuronal noradrenaline uptake by desipramine (Esler et al. 1991b), and there is no intraneuronal processing of the radiotracer to tritiated DHPG (Kaye et al. 1993).

Radiotracer imaging scans

The integrity of sympathetic innervation of the heart can be assessed directly using a variety of imaging methods. Positron emission tomography (PET) scanning following injection of 6-[^{18}F]fluorodopamine (6F-DOPA) (Goldstein et al. 1993) or [^{11}C]hydroxyephedrine (Law et al. 1997, Caldwell et al. 1998) and scintigraphy or single-photon emission computed tomography after injection of iodine-123 MIBG (Wieland et al. 1980, Kline et al. 1981) have been widely used to quantify cardiac sympathetic innervation. Given that entry and subsequent labelling of vesicles is dependent on transport of the radioactive drug by the uptake-1 process, these imaging methodologies do provide an index of the efficiency of neuronal noradrenaline uptake. Use of these agents to estimate sympathetic activity per se (i.e. sympathetic nerve firing and noradrenaline turnover) is more problematic. MIBG and [^{11}C] hydroxyephedrine, unlike noradrenaline, are not stored in the neurotransmitter vesicles and are not subject to electrically coupled vesicular release. 6F-DOPA is more satisfactory in this regard, as the tracer is converted to 6F-noradrenaline after it is taken up into sympathetic nerves.

6F-DOPA has been successfully used to demonstrate cardiac sympathetic denervation in patients with pure autonomic failure and Parkinson's disease (Goldstein et al. 2000). Interestingly, in this study by Goldstein and colleagues, the concentration of 6F-DOPA-derived radioactivity positively correlated with the extraction of ^{3}H-noradrenaline across the heart and the coronary sinus–arterial plasma concentration differences of both DOPA and DHPG. MIBG studies in patients with Parkinson's disease have yielded similar results (Orimo, 1999; Braune, 1999; Takatsu, 2000). Moreover, quantification of cardiac MIBG uptake has proven a valuable tool in differentiating between patients with Parkinson disease and patients with other neurodegenerative disorders, such as multiple system atrophy (Braune, 2001 #82). In agreement with the neurochemical methods outlined earlier, MIBG imaging has been used to demonstrate a deficiency in noradrenaline transporter function in patients with heart failure (Merlot et al. 1992) and after the sympathetic nerve section and degeneration that accompanies cardiac transplantation (Glowniak et al. 1989). Interestingly, given the effectiveness of β-adrenergic blockade in improving mortality and morbidity in patients with heart failure (Packer et al. 1996), heart-mediastinum MIBG ratios are improved following carvedilol treatment in patients with diopathic cardiomyopathy (Gerson et al. 2002).

Adrenaline secretion

Adrenaline secretion by the adrenal medulla can be gauged from plasma adrenaline concentration measurements, and from adrenaline secretion rates measured by isotope dilution. Although adrenaline in certain contexts is released from sympathetic nerves as a cotransmitter, this neuronally released adrenaline makes trivial contribution to the adrenaline plasma pool.

An important principle is that the sympathetic nervous system and the adrenal medulla do not necessarily respond to stimuli as a homogeneous unit; the responses are not always congruent and, in fact, can be directionally opposite (Table 26.1) (Esler et al. 1990). Examples are adrenaline secretion provoked by hypoglycaemia (which is proportionally much greater than the accompanying minor sympathetic nervous activation), adrenaline secretion with mental stress (accompanied by sympathetic inhibition in one outflow, to the skeletal muscle vasculature), sympathetic activation with ageing (adrenaline secretion is reduced), sympathetic activation in essential hypertension (adrenaline secretion is unremarkable) and the pronounced secretion of adrenaline during vasovagal syncope (accompanied by sympathetic inhibition) (Esler et al. 1990) (Table 26.1).

Brief overview of clinical impact of the spillover methodology

Heart failure

The cardiac sympathetic nerves are preferentially stimulated in severe heart failure (Esler et al. 1990, Hasking et al. 1986). The level of sympathetic nervous drive to the failing heart in patients with severe heart failure has been demonstrated to be a major determinant of prognosis, patients with the highest cardiac sympathetic activity having greatly reduced survival (Kaye et al. 1995). These findings provided a theoretical underpinning for the testing of β-adrenergic blocking drugs (Esler et al. 1997, Packer et al. 1996), now part of conventional heart failure therapy.

Essential hypertension

The sympathetic nervous system is commonly activated in patients with essential hypertension. Analysis of regional sympathetic nervous system function has demonstrated activation of the sympathetic nervous outflows to the heart, the kidneys and skeletal muscle vasculature (Esler et al. 1990, Grassi et al. 1998, Grassi and Esler 1999, Esler 2004). The sympathetic stimulation present in human hypertension no doubt contributes to the blood pressure elevation, a view reinforced by recent data describing a substantial and sustained reduction in both blood pressure (Krum et al. 2009) and central sympathetic outflow (Schlaich et al. 2009) in patients with severe and treatment-resistant hypertension following percutaneous catheter-based sympathetic denervation of the kidney. The sympathetic nervous activation also seems to have adverse consequences going beyond initiating the blood pressure elevation. A trophic effect of cardiac sympathetic activation on cardiac myocyte growth is also likely; left ventricular hypertrophy is commonest in essential hypertension patients with the highest levels of cardiac sympathetic activity (Schlaich et al. 2003), in whom a blood pressure-independent contribution to left ventricular mass is evident. Importantly, even in young overweight-obese subjects,

prior to the development of hypertension, the degree of sympathetic nervous activation is predictive of subclinical organ damage to the heart, kidney and endothelium (Lambert et al. 2010). Given this common neural pathophysiology of essential hypertension, antihypertensive drugs suppressing sympathetic outflow, the imidazoline receptor-binding agents such as moxonidine and rilmenidine (Sannajust and Head 1994) would appear to be under-utilized in contemporary care of hypertensive patients, in which antagonism of the renin-angiotensin system is the dominant therapy.

Syndromes of autonomic nervous failure

Differentiating between the various syndromes of autonomic failure causing postural hypotension and syncope can be difficult, specifically in making the diagnostic distinction between pure autonomic failure, where there is loss of postganglionic sympathetic fibres, and multiple system atrophy, where the peripheral sympathetic innervation is preserved but central nervous system degeneration has caused a loss of central integration of the circulatory reflexes. Neurochemical techniques targeting the sympathetic nerves of the heart can reliably discriminate between these syndromes of autonomic nervous failure. When scanning and noradrenaline spillover techniques demonstrate the presence and normal functioning of the cardiac sympathetic nerves, as is seen in multiple system atrophy, pure autonomic failure is reliably excluded (Meredith et al. 1991b, Goldstein et al. 1997). Further discrimination between these and other neurocirculatory disorders may be achieved through combination of direct nerve recording (microneurography) coupled with analysis of sympathetic nerve proteins in forearm vein tissue (Fig. 26.2). For instance, in patients with the postural orthostatic tachycardia syndrome (POTS) a recent report by our group was able to demonstrate that the exaggerated heart rate and sympathetic nervous reactivity to head up tilt in POTS was associated with reduced NET protein extracted from forearm vein biopsies (Lambert et al. 2008).

Psychogenic heart disease

Severe acute mental stress can serve as a trigger for heart attacks. The truth of this is contested, but the marked increase in non-traumatic sudden death during earthquakes is one indisputable example (Leor et al. 1996). Adverse cardiac events occurring during panic attacks are analogous (Mansour et al. 1998). In patients with the metabolic syndrome and elevated blood pressure chronic mental stress modulates the pattern of sympathetic activity, which, in turn, may confer greater cardiovascular risk associated with increased neurotransmitter release during bursts of sympathetic activity (Lambert et al. 2010). Two mechanisms by which acute mental stress mediates heart risk are atherosclerotic plaque rupture from increased shear stress in the arterial wall, and the development of neural, sympathetically-mediated cardiac arrhythmias

Major depressive disorder (MDD) is also a major risk factor for coronary heart disease, no less important than hypercholesterolemia or diabetes (Musselman et al. 1998). The mechanism is uncertain, but in a subset (approximately 25%) of patients with untreated MDD sympathetic nervous activity in the heart is extraordinarily high (Barton et al. 2007), cardiac noradrenaline spillover values being comparable to that observed in patients without depressive illness who unexpectedly developed ventricular arrhythmias (Meredith et al. 1991a). β-adrenergic blockade is life-saving in cardiac failure. Perhaps there will be a future place for anti-adrenergic cardiac protection also in MDD, especially in drug-resistant patients with depression.

References

Akselrod, S., Gordon, D., Madwed, J. B., Snidman, N. C., Shannon, D. C., Cohen, R. J. (1985). Hemodynamic regulation: investigation by spectral analysis. *Am. J Physiol.* **249**(4 Pt 2), H867–75.

Barton, D. A., Dawood, T., Lambert, E. A., *et al.* (2007). Sympathetic activity in major depressive disorder: identifying those at increased cardiac risk? *J Hypertens.* **25**(10), 2117–24.

Bradley, T., Hjemdahl, P. (1984). Further studies on renal nerve stimulation induced release of noradrenaline and dopamine from the canine kidney *in situ*. *Acta Physiol. Scand.* **122**, 369–79.

Braune, S., Reinhardt, M., Schnitzer, R., Riedel, A., Lucking, C. H. (1999). Cardiac uptake of [123I]MIBG separates Parkinson's disease from multiple system atrophy. *Neurology* **53**(5), 1020–5.

Brown, G. L., Gillespie, J. S. (1957). The output of sympathetic transmitter from the spleen of the cat. *J Physiol* 29;**138**(1):81–102.

Caldwell, J. H., Kroll, K., Li, Z., Seymour, K., Link, J. M., Krohn, K. A. (1998). Quantitation of presynaptic cardiac sympathetic function with carbon-11-meta-hydroxyephedrine. *J Nucl. Med.* **39**(8), 1327–34.

Chang, P. C., van der Krogt, J. A., van Brummelen, P. (1987). Demonstration of neuronal and extraneuronal uptake of circulating norepinephrine in the forearm. *Hypertension* **9**(6), 647–53.

Chidsey, C. A., Braunwald, E. (1966). Sympathetic activity and neurotransmitter depletion in congestive heart failure. *Pharmacol. Rev.* **18**(1), 685–700.

Cousineau, D., Goresky, C. A., Bach, G. G., Rose, C. P. (1984). Effect of beta-adrenergic blockade on in vivo norepinephrine release in canine heart. *Am. J Physiol.* **246**(2 Pt 2), H283–92.

DeQuattro, V., Miura, Y., Lurvey, A., Cosgrove, M., Mendez, R. (1975). Increased plasma catecholamine concentrations and vas deferens norepinephrine biosynthesis in men with elevated blood pressure. *Circ. Res.* **36**(1), 118–26.

Eckberg, D. L. (1997). Sympathovagal balance: a critical appraisal. *Circulation* **96**(9), 3224–32.

Eisenhofer, G., Goldstein, D. S., Ropchak, T. G., Nguyen, H. Q., Keiser, H. R., Kopin, I. J. (1988). Source and physiological significance of plasma 3,4-dihydroxyphenylglycol and 3-methoxy-4-hydroxyphenylglycol. *J Auton. Nerv. Sys.* **24**, 1–14.

Eisenhofer, G., Meredith, I. T., Ferrier, C., *et al.* (1991a). Increased plasma dihydroxyphenylalanine during sympathetic activation in humans is related to increased norepinephrine turnover. *J Lab. Clin. Med.* **117**(4), 266–73.

Eisenhofer, G., Smolich, J. J., Cox, H. S., Esler, M. D. (1991b). Neuronal reuptake of norepinephrine and production of dihydroxyphenylglycol by cardiac sympathetic nerves in the anesthetized dog. *Circulation* **84**(3), 1354–63.

Eisenhofer, G., Esler, M. D., Meredith, I. T., *et al.* (1992a). Sympathetic nervous function in human heart as assessed by cardiac spillovers of dihydroxyphenylglycol and norepinephrine. *Circulation* **85**(5), 1775–85.

Eisenhofer, G., Smolich, J. J., Esler, M. D. (1992b). Increased cardiac production of dihydroxyphenylalanine (DOPA) during sympathetic stimulation in anaesthetized dogs. *Neurochem. Int.* **21**(1), 37–44.

Eisenhofer, G., Friberg, P., Rundqvist, B., *et al.* (1996). Cardiac sympathetic nerve function in congestive heart failure. *Circulation* **93**(9), 1667–76.

El-Osta, A. (2004). Coordination of epigenetic events. *Cell Mol. Life. Sci.* **61**(17), 2135–6.

Engelman, K., Portnoy, B., Lovenberg, W. (1968). A sensitive and specific double-isotope derivative method for the determination of catecholamines in biological specimens. *Am. J Med. Sci.* **255**, 259–68.

Esler, M. (2004). Looking at the sympathetic nervous system as a primary source. In: Zanchett A, Robertson JIS, Birkenhage WH, editors. *Handbook of Hypertension: Hypertension research in the Twentieth Century.* Amsterdam: Elsevier; p.81–103.

Esler, M., Jackman, G., Bobik, A., *et al.* (1979). Determination of norepinephrine apparent release rate and clearance in humans. *Life Sci.* **25**, 1461–70.

Esler, M., Jackman, G., Bobik, A., *et al.* (1981). Norepinephrine kinetics in essential hypertension. Defective neuronal uptake of norepinephrine in some patients. *Hypertension* **3**(2), 149–56.

Esler, M., Blombery, P., Leonard, P., Jennings, G., Korner, P. (1982). Radiotracer methodology for the simultaneous estimation of total and renal sympathetic nervous system activity in humans. *Clin. Sci.* **63**, 285S–7S.

Esler, M., Jennings, G., Korner, P., Blombery, P., Sacharias, N., Leonard, P. (1984). Measurement of total and organ-specific norepinephrine kinetics in humans. *Am. J Physiol.* **247**, E21–E8.

Esler, M., Jennings, G., Lambert, G., Meredith, I., Horne, M., Eisenhofer, G. (1990). Overflow of catecholamine neurotransmitters to the circulation: source, fate, and functions. *Physiol. Rev.* **70**(4), 963–85.

Esler, M., Eisenhofer, G., Dart, A., *et al.* (1991a). Adrenaline release by the human heart. *Clin. Exp. Pharmacol. Physiol.* **18**(2), 67–70.

Esler, M. D., Wallin, G., Dorward, P. K., *et al.* (1991b). Effects of desipramine on sympathetic nerve firing and norepinephrine spillover to plasma in humans. *Am. J Physiol.* **260**(4 Pt 2), R817–23.

Esler, M., Kaye, D., Lambert, G., Esler, D., Jennings, G. (1997). Adrenergic nervous system in heart failure. *Am. J Cardiol.* **80**(11A), 7L–14L.

Esler, M., Hastings, J., Lambert, G., Kaye, D., Jennings, G., Seals, D. R. (2002a). The influence of aging on the human sympathetic nervous system and brain norepinephrine turnover. *Am. J Physiol. Regul. Integr. Comp. Physiol.* **282**(3), R909–16.

Esler, M., Lambert, G., Kaye, D., Rumantir, M., Hastings, J., Seals, D. R. (2002b). Influence of ageing on the sympathetic nervous system and adrenal medulla at rest and during stress. *Biogerontology* **3**(1–2), 45–9.

Gerson, M. C., Craft, L. L., McGuire, N., Suresh, D. P., Abraham, W. T., Wagoner, L. E. (2002). Carvedilol improves left ventricular function in heart failure patients with idiopathic dilated cardiomyopathy and a wide range of sympathetic nervous system function as measured by iodine 123 metaiodobenzylguanidine. *J Nucl. Cardiol.* **9**(6), 608–15.

Glowniak, J. V., Turner, F. E., Gray, L. L., Palac, R. T., Lagunas-Solar, M. C., Woodward, W. R. (1989). Iodine-123 metaiodobenzylguanidine imaging of the heart in idiopathic congestive cardiomyopathy and cardiac transplants. *J Nucl. Med.* **30**(7), 1182–91.

Goldstein, D. S., Udelsman, R., Eisenhofer, G., Stull, R., Keiser, H R., Kopin, I. J. (1987). Neuronal source of plasma dihydroxyphenylalanine. *J Clin. Endocrinol. Metab.* **64**, 856–61.

Goldstein, D. S., Brush, J., Eisenhofer, G., Stull, R., Esler, M. (1988a). *In vivo* measurement of neuronal uptake of norepinephrine in the human heart. *Circulation* **78**, 41–8.

Goldstein, D. S., Eisenhofer, G., Stull, R., Folio, C. J., Keiser, H. R., Kopin, I. J. (1988b). Plasma dihydroxyphenylglycol and the intraneuronal disposition of norepinephrine in humans. *J Clin. Invest.* **81**, 213–20.

Goldstein, D. S., Eisenhofer, G., Dunn, B. B., *et al.* (1993). Positron emission tomographic imaging of cardiac sympathetic innervation using 6-[18F]fluorodopamine: initial findings in humans. *J Am. Coll. Cardiol.* **22**(7), 1961–71.

Goldstein, D. S., Holmes, C., Cannon, R. O., 3rd, Eisenhofer, G., Kopin, I. J. (1997). Sympathetic cardioneuropathy in dysautonomias. *N Engl. J Med.* **336**(10), 696–702.

Goldstein, D. S., Holmes, C., Li, S. T., Bruce, S., Metman, L. V., Cannon, R. O., 3rd. (2000). Cardiac sympathetic denervation in Parkinson disease. *Ann. Intern. Med.* **133**(5), 338–47.

Grassi, G., Esler, M. (1999). How to assess sympathetic activity in humans. *J Hypertens.* **17**(6),719–34.

Grassi, G., Colombo, M., Seravalle, G., Spaziani, D., Mancia, G. (1998). Dissociation between muscle and skin sympathetic nerve activity in essential hypertension, obesity, and congestive heart failure. *Hypertension* **31**(1), 64–7.

Hagbarth, K. E., Vallbo, A. B. (1968). Pulse and respiratory grouping of sympathetic impulses in human muscle-nerves. *Acta Physiol. Scand.* **74**(1), 96–108.

Hasking, G. J., Esler, M. D., Jennings, G. L., Burton, D., Johns, J. A., Korner, P. I. (1986). Norepinephrine spillover to plasma in patients with congestive heart failure: evidence of increased overall and cardiorenal sympathetic nervous activity. *Circulation* **73**(4), 615–21.

Kahan, T., Taddei, S., Pedrinelli, R., Hjemdahl, P., Salvetti, A. (1992). Nonadrenergic sympathetic vascular control of the human forearm in hypertension: possible involvement of neuropeptide Y. *J Cardiovasc. Pharmacol.* **19**(4), 587–92.

Kaye, D. M., Esler, M., Kingwell, B., McPherson, G., Esmore, D., Jennings, G. (1993). Functional and neurochemical evidence for partial cardiac sympathetic reinnervation after cardiac transplantation in humans. *Circulation* **88**, 1110–8.

Kaye, D. M., Lefkovits, J., Jennings, G. L., Bergin, P., Broughton, A., Esler, M. D. (1995). Adverse consequences of high sympathetic nervous activity in the failing human heart. *J Am. Coll. Cardiol.* **26**,1257–63.

Kaye, D. M., Vaddadi, G., Gruskin, S. L., Du, X. J., Esler, M. D. (2000). Reduced myocardial nerve growth factor expression in human and experimental heart failure. *Circ. Res.* **86**(7), E80–4.

Khan, M. H., Sinoway, L. I., MacLean, D. A. (2002). Effects of graded LBNP on MSNA and interstitial norepinephrine. *Am. J Physiol. Heart. Circ. Physiol.* **283**(5), H2038–44.

Kingwell, B. A., Thompson, J. M., Kaye, D. M., McPherson, G. A., Jennings, G. L., Esler, M. D. (1994). Heart rate spectral analysis, cardiac norepinephrine spillover, and muscle sympathetic nerve activity during human sympathetic nervous activation and failure. *Circulation* **90**(1), 234–40.

Kline, R. C., Swanson, D. P., Wieland, D. M., *et al.* (1981). Myocardial imaging in man with I-123 meta-iodobenzylguanidine. *J Nucl. Med.* **22**(2), 129–32.

Krum, H., Schlaich, M., Whitbourn, R., *et al.* (2009). Catheter-based renal sympathetic denervation for resistant hypertension: a multicentre safety and proof-of-principle cohort study. *Lancet* **373**(9671), 1275–81.

Lambert, E., Eikelis, N., Esler, M., *et al.* (2008). Altered sympathetic nervous reactivity and norepinephrine transporter expression in patients with postural tachycardia syndrome. *Circ. Arrhythm. Electrophysiol.* **1**(2), 103–9.

Lambert, E., Dawood, T., Straznicky, N., *et al.* (2010). Association between the sympathetic firing pattern and anxiety level in patients with the metabolic syndrome and elevated blood pressure. *J Hypertens* **28**(3):543–50.

Lambert, E. A., Ika Sari, C., Dawood, T., *et al.* (2010). Sympathetic nervous system activity is associated with obesity-induced subclinical organ damage in young adults. *Hypertension* **56**(3), 351–8.

Lambert, G. W., Kaye, D. M., Vaz, M., *et al.* (1995). Regional origins of 3-methoxy-4-hydroxyphenylglycol in plasma: effects of chronic sympathetic nervous activation and denervation, and acute reflex sympathetic stimulation. *J Auton. Nerv. Syst.* **55**(3), 169–78.

Law, M. P., Osman, S., Davenport, R. J., Cunningham, V. J., Pike, V. W., Camici, P. G. (1997). Biodistribution and metabolism of [N-methyl-11C]m-hydroxyephedrine in the rat. *Nucl. Med. Biol.* **24**(5), 417–24.

Leor, J., Poole, W. K., Kloner, R. A. (1996). Sudden cardiac death triggered by an earthquake. *N Engl. J Med.* **334**(7), 413–9.

Mansour, V. M., Wilkinson, D. J., Jennings, G. L., Schwarz, R. G., Thompson, J. M., Esler, M. D. (1998). Panic disorder: coronary spasm as a basis for cardiac risk? *Med. J Aust.* **168**(8), 390–2.

Meredith, I. T., Broughton, A., Jennings, G. L., Esler, M. D. (1991a). Evidence for a selective increase in resting cardiac sympathetic activity in some patients suffering sustained out of hospital ventricular arrhythmias. *New Engl. J Med.* **325**, 618–24.

Meredith, I. T., Esler, M. D., Cox, H. S., Lambert, G. W., Jennings, G. L., Eisenhofer, G. (1991b). Biochemical evidence of sympathetic denervation of the heart in pure autonomic failure. *Clin. Auton. Res.* (3), 187–94.

Meredith, I. T., Eisenhofer, G., Lambert, G. W., Jennings, G. L., Thompson, J., Esler, M. D. (1992). Plasma norepinephrine responses to head-up tilt are misleading in autonomic failure. *Hypertension* **19**(6 Pt 2), 628–33.

Meredith, I. T., Eisenhofer, G., Lambert, G. W., Dewar, E. M., Jennings, G. L., Esler, M. D. (1993). Cardiac sympathetic nervous activity in congestive heart failure. Evidence for increased neuronal norepinephrine release and preserved neuronal uptake. *Circulation* **88**(1), 136–45.

Merlot, P., Dubois-Rande, J. L., Adnot, S., *et al.* (1992). Myocardial beta-adrenergic desensitization and neuronal norepinephrine uptake function in idiopathic dilated cardiomyopathy. *J Cardiovasc. Pharmacol.* **19**(1), 10–6.

Micutkova, L., Krepsova, K., Sabban, E., Krizanova, O., Kvetnansky, R. (2004). Modulation of catecholamine-synthesizing enzymes in the rat heart by repeated immobilization stress. *Ann. N Y Acad. Sci.* **1018**, 424–9.

Morris, M. J., Russell, A. E., Kapoor, V., *et al.* (1986). Increases in plasma neuropeptide Y concentrations during sympathetic activation in man. *J Auton. Nerv. Syst* **17**(2), 143–9.

Morris, M. J., Cox, H. S., Lambert, G. W., *et al.* (1997). Region-specific neuropeptide Y overflows at rest and during sympathetic activation in humans. *Hypertension* **29**(1 Pt 1), 137–43.

Musselman, D. L., Evans, D. L., Nemeroff, C. B. (1998). The relationship of depression to cardiovascular disease: epidemiology, biology, and treatment. *Arch. Gen. Psychiatry.* **55**(7), 580–92.

Nagatsu, T., Levitt, M., Udenfriend, S. (1964). Tyrosine hydroxylase. The initial step in norepinephrine biosynthesis. *J Biol. Chem.* **239**, 2910–7.

O'Connor, D. T., Bernstein, K. N. (1984). Radioimmunoassay of chromogranin A in plasma as a measure of exocytotic sympathoadrenal activity in normal subjects and patients with pheochromocytoma. *N Engl. J Med.* **311**(12), 764–70.

Orimo, S., Ozawa, E., Nakade, S., Sugimoto, T., Mizusawa, H. (1999). (123) I-metaiodobenzylguanidine myocardial scintigraphy in Parkinson's disease. *J Neurol. Neurosurg. Psychiatry* **67**(2), 189–94.

Packer, M., Bristow, M. R., Cohn, J. N., *et al.* (1996). The effect of carvedilol on morbidity and mortality in patients with chronic heart failure. U.S. Carvedilol Heart Failure Study Group. *N Engl. J Med.* **334**(21), 1349–55.

Petersson, M. J., Rundqvist, B., Johansson, M., *et al.* (2002). Increased cardiac sympathetic drive in renovascular hypertension. *J Hypertens.* **20**(6), 1181–7.

Robertson, D., Johnson, G. A., Robertson, R. M., Nies, A. S., Shand, D. G., Oates, J. A. (1979). Comparative assessment of stimuli that release neuronal and adrenomedullary catecholamines in man. *Circulation* **59**(4), 637–43.

Rumantir, M. S., Kaye, D. M., Jennings, G. L., Vaz, M., Hastings, J. A., Esler, M. D. (2000). Phenotypic evidence of faulty neuronal norepinephrine reuptake in essential hypertension. *Hypertension* **36**(5), 824–9.

Rundquist, B., Eisenhofer, G., Dakak, N. A., Elam, M., Waagstein, F., Friberg, P. (1993). Cardiac noradrenergic function one year following cardiac transplantation. *Blood Press.* **2**(4), 252–61.

Runkel, F., Bruss, M., Nothen, M. M., Stober, G., Propping, P., Bonisch, H. (2000). Pharmacological properties of naturally occurring variants of the human norepinephrine transporter. *Pharmacogenetics* **10**(5), 397–405.

Sannajust, F., Head, G. A. (1994). Involvement of imidazoline-preferring receptors in regulation of sympathetic tone. *Am. J Cardiol.* **74**(13), 7A–19A.

Schildkraut, J. J. (1965). The catecholamine hypothesis of affective disorders: A review of supporting evidence. *Am. J Psychiatry* **122**, 509–22.

Schlaich, M.P., Kaye, D. M., Lambert, E., Sommerville, M., Socratous, F., Esler, M. D. (2003). Relation between cardiac sympathetic activity and hypertensive left ventricular hypertrophy. *Circulation* **108**(5), 560–5.

Schlaich, M. P., Lambert, E., Kaye, D. M., *et al.* (2004). Sympathetic augmentation in hypertension: role of nerve firing, norepinephrine reuptake, and Angiotensin neuromodulation. *Hypertension* **43**(2), 169–75.

Schlaich, M. P., Sobotka, P. A., Krum, H., Lambert, E., Esler, M. D. (2009). Renal sympathetic-nerve ablation for uncontrolled hypertension. *N Engl. J Med.* **361**(9), 932–4.

Shannon, J. R., Flattem, N. L., Jordan, J., *et al.* (2000). Orthostatic intolerance and tachycardia associated with norepinephrine-transporter deficiency. *N Engl. J Med.* **342**(8), 541–9.

Takatsu, H., Nishida, H., Matsuo, H., *et al.* (2000). Cardiac sympathetic denervation from the early stage of Parkinson's disease: clinical and experimental studies with radiolabeled MIBG. *J Nucl. Med.* **41**(1), 71–7.

Tidgren, B., Hjemdahl, P. (1989). Renal responses to mental stress and epinephrine in humans. *Am. J Physiol.* **257**(4 Pt 2), F682–9.

Vaddadi, G., Esler, M. D., Dawood, T., Lambert, E. (2011). Persistence of muscle sympathetic nerve activity during vasovagal syncope. *Eur. Heart J.* **31**(16), 2027–33.

von Euler, U. S. (1946). A specific sympathetic ergone in adrenergic nerve fibres (sympathin) and its relation to adrenaline and noradrenaline. *Acta Physiologica Scandinavica* **12**, 73–97.

von Euler, U. S., Hellner, S., Purkhold, A. (1954). Excretion of noradrenaline in the urine in hypertension. *Scan. J Clin. Lab. Invest.* **6**, 54–9.

Weinshilboum, R. M., Raymond, F. A., Elveback, L. R., Weidman, W. H. (1973). Serum dopamine-beta-hydroxylase activity: sibling-sibling correlation. *Science* **181**(103), 943–5.

Wieland, D. M., Wu, J., Brown, L. E., Mangner, T. J., Swanson, D. P., Beierwaltes, W. H. (1980). Radiolabeled adrenergi neuron-blocking agents: adrenomedullary imaging with [131I]iodobenzylguanidine. *J Nucl. Med.* **21**(4), 349–53.

Wilkinson, D. J., Thompson, J. M., Lambert, G. W., *et al.* (1998). Sympathetic activity in patients with panic disorder at rest, under laboratory mental stress, and during panic attacks. *Arch. Gen. Psychiatry* **55**(6), 511–20.

Zweifler, A. J., Julius, S. (1982). Increased platelet catecholamine content in pheochromocytoma: a diagnostic test in patients with elevated plasma catecholamines. *N Engl. J Med.* **306**(15), 890–4.

CHAPTER 27

Autonomic function and the gastrointestinal tract

D.G. Thompson and D.L. Wingate

Historical

In 1901, Langley stated that there were four divisions of the autonomic nervous system: 'sympathetic, cranial, sacral, and enteric'. The enteric division was the focus of intense interest in the closing decades of the 20th century, after many years of neglect. Meissner established the existence of the submucous plexus in 1857 and Auerbach identified the myenteric plexus in 1864. Controversy over whether these were indeed networks of nerves continued for more than a century, and attempts to define their function met with little success. In 1899, Bayliss and Starling demonstrated that the peristaltic reflex is mediated by the intrinsic innervation of the gut wall, but this was not, until many years later, related mechanistically to neuroanatomy and neurophysiology. Obstacles to progress included the belief that the autonomic nervous system was binary (sympathetic, parasympathetic) and relied upon two transmitters, acetylcholine and adrenaline, according to the Dale concept of 'one nerve, one transmitter'. The plexi were viewed as, at best, interruptions in the sympathetic and parasympathetic pathways that allowed neurons to be labelled as 'preganglionic' or 'postganglionic'; the postganglionic fibres in the gut were still considered to be sympathetic or parasympathetic components.

In the 20th century, advances came from several directions:

- Developments in physiology—in 1921, Walter Alvarez demonstrated the inherent electrical rhythmicity of the gastrointestinal musculature, and that the timing of contractile events is dictated by pacemaking activity in the gut wall. But, while pacemakers mark moments when smooth muscle contraction *may* occur, contraction is not the automatic response to a pacemaking wave, and this implies an additional level of control. In the 1960s, Code and others (Bass 1997, Szurszewski et al. 1970) used enteric electromyography in conscious animals to document stereotypic patterns of enteric motor activity.

- Developments in pharmacology—by the mid 20th century, the enormous complexity of enteric neurotransmission had become clear, starting with the pharmacological discovery of the non-adrenergic, non-cholinergic (NANC) transmitter, postulated by Burnstock to be adenosine triphosphate (ATP) (Burnstock et al. 1970). Serotonin, identified in the myenteric plexus (Goodrich et al. 1980), was a rival candidate. These advances were overtaken by the explosion of neuropeptide research, from which emerged the realization that there are many transmitter peptides within the ENS, identical to those found in the central nervous system, and that many so-called 'gut hormones' had primarily local (paracrine or neurocrine) rather than distant (endocrine) activity.

The situation today

In man, the major obstacle to further progress remains the difficulty of physiological study of the intact human digestive tract. Even such an apparently simple function as propulsion of luminal content is highly complex; the transit speed of material through the digestive tract ranges from a few seconds in the oesophagus to many hours in the colon. Moreover, the content is transformed as it passes through the bowel by the processes of exocrine secretion, mechanical and chemical digestion, and absorption (Fig. 27.1).

Motility as an exemplar of autonomic control of gut function

In the sections that follow, there is an emphasis on neural control of the motor activity (or motility) of the gut with an apparent neglect of other physiological functions such as secretion, absorption, and blood flow. This reflects the fact it is at present easier to study neural control of the gut *in vivo* via transient changes in contractile activity than other aspects of gut physiology. The same is true of the pathophysiology; only the motor consequences of autonomic dysfunction have been clearly identified in clinical practice.

Innervation of the digestive tract

It is important to understand that the digestive tract is innervated in a manner that is unique in the human body. The gut itself has its own intrinsic innervation, the ENS. Equally unusual, the extrinsic innervation of the digestive tract is diverse and multiple. In addition to spinal innervation (the classic sympathetic innervation) the great majority of the gastrointestinal tract receives innervation (largely sensory but also some motor) from the 10th cranial nerve (vagus nerve).

The autonomic control of the gut can be best understood when it is appreciated that the *intrinsic* innervation, the ENS (ENS), is largely autonomous (Grundy et al. 1996). It functions effectively to regulate digestive function and ensure digestion with little need for intervention by the central nervous system (CNS). The overall demands of

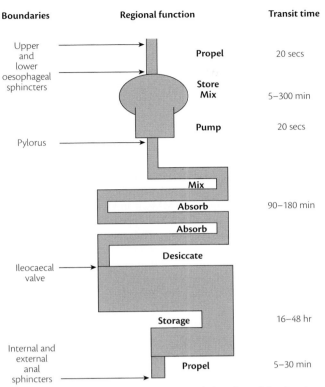

Fig. 27.1 Schematic summary of the anatomy and physiology of the digestive tract, and the time taken for material to pass through the different regions of the gut.

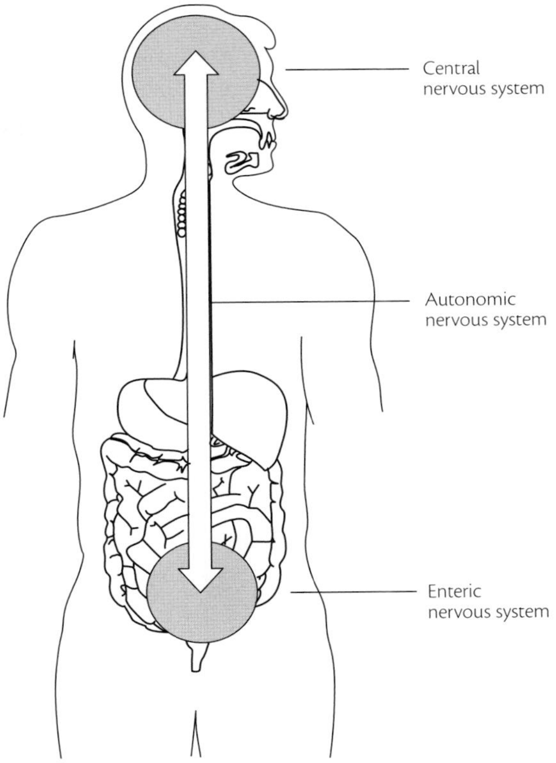

Fig. 27.2 Functional components of gut neural control: (a) block diagram of relationship between neural networks (b) details of parasympathetic and sympathetic innervation of the enteric nervous system.

the organism do however require more subtle co-ordination between the digestive tract and other body systems, and this is achieved by communication between the ENS and CNS along *extrinsic* autonomic neurons (Fig. 27.2).

Intrinsic innervation: the enteric nervous sytem

Morphology

The ENS consists of two interconnecting neurone networks within the gut wall, the myenteric plexus of Auerbach, and the submucosal plexus of Meissner. The latter, located between the circular smooth muscle and the submucosa, is mainly responsible for regulating the absorptive and secretory activity of the mucosa and the neural modulation of the gut immune system. Neural modulation of these functions is not easily studied *in vivo* and consequently clinically relevant knowledge remains fragmentary. More is known about the myenteric plexus, situated between the longitudinal and circular smooth muscle coats, as it is concerned with the regulation of gut motility. Both electrical transients and luminal pressure change can be recorded that correspond to muscle activity, making it possible to describe the patterns of motor activity corresponding to neural activation and inhibition.

The structure of the two plexuses is relatively simple. Cell bodies are grouped in ganglia, interconnected by axon bundles. The neuronal population is diverse, comprising primary afferents from the gut wall and the mucosal surface, primary efferents that regulate effector cells, and interneurons. This density and diversity of neurons confer the properties of a neural network on the ENS,

particularly the capacity for implementing 'programmes' of function in response to changes in luminal environment.

The ganglia of the ENS are also the location for synaptic communication with the long neurons of the extrinsic neurons of the autonomic nervous system. In this respect, the classical nomenclature of 'pre-ganglionic' and 'postganglionic' for gut autonomic nerves was technically correct.

Basic physiology and the enteric nervous system

Peristalsis

The concept of 'The Law of the Intestine' proposed by Bayliss and Starling in 1899 was the first description of the physiology of peristalsis. They studied the effect of placing a bolus of material in the lumen of the *in vivo* canine intestine, and showed that it stimulated a wave of contraction that propelled it aborally along the bowel. From this, they concluded that distending the bowel by a bolus of material produced muscular contraction behind the bolus, and relaxation in front, thus propelling the bolus onwards. Thereby they deduced, correctly, that the nerves responsible for peristalsis resided in the gut wall.

It is now clear that the circuitry for the peristaltic reflex resides within the intrinsic intramural plexuses. The digestive tube peristaltic machinery is functionally composed of a series of overlapping segments, each containing the primary afferents, efferents, and interneurons required for peristalsis. These neuronal networks are connected by 'forward feed' neurons to the adjacent functional segment, so that a bolus can be passed from segment to segment.

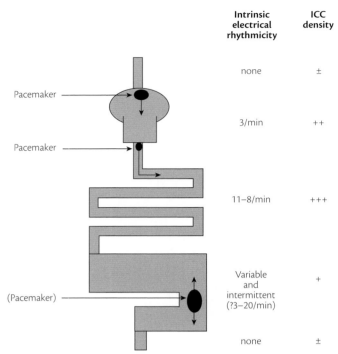

	Intrinsic electrical rhythmicity	ICC density
Pacemaker	none	±
Pacemaker	3/min	++
	11–8/min	+++
(Pacemaker)	Variable and intermittent (?3–20/min)	+
	none	±

Fig. 27.3 Electrical rhythmicity of different regions of the gut, and the associated density of distribution of interstitial cells of Cajal (ICC).

The timing of peristalsis is dictated by the electrical rhythmicity of the smooth muscle layers, the frequency of which varies from region to region. It was originally believed that the regular electrical oscillation of depolarization and repolarization in the muscle layer reflected the biological properties of the smooth muscle cells, but it is now clear that the oscillation frequency is provided by specialized cells in the musculature known as the interstitial cells of Cajal and which act as an interface between the motor nerves and the smooth muscle.

In the proximal intestine the frequency of the pacemaker would permit at least 12 opportunities for contraction every minute. If this happened, 12 peristaltic waves would sweep through the entire bowel in a couple of minutes. As this does not happen, it can be deduced that the motor neural input into the smooth muscle is largely *inhibitory*. Discrete motor programmes that have specific functions in delaying transit, and mixing luminal content to allow digestion, absorption, and storage to take place, confer this inhibition.

The migrating motor complex

The real time recording of pressure transients with intraluminal sensors is now an established clinical technique in the oesophagus and small bowel. In these regions, contractions of the gut wall occlude the lumen, and are easily detected by force transducers placed within the lumen. Digital electronic technology permits continuous recording from multiple sensors for 24 hours or more, and miniature data loggers enable data capture in ambulant subjects (Lindberg et al. 1990). This has enabled the documentation of periodic activity and circadian variations in the integrated motor patterns of the gut.

V.N. Boldyreff, who was one of Pavlov's research students, was the first to describe the 'periodic' nature of motor activity in the fasting gut at the beginning of the 20th century (Wingate 1981). J.H. Szurszewski described a regular period variation of motor activity in the canine small bowel that migrated slowly along the length of the bowel (Szurszewski 1969). The concept was further refined in the next few years, and the periodic sequence was divided into three successive phases (Code and Marlett 1975). In Phase I, there is no contractile activity. In phase II, contractile activity is sporadic. Phase III is the most easily identified by pressure manometry; it consists of a sequence of contractions, each one linked to successive electrical slow waves, that lasts for 3–8 minutes. In terms of neural input into the smooth muscle, Phase I represents a period of maximal inhibition, while Phase III represents the complete removal of inhibition. Collectively, the three phases are known as the migrating motor complex (MMC), and if the activity of the gut is recorded from sensors the MMC appears to migrate along the entire length of the intestine (Fig. 27.4), although individual contractions of course do not. The period between each phase of the MMC cycle is about 90 minutes, although this is extremely variable (Thompson et al. 1980), and the migration velocity, again variable, is in the order of 5 centimetres per minute.

The MMC is the most clearly defined integrated motor programme attributable to the ENS. The evidence for this can be summarized briefly, as follows:

- MMC activity is invariably **present** in the undamaged *in vivo* gut (Fig. 27.5a).

- Phase III is **abnormal** in enteric neuropathy (e.g. Chagas' disease [Fig. 27.5]) and **absent** in the rare condition of visceral aganglionosis.

- MMC activity is **preserved** in small bowel transplantation in which, of necessity, all extrinsic neurons are sectioned (Wallin et al. 1992).

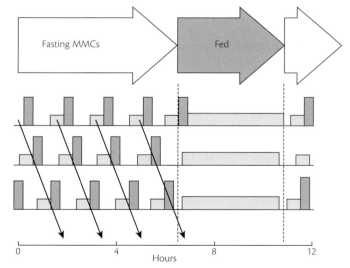

Fig. 27.4 Summary of the intensity of physiological small bowel motor activity at three different sites over 12 hours that include one meal. Low shaded areas represent the irregular activity of Phase II, and vertical bars the regular contractile activity of Phase III. This illustrates the periodic repetition of fasting activity as a motor complex, and the apparent migration down the bowel. Regular periodicity of the MMC, as depicted here, is commonly seen in laboratory animals under controlled conditions, but in man, the periodicity of the MMC is very variable between and within subjects.

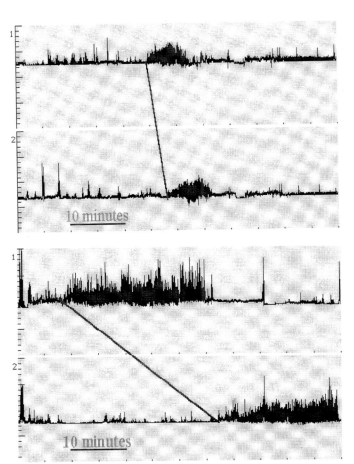

Fig. 27.5 **(a)** The characteristic cluster of regular contractions marking Phase III of the migrating motor complex recorded in a healthy adult at two sites 15 cm apart in the proximal small bowel. The diagonal line illustrates the aboral migration along the bowel. At each recording site, Phase III is preceded by the irregular contractions of Phase II. The motor quiescence of Phase I that follows Phase III is readily apparent in this recording in an ambulant subject, but the deflections that follow Phase III are simultaneous at each recording site, indicating that these are due to changes in intra-abdominal pressure caused by body movements. **(b)** A similar recording in a patient suffering from Chagas' disease (courtesy D.L. Wingate). Note the prolongation of the clustered contractions. The decreased slope of the diagonal line illustrates the reduced velocity of aboral migration.

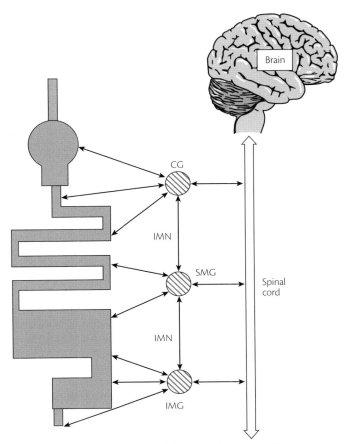

Fig. 27.6 Schematic representation of the prevertebral ganglia (CG, coeliac ganglion; SMG, superior mesenteric ganglion; IMG, inferior mesenteric ganglion) and the intermesenteric nerves (IMN). This illustrates not only the path of spinal autonomic nerves, but also the route through the intermesenteric nerves that enables the rapid transmission of information between remote areas of the bowel.

In man, the MMC appears to be important in preventing the retrograde spread of colonic bacteria (Vantrappen et al. 1977, Kellow 1987). Clinically, the MMC is the major indicator of the integrity of the ENS.

Extrinsic innervation: the prevertebral ganglia

The three prevertebral ganglia—coeliac, superior mesenteric, and inferior mesenteric (Fig. 27.6)—are anatomically separate from the gut and can be considered primarily as relay stations for sympathetic fibres running between gut and spinal cord. Additionally, however, they function as relay stations, for the rapid transmission of information between remote areas of the gut, mediating intestino-intestinal reflexes (Kreulen et al. 1979) and the induction of ileus throughout the gut in response to local injury.

Extrinsic innervation: the gut-brain-gut pathways

The conventional view of the extrinsic innervation of the gut is that it is comprised of parasympathetic and sympathetic efferent neurons, and is therefore mainly a system which modulates motor activity. This is now known to be erroneous (Aziz and Thompson 1998). Most extrinsic fibres are afferent, and serve to continually transmit information to the CNS on the functional status of the digestive tract. The extrinsic innervation therefore forms a functional 'gut-brain-gut axis' (Fig. 27.7).

Afferent innervation: gut to brain pathways

The sensory information is conveyed to the CNS via two anatomically and functionally distinct pathways, vagal and spinal pathways.

Vagal innervation conveys physiological information to the CNS from mucosal receptors that are touch and chemosensitive, and nerve endings that encode stretch, presumably as a result of mural deformation. Vagal innervation of the gut extends down to the mid colon and synapse in the dorsal vagal complex in the brain stem. The pattern of afferent traffic in the vagus encodes the physiological state within the gut, in particular the presence or absence of food. Healthy humans do not normally perceive the types of stimuli that

The autonomic nervous system: The gut-brain-gut axis

Parasympathetic		Sympathetic	
Vagus nerves *Pelvic nerves*		*Spinal cord*	
Afferent	Efferent	Afferent	Efferent
Physiological stimuli	*Excitatory*	*Noxious stimuli*	*Inhibitory*
• Mucosal touch	to motor and exocrine function	• Excess distention	to motor and exocrine function
• Muscle tension		• Ischaemia	
• Luminal content		• Mucosal damage	

Fig. 27.7 Summary of the parasympathetic and sympathetic systems that link the central and enteric nervous systems.

alter vagal input to the brainstem, implying that the input does not—at least in health—reach the cerebral cortex (Fig. 27.8) although brainstem signals do ascend to the hypothalamus to influence hunger/feeding behaviour.

Spinal afferents mediate conscious stimuli and nociception. The nerve endings are located on the mesenteric surface of the bowel, and respond primarily to distension of the gut wall and its metabolic state, particularly acidosis. They also respond to direct stimulation, and are almost certainly responsible via additional synaptic relay in the prevertebral ganglia for the ileus that follows injury to the bowel. These afferent fibres mediate pain arising in the gut, and, unlike vagal traffic, this information is relayed to the cerebral cortex; positron emission tomography has been used in man to demonstrate cortical activation by painful distension of the gut (Aziz et al. 1995, Silverman et al. 1997). It is plausible that in painful functional disorders of the gut, the threshold of these afferents might be lowered so that they respond to distension levels that are within the physiological range (Aziz et al. 1995).

Efferent innervation: brain to gut pathways

The classic concept of the extrinsic innervation was that it controlled the motor activity of the gut, with the two divisions, parasympathetic and sympathetic, being respectively excitatory and inhibitory

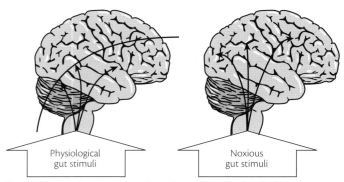

Fig. 27.8 Normally, information relayed from the gut reaches the brainstem, hindbrain, and midbrain, but not the cerebral cortex (left). Noxious stimuli are relayed to the cortex (right).

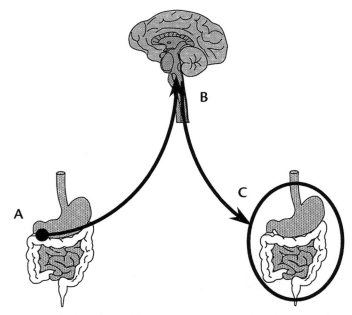

Fig. 27.9 The dependence of the motor response to a meal on the vago-vagal transmission of information. The arrival of a meal in the foregut is detected by gastric and duodenal sensory nerve terminals **(A)** that respond to volume and chemical stimulation, and this information is transmitted to the dorsal vagal complex **(B)**. From there it passes through the efferent vagus to the effector organs of the gut **(C)** initiating a fed pattern of motor activity (Fig. 27.4), increased bile flow, and exocrine pancreatic secretion.

and with acetylcholine and noradrenaline as the respective neurotransmitters. As indicated above, this view is now known to be excessively simplistic.

The contemporary approach to the neural control of the gut is exemplified by one aspect of vagal activity, its role in transforming the function of the upper gut from a fasting to a postprandial pattern. Although the ENS has primary afferent neurons, the sensors that detect the arrival of food in the gut are chemosensitive vagal receptors that have no direct input into the ENS. The arrival of food in the gut is signalled to the ENS by information that is relayed by afferent fibres to the dorsal vagal complex (Ewart and Wingate 1984) and thence by vagal efferent fibres to the ENS (Fig. 27.9). Temporary vagal blockade in conscious dogs causes a reversion from the postprandial pattern to the fasting pattern, and this effect is abolished when the vagal blockade is removed (Chung and Diamant 1987). Patients who were deliberately submitted to truncal vagotomy for the relief of duodenal ulcer disease or who suffer vagal damage in neurological disease show similar attenuation of the postprandial response, which probably explains the consequent meal-stimulated diarrhoea (Thompson et al. 1982).

Central nervous system control of gut function

The control over the operations of the digestive tract is shared between CNS and ENS (Fig. 27.10). The CNS has a major influence on conscious gut-related behaviour, such as swallowing and defaecation, which require complex body synchronization. For example, the conscious urge to defecate is prompted by a cue from rectal receptors that respond to rectal filling. The decision to defecate is dependent on the conscious perception of a suitable opportunity, and body movements leading to a squatting posture. The actual

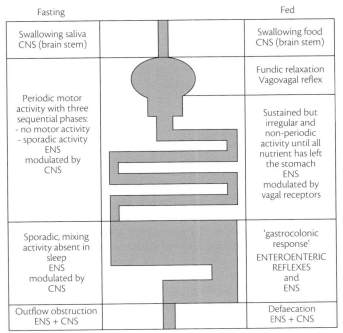

Fasting			Fed
Swallowing saliva CNS (brain stem)			Swallowing food CNS (brain stem)
			Fundic relaxation Vagovagal reflex
Periodic motor activity with three sequential phases: - no motor activity - sporadic activity ENS modulated by CNS			Sustained but irregular and non-periodic activity until all nutrient has left the stomach ENS modulated by vagal receptors
Sporadic, mixing activity absent in sleep ENS modulated by CNS			'gastrocolonic response' ENTEROENTERIC REFLEXES and ENS
Outflow obstruction ENS + CNS			Defaecation ENS + CNS

Fig. 27.10 Summary of the regional motor activity, and the relative control exerted by the central nervous system (CNS) and the enteric nervous system (ENS).

expulsion of stool requires the synergy of pelvic musculature and sphincters with both CNS and ENS input.

The CNS can also modulate those enteric functions that normally lie within the unconscious domain of the ENS. The function of the stomach, small bowel and colon can all be altered under conditions of psychological stress. In this paradigm, the participation of the CNS is essential for the perception of stressors and the subsequent transmission along autonomic pathways (Thompson et al. 1982).

An important advance in the understanding of gut function in recent years has been the development of systems for prolonged monitoring. Miniature strain gauges, digital logging, and computer analysis of large volumes of data are now incorporated into systems that permit continuous observation of different regions of the gut for 24 hours or longer. These studies have revealed a circadian modulation of gut function that is evident in both the small intestine (Fig. 27.11) and the colon. From these studies it can be inferred that it is brain-gut interaction that is being modulated in this way, and that the major influence is CNS arousal (Kumar et al. 1990). During sleep, the small bowel is mostly quiescent, but the regular contractions of Phase III nevertheless remain (Kumar et al. 1989). The colon appears to be virtually inert during sleep, but activity returns on waking (Narducci et al. 1987).

Autonomic dysfunction and the gastrointestinal tract

In the context of gastrointestinal pathology in most of the world, overt autonomic failure of the gut is exceedingly uncommon. Suspected autonomic dysfunction is more common, but the incidence is sporadic, the aetiology is diverse, and there is as yet still no agreed taxonomy.

Clinical descriptions of gut autonomic failure are extensive, but obscured by limited confirmation. The classification of such disorders into 'neuropathy' or 'myopathy' is overly simplistic. Manometric studies that appear to show an inert bowel have been attributed to 'myopathy' (Summers et al. 1983), but may only reflect a dilated bowel, where contractions do not occlude the lumen and are not detected by intraluminal sensors. One useful fact to assist distinction between such disorders is that the neural input to the smooth muscle in the pacemaker-driven regions of the gut is largely inhibitory. Thus enteric neuropathies are generally

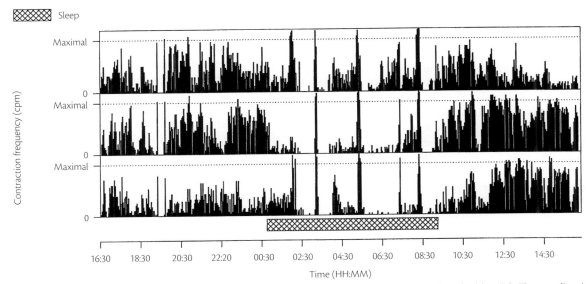

Fig. 27.11 Histogram of the minute by minute incidence of contractions over 24 hours at three sites of the small bowel in a healthy adult. The recording sites were 15 cm proximal to the ligament of Treitz (above), at the ligament of Treitz (centre) and 15 cm distal to it (below). The transient peaks at the maximal contractile frequency (10/minute) mark phase III of the migrating motor complex. During sleep, show as the hatched bar, phase II activity disappears but phase III continues.

marked by an *increase* in contractile activity (Stanghellini et al. 1987). Clinically, increased motor activity is most easily detected during sleep, when the bowel is normally relatively quiescent.

Clinical manifestations of enteric neuropathy

The major clinical manifestation of ENS dysfunction is the condition known as intestinal pseudo-obstruction (Stanghellini et al. 1987). This can be localized, as in achalasia of the cardia and Hirschsprung's disease, or generalized, when the entire bowel is involved. The clinical picture mimics that of mechanical obstruction, with distension, abdominal pain, constipation and vomiting. Often the diagnosis is only achieved after laparotomy fails to identify suspected true obstruction.

Usually, the clinical pattern of pseudo-obstruction is of slow progressive symptom development and patients may remain in a stable condition for prolonged periods. One common consequence of ENS impairment is, as might be predicted, a bacterial overgrowth of the small intestine, a consequence of disturbance of the migrating motor complex which normally maintains the small intestine free of bacteria and prevents the orad migration of colonic flora. When motor patterns are abnormal, this protective mechanism fails, and the small bowel is colonized (Vantrappen et al. 1977). This leads to bacterial metabolism of nutrients and breakdown of bile in the bowel lumen with resulting malabsorption and diarrhoea.

Regional disorders of the enteric nervous system

Achalasia of the cardia is a neuropathy of the lower smooth muscle section of the oesophagus, including the lower oesophageal sphincter, which leads to failure of inhibition of the sphincter and aperistalsis of the oesophageal body. The incidence is said to be about 1 per 100,000 of the population; the true incidence is unknown but certainly higher, as many cases, particularly if the neuropathy is incomplete, remain undiagnosed. The classical presentation is dysphagia due to failure of relaxation of the lower oesophageal sphincter and weakened peristalsis of the lower oesophagus. As the condition advances motor function fails, the oesophagus becomes dilated and meal residues fail to be cleared. Very infrequently, achalasia may be the prodrome of generalized enteric neuropathy. The only treatment for achalasia is to disrupt lower oesophageal sphincter, circumferential rupture by pneumatic dilatation, or by botulinism toxic injection. Surgical myotomy is rarely necessary.

Hirschsprung disease classically presents as childhood constipation due to an aganglionic segment of the colon (Rogawski et al. 1978) producing a functional obstruction to defaecation, and consequent dilatation of the colon proximal to the aperistaltic segment. It normally presents in infancy, symptoms occasionally are delayed into adulthood. The condition occurs as a result of failure of migration of enteric neurons to the entire gastrointestinal tract at the time of gut development, the most distal colon being the most vulnerable region for aganglionosis, hence the clinical presentation. Clinical diagnosis is usually made by demonstrating failure of the normal relaxation of the internal anal sphincter on rectal distension and localized increase of acetylcholinesterase activity in extrinsic nerve fibres in affected tissue on biopsy. Treatment is by resection of the affected area.

Generalized disorders of the enteric nervous system

Worldwide the most common generalized disease of the ENS is *Chagas' disease*, also known as South American trypanosomiasis. At the present time, there are an estimated 10 million patients still suffering from the disease despite major improvements in public health and reduction in its incidence. The causative pathogen is the protozoan parasite *Trypanosoma cruzii*, but the clinical manifestation is in fact the result of autoimmune disease. The vector is the Reduvid beetle that normally lives in unplastered walls. When the beetle bites a victim, it also defecates on the lesion so expelling the parasite. Rubbing the lesion ensures the introduction of the trypanosome into the blood stream.

The neuropathic stage of the disease starts with the production of anti-trypanosomal antibodies, which cross-react with a surface antigen on autonomic neuronal cell bodies (dos Santos et al. 1979) and it is this antibody-antigen fusion that induces the neuropathy. Clinically the gastrointestinal manifestations are of oesophageal and colonic failure. The presentation is often identical to that of achalasia of the cardia, with dysphagia, oesophageal dilatation, and eventually the aspiration of retained food. Megacolon also occurs, presenting with distension and constipation. Clinical small bowel involvement is a late manifestation and marked by distension and diarrhoea due to bacterial overgrowth (Aprile et al. 1995) consequent upon damage to the myenteric plexus in the small bowel (Costa and Alcantagar 1966). No important abnormality of gastric emptying has been demonstrated, although some changes can be found (Troncon and Iazigi 1992).

As might be expected, in the small intestine the pathophysiology is an abnormality of the MMC. Phase III is prolonged in duration from about 6 minutes to as much as 20 minutes, and the velocity with which it appears to migrate along the bowel is about 25% of the normal velocity (Fig 27.5).

With the exception of Chagas' disease, clinical enteric neuropathy is not only very uncommon but also its manifestations are diverse. The commonest age of presentation is in infancy or childhood (Hyman et al. 1988, Fell et al. 1996). Familial cases occur (Camilleri et al. 1991), but most appear to be isolated. In adults, enteric neuropathies are most commonly found in association with small cell bronchial carcinoma (Chinn and Schuffler 1988, Sodhi et al. 1989) and, as in Chagas' disease, appear to be the manifestation of an autoimmune process associated with circulating anti-neuronal (anti-Hu) antibodies (Smith et al. 1997). Histological confirmation of the diagnosis was usually lacking because it requires a full-thickness small bowel biopsy, but this is now possible with the advent of laparoscopic techniques. Antroduodenal (Hyman et al. 1988) or small bowel manometry (Quigley et al. 1997) shows evidence of enteric neuronal dysfunction, supporting the view that there is a stereotypic disruption of the small bowel fasting motility programme in enteric neuropathy.

Management of patients with pseudo-obstruction as a result of enteric neuropathy is difficult. Resection of 'non-functioning bowel' should only be undertaken with caution and after much thought; the neuropathy is usually more extensive than clinical evidence would suggest and the consequences of reconstructing the bowel are difficult to predict. Malnutrition is the major problem; and long-term parenteral nutrition is often required. Pain is a frequent problem, probably due to intestinal distension, as a result of propulsive dysfunction and opiate analgesia is often used, but this in turn worsens the propulsive failure. 'Prokinetic' drugs, such as substituted benzamides, are usually of little help. Small bowel transplantation is now a treatment option, but only as a last resort and in those in whom parenteral nutrition is, for whatever reason, impossible to initiate or no longer possible to maintain.

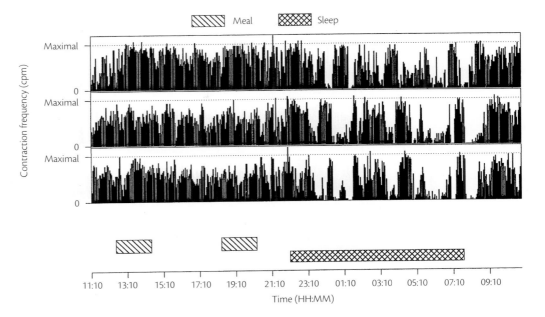

Fig. 27.12 Histogram of small bowel motor activity in a 28-year-old woman suffering from a familial enteric neuropathy. Compared with a healthy individual (see Fig. 27.11), there is an overall increase in the incidence of contractions, while the nocturnal Phase III peaks of maximal activity are prolonged in duration, and migrate more slowly. The motor abnormalities in this patient are identical with those found in Chagas' disease (see Fig. 27.5b).

Parkinson's disease is often complicated by gastrointestinal symptoms, particularly constipation. This was originally attributed to the side-effects of medication, but it now seems that the disease can also directly involve the ENS; Loewy bodies have been identified in the myenteric plexus of the oesophagus and colon (Kupsky et al. 1987).

Disorders of extrinsic innervation

There is little doubt that the gastrointestinal tract is disturbed in widespread dysautonomia syndromes. In severe Type 1 diabetes, gastroparesis-diminished gastric motor activity with consequent stasis—is common (Ewing and Clarke 1986) and is one of the early manifestations of diabetic autonomic neuropathy (Reid et al. 1992), even though it is often asymptomatic and only detected by gamma scintigraphy. In any Type 1 diabetic who complains of epigastric fullness, nausea, and vomiting, it is likely that the deficit is in the emptying of solids (Dooley et al. 1988); due to both diminished motor activity in the gastric antrum, and to the absence of gastric MMC activity. Gastric MMCs are required to empty solid residues; in diabetic gastroparesis, these accumulate and can lead to the formation of bezoars. Gastroparesis also makes diabetic control more difficult, furthermore hyperglycaemia itself exacerbates gastroparesis. Therapy is primarily directed towards better diabetic control. Drug treatment of delayed gastric emptying has been shown to confer some benefit (Annese et al. 1997), in particular with the macrolide antibiotic erythromycin (Tack et al. 1992), which attaches to motilin receptors in the stomach and duodenum and stimulates the genesis of MMC activity. The benefit is usually short-lived, however, due to tachyphylaxis, but it does provide an opportunity to improve diabetic control. The 'diabetic bowel' is a well-known phenomenon, marked by chronic diarrhoea and evidence of small intestinal bacterial overgrowth (Rosa-e-Silva et al. 1996). The nature of the bowel neuropathy, that is likely to be the cause of the problem remains uncertain (Yoshida et al. 1988).

In the primary 'idiopathic' autonomic failure syndromes, such as multiple system atrophy, there is widespread involvement of gut function (Camilleri et al. 1990) although precise data, especially on motility, are few (Suarez et al. 1994).

Other disorders

Several of the maladies of unknown nature that present with abdominal symptoms and are currently entitled 'functional disorders' may prove to be neuropathic. Of particular interest in this respect, not least because of its high prevalence, is irritable bowel syndrome. Progress has been hampered by the absence of an objective marker for the syndrome; the diagnosis at present depends upon the clinician's judgment of whether a combination of symptoms falls within the diagnostic category. About one quarter of all cases are reported to be the sequel of an acute gastroenteritis (McKendrick and Read 1994), and there is accumulating evidence that one component of its pathology may be a mild sensory neuropathy with a lowered sensory threshold of visceral afferents and exaggerated visceral perception in the central nervous system (Mertz et al. 1995). Concomitant motor response abnormalities have been shown in small bowel motor activity (Fig. 27.13) and colon (Kumar and Wingate 1985, Kellow et al. 1988, Narducci et al. 1985), and increased cortical representation of gastrointestinal signals has been reported (Silverman et al. 1997).

Conclusion

Our concepts of gut autonomic neural physiology have now advanced to provide a clearer understanding of its extrinsic control and the autonomy of the ENS. Clinically, specific types of dysfunction probably exist according to the neuronal population affected but, with the exception of Chagas' disease, there is still little information. The development of newer brain imaging techniques which permit *in vivo* analysis of intact man, together with easier access to biopsy material should now lead to a more rational classification of gut dysautonomia and the development of clearer management protocols.

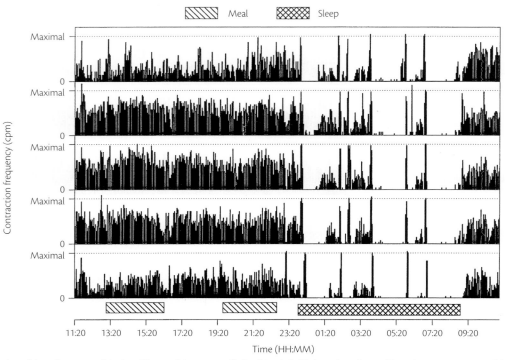

Fig. 27.13 Histogram of small bowel motor activity in a 42-year-old woman suffering from irritable bowel syndrome. Note the excess motor activity during the day and the normal activity during sleep.

References

Annese, V., Lombardi. G., Frusciante, V., Germani, U., Andriulli, A., Bassotti, G. (1997). Cisapride and erythromycin prokinetic effects in gastroparesis due to type 1 (insulin-dependent) diabetes mellitus. *Aliment Pharmacol. Ther.* **11**, 599–603.

Aprile, L. R., Troncon, L. E., Meneghelli, U. G., de Oliveira, R. B. (1995). [Small bowel bacterial overgrowth syndrome in chagasic megajejunum: report of 2 cases (see comments)]. [Portuguese]. *Arquivos de Gastroenterologia* **32**, 71–8.

Aziz, Q., Furlong, P. L., Barlow, J., *et al.* (1995). Topographic mapping of cortical potentials evoked by distension of the human proximal and distal oesophagus. *Electroencephalography & Clinical Neurophysiology* **96**, 219–28.

Aziz, Q., Thompson, D.G. (1998). Brain-gut axis in health and disease. *Gastroenterology* **114**, 559–78.

Bass, P. (1997). Electric activity of smooth muscle in the gastrointestinal tract. *Gastroenterology* **49**, 391–4.

Burnstock, G., Campbell, G., Satchell, D., Smythe, A. (1970). Evidence that adenosine triphosphate or a related nucleotide is the transmitter substance released by non-adrenergic inhibitory nerves in the gut. *Br. J Pharmacol.* **40**, 668–88.

Camilleri, M., Fealey, R. D. (1990). Idiopathic autonomic denervation in eight patients presenting with functional gastrointestinal disease. A causal association? *Dig. Dis. Sci.* **35**, 609–16.

Camilleri, M., Carbone, L. D., Schuffler, M. D. (1991). Familial enteric neuropathy with pseudoobstruction. *Dig. Dis. Sci.* **36**, 1168–71.

Chinn, J. S., Schuffler, M. D. (1988). Paraneoplastic visceral neuropathy as a cause of severe gastrointestinal motor dysfunction. *Gastroenterology* **95**, 1279–86.

Chung, S. A., Diamant, N. E. (1987). Small intestinal motility in fasted and ostprandial states: effect of transient vagosympathetic blockade. *Am. J Physiol.* **252**, G301–8.

Code, C. F., Marlett, J. A. (1975). The interdigestive myo-electric complex of the stomach and small bowel of dogs. *J Physiol. (Lond)* **246**, 289–309.

Costa, R. D., Alcantagar, F. G. de (1966). [Submucous and myenteric plexuses of the human ileum in Chagas' disease]. [Portuguese]. *Revista Brasileira de Medicina* **23**, 399–400.

Dooley, C. P., el Newihi, H. M., Zeidler, A., Valenzuela, J. E. (1988). Abnormalities of the migrating motor complex in diabetics with autonomic neuropathy and diarrhea. *Scand. J Gastroenterol.* **23**, 217–23.

Ewart, W. R., Wingate, D. L. (1984). Central representation of arrival of nutrient in the duodenum. *Am. J Physiol.* **246**, G750–6.

Ewing, D. J., Clarke, B. F. (1986). Autonomic neuropathy: its diagnosis and prognosis. *Clin. Endocrinol. Metab.* **15**, 855–88.

Fell, J. M., Smith, V. V., Milla, P. J. (1996). Infantile chronic idiopathic intestinal pseudo-obstruction: the role of small intestinal manometry as a diagnostic tool and prognostic indicator. *Gut* **39**, 306–11.

Goodrich, J.T., Bernd, P., Sherman, B., Gershon, M. D. (1980). Phylogeny of enteric serotonergic neurons. *J Comp. Neurol.* **190**, 15–28.

Grundy, D., Enck, P., Wood, J. D. (1996). Little brain—big brain. IV: Munich, 30 October to 3 November 1995. *Neugastroenterol Motil* **8**, 153–5.

Hyman, P. E., McDiarmid, S. V., Napolitano, J., Abrams, C. E., Tomomasa, T. (1988). Antroduodenal motility in children with chronic intestinal pseudo-obstruction. *J Pediatr.* **112**, 899–905.

Kellow, J. E., Gill, R. C., Wingate, D. L. (1987). Modulation of human upper gastrointestinal motility by rectal distension. *Gut* **28**, 864–8.

Kellow, J. E., Phillips, S. F., Miller, L. J., Zinsmeister, A. R. (1988). Dysmotility of the small intestine in irritable bowel syndrome. *Gut* **29**, 1236–43.

Kreulen, D. L., Szurszewski, J. H. (1979). Reflex pathways in the abdominal prevertebral ganglia: evidence for a colo-colonic inhibitory reflex. *J Physiol. (Lond)* **295**, 21–32.

Kumar, D., Soffer, E. E., Wingate, D. L., Britto, J., Das-Gupta, A., Mridha, K. (1989). Modulation of the duration of human postprandial motor activity by sleep *Am. J Physiol.* **256**, G851–5.

Kumar, D., Thompson, P. D., Wingate, D. L. (1990). Absence of synchrony between human small intestinal migrating motor complex and rectalmotor complex. *Am. J Physiol.* **258**, G171–2.

Kumar, D., Wingate, D. L. (1985). The irritable bowel syndrome: a paroxysmal motor disorder. *Lancet* **2**, 973–7.

Kupsky, W. J., Grimes, M. M., Sweeting, J., Bertsch, R., Cote, L. J. (1987) Parkinson's disease and megacolon: concentric hyaline inclusions (Lewy bodies) inenteric ganglion cells. *Neurology* **37**, 1253–5.

Lindberg, G., Iwarzon, M., Stal, P., Seensalu. R. (1990). Digital ambulatory monitoring of small-bowel motility. *Scand. J Gastroenterol.* **25**, 216–24.

McKendrick, M. W., Read, N. W. (1994). Irritable bowel syndrome—post salmonella infection. *J Infect.* **29**, 1–3.

Mertz, H., Naliboff, B., Munakata, J., Niazi, N., Mayer, E. A. (1995). Altered rectal perception is a biological marker of patients with irritable bowel syndrome [published erratum appears in *Gastroenterology* (1997) 113, 1054]. *Gastroenterology* **109**, 40–52.

Narducci, F., Bassotti, G., Gaburri, M., Morelli, A. (1987). Twenty four hour manometric recording of colonic motor activity in healthy man. *Gut* **28**, 17–25.

Narducci, F., Snape, W. J. J., Battle, W. M., London, R. L., Cohen, S. (1985). Increased colonic motility during exposure to a stressful situation. *Di.g Dis. Sci.* **30**, 40–4.

Quigley, E. M., Deprez, P. H., Hellstrom P., *et al.* (1997). Ambulatory intestinal manometry: a consensus report on its clinical role. *Dig. Dis. Sci.* **42**, 2395–400.

Reid, B., DiLorenzo, C., Travis, L., Flores, A. F., Grill, B. B., Hyman, P. E. (1992). Diabetic gastroparesis due to postprandial antral hypomotility in childhood. *Pediatrics* **90**, 43–6.

Ribeiro dos Santos, R., Marquez, J. O., Von Gal Furtado, C. C., Ramos de Oliveira, J. C., Martins, A. R., Koberle, F. (1979). Antibodies against neurons in chronic Chagas' disease. *Tropenmedizin und Parasitologie* **30**, 19–23.

Rogawski, M. A., Goodrich, J. T., Gershon, M. D., Touloukian, R. J. (1978). Hirschsprung's disease: absence of serotonergic neurons in the aganglionic colon. *J Pediatr. Surg.* **13**, 608–15.

Rosa-e-Silva, L., Troncon, L. E., Oliveira, R. B., Fossa, M. C., Braga, F. J., Gallo Junior, L. (1996) Rapid distal small bowel transit associated with sympathetic denervation in type I diabetes mellitus *Gut* **39**, 748–56.

Silverman, D. H., Munakata, J. A., Ennes, H., Mandelkern, M. A., Hoh, C. K., Mayer, E. A. (1997). Regional cerebral activity in normal and pathological perception of visceral pain. *Gastroenterology* **112**, 64–72.

Smith, V. V., Gregson, N., Foggensteiner, L., Neale, G., Milla, P. J. (1997). Acquired intestinal aganglionosis and circulating autoantibodies without neoplasia or other neural involvement. *Gastroenterology* **112**, 1366–71.

Sodhi, N., Camilleri, M., Camoriano, J. K., Low, P. A., Fealey, R. D., Perry, M. C. (1989). Autonomic function and motility in intestinal pseudoobstruction caused by paraneoplastic syndrome. *Dig. Dis. Sci.* **34**, 1937–42.

Stanghellini, V., Camilleri, M., Malagelada, J. R. (1987). Chronic idiopathic intestinal pseudo-obstruction: clinical and intestinal manometric findings. *Gut* **28**, 5–12.

Suarez, G. A., Fealey, R. D., Camilleri, M. (1994). Idiopathic autonomic neuropathy: clinical, neurophysiologic, and follow-up studies on 27 patients. *Neurology* **44**, 1675–82.

Summers, R. W., Anuras, S., Green, J. (1983). Jejunal manometry patterns in health, partial intestinal obstruction, and pseudoobstruction. *Gastroenterology* **85**, 1290–1300.

Szurszewski, J. H. (1969). A migrating electric complex of canine small intestine. *Am. J Physiol.* **217**, 1757–63.

Szurszewski, J. H., Elveback, L. R., Code, C. F. (1970). Configuration and frequency gradient of electric slow wave over canine small bowel. *Am. J Physiol.* **218**, 1468–73.

Tack, J., Janssens, J., Vantrappen, G., *et al.* (1992). Effect of erythromycin on gastric motility in controls and in diabetic gastroparesis. *Gastroenterology* **103**, 72–9.

Thompson, D. G., Ritchie, H. D., Wingate, D. L. (1982). Patterns of small intestinal motility in duodenal ulcer patients before and after vagotomy. *Gut* **23**, 517–23.

Thompson, D. G., Wingate, D. L., Archer, L., Benson, M. J., Green, W. J., Hardy, R. J. (1980). Normal patterns of human upper small bowel motor activity recorded by prolonged radiotelemetry. *Gut* **21**, 500–6.

Troncon, L. E., Iazigi, N. (1992). Scintigraphic study of the gastrointestinal transit of a liquid meal in patients with chronic Chagas' disease. *Braz. J Med. Biol. Re.s* **25**, 145–8.

Vantrappen, G., Janssens, J., Hellemans, J., Ghoos, Y. (1977). The interdigestive motor complex of normal subjects and patients with bacterial overgrowth of the small intestine. *J Clin. Invest.* **59**, 1158–66.

Wallin, C., Engqvist, A., Lindberg, G., Veress, B., Reichard, H. (1992). Transplantation of the small intestine can be suitable in patients with pseudoobstruction. *Lakartidningen* **89**, 309–10.

Wingate, D. L. (1981). Backwards and forwards with the migrating complex. *Dig. Dis. Sci.* **26**, 641–66.

Yoshida, M. M., Schuffler, M. D., Sumi, S. M. (1988). There are no morphologic abnormalities of the gastric wall or abdominal vagus in patients with diabetic gastroparesis. *Gastroenterology* **94**, 907–14.

CHAPTER 28

Postprandial hypotension in autonomic disorders

Christopher J. Mathias and Karen Jones

Introduction

It is now recognized that postprandial hypotension occurs frequently and represents a generally underestimated source of morbidity (and possibly mortality) in patients with autonomic disorders, as well as apparently 'healthy' elderly and nursing home residents. In normal subjects, food ingestion results in a number of hormonal, neural, and regional haemodynamic changes, and the release of a variety of pancreatic and gastrointestinal peptides may affect the cardiovascular system either directly or indirectly through modulation of autonomic nervous activity. Following a meal there is a substantial redistribution of blood into the splanchnic circulation as splanchnic blood flow increases to ~20% of total blood volume (Jansen and Lipsitz 1995). In healthy, young subjects the postprandial increase in splanchnic flow is compensated for by compensatory increases in heart rate and sympathetic activity so that there is little, if any, change in systemic blood pressure (Jansen and Lipsitz 1995). In contrast, in patients with disturbances of autonomic function, ingestion of food may frequently lower blood pressure substantially.

Postprandial hypotension as a clinical problem was first reported by Seyer-Hansen (1977) in a 65-year-old man with autonomic failure and parkinsonism, who suffered from meal-related symptoms of severe dizziness and visual disturbance and in whom hypotension could be provoked by oral glucose. Studies by Robertson et al. (1981), in a group of patients with autonomic dysfunction, confirmed a profound fall in both systolic and diastolic blood pressure after food ingestion. In these studies, the patients were seated and it was unclear to what degree the upright posture contributed to the hypotension.

Postprandial hypotension, currently defined as a fall in systolic blood pressure of > 20 mmHg, occurring within 2 hours of a meal, or a decrease in blood pressure < 90 mmHg when the baseline blood pressure is ≥ 100 mmHg (Mathias 1991, Jansen and Lipsitz 1995, Jansen et al. 1995) can be a major clinical problem in some patients with autonomic failure (Vloet et al. 2005, Jansen et al. 1995, Fisher et al. 2005). In this chapter the pathophysiology of postprandial hypotension, particularly neural, haemodynamic, gastrointestinal, humoral, and biochemical mechanisms, will be initially discussed, followed by current approaches to management of this condition.

Haemodynamic responses to food ingestion

In normal subjects, food ingestion in either the seated or the supine position usually causes minimal, or no, change in blood pressure. When given a standardized meal (450 kcal, containing carbohydrate, protein, and fat) in the supine position, there is a modest rise in heart rate together with an elevation in stroke volume and cardiac output (Mathias et al. 1989a). Forearm muscle blood flow falls, reflecting an elevation in forearm vascular resistance. There are no changes in the cutaneous circulation. There is a fall in calculated peripheral vascular resistance (Fig. 28.1a), presumably because of a large increase in splanchnic blood flow, as has been demonstrated by non-invasive measurements of a major splanchnic vessel, the superior mesenteric artery (Fig. 28.1b). Plasma noradrenaline levels rise, indicative of an overall increase in sympathetic nervous activity, while there are no changes in plasma adrenaline levels (Kooner et al. 1989). Plasma renin activity levels double. There is an increase in muscle sympathetic nerve activity, as measured by microneurographic techniques, after ingestion of a nutrient such as glucose (Berne et al. 1989) (Fig. 28.2). Studies using noradrenaline spillover techniques indicate that skeletal muscle and the kidneys are major sites of sympathetic activation postprandially, while cardiac spillover is unaltered (Cox et al. 1995) (Fig. 28.3). Hence, it appears that the nervous and endocrine systems, among others, exert multiple adjustments that result in the maintenance of blood pressure in normal individuals.

In patients with autonomic failure, even in the supine position, there is a substantial fall in blood pressure that occurs within 10–15 minutes of meal ingestion, reaching a nadir within 60 minutes (Fig. 28.4). There are usually modest, or no, changes in heart rate, particularly if there is associated cardiac parasympathetic denervation. Superior mesenteric artery blood flow rises to a comparable extent to that in normal subjects, but there are no changes in blood flow to the skin and forearm vasculature, and no significant increase in cardiac output, indicative of impairment in the haemodynamic adjustments required to counteract splanchnic vasodilatation (Mathias et al. 1989a, Kooner et al. 1990). In patients with multiple system atrophy (MSA) and postprandial hypotension, oral glucose fails to decrease calf venous capacitance when compared with patients without postprandial hypotension or healthy controls, a potential factor contributing to postprandial

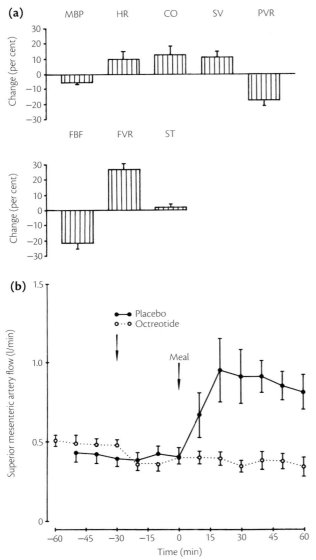

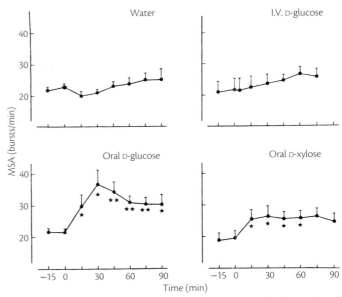

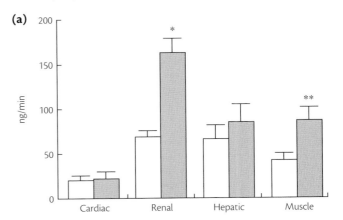

Fig. 28.2 Muscle nerve sympathetic activity (MNSA) expressed as the number of bursts per minute in normal subjects after ingestion of either 300 ml of water orally, D-glucose (0.35 g/kg body weight i.v.), 100 g of D-glucose and 75.6 g of D-xylose orally, * $p < 0.05$; ** $p < 0.01$. With permission from Berne, C., Fagius, J., and Niklasson, F. (1989) *J. Clin. Invest.* **84**, 1403–9.

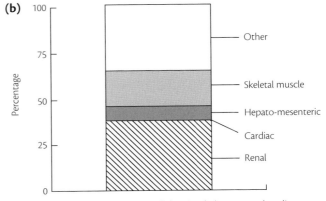

Fig. 28.1 (a) Maximum percentage change in mean blood pressure (MBP), heart rate (HR), cardiac output (CO), stroke volume (SV), calculated peripheral vascular resistance (PVR), forearm muscle blood flow (FBF), calculated forearm vascular resistance (FVR), and skin temperature to the index finger (ST) in six normal subjects in the first hour after food ingestion. Vertical bars indicate ± SEM. **(b)** Superior mesenteric artery blood flow in normal subjects before and after a balanced liquid meal, when given either saline placebo (continuous line, filled circles) or 50 g of octreotide (dotted line, open circles), both subcutaneously. Kooner, J. S., Peart, W. S., and Mathias, C. J. (1989). The peptide release inhibitor Octreotide (SMS 201-995), prevents the haemodynamic changes following food ingestion in normal human subjects. Q. *J. Exp. Physiol.* **74**, 569–72, with permission from Wiley.

Fig. 28.3 (a) Preprandial and postprandial regional plasma noradrenaline spillover, indicating sympathetic nervous system activation in normal subjects. The open histograms indicate the values while fasting, and the filled histograms postprandially, in different vascular beds. The percentage changes are indicated in **(b)**. There is greater activation in the renal and skeletal muscle vasculature than in cardiac or hepatic regions. Reprinted from *J. Autonom. Nerv. Syst.* **56**, Vaz, M., Cox, H. S., Kaye, D. M., Turner, A. G., Jennings, G. L., and Esler, M. D. Fallibility of plasma noradrenaline measurements in studying postprandial sympathetic nervous responses, 97–104, Copyright 1995, with permission from Elsevier.

hypotension (Takamori et al. 2007). Plasma noradrenaline and adrenaline levels remain unchanged, consistent with the inability of these patients to activate the sympathetic nervous system. Postural change after food ingestion often results in a fall in blood pressure to even lower levels and has the capacity to enhance symptoms of impaired cerebral perfusion markedly (Mathias et al. 1991). While orthostatic hypotension has been considered a risk factor for postprandial hypotension, it is now recognized that the two disorders are additive rather than synergistic (Maurer et al. 2000).

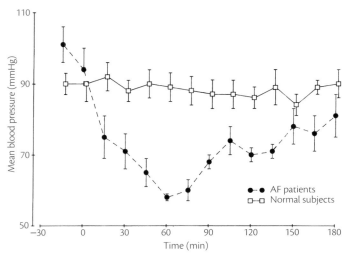

Fig. 28.4 Percentage change in mean blood pressure in a group of patients with chronic autonomic failure (dashed line, filled circles) and in normal subjects (continuous line, open squares) before and after food ingestion at time 0. The bars indicate means ± SEM. Reprinted from *J. Neurol. Sci.*, **94**, Mathias, C. J., Da Costa, D. F., Fosbraey, P., et al. Cardiovascular, biochemical and hormonal changes during food induced hypotension in chronic autonomic failure, 255–69, Copyright 1989, with permission from Elsevier.

The magnitude of the postprandial fall in systolic blood pressure appears to be greater in pure autonomic failure (PAF) than in MSA (Mathias et al. 1991) (Fig. 28.5). Whether this reflects differences in the lesion (peripheral in PAF and central in MSA), a differential ability to release vasodilatatory and vasoconstrictor substances, or supersensitivity of target organs to vasoactive substances, remains uncertain. The severity of the autonomic lesion may be of importance; thus in

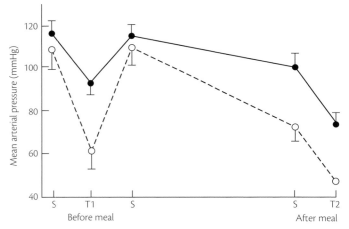

Fig. 28.5 Average levels of mean arterial blood pressure (with standard error of mean) in patients with multiple system atrophy (MSA, ●—●) and pure autonomic failure (PAF, ○—○) before a meal while supine (S) and during head-up tilt to 45° (T1), while supine for 45 minutes postprandially, and before and during retilting (T2 on right, after meal). There is a greater postprandial fall in blood pressure while supine in PAF. After the meal the blood pressure falls to lower levels in both MSA and PAF. The lower pressure, and presumed reduction in cerebral perfusion, is likely to account for the increase in postural symptoms after a meal. Reproduced from *J. Neurol. Neurosurg. Psychiat.*, Mathias, C. J., Holly, E., Armstrong, E., Shareef, M., and Bannister, R., **54**, 726–30, 1991, with permission from BMJ Publishing Group Ltd.

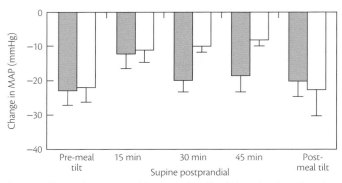

Fig. 28.6 Changes in mean arterial pressure (MAP) + SEM on head-up tilt and after standard liquid meal ingestion in two subgroups with multiple system atrophy, the cerebellar (MSA-C) (filled histograms) and the parkinsonian (MSA-P) (open histograms). The difference between the groups while supine postprandially was significant at 30 and 45 minutes. Although there is less supine postprandial hypotension in MSA-P, the postural fall was similar in both groups pre- and post-meal. Reprinted from *Parkinsonism Relat Disord*, **4**, Smith GD, Von Der Thusen J, and Mathias CJ. Comparison of the blood pressure response to food in two clinical subgroups of multiple system atrophy (Shy-Drager syndrome), 113–117, copyright 1998, with permission from Elsevier.

MSA, where the disorder is progressive, autonomic nervous system impairment may be less severe later in the course of the disease, which may account for the difference from PAF; longitudinal studies evaluating postprandial blood pressure as the disease in MSA progresses have hitherto not been described. There also appear to be differential responses to food ingestion within the MSA groups so that the cerebellar form has a greater degree of supine postprandial hypotension than the parkinsonian form (Fig. 28.6) (von der Thusen et al. 1996); this may be related to differences in the central autonomic areas affected in these groups. In the cerebellar form of MSA, where the lesions are more rostral, in addition to neurons affecting motor control, centres influencing cardiovascular autonomic regulation are more likely to be impaired than in the parkinsonian form. Similar differences between the cerebellar and parkinsonian forms of MSA have been reported with exercise-induced hypotension (Smith and Mathias 1996). These recent observations indicate the importance of clear identification of the autonomic disorder, and especially in MSA even the subgroup, when pathophysiological studies are reported.

Gastric and small intestinal motility

The gut is richly innervated by autonomic nerves and in patients with autonomic failure there is a high prevalence of disordered gastrointestinal motility, affecting various segments of the tract (Mathias 1996, Hardoff et al. 2001, Jost 2009). The latter may be associated with delayed and/or more rapid gastric emptying and small intestinal transit (Davies et al. 1996, Jost 2009). In many, there is evidence of cardiac vagal denervation, favouring vagal impairment of the upper gut and the potential for 'dumping'. In the classical 'dumping syndrome' which is well recognized as a complication of gastric drainage procedures and truncal vagotomy, patients experience symptoms including weakness, sweating, tachycardia, palpitations, and occasionally exhibit a modest fall in blood pressure soon after meal ingestion, especially if the latter contains a high carbohydrate load and meals are consumed in the erect posture. In this 'early' dumping syndrome, the rapid entry of a hyperosmotic (often carbohydrate) load into the jejunum is thought to cause fluid absorption within the gut, resulting in a reduction in plasma volume and an increase in raising the haematocrit, which would normally be opposed by an increase in sympathetic activity, thus accounting for some of the symptoms. In contrast, in autonomic failure there are no changes in plasma osmolality or the haematocrit after food, making it less likely that fluid translocation into the gut, either as a result of osmotic changes or for other reasons, results in contraction in plasma volume as in the early dumping syndrome (Mathias et al. 1989a).

The onset of the postprandial fall in blood pressure and rise in heart rate usually occurring soon after a meal, with a maximum response at 30–60 minutes (Jansen and Lipsitz 1995), suggests a relationship to the delivery of nutrients into the small intestine. While it was traditionally believed that the rate of gastric emptying played a minor, if not insignificant, role in postprandial hypotension, several recent studies (Jones et al. 1998, Jones et al. 2001, O'Donovan et al. 2002, Berry et al. 2003, Russo et al. 2003, O'Donovan et al. 2004, Gentilcore et al. 2005a, Gentilcore et al. 2005b, Jones et al. 2005, O'Donovan et al. 2005) have demonstrated that the hypotensive response to meals is triggered by the interaction of nutrients with the small intestine. Nutrient-mediated feedback arising from the small intestine plays a major role in the regulation of gastric emptying in health (Heddle et al. 1989). As a result of this feedback, which is influenced by the length (Lin et al. 1989, Lin et al. 1990a) and possibly the region (Lin et al. 1990b) of small intestine exposed, nutrients empty from the stomach at an overall rate of 1–4 kcal/minute (Brener et al. 1983). In an initial cross-sectional study of patients with type 2 diabetes, following ingestion of 75 g glucose in 350 ml water, the magnitude of the hypotensive response was greater when gastric emptying was relatively more rapid (Fig. 28.7) (Jones et al. 1998). In healthy older subjects, glucose infused intraduodenally at a rate of 3 kcal/minute, induced a substantially greater fall in blood pressure and rise in heart rate than at a rate of 1 kcal/minute (O'Donovan et al. 2002), establishing that the rate of small intestinal glucose delivery is a major determinant of the blood pressure response. It was suggested

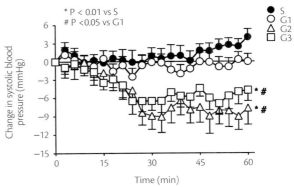

Fig. 28.8 Change in systolic blood pressure from baseline in response to intraduodenal saline (●) and glucose at a rate of either 1 kcal/min (○), 2 kcal/min (△) or 3 kcal/min (□), in healthy older subjects. Data are mean values ± SEM (n = 12). Systolic blood pressure treatment effect: * p < 0.01 'S' compared with 'G2' and 'S' compared 'G3', # p < 0.05 'G1' compared with 'G2' and 'G1' compared with 'G3'. With permission from Vanis L, Gentilcore D, Rayner CK, Wishart JM, Horowitz M, Feinle-Bisset C, Jones KL. Effects of small intestinal glucose load on blood pressure, splanchnic blood flow, glycemia and GLP-1 release in healthy older subjects. *Am J Physiol Regul Integr Comp Physiol* 2011 **300**:R1524–R1531.

(O'Donovan et al. 2002) that there is a 'threshold' small intestinal glucose load that must be exceeded to elicit a reduction in blood pressure and this appears to be the case. In a recent study, also in healthy older subjects (Vanis et al. 2009), the fall in blood pressure in response to intraduodenal glucose at 2 kcal/minute was comparable to 3 kcal/minute, while infusion at a rate of 1 kcal/minute had no effect compared with saline, suggesting that this threshold may be between 1 kcal/minute and 2 kcal/minute (Fig. 28.8) (Vanis et al. 2009). In healthy older subjects, intraduodenal infusions of glucose at a constant load (~3 kcal/minute), but varying concentrations (4.1%, 8.3% and 16.7%), lead to comparable falls in blood pressure (Gentilcore et al. 2006a) indicating that the hypotensive effect of intraduodenal glucose is dependent on load and not concentration. The effects of direct infusion of nutrients into the small intestine on blood pressure in patients with autonomic disorders have not been reported, but there are limited data that in patients with postprandial hypotension the effects of intraduodenal glucose are greater (van Orshoven et al. 2008). In two patients with symptomatic postprandial hypotension, intraduodenal glucose infusion at 3 kcal/minute induced falls in blood pressure of 92 mmHg and 28 mmHg (van Orshoven et al. 2008).

Gastric distension

'Intragastric' mechanisms, apparently related to gastric distension, have profound effects on the cardiovascular response to food (Shannon et al. 2002, van Orshoven et al. 2004, Jones et al. 2005, Gentilcore et al. 2008b). In healthy young and older subjects, proximal gastric distension with a balloon linked to a so-called 'barostat' increases blood pressure, heart rate, and musclular sympathetic nerve activity (MSNA)—the 'gastrovascular' reflex (van Orshoven et al. 2004). The latter is significantly attenuated in healthy older subjects. Rapid consumption of 480 ml water before a meal attenuates the fall in systolic blood pressure in patients with postprandial hypotension and autonomic failure; from −43 ± 36 mmHg to −22 ± 10 mmHg (Shannon et al. 2002), while in another study, 350 ml of tap water reduced the postprandial fall in blood pressure after a meal in patients with MSA, who had intractable orthostatic

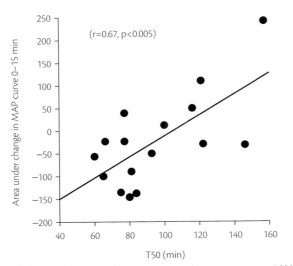

Fig. 28.7 Relationship between the area under the change in mean arterial blood pressure (MAP) curve between t = 0–15 minutes and the 50% emptying time (T50) of 75 g glucose in one patient with type 2 diabetes (n = 16). Reproduced with permission, from Jones, K. L., Tonkin, A., Horowitz, M., et al., 1998, *Clinical Science*, 94, 65–70, © the Biochemical Society.

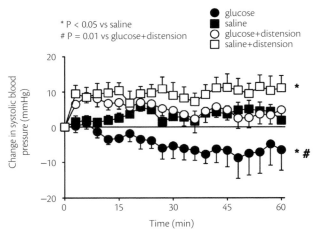

Fig. 28.9 Change in systolic blood pressure from baseline and in response to 'glucose' (●), 'saline' (■), 'glucose+distension' (○), and 'saline+distension' (□) in healthy older subjects. Data are mean values ± SEM (n = 8). Systolic blood pressure treatment effect: * p < 0.05 'saline' compared with 'glucose' and 'saline' compared with 'saline+distension'; # p = 0.01 'glucose' compared with 'glucose+distension'. With permission from The American Physiological Society (Vanis et al. 2010)..

hypotension and postprandial hypotension (Deguchi et al. 2007). More recently, gastric distension induced by intragastric water infusion (500 ml) has been shown to markedly attenuate the fall in blood pressure induced by intraduodenal glucose (Gentilcore et al. 2008b) and intraduodenal glucose delivered at an identical rate to that of gastric emptying of glucose induces a greater fall in blood pressure (Gentilcore et al. 2009) in healthy older persons. Moreover, the fall in blood pressure induced by intraduodenal glucose is markedly attenuated by concurrent gastric distension with a barostat balloon placed in the proximal stomach (at 8 mmHg above minimum distending pressure) in healthy older subjects (Vanis et al. 2010) (Fig. 28.9). That the effects of intraduodenal glucose appear to be potentiated in patients with postprandial hypotension (van Orshoven et al. 2008) support the concept of a protective role of gastric distension in postprandial hypotension.

It has also been demonstrated, in healthy older subjects, that the maximum fall in blood pressure is less when glucose (either 25 g or 75 g) is ingested in a volume of 600 ml compared with 200 ml (Jones et al. 2005), which was shown to be related closely to an increase in proximal, but not distal, gastric content (Jones et al. 2005). This suggests that the beneficial effect on blood pressure may be dependent on the site of gastric distension, as determined by intragastric meal distribution (which is influenced by meal volume, composition, and posture) (Horowitz et al. 1993).

Meal volume (load)

The magnitude of the postprandial reduction in blood pressure appears to be greater with increased carbohydrate content (Puvi-Rajasingham et al. 1996, Vloet et al. 2001). In 12 elderly patients with postprandial hypotension, the magnitude and duration of the fall in systolic blood pressure were progressively greater with 200 ml drinks containing 25 g vs 65 g vs 125 g glucose. However, in this study gastric emptying was not measured and the observed effects may potentially be accounted for by differences in the rate of nutrient delivery (Vloet et al. 2001). In patients with primary autonomic failure, when daily isocaloric mixed meals were

consumed as either three 'large' meals, when compared with six 'small' meals, the postprandial fall in blood pressure was less with the latter (Puvi-Rajasingham et al. 1996).

Meal composition, timing and temperature

The hypotensive response to food was traditionally believed to be greatest following ingestion of carbohydrate when compared with other macronutrients (fat and protein) (Jansen et al. 1990) but this is now recognized to be incorrect (Gentilcore et al. 2008a). In patients with autonomic failure, ingestion of a largely solid, balanced meal causes a similar fall in blood pressure when compared with the effects of an isocaloric, balanced liquid meal, indicating that meal consistency (solids are ground into small particles before emptying from the stomach) is not a major determinant of the hypotensive response. The outcome of a series of studies using different food components, which were isocaloric, isovolumic, and wherever possible isotonic, was indicative of major differences in the hypotensive effects of different food components in these patients (Mathias et al. 1989b). After glucose, the onset and duration of hypotension appeared similar to that observed after a balanced meal. In contrast, fat had slower, smaller, and less sustained, hypotensive effects while an elemental protein meal caused virtually no change in blood pressure. These studies did not take into account the potential effects of differences in gastric emptying and, hence, both gastric distension and small intestinal nutrient exposure. More recent studies in healthy elderly subjects have demonstrated that the magnitude of the falls in blood pressure induced by oral fat and carbohydrate (Visvanathan et al. 2006) and intraduodenal glucose, fat, and protein, are comparable, although the hypotensive response to fat and protein occurs later (Fig 28.10) (Gentilcore et al. 2008a), presumably reflecting variations in the rate of digestion (i.e. it is likely that the hypotensive response is induced by fatty acids and amino acids respectively for fat and protein), although this has not been evaluated formally.

As stated earlier, the hypotensive effects of oral glucose are not mediated by its hyperosmolality (Gentilcore et al. 2006a). In patients with autonomic failure (Mathias et al. 1989b) (Fig 28.11)

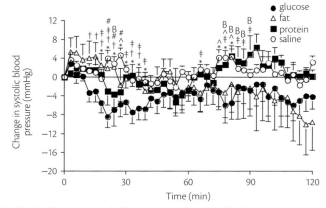

Fig. 28.10 Change in systolic blood pressure from baseline during intraduodenal infusion of glucose, fat, protein, and saline in healthy older subjects Data are mean values ± SEM (n = 8). * p < 0.05 for glucose compared with saline; † p < 0.05 for glucose compared with fat; ‡ p < 0.0001 for glucose compared with protein; ^ p < 0.05 for fat compared with saline; # p< 0.05 for protein compared with saline; ꝏ<p < 0.05 for fat compared with protein. With permission from Gentilcore, D., Hausken, T., Meyer, J. H., et al. (2008a), *Am J Clin Nutr*, **87**: 156–161.

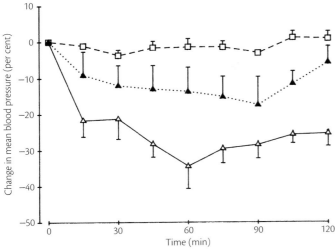

Fig. 28.11 Percentage change in mean blood pressure in eight normal subjects after oral glucose (dashed line, open squares) and in six chronic autonomic failure patients after glucose (continuous line, open triangles) and xylose (dotted line, filled triangles). Results are mean values ± SEM as vertical bars. The difference between the fall in blood pressure after glucose and xylose in the autonomic failure patients, calculated as the area under the curve, is highly significant (p < 0.01). Reproduced with permission, from Mathias, C. J., Da Costa, D. F., McIntosh, C. M. et al. 1989, *Clinical Science*, **77**, 85–92, © the Biochemical Society.

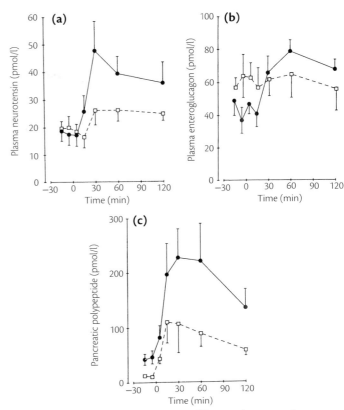

Fig. 28.12 Levels of **(a)** plasma neurotensin, **(b)** enteroglucagon, and **(c)** pancreatic polypeptide in patients with chronic autonomic failure (continuous line, filled circles) and in normal subjects (dashed line, open squares) before and after food ingestion at time 0. The vertical bars are ± SEM. Reproduced with permission, from Mathias, C. J., Da Costa, D. F., McIntosh, C. M. et al. 1989, *Clinical Science*, **77**, 85–92, © the Biochemical Society.

and in healthy older subjects (Vanis et al. unpublished observation) an isocaloric, isosmotic, and isovolumic solution of the carbohydrate, xylose, causes much smaller falls in blood pressure probably because it is digested much more slowly.

The timing and temperature of meals appears to be important. In elderly patients with postprandial hypotension, the magnitude of the fall in blood pressure is substantially greater after identical meals consumed at breakfast or lunch when compared with meals consumed later in the day (Vloet et al. 2003). In the healthy elderly, meals consumed at a higher temperature (~50°C) induce a modestly greater fall in blood pressure than cooler (~5°C) meals (Kuipers et al. 1991). The mechanisms mediating these effects remains to be determined.

Neural and humoral mechanisms

Food ingestion is associated with the release of pancreatic and gastrointestinal hormones, some of which are released into the circulation to exert distant effects, while others may act locally. Information about the neural/humoral pathways that mediate the postprandial fall in blood pressure is limited. A number of hormones have been measured in both normal subjects and in patients with autonomic failure before and after food ingestion. Changes in plasma levels of gastrin, vasoactive intestinal polypeptide, somatostatin, and cholecystokinin-8 are similar in both groups (Mathias et al. 1989a). Glucagon, pancreatic polypeptide, and neurotensin levels rise to a greater extent in patients with autonomic failure (Fig. 28.12) (Mathias et al. 1989b); the first two do not have vasodilatatory or negative cardiac inotropic effects and are unlikely to contribute to the hypotension. Neurotensin has potential vasodilatatory effects; however, the haemodynamic studies indicated that it was unlikely that postprandial hypotension resulted from its systemic effects. The studies utilizing peripheral venous measurements described above have limitations, as release of peptides and

related substances from enteric regions may exert significant autonomic and vascular effects locally without changes reflected in the periphery. An example is a study in humans indicating that feeding almost doubles neuropeptide Y (NPY) overflow in the hepatomesenteric region independently of noradrenaline spillover, but without similar changes in NPY concentration in peripheral blood (Morris et al. 1997). The vasodilatory peptide, calcitonin-generelated peptide (CGRP), has also been implicated in postprandial hypotension. In older subjects, increases in CGRP levels after oral glucose have been shown to be significantly related to blood pressure reductions (Edwards et al. 1996) so that greater increments in CGRP were observed in older subjects who experienced decreases in blood pressure of > 15 mmHg when compared with young or middle-aged subjects (Edwards et al. 1996). Further studies are required.

Intravenous administration of hypertonic glucose (25–50 ml of 50% solution) lowers blood pressure rapidly in patients with tetraplegia and autonomic failure, but this effect is transient (Mathias et al. 1987). The effects of oral glucose on blood pressure appear to be unrelated to its increasing plasma concentration, as intravenous infusions of glucose, despite resulting in higher plasma levels, do not lower blood pressure to the same extent as after oral glucose (Jansen and Hoefnagels 1987). Of the various peptides, the cardiovascular autonomic effects of insulin have been studied in most detail. In normal subjects, exogenous insulin does not lower blood pressure, but increases sympathetic nerve activity and elevates plasma noradrenaline levels (Fagius et al. 1986); these changes occur even in adrenalectomized patients, excluding a role for the adrenal medulla. Whether these effects of insulin are through an action on the brain (as suggested by animal studies; Muntzel et al. 1994) or directly through causing vasodilatation, is uncertain. Vasodilatatory effects of insulin may occur in various vascular regions. When normal subjects were given a high-fat meal without an insulin infusion, or in combination with an insulin infusion to raise insulin levels to those observed after a high carbohydrate meal (Kearney et al. 1996a), changes were observed in both the skeletal musculature and splanchnic circulation. Vasodilatation in calf muscle did not occur after the meal alone, but when combined with insulin; there were similar changes in calf muscle vascular resistance. Superior mesenteric artery blood flow responses were similar, with dilatation (consistent with the effects of exogenous insulin observed without a meal), but vascular resistance was greater when insulin was infused. This suggests that the vasodilatation induced by insulin occurs in both the skeletal muscle and splanchnic vasculature in normal man.

In normal subjects, the somatostatin analogue, octreotide, is effective in preventing the release of pancreatic and gut hormones in response to various stimuli, including food and alcohol ingestion (Fig. 28.13). Octreotide has to be administered subcutaneously and causes an initial but transient elevation in blood pressure that occurs only in autonomic failure patients and not in normal subjects; the reasons for this are uncertain and include pressor supersensitivity, possibly to the venoconstrictor effects of octreotide. Octreotide is effective in preventing both glucose and food-induced hypotension in autonomic failure (Fig. 28.14) (Hoeldtke et al. 1986, Raimbach et al. 1989) and attenuates the rise in insulin, neurotensin, and a range of other hormones in response to food (Fig. 28.15). However, octreotide has no effect on cardiac output, muscle or skin blood flow, suggesting that it prevents postprandial hypotension largely by its effects on the splanchnic vasculature. This has been confirmed by non-invasive measurement of superior mesenteric artery blood flow, which rises markedly after a liquid meal but is unchanged after pretreatment with octreotide (Kooner et al. 1990). This emphasizes the role of the splanchnic circulation and of vasodilatatory gut hormones in postprandial hypotension.

Recent studies in animals (Barragan et al. 1996) and humans (Edwards et al. 1998, Gentilcore et al. 2005a) suggest that glucagon-like peptide-1 (GLP-1) may play a role in postprandial hypotension. GLP-1, which is released predominantly from the distal small intestine, together with glucose-dependent insulinotropic peptide (GIP), which is released proximally (the so-called 'incretin' hormones), account for the substantially greater insulin response to enteral, compared with intravenous, glucose (Holst and Gromada 2004). Amongst its physiological properties (assessed using the specific antagonist, exendin 9–39) GLP-1 slows gastric emptying, suppresses glucagon, stimulates glucose-dependent insulin secretion leading to reductions in fasting and postprandial glycaemia (Schirra et al. 2009, Deane et al. 2010). In addition to these effects, pharmacological doses of GLP-1 markedly delay gastric emptying and reduce appetite (Little et al. 2006). In healthy young subjects subcutaneous administration of GLP-1 increases heart rate and mean arterial blood pressure (GLP-1: 83 ± 5 mmHg vs saline: 77 ± 4 mmHg; p <0.05) (Edwards et al. 1998). In healthy elderly subjects, the α-glucosidase inhibitor, acarbose, used in the management of

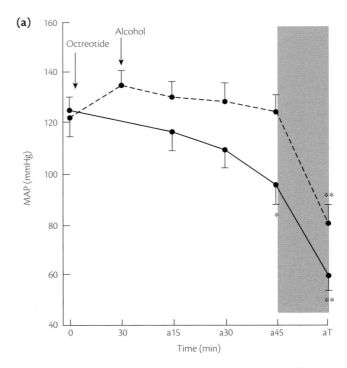

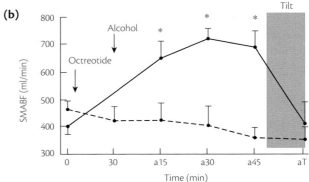

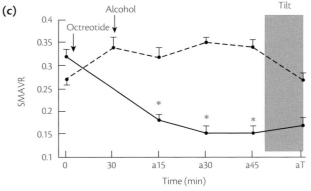

Fig. 28.13 (a) Mean arterial blood pressure (MAP) before and after alcohol ingestion alone without octreotide (continuous line) and after pretreatment with octreotide (interrupted line), 15, 30, and 45 minutes (a15, a30, a45) after alcohol ingestion. Blood pressure falls after alcohol alone while supine, and to lower levels during tilt (aT), unlike when ingested after pretreatment with octreotide. (b) Superior mesenteric artery blood flow (SMABF), and (c) superior mesenteric artery vascular resistance (SMAVR), before and after alcohol ingestion alone (continuous line) and after pretreatment with octreotide (interrupted line). The fall in SMABF after tilt is greater after alcohol alone (aT). The rise in SMABF is prevented by octreotide. * p < 0.05; ** p < 0.001. From Chaudhuri et al. 1995, with permission.

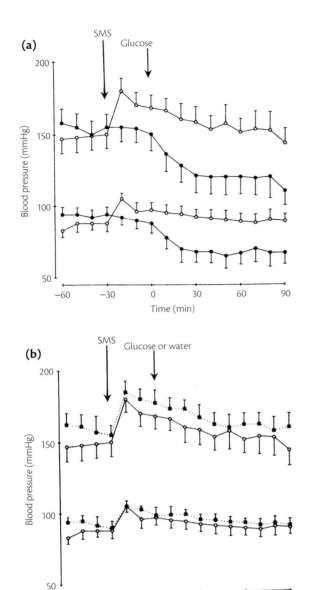

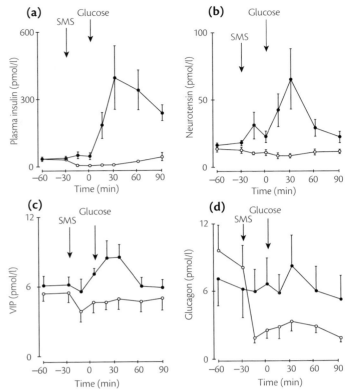

Fig. 28.15 Changes in plasma levels of **(a)** insulin, **(b)** neurotensin, **(c)** vasoactive intestinal polypeptide (VIP), and **(d)** glucagon in patients with chronic autonomic failure after placebo (filled circles) or octreotide (SMS 201–995) (open circles), given at −30 minutes followed by oral glucose at 0 minutes. Results are mean values ± SEM. From Raimbach et al. 1989, with permission.

Fig. 28.14 **(a)** Systolic and diastolic blood pressure and heart rate in patients with chronic autonomic failure on two occasions when given oral glucose at time 0 with pretreatment at −30 minutes with either octreotide (SMS 201–995) 50 µg (open circles) or saline placebo (filled circles) both subcutaneously. **(b)** Systolic and diastolic blood pressure in patients with chronic autonomic failure given octreotide (SMS 201–995) 50 µg subcutaneously at −30 minutes followed at 0 minutes by either oral glucose (open circles) or an equivalent amount of water (filled squares). Reproduced with permission, from Raimbach, S. J., Cortelli, P., Kooner, J. S., Bannister, R., Bloom, S. R., and Mathias, C. J., 1989, *Clinical Science.* **77**, 623–8, © the Biochemical Society.

type 2 diabetes (Breuer 2003) attenuates the fall in blood pressure induced by oral sucrose and markedly stimulates the release of GLP-1, and this is temporally associated with slowing of gastric emptying (Gentilcore et al. 2005a). Beneficial effects of acarbose on postprandial hypotension have also been observed in patients with diabetes (Sasaki et al. 2001, Maule et al. 2004), in elderly patients with postprandial hypotension (Jian and Zhou 2008), and in patients with autonomic failure (Shibao et al. 2007). GLP-1 analogues have

recently become available for the management of type 2 diabetes. While a modest reduction in systolic blood pressure has been reported with the use of these agents (e.g. exenatide and liraglutide), it is not clear whether measurements were performed in the fasted or postprandial states.

In patients with autonomic failure, exogenous insulin lowers blood pressure substantially, even in the absence of changes in blood glucose (Mathias et al. 1987; Brown et al. 1989). Bolus intravenous insulin (0.15 units/kg) causes hypotension (Fig. 28.16), but without dilatation in forearm muscle or cutaneous vascular beds. When administered with an euglycaemic clamp, blood pressure falls independently of changes in blood glucose and without changes in cardiac output and forearm muscle or skin blood flow, thus favouring an effect on a large vascular bed such as the splanchnic circulation. In autonomic failure, it is likely that insulin causes splanchnic vasodilatation and lowers blood pressure, in the absence of a compensatory increase in sympathetic nerve activity. This is consistent with the ability of insulin to lower blood pressure in diabetics with autonomic neuropathy (Chapter 53). As discussed, patients with PAF often have a greater degree of postprandial hypotension than those with MSA (Mathias et al. 1991); plasma glucose and insulin levels before a meal are similar in both groups (Fig. 28.17). After a meal, however, glucose levels are similar, but there is a greater rise in postprandial insulin levels in PAF that may potentially account for the greater degree of postprandial hypotension in PAF (Armstrong and Mathias 1991). While the above

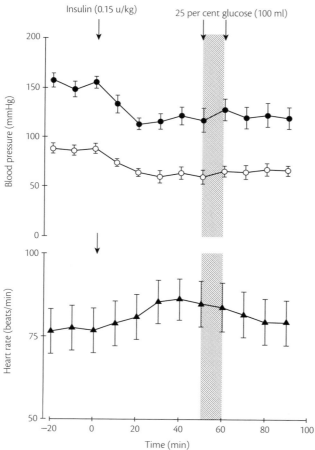

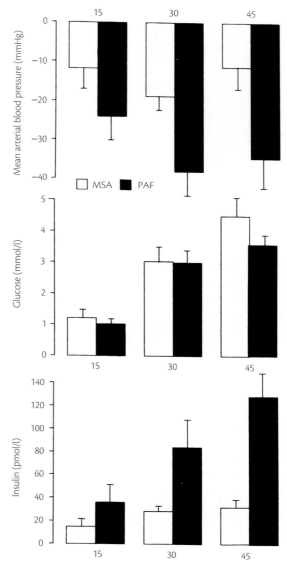

Fig. 28.16 Systolic (filled circles) and diastolic (open circles) blood pressure and heart rate in five patients with chronic autonomic failure before and after intravenous insulin. Both systolic and diastolic blood pressure fall within 10 minutes. Hypoglycaemia occurred at around 30 minutes and did not result in a further fall in blood pressure. Blood pressure remained low even after reversal of hypoglycaemia with 25% glucose infused over 10 minutes. Reproduced from *BMJ*, Mathias, C. J., Da Costa, D. F., Fosbraey, P., Christensen, N. J., and Bannister, R. **295**, 161–3, 1987, with permission from BMJ Publishing Group Ltd.

Fig. 28.17 Fall in mean blood pressure in patients with multiple system atrophy (open histograms, MSA) and patients with pure autonomic failure (filled histograms, PAF) at intervals of 15, 30, and 45 minutes after a balanced liquid meal ingested in the supine position. The middle panel indicates the changes in plasma glucose, and the lower panel in plasma insulin, at similar time points. In PAF there is a greater fall in blood pressure than in MSA. The rise in plasma glucose levels appears similar, while the rise in plasma insulin levels are considerably greater in PAF.

observations are of interest, there is also evidence to suggest that the role for insulin in postprandial hypotension, if any, may well be modest. In particular, in the elderly, intravenous glucose, resulting in substantial insulin secretion, does not affect blood pressure (Jansen and Hoefnagels 1987) and postprandial hypotension occurs in patients with type 1 diabetes who are insulin deficient (Gentilcore et al. 2006b).

Nitric oxide (NO) released endogenously by the action of NO synthase on L-arginine (Moncada and Higgs 1991), acts as a vasodilator and is an important neurotransmitter in the gastrointestinal tract (Su et al. 2001). The role of NO mechanisms can be optimally addressed by the use of specific inhibitors of its production, such as NG-nitro-L-arginine-methyl-ester (L-NAME) (Su et al. 2001) and NG-methyl-L-arginine (L-NMMA) (Alemany et al. 1997). In healthy older subjects, the fall in blood pressure induced by oral glucose, has been shown to be mediated by NO mechanisms, apparently unrelated to changes in gastric emptying (Gentilcore et al. 2005b), while studies in animals indicate that NO mechanisms are important in the regulation of splanchnic blood flow, for example in pigs L-NMMA attenuates the meal-induced increase in

mesenteric blood flow (Alemany et al. 1997), while in rats, intestinal arteriolar distension induced by topical application of glucose is blocked by L-NAME (Matheson et al. 1997). Hence, a role for NO in the regulation of splanchnic blood flow in humans is also likely.

The rise in MSNA in response to oral glucose has been shown to be attenuated in the elderly when compared with young subjects (Fagius et al. 1996). The reduction in MSNA is consistent with studies evaluating heart rate spectral analysis that have demonstrated that the increase in sympathetic activity is less in elderly patients with postprandial hypotension when compared with young or elderly subjects without postprandial hypotension (Imai et al. 1998, Ryan et al. 1992). Moreover, the rise in catecholamines (a marker of sympathetic activity), observed following a meal, are reduced in patients with essential hypertension and postprandial hypotension compared with patients without postprandial hypotension (Mitro et al. 2001). In contrast, when the stomach is bypassed (i.e. during intraduodenal glucose infusion), there is no difference in MSNA between healthy young and older subjects despite greater falls in blood pressure in the elderly (van Orshoven et al. 2008), supporting the hypothesis that gastric distension is important in mediating postprandial hypotension. As stated earlier, the rise in MSNA induced by gastric distension is significantly attenuated in healthy older subjects (van Orshoven et al. 2004), and other factors such as the release of gastrointestinal hormones also play a role.

Investigation of postprandial hypotension

This is described in Chapter 22.

Management of postprandial hypotension

A better understanding of the pathophysiological mechanisms have increased therapeutic possibilities to limit the problems caused by postprandial hypotension; however, treatment remains suboptimal and must be individualized (Mathias, 1997) (Table 28.1). It should be recognized that no studies have examined the relationship between symptoms and the magnitude of the postprandial fall in blood pressure. The patient should be made aware of food-induced hypotension and provided with appropriate information concerning the composition, size, and frequency of meals as well as the potential benefits of gastric distension. Carbohydrate may increase vulnerability to postural hypotension, especially if refined carbohydrate is used, and dietetic advice about different foods and their composition is needed. The benefit of taking the same caloric intake, but spread as smaller meals given more frequently has been documented as being helpful (Puvi-Rajasingham and Mathias 1996). Food ingestion enhances postural hypotension (Fig. 28.6) and, especially after large meals patients should be cautious about

Table 28.1 Some of the approaches used to prevent or reduce postprandial hypotension

Advice
◆ Have smaller meals, more frequently
◆ Caution with hot meals
◆ Employ strategies to slow small intestinal nutrient delivery and absorption e.g. add guar
◆ Maximize gastric distension during a meal e.g. water preload
◆ Reduce refined carbohydrate
◆ Avoid alcohol
◆ Caution with standing or walking after meals

Drugs
◆ Acarbose or other α-glucosidase inhibitors
◆ Octreotide or other somatostatin analogues
◆ Indomethacin
◆ Caffeine
◆ Denopamine and midodrine
◆ l-Dihydroxyphenylserine
◆ Frusemide withdrawal

standing or walking. Many are aware that their tolerance to even small amounts of alcohol is low, which is not surprising given that alcohol lowers blood pressure and enhances postural hypotension, probably through its vasodilatatory effects, including those on the splanchnic vasculature (Ray Chaudhuri et al. 1994). Diuretics (e.g. frusemide) should be withdrawn if possible as their use exacerbates the postprandial fall in blood pressure (van Kraaij et al. 1999, Mehagnoul-Schipper et al. 2002).

Various drugs have been used. In the initial studies of Robertson et al. (1981), single doses of propranolol, diphenhydramine, cimetidine, and indomethacin were evaluated. Propranolol (40 mg orally) had no beneficial effect and may even have worsened postprandial hypotension. The H_1 antihistamine, diphenhydramine, and the H_2 blocker, cimetidine, also had no effect. The hypotensive response to food was attenuated by indomethacin (50 mg orally), suggesting that vasodilatatory prostaglandins or arachidonic acid metabolites may be responsible. Long-term studies in postprandial hypotension have not been reported with indomethacin or any other non-steroidal anti-inflammatory drug; however, it has the well-recognized potential to induce gastrointestinal erosions and bleeding.

Data relating to the use of caffeine as a potential treatment for postprandial hypotension are inconsistent. Caffeine raises blood pressure in normal subjects by stimulating the sympathetic or renin–angiotensin system and it was reported to be highly effective in preventing postprandial hypotension in autonomic failure (Onrot et al. 1985). The latter occurred independently of stimulation of the sympathetic and renin–angiotensin systems, and a postulated mechanism was blockade of vasodilatatory adenosine receptors. Similarly, in elderly subjects, caffeine, in doses of 100–200 mg, reduced the magnitude of the fall in blood pressure and associated symptoms (Heseltine et al. 1991a, Heseltine et al. 1991b). In contrast, Lipsitz et al. (1994) found no benefit of caffeine in elderly patients with postprandial hypotension. When administered to patients with PAF or MSA in single doses of 250 mg and 500 mg, and also on a regular basis, there was neither objective nor subjective evidence of benefit (Armstrong et al. 1990). Whether patients with incomplete autonomic lesions (in whom the residual sympathetic or renin–angiotensin systems may be stimulated) are likely to benefit, remains to be elucidated.

An effective drug in preventing postprandial hypotension is the somatostatin analogue, octreotide (Hoeldtke et al. 1986, Jansen et al. 1988, 1989) (Fig. 28.18). This was first used by Hoeldtke et al. (1986) and, as discussed, is a synthetic, long-acting peptide-release inhibitor. It is effective in autonomic failure in reducing glucose-induced and alcohol-induced hypotension (Raimbach et al. 1989, Ray Chaudhuri et al. 1995) probably by reducing splanchnic vasodilatation. Octreotide can be given in small doses, ranging from 25 g to 50 g two or three times daily, ideally about half an hour before meal ingestion. Its disadvantages include its subcutaneous administration and local discomfort because of its low pH; it also may induce nausea, abdominal colic, and diarrhoea, the last especially after a fatty meal. Its longer-term side-effects (such as cholelithiasis), although well charted in various endocrine conditions where larger doses usually are used, are less clear in autonomic failure. In one of our patients with PAF hyperglycaemia occurred, necessitating oral hypoglycaemics, while in two others intermittent hypoglycaemia was a possibility; the precise cause and relationship was unclear.

Beneficial effects of octreotide have been demonstrated on hypotension induced by postural change and even by exercise

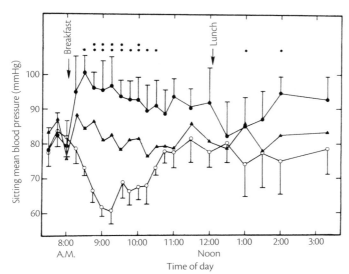

Fig. 28.18 Sitting mean blood pressure after breakfast and lunch in six patients with autonomic failure of different aetiology, when given placebo (open circle) or two different doses of the somatostatin analogue SMS 201–995 (octreotide, filled circles, 0.4 µg/kg and filled triangles, 0.2 µg/kg). For comparisons of drug and placebo, * p < 0.05 and ** p < 0.001. SEM for low doses of drug are omitted for clarity. Reprinted from *The Lancet*, **328**, Hoeldtke, R. D., O'Dorisio, T. M., and Boden, G., Treatment of autonomic neuropathy with a somatostatin analogue SMS-201-995, 602–5, Copyright 1986, with permission from Elsevier.

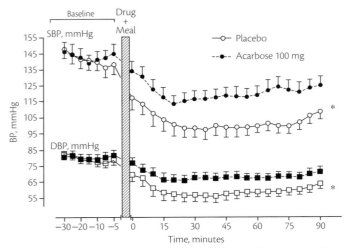

Fig. 28.19 Change in systolic (circles) and diastolic (squares) blood pressure from baseline before and after a solid mixed meal with and without 100 mg acarbose in patients with autonomic failure and postprandial hypotension. Data are mean values ± SEM (n = 9). * p < 0.01. With permission from Shibao, C., Gamboa, A., Diedrich, A., et al. (2007). Acarbose, an alpha-glucosidase inhibitor, attenuates postprandial hypotension in autonomic failure. *Hypertension* **50**(1):54–61.

(Armstrong and Mathias 1991, Smith et al. 1995), although these effects may be modest. A further question concerns whether it might enhance nocturnal hypertension in autonomic failure. This has been addressed using 24-hour ambulatory blood pressure profiling, and indicates a favourable effect, with a reduction in nocturnal hypertension (Alam et al. 1995). Octreotide has been superseded by other somatostatin analogues, including preparations with a much longer duration of action and a lower prevalence of adverse effects (Hoeldtke et al. 2007, Colao et al. 2010). Octreotide LAR (long acting release) has been used to treat orthostatic hypotension in patients with autonomic failure and should benefit postprandial hypotension, but the possibility of supine hypertension and post postprandial hyperglycaemia need consideration (Hoeldtke RD et al. 2007). While these drugs are now used widely in the management of a number of disorders (e.g. acromegaly, carcinoid syndrome), there are no reports relating to their use in the management of postprandial hypotension.

There has been recent increasing interest in the use of alpha-glucosidase inhibitors (e.g. acarbose and voglibose), as a potential therapy for postprandial hypotension (Sasaki et al. 2001, Maule et al 2004, Gentilcore et al. 2005a, Maruta et al. 2006, Shibao et al. 2007, Jian and Zhou 2008). In healthy older subjects 100 mg of acarbose reduces the magnitude of the fall in blood pressure after both oral (Gentilcore et al. 2005a) and intraduodenal (Gentilcore et al. 2010) sucrose. Randomized trials in elderly patients with postprandial hypotension (Jian and Zhou 2008) and autonomic failure (Shibao et al. 2007) (Fig 28.19) indicate that acarbose is effective in reducing postprandial hypotension. Acarbose, however, is not without side-effects such as diarrhoea and flatulence that may limit its use.

That the rate of nutrient delivery is an important determinant of the hypotensive response to a meal (Jones et al. 1998, O'Donovan et al. 2002), while gastric distension attenuates the fall in blood pressure, suggests that strategies aimed at slowing gastric emptying and small intestinal absorption while maximizing gastric distension, would be beneficial in the management of patients with postprandial hypotension. In healthy elderly subjects (Jones et al. 2001) (Fig. 28.20) and patients with type 2 diabetes (Russo et al. 2003),

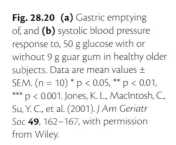

Fig. 28.20 **(a)** Gastric emptying of, and **(b)** systolic blood pressure response to, 50 g glucose with or without 9 g guar gum in healthy older subjects. Data are mean values ± SEM. (n = 10) * p < 0.05, ** p < 0.01, *** p < 0.001. Jones, K. L., MacIntosh, C., Su, Y. C., et al. (2001). *J Am Geriatr Soc* **49**, 162–167, with permission from Wiley.

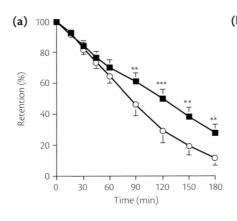

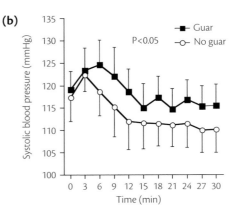

the addition of guar, a naturally occurring polysaccharide, attenuates the magnitude of fall in blood pressure after oral glucose by slowing gastric emptying and small intestinal absorption. Unfortunately, guar is unpalatable and may have gastrointestinal side-effects.

The splanchnic circulation may be targeted in other ways (Mathias 1997), such as through the known effects of vasopressin on the portal circulation. This provides another possible approach in postprandial hypotension, as demonstrated in five patients with MSA in whom infusion of vasopressin prevented glucose-induced hypotension (Hakusui et al. 1991). Analogues such as glypressin (Chapter 47) may also be of value.

There are data to suggest that sympathomimetics may be useful in the management of postprandial hypotension. A combination of the α-adrenergic agonist midodrine, and the β₁-adrenergic agonist, denopamine, successfully reduced glucose-induced hypotension in eight patients with autonomic failure (Hirayama et al. 1993). When given alone, neither drug had a beneficial effect. The combination resulted in an increase in peripheral vascular resistance (presumably through midodrine) and an elevation of cardiac output (probably through denopamine), thus correcting the two major haemodynamic abnormalities contributing to postprandial hypotension. These patients were also placed on long-term treatment, with continuing benefits and no adverse effects.

The prodrug dihydroxyphenylserine (DOPS; in the racaemic, DL form), has been shown to reduce postprandial hypotension in both PAF and MSA patients; there was probably a greater response in PAF (Freeman et al. 1996). The mechanisms by which DOPS reduces hypotension are discussed in Chapters 47 and 49.

Effects of food in other groups of patients, some with autonomic dysfunction

Postprandial hypotension has been reported in a number of other patient groups. Literature relating to these patients is discussed in this section.

Patients on ganglionic blockers and following splanchnic denervation

The hypotensive effect of food appears to have been first recorded by Smirk (1953) in hypertensive patients after the ganglionic blocker, pentolinium, was used. He observed a fall in pressure in the lying, sitting, and standing position after lunch. Whether postprandial hypotension occurs after other antihypertensive sympatholytic drugs known to cause postural hypotension, such as reserpine, debrisoquine, guanethidine, and bethanidine, is not clearly documented.

Insulin lowers blood pressure when given to normal subjects after a ganglionic blocker (hexamethonium) (di Salvo et al. 1956). Insulin-induced hypotension has been recorded in patients after splanchnic denervation from T7 to L3 inclusive, performed for the relief of severe hypertension (French and Kilpatrick 1955). It is likely in both groups that splanchnic vasodilatation not accompanied by appropriate compensatory sympathetic nervous activity was responsible for the fall in blood pressure.

Diabetes mellitus

Studies in patients with type 2 diabetes indicate that postprandial hypotension occurs in 20–44% (Jones et al. 1998). Insulin lowers blood pressure in diabetic patients with autonomic neuropathy and baroreceptor abnormalities and can provoke or enhance postural hypotension (Miles and Hayter 1968) (Chapter 49). In postprandial hypotension in diabetics with autonomic neuropathy, it has been difficult to separate the effects of food itself from that of insulin. Observations of Hoeldtke et al. (1986), however, demonstrating that the beneficial effects of octreotide to reduce postprandial hypotension in diabetic autonomic neuropathy were not reversed by insulin administration, and that postprandial hypotension occurs in patients with type 1 diabetes who are, by definition, insulin deficient, suggest that other factors, than postprandial insulin release, are important mediators of this condition.

The elderly

Postprandial hypotension is now recognized as occurring in a significant number (~20–40%) of the elderly, especially in patients over 80 years of age (Chapter 70). Food predominantly lowers systolic blood pressure but there are also falls in diastolic pressure. It is unclear whether this is related to autonomic failure associated with aging, or to a combination of other factors that include impairment of hormonal responses, baroreceptor activity, and cardiac function. A range of studies indicates that some of the mechanisms responsible for postprandial hypotension in autonomic failure are similar in the elderly; so also are some of the therapeutic approaches, including the administration of octreotide and acarbose.

Cerebrovascular and coronary artery disease

Patients with cerebrovascular and coronary artery disease do not necessarily have an autonomic deficit, but when on vasoactive drugs they may be prone, because of their regional vascular deficits, to potentially deleterious effects induced by food ingestion. In the presence of carotid artery stenosis an even modest fall in blood pressure may critically impair cerebral perfusion, resulting in a transient ischaemic attack or a stroke; the former has been reported in a single case report (Kamata et al. 1994). Relatively recent studies indicate that in patients with haemodynamically significant unilateral and bilateral carotid artery stenosis (with over 80% luminal occlusion), the autonomic control of the circulation is impaired, with postural hypotension occurring in over 50% (Akinola et al. 1997). It remains to be determined whether food-induced hypotension further compromises cardiovascular control in such patients.

In patients with coronary artery disease, the increased cardiac workload following food ingestion may contribute to angina and, possibly, to myocardial infarction. In his original description in 1772, Heberden noted that angina was exacerbated by exercise, particularly after food. It has been suggested that the composition of food is of importance, so that carbohydrate is more likely to induce myocardial ischaemia and reduce exercise capacity than a fat or protein meal (Baliga et al. 1997a) (Fig. 28.21). This may be related to variations in sympathetic activation and an interaction with peptides released by different components in food. Whether there are differences in the efficacy of anti-anginal drugs in preventing postprandial exacerbations of angina is unclear—and/or adrenergic blockers may be effective if they prevent sympathetically mediated cardiac work. However, if non-adrenergic vasoconstrictor substances play an important intracoronary role, vasodilatation induced by calcium-channel agonists, such as nifedipine, may counteract food-induced myocardial ischaemia; alternatively, preventing peptide release may be beneficial as has been demonstrated with octreotide (Baliga et al. 1996).

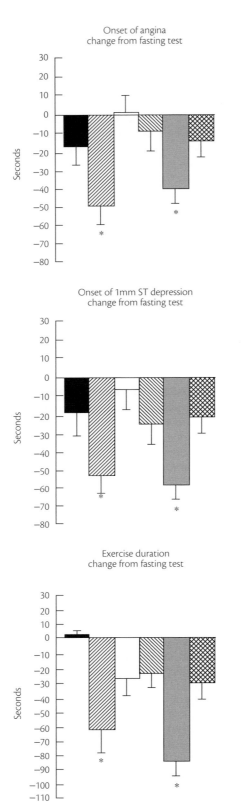

Fig. 28.21 Time differences to onset of angina, 1 mm ST segment depression, and exercise duration after water (black bars), carbohydrate (slashed upwards), fat (white bars), protein (slashed downwards), balanced meal (fine stippled bars), and xylose (boxed bars) compared with corresponding values during exercise in the fasting state in patients with postprandial angina. * p = 0.05. Carbohydrate, either alone or in a mixed balanced meal, was more likely to provoke or worsen angina than other food components. From Baliga et al. 1997a, with permission.

Cardiac transplantation

In cardiac transplantees there may be partial or complete cardiac autonomic denervation. In these patients the heart rate and cardiac output response to a high carbohydrate meal is preserved, while the cardiac response appears to be attenuated if a high-fat meal has been administered (Kearney et al. 1996b). The reasons for the rise in heart rate with both meals warrant explanation. In normal subjects there is no rise in noradrenaline spillover post-meal, excluding an increase in cardiac sympathetic activation (Cox et al. 1995), and suggesting that heart rate changes may be mediated through parasympathetic (vagal) withdrawal. However, the cardiac transplantees were vagally denervated, excluding this possibility. This therefore favours humoral factors, either adrenergic or non-adrenergic, especially if their effects were enhanced in the presence of denervation supersensitivity, as has been demonstrated with isoprenaline (Yusuf et al. 1987). Postprandial hypotension did not occur in the transplantees with either meal. With both meals there was an attenuation of the expected postprandial dilatation in the superior mesenteric artery for reasons that are unclear. The studies suggest that neurogenic dysfunction in one region may be compensated for in various ways, in other regions.

Neurodegenerative disorders

The hypotensive effects of food ingestion in a group of patients with Parkinson's disease were described by Micieli et al. (1987); the patients also had postural hypotension, raising the possibility that some had MSA. In a further study in Parkinson's disease without postural hypotension, and with normal autonomic function (Thomaides et al. 1993), postprandial hypotension also was observed. When comparisons were made with PAF and MSA, however, the degree of supine hypotension was less, and furthermore, food did not induce or accentuate post-meal postural hypotension. Whether postprandial hypotension occurs in other parkinsonian syndromes (such as progressive supranuclear palsy) has not been studied systematically. In Alzheimer's disease, 7 out of 10 patients had hypotension between 20 minutes and 120 minutes after food ingestion; none had postural hypotension, making it unlikely that they had underlying autonomic failure (Idiaquez et al. 1997).

Tetraplegia and paraplegia

Patients with complete cervical spinal cord transection cannot activate sympathetic activity in response to agents with vasodilatatory properties (Chapter 66). Exogenous insulin lowers blood pressure in tetraplegics (Mathias et al. 1979); the fall appears to be smaller than in patients with autonomic failure, although no direct comparison has been performed. In tetraplegics, using a similar protocol to those with autonomic failure, ingestion of food causes only modest falls in systolic and diastolic blood pressure, with a rise in heart rate in the supine position (Baliga et al. 1997b). The reason for the difference from PAF and MSA patients is unclear, and could include the ability of the intact vagus to increase heart rate and cardiac output and, thus, partially buffer the fall in blood pressure. In these tetraplegics, forearm venous plasma noradrenaline did not change after food. However, this does not exclude localized activation of spinal reflexes induced by stimulation of intestinal afferents, as changes in peripheral levels of noradrenaline may not occur because the liver is a major extractor of noradrenaline (Eisenhofer et al. 1995). In the tetraplegics, postural hypotension post-meal was not enhanced, unlike that observed in PAF and MSA. A case study of postprandial hypotension reported in a patient with thoracic paraplegia (Catz et al. 1992), but not in tetraplegia, suggested the fall in postprandial blood pressure may be due to a thoracic rather than cervical spinal cord lesion. This was confirmed in a more recent study comparing patients with C4–C7 tetraplegia and T4–T6 paraplegia (Catz et al. 2007), only significant reductions in blood pressure after a mixed liquid drink in the paraplegics indicating that the hypotensive response to a meal is mediated via the thoracic and not cervical spinal cord.

Dopamine-beta-hydroxylase deficiency

Patients with dopamine-beta-hydroxylase (DBH) deficiency are unable to synthesize either noradrenaline or adrenaline and have severe postural hypotension with selective sympathetic adrenergic failure (Chapter 46). Food ingestion does not lower their blood pressure (Mathias et al. 1990), unlike patients with PAF and MSA. The DBH deficiency patients differ from PAF and MSA in their ability to release dopamine, and presumably other vasoactive chemicals, from otherwise intact sympathetic nerve endings. It remains to be resolved whether their ability to release dopamine (which could affect the heart and vasculature) and other vasoconstrictors (such as NPY and adenosine triphosphate) from nerve terminals accounts for their resistance to postprandial hypotension.

Tabes dorsalis with an afferent lesion

We have studied one patient with tabes dorsalis who, on detailed autonomic testing, had evidence of an afferent baroreceptor lesion without impairment of central and peripheral sympathetic pathways (Mathias and Bannister, unpublished observations). He had pronounced hypotension after food, suggesting that the lesion, which probably also involved afferents from the gut, blocked the normal activation of corrective reflexes and thus contributed to the fall in blood pressure after food.

Conclusion

Postprandial hypotension occurs frequently in patients with autonomic dysfunction and is associated with increased morbidity and mortality. The mechanisms mediating the condition are not completely understood; however, changes in sympathetic nerve activity, splanchnic blood flow, small intestinal nutrient delivery and absorption, gastric distension, and the release of gastrointestinal hormones are all thought to play a role. Treatment strategies are currently suboptimal and although there have been many advances, further research in this area is required.

References

Akinola A. B., Mathias, C. J., Mansfield, A. *et al.* (1997). Altered neural control of the cardiovascular system in unilateral and bilateral carotid artery stenosis. *Clin. Auton. Res.* **7**, 105–6.

Alam, M., Smith, G. D. P., Bleasdale-Barr, K., Pavitt, D. V., and Mathias, C. J. (1995). Effects of the peptide release inhibitor, Octreotide, on daytime hypotension and on nocturnal hypertension in primary autonomic failure. *J. Hypertension* **13**, 1664–9.

Alemany, C. A., Oh, W., and Stonestreet, B. S. (1997). Effects of nitric oxide synthesis inhibition on mesenteric perfusion in young pigs. *Am J Physiol* **272**, G612–616.

Armstrong, E., Watson, L., Hardman, T. C., Bannister, R., and Mathias, C. J. (1990). Effect of oral caffeine on post-prandial and postural hypotension, before and after food ingestion, in primary autonomic failure. *J. Autonom. Nerv. Syst.* **31**, 174–5.

Armstrong, E. and Mathias, C. J. (1991). The effects of the somatostatin analogue, Octreotide, on postural hypotension, before and after food ingestion, in primary autonomic failure. *Clin. Auton. Res.* **1**, 135–40.

Baliga, R. R., Burden, L., Mandeep, S. K., Rampling, M. W., and Kooner, J. S. (1997a). Effects of components of meals (carbohydrate, fat, protein) in causing postprandial exertional angina pectoris. *Am. J. Cardiol.* **79**, 1397–400.

Baliga, R. R., Burden, L., and Kooner, J. S. (1996). Octreotide prevents post-prandial angina pectoris and improves exercise capacity after food ingestion. *Circulation* **94**, 8.

Baliga, R. R., Catz, A. B., Watson, L. P., Short, D. J., Frankel, H. L., and Mathias, C. J. (1997b). Cardiovascular and hormonal responses to food ingestion in humans with spinal cord transection. *Clin. Auton. Res.* **7**, 137–41.

Barragan, J. M., Rodriguez, R. E., Eng, J., and Blazquez, E. (1996). Interactions of exendin-(9–39) with the effects of glucagon-like peptide-1-(7–36) amide and of exendin-4 on arterial blood pressure and heart rate in rats. *Regul Pept* **67**, 63–68.

Berne, C., Fagius, J., and Niklasson, F. (1989). Sympathetic response to oral carbohydrate administration. Evidence from micro-electrode recordings. *J. Clin. Invest.* **84**, 1403–9.

Berry, M. K., Russo, A., Wishart, J. M., *et al.* (2003). Effect of solid meal on gastric emptying of, and glycemic and cardiovascular responses to, liquid glucose in older subjects. *Am J Physiol Gastrointest Liver Physiol* **284**, G655–662.

Brener, W., Hendrix, T. R., and McHugh, P. R. (1983). Regulation of the gastric emptying of glucose. *Gastroenterology* **85**, 76–82.

Breuer, H. W. (2003). Review of acarbose therapeutic strategies in the long-term treatment and in the prevention of type 2 diabetes. *Int J Clin Pharmacol Ther* **41**, 421–40.

Brown, R. T., Polinsky, R. J., and Bancom, C. E. (1989). Euglycemic insulin-induced hypotension in autonomic failure. *Clin. Neuropharmacol.* **12**, 227–31.

Catz, A., Bluvshtein, V., Pinhas, I., *et al.* (2007). Hemodynamic effects of liquid food ingestion in mid-thoracic paraplegia: is supine postprandial hypotension related to thoracic spinal cord damage? *Spinal Cord* **45**, 96–103.

Catz, A., Mendelson, L., and Solzi, P. (1992). Symptomatic postprandial hypotension in high paraplegia. Case report. *Paraplegia* **30**, 582–86.

Colao, A., Faggiano, A., and Pivonello, R. (2010) Somatostatin analogues: treatment of pituitary and neuroendocrine tumors. *Prog Brain Res* **182**, 281–94.

Cox, H. S., Kaye, D. M., Thompson, J. M. *et al.* (1995). Regional sympathetic nervous activation after a large meal in humans. *Clin. Sci.* **89**, 145–54.

Davies, K. N., King, D., Billington, D., and Barrett, J. A. (1996). Intestinal permeability and orocaecal transit time in elderly patients with Parkinson's disease. *Postgrad Med J* **72**, 164–67.

Deane, A. M., Nguyen, N. Q., Stevens, J. E., *et al.* (2010) Endogenous glucagon-like peptide-1 slows gastric emptying in healthy subjects, attenuating postprandial glycemia. *J Clin Endocrinol Metab* **95**, 215–21.

Deguchi, K., Ikeda, K., Sasaki, I., *et al.* (2007). Effects of daily water drinking on orthostatic and postprandial hypotension in patients with multiple system atrophy. *J Neurol* **254**, 735–40.

Edwards, B. J., Perry, H. M., 3rd, Kaiser, F. E., *et al.* (1996). Relationship of age and calcitonin gene-related peptide to postprandial hypotension. *Mech Ageing Dev* **87**, 61–73.

Edwards, C. M., Todd, J. F., Ghatei, M. A., and Bloom, S. R. (1998). Subcutaneous glucagon-like peptide-1 (7–36) amide is insulinotropic and can cause hypoglycaemia in fasted healthy subjects. *Clin Sci (Lond)* **95**, 719–24.

Eisenhofer, G., Aneman, A., Hooper, D., Holmes, C., Goldstein, D., and Friberg, P. (1995). Production and metabolism of dopamine and norepinephrine in mesenteric organs and liver of swine. *Am. J. Physiol.* **268**, G641–49.

Fagius, J., Ellerfelt, K., Lithell, H., and Berne, C. (1996). Increase in muscle nerve sympathetic activity after glucose intake is blunted in the elderly. *Clin Auton Res* **6**, 195–203.

Fagius, J., Niklasson, F., and Berne, C. (1986). Sympathetic outflow in human muscle nerves increases during hypoglycaemia. *Diabetes* **35**, 1124–9.

Fisher, A. A., Davis, M. W., Srikusalanukul, W., and Budge, M. M. (2005). Postprandial hypotension predicts all-cause mortality in older, low-level care residents. *J Am Geriatr Soc* **53**, 1313–20.

Freeman, R., Young, J., Landsberg, L., and Lipsitz, L. (1996). The treatment of postprandial hypotension in autonomic failure with 3,4-DL-threo-dihydroxyphenylserine. *Neurology* **47**, 1414–20

French, E. B. and Kilpatrick, R. (1955). The role of adrenaline in hypoglycemic reactions in man. *Clin. Sci.* **14**, 639–51.

Gentilcore, D., Bryant, B., Wishart, J. M., *et al.* (2005a). Acarbose attenuates the hypotensive response to sucrose and slows gastric emptying in the elderly. *Am J Med* **118**, 1289.

Gentilcore, D., Doran, S., Meyer, J. H., Horowitz, M., and Jones, K. L. (2006a). Effects of intraduodenal glucose concentration on blood pressure and heart rate in healthy older subjects. *Dig Dis Sci* **51**, 652–56.

Gentilcore, D., Hausken, T., Meyer, J. H., *et al.* (2008a). Effects of intraduodenal glucose, fat, and protein on blood pressure, heart rate, and splanchnic blood flow in healthy older subjects. *Am J Clin Nutr* **87**, 156–61.

Gentilcore, D., Jones, K. L., O'Donovan, D. G., and Horowitz, M. (2006b). Postprandial hypotension—novel insights into pathophysiology and therapeutic implications. *Curr Vasc Pharmacol* **4**, 161–71.

Gentilcore, D., Meyer, J. H., Rayner, C. K., Horowitz, M., and Jones, K. L. (2008b). Gastric distension attenuates the hypotensive effect of intraduodenal glucose in healthy older subjects. *Am J Physiol Regul Integr Comp Physiol* **295**, R472–477.

Gentilcore, D., Nair, N. S., Vanis, L., *et al.* (2009). Comparative effects of oral and intraduodenal glucose on blood pressure, heart rate, and splanchnic blood flow in healthy older subjects. *Am J Physiol Regul Integr Comp Physiol* **297**, R716–722.

Gentilcore, D., Vanis, L., Rayner, C. K., Horowitz, M., and Jones, K. L. (2010). Effects of intraduodenal acarbose on blood pressure, heart rate and splanchnic blood flow in healthy older subjects. *JAGS* **58**(Supp 1), S280.

Gentilcore, D., Visvanathan, R., Russo, A., *et al.* (2005b). Role of nitric oxide mechanisms in gastric emptying of, and the blood pressure and glycemic responses to, oral glucose in healthy older subjects. *Am J Physiol Gastrointest Liver Physiol* **288**, G1227–1232.

Hakusui, S., Sugiyama, Y., Iwase, S. *et al.* (1991). Postprandial hypotension: microneurographic analysis and treatment with vasopressin. *Neurology* **41**, 712–15.

Hardoff, R., Sula, M., Tamir, A., *et al.* (2001). Gastric emptying time and gastric motility in patients with Parkinson's disease. *Mov Disord* **16**, 1041–47.

Heberden, W. (1772). Some account of a disorder of the breast. *Medical Transactions* (published by the College of Physicians in London) **2**, 59–67.

Heddle, R., Collins, P. J., Dent, J., *et al.* (1989). Motor mechanisms associated with slowing of the gastric emptying of a solid meal by an intraduodenal lipid infusion. *J Gastroenterol Hepatol* **4**, 437–47.

Heseltine, D., Dakkak, M., Woodhouse, K., Macdonald, I. A., and Potter, J. F. (1991a). The effect of caffeine on postprandial hypotension in the elderly. *J Am Geriatr Soc* **39**, 160–64.

Heseltine, D., el-Jabri, M., Ahmed, F., and Knox, J. (1991b). The effect of caffeine on postprandial blood pressure in the frail elderly. *Postgrad Med J* **67**, 543–47.

Hirayama, M., Watanabe, H., Koike, Y. *et al.* (1993). Treatment of postprandial hypotension with selective ₁ and ₁ adrenergic agonists. *J. autonom. nerv. Syst.* **45**, 149–54.

Hoeldtke, R. D., O'Dorisio, T. M., and Boden, G. (1986). Treatment of autonomic neuropathy with a somatostatin analogue, SMS 201–995. *Lancet* **ii**, 602–5.

Hoeldtke R. D., Bryner K. D., Hoeldtke M. E., Hobbs G.. (2007) Treatment of autonomic neuropathy, postural tachycardia and orthostatic syncope with octreotide LAR. *Clin Auton Res.* **217**, 334–40.

Holst, J. J., and Gromada, J. (2004). Role of incretin hormones in the regulation of insulin secretion in diabetic and nondiabetic humans. *Am J Physiol Endocrinol Metab* **287**, E199–206.

Horowitz, M., Jones, K., Edelbroek, M. A., Smout, A. J., and Read, N. W. (1993). The effect of posture on gastric emptying and intragastric distribution of oil and aqueous meal components and appetite. *Gastroenterology* **105**, 382–90.

Idiaquez, J., Rios, L., and Sandoval, E. (1997). Post-prandial hypotension in Alzheimer's disease. *Clin. Auton. Res.* **7**, 119–20.

Imai, C., Muratani, H., Kimura, Y., *et al.* (1998). Effects of meal ingestion and active standing on blood pressure in patients > or = 60 years of age. *Am J Cardiol* **81**, 1310–1314.

Jansen, R. W., Connelly, C. M., Kelley-Gagnon, M. M., Parker, J. A., and Lipsitz, L. A. (1995). Postprandial hypotension in elderly patients with unexplained syncope. *Arch Intern Med* **155**, 945–52.

Jansen, R. W., Lenders, J. W., Peeters, T. L., van Lier, H. J., and Hoefnagels, W. H. (1988). SMS 201–995 prevents postprandial blood pressure reduction in normotensive and hypertensive elderly subjects. *J Hypertens Suppl* **6**, S669–672.

Jansen, R. W., Peeters, T. L., Lenders, J. W., *et al.* (1989). Somatostatin analog octreotide (SMS 201–995) prevents the decrease in blood pressure after oral glucose loading in the elderly. *J Clin Endocrinol Metab* **68**, 752–56.

Jansen, R. W., Peeters, T. L., Van Lier, H. J., and Hoefnagels, W. H. (1990). The effect of oral glucose, protein, fat and water loading on blood pressure and the gastrointestinal peptides VIP and somatostatin in hypertensive elderly subjects. *Eur J Clin Invest* **20**, 192–98.

Jansen, R. W., and Hoefnagels, W. H. (1987). Influence of oral and intravenous glucose loading on blood pressure in normotensive and hypertensive elderly subjects. *J Hypertens* **5**, S501–S503.

Jansen, R. W., and Lipsitz, L. A. (1995). Postprandial hypotension: epidemiology, pathophysiology, and clinical management. *Ann Intern Med* **122**, 286–95.

Jian, Z. J., and Zhou, B. Y. (2008). Efficacy and safety of acarbose in the treatment of elderly patients with postprandial hypotension. *Chin Med J (Engl)* **121**, 2054–59.

Jones, K. L., MacIntosh, C., Su, Y. C., *et al.* (2001). Guar gum reduces postprandial hypotension in older people. *J Am Geriatr Soc* **49**, 162–67.

Jones, K. L., O'Donovan, D., Russo, A., *et al.* (2005). Effects of drink volume and glucose load on gastric emptying and postprandial blood pressure in healthy older subjects. *Am J Physiol Gastrointest Liver Physiol* **289**, G240–248.

Jones, K. L., Tonkin, A., Horowitz, M., *et al.* (1998). Rate of gastric emptying is a determinant of postprandial hypotension in non-insulin-dependent diabetes mellitus. *Clin Sci (Lond)* **94**, 65–70.

Jost, W. H. (2010). Gastrointestinal dysfunction in Parkinson's Disease. *J Neurol Sci* **289**, 69–73.

Kamata, T., Yokota, T., Furukawa, T., and Tsukagoshi, H. (1994). Cerebral ischaemic attack caused by post-prandial hypotension. *Stroke* **25**, 511–13.

Kearney, M. T., Cowley, A. J., Stubbs, T. A., Perry, A. J., and Macdonald, I. A. (1996b). Central and peripheral haemodynamic responses to high carbohydrate and high fat meals in human cardiac transplant recipients. *Clin. Sci.* **90**, 473–83.

Kearney, M. T., Cowley, A. J., Stubbs, T. A., and Macdonald, I. A. (1996a). Effect of a physiological insulin infusion on the cardiovascular responses to a high fat meal: evidence supporting a role for insulin in modulating postprandial cardiovascular homoestasis in man. *Clin. Sci.* **91**, 415–23.

Kooner, J. S., Armstrong, E., Bannister, R., Peart, W. S., and Mathias, C. J. (1990). Octreotide (SMS 201–995) prevents superior mesenteric artery vasodilatation and post-prandial hypotension in human autonomic failure. *Br. J. Clin. Pharmacol.* **29**, 154P.

Kooner, J. S., Peart, W. S., and Mathias, C. J. (1989). The peptide release inhibitor Octreotide (SMS 201–995), prevents the haemodynamic changes following food ingestion in normal human subjects. *Q. J. Exp. Physiol.* **74**, 569–72.

Kuipers, H. M., Jansen, R. W., Peeters, T. L., and Hoefnagels, W. H. (1991). The influence of food temperature on postprandial blood pressure reduction and its relation to substance-P in healthy elderly subjects. *J Am Geriatr Soc* **39**, 181–84.

Lin, H. C., Doty, J. E., Reedy, T. J., and Meyer, J. H. (1989). Inhibition of gastric emptying by glucose depends on length of intestine exposed to nutrient. *Am J Physiol* **256**, G404–411.

Lin, H. C., Doty, J. E., Reedy, T. J., and Meyer, J. H. (1990a). Inhibition of gastric emptying by acids depends on pH, titratable acidity, and length of intestine exposed to acid. *Am J Physiol* **259**, G1025–1030.

Lin, H. C., Doty, J. E., Reedy, T. J., and Meyer, J. H. (1990b). Inhibition of gastric emptying by sodium oleate depends on length of intestine exposed to nutrient. *Am J Physiol* **259**, G1031–1036.

Lipsitz, L. A., Jansen, R. W. M. M., Connelly, C. M., Kelley-Gagnon, M. M., and Parker, A. J. (1994). Haemodynamic and neurohumoral effects of caffeine in elderly patients with symptomatic postprandial hypotension: a double-blind, randomized, placebo-controlled study. *Clin. Sci.* **87**, 259–67.

Little, T. J., Pilichiewicz, A. N., Russo, A., *et al.* (2006). Effects of intravenous glucagon-like peptide-1 on gastric emptying and intragastric distribution in healthy subjects: relationships with postprandial glycemic and insulinemic responses. *J Clin Endocrinol Metab* **91**, 1916–23.

Maruta, T., Komai, K., Takamori, M., and Yamada, M. (2006). Voglibose inhibits postprandial hypotension in neurologic disorders and elderly people. *Neurology* **66**, 1432–34.

Matheson, P. J., Wilson, M. A., Spain, D. A., *et al.* (1997). Glucose-induced intestinal hyperemia is mediated by nitric oxide. *J Surg Res* **72**, 146–54.

Mathias, C. J. (1991). Postprandial hypotension. Pathophysiological mechanisms and clinical implications in different disorders. *Hypertension* **18**, 694–704.

Mathias, C. J. (1996). Gastrointestinal dysfunction in multiple system atrophy. *Semin. Neurol.* **16**, 251–5.

Mathias, C. J. (1997) Pharmacological manipulation of human gastrointestinal blood flow. *Fund. Clin. Pharmacol.* **11**, 29–34.

Mathias, C. J., Bannister, R., Cortelli, P. *et al.* (1990). Clinical, autonomic and therapeutic observations in two siblings with postural hypotension and sympathetic failure due to an inability to synthesize noradrenaline from dopamine because of a defiency of dopamine hydroxylase. *Q. J. Med.,* **278**, 617–33

Mathias, C. J., Da Costa, D. F., Fosbraey, P., Christensen, N. J., and Bannister, R. (1987). Hypotensive and sedative effects of insulin in autonomic failure. *BMJ.* **295**, 161–3.

Mathias, C. J., Da Costa, D. F., Fosbraey, P., *et al.* (1989a). Cardiovascular, biochemical and hormonal changes during food induced hypotension in chronic autonomic failure. *J. Neurol. Sci.* **94**, 255–69.

Mathias, C. J., Da Costa, D. F., McIntosh, C. M. *et al.* (1989b). Differential blood pressure and hormonal effects after glucose and xylose ingestion in chronic autonomic failure. *Clin. Sci.* **77**, 85–92.

Mathias, C. J., Frankel, H. S., Turner, R. C., and Christensen, N. J. (1979). Physiological responses to insulin hypoglycaemia in spinal man. *Paraplegia* **17**, 319–26.

Mathias, C. J., Holly, E., Armstrong, E., Shareef, M., and Bannister, R. (1991). The influence of food on postural hypotension in three groups with chronic autonomic failure—clinical and therapeutic implications. *J. Neurol. Neurosurg. Psychiat.* **54**, 726–30.

Maule, S., Tredici, M., Dematteis, A., Matteoda, C., and Chiandussi, L. (2004). Postprandial hypotension treated with acarbose in a patient with type 1 diabetes mellitus. *Clin. Auton. Res.* **14**, 405–407.

Maurer, M. S., Karmally, W., Rivadeneira, H., Parides, M. K., and Bloomfield, D. M. (2000). Upright posture and postprandial hypotension in elderly persons. *Ann. Intern. Med.* **133**, 533–36.

Mehagnoul-Schipper, D. J., Colier, W. N., Hoefnagels, W. H., Verheugt, F. W., and Jansen, R. W. (2002). Effects of furosemide versus captopril on postprandial and orthostatic blood pressure and on cerebral oxygenation in patients > or = 70 years of age with heart failure. *Am. J Cardiol.* **90**, 596–600.

Micieli, G., Martignoni, E., Cavallini, A., Sandrini, G., and Nappi, G. (1987). Postprandial and orthostatic hypotension in Parkinson's disease. *Neurology* **37**, 386–93.

Miles, D. W. and Hayter, C. J. (1968). The effects of intravenous insulin on the circulatory responses to tilting in normal and diabetic subjects with special reference to baroreceptor reflex block and atypical hypoglycaemic reactions. *Clin. Sci.* **34**, 419–30.

Mitro, P., Feterik, K., Lenartova, M., *et al.* (2001). Humoral mechanisms in the pathogenesis of postprandial hypotension in patients with essential hypertension. *Wien Klin Wochenschr* **113**, 424–32.

Moncada, S., and Higgs, E. A. (1991). Endogenous nitric oxide: physiology, pathology and clinical relevance. *Eur J Clin Invest* **21**, 361–74.

Morris, M. J., Cox, H. S., Lambert, G. W., *et al.* (1997). Region-specific neuropeptide Y overflows at rest and during sympathetic activation in humans. *Hypertension.* **29**, 137–43.

Muntzel, M., Morgan, D. A., Mark, A. L., and Johnson, A. K. (1994). Intracerebroventricular insulin produces non-uniform increases in sympathetic nerve activity. *Am. J. Physiol.* **267**, R1350–5.

O'Donovan, D., Feinle, C., Tonkin, A., Horowitz, M., and Jones, K. L. (2002). Postprandial hypotension in response to duodenal glucose delivery in healthy older subjects. *J Physiol.* **540**, 673–79.

O'Donovan, D., Feinle-Bisset, C., Chong, C., *et al.* (2005). Intraduodenal guar attenuates the fall in blood pressure induced by glucose in healthy older adults. *J Gerontol A Biol Sci Med Sci* **60**, 940–46.

O'Donovan, D., Horowitz, M., Russo, A., *et al.* (2004). Effects of lipase inhibition on gastric emptying of, and on the glycaemic, insulin and cardiovascular responses to, a high-fat/carbohydrate meal in type 2 diabetes. *Diabetologia* **47**, 2208–2214.

Onrot, J., Goldberg, M. R., Biaggioni, I., Hollister, A. S., Kincaid, D., and Robertson, D. (1985). Haemodynamic and humoral effects of caffeine in autonomic failure. Therapeutic implications for post-prandial hypotension. *New Engl. J. Med.* **313**, 549–54.

Puvi-Rajasingham, S., and Mathias, C. J. (1996). Effect of meal size on the blood pressure before and after postural change in primary autonomic failure. *Clin. Auton. Res.* **6**, 1–6

Raimbach, S. J., Cortelli, P., Kooner, J. S., Bannister, R., Bloom, S. R., and Mathias, C. J. (1989). Prevention of glucose-induced hypotension by the somatostatin analogue Octreotide (SMS 201–995) in chronic autonomic failure haemodynamic and hormonal changes. *Clin. Sci.* **77**, 623–8.

Ray Chaudhuri, K., Maule, S., Thomaides, T., Pavitt, D., and Mathias, C. J. (1994). Alcohol ingestion lowers supine blood pressure, causes splanchnic vasodilatation and worsens postural hypotension in primary autonomic failure. *J. Neurol.* **241**, 145–52.

Ray Chaudhuri, K., Thomaides, T., Watson, L., and Mathias, C. J. (1995). Octreotide reduces alcohol-induced hypotension and orthostatic symptoms in primary autonomic failure. *Q. J. Med.* **88**, 719–25.

Robertson, D., Wade, D., and Robertson, R. M. (1981). Post-prandial alterations in cardiovascular haemodynamics in autonomic dysfunction states. *Am. J. Cardiol.* **48**, 1048–52.

Russo, A., Stevens, J. E., Wilson, T., *et al.* (2003). Guar attenuates fall in postprandial blood pressure and slows gastric emptying of oral glucose in type 2 diabetes. *Dig Dis Sci* **48**, 1221–29.

Sasaki, E., Goda, K., Nagata, K., *et al.* (2001). Acarbose improved severe postprandial hypotension in a patient with diabetes mellitus. *J Diabetes Complications* **15**, 158–61.

Schirra, J., Nicolaus, M., Woerle, H. J., *et al.* (2009). GLP-1 regulates gastroduodenal motility involving cholinergic pathways. *Neurogastroenterol Motil* **21**, 609–618, e621–602.

Seyer-Hansen, K. (1977). Post-prandial hypotension. *BMJ* **2**, 1262.

Shannon, J. R., Diedrich, A., Biaggioni, I., *et al.* (2002). Water drinking as a treatment for orthostatic syndromes. *Am J Med* **112**, 355–60.

Shibao, C., Gamboa, A., Diedrich, A., *et al.* (2007). Acarbose, an alpha-glucosidase inhibitor, attenuates postprandial hypotension in autonomic failure. *Hypertension* **50**, 54–61.

Smirk, F. M. (1953). Action of a new methonium compound in arterial hypotension, M & B 205A. *Lancet* **i**, 457.

Smith, G. D. P., Alam, M., Watson, L. P., and Mathias, C. J. (1995). Effects of the somatostatin analogue, octreotide, on exercise induced hypotension in human subjects with chronic sympathetic failure. *Clin. Sci.* **89**, 367–73.

Smith, G. D. P., and Mathias, C. J. (1996). Differences in the cardiovascular responses to supine exercise and to standing post-exercise in two clinical subgroups of the Shy–Drager syndrome (multiple system atrophy). *J. Neurol. Neurosurg. Psychiat.* **61**, 297–303.

Su, Y. C., Vozzo, R., Doran, S., *et al.* (2001). Effects of the nitric oxide synthase inhibitor NG-nitro-L-arginine methyl ester (L-NAME) on antropyloroduodenal motility and appetite in response to intraduodenal lipid infusion in humans. *Scand J Gastroenterol* **36**, 948–54.

Takamori, M., Hirayama, M., Kobayashi, R., *et al.* (2007). Altered venous capacitance as a cause of postprandial hypotension in multiple system atrophy. *Clin Auton Res* **17**, 20–25.

Thomaides, T., Bleasdale-Barr, K. Chaudhuri, K. R., Pavitt, D. V., Marsden, C. D., and Mathias, C. J. (1993). Cardiovascular and hormonal responses to liquid food challenge in idiopathic Parkinsons disease, multiple system atrophy and pure autonomic failure. *Neurology* **43**, 900–4.

Vanis, L., Gentilcore, D., Hausken, T., *et al.* (2010). Effects of gastric distension on blood pressure and superior mesenteric artery blood flow responses to intraduodenal glucose in healthy older subjects. *Am J Physiol Regul Integr Comp Physiol.* (in press)

Vanis, L., Gentilcore, D., Rayner, C. K., Horowitz, M., Feinle-Bisset, C., and Jones K. L. (2009). Effects of glucose load on blood pressure, heart rate and splanchnic blood flow in healthy elderly. *JNHA* **13**(Suppl 1), S478.

Vaz, M., Cox, H. S., Kaye, D. M., Turner, A. G., Jennings, G. L., and Esler, M. D. (1995). Fallibility of plasma noradrenaline measurements in studying postprandial sympathetic nervous responses. *J. Autonom. Nerv. Syst.* **56**, 97–104.

Visvanathan, R., Horowitz, M., and Chapman, I. (2006). The hypotensive response to oral fat is comparable but slower compared with carbohydrate in healthy elderly subjects. *Br J Nutr* **95**, 340–45.

Vloet, L. C., Mehagnoul-Schipper, D. J., Hoefnagels, W. H., and Jansen, R. W. (2001). The influence of low-, normal-, and high-carbohydrate meals on blood pressure in elderly patients with postprandial hypotension. *J Gerontol A Biol Sci Med Sci* **56**, M744–748.

Vloet, L. C., Pel-Little, R. E., Jansen, P. A., and Jansen, R. W. (2005). High prevalence of postprandial and orthostatic hypotension among geriatric patients admitted to Dutch hospitals. *J Gerontol A Biol Sci Med Sci* **60**, 1271–77.

Vloet, L. C., Smits, R., and Jansen, R. W. (2003). The effect of meals at different mealtimes on blood pressure and symptoms in geriatric patients with postprandial hypotension. *J Gerontol A Biol Sci Med Sci* **58**, 1031–35.

Yusuf, S., Theodropoulos, S., Mathias, C. J. *et al.* (1987). Increased sensitivity of the denervated transplanted human heart to isoprenaline both before and after beta-adrenergic blockade. *Circulation* **75**, 696–704.

di Salvo, R. J., Bloom, W. L., Brost, A. A., Ferguson, W. F., and Ferris, E. B. (1956). A comparison of the metabolic and circulatory effects of epinephrine, norepinephrine and insulin hypoglycaemia with observations on the influence of autonomic blocking agents. *J. Clin. Invest.* **35**, 568–77.

van Kraaij, D. J., Jansen, R. W., Bouwels, L. H., and Hoefnagels, W. H. (1999). Furosemide withdrawal improves postprandial hypotension in elderly patients with heart failure and preserved left ventricular systolic function. *Arch Intern Med* **159**, 1599–1605.

van Orshoven, N. P., Oey, P. L., van Schelven, L. J., *et al.* (2004). Effect of gastric distension on cardiovascular parameters: gastrovascular reflex is attenuated in the elderly. *J Physiol* **555**, 573–83.

van Orshoven, N. P., van Schelven, L. J., Akkermans, L. M., *et al.* (2008). The effect of intraduodenal glucose on muscle sympathetic nerve activity in healthy young and older subjects. *Clin Auton Res* **18**, 28–35.

von der Thusen, J. H., Smith, G. D. P., Bleasdale-Barr, K., and Mathias, C. J. (1996). Differences in postprandial hypotension in two subtypes with human central autonomic failure (Shy–Drager syndrome/multiple system atrophy). *J. Physiol.* **495**, 129P.

CHAPTER 29

Cardiovascular effects of water ingestion in autonomic failure

Timothy M. Young and Christopher J. Mathias

Introduction

Remarkably for such a fundamental process as water drinking, the pressor effects of water ingestion have only recently been described. The first suggestion that water ingestion could increase blood pressure in autonomic failure was reported in 1983 with improvement of orthostatic symptoms in a subject with autonomic failure who drank large quantities of seawater. (Frewin and Bartholomeusz 1983). A pressor effect of water alone in autonomic failure was only confirmed prior to the new millennium with the first report of the pressor effect of drinking 480 ml of tap water (Jordan et al. 1999; Mathias, 2000a). Jordon et al. observed that in seated young healthy subjects there was no change in blood pressure (BP) in following water ingestion. Older healthy subjects showed an 11 mm Hg rise in systolic BP following ingestion of the same volume of water. A more substantial rise in systolic BP was observed in seated subjects with chronic autonomic failure. In some the increase was in excess of 30 mm Hg. The pressor effects described above began a few minutes after ingestion of water and peaked around 20 minutes. As tap water contains small quantities of cations, which could conceivably be a factor in pressor responses, the effects of similar volumes of distilled water were studied in patients with severe sympathetic denervation due to pure autonomic failure (PAF) (Cariga and Mathias 2001) and in multiple system atrophy (MSA) (Young and Mathias 2004a). Distilled water also resulted in a pressor effect of similar magnitude and time course to that observed with tap water. While the pressor effects of oral water are likely to last for no more than about an hour, the potential of water ingestion as a therapy for orthostatic hypotension was suggested (Mathias 2000a). Oral ingestion of 480 ml of distilled water in MSA and PAF has been shown both to alleviate the reduction in BP on subsequent standing (Shannon et al. 2002) and symptoms of orthostatic hypotension whilst standing (Young and Mathias 2004a). Suggestions of a smaller rise in BP have been made in patients with spinal cord injury following water ingestion (Tank et al. 2003). Interestingly possible improvements in orthostatic tolerance in intermittent autonomic dysfunction such as vasovagal syncope and in normal subjects exposed to negative lower body pressure in upright posture or blood donation (Lu et al. 2003, Schroeder et al. 2002, Hanson and France 2004).

Water ingestion thus has cardiovascular effects in both normal and diseased man. The mechanisms of the pressor response remain unclear. Better understanding of the aetiology of the water pressor effect would be likely to aid both understanding of the pathophysiology of autonomic failure, and the treatment of orthostatic hypotension, which can be so debilitating in these patients. As alluded to above, patients with other causes of orthostatic intolerance such as postural orthostatic tachycardia syndrome (PoTS) and vasovagal syncope and hypotension related to exercise or food may also benefit both by oral ingestion of water, although more confirmatory studies are needed in this regard. Finally, it should be remembered that the importance of the cardiovascular effects of water drinking potentially extends well beyond the field of autonomic medicine. Even the small increases in blood pressure noted in older 'healthy' subjects after water drinking could be significant in the long term in the Western world where hypertension is endemic—certainly the very limited studies available so far would suggest a transient effect greater than that seen with the addition of table salt to food, which has been targeted extensively as a cause of hypertension in the past few decades. In addition, early phase drug trials incorporate the ingestion of water with study medication as if it were inert, yet subsequently monitor cardiovascular responses including heart rate and postural hypotension. That water ingestion has very real cardiovascular effects has now been established; to attempt to unravel the mechanisms by which water exerts these effects is now therefore an important step.

Physiology of water ingestion

Water drinking is a fundamental aspect of animal life. In man typically 2–3 litres of fluid is ingested each day, either in response to thirst stimuli or as a result of direct volition. The volume of the typical stomach is typically only 50 ml when empty but can expand to a capacity of approximately 1 litre after a meal (Sherwood 2004), although this varies considerably with age and body size. The stomach is distensible to a point, although ingested volumes much in excess of 500 ml typically start to lead to sensations of fullness or discomfort (Penagini et al. 1998) and usually give rise to a sensation of satiety inhibiting further intake until the contents is reduced by gastric emptying. Usually fluid is taken in the form of hypotonic solutions (e.g. tap water, tea, carbonated beverages), often taken in association with eating. The mix of ingested fluid and food is termed chyme. The fluid:food ratio of chyme and its volume can significantly influence gastric emptying. This is important because the tight junctions of the gastric mucosa markedly limit the absorption of water while the chyme is still within the stomach. Once the chyme clears the pyloric junction and enters the vast surface area of the permeable small intestine, water absorption from the gut lumen to the extracellular and then intracellular spaces is rapid. The marked differences in gastric emptying between water and mixed meal ingestion is illustrated in Fig. 29.1 in normal subjects, using scintigraphy, which has now largely superseded other radiological methods (Lawaetz et al. 1989, Lin et al. 2005). The situation is slightly more complex for mixed meal/fluid ingestion as the different components tend to be released from the stomach to the small intestine at different rates, with fluids often preceding the solid components (Lin et al. 2005). Furthermore the volume and tonicity of chyme may be significantly altered by secretions and absorption, additional components in determining gastric emptying.

There is a basic peristaltic reflex in the gut whereby local luminal dilation results in an ascending muscular excitation pathway and descending inhibition. The higher co-ordination of the movement of chyme from the stomach to small intestine is provided by a vagally mediated reflex originating in the brainstem, while additional control is provided by a prevertebral reflex arc responding to stomach visceral afferents (Thompson 2003). Normally a vagally mediated reflex on ingestion inhibits the periodic migrating motor complex, which periodically propagates distally from the stomach in the fasted state. For water ingestion in normal subjects, the net result is a fairly rapid gastric emptying as shown in the upper graph of Fig. 29.1. Greater stomach volumes are emptied more rapidly (Noakes et al. 1991, Doran et al. 1998).

Upon gastric emptying, chyme enters the duodenum (the portion of the intestine from the pyloric sphincter to the ligament of Treitz), being 20–30 cm in length. It is highly permeable with

evidence suggesting that pure water is ingested at least as fast as isotonic 6% carbohydrate-electrolyte drink, possibly because the duodenum tends to bring the chyme towards isotonicity by means of secretions/absorption (Lambert et al. 1997). These results suggest that the rate of tracer accumulation in the blood after ingestion of different volumes of test drinks is not a reliable indication of the availability of the ingested fluid, but gives at least a qualitative measure of the sum of the effects of gastric emptying and intestinal water absorption (Lambert et al. 1997).

Although the physiology of gastric emptying has been extensively studied in normal subjects, the situation in autonomic failure is less clear, with initial evidence suggestive of accelerated gastric emptying in PAF (Mathias and Bannister 2001). However, the possibility of slowing of gastric emptying in primary autonomic failure has recently been reported (Maule et al. 2002). These authors used $^{13}CO_2$-octanoid acid breath test (OBT) and electrogastrogram (EGG) to assess gastric emptying following a standard test meal of one scrambled egg, two slices of bread, 50 g ham and 10 g butter in 3 PAF and 9 MSA subjects. The egg yolk was labelled with 0.1 ml of $^{13}CO2$-octanoid acid. 13C-octanoid acid is rapidly absorbed in the duodenum, but not stomach, and metabolized in the liver; following oxidation, the resulting $^{13}CO2$ is excreted in the breath. Breath samples were collected at baseline and at 15-minute intervals analysed by isotope-selective non-dispersive infrared spectrometry. Half-time gastric emptying (t½) was thus calculated with t½ ≤144 minutes considered normal. Gastric emptying was found to be delayed in 5/9 MSA and 1/3 PAF. In contrast 2/3 PAF had relatively fast gastric emptying with gastric emptying t ½ of 97 and 80 minutes. EGG found normogastria in 6/9 MSA and bradigastria in 3/9. In PAF, 2/3 showed bradigastria and 1/3 (same subject with gastric emptying t ½ of 80 minutes) showed tachigastria.

Thus the gastric emptying rates in MSA and PAF appears to be abnormal in many cases, but whether this is consistently delayed or accelerated is not clear at present. In particular it should be noted that the study by Maule et al. utilized oral food and the gastric emptying with water may well be different as with normal subjects.

Cardiovascular autonomic responses to water ingestion

Normal subjects

In most studies 480–500 ml of water have been ingested rapidly over a few minutes, with measurements made in the seated position. In young normal subjects aged 25–40 years, blood pressure did not change after water ingestion (Jordan et al. 2000, Scott et al. 2001, Routledge et al. 2002). Young normal individuals do appear to have a significant reduction in heart rate following water ingestion, with a peak effect 20–25 minutes post-ingestion (Routledge et al. 2002). Older normal individuals (mean age 57 years) have shown an increase in blood pressure with systolic pressure increasing by 11 ± 2 mm Hg, after 35 minutes, heart rate fell by 5.4 ±1 bpm after 20 minutes Fig. 29.2 (Jordan et al. 2000). This pressor response began within 5 minutes of ingestion, reached a peak at 30–35 minutes and waned after 90 minutes. In elderly normal subjects (70 ± 5 years) without autonomic dysfunction, 400 ml of water ingested over 10 minutes resulted in negligible increase in seated systolic and diastolic blood pressure (Imai et al. 1998). Similarly aged subjects showed some increase in seated blood pressure following ingestion of 379 ml of water ingested within 3 minutes although this did not reach significance (Visvanathan et al. 2004).

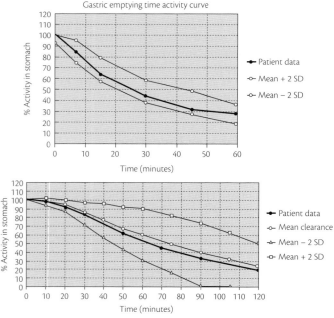

Fig. 29.1 Measurement of gastric emptying in normal subjects following ingestion of 300 ml water (above) or a similar volume of mixed meal (120 ml water, 2 large scrambled eggs, a piece of toast and a teaspoon of butter) (below) at time '0' by use of by gamma scintigraphy. With kind permission from Springer Science+Business Media: *Digestive Diseases and Sciences, Measurement of Gastrointestinal Transit*, **50**, 2005, 989–1004, Lin HC, Prather C, Fisher RS, et al.

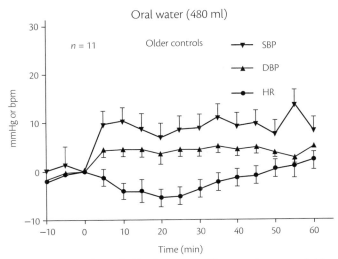

Fig. 29.2 Systolic and diastolic blood pressure and heart rate in a group of older normal subjects (mean age 57 years) before and after ingestion of 480 ml Nashville tap water. Jordan J, Shannon JR, Black BK, Ali Y, Farley M, Costa F et al. (2000) The pressor response to water drinking in humans: a sympathetic reflex? *Circulation* **101**: 504–509, with permission from Wolters Kluwer Health.

Following water ingestion plasma noradrenaline levels rose in younger subjects (without a pressor response) and also in older normal subjects (with a pressor response). In young normal individuals muscular sympathetic nerve activity (MSNA) was measured by microneurography; it increased 20 minutes after water ingestion, peaked at 30 minutes and returned to control levels at 50 minutes, with a corresponding increase in calf vascular resistance, peaking at 40 minutes post-ingestion (Scott et al. 2001). This was not reproduced in a further study of normal young subjects (Endo et al. 2002) where a transient pressor response and increase in MSNA occurred only whilst drinking. In view of possible sympathetic activation, the effects of water drinking on thermogenesis in normal subjects have been studied (Boschmann et al. 2003). It was found that drinking 500 ml of water increased metabolic rate by 30% within 10 minutes with a peak after 30–40 minutes. β-adrenoceptor blockade appeared to attenuate this effect. Only 40% of the energy expenditure was used to increase the water from room temperature to body temperature.

A possible mechanism for the pressor response to water is reflex sympathetic activation resulting from gastric distension. In normal subjects, graded gastric balloon distension causes a rise in MSNA and blood pressure (Rossi et al. 1998). In normal subjects, oral water raises MSNA but not blood pressure (Scott et al. 2001). However, in a later study also in normal subjects, water caused an initial transient rise in blood pressure and heart rate but a decrease in MSNA (Endo et al. 2002). In this study MSNA did not rise above the baseline after water ingestion, in contrast to the earlier study by Scott et al. 2001. Furthermore, the same volume of water administered by a stomach tube over 20 minutes caused no change in either MSNA or blood pressure.

The discrepancy in pressor response between normal young subjects (no pressor response) and older subjects has been hypothesized to be related to the reflex bradycardia which younger but not older subjects produce in response to oral water. This may serve to buffer any pressor mechanisms activated by water ingestion in younger subjects (Routledge et al. 2002). It was further postulated that older subjects have reduced cardiac vagal buffering ability as demonstrated by the presence of a pressor response but no HR

change following water ingestion in 4 patients with denervated hearts (post heart transplant). It should be noted however that these post-transplant patients would have been closer in age to the older individuals described earlier, with ages between 50 years and 62 years, and medication may have been a further confounding factor in the response. It has been proposed that water drinking does raise sympathetic activity and that the increase in sympathetic activity only generates a pressor response in the setting of impaired baroreflex function and/or increased vascular sensitivity, e.g., in the elderly and/or in those with autonomic dysfunction, e.g., autonomic failure (May and Jordan, 2010).

Primary autonomic failure

The pressor effects of water ingestion have been studied in two groups with primary autonomic failure—PAF and MSA. In PAF, the autonomic nervous system only is involved with a peripheral postganglionic sympathetic lesion. In MSA, there are associated neurological deficits (parkinsonian and cerebellar signs), and the lesion is predominantly central and preganglionic (Mathias 2000b). Blood pressure rose by 37 ± 7/14 ± 3 mmHg in PAF and 33 ± 5/16 ± 3 mmHg in MSA (Jordan et al. 2000). However, scrutiny of the physiological responses to autonomic testing in their patients with PAF suggested that sympathetic denervation might not have been complete. Furthermore, in a study of 13 patients with Parkinson's disease and orthostatic hypotension due to autonomic failure (confirmed on physiological testing) studied while supine, there was no change in blood pressure after ingestion of water (Senard et al. 1999). To evaluate this factor, Cariga and Mathias (2001) studied 14 patients with PAF with severe orthostatic hypotension, all of whom had substantial sympathetic denervation, as based on a series of physiological and biochemical studies. In the original studies Nashville tap water was used and therefore distilled water was used to exclude the potential effects of even small amounts of vasopressor substances as PAF are known to have enhanced pressor sensitivity (see Chapter 39). After water ingestion, blood pressure rose after a few minutes, peaked at 40 minutes and remained elevated for 35 minutes before returning to basal levels at 50 minutes (Figs 29.3 and 29.4).

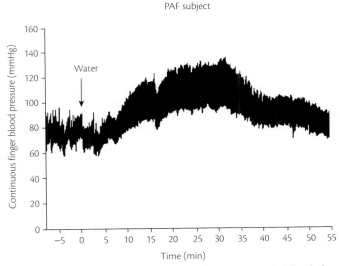

Fig. 29.3 Blood pressure changes in a patient with pure autonomic failure before and after 500 ml distilled water ingested at time '0'. Blood pressure is measured continuously using the Portapres. Reproduced with permission, from Cariga P, Mathias CJ, (2001). *Clinical Science*, **101**, 313–319 © the Biochemical Society.

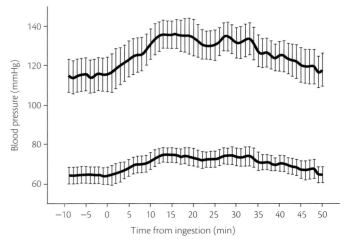

Fig. 29.4 Systolic and diastolic blood pressure ± SEM) in 14 patients with pure autonomic failure, before and after oral ingestion of 500 ml distilled water at time '0' . Reproduced with permission, from Cariga P, Mathias CJ, (2001). *Clinical Science*, **101**, 313–319 © the Biochemical Society.

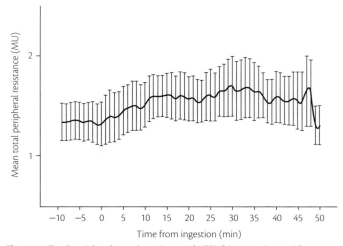

Fig. 29.5 Total peripheral vascular resistance (± SEM) in 14 patients with pure autonomic failure, before and after oral ingestion of 500 ml distilled water at time '0'. Reproduced with permission, from Cariga P, Mathias CJ, (2001). *Clinical Science*, **101**, 313–319 © the Biochemical Society.

Systolic blood pressure increased by 18 mmHg (range 7–64) and diastolic by 9mm Hg (range 5–37). Heart rate fell by 4 bpm. In a further study comparing PAF and MSA (Young and Mathias 2004a), similar changes were noted but with different time courses in the two groups; blood pressure rose significantly within 5 minutes in PAF, but took longer up to 14 minutes in MSA. In neither the original nor in the confirmation studies were plasma noradrenaline levels measured before and after water ingestion in the autonomic failure patients.

Regional haemodynamic measurements

Continuous measurement of cardiac function and regional haemodynamics measured in PAF (Cariga and Mathias 2001, Young and Mathias 2004a), have provided insight into the pressor mechanisms. After water ingestion there was a small fall in heart rate (5 ± bpm) with no change in ejection fraction, stroke volume or cardiac output. However, calculated total peripheral vascular resistance rose, favouring vasoconstriction as the haemodynamic mechanism responsible for the blood pressure rise Figs 29.5 and 29.6. Similar findings were observed when 500 ml of distilled water was infused directly into the stomach of a patients with PAF via a gastrostomy tube Fig. 29.7.

The time course of the rise in blood pressure and total peripheral vascular resistance after water ingestion in PAF is slow (over minutes), with an even later rise in MSA (Young and Mathias 2004a). This is considerably slower than after activation of reflexes that are known to raise blood pressure. In tetraplegics with high spinal cord lesions, activation of viscera (such as the urinary bladder and large bowel), or induction of skeletal muscle spasms, results in autonomic dysreflexia with a rapid rise in blood pressure, often within a few seconds, as a result of activation of spinal sympathetic reflexes below the segmented level of lesion (Mathias et al. 1976a). Humoral factors do not appear to contribute, which is consistent with the speed of rise and blood pressure. On discontinuing the provocative stimulus, blood pressure falls over a few minutes rather than rapidly, probably because of a combination of impaired baroreflex activity and pressor supersensitivity (Mathias et al. 1976b).

The response to water ingestion recently has been reported in tetraplegics in whom central sympathetic outflow is interrupted but vagal efferents preserved (Tank et al. 2003). The pressor response to water varied; mean supine finger blood pressure rose from 123 ± 8/165 ± 4 to 138 ± 8/73 + 4 mmHg after 40 minutes, while heart rate fell from 64 ± 2 to 60 ± 2 bpm. In some there was no pressor response. The reasons for this are unclear. In this study, the patients were studied supine, with the upper body at 15°; in previous studies patients were seated. The pressor response to water, without a gravitational stimulus, would be expected to be as great or greater, if sympathetic activation was responsible, especially in tetraplegics who are known to respond briskly to such stimuli. The latency of the response was unlike that of autonomic dysreflexia, and similar to the slower time course in autonomic failure, raising the probability that similar mechanisms accounted for the pressor response to water in the different groups.

Mechanisms of the pressor effect of water ingestion

The exact mechanism by which water ingestion results in a pressor response remains uncertain. Various factors are important in determining blood pressure; these include cardiac output, tone in resistance vessels (influenced by either circulating or locally produced constrictor or dilator substances), the state of capacitance vessels, intravascular volume and overall fluid status. The sympathetic nervous system acting on a beat-by-beat basis through the baroreceptor reflex to allow rapid adjustment of blood pressure. There have been various studies attempting to determine the precise mechanisms by which water exerts its pressor effect.

Effects of water temperature and volume

To determine if there was temperature and volume dependency, four subjects with autonomic failure were studied (Jordan et al. 2000). There was no difference in the pressor response when water at either 9°C or 24°C was administered. The pressor response was related to the volume ingested, as systolic blood pressure increased by up to 50 mm Hg after 480 ml water, and by 30 mm Hg after 240 ml when studied in four subjects with chronic autonomic failure, raising the possibility of reflex sympathetic activation from stomach distension in the generation of the pressor response. Studies in healthy animals and humans have demonstrated that

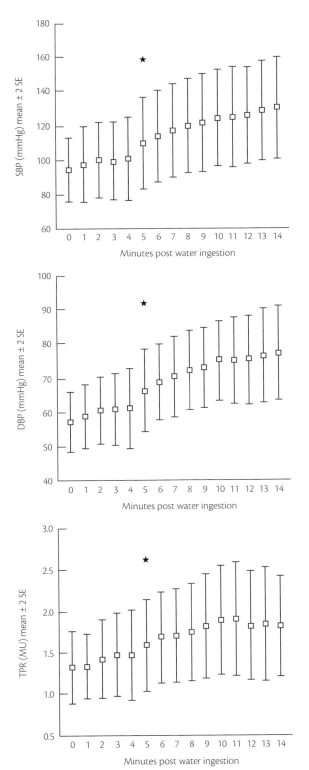

Fig. 29.6 Continuous Portapres monitoring of systolic (SBP) and diastolic (DBP) blood pressure following oral water ingestion in 7 patients with pure autonomic failure, demonstrating the relationship between increased total peripheral resistance (calculated through Modelflow analysis) and BP rise. Reproduced from *Journal of Neurol, Neurosur and Psych*, Young TM, Mathias CJ, **75**, 1737–4, 2004 with permission from BMJ Publishing Group Ltd.

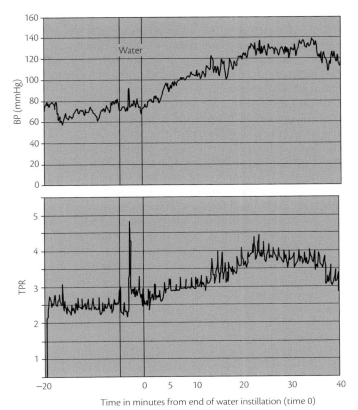

Fig. 29.7 Systolic blood pressure (top graph) and total peripheral resistance (lower graph) recorded via Portapres in a patient with pure autonomic failure with 500 ml of distilled water instilled directly into stomach via gastrostomy tube at time point '0'. Reprinted from *Autonomic Neuroscience: Basic and Clinical*, **113**, Young TM, Mathias CJ, Pressor effect of water instilled via gastrostomy tube in pure autonomic failure, 79–81, copyright 2004, with permission from Elsevier.

graded gastric balloon distension causes a rise in MSNA and blood pressure (Rossi et al. 1998). However, in normal subjects, oral water ingestion was shown to raise MSNA but not elevate blood pressure (Scott et al. 2001). Conflicting results were later shown in another group of normal young subjects where oral water ingestion caused an initial transient rise in blood pressure and heart rate but a decrease in MSNA (Endo et al. 2002). In that study the same volume of water administered by a stomach tube over 20 minutes, caused no change in either MSNA or blood pressure, raising the possibility that the initial pressor response resulted from the pharyngeal/oesophageal phase of water drinking. The degree of distension may be a factor in explaining this discrepancy—it is known that excessive dilatation the stomach may result in extreme bradycardia and even hypotension presumably via vasovagal mechanisms (Hmouda et al. 1994). The swallowing stage of drinking does not appear to be involved in generating the pressor effect in chronic autonomic failure, with a pressor effect to water having been demonstrated when water is instilled directly into the stomach of a patient with PAF (Young and Mathias 2004b) or MSA (Lipp et al. 2005).

Recent comparisons between haemodynamic responses to gastric distension with a barostat have been made in 8 young and 8 older normal subjects (van Orshoven et al. 2004). In this study the older subjects tended to show a higher increase in mean arterial pressure, heart rate and total peripheral arterial resistance despite showing a significantly attenuated increase in MSNA compared with the young subjects. The older subjects reported less symptoms of stomach distension, although there was no significant difference in stomach compliance between the young and older subjects. Possible reasons for these results might include the known reduction in central arterial compliance with ageing suggesting that even the attenuated increase in MSNA seen in the older group could still result in a significant pressor effect. An alternative possibility would be that the attenuation of sympathetic outflow in response to gastric distension in older normal subjects and in autonomic failure alters the local effect of locally released vasoactive substances akin to the known vasopressor supersensitivity known to occur in PAF.

That volume alone is insufficient to produce a pressor effect is clear from the fact that food consumption is associated with post-prandial hypotension in chronic autonomic failure. There are several possible factors in explaining the discrepancy in blood pressure response to ingestion of food or water. Food, especially carbohydrates, results in splanchnic circulation vasodilation in autonomic failure as a result of insulin release and subsequent nitric oxide release. Secondly the presence of food substantially slows gastric emptying and thus delays the absorption of water from the small bowel (Fig. 29.1). Furthermore, intragastric and intraduodenal water infusion induced an identical pressor response in sinoaortic-denervated mice (McHugh et al. 2010), suggesting that the afferent structure responding to water is likely located distally from the stomach (May and Jordan, 2010). Final additional factors such as osmoceptor activation would be more likely with relatively hypotonic chyme following water ingestion alone.

Effects of water osmolality

The first publication suggesting that water ingestion may lead to pressor response in chronic autonomic failure described a patient who had noted that the ingestion of seawater improved their postural hypotension symptoms (Frewin and Bartholomeusz 1983). Subsequent investigations confirmed that a pressor effect occurs in chronic autonomic failure after ingestion of either tap water (Jordan et al. 1999) or distilled water (Cariga and Mathias 2001, Young and Mathias 2004a). In dogs, data have suggested that gastric distension with saline results in a pressor response, but that the magnitude of BP increase is twice as great when distilled water is used (Haberich 1968). In humans hypo-osmolar water infused through a nasogastric tube induces greater sweating than isomolar saline, and it had been suggested that this might reflect greater sympathetic activation by hypo-osmolar solutions (Haberich 1968). More recently the possible effects of osmolarity have been studied in MSA (Lipp et al. 2005). A total of 10 patients were studied in a semi supine position with 500ml of either normal saline (iso-osmotic) or distilled water (hypo-osmotic) infused into the stomach over 5 minutes through a nasogastric tube. There was fairly marked variability in response. However, there was a significant difference in the BP response between the two groups, with distilled water but not saline producing a pressor effect between 10 minutes and 40 minutes post-ingestion. Similar findings are evident in sinoaortic-denervated mice (McHugh et al. 2010). Moreover, addition of sodium chloride to drinking water attenuated the pressor response in autonomic failure patients (Raj et al. 2006). These findings have led to the hypothesis that hypoosmolarity is the stimulus for the water-induced pressor response (or osmopressor response; May and Jordan, 2010). These authors

propose that water ingestion results in particularly large osmolality changes in the portal tract and in the liver which are detected by osmosensitive afferent neurons (May and Jordan, 2010). Consequently, the water osmopressor response is instigated via a spinal reflex-like mechanism, requiring transient receptor potential vanniloid 4 (Trpv4) channels (McHugh et al. 2010; May and Jordan, 2010). The authors propose that the spinal reflex-like mechanism is supported by the observation that heart rate decreases with water drinking, whereas heart rate variability increases (May and Jordan, 2011) and that spinal sympathetic activation induced by bladder distention elicits hypertension and bradycardia in patients with high spinal cord injury, albeit at a shorter latency compared to the pressor effect of water (see Chapter 66).

Vasoactive neurohumoral substances

The pressor effect to water occurs after a latency of at least 5 minutes, raising the possibility of local or systemic vasoconstrictor substances in its aetiology. Systemic circulating hormones, such as vasopressin and angiotensin-II are powerful vasoconstrictors. However, in normal subjects, plasma vasopressin and renin activity did not change following water ingestion, and levels were not reported in autonomic failure except for plasma renin, which was reported unchanged in two subjects with autonomic failure (Jordan et al. 2000). Plasma noradrenaline levels increased after water ingestion in both young and older normal subjects (Jordan et al. 2000 and Scott et al. 2001), but there was no correlation between the rise in plasma noradrenaline levels and the changes in blood pressure. Younger normal subjects do not change BP in response to oral water despite a rise in plasma noradrenaline (Scott et al. 2001). The increase in circulating plasma noradrenaline in these subjects following water ingestion are more likely to reflect the increase in sympathetic nerve activity suggested by increased MSNA than have direct vascular effects (Scott et al. 2001). Plasma noradrenaline increased in autonomic failure patients and this coincided with the time of the greatest blood pressure elevation (30 min) (Raj et al. 2006).

Locally released vasoactive substances also warrant discussion in the context of water ingestion. Inhibition of vasodilators or increased levels of vasoconstrictors such as endothelin could theoretically cause locally mediated pressor effects. It is known that distension of an isolated rat stomach results in release of somatostatin and reduced release of gastrin (Li 2003). Both somatostatin and intrinsic cholinergic pathways were involved distention-induced inhibition of gastrin release. Although the affect of water ingestion on these hormones in man is not known, the combination of release of somatostatin and reduced release of gastrin is interesting as somatostatin causes splanchnic arteriolar vasoconstriction by protein kinase C (PKC)-dependent vasoconstrictors, possibly via somatostatin receptor type 2 (SSTR2) receptors (Reynaert and Geerts 2003), and enhances endothelin-1-induced vasoconstriction (Huang et al. 2002). Gastrin on the other hand is a vasodilator. Gastrin is released by gastrin-releasing peptide, which has recently been shown to be a potent systemic vasodilator in healthy human subjects (Clive et al. 2001). The effects of gastrin on blood pressure are not as clear, although pentagastrin, a synthetic analogue, appears to increase BP and HR in man (Tavernor et al. 2000). The situation in chronic autonomic failure is complicated by the fact that basal gastrin and release following hypoglycaemia may be increased in PAF, but reduced in MSA (Polinsky et al. 1988)

Pharmacological studies

Pharmacological studies have been used at both ganglionic and presynaptic sympathetic levels. The possibility that residual sympathetic nerve activity may have been a factor in generating the pressor effect to water has been studied with trimethaphan ganglionic block (Jordan et al. 2000). Plasma noradrenaline was measured in two MSA patients, before and after ganglionic blockade. In both MSA subjects plasma noradrenaline levels fell, indicating suppression of residual sympathetic nerve activity. In neither was there a pressor response when water was administered after ganglionic blockade. The lack of a pressor response to water in MSA after ganglionic blockade raised further the possibility of activation of sympathetic neural mechanisms. Further evidence in normal subjects was considered to favour this, as the pressor response to water was also absent after ganglionic blockade (Jordan et al. 2000). However, this was performed only in younger subjects, who did not have a pressor response to water. Furthermore the pressor response is clearly seen in PAF subjects with extensive sympathetic denervation (Cariga and Mathias 2001) further supporting the concept that a pressor response only occurs in the setting of impaired autonomic cardiovascular function (May and Jordan, 2010).

Yohimbine acts on α_2-presynaptic receptors resulting in noradrenaline release and thus its effect is dependent on the integrity of sympathetic nerve terminals. In patients with primary autonomic failure there was a correlation between the pressor response to yohimbine and to water, suggesting that those with less sympathetic denervation had a greater pressor response (Jordan et al. 2000). This would be in keeping with a previous report where it was observed that patients with PAF with the greatest increase in blood pressure after water had a normal or even exaggerated pressor response (Jordan et al. 1999). This also implies the reverse, that patients with substantial sympathetic failure are less likely to have a pressor response to water. However, in later studies (Cariga and Mathias 2001) a marked pressor response to water ingestion also occurred in PAF with marked sympathetic dysfunction. Furthermore, in spinal cord injury tetraplegics, who have preserved sympathetic nerve terminals and have exaggerated pressor responses to vasoactive drugs and a range of visceral and other stimuli (see Chapter 66); the pressor response to water was similar or less than patients with autonomic failure. This suggests that other possibilities are needed to explain the pressor response. Finally it should be noted that Yohimbine is not a pure α_2-antagonist. It also displays partial agonist activity at cloned human 5-HT1A receptors, significant affinity for 5-hydroxytryptamine type 1B (5-HT1B) and type 1D (5-HT1D) receptors and antagonist properties at dopaminergic D2 receptors (Millan et al. 2000). Of these the D2 effect might be especially significant given the known action of other D2 antagonists such as domperidone and gastric motility and blood flow.

Correction of fluid depletion

For a variety of reasons fluid depletion is more likely to occur in patients with autonomic failure. Tubular absorption of sodium and other solutes, is influenced by sympathetic nerve activity, and may account for the urinary sodium and water loss in such patients (DiBona and Wilcox 2002). When supine patients with autonomic failure often develop raised blood pressure, sometimes to a marked extent. This in turn increases renal perfusion pressure and probably contributes to recumbency-induced polyuria (Schalekamp

1985, Kooner et al. 1987). Overnight, if lying flat their body weight can fall by 1–1.5 kg, which worsens both the symptoms and degree of orthostatic hypotension in the morning (Mathias et al. 1986). Correction of this deficit is the basis for nocturnal use of the vasopressin-2 agonist desmopressin, which reduces water loss, overnight weight loss, improves morning orthostatic hypotension as well as reducing symptoms (Mathias et al. 1986, Mathias and Young 2003).

An important consideration when considering possible correction of fluid depletion is the speed with which water is absorbed from the gut, given that the pressor effect is observed as rapidly as 5 minutes post-ingestion. As significant volumes of water are not absorbed into the portal circulation until water leaves the stomach to enter the duodenum, gastric emptying is a key concept. In normal subjects, the emptying half time of 800 ml of water is 21 minutes (Ploutz-Snyder et al. 1999), as measured with magnetic resonance imaging. With smaller volumes of 500 ml this is likely to be different. In normal subjects, water alone increases portal blood flow, measure by Doppler sonography (Host et al. 1996). Extrapolating from studies in normal subjects, who are well hydrated, may be erroneous if compared to relatively dehydrated autonomic failure patients. In normal subjects, hydration is recognized as reducing orthostatic responses. Gastric emptying in autonomic failure appears more rapid than in normal subjects (Mathias and Bannister 2001), and absorption of even a small fluid volume could create a sufficient pressor effect in patients because of impaired baroreflex function. In studies on rehydration after fluid restriction, the importance of extravascular hydration was thought to be of greater importance than intravascular hydration, in determining orthostatic tolerance (Harrison et al. 1986).

Water ingestion initially may raise plasma volume, but it is likely that redistribution then occurs with subsequent movement of fluid from intravascular into extravascular spaces. Saline has advantages over water alone, because it is stored extracellularly and causes greater explosion of both extra and intravascular spaces (Harrison 1986). This explains the benefit of saline drinking in autonomic failure (Frewin and Bartholomeusz 1983), although ingestion of salt and water often causes side effects, including diarrhoea. Recent work on the effects of different osmolarities of water however suggests that hypo-osmolar water produces a greater pressor response on ingestion in MSA than isotonic saline (Lipp et al. 2005). The haematocrit, as a measure of plasma volume was measured in normal subjects before, 30 and 60 minutes after water ingestion (Jordan et al. 2000). No significant changes in the haematocrit were observed, seemingly excluding increases in intravascular volume as a factor. A variety of factors can influence interpretation of haematocrit in this context, especially in subjects with denervation (DiBona and Wilcox 2002). Furthermore, the pressor effect of water occurred after 5 minutes and peaked at 30 minutes making it likely that water redistribution had occurred when the first measurements were made post-water ingestion. To measure the direct effects of plasma expansion, intravenously administered 5% dextrose was infused into five PAF, but over a 60-minute period (Jordan et al. 2000). After infusion plasma volume increased by 5.3% and blood pressure by 18 mm Hg, compared with 52 mm Hg with oral water. Patients with autonomic failure usually have a brisk pressor response to intravenous fluid replacement, although normal saline usually is used for rehydration and to raise blood pressure. However, carbohydrate is known to lower blood pressure in autonomic failure (Mathias et al. 1989), and the potential hypotensive effect of dextrose may have negated the pressor effect of this volume of water intravenously. Finally the time course of water infusion in this study is difficult to interpret, as the time taken to fully absorb ingested water into the systemic circulation in PAF is not known.

The reasons for the differential responses to water ingestion in young and older normal subjects remain unclear. Older subjects are more likely to have a degree of refractoriness of their renal tubules to vasopressin, and thus may be relatively less fluid replete than younger individuals. However, other factors, greater vascular responses to pressor stimuli, or less effective baroreceptor reflexes are also possible. This also may account for the pressor response to water (13–29 mmHg) observed in four cardiac transplant recipients who lacked cardiac autonomic innervation (Routledge et al. 2002). The pressor response to gastric distension with a barostat appears to be greater in older individuals despite an attenuation in MSNA increase compared with younger individuals. Reduced compliance of central arteries with ageing may explain this apparent discrepancy.

The beneficial effects of water ingestion in autonomic failure

The early observations of the pressor effect of water prompted suggestions of potential therapeutic effects on orthostatic and post-prandial and exercise-induced hypotension, in autonomic failure (Mathias 2000). Subsequent studies have confirmed the therapeutic potential of water ingestion. In autonomic failure, water ingestion raises standing blood pressure (83 ± 6/53 ± 3mm Hg pre water to 114 ± 30/66 ± 18), 35 minutes after water when measurements were made 1 minute after standing (Shannon et al. 2002). Postprandial hypotension (43/20 mm Hg after 90 minutes) was reduced when water was ingested immediately before a meal (22/12 mm Hg after 90 minutes). In a further study comparing PAF and MSA, similar observations have been made in relation to the effectiveness of water in reducing orthostatic hypotension in the different groups; furthermore, in this study there was objective evidence of a reduction in orthostatic symptoms (Young and Mathias 2004). The effects of repeated water ingestion are not known. Topping up with subsequent smaller drinks of water maintains a large gastric volume thus keeping gastric emptying at a high rate in healthy subjects (Noakes et al. 1991). It is not known whether 'topping' up with subsequent small drinks of water can prolong the pressor effect in autonomic failure. However, water ingestion does not appear to raise blood pressure, supine or standing, in Parkinson's disease with autonomic failure (Senard et al. 1999) and its effects in the other diseases causing orthostatic hypotension requires further study.

Haemodynamic effects of water ingestion in other autonomic diseases

Water ingestion may benefit disorders such as neurally mediated syncope and the postural tachycardia syndrome where there is intermittent autonomic dysfunction. Vasovagal syncope is the most common form of autonomically-mediated syncope (AMS; Mathias et al. 2000) with cardio-inhibitory, vasodepressor and mixed components. Oral water drinking was suggested as a treatment in children with vasodepressor syncope (Younoszai et al. 1998). In normal subjects water ingestion increases orthostatic

tolerance (by up to 5 minutes) when tested with a combination of head-up tilt (to 60°) and lower body negative pressure (at levels of –20, –40 and –60 mm Hg for 10 minutes each, or until pre-syncope occurred) (Schroeder et al. 2000). Water increased peripheral vascular resistance and reduced the fall in stroke volume. Thus, water may benefit subjects with vasovagal syncope prone to episodes especially whilst standing still or in hot weather.

In the postural orthostatic tachycardia syndrome (PoTS) there is a substantial rise in heart rate (of over 30 bpm), usually without a fall in blood pressure, on sustaining an upright posture. Following water ingestion standing levels of blood pressure were not affected, but standing heart rate was lowered, from 123 ± 23 bpm after 3 minutes of standing pre water, to 108 ± 21 bpm after water (Shannon et al. 2002). The effects of water ingestion on symptoms however, were not reported.

Conclusion

Substantial data now clearly indicate that ingestion of 480–500 ml of water results in a pressor response in older normal subjects and an even greater response in autonomic failure due to PAF and MSA while not changing blood pressure in young normal subjects. A variable pressor response also occurs in tetraplegics with high spinal cord lesions. The mechanisms of this pressor response to water remain unclear. However, water is effective in autonomic failure in reducing both orthostatic and postprandial hypotension and also improves symptoms resulting from orthostatic hypotension. Longer-term effects remain to be established, especially in MSA where an expected later diuresis might offset some of these early benefits.

Water ingestion may be of benefit in both PoTS and vasovagal syncope. In vasovagal syncope, increasing salt intake and fluid is of benefit in reducing presyncope and syncope. In the postural tachycardia syndrome, hypovolaemia is one of the factors that may be contributory. Water does not result in a pressor effect in PoTS, but attenuates the postural rise in HR. Whether this is likely to be more effective in the postural tachycardia syndrome where symptoms are directly related to the head-up postural change, as compared with neurally mediated syncope when a variety of events may trigger a depressor response, remains to be determined.

Although much work has been performed over the past few years in both confirming and investigating the aetiology of the pressor effect of water, the role of osmoreceptors in normal and orthostatic intolerance (especially AMS) need to be further explored (May and Jordan, 2010) as well as the measurement of vasoactive neurohumoral substances resulting from water ingestion in both normal subjects and those with autonomic failure. Improved understanding of the pressor effect would be of benefit in aiding better understanding of the pathophysiology of autonomic failure. In addition, the pressor effects observed in older subjects prompt the important question of the possible role water ingestion may play in hypertension, an endemic problem in our ageing population.

References

Boschmann, M., Steiniger, J., Hille, U., *et al.* (2003). Water-Induced Thermogenesis *J Clin. Endocrinol. Metab.* **88**, 6015–6019.

Cariga, P., Mathias, C. J. (2001). Haemodynamics of the pressor effect of oral water in human sympathetic denervation due to autonomic failure. *Clin. Sci.*, **101**, 313–319.

Clive, S., Jodrell, D., Webb, D. (2001). Gastrin-releasing peptide is a potent vasodilator in humans. *Clin. Pharmacol. Ther.* **69**, 252–9.

DiBona, G. F., Wilcox, C. S. (2002). The kidney and the sympathetic nervous system. In: *Autonomic Failure: A Textbook of Clinical Disorders of the Autonomic Nervous System*. Eds. Mathias, C. J., Bannister, R. 4th Edition. Oxford University Press, Oxford. pp. 143–50.

Doran, S., Jones, K. L., Andrews, J. M., *et al.* (1998). Effects of meal volume and posture on gastric emptying of solids and appetite. *Am. J Physiol.* **275**, R1712–R1718.

Endo, Y., Yamauchi, K., Tsutsui, Y., Ishihara, Z., Yamazaki, F., Sagawa, S., Shiraki, K. (2002). Changes in blood pressure and muscle sympathetic nerve activity during water drinking in humans. *Jap. J Physiol.* **52**, 421–7.

Frewin, D. B., Bartholomeusz, F. D. (1983) Sea water, a novel self-medication for orthostatic hypotension. *Med. J Aust.* **2**, 521–22.

Haberich, F. J. (1968). Osmoreception in the portal circulation. *Fed. Proc.* **27**, 1137–41.

Hanson, S. A., France, C. R. (2004). Predonation water ingestion attenuates negative reactions to blood donation. *Transfusion* **44**, 924–28.

Harrison, M. H., Hill, L. C., Spaul, W. A., Greenleaf, J. E. (1986). Effect of hydration on some orthostatic and haematological responses to head-up tilt. *Eur. J Appl. Physiol.* **55**: 187–94.

Hmouda, H., Jemni, L., Jeridi, G., Ernez-Hajri, S. (1994). Ammar H. Unusual presentation of gastric dilatation. Dramatic complete atrioventricular block. *Chest* **106**(2), 634–6.

Host, U., Kelbaek, H., Rasmusen, H., Court-Payen, M., Juel Christensen, N., Pedersen-Bjergaard, U., Lorenzen, T. (1996). Haemodynamic effects of eating: the role of meal composition. *Clin. Sci.* **90**, 269–76.

Huang, H. C., Lee, F. Y., Chan, C. C., *et al.* (2002). Effects of somatostatin and octreotide on portal-systemic collaterals in portal hypertensiverats. *J Hepatol.* **36**, 163–8.

Imai, C., Muratani, H., Kimura, Y., Kanzato, N., Takishita, S., Fukiyama, K. (1998). Effects of meal ingestion and active standing on blood pressure in patients ≥60 years of age. *Am. J Cardiol.* **81**, 1310–1314.

Jordan, J., Shannon, J. R., Black, B. K., *et al.* (2000). The pressor response to water drinking in humans: a sympathetic reflex? *Circulation* **101**, 504–509.

Jordan, J., Shannon, J. R., Grogan, E., Biaggioni, I., Robertson, D. (1999). A potent pressor response elicited by drinking water. *Lancet* **353**, 723.

Kooner, J. S., da Costa, D. F., Frankel, H. L., Bannister, R., Peart, W. S., Mathias, C. J. (1987). Recumbency induces hypertension, diuresis and natriuresis in autonomic failure but diuresis alone in tetraplegia. *J Hypertension* **5**; suppl 5, 327–29.

Lambert, G. P., Chang, R. T., Xia, T., Summers, R. W., Gisolfi, C. V. (1997). Absorption from different intestinal segments during exercise. *J Appl. Physiol.* **83**, 204–212.

Lawaetz, O., Dige-Petersen, H. (1989). Gastric emptying of liquid meals:validation of the gamma camera technique. *Nucl. Med. Commun.* **10**, 353–64.

Li, Y. Y. (2003). Mechanisms for regulation of gastrin and somatostatin release from isolated rat stomach during gastric distention *World J Gastroenterol.* **9**(1), 129–33.

Lin, H. C., Prather, C., Fisher, R. S., *et al.* (2005). Measurement of Gastrointestinal Transit. *Digestive Diseases and Sciences*, 50 No/6:989–1004.

Lipp, A., Tank, J., Franke, G., Arnold, G., Luft, F. C., Jordan, J. (2005). Osmosensitive mechanisms contribute to the water drinking-induced pressor response in humans. *Neurology* **65**, 905–907.

Lu, C., Diedrich, A., Tung, C., *et al.* (2003). Water ingestion as prophylaxis against syncope. *JAMA* **108**(21), 2660–65.

Mathias, C. J. (2000a). A 21st century water cure. *Lancet* **356**, 1046–48.

Mathias, C. J. Disorders of the autonomic nervous system (2000b).In: *Neurology in Clinical Practice*. 3rd edition. Eds. W. G Bradley, R. B Daroff, G. M Fenichel, C. D Marsden. Butterworth-Heinemann, Boston, USA. pp. 2131–65

Mathias, C. J., Bannister, R. (2001). Postprandial hypotension in autonomic disorders. In: Mathias, C. J, Bannister, R., eds. *Autonomic Failure: A Textbook of Clinical Disorders of the Autonomic Nervous System*, 4th edn. Oxford University Press, Oxford, pp. 283–95.

Mathias, C. J., Christensen, N. J., Corbett, J. L., Frankel, H. L., Spalding, J. M. K. (1976a). Plasma catecholamines during paroxysmal neurogenic hypertension in quadriplegic man. *Circ. Res.* **39**, 204–208.

Mathias, C. J., Fosbraey, P., da Costa, D. F., Thornley, A., Bannister, R. (1986). The effect of desmopressin on nocturnal polyuria, overnight weight loss and morning postural hypotension in patients with autonomic failure. *Br. Med. J* **293**, 353–54.

Mathias, C. J., Frankel, H. L., Christensen, N. J., Spalding, J. M. K. (1976b). Enhanced pressor response to noradrenaline in patients with cervical spinal cord transection. *Brain* **99**, 757–70.

Mathias, C. J., Frankel, H. L. (1983). Clinical manifestations of malfunctioning sympathetic mechanisms in tetraplegia. *J Auton. Nerv. Syst.* **7**: 303–12.

Mathias, C. J., Young, T. M. (2003). Plugging the leak—benefits of the vasopressin-2 agonist, desmopressin in autonomic failure. *Clin. Auton. Res.* **13**: 85–87.

Mathias, C. J., da Costa, D. F., McIntosh, C. M., *et al.* (1989). Differential blood pressure and hormonal effects following glucose and xylose ingestion in chronic autonomic failure. *Clin. Sci* **77**, 85–92.

Maule, S., Lombardo, L., Rossi, C., *et al.* (2002). Helicobacter pyloriinfection and gastric function in primary autonomic neuropathy *Clin. Auton.* **12**, 193–96.

May, M., Jordan, J. (2011). The osmopressor response to water drinking. *Am. J. Physiol. Regul. Integr. Comp. Physiol.* **300**(1), R40–6.

McHugh, J., Keller, N. R., Appalsamy, M., *et al.* (2010). Portal osmopressor mechanism linked to transient receptor potential vanilloid 4 and blood pressure control. *Hypertension* **55**, 1438–43.

Millan, M. J., Newman-Tancredi, A., Audinot, V., *et al.* (2000). Agonist and antagonist actions of yohimbine as compared to fluparoxan at alpha(2)-adrenergic receptors (AR)s, serotonin (5-HT)(1A), 5-HT(1B), 5-HT(1D) and dopamine D(2) and D(3) receptors. Significance for the modulation of frontocortical monoaminergic transmission and depressive states. *Synapse* **35**(2), 79–95.

Noakes, T. D., Rehrer, N. J., Maughan, R. J. (1991). The importance of volume in regulating gastric emptying. *Med. Sci. Sports Exerc.* **23**(3), 307–13.

Penagini, R., Hebbard, G., Horowitz, M., Dent, J., Bermingham, H., Jones, K., Holloway, R. H. (1998). Motor function of the proximal stomach and visceral perception in gastro-oesophageal reflux disease. *Gut* **42**, 251–57.

Ploutz-Snyder, L., Foley, J., Ploutz-Snyder, R., Kanaley, J., Sagendorf, K., Meyer, R. (1999). *Eur. J Applied Physiol. and Occupational Physiol.* **79**, 212–20.

Polinsky, R. J., Taylor, I. L., Weise, V., Kopin, I. J. (1988). Gastrin responses in patients with adrenergic insufficiency. *J Neurol. Neurosurg. Psychiatry* **51**(1), 67–71.

Raj, S. R., Biaggioni, I., Black, B. K., *et al.* (2006). Sodium paradoxically reduces the gastropressor response in patients with orthostatic hypotension. *Hypertension* **48**, 329–34.

Reynaert, H., Geerts, A. (2003). Review article: pharmacological rationale for the use of somatostatin and analogues in portal hypertension. *Aliment Pharmacol. Ther.* **18**, 375–86.

Rossi, P., Andriesse, G. I., Oey, P. L., Wieneke, G. H., Roelofs, J. M., Akkermans, L. M. (1998). Stomach distension increases efferent muscle sympathetic nerve activity and blood pressure in healthy humans. *J Neurol. Sci.* **161**, 148–55.

Routledge, H. C., Chowdhary, S., Coote, J. H., Townend, J. N. (2002). Cardiac vagal response to water ingestion is normal human subjects. *Clin. Sci.* **103**, 157–62.

Schalekamp, M. A. D. H., Man in't Veld, A. J., Wenning, G. J. (1985). The second Sir George Pickering Memorial Lecture: What regulates whole body autoregulation? Clinical observations. *J Hypertens.* **3**, 97–107.

Schroeder, C., Bush, V. E., Norcliffe, L. J., Luft, F. C., Tank, J., Jordan, J., Hainsworth, R. (2002). Water drinking acutely improves orthostatic tolerance in healthy subjects. *Circulation* **106**, 2806–11.

Scott, E. M., Greenwood, J. P., Gilbey, S. G., Stoker, J. B., Mary, D. A. (2001). Water ingestion increases sympathetic vasoconstrictor discharge in normal human subjects. *Clin. Sci.* **100**, 335–42

Scott, E. M., Greenwood, J. P., Stoker, J. B., Gilbey, S. G., Mary, D. A. (2000). Water Drinking and Sympathetic Activation. *Lancet* **356**, 2013.

Senard, J-M., Bretel, C., Carel, C., Tran, M-A., Montastruc, J. L. (1999). Water drinking and the heart. *Lancet* **353**, 1971.

Shannon, J. R., Diedrich, A., Biaggioni, I., *et al.* (2002). Water drinking as a treatment for orthostatic syndromes. *Am. J Med.* **112**, 355–60.

Sherwood, L. (2004). *Human Physiology - from cells to systems* (International Student Edition, 5th Ed). Brooks/Cole p. 604

Tank, J., Schroeder, C., Stoffels, M., Diedrich, A., Sharma, A. M., Luft, F. C., Jordan, J. (2003). Pressor effect of water drinking in tetraplegics patients may be a spinal reflex. *Hypertension* **41**, 1234–39.

Tavernor, S. J., Abduljawad, K. A., Langley, R. W., Bradshaw, C. M., Szabadi, E. (2000). Effects of pentagastrin and the cold pressor test on the acoustic startle response and pupillary function in man. *J Psychopharmacol.* **14**(4), 387–94.

Thompson, D. G. (2003). Structure and Function of the gut p. 14.01.01.01 in *Oxford Testbook of Medicine* 4th Ed Warrell, D., Cox, T. M., Firth, J. D., Benz, E. J. Eds, Oxford University Press: Oxford.

Visvanathan, R., Chen, R., Horowitz, M., Chapman, I. (2004). Blood pressure responses in healthy older people to 50 g carbohydrate drinks with differing glycaemic effects. *Br. J Nutrition* **92**, 335–40.

Young, T. M., Mathias, C. J. (2004a).The Effects of Water Ingestion on Orthostatic Hypotension in multiple system atrophy and pure autonomic failure. *Journal of Neurology, Neurosurgery and Psychiatry* **75**(12), 1737–41.

Young, T. M., Mathias, C. J. (2004b). Pressor effect of water instilled via gastrostomy tube in pure autonomic failure. *Autonomic Neuroscience: Basic and Clinical* **113**, 79–81.

Younoszai, A. K., Franklin, W. H., Chan, D. P., Cassidy, S. C., Allen, H. D. (1998). Oral fluid therapy. A promising treatment for vasodepressor syncope. *Arch. Pediatr. Adolesc. Med.*; **152**, 163–68.

van Orshoven, N. P., Oey, P. L., van Schelven, L. J., Roelofs, J. M. M., Jansen, P. A. F., Akkermans, L. M. (2004). Effect of gastric distension on cardiovascular parameters: gastrovascular reflex is attenuated in the elderly. *J Physiol.*; **555**, 573–83.

CHAPTER 30

Exercise-induced hypotension in autonomic disorders

Antonio Claudio Lucas da Nóbrega,
David A. Low and Christopher J. Mathias

Introduction

Physical exercise causes a plethora of physiological responses, including somatic and autonomic neural activation, hormonal changes, and cardiorespiratory adjustments. In normal individuals, systolic blood pressure increases during dynamic contractions as a consequence of a proportionally greater increase in cardiac output alongside the fall in total peripheral vascular resistance (Shepherd 1987). These haemodynamic adjustments occur with a marked increase in arterial blood inflow to exercising muscles and depend on sympathetic activation that plays a pivotal role in increasing heart rate, enhancing myocardial inotropism, constricting vascular beds of relatively quiescent organs, and modulating metabolic vasodilatation in contracting muscle groups.

In contrast to healthy individuals where exercise normally raises blood pressure, patients with autonomic failure may lower their blood pressure during dynamic exercise. Exercise-induced hypotension (EIH) was originally reported as a clinical problem in 1961 by John Shepherd and his colleagues (Marshall et al. 1961) studying six patients with 'idiopathic orthostatic hypotension' and one who had undergone thoracolumbar sympathectomy. They were subjected to pedaling at a 'mild' intensity while in the supine position and a 'pronounced fall in blood pressure was observed during and immediately after the exercise indicating that there was a major disturbance in the control of blood pressure even in circumstances in which gravitational factors were excluded' (Fig. 30.1). Subsequent studies indicated that EIH is a clinical problem that can complicate management in many autonomic disorders (Smith et al. 1995a, Smith et al. 1996a, Smith et al. 1998, Akinola et al. 2001).

This chapter will consider the haemodynamic responses to exercise, the neural and haemodynamic pathophysiological mechanisms responsible for exercise-induced hypotension, and discuss clinically useful interventions and therapeutic measures. We shall focus on subjects with primary chronic autonomic failure (pure autonomic failure [PAF], and multiple system atrophy [MSA]), consider the implications of exercise in other autonomic disorders, and draw attention to differentiating these patients from others without autonomic dysfunction but in whom clinical conditions may cause blood pressure to decrease during exercise. *Exercise-induced hypotension* is defined as a ≥10 mmHg fall in systolic blood pressure during exercise and should be regarded as the end of a spectrum of possible pressure responses to exercise, ranging from expected increases in systolic pressure, proportional to the exercise workload, in normal subjects, to these precipitous decreases in systolic blood pressure in patients with autonomic dysfunction. It is a different phenomenon from *post-exercise hypotension*, which is defined as ≥5 mmHg fall in blood pressure *after* exercise has stopped and is quite commonly observed (Kenney and Seals 1993, Forjaz et al. 2000, Halliwill 2001, Charkoudian et al. 2003).

Haemodynamic responses to exercise

The capacity to perform physical exercise is a major functional characteristic of the human body. Exercise is a significant physiological stress because of the increased metabolic demand from muscle contractions and the associated heat production. Therefore, exercise provokes complex physiological adjustments that enhance oxygen and micronutrient delivery to working muscles and maintain homeothermia, collectively known as acute effects or physiological responses to exercise, the magnitude of which are proportional to exercise intensity. As exercise is a physiological burden, it is not surprising that repetitive and regular bouts of exercise trigger morphological and functional adaptations after a few weeks (Nobrega 2005), which are known as chronic effects of exercise (Thompson et al. 2001). The main consequence of many of these physiological adaptations is an increased capacity to exercise and less severe acute responses to the same workload.

Skeletal muscle contraction is the basic functional unit of physical exercise. When muscular contraction causes movement about a joint it is called a dynamic (isotonic) contraction as opposed to a static (isometric) contraction where muscle activation—energy expenditure, heat release and tension development—occurs without external work (Asmussen 1981). Whenever the developed tension is greater than the imposed load, the muscle shortens along its longitudinal axis, producing a concentric dynamic contraction. However, when the developed muscle tension is lower than the external load, the muscle is stretched, producing an eccentric contraction. The latter is common for anti-gravitational or postural muscles when one sits or lies down, or lowers an object towards the ground, allowing gravitational acceleration to cause the movement

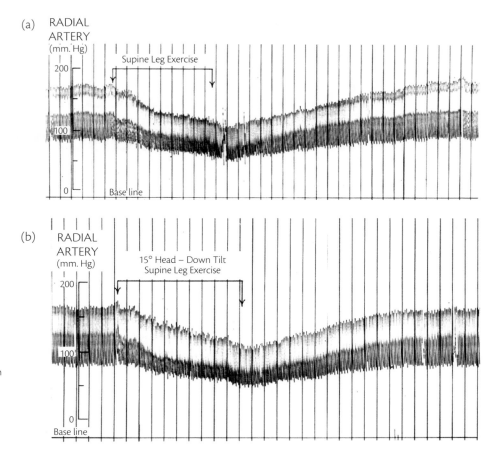

(a) RADIAL ARTERY (mm. Hg)

Supine Leg Exercise

Base line

(b) RADIAL ARTERY (mm. Hg)

15° Head – Down Tilt Supine Leg Exercise

Base line

Fig. 30.1 Original blood pressure tracing of one subject with exercise-induced hypotension. With permission from Marshall, R.J., Schirger, A., and Shepherd, J.T. (1961). Blood pressure during supine exercise in idiopathic orthostatic hypotension. *Circulation.* **24**, 76–81.

but slowing it down by muscular action. Regardless of the type of contraction, metabolic demand increases generating local metabolic factors within exercising skeletal muscle that provoke arteriolar vasodilatation. The increase in muscle blood flow is, however, partially counteracted by the augmented intramuscular pressure during contraction (Wesche 1986); therefore, during static exercise the increase in muscle blood flow is somewhat attenuated in comparison with during dynamic exercise, where mean muscle blood flow is greatly increased and adopts an intermittent profile (Asmussen 1981). It has also recently been shown that at the onset of dynamic exercise, the compression of intramuscular arterioles during the initial contraction can elicit rapid vasodilatation following that contraction (e.g. during the subsequent relaxation) through a mechanosensitive response (Clifford 2007, Kirby et al. 2007).

In addition to the direct mechanical influence of muscle tension, the magnitude of the increase in muscle blood flow depends on a complex interaction between vasodilatatory and vasoconstrictor factors released by surrounding muscle fibres and endothelium, as well as the action of noradrenaline secreted from sympathetic nerve terminals (Fig. 30.2). One important feature of the mechanisms involved with the blood flow response in active muscle during exercise is that although sympathetic nerve activity is increased, it has a diminished constrictive effect, an action termed 'functional sympatholysis' (Remensnyder et al. 1962). This reduced vasoconstrictor responsiveness may result from a prejunctional reduction in neurotransmitter release as well as from postjunctional interference with the action of noradrenaline on smooth muscle cells

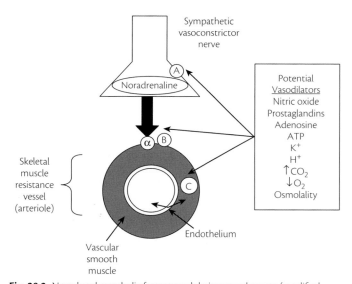

Fig. 30.2 Neural and metabolic factors modulating vascular tone (modified from Halliwill 2001) depicting the possible mechanisms of action of endothelium-derived relaxing factors causing 'functional sympatholysis'. **A:** Presynaptic modulation of noradrenaline release; **B:** modulation of the postsynaptic effect of noradrenaline on α-receptors on vascular smooth muscle, and **C:** intracellular modulation of contractile properties of vascular smooth muscle. With permission from Halliwill, J.R. (2001) Mechanisms and clinical implications of post-exercise hypotension in humans. *Exerc. Sport. Sci. Rev.* **29**, 65–70.

(Rosenmeier et al. 2003). Regardless of the mechanism(s) involved, functional sympatholysis represents only a partial inhibition of the vasoconstrictor effect of adrenergic nerve activation on vascular smooth muscle, since there is ongoing sympathetic restraint of blood flow to the active muscles as shown by increases in arteriolar blood flow to exercising muscle on, either, interruption of sympathetic outflow or antagonism of α-receptors (Thomas and Segal 2004).

The circulation is a closed system and increased muscle blood flow during exercise therefore causes a proportional increase in venous return and cardiac output. Although the heart is regarded as the 'master' of the circulation, it actually 'serves' the peripheral circulation, since tissues and organs determine their blood flow simply by increasing their metabolic demand, causing an overall increase in total flow (i.e. cardiac output) (Rowell, 1993). Nevertheless, autonomic modulation of the heart and circulation plays a key role in determining adjustments at the onset and offset of exercise, by integrating, and amplifying the magnitude of the haemodynamic responses. Consequently, impaired autonomic function itself does not prevent a person from exercising completely, but patients with severe autonomic failure may be limited to only light and short bouts of physical effort because of EIH, as discussed below.

During exercise, metabolic vasodilatation in contracting muscle groups (i.e. skeletal muscles in exercising limbs, the myocardium, and respiratory muscles) is accompanied by a redistribution of cardiac output to active muscles through neurally mediated vasoconstriction in non-exercising muscles and in the splanchnic and renal circulations (Thomas and Segal, 2004). Overall, these effects reduce total peripheral resistance, particularly during high-intensity dynamic exercise of large muscle groups. Blood flow to the skin decreases initially as part of neural adrenergic activation, but as exercise continues and core temperature rises, skin blood flow increases and sweating is activated by central homeothermic mechanisms (Kenney and Johnson, 1992, Shibasaki et al. 2006). Global blood flow to the brain is controlled via adjustments in systemic haemodynamics (i.e. perfusion pressure) (Van Lieshout et al. 2003, Ogoh et al. 2005, Ogoh et al. 2008) and through local vascular regulation (i.e. cerebral autoregulation) (Paulson et al. 1990, Panerai 2008), where arterial carbon dioxide partial pressure (pCO_2) plays a major role. During exercise, cerebral perfusion, evaluated using the 133-xenon clearance technique, or blood velocity in basal cerebral arteries, is increased (Secher et al. 2008). Alongside increases in global cerebral blood flow during exercise, there is also regional redistribution with increased flow to active areas such as the primary and supplementary motor and insular cortices (Herholz et al. 1987, Williamson et al. 1997).

In normal individuals, cardiac output is typically increased during dynamic contractions, although the mechanisms involved vary depending on exercise intensity and body position (Rowell 1993). During progressive exercise, such as during a conventional stress test, cardiac output increases initially by a proportionally greater contribution from stroke volume, whereas the increase in heart rate plays a progressively more important role after 50% of maximal exercise intensity when stroke volume has already reached, or is approaching, its maximum (Vella and Roberds 2005, Gonzalez-Alonso 2008). When dynamic exercise is performed in a recumbent or supine position, venous return is facilitated and stroke volume is higher than in the sitting or standing position; thus, cardiac output increases through a greater contribution from

the chronotropic response (Bevegard et al. 1966, Thadani and Parker 1978, Miyamoto et al. 1983). Cardiac output increases and total peripheral resistance decreases during dynamic contractions and the blood pressure response to exercise thus depends on the relative magnitude of these responses.

During static contractions in subjects with normal left ventricular function, blood pressure rises due to increases in cardiac output (peripheral resistance does not change), which in turn depends on the positive chronotropic response, since stroke volume remains at resting values. When the heart rate response to static contraction is blunt, stroke volumes increases, leading to the normal increase in cardiac output and blood pressure (Nobrega et al. 1997). A similar compensatory mechanism operates also during dynamic exercise where the blood pressure response occurs by a lack of the normal fall in peripheral vascular resistance, when the increase in cardiac output is inhibited by restricting venous return (Nobrega et al. 1995).

Reflex control of the circulation during exercise

There is a close relationship between exercise intensity and the magnitude of the haemodynamic responses to exercise. These haemodynamic adjustments are co-ordinated by reflex autonomic networks and nuclei in the brainstem that integrate afferent input from both 'activating' and 'modulatory' mechanisms (Fig. 30.3). The activating neural mechanisms (central command and ergoreflex) represent specific stimuli related to exercise itself and provide information about the intensity of the effort, whereas the modulatory mechanisms, such as the cardiopulmonary and arterial baroreflexes, participate continuously, not only during exercise, in the regulation of cardiovascular function and interact with activating mechanisms to produce the typical autonomic and haemodynamic responses to physical exercise (Smith et al. 2006). Central command represents the parallel activation of somatic and autonomic nuclei within the central nervous system. Although the precise group of nuclei comprising the role of central command is still undefined, the insular and anterior cingulate cortices, as well as the thalamic region, appear involved (Critchley et al. 2000, Williamson et al. 1997).

As a control system, the magnitude of central command's signal is proportional to the volitional component of exercise. The exercise pressor reflex is a typical feedback mechanism involving the reflex activation of type III and IV sensory fibres by mechanical and metabolic receptors within active muscles (Kaufman and Hayes 2002). Both central command and the exercise pressor reflex send neural input to the cardiovascular control center in the brainstem, which in turn cause the appropriate autonomic adjustments (Mitchell 1990). As part of these autonomic adjustments, both central command and the exercise pressor reflex interact and 'reset' the arterial baroreflex, in direct relation to exercise intensity, allowing the arterial baroreflex to regulate prevailing blood pressure evoked by the exercise (Rowell and O'Leary 1990, Raven et al. 2006). The general pattern of efferent autonomic adjustment during exercise combines sympathetic adrenergic activation and parasympathetic withdrawal. The reverse occurs when muscular contractions cease. The kinetics of the two branches are substantially different as faster responses depend on parasympathetically mediated vagal tone changes, whereas slower and more sustained responses are mainly sympathetically mediated (Fig. 30.4). In healthy subjects, the heart rate response observed in the first few seconds after the onset of

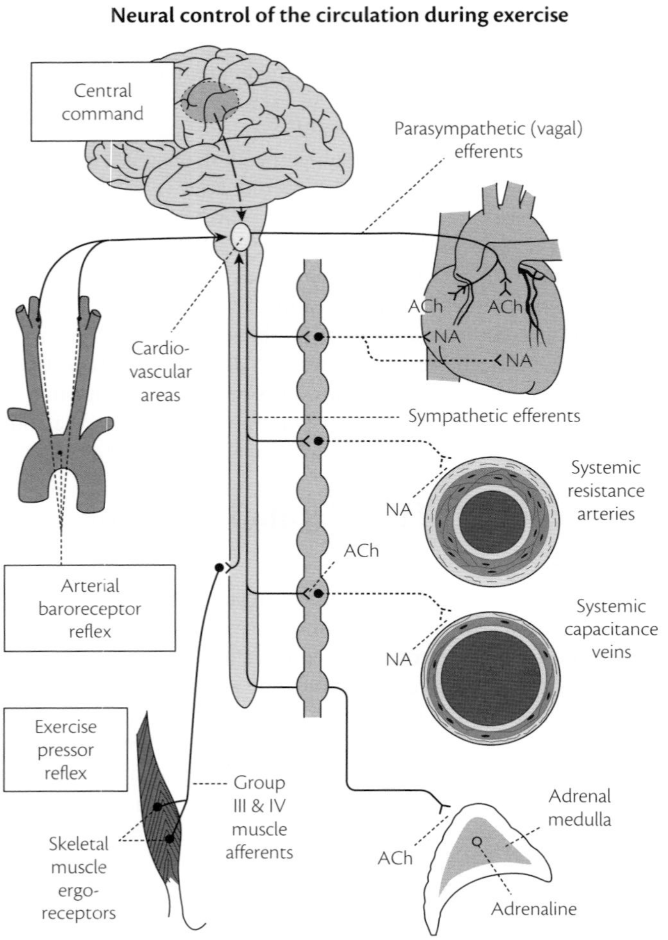

Neural control of the circulation during exercise

![Neural control of the circulation during exercise diagram with central command, cardiovascular areas, parasympathetic vagal efferents, sympathetic efferents, arterial baroreceptor reflex, exercise pressor reflex, skeletal muscle ergoreceptors, Group III & IV muscle afferents, systemic resistance arteries, systemic capacitance veins, adrenal medulla]

Fig. 30.3 Neural control of the circulation during exercise. Neural signals originating from the brain (central command) and skeletal muscle (exercise pressor reflex) activate the autonomic nervous system along with modulatory signals from the aorta and carotid arteries (arterial baroreflex). The alterations in autonomic outflow (increased sympathetic and decreased parasympathetic activity) induce changes in heart rate and contractility, changes in the diameter of resistance and capacitance vessels within peripheral tissue beds, and release of adrenaline from the medulla of the adrenal gland. As a result, changes in heart rate, stroke volume, and systemic vascular resistance mediate alterations in mean arterial pressure appropriate for the intensity and modality of exercise. ACh, acetylcholine; NA, noradrenaline. With permission from Smith, S.A., Mitchell, J.R., and Garry, M.G. (2006), *The mammalian exercise pressor reflex in health and disease*, Wiley.

dynamic exercise is mediated by both central command and the exercise pressor reflex (Williamson et al. 1995) and is achieved via vagal withdrawal (Araujo et al. 1992). Accordingly, the initial chronotropic response to the onset of exercise, as well as heart rate recovery in the first minutes after exercise has ceased, have been used to evaluate the functional integrity of parasympathetic modulation of heart rate.

Mechanisms of exercise-induced hypotension in autonomic failure

During dynamic exercise in healthy individuals, systolic blood pressure increases in proportion to exercise intensity, whereas diastolic blood pressure usually does not change more than ~10 mmHg and in fact typically decreases due to the decrease in

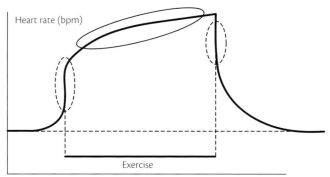

Fig. 30.4 Heart rate response to dynamic exercise. The interrupted-line circles show the instantaneous increase/decrease at the onset/offset of exercise that are mediated by inhibition/reactivation of parasympathetic tone. The continuous-line circle shows the progressive increase in heart rate that depends mainly on increasing sympathetic activation.

total peripheral resistance. Mean arterial blood pressure increases due to increased cardiac output and neurally mediated sympathetic vasoconstriction of inactive muscle groups, the visceral circulation and restriction of metabolic vasodilatation of active muscles (Shepherd, 1987, Rowell 1993). In PAF, patients may present with as low as 20% of sympathetic postganglionic neurons in the inter-mediolateral columns of the spinal cord (Johnson et al. 1966, Oppenheimer 1980), a marked reduction of sympathetic efferent nerve impulse activity by direct intraneural recordings (Dotson et al. 1990) and low noradrenaline levels (Bannister and Mathias 1999). In contrast to PAF, MSA patients have functional integrity of postganglionic sympathetic efferent neurons and spontaneous bursts of sympathetic nerve impulses may be recorded (Dotson et al. 1990). In MSA, however, patients have a central lesion that inhibits preganglionic sympathetic nerve activity (Matthews 1999). Regardless of the site of the lesion in these individuals, PAF and MSA patients are unable to increase plasma noradrenaline during exercise (Smith et al. 1995, Akinola et al. 1999). Considering that the exercise pressor response depends to a major extent on sympathetic activation, it is not surprising that these patients do not sufficiently elevate their blood pressure during exercise, with PAF patients showing a greater fall in blood pressure during exercise than MSA patients (Smith et al. 1995a, Akinola et al. 2001) (Fig. 30.5). Isolated dopamine-beta-hydroxylase (DBH) deficiency patients, individuals without the enzyme responsible for converting dopamine to noradrenaline, typically show undetectable plasma adrenaline and noradrenaline (Mathias et al. 1990), but plasma dopamine is elevated and rises further with exercise leading to some degree of vasoconstriction that is sufficient to prevent a blood pressure fall (Smith et al. 1995a). Therefore, patients with DBG deficiency show little change in blood pressure during dynamic exercise (Smith et al. 1995a, Smith and Mathias 1995).

The mechanisms involved in exercise-induced hypotension in autonomic failure could involve a smaller increase, or the absence of an increase, in cardiac output and/or a disproportional decrease in peripheral vascular resistance. The latter could be due to a lack of arteriolar vasoconstriction in non-exercising muscle groups and/or splanchnic and renal circulations. Some studies measuring the hemodynamic responses to exercise in autonomic failure patients have shown an association between the impaired plasma noradrenaline elevation and blunted heart rate responses with the

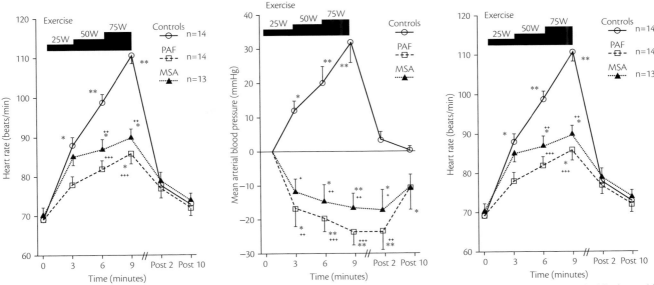

Fig. 30.5 Changes in mean arterial pressure, heart rate, and plasma noradrenaline concentrations before, during, and after exercise in three groups: healthy (controls), and subjects with pure autonomic failure (PAF), and multiple system atrophy (MSA), Significant changes from baseline: * = p <0.05, ** = p <0.01; significant differences between controls and subjects with PAF or MSA: + = p <0.05; ++ = p <0.01; +++ = p<0.0001. Modified from Akinola et al. 2001, with permission.

fall in blood pressure, suggesting a role for a lack of increase in cardiac output in exercise-induced hypotension (Akinola et al. 2001). However, a more comprehensive analysis of the cardiovascular responses to exercise demonstrated that stroke volume may compensate for the blunted chronotropic response in

autonomic failure leading to a normal increase in cardiac output (Smith et al. 1995a) (Fig. 30.6). This effect was probably due to the Frank–Starling mechanism, which is an intrinsic characteristic of the heart that enables ventricular ejection performance to increase when ventricular filling increases (Rowell 1993). Considering that

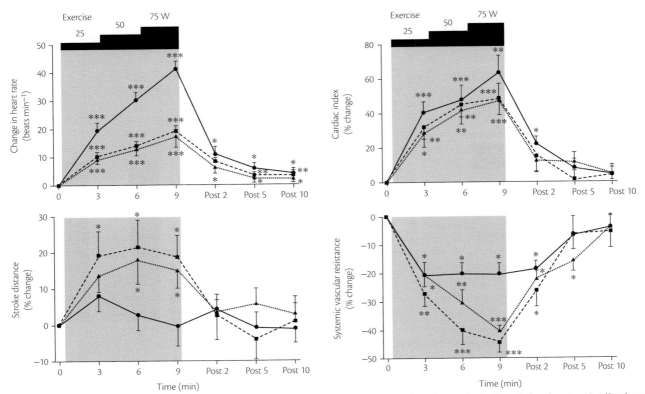

Fig. 30.6 Changes in systolic blood pressure, heart rate, cardiac index, stroke distance, and systemic vascular resistance during (Exercise) and post-supine (Post) exercise in normal subjects (circles), and subjects with multiple system atrophy (triangles) and pure autonomic failure (squares). Significant changes from baseline: * p < 0.05; ** p < 0.001; *** p < 0.0001. With permission from Smith, G.D., Watson, L.P., Pavitt, D.V., and Mathias, C.J. (1995). Abnormal cardiovascular and catecholamine responses to supine exercise in human subjects with sympathetic dysfunction. *J. Physiol.* **484**, 255–65, Wiley.

cardiac output increases typically, a greater than normal decrease in systemic vascular resistance is the major mechanism responsible for exercise-induced hypotension in autonomic failure (Smith et al. 1995a) (Fig. 30.6). Impaired splanchnic vasoconstriction may contribute to increased systemic vascular conductance at the early stages of exercise (Puvi-Rajasingham et al. 1997) (Fig. 30.7), whereas lack of proper restraint of metabolic vasodilatation in active muscles, through attenuated elevations in sympathetic nerve activity may lower systemic vascular resistance and blood pressure to a greater extent than in control subjects (Puvi-Rajasingham et al. 1997, Schrage et al. 2004). Various investigations have also examined the potential role of neurohumoral, metabolic, and biochemical factors in causing exercise-induced hypotension in autonomic failure. These have ruled out any important contribution of plasma lactate (Akinola et al. 2001), nitric oxide (Akinola et al. 1999), insulin, renin, C-peptide, and growth hormone (Smith et al. 1996b), reinforcing the key role of impaired sympathetic neural activity causing inadequate compensatory vasoconstriction in exercise-induced hypotension.

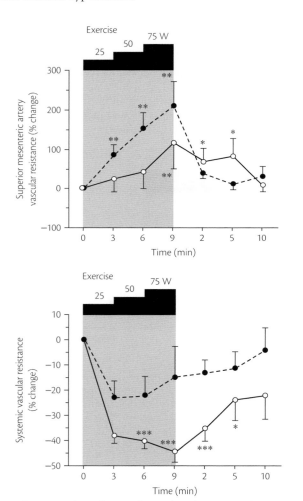

Fig. 30.7 Percentage change in systemic vascular resistance, superior mesenteric artery blood flow, and vascular resistance during (Exercise; at 25, 50 and 75 W) and after exercise in controls (closed circles) and in subjects with autonomic failure (open circles). Significant changes from baseline: * p < 0.05, ***p< 0.0005. Adapted from Puvi-Rajasingham, S., Smith, G.D., Akinola, A., and Mathias, C.J. (1997). Abnormal regional blood flow responses during and after exercise in human sympathetic denervation. *J. Physiol.* **15**, 841–9.

Exercise-induced hypotension: static versus dynamic exercise

Static (isometric) exercise produces a marked pressor response; therefore, it can be a very useful test in the investigation of sympathetic function in autonomic disorders (Mathias and Banister 1999). The increase in blood pressure is vastly attenuated, if not absent, in patients with autonomic disorders (Khurana and Setty 1996; Mathias and Banister 1999) (Fig. 30.8). Similar to during dynamic exercise, the ability of MSA and PAF patients to constrict non-exercising vascular beds is reduced, including the splanchnic vasculature, which prevents or limits the pressor response during static exercise (Fig. 30.9). Increases in cardiac output of a similar magnitude to healthy controls are still evident. During static exercise, there is a reduced muscle arteriolar vasodilatation relative to dynamic exercise, because of a lower metabolic demand and direct mechanical compression of the muscle vasculature during the isometric contraction, which results in an attenuation of the fall in total peripheral resistance (Lewis et al. 1983, Lewis et al. 1985, Kaufman and Hayes 2002). Consequently, this relatively lower requirement for muscle perfusion, typically of a smaller muscle mass during static exercise, may limit the depressor effect of a lack of sympathoexcitation in autonomic failure patients and thus result in the relative lack of change in blood pressure, rather than a precipitous fall, during isometric exercise.

Clinical significance and differential aetiological diagnosis of exercise-induced hypotension

The lack of an increase or a decrease in blood pressure during dynamic exercise can compromise the ability to generate adequate blood flow potentially leading to reduced physical capacity, fatigue, dizziness, and syncope in both healthy and vasodepressor patients (Sneddon et al. 1994, Colivicchi et al. 2002, Krediet et al. 2004, 2005,

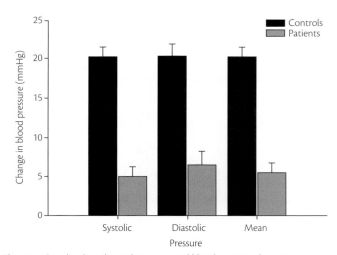

Fig. 30.8 Systolic, diastolic, and mean arterial blood pressure changes after 4 minutes of isometric exercise (30% MVC) in 71 control and 53 dysautonomic patients (pure autonomic failure, multiple system atrophy, diabetic dysautonomia and miscellaneous dysfunction). With kind permission from Springer Science+Business Media: *Clinical Autonomic Research*, The value of the isometric hand-grip test-studies in various autonomic disorders, **6**, 1996, 211–218, Khurana RK and Setty A.

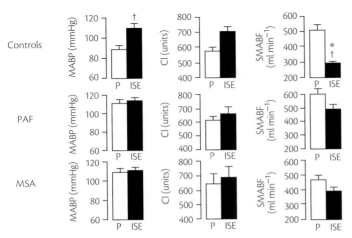

Fig. 30.9 Mean arterial blood pressure (MABP), cardiac index (CI; roke distance x heart rate; continuous wave Doppler ultrasound) and superior mesenteric artery blood flow (SMABF) before (P) and during 2 minutes of isometric exercise (ISE; 33% MVC) in controls, pure autonomic failure (PAF) and multiple system atrophy (MSA) patients. † = p <005 versus Pre; * = p <0.01 versus PAF and MSA; ** = p < 0.001 versus controls. With permission from Chaudhuri KR, Thomaides T & Mathias CJ (1992). Abnormality of superior mesenteric artery blood flow responses in human sympathetic failure. *The Journal of Physiology* **457**, 477–489, Wiley.

Whyte et al. 2004). Syncope usually occurs whenever there is a dramatic and sudden drop in systemic blood pressure and cerebral perfusion, however, syncopal symptoms tend to be less common in patients with autonomic failure, who may adapt to low cerebral perfusion due to chronic hypotension throughout the day, especially in orthostatic or sitting positions and after meals (Frongillo et al. 1995). Therefore, patients with autonomic failure may not present any specific sign or symptom of hypotension during exercise, despite severe reductions in blood pressure.

The first approach to individuals presenting with exercise-induced hypotension is a default medical history and physical exam in order to differentiate between occasional episodes of hypotension and an irreversible progressive pathological condition. For example, highly motivated healthy subjects may reach intense lactic metabolism at peak exercise causing relatively greater arteriolar vasodilatation than the increase in cardiac output, and thus a lack of further increase or even a decrease in arterial blood pressure as exercise continues near maximal effort (Gonzalez-Alonso and Calbet 2003). In the absence of any other changes, such as electrocardiographic changes or chest pain complaints, this episode of arterial hypotension should be regarded as a physiological phenomenon without any further clinical relevance. Conversely, patients with known coronary artery disease that present with arterial hypotension during an episode of chest pain and electrocardiographic changes, suggestive of myocardial ischaemia while performing an exercise test, have an increased risk of cardiac events (Dubach et al. 1988). In this case, the mechanism is believed to typically depend on the inability to increase cardiac output to match metabolic vasodilatation, but at least one study has shown above normal vasodilatation along with normal or even increased cardiac output underlying EIH in patients with coronary artery disease (Lele et al. 1994). In these patients, successful angioplasty typically results in resolution of symptoms and abnormal hemodynamic responses during exercise, suggesting that a reflex originating within the heart is responsible for the exercise-induced

hypotension in these patients. This is different from patients with chronic autonomic dysfunction where blood pressure often progressively decreases from the onset of even mild to moderate exercise (Fig. 30.4).

Syncope during physical exertion is not only alarming for the patient but is also an important diagnostic challenge for the physician as it may anticipate sudden death or may be a consequence of benign factors (O'Connor et al. 1999, Krediet et al. 2004). A key question in the initial clinical evaluation is to determine whether syncope occurred *during* exercise or *after* exertion had stopped, as the latter carries a very low probability of heart disease as the cause. Therefore, in evaluating patients with single or recurrent episodes of exercise-related syncope, it is imperative to search for either structural or arrhythmic cardiac diseases (Marvin et al. 1935, McKenna et al. 1981, O'Connor et al. 1999). When syncope occurs during exercise and the presence of heart disease or metabolic disorders have been excluded, neurally mediated reflexes should be considered (Abe et al. 1997, Krediet et al. 2005), although classical vasovagal syncope is more common after exercise has ceased. In subjects with vasovagal syncope there is a smaller increase in plasma noradrenaline and a greater fall in systemic vascular resistance than healthy controls during supine exercise, although these differences are less pronounced than in patients with PAF (Smith et al. 1996a). It is important to note here however that patients with primary autonomic failure can have prolongation of QT intervals (Lo et al. 1996), which can identify patients at risk of developing ventricular fibrillation and sudden cardiac death (Schwartz and Wolf 1978). In addition, ST depression has also been recorded in a patient with PAF, suggesting the presence of myocardial ischaemia (Asahina et al. 2006). Although the mechanism responsible for the exercise-induced ischaemia concomitant with hypotension in this one patient was unclear, it calls attention to the possibility that circulating hormonal vasoconstrictor factors released during exercise combined with arterial hypotension could cause myocardial ischaemia in patients with autonomic failure, even in the absence of chest pain and significant obstruction on coronary angiogram (Asahina et al. 2006).

Another group of conditions that cause hypotension during physical effort includes allergic or anaphylactic reactions associated with exercise (Sheffer and Austen 1980). Food-dependent exercise-induced anaphylaxis is a subset form of food allergy induced by physical exercise (Morita et al. 2007). Symptoms are typically generalized urticaria, and severe allergic reactions such as shock or hypotension. Symptoms generally occur within 2 hours of eating specific food types and engaging in vigorous exertion, although milder exercise may also induce these symptoms. Several food items may be responsible for the causing of food-dependent exercise-induced anaphylaxis, including vegetables (especially tomatoes), wheat, and others such as shellfish, hazelnuts, fruits, and eggs. Aspirin has also been known to be an additional exacerbating factor (Morita et al. 2007).

Exercise-induced hypotension in different autonomic disorders

The presence of coronary artery disease may be associated with exercise-induced arterial hypotension with prognostic implications (Lele et al. 1994, Dubach et al. 1988). In this situation, blood pressure increases from the beginning of exercise and hypotension

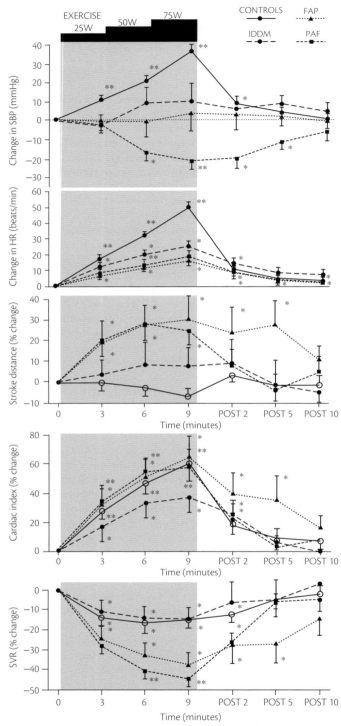

Fig. 30.10 Change in systolic blood pressure (SBP), heart rate (HR), stroke distance, cardiac index, and systemic vascular resistance (SVR) during and after (post) supine exercise, in controls, insulin-dependent diabetes mellitus (IDDM), familial amyloid polyneuropathy (FAP), and pure autonomic failure (PAF) patients. Significant changes from baseline: * p <0.05 and ** p <0.001. Reprinted from *J. Auton. Nerv. Syst.* **73**, Smith, G.D., Watson, L.P., and Mathias, C.J., Differing haemodynamic and catecholamine responses to exercise in three groups with peripheral autonomic dysfunction: insulin-dependent diabetes mellitus, familial amyloid polyneuropathy and pure autonomic failure, 125–34, Copyright 1998 with permission from Elsevier.

tends to occur at a certain point during exercise usually coincident with the development of myocardial ischaemia (Dubach et al. 1988). Other structural heart diseases such as aortic stenosis (Marvin et al. 1935) and hypertrophic cardiomyopathy (McKenna et al. 1981) may cause arterial hypotension during exercise due to obstructed left ventricular outflow.

Subjects with primary or secondary autonomic failure have a different profile of blood pressure response during exercise from the sudden drop occasionally seen in patients with heart disease. The presence of autonomic denervation impairs the physiological splanchnic vasoconstriction and the modulation of metabolic vasodilatation in active muscles failing to restrain the drop in systemic vascular resistance, thus leading to a progressive and continuous decrease in blood pressure from the beginning of exercise (Puvi-Rajasingham et al. 1997, Schrage et al. 2004). This response tends to be more severe in patients with PAF and somewhat less

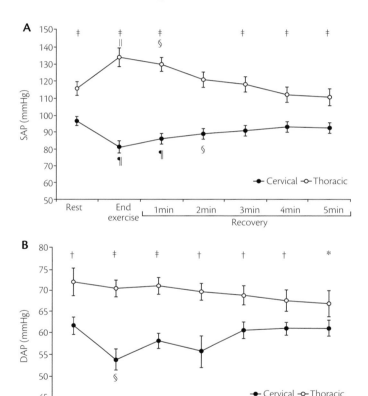

Fig. 30.11 A: Systolic (SAP) and **B:** diastolic (DAP) blood pressure responses to and post-exercise in subjects with thoracic and cervical spinal cord injury (SCI). Resting seated SAP and DAP were significantly higher in subjects with thoracic than those with cervical SCI. At the end of exercise, SAP increased and DAP was unchanged in the subjects with thoracic SCI, whereas SAP and DAP both decreased in subjects with cervical SCI. During recovery from exercise, blood pressures began to return to the resting levels in both groups, but were consistently elevated in subjects with thoracic compared with cervical SCI. * p <0.05; † p <0.01; ‡ p <0.001 cervical versus thoracic; § p <0.05; ‡ p <0.01; p <0.001 within-group comparison against the resting condition. Note the change in scale in the lower panel. Reprinted from *Arch. Phys. Med. Rehabil.* **87**, Claydon, V.E., Hol, A.T., Eng, J.J., and Krassioukov, A.V., Cardiovascular responses and postexercise hypotension after arm cycling exercise in subjects with spinal cord injury, 1106–14, Copyright 2006, with permission from Elsevier.

intense in MSA (Fig. 30.5). Other conditions associated with sympathetic autonomic dysfunction, such as DBH deficiency (Smith and Mathias 1995, Smith et al. 1995a) and familial amyloid polyneuropathy present little blood pressure change during exercise (Smith et al. 1998a) (Fig. 30.10). As such, a smaller increase in heart rate associated with a compensated elevation in stroke volume is observed, leading to a normal increase in cardiac output in these latter conditions (Fig. 30.10). Since systemic vascular resistance drops to lower levels than in healthy subjects, but not as much as in PAF, the overall effect is the greatest decrease in blood pressure in PAF and little change in blood pressure in DBH deficiency and familial amyloid polyneuropathy (Fig. 30.10).

In patients with insulin-dependent diabetes mellitus there may be a more complex situation where myocardial dysfunction can be associated with autonomic impairment. Accordingly, the chronotropic response to exercise is inhibited, but stroke volume does

increase, albeit slightly, in a compensatory manner, overall not allowing for the increase in cardiac output as in PAF and MSA (Fig. 30.10). However, because systemic vascular resistance does not decrease as much as in PAF or MSA, blood pressure does not decrease; it may increase to some degree during exercise (Smith et al. 1998a).

Exercise-induced hypotension may present in spinal cord injury (SCI) (King et al. 1994, Claydon et al. 2006, Takahashi et al. 2004). The haemodynamic responses to exercise in SCI depend mainly on the type of contraction—dynamic or static—and the level of injury. In addition, the degree to which the altered responses to exercise are observed in these subjects, compared with normal controls is also modified by the completeness and morphology of the injury (Winchester et al. 2000). During dynamic exercise, the lack of central control of sympathetic activity impairs the capacity to increase adrenergic tone and thus, to restrain metabolic vasodilatation and

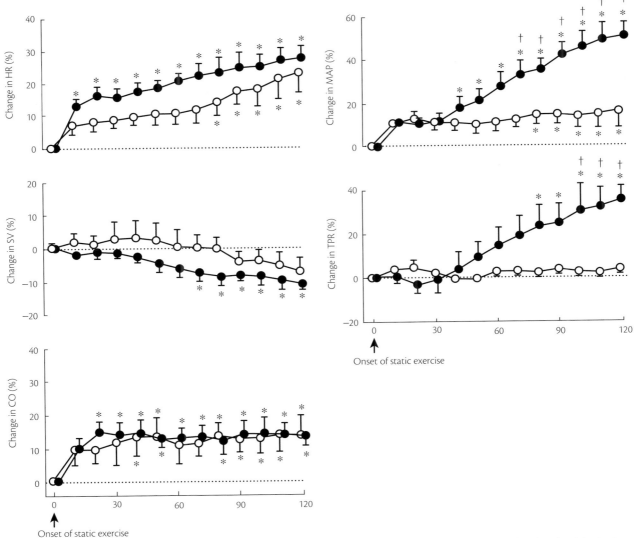

Fig. 30.12 Time courses of the relative changes in heart rate (HR), stroke volume (SV), cardiac output (CO), mean arterial pressure (MAP), and total peripheral resistance (TPR) during static arm exercise at 35% of MVC in control (n = 6) and tetraplegic subjects (n = 6). Baseline cardiovascular values before exercise were defined as 0% control levels in each subject. Their relative percentage changes from the control levels were calculated during static exercise. * Significant difference from baseline control levels (p < 0.05). † Significant difference between the two groups at an individual time point (p < 0.05). With permission from The American Physiological Society (Takahashi et al. 2004).

venous pooling below the lesion, resulting in a reduced venous return and left ventricular filling (King et al. 1994). These effects are typically evident in those subjects with high cervical lesions where blood pressure can decrease (Claydon et al. 2006) (Fig. 30.11). On the contrary, during static contractions in high cervical lesions, where cardiac output increases due to heart rate elevation, despite a possible decrease in stroke volume, blood pressure is elevated at the onset of exercise (Fig. 30.12). However, during a sustained static contraction, the lack of increase in peripheral vascular resistance as a consequence of the severed connections between supraspinal and lower sympathetic neurons prevents a further increase in blood pressure (Fig. 30.12). In some patients with cervical SCI heart rate may not increase during static contraction, but blood pressure may be slightly elevated and this effect has been suggested to be evidence of reflex activation of sympathetic nerve activity at the spinal level through muscle ergoreceptors (Yamamoto et al. 1999). Overall, these responses are part of the haemodynamic adjustments to exercise performed by the upper limbs. In SCI at or above T6 autonomic dysreflexia can occur in response to noxious or non-noxious stimuli below the lesion. Autonomic dysreflexia increases systolic blood pressure >20 mmHg and subsequently causes neurally mediated reflexes above the lesion to lower blood pressure, such as, vasodilation and sweating and vasoconstriction below the lesion (Alexander et al. 2009).

Management of exercise-induced hypotension

Two key aims in the treatment of autonomic impairments are to reduce orthostatic hypotension and increase mobility of independence. This latter aim can be substantially reduced if EIH is a problem even while orthostatic hypotension is successfully

reduced. Reducing EIH in patients with autonomic failure is likely to improve exercise tolerance and may also reduce fatigue (Butler et al. 2004). Therefore, daily activities should be better tolerated, increasing quality of life and facilitating the engagement of regular exercise, which per se, increases plasma volume, muscle mass and muscle tone, enhancing orthostatic tolerance and, at the same time, decreasing cardiovascular risk.

Non-pharmacological measures

A range of non-pharmacological measures are available that can prevent severe blood pressure falls during exercise. Pre-emptive actions should be taken, such as ensuring adequate previous hydration, avoiding food intake for several hours before exercise and performing exercise in sitting or supine positions, as exercising in the orthostatic position worsens hypotension. Physical manoeuvres such as muscle tensing and abdominal compression, as well as devices such as lower limb elastic stockings and abdominal binders, can decrease venous pooling and reduce orthostatic hypotension (Mathias 2003, Smit et al. 2004, Krediet et al. 2007). Furthermore, increasing daily salt intake is effective in preserving blood volume and reducing symptoms of orthostatic intolerance (Cooper and Hainsworth 2002, Jacob et al. 1997). Ingestion of water has been shown to have a potent pressor effect (Mathias 2000) and although EIH is unaffected, blood pressure during exercise is increased and post-exercise hypotension is ameliorated after ingestion in autonomic failure patients (Humm et al. 2008) (Fig. 30.13).

Pharmacological measures

Unlike postprandial hypotension, where artificially directed drugs such as octreotide are effective, there are limitations to pharmacological treatment in EIH. Smith et al. (1995b) tested the effect of the subcutaneous administration of the somatostatin analogue,

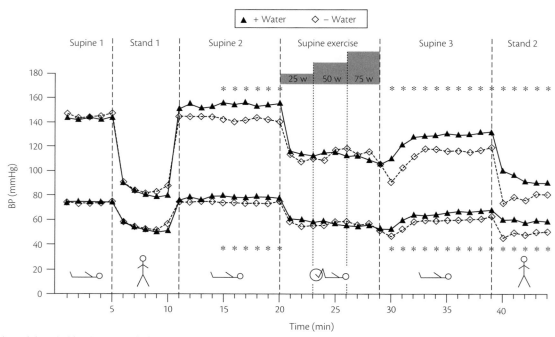

Fig. 30.13 Systolic and diastolic blood pressures (BP) during incremental supine exercise. Eight patients with pure autonomic failure (PAF) drank 480 ml of distilled water immediately after Stand 1 and before Supine 2. * p < 0.05 versus no water. Reproduced from the *Journal of Neurology, Neurosurgery and Psychiatry*, Humm, A.M., Mason, L.M. and Mathias, C.J., **79**, 1160–1164, Copyright 2008, with permission from BMJ Publishing Group Ltd.

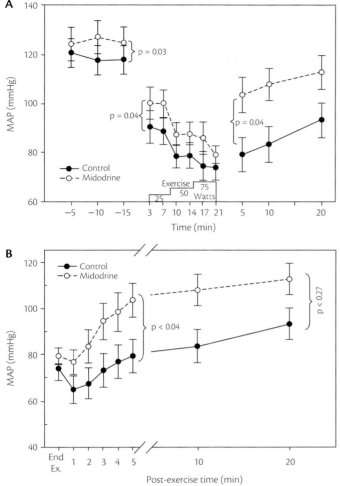

Fig. 30.14 Effects of midodrine on the mean arterial blood pressure (MAP) response before, during, and after supine cycling. MAP was higher at rest after midodrine (p = 0.03), but the rate of decrease in MAP during cycling was similar (p = 0.14; **A**). Recovery of MAP after cycling was faster in the midodrine trial over the first 5 min (p = 0.04; **B**). Over minutes 5–20 of recovery MAP was higher (p = 0.008), but the increase was similar (p = 0.27) between trials. With permission from The American Physiological Society (Adapted from Schrage et al. 2004).

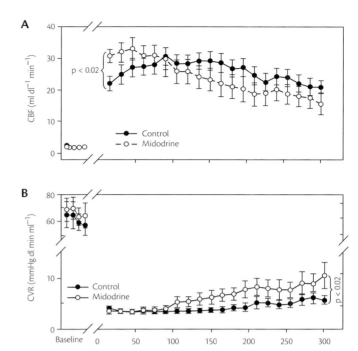

Fig. 30.15 A: Calf blood flow (CBF) and **B:** calf vascular resistance (CVR) before and after ischaemic calf exercise during control and midodrine trials. CBF was measured at rest and 5 minutes after ischaemic calf exercise. Baseline CBF was similar between trials (p = 0.79). After ischaemic exercise, CBF increased ~15-fold in both trials (p < 0.0001), which was similar between trials (p = 0.44). However, after midodrine CBF returned toward baseline levels faster (p = 0.02). CVR was similar at baseline (p = 0.96) and decreased similarly (p = 0.49) after ischaemic exercise. However, after midodrine CVR returned towards baseline levels faster (p = 0.02; **B**). With permission from The American Physiological Society (Adapted from Schrage et al. 2004).

octreotide, on exercise-induced hypotension in patients with PAF and MSA. Despite some positive effect on absolute values of blood pressure before and after exercise, octreotide did not improve EIH in the supine position, suggesting that octreotide-sensitive vasodilatory peptides are less likely to contribute to the blood pressure fall during exercise. Midodrine, an α_1-adrenergic agonist, reduces orthostatic hypotension in patients with autonomic failure (Low et al. 1997) and its effect on EIH was investigated in an uncontrolled open protocol by Schrage et al. (2004). The haemodynamic responses to supine cycling were recorded before and 1 hour after a single dose of 10 mg of midodrine, since the level of the active form of midodrine (desglymidodrine) reaches peak blood concentrations approximately 1 hour after ingestion of the tablet and raises supine blood pressure 35 mmHg for 2–3 hours (Wright et al. 1998). Midodrine increased blood pressure during and after exercise, but the exercise-induced hypotension was unaffected (Schrage et al. 2004) (Fig. 30.14). This pressor effect was due to an increase in peripheral vascular resistance, mainly on active muscles (Fig. 30.15).

Although midodrine had no specific effect on EIH, the increase in blood pressure overall may be beneficial in reducing fatigue (Butler et al. 2004). In support of this hypothesis, the use of midodrine (10 mg) in patients with spinal cord injury (C6–C8), reduced ratings of perceived exertion and increased oxygen uptake, as well as blood pressure, at peak exercise (Nieshoff et al. 2004), supporting the use of midodrine as a potentially useful option for the pharmacological treatment of exercise-induced hypotension. However, the effect of long-term treatment with midodrine on EIH caused by daily activity is yet to be tested.

References

Abe, H., Iwami, Y., Nakashima, Y., Kohshi K. and Kuroiwa, A. (1997). Exercise-induced neurally mediated syncope. *Jpn. Heart. J.* **38**, 535–9.

Akinola, A. B., Land, J. M., Mathias, C. J. *et al.* (1999). Contribution of nitric oxide to exercise-induced hypotension in human sympathetic denervation. *Clin. Auton. Res.* **9**, 263–9.

Akinola, A. B., Smith, G. D., Mathias, C. J. *et al.* (2001). The metabolic, catecholamine and cardiovascular effects of exercise in human sympathetic denervation. *Clin. Auton. Res.* **11**, 251–7.

Alexander, M. S. *et al.* (2009). International standards to document remaining autonomic function after spinal cord injury. *Spinal Cord.* **47**, 36–43.

Araujo, C. G., Nobrega, A. C. L. and Castro, C. L. (1992) Heart rate responses to deep breathing and 4-seconds of exercise before and after pharmacological blockade with atropine and propranolol. *Clin. Auton. Res.* **2**, 35–40.

Asahina, M., Hiraga, A., Hayashi, Y. *et al.* (2006). Ischemic electrocardiographic change induced by exercise in a patient with chronic autonomic failure. *Clin. Auton. Res.* **16**, 72–5.

Asmussen, E. (1981). Similarities and dissimilarities between static and dynamic exercise. *Circ Res.* **48**, I3–10.

Babai, L., Szigeti, Z., Parratt, J. R., and Vegh, A. (2002). Delayed cardioprotective effects of exercise in dogs are aminoguanidine sensitive: possible involvement of nitric oxide. *Clin. Sci. (Lond).* **102**, 435–45.

Bannister, R. and Mathias, C. J. (1999). Clinical features and evaluation of the primary chronic autonomic failure syndromes. In *Autonomic Failure: A Textbook of Clinical Disorders of the Autonmic Nervous System,* (eds. C.J. Mathias and R.Bannister), pp. 307–316. Oxford University Press, New York.

Behling, A., Moraes, R. S., Rohde, L. E., Ferlin, E. L., Nobrega, A. C., and Ribeiro, J. P. (2003). Cholinergic stimulation with pyridostigmine reduces ventricular arrhythmia and enhances heart rate variability in heart failure. *Am. Heart J.* **146**, 494–500.

Bevegard S., Freyschuss U. and Strandell T.. (1966). Circulatory adaptation to arm and leg exercise in supine and sitting position. *J Appl Physiol* **21**, 37–46.

Butler, J. E., Ribot-Ciscar, E., Zijdewind, I., and Thomas, C. K. (2004). Increased blood pressure can reduce fatigue of thenar muscles paralyzed after spinal cord injury. *Muscle. Nerve.* **29**, 575–84.

Castro, R. R., Porphirio, G., Serra, S. M., and Nóbrega, A. C. (2004). Cholinergic stimulation with pyridostigmine protects against exercise induced myocardial ischaemia. *Heart.* **90**, 1119–23.

Charkoudian, N., Halliwill, J. R., Morgan, B. J., Eisenach, J. H., and Joyner M. J. (2003). Influences of hydration on post-exercise cardiovascular control in humans. *Physiol.* **15**, 635–44.

Christ-Roberts, C. Y., and Mandarino, L. J. (2004). Glycogen synthase: key effect of exercise on insulin action. *Exerc. Sport. Sci. Rev.* **32**, 90–4.

Claydon, V. E., Hol, A. T., Eng, J. J., and Krassioukov, A. V. (2006). Cardiovascular responses and postexercise hypotension after arm cycling exercise in subjects with spinal cord injury. *Arch. Phys. Med. Rehabil.* **87**, 1106–14.

Clifford, P. S. (2007). Skeletal muscle vasodilatation at the onset of exercise. *J Physiol* **583**, 825–33.

Colivicchi, F., Ammirati, F., Biffi. A., Verdile, L., Pelliccia, A., Santini, M. (2002). Exercise-related syncope in young competitive athletes without evidence of structural heart disease. Clinical presentation and long-term outcome. *Eur Heart J.* **23**, 1125–30.

Cooper, V. L. and Hainsworth, R. (2002). Effects of dietary salt on orthostatic tolerance, blood pressure and baroreceptor sensitivity in patients with syncope. *Clin Auton Res.* **12**, 236–41.

Dotson, R., Ochoa, J., Marchettini, P. and Cline M. (1990). Sympathetic neural outflow directly recorded in patients with primary autonomic failure: clinical observations, microneurography, and histopathology. *Neurology.* **40**, 1079–85.

Dubach, P., Froelicher, V. F., Klein, J., Oakes, D., Grover-McKay, M., and Friis, R. (1988). Exercise-induced hypotension in a male population. Criteria, causes, and prognosis. *Circulation.* **78**, 1380–7.

Endo, A., Kinugawa, T., Ogino, K. *et al.* (2000). Cardiac and plasma catecholamine responses to exercise in patients with type 2 diabetes: prognostic implications for cardiac-cerebrovascular events. *Am. J. Med. Sci.* **320**, 24–30.

Forjaz, C. L., Tinucci, T., Ortega, K. C., Santaella, D. F., Mion D. Jr., and Negrao, C. E. (2000). Factors affecting post-exercise hypotension in normotensive and hypertensive humans. *Blood. Press. Monit.* **5**, 255–62.

Frongillo, D., Stocchi, F., Buccolini, P. *et al.* (1995). Ambulatory blood pressure monitoring and cardiovascular function tests in multiple system atrophy. *Fundam. Clin. Pharmacol.* **9**, 187–96.

Gonzalez-Alonso, J. (2008). Point: Stroke volume does/does not decline during exercise at maximal effort in healthy individuals. *Journal of Applied Physiology* **104**, 275–76; discussion 279–280.

Gonzalez-Alonso, J. and Calbet, J. A. (2003). Reductions in systemic and skeletal muscle blood flow and oxygen delivery limit maximal aerobic capacity in humans. *Circulation* **107**, 824–30.

Halliwill, J. R. (2001) Mechanisms and clinical implications of post-exercise hypotension in humans. *Exerc. Sport. Sci. Rev.* **29**, 65–70.

Haskell, W. L. (1994). Health consequences of physical activity: understanding and challenges regarding dose-response. *Med. Sci. Sports Exerc.* **26**, 649–60.

Herholz, K., Buskies, W., Rist, M., Pawlik, G., Hollmann, W., and Heiss, W. D. (1987). Regional cerebral blood flow in man at rest and during exercise. *J. Neurol.* **234**, 9–13.

Holten, M. K., Zacho, M., Gaster, M., Juel, C., Wojtaszewski, J. F., and Dela, F. (2004) Strength training increases insulin-mediated glucose uptake, GLUT4 content, and insulin signaling in skeletal muscle in patients with type 2 diabetes. *Diabetes.* **53**, 294–305.

Humm, A. M., Mason, L. M. and Mathias, C. J. (2008). Effect of water drinking on cardiovascular responses to supine exercise and on orthostatic hypotension after exercise in pure autonomic failure. *Journal of Neurology, Neurosurgery and Psychiatry.* **79**, 1160–64.

Jacob, G., Shannon, J. R., Black, B., Biaggioni, I., Mosqueda-Garcia, R., Robertson, R. M., Robertson, D. (1997). Effects of volume loading and pressor agents in idiopathic orthostatic tachycardia. *Circulation.* **15**, 575–80.

Johnson, R. H., Lee Gde, J., Oppenheimer, D. R., and Spalding, J. M. (1966). Autonomic failure with orthostatic hypotension due to intermediolateral column degeneration. A report of two cases with autopsies. *Q. J. Med.* **35**, 276–92.

Jorgensen, L. G., Perko, G., and Secher, N. H. (1992). Regional cerebral artery mean flow velocity and blood flow during dynamic exercise in humans. *J. Appl. Physiol.* **73**, 1825–30.

Kantor, M. A., Cullinane, E. M., Sady, S. P., Herbert, P. N., and Thompson, P. D. (1987). Exercise acutely increases high density lipoprotein-cholesterol and lipoprotein lipase activity in trained and untrained men. *Metabolism.* **36**, 188–92.

Kaufman, M. P. and Hayes, H. G. (2002). The exercise pressor reflex. *Clin. Auton. Res.* **12**, 429–39.

Kaufman, M. P., Longhurst, J. C., Rybicki, K. J., Wallach, J. H., and Mitchell, J. H. (1983). Effects of static muscular contraction on impulse activity of groups III and IV afferents in cats. *J. Appl. Physiol.* **55**, 105–12.

Kenney, M. J., and Seals, D. R. (1993). Postexercise hypotension. Key features, mechanisms, and clinical significance. *Hypertension.* **22**, 653–64.

Kenney, W. L. and Johnson, J. M. (1992). Control of skin blood flow during exercise. *Med Sci Sports Exerc* **24**, 303–312.

Khurana, R. K. and Setty, A. (1996). The value of the isometric hand-grip test—studies in various autonomic disorders. *Clin. Auton. Res.* **6**, 211–18.

King, M. L., Lichtman, S. W., Pellicone, J. T., Close, R. J., and Lisanti P. (1994). Exertional hypotension in spinal cord injury. *Chest.* **106**, 1166–71.

Kirby, B. S., Carlson, R. E., Markwald, R. R., Voyles, W. F. and Dinenno, F. A. (2007). Mechanical influences on skeletal muscle vascular tone in humans: insight into contraction-induced rapid vasodilatation. *J Physiol* **583**, 861–74.

Krediet, C. T., Wilde, A. A., Wieling, W., and Halliwill, J. R. (2004). Exercise related syncope, when it's not the heart. *Clin. Auton. Res.* **14**, 25–36.

Krediet, C. T., Wilde, A. A., Halliwill, J. R., Wieling, W. (2005). Syncope during exercise, documented with continuous blood pressure monitoring during ergometer testing. *Clin Auton Res.* **15**, 59–62.

Krediet, C. T., Go-Schon, I. K., Kim, Y. S., Linzer, M., Van Lieshout, J. J., and Wieling, W. (2007). Management of initial orthostatic hypotension: lower body muscle tensing attenuates the transient arterial blood pressure decrease upon standing from squatting. *Clin. Sci. (Lond)* **113**, 401–7.

La Rovere, M. T., Bigger, J. T. Jr., Marcus, F. I., Mortara, A., and Schwartz, P. J. (1998). Baroreflex sensitivity and heart-rate variability in prediction of total cardiac mortality after myocardial infarction. ATRAMI (Autonomic Tone and Reflexes After Myocardial Infarction) Investigators. *Lancet.* **14**, 478–84.

Lele, S. S., Scalia, G., Thomson, H. *et al.* (1994). Mechanism of exercise hypotension in patients with ischemic heart disease. Role of neurocardiogenically mediated vasodilatation. *Circulation.* **90**, 2701–9.

Lewis, S. F., Snell, P. G., Taylor, W. F., *et al.* (1985). Role of muscle mass and mode of contraction in circulatory responses to exercise. *J. Appl. Physiol.* **58**, 146–51.

Lewis, S. F., Taylor, W. F., Graham, R. M., Pettinger, W. A., Schutte, J. E., and Blomqvist, C. G. (1983). Cardiovascular responses to exercise as functions of absolute and relative work load. *J. Appl. Physiol.* **54**, 1314–23.

Lo, S. S., Mathias, C. J., and Sutton, M. S. (1996). QT interval and dispersion in primary autonomic failure. *Heart* **75**, 498–501.

Low, P. A., Gilden, J. L., Freeman, R., Sheng, K. N., and McElligott, M. A. (1997). Efficacy of midodrine vs placebo in neurogenic orthostatic hypotension. A randomized, double-blind multicenter study Midodrine Study Group [see comment]. *JAMA* **277**, 1046–51. [Corrigenda. *JAMA* 3: August 1997, p. 388.]

Marshall, R. J., Schirger, A., and Shepherd, J. T. (1961). Blood pressure during supine exercise in idiopathic orthostatic hypotension. *Circulation.* **24**, 76–81.

Marvin, H. M., and Sullivan, A. G. (1935). Clinical observations upon syncope and sudden death in relation to aortic stenosis. *Am. Heart. J.* **10**, 705–35.

Mathias, C. J. (2000). A 21st century water cure. *The Lancet.* **356**, 1046–48.

Mathias, C. J. (2003). Autonomic diseases: management. *J Neurol Neurosurg Psychiatry* **74** suppl 3, iii42–47.

Mathias, C. J., Bannister, R. B., Cortelli, P., *et al.* (1990). Clinical, autonomic and therapeutic observations in two siblings with postural hypotension and sympathetic failure due to an inability to synthesize noradrenaline from dopamine because of a deficiency of dopamine beta hydroxylase. *Q J Med.* **75**, 617–33.

Matthews, M. R. (1999). Autonomic ganglia and preganglionic neurons in autonomic failure. In *Autonomic Failure: A Textbook of Clinical Disorders of the Autonmic Nervous System,* (eds. C.J. Mathias and R.Bannister), pp. 329–39. Oxford University Press, New York.

McKenna, W., Deanfield, J., Faruqui, A., England, D., Oakley, C., and Goodwin, J. (1981). Prognosis in hypertrophic cardiomyopathy: role of age and clinical electrocardiographic and haemodynamic feature. *Am. J. Cardiol.* **47**, 532–8.

Mitchell, J. H. (1990). J.B. Wolffe memorial lecture. Neural control of the circulation during exercise. *Med. Sci. Sports Exerc.* **22**, 141–54.

Miyamoto, Y., Higuchi, J., Abe, Y., Hiura, T., Nakazono, Y. and Mikami, T. (1983). Dynamics of cardiac output and systolic time intervals in supine and upright exercise. *J Appl Physiol* **55**, 1674–81.

Morita, E., Kunie, K., Matsuo, H. (2007). Food-dependent exercise-induced anaphylaxis. *J Dermatol. Sci.*, **47**, 109–17.

Morrison, W. L., and Petch, M. C. (1987). Exercise-induced hypotension. *Lancet.* **24**, 969.

Nieshoff, E. C., Birk, T. J., Birk, C. A., Hinderer, S. R., and Yavuzer, G. (2004). Double-blinded, placebo-controlled trial of midodrine for exercise performance enhancement in tetraplegia: a pilot study. *J. Spinal. Cord. Med.* **27**, 219–25.

da Nobrega, A. C. (2005). The subacute effects of exercise: concept, characteristics, and clinical implications. *Exerc. Sport Sci. Rev.* **33**, 84–7.

O'Connor, F. G., Oriscello, R. G., and Levine, B. D. (1999). Exercise-related syncope in the young athlete: reassurance, restriction or referral? *Am. Fam. Physician.* **60**, 2001–8.

Ogoh, S., Brothers, R. M., Barnes, Q., Eubank, W. L., Hawkins, M. N., Purkayastha, S., A OY and Raven, P. B. (2005). The effect of changes in cardiac output on middle cerebral artery mean blood velocity at rest and during exercise. *J Physiol.* **569**, 697–704.

Ogoh, S., Brothers, R. M., Eubank, W. L. and Raven, P. B. (2008). Autonomic neural control of the cerebral vasculature: acute hypotension. *Stroke; a journal of cerebral circulation* **39**, 1979–87.

Oppenheimer, D. R. (1980). Lateral horn cells in progressive autonomic failure. *J. Neurol. Sci.* **46**, 393–404.

Panerai, R. B. (2008). Cerebral autoregulation: from models to clinical applications. *Cardiovascular engineering (Dordrecht, Netherlands)* **8**, 42–59.

Paulson, O. B., Strandgaard, S. and Edvinsson, L. (1990). Cerebral autoregulation. *Cerebrovascular and brain metabolism reviews* **2**, 161–92.

Puvi-Rajasingham, S., Smith, G. D., Akinola, A., and Mathias, C. J. (1997). Abnormal regional blood flow responses during and after exercise in human sympathetic denervation. *J. Physiol.* **15**, 841–9.

Radice, M., Rocca, A., Bedon, E., Musacchio, N., Morabito, A., and Segalini, G. (1996). Abnormal response to exercise in middle-aged NIDDM patients with and without autonomic neuropathy. *Diabet. Med.* **13**, 259–65.

Raven, P. B., Fadel, P. J. and Ogoh, S. (2006). Arterial baroreflex resetting during exercise: a current perspective. *Exp Physiol* **91**, 37–49.

Remensnyder, J. P., Mitchell, J. H., and Sarnoff, S. J. (1962). Functional sympatholysis during muscular activity. Observations on influence of carotid sinus on oxygen uptake. *Circ. Res.* **11**, 370–80.

Ronsen, O., Haugen, O., Hallen, J., and Bahr, R. (2004). Residual effects of prior exercise and recovery on subsequent exercise-induced metabolic responses. *Eur. J. Appl. Physiol.* **92**, 498–507.

Rosenmeier, J. B., Dinenno, F. A., Fritzlar, S. J., and Joyner, M. J. (2003). Alpha1- and alpha2-adrenergic vasoconstriction is blunted in contracting human muscle. *J. Physiol.* **15**, 971–6.

Rowell, L. B. (1993). *Human Cardiovascular Control.* Oxford University Press, New York.

Rowell, L. B. and O'Leary, D. S. (1990). Reflex control of the circulation during exercise: chemoreflexes and mechanoreflexes. *Journal of Applied Physiology* **69**, 407–418.

Schrage, W. G., Eisenach, J. H., Dinenno, F. A. *et al.* (2004). Effects of midodrine on exercise-induced hypotension and blood pressure recovery in autonomic failure. *J. Appl. Physiol.* **97**, 1978–84.

Schwartz, P. J. and Wolf, S. (1978). QT interval prolongation as predictor of sudden death in patients with myocardial infarction. *Circulation* **57**, 1074–7.

Secher, N. H., Seifert, T. and Van Lieshout, J. J. (2008). Cerebral blood flow and metabolism during exercise: implications for fatigue. *Journal of Applied Physiology* **104**, 306–314.

Sheffer, A. L., and Austen, K. F. (1980) Exercise-induced anaphylaxis. *J. Allergy Clin. Immunol.* **66**, 106–11.

Shepherd, J. T. (1987). Circulatory response to exercise in health. *Circulation.* **76**, VI3–10.

Shibasaki, M., Wilson, T. E. and Crandall, C. G. (2006). Neural control and mechanisms of eccrine sweating during heat stress and exercise. *Journal of Applied Physiology* **100**, 1692–1701.

Singer, W., Sandroni, P., Opfer-Gehrking, T.L. *et al.* (2006). Pyridostigmine treatment trial in neurogenic orthostatic hypotension. *Arch. Neurol.* **63**, 513–8.

Smit, A. A., Wieling, W., Fujimura, J. *et al.* (2004). Use of lower abdominal compression to combat orthostatic hypotension in patients with autonomic dysfunction. *Clin. Auton. Res.* **14**, 167–75.

Smith, G. D., Alam, M., Watson, L. P., and Mathias, C. J. (1995b). Effect of the somatostatin analogue, octreotide, on exercise-induced hypotension in human subjects with chronic sympathetic failure. *Clin. Sci. (Lond).* **89**, 367–73.

Smith, G. D., Watson, L. P., Pavitt, D. V., and Mathias, C. J. (1995a). Abnormal cardiovascular and catecholamine responses to supine exercise in human subjects with sympathetic dysfunction. *J. Physiol.* **255–65.**

Smith, G. D., Watson, L. P., and Mathias, C. J. (1996a). Cardiovascular and catecholamine changes induced by supine exercise and upright posture in vasovagal syncope. Comparisons with normal subjects and subjects with sympathetic denervation. *Eur. Heart. J.* **17**, 1882–90.

Smith, G. D., Watson, L. P., and Mathias, C. J. (1996b). Neurohumoral, peptidergic and biochemical responses to supine exercise in two groups with primary autonomic failure: Shy-Drager syndrome/multiple system atrophy and pure autonomic failure. *Clin. Auton. Res.* **6**, 255–62.

Smith, G. D., Watson, L. P., and Mathias, C. J. (1998). Differing haemodynamic and catecholamine responses to exercise in three groups with peripheral autonomic dysfunction: insulin-dependent diabetes mellitus, familial amyloid polyneuropathy and pure autonomic failure. *J. Auton. Nerv. Syst.* **73**, 125–34.

Smith, G. D., and Mathias, C. J. (1995). Postural hypotension enhanced by exercise in patients with chronic autonomic failure. *Qjm.* **88**, 251–6.

Smith, S. A., Mitchell, J. R., and Garry, M. G. (2006). The mammalian exercise pressor reflex in health and disease. *Exp. Physiol.* **91**, 89–102.

Sneddon, J. F., Scalia, G., Ward, D. E., McKenna, W. J., Camm, A. J., Frenneaux, M. P. (1994). Exercise induced vasodepressor syncope. *Br Heart J.* **71**, 554–57.

Takahashi, M., Sakaguchi, A., Matsukawa, K., Komine, H., Kawaguchi, K., and Onari, K. (2004). Cardiovascular control during voluntary static exercise in humans with tetraplegia. *J. Appl. Physiol.* **97**, 2077–82.

Thadani, U. and Parker, J. O. (1978). Hemodynamics at rest and during supine and sitting bicycle exercise in normal subjects. *Am J Cardiol* **41**, 52–59.

Thomas, G. D., and Segal, S. S. (2004). Neural control of muscle blood flow during exercise. *J. Appl. Physiol.* **97**, 731–8.

Thompson, P. D., Crouse, S. F., Goodpaster, B., Kelley, D., Moyna, N., and Pescatello, L. (2001). The acute versus the chronic response to exercise. *Med. Sci. Sports. Exerc.* **33**, S438–45; discussion S52–3.

Van Lieshout, J. J., Wieling, W., Karemaker, J. M. and Secher, N. H. (2003). Syncope, cerebral perfusion, and oxygenation. *Journal of Applied Physiology* **94**, 833–48.

Vella, C. A. and Robergs, R. A. (2005). A review of the stroke volume response to upright exercise in healthy subjects. *Br J Sports Med* **39**, 190–95.

Wesche, J. (1986). The time course and magnitude of blood flow changes in the human quadriceps muscles following isometric contraction. *J Physiol* **377**, 445–62.

Whyte, G., Stephens, N., Budgett, R., Sharma, S., Shave, R. E., McKenna, W. J. (2004). Exercise induced neurally mediated syncope in an elite rower: a treatment dilemma. *Br J Sports Med.* **38**, 84–5.

Williamson, J. W., Fadel, P. J. and Mitchell, J. H. (2006). New insights into central cardiovascular control during exercise in humans: a central command update. *Exp Phys.* **91**, 51–58.

Williamson, J. W., Nobrega, A. C., McColl, R., *et al.* (1997). Activation of the insular cortex during dynamic exercise in humans. *J. Physiol.* **503**, 277–83.

Williamson, J. W., Nobrega, A. C., Winchester, P. K., Zim, S., and Mitchell, J. H. (1995). Instantaneous heart rate increase with dynamic exercise: central command and muscle-heart reflex contributions. *J. Appl. Physiol.* **78**, 1273–9.

Winchester, P. K., Williamson, J. W., and Mitchell, J. H. (2000). Cardiovascular responses to static exercise in patients with Brown-Séquard syndrome. *J. Physiol.* **15**, 193–202.

Wright, R. A., Kaufmann, H. C., Perera, R., Opfer-Gehrking, T. L., McElligott, M. A., Sheng, K. N., and Low, P. A. (1998). A double-blind, dose-response study of midodrine in neurogenic orthostatic hypotension. *Neurology* **51**, 120–4.

Yamamoto, M., Tajima. F., Okawa, H., Mizushima, T., Umezu, Y., and Ogata, H. (1999). Static exercise-induced increase in blood pressure in individuals with cervical spinal cord injury. *Arch. Phys. Med Rehabil.* **80**, 288–93.

CHAPTER 31

Evaluation of sudomotor function

Phillip A. Low and Robert D. Fealey

Introduction

Anatomy and physiology of sweating

Thermoreceptors are present in the preoptic-anterior hypothalamus area, in skin, in viscera, and in spinal cord. In addition to the spinothalamic tract, other afferent pathways ascend as multisynaptic fibres diffusely in lateral spinal cord, to reticular formation of brainstem, and finally to hypothalamus and thalamus. These signals are integrated in the posterior hypothalamus where a set-point is established.

Efferent pathways as crossed and uncrossed fibres from the hypothalamus travel via the tegmentum of the pons and the lateral reticular substance of the medulla to the intermediolateral column. Many of these fibre connections are polysynaptic.

The intermediolateral column neurons are cholinergic and synapse with paravertebral sympathetic ganglia from whence postganglionic sympathetic cholinergic sudomotor axons supply eccrine sweat glands. There are about 5000 preganglionic neurons per segment of thoracic cord in humans, and there is an attrition rate of 5–7% per decade (Low et al. 1977).

There are less precise sudomotor than sensory dermatomes since a single ganglion receives fibres from 5–6 preganglionic levels and skin is multi-innervated. Approximate sudomotor dermatomes are: T1–2, ipsilateral face; T2–6, upper limb; T5–12, trunk; T10–L3, lower limb. As a rule, concordance of sudomotor dermatomes is good once postganglionic fibres enter the nerve trunk but poor proximal to that.

There are two types of sweat glands, eccrine and apocrine (Ogawa and Low 1993). The eccrine sweat glands are simple, tubular glands that extend down from the epidermis to the lower dermis. The lower portion is a tightly coiled secretory apparatus consisting of two types of cells. One is a dark basophilic cell that secretes mucous material and the other a light acidophilic cell that is responsible for the passage of water and electrolytes. Surrounding the secretory cells are myoepithelial cells, which are thought to aid the expulsion of sweat by contraction. These glands receive a rich supply of blood vessels and sympathetic nerve fibres, but are unusual in that sympathetic innervation is cholinergic. The full complement of eccrine glands develops in the embryonic state (Kuno 1956). No new glands develop after birth.

The postganglionic sweat response fails progressively with increasing age (Low 1997a). We evaluated 357 normal subjects of 10–83 years, of age, evenly distributed by age and gender. There is a proximo-distal gradient of severity. All lower extremity sites, measured by the quantitative sudomotor axon reflex test (QSART), underwent a significant reduction with age ($p < 0.001$) with a slope of 0.02 µl/cm^2/year for proximal leg and foot and 0.03 µl/cm^2 for the distal leg. The sweat loss is associated with a loss of cholinergic unmyelinated fibre stained with the panaxonal marker protein gene product 9.5 (PGP9.5) and acetylcholinesterase (AChE) (Abdel-Rahman et al. 1992).

The distribution of eccrine glands shows area differences (Kuno 1956), with the greatest density in the palms and soles. They vary in density from 400/mm^2 on the palm to about 80/cm^2 on the thighs and upper arm and least in the back. The total numbers are approximately 2–5 million (Kuno 1956), and they weigh about 30–40 µg each (Sato and Sato 1983). Although sweat gland density is highest on the palms and soles, these areas are much less activated during thermoregulatory sweating compared with head and trunk sweat glands (Ogawa 1975, Shih and Lin 1979, Kerassidis 1994). These areas, however, are regularly responsive to emotional sweat stimuli, which are thought to arise in anterior cingulate, orbital-fronto, and limbic cortices, and project eventually to the spinal cord autonomic centres.

The physiology of the human sweat response is known from the detailed *in vitro* studies of Sato et al. (Sato et al. 1993). Acetylcholine secretion results in the production of an ultrafiltrate (isotonic) by the secretory coil. Directly collected sweat has identical Na$^+$ and K$^+$ values to plasma. Reabsorption of sodium ions by the eccrine sweat duct results in hypotonic sweat. Directly collected sweat from the proximal duct is hypotonic (Na$^+$, 20–80 mM; K$^+$, 5–25 mM) (Sato and Sato 1983). Extracellular Ca^{2+} is important since removal of periglandular Ca^{2+} with [ethylene-bis(oxy-ethylenenitrilo)] tetraaceic acid (EGTA) completely inhibits sweat secretion, while the calcium ionophore A23187 strongly and persistently stimulates sweating (Sato and Sato 1983). Magnesium ions appear to be unimportant.

Sato and Sato (1983) made additional key observations on isolated human eccrine sweat gland regulation. The regulation of sweating is cholinergic and muscarinic since it is completely inhibited by atropine. Sudomotor function is metabolically active. It is inhibited by cold (4°C) and involves active transport, being inhibited by ouabain and by the metabolic inhibitors, cyanide or dinitrophenol (DNP). The prostaglandin, PGE_1, has sudorific effect *in vitro* comparable to acetylcholine and was thought to act via cyclic adenosine monophosphate (cAMP). Microtubules may be important since vinblastine strongly but reversibly inhibits sweating. Endogenous cAMP appears to be the second messenger, since theophylline, by inhibiting phosphodiesterase, markedly increases the sweat response.

The major function of the sweat gland in humans is thermoregulatory. With repeated episodes of profuse sweating, the salt content of the sweat declines progressively. In the individual acclimatized to a hot climate, the salt content is reduced, probably reflecting an increase of mineralocorticoids in response to thermal stress (Kuno 1956).

The long efferent course of autonomic sudomotor fibres can be interrupted by autonomic disorders, both central and peripheral, and results in an impairment of the sweat response. This impairment can be evaluated using the thermoregulatory sweat test (TST). The postganglionic fibres can be evaluated using the QSART and related tests.

Tests of sudomotor function

Quantitative sudomotor axon reflex test

The principle of the QSART can be seen in Fig. 31.1. When postganglionic sympathetic terminals are stimulated, an antidromic impulse occurs, reaches a branch-point, then travels orthodromically to release acetylcholine from a nerve terminal. Acetylcholine traverses the neuroglandular junction and binds to M_3 muscarinic receptors on eccrine sweat glands (Torres et al. 1991) to evoke the sweat response. Acetylcholinesterase in subcutaneous tissue cleaves acetylcholine to acetate and choline, resulting in its inactivation and cessation of the sweat response. Other neurotransmitters, such as calcitonin-gene-related polypeptide (CGRP) play an important subsidiary role. To avoid direct stimulation of the sweat gland, the stimulus and recording compartments are anatomically separated within a multi-compartmental sweat cell, with the recording compartment in the centre, surrounded by the stimulus compartment, separated by an air-gap (Fig. 31.2). The stimulus is iontophoresed acetylcholine and a constant current of 2 mA for 5 minutes is delivered. The sweat response is measured by a sudorometer, which determines the sweat volume. The same response can be evoked by

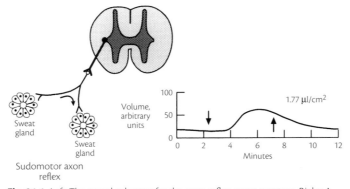

Fig. 31.1 Left: The neural substrate for the axon-reflex sweat response. Right: A representative axon-reflex sweat response. With kind permission from Springer Science+Business Media: *Clinical Autonomic Research*, In vivo studies on receptor pharmacology of the human eccrine sweat gland, **2**, 1992, 29–34, Low PA, Opfer-Gehrking TL, Kihara M.

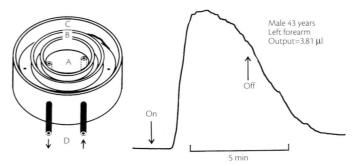

Fig. 31.2 Multicompartmental sweat cell (left) and evoked sweat response (right). The capsule is strapped on to skin, and acetylcholine (compartment C) is iontophoresed using a constant current generator with the anode connected to compartment C. Axon reflex evoked sweat response in compartment A is evaporated off by a stream of nitrogen at a controlled flow rate and quantitated dynamically by a sudorometer. Compartment B and associated ridges prevent diffusion and leakage of acetylcholine. With permission from Low PA, Zimmerman BR, Dyck PJ (1986), *Muscle and Nerve*, Wiley.

electrical stimulation, but requires high stimulus intensity and long duration pulses, in order to activate these C-fibres (Namer et al. 2004). Electrically evoked sweat response has a much shorter latency and is quite painful (Namer et al. 2004).

The tests are sensitive and reproducible in controls (Low 1997b) and in patients with diabetic neuropathy (Low et al. 1986, Low 1997b). Tests repeated on two different days regress with a high coefficient of regression. Tests repeated daily to the identical site may evoke local skin alterations, possibly to the sweat duct after about the third or fourth repetition, but this 'tolerance' is highly variable. The coefficient of variation is 8% (Low et al. 1983).

The recordings are symmetrical so that in normal individuals, the left side is not significantly different to the right (Low 1997b). We routinely record from the left but will study the right side when clinically warranted (e.g. following left sural nerve biopsy, or with unilateral symptoms). Four standard recording sites are the medial forearm, the proximal leg, distal leg, and the proximal foot (on a flat surface over the extensor digitorum brevis muscle). The innervation of the forearm, proximal leg, distal leg, and proximal foot are by ulnar, peroneal, saphenous, and sural (mainly) nerves, respectively.

The most common abnormality is a loss of sweat volume. A length-dependent neuropathy is typically associated with a loss of sweat volume that is maximal distally (Fig. 31.3). Acute preganglionic nerve lesions result in anhidrosis on the thermoregulatory sweat test, with normal QSART. With long-standing preganglionic denervation, QSART volumes are also reduced. For instance, postganglionic sudomotor failure occurred at the forearm in 50% each of pure autonomic failure (PAF) (postganglionic) and multiple system atrophy (MSA) (preganglionic) patients and at the foot in 69% and 66% of PAF and MSA patients, respectively (Cohen et al. 1987).

Since QSART volumes vary with age and gender (Low 1997a), we developed a composite autonomic scoring scale (CASS) that corrects for the confounding effects of age and gender (Low 1993). The sudomotor subset is scored for 0 (no deficit) to 3 (maximal deficit).

QSART in disorders of sweating

QSART recordings have been performed in many disorders, including diabetic neuropathy (Low et al. 1986), Sjögren's syndrome,

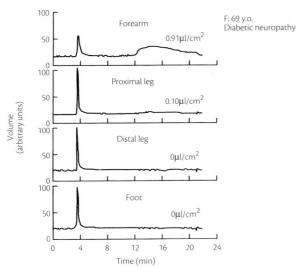

Fig. 31.3 Quantitative sudomotor axon reflex test volumes are normal over forearm and reduced over the entire lower extremity in a patient with autonomic neuropathy.

Lambert–Eaton myasthenic syndrome, distal small fibre neuropathy (Stewart et al. 1992), atopic dermatitis, ageing, idiopathic autonomic neuropathy (Suarez et al. 1994), and distal small fibre neuropathy (Stewart et al. 1992), acute panautonomic neuropathy (Suarez et al. 1994) and Parkinson's disease (PD) and related extrapyramidal and cerebellar disorders (Sandroni et al. 1991), a gamut of neuropathies (Low and McLeod 1997), in MSA and PAF (Cohen et al. 1987), chronic idiopathic anhidrosis (Low et al. 1985), and in studying the pharmacology of sweating (Low et al. 1992).

We have reported data based on 26 patients with PAF, 60 patients with PD, 70 patients with mild MSA (MSA-I), 100 patients with classic MSA (MSA-II), and 51 patients with PD with associated autonomic failure (PD-AF). All cases have been evaluated by a neurologist, and quantitative tests of autonomic function to evaluate the severity and distribution of sudomotor, cardiovagal, and adrenergic function were undertaken, and a CASS was derived, which corrects for the confounding effects of age and gender. In an initial study, confined to MSA and PAF patients (Cohen et al. 1987), there was no difference in percentage anhidrosis on thermoregulatory sweat test (TST; >70% anhidrosis). QSART indicated postganglionic sudomotor impairment in the lower extremity in more than 65% of both MSA and PAF patients. In a study on the sensitivity and specificity of CASS in the diagnosis of autonomic failure, we compared MSA (n = 18), autonomic neuropathy, PD (n = 20), and common neuropathy (without clinical autonomic failure), CASS for MSA, autonomic neuropathy, and PD were 8.5 ± 1.3, 8.6 ± 1.2, and 1.5 ± 1.1, respectively. All patients with MSA had scores greater than 4 and all patients with PD, less than 4; with 89% of MSA patients having scores above 7.

However, in a review of a larger group of patients referred to the autonomic laboratory (Sandroni et al. 1991), comprising PD (n = 35), PD-AF (n = 54), MSA-I (n = 73), and MSA-II (n = 75), a range of autonomic failure was found. Clinical autonomic failure was 11%, 83%, 89%, and 100% for PD, PD-AF, MSA-I, and MSA-II, respectively. QSART was reduced in the lower extremity in 40%, 55%, 66%, and 70%, respectively. Corresponding values for percentage anhidrosis on TST were 39%, 63%, 72%, and

85%, respectively. A similar gradation in cardiovagal and adrenergic function was also found. This gradation seems to translate into outcome. Time in years to evolve from onset to Hoehn–Yahr stage IV was 9.5, 5.1, 4.8, and 3.4 years, respectively. The conclusion was that MSA and PAF are definable, but that it is important to recognize gradations, and that autonomic function tests are helpful in defining these intermediate types.

There is some evidence that patients with neuropathic pain can have a switch back to adrenergic regulation of sudomotor innervation. Patients with complex regional pain syndrome type I (CRPS I) were found to have supersensitivity to α-adrenergic stimulation (Chemali et al. 2001). These workers compared the sweat response to iontophoresis of an α-adrenergic agent (phenylephrine) in 4 patients with acute CRPS I and 3 patients with resolved CRPS I with that in 9 control subjects using QSART. A significantly higher sweat response was observed in the affected limb of patients with acute CRPS I compared to their unaffected limb (p = 0.03), to control subjects (p > 0.018), and to the affected or unaffected limbs of patients with resolved CRPS I (p = 0.02), whose sweat response was not significantly different from that of control subjects. They concluded that the abnormal response in patients with acute CRPS I was most likely mediated by an axon reflex and that α-adrenoceptor supersensitivity occurs in the presynaptic portion of the postganglionic sudomotor axon.

The nicotinic (indirect or axon-reflex) versus the muscarinic (direct) response in normal subjects and patients with diabetic neuropathy has been compared (Kihara et al. 1993). Using a specially designed multi-compartmental sweat cell and dual sudorometers, we were able to record the evoked the direct and indirect responses simultaneously. In control subjects, sudorometric direct recordings were consistently larger than axon-reflex mediated responses. There was no difference in sweat droplet density by sex, but the size of droplets was larger in males. In diabetic patients, 3 of 23 had absent axon-reflex but preserved direct responses. Patients with mild neuropathy had an overrepresentation of large-diameter droplets in the silastic imprints, while patients with severe neuropathy had a markedly reduced density and small-diameter droplets.

Thermoregulatory sweat test

TST provides a sweat stimulus via raised blood and mean skin temperature. The efferent sympathetic response is mediated by preganglionic centres including the hypothalamus, bulbospinal pathways, the intermediolateral cell columns, and white rami; postganglionic paths include the sympathetic chain and postganglionic sudomotor nerves to sweat glands.

The TST conducted in the Mayo Thermoregulatory Laboratory is a modification of Guttmann's quinizarin sweat test (Guttmann 1947). Unclothed subjects lie supine on a cart and the exposed body surface (exclusive of eyes, nose, mouth, and genitalia) is covered with an indicator powder mixture (alizarin red, sodium carbonate, and cornstarch) (Fealey et al. 1989, Fealey 1996). Subjects are totally enclosed in the sweat cabinet for 45–65 minutes (air temperature 44–50°C, relative humidity 35–45%) and skin temperature is carefully maintained between 39°C and 40°C via overhead infrared heaters. This skin temperature range is critical to recruiting a maximal central response yet is not so high as to cause skin injury, direct sweat gland activation, or somatosympathetic reflex sweating below the level of the lesion (i.e. in complete cervical cord transection). The humidity is regulated to be moderate and the heating time no greater than 70 minutes, in order to avoid hydromeiosis (Fealey 1996). The oral temperature is monitored continuously and must rise to at least 38.0°C or by 1.0°C above baseline temperature, whichever yields the higher value. For normal subjects, the mean temperature rise during the TST is 1.2°C and the average heating time 45 minutes. All normal individuals show relatively uniform sweating over the entire anterior body surface, with characteristic areas of heavier or lighter sweating (Fealey 1996). It is essential to review the patient's list of medications and, if possible, discontinue those with strong anticholinergic side effects for 48 hours prior to testing. Testing during the early stages of a febrile response or within 4 hours of a dose of a mu-opioid agonist may produce an abnormal (anhidrotic) test result that is simply related to failing to raise core temperature to the elevated 'set-point' temperature produced by fever and opioids. Retesting when afebrile or when off opioids for 12–24 hours will resolve this issue.

The sweat distribution is documented by digital photography of the body surface and colour digital pictures are made on standard anatomical drawings for use in report generation. The digital images are also processed by a colour pixel counter to derive an accumulative value for the area of anhidrosis and the percentage of anhidrosis (TST% or %ANH). Alternatively a planimeter (LASICO, model 1252M, resolution = 0.005 cm^2) can be used, with measurement of areas directly from the anatomical drawing. TST% is the measured area of anhidrosis divided by the area of the anatomic figure, multiplied by 100. Normal sweat distributions and TST% have been published (Fealey et al. 1989, Fealey 1996).

Thermoregulatory sweat test in disorders of sweating

Widespread anhidrosis is characteristic of MSA and PAF (Chapter 39). Cohen et al. (Cohen et al. 1987) found median values of body surface anhidrosis (TST%) of 97% and 91%, respectively. Representative sweat distributions are shown in Fig. 31.4.

We have shown that the severity of clinical autonomic failure in patients with extrapyramidal and cerebellar system disorders regressed significantly with TST% (Sandroni et al. 1991). The orthostatic blood pressure decrement and TST% were found to have a near identical rank order of severity by disease category, being milder for Parkinson's disease and progressive supranuclear palsy and severe for MSA.

In 2001, we reviewed the thermoregulatory sweat tests, over the prior 3 year period, of all patients having a clinical diagnosis of either MSA or PD (Fealey 2001a, 2001b). All patients were independently diagnosed by Movement Disorder and/or Autonomic Disorder Specialist. The clinical diagnosis made use of clinical autonomic symptoms but not the autonomic test results but otherwise followed published consensus criteria regarding the diagnosis of probable MSA and PD. QSART results were available on 129 of the 143 patients. Digital photos, digitized body images, percentage of anterior body surface anhidrosis on TST, and sweat volume outputs at each QSART site were analyzed.

The following criteria were used to determine the site of autonomic involvement:

◆ a preganglionic lesion—normal QSART volume in an area of complete anhidrosis on TST

◆ a mixed (preganglionic and postganglionic) lesion—reduced but not absent QSART in an area of complete anhidrosis on TST

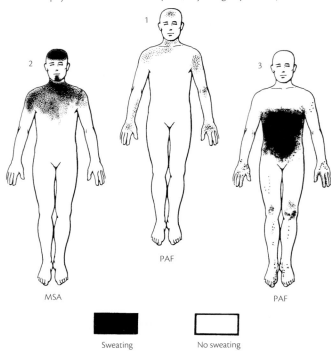

Thermoregulatory sweating abnormalities
in pure autonomic failure (PAF) and multiple system atrophy with autonomic failure (MSA; Shy–Drager syndrome)

Sweating   No sweating

Fig. 31.4 Thermoregulatory sweat test results showing characteristic anhidrosis in patients with multiple system atrophy and pure autonomic failure. Cohen J, Low P, Fealey R, Sheps S, Jiang NS (1987). *Annals of Neurology*, **22**, 692–99, with permission from Wiley.

◆ a postganglionic lesion—similar reduction of QSART and TST sweat output in the same area

◆ normal sweating—both TST and QSART normal at a given site.

Mean percentage of body surface anhidrosis (%ANH) and QSART volumes were compared in MSA and PD patients using independent t-statistic. Highly significant differences were found between MSA (n = 91) and PD (n = 43) patients in percentage of body surface anhidrosis (70% vs 8%, p <0.0001). QSART volumes were moderately reduced at the forearm, proximal leg, and distal leg in MSA compared with PD (p <0.007) but were no different in the foot (p = 0.09). The frequency and distribution of preganglionic sudomotor failure at all QSART sites was highly associated with MSA (p <0.0001 for all sites) compared to PD. A review of these PD and MSA patients is currently underway to ascertain their clinical course and accuracy of diagnosis and predictions made in 2001 (Fealey, manuscript in preparation).

These observations emphasize the important necessity of %ANH. This study and an earlier one (Sandroni et al. 1991) found that %ANH is a powerful discriminator of MSA from PD and contrasts with a recent report (Riley and Chelimsky 2003), which concluded that autonomic tests did not discriminate. Remarkably this study did not evaluate %ANH.

Sweat distributions that may portend the occurrence of generalized autonomic failure include regional anhidrosis of the lower legs or of the lower abdomen and legs. Many have some sweating of the distal feet and preserved postganglionic sweat responses (QSART) in areas of TST anhidrosis (the combination of which suggests a preganglionic lesion) (Fig. 31.5). Patients who are clinically PD often have normal sweating or mild distal impairment of sweating on both TST and QSART.

A recent review of TST data for 2004 continues to show marked differences in %ANH for MSA versus PD, mean values of 69% versus 7% (Fealey, unpublished observations).

In 2004, Thaisetthawatkul and colleagues reviewed the Mayo Clinic experience with autonomic dysfunction in diffuse Lewy body disease (DLBD) (Thaisetthawatkul et al. 2004). Twenty patients with DLBD evaluated from 1995 to 2000 were compared with 20 age-matched MSA and PD patients evaluated from 1999 to 2002. Disease characteristics, autonomic symptoms, and function tests on the CASS and the TST distributions and %ANH were analysed using analysis of variance, Fisher exact test, and Student t-test. As pathological studies have indicated different anatomical sites of autonomic neuronal degeneration in MSA versus PD versus PAF, at least early on, and prognosis and treatment responses vary with the diagnosis, combined TST/QSART determinations may help to identify early cases of each category, allowing for better predictability of prognosis and response to current and future treatment strategies.

Focal primary hyperhidrosis (essential hyperhidrosis) is a common disorder of excessive sweating of body regions concerned with emotional sweating, like the palms and soles. Such patients have sweat drippage at normal core temperatures from these areas in response to emotional stimuli. Thermoregulatory sweating is usually normal in these patients (Shih and Lin 1979, Atkinson and Fealey 2003). The excessive sweating can be demonstrated via deterite/filter paper, ventilated capsule techniques or by indicator powder and digital photographs of the sweat distribution.

Sympathetic skin response

Skin potential recordings can be used to detect sympathetic sudomotor deficit in the peripheral neuropathies and central autonomic disorders (Shahani et al. 1984, Schondorf 1997). The recording electrodes are commonly electrode pairs 1 cm in diameter applied to the dorsal and ventral surfaces of the foot, the hand, or the thighs. The stimulus might be an inspiratory gasp, a cough, a loud noise, or an electric shock. The sources of the skin potential are the sweat gland and the epidermis (Edelberg 1967). It is important to recognize that sudomotor function and skin potential evaluate similar but not identical functions. Human studies have been limited to pharmacological dissection in very few subjects. A reasonable interpretation of studies in mammals, including humans, are that a component of the skin potential (early fast changes) is related to sweating, but that the later changes are due to skin potential changes. The latter can occur in patients who have congenital absence of sweat glands (Lloyd 1961, Shaver et al. 1962).

The major advantage of the method is its simplicity so that it can be used in any neurophysiology laboratory. The disadvantages are its enormous variability and the tendency of the responses to habituate although claims for low coefficient of variation have appeared (Levy et al. 1992). The responses vary with the recording system, composition of the electrolyte paste, stimulus frequency, age, temperature, stress, status of central structures, and the effects of hormones and drugs (Low 1984).

Following peripheral nerve section, skin potentials are no longer obtainable in the affected dermatome on direct and reflex stimulation. There was usually associated hypothermia and anhidrosis. Following sympathectomy, skin potentials are also lost, but only temporarily, returning in 4–6 months (Sourek 1965).

There is general agreement that a loss of sympathetic skin response (SSR) is abnormal. There is some controversy as to whether a reduction of skin potential or a reduction in latency are reliable abnormalities. There is some evidence that unmyelinated fibres conduct without slowing or not at all (Tzeng et al. 1993). The test has been reported to correlate well with QSART (Maselli et al. 1989), but in our experience it is often present when QSART is clearly impaired. Potentials are reported to become reduced with ageing (Drory and Korczyn 1993).

Sympathetic skin response in disorders of sweating

SSR has been utilized in the evaluation of the peripheral neuropathies, especially diabetic neuropathy (Knezevic and Bajada 1985). The SSR deficit in amplitude and volume is reported to worsen with increasing duration of diabetes and correlates with sweatspot values (Levy et al. 1992) and clinical neuropathy (Braune and Horter 1996). Both amplitude reduction and latency prolongation were seen and abnormalities may precede clinical neuropathy (Braune and Horter 1996). SSR in the foot is abnormal or absent in the majority of patients with well-established neuropathy (Niakan and Harati 1988). For instance, in a study of 72 diabetic patients with electrophysiologically confirmed sensorimotor peripheral neuropathy, SSR was absent in 83%. A statistically significant correlation was found between the Valsalva test abnormality, the degree of peripheral neuropathy, and the SSR (Niakan and Harati 1988).

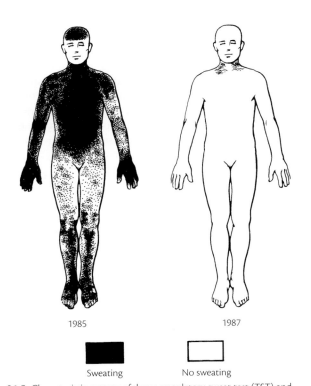

1985   1987

■ Sweating   □ No sweating

Fig. 31.5 Characteristic pattern of thermoregulatory sweat test (TST) and quantitative sudomotor axon reflex test (QSART) responses in a patient with early multiple system atrophy. Note the preservation of axon reflex sweating (QSART) in areas of near complete anhidrosis on TST. Also note the sweat level on the trunk. The combined TST and QSART result is suggestive of a spinal cord lesion affecting the intermediolateral cell columns.

Its sensitivity and specificity to detect early abnormalities or to detect improvement in clinical trials have not been established.

SSR are reported to be asymmetrical in amplitude or latency in patients with peripheral complex regional pain syndrome (CARP I), previously known as reflex sympathetic dystrophy (Drory and Korczyn 1995). These reports documented either an increase or reduction in amplitude, and suggested that the changes supported the involvement of sympathetic dysfunction in CARP I. Asymmetry should be interpreted with caution in patients who have central nervous system involvement, since lesions of the central pathways are known to cause asymmetry (Korpelainen et al. 1993).

SSR in patients with PD and MSA have been compared. The frequency of abnormalities in PD is relatively modest, occurring in 8–38% of patients (Wang et al. 1993). These changes are dramatically more marked in patients with MSA or PAF (Baser et al. 1991) where abnormalities are present in at least two-thirds of patients.

Sweat imprint

Kennedy and colleagues have systematically measured the number and size of sweat droplets activated in response to direct chemical stimulation (Kennedy et al. 1984a, Kennedy et al. 1984b). The workers used a silastic imprint material that hardens over 1or 2 minutes, the hardening time varying with the composition of the silastic. They stimulated sweating by a number of methods in the experimental animal and in humans. The most reliable method was the iontophoresis of pilocarpine (Kennedy et al. 1984a, Kennedy et al. 1984b). They recorded from the same population of sweat glands. The method appears to detect sweat gland failure reliably in diabetic neuropathy.

Sweat imprint in disorders of sweating

In a study of 81 diabetic and 30 control subjects, these workers found that many diabetic patients had a reduced number of excitable sweat glands and a low volume of sweat per square centimetre of skin. The results of the sweat tests correlated best with the clinically determined perception of pain from pin-prick. The similar degree of involvement of sudomotor axons and pain-conveying axons may be related to the known similarity in size and reinnervation patterns. There was poor correlation of the sweating deficiency with α motor conduction velocity and with denervation of foot muscles, as determined by the evoked muscle action potential. In another report, where both the silastic sweat imprint and an evaporimeter were used (Kennedy and Navarro 1989) in 357 type I diabetic patients, the number of active sweat glands was below normal in the hands of 24% of patients and in the feet of 56%, in the foot, while the sweat evaporation rate was low in 17% and 40% of patients, respectively. Computerized analysis of the molds, which allowed automatic sweat gland counts and estimations of the secretion volume of each sweat gland, detected abnormalities in 36% and 60% of patients. The silastic imprint technique was found to be a sensitive test for detection of sympathetic nerve involvement, even in asymptomatic patients with normal clinical and nerve conduction examinations. Its sensitivity and accuracy has been enhanced by the computerized analysis of the molds.

Clinical syndromes: anhidrosis

There are many neurological and some non-neurological causes of anhidrosis and hyperhidrosis. Table 31.1 summarizes the causes, with examples, sites of the lesion, and proposed mechanisms of the major causes of anhidrosis. Some characteristic patterns are seen (Fealey 1997). Distal anhidrosis is commonly seen in the peripheral neuropathies and is almost invariably due to postganglionic denervation. When more widespread anhidrosis occurs (e.g. in some cases of amyloid and in diabetic neuropathy), there could be a component of preganglionic anhidrosis.

Global anhidrosis may be central (as in MSA) or peripheral (as in acute panautonomic neuropathy and Tangier disease). Global anhidrosis with sparing of hands and feet is usually central and may occur not infrequently in MSA.

Lesions of peripheral nerves (root, plexus, trunk, or twigs) usually result in sweat impairment of dermatomal distribution. The anhidrosis resulting from 2nd thoracic sympathectomy has been well described (Fealey 1997). A complete interruption of sympathetic efferent pathways from the hypothalamus to the intermediolateral column of the spinal cord results in hemi-anhidrosis.

Table 31.1 Causes and pattern of anhidrosis with examples and proposed mechanisms

Causes	Examples	Pattern	Mechanism
Primary autonomic failure	Multiple system atrophy	Global with acral sparing; segmental affecting lower body	Preganglionic denervation
	Pure autonomic failure	Segmental often with differing levels on left and right	Postganglionic denervation
Central nervous system disease	Brain tumour	Segmental, global or regional	Preganglionic denervation
	Strokes		
	Traumatic spinal cord injury		
Peripheral nervous system disease	Distal small fibre neuropathy	Distal	Postganglionic denervation
	Diabetic neuropathy	Variable	Postganglionic denervation
	Panautonomic neuropathy	Global or regional often with small "islands" of sweating	Postganglionic denervation
	Chronic idiopathic anhidrosis		Sweat gland for some cases of chronic idiopathic anhidrosis
Iatrogenic	Anticholinergic medications	Global	Sweat gland postganglionic
	Sympathectomy	Regional typically	
Skin lesions	Leprosy	Multifocal	Nerve terminals
	Radiation injury	Focal	Sweat gland injury

However, most lesions of brainstem or spinal cord (such as syringomyelia or neoplasms) result in incomplete hemi-anhidrosis since sympathetic efferent bundles are not well compacted.

Skin lesions of various types may damage sweat glands or plug sweat ducts resulting in anhidrosis sometimes with associated compensatory hyperhidrosis of remaining sweat glands.

Clinical syndromes: hyperhidrosis

Hyperhidrosis may result from lesions of the brain, spinal cord, or peripheral nerves. It can also occur in non-neurological disorders (Table 31.2). Examples of the latter include phaeochromocytoma, thyrotoxicosis, or with lymphomas and certain chronic infectious illnesses, where the neural pathways are intact but the central drive is increased or there is overactivity of certain humoral factors, such as thyroxine, catecholamines, cytokines, or vasoactive intestinal polypeptide.

Damaged peripheral nerves, especially small-diameter fibres, are prone to fire spontaneously. Factors enhancing spontaneous activity include increased sympathetic drive, α-adrenergic activation, mechanostimulation, and nerve microenvironmental perturbations, such as hyperkalaemia. The peripheral neuropathies, especially the toxic and certain metabolic ones (e.g. thallium, arsenic, acrylamide poisoning, and painful diabetic neuropathy), usually have a phase of distal hyperhidrosis, coldness, and pain. Nerve root or plexus irritation may result in a phase of hyperhidrosis followed by an anhidrotic lesion with surrounding hyperhidrosis. A less-pronounced perilesional hyperhidrosis may occur with spinal cord lesion at the edge of the sensory loss, suggesting that central mechanisms may also be involved.

Gustatory sweating following a partial nerve lesion may occur in diabetic neuropathy. The sweating is thought to result from fibre damage with misdirected regeneration, so that a taste stimulus results in excessive sweating. A cardinal feature of reflex sympathetic dystrophy is increased sympathetic traffic with hyperhidrosis.

When a large portion of eccrine sweat glands are denervated, peripherally or centrally, the remaining glands undergo increased sweat secretion and compensatory hyperhidrosis results. This phenomenon may occur with central structural lesions as in cerebral infarction, brain tumours, or following head trauma. Peripheral denervation following extensive sympathectomy also may result in compensatory hyperhidrosis. Extensive sweat gland disease also may impose an increased secretory burden on remaining sweat glands.

Essential or primary hyperhidrosis is a distressing condition, characterized by excessive sweating of eccrine sweat glands. The sites affected are mainly the hands, axillae, and feet. Onset is early, especially pronounced by the teens, and becomes less by the fourth or fifth decade. The volume of sweat output can be extremely high and can exceed 30 ml/hour. Clinically, the sites are confined to those mentioned above, but quantitatively there may be generalized hyperhidrosis. Some cases are clinically generalized or confined to craniofacial sweating. The pathophysiology appears to be an exaggerated response to emotional sweating. There is increased sympathetic drive and possibly hypertrophied sweat glands. Patients may be introverted and anxious but often levels of manifest anxiety are not elevated. The constant dripping causes social distress. Maceration of skin is not uncommon. A positive family history is present in 25–50% of the patients. It likely has an autosomal dominant inheritance with incomplete penetrance (Khurana 1997, Eisenach et al. 2005).

Treatment is unsatisfactory, consisting of local treatments, medications, and surgical procedures; the latter commonly done for severe cases of palmar hyperhidrosis. Local treatment with iontophoresis of tap water can half the sweat secretion. However, it does so by the plugging up of sweat pores, although the accumulation of hydrogen ions in the duct or pore may also inhibit secretion. The local application of 20% aluminum chloride hexahydrate in 95% ethyl alcohol yields comparable results. Botulinum toxin will block the autonomic transmission in sympathetic cholinergic fibres to sweat glands. Axillary hyperhidrosis may be the most amenable to botulinum toxin treatment although it is also in wide use for palmar-plantar hyperhidrosis. Repeat injections of toxin are needed on the average of every 4–7 months. Other local topical therapy has included aluminum chloride, formalin, glutaraldehyde,

Table 31.2 Causes of hyperhidrosis

Cause	Examples	Pattern	Mechanism
Primary	Primary hyperhidrosis	Acral and axillary	Probably central (premotor cortex) with overactivity of sympathetic fibres passing through the T2–3 ganglia
Systemic or neoplastic	Thyroxicosis	Generalized	Inappropriate hormone or catecholamines induced thermogenesis
	Phaeochromocytoma	Generalized	Altered set-point; altered prostaglandin E2; thermogenic cytokines (interleukins, tumour necrosis factor); activation of 'pyrogenic' vagal afferent pathways by complement factors
	Malignancy		
Central nervous system disease	Shapiro's syndrome	Generalized	Triggered by much lower hypothalamic 'set-point' temperature
	Idiopathic paroxysmal hyperhidrosis	Commonly head and upper torso	Multifactorial central causes
Peripheral nervous system disease	Painful peripheral neuropathies	? acral hyperhidrosis	Unknown
	Perilesional hyperhidrosis	Focal or radicular loss with surrounding radicular or segmental hyperhidrosis	Unknown;? somatosympathetic or sympatho-sympathetic reflex
	Compensatory hyperhidrosis		Aberrant regeneration of cholinergic salivatory nerves
	Gustatory sweating	Hyperhidrotic islands of sweat on face with eating	
Iatrogenic	Medications and drugs	Upper body or generalized	Unknown

and topical propantheline bromide. Talc, starch, and other powders have been suggested to absorb excessive sweat. Scopolamine patches have also been used successfully in some patients.

Drug treatment of hyperhidrosis is unsatisfactory but can provide partial improvement for a few hours. Drugs that have been used include anticholinergics such as glycopyrrolate and propantheline and α-adrenergic blocking agents such as phenoxybenzamine. Other drugs have included methantheline bromide, alone or in combination with ergoloid mesylates, mecamylamine, atropine, and propoxyphenel. Other agents that have been used include dibenamine, piperoxan, and phentolamine and compounds of belladonna, ergotamine, and phenobarbital.

A number of approaches to surgical sympathectomy are in use. All modern approaches lesion the sympathetic outflow below T1. Surgical approaches include the bilateral suction-assisted lipolysis technique, bilateral upper dorsal sympathectomy via the supraclavicular approach, thoracoscopic sympathicolysis, and percutaneous radiofrequency upper thoracic sympathectomy. Sympathetic ganglion blockade has been suggested as an alternative. Compensatory and gustatory sweating were the most frequently stated reasons for dissatisfaction.

References

Abdel-Rahman, T. A., Collins, K. J., Cowen, T., Rustin, M. (1992). Immunohistochemical, morphological and functional changes in the peripheral sudomotor neuro-effector system in elderly people. *J Auton. Nerve. Syst.*, 37, 187–97.

Atkinson, J. L., Fealey, R. D. (2003). Sympathotomy instead of sympathectomy for palmar hyperhidrosis: minimizing postoperative compensatory hyperhidrosis. *Mayo Clin. Proc.*, 78, 167–72.

Baser, S. M., Meer, J., Polinsky, R. J., Hallett, M. (1991). Sudomotor function in autonomic failure. *Neurology*, 41, 1564–66.

Braune, H. J., Horter, C. (1996). Sympathetic skin response in diabetic neuropathy: a prospective clinical and neurophysiological trial on 100 patients. *J Neurol. Sci.*, 138, 120–24.

Chemali, K. R., Gorodeski, R., Chelimsky, T. C. (2001). Alpha-adrenergic supersensitivity of the sudomotor nerve in complex regional pain syndrome. *Ann. Neurol.*, 49, 453–59.

Cohen, J., Low, P., Fealey, R., Sheps, S., Jiang, N. S. (1987). Somatic and autonomic function in progressive autonomic failure and multiple system atrophy. *Ann. Neurol.*, 22, 692–99.

Drory, V. E., Korczyn, A. D. (1993). Sympathetic skin response: age effect. *Neurology*, 43, 1818–20.

Drory, V. E., Korczyn, A. D. (1995). The sympathetic skin response in reflex sympathetic dystrophy. *J. Neurol. Sci.*, 128, 92–95.

Edelberg, R. (1967). Electrical properties of the skin. In CC Brown, ed. *Methods in Psychophysiology*, pp. 1–52. Williams and Wilkins, Baltimore.

Eisenach, J. H., Atkinson, J. L., Fealey, R. D. (2005). Hyperhidrosis: evolving therapies for a well-established phenomenon. *Mayo Clin Proc*, 80, 657–66.

Fealey, R. D. (1996). Thermoregulatory sweat test. In JR Daube, ed. *Clinical Neurophysiology*, pp. 396–402. F. A. Davis Co., Philadelphia.

Fealey, R. D. (1997). Thermoregulatory sweat test. In PA Low, ed. *Clinical Autonomic Disorders: Evaluation and Management*, pp. 245–57. Lippincott-Raven, Philadelphia.

Fealey, R. D. (2001a). Combined use of the Thermoregulatory Sweat Test and the Quantitative Sudomotor Axon Reflex Test clearly distinguishes autonomic failure due to multiple system atrophy from the dysautonomia of Parkinson's disease. *Neurology*, 56, A422.

Fealey, R. D. (2001b). Use of the Thermoregulatory Sweat Test in the evaluation of patients with autoimmune autonomic neuropathy and early multiple system atrophy syndromes. *Japanese Journal of Perspiration Research*, 8, 37–40.

Fealey, R. D., Low, P. A., Thomas, J. E. (1989). Thermoregulatory sweating abnormalities in diabetes mellitus. *Mayo Clin Proc*, 64, 617–28.

Guttmann, L. (1947). The management of the quinizarin sweat test (QST). *Postgrad. Med. J*, 23, 353–66.

Kennedy, W. R., Navarro, X. (1989). Sympathetic sudomotor function in diabetic neuropathy. *Arch. Neurol.*, 46, 1182–86.

Kennedy, W. R., Sakuta, M., Sutherland, D., Goetz, F. C. (1984a). Quantitation of the sweating deficit in diabetes mellitus. *Ann/Neurol.*, 15, 482–88.

Kennedy, W. R., Sakuta, M., Sutherland, D., Goetz, F. C. (1984b). The sweating deficiency in diabetes mellitus: methods of quantitation and clinical correlation. *Neurology*, 34, 758–63.

Kerassidis, S. (1994). Is palmar and plantar sweating thermoregulatory? *Acta Physiologica Scandinavica*, 152, 259–63.

Khurana, R. (1997). Acral sympathetic dysfunction and hyperhidrosis. In PA Low, ed. *Clinical Autonomic Disorders: Evaluation and Management*, pp. 809–18. Lippincott-Raven, Philadelphia.

Kihara, M., Opfer-Gehrking, T. L., Low, P. A. (1993). Comparison of directly stimulated with axon reflex-mediated sudomotor responses in human subjects and in patients with diabetes. *Muscle and Nerve*, 16, 655–60.

Knezevic, W., Bajada, S. (1985). Peripheral autonomic surface potential. A quantitative technique for recording sympathetic conduction in man. *J Neurol. Sci.*, 67, 239–51.

Korpelainen, J. T., Tolonen, U., Sotaniemi, K. A., Myllyla, V. V. (1993). Suppressed sympathetic skin response in brain infarction. *Stroke*, 24, 1389–92.

Kuno, Y. (1956) *Human Perspiration*, Charles C. Thomas, Springfield, IL.

Levy, D. M., Reid, G., Rowley, D. A., Abraham, R. R. (1992). Quantitative measures of sympathetic skin response in diabetes: relation to sudomotor and neurological function. *JNNP*, 55, 902–08.

Lloyd, D. (1961). Action potential and secretory potential of sweat glands. *Proc. Natl. Acad. Sci. U S A*, 47, 351–62.

Low, P. A. (1984). Quantitation of autonomic function. In PJ Dyck, PK Thomas, EH Lambert and R Bunge, eds. *Peripheral Neuropathy*, pp. 1139–65. W. B. Saunders, Philadelphia.

Low, P. A. (1993). Composite autonomic scoring scale for laboratory quantification of generalized autonomic failure. *Mayo Clin Proc*, 68, 748–52.

Low, P. A. (1996). Diabetic autonomic neuropathy. *Semin. Neurol.* 16, 143–51.

Low, P. A. (1997a). The effect of aging on the autonomic nervous system. In P.A. Low, ed. *Clinical Autonomic Disorders: Evaluation and Management*, pp. 161–75. Lippincott-Raven, Philadelphia.

Low, P. A. (1997b). Laboratory evaluation of autonomic function. In P.A. Low, ed. *Clinical Autonomic Disorders: Evaluation and Management*, pp. 179–208. Lippincott-Raven, Philadelphia.

Low, P. A., Caskey, P. E., Tuck, R. R., Fealey, R. D., Dyck, P. J. (1983). Quantitative sudomotor axon reflex test in normal and neuropathic subjects. *Ann. Neurol.*, 14, 573–80.

Low, P. A., Fealey, R. D., Sheps, S. G., Su, W. P., Trautmann, J. C., Kuntz, N. L. (1985). Chronic idiopathic anhidrosis. *Ann. Neurol.*, 18, 344–48.

Low, P. A., McLeod J. G. (1997). Autonomic neuropathies. In PA Low, ed. *Clinical Autonomic Disorders: Evaluation and Management*, pp. 463–86. Lippincott-Raven, Philadelphia.

Low, P. A., Okazaki, H., Dyck, P. J. (1977). Splanchnic preganglionic neurons in man. I. Morphometry of preganglionic cytons. *Acta Neuropathologica*, 40, 55–61.

Low, P. A., Opfer-Gehrking, T. L., Kihara, M. (1992). In vivo studies on receptor pharmacology of the human eccrine sweat gland. *Clin. Autom. Res.*, 2, 29–34.

Low, P. A., Zimmerman, B. R., Dyck, P. J. (1986). Comparison of distal sympathetic with vagal function in diabetic neuropathy. *Muscle and Nerve*, 9, 592–96.

Maselli, R. A., Jaspan, J. B., Soliven, B. C., Green, A. J., Spire, J. P., Arnason, B. G. W. (1989). Comparison of sympathetic skin response with quantitative sudomotor axon reflex test in diabetic neuropathy. *Muscle and Nerve, 12*, 420–23.

Namer, B., Bickel, A., Kramer, H., Birklein, F., Schmelz, M. (2004). Chemically and electrically induced sweating and flare reaction. *Autonomic Neuroscience-Basic & Clinical, 114*, 72–82.

Niakan, E., Harati, Y. (1988). Sympathetic skin response in diabetic peripheral neuropathy. *Muscle and Nerve, 11*, 261–64.

Ogawa, T. (1975). Thermal influence on palmar sweating and mental influence on generalized sweating in man. *Jpn. J Physiol., 25*, 525–36.

Ogawa, T., Low, P. A. (1993). Autonomic regulation of temperature and sweating. In P.A. Low, ed. *Clinical Autonomic Disorders: Evaluation and Management*, pp. 79–91. Little, Brown and Company, Boston.

Riley, D. E., Chelimsky, T. C. (2003). Autonomic nervous system testing may not distinguish multiple system atrophy from Parkinson's disease. *JNNP, 74*, 56–60.

Sandroni, P., Ahlskog, J. E., Fealey, R. D., Low, P. A. (1991). Autonomic involvement in extrapyramidal and cerebellar disorders. *Clin. Auton. Res., 1*, 147–55.

Sato, K., Ohtsuyama, M., Sato, F. (1993). Normal and abnormal eccrine sweat gland function. In P.A. Low, ed. *Clinical Autonomic Disorders: Evaluation and Management*, pp. 93–104. Little, Brown and Company, Boston.

Sato, K., Sato, F. (1983). Individual variations in structure and function of human eccrine sweat gland. *Am. J Physiol., 245*, R203–R08.

Schondorf, R. (1997). Skin potentials: normal and abnormal. In P.A. Low, ed. *Clinical Autonomic Disorders: Evaluation and Management*, pp. 221–32. Lippincott-Raven, New York.

Shahani, B. T., Halperin, J. J., Boulu, P., Cohen, J. (1984). Sympathetic skin response—a method of assessing unmyelinated axon dysfunction in peripheral neuropathies. *JNNP, 47*, 536–42.

Shaver, B. A., Brusilow, S. W., Cooke, R. E. (1962). Origin of the galvanic skin response. *Proc. Soc. Exp. Biol. Med., 110*, 559–64.

Shih, C. J., Lin, M. T. (1979). Thermoregulatory sweating in palmar hyperhidrosis before and after upper thoracic sympathectomy. *J Neurosurg., 50*, 88–94.

Sourek, K. (1965) *The Nervous Control of Skin Potentials in Man*, Rozpravy Ceskoslovenske Akademie Ved Roenik 75-Sesit 1, Prague.

Stewart, J. D., Low, P. A., Fealey, R. D. (1992). Distal small fibre neuropathy: results of tests of sweating and autonomic cardiovascular reflexes. *Muscle and Nerve, 15*, 661–65.

Suarez, G. A., Fealey, R. D., Camilleri, M., Low, P. A. (1994). Idiopathic autonomic neuropathy: Clinical, neurophysiologic, and follow-up studies on 27 patients. *Neurology, 44*, 1675–82.

Thaisetthawatkul, P., Boeve, B. F., Benarroch, E. E., *et al.* (2004). Autonomic dysfunction in dementia with Lewy bodies. *Neurology, 62*, 1804–09.

Torres, N. E., Zollman, P. J., Low, P. A. (1991). Characterization of muscarinic receptor subtype of rat eccrine sweat gland by autoradiography. *Brain Research, 550*, 129–32.

Tzeng, S. S., Wu, Z. A., Chu, F. L. (1993). The latencies of sympathetic skin responses. *European Neurology, 33*, 65–68.

Wang, S. J., Fuh, J. L., Shan, D. E., *et al.* (1993). Sympathetic skin response and r-r interval variation in parkinson's disease. *Movement Disorders, 8*, 151–57.

CHAPTER 32

Treatment of hyperhidrosis

Markus Naumann and Christopher J. Mathias

Introduction

Hyperhidrosis may be defined as excessive sweating beyond what is required to return elevated body temperature to normal. It may be primary (idiopathic or essential), or secondary to an underlying medical conditions (endocrine, metabolic), or the result of drugs. Hyperhidrosis can be focal (localized) or generalized, with the former commonly affecting the axillae, palms, soles of the feet, and the face (facial hyperhidrosis). The main causes for focal and generalized hyperhidrosis are shown in Table 32.1. In some there is a genetic predisposition to primary hyperhidrosis and it often manifests itself in childhood or puberty (Kaufmann et al. 2003, Li et al. 2007, Yamashita et al. 2009). It is thought to link to chromosome 14q11.2–q13 (Higashimoto et al. 2006). The prevalence of focal hyperhidrosis has been estimated to be 7.2 per 10,000 in a study from Taiwan (Chu et al. 2010) and is not known or underestimated in other populations. A pilot study of young Israelis reported an incidence of 1% (Adar et al. 1977). A recent representative survey of the US population found a prevalence of 2.8% (Strutton et al. 2003).

Hyperhidrosis is frequently chronic and can lead to significant disruption in both social and professional life, leading to a marked negative impact on the patient's quality of life (QOL). Patients find the symptoms embarrassing and often complain that the anticipation of sweating leads to avoidance of certain activities (Hamm et al. 2006). In particular, axillary sweating causes social embarrassment and can cause staining and rotting of clothes. In addition, profuse sweating can also result in malodour, and in severe cases can lead to painful skin maceration, which can, in turn, lead to secondary infection, such as tinea pedis, viral verrucae, and dermatitis.

The effects of hyperhidrosis have been assessed on various QOL scales, such as the Dermatology Life Quality Index (DLQI) (a simple, practical method of scoring the impact of skin disease using 10 questions, each with four possible answers) and the Hyperhidrosis Impact Questionnaire© (HHIQ). The DLQI is a validated measure that allows comparison of hyperhidrosis to other dermatological conditions, whereas the HHIQ focuses specifically on how hyperhidrosis affects patients. Studies using both scales have shown that hyperhidrosis has a significant impact on a patient's life. However, there is still a low awareness of it as a true medical condition and a lack of information on the treatment options available.

Diagnosis of focal hyperhidrosis

The diagnosis of primary focal hyperhidrosis should be made only after excluding secondary causes of excessive sweating (Walling 2011) (Table 32.1). In the presence of unilateral or asymmetric presentation, particular care must be taken to rule out a neurological lesion or malignancy. The line between 'normal' sweating and hyperhidrosis is poorly defined and objective evaluations of the disease are needed before treatment can be justified and evaluated. Subjective measurements can be used, as well as objective assessments such as gravimetric assessment of sweat production and Minor's iodine starch test especially in focal hyperhidrosis. In generalized hyperhidrosis the detection of sweat production during the thermoregulatory sweat test, when body temperature is ideally raised by a degree centigrade (Chapter 21) can be enhanced by using indicator dyes such as ponso red or alizarin red when sprinkled on the skin they turn from pale pink to bright red on exposure to moisture (Fig. 32.1). However, one of the main criteria for determining whether treatment is justified is the effect of the condition on the patient's QOL (Finlay 1997). In a study of axillary hyperhidrosis, there was a nearly five-fold increase in sweat production in patients when compared with controls (Hund et al. 2001). Minor's iodine starch test may be useful in mapping areas of

Table 32.1 Causes of hyperhidrosis

Generalized	
Environment	Heat, humidity, exercise
Febrile disease, systemic diseases	Acute and chronic infections, malignancy, cardiovascular disorders, shock and syncope, respiratory failure, intense pain, alcohol, drug withdrawal
Metabolic	Thyrotoxicosis, diabetes mellitus, hypoglycaemia, gout, phaeochromocytoma, hyperpituitarism, acromegaly, carcinoid tumor, menopause
Neurological	Riley–Day syndrome, hypothalamic lesions, Parkinson´s disease
Drugs	Propranolol, physostigmine, pilocarpine, tricyclic antidepressants, SSRIs such as Venlafaxine
Focal	
Extrinsic	Heat, olfactory
Gustatory	Citric acid, coffee, chocolate, peanut butter, spicy food
Neurological/ behavioural	Central or peripheral nervous system lesions that cause localized anhidrosis can cause compensatory sweating in other areas (stroke, spinal cord lesions, neuropathy, Ross syndrome and Holmes–Adie syndrome), Frey syndrome (gustatory hyperhidrosis); eccrine nevus
	Anxiety disorders

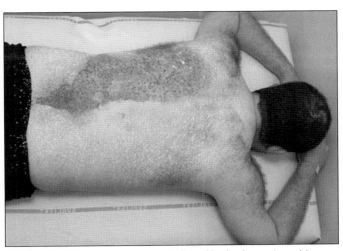

Fig. 32.1 Areas of excessive sweating as indicated by the dye turning red, in a patient with the Holmes–Adie syndrome, where there are areas of anhidrosis even during raising temperature by 1°C resulting in regional compensatory hyperhidrosis that involve large areas of the left back.

excessive sweating prior to injection with botulinum toxin or local surgery (Naumann and Lowe 2001, Rompel and Scholz 2001).

The following criteria have been recommended for establishing the diagnosis of primary focal hyperhidrosis (Hornberger et al. 2004):

♦ Focal, visible, excessive sweating of at least 6 months' duration without apparent cause with at least two of the following characteristics:

   • bilateral and relatively symmetric

   • impairs daily activities

   • frequency of at least one episode per week

   • age of onset less than 25 years

   • positive family history

   • cessation of focal sweating during sleep.

Treatment

Generalized hyperhidrosis

Systemic medication is the domain of treating generalized hyperhidrosis whereas botulinum toxin or topical agents are primarily indicated in cases of focal hyperhidrosis. Low dose pharmacotherapy includes the anticholinergic probanthine (15 or 30 mg tds) and the sympatholytic clonidine (25 or 50 µg tds) (Conrad et al. 1983, Namer et al. 1986, Canaday and Stanford 1995, Torch 2000). Higher doses result in greater side-effects, which include hypostomia, common to both drugs. A variety of anticholinergic drugs, ranging from oxybutinin to glycopyrolate, have been used with varying side-effects, including a dry mouth, focusing difficulty, and constipation. Beta-blockers and the selective serotonin reuptake inhibitors (SSRIs) may have a role in anxiety-related hyperhidrosis (Böni 2002); there is a role for cognitive behavioural therapy in some patients (Davidson et al. 2002, Shenefelt 2003, Davidson 2006).

Focal hyperhidrosis

Axillary hyperhidrosis

Locally applied medication is the least invasive treatment, and should be used as first-line therapy. Topical use of aluminium salts

is the preferred method and is often effective particularly in moderate hyperhidrosis, when used in the evening before going to bed. They are thought to mechanically obstruct the eccrine sweat gland, although atrophy of the secretory cells is also thought to contribute to the effect following long-term use (Quinton 1983). Two small controlled studies and two larger observational studies have demonstrated the efficacy of topical aluminium chloride hexahydrate in the treatment of axillary hyperhidrosis (Rayner et al. 1980, Glent-Madsen et al. 1988, Scholes et al. 1978). Treatment response was assessed using patient self-reported severity of sweating and/or gravimetry. It was generally well tolerated. The most frequent side-effect was local skin irritation.

Oral anticholinergic drugs can be used to treat hyperhidrosis, although response to treatment is variable and systemic side-effects are common, such as dry mouth and blurred vision. Other drugs such as glycopyrrolate (glycopyrronium bromide), phenoxybenzamine, an α-adrenergic blocking agent, and indomethacin may be of some benefit in selected cases but can generally not be recommended.

Botulinum toxin type A has substantial benefit in the treatment of axillary hyperhidrosis (Fig. 32.2), and is the treatment of choice if topical treatment is ineffective. Botulinum toxin is produced by the anaerobic bacillus *Clostridium botulinum* and is the cause of the clinical signs and symptoms of botulism. Its mechanism of action is to inhibit the release of acetylcholine at the presynaptic membrane of cholinergic neurons (Moore and Naumann 2003). This is achieved by the injection of the drug in areas of excessive sweating,

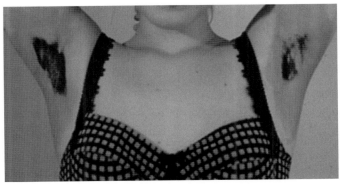

(a)

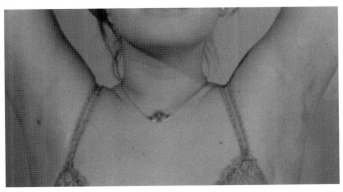

(b)

Fig. 32.2 Axillary hyperhidrosis before **(a)** and after **(b)** focal intradermal application of botulinum toxin (Minor´s iodine starch test indicates areas of sweating [dark]). With permission from Naumann et al, *Arch Dermatol* 1998;**134**:301–301. Copyright © 1998 American Medical Association. All rights reserved.

causing a localised, long-lasting but reversible decrease in cholinergic transmission.

Many prospective observational, and a few placebo-controlled studies have enrolled more than 700 patients to study the safety and efficacy of botulinum toxin (Naumann and Lowe 2001, Heckmann et al. 2001, Odderson 2002, Naver et al. 2000, Schnider et al. 1999, Tan and Solish 2002, Whatling and Collin 2001). In the largest of the studies, 320 patients were randomized to receive either botulinum toxin A or placebo in both axillae (Naumann and Lowe 2001). Patients were followed for 16 weeks and treatment responders were defined as patients achieving greater than 50% reduction in sweat production by gravimetry. A total of 82% of patients were treatment responders, with an average reduction in sweat production of 69%. Side-effects were minimal. An open label continuation study allowed 207 patients to receive up to three further botulinum A injections over the following 12 months. This study showed a sustained response of 7 months on average, although a substantial proportion of patients had a benefit of up to 16 months after botulinum toxin injection (Naumann et al. 2003). The efficacy of botulinum toxin type A in axillary hyperhidrosis has been shown in a multicentre trial in 145 patients previously unresponsive to topical therapy where a significant (p <0.001) decrease in sweat production compared with placebo occurred 2 weeks post-injection and was maintained for 24 weeks after injection (Heckmann et al. 2001). Treatment was well tolerated and 98% of patients indicated that they would recommend botulinum toxin therapy to others.

Palmar hyperhidrosis

The oral agents discussed under axillary hyperhidrosis are also applicable for patients presenting with palmar hyperhidrosis.

Tap-water iontophoresis using has been shown to be an effective treatment for palmar hyperhidrosis, in small controlled studies (Reinauer et al. 1993). The reduction in sweating lasted 3–4 days. The procedure is well tolerated and is usually repeated five to six times a week until sweating has been reduced to an acceptable level, whereupon maintenance treatment has to be continued once or twice weekly. Iontophoresis is thought to work by blockage of the sweat gland at the stratum corneum level, although structural changes have not been shown. It has also been suggested that the mechanism of action is due to interruption of the stimulus-secretion-coupling that then leads to a functional disturbance of sweat secretion. However, iontophoresis can cause discomfort (burning and tingling) and skin irritation, including erythema and vesicle formation, and incorrect use can cause burns at the sites of minor skin injury as well as cutaneous necrosis.

Botulinum toxin type A is also beneficial for palmar hyperhidrosis (Fig. 32.3). A few controlled, and several observational studies were performed to assess its efficacy, tolerability, and safety (Naver et al. 2000, Naumann et al. 1998, Lowe et al. 2002, Saadia et al. 2001, Schnider et al. 1997, Ito et al. 2011). The response rates exceeded 90% and the duration of euhidrosis generally exceeded the length of the trial. The only notable side-effect was mild and transient weakness of the intrinsic hand muscles. This complication was well tolerated, but patients must be clearly informed that fine motor control of the hand may be compromised. A major problem during initiation of treatment is intense pain associated with injections into the densely innervated skin of the palm. Local or regional pain management is recommended. The topical anaesthetic agent

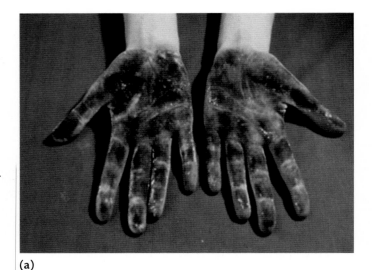

(a)

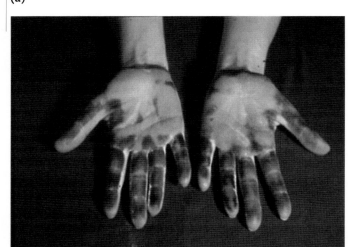

(b)

Fig. 32.3 Palmar hyperhidrosis before **(a)** and after **(b)** focal intradermal application of botulinum toxin (Minor´s iodine starch test indicates areas of sweating [dark]). With permission from Naumann et al, *Arch Dermatol* 1998;**134**:301–301. Copyright © 1998 American Medical Association. All rights reserved.

EMLA was less effective than other methods including application of ice immediately before injection, nerve blocks, and intravenous regional anaesthesia (Bier's block).

Endoscopic thoracic sympathectomy has been used to treat palmar hyperhidrosis (Herbst et al. 1994, Meagher et al. 2001, Chuang et al. 2002) with over 20 case series involving more than 14,000 patients published. These series lack uniformity in patient inclusion criteria, particularly in grading severity of disease, surgical technique and the level of the procedure (T2 only, T2–T3, T2–T4, or lower T1–T4). The reported primary success rate for endoscopic thoracic sympathectomy exceeds 95%, but follow up was usually short term. Relapse rates vary between 0% and 16%. Acute complications occurring in less than 2% of cases include pneumothorax, haemothorax, bleeding from intercostals vessels, atelectasis, pneumonia, wound infection, and persisting intercostal pain. The reported rates of long-term complications including Horner's syndrome, compensatory hyperhidrosis (24–100%) (Fig. 32.4a, b, c), and gustatory hyperhidrosis vary widely, perhaps

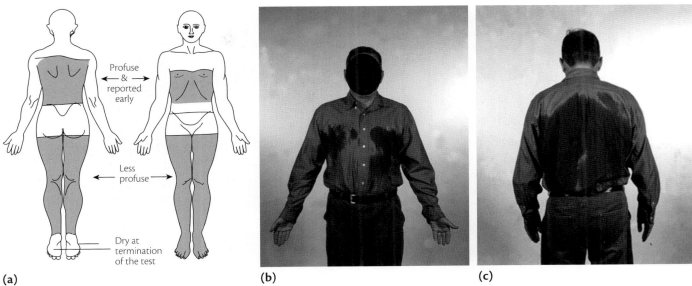

Fig. 32.4 Manikin with areas of anhidrosis (upper limbs and palms) and severe compensatory hyperhidrosis **(a)** in innervated areas as demonstrated in a patient post-endoscopic thoracic sympathectomy **(b, c)**.

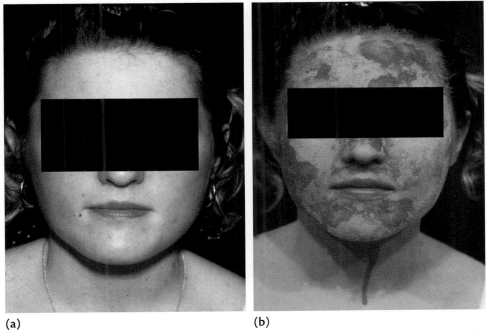

Fig. 32.5 Patient recovering from an acute autonomic neuropathy with aberrant re-innervation resulting in gustatory hyperhidrosis causing dripping over the chin and neck. The left panel is with the powder dye in the pre moisture exposed phase, a pale pink changing to a vivid red on exposure to moisture.

because of a lack of standardized methods of follow-up. Compensatory hyperhidrosis can be extremely disabling and is refractory to most approaches used in the treatment of generalized hyperhidrosis.

Other types of focal hyperhidrosis

Only a few studies have addressed the treatment of *plantar hyperhidrosis,* perhaps because it is less common or perceived as less problematic than axillary or palmar hyperhidrosis. One large observational study supported topical aluminium chloride hexahydrate (Benohanian et al. 1998). Of 139 patients enrolled, 84% had a good or excellent response to 30–40% aluminium chloride in a salicylic acid gel. In five observational studies of tap water iontophoresis, the response rate was 90–100%. There are no published controlled studies of botulinum toxin in plantar hyperhidrosis, but it is recognized that the response rate is slightly lower than in palmar hyperhidrosis, presumably because a thicker stratum corneum makes intradermal injection more difficult.

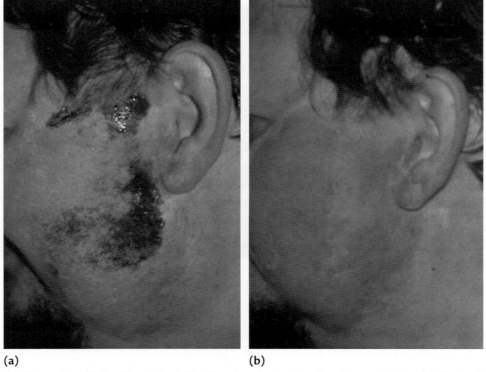

(a)   **(b)**

Fig. 32.6 Gustatory sweating (Frey syndrome) before **(a)** and after **(b)** focal intradermal application of botulinum toxin (Minor´s iodine starch test indicates areas of sweating [dark]). *Ann Neurol* 1997;**42**:973–975, K. V. Toyka, K. Reiners, M. Naumann, M. Zellner, with permission from Wiley.

Approximately 50% of patients with palmar and plantar hyperhidrosis who undergo endoscopic thoracic sympathectomy for excessive palmar sweating also have a reduction in plantar hyperhidrosis.

Frontal hyperhidrosis has been successfully treated with botulinum toxin type A, with a reduction in sweating of approximately 75% seen for a period of at least 5 months (Kinkelin et al. 2000) (Fig. 32.5a, b). Data on the efficacy and safety of endoscopic thoracic sympathectomy for craniofacial hyperhidrosis is limited. This option should be restricted to selected patients who are unable to tolerate other therapies and for whom the burden of hyperhidrosis is severe.

Botulinum toxin type A is also widely used with excellent efficacy for gustatory sweating (Frey's syndrome) (Fig. 32.6) and some recommend this option as first-line treatment (Laskawi and Rohrbach 2002, Naumann et al. 1997). In six observational series of botulinum toxin A for gustatory hyperhidrosis, 163 of 165 patients responded with a duration of 5–17 months. Its use has also been suggested in the treatment of Ross Syndrome (progressive segmental anhidrosis) to treat areas of compensatory hyperhidrosis (Laskawi and Rohrbach 2002).

References

Adar, R., Kurchin, A., Zweig, A., and Mozes, M. (1977). Palmar hyperhidrosis and its surgical treatment: a report of 100 cases. *Ann Surg.* **186**, 34–41.

Benohanian, A., Dansereau, A., Bolduc, C., and Bloom, E. (1998). Localized hyperhidrosis treated with aluminum chloride in a salicylic acid gel base. *Int J Dermatol.* **37**, 701–708.

Böni, R. (2002). Generalized hyperhidrosis and its systemic treatment. In: Kreyden OP, Böni R, Burg G, eds. *Hyperhidrosis and botulinum toxin in dermatology.* **20**, 44–7. Basel, Karger.

Campanati, A., Penna, L., Menotta, L. *et al.* (2003). Quality of life assessment in patients suffering from hyperhidrosis and its modification after treatment with botulinum toxin: Results of an open study. *Clin Ther.* **25**, 298–308.

Canaday, B. R., Stanford, R. H. (1995). Propantheline bromide in the management of hyperhidrosis associated with spinal cord injury. *Ann Pharmacother.* **29**, 489–92.

Chu, D., Chen, R. C., Lee, C. H., Yang, N. P., and Chou, P. (2010). Incidence and frequency of endoscopic sympathectomy for the treatment of hyperhidrosis palmaris in Taiwan. *Kaohsiung J Med Sci.* **26**, 123–9.

Chuang K-S., Liu J-C.. (2002). Long-term assessment of percutaneous stereotactic thermocoagulation of upper thracic ganglionectomy and sympathectomy for palmar and craniofacial hyperhidrosis in 1742 cases. *Neurosurgery* **51**, 963–70.

Conrad, F., Baumgartner, H., Wiedermann, C., and Klein, G. (1983). Clonidine and hyperhidrosis. *Ann Intern Med.* **99**, 570.

Davidson, J. R. (2006). Pharmacotherapy of social anxiety disorder: what does the evidence tell us? *J Clin Psychiatry* **67**, 20–6.

Davidson, J. R., Foa, E. B., Connor, K. M., and Churchill, L. E. (2002). Hyperhidrosis in social anxiety disorder. *Prog Neuropsychopharmacol Biol Psychiatry.* **26**, 1327–31.

Finlay, A.Y. (1997). Quality of life measurement in dermatology: a practical guide. *Br J Dermatol.* **136**, 305–14.

Glent-Madsen, L., Dahl, J. C. (1988). Axillary hyperhidrosis. Local treatment with aluminium-chloride hexahydrate 25% in absolute ethanol with and without supplementary treatment with triethanolamine. *Acta Derm Venereol.* **68**, 87–89.

Hamm, H., Naumann, M. K., Kowalski, J. W., Kütt, S., Kozma, C., and Teale, C. (2006). Primary focal hyperhidrosis: disease characteristics and functional impairment. *Dermatology* **212**, 343–53.

Heckmann, M., Ceballos-Baumann, A. O., and Plewig, G. (2001). Botulinum toxin A for axillary hyperhidrosis (excessive sweating). *N Engl J Med.* **344**, 488–93.

Herbst, F., Plas, E. G., Fugger, R., Fritsch, A. (1994). Endoscopic thoracic sympathectomy for primary hyperhidrosis of the upper limbs. A critical analysis and long-term results of 480 operations. *Ann Surg.* **220**, 86–90.

Higashimoto, I., Yoshiura, K., Hirakawa, N., *et al.* (2006). Primary palmar hyperhidrosis locus maps to 14q11.2-q13. *Am J Med Genet A.* **15**, 567–72.

Hornberger, J., Grimes, K., Naumann, M. *et al.* (2004). Recognition, diagnosis, and treatment of primary focal hyperhidrosis. *J Am Acad Dermatol.* **51**, 274–86.

Hund, M., Kinkelin, I., Naumann, M., and Hamm, H. (2001). Definition of Axillary Hyperhidrosis by Gravimetric Assessment. *Archives Dermatol.* **138**, 539–41.

Ito, K., Yanagishita, T., Ohshima, Y., Tamada, Y., and Watanabe, D. (2011). Therapeutic effectiveness of botulinum toxin type A based on severity of palmar hyperhidrosis. *J Dermatol.* May 4. doi: 10.1111/j.1346–8138.2011.01214.x. [Epub ahead of print]

Kaufmann, H., Saadia, D., Polin, C., Hague, S., Singleton, A., and Singleton, A. (2003). Primary hyperhidrosis—evidence for autosomal dominant inheritance. *Clin Auton Res.* **13**, 96–8.

Kinkelin, I., Hund, M., Naumann, M., and Hamm, H. (2000). Effective treatment of frontal hyperhidrosis with botulinum toxin A. *Br J Dermatol.* **143**, 824–7.

Laskawi, R., Rohrbach, S. (2002). Frey's syndrome—Treatment with botulinum toxin. In: Kreyden OP, Boni R, Burg G, eds. *Hyperhidrosis and botulinum toxin in Dermatology* **30**, 170–77, Karger, Basel.

Li, X., Chen, R., Tu, Y. R., *et al.* (2007). Epidemiological survey of primary palmar hyperhidrosis in adolescents. *Chin Med J (Engl).* **20**, 2215–7.

Lowe, N.J., Yamauchi, P.S., Lask, G.P., Patnaik, R., and Iyer, S. (2002). Efficacy and safety of botulinum toxin type a in the treatment of palmar hyperhidrosis: a double-blind, randomized, placebo-controlled study. *Dermatol Surg.* **28**, 822–27.

Meagher, R.J., Narayan, R.K., Furukawa, S., Garza, J., and Ruchinskas, R. (2001). Endocsopic thoracic sympathectomy for essential hyperhidrosis: outcomes analysis in 50 patients. *Neurosurgery.* **49**, 539.

Moore, A. P., Naumann, M. (2003). *Handbook of botulinum toxin.* Blackwell Science.

Namer, I. J., Kansu, T., and Zileli, T. (1986). [Idiopathic localized paroxysmal hyperhidrosis. Treatment with clonidine]. *Rev Neurol (Paris).* **142**, 706–9.

Naumann, M., Hamm, H., and Lowe, N. J. (2002). (on behalf of the BOTOX hyperhidrosis clinical study group). Effect of botulinum toxin type A on quality of life measures in patients with excessive axillary sweating: a randomised controlled trial. *Br J Dermatol.* **147**, 1–9.

Naumann, M., Hofmann, U., Bergmann, I., Hamm, H., Toyka, K. V., and Reiners, K. (1998). Focal hyperhidrosis: effective treatment with intracutaneous botulinum toxin. *Arch Dermatol.* **134**(3), 301–304.

Naumann, M., Lowe, N. J. (2001). Botulinum toxin type A in treatment of bilateral primary axillary hyperhidrosis: randomised, parallel group, double blind, placebo controlled trial. *BMJ.* **323**, 596–9.

Naumann, M., Lowe, N., Kumar, C., and Hamm, H. (2003). Botulinum toxin type A is a safe an effective treatment for axillary hyperhidrosis over 16 months. *Arch Dermatol.* **139**, 731–6.

Naumann, M., Zellner, M., Toyka, K., and Reiners, K. (1997). Treatment of gustatory sweating with botulinum toxin. *Ann Neurol.* **42**, 973–5.

Naver, H., Swartling, C., and Aquilonius, S. M. (2000). Palmar and axillary hyperhidrosis treated with botulinum toxin: one-year clinical follow-up. *Eur J Neurol.* **7**, 55–62

Odderson, I. R. (2002). Long-term quantitative benefits of botulinum toxin type A in the treatment of axillary hyperhidrosis. *Dermatol Surg.* **28**, 480–3.

Park, E. J., Han, K. R., Choi, H., Kim do W., and Kim C. (2010). An epidemiological study of hyperhidrosis patients visiting the Ajou University Hospital hyperhidrosis center in Korea. *J Korean Med Sci.* **25**, 772–5.

Proebstle, T. M., Schneiders, V., and Knop, J. (2002). Gravimetrically controlled efficacy of sucorial curettage: a prospective study for treatment of axillary hyperhidrosis. *Dermatol Surg.* **28**, 1022–6.

Quinton, P. M. (1983). Sweating and its disorders. *Ann Rev Med.* **34**, 429–520.

Rayner, C. R. W., Ritchie, I. D., and Stark, G. P. (1980). Axillary hyperhidrosis, 20% aluminium chloride hexahydrate, and surgery. *BMJ* 1168.

Reinauer, S., Neusser, A., Schauf, G., and Hölzle, E. (1993). Iontophoresis with alternating current and direct current offset (AC/DC iontophoresis): a new approach for the treatment of hyperhidrosis. *Br J Dermatol* **129**, 166–9.

Rompel, R., Scholz, S. (2001). Subcutaneous curettage vs. injection of botulinum toxin A for treatment of axillary hyperhidrosis. *J Eur Acad Dermatol Venereol.* **15**, 207–11.

Saadia, D., Voustianiouk, A., Wang, A. K., and Kaufmann, H. (2001). Botulinum toxin type A in primary palmar hyperhidrosis: randomized, single-blind, two-dose study. *Neurology.* **57**, 2095–9.

Schnider, P., Binder, M., Auff, E., Kittler, H., Berger, T., and Wolff, K. (1997). Double-blind trial of botulinum A toxin for the treatment of focal hyperhidrosis of the palms. *Br J Dermatol.* **136**, 548–52.

Schnider, P., Binder, M., Kittler, H., *et al.* (1999). A randomized, double-blind, placebo-controlled trial of botulinum A toxin for severe axillary hyperhidrosis. *Br J Dermatol.* **140**, 677–80.

Scholes, K. T., Crow, K. D., Ellis, J. P., Harman, R. R., and Saihan E. M. (1978). Axillary hyperhidrosis treated with alcoholic solution of aluminium chloride hexahydrate. *Br Med J.* **2**, 84–85.

Shenefelt, P. D. (2003). Biofeedback, cognitive-behavioral methods, and hypnosis in dermatology: is it all in your mind? *Dermatol Ther.* **16**, 114–22.

Strutton, D., Kowalski, J. (2003). U.S. prevalence of hyperhidrosis: results from a national consumer panel. *Scienfitic Poster American Dermatology Meeting.*

Swartling, C., Naver, H., and Lindberg, M. (2001). Botulinum A toxin improves life quality in severe primary focal hyperhidrosis. *Eur J Neurol.* **8**, 247–52.

Tan, S. R., Solish, N. (2002). Long-term efficacy and quality of life in the treatment of focal hyperhidrosis with botulinum toxin A. *Dermatol Surg.* **28**, 495– 99.

Torch, E. M. (2000). Remission of facial and scalp hyperhidrosis with clonidine hydrochloride and topical aluminum chloride. *South Med J.* **93**, 68–9.

Walling, H. W. (2011). Clinical differentiation of primary from secondary hyperhidrosis. *J Am Acad Dermatol.* **64**, 690–5.

Whatling, P. J., Collin, J. (2001). Botulinum toxin injection is an effective treatment for axillary hyperhidrosis. *Br J Surg.* **88**, 814–5.

Yamashita, N., Tamada, Y., Kawada, M., Mizutani, K., Watanabe, D., and Matsumoto, Y. (2009).Analysis of family history of palmoplantar hyperhidrosis in Japan. *J Dermatol.* **36**, 628–31.

Zacherl, J., Huber E. R., Imhof, M., Plas, E. G., Herbst, F., and Fugger, R. (1998). Long-term results of 630 thoracoscopic sympathicotomies for primary hyperhidrosis: the Vienna experience. *Eur J Surg Suppl.* **580**, 43–46.

CHAPTER 33

Assessment of sleep disturbances in autonomic failure

Sudhansu Chokroverty

Introduction

There is an intimate relationship between the autonomic nervous system (ANS) from the anatomical and functional points of view. Profound functional changes occur in circulation, respiration, thermal regulation, gastrointestinal, and urogenital systems during sleep due to alterations in autonomic outflow. Thus, sleep has a profound effect on the function of the ANS, and dysfunction of the ANS may have significant impact on human sleep and respiration during sleep. It is therefore, logical to expect sleep disorder and sleep-related breathing disorders in patients with autonomic failure (AF). Sleep and sleep-disordered breathing (SDB) in conditions associated with AF should be easy to understand when one also remembers that the peripheral respiratory receptors and central respiratory and hypnogenic neurons located in the lower brainstem and ventrolateral preoptic (VLPO) hypothalamic regions are linked intimately by the ANS. This chapter is concerned with an assessment of sleep and respiratory disturbances in AF, including the influence of the ANS on cardiac rhythm during sleep. A basic familiarity with the central autonomic network (CAN) (Loewy and Spyer 1990), the stages of sleep, the control of breathing during sleep and wakefulness, and the interrelationship between the CAN and the neuronal network controlling breathing is a prerequisite to an understanding of sleep and breathing dysfunction in AF.

Central autonomic network

The general organization of the ANS includes CAN (Loewy and Spyer 1990), sympathetic and parasympathetic efferents, autonomic afferents, and the enteric nervous system. The CAN includes the nucleus tractus solitarius (NTS), the single most important relay station for general visceral and taste afferents. The NTS receives afferents from the cardiovascular and the respiratory systems for autonomic control of cardiac rhythm, circulation and respiration. Lower brainstem hypnogenic neurons are also located in the region of the NTS. The NTS has ascending projections to the insular, anterior cingulate and orbitofrontal cortex, amygdala, hypothalamus, periaqueductal gray matter, and parabrachial

nucleus of the pons. The NTS sends descending projections to the ventrolateral medulla and the preganglionic sympathetic neurons in the column of the intermediolateral spinal cord, parasympathetic neurons and fibres responsible for baroreflex, chemoreflex, cardiorespiratory, and gastrointestinal reflexes. Through these ascending and descending reciprocal connections (Figs 33.1 and 33.2) between the NTS, ventral medulla and other regions of the

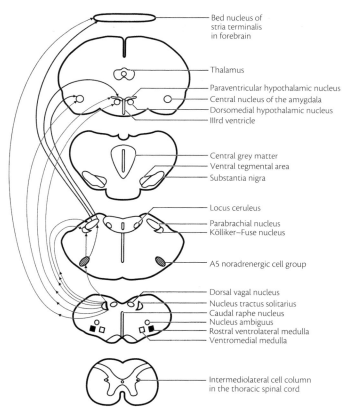

Fig. 33.1 Central autonomic network: ascending projections (schematic). (Modified from Loewy and Spyer (1990); reproduced with permission from Chokroverty (1991) and the American Academy of Neurology.)

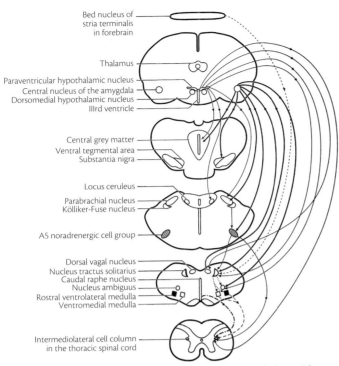

Bed nucleus of
stria terminalis
in forebrain

Thalamus

Paraventricular hypothalamic nucleus
Central nucleus of the amygdala
Dorsomedial hypothalamic nucleus
IIIrd ventricle

Central grey matter
Ventral tegmental area
Substantia nigra

Locus ceruleus

Parabrachial nucleus
Kölliker-Fuse nucleus

A5 noradrenergic cell group

Dorsal vagal nucleus
Nucleus tractus solitarius
Caudal raphe nucleus
Nucleus ambiguus
Rostral ventrolateral medulla
Ventromedial medulla

Intermediolateral cell column
in the thoracic spinal cord

Fig. 33.2 Central autonomic network: descending projections (schematic). (Modified from Loewy and Spyer (1990); reproduced with permission from Chokroverty (1991) and the American Academy of Neurology.)

brainstem, and hypothalamic preoptic hypnogenic and respiratory neurons, the CAN orchestrates the ANS, sleep, respiration, circulation, and other body systems to maintain the homeostasis.

An overview of sleep

Sleep scientists define sleep on the basis of behavioural criteria (e.g. lack of mobility or slight mobility, closed eyes, a markedly reduced response to external stimulation, a characteristic sleeping posture, and a reversibly unconscious state) and physiological criteria (e.g. recordings obtained by electroencephalography [EEG], electrooculography [EOG], and electromyography [EMG]). Based on physiological observations, two types of sleep have been recognized (Chokroverty 2003): non-rapid eye movement (NREM) comprising 75–80%, and rapid eye movement (REM) or paradoxical sleep, comprising 20–25% of sleep time in adults. According to the standard traditional criteria, four stages of NREM sleep (Stages 1–4) have been established based mainly on the EEG criteria. This traditional staging has recently been slightly modified by the new American Academy of Sleep Medicine (AASM) scoring criteria (Iber et al. 2007), which combine stages 3 and 4 into one stage (N3), dividing NREM into N1, N2, N3. The hallmark of REM sleep is presence of rapid eye movements in all directions and the marked absence of muscle activities in the chin EMG. Tonic REM sleep is characterized by a desynchronized EEG and muscle atonia, and phasic REM sleep is characterized by REMs as well as phasic swings in blood pressure and heart rate, irregular respiration, and phasic tongue movements. A few periods of apnoea or hypopnoea may arise during normal REM sleep. In normal individuals, the REM sleep begins 60–90 minutes after sleep onset and recurs in a cyclic manner every 90–100 minutes throughout the night.

Based on the ablation and stimulation experiments, single unit recordings, immunocytochemistry, C-*fos* staining and neuropathological findings, it is believed that NREM or synchronized sleep results from a combination of two factors (Steriade and McCarley 2005, Chokroverty and Montagna, 2009):

◆ disfacilitation of the ascending reticular activating system

◆ activation of the hypnogenic neurons located primarily in the VLPO area of the hypothalamus as well as in the region of the NTS in the dorsomedial medulla.

The original concept of a reciprocal interaction model for REM sleep generation has recently been revised, which suggests that there are anatomically distributed and neurochemically interpenetrated REM "on" and REM "off" cells in the brainstem. The interaction and oscillation between the cholinergic REM-promoting and aminergic REM-inhibiting neurons generate the REM-NREM cycle (Steriade and McCarley 2005). In the latest modification of the reciprocal interaction model, McCarley (2007) suggested that in addition to cholinergic excitation of pontine reticular formation (PRF), an activation of γ-aminobutyric acid (GABA) neurons in the PRF causing inhibition of REM "off" neurons, may also play a role in REM sleep generation. Muscle hypotonia or atonia during REM sleep is thought to depend on inhibitory postsynaptic potentials generated by dorsal pontine interneurons sending descending axons. A pathway from the peri-locus coeruleus alpha region ventral to the locus coeruleus to the lateral tegmental reticular tract and then to the medial medullary region (e.g. nucleus magnocellularis and paramedianus) and the reticulospinal tract projecting to the anterior horn cells of the spinal cord, controls REM sleep induced muscle atonia. An experimental lesion in the peri-locus coeruleus alpha region as well as the medial medullary region produced REM sleep without muscle atonia. In humans, REM behaviour disorder causing dream-enacting behaviour associated with REM sleep without muscle atonia, a structural or functional alteration of the pathway maintaining muscle atonia during REM sleep is most likely responsible for such disorders. Recently, there are two other models proposed for REM sleep generation. In the model proposed by Luppi's group (Luppi et al. 2011), active neurons during REM sleep are identified in a small area in dorsolateral pontine tegmentum of rats, called sublaterodorsal (SLD) nucleus (corresponding to dorsal sub-coeruleus or peri-locus coeruleus alpha in cats). In this model, there is also a kind of reciprocal interaction of glutamatergic (REM-on neurons) and GABA-ergic (REM-off neurons) localized within SLD. The onset of REM sleep is due to activation of REM-on glutamatergic neurons from the SLD. During NREM sleep and wakefulness, these neurons in SLD would be hyperpolarized by tonic GABA-ergic input from GABA-ergic off neurons located in the SLD, deep mesencephalic and pontine reticular nuclei, and ventrolateral periaqueductal gray as well as aminergic REM-off neurons. In the other model proposed by Saper's group (Lu and co-workers 2006), there is a kind of flip-flop switch between GABA-ergic REM-off neurons in ventrolateral periaqueductal gray and lateral pontine tegmentum, and GABA-ergic REM-on neurons in SLD and a dorsal extension of SLD, termed the pre-coeruleus. Finally, the recently described hypocretin (orexin) peptidergic system (DeLecea et al. 1998, Sakurai et al. 1998), located in the lateral hypothalamic region and peri-fornical area with its widespread ascending and descending projections to aminergic, cholinergic, glutamatergic, and other neurotransmitter systems is thought to play a role in the control of sleep and wakefulness.

Autonomic nervous system and sleep

There are several changes in the autonomic functions during sleep affecting particularly the cardiovascular and the respiratory systems (Loewy and Spyer 1990). The neural regulation of the heart predominantly involves the sympathetic and parasympathetic divisions of the ANS but to an extent involves the whole CNS axis. The limbic–hypothalamic region, by controlling the central autonomic network (Loewy and Spyer 1990), affects cardiac rhythm. Sympathetic preganglionic neurons in the intermediolateral column of the spinal cord and the parasympathetic preganglionic neurons in the nucleus ambiguus and dorsal motor nucleus of the vagus, along with the extensive connections with the central autonomic network and the peripheral afferent inputs to the central autonomic network, control the cardiovascular regulation in wakefulness and sleep (Loewy and Spyer 1990). Based on animal experiments and human studies, it is known that heart rate slows during NREM sleep due to tonic increase in parasympathetic activity. There is further slowing of the heart rate during REM sleep due to combination of two factors: persistence of parasympathetic predominance and an additional decrease of sympathetic activity. Similarly, the blood pressure falls during NREM with further fall during REM sleep due to the same mechanism. Blood pressure and heart rate are unstable during phasic REM due to phasic inhibition of the vagus and phasic activation of sympathetic tone, resulting from changes in the brainstem neural activity. The reduction in cardiovascular hemodynamic activities in normal sleep, involving the heart rate, peripheral vascular resistance, blood pressure, blood flow, and cardiac output, becomes critical in patients with cardiopulmonary diseases (e.g. ischaemic heart disease, congestive cardiac failure, pulmonary emphysema, and chronic obstructive pulmonary disease).

Control of breathing during sleep and wakefulness

The anatomical relationship suggests a close functional interdependence between the central autonomic network, the respiratory and hypnogenic neurons. Two separate and independent controlling systems are responsible for breathing (Chokroverty and Montagna 2009): the metabolic or automatic system and a voluntary or behavioural system. Both voluntary and metabolic systems operate during wakefulness but respiration during sleep depends upon the inherent rhythmicity of the automatic respiratory control system located in the medulla. These two controlling systems are complimented by a third system, the reticular arousal system exerting a tonic influence on the brainstem respiratory neurons (McNicholas et al. 1983).

Upper brainstem respiratory neurons located in the rostral pons in the region of parabrachial and Kölliker–Fuse nuclei (pneumotaxic centre), and in the dorsolateral region of the lower pons (apneustic centre) influence the automatic respiratory neurons. The medullary (automatic) respiratory neurons consist of two principal groups (Berger et al. 1977): the dorsal respiratory group located in the NTS responsible predominantly, but not exclusively, for inspiration, and the ventral respiratory group located in the

region of the nucleus ambiguus and retroambigualis, responsible for both inspiration and expiration (Fig. 33.3). The ventral respiratory group contains the Bötzinger complex in the rostral region and pre-Bötzinger region immediately below the Bötzinger complex responsible mainly for the automatic respiratory rhythmicity as these neurons have intrinsic pacemaker activity. These respiratory premotor neurons send axons which decussate below the obex and descend in the reticulospinal tracts in the ventrolateral spinal cord to synapse with spinal respiratory motor neurons innervating the various respiratory muscles. Tonic inputs from the peripheral and central structures converge on the medullary respiratory neurons. Fig. 33.4 shows schematically the effects of various brainstem and vagal transections on the ventilatory patterns.

The voluntary breathing system originating in the cerebral cortex (forebrain and limbic system) controls respiration during wakefulness in addition to participating in non-respiratory functions. The system descends partly to the automatic medullary controlling system and integrates in part there but mostly descends with the corticobulbar and corticospinal tracts to the spinal respiratory motor neurons where the fibres finally integrate with the reticulospinal fibres originating from the automatic medullary respiratory neurons.

The control of respiration during NREM sleep in normal individuals is entirely dependent upon the automatic control system.

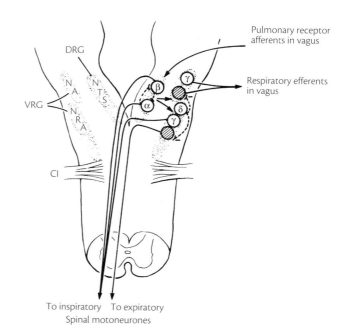

Fig. 33.3 Medullary respiratory neurons, cell types, and interconnections are shown schematically. DRG, dorsal respiratory group; VRG, ventral respiratory group; NTS, nucleus tractus solitarius; NA, nucleus ambiguus; NRA, nucleus retroambigualis; CI, first cervical dorsal root; subscripts α, β, γ, δ, inspiratory cell subtype designations. The DRG located in the ventrolateral NTS is the site where vagal sensory information is first incorporated into a respiratory motor response. The DRG drives the VRG and some spinal inspiratory motoneurons. The VRG is composed of NA and NRA. Vagal respiratory motoneurons arise from NA. Axons from NRA project to some spinal inspiratory and probably all spinal expiratory motoneurons. Inspiratory cells are indicated by open circles, and expiratory by hatched circles. Dashed lines indicate some of the hypothesized intramedullary neural interconnections. With permission from Berger, A. J., Mitchel, R. A., and Severinghaus, J. N. (1977). Regulation of respiration. *New Engl. J. Med.* **297**, 138–43, copyright MMS.

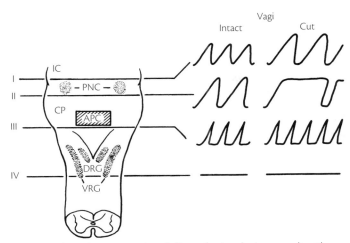

Fig. 33.4 Schematic representation of effects of various brainstem and vagal transections on the ventilatory pattern of the anaesthetized animal. IC, inferior colliculus; PNC, pneumotaxic centre; CP, cerebellar peduncle; APC, apneustic centre; DRG, dorsal respiratory group; VRG, ventral respiratory group. On the left is a representation of the dorsal surface of the lower brainstem and, on the right, a representation of tidal volume with inspiration upwards. Transection I, just rostral to the PNC, does not affect normal breathing, but, in combination with vagotomy, slow deep breathing results. Transection II, isolating the PNC from the lower brainstem, causes slow deep breathing with the vagi intact, and either apneusis (sustained inspiration) or apneustic breathing (rhythmic respiration with marked increase in inspiratory time) when the vagi are cut. Transection III, isolating structures rostral to the medulla, results in most cases in a regular gasping breathing that is generally not affected by vagotomy. Transection IV, at the medullospinal junction, results in respiratory arrest. With permission from Berger, A. J., Mitchel, R. A., and Severinghaus, J. N. (1977). Regulation of respiration. *New Engl. J. Med.* **297**, 138–43, copyright MMS.

The ventilation, tidal volume, and respiratory rate decrease in NREM sleep. Ventilatory responses to hypercapnia and hypoxia are attenuated during NREM sleep in normal individuals. These findings suggest decreased sensitivity of the central chemoreceptors subserving medullary respiratory neurons. In REM sleep respiration is rapid and erratic; tonic and phasic activities in the intercostal and upper airway muscles decrease while phasic activity is maintained in the diaphragm but the tonic activity in the diaphragm is reduced. There is some uncertainty about the ventilatory responses to CO_2 and hypoxia in REM sleep. Compared with the responses during NREM sleep the hypercapnic and hypoxic ventilatory responses in the adult human are reduced during REM sleep. The voluntary respiratory control system may be active during some part of REM sleep. Thus, in normal individuals, respiration is vulnerable during sleep; mild respiratory irregularities and pauses may occur in normal individuals, but in disease states these may assume a pathological significance.

Sleep and respiratory disturbances in autonomic failure

AF may be classified into primary and secondary AF. Primary AF (without known cause) includes pure AF without any somatic neurological deficits (Bradbury–Eggleston syndrome), multiple system atrophy (MSA or the Shy–Drager syndrome) (see introductory chapter on the Classification of Autonomic Disorders), some cases of postural tachycardia syndrome (POTS), familial dysautonomia

and autoimmune autonomic neuropathy or acute pandysautonomia. The best-known condition with AF in which sleep and respiratory disturbances have been reported and well described is MSA or the Shy–Drager syndrome. Familial dysautonomia, a recessively inherited disease with AF, is also known to be associated with disturbances of breathing and sleep. A large number of neurological and general medical disorders are associated with prominent secondary AF. In many patients with diabetic autonomic neuropathies, amyloidotic neuropathy, and Guillain–Barré syndrome, sleep and sleep-related respiratory disturbances have been noted. In many neurological conditions, sleep and respiratory disturbances secondary to the structural lesions involving the central hypnogenic or respiratory neurons have been described.

In this section an assessment of sleep and respiratory disturbances in MSA will be given. In addition, a brief account will also be presented of the following conditions in which sleep disturbances or sleep-related breathing disorders may be the prominent features: familial dysautonomia, diabetic autonomic neuropathy, neurodegenerative diseases with AF (e.g. Parkinson's disease [PD] and diffuse Lewy body disease [DLBD]), and fatal familial insomnia, a rare prion disease with severe sleep disturbances and dysautonomia. Finally, sleep, cardiac arrhythmia, sudden cardiac death, and autonomic deficits in obstructive sleep apnoea syndrome will be briefly reviewed.

Primary autonomic failure

Multiple system atrophy (Shy–Drager syndrome)

Since the original description by Shy and Drager (1960) of a neurodegenerative disorder characterized by AF and MSA, there have been numerous reports (Chokroverty et al. 1969, Bannister and Oppenheimer 1972, Bannister et al. 1981, Wenning et al. 2003, Chokroverty and Montagna, 2009) of the condition that has generally come to be known as MSA, which is the term suggested in a consensus statement (1996) and second statement later (Gilman et al. 2008) to replace the term Shy–Drager syndrome). Patients with this syndrome frequently manifest sleep and respiratory disturbances, particularly in the later stage of the illness. Further clinical details are given in Chapter 41. Based on the presence of a distinctive pathological finding of oligodendrological cytoplasmic inclusions and other evidence Wenning et al. (2008) recently hypothesized that MSA is a primary oligodendrogliopathy.

Sleep dysfunction is very common in MSA and includes insomnia with sleep fragmentation, REM behaviour disorder and sleep related respiratory dysrhythmias. REM behaviour disorder (RBD) is very common and present in 80– 95% of patients with MSA (Plazzi et al. 1997, Boeve et al. 2007, Iranzo et al. 2009, Boeve 2010). The characteristic clinical features of RBD include intermittent loss of REM-related muscle atonia and the appearance of a variety of abnormal motor activities during sleep. The patient presents a violent dream-enacting behaviour during REM sleep often causing self-injury or injury to the patient's bed partner. RBD may precede the illness or may present concomitantly or after the onset of MSA (Boeve et al. 2007, Iranzo et al. 2009). Positron emission tomography (PET) and single photon emission computed tomography (SPECT) studies by Gilman et al. (2003) suggested that RBD in MSA is related to nigrostriatal dopaminergic deficit. In other cases, RBD and MSA may be due to the neuropathological changes in the brainstem REM-generating neurons. Sleep-related respiratory dysrhythmias associated with repeated arousals and hypoxaemia are the most common and life-threatening disorders in MSA, and present in almost 100% of the cases in the advanced stages of the illness. Clinical manifestations due to respiratory dysfunction may consist of daytime hypersomnolence resulting from severe nocturnal sleep disruption, early morning headache, daytime fatigue, intellectual deterioration, primary hypertension, cor pulmonale, congestive cardiac failure, and cardiac arrhythmias. Sudden nocturnal death in some patients with MSA may be due to respiratory arrest or cardiac arrhythmia. Polysomnographic study may show the following: a reduction of total sleep time, decreased sleep efficiency, increased number of awakenings during sleep, a reduction of slow-wave and REM sleep, absence of muscle atonia in REM sleep in those with REM behaviour disorder, and a variety of respiratory dysrhythmias, as described below.

The spectrum of respiratory dysrhythmias (schematically shown in Fig. 33.6) consists of (Chokroverty and Montagna, 2009):

◆ central, upper-airway obstructive, and mixed apnoeas associated with oxygen desaturation during NREM stages 1 and 2 and REM sleep

◆ dysrhythmic breathing (irregular rate, rhythm, and amplitude of respiration with and without oxygen desaturation becoming worse in sleep) (McNicholas et al. 1983, Chokroverty and Montagna, 2009), Cheyne–Stokes pattern and Cheyne–Stokes variant (hypopnoea substitutes apnoea) pattern of breathing becoming worse in sleep

◆ transient occlusion of the upper airway or transient uncoupling of the intercostal and diaphragmatic muscle activities

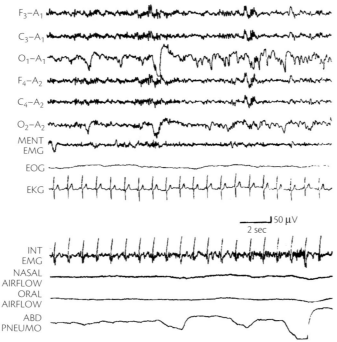

Fig. 33.5 A portion of a polygraphic recording in a patient with multiple system atrophy showing mixed apnoea associated with oxygen desaturation. Reproduced with permission from Chokroverty S., 'Sleep, Breathing and Neurologic Disorders' in *Sleep Disorders Medicine: Basic Science, Technical Considerations, and Clinical Aspects*, pp. 436–498, Copyright Elsevier (2009).

◆ prolonged periods of central apnoea accompanied by mild oxygen desaturation in relaxed wakefulness as if the respiratory centre forgot to breathe (Chokroverty et al. 1978, 1984, Guilleminault et al. 1981, Munschauer et al. 1990)

◆ periodic breathing in the erect posture accompanied by postural fall of blood pressure

◆ inspiratory gasps and apneustic-like breathing

◆ nocturnal stridor due to posterior cricoarytenoid atrophy or laryngeal dystonia (Merlo et al. 2002, Bannister et al. 1981, Munschauer et al. 1990, Sadaoka et al. 1996).

The nocturnal stridor can be inspiratory, expiratory or both and cause excessive snoring and upper airway obstruction during sleep. Stridor may give rise to a striking noise which may be likened to a noise resembling "donkey braying". Less commonly, apneustic breathing, inspiratory gasping, or Cheyne–Stokes breathing may occur. Impaired hypoxic or hypercapnic ventilatory responses and mouth occlusion pressure response in some patients suggested impairment of the metabolic respiratory system (McNicholas et al. 1983, Chokroverty and Montagna 2009) while normal hypercapnic and hypoxic ventilatory responses in some patients in the presence of an abnormal respiratory pattern indicated that the chemoreceptor control and respiratory pattern generator are probably subserved by different population of neurons with selective vulnerability of these neurons in MSA (Lockwood 1976, Chokroverty and Montagna 2009). Post-mortem findings of marked loss of neurons in the pontine tegmentum and medullary reticular formation including neurons around the nucleus tractus solitarius in those MSA patients with sleep-related respiratory dysrhythmias confirmed involvement of the respiratory neurons in the brainstem (Chokroverty et al. 1978 Munschauer et al. 1990).

Sleep disruption in MSA may result from both direct and indirect pathogenetic mechanisms and include:

◆ direct involvement of the medullary respiratory neurons

◆ involvement of the arousal system (ascending reticular activating system), and severe compromise of the wakefulness stimulus

◆ involvement of the respiratory and non-respiratory motor neurons in the brainstem (e.g. the nucleus ambiguous and hypoglossal nuclei) causing laryngeal abductor paresis, and pharyngeal and genioglossal weakness causing upper airway obstructive apnoea

◆ involvement of the respiratory motor neurons in the cervical and thoracic spinal cord, thereby reducing impulse traffic along the phrenic and intercostal nerves to the diaphragm and the intercostal muscles

◆ interference with the forebrain, midbrain and pontine inputs to the medullary respiratory neurons causing dysrhythmic and apneustic breathing

◆ involvement of the direct projections from the hypothalamus and the central nucleus of amygdala to the respiratory neurons in the NTS and nucleus ambiguous

◆ involvement of the vagal afferens from the lower and upper airway receptors thus reducing the input to these central respiratory neurons causing respiratory dysrhythmia

◆ sympathetic denervation of the nasal mucosa causing increased nasal resistance promoting upper airway obstructive apnoea

◆ SPECT findings by Gilman et al. (2003) suggesting decreased pontine cholinergic projections to the thalamus contributing to obstructive sleep apnoea in MSA.

Finally, in a series of post-mortem studies of brains obtained from patients with MSA, Benarroch and colleagues reported depletion of catecholaminergic neurons in the ventrolateral medulla (Benarroch et al. 1998), cholinergic neurons in the medullary arcuate nucleus (Benarroch et al. 2001), corticotrophin releasing factor (CRF) neurons (Benarroch and Schmeichel 2001), in the putative pontine micturition centre, mesopontine cholinergic neurons in the pedunculopontine and laterodorsal tegmental nucleus (Benarroch et al. 2003a), ventrolateral medullary neurokinin-1 receptor-like-immunoreactive (NK-1-L-I) neurons (Benarroch et al. 2003b), chemosensitive glutamatergic and serotonergic neurons in the arcuate nucleus in the ventral medullary surface as well as serotonergic neurons in the medullary raphe (Benarroch et al. 2007), serotonergic neurons in the pontomedullary raphe neurons (Benarroch et al. 2004), in the ventrolateral nucleus ambiguus innervating the heart and dorsal vagal nucleus innervating enteric neurons (Benarroch et al. 2006), as well as loss of hypocretin (Orexin) hypothalamic neurons (Benarroch 2007). Loss of these cell groups may contribute to the respiratory disturbances including loss of automatic respiration and other autonomic dysfunction involving various systems in MSA (Benarroch 2007).

Vetrugno et al. (2004) performed video-polysomnographic (PSG) study in 19 consecutive MSA patients and documented RBD in 100%, stridor in 42%, obstructive sleep apnoea in 37%, and periodic limb movements in sleep (PLMS) in 88% of cases. In 39 consecutive MSA patients, Plazzi et al. (1997) documented RBD in 90% of patients. RBD preceded in 44%, concomitantly appeared in 26%, and followed the onset of MSA symptoms in 30% of cases. They also noted obstructive sleep apnoea, stridor and PLMS in some patients. RBD can sometimes progress into status dissociatus (Vetrugno et al. 2009). Ghorayeb et al. (2002) based on a standard sleep questionnaire reported a variety of sleep disorders in 70% of 57 patients in an unselected group with MSA: sleep fragmentation (52.5%), vocalization (60%), RBD (47.5%), and nocturnal stridor (19%). The severity of motor symptoms, disease duration, comorbid depression and the duration of levodopa treatment correlated with sleep problems. Silber and Levine (2000) reviewed 42 patients with MSA (17 with nocturnal stridor and 25 without stridor). They concluded that the survival is shorter in those with stridor than in those without stridor. There are other reports of stridor, particularly nocturnal in MSA, and in some patients sudden nocturnal death was presumably related to laryngeal obstruction. Iranzo et al. (2000) in a prospective study of laryngeal function in 20 patients with MSA reported sleep disturbance in all and vocal cord abduction dysfunction in 14 (70%). Continuous positive airway pressure (CPAP) in 3 patients eliminated laryngeal stridor and obstructive apnoeas. In later studies, Iranzo et al. (2004) reported beneficial effect of long-term CPAP therapy followed for months in 13 MSA subjects with stridor. In addition to improvement in sleep quality, they found similar median survival in patients with and without stridor. Ghorayeb et al. (2005) in a study of 22 MSA patients with stridor and sleep-related breathing disorders found 3 with OSA without stridor and 15 with stridor alone or accompanied by apnoea. Twelve patients had CPAP treatment. Of these 12 patients, two died shortly after CPAP titration and one died 17 months later. Five patients discontinued the use of CPAP because of discomfort and four continued with CPAP with improvement of sleep and daytime alertness. The authors concluded that the severity of motor impairment at the time of initial CPAP is the most significant limiting factor for long-term CPAP acceptance. In a recent study Freilich and co-workers (2010) noted increased sleep disturbances and an attenuated heart rate response to arousal from sleep in patients with AF.

Postural orthostatic tachycardia syndrome

Postural orthostatic tachycardia syndrome (POTS), also known as orthostatic intolerance syndrome is a recently described entity that is still in search of an identity, and the clinical manifestations are still evolving. Sleep dysfunction is often an important component of the clinical features, but has largely been neglected in the literature (Chokroverty et al. 2001). The fundamental manifestations of POTS include symptoms of orthostatic intolerance accompanied by a heart rate of 120 beats per minute or more, or a heart rate increment of 30 beats or more per minute on changing from supine to upright position within 5 minutes of standing or head-up tilt. The symptoms of orthostatic intolerance consist of dizziness, faint feelings, palpitations, nausea, tremulousness, anxiety, and visual blurring on standing without significant orthostatic hypotension. The other symptoms include extreme fatigue, diffuse muscle aches and pains, upper and lower gastrointestinal symptoms, as well as sleep dysfunction. Patients may complain of sleep onset or maintenance insomnia whereas others may have daytime hypersomnolence or circadian rhythm disorders. Some patients may complain of fatigue, which is a very common manifestation in these patients, and may be difficult to differentiate from excessive daytime sleepiness. Sleep onset and maintenance insomnia in patients with POTS may be related to PLMS, inadequate sleep hygiene, diffuse muscle aches and pains, and anxiety. Daytime hypersomnolence may be secondary to sleep deprivation at night as well as depression in some patients. Circadian rhythm disorder suggests a dysfunction of the circadian clock in the suprachiasmatic nuclei. It is important to pay attention to sleep dysfunction in these patients as treatment combining pharmacological therapy (short-term hypnotics or selective serotonin reuptake inhibitors) or non-pharmacological treatment (sleep hygiene, stimulus control, relaxation measures, and appropriately timed bright light exposure) may be beneficial in these patients. An adequate number of patients with POTS have not been studied to understand the pathophysiology of sleep dysfunction in these patients.

Familial dysautonomia

Familial dysautonomia, also known as Riley–Day syndrome, is a recessively inherited disorder confined to the Jewish population and presenting in childhood. The clinical manifestations comprise autonomic, neuromuscular, cardiovascular, skeletal, renal, and respiratory abnormalities. Patients show a characteristic absence of the fungiform papillae of the tongue. Other features include defective lacrimation and sweating, vasomotor instability, fluctuation of blood pressure (postural hypotension and paroxysmal hypertension), relative insensitivity to pain, and absent muscle stretch reflexes. Most patients have a mild respiratory and sleep disorder associated with both central and obstructive sleep apnoeas (Gadoth et al. 1983). The sleep abnormalities include increased arousals and awakenings; prolonged sleep onset; prolonged REM sleep onset but reduced total REM sleep time; and apnoeas during sleep.

The patients with familial dysautonomia often show severe breath-holding spells due to defective responses of central respiratory neurons to changes in PaCO2. Guilleminault et al. (1981) and McNicholas et al. (1983) found an irregular pattern of breathing in patients with familial dysautonomia similar to that noted in Shy–Drager syndrome. Oesophageal reflux during sleep causing frequent awakenings was noted in one patient by Guilleminault et al. (1981). Recently an infant with familial dysautonomia with episodic somnolence lasting for 4–15 hours during the neonatal period was reported (Casella et al. 2005). The diagnosis of familial dysautonomia was confirmed by the demonstration of mutations in the I kappa B kinase complex-associated protein gene with the identification of IVS 20, which is responsible for more than 99.5% of known Ashkenazi Jewish patients with familial dysautonomia.

Secondary autonomic failure (those associated with other medical and neurological disorders)

Diabetic autonomic neuropathy

Autonomic neuropathies have been described in many neurological and medical disorders. However, the sleep and respiratory functions have not been studied well in most of these conditions. In diabetic polyneuropathies there have been reports of disturbances of sleep and respiration. Similar disturbances have been described in some patients with AF associated with amyloidosis and Guillain–Barré syndrome, and paraneoplastic autonomic neuropathy.

Central or upper airway obstructive apnoeas have been described in several patients with diabetes mellitus and autonomic neuropathy (Guilleminault et al. 1981). Bottini et al. (2003) described obstructive sleep apnoea/hypopnoea with a frequency of more than 30% in adult non-obese diabetics with autonomic neuropathy independent of the severity of their dysautonomia.

Neurodegenerative disease with autonomic failure and sleep dysfunction

Two neurodegenerative diseases, PD and DLBD, are associated with AF and sleep disturbances, and are considered synucleinopathies, which are a group of disorders with abnormal deposition of alpha synuclein in the cytoplasm of neurons or glial cells.

Parkinson's disease with autonomic failure

Sleep dysfunction is present in 70–90% of patients with PD, with progressive impairment with the progression of the disease. Sleep onset and maintenance insomnia is very common. There are several nocturnal motor abnormalities noted, such as RBD, PLMS, sleep-onset blinking, REM-onset blepharospasm, and intrusion of REMs into NREM sleep. Another characteristic feature in patients with PD is daytime hypersomnolence and irresistible sleep attacks, which may be due to a combination of the intrinsic disease process and dopaminergic medications.

Sleep-related respiratory dysfunction in PD patients is more common than in age-matched controls. It may be related to impairment of breathing control, impaired respiratory muscle function due to rigidity and faulty autonomic control of lungs, fluctuating muscle functioning, laryngeal spasm associated with off-states, or upper airway dysfunction with tremor-like oscillations (Hening et al. 2009). Obstructive, central, and mixed apnoeas have also been described in PD patients. Patients with PD may have stridor or laryngeal spasms associated with off-state or dystonia episodes (Vas et al. 1965, Corbin and Williams 1987); abnormal vocal cord function with regular rhythmic movements or irregular jerky movements in the glottic area may also produce changes of air flow contributing to intermittent airway closure (Vincken et al. 1984). Similar activity persisting during sleep can lead to obstructive sleep apnoea or upper airway resistance syndrome (Efthimiou et al. 1986). It should be noted that patients with parkinsonism and autonomic impairment more often develop sleep apnoea and related respiratory abnormalities, including central and obstructive apnoeas and nocturnal hypoventilation than those without dysautonomia. In the presence of sleep apnoea, patients with autonomic impairment are probably more likely than other patients to have nocturnal cardiac arrhythmias.

Another important sleep disturbance in PD is the emergence of REM behaviour disorder, and the frequency of RBD in PD is approximately 33–60% (Gagnon et al. 2002). RBD is very common in patients with synucleinopathies such as DLBD, MSA, and PD. Schenck et al. (1996) originally reported that 38% of patients with idiopathic RBD developed PD within 4 years, and in a later (2002) report, this figure increased to 65% of idiopathic RBD patients that developed PD after a mean of 13 years. This pattern has been noted in several other reports (Boeve et al. 2007, Boeve 2010, Iranzo et al. 2009). RBD thus may precede, appear concomitantly, or appear after the onset of PD, and the condition can be diagnosed by history and video-polysomnographic study. RBD patients often show subtle motor, cognitive, autonomic, olfactory, and visual changes that are associated with PD (Gagnon et al. 2006, Postuma et al. 2009, 2011). Reduced cardiac iodine-123 (^{123}I) uptake suggesting loss of sympathetic terminals in idiopathic RBD is consistent with a similar deficit in PD (Miyamoto et al. 2006).

Diffuse Lewy body disease and autonomic failure

The core diagnostic features of DLBD include fluctuating cognition, recurrent visual hallucinations, and parkinsonian features (e.g. rigidity, postural instability, and akinesia or bradykinesia), coupled with other features such as repeated falls, neuroleptic sensitivity, and RBD. According to the criteria developed by McKeith et al. (2006), supporting features of DLBD include syncope. Symptomatic orthostatic hypotension including syncope occurs in up to 30% of patients with DLBD (Wenning et al. 1999, Thaisetthawatkul et al. 2004), sometimes as the presenting feature (Larner et al. 2000). Other dysautonomic features in DLBD may include urogenital disturbance. Sleep dysfunction in DLBD includes RBD (present in 50–80% of patients with DLBD), which often precedes the onset of the illness (Boeve et al. 2007), sleep apnoea, nocturnal visual hallucinations, insomnia, and daytime hypersomnolence. Excessive daytime sleepiness, hallucinations, and RBD may occur in both DLBD and narcolepsy; however, Baumann et al. (2004) found normal levels of hypocreatin-1 in the cerebrospinal fluid in 10 patients with DLBD. In narcolepsy-cataplexy patients, levels of hypocreatin-1 in the cerebrospinal fluid are generally low.

Fatal familial insomnia

Fatal familial insomnia (FFI) is a rare autosomal dominant prion disease akin to Creutzfeldt–Jakob disease (Chokroverty and Montagna 2009) with onset in adults. The term 'prion' refers to a proteinaceous infectious particle resistant to inactivation by most standard procedures. The major clinical findings include progressive insomnia, motor abnormalities in the form of spontaneous and reflex myoclonus, ataxia, dysarthria, and hyperreflexia, neuroendocrine abnormalities, and dysautonomia. Insomnia is progressive with worsening within a few months. The autonomic dysfunction is manifested by sympathetic hyperreflexia as evidenced by hypertension, tachycardia, tachypnoea, hyperhidrosis, and urinary dysfunction and impotence. Tests for parasympathetic function are normal. Neuroendocrine dysfunction is characterized by elevated plasma cortisol and catecholamines, reduced circadian oscillations of cortisol and failure of rise of melatonin during darkness, and absence of a tight relationship between slow-wave sleep and rise of growth hormone and prolactin. There is no evidence of dementia but neuropsychological tests may show frontal lobe type dysfunction. The most prominent finding in the polysomnographic recording is progressive decrement of NREM and REM sleep to only brief NREM sleep. EEG shows diffuse background slowing and periodically recurring spikes in some cases in the later stage. Cerebral evoked potentials, brain computerized tomography and magnetic resonance imaging are normal. PET scan shows glucose hypometabolism in the thalamus.

The course of the illness is relentlessly progressive, lasting for 1–4 years. In the final stage, the patients display random myoclonus and dream-like hallucinatory behaviour in wakefulness. In the final terminal months, sleeplessness gives way to stupor and coma.

Neuropathological findings consist of degeneration and loss of neurons in the dorsomedial and anterior thalamic nuclei with normal hypothalamus and brainstem reticular formation. Frontal and temporal cortex shows mild to moderate gliosis. DNA analysis shows that FFI results from a point mutation at codon 178 and a polymorphism on codon 129 on the prion gene on chromosome 20.

Sleep and cardiac arrhythmias

Several studies have been obtained in normal individuals using Holter monitoring to understand the effect of sleep on cardiac rhythm (Parish and Shepard 1990). The most frequent nocturnal dysrhythmia is sinus arrhythmia, which is noted in 50% of young individuals (Parish and Shepard 1990). One-third of them had sinus pauses lasting from 1.8 seconds to 2 seconds, and in another 6% there were episodes of atrioventricular block. In young healthy adults, sinus arrest has been noted lasting up to 9 seconds during REM sleep without associated apnoeas or significant oxygen desaturation (Parish and Shepard 1990).

Although human studies revealed contradictory results about the effect of sleep on ventricular arrhythmia, the majority (Verrier and Kirby 1988) showed an antiarrhythmic effect of sleep on ventricular premature beats. This seems to be due to enhanced parasympathetic tone during sleep conferring protection against ventricular arrhythmia and sudden cardiac death.

There are also several reports of ventricular arrhythmias occurring during arousal from sleep. A classic example was a 14-year-old girl who was awakened from sleep by a loud auditory stimulation with ventricular tachyarrhythmia (Verrier and Kirby 1988). This was thought to be due to an increase of sympathetic activity as the episodes could be prevented by propranolol, a beta-blocker.

In patients with ischaemic heart disease, 24-hour Holter monitoring may reveal several different electrocardiographic (ECG) changes during sleep: ST segment depression and T-wave inversion. Nocturnal cardiac ischaemia associated with ST segment depression or elevation has been noted in some middle-aged men and also in postmenopausal women during sleep.

Sleep and sudden cardiac death

Muller et al. (1987) analysed the time of sudden cardiac death in 2203 individuals dying out of hospital in 1983. There was low incidence during the night and high incidence from 7 a.m. to 11 a.m. This pattern is similar to the incidence of non-fatal myocardial infarction and episodes of myocardial ischaemia, which are more likely to occur in the morning. One suggestion is that the sudden cardiac death may result from a primary arrhythmic event. It is known that in the morning there is increased sympathetic activity, which may increase myocardial electrical instability giving rise to fatal arrhythmia. Besides myocardial infarction as a risk factor for sudden cardiac death, another clinical entity, known as the congenital long QT syndrome (CLQTS), may cause syncope or sudden death. In CLQTS, ECG shows a prolonged QT interval with abnormal T and U waves, and torsade de pointes (polymorphic ventricular tachycardia).

Another cause of sudden death in young adults in the Western literature is the Brugada syndrome described in 1992 (Antzelevitch et al. 2006). Patients with Brugada syndrome present with characteristic ECG abnormalities of atypical right-bundle branch block and ST segment elevation over the right precordial leads. They have life-threatening ventricular tachyarrhythmias without any structural cardiac lesions; an involvement of the ANS is suggested and abnormal ^{123}I-meta-iodobenzyl guanidine (MIBG) SPECT uptake in Brugada syndrome indicating presynaptic sympathetic dysfunction of the heart has been reported by Wichter et al. (2002). The Brugada syndrome has a genetic basis and is linked to mutation in SCN5A, the gene encoding the alpha-subunit of the sodium channel. The ideal treatment suggested for this syndrome is implantation of a cardioverter defibrillator. Sudden unexplained nocturnal death syndrome (SUNDS) is a disorder found in South East Asia with abnormal electrocardiographic findings similar to those noted in Brugada syndrome. It has been suggested that both SUNDS and Brugada syndrome may have a common genetic and biophysical basis (Vatta et al. 2002).

Cardiac arrhythmias, autonomic deficits, and obstructive sleep apnoea syndrome

Several varieties of cardiac dysrhythmias are noted in patients with obstructive sleep apnoea syndrome (OSAS) (Parish and Shepard 1990). These arrhythmias are determined by the changes in autonomic nervous system. The most common is bradytachyarrhythmia alternating during apnoea and immediately after termination of apnoea. The other dysrhythmias consist of: sinus bradycardia with less than 30 beats per minute; sinus pauses lasting for 2–13 seconds; second-degree heart block; and ventricular ectopic beats including complex and multifocal ectopic beats, and ventricular tachycardia. There is a clear relationship between the level of oxygen saturation (SaO_2) and premature ventricular complex, and sleep apnoea syndrome. Patients with SaO_2 below 60% are the most vulnerable. Hoffstein and Mateika (1994), using nocturnal polysomnography (PSG), prospectively studied 458 patients with OSAS. They found a high prevalence (58%) of cardiac arrhythmias in these patients, and those with arrhythmias had more severe apnoea and nocturnal hypoxaemia than those without arrhythmias.

Earlier studies thus showed a higher prevalence than more recent epidemiological studies suggested. Roche et al. (2003) performed a prospective study in 147 consecutive patients referred for assessment of OSAS. The authors found OSAS in over 45% with apnoea-hypopnoea index (AHI) ≥ 10. They found significantly more nocturnal paroxysmal asystole in OSAS patients (10.6% vs 1.2%). They further noted that the number of episodes of bradycardia and pauses increased with severity of OSAS syndrome. CPAP treatment followed for 1 year showed amelioration of arrhythmic events in patients with OSAS, indicating usefulness of CPAP treatment. The ANS dysfunction was implicated in cardiovascular mortality and morbidity in OSAS (e.g. diurnal hypertension, left ventricular failure, high risk of coronary or cerebral events) (Ito et al. 2005). CPAP treatment can prevent the cardiovascular risk associated with ANS function. Gami et al. (2005) after reviewing the PSG and death certificates of 112 Minnesota residents who had died suddenly from cardiac causes during the period from July 1987 to July 2003 concluded that OSAS patients had a peak sudden death from cardiac causes during sleeping hours contrasting with the nadir of sudden death in those without OSAS and in general population. Peltier et al. (2007) recruited 32 patients with complaints of excessive daytime somnolence and snoring, and performed PSG and 2-hour oral glucose tests as well as autonomic testing consisting of heart rate response to deep breathing, Valsalva manoeuvre, tilt-up and quantitative sudomotor axon reflex testing (QSART). They found that 19 of 24 patients with OSAS had abnormal glucose tolerance, and cardiac autonomic function was more strongly associated with impaired glucose regulation than OSAS. They concluded that cardiovagal and adrenergic dysfunction are responsible for cardiovascular adverse consequences in OSAS but the question remains whether impaired glucose regulation in such patients may have been responsible for such ANS dysfunction. There is a complex relationship between OSAS, autonomic function and glucose regulation, and larger studies are needed to resolve these issues.

Laboratory diagnosis of sleep and respiratory dysfunction in autonomic failure

The diagnosis of primary and secondary AF is based on a combination of clinical manifestations, documentation of autonomic dysfunction, and exclusion of other causes of dysautonomia and somatic neurological diseases. CT, MRI, PET using fluorodopa, EMG and nerve conduction study, cerebrospinal fluid examination, and routine EEG in addition to special autonomic function studies may be necessary to establish the diagnosis. EMG of the external urethral or anal sphincter muscles may be helpful in the diagnosis of some suspected cases of MSA by showing evidence of denervation and reinnervation. Once the diagnosis of MSA or other secondary AF is made, further studies are necessary in patients suspected of sleep and respiratory dysrhythmia to diagnose and treat the specific disturbance. A thorough history and physical examination including otolaryngological examination to detect laryngeal and oropharyngeal muscle weakness should precede the special studies described.

Polysomnographic study

For the assessment of sleep and respiratory dysfunction in AF, it is important to obtain a complete PSG study. To assess the severity of the sleep and respiratory disturbances, and to fully understand the structure of sleep, all-night recordings should be obtained. The study should include simultaneous recordings of multiple channels of EEG, EMG of submental and tibialis anterior muscles (if RBD is suspected, multiple cranial, upper and lower limb muscles should be included), ECG, electrooculogram, respiratory recordings, and continuous oxygen saturation by an oximeter. Respiration can be monitored by oronasal thermistors or preferably by nasal pressure transducer to detect airflow and by use of an abdominal pneumograph or inductive plethysmograph (Respitrace) to detect respiratory effort. Inclusion of video PSG study may be needed in some patients to diagnose REM behaviour disorder, which may occur in patients with MSA, and PD, and DLBD.

The importance of studying the sleep architecture is that sleep may accentuate respiratory abnormalities, and respiratory dysfunction may affect sleep structure adversely; both these factors may alter the long-term course of the illness. A 24-hour ambulatory recording of sleep and breathing may also be obtained to assess their circadian variation.

Multiple sleep latency test

Multiple sleep latency test (MSLT) is an objective test for assessment of daytime pathological sleepiness. It may help in assessing the severity of daytime hypersomnolence and for monitoring the effect of treatment. In this recording, 4 or 5 daytime tests at 2-hour intervals, each time lasting for 20 minutes, are obtained. The patients are encouraged to remain awake in between the recordings and the recording must follow a standardized protocol to validate the results of the tests adequately. Sleep onset latency and sleep onset REM are noted. Sleep onset latency of 8 minutes or less is indicative of pathological sleepiness.

Maintenance of wakefulness test

Maintenance of wakefulness test (MWT) is a variant of MSLT measuring the subject's ability to stay awake. It also consists of 4 to 5 trials of remaining awake recording every 2 hours. Each trial is terminated if no sleep occurs after 40 minutes or immediately after three consecutive epochs of stage 1 NREM or the first epoch of any other stage of sleep. If the mean sleep latency is less than 8 minutes, it is then considered an abnormal test and values greater than this but less than 40 minutes are of uncertain significance. The MWT is less sensitive than the MSLT as a diagnostic test but is more sensitive in assessing the effect of treatment (e.g. CPAP titration in OSAS).

Pulmonary function tests

In order to exclude intrinsic bronchopulmonary disease contributing to respiratory dysfunction in AF, one should obtain pulmonary function tests (PFT) to assess respiratory and ventilatory muscle function. PFTs include measurements of lung volumes (quantities of air within the lungs), lung capacities (derived from lung volume) and blood gases (PaO_2 and $PaCO_2$). Spirometry measures most of the lung volumes and capacities except residual volume (RV), functional residual capacity (FRC) and total lung capacity (TLC), which require non-spirometric techniques (e.g. gas dilution technique). Important spirometric measurements include forced vital capacity (FVC), forced expiratory volume in one second (FEV_1) and the ratio of FEV_1 and FVC. Values are expressed as percentage predicted. The maximum static inspiratory and expiratory pressures should also be measured. These are more important than the dynamic measurements in detecting respiratory muscle weakness. To measure the chemical control of breathing, hypercapnic or hypoxic ventilatory and mouth occlusion pressure (Po.1) responses, with or without load, should be studied. Mouth occlusion pressure reflects central respiratory drive and inspiratory muscle strength independent of pulmonary mechanical factors. These measurements may be impaired in patients with dysfunction of the metabolic respiratory control system.

Electromyography of respiratory muscles

Electrical activity of the respiratory and upper airway including genioglossus and laryngeal muscles may be obtained to assess ventilatory activity and upper airway muscle tone. Laryngeal EMG is important in patients suspected of laryngeal paresis.

Electrocardiogram

ECG recording is essential in patients with suspected cardiac dysrhythmia or in those at high risk for developing such arrhythmias. Continuous monitoring of ECG by Holter monitoring for one or more days is required in some patients. This will give an indication about the circadian variation of the heart rate as well as the circadian influence on the cardiac dysrhythmias.

Treatment of sleep dysfunction and sleep disordered breathing in autonomic failure

Specific treatment of neurological disorders causing AF is beyond the scope of this chapter. In the absence of an adequate understanding of the pathogenesis and the lack of a definite aetiological agent causing MSA or other neurodegenerating diseases, treatment remains unsatisfactory and consists of symptomatic measures only. MSA is an inexorably progressive neurological disease pursuing a relentless course despite improvement of orthostatic hypotension and other dysautonomic manifestations following symptomatic treatment that may improve the quality of life temporarily. Treatment of sleep dysfunction in AF should include measures to address sleep related respiratory dysrhythmias and other types of sleep dysfunction. The major disability impairing the quality of life in AF is related to the sleep dysfunction resulting from sleep-related respiratory dysrhythmias which will be discussed below. For improving the quality of sleep, general sleep hygiene measures (Table 33.1) should be instituted in all patients. Most cases of RBD respond dramatically to a small dose of clonazepam (e.g. 0.5–2 mg at night). Some patients who do not respond to clonazepam may benefit from nightly dose of melatonin or pramipexole. In addition, preventive measures to protect patients from injuring themselves or others should be instituted in patients with RBD. Sleep has not been consistently improved in patients with Parkinson's disease following anti-Parkinsonian medication. Adjustment in the timing and choice of medication may be helpful in those patients with re-activation of parkinsonian symptoms during sleep at night. In some patients, dopamine agonists or longer-acting preparations of levodopa at bedtime may be helpful. Antihistamines such as diphenhydramine may promote sleep in addition to the modest anti-parkinsonian effect. A small dose of levodopa/carbidopa with a second dose later at night when the patient awakens may sometimes help those with insomnia.

Treatment of sleep-related respiratory dysrhythmia

The pathogenesis of sleep-related respiratory dysrhythmias in MSA and other disorders of AF is not clearly understood; therefore, the treatment remains difficult. Repeated hypoxemias during sleep are potentially harmful, not only to the immediate health of the patient but also to the long-term course of the illness. It is, therefore, important to diagnose and assess the type of respiratory dysrhythmia and take appropriate measures to ameliorate the disability. Improvement of the quality of life and prevention of life-threatening cardiac arrhythmias, pulmonary hypertension, and congestive cardiac failure should be the aim of treatment. Treatment should be directed at treating the upper airway obstructive sleep apnoea, central sleep apnoea including Cheyne–Stokes breathing and alveolar hypoventilation in patients with AF. Treatment includes general measures, pharmacological treatment, mechanical and surgical treatment as well as botulinum toxin injection.

General measures

Reduction or elimination of the risk factors that may enhance the sleep-related respiratory dysrhythmias constitutes the fundamental general principles. The patient must avoid alcohol and sedative–hypnotic drugs, which may further depress the respiratory centre. The role of alcohol and sedative–hypnotic drugs in disrupting the sleep architecture and in increasing the frequency and duration of sleep apnoeas is well established but the mechanism is not known. These agents may depress genioglossal muscle activity, thus selectively promoting upper airway obstructive apnoea.

Pharmacological treatment

Ideally, pharmacological treatment should be directed towards agents that will change the respiratory centre motor output selectively to stimulate the upper airway muscles to overcome the hypotonia of the genioglossal and other upper airway muscles, and so prevent central and obstructive apnoea. By correcting apnoea these agents might then improve the sleep architecture. However, no such selective and ideal agents have yet been found. Protriptyline, a non-sedating tricyclic antidepressant, and medroxyprogesterone acetate have been used with some success in patients with mild-to-moderate obstructive sleep apnoea. Acetazolamide has been used to treat central apnoea in MSA. However, one must be cautious because of the danger of increasing orthostatic hypotension resulting from diuresis and natriuresis. Unfortunately, these pharmacological agents have not been very helpful in patients with MSA because the natural history of the illness shows relentless progression despite treatment.

Mechanical treatment

CPAP treatment delivered through the nose has been the most significant recent development in the treatment of patients with OSAS. This treatment may be tried in patients with MSA showing predominantly obstructive or mixed sleep apnoea. One should use

Table 33.1 Sleep hygiene measures

◆ Keep a regular sleep–wake schedule, including weekends
◆ Avoid caffeinated beverages after lunch
◆ Avoid smoking, especially in the evening
◆ Avoid alcohol near bedtime
◆ Restrict sleep to amount needed to feel rested
◆ Do not go to bed hungry
◆ Adjust bedroom environment
◆ Do not engage in planning the next day's activities at bedtime
◆ Exercise regularly for about 20–30 minutes, preferably 4–5 hours before bedtime and not immediately before bedtime

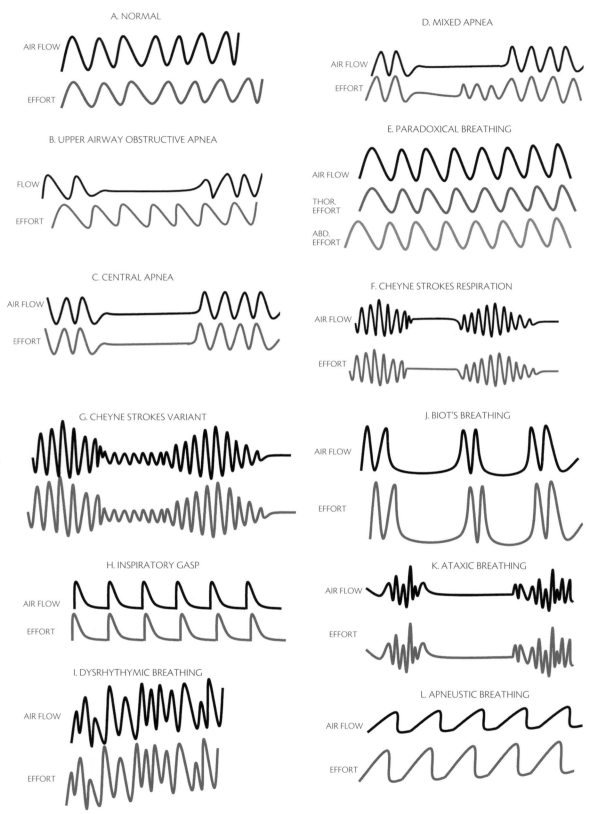

Fig. 33.6 Schematic diagram to show different types of breathing patterns in neurologic illnesses. (a) Normal breathing pattern. (b) Upper airway obstructive apnea. (c) Central apnea. (d) Mixed apnea (initial central followed by obstructive apnea). (e) Paradoxical breathing. (f) Cheyne-Stokes breathing. (g) Cheyne-Stokes variant pattern. (h) Inspiratory gasp. (i) Dysrhythmic breathing. (j) Biot's breathing (a special type of ataxic breathing characterized by 2–3 breaths of nearly equal volume followed by a long period of apnea). (k) Ataxic breathing. (l) Apneustic breathing. Reproduced with permission from Chokroverty S., 'Sleep, Breathing and Neurologic Disorders' in *Sleep Disorders Medicine: Basic Science, Technical Considerations, and Clinical Aspects*, pp. 436–498, Copyright Elsevier (2009).

the lowest pressure that will be effective in decreasing the number and duration of apnoeic events. Some patients may need bilevel positive airway pressure (BiPAP) where the inspiratory and the expiratory pressure can be altered independently. CPAP uses same pressure during inspiration/expiration but in BiPAP, the expiratory pressure can be lowered and this is more comfortable in some patients who cannot tolerate CPAP. If nasal CPAP or BiPAP shows a good response during PSG study in the laboratory, then this treatment may be considered in patients with moderate to severe obstructive or mixed sleep apnoea. There are several types of home CPAP or BiPAP units available for this purpose. In patients with obstructive sleep apnoea, following CPAP or BiPAP treatment there is dramatic improvement in apnoea–hypopnoea index along with amelioration of daytime hypersomnolence and correction of oxygen desaturation. However, it should be noted that the PSG study will show REM rebound with increased REM density and reduction of REM latency along with marked increase of slow-wave sleep. The long-term effect of CPAP or BiPAP treatment in the usual patients of OSAS is probably beneficial but cannot be stated definitely without prolonged follow-up, and the mechanism of its action is not definitely known. Recently Iranzo et al. (2000, 2004) and Ghorayeb et al. (2002, 2005) showed improvement in sleep quality after short-term and in some cases long-term CPAP or BiPAP treatment. Severity of the motor symptoms in MSA is a limiting factor for long-term adherence (compliance) and therefore, the best candidates are those at the relatively early stage of the illness. The natural history of the illness, however, is one of relentless progression despite some improvement of dysautonomic symptoms and sleep quality.

Surgical treatment

Tracheostomy remains the only effective treatment used as an emergency measure in patients with severe respiratory dysfunction accompanied by marked hypoxaemia and cyanosis, and in patients with sudden respiratory arrest after resuscitation by intubation. Tracheostomy is also the only form of treatment used successfully in patients with severe laryngeal stridor due to laryngeal abductor paralysis. An attempt should be made to wean a patient from a tracheostomy but the weaning procedure may be difficult in patients with MSA because of the progressive course of the illness. The decision to perform tracheostomy in a progressive neurodegenerative disease with AF with an overall unfavourable prognosis must be carefully weighed before pursing this therapy. Palliative measures, however, should be used to improve the patient's quality of life temporarily.

Several other surgical techniques, such as vocal cord lateralization, cordectomy, and arytenoidectomy have been used in a limited number of cases of MSA with stridor, bilateral vocal cord abductor paralysis, and sleep apnoea, with some success (see Iranzo et al. 2000). It should be noted that these surgical procedures are associated with an increased risk of aspiration, hoarseness, severe hypotension, and respiratory depression.

Botulinum toxin

Marlo et al. (2002) used unilateral botulinum toxin into the thyroarytenoid muscle in two patients with laryngeal dystonia causing stridor in MSA who had some improvement in their symptoms.

Despite considerable advances in our understanding in MSA and the sleep and respiratory disturbances observed in this illness, an effective treatment for the respiratory dysrhythmias continues to elude us. In AF other than MSA causing sleep and respiratory disturbances, similar lines of treatment may be tried.

References

Antzelevitch, C. (2006). Brugada syndrome. *Pacing Clin. Electrophysiol*, **29**, 1130–59.

Bannister, R. and Oppenheimer, D. R. (1972). Degenerative disease of the nervous system associated with autonomic failure. *Brain* **95**, 457–74.

Bannister, R., Gibson, W., Michaels, L., and Oppenheimer, D. R. (1981). Laryngeal abductor paralysis in multiple system atrophy. *Brain* **104**, 351–68.

Baumann, C. R., Dauvilliers, Y., Mignot, E., Bassetti, CL. (2004). Normal CSF hypocretin-1 (orexin-A) levels in dementia with Lewy bodies associated with excessive daytime sleepiness. *European Neurol* **52**, 73–6.

Benarroch, E. E., Smithson, I. L., Low, P. A., et al. (1998). Depletion of catecholaminergic neurons of the rostral ventrolateral medulla in multiple systems atrophy with autonomic failure. *Ann. Neurol.* **43**(2), 156–63.

Benarroch, E. E., Schmeichel, A. M., Low, P. A., et al. (2008). Loss of A5 noradrenergic neurons in multiple system atrophy. *Acta Neuropathol.* **115**(6), 629–34.

Benarroch, E. E., Schmeichel, A. M., Parisi, J. E. (2001). Depletion of cholinergic neurons of the medullary arcuate nucleus in multple system atrophy. *Autonomic Neuroscience* **87**(2–3), 293–9.

Benarroch, E. E., Schmeichel, A. M. (2001). Depletion of corticotrophin-releasing factor neurons in the pontine micturition area in multiple system atrophy. *Ann Neurol* **50**(5), 640–5.

Benarroch, E. E., Schmeichel, A. M., Parisi, J. E. (2003a). Depletion of mesopontine cholinergic and sparing of raphe neurons in multiple system atrophy. *Neurology* **59**(6), 944–6.

Benarroch, E. E., Schmeichel, A. M., Low, P. A., et al. (2003b). Depletion of ventromedullary NK-1 receptor-immunoreactive neurons in multiple system atrophy. *Brain* **126**(pt 10), 2183–90.

Benarroch, E. E., Schmeichel, A. M., Low, P. A., et al. (2007). Depletion of putative chemosensitive respiratory neurons in the ventral medullary surface in multiple system atrophy. *Brain* **130**(2), 469–75.

Benarroch, E. E., Schmeichel, A. M., Low, P. A., et al. (2004). Involvement of medullary serotonergic groups in multiple system atrophy. *Ann. Neurol.* **55**(3), 418–22.

Benarroch, E. E., Schmeichel, A. M., Sandroni, P., et al. (2006). Involvement of vagal autonomic nuclei in multiple system atrophy and Lewy body disease. *Neurology* **66**, 378–83.

Benarroch, E. E., Schmeichel, A. M., Sandroni, P., et al. (2007). Involvement of hypocreatin neurons in multiple system atrophy. *Acta Neurophathol* **113**(1), 75–80.

Benarroch, E. E. (2007). Brainstem respiratory chemosensitivity: new insights and clinical implications. *Neurology* **68**, 2140–43.

Berger, A. J., Mitchel, R. A., and Severinghaus, J. N. (1977). Regulation of respiration. *New Engl. J. Med.* **297**, 138–43.

Boeve, B. F., Silber, M. H., Saper, C. B., et al. (2007). Pathophysiology of REM sleep behaviour disorder and relevance to neurodegenerative disease. *Brain* **130**, 2770–88.

Boeve, B. F. (2010). REM Sleep Behaviour Disorder. Updated review of the core features, the REM sleep behaviour disorder-neurodegenerative disease association, evolving concepts, controversies, and future directions. *Ann. NY Acad. Sci.* **1184**, 15–54.

Bottini, P., Dottorini, M. L., Cristina Cordoni, M., et al. (2003). Sleep-disordered breathing in non-obese diabetic subjects with autonomic neuropathy. *Eur. Respir. J* **22**, 654–60.

Casella, E. B., Bousso, A., Corvello, C. M., et al. (2005). Episodic somnolence in an infant with Riley-Day syndrome. *Pediatr Neurol*, **32**, 273–4.

Chokroverty, S. (1991). Functional anatomy of the autonomic nervous system: autonomic dysfunction and disorders of the CNS. In *Correlative neuroanatomy and neuropathology for the clinical neurologist.* American Academy of Neurology Course No. 144. American Academy of Neurology, Minneapolis.

Chokroverty, S. (2003). An overview of normal sleep. In *Sleep and Movement Disorders,* (eds. S. Chokroverty, W. Hening, A. Walters), Elsevier/Butterworth, Philadelphia.

Chokroverty, S., Montagna, P. (2009). Sleep, breathing and neurological disorders. In *Sleep disorders medicine: basic science, technical considerations and clinical aspects,* 3nd edition, (ed. S. Chokroverty), Saunders/Elsevier, Philadelphia.

Chokroverty, S., Barron, K. D., Katz, F. M., Del Greco, F., and Sharp, J. T. (1969). The syndrome of primary orthostatic hypotension. *Brain* **92,** 743–68.

Chokroverty, S., Sharp, J. T., and Barron, K. D. (1978). Periodic respiration in erect posture in Shy–Drager syndrome. *J. Neurol. Neurosurg. Psychiat.* **41,** 980–6.

Chokroverty, S., Sachdeo, R., and Masdeu, J. (1984). Autonomic dysfunction and sleep apnoea in olivopontocerebellar degeneration. *Arch. Neurol.* **41,** 926–31.

Chokroverty, S., Khurana, R., Bhatt, M., *et al.* (2001). Sleep disturbance in postural tachycardia syndrome (POTS), an entity in search of an identity. *Neurology,* **56**(suppl 3), A426 (abstract).

Consensus statement on the definition of orthostatic hypotension, pure autonomic failure, and multiple system atrophy. (1996). *Neurology* **46,** 1470.

Corbin, D. O., Williams, A. C. (1987). Stridor during dystonic phases of Parkinson's disease [letter]. *J Neurol. Neurosurg. Psychiatry* **50,** 821–22.

De Lecea, L., Kilduff, T. S., Peyson, C., *et al.* (1998). The hypocretins : hypothalamus-specific peptices with neuroexcitatory activity. *Proc. Natl. Acad. Sci. USA* **95,** 322–27.

Efthimiou, J., Ellis, S. J., Hardie, R. J., Stern, G. M. (1986). Sleep apnoea in idiopathic and postencephalitic Parkinsonism. In: Yahr, M. D., Bergmann, K. J., eds. *Parkinson's Disease (Advances in Neurology 45).* New York: Raven Press, 275–76.

Freilich, S., Goff, E. A., Malaweera, A. S., *et al.* (2010). Sleep architecture and attenuated heart rate response to arousal from sleep in patients with autonomic failure. *Sleep Med* **11,** 87–92.

Gadoth, N., Solol, J., and Lavie, P. (1983). Sleep structure and nocturnal disordered breathing in familial dysautonomia. *J. Neurol. Sci.* **60,** 117–25.

Gagnon, J. F., Bedard, M. A., Fantini, M. L., *et al.* (2002). REM sleep behaviour disorder and REM sleep without atonia in Parkinson's disease. *Neurology* **59,** 585–9.

Gagnon, A. F., Postuma, R. B., Mazza, S., *et al.* (2006). Rapid-eye-movement sleep behaviour disorder and neurodegenerative diseases. *Lancet Neurol.* **5,** 424–32.

Gami, A. S., Howard, D. E., Olson, E. J., Somers, V. K. (2005). Day-night pattern of sudden death in obstructive sleep apnoea. *N Engl. J Med.,* **352,** 1206–14.

Ghorayeb, J., Yekhlef, F., Bioulac, B., Tison, F. (2005). Continuous positive airway pressure for sleep-related breathing disorders in multiple system atrophy: long-term acceptance. *Sleep Med* **6,** 359–62.

Ghorayeb, I., Yekhef, F., Chrysotome, V., *et al.* (2002). Sleep disorders and their determinants in multiple system atrophy. *J Neurol. Neurosurg. Psychiatry* **72,** 798–800.

Gilman, S., Chervin, R. D., Koeppe, R. A., *et al.* (2003). Obstructive sleep apnoea is related to a thalamic cholinergic deficit in MSA. *Neurology* **61,** 35–9.

Gilman, S., Wenning, G. K., Low, P. A., *et al.* (2008). Second consensus statement on the diagnosis of multiple system atrophy. *Neurology* **71,** 670–76.

Guilleminault, C., Briskin, J. G., Greenfield, M. S., and Silvestri, R. (1981). The impact of autonomic nervous system dysfunction on breathing during sleep. *Sleep* **4,** 263–78.

Hening, W. A., Allen, R., Walters, A. S., Chokroverty, S. (2009). Motor functions and dysfunctions of sleep. In: Chokroverty, S. (ed): *Sleep Disorders Medicine: Basic Science, technical considerations and clinical aspects.* Philadelphia: Saunders/Elsevier/Butterworth.

Hoffstein, V. and Mateika, S. (1994). Cardiac arrhythmias, snoring and sleep apnoea. *Chest* **106,** 466–71.

Iber, C., Ancoli-Israel, S., Chesson, A. L., Jr., Quan, S. F. (2007). *The AASM manual for the scoring of sleep and associated events.* American Academy of Sleep Medicine, Westchester, IL.

Iranzo, A., Santamaria, J., Tolosa, E., *et al.* (2004). Long-term effect of CPAP in the treatment of nocturnal stridor in multiple system atrophy, *Neurology,* **63,** 930–2.

Iranzo, A., Santamaria, J., Tolosa, E., on behalf of the Barcelona Multiple System Atrophy Group. (2000). Continuous positive airway pressure eliminates nocturnal stridor in multiple system atrophy. *Lancet,* **356,** 1329–30.

Iranzo, A., Santamaria, J., Tolosa, E. (2009). The clinical and pathophysiological relevance of REM sleep behaviour disorder in neurodegenerative disease. Clinical Review. *Sleep Med. Rev.* **13,** 385–401.

Ito, R., Hamada, I. I., Yokoyama, A., *et al.* (2005). Successful treatment of obstructive sleep apnoea syndrome improves autonomic nervous system dysfunction. *Clin. Ex. Hypertens.,* **27,** 259–61.

Larner, A. J., Mathias, C. J., Rossor, M. N. (2000). Autonomic failure preceding dementia with Lewy bodies. *J Neurol.* **247,** 229–31.

Lockwood, A. H. (1976). Shy–Drager syndrome with abnormal respirations and antidiuretic hormone release. *Arch. Neurol.* **33,** 292–5.

Loewy, A. D. and Spyer, K. M. (1990). *Central regulation of autonomic functions.* Oxford University Press, Oxford.

Lu, J., Sherman, D., Devor, M., Saper, C. B. (2006). A putative flip-flop switch for control of REM sleep. *Nature* **441,** 589.

Luppi, P-H., Clement, O., Sapin, E., *et al.* (2011). The neural network responsible for paradoxical sleep and its dysfunctions causing narcolepsy and rapid eye movement (REM) behavior disorder. *Sleep Med Rev.,* **15,** 153–63.

Mackenzi, I. A. (2000). Dementia with Lewy Bodies, *Neuroscience News,* **3,** 28.

McCarley, R. W. (2007). Neurobidogy of REM and NREM Sleep, *Sleed Med* **8,** 302–30.

McKeith, I. G. (2006). Consensus guidelines for the clinical and pathologic diagnosis of dementia with Lewy bodies (DLB): report of the Consortium on DLB International Workshop. *J Alzheimers Dis.,* **9**(Suppl 3), 417–23.

McNicholas, W. T., Rutherford, R., Grossman, R., Moldofsky, H., Zamel, N., and Phillipson, E. A. (1983). Abnormal respiratory pattern generation during sleep in patients with autonomic dysfunction. *Am. Rev. Respir. Dis.* **128,** 429–33.

Merlo, I. M., Occhini, A., Pacchetti, C., Alfonsini, E. (2002). Not paralysis, but dystonia causes stridor in multiple system atrophy. *Neurology,* **58,** 649–52.

Miyamoto, T., Miyamoto, M., Inoue, Y., *et al.* (2006). Reduced cardiac 123I-MIBG scintigraphy in idiopathic REM sleep behavior disorder. *Neurology.,* **67,** 2236–8.

Muller, J. E., Ludmer, P. L., Willich, S. N. *et al.* (1987). Circadian variation in the frequency of sudden cardiac death. *Circulation* **75,** 131–8

Munschauer, F. E., Loh, L., Bannister, R., and Newsom-Davis, J. (1990). Abnormal respiration and sudden death during sleep in multiple system atrophy with autonomic failure. *Neurology* **40,** 677–9.

Parish, J. M. and Shepard, J. W., Jr (1990). Cardiovascular effects of sleep disorders. *Chest* **97,** 1220–6.

Peltier, A. C., Consens, F. B., Sheikh, *et al.* (2007). Autonomic dysfunction in obstructive sleep apnoea is associated with impaired glucose tolerance. *Sleep Med* **8,** 149–55.

Plazzi, G., Corsini, R., Provini, F., *et al.* (1997). REM sleep behaviour disorders in multiple system atrophy. *Neurology,* **48,** 1094–7.

Postuma, R. B., Gagnon, J. F., Vendetta, M., Montplaisir, J. Y. (2009). Markers of neurodegeneration in indiopathic rapid eye movement sleep behaviour disorder and Parkinson's disease. *Brain* **132**, 3298–3307.

Postuma, R. B., Gagnon, J. F., Vendette, M., *et al.* (2011). Olfaction and color vision identify impending neurodegeneration in rapid eye movement sleep behavior disorder. *Ann. Neurol.*, **69**, 811–8.

Roche, F., Xuong, A. N., Court-Fortune, I., *et al.* (2003). Relationship among the severity of sleep apnoea syndrome, cardiac arrhythmias, and autonomic imbalance. *Pacing Clin. Electrophysiol.*, **26**, 669–77.

Sadaoka T., Kakitsuba, N., Fujiwara, Y. *et al.* (1996). Sleep-related breathing disorders in patients with multiple system atrophy and vocal fold palsy. *Sleep* **19**, 479–84.

Sakurai, T., Amemiya, A., Ishii, M., *et al.* (1998). Orexins and orexin receptors : a family of hypothalamic neuropeptides and G protein-coupled receptors that regulate feeding behaviour. *Cell* **92**, 573–85.

Schenck, C. H. and Mahowald, M. W. (1996). Delayed emergence of a parkinsonian disorder in 38% of 29 older males initially diagnosed with idiopathic REM sleep behaviour disorder. *Neurology* **46**, 388–93.

Schenck, C. H., Mahowald, M. W. (2002). REM sleep behaviour disorder: Clinical, developmental, and neuroscience perspectives 16 years after its formal identification in sleep. *Sleep* **25**, 120–38.

Schmeichel, A. M., Buchhalter, L. C., Low, P. A., *et al.* (2008). Mesopontine cholinergic neuron involvement in Lewy body dementia and multiple system atrophy. *Neurology* **70**(5), 368–73.

Shy, G. M. and Drager, G. A. (1960). A neurological syndrome associated with orthostatic hypotension. *Arch. Neurol., Chicago* **2**, 511–27.

Silber, M. H., Levine, S. (2000). Stridor and death in multiple system atrophy. *Mov. Disord.* **15**, 699–704.

Steriade, M., McCarley, R. W. (2005). *Brain Control of Wakefulness and Sleep*, ed. 2. New York: Kluwer Academic?plenum Publishers.

Thaisetthawatkul, P., Boeve, B. F., Benarroch, E. E., *et al.* (2004). Autonomic dysfunction in dementia with Lewy bodies. *Neurology* **62**, 1804–9.

Vas, C. J., Parsonage, M., Lord, O. C. (1965). Parkinsonism associated with laryngeal spasm. *J Neurol. Neurosurg. Psychiatr.* **28**, 401–03.

Vatta, M., Dumaine, R., Varghese, G., *et al.* (2002). Genetic and biophysical basis of sudden unexplained nocturnal death syndrome (SUNDS), a disease allelic to Brugada syndrome. *Hum. Mol. Genet.*, **11**, 337–45.

Verrier, R. L. and Kirby, D. A. (1988). Sleep and cardiac arrhythmias. *Ann. New York Acad. Sci.* **533**, 238–51.

Vetrugno, R., Provini, F., Cortelli, P., *et al.* (2004). Sleep disorders in multiple system atrophy: a correlative video-polysomnographic study. *Sleep Med.*, **5**, 21–30.

Vetrugno, R., Alessandria, M., D'Angelo, R., *et al.* (2009). Status dissociatus evolving from REM sleep behaviour disorder in multiple system atrophy. *Sleep Med.* **10**, 247–52.

Vincken, W. G., Gauthier, S. G., Dollfuss, R. E., *et al.* (1984). Involvement of upper airway muscles in extrapyramidal disorders. *New Eng. J Med.* **311**, 438–42.

Wenning, G. K., Gesser, F., Stampler-Kountchev, M., Tison, F. (2003). Multiple system atrophy: an update. *Mov. Disord.*, Vol. 18 (Suppl. 6), pp. S34–42.

Wenning, G. K., Scherfler, C., Granata, R., *et al.* (1999). Time course of symptomatic orthostatic hypotension and urinary incontinence in patients with postmortem confirmed Parkinsonian syndromes: a clinicopathological study. *J Neurol. Neurosurg. Psychiatry* **67**, 620–3.

Wenning, G. K., Stefanova, N., Jellinger, K. A., *et al.* (2008). Multiple system atrophy: a primary oligodendrogliopathy. *Ann. Neurol.* **64**, 239–46.

Wenning, G. K., Tison, F., Ben Shlomo, Y., *et al.* (1997). Multiple system atrophy: a review of 203 pathologically proven cases. *Mov. Disord.* **12**, 133.

Wichter, T., Matheja, P., Eckardt, L., *et al.* (2002). Cardiac autonomic dysfunction in Brugada syndrome. *Circulation*, **105**, 702–6.

CHAPTER 34

Vestibular and autonomic interaction

Linda Luxon and Waheeda Pagarkar

Key points

- Vestibular dysfunction or stimulation may be associated with autonomic symptoms and autonomic disorders may cause dizziness.
- Vestibular autonomic interactions are mediated by a network of neural pathways between the vestibular nuclei and centres such as the parabrachial nucleus and the nucleus of the tractus solitarius.
- Autonomic responses to vestibular stimuli are mediated by vestibular connections to the medullary centres of cardiorespiratory control and vomiting.
- Vestibulo-autonomic interactions are prominent in clinical conditions such as motion sickness and in the relationship between migraine, anxiety, and dizziness

An interaction between the vestibular and autonomic systems has long been suspected. Jones (1918) noted that caloric stimulation, seasickness and acute vestibular dysfunction all produce similar autonomic manifestations. It is now well recognized that vestibular stimulation, be it pathological or physiological, is commonly accompanied by autonomic symptoms that may be as unpleasant as the dizziness itself, a classic example being motion sickness. Dizziness and vertigo frequently evoke affective changes, mediated by vestibulo-autonomic interactions, and psychological disorders such as anxiety and panic, which cause autonomic system stimulation, are associated with vestibular symptoms. In addition, movement and exercise produce demands on the cardiorespiratory system and it is logical to assume that, close integration between vestibular and autonomic circuits serves to bring about a coordinated cardiorespiratory response to movement. Vestibulo-autonomic interactions occur in a variety of conditions as outlined in Table 34.1. This review will explore vestibular autonomic links from a neuro-otological perspective and discuss their clinical implications.

Neural pathways for vestibulo-autonomic interactions

A general schema of vestibular connections mediating autonomic responses is outlined in Fig. 34.1. Ascending vestibulo-autonomic pathways connect the vestibular nuclei to the parabrachial nucleus (PBN), whereas descending vestibulo-autonomic pathways connect them to the medullary centres mediating cardiorespiratory changes and vomiting. There is a convergence of both visceral and vestibular information in the PBN, nucleus tractus solitarius (NTS) and ventrolateral medullary reticular formation, and this integration of information provides a central representation of gravitoinertial forces. The NTS receives afferent inputs from somatic, cranial, visceral and vestibular afferents and projects to the medullary raphe nucleus and ventrolateral medullary reticular formation, which in turn project on to sympathetic preganglionic neurons, to mediate sympathetic responses. The NTS influences parasympathetic output by projections to nucleus ambiguous and dorsal motor nucleus of the vagus nerve. Connections of the PBN with the amygdala and insular cortex mediate affective responses of vestibular dysfunction and those with the locus coeruleus mediate alerting responses (e.g. to caloric stimulation). The cerebellum appears to play a part in modulating the brainstem autonomic reflexes just as it has a regulatory role in vestibulo-ocular reflexes (Balaban 1996, Balaban 2004).

Vestibular dysfunction and autonomic control

Acute unilateral vestibular dysfunction produces both autonomic symptoms attributed to responses of the gastrointestinal tract and the nervous system (e.g. nausea, malaise, drowsiness, abdominal awareness, anxiety, distress, dread, reduced vigilance) and autonomic signs (e.g. changes in salivation, gastric motility, vomiting, endocrine responses, cold sweating, pallor, increased blood flow to skeletal muscles, and changes in heart rate). Most autonomic symptoms (e.g. vomiting) gradually resolve as vestibular compensation occurs, but others such as nausea and malaise often continue, and the reason for this is not clear. Just as referred pain is due to convergence of visceral and somatic afferents on common spinal segments, similarly convergence of vestibular and autonomic information in the brainstem may mediate referred symptoms from the vestibular system to visceral sites (e.g. vomiting) (Balaban 1999).

Autonomic responses accompanying vestibular tests

Caloric testing activates a number of cortical and subcortical structures, which receive visual, optokinetic and proprioceptive projections,

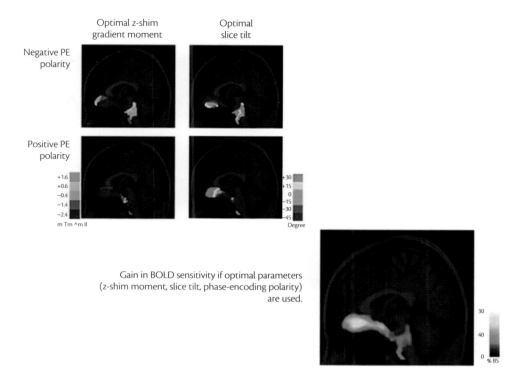

Negative PE polarity — Optimal z-shim gradient moment — Optimal slice tilt

Positive PE polarity

+1.6
+0.6
−0.4
−1.4
−2.4
m Tm ^m II

+30
+15
0
−15
−30
−45
Degree

Gain in BOLD sensitivity if optimal parameters (z-shim moment, slice tilt, phase-encoding polarity) are used.

30
40
0
% BS

Plate 1 Compensatory measures required to optimize functional magnetic resonance imaging (fMRI) signal acquisition from orbitofrontal cortex and brainstem (Weiskopf et al. 2005, Deichmann et al. 2002, 2003). The values are based on group means from five subjects scanned using T2* sensitive echoplanar imaging (EPI) on a Siemens 3T Allegra scanner. The four smaller figures show respectively the optimal slice tilt and z-shim moments for either a positive or negative phase encoding (PE) polarity. The signal (blood oxygenation level dependent [BOLD]) sensitivity gain is determined in comparison with a standard EPI (tilt 0º, z-shim moment = 0, PE positive). See also Fig. 12.2. Reprinted from *Neuroimage* **1**;33(2) Weiskopf N, Hutton C, Josephs O, Deichmann, Optimal EPI parameters for reduction of susceptibility-induced BOLD sensitivity losses: a whole-brain analysis at 3 T and 1.5 T. R., 493–504, Copyright 2006, with permission from Elsevier.

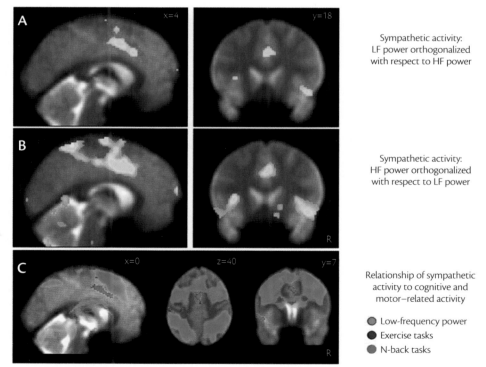

Sympathetic activity: LF power orthogonalized with respect to HF power

Sympathetic activity: HF power orthogonalized with respect to LF power

Relationship of sympathetic activity to cognitive and motor–related activity

● Low-frequency power
● Exercise tasks
● N-back tasks

Plate 2 Functional magnetic resonance imaging (fMRI) study of sympathetic influences on heart rate variability. Subjects were scanned using fMRI performing a cognitive task (n-back) at two levels of difficulty, and two levels of an exercise task, while echocardiography was continuously acquired during scanning. Post hoc analyses enabled extraction of a timeline for sympathetic (low frequency, LF) power in heart rate variability, which could be related to changes in regional brain activity, controlling for the task performance and high frequency (HF, parasympathetic) influences on heart rate. **A** and **B**: The location of brain activity correlated with cardiac sympathetic influences, respectively keeping and losing variance shared with parasympathetic changes. **C**: The activation of dorsal cingulate and insula cortices can be anatomically distinguished from activity related to cognitive work or motor task performance. These group data sets are plotted on sections of a mean functional (echoplanar T2*) image from the group illustrating the anatomical resolution of fMRI and the caudal orbitomedial area of signal loss due to susceptibility artefact. See also Fig. 12.5. Reprinted from Critchley HD et al., Dolan RJ, Human cingulate cortex and autonomic control: converging neuroimaging and clinical evidence. *Brain*. 2003, **126**(Pt 10):2139–52, by permisssion of Oxford University Press.

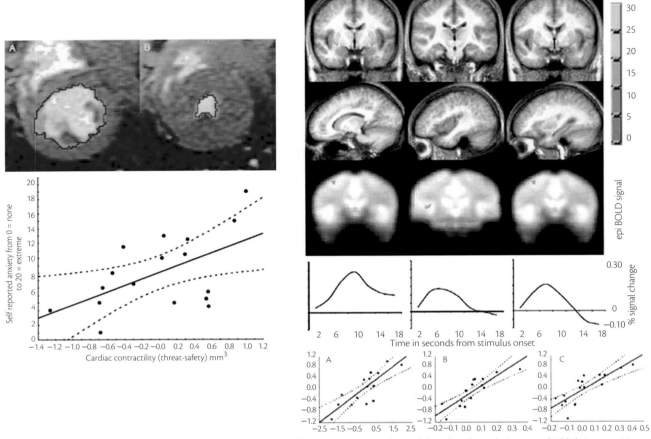

Plate 3 Heart–brain correlations during stress. Correlations between regional brain activity and cardiac end diastolic volume during stress, highlighting a positive relationship between amygdala insula and prefrontal activity and cardiac filling induced autonomically by anticipatory fear. The figure to the left shows cross-sectional magnetic resonance image of the left ventricle at **(A)** maximum diastole and **(B)** maximal systole. The scatter plot beneath relates measured cardiac contractility with self-report measures of anxiety in threat versus safety conditions. The figures to the right illustrate clusters of brain activation during threat in **(A)** amygdala, **(B)** insula and **(C)** prefrontal cortex positively associated with cardiac contractility to the threat of shock. The first two rows display the location and size of the clusters, with the colour of the cluster indexing the size of the effect. The third row is composed of the same clusters superimposed on an averaged EPI BOLD signal indicating adequate signal coverage for each cluster. The fourth row is the averaged haemodynamic response function to the threat condition for each cluster. The last row contains the scatter plots for each cluster with the difference in cardiac contractility (threat minus safety) on the x axis and the difference in percentage signal change (threat minus safety) for each cluster. See also Fig. 12.6. With permission from Dalton KM, Kalin NH, Grist TM, Davidson RJ. 2005. *J Cogn. Neurosci.* MIT Press.

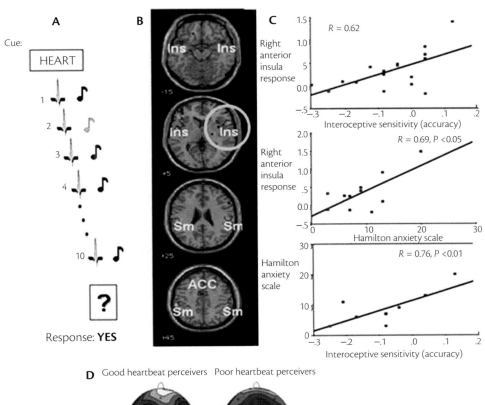

A

Cue:

HEART

1
2
3
4

10

Response: **YES**

B

C

Right anterior insula response

$R = 0.62$

Interoceptive sensitivity (accuracy)

Right anterior insula response

$R = 0.69, P < 0.05$

Hamilton anxiety scale

Hamilton anxiety scale

$R = 0.76, P < 0.01$

Interoceptive sensitivity (accuracy)

D Good heartbeat perceivers   Poor heartbeat perceivers

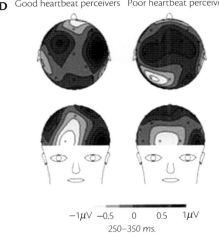

−1μV −0.5   0   0.5   1μV
250–350 ms.

Plate 4 Interoception and feeling states neural activity during interoceptive awareness. Healthy individuals were scanned while they performed a heartbeat detection task (adapted from that used in Wiens et al. 2000) in which they judged the timing of their own heartbeats to auditory tones (triggered by their heartbeats). **A:** Subjects were cued to attend to their heart then a series of 10 tones would be played that were either synchronous with their finger pulse, or delayed by 500 ms. Individuals made the judgement at the end of each trial of 10 beats. In a control condition ('note'), subjects attended only to the quality of the notes, identifying the presence of a subtle change in note pitch in the sequence. **B:** Activity when attending to heartbeat timing was enhanced (relative to the exteroceptive 'note' task) in bilateral insula, bilateral somatomotor and anterior cingulate cortices. **C:** Only activity in right anterior insula correlated with conscious awareness of the timing of heartbeats i.e. interoceptive sensitivity (performance accuracy on the task, relative to the control condition). Across individuals, there were significant correlations between activity of right anterior cortex, interoceptive sensitivity and day-to-day experience of anxiety symptoms, consistent with a proposal that right anterior insula is a substrate for feeling states generated from afferent visceral responses. **D:** Beneath shows a figure from Pollatos and Schandry (2004) showing a right prefrontal brain potential time locked 250–300 ms after the echocardiograph R wave of each heartbeat. With permission from Wiens S, Mezzacappa ES, Katkin ES. (2001). Heartbeat detection and the experience of emotions. *Cognition and Emotion* **14**:417–427, reprinted by permission of the publisher (Taylor and Francis Group, http://informaworld.com). See also Fig. 12.7. Figure D from Pollatos O, Schandry R. 2004. Accuracy of heartbeat perception is reflected in the amplitude of the heartbeat-evoked brain potential. *Psychophsyiology* **41**:476–482, Wiley.

A *Visual presentation during task*

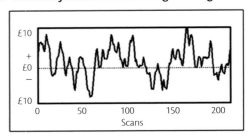

B *Random function determining winnings*

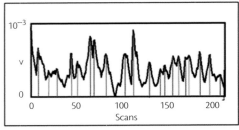

C *EDA in one individual during task*

D *Activity covarying with EDA*

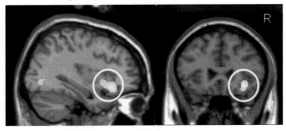

Right anterior insula/orbitofrontal cortex

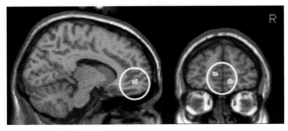

Bilateral ventromedial prefrontal cortex

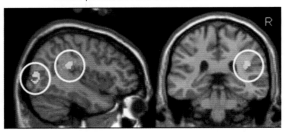

Inferior parietal lobe and extrastriate cortex

Plate 5 Regional activity relating to electrodermal activity during gambling task performance. **A:** Six subjects were scanned using functional magnetic resonance imaging performing a decision-related gambling task. In individual trials, the subject was presented with pairs of playing cards and was required to respond to one or other in order to win money. Immediate feedback was given (tick/cross replacing the question mark) indicating if the individual had won or lost money, and the level of overall winnings modified accordingly. **B:** Unknown to the subject, feedback (wins/losses) on any particular trial was predetermined by a binomial random walk. **C:** Performing the task produced individualized fluctuations in electrodermal activity (EDA) recorded throughout the task (black line). In a covariance analysis these continuous data were used to examine activity covarying with EDA. Also, peaks in EDA responses were identified (illustrated in red) and used in an event-related analysis. **D:** Brain regions covarying with EDA. Significant group activity is mapped on parasagittal and coronal sections of a template brain and is observed in anterior insula and ventromedial prefrontal cortices, extrastriate visual cortex, and right parietal lobe. See also Fig. 12.8. With permission from Critchley (2000a).

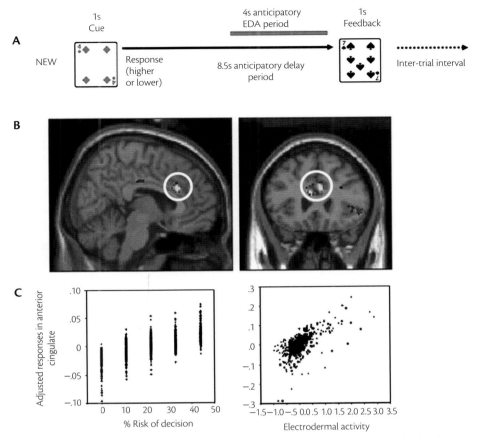

Plate 6 Modulation of delay-period activity by risk and anticipatory electrodermal activity arousal. **A:** Diagram of individual trial. Subjects made a response to a cue card, judging if next (feedback) card would be higher or lower. Activity during the delay period before outcome was examined for modulation by riskiness of decision and by anticipatory electrodermal activity (EDA) response (mean EDA in 4 seconds prior to outcome feedback). **B** and **C:** Activity within anterior cingulate was modulated as function of both risk and EDA. From Critchley et al. 2001a, with permission. Damage to both dorsolateral prefrontal and anterior cingulate cortices has previously been observed to diminish EDA response magnitude (Zahn et al. 1999 Tranel 2000). The neuroimaging findings strongly implicate anterior cingulate cortex in the integration of cognitive processes (e.g. processing risk and expectancy) with EDA and other bodily states of arousal. The role of the dorsolateral prefrontal activation in these studies may reflect a more selective relationship between contextual control of bodily arousal during cognitive processing related to expectation, action, and experience. See also Fig. 12.9. Reprinted from *Neuron*, **29**, Critchley HD, Mathias CJ, Dolan RJ., Neural activity relating to reward anticipation in the human brain, 537–545, Copyright 2001, with permission from Elsevier.

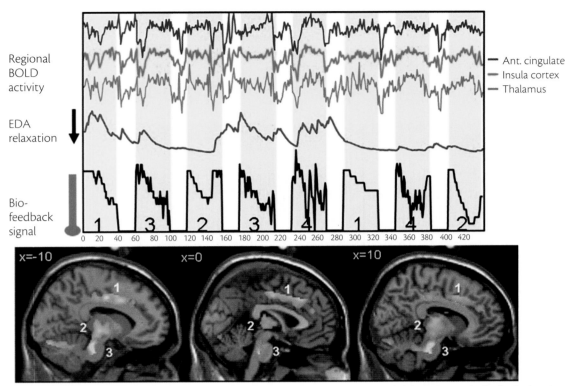

Plate 7 Brain activity during biofeedback relaxation magnetic resonance imaging study. Subjects were scanned while performing biofeedback relaxation tasks, which differed either in the sensitivity or in the accuracy of the feedback signal. Compared with rest, performance of biofeedback tasks was associated with activity in a distributed network of cortical, subcortical and brainstem regions, including many putative autonomic control centres. The upper figure shows the relationship of regional brain activity, measured electrodermal activity (EDA) and the quality of the biofeedback signal during imaging. The figure below shows group activity plotted on a parasagittal section of a template brain illustrating involvement of cingulate, thalamus, hypothalamus pons and cerebellum in biofeedback task performance. The figure to the right illustrates increased activity within anterior cingulate cortex in association with decreasing EDA arousal across the whole experiment. See also Fig. 12.10. Reprinted from *Neuroimage*, **6**, Critchley HD, Melmed RN, Featherstone E, Mathias CJ, Dolan RJ, Volitional control of autonomic arousal: a functional magnetic resonance study, 909–19, Copyright 2002, with permission from Elsevier.

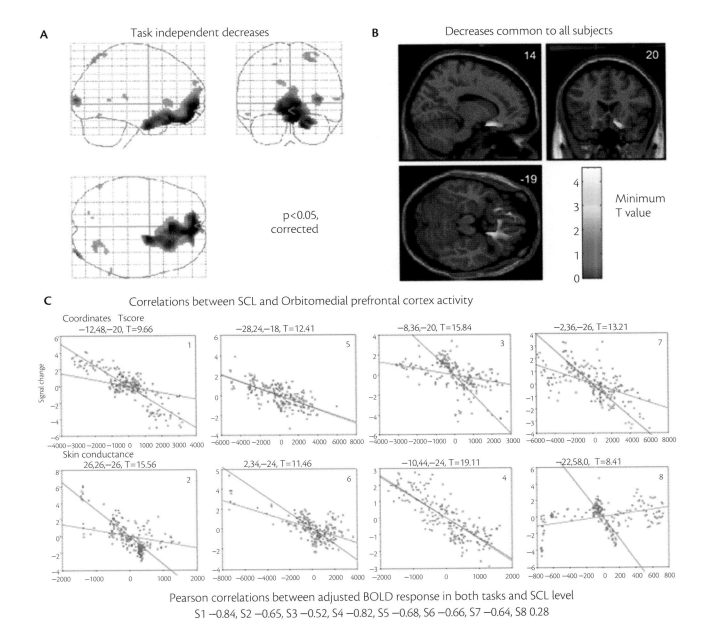

A Task independent decreases

p<0.05, corrected

B Decreases common to all subjects

14
20
−19

4
3
2
1
0
Minimum T value

C Correlations between SCL and Orbitomedial prefrontal cortex activity

Coordinates Tscore
−12,48,−20, T=9.66

−28,24,−18, T=12.41

−8,36,−20, T=15.84

−2,36,−26, T=13.21

Signal change
Skin conductance

26,26,−26, T=15.56

2,34,−24, T=11.46

−10,44,−24, T=19.11

−22,58,0, T=8.41

Pearson correlations between adjusted BOLD response in both tasks and SCL level
S1 −0.84, S2 −0.65, S3 −0.52, S4 −0.82, S5 −0.68, S6 −0.66, S7 −0.64, S8 0.28

Plate 8 Regional brain activity associated with decreases in skin conductance level. (A) Regional brain activity related to task-independent decreases in skin conductance level (SCL). Decreases in SCL were associated with increased activity in VMPFC and OFC. A conjunction analysis was used to identify regional activity negatively correlating with across both biofeedback relaxation and arousal tasks ($P < 0.05$, corrected). (B) Regional brain activity associated with decreases in tonic skin conductance level common across all subjects (conjunction analysis associated with decreases in skin conductance), presented on a normalized template brain scan ($P < 0.05$, corrected). The scale represents the minimum t value shared by all eight subjects contributing to the conjunction analysis. Common brain activity was found in VMPFC and OFC. (C) Plots of individual subjects' data showing correlations between skin conductance and ventromedial and orbitofrontal BOLD activity during biofeedback relaxation (light dots) and arousal tasks (dark dots). Data are plotted for the peak voxels of activity identified in first-level individual subject analyses. Pearson correlations showed significant negative correlation between adjusted VMPFC and OFC BOLD responses and task-independent SCL activity in the eight subjects. See also Fig. 12.11. Copyright from Nagai et al. (2004) with permission from Elsevier.

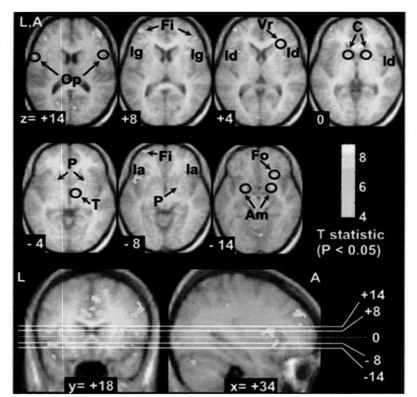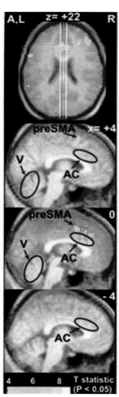

Plate 9 Brain activity related to air hunger. Statistical maps of significant brain activation associated with periods of air hunger for the group (same T statistic map as in Fig. 12.4) superimposed onto the group mean structural image. Selected axial slices are displayed illustrating the effect size of regions of interest: insula, prefrontal cortex, basal ganglia, and amygdala. 'L, A' indicates left anterior. Horizontal slices are depicted on a coronal image and sagittal image. Relevant local maxima are labelled: Am, amygdala; C, caudate; Fi, inferior frontal gyrus; Fo, orbital frontal gyrus; Ia, insula (agranular); Id, insula (dysgranular); Ig, insula (granular); Op, operculum; P, putamen; T, thalamus; Vr, vertical ramus lateral fissure. See also Fig. 12.12. With permission from the American Physiological Society (Evans *et al.* 2002).

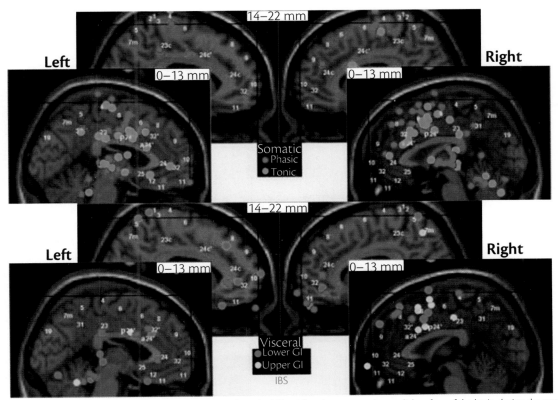

Plate 10 Viscerosensory stimulation. The centre of each reported regional cerebral blood flow increase on the medial surface of the brain during the experience of phasic or tonic somatic pain (top) and during the experience of visceral pain (bottom) in the lower or upper gastrointestinal (GI) tract. Responses to lower GI distension in patients with irritable bowel syndrome are shown in purple. The responses are plotted onto the standard MNI brain provided with SPM99 and the Brodmann's areas shown. The ACC is divided into perigenual (24), anterior midcingulate (a24') and posterior midcingulate (p24'). See also Fig. 12.13. With permission from Derbyshire SW. 2003. Visceral afferent pathways and functional brain imaging. *Scientific World Journal.* **3**:1065–80.

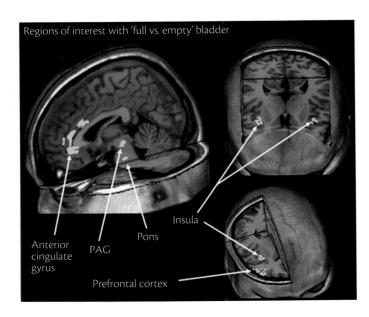

Plate 11 Brain activity related to urinary control. Summary of regions of interest comparing 'full versus empty' bladder conditions based on the coordinates published in five positron emission tomography studies: Athwal et al. 2001, Blok et al. 1997, Blok et al. 1998, Nour et al. 2000, Matsuura et al. 2002. See also Fig. 12.14. With permission from Kavia RB, Dasgupta R, Fowler CJ. 2005. Functional imaging and the central control of the bladder. *J Comp. Neurol.* **493**:27–32, Wiley.

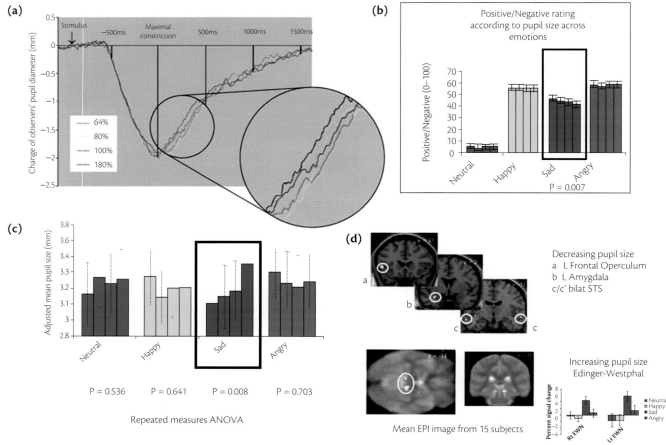

Plate 12 Pupillary contagion during emotional processing. **(a)** Subjects' mean pupil response to a 500 ms stimulus presentation, illustrating the pupillary light response beginning approximately 200 ms after stimulus onset and peaking 200 ms after stimulus offset, followed by a gradual return to baseline. **(b)** Mean ratings for each of the facial expressions according to emotion and pupil size (64% to 180% left to right). 1) Modulus of the positive/negative rating on a 0–100 absolute scale. Small pupils in expressions of sadness are rated as significantly more negative (*—repeated measures ANOVA $F_{(3,30)}$ = 4.340, p = 0.007, Contrasts, 64% vs 100% $F_{(1,30)}$ = 5.481, p = 0.026, 64% vs 180% $F_{(1,30)}$ = 9.311, p = 0.005, 80% vs 180% $F_{(1,30)}$ = 5.377, p = 0.027) than those with larger pupils. **(c)** Subject's mean pupil size in the 500 ms window following maximal pupillary constriction for neutral, happy, sad, and angry facial expressions. Pupil size is plotted in response to observed pupil areas 64%, 80%, 100% and 180% of the original image (from left to right). Observers' own pupil size was significantly smaller when viewing sad faces with small pupils than when viewing those with larger pupils (Repeated measures ANOVA F = 5.04, p = 0.008) with significantly smaller pupil size when viewing sad faces with pupil area 64% (* p = 0.002), 80% (* p = 0.005) and 100% (* p = 0.049) of the original compared with images with pupils 180% of the area of the original image. The horizontal line indicates subjects' mean pupil size across all trials. **(d)** Prefrontal lateral temporal and amygdala brain regions showing a significant correlation with linearly decreasing pupil size in the context of expressions of sadness. All regions shown are significant at the p ≤ 0.001, uncorrected. Midbrain regions showing a significant correlation with linearly increasing pupil size in the context of expressions of sadness. Both regions shown are significant at the p ≤ 0.001 uncorrected. Percent signal change for the right and left brainstem regions plotted against emotional expression. Increasing pupil size effects a significantly greater percentage signal change in sad facial expressions than the other emotional expressions in both brainstem regions shown. See also Fig. 12.15. Harrison N, Singer T, Rotshtein P, Dolan RJ, Critchley HD, Pupil size modulates the empathic experience of sadness. *Social Cognitive and Affective Neuroscience* (SCAN) 2006 **1**, 1–13, by permission of Oxford University Press.

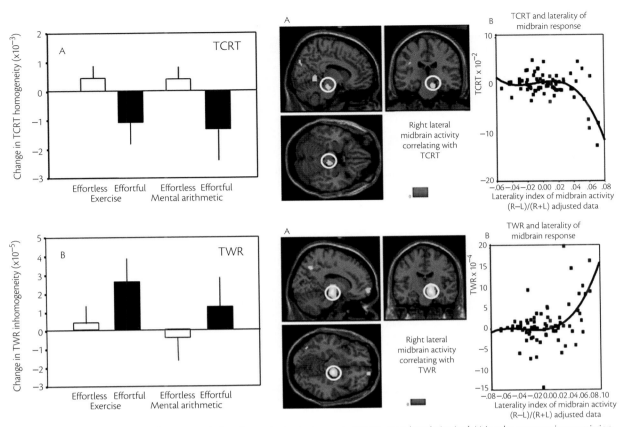

Plate 13 Lateral shift in midbrain activity predicting stress-induced proarrhythmic changes in ECG T-waves (repolarization). Using the same positron emission tomography design illustrated in Fig. 12.4, 10 cardiac patients were scanned with simultaneous 12-lead ECG monitoring. Complementary measures of T-wave changes indicative of proarrhythmic electrical inhomogeneity of myocardial repolarization were derived (decreased TCRT and increased TWR) and shown to be enhanced by cognitive and physical effort (figures to left). The same measures were predicted by right-left right shifts in the activity of the midbrain. The data suggest that a lateralized imbalance in the autonomic drive to the heart, originating in functional imbalance at the level of a midbrain autonomic relay, may predispose to stress-induced arrhythmia and sudden cardiac death. Middle figures illustrate this correlation with midbrain activity across the group, and the effect is plotted for each measure in scatter plots to the right. See also Fig. 12.16. Critchley HD, Taggart P, Sutton PM, Holdright DR, Batchvarov V, Hnatkova K, Malik M, Dolan RJ., Mental stress and sudden cardiac death: asymmetric midbrain activity as a linking mechanism, *Brain*, 2005, **128**:75–85, by permission of Oxford University Press.

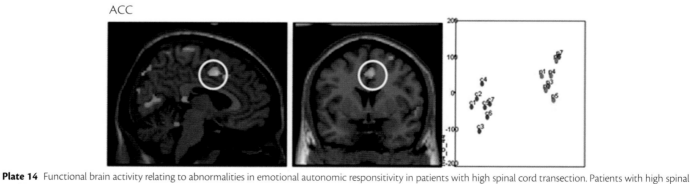

Plate 14 Functional brain activity relating to abnormalities in emotional autonomic responsitivity in patients with high spinal cord transection. Patients with high spinal cord lesions, compared with healthy controls, showed abnormal fear conditioning with heightened activity in pain processing regions, suggesting upregulation of pain systems. When exposed to the threat of pain, they showed attenuated activity within medial orbitofrontal/subgenual cingulate and motor cingulate cortices (top two panels) To the left, the anatomical location of differences in activity is plotted on orthogonal sections of a template brain and to the right responses for threat-related activity is shown for controls (blue) and patients (red). The bottom two panels illustrate enhanced activity in pain reactive regions to the threat of pain in spinal lesioned subjects (i.e. the periaqueductal grey matter and a midcingulate region). These data show an impact on emotional systems of the relative loss of autonomic control and afferent spinal visceral information consequent upon upper thoracic or cervical spinal damage. See also Fig. 12.17. Nicotra A, Critchley HD, Mathias CJ, Dolan RJ, Emotional and autonomic consequences of spinal cord injury explored using functional brain imaging. *Brain.* 2005, **129** (3): 718–728, by permission of Oxford University Press.

(a)

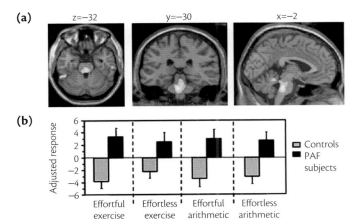

z=−32   y=−30   x=−2

(b)

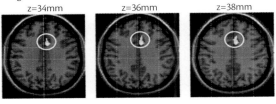

□ Controls
■ PAF subjects

(c) Interaction with effort: Anterior cingulate activity greater in PAF subjects during effortful versus effortless tasks

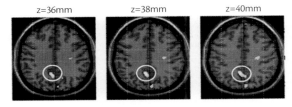

z=34mm   z=36mm   z=38mm

(d) Interaction with effort: Medial parietal/posterior cingulate activity greater in controls during effortful versus effortless tasks

z=36mm   z=38mm   z=40mm

Plate 15 Regional activity differences in patients with pure autonomic failure (PAF). Patients with PAF, a peripheral autonomic denervation, and matched controls were scanned using positron emission tomography during performance of effortful cognitive (mental arithmetic) and physical (isometric exercise) stress tasks and low grade, effortless, control conditions. Consistent with their diagnosis, patients with PAF did not show significant increases in blood pressure or heart rate. **(a)** Independent of task, patients with PAF showed significantly increased blood flow relative to controls in dorsal pons, consistent with increased autoregulatory activity in absence of continuous negative feedback of autonomic responses. The figure plots this group difference in activity on axial coronal and parasagittal sections of a template brain, together with **(b)** bar graphs of the adjusted blood flow responses for the four-task conditions for the patient groups. **(c)** In the absence of autonomic responses during effortful cognitive and physical behaviours, patients with PAF had significantly greater activity than controls in right anterior cingulate (beyond that seen in association with autonomic arousal [see Fig. 12.3B]), suggestive of a context-specific increase in activity in the absence of negative feedback of autonomic arousal. **(d)** In contrast, decreased activity in posterior cingulate/medial parietal cortex was observed in the patients with PAF during effortful behaviour, independent of task modality. The anatomical locations of these second-order differences are illustrated on axial sections of a template brain. See also Fig. 12.18. Reprinted by permission from Macmillan Publishers Ltd: *Nature Neurosci*, Critchley HD, Mathias CJ, Dolan RJ. Copyright (2001).

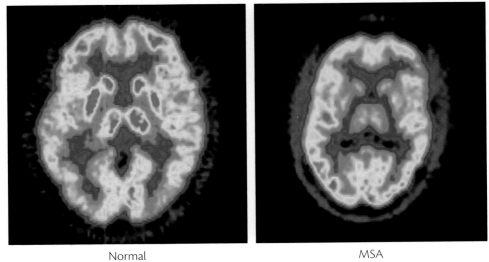

Normal   MSA

Plate 16 ^{18}F-fluorodeoxyglucose positron emission tomography images of regional cerebral glucose metabolism. The multiple system atrophy (MSA) case shows reduced resting basal ganglia function. See also Fig. 40.2.

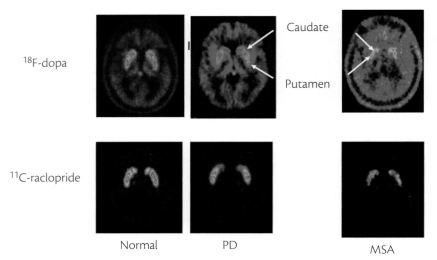

Plate 17 F-DOPA and ¹¹C-raclopride positron emission tomography images of dopamine storage capacity and D2 receptor binding. The multiple system atrophy (MSA) case shows reduced caudate and putamen 6F-DOPA and ¹¹C-raclopride uptake. Caudate 6F-DOPA uptake and striatal ¹¹C-raclopride binding are preserved in Parkinson's disease (PD). See also Fig. 40.3.

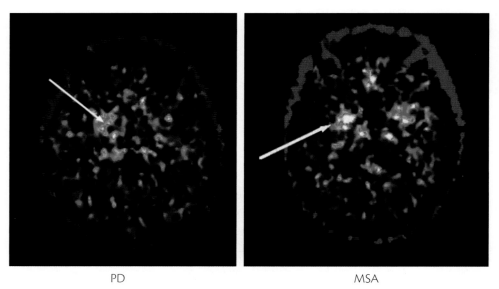

Plate 18 ¹¹C-PK11195 positron emission tomography images of microglial activation in Parkinson's disease (PD) and multiple system atrophy (MSA). Both conditions show increased basal ganglia uptake but this is more extensive in MSA. See also Fig. 40.5. Courtesy of A Gerhard.

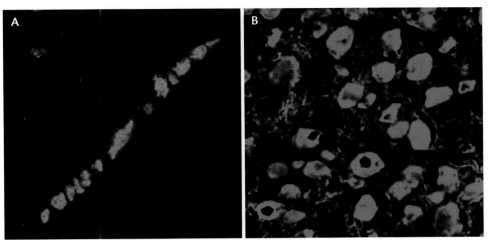

Plate 19 Binding of antineuronal nuclear antibody type 1 (ANNA-1) antibodies to autonomic ganglia neurons. Human ANNA-1 antibodies bound to rabbit autonomic tissues were detected by indirect immunofluorescence. ANNA-1 binds to the nuclei and cytoplasm of **(A)** enteric neurons in myenteric plexus and **(B)** sympathetic neurons in superior cervical ganglia. See also Fig. 52.1.

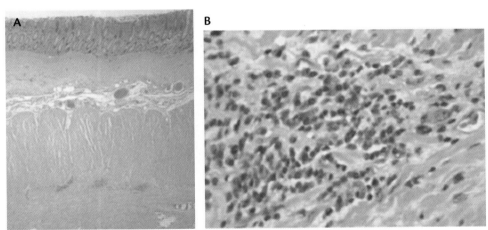

Plate 20 Lymphoplasmacytic infiltration of myenteric plexus ganglia in a bowel section from a patient with paraneoplastic enteric neuropathy. **A:** A full thickness view of the colon shows normal mucosa and submucosa. There is a chronic inflammatory infiltrate between the longitudinal and circular layers of the muscularis propria. (H&E, 20x). **B:** A dense lymphoplasmacytic infiltrate is noted in the location of the myenteric plexus. Ganglion cells can be seen surrounded by inflammation (H&E, 400x). See also Fig. 52.2. With permission from Jun, S., Dimyan, M., Jones, K. D. and Ladabaum, U. (2005), *Neurogastroenterology & Motility*, Wiley.

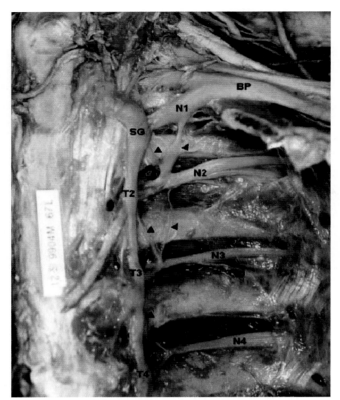

Plate 21 An anatomical dissection of the rami communicantes of the thoracic sympathetic ganglia. See also Fig. 72.2. Reprinted from *European Journal of Cardio-thoracic Surgery*, **27**, Cho HM, Lee DY and Sung SW, Anatomical variations of rami communicantes in the upper thoracic sympathetic trunk, 320–324, Copyright (2005), with permission from Elsevier.

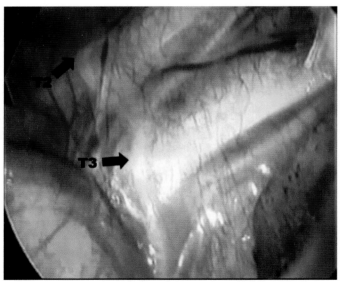

Plate 22 A view of the sympathetic chain through the thoracoscope demonstrating the second and third sympathetic ganglia (arrows). See also Fig. 72.3. Photograph courtesy of Mr Trevor Paes, FRCS.

Table 34.1 Clinical spectrum of vestibular autonomic interactions

Scenario	Clinical condition	Mechanism of signs and symptoms
Vestibular dysfunction causing associated autonomic symptoms	◆ Peripheral vestibular dysfunction (e.g. vestibular neuritis)	Nausea and vomiting due to vestibular connections with nuclei controlling respiratory and gastric efferent nerves
Vestibular stimulation presenting with predominantly autonomic symptoms	◆ Motion sickness	Sensory conflict causing activation of vestibular autonomic connections
Vestibular influence on autonomic functions (e.g. blood pressure, respiration, and sleep)	◆ Orthostatic hypotension with ageing? ◆ Obstructive sleep apnoea?	Vestibular connections with medullary cardiorespiratory centres
Vestibular disorder with possible autonomic etiology	◆ Menière's disease	Parasympathetic dysfunction?
Neurological diseases involving both vestibular and autonomic systems	◆ Migraine ◆ Multisystem atrophy	'Trigeminal-vascular reflex', chemical mediators Dysfunction of central vestibular and autonomic pathways
Interaction between vestibular and psychiatric conditions	◆ Vestibular dysfunction triggering anxiety and agoraphobia	Shared neural circuits between central vestibular pathways and centres controlling autonomic function (e.g. amygdala, locus coeruleus)
Autonomic disturbance causing vestibular symptoms	◆ Orthostatic hypotension	Dizziness due to reduced cerebral blood flow
Conditions with possible overlap in vestibular and autonomic symptomatology	◆ Drop attacks ◆ Cervical vertigo	Sudden loss of muscle tone, Drop in blood pressure Neck proprioceptors involved? Cervical sympathetic fibres involved?

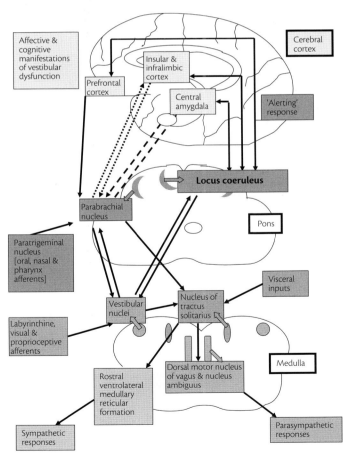

Fig. 34.1 Neural connections mediating vestibulo-autonomic responses. Adapted from Balaban and Porter 1998, with permission.

as demonstrated by functional magnetic resonance imaging (fMRI) (Suzuki et al. 2001). This test may induce nausea and vomiting, but no consistent changes in heart rate or blood pressure are noted except for those secondary to respiration (Costa et al. 1995, Jauregui-Renaud et al. 2000). Hallpike and coworkers (1951) were the first to report an increased duration of caloric responses and directional preponderance in 'neurotic' patients. It is now well established that mental alerting improves the response of caloric nystagmus and anxiety influences the gain of the vestibulo-ocular reflex. (Davis and Mann 1987, Yardley et al, 1995, Wuyts et al. 2003) On the contrary, an experienced test subject can completely suppress caloric nystagmus, even in response to ice water (e.g. trained ice skaters) (McCabe 1960). This habituation of the vestibular response is considered to be primarily consequent upon cerebellar function and neural plasticity (Boyden et al. 2004) Mental alerting, in this situation, may release the suppression of nystagmus. This arousal response is mediated through neuronal circuits involving the higher autonomic control centres—the locus coeruleus and noradrenergic pathways that connect to the cortex, amygdala and the vestibular nuclei (Fig. 34.1).

Conventional rotation chair tests infrequently result in distressing nausea necessitating discontinuation of the test, but, autonomic symptoms are a limiting factor in off-vertical axis rotation (OVAR) and this may be related to the tilt of the rotational axis and an unfamiliar combination of otolithic and semicircular canal inputs. Keeping ambient temperature less than 65°F and limiting the test time helps to reduce the unpleasant side effects (Furman 1998).

Optokinetic testing causes sensory conflict or visuo-vestibular mismatch, and this may provoke autonomic symptoms as explained in the section on motion sickness.

Motion sickness—the overlap between vestibular and autonomic symptoms

Motion sickness demonstrates most clearly the inter-relationship between autonomic and vestibular pathways. This condition reflects a group of primarily autonomic symptoms that are produced in response to movement or perceived movement in the environment. It is caused due to activation of the vestibulo-autonomic pathways during an unfamiliar body motion or visual movement. Common triggers are travel in automobiles, aircraft, or exposure to moving visual scenes (cinerama sickness, simulator sickness). Motion sickness is generated by signals from the vestibular system, as evidenced from animal studies and by the observation that labyrinthine defective subjects are typically not susceptible to the malady (Money and Friedberg 1964, Kennedy et al. 1968). Of note, vestibular function is essential for motion sickness (even that provided by visual stimuli) (Cheung et al. 1991), but visual signals are not essential, as the blind can also suffer these symptoms (Graybiel 1970).

Theories of motion sickness

Reason (1978) proposed that the generation of motion sickness is related to *sensory conflict*. The 'normal' learned relationship between motor commands and sensory inputs, is stored within the brain and any incoming sensory information is then compared with previous sensorimotor experience. Motion sickness ensues when multiple sensory inputs provide repeated contradictory information causing *intersensory conflict* or provide information that is at variance with previous sensorimotor experience. As motion sickness involves comparison between current and previous sensory inputs, adaptation to the triggering stimuli is possible.

A variant of the sensory conflict theory is that motion sickness occurs only when *the subjective vertical as determined by previous experience differs from the sensed vertical*, as determined on basis of incoming sensory information (Bles et al. 1998). This explains the occurrence of the Coriolis effect, which is the disorientating and nauseating sensation brought on by head tilt during constant velocity rotation, it also explains the milder pseudo-Coriolis effect induced by head tilts during pure optokinetic/somatosensory rotatory stimulation. Proponents of this theory believe that the degree of motion sickness can be modified by providing simultaneous incongruent or congruent visual/somatosensory information (Bles 1998).

The *postural instability theory* proposes that motion sickness stems from prolonged unstable control of body posture that may accompany exposure to novel motion environments. Reductions on the demand for postural control (e.g. lying down) should thus reduce severity of motion sickness (Riccio and Stoffregen 1991). Although it has been shown that postural instability precedes and predicts the onset of motion sickness, evidence for this theory is not consistent (Stoffregen and Smart 1998, Warwick-Evans et al. 1998).

More recently, it was proposed that acetylcholine may mediate the symptoms associated with motion sickness (Eisenman 2009). Motion stimulation activates the primary vestibular afferents leading to activation of secondary vestibulo-cerebellar fibres, some of which are cholinergic. The acetylcholine, once released from these synaptic terminals diffuses into the cerebrospinal fluid in the 4th ventricle and activates the cholinergic receptors in the autonomic and emetic centres within the dorsal brainstem to produce the symptoms of motion sickness. The acetylcholine would also initiate a positive feedback loop through the vestibular nuclei where it facilitates transmission and reinforces the vestibulo-cerebellar activity.

Motion sickness may have a phylogenetic role in that it may occur as an emetic 'poison response'—a protective mechanism against unnatural motions. It has, therefore, been suggested that motion sickness has a protective role in inducing an individual to remain sedentary during abnormal motion (Yates et al. 1998). Susceptibility to motion sickness differs and genetic factors, perceptual ability and biofeedback may influence individual response.

Neural pathways mediating motion sickness

Vomiting in motion sickness involves coordinated action of the major respiratory and upper airway muscles, along with retrograde contractions of the gastrointestinal tract and stomach relaxation. The latter gastrointestinal components are not essential for motion sickness, as retching and expulsion appear to be mediated by respiratory pump muscles. In fact, motion sickness related vomiting can occur in dogs after the sympathetic and parasympathetic nerve supplies to the gut are severed (Wang et al. 1957). The neuronal circuits presumed to be involved in motion sickness vomiting are shown in Fig. 34.2 (Yates et al. 1995; Money et al. 1996).

Clinical features of motion sickness

Symptoms of motion sickness are related to stomach emptying, which is parasympathetically mediated and the accompanying stress, which is sympathetically mediated. Abdominal sensations,

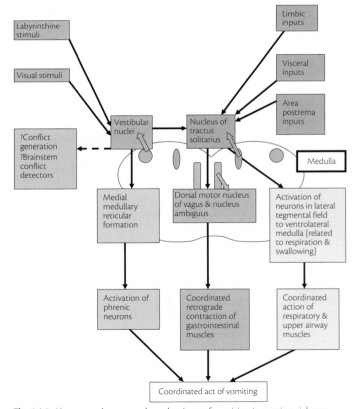

Fig. 34.2 Known and presumed mechanisms of vomiting in motion sickness. Adapted from Yates 1998, with permission.

malaise and drowsiness, nausea, repetitive swallowing, retching, and vomiting are common (Money et al. 1996). Motion sickness is thought to be less common with vestibular habituation (e.g. in skaters) (Tanguy et al. 2008). The nausea and vomiting are thought to correlate with an increase in plasma vasopressin, which serves to reabsorb water from the kidneys and to alter visceral blood flow, and may, therefore, help to counter the fluid loss in emesis. The inferior frontal gyrus may play a role in generating the nausea (Miller et al. 1996). Primary changes in blood pressure and heart rate variability are uncommon, though these may occur secondary to changes in respiration. Thus, there appears to be a selective activation of the autonomic system during motion sickness. The stress response, produced by an increase in plasma adrenocorticotrophic hormone (ACTH), cortisol, adrenaline, noradrenaline, manifests as a sense of anxiety, distress, dread, pallor, and cold sweating. Other autonomically mediated endocrine responses, such as decreased thyroid stimulating hormone (TSH), increased growth hormone, prolactin, and beta-endorphin have been noted.

Management of motion sickness is targeted towards control of vomiting. The anti-emetic action of currently used antihistaminics and antimuscarinics is thought to be mediated by suppression of activity in the vestibular nuclei. A recent systematic review concluded that scopolamine (anticholinergic drug acting on muscarinic receptors) is effective in preventing motion sickness. Other drugs (zamafenacin, meclizine, flunarizine), biofeedback and complementary medical therapies, such as acupressure and acupuncture, have been tried, but there are no randomized controlled trials to compare their effectiveness with scopolamine (Spinks et al. 2004). More recently there is evidence that serotonin agonist, rizatriptan, reduces vestibular-induced motion sickness in migraineurs (Furman 2010).

Autonomic disturbances in altered gravity environments

Unlike on earth, head tilt during spaceflight (zero gravity environment) activates the canals, but not the otoliths, producing sensory conflict with the expected pattern of stimulation. Adaptation from this sensory conflict involves reinterpretation of otolithic signals as translational rather than tilt or translational. This concept is called the *tilt-translational* hypothesis (Parker 1998). Sustained zero gravity environment in the first few days causes sympathetic deficiency—decreased orthostatic tolerance, decreased catecholamines and a decrease in blood volume, but significant changes in heart rate and blood pressure are not common (Previc 1996). Space motion sickness (SMS) occurs after 2–3 days and adaptation to the abnormal environment is usually complete in a week (Jennings 1998). Symptoms of SMS are similar to terrestrial motion sickness, with some differences; in SMS, nausea, pallor and sweating are absent and Coriolis effects are not disturbing, but symptoms last longer. As compared to activation of both parasympathetic and sympathetic systems in terrestrial motion sickness, it is thought that only parasympathetic activation occurs in SMS.

On return to earth, many astronauts suffer post-spaceflight orthostatic intolerance (PSOI)—they are unable to maintain blood pressure in the standing position. This is thought to be due to attenuation of the vestibular-autonomic responses and the use of non labyrinthine inputs, such as visual and visceral activity to replace the conflicting vestibular inputs during spaceflight.

Recovery from PSOI depends on substitution of the non labyrinthine inputs with those from the vestibular labyrinth, mediated by the cerebellar vermis, which is known to modulate neural plasticity (Yates et al. 2003).

Vestibular influence on cardiovascular control

Evidence in animals

Electrical stimulation of the vestibular nerve, as well as natural vestibular stimulation, changes the activity of sympathetic nerves in the heart, kidney and splanchnic vessels, causing a redistribution of blood flow within the circulation (Yates 1996). Doba and Reis (1974) showed that transection of the eighth nerves in anaesthetized and paralysed cats caused a greater drop in blood pressure during nose up pitch than in vestibular intact animals. Moreover, vestibular mediated sympathetic circulatory responses produce precise effects (hindlimb vasodilatation and forelimb vasoconstriction). This sympathetic patterning may be a complementary autonomic response to motor activation consequent upon an unexpected postural changes (e.g. righting response) (Kerman et al. 2000a, 2000b). Vestibular lesions in animals produce a deficient control of blood pressure during movement, but compensatory changes occur when non-labyrinthine inputs are used to judge body position. This adaptive change is possibly mediated by the cerebellum, in line with adaptive changes, which occur in vestibulo-ocular reflex responses (Yates et al. 2000).

Evidence in humans

As the vestibular system detects changes in posture, it is likely to be involved in homeostatic responses to posture change and there is evidence to suggest that this may occur as a result of activation of both sympathetic and parasympathetic responses. Standing from a supine position causes pooling of blood in the lower half of the body and decreased cardiac output. Head down neck flexion in prone subjects produces a decrease in calf and forearm blood flow, as would occur to redistribute blood flow during orthostatic hypotension (Essandoh et al. 1988), and an increase in muscle sympathetic nerve activity (Ray and Monahan 2002). The vestibulo-sympathetic reflex that mediates these responses is a robust and independent reflex that acts synergistically with sympathetic reflexes mediated by both thermal and mental stress and arterial chemoreceptors (Monahan and Ray 2002, Carter et al. 2002, Wilson and Ray 2004). It is attenuated with ageing and this may contribute to the increased prevalence of orthostatic hypotension in the elderly (Ray and Monahan 2002). Moreover, compared with controls, patients with bilateral vestibular hypofunction have lower cardiovascular responses during linear acceleration, supporting a role for vestibular influence on blood pressure (Yates et al. 1999).

There is also evidence to suggest the existence of a parasympathetically mediated short latency response, which results in increased heart rate with rapid change in posture, before the baroreceptor mediated reflex comes into play. Absence of this rapid response may contribute to the malaise seen in patients with vestibular disease (Radtke et al. 2003). The otoliths appear to be more important than semicircular canals in mediating vestibulo-cardiac reflexes (Watenpaugh et al. 2002, Ray and Carter 2003). The neural circuits involved in vestibulo-sympathetic control are shown in Fig. 34.3.

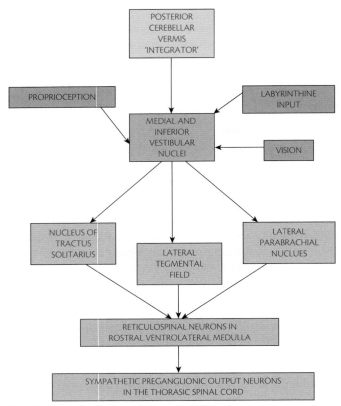

Fig. 34.3 Neural circuits for vestibular control of blood pressure.

Vestibular influence on respiratory control

Changes in posture can affect the respiratory system by:

♦ changing the resting length of the diaphragm

♦ reducing airway patency as the tongue falls backwards

♦ stimulating the pulmonary receptors and respiratory muscle stretch receptors.

Conversely, respiratory muscles may be involved in stabilizing posture during perturbation, as well as improving venous return to the heart. It may be postulated that the function of vestibulo-respiratory connections is to optimize ventilation in response to change in posture, improve venous return and aid in postural responses (Yates and Miller 1998).

Evidence in animals

Electrical stimulation of the vestibular nerve causes discharge in respiratory related motor neurons, which is reduced when vestibular inputs are eliminated. Similarly, head rotations are known to alter upper airway and respiratory pump muscle activity, even when non-labyrinthine inputs are excluded (Yates et al. 2002, Miller and Yates 1996).

Evidence in humans

The semicircular canals, but not otoliths mediate increased ventilation in humans (Monahan et al. 2002). In acute unilateral vestibular lesions, the vestibular modulation of breathing following reorientation of the head and trunk to the upright position is reduced (Jáuregui-Renaud et al. 2005). The vestibular mediated respiratory

response is impaired by ageing, implying that the immediate increase in ventilation during non-stationary exercise may be blunted (Kuipers et al. 2003). Although there is no evidence that vestibular hypofunction may cause respiratory difficulties, it is known that vestibular stimulation by rocking produces entrainment of respiration and reduction of obstructive sleep apnoea in infants, although the role of cutaneous stimulation has been difficult to exclude in these studies (Farrimond 1990, Sammon and Darnall 1994).

Neural pathways mediating vestibular influence on respiratory system

Pathways subserving vestibular respiratory reflexes are complex and have not been completely elucidated. Vestibular inputs from the medial and inferior vestibular nuclei feed into the ventral respiratory group (VRG) pre-motor neurons in the medulla, which along with the dorsal group are involved in the cyclic excitation and inhibition of the spinal motor neurons producing coordinated activity of respiratory muscles. The VRG neurons connect with respiratory motoneurons. However, ablative studies suggest that apart from VRG, other direct vestibular pathways may play a part in modulating respiratory activity (Yates et al. 1995).

Vestibular system and sleep

Nuclei involved in sleep regulation—raphe nuclei, locus coeruleus and reticular formation—receive vestibular inputs, and, in particular the otoliths project on to the pontine reticular formation. This may explain why rocking, car riding, and other body movements are conducive to sleep. The typical eye movements during rapid eye movement (REM) sleep are partly mediated through vestibulo-ocular connections and sleep atonia is mediated by vestibulo-reticular connections. REM sleep also causes pupillary dilatation, a change in blood pressure and heart rate that are abolished by lesions of the vestibular nuclei. Thus, autonomic influences during REM sleep are modulated by the vestibular system, but sleep patterns in patients with vestibular lesions have not been studied (Yates 1998).

Autonomic disorder in Menière's disease

Autonomic dysfunction is proposed as one of the aetiopathogenetic factors of Menière's disease (MD). Although a number of studies have indicated both parasympathetic and sympathetic dysfunction in MD, a causal role for autonomic dysfunction in the aetiology of MD remains to be established. Abnormal autonomic function on the side of MD was detected during the attack as well as in the interval stage, using the mecholyl test and pupillometry (Uemura et al. 1980). Studies of the pupillary response have suggested a parasympathetic defect on the affected side during the attack stage, and this was unrelated to the labyrinthine defect (Inoue et al. 1988, Guidetti and Botti 1991). Other studies have indicated blunting of the sympathetic orthostatic response in the interval stage (Yamada et al. 1999) and a disturbance of equilibrium, associated with various sympathetic and parasympathetic stimuli (carotid sinus pressure, injection of adrenaline, atropine) (Tokita et al. 1971). Sympathetic overactivity has been reported during the attack stage, but it is not known if this was a cause or effect of the attack (Kawasaki 1993). In a study evaluating symptoms, several patients with dysautonomia presented with symptoms of MD, and responded to increased fluid and sodium intake, indicating an autonomic aetiology for MD (Pappas and Banyas 1991, Pappas 2003). Overall, there is evidence of a parasympathetic defect on the affected side in MD and some evidence that dysautonomia may present with symptoms similar to those of MD. However, the exact role of autonomic disturbance in the pathogenesis of MD remains unclear.

Drop attacks in MD are postulated to result from a reflex loss of vestibulo-spinal postural control, consequent upon sudden changes in endolymphatic fluid pressure, causing non-physiological stimulation of the utricle or saccule. Drop attacks can also occur in other conditions, such as a loss of orthostatic blood pressure control especially in the elderly. A differential diagnosis of these attacks, especially in the elderly, will involve careful exclusion of pathology in the autonomic system, and also other neurological pathology.

Migraine—the overlap between vestibular and autonomic symptoms

Migraine is a chronic condition with recurrent headaches, aura, and autonomic dysfunction. There is an increased prevalence of dizziness, motion sickness, and anxiety in migraine, which are considered to be mediated by autonomic pathways.

Autonomic disturbances in migraine

Pain innervation of the intracranial structures is subserved by the ophthalmic division of the trigeminal nerve. The afferent nerve endings from the meninges terminate in bipolar neurons within the trigeminal ganglion, which synapse proximally with the nucleus trigeminalis caudalis, extending to the dorsal C1–C2 segment. The quintothalamic tract carries pain sensations from the trigeminal nucleus to the thalamus and cortex (Goadsby 1996).

The pathogenesis of migraine headache is not completely understood (Fig. 34.4). It is thought to be related to the vasodilatation of the large cranial vessels, mediated by the trigeminal-parasympathetic reflex. The trigeminal neurons are stimulated by a variety of endogenous (cortical spreading depression [CSD]) and exogenous (e.g. food) factors. CSD is important in mediating migraine aura. Trigeminal neurons on stimulation release vasodilators (calcitonin-gene-related peptide [CGRP], neurokinin A [NKA], substance P) that mediate a sterile inflammation around cranial arteries. The chemical mediators lower the sensitivity of perivascular nerve fibres and the central trigeminal neurons and mediate the parasympathetic vasodilatation of the large cranial vessels, causing headache. This sensitization explains a disproportionate increase in migrainous pain in response to small increases in intracranial pressure such as bending and the cutaneous allodynia (or painful perception of non nociceptive stimuli). Serotonin from the dorsal raphe nucleus and norepinephrine from the nucleus raphe magnus are proposed to modulate the trigeminal-parasympathetic reflex and influence central pain pathways. A network of cortical and subcortical structures (e.g. periaqueductal gray) with modulatory nociceptive/anti-nociceptive functions may be activated in migraine (Goadsby 1996, Welch 2003, Waeber and Moskowitz 2005).

Autonomic symptoms such as increased lacrimation, rhinorrhoea, facial flushing, (mediated by the trigeminal parasympathetic reflex), pallor, diaphoresis, nausea, vomiting and diarrhoea, commonly occur in migrainous attacks. Rarely, cardiac arrhythmias, including asystole, have been reported and autonomic function

tests have demonstrated abnormalities (Buchhalter et al. 2001, Avnon et al. 2004). Cyclical vomiting is considered a migrainous variant; many children with the condition develop migraine in their later years (Dignan 2001).

Migraine and dizziness—autonomic links

There is evidence to suggest that the association between migraine and vertigo is more than coincidence. In a study of 363 patients with vertigo, 32% had migraine and in the absence of any additional pathology, the incidence of vestibular abnormalities was higher in the migraineurs compared with non-migraineurs (Savundra et al. 1997). In a separate study, incidence of migraine was 1.6 times higher in a dizziness clinic, as compared to an age and sex matched population in an orthopaedic clinic (Neuhauser et al. 2001). In a study of patients with unclassified vertigo, the incidence of migraine was found to be 33% (Aragones et al. 1993). In the seminal paper of Kayan and Hood (1984), vestibular symptoms occurred in 54% and vertigo in 26% of migraineurs. Migrainous vertigo (MV) has been proposed as a distinct entity, with well defined diagnostic criteria (Neuhauser et al. 2001).

A pathophysiological model for MV has been proposed by Furman et al. (2003) (Fig. 34.4). The vestibular nuclei have reciprocal connectivity with the trigeminal caudalis that mediates the parasympathetic vasodilatation in migraine; hence, vestibular processing can be simultaneously altered, causing vertigo. Dizziness during migraine attacks could also have a peripheral origin as the inner ear is innervated by trigeminal afferents. The vasodilatory peptides released by the trigeminal and eighth nerve fibres in the inner ear and acting on neural and vascular elements, could contribute to migraine related dizziness. Central vestibular activation can alter monoaminergic pathways through the dorsal raphe nucleus. This, in turn, can trigger migraine related symptoms and modulate activity in pain and anxiety related pathways.

MV may be temporally dissociated from the headaches. It may occur both with and without headaches and may be spontaneous or positional. It may be associated with photophobia, phonophobia, and visual aura, which are pointers to the diagnosis. Neuro-otological evaluation and tests may reveal nonspecific central and/or peripheral abnormalities, but not infrequently no fixed vestibular deficit is defined.

Migraine and motion sickness

Migraine sufferers are independently more susceptible to motion induced and visually triggered sickness. The former may be linked to vestibular dysfunction caused by episodic ischaemia of the labyrinth/brainstem, trigeminal-vascular modulation of blood flow to the labyrinth, or the abnormal central processing of vestibular inputs that is known to occur in migraine sufferers and the latter to abnormal visual processing. It is proposed that once symptoms begin, the gastrointestinal neurons in the brainstem have a low threshold of excitation causing a rapid escalation of nausea during migraine (Drummond 2005).

Migraine and anxiety

Panic is more common in migraineurs and the presence of anxiety in patients with migraine predicts a worse prognosis. (Guidetti et al. 1998, Breslau et al. 2001) Migraine-anxiety links are further explored in the section on migraine anxiety related dizziness.

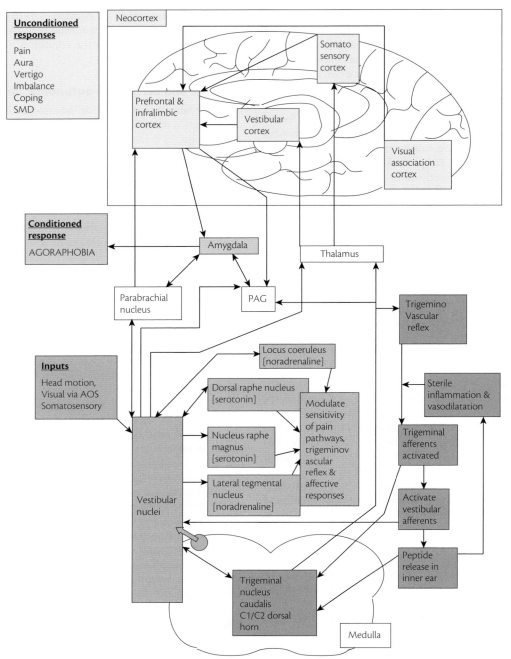

Fig. 34.4 Neural circuits involved in migraine, anxiety and dizziness. If seen in conjunction with Figs 34.1 and 34.2, the visceral responses to vestibular stimuli, migraine, and anxiety can be understood. AOS, accessory optic system; PAG, periaqueductal grey; SMD, space and motion discomfort. Adapted from Furman 2005, with permission.

Migraine and autonomic links—implications for management

From the above discussion, it is apparent that autonomic links are important in the pathogenesis, symptoms and associations of migraine. A variety of drugs acting at various steps in the pathogenesis could have a place in treatment of acute attacks and prophylaxis. Triptans, which are 5-hydroxytryptamine (5-HT) agonists act by promoting vasoconstrictor action of the 5-HT 1B-receptors at peripheral trigeminal nerve endings (thereby inhibiting CGRP release) and 5-HT 1D receptors centrally, within the trigeminal neurons. Prophylactic medications like pizotifen and methysergide act by inhibiting the vascular 5-HT 2-receptors in preventing release of inflammatory mediators. Anticonvulsants (e.g. valproate) act by promoting inhibitory γ-aminobutyric acid (GABA) transmission and regulating the voltage dependant sodium or calcium channels that decrease trigeminal neurotransmission. This action is shared by tricyclics, which also act on N-methyl-D-aspartate (NMDA) receptors (Waeber and Moskowitz 2003). There is little evidence for effective treatment of migrainous vertigo, but medications for treatment of acute migraine attacks and for prophylaxis are used—propranolol, pizotifen, flunarizine, and acetazolamide.

Anxiety and dizziness—the autonomic link

Clinical evidence of balance-anxiety-autonomic link

Any of us who experience acute vertigo will not forget the accompanying feeling of fear, anxiety, and dread. Vestibular dysfunction can evoke low grade emotional responses (prolonged motion sickness causing malaise and disgust) as well as acute panic (patients with Menière's disease and benign paroxysmal positional vertigo [BPPV]). A questionnaire based study of general practice patients indicated that half of the respondents who were dizzy reported anxiety or avoidance behaviour or both (Yardley et al. 1998). In a community questionnaire survey of dizzy patients, approximately 65% reported panic attacks and 25% met criteria for a panic disorder. Patients whose panic was associated with dizziness reported high level of agoraphobia and occupational disability (Yardley et al. 2001). Psychological factors contribute to poor compensation from vestibular dysfunction and recurrence of symptoms in compensated vestibular lesions. Poor recovery in turn produces anxiety, perpetuating a vicious cycle. One study showed that persistence of vertigo 1 year after vestibular neuritis correlated with presence of anxiety rather than the extent of vestibular dysfunction (Godemann et al. 2005).

There is considerable individual variation in anxiety response to vestibular dysfunction and some susceptibility is attributed to genetic factors (anxiety proneness), somatization (tendency to be preoccupied by medical symptoms from various organs), and obsessive compulsive personality disorder (Jacob et al. 2003). Symptoms of anxiety induced by vestibular disorders include anxious thoughts and somatic symptoms due to autonomic activation (palpitations, sweating, trembling, nausea, abdominal distress, and hot flashes) and hyperventilation (shortness of breath, chest pain, dizziness, depersonalization, and paraesthesia). Increased body sway and nystagmus are seen after hyperventilation in patients with compensated vestibular lesions. Somatic symptoms predominate in a panic attack. Some patients with panic disorder will avoid exposure to triggering situations, and are said to have panic with agoraphobia (fear of situations from which escape seems impossible or help may not be available).

Clinical types of balance anxiety links (Jacob et al. 2003)

Psychosomatic interactions

Vestibular function is affected by psychological factors (i.e. anxiety, sleep deprivation, and psychological arousal). The arousal response in anxiety can alter the gain of vestibular responses (e.g. increased responses to caloric stimulation) and can trigger vestibular dysfunction.

Somatopsychic mechanism

Vestibular dysfunction can cause anxiety, fatigue, reduced concentration (as increased attention is devoted to maintaining balance) and depression (due to restrictions on lifestyle), which may manifest in absence of vestibular complaints. A vicious cycle can ensue with negative cognitive thoughts (fear that dizziness will recur), social withdrawal, and employment issues further promoting psychological symptoms.

Sensory integration of the visual, proprioceptive and vestibular inputs provides an opportunity for a sensory mismatch (i.e. disparity among these inputs). Some disparity can occur in normal individuals (e.g. designed mismatch) such as in amusement park rides. With vestibular dysfunction, mismatch occurs between the senses and there is increased dependence on non-vestibular inputs to replace the misleading vestibular cues. This acts as a drive for the brain to alter its patterns of sensory integration giving rise to space and motion sensitivity (SMS) (i.e. increased sensitivity to misleading or degraded visual and sensory clues such as rapid head turns and optic flow stimuli [crowds]). SMS can lead to situationally specific symptoms or space and motion discomfort (SMD), defined as inadequate visual and kinaesthetic information for normal spatial orientation. Patients feel uncomfortable in places like glass elevators, supermarkets, railway stations, and on escalators. Some of them develop a fear of the trigger situations (e.g. motorist disorientation syndrome, supermarket syndrome) and major avoidance behaviour, to the extent that normal functioning is affected and this is described as space and motion phobia (SMP) (Furman and Jacob 2001). Patients with anxiety and prominent SMD have increased sensitivity to optic flow stimuli and agoraphobics, known to have a high degree of SMD exhibit surface dependent sway pattern on dynamic posturography (Jacob et al. 1995). The avoidance behaviour is an adaptive response to prevent the unpleasant somatic manifestations accompanying the triggering conditions and poses a major hurdle for recovery from vestibular dysfunction, as patients tend not to expose themselves to stimuli necessary for rehabilitation e.g. physical exercises and stray visual stimuli (Furman et al. 1998).

Psychiatric dizziness

Psychiatric dizziness refers to dizziness as a defining symptom of a psychiatric disorder (e.g. panic). In these patients, dizziness between panic attacks may be a predictor of vestibular abnormality.

Common neural connections

Vestibular dysfunction and psychiatric symptoms are mediated by common neural mechanisms (e.g. anxiety is a reaction to vestibular dysfunction, just as palpitations occur with exercise).

Migraine anxiety related dizziness

From the previous discussions, it is clear that a significant co-morbidity exists between migraine, anxiety and dizziness and the term migraine anxiety related dizziness (MARD) denotes a subgroup of patients who suffer from a combination of the three symptoms. Balaban and Thayer (2001) and Furman et al. (2005) have published excellent reviews on the mechanisms of migraine, balance and anxiety links. Pathophysiology of MARD is explained by pathways involving migrainous vertigo and shared neural circuits between anxiety and vertigo with a central role for the PBN network.

Neural pathways mediating the migraine-anxiety-balance—autonomic link

The following points are worthy of note (Fig. 34.4):

♦ The central autonomic regulation is influenced by the insular cortex, which has connections with the prefrontal cortex, amygdala, hippocampus, and hypothalamus. These areas are involved in emotional responses and conditioned responses and have connections with the parabrachial nucleus and the NTS. The NTS receives afferent connections from the vestibular nuclei, which in turn have reciprocal connections with the PBN (Fig. 34.1). The connectivity of the PBN enables it to mediate a volley of autonomic and respiratory responses (changes in heart rate, blood pressure, hyperventilation, and hormonal stress responses) in response to triggers for panic, including asymmetric vestibular input, unpleasant visceral stimuli (vomiting), nociceptive stimuli (migraine) and visual, auditory, somaesthetic stimuli from the thalamocortical pathways. It is now easy to recognize how vestibular mismatch can cause anxiety, how anxiety produces autonomic responses and how these unpleasant responses affect conditioned avoidance. Reciprocal connections within the neural circuits serve to match afferent stimuli with previous experience in an aversive context.

◆ The locus coeruleus (which has reciprocal connections with the prefrontal cortex and vestibular nuclei) mediates the effects of vigilance, alerting and anxiety on vestibular reflexes through noradrenergic pathways. Connections of the dorsal raphe nucleus, through serotonergic transmission, act synergistically to increase arousal (Jacob et al. 1996).

◆ Migraine is linked to the balance anxiety circuit by connections through the periaqueductal gray. This area receives input from the vestibular nuclei, insular and prefrontal orbital cortex and projects to the trigeminal nucleus caudalis. It has reciprocal connections with the amygdala. Activation of these circuits can produce affective changes, coping strategies, and serve as a stimulus for phobic avoidance. These additive effects may differ in individuals, accounting for differences in susceptibility to avoidance behaviour and agoraphobia.

◆ Panic is thought to be due to a state of brainstem autonomic dysregulation creating irritable foci in the locus coeruleus, dorsal raphe nucleus, and medullary chemoreceptors that mediate respiratory and cardiovascular alterations. Vestibular dysfunction, by virtue of connections with these nuclei can trigger panic attacks and facilitate SMD (Jacob et al. 1996).

Clinical implications for management

The close overlap and co-morbidity between migraine, dizziness, and anxiety implies that it is important to look for the other two symptoms when one of them is present. Patients referred to specialty clinics may have only one aspect of the disorder recognized and addressed, a frustrating experience for both the clinician and patient. A common feature of MARD is visual dependence, causing SMD. Management of MARD should be aimed at each component, and is likely that treatment aimed at a common pathological mechanism may result in improvement of more than one component (e.g. treatment of panic attacks resolves the dizziness associated with panic and treatment of migraine may alleviate both the headache and dizziness) (Furman et al. 2005).

Autonomic vertigo

A discussion of vestibulo-autonomic interactions would not be complete without elaborating on vestibular manifestations of autonomic dysfunction. *Orthostatic hypotension* classically causes light-headedness due to reduced cerebral blood flow, but vertigo is also reported (Pappas 2003). Its mechanism may be related to

ischaemia of the vestibular nuclei, which are particularly sensitive to ischaemia (Luxon 1990). Vertigo can be produced by *disorders affecting the central or peripheral autonomic system*. Diabetes, and uraemia cause *autonomic neuropathy* but the exact mechanism is uncertain. Exertional dizziness may be a clinical manifestation of autonomic nervous system dysregulation (Staab et al. 2002). *Cervical vertigo* is a commonly diagnosed entity, in which vertigo is thought to be mediated by damage to the neck afferents from cervical pathology/trauma such as whiplash injury. The definition and aetiology of this condition remains controversial, but over-excitation of the cervical sympathetic nerves has been postulated to contribute to symptoms of vertigo, although there is little evidence to support this (Hinoki 1984). Another condition with autonomic involvement is multiple system atrophy (MSA), a neurodegenerative disease of undetermined origin, which is also associated with parkinsonian features, cerebellar, and pyramidal dysfunction. Dizziness in MSA can occur due to orthostatic hypotension, as well as due to involvement of the central vestibular pathways in the cerebellum and brainstem (Wang and Young 2003)

Summary

The convergence of afferent vestibular, visual, proprioceptive and visceral information in the brainstem nuclei and neural connections between vestibular, somatic, autonomic, and cortical centres mediate autonomic responses to physiological and pathological vestibular inputs. The unpleasant visceral symptoms that accompany vestibular dysfunction—nausea, vomiting, and the psychological disturbances that impact on the management and outcome of vestibular disorders, are mediated by vestibular autonomic connections. The vestibular system regulates cardiovascular homeostatic responses to change in posture, and generates motion sickness—a poison response to unnatural motions through its autonomic circuits. The close relationship between migraine, dizziness, and anxiety based on vestibulo-autonomic interactions has important clinical and therapeutic implications. Although current knowledge of overlap between vestibular and autonomic symptoms is supported by a number of animal experiments and clinical studies, it is bridged by hypotheses and presumptions that remain to be verified. This creates the opportunity for further research into a number of areas that could provide a clearer insight into the maze of vestibular and autonomic interactions.

References

Aragones, J., Fortes–Rego, J., Fuste, J., Cardozo, C. (1993). Migraine: an alternative in the diagnosis of unclassified vertigo. *Headache*, **33**, 125–8.

Avnon, Y., Nitzan, M., Sprecher, E., Rogovski, Z., Yarnitsky, D. (2004). Autonomic asymmetry in migraine: augmented parasympathetic activation in left unilateral migraineurs. *Brain*, 127, 2099–108.

Balaban, C. (1996). The role of the cerebellum in vestibular-autonomic regulation. In B. Yates & A. Miller Eds. *Vestibular autonomic regulation*, pp. 127–44. CRC press, Boca Raton (FL).

Balaban C. (1999). Vestibular autonomic regulation (including motion sickness and the mechanism of vomiting). *Curr. Opin. Neurol.*, **12**, 29–33.

Balaban, C. (2004). Projections from the parabrachial nucleus to the vestibular nuclei: potential substrates for autonomic and limbic influences on vestibular responses. *Brain Research*, **996**, 126–37.

Balaban, C., Porter, J. (1998). Neuroanatomic substrates for vestibulo-autonomic interactions. *J Vestibular Res.*, **8**, 7–16.

Balaban, C., Thayer, J. (2001). Neurological basis for balance –anxiety links. *J Anxiety Dis.*, **15**, 53–79.

Bles,W. (1998). Coriolis effects and motion sickness modeling. *Brain Res. Bull.*, **47**, 543–49.

Bles, W., Bos, J., de Graaf, B., Groen, E., Wertheim, A. (1998). Motion sickness: only one provocative conflict? *Brain Res. Bull.*, **47**, 481–7.

Boyden, E., Katoh, A., Raymond, J. (2004). Cerebellum dependent learning: the role of multiple plasticity mechanisms. *Ann. Rev. Neurosci.*, **27**, 581–609.

Breslau, N., Schultz, L., Stewart, W., Lipton, R., Welch, K. (2001), Headache types and panic disorder: directionality and specificity. *Neurology*, **56**, 350–4.

Buchhalter, J., Berland, G., Konkol, R., Silka, M. (2001). Migraine-associated vomiting and asystole in a child. *Headache*, **41**, 88–91.

Carter, J., Ray, C., Cooke, W. (2002). Vestibulosympathetic activity during mental stress. *J Appl. Physiol.*, **93**, 1260–4.

Cheung, B., Howard, I., Money, K. (1991). Visually-induced sickness in normal and bilaterally labyrinthine-defective subjects. *Aviation Space and Environmental Medicine*, **62**, 527–31.

Costa, F., Lavin, P., Robertson, D., Biaggoni, I. (1995). Effect of neurovestibular stimulation on autonomic regulation. *Clin. Auton. Res.*, **5**, 289–93.

Davis, R., Mann, R. (1987). The effects of alerting tasks on caloric induced vestibular nystagmus. *Ear and Hearing*, **8**, 58–60.

Dignan, F., Symon, D., AbuArafeh, I., Russell, G. (2001). The prognosis of cyclical vomiting syndrome. *Arch. Dis. Child.*, **84**, 55–7.

Doba, N., Reis, D. (1974). Role of the cerebellum and vestibular apparatus in regulation of orthostatic reflexes in the cat. *Circulation Res.*, **40**, 9–18.

Drummond, P. (2005). Triggers of motion sickness in migraine sufferers. *Headache*, **45**, 653–6.

Eisenman, L. (2009). Motion sickness may be caused by a neurohumoral action of acetylcholine. Medical *Hypotheses*, **73**, 790–3.

Essandoh, L., Duprez, D., Shepherd, J. (1988). Reflex constriction of human resistance vessels to head down neck flexion. *J Appl. Physiol.*, **64**, 767–70.

Furman, J., Marcus, D., Balaban, C. (2003). Migrainous vertigo: development of a pathogenetic model and structured diagnostic interview. *Curr. Opin. Neurol.*, **16**, 5–13.

Farrimond, T. (1990). Sudden infant death syndrome and possible relation to vestibular function. *Perceptual and Motor Skills*, **71**, 419–23.

Furman, J., Jacob, R. (2001). A clinical taxonomy of dizziness and anxiety in the otoneurological setting. *J Anxiety Disord.*, **15**, 9–26.

Furman, J., Jacob, R., Redfern, M. (1998). Clinical evidence that the vestibular system participates in autonomic control. *J Vestibular Res.*, **8**, 27–34.

Furman, J., Balaban, C., Jacob, R., Marcus, D. (2005). Migraine-anxiety related dizziness (MARD): a new disorder? *JNNP*, **76**, 1–8.

Furman, J., Marcus, D., Balaban, C. (2010). Rizatriptan reduces vestibular-induced motion sickness in migraineurs. *J Headache Pain.* Sep 23. (Epub ahead of print).

Goadsby, P. (1996). Diagnosis and management of migraine. *Br. Med. J*, **312**, 1279–83.

Godemann, F., Siefert, K., Hantschke-Bruggemann, M., Neu, P., Seidl, R., Strohle, A. (2005). What accounts for vertigo one year after neurititis vestibularis—anxiety or a dysfunctional vestibular organ?. *J Psychiatric Res.*, **39**, 529–34.

Graybiel, A. (1970). Susceptibility to acute motion sickness in blind persons. *Aerospace Medicine*, **41**, 650–3.

Guidetti, G., Botti, M. (1991). Pupillometry in Meniere's disease. *Reviews of Laryngology Otology and Rhinology (Bord)*, **112**, 133–6.

Guidetti, V., Galli, F., Fabrizi, P., *et al.* (1998) Headache and psychiatric comorbidity: clinical aspects and outcome in an 8—year follow up study. *Cephalalgia*, **18**, 455–62.

Hallpike, C., Harrison, M., Slater, E. (1951). Abnormalities of the caloric test results in certain varieties of mental disorder. Acta *Otolaryngologica*, **39**, 151–9.

Hinoki, M. (1984). Vertigo due to whiplash injury: a neurotological approach. *Acta Otolaryngologica Supplement*, **419**, 9–29.

Inoue, H., Uemera T. (1988). Sluggishness of pupillary light contraction in patients with Meniere's disease. *Acta Otolaryngologica*, 105, 582–86.

Jacob, R., Furman, J., Perel, J. (1996). Panic phobia and vestibular dysfunction, In B Yates & A Miller Eds. *Vestibular autonomic regulation*, pp.197–227. CRC press, Boca Raton (FL).

Jacob, R., Furman, J., Cass, S. (2003). Psychiatric consequences of vestibular dysfunction. In L Luxon, A Martini, J Furman & D Stephens Eds. *Textbook of Audiological Medicine*, pp. 869–87. Martin Dunitz, London.

Jáuregui-Renaud, K., Villanueva, P., del Castillo, M. (2005). Influence of acute unilateral vestibular lesions on the repiratory rhythm after active change of posture in human subjects. *J Vestibular Res.*, **15**, 41–8.

Jauregui-Renaud, K., Yarrow, K., Oliver, R., Gresty, M., Bronstein, A. (2000). Effects of caloric stimulation on respiratory frequency and heart rate and blood pressure variability. *Brain Research Bulletin*, **53**, 17–23.

Jennings, R. (1998). Managing space motion sickness. *J Vestibular Res.*, **8**, 67–70.

Jacob, R., Redfern, M., Furman, J. (1995). Optic flow induced sway in anxiety disorders associated with space and motion discomfort. *J Anxiety Disorders*, **9**, 411–25.

Jones, I. (1918). *Equilibrium and vertigo*, pp. 1–444. JB Lippincott, Philadelphia.

Kayan, A., Hood, J. (1984). Neurootological manifestations of migraine. *Brain*, **107**, 1123–42.

Kawasaki, Y. (1993). Autonomic nervous function of vertiginous patients-assessment of spectral analysis of heart rate variability. *Nippon Jibiinkoka Gakkai Kaiho*, **96**, 444–56.

Kennedy, R., Graybeil, A., McDonough, R., Beckwith, F. (1968). Symptomatology under storm conditions in the North Atlantic in control subjects and in persons with bilateral labyrinthine defects. *Acta Otolaryngologica*, **66**, 533–40.

Kerman, I., Emanuel, B., Yates, B. (2000a). Vestibular stimulation leads to distinct hemodynamic patterning. *American Journal of Physiology—Regulatory, Integrative and Comparative Physiology*, **279**, R118–25.

Kerman, I., McAllen, R., Yates, B. (2000b). Patterning of sympathetic nerve activity in response to vestibular stimulation. *Brain Res. Bull.*, **53**, 11–6.

Kuipers, N., Sauder, C., Ray, C. (2003). Aging attenuates the vestibulorespiratory reflex in humans. *J Physiol.*, **548**, 955–61.

Luxon, L. (1990). Signs and Symptoms of Vertebrobasilar Insufficiency. In: Hofferberth, B. Ed. *Vascular Brain Stem Diseases*, pp. 93–111. Karger, Basel.

McCabe, B. (1960). Vestbular suppression in figure skaters. Trans *American Academy of Ophthalmology and Otolaryngology*, **64**, 264–68.

Miller, A., Yates, B. (1996). Vestibular effects on respiratory activity. In B. Yates & A. Miller Eds. *Vestibular autonomic regulation*, pp.113–25. CRC press, Boca Raton (FL).

Mcloed, J., Tuck, R. (1987). Disorders of the autonomic nervous system, part 1: pathophysiology and clinical features. *Ann. Neurol.*, **21**, 419–30.

Miller, A., Rowley, H., Roberts, T., Kucharczyk, J. (1996). Human cortical activity during vestibular- and drug-induced nausea detected during magnetic source imaging. *Ann. N Y Acad. Sci.*, **781**, 670–72.

Monahan, K., Ray, C. (2002). Interactive effect of hypoxia and otolith organ engagement on cardiovascular regulation in humans. *J Appl. Physiol.*, **93**, 576–80.

Monahan, K., Sharpe, M., Drury, D., Ertl, A., Ray, C. (2002). Influence of vestibular activation on respiration in humans. *American Journal of Physiology—Regulatory, Integrative and Comparative Physiology*, **282**, R689–94.

Money, K., Friedberg, J. (1964). The role of the semicircular canals in causation of motion sickness and nystagmus in the dog. *Can. J Physiol. Pharmacol.*, **42**, 793–801.

Money, K., Lackner, J., Cheung, R. (1996). The autonomic nervous system and motion sickness. In B. Yates & A. Miller Eds. *Vestibular autonomic regulation*, pp.147–73. CRC press, Boca Raton (FL).

Neuhauser, H., Leopold, M., Brevern, M., Arnold, G., Lempert, T. (2001). The interrelations of migraine, vertigo and migrainous vertigo. *Neurology*, 56, 684–6.

Pappas, D. (2003). Autonomic related vertigo. *Laryngoscope*, 113, 1658–71.

Pappas, D., Banyas, J. (1991). A newly recognized etiology of Meniere's syndrome. *Acta Otolaryngologica supplement*, 485, 104–7.

Parker, D. (1998). The relative roles of the otoliths organs and semicircular canals in producing space motion sickness. *J Vestibular Res.*, 8, 57–59.

Previc, F. (1996). Disturbances from exposure to altered gravitational environments. In B. Yates & A. Miller Eds. *Vestibular autonomic regulation*, pp.175–95. CRC press, Boca Raton (FL).

Radtke, A., Popov, K., Bronstein, A., Gresty, M. (2003). Vestibulo-autonomic control in man: short and long latency vestibular effects on the cardiovascular function. *J Vestibular Res.*, 13, 25–37.

Ray, C., Carter, J. (2003). Vestibular activation of sympathetic nerve activity. *Acta Physiologica Scandinavica*, 177, 313–9.

Ray, C., Monahan, K. (2002). Aging attenuates the vestibulosympathetic reflex in humans. *Circulation*, 105, 956–61.

Reason, J. (1978). Motion sickness adaptation: a neural mismatch model. *J R Soc. Med.*, 71, 819–29.

Riccio, G., Stoffregen, T. (1991). An ecological theory of motion sickness and postural stability. *Ecological Psychology*, 3, 195–240.

Sammon, M., Darnall, R. (1994). Entrainment of respiration to rocking in premature infants: coherence analysis. *J Appl. Physiol.*, 77, 1548–54.

Savundra, P., Carroll, J., Davies, R., Luxon, L. (1997). Migraine–associated vertigo. *Cephalalgia*, 17, 505–10.

Spinks, A., Wasiak, J., Bernath, V. (2004). Scopolamine for preventing and treating motion sickness. *Cochrane Database Syst. Rev.*, 3, CD002851.

Staab, J., Ruckenstein, R., Solomon, D., Shepard, N. (2002). Exertional dizziness and autonomic dysregulation. *Laryngoscope*, 112, 1346–50.

Stoffregen, T., Smart, L. (1998). Postural instability precedes motion sickness. *Brain Res. Bull.*, 47, 437–48.

Suzuki, M., Kitano, H., Ito, R. *et al.* (2001). Cortical and subcortical vestibular response to caloric stimulation detected by functional magnetic resonance imaging. *Brain Res. Cogn. Brain. Res.*, 12, 441–9.

Tanguy, S., Quarck, G., Etard, O., Gauthier, A., Denise, P. (2008). Vestibulo-ocular reflex and motion sickness in figure skaters. *Eur. J Appl. Physiol.*, Aug 30 EPUB.

Tokita,T., Aoki, S., Miyata, H., Suzuki, S. (1971). The loading equilibrium examination for the etiologic diagnosis of Menière's disease. *Acta Otolaryngologica*, 72, 107–117.

Uemura, T., Itoh, M., Kikuchi, N. (1980). Autonomic dysfunction on the affected side in Meniere's disease. *Acta Otolaryngologica*, 89, 109–117.

Waeber, C., Moskowitz, M. (2003). Therapeutic implications of central and peripheral neurologic mechanisms in migraine. *Neurology*, 61:S9–S20.

Waeber, C., Moskowitz, M. (2005). Migraine as an inflammatory disorder. *Neurology*, 64, S9–S15.

Wang, S., Young, Y. (2003). Multiple system atrophy manifested as dizziness and imbalance: a report of two cases. *European Archives of Otorhinolaryngology*, 260, 404–7.

Wang, S., Chinn, H., Renzi, A. (1957). Experimental motion sickness in dogs: Role of abdominal visceral afferents. *Am. J Physiol.*, 190, 578–80.

Warwick-Evans, L., Symons, N., Fitch, T., Burrows, L. (1998). Evaluating sensory conflict and postural instability. Theories of motion sickness. *Brain Res. Bull.*, 47, 465–9.

Watenpaugh, D., Cothron, A., Wasmund, S. *et al.* (2002). Do vestibular otoliths organs participate in human orthostatic blood pressure control? *Autonomic Neuroscience*, 100, 77–83.

Welch, K. (2003). Contemporary concepts of migraine pathogenesis. *Neurology*, 61, S2–S8.

Wilson, T., Ray, C. (2004). Effect of thermal stress on the vestibulosympathetic reflexes in humans. *J Appl. Physiol.*, 97, 1367–70.

Wuyts, F., Furman, J., Van de Heyning, P. (2003). Instrumentation and principles of vestibular testing. In L. Luxon, A. Martini, J. Furman & D. Stephens Eds. *Textbook of Audiological Medicine*, pp. 717–34. Martin Dunitz, London.

Yamada, M., Keisuke, M., Ito, Y., Furuta, M., Sawai, S., Miyata, H. (1999). Autonomic nervous function in patients with Meniere's disease evaluated by power spectral analysis of heart rate variability. *Auris, Nasus, Larynx*, 26, 419–26.

Yardley, L., Owen, N., Nazareth, I., Luxon, L. (1998). Prevalance and presentation of dizziness in a general practice community sample of working age people. *Br. J Gen. Pract.*, 48, 1131–5.

Yardley, L., Owen, N., Nazareth, I., Luxon, L. (2001). Panic disorder with agoraphobia associated with dizziness: Characteristic symptoms and psychological sequelae. *Journal of Nervous and Mental Disease*, 189, 321–7.

Yardley, L., Watson, S., Britton, Lear, S., Bird, J. (1995). Effects of anxiety, arousal and mental stress on the vestibule-ocular reflex. *Acta Otolaryngologica*, 115, 597–602.

Yates, B. (1996). Vestibular influences on cardiovascular control. In B. Yates & A. Miller Eds. *Vestibular autonomic regulation*, pp.97–111. CRC press, Boca Raton (FL).

Yates, B., Siniaia, M., Miller, A. (1995). Descending pathways necessary for vestibular influences on sympathetic and inspiratory outflow. *Am. J Physiol.*, 268, 1381–5.

Yates, B., Aoki, M., Burchill, P., Bronstein, A., Gresty, M. (1999). Cardiovascular responses elicited by linear acceleration in humans. *Exp. Brain Res.*, 125, 476–84.

Yates, B., Balaban, C., Miller, A., Endo, K., Yamaguchi, Y. (1995). Vestibular inputs to the lateral tegmental field of the cat: potential role in autonomic control. *Brain Research*, 689, 197–206.

Yates, B., Miller, A. (1998). Physiological evidence that the vestibular system participates in autonomic and respiratory control. *J Vestibular. Res*, 8, 17–25.

Yates, B., Holmes, M., Jian, B. (2000). Adaptive plasticity in vestibular influences on cardiovascular control. *Brain Res. Bull.*, 53, 3–9.

Yates, B. (1998). Autonomic reaction to vestibular damage. *Otolaryngology—Head and Neck Surgery*, 119, 106–112.

Yates, B., Holmes, M., Jian, B. (2003). Plastic changes in processing of graviceptive signals during spaceflight potentially contribute to postflight orthostatic intolerance. *J Vestibular Res.*, 13, 395–404.

Yates, B., Miller, A., Lucot, J. (1998). Physiological basis and pharmacology of motion sickness: An update. *Brain Res. Bull.*, 47, 395–406.

CHAPTER 35

Epilepsy and the overlap with autonomic disorders

John S. Duncan and Helen J. Cross

Introduction

The thrust of this chapter is the differential diagnosis of epileptic seizures. There are a wide range of epileptic seizures and syndromes, with some age specific variations in the range of differential diagnoses. Autonomic dysfunction, with resultant presyncopal and syncopal symptoms, and epilepsy are differential diagnoses in a variety of clinical presentations. Patients may present with more than one dominant form of episode, so the approach taken is to consider the principal differential diagnoses of the common dominant presenting themes. As there are some differences to the common presentations and differential diagnoses in adults, infants and children, we consider these groups separately but recognize that there are considerable similarities and overlap.

The key to making a correct diagnosis is a detailed history from the individual patient and from a reliable witness who has seen the episodes in question. In individuals attending clinics with "first seizures" it is generally concluded that not more than 25% of patients are thought to have an epileptic seizure (Day et al. 1982, Chadwick and Smith 2002). The most common diagnostic error is to diagnose a syncopal episode as an epileptic seizure (Hoefnagels et al. 1991, Lempert et al. 1994, Sheldon et al. 2002). Undue reliance is often placed on investigations, particularly the EEG and MRI. Inappropriate weight is often placed on EEG findings that are "compatible with epilepsy".

It is a sound aphorism that the diagnosis of epilepsy is made on the history, and the role of the EEG is to assist in the subsequent classification of the type of epileptic seizures and the epilepsy syndrome, regardless of the age of the individual. The role of MRI is not to diagnose epilepsy, but in those with a diagnosis of that condition, to identify if there is an underlying structural cerebral abnormality.

There is considerable scope for misdiagnosis or of inaccurate diagnosis of epilepsy and epilepsy syndrome, which can have very serious consequences. In tertiary referral practice it is estimated that in 26% of those with a diagnosis of refractory epilepsy the diagnosis is incorrect or inaccurate (Smith et al. 1999).

The consequences of misdiagnosis are profound: an individual may have taken ineffective medication for years with adverse effects including teratogenesis if taken in pregnancy, and been denied a driving license and leisure, sporting and employment opportunities. Further, a treatable condition may have gone untreated. Whilst the range of differential diagnoses is large, in adults presenting with episodes of loss of awareness the most common are syncope, cardiac arrhythmias and dissociative episodes.

When taking the history it is suggested to firstly allow the individual and witnesses to give their own freehand account of the points that they consider most important, and to then go through the salient points in a systematic manner. It is not uncommon that a dramatic event leads to the individual seeking advice and that minor events have also occurred for some time but not been of sufficient concern to cause help to be sought. Such minor events may produce vital diagnostic clues and so need to be specifically enquired for. For example, a greying out of vision and unsteadiness on prolonged standing, which is likened to the head rush that occurs when rising up quickly from a crouch, suggests presyncope. In contrast, episodes of an epigastric rising sensation, déjà vu and premonition suggest temporal lobe onset focal seizure; brief blank spells and flurries of upper limb jerks in the first hour after waking suggest a generalized epilepsy.

In those who have had repeated episodes, a videotape recording of an episode is frequently invaluable, conveying more information that can be relayed by even the most careful witness, and being entirely objective. It is not uncommon for witnesses (including carers) to relate important details, such as which arm was stiff and extended and which was juddering, incorrectly (Samuel and Duncan 1994). As video cameras (particularly on mobile telephones) and Internet communications become increasingly prevalent, this is becoming more of a practical proposition and it is commonplace for individuals to send video recordings into the clinic.

The clinical examination is usually less rewarding than the history, but is still important. In addition to determining if there are any focal neurological deficits, or evidence of raised intracranial pressure, the individuals' mood and mental state need to be assessed. The skin should be examined to look for evidence of a neurocutaneous syndrome, and blood pressure should be checked. If an individual presents with episodes of loss of awareness or falling, a cardiac examination and checking of lying and standing blood pressure is indicated.

Differential diagnosis of epilepsy in adults

Epileptic seizures need to be considered in the differential diagnosis of a range of clinical presentations. These are principally:

◆ Loss of awareness

◆ Generalized convulsive movements

◆ Drop attacks

◆ Transient focal motor attacks

◆ Transient focal sensory attacks

◆ Facial muscle and eye movements

◆ Psychic experiences

◆ Aggressive or vocal outbursts

◆ Episodic phenomena in sleep

◆ Prolonged confusional or fugue states.

The principal differential diagnoses for each presenting clinical scenario follow, with brief explanatory text the key diagnostic features of each diagnosis.

Loss of awareness

Whatever the cause, the patient may have amnesia for both the event and its exact circumstances. The three main causes are: syncope, epilepsy, and cardiac arrhythmias. Transient cerebral ischaemia due to vascular abnormalities is less common. Microsleeps (very short daytime naps) may occur with any cause of severe sleep deprivation or disruption. Other causes of diagnostic confusion are much less common and include: hypoglycaemia or other intermittent metabolic disorders, structural anomalies of the skull base affecting the brainstem, or lesions affecting the circulation of the cerebrospinal fluid.

Syncope

Syncope is the commonest cause of episodes of loss of awareness. Simple faints or vasovagal syncopal attacks can usually be related to identifiable precipitants. Most often they occur on getting up quickly, or standing for prolonged periods, particularly if associated with peripheral vasodilation (e.g. during hot, stuffy weather, crowded trains or rooms, or are related to drug or alcohol use). Frightening, emotional or unpleasant scenes, and painful stimuli may also be triggers, due to increased vagal activity.

There are various other causes of syncopal attacks, and classification depends on terminology. Cough and micturition syncope are well recognized. Changes in intrathoracic pressure (cough syncope), impaired baroreceptors due to atheroma of the carotid (carotid sinus syncope), cardiac arrhythmias, or autonomic disturbances may also lead to cerebral hypoperfusion and fainting. As these may not be due to vasovagal reflex changes, the typical aura of a vasovagal syncope may not be present.

Epilepsy

Several types of epileptic seizure may present with loss of awareness as the only reported feature. These include absences, complex partial, tonic or atonic seizures. Typical absences involve arrest of activity, reduced or lost awareness, eyelid blinking or twitching, and sometimes small myoclonic facial or limb jerks, or brief facial automatisms such as lip smacking or chewing. Typical absences are usually brief but often occur many times per day. There may also be isolated myoclonic jerks. Atonic seizures usually give rise to drop attacks but may appear to cause blank spells if the patient is sat or lying down and so cannot fall. Complex partial seizures may cause loss of awareness with few if any other features. Detailed enquiry must always be made for any associated psychic or motor phenomena that may raise the possibility of a seizure disorder.

Cardiac disorders

There are often prodromal features similar to simple syncope, as well as palpitations, chest pain, shortness of breath or other features of cardiovascular insufficiency. Attacks due to transient complete heart block or asystole are abrupt and short with rapid loss of consciousness. Lack of cardiac output may also be due to short episodes of ventricular tachycardia or fibrillation. Prolongation of the QT interval may lead to such events. Attacks may be preceded by palpitations, extreme fatigue or presyncopal features.

Mitral valve prolapse and aortic stenosis may present with episodic loss of awareness due to fluctuating cardiac output or associated arrhythmias. Aortic stenosis and hypertrophic cardiomyopathy is especially prone to present with episodes of sudden collapse with loss of awareness during exercise. A cardiological opinion should be sought if there is the possibility of cardiac dysfunction causing episodes of loss of awareness, falls or convulsions. A 12-lead ECG should be carefully inspected, particularly for evidence of prolongation of the QT interval and consideration given to prolonged ECG monitoring with an implanted ECG loop recorder (Zaidi et al. 1999).

Microsleeps

Any cause of sleep deprivation may lead to brief day-time naps, sometimes lasting for only a few seconds. Impaired quality of sleep may also be a factor. The most important is obstructive sleep apnoea. Microsleeps are a common problem when driving, particularly on featureless straight roads and are the cause of many road traffic accidents. There are usually clear warning signs such as the driver feeling a need to close their eyes, yawn, turn the radio volume up and opening the windows. These events are of legal significance as a driver who continues to drive despite such warning signs and who causes an accident is likely to be prosecuted for dangerous driving and face a custodial sentence. Narcolepsy can present with short periods of suddenly falling asleep during the day. Systematic enquiry should be made for other symptoms of the narcolepsy-cataplexy syndrome, such as loss of body tone precipitated by emotion or laughter, sleep paralysis, and hypnogogic hallucinations.

Panic attacks

Panic attacks usually present with feelings of fear and anxiety, associated with autonomic changes and hyperventilation. This leads to dizziness or light-headedness, orofacial and/or peripheral paraesthesia (which may be asymmetric), carpopedal spasm, twitching of the peripheries, blurred vision, or nausea. Occasionally these preludes may be forgotten, and attacks present with loss of awareness. Often (but not always) there is a clear precipitant, such as a particular situation. None of these features are consistent, however, and differentiation from epilepsy can be difficult.

Hypoglycaemia

Hypoglycaemic attacks causing loss of consciousness are extremely rare except in patients with treated diabetes mellitus. Very occasional cases may be seen due to insulin secreting tumours. There is usually a clear history of events occurring if meals are delayed or

Table 35.1 Checklist of possible seizure-related symptoms to enquire for when considering a possible diagnosis of epilepsy

1. Have there been any presyncopal symptoms at other times, and is there any similarity between these and the onset of an episode of loss of awareness? Are such symptoms at all similar to those experienced on rising quickly from a crouch?

2. Have there been any spontaneous and otherwise unexplained paroxysmal symptoms?

In particular:

Sudden falls

Involuntary jerky movements of limbs whilst awake

Blank spells

Unexplained incontinence of urine with loss of awareness, or in sleep

Odd events occurring in sleep, e.g. fall from bed, jerky movements, automatisms

Episodes of confused behaviour with impaired awareness, recollection

Possible simple partial seizures

Epigastric rising sensation

Déjà vu

Premonition

Fear

Elation, Depression

Depersonalization, derealization

Inability to understand or express language (written or spoken)

Loss of memory, disorientation

Olfactory, gustatory, visual, auditory hallucination

Focal motor or Somatosensory deficit, or positive symptoms (jerking, tingling).

missed and prodromal symptoms of anxiety, sweating, and unease that recede with taking glucose.

Other neurological disorders

If a head injury causes loss of consciousness, there is amnesia. In accidental head injury, particularly road traffic accidents, it may be difficult to distinguish amnesia caused by the injury from cases in which there was a loss of consciousness that caused the accident. Isolated episodes of loss of awareness may also be caused by abuse of psychotropic drugs or other substances.

Dissociative seizures

Dissociative seizures (previously known as non-epileptic attack disorder (NEAD)), or pseudoseizures typically give rise episodes of two broad types:

(a) attacks involving motor phenomena

(b) attacks of lying motionless.

The latter are often prolonged, continuing for several minutes or sometimes hours. Such behaviour is very rare in epileptic seizures: there will nearly always be other positive phenomena in epileptic attacks that last for more than a few minutes. In addition, attacks are often triggered by external events or stress. Patients with dissociative seizures often have a history of abnormal illness behaviour. Dissociative seizures are much commoner in females than males, and usually commence in adolescence or early adulthood (Table 2).

Generalized convulsive movements

Epilepsy

A generalized convulsion is generally the most readily diagnosed epileptic phenomenon. Classically, there is a cry, generalized stiffening of body and limbs, followed by rhythmic jerking of all four limbs, associated with loss of awareness, eyes staring blankly, tongue biting and urinary incontinence. The generalized convulsive movements usually last for a minute or so, and as the attack

Table 35.2 Differentiation of epileptic seizures and dissociative seizures

	Epileptic seizure	Dissociative seizures
Precipitating cause	Rare	Common, emotional & stress related
When alone or asleep	Common	May be reported
Onset	Usually short	May be short or over several minutes
Aura	Various, usually stereotyped	Fear, panic, altered mental state
Speech	Cry, grunt at onset; muttering, words in automatisms	Semi-voluntary, often unintelligible
Movement	Atonic; tonic; if clonic, synchronous small amplitude jerks	Asynchronous flailing of limbs; pelvic thrusting; opisthotonous
Injury	Tongue biting, fall; directed violence rare	May bite tongue, cheeks, lip, hands, throw self to ground. Directed violence not uncommon
Consciousness	Complete loss in generalized tonic-clonic; may be incomplete in complex partial	Variable, often inconsistent with seizure type
Response to stimulation	None in generalized tonic-clonic; may respond in complex partial and post-ictally	Often reacts and this may terminate episode
Incontinence	Common	Sometimes
Duration	Few minutes	Few minutes, may be prolonged
Recovery	Depends on seizure type. Few minutes and more prolonged confusion	May be rapid or very prolonged

proceeds the jerking slows in frequency and increases in amplitude. There is often tachycardia, apnoea, cyanosis, and afterwards irregular breathing followed by confusion, headache and sleepiness.

Syncope with secondary jerking movements

People who faint often have myoclonic twitches of the extremities that last for less than one minute (Lempert et al. 1994). This may be associated with limb posturing and stiffening. With prolonged cerebral hypoperfusion, as may occur if the person is held upright by well-meaning bystanders, or an aircraft seat, these may be more prominent and prolonged, and be reported as "a convulsion". Incontinence of urine may occur, particularly if the bladder is full. Tongue biting may occur if the tongue is caught between the teeth as the individual falls to the ground.

Primary cardiac or respiratory abnormalities presenting with secondary anoxic seizures

Episodes of complete heart block or transient asystole may have syncopal features followed by collapse to the ground and secondary anoxic seizures. More commonly there is an abrupt collapse with no warning and the person is observed to be pale and witnesses commonly remark that "they thought the person was dead". The attacks last for less than one minute, but may be followed by a prolonged period of confusion, particularly in elderly patients. There should be a low threshold for obtaining a cardiological opinion in such cases and consideration given to insertion of an implanted ECG loop recorder (Zaidi et al. 1999).

Involuntary movement disorders and other neurological conditions

There is no alteration in consciousness. The best known is paroxysmal kinesiogenic choreoathetosis. Attacks are usually precipitated by sudden specific movements. They last a few seconds to minutes. Paroxysmal dystonia can present with attacks that last for minutes to hours. Patients with involuntary movement disorders such as idiopathic torsion dystonia may show severe acute exacerbations that may mimic convulsive movements.

Patients with mental retardation often have stereotyped or repetitive movements, which may include head banging or body rocking, and more subtle movements which may be difficult to differentiate from complex partial seizures.

Hyperekplexia

Hyperekplectic attacks are characterized by excessive startle, may cause stiffening, and collapse with a sudden jerk of all four limbs. Attacks are provoked by sudden unexpected stimuli, usually auditory. Hyperekplexia needs to be distinguished from seizures induced by startle, which commonly have the features of a frontal lobe epilepsy.

Dissociative seizures

Dissociative seizures involving prominent motor phenomena are commoner than those with arrest of activity. Movements are varied but often involve semi-purposeful thrashing of all four limbs, waxing and waning over many minutes, distractibility or interaction with the environment, prominent pelvic movements and back arching (Table 2). Dissociative seizures may be difficult to differentiate from complex partial seizures of frontal lobe origin, which can present with very bizarre motor attacks. The key feature of the latter is that the episodes are usually stereotyped and occur during both wake and sleep.

Drop attacks

Any cause of loss of awareness may proceed to a sudden collapse or drop attack. Epilepsy, syncope and other cardiovascular disorders are the commoner causes of drop attacks.

Epilepsies

Sudden drop attacks are common in patients with mental retardation and secondary generalized epilepsies. The falls may be tonic or atonic or atonic in nature and frequently cause severe facial injuries if the individual falls forwards.

Cardiovascular

If cerebral hypoperfusion is sufficient to cause sudden collapse there is usually loss of awareness, but a drop attack may be the dominant presenting symptom.

Movement disorders

Most movement disorders that cause drop attacks have other more prominent features which make the diagnosis clear (e.g. Parkinson's disease). Paroxysmal kinesiogenic choreoathetosis may cause drop attacks if there is lower limb involvement.

Brainstem, spinal or lower limb abnormalities

There are usually fixed neurological signs that give a clue towards a diagnosis in this area. Tumours of the third ventricle, such as colloid cysts, may present with sudden episodes of collapse. Spinal cord vascular abnormalities may present with abrupt episodes of lower limb weakness leading to falls, without impairment of awareness.

Cataplexy

Cataplexy usually occurs in association with narcolepsy, although it may be the presenting clinical feature. There is no loss of consciousness with attacks. Attacks may be precipitated by emotion, especially laughter. Often there is only loss of tone in the neck muscles, with slumping of the head rather than complete falls.

Metabolic disorders

Periodic paralysis due to sudden changes in serum potassium is rare. The condition may be familial or associated with other endocrine disorders or drugs. Usually there is a gradual onset, and the attacks last for hours.

Idiopathic drop attacks

These attacks are most common in middle aged females. They take the form of a sudden fall without loss of consciousness. Characteristically the patients remember falling and hitting the ground. Recovery is instantaneous, but injury may occur.

Vertebrobasilar ischaemia

This condition is over-diagnosed and probably accounts for very few drop attacks. Typically, the attacks occur in the elderly, with evidence of vascular disease and cervical spondylosis. The attacks may be precipitated by head turning or neck extension resulting in distortion of the vertebral arteries and are of sudden onset, with features of brainstem ischaemia such as diplopia, vertigo, and bilateral facial and limb sensory and motor deficits.

Transient focal motor attacks

The commonest cause of transient focal motor attacks is epilepsy. Tics may develop in adolescence. Paroxysmal movement disorders are rare, although unilateral paroxysmal kinesiogenic choreoathetosis may mimic motor seizures. Transient cerebral ischaemia usually presents with negative phenomena. Tonic spasms of multiple sclerosis are usually seen once other features of the illness have become apparent, but may be a presenting feature.

Focal motor seizures

Focal motor seizures may involve jerking and posturing of one extremity, or reflect the spread of epileptic activity along the primary motor cortex. There is often associated paraesthesia. There may be localized transient weakness following the attack for seconds or minutes, sometimes longer. Seizures arising in many different brain regions may cause dystonic posturing.

Epilepsia partialis continua is a rare form of epilepsy that often causes diagnostic confusion. There is very frequent focal motor activity such as jerking of the hand or part of the face. This can persist for hours or days, continue into sleep, and may go on for years. The movements often become slow and pendulous, with some associated dystonic posturing.

Tics

Tics usually present with stereotyped movements in childhood or adolescence, sometimes restricted to one particular action (e.g. eye blinking) but may be multiple in nature. Tics may be confused with myoclonic jerks. They can be suppressed voluntarily, although to do so leads to a rise in psychological tension and anxiety that is then relieved by the patient allowing the tics to occur. Repetitive tics and stereotypies are particularly common in those with intellectual disability.

Transient cerebral ischaemia

Transient ischaemic attacks (TIAs) usually present with negative phenomena, i.e. loss of use of a limb, hemiplegia or other deficits, although positive phenomena such as paraesthesiae may occur. Transient ischaemic attacks may last for a few minutes, but may persist for up to 24 hours. TIAs are not usually stereotyped or repeated with the frequency of epileptic seizures, and there are usually associated features to suggest vascular disease.

Tonic spasms of multiple sclerosis

These spasms usually occur in the setting of known multiple sclerosis, but may be the presenting feature, although other evidence of multiple sclerosis may be found on examination and investigation. The spasms may last for several seconds, sometimes longer than one minute.

Paroxysmal movement disorders

Paroxysmal kinesiogenic choreoathetosis may present with focal motor attacks that are very similar to epileptic seizures. Tremor may occur in a variety of movement disorders and is usually sufficiently persistent to make the non-epileptic nature clear, but may be difficult to distinguish from certain forms of epilepsia partialis continua. Myoclonus of subcortical origin may be suspected from the distribution of involved muscles (e.g. spinal myoclonus may be restricted to specific segments, either unilateral or bilateral). Peripheral nerve entrapment usually presents with weakness but occasionally can present with episodic jerks or twitches.

Transient focal sensory attacks

Somatosensory attacks

Epileptic seizures involving the primary sensory cortex are less common than motor seizures, and may cause spreading paraesthesia.

Seizures involving the second sensory areas or mesial frontal cortex may cause sensory symptoms. There are usually other epileptic features due to involvement of adjacent or related brain structures. Transient sensory phenomena may also be seen in peripheral nerve compression or other abnormalities of the ascending sensory pathways, hyperventilation or panic attacks and in TIAs. TIAs are not usually stereotyped or repeated with the frequency of epileptic seizures, and there are usually associated features to suggest vascular disease.

Lesions of sensory pathways cause persistent symptoms, but diagnostic confusion may arise in the early natural history, when complaints are intermittent, or if they are posture related. Hyperventilation may be associated with unilateral and localized areas of paraesthesia (e.g. one arm). Intermittent sensory illusions may be experienced in relation to amputated or anaesthetic limbs. Migrainous episodes may also cause localized areas of paraesthesia, but usually have the distinction of a gradual evolution of sensory phenomena, both positive and negative, and associated features of migraine.

Transient vestibular symptoms

Acute attacks of vertigo may occasionally be due to a seizure in parietal or temporal lobes. In these cases there are generally associated features that point to cerebral involvement, such as a focal somatosensory symptoms, déjà vu, or disordered perception. Peripheral vestibular disease is a much more common cause and may give rise to paroxysmal rotational vertigo and perception of linear motion and there are often also other symptoms of auditory and vestibular disease such as: deafness, tinnitus, pressure in the ear and relation to head position.

Visual symptoms

Migraine is a common cause of episodic visual phenomena. The evolution is usually gradual, over several minutes, with fortification spectra, and associated photophobia, nausea and headache. Epileptic phenomena are usually much shorter, evolving over seconds, and the visual hallucinations are more commonly of coloured blobs, rather than jagged lines.

Facial muscle and eye movements

Facial movements may occur in a variety of neurological conditions including partial seizures, tics, dystonias or other paroxysmal movement disorders, especially drug induced dyskinesias and hemifacial spasm, as well as psychological disorders.

Partial seizures

Benign rolandic epilepsy usually presents with seizures in childhood affecting the face, often with unilateral grimacing, hemicorporeal sensory and motor phenomena, or secondarily generalized seizures occurring in sleep. Focal motor seizures may cause twitching of one side of the face that may be restricted to specific areas.

Complex partial seizures may cause automatisms with lip smacking, chewing, swallowing, sniffing or grimacing, with amnesia and impaired awareness. If these features are due to seizure activity the attacks are usually relatively infrequent, whereas with dystonia or other movement disorders episodes are likely to occur many times per day.

Movement disorders

Hemifacial spasm typically presents in the elderly or middle aged with clusters of attacks that initially involve the eye but subsequently spread to the rest of that side of the face. Facial weakness may develop that persists between attacks.

Bruxism may occur either during the day or in sleep, especially in children with learning disability. Episodes are usually more prolonged than with the automatisms of complex partial seizures, and there are no associated features to suggest an epileptic basis.

As with dystonia and other movement disorders affecting the face there may be evidence of involvement elsewhere, and attacks are usually more frequent than is seen with isolated seizures.

Other neurological disorders

Defects of eye movement control are common in patients with a wide range of neurological disorders. There are usually associated features that indicate a non-epileptic basis. Bizarre eye movements also occur in blindness and may be mistaken for epileptic activity. Careful examination is required to ascertain the precise features of the eye movement disorder, and in particular any precipitating factors or features of cerebellar or brainstem disease.

Psychic experiences

Intermittent psychic phenomena can be seen in partial seizures (especially of temporal lobe origin), migraine, panic attacks, transient cerebral ischaemia, drug induced flash-backs, or with illusions associated with loss of a sensory modality as well as psychotic illnesses.

Epilepsy

Partial seizures of temporal lobe origin are especially likely to be manifest by auras involving psychic phenomena. The most common are fear, déjà vu, memory flashbacks, visual, olfactory or auditory hallucinations. Other manifestations include altered perception of the environment with a distancing from reality or change in size or shape of objects; altered language function; emotions such as sadness, elation, and sexual arousal.

Psychic experiences may have some relation to past experiences. They are usually recalled as brief scenes, sometimes strung together into a sequence. They usually lack clarity, for example a patient may describe an illusion of someone standing in front of them who they know, but they cannot name them or describe them in detail. A rising epigastric sensation may occur alone or in association with such experiences. Elemental visual phenomena, such as flashing lights, are more often seen in occipital lobe epilepsy.

Migraine

Migrainous psychic phenomena may involve an initial heightening of awareness. The principal features are usually visual illusions that may be elemental or complex. They rarely have the same intense emotional components of temporal lobe illusions or hallucinations. The time course is usually more prolonged than with partial seizures, with an evolution over several minutes and there are associated features of a pounding headache, photophobia and nausea or vomiting. There may be recognized precipitants, and there is often a relevant family history.

Panic attacks

These are usually associated with feelings of fear and anxiety. Hyperventilation may lead to dizziness and light-headedness. There are often unpleasant abdominal sensations similar to the epigastric aura of partial seizures. The evolution, associated increases in heart rate and respiration, longer time course and history of precipitating factors usually make the diagnosis clear, but

distinction from temporal lobe seizures may be difficult (Ref Thompson).

Drug induced flashbacks

These share many of the qualities of psychic temporal lobe seizures. They are individualized hallucinations usually related to the circumstances of the drug abuse, often with emotional content of fear or anxiety. A careful history should be taken for substance abuse, especially LSD, Psilocibine, peyote and mescaline.

Hallucinations or illusions caused by loss of a primary sense

Hallucinations and illusions of an absent limb are well recognized in amputees. Similarly, people who lose sight either in the whole or part field may experience visual hallucinations or illusions in the blind field. Such phenomena can be elemental or complex and include evolving scenes. Similar experiences can occur with deafness.

Such experiences due to the loss of a primary sense present particular diagnostic difficulty when they occur in the setting of a structural lesion, which could result in both phenomena. An occipital infarction, for example, could cause visual loss and could also give rise to epileptic seizures. Often the hallucinations due to sensory loss are more prolonged, lasting for minutes or hours, but can be brief.

Psychotic hallucinations and delusions

Hallucinations and delusions are the hallmark of psychotic illnesses. The following features would suggest a psychiatric rather than epileptic basis: complex nature with an evolving or argued theme, auditory nature involving instructions or third person language, paranoid content or associated thought disorder. Psychotic episodes are usually longer-lasting than isolated epileptic seizures, although intermittent psychosis may have a similar time course to nonconvulsive status. Persistent mood changes may be a helpful guide, but even short temporal lobe seizures may be followed by mood changes lasting for hours or days. Furthermore, flurries of epileptic attacks may themselves cause an organic psychosis lasting for several days. Ruminations and pseudo-hallucinations, in which the patient retains some insight, may occur in affective disorders.

Dissociative seizures

Dissociative seizures may be associated with reports of hallucinations and illusions. Initially the symptoms may seem plausible, but should be suspected if they are florid and multiple in type (e.g. auditory, olfactory and visual at different times) with evolving stories or patterns of expression.

Aggressive or vocal outbursts

These are rarely epileptic in nature if they occur in isolation. They are especially common in adults and children with mental retardation. In this setting there is organic brain disease that could lower the overall seizure threshold. A not infrequent forensic issue is the occurrence of violent, or other, crimes in patients with epilepsy, in which it is a defence claim that the crime was committed in a state of automatism. Certain features are strong evidence against an epileptic basis to the attack:

- Absence of a prior history of epilepsy with automatisms
- Premeditation and evidence of planning or preparation
- Directed violence

◆ Evidence of complicated and organized activity during the episode

◆ Recall of events during the episode

◆ Witness accounts not indicative of a disturbance of consciousness

◆ Subsequent attempts at escape or concealment of evidence.

Episodic phenomena in sleep

Attacks occurring during sleep present particular diagnostic difficulties because they are often poorly witnessed, and the patient may have little, if any, recall of the event or the preceding circumstances.

Normal physiological movements

Whole body jerks commonly occur in normal subjects on falling asleep. Fragmentary physiological myoclonus usually involves the peripheries or the face, and occurs during stages 1 and 2 and REM sleep.

Periodic movements of sleep may be an age related phenomenon, being seen in less than 1% of young adults, but occurring with increasing frequency during middle and old age such that they are present in perhaps half the elderly population. Typically these movements occur at regular intervals of 10–60 seconds and may occur in clusters over many minutes.

Frontal lobe epilepsy

Frontal lobe seizures may display specific sleep related characteristics causing diagnostic confusion. Such attacks are often frequent, brief, bizarre, and may only occur during sleep. Attacks may include apnoea, dystonic, myoclonic, or choreiform movements that may be unilateral or bilateral, and some retention of awareness. The attacks are scattered throughout the night, and usually arise from non-REM sleep. Frequency is highly variable, but some patients have more than 20 attacks in a night. An important clue to the diagnosis is the occurrence of additional secondary generalized seizures and seizures occurring in wakefulness.

Other epilepsies

Seizures arising in other brain regions may present with nocturnal attacks. Patients may be aroused by an aura, although often this is not recalled when attacks arise from sleep. Complex automatisms, in which patients get out of bed and wander around may cause confusion with parasomnias. With nocturnal seizures of any type the partner is frequently awoken by particular components, such as vocalization and does not witness the onset. Generalized tonic-clonic seizures not uncommonly occur on or shortly after awakening.

Pathological fragmentary myoclonus

Excessive fragmentary myoclonus persisting into sleep stages 3 and 4 may be seen with any cause of disrupted nocturnal sleep.

Restless leg syndrome

The restless leg syndrome is characterized by an urge to move the legs, especially in the evening when lying or sitting. It may be associated with various unpleasant paraesthesiae. All patients with restless legs have periodic movements of sleep. These may be severe and can also occur during wakefulness. In addition there may be a variety of brief daytime dyskinesias.

Non-REM parasomnias

These involve night terrors or sleep walking. They usually present in childhood or adolescence, and are often familial. The attacks arise from slow wave sleep, typically at least thirty minutes, but not more than four hours, after going to sleep and the timing is often consistent. Attacks may be spaced out by months or years and rarely occur more than once per week, and usually no more than one attack occurs in a single night. They are more likely after stressful events, or when sleeping in a strange bed.

Night terrors involve intense autonomic features (sweating, flushing, palpitations) and a look of fear. Patients may recall a frightening scene or experience, but do not usually recount a vivid dream prior to the attacks. Certainly children do not recall events. They may be difficult to arouse, and confused for several minutes. Vocalizations are common. Sleepwalking may involve getting out of bed and performing complex tasks. Sometimes it is possible to lead the patient back to bed without awakening. They may respond if spoken to, but their speech is usually slow or monosyllabic. Brief, abortive episodes are commoner, involving sitting up in bed with fidgeting and shuffling (mimicking a complex partial seizure). Non-REM parasomnias may cause self-injury but rarely directed aggression. They are associated with enuresis.

REM parasomnias

REM parasomnias usually occur in middle age or the elderly, and show a marked male predominance. They more often occur in the later portion of sleep. During REM sleep patients may have an increase in the frequency or severity of fragmentary myoclonus, thrash about, call out, display directed violence, or appear to enact vivid dreams. Attacks may last from seconds to minutes. If awoken, patients may recall part of these dreams. Although REM sleep behaviour disorders may occur in healthy elderly subjects they are also seen in association with drugs (e.g. tricyclics) or alcohol, or central nervous system diseases such as multisystem atrophy. The possibility of REM sleep disorders needs to be considered both at initial presentation, and also in patients known to have central nervous system disorders.

Sleep apnoea

Patients with sleep apnoea usually present with day-time hypersomnolence. However, the apnoeic episodes may cause episodic grunting, flailing about or other restless activity that appears to mimic nocturnal epilepsy. Occasionally the resultant hypoxia leads itself to secondary seizures.

Other movements in sleep

Nocturnal body rocking may occur in patients with learning disability, or following head injuries. In patients with many different forms of day-time dyskinesias, similar movements may occasionally occur during overnight sleep, usually in the setting of brief arousals.

Prolonged confusional or fugue states

Epileptic seizures usually last for seconds or minutes. After generalized tonic-clonic seizures (or less often complex partial seizures) there may be confusion lasting for many minutes, but rarely more than an hour. Such episodes only present diagnostic difficulty if the initial seizure is unwitnessed. Nevertheless, epileptic states can last for longer periods of time, as can other types of cerebral disorder and the differential diagnosis of prolonged epileptic confusional states (non-convulsive status) should include: acute encephalopathy, nonconvulsive status epilepticus, transient global amnesia, intermittent psychosis, and dissociative seizures.

Acute encephalopathy

Virtually any severe metabolic disturbance may cause an acute encephalopathy (e.g. diabetic ketoacidosis, hypoglycaemia, respiratory, renal or hepatic failure, drug ingestion, hyperpyrexia, sepsis). Transient metabolic disturbances are most often seen in treated diabetes mellitus due to insulin induced hypoglycaemia. Occasionally metabolic disorders may present with exacerbations with symptoms lasting for hours or days that give the appearance of an episodic condition. These include: porphyria and urea cycle enzyme defects.

Acute neurological conditions also need to be considered, particularly: encephalitis, meningitis, other intracranial infection, head injury, cerebral infarction or haemorrhage. Drug abuse may cause isolated episodes or recurrent bouts, related to intoxications.

Non-convulsive status epilepticus

Patients with complex partial seizures, typical or atypical absences may present with prolonged confusional states due to complex partial epilepticus or absence status. Such attacks may be the first manifestation of the seizure disorder, or occur in the setting of known epilepsy.

Intermittent psychosis

Although usually more sustained, psychiatric disorders may present with episodes of delusions, hallucinations or apparent confusion, lasting for hours or days.

Transient global amnesia

These episodes typically commence acutely, and last for minutes or hours and involve both retrograde and anterograde amnesia. Patients may perform complex activities, but afterwards have no recall of them. There is a lack of other neurological features to the attacks, and consciousness appears to be preserved. The attacks may involve bilateral medial temporal dysfunction, which in some patients may be on the basis of ischaemia, whilst some may have an epileptic basis.

Hysterical fugue

A fugue state may arise without an organic physical cause, as a conversion symptom. These episodes may be brief or very prolonged, lasting for days or even weeks. If seen at the time of episode inconsistencies are often found on examination of the mental state. In some cases, the question of malingering arises, most commonly in a situation in which the person's state prevents questioning by Law Officers. The diagnosis is more difficult to identify if the patient is only seen subsequently. The matching of witness accounts and the apparent sequence of events is essential, but it may remain difficult to come to a firm conclusion. In this situation, there is sometimes a forensic aspect, typically when the person concerned is alleged to have committed a crime and they profess to have no memory of the events.

Differential diagnosis of epilepsy in children

There is a range of possible differential diagnoses when considering the child with a "funny turn". The considerations will vary depending on certain key features of the event, as well as the age of the child. The history is key to any diagnosis, and is likely to be far more useful than any investigation that can be requested. Always seek the initial event—a trigger or warning, however young the child.

There may be a typical behaviour prior to any event or a slightly older child may be able to relate a feeling prior to or during the event. A description of each change in the child should be sought, and the evidence of loss or not of awareness. Other important aspects of the history are medications taken, developmental history and past medical history, but information from these will only be supplementary to the history of the events themselves. There are a limited but well-defined number of possibilities within the differential diagnosis of epilepsy in childhood; however a lack of awareness of such alternatives remains the major reason for error and the premature, possible misdiagnosis, of epilepsy (Table 3). A difference from the approach with adults is the prominence of the child's age as being a factor in deciding the likely differential diagnosis.

Table 35.3 Differential diagnoses of epilepsy in children

Syncope & related disorders	
◆ Disorders of orthostatic control	Reflex syncope
◆ Respiratory syncope	Reflex & expiratory apnoeic syncope
	'Fainting lark'
◆ Cardiac syncope	Upper airway obstruction
	Arrhythmias
	Complete heart block
	Wolff-Parkinson-White
◆ Brainstem syncope	Tumour
	Brain stem herniation or compression
◆ Other	Anoxic epileptic seizures
Neurological	Tics
	Myoclonus
	Paroxysmal dystonia
	Sandifer syndrome
	Paroxysmal dyskinesias
	Cataplexy
	Benign paroxysmal vertigo/torticollis
	Migraine
	Alternating hemiplegia
	Eye movement disorders
	Overflow movements
	Hyperekplexia
Behavioural/psychiatric	Daydreams
	Dissociative states
	Self-gratification behaviour
	Hyperventilation
	Panic/anxiety
	Non epileptic attack disorder
	Fabricated attacks
	Pseudosyncope
	Stereotypies/ritualistic behaviour
Parasomnias	Sleep myoclonus
	Headbanging
	Confusional arousal
	REM sleep disorder/night terrors

The child under the age of 12 months

In a child of this age, it may be very difficult to determine the true nature of an event when taking the history for the first time, and there is likely to be considerable anxiety on the part of carers. Key questions in the evaluation will include whether the event related to any particular activity—for example, feeding may suggest reflux, history of medication ingestion may suggest dystonic reaction, and events exclusive to sleep in a developmentally normal child may suggest benign sleep myoclonus. Further it is important to determine the major motor component, whether hypertonia, hypotonia or dystonia, and whether it is repetitive or sustained. Repetitive jerks may imply seizures, although again seen only from sleep may suggest sleep myoclonus. Repetitive infantile spasms, a specific seizure type seen in this age group will involve stereotyped episodes of flexion of the trunk, with adduction of the limbs occurring in clusters. However they may be more subtle involving eye change and head nod only. Sudden sustained hypertonia may give a clue to hyperekplexia or brainstem syncope.

The presence or absence of semi-purposeful movements may suggest retained awareness as well as whether the child has behavioural arrest with or without eye movement, and whether they can be distracted. Distress may suggest awareness, although may be seen following an event (particularly in between infantile spasms within a cluster) or during seizures (manifest as fear). Colour change may also be important; pallor or cyanosis may be seen in cardiac arrythmias; cyanotic attacks are commonly associated with reflux. Flushing and other autonomic features may be seen with repetitive movement in self-gratification behaviour. If the event can be interrupted, it may suggest a non-epileptic event.

In the toddler (age 1 to 3 years)

Again, whether the events are related to any particular activity may give a clue as to the nature of the episode. Obviously recurrent events with change in tone/loss of awareness in association with high fever may be febrile seizures. The seizures are usually seen in association with the abrupt rise in temperature, to >39°C. The temperature is thereafter usually sustained for a period.

From sleep, parasomnias are very common at this age and in some instances mimic seizures. Night terrors usually occur at a specific time each night, and during which the child may appear unreachable. There is normally no recollection of the event. Confusional arousals may also cause alarm as the child is inaccessible. If events are always triggered by adverse or noxious events, breath holding/reflex anoxic seizures should be considered. These may be quite profound, with a hypoxic seizure at the end. Abnormal movements, particularly of the head and neck in association with feeding may suggest Sandifer syndrome—a movement disorder associated with reflux, thought to be induced by an attempted change intrathoracic pressure to relieve pain from oesophagitis.

Often, this age group may also have distal movements associated with excitement, otherwise known as overflow movements, which are completely benign. Stereotypic movements or ritualistic behaviours may be seen in children with developmental delay or communication disorders at any time, but particularly in relation to excitement, stress or boredom. Sudden loss of tone in association with emotion could be cataplexy, and must always be thought of in the differential diagnosis of drop attacks, particularly in the absence of other apparent seizure types. Cataplexy is underdiagnosed in childhood.

The differential diagnosis for drop attacks associated with increased tone includes reflex/expiratory syncope, tonic/tonic clonic seizure, and hyperekplexia. Intermittent dystonia, particularly of the neck in an otherwise normal child may suggest benign paroxysmal torticollis. Intermittent unsteadiness with nystagmus may imply benign, paroxysmal vertigo, a paroxysmal condition of unknown aetiology in which children usually stop having attacks by the age of 5 years.

Repetitive short duration rhythmic movement over short period or with greater duration between may imply seizures, although repetitive short movements predominantly of the face may be tics. Semi-purposeful movements at any time may give a clue as to the state of awareness as with infants.

A child staring unresponsively, with or without minor movement may imply seizures but day dreaming is by far more common, and can be quite profound. Inability to be brought round using voice may not necessarily imply seizures; however it is more reliable to see whether they can be brought around by touch, and whether they occur in any environment. Daydreaming is far more common in school-age children.

Colour change may have an implication as with children under one year; reflex anoxic seizures and self-gratification behaviour are seen in this age group, the former being more common in this than in the younger age group. The majority cease by age 5 years.

In the older child

Parasomnias are very common in this age group and often mimic seizures. However, as with adult frontal lobe epilepsy, seizures can take a very bizarre format and it can be quite difficult to differentiate between the two.

Paroxysmal movement disorders may become apparent at this age; abnormal movement specifically related to initiation of movement with retention of awareness may suggest a movement disorder such as paroxysmal kinaesogenic choreoathetosis – there is also often a family history. They may also suggest a paroxysmal dystonia. Again stereotypic movements/ritualistic behaviours may be seen in children with developmental delay/communication disorders at any time, but particularly at times of excitement, stress or boredom.

Cataplectic attacks may also be seen at this age and be misdiagnosed, so one should be alerted to drop attacks, particularly initiated by emotion and seen in the absence of other epileptic attacks. The major motor component being hypertonia may suggest reflex/expiratory syncope, a tonic/tonic clonic seizure, or hyperekplexia. Where it is hypotonia the differential may lie between syncope, cataplexy, or 'akinetic' epileptic attack. Intermittent unsteadiness, again without change of awareness may suggest intermittent ataxia; in the episodic ataxias epileptic attacks may also be seen as part of the phenotype. Repetitive movement, particularly of short duration of the upper body may suggest tics—preceded by a period of hypertonia with loss of awareness, the diagnosis is likely to be a generalized tonic clonic seizure.

Episodes of staring unresponsively, particularly if only seen within the educational setting, are far more likely to be episodes of daydreaming than true absence seizures. Commonly parents are concerned as they feel they cannot distract the children by calling—this does not necessarily suggest loss of awareness as children are able to 'switch off' quite profoundly. Often the indication is they respond to touch. Typical absence seizures occur frequently, and in any situation, being of relatively short duration (5–10s).

Untreated individuals are likely to demonstrate an attack if asked to hyperventilate (by blowing) in the clinic situation.

As in adults, true 'rage' attacks in isolation are rarely, if ever epileptiform in origin. Typically they are seen in children with learning difficulties, but are not unseen in children with very specific learning problems that have not yet been recognized. The children may become aggressive and destructive, and may have little, if any recollection of the event.

Pallor or cyanosis may be seen in cardiac arrhythmias. Pallor is likely to be seen in association with any syncope. Flushing may be seen with self-gratification behaviour; in this age group this is more commonly seen in the learning disability population.

In the older child it is imperative to ask whether they can describe any phenomenology, indicating awareness or event clues to the nature of the event. Too often we are keen to ask parents and presume a child may have little to contribute. A feeling prior to the event, whether abdominal or visual symtomatology may suggest seizures (the latter may be quite descriptive); buzzing in the ears and light-headedness may suggest vaovagal syncope—the latter is rare under the age of 10 years so if in younger children, this is suspected, or episodes of collapse are related to exercise cardiac referral should be arranged as a cardiac arrythmia should be suspected.

A particular seizure disorder seen in the 2–7 year old age group, associated with autonomic symptoms, is Panayiotopoulos syndrome—benign epilepsy with occipital paroxysms. Typically a child may present with a prolonged period of unresponsiveness associated with vomiting; often they are not recognized as an epileptic seizure and admitted to hospital, treated as encephalitis. There may however, on further observation or direct questioning if events are recurrent, evidence of other autonomic features including pupillary change and hypersalivation. Often there may only be one such event—an EEG may show multifocal or generalized spikes, although occipital spikes are seen in around 40% in the first EEG increasing to 75% with further recordings, and fixation off sensitivity may be diagnostic. The condition has an extremely good prognosis with limited duration of treatment, if any, required.

References

Chadwick, D., Smith, D. F. (2002). The misdiagnosis of epilepsy. *BMJ* 2;324(7336), 495–6.

Day, S. C., Cook, E. F., Funkenstein, H., Goldman, L. (1982). Evaluation and outcome of emergency room patients with transient loss of consciousness. *Am J Med* **73**, 15–23.

Hoefnagels, W. A., Padberg, G. W., Overweg, J., Van der Velde, E. A., Roos, R. A. (1991). Transient loss of consciousness: the value of the history for distinguishing seizure from syncope. *J Neurol* **238**, 39–43.

Lempert, T., Bauer, M., Schmidt, D. (1994). Syncope: a videometric analysis of 56 episodes of transient cerebral hypoxia. *Ann Neurol* **36**, 233–7.

Samuel, M., Duncan, J. S. (1994). The use of the hand-held video camcorder in the evaluation of seizures. *J Neurol Neurosurg Psychiat* **57**, 1417–8.

Sheldon, R., Rose, S., Ritchie, D., *et al.* (2002). Historical criteria that distinguish syncope from seizures. *JACC* **40**, 142–8.

Smith, D., Defalla, B. A., Chadwick, D. W. (1999). The misdiagnosis of epilepsy and the management of refractory epilepsy in a specialist clinic. *QJM* **92**, 15–23.

Zaidi, A., Clough, P., Mawer, G., Fitzpatrick, A. (1999). Accurate diagnosis of convulsive syncope: role of an implantable subcutaneous ECG monitor. *Seizure* **8**, 164–186.

CHAPTER 36

Pupil abnormality in autonomic disorders

Detection and occurrence

F.D. Bremner and S.E. Smith

Introduction

This chapter describes the assessment of pupil function and the occurrence of pupil disturbance in disorders of the autonomic nervous system. The anatomical innervation of the muscles that determine pupil size is two-fold. Pupillary constriction is produced by contraction of the circular sphincter pupillae muscle, which is situated close to the pupillary margin of the iris. Its innervation is cholinergic and is derived from the parasympathetic system via the third (IIIrd) cranial nerve. The cholinoceptors involved are muscarinic, predominantly of the M_3 subtype. Pupillary dilatation is produced by contraction of the dilator pupillae muscle, the fibres of which are arranged radially within the substance of the iris. Its innervation is noradrenergic and comes from the sympathetic system via the cervical sympathetic chain and the long ciliary nerves. The adrenoceptors involved are alpha, probably of the α_1-subtype. At any one moment the size of the pupil depends on a balance of constrictor and dilator function.

Pupil constriction

Contraction of the sphincter pupillae constricts the pupil during the reflex responses to light and accommodation (near). Both reflexes involve activation of parasympathetic preganglionic neurons, the cell bodies of which lie in the Edinger–Westphal nuclei, a pair of slim columns of small cells situated dorsorostrally to the main mass of the oculomotor nuclear complex in the midbrain. These preganglionic neurons pass uncrossed in the superficial part of the IIIrd cranial nerve to the ciliary ganglion, which lies about 10 mm in front of the superior orbital fissure in the loose fatty tissue of the orbital cavity. This ganglion contains cell bodies of the postganglionic parasympathetic fibres, the axons of which travel forward to the iris sphincter and ciliary muscle via the short ciliary nerves that penetrate the eyeball at its posterior pole. Fibres subserving pupil constriction comprise only about 3% of the parasympathetic outflow from the ciliary ganglion; the majority subserve accommodation, in accordance with the relatively greater bulk of the ciliary compared with the sphincter muscle.

The course of the light reflex pathway from the retina to the sphincter is illustrated in Fig. 36.1 Afferent impulses for visual perception and pupil constriction diverge in the posterior third of the optic tracts. The visual fibres relay in the lateral geniculate bodies, whereas the pupillary fibres leave the optic tracts and synapse in the pretectal nuclei in the midbrain. Fibres from these nuclei carry pupillomotor impulses to the Edinger–Westphal nuclei of both sides. In man, this crossing, together with the preceding one at the optic chiasm, is essentially symmetrical. Thus, illumination

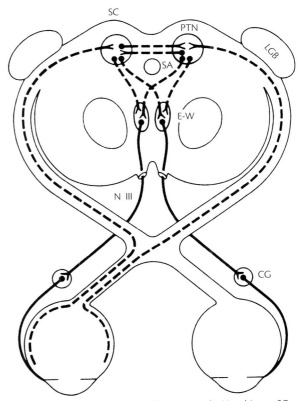

Fig. 36.1 The light reflex pathway from the retina to the iris sphincter. SC, superior colliculus; PTN, pretectal nucleus; LGB, lateral geniculate body; SA, Sylvian aqueduct; E-W, Edinger–Westphal nucleus; N III, oculomotor nerve; CG, ciliary ganglion. With kind permission from Springer Science+Business Media: *The Pupil.* 1985, Alexandridis E.

of only one eye produces reflex constriction of both pupils of approximately equal magnitude. In some individuals a small imbalance may result in a greater constriction of the direct over the consensual pupil (contraction anisocoria), but this difference is rarely if ever detectable clinically.

During fixation on a near object, the pupil constricts in association with accommodation produced by ciliary muscle contraction and convergence elicited by contraction of the medial rectus muscles. The light and near reflexes share a common neuronal path only from the Edinger–Westphal nucleus onward. Prior to that, the near reflex pathway descends from the occipital cortex, bypassing the pretectal nucleus on its way to the Edinger–Westphal nucleus. As the fibres approach the nucleus they are probably situated more ventrolaterally than the light reflex fibres for they are often spared in patients in whom pineal or collicular tumours have abolished the light reflex by pressure on the dorsal midbrain.

The postganglionic nerves release acetylcholine to activate muscarinic receptors on the sphincter pupillae. Parasympathomimetic agents such as pilocarpine, applied topically, have a similar action. A small number of muscarinic receptors are present on the dilator, which may relax the radial smooth muscle fibres during pupil constriction.

Pupil dilatation

Dilatation of the pupil in darkness and during arousal is elicited by two mechanisms: central inhibition of the Edinger–Westphal nucleus and activation of the peripheral sympathetic innervation of the radial smooth muscle fibres of the dilator pupillae. The central inhibition is said to be via sympathetic fibres from the posterior hypothalamus to the oculomotor nucleus (Lowenstein and Loewenfeld 1950).

The peripheral sympathetic pathway comprises three parts (Fig. 36.2). The first neuron arises in the hypothalamus and receives drive from higher centres including the cerebral cortex. From the hypothalamus the fibres descend uncrossed through the brainstem to the ciliospinal centre of Budge in the intermediolateral columns at the level of the last cervical and the first two thoracic segments of the cord. This centre contains the cell bodies of the preganglionic neurons, which form the second stage of the pathway. Their axons leave the cord by the ventral roots of the first two thoracic segments and enter the cervical sympathetic trunk. They traverse

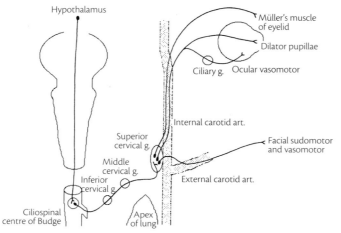

Fig. 36.2 The peripheral sympathetic pathway subserving pupil dilatation.

the inferior and middle cervical ganglia before reaching the superior cervical ganglion near the bifurcation of the internal and external carotid arteries. Since these preganglionic fibres pass close to the apex of the lung, the sympathetic pathway to the pupil may be interrupted by malignancy in this area. Within the superior cervical ganglion they synapse with the cell bodies of the postganglionic nerves, which form the third stage of the pathway. Fibres that subserve pupil dilatation, retraction of the eyelids by Müller's (smooth) muscle, and local vasomotor and sudomotor function leave the ganglion and follow the course of the internal carotid artery into the cranium. The pupil fibres join the trigeminal nerve and approach the orbit in its ophthalmic branch, entering via the superior orbital fissure. They continue in its nasociliary division and enter the eye in the long ciliary nerves. In man, some of the fibres traverse, but do not synapse in, the ciliary ganglion.

The postganglionic nerves release noradrenaline, which stimulates α_1-adrenoceptors on the dilator muscle. Sympathomimetic agents such as phenylephrine and adrenaline applied topically have similar actions. A small number of β-adrenoceptors is present on the sphincter pupillae, which relax these circular fibres during pupil dilatation. As with the cholinergic reciprocal innervation, there is no indication that these are of physiological significance and they do not mediate a change in pupil function in patients receiving topical β-adrenoceptor blocking drugs for the treatment of glaucoma.

Pupil measurement

Simple inspection of the pupil combined with registration of light and near reflexes is usually adequate for most clinical purposes. All neurologists in training learn to recognize the principal features of anisocoria, impaired reflexes, the tonic pupil, light-near dissociation, and Horner's syndrome. When the clinical disorder involves only one pupil, availability of a normal pupil for comparison means that relatively minor disturbances can be detected without too much difficulty. In bilateral disorders, however, no comparator is available and the detection of abnormality can be much more difficult, particularly in that all aspects of pupil function are subject to substantial variability within and between individuals. Small pupils in darkness may, for example, be abnormal in one subject yet quite normal in another, depending on the age of the patient and other circumstances. Flash photography has proved useful in the detection of abnormality, particularly in relation to diabetes, though of course only static measurements can be obtained.

Infrared video pupillography can provide accurate and repeatable dynamic measurements of the pupil, and it permits recording of light, near and psychosensory reflexes with elucidation of their characteristics. For research purposes this technology is essential. The most recent methods involve use of an infrared video camera, the image from which is automatically analysed by dedicated computer software. Several modern dynamic pupillometers are available commercially. Pupil findings reported here have all been obtained by video pupillography.

Physiological pupil function tests
Resting diameter

The size of the healthy pupil at rest in darkness is determined by the amount of central inhibition of the parasympathetic outflow and the level of sympathetic drive. It is age dependent, being small in infancy but gradually increasing to a peak diameter in adolescence (Miller 1985). Thereafter the diameter decreases linearly at about 0.4 mm per decade. Its confidence intervals are large, however, and the normal range when defined by such intervals includes at least 1.5 mm on either side of the expected value (Table 36.1, Fig. 36.3). Within individuals repeated measurements show coefficients of variation of only 3–4%, indicating that in darkness, at least under laboratory conditions, the measurement is remarkably reproducible.

Static measurement of the pupil diameter in bright light can be used as an indicator of the integrity of the light reflex. In the light, for example, an abnormally large pupil may indicate the presence of parasympathetic impairment, whereas in darkness when parasympathetic drive is at a minimum no such abnormality may be apparent. The reverse holds true if sympathetic drive is impaired. Thus, in bright light the pupil will be normally small, whereas in darkness it will fail to dilate and therefore remain abnormally small.

Anisocoria

In most healthy subjects the pupils are approximately equal in size. In darkness, 5% of healthy subjects, however, have anisocoria of 0.7 mm or more; in 1% it is 1.0 mm or more. In the light, these figures are 0.4 and 0.6 mm respectively. Such differences in diameter can be detected clinically. The most important characteristic

Table 36.1 Normal values with 95% confidence intervals for darkness pupil diameter. Taken from measurements on 315 healthy subjects

Age (years)	Diameter (mm)	Range
20	7.4	5.8–9.0
30	7.0	5.4–8.6
40	6.6	4.9–8.2
50	6.1	4.5–7.8
60	5.7	4.1–7.3
70	5.3	3.6–6.9
80	4.8	3.2–6.5

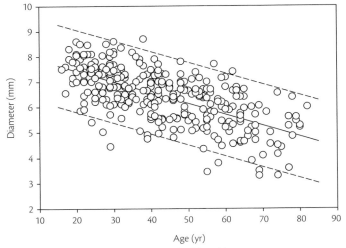

Fig. 36.3 Darkness pupil diameter in 315 healthy subjects.

of such physiological anisocoria is that the pupils react to light and near approximately symmetrically. Pathological anisocoria can be distinguished from physiological anisocoria by examination in darkness and in light and by pharmacological tests. An appropriate flow chart for this examination has been published by Czarnecki et al. (1979).

Light reflex

Normal reflex responses to light are dependent on both intact afferents (from the retina and optic nerve) and intact efferents (in the parasympathetic nerve). Pupillographic recordings of the normal reflex response to a flash of light (Fig. 36.4) show that after a latent period of approximately 0.25 seconds the pupil constricts very rapidly, reaching a minimum diameter after about 1 second. Thereafter redilatation occurs, usually at a rate that is substantially slower than the constriction phase. The roles of the various autonomic components to this reflex were determined originally by Lowenstein and Loewenfeld (1950) and they are indicated in the illustration. All other things being equal, the amplitude of the reflex provides a measure of the parasympathetic drive to the pupil. Reduced stimuli result in smaller reflexes with slower responses. The amplitude of the light reflex response to bright stimuli shows an individual coefficient of variation of about 10%. Dynamic measurements of the reflex permit derivation of latency, constriction time, and constriction and dilatation velocities. In practice such derivatives have only limited value because they are all strongly dependent on the amplitude of the reflex and they are less reproducible. Redilatation velocities are discussed below.

Near reflex

When a subject changes fixation from far to near there is a pupil constriction that accompanies accommodation and convergence. These three functions are associated but they are not interdependent, animal experiments showing that focal electrical stimulation in the brain can elicit each function independently. The time course and amplitude of the pupil near reflex can be measured with video pupillography but it often provides a less useful indicator of parasympathetic function than does the light reflex because it depends on voluntary effort. An absent near reflex may therefore reflect either impaired parasympathetic function or reduced accommodative effort. By contrast, when the near reflex exceeds the light reflex (light-near dissociation) this can be an important diagnostic sign in certain autonomic neuropathies.

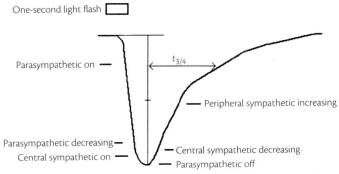

Fig. 36.4 Pupillographic diagram of a light reflex to show the $t_{3/4}$ measure of redilatation time. The presumed activity of the autonomic nervous system in shaping the reflex is shown.

Redilatation time

Inspection of the shape of the light reflex curve (Fig. 36.4) indicates that recovery takes longer than contraction. Redilatation is rapid at first; this phase represents offset of the parasympathetic drive which caused the contraction. Thereafter redilatation is slower and its rate is largely dependent on the peripheral sympathetic drive to the dilator muscle. Studies with α-adrenoceptor antagonists (Smith and Smith 1990) have shown that the time to three-quarter dilatation ($t_{3/4}$) closely reflects the degree of sympathetic drive. Further studies in healthy subjects reveal that this redilatation time is not influenced by age or starting pupil diameter, but it increases linearly with the amplitude of the light reflex (Fig. 36.5). Values of ($t_{3/4}$) greater than the 97.5 percentile indicate significant redilatation lag and signal the presence of sympathetic dysfunction. The test has an individual coefficient of variation of about 20%.

A simpler photographic method for detection of redilatation lag in patients with unilateral Horner's syndrome was introduced by Thompson (1977a). In this method, binocular photographs are taken at 5 seconds and 15 seconds after putting out the room lights, allowing the pupils to dilate. If there is more anisocoria in the 5 seconds photograph than in the 15 seconds one, the subject has relative redilatation lag. The 5 seconds photograph corresponds approximately to the $t_{3/4}$ time.

Hippus

In bright light the pupils of the healthy subject constrict briskly and then partly redilate as retinal adaptation to the light occurs. Thereafter pupil size oscillates slowly, a phenomenon known as hippus (Lowenstein and Loewenfeld 1969). This pupillary unrest is always synchronous in the two eyes and is therefore likely to be central in origin. Fourier analysis indicates that it comprises mostly low frequency waves of less than 0.2 Hz.

Hippus does not occur in darkness, but unrest will occur if the subject is sleepy. Such 'fatigue waves' are, however, of much larger amplitude and slower frequency than hippus. The occurrence of undue unrest in darkness has been used to detect narcolepsy (Yoss et al. 1969, Wilhelm et al. 1998 and 2001).

Psychosensory dilatation

When a subject is aroused, alarmed or afraid, the pupils dilate. Central inhibition of the parasympathetic outflow, peripheral

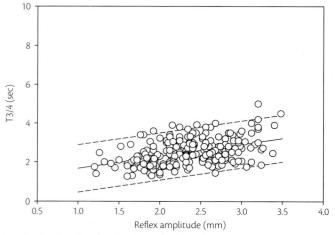

Fig. 36.5 Pupil redilatation time in 225 healthy subjects.

sympathetic drive, and circulating adrenaline may all contribute. The binocular response can be measured by pupillography in background light to a stimulus such as a loud noise. Though its absence can indicate a sympathetic deficit, the test has poor reproducibility and is therefore unreliable.

Pharmacological pupil function tests

These are a useful supplement to clinical signs and physiological tests. Pupil responses to drugs, however, show great interindividual variability, which is in part due to different amounts of tear formation in response to eyedrop instillation, in part to variable transcorneal penetration, and in part to variable drug binding by ocular melanin in the iris itself. Thus dark eyes tend to respond less than light eyes, which have less melanin. Care must be used in the interpretation of pharmacological tests in patients with generalized autonomic neuropathy in which condition tear formation is often impaired and even the integrity of the cornea compromised. In this situation topically applied drugs traverse the cornea more readily and they have therefore greater bioavailability with resultant enhanced pharmacological effects.

Drug effects on the pupil are often long lasting, in part due to melanin binding, so that in practice at least 48 hours should elapse between repeated drug tests. Experiments with miotic agents should be performed in darkness, whereas the action of mydriatics is best recorded in the light.

Denervation supersensitivity

An organ deprived of its innervation becomes supersensitive to the transmitter normally released from those nerves. This 'up-regulation' is thought to be mediated by an increase in the number and activity of receptors on the end organ and it extends to other agonists or mimetics active at those receptors. It occurs not only with complete lesions of the postganglionic nerve, but also to a lesser degree with partial lesions, lesions more proximal in the nerve pathway, and even with functional non-anatomical deficits. The change in sensitivity is now understood to be one end of a regulatory spectrum, the other end of which is the decreased sensitivity or 'down-regulation' that follows excessive excitation. Thus, prolonged topical treatment with pilocarpine reduces responsiveness of the sphincter pupillae, and a phaeochromocytoma that secretes large amounts of noradrenaline and adrenaline into the circulation can induce bilateral Horner's syndrome.

Cholinergic tests

A large pupil with poor light and near responses may result from a parasympathetic deficit (e.g. a IIIrd nerve palsy or Holmes–Adie syndrome), from local iris sphincter trauma, or from cholinolytic (atropine-like) drug treatment. The former can be distinguished from the latter two with a muscarinic agonist such as pilocarpine. The denervated pupil will show supersensitivity whereas the damaged or atropinized pupil will not constrict. Thompson (1977b) recommended the use of pilocarpine 0.125% (others use 0.1%), which usually gives only a very slight response in the healthy pupil. He found that 80% of unilateral Holmes–Adie pupils constricted by at least 0.2 mm more than their consensual pupils, the peak effects occurring at about 1 hour after instillation.

A supersensitive response indicates dysfunction anywhere from the midbrain to the nerve endings in the sphincter pupillae

(Ponsford et al. 1982, Jacobson 1990). A positive test is therefore not diagnostic for a particular lesion locus.

Sympathetic tests

There is a wider range of drug tests for sympathetic deficits. Cocaine, phenylephrine, or apraclonidine are used to establish whether a small pupil is caused by sympathetic dysfunction, and hydroxyamphetamine, pholedrine or tyramine can help to locate the lesion.

Cocaine 4% (10% is used in the USA) dilates the normal pupil by blocking reuptake of noradrenaline back into the nerve ending, which then accumulates at the receptor site. In Horner's syndrome, either preganglionic or postganglionic, less noradrenaline is released and less accumulates. As a result, there is a relative failure of mydriatic response.

Phenylephrine 1% and apraclonidine 0.5–1% are weak sympathomimetics, which show negligible effects in healthy eyes but dilate the supersensitive pupil in the presence of a sympathetic deficit. In Horner's syndrome they therefore produce exaggerated mydriasis. As with cocaine, however, the altered response is most readily detected when the condition is unilateral and there is a control pupil for comparison. In bilateral deficits comparisons can be made only against control experiments using the same ambient conditions; the wide range of normal responsiveness makes the tests of only limited usefulness.

Hydroxyamphetamine (0.5 or 1%), pholedrine (0.5%) and tyramine (2.5%) are indirect-acting sympathomimetics, which dilate the pupil by displacing noradrenaline from its storage sites in sympathetic nerve endings. None of them has significant direct action on the receptors. If the postganglionic sympathetic nerve is damaged, these agents cause less mydriasis than normal as there is less transmitter available to release. If the lesion is preganglionic or central in origin, these agents give a normal or somewhat enhanced mydriasis as the postganglionic nerves have normal transmitter stores, which after release act on supersensitive receptors. Such agents can therefore be used to locate the lesion. If the anisocoria is reduced, the lesion is preganglionic; if the anisocoria is enhanced, the lesion is postganglionic. The response to hydroxyamphetamine 0.5% is weakly age dependent. Most experience with indirect-acting sympathomimetics in the localization of lesions in Horner's syndrome has been gained with this drug (Cremer et al. 1990). Pholedrine appears to have exactly similar actions (Bates et al. 1995).

Pupil disorders

Tonic pupils

In the acute stage, lesions of the parasympathetic cause internal ophthalmoplegia. Subsequently, however, in many conditions some degree of reinnervation often occurs and then pupil constrictor and particularly ciliary muscle activity may recover. For reasons that are ill understood, these muscles then respond to light and near more slowly than normal; the pupil is then said to be tonic. A variety of inflammatory, infective, malignant, and traumatic conditions can cause tonic pupils, but the most common condition associated with these pupils is Holmes–Adie syndrome. The term 'Adie pupil' should be avoided because it confuses two separate phenomena: an abnormally behaving pupil on the one hand, and a pathological syndrome on the other.

Holmes–Adie syndrome

Holmes–Adie syndrome is a benign condition in which idiopathic pathology in the ciliary ganglion is accompanied by loss of deep tendon limb reflexes (Holmes 1931, Adie 1932). The condition, more common in women than in men in the ratio of about 2:1, is often of sudden onset, usually in the second, third or fourth decades of life. At the outset the affected pupil is large and there is total absence of light and near responses. Corneal sensation may be blunted from involvement of sensory nerves, some of which pass through the ciliary ganglion.

The affected pupil remains larger than its fellow for about 2–6 months (Thompson 1977b). After a few weeks some reinnervation occurs, the pupil becomes progressively smaller and it develops slow tonic but usually very limited reactions to light and larger exaggerated responses to near. This light–near dissociation, which persists, occurs because much of the nerve regeneration is aberrant, a proportion of the large excess of fibres destined for the ciliary muscle (originally more than 95% of the total) now innervate the sphincter pupillae. Slit-lamp examination shows a pupil of irregular outline with segmental iris palsy. Ultimately, the affected pupil becomes very small and at this stage may be hard to distinguish from an Argyll Robertson pupil. The crucial difference is that near responses of Holmes–Adie pupils always remain tonic, whereas those of Argyll Robertson pupils are brisk. The pupil becomes supersensitive to topical pilocarpine.

At onset, the condition usually affects only one eye, though the second one may become affected later. Thompson (1977b) has estimated that involvement of the other eye occurs in about 4% of patients per annum. Consequently, anisocoria is usually present even after involvement of the second eye. If both eyes are thought to have been affected at the same time and there is no or little anisocoria, then the diagnosis is unlikely to be Holmes–Adie syndrome.

In most cases the condition is benign, visual symptoms gradually decline and the loss of tendon reflexes is without consequence. In our experience, at least half the patients with this condition have never been aware of it until an optometrist has drawn attention to it. Holmes–Adie syndrome may therefore be rather more common than is usually supposed and the presence of either one or two tonic pupils in a patient with generalized neuropathy does not necessarily mean that the generalized neuropathy is causative. A small proportion of patients have persistent visual symptoms, usually from difficulty accommodating from far to near or vice versa.

A further small proportion of patients develop segmental hypohidrosis (Ross 1958), which can progress to disabling difficulty with temperature regulation and compensatory hyperhidrosis in the unaffected skin areas. In our experience, two thirds of patients with Ross' syndrome have bilateral tonic pupils, one third having only a unilateral tonic pupil. There is more recent evidence from patients with long-standing Holmes–Adie syndrome that sweating deficits are much more common than previously supposed (Bacon and Smith 1993). These and other workers (Hope-Ross et al. 1990) have reported that some patients have impaired cold-pressor responses and reduced Valsalva reflexes, although the vasomotor sympathetic deficit was not enough to cause postural hypotension. It remains to be elucidated whether these cohorts of patients represent a distinct group pathologically or whether they reflect merely the longevity of a potentially widespread neurological disorder.

Argyll Robertson pupils

Pupil dysfunction occurs in some conditions from disinhibition of the Edinger–Westphal nuclei, which results in miotic pupils. Such is the case in Argyll Robertson pupils of neurosyphilis. In this condition the pupils are small and irregular in outline. The light reflexes are reduced or absent, whereas the near response is well preserved and brisk in onset and offset. The pupil abnormality is thought to be due to pathology close to and slightly anterior to the oculomotor nucleus in the midbrain (Lowenstein and Loewenfeld 1969). Such a lesion would destroy the terminal branches of both the crossed and uncrossed pretectal fibres subserving the light reflex, but would spare the more ventrally situated supranuclear pathways for the near reaction. Other inhibitory inputs from higher brain centres would also be interrupted, thereby disinhibiting the parasympathetic motor nuclei. As mentioned above, Argyll Robertson pupils may look very like long-standing Holmes–Adie pupils but they may be distinguished by the speed of the near reaction.

Miosis

Other situations in which the pupils are small from central disinhibition are fatigue, sleep (natural or drug-induced), and narcolepsy. In this condition of chronic hypersomnia the pupils show normal responses to light and near but in darkness they are abnormally small and show large spontaneous oscillations in diameter. Treatment with centrally active sympathomimetics of the amphetamine type reverses the miosis and the fatigue waves.

Horner's syndrome

In Horner's syndrome sympathetic dysfunction leads to partial or complete inactivity of the dilator pupillae. The affected pupil is therefore small, it fails to dilate in darkness and, although the constrictor response to light or near is normal, the subsequent redilatation is slow—there is 'redilatation lag' and the $t_{3/4}$ time is prolonged. A typical pupillogram of Horner's syndrome is shown in Fig. 36.6. In this patient, a 44-year-old woman with a dissecting carotid aneurysm, the light reflexes are normal in amplitude but there is redilatation lag on the affected side ($t_{3/4} = 5.3$ seconds vs 2.3 seconds on the normal side).

In our experience, patients with unilateral Horner's syndrome always show relative darkness miosis and redilatation lag on the affected side. The degree of miosis, however, was such that in only 35/176 cases of known Horner's syndrome were the affected pupils smaller than those of an age-matched healthy population. As a test of abnormality darkness miosis had 19.9% sensitivity and 96.9% specificity. By contrast, the $t_{3/4}$ redilatation time gave 80.0% sensitivity and 93.9% specificity. The latter is therefore the more useful detector of the condition in patients with suspected bilateral sympathetic loss.

Irritation of sympathetic nerves anywhere from the brainstem to the iris dilator can cause intermittent unilateral or bilateral mydriasis, the 'springing pupil', sometimes associated with hyperhidrosis. In some of these patients the pupil may be distorted in shape during an attack, one part of the iris being elongated towards the periphery; the condition is referred to as 'tadpole pupil'. Attacks often occur towards evening and may be associated with tiredness and a sudden change in ambient illumination. The condition is usually totally benign, but Horner's syndrome is occasionally found.

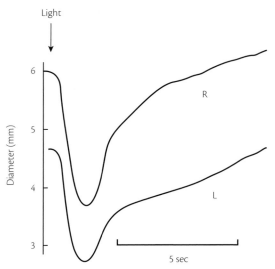

Fig. 36.6 Pupillogram of 44-year-old woman with L-sided unilateral Horner's syndrome caused by a dissecting carotid aneurysm, showing redilatation lag on the affected side. $t_{3/4}$ values—R: 2.3 seconds; L: 5.3 seconds.

An intact sympathetic innervation of the eye is necessary for the formation of ocular melanin in neonates. Congenital unilateral Horner's syndrome is therefore accompanied by heterochromia iridis, the iris on the affected side being paler than that on the normal side. Whether or not heterochromia occurs in long-standing acquired Horner's syndrome has long been debated and is still uncertain.

Pupil abnormalities in generalized autonomic neuropathies and autonomic failure

On theoretical grounds, combined failure of both parasympathetic and sympathetic innervation should result in a pupil of mid-size that does not respond to light or near. In practice this occurs almost exclusively in acute and subacute dysautonomia. Recent observations suggest that pupil abnormality in both acute and chronic cases may result from widespread autonomic ganglionopathy and it is strongly linked to the presence of autoantibodies to ganglionic cholinoceptors (Vernino et al. 2000, Goldstein et al. 2002, Klein et al. 2003). In our experience (Bremner and Smith, unpublished observations) patients with chronic forms of autonomic failure often show pupil abnormality, but most frequently this presents as either predominant parasympathetic or predominant sympathetic dysfunction. The following data are taken from a survey of 145 cases of varying aetiology.

Acute and subacute dysautonomia

All of the five cases of acute and subacute dysautonomia seen had abnormal pupils, though in only one of them were the pupils of mid-size and completely unreactive, as predicted theoretically. His pupils were supersensitive to both phenylephrine and pilocarpine, the latter drug producing also 3 dioptres of myopia, indicating that the ciliary muscle was also affected. These findings are consistent with those in about 75 published case reports. Two of our cases had bilateral Horner's syndrome and one bilateral tonic pupils without light-near dissociation.

Amyloidosis

Generalized autonomic dysfunction is common in familial and acquired amyloidosis. Out of 21 patients seen, 20 had pupil abnormality, a frequency (95.2%) that does not differ significantly from 100%. Bilateral Horner's syndrome was found in 10 of these patients (Fig. 36.7); 6 had bilateral tonic pupils, the prevalent abnormality depending presumably on whether amyloid material was deposited mostly in sympathetic (Davies and Smith 1999) or parasympathetic (Witschel and Mobius 1974) nerves and ganglia. These are of course not mutually exclusive and it is to be expected that many of these eyes are subject to both sympathetic and parasympathetic loss. Unfortunately pharmacological tests are usually unreliable because of impaired tear formation.

Diabetes mellitus

Small pupils for age have long been recognized as a characteristic sign in diabetes mellitus (Smith et al. 1978, Hreidarsson 1982). In our present series, altogether 22 of 28 patients (78.6%) had abnormal pupils. The most common abnormality, darkness miosis, was present in 14 patients (Fig. 36.8). Eight patients had bilateral Horner's syndrome (as for example in Fig. 36.9) and 6 had bilateral tonic pupils. Interpretation of the latter is, however, difficult because immobility of the diabetic iris may be multifactorial. First, there may be autonomic nerve damage occurring as a result of the disease. Secondly, if the patient has had laser treatment for retinopathy the parasympathetic nerves can be further damaged. In our survey, such patients were excluded. Thirdly, there may be rubeosis, a proliferative iridopathy with neovascularization sufficient to stiffen the structure of the iris and further reduce its mobility. In the individual case it can be hard to discern the precise contribution of these factors.

Significant associations between small pupils and a wide range of diabetic complications have been recorded: cardiovascular autonomic dysfunction (Smith and Smith 1983), peripheral sensory loss (Smith et al. 1978, Hreidarsson 1982), retinopathy (Hayashi and Ishikawa 1979) and nephropathy (Hreidarsson 1982). Patients are more likely to have pupil abnormality if their hyperglycaemia

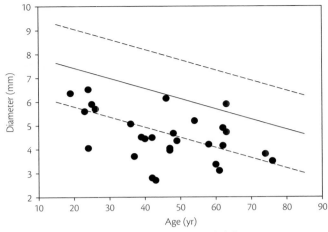

Fig. 36.8 Darkness pupil diameter in 28 patients with diabetes.

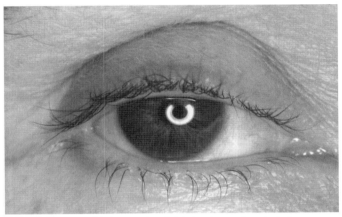

Fig. 36.9 Right eye of diabetic patient (F.42) showing ptosis and miosis.

has been of marked degree and duration (Hreidarsson 1982, Smith and Smith 1983). In such a long-standing multifactorial condition such associations are to be expected. Acute hyperglycaemia may cause miosis that reverses when normoglycaemia is established (Hreidarsson 1981, Boutros and Insler 1984).

Pure autonomic failure

The pupils of patients with pure autonomic failure (PAF) have been little studied in the past and in most reports of individual cases usually found to be normal. In our series 16 of 33 patients had bilateral Horner's syndrome (Fig. 36.10), as do many patients with autonomic neuropathy of amyloid or diabetic origin. Bilateral redilatation lag, upon which our deduction rests, is hard to detect clinically; the condition may thereby have been missed. Overall 67% of the patients had abnormal pupils.

Multiple system atrophy

In patients with multiple system atrophy (MSA) the pupils are often remarkably normal (Thomas and Schirger 1970) even when there is evidence of severe autonomic damage affecting the cardiovascular system and the urinary tract. In some patients the resting pupil may be larger than normal in the dark, but its reflex responses to light and near are usually preserved. The reasons for this are not

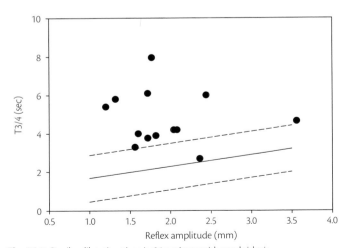

Fig. 36.7 Pupil redilatation time in 21 patients with amyloidosis.

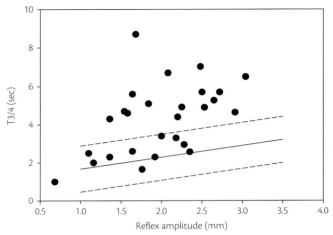

Fig. 36.10 Pupil redilatation time in 28 patients with pure autonomic failure (PAF).

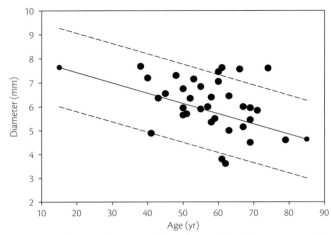

Fig. 36.11 Darkness pupil diameter of 34 patients with multiple system atrophy (MSA).

known and are hard to determine, particularly in that many of these cases are under treatment with dopaminergic and anticholinergic drugs, which can themselves influence the pupil. In patients free of drug effects, the unique preservation of the pupillary reflexes presumably indicates that the midbrain centres involved are unaffected by the disease process, unlike those concerned with cardiovascular and genitourinary regulation. More detailed studies of the relevant pathology are needed to resolve this apparent enigma.

Pupil abnormality is occasionally found. In their original description of this condition, Shy and Drager (1960) described iris atrophy and anisocoria in both of their two patients. One of them had ptosis and miosis in one eye and had reduced reactions to light and near. Anisocoria appears frequently in subsequent reports (Micieli et al. 1995). These and some other patients may have had unilateral Horner's syndrome (Sobue et al. 1992) and there are reports of alternating Horner's syndrome (Tan et al. 1990), though the origin of this and the nature of the mechanism involved is obscure.

In our series, 26 of 34 patients had completely normal pupils. Seven had unilateral Horner's syndrome and three other patients had a minor degree of anisocoria, though as a sole finding statistically this is of no significance. There were no cases of bilateral Horner's syndrome or bilateral pupillotonia. As a diagnostic test for the distinction between PAF and MSA, the occurrence of bilateral Horner's syndrome or bilateral pupillotonia has 54.5% sensitivity and 100% specificity for PAF.

Inherited sympathetic neuropathy

We have seen two sibling pairs who have a generalized sympathetic neuropathy. Both pairs, that with dopamine -beta-hydroxylase deficiency (Mathias et al. 1990, Smith and Smith 1999) and the other of unknown aetiology, had bilateral Horner's syndrome and adrenoceptor supersensitivity. These findings are consistent with other published reports.

Other conditions

Pupil abnormality has been widely reported in patients with paraneoplastic syndromes of various kinds. In Lambert–Eaton myasthenic syndrome (LEMS) bilateral tonic pupils, absent or sluggish reactions to light, or prolonged pupil cycle times have been described in a number of cases (Waterman 2001).

Pupil abnormality occurs also in other paraneoplastic syndromes. Bilateral tonic pupils with pilocarpine supersensitivity has been reported in infants with neuroblastoma and in adults with presumed antiHu-mediated neuropathies associated with small cell lung carcinoma (Casas Parera et al. 1998), and other neoplasms. Our survey included five cases (two with LEMS), four of whom had pupil abnormality.

Generalized autonomic neuropathy is a common complication of Sjögren's syndrome. In this situation unilateral or bilateral tonic pupils occur, usually with light-near dissociation (Tajima et al. 1997, Goto et al. 2000). Our survey included two out of three cases with bilateral tonic pupils. Similar findings have been reported in patients with sicca syndrome on whom a definitive diagnosis of Sjögren's syndrome had not yet been made (Wright et al. 1999). In a recent report, a large cohort of patients with Sjögren's syndrome has been divided into seven groups according to the spectrum of clinical features. In this study pupil abnormality is significantly associated with sensory ataxic neuropathy and autonomic neuropathy (Mori et al. 2005).

Conclusion

The findings of our study indicate that pupil abnormality is common in patients with generalized autonomic neuropathy or autonomic failure, much more common than hitherto supposed from many published case reports, perhaps because in many patients a pupillary sympathetic deficit can only be recognized reliably with pupillography. The exception to this general picture is MSA in which most patients have normal pupils despite widespread autonomic dysfunction elsewhere in the body.

Acknowledgement

Dr Shirley Smith made major contributions to earlier editions of this chapter. We have drawn upon them and acknowledge her help with gratitude.

References

Adie, W. J. (1932). Tonic pupils and absent tendon reflexes: a benign disorder sui generis. Its complete and incomplete forms. *Brain* **55**, 98–113.

Alexandridis, E. (1985). *The Pupil*. Springer Verlag, New York.

Bacon, P. J. and Smith, S. E. (1993). Cardiovascular and sweating dysfunction in patients with Holmes-Adie Syndrome. *JNNP*, **56**, 1096–102.

Bates, A., Chamberlain, S., Champion, M., *et al.* (1995). Pholedrine: a substitute for hydroxyamphetamine as diagnostic eyedrop test in Horner's syndrome. *JNNP*, **58**, 215–7.

Boutros, G. and Insler, M. S. (1984). Reversible pupillary miosis during a hyperglycaemic episode: case report. *Diabetologia*, **27**, 50–1.

Casas Parera, I., Fischman, D., Paz, L., Lehkuniec, E. and Muchnik, S. (1998). [Paraneoplastic neuropathy with positive anti-Hu]. *Medicina (Buenos Aires)*, **58**, 197–201.

Cremer, S. A., Thompson, H. S., Digre, K. B. and Kardon, R. H. (1990). Hydroxyamphetamine mydriasis in Horner's syndrome. *Am. J Ophthalmol.*, **110**, 71–6.

Czarnecki, J. S., Pilley, S. F. and Thompson, H. S. (1979). The analysis of anisocoria. The use of photography in the clinical evaluation of unequal pupils. *Can. J Ophthalmol.* **14**, 297–302.

Davies, D. R. & Smith, S. E. (1999). Pupil abnormality in amyloidosis with autonomic neuropathy. *JNNP*, **67**, 819–22.

Goldstein, D. S., Holmes, C., Dendi, R., Li, S-T., Brentzel, S. and Vernino, S. (2002). Pandysautonomia associated with impaired ganglionic neurotransmission and circulating antibody to the neuronal nicotinic receptor. *Clin. Auton. Res*, **12**, 281–5.

Goto, H., Matsuo, H., Fukudome, T., Shibnya, M., Ohnishi, A. and Nakamura, H. (2000). Chronic autonomic neuropathy in a patient with primary Sjögren's syndrome. *JNNP*, **69**, 135.

Hayashi, M. and Ishikawa, S. (1979). Pharmacology of papillary responses in diabetics—correlative study of the responses and grade of retinopathy. *Jpn. J Ophthalmol.*, **23**, 65–72.

Holmes, G. (1931). Partial iridoplegia associated with symptoms of other diseases of the nervous system. *Transactions of the Ophthalmological Society of the UK*, **51**, 209–28.

Hope-Ross, H., Buchanan, T. A. S., Archer, D. B. and Allen, J. A. (1990). Autonomic function in Holmes- Adie syndrome. *Eye*, **4**, 607–12.

Hreidarsson, A. B. (1981). Acute, reversible autonomic nervous system abnormalities in juvenile insulin-dependent diabetes. A pupillographic study. *Diabetologia*, **20**, 475–81.

Hreidarsson, A. B. (1982). Pupil size in insulin-dependent diabetes. *Diabetes*, **31**, 442–8.

Jacobson, D. M. (1990). Pupillary responses to dilute pilocarpine in preganglionic 3rd nerve disorders. *Neurology*, **40**, 804–8.

Klein, C. M., Vernino, S., Lennon, V. A., Sandroni, P. and Fealey, R. D. (2003). The spectrum of autoimmune autonomic neuropathies. *Ann. Neurol.*, **53**, 752–8.

Lowenstein, O. and Loewenfeld, I. E. (1950). Mutual role af sympathetic and parasympathetic in shaping of the pupillary reflex to light. Pupillographic studies. *Arch. Neurol. Psychiatry*, **64**, 341–77.

Lowenstein, O. and Loewenfeld, I. E. (1969). The Pupil. In H Davson, ed.*The Eye*, Vol.3, pp.255–337. Academic Press, New York.

Mathias, C. J., Bannister, R. B., Cortelli, P., Heslop, K., Polak, J. M., Raimbach, S. *et al* (1990). Clinical, autonomic and therapeutic observations in two siblings with postural hypotension and sympathetic failure due to an inability to synthesise noradrenaline from dopamine because of a deficiency of dopamine beta hydroxylase. *Q J Med.*, **75**, 617–33.

Micieli, G., Tassorelli, C., Martignoni, E., Marcheselli, S., Rossi, F. and Nappi, G. (1995). Further characterization of autonomic involvement in multiple system atrophy: a pupillometric study. *Functional Neurology*, **10**, 273–80.

Miller, N. R. (1985). The autonomic nervous system: pupillary function, accommodation and lacrimation. In NR Miller, ed. *Walsh and Hoyt's Clinical Neuro-Ophthalmology*, (4th edn.), Vol.2, pp. 385–556. Williams & Wilkins, Baltimore.

Mori, K., Iijima, M., Koike, H., *et al.* (2005). The wide spectrum of clinical manifestations in Sjögren's syndrome-associated neuropathy. *Brain*, **128**, 2518–34.

Ponsford, J. R., Bannister, R. and Paul, E. A. (1982). Methacholine papillary responses in third nerve palsy and Adie's syndrome. *Brain*, **105**, 583–97.

Ross, A. T. (1958). Progressive selective sudomotor degeneration. *Neurology*, **8**, 809–17.

Shy, G. M. and Drager, G. A. (1960). A neurological syndrome associated with postural hypotension: a clinical-pathologic study. *Arch. Neurol.*, **2**, 511–27.

Smith, S. A., Smith, S. E. (1999). Bilateral Horner's syndrome: detection and occurrence. *JNNP*, **66**, 48–51.

Smith, S. A. and Smith, S. E. (1983). Evidence for a neuropathic aetiology in the small pupil of diabetes mellitus. *Br. J Ophthalmol.*, **67**, 89–93.

Smith, S. A. and Smith, S. E. (1990). The quantitative estimation of pupillary dilatation in Horner's syndrome. In A Huber, ed. *Sympathicus und Auge*; Proc. JF Horner Centenary Symposium. pp.152–65. Ferdinand Enke Verlag, Stuttgart.

Smith, S. E., Smith, S. A., Brown, P. M., Fox, C. and Sonksen, P. H. (1978). Pupillary signs in diabetic autonomic neuropathy. *BMJ*, **2**, 924–7.

Sobue, G., Terao, S-i., Kachi, T., *et al.* (1992). Somatic motor efferents in multiple system atrophy with autonomic failure: a clinico-pathological study. *J Neurol. Sci.*, **112**, 113–25.

Tajima, Y., Tsukishima, E., Sudo, K., Aimoto, Y. and Tashiro, K. (1997). [A case of Sjögren syndrome associated with multiple mononeuritis and dysautonomia including bilateral tonic pupils.] *Brain and Nerve*, **49**, 825–8.

Tan, E., Kansu, T., Saygi, S. and Zileli, T. (1990). Alternating Horner's syndrome. A case report and review of the literature. *Neuro-Ophthalmology*, **10**, 19–22.

Thomas, J. E. and Schirger, A. (1970). Idiopathic orthostatic hypotension. A study of its natural history in 57 neurologically affected patients. *Arch Neurol.*, **22**, 289–93.

Thompson, H. S. (1977a). Diagnosing Horner's syndrome. *Transactions of the American Academy of Ophthalmology and Otolaryngology*, **83**, 840–2.

Thompson, H. S. (1977b). Adie's syndrome: some new observations. *Transactions of the American Ophthalmological Society*, **75**, 587–626.

Vernino, S., Low, P. A., Fealey, R. D., Stewart, J. D., Farrugia, G. and Lennon, V. A. (2000). Autoantibodies to ganglionic receptors in autoimmune autonomic neuropathies. *N Engl. J Med.*, **343**, 847–55.

Waterman, S. A. (2001). Autonomic dysfunction in Lambert-Eaton myasthenic syndrome. *Clin. Auton. Res.*, **11**, 145–54.

Wilhelm, B., Giedke, H., Ludtke, H., Bittner, E., Hofmann, A. and Wilhelm, H. (2001). Daytime variations in central nervous system activation measured by a pupillographic sleepiness test. *J Sleep Res.*, **10**, 1–7.

Wilhelm, B., Ludtke, H., and Wilhelm, H. (1998). Pupillographic sleepiness testing in hypersomniacs and normals. *Graefes Archives for Clinical and Experimental Ophthalmology*, **236**, 725–9.

Witschel, H. and Mobius, W. (1974). Augenveränderungen bei generalisierter Amyloidose. *Klinische Monatsblätter Augenheilkunde*, **165**, 610–6.

Wright, R. A., Grant, I. A. and Low, P. A. (1999). Autonomic neuropathy associated with sicca complex. *J Auton. Nerv. Syst.*, **75**, 70–6.

Yoss, R. E., Moyer, N. J. and Ogle, K. N. (1969). The pupillogram and narcolepsy. *Neurology*, **19**, 921–8.

CHAPTER 37

Investigation and treatment of bladder dysfunction in diseases affecting the autonomic nervous system

Soumendra N. Datta and Clare J. Fowler

Introduction

The lower urinary tract is largely innervated by autonomic fibres and consequently disturbances of bladder function are common in patients with diseases of the autonomic nervous system. Poor bladder emptying, frequency of micturition, and incontinence can be either presenting symptoms of autonomic nervous system failure or occur as troublesome problems in patients with established disease. Investigation of such complaints using urodynamic or neurophysiological methods may be carried out for the purpose of establishing a neurological diagnosis, particularly if some local structural disorder could produce similar symptoms or with a view to introducing treatment. The management of urinary dysfunction arising from autonomic failure is mostly symptomatic and many of the treatments now available are highly effective and do not require surgical input. However, in patients who have pain, haematuria, or recurrent urinary tract infections, a urological opinion should be obtained.

Methods of investigation

Urodynamic studies

Urodynamic studies include various tests devised to investigate the storage and emptying functions of the lower urinary tract. Although of value in providing descriptive information about the pathophysiological behaviour of the bladder, such tests cannot be expected to provide a diagnosis in neurological terms. Furthermore, very similar findings may occur in urological and neurological disease.

Tests range from simple charting of voided volumes over a 24-hour period to complex studies involving the simultaneous recording of the intravesical pressure, intra-abdominal pressure, urinary flow, and sphincter electromyography.

Urine dipstick and midstream urine specimen

A simple cheap, effective and bedside method for screening for haematuria, glucose and infection can be done by a urine dipstick. Should this be positive, microscopy and bacterial culture and

sensitivity should be carried out. Uncomplicated urinary tract infections diagnosed by positive leukocyte esterase and nitrite tests can often be treated without culture.

Voiding diary

A voiding diary filled out over a few days is a simple, objective and non-invasive measure that will give an indication of the problem and severity of the patient's symptoms. There is evidence which shows that a 4-day diary is as good in terms of reliability, as a 7-day diary but with better patient compliance (Schick et al. 2003). The number of voids, nocturia and leak episodes can then be readily assessed and comparisons made of the frequency of those events following treatment. In addition, advice based on the readings can be offered on optimizing the timing of medication, and reducing fluid intake during the most symptomatic periods.

Uroflowmetry and post-micturition studies

Measurement of the urinary flow rate and the post-micturition urinary volume are useful initial screening tests. Flow meters provide a graphic trace of urinary flow (Fig. 37.1), with automated measurements of maximum flow rate, voided volume, and the time taken to complete micturition. Urinary flow rates can only be assessed properly if the patient voids at least 150 ml. Nomograms adjusted for age, sex, and the voided volume can be used to interpret the results.

After voiding, the residual urine can be measured either by passing a urethral catheter into the bladder or by ultrasound (Fig. 37.2A). Small, relatively inexpensive hand-held ultrasound device (as shown in Fig. 37.2B) are now available and many specialist nurse continence advisors have access to one.

If the patient voids with a normal flow rate and has a residual of less than 50 ml, a significant abnormality of function and innervation of the bladder is unlikely.

Cystometry—filling and voiding

Cystometry involves monitoring the detrusor pressure while the bladder is filled and during voiding. Intravesical pressure is

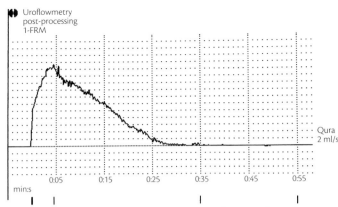

Fig. 37.1 Normal uroflowmetry. Qura is the urinary flow rate. The maximum flow rate is 22 ml/s and the trace is smooth, indicating an uninterrupted urine flow.

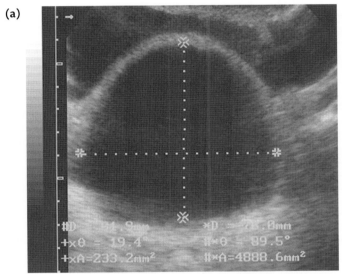

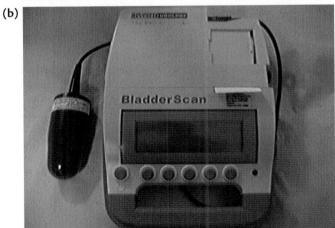

Fig. 37.2 A Ultrasound image of bladder. Cursors are placed on the image and, after measurement in three planes, the volume of urine is estimated assuming the bladder to be nearly spherical. **B** Portable handheld ultrasound scanner—can be used easily to measure residual volumes.

measured using a fine catheter (1 mm diameter) passed into the bladder alongside a larger Nelaton catheter (3 mm diameter) which is used to fill the bladder at a controlled rate. Rectal pressure provides a measure of intra-abdominal pressure and is recorded by means of another fine catheter inserted into the rectum. The urodynamic machine calculates the detrusor pressure by subtraction of the rectal pressure from the total intravesical pressure.

The filling phase of cystometry is most useful in the investigation of patients with symptoms of urgency and frequency and incontinence. Normally during filling there is only a small rise in the detrusor pressure, which occurs when the bladder is nearly full (Fig. 37.3). Abnormal detrusor contractions may be recorded during filling (Fig. 37.4) and if they occur in a patient with known neurological disease the patient is said to have 'neurogenic detrusor overactivity'. This replaces the former term 'detrusor hyper-reflexia', according to recent recommendations of the International Continence Society (Abrams et al. 2002).

Detrusor overactivity occurs very commonly in patients with spinal cord disease but may also occur in patients with parkinsonism or cerebral disease. However, exactly the same appearance may be seen in patients who do not have neurological disease and then the activity is called 'idiopathic detrusor overactivity'. Thus, the cause of bladder overactivity cannot be deduced from urodynamic studies and its correct classification depends on the clinician recognizing the underlying neurological disease. Urinary symptoms reported by patients with detrusor overactivity include frequency, urgency, and urge incontinence.

Pressure-flow studies during micturition are useful in the investigation of patients with difficulty voiding and incomplete emptying. Analysis of the urinary flow and the detrusor pressure sustained during voiding may show that a low urine flow rate is due either to a failure of detrusor contraction or to obstructed outflow. An abnormality of the parasympathetic innervation of the bladder will result in weak, poorly sustained detrusor contractions during attempts to void, a low urinary flow rate, and possibly a raised post-micturition residual volume. By contrast, a local urological abnormality such as prostatic hypertrophy (Fig. 37.5) may cause poor urine flow but with a high detrusor pressure. The literature on the cystometric findings in urological and neuro-urological disease is extensive, and reference to recent textbooks is recommended for further reading (Abrams 1997).

Any interruption of the neural connections between the pons and the sacral cord causes a loss of the coordinated activity of the bladder and sphincter (Table 37.1, see also Chapter 19) so that instead of the sphincter relaxing with the initiation of micturition, the bladder may contract spontaneously due to detrusor overactivity and the sphincter contract at the same time. This disorder is known as 'detrusor-sphincter dyssynergia' and may be demonstrated by simultaneous recordings of sphincter electromyographic (EMG) activity and urine flow rate. However, most centres with a particular interest in the urological problems of patients following spinal cord injury use video-urodynamics, which uses fluoroscopy during cystometry. This provides the opportunity to visualize the upper renal tracts and detect the potentially serious problem of ureteric reflux, together with the possibility of observing the voiding phase and seeing the precise location of any outflow obstruction, thus making redundant the need to record simultaneous EMG.

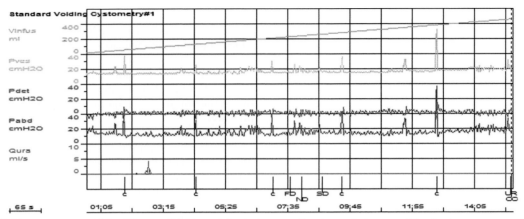

Fig. 37.3 A 'stable' bladder on cystometry. Vinfus, filling rate; Pabd, intra-abdominal pressure; Pves, intravesical pressure; Pdet, the detrusor pressure, is derived by subtracting Pabd from Pves. This trace shows the detrusor pressure rising to less than 10 cm of water on filling to 450 ml. The sudden increase in Pves, which also occurs in Pabd occurred when the subject was asked to cough.

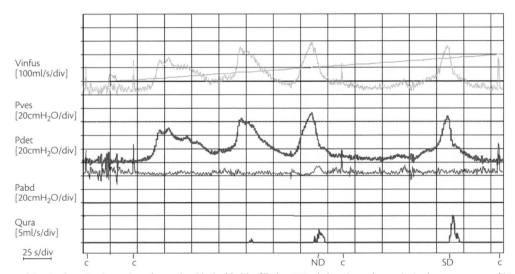

Fig. 37.4 Detrusor overactivity. At about 5 minutes into the study with the bladder filled to 200 ml, there is an abrupt rise in detrusor pressure (60 cm water), which the patient was unable to suppress.

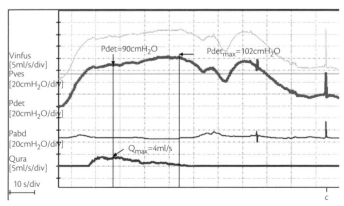

Fig. 37.5 Obstructed voiding. There is a detrusor pressure of 90 cmH$_2$O associated with max flow rate of 4 ml/second.

Neurophysiological investigation of the urogenital tract

EMG of the urethral sphincter as described above, as part of a urodynamic study is now rarely performed. However, concentric needle electrode EMG of the anal or urethral sphincter is still used in some centres to capture tonically firing individual motor units, examining for changes of denervation and chronic reinnervation (Fig. 37.6). This was proposed as being of value in recognizing multiple system atrophy (MSA) (Palace et al. 1997) but there is some controversy about the specificity and sensitivity of this test.

Table 37.1 Pathophysiological consequences on bladder function of spinal cord dysfunction

◆ Detrusor overactivity
◆ Detrusor-sphincter dyssynergia
◆ Incomplete bladder emptying

(a) Quantitative EMG

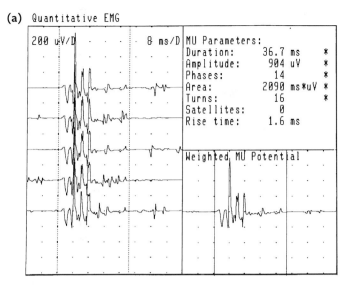

(b) Quantitative EMG

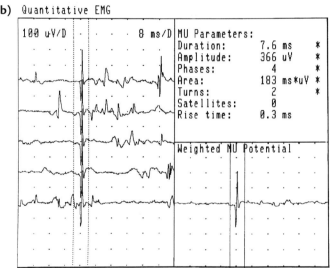

Fig. 37.6 (a) An abnormally prolonged motor unit recorded from the anal sphincter of a patient with multiple system atrophy using a trigger and delay line. The unit is shown on the left in a falling leaf display and the inset shows the 'weighed motor potential'. The cursors have been set to show its duration of 36.7 ms. **(b)** A normal duration motor unit, recorded and displayed in the same way as in Fig 37.5.

(Valldeoriola et al. 1995, Vodusek 2001). Inevitably the result depends very much on the method used to capture and analyse the motor units (Podnar and Fowler 2004).

Other neurophysiological investigations that have been used to examine the innervation of the pelvic floor and lower urinary tracts suffer mostly from the defect that they test only the somatic innervation of the region. It is possible to record sacral reflex latencies electrophysiologically (i.e. recordings made from striated muscle structures in the pelvic floor in response to stimulation of the dorsal nerve of the penis/clitoris) and although the latency of responses may be abnormal in a patient with a cauda equina lesion or peripheral neuropathy, the test only examines conduction in the large myelinated fibres innervating the region, not the unmyelinated fibre autonomic innervation. Likewise, the pudendal evoked potential

can be delayed in patients with spinal cord disease and urogenital dysfunction, but there is usually other clinical evidence of such a problem, and the test is very rarely diagnostic (Delodovici and Fowler 1995). A similar criticism can be made of measurement of the latency of pelvic floor muscle contraction in response to cortical magnetic stimulation.

Sympathetic skin responses recorded from the genital region do, however, give information about local sympathetic innervation. Using the same technique as is used to record the responses from the hands or the feet, surface electrodes can be attached to the perineum or genitalia and record either spontaneous ongoing activity or the response to stimulation of a distant nerve (Ertekin et al. 1995). Unfortunately, no significance can be attached to a low amplitude response and only an absent response can be considered definitely abnormal.

Treatments

Treatment of neurogenic bladder disorders

When a patient with neurological disease complains of urinary urgency and frequency it is reasonable to assume the pathophysiological basis of the symptoms is detrusor overactivity and prescribe anticholinergic medication. However, this course of action overlooks the possible contribution that incomplete bladder emptying may be making to the problem. In several of the neurological disorders that affect the innervation of the bladder, both detrusor overactivity and incomplete bladder emptying occur, although symptoms from the latter may be relatively minor. A constant residual urine volume in the bladder is likely to act as a stimulus for detrusor overactivity so that urgency and frequency will persist as long as the bladder is not emptied. For this reason it has been proposed that measurement of the post-micturition residual volume be made in all patients with neurogenic incontinence (Fowler 1996). If this is in excess of 100 ml, it will be necessary for the patient to achieve better bladder emptying before anticholinergics can be effective, particularly since drugs with anticholinergic action may exacerbate poor bladder emptying. An algorithm for bladder management which requires minimal investigation is outlined in Fig. 37.7. If the patient fails to report sustained improvement after starting anticholinergic medication, the post-micturition residual volume should be re-measured.

Clean intermittent self-catheterization

Incomplete bladder emptying may result from a disturbance of the parasympathetic innervation of the detrusor or poorly co-ordinated detrusor–sphincter activity and is best managed by clean intermittent self-catheterization (CISC). Introduced for the treatment of urinary dysfunction in patients with spinal injuries, the technique has since greatly improved the management of patients with urinary dysfunction resulting from various different neurological causes. In general the greatest symptomatic improvement can be expected in those patients with large residual volumes and good bladder capacity.

A specialist nurse or continence advisor, or if necessary their carer, is the most suitable person to instruct the patient in the technique. In general, female patients find the procedure more difficult initially and usually require a mirror to help locate the urethral orifice. However once learnt, even blind or partial sighted patients can become proficient. Most patients performing CISC will void a

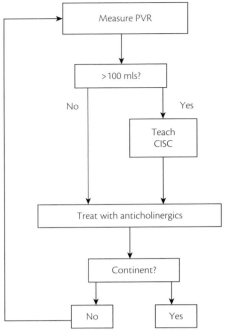

Fig. 37.7 Algorithm for management of neurogenic incontinence. In a patient with known neurological disease with urinary symptoms of urgency and frequency, detrusor overactivity requiring treatment with an anticholinergic can reasonably be assumed to be the underlying cause. An essential measurement is the post-micturition residual urine volume since if this is raised urine in the bladder will act as a constant stimulus, causing continued bladder contractions. Clean intermittent self-catheterization (CISC) can be highly effective in emptying the bladder and thus reducing symptoms.

variable amount before passing the catheter but after commencing anticholinergic medication, effective voiding may be so reduced that the patient relies more on their intermittent self-catheterization. Frequency of catheterization will best be determined by the patient, but initially they should be advised to perform the procedure three or four times a day, ensuring that the residuals are kept lower than 500 ml. Contact and support by the specialist nurse, particularly in the early stages of learning the technique, increases the patient's confidence, and careful follow-up ensures compliance to a prescribed regimen. Asymptomatic bacteriuria is a common finding in those using CISC, and is not an indication for antibiotic treatment.

Catheter technology has advanced significantly in recent years. Various innovative features have been incorporated into the design although mostly only into single use catheters, which unfortunately increases the cost. The new catheters are all of single lumen design, manufactured from different materials, and of differing lengths and diameters. Catheters choice depends on various factors such as ease of use and storage, discomfort and minimization of damage on insertion, and the risk of urinary tract infection. Trauma and discomfort are reduced by using gel on the catheter, although many of those which recently became available are hydrophilically coated so that on contact with water they develop a highly lubricated surface; some now come packed 'pre-wetted'. Convenience of use has been improved as they are now disposable and can be hidden away in a small bag. Those for use in women can even be compacted into a tube similar in size to a lipstick container.

The continence advisor or specialist nurse can advise on the types of catheter available and put the patient in touch with suppliers.

Anticholinergic medication

Detrusor overactivity is best treated by drugs with anticholinergic properties which act as antagonists to the action of acetylcholine. The postganglionic parasympathetic receptors on the detrusor are muscarinic. Recent radioligand studies with competitive antagonists in the detrusor have indicated a receptor population of 71% M_2, 22% M_3 and 7% M_1. In the urothelium 75% of sites are M_2 receptors, with 25% being M_3/M_5 receptors (Mansfield et al. 2005). The minority M_3 receptor is thought to cause direct muscle contraction of the detrusor (Chess-Williams et al. 2001), while the role for the M_2 receptor in the detrusor is thought to be modulatory. The M_2 receptor has been found to mediate bladder contractions in patients with neurogenic detrusor overactivity (Pontari et al. 2004) and thus may play a greater role in disease states. Muscarinic receptors are also present in other organ systems such as the brain, heart, eye and smooth muscle and blockade of acetylcholine at these sites results inevitably in side-effects, which commonly include a dry mouth, impaired accommodation, and constipation.

Oxybutynin (2.5 mg two or three times a day) is often highly effective if the patient has detrusor overactivity. It has a smooth muscle relaxant effect in addition to anticholinergic action. Tolteridine XL (10 mg once a day) can be used as an alternative as it is been shown to have fewer side-effects together with greater efficacy and its extended release profile allows it to be taken once daily (Sussman and Garely 2002), although both medications have the expected side-effects of non-selective anticholinergics. Newer anticholinergics, solifenacin (M_2/M_3 receptor selective) and darifenacin (M_3 receptor selective) have recently been introduced and appear to be clinically effective, but are by no means free of side-effects, with further evaluation in neurogenic detrusor overactivity still required. Few of these agents have had specific trials in patients with neurogenic detrusor overactivity. The details of these various medications are given in Table 37.2.

Other medication to treat urinary symptoms

Duloxetine, a 5-hydroxytryptamine (5-HT) and noradrenaline reuptake inhibitor has recently been licensed and introduced in the European Union, with the main indication being stress urinary incontinence. The mechanism of action, based on experimental data from a cat model, is thought to be via augmentation of striated urethral sphincter activity (Thor and Katofiasc 1995). Duloxetine acts by increasing serotonin and norepinephrine stimulation of the 5-HT$_2$ and α_1-adrenergic receptors, respectively (Wong et al.1993) in the anterior horn cells in Onuf's nucleus and thereby up-regulates glutamate induced activity of the pudendal nerve.

Four randomized, double-blind, placebo controlled trials on duloxetine, with similar study design and study population, have been published in the literature. Taken together there was a 52–54% improvement in incontinence episode frequency (IEF) sustained between 4 weeks and 12 weeks in the duloxetine group compared with 22–33% improvement in the placebo group (Zinner 2005). There were significant improvements in quality of life scores. Nausea is the most frequent side-effect in all of the four studies.

Table 37.2 Medication for neurogenic detrusor overactivity

Generic name	Trade name	Dose (mg)	Frequency	Receptor subtype selectivity	Elimination half life of drug (hours)
Propantheline	Pro-banthine	15	TDS	Non-selective	<2
Tolterodine tartrate	Detrusitol	2	BD	Non-selective	2.4
Tolterodine tartrate XL	Detrusitol XL	4	OD	Non-selective	8.4
Trospium chloride	Regurin	20	BD	Non-selective (does not cross blood–brain barrier)	20
Oxybutynin chloride	Ditropan	2.5–5	BD–QDS	Non-selective	2.3
Oxybutynin chloride XL	Lyrinel XL	5–30	OD	Non-selective	13.2
Propiverine hydrochloride	Detrunorm	15	OD–QDS	Non-selective	4.1
Darifenacin	Emselex	7.5–15	OD	Selective muscarinic M_3 receptor antagonist	3.1
Solifenacin	Vesicare	5–10	OD	Selective muscarinic M_2 and M_3 receptor selectivity	40–68

BD, twice a day; OD, once a day; QDS, four times a day

DDAVP (1-deamino-8-D-arginine vasopressin)

The synthetic antidiuretic hormone desmopressin (Desmospray®) was initially introduced for the treatment of diabetes insipidus but has become widely accepted as a treatment for nocturnal enuresis in children. Desmospray® has also been used to treat patients with multiple sclerosis who are troubled by night-time frequency and some of these patients have taken to using it during the day if they particularly require a 4–6-hour period free from urinary urgency (ref needed). This is safe provided that the patient understands the importance of only using the medication once in 24 hours.

Patients with autonomic failure are often troubled by night-time frequency, possibly as a result of progressive daytime hypotension causing poor renal profusion. Desmopressin may lessen nocturnal frequency in these patients and seems to have an added beneficial effect in the management of postural hypotension (Chapter 47). It is now available in a tablet form. Whereas a metered dose of 10 µg is administered from the nasal spray, the tablets contain either 0.1 mg or 0.2 mg of desmopressin, the higher dose being necessary because of enzymatic degradation when the substance is taken orally.

Capsaicin and resiniferatoxin—the vanilloids

An alternative approach to lessening detrusor overactivity if patients have spinal cord disease has been the use of intravesical vanilloids. Following a spinal cord lesion that disconnects the sacral cord from the pontine micturition centre, a new segmental reflex emerges at the sacral level of the cord, the afferents of which are unmyelinated C-fibres (Chapter 19). Although these fibres are present in the neurologically intact, they are usually quiescent unless activated by irritations such as bacterial infection. The principle for using intravesical vesical vanilloids is to deafferent the bladder through the selective C-fibre neurotoxic effect of these substances (Fowler 2000).

Intravesical capsaicin was tried first, and although evidence has accumulated of a significant therapeutic effect (de Seze et al. 1999), use of the agent was largely abandoned because it was not licensed and could cause considerable discomfort when instilled. However, intravesical resiniferatoxin (RTX), an ultra-potent capsaicinoid (Appendino and Szallasi 1997) thought to have the same neurotoxic effect on bladder afferents, was much less pungent.

Unfortunately, the efficacy of this substance in formal clinical trials has not been demonstrated due to a number of factors, and its pharmaceutical future is uncertain.

Further work with capsaicin showed that if glucidic acid rather than 30% alcohol was used as the diluent, the solution was much less irritant (de Seze et al. 2004). A randomized controlled trial that compared the efficacy and tolerability of capsaicin in glucidic acid and RTX in 10% alcohol in patients with neurogenic bladder overactivity concluded that the formulations were highly comparable in relieving symptoms of neurogenic detrusor overactivity (de Seze et al. 2004). Intravesical capsaicin in glucidic acid is still offered as a treatment option in parts of France.

Botulinum toxin

Intradetrusor injections of botulinum neurotoxin type A (BoNT/A) were first described by Schurch et al. in 2000 (Schurch et al. 2000) and since then urologists worldwide have started to use the treatment for patients with intractable neurogenic detrusor overactivity. A large prospective study confirmed the efficacy in this patient group (Reitz et al. 2004) and recently the results of a placebo controlled trial were published (Schurch and de Seze 2004).The treatment has mostly been used in neurological patients with spinal cord injury or multiple sclerosis, and it is usually the case that such patients have reached a point of needing to perform CISC by the time BoNT/A injections are being considered. Following treatment in neurological patients CISC is almost always necessary so that being able or willing to perform this is a requirement before BoNT/A treatment can be considered.

Within a few days of the injections patients report a significant reduction in their sense of urinary urgency (Rapp et al. 2004), and cystometric studies show highly significant improvements at 3 months in maximum cystometric capacity, maximum detrusor pressure during voiding, volume at first reflex detrusor contraction, and bladder compliance, which was maintained at 9 months after treatment (Reitz et al. 2004). The benefit of injections lasts for 9–11 months, and subsequent injections appear to be as equally effective as the first one (Grosse et al. 2005).

It was first thought that BoNT/A acted by blocking the presynaptic release of acetylcholine and thus simply temporarily paralysed the detrusor; however, the benefits seem to exceed expectations. It is now thought likely that that BoNT/A is preventing the release of other neurotransmitters such as adenosine triphosphate (Khera et al. 2004), which are thought to be important in the afferent arm of reflex bladder contractions.

As originally described, the technique used a rigid cystoscope through which to give the injections, which in men at least, requires general anaesthesia. At our centre, however, we have introduced a minimally invasive local anaesthetic technique using a fine-gauge needle through a flexible cystoscope (Harper et al. 2003), so that the treatment may be given in 20 minutes as an outpatient procedure.

Most recently, studies have been reported on the effect of this treatment in idiopathic detrusor overactivity and in our own centre we have found it to be equally efficacious (Popat et al. 2005). It therefore appears to be a suitable treatment for the overactive bladder whatever the cause, and the limitation of its use in neurological patients will probably depend on their concomitant neurological disability.

Bladder dysfunction resulting from specific conditions

Spinal cord pathology

Spinal cord pathology resulting from traumatic injury, demyelination, or neoplastic changes causes a severe disruption of bladder function. This is because the efferent and afferent spinal pathways that pass between the pontine micturition centre and sacral spinal cord are interrupted. In health these pathways are important in maintaining the bladder as a low-pressure, compliant organ during filling and co-ordinating the relaxation of the striated muscle of the urethral sphincter preceding a detrusor contraction during voiding. With loss of this modulating activity the bladder becomes overactive and emptying can also be affected both by poorly sustained detrusor contractions and detrusor sphincter dyssynergia (Chapter 19). In patients following spinal cord injury, upper-tract disease can ensue, leading to renal failure unless effective preventive measures are taken. However, in patients with progressive neurological disease upper-tract involvement is fortunately uncommon and effective management of incontinence for most patients, particularly those less severely disabled, can be achieved by following the algorithm shown in Fig. 37.7.

Multiple system atrophy

Urinary and sexual symptoms are a pronounced feature of patients with MSA. Erectile dysfunction (ED) is frequently the first symptom of the disease in men. In a retrospective study of 71 male patients, ED preceded the onset of bladder symptoms in 58%, and the onset of orthostatic hypotension in 91% (Kirchhof et al. 2003). Two earlier reports had showed that urinary symptoms predate symptoms of postural hypotension by several years (Beck et al. 1994, Sakakibara et al. 2000) and it has been long known that in approximately 60% of patients genitourinary symptoms precede those of parkinsonism (Beck et al. 1994, Chandiramani et al. 1997).

Initial urinary symptoms include urgency, frequency of micturition, nocturia, and a reduced urinary stream. These symptoms are also typical of the much more common condition of prostatic hypertrophy, and men with MSA have not infrequently had a prostate resection without benefit (Chandiramani et al. 1997). Likewise, women have undergone surgery for stress incontinence with a poor

outcome before the underlying neurological disorder has been recognized.

The explanation for ED as a premonitory symptom is far from certain but on the evidence available it seems unlikely to be secondary to hypotension and may reflect degeneration in the parasympathetic or dopaminergic pathways. It has been suggested that detrusor overactivity in MSA may result from the degeneration of areas in the midbrain and basal ganglia (Benarroch 2003), and the poorly contracting bladder seen in the later stages of the disease may be due to progressive degeneration of the intermediolateral columns of the cord and the loss of cells from preganglionic neurons of the thoracolumbar and sacral spinal segments. As the strength of detrusor contractions diminishes, the bladder fails to empty and large post-micturition residual volumes develop. Upper-tract urinary complications are rare, possibly because the residual urine remains at a low pressure. The urethral and anal sphincters are innervated by motor neurons whose cell bodies lie in Onuf's nucleus in the ventral horn of the spinal cord at S2, S3 and S4, which also undergoes selective degeneration (Mannen et al. 1982). Thus, a patient with MSA may have detrusor overactivity, incomplete bladder emptying, and a weak sphincter, all factors likely to cause incontinence. It may be because the neural control of the bladder is affected at several different sites within the nervous system that incontinence occurs early and is so severe in patients with MSA.

The loss of anterior horn cells in Onuf's nucleus in MSA, demonstrated by early histopathology studies (Sung et al. 1979, Mannen et al. 1982) is the basis for the use of sphincter EMG to recognize this condition. Motor units recorded from the anal and urethral sphincter with a concentric needle electrode may show marked changes of reinnervation, being abnormally prolonged. The mean duration of 10 motor units was proposed as a test used to distinguish between patients with idiopathic Parkinson's disease and patients with MSA who present with atypical parkinsonism (Eardley et al. 1989, Palace et al. 1997), as Onuf's nucleus is preserved in idiopathic Parkinson's disease.

This has recently become a subject of some debate, although one paper concluded that both specificity and sensitivity is high if thresholds for detecting abnormality are set optimally (Tison et al. 2000). Another study demonstrated that, when sphincter EMG is combined with investigations with a similar specificity, such as the clonidine–growth hormone test, the accuracy becomes very high (Lee et al. 2002). A recent review concluded that anal sphincter EMG obtained within 5 years of onset should be tentatively accepted as a criterion for 'laboratory supported MSA' (Vodusek 2001).

The abnormalities that occur may be extreme although detecting them quite method dependant, since automated methods of motor unit selection may miss the highly prolonged duration units (Podnar and Fowler 2004). However, EMG changes of reinnervation are not specific and results from women who have had multiple births or patients who have undergone anal surgery must be interpreted with caution. Also, the test is not specific for MSA among other neurodegenerative conditions such as progressive supranuclear palsy (Valldeoriola et al. 1995, Vodusek 2001).

Treatment of urinary dysfunction in patients with MSA can be effective until the late stages of the disease—initially detrusor overactivity is the predominant abnormality and, if there is no significant residual, anticholinergic medication alone may then be helpful. In the later stages of the disease a high post-micturition residual volume may develop, and volumes in excess of 200 ml are not unusual (Beck et al. 1994, Chandiramani et al. 1997). The algorithm shown in Fig. 37.5 should be followed if possible. Desmopressin nasal spray administered at night is valuable in reducing nocturia and treating nocturnal enuresis. However, with progression of the disease a stage may be reached when an indwelling catheter becomes necessary. A suprapubic catheter is recommended at this stage as it is easy to change by the caregiver and prevents erosion and destruction of the urogenital anatomy.

Parkinson's disease

The concept of PD as a disease restricted to nigrostriatal degeneration resulting in only motor symptoms is now being revised as our understanding of the 'vegetative' and cognitive consequences of the wide spread dopaminergic and non-dopaminergic cell loss grows (Lang and Obeso 2004). Bladder symptoms can be marked in PD but the nature of the bladder dysfunction is different from that which occurs in MSA.

The prevalence of severe urinary symptoms has been estimated to be 27–39% (Araki and Kuno 2000, Campos-Sousa et al. 2003) and the severity of urinary symptoms is related to the neurological disability (Araki et al. 2000) and stage of disease (Sakakibara et al. 2001). The main complaints are urgency (33–54%) and frequency (16–36%), and urge incontinence if there is poor mobility that complicates their bladder symptoms (Araki and Kuno 2000, Campos-Sousa et al. 2003).

In animal studies, the basal ganglia have been shown to exert an inhibitory effect on the bladder, and loss of this central inhibition may explain the occurrence of detrusor overactivity in patients with idiopathic PD. Studies have been performed to examine the relationship between detrusor overactivity and the effect of anti-parkinsonian drugs in patients undergoing cystometric studies in both 'on' and 'off' states, with somewhat conflicting results over the years.

However, a recent study of 18 patients with advanced PD who showed 'on-off' phenomenon, showed that a single dose of levodopa (L-3,4-dihydroxyphenylalanine [L-dopa]) worsened storage function with increased urgency, detrusor overactivity and decreased maximum cystometric capacity but improved voiding allowing unchanged maximum flow rate but a decrease in the residual volumes (Uchiyama et al. 2003).

It has been proposed that there may be a failure of relaxation of the urethral sphincter in patients with PD, and in men apomorphine injections or oral L-dopa may be helpful in deciding whether urinary symptoms might be due to PD or prostatic enlargement. Following apomorphine injections, urinary flow rates increased and residual volumes decreased (Christmas et al. 1988).

Poor voiding in men with PD does present a difficult management problem, however, and there may be a combination of both neurogenic detrusor overactivity and prostatic obstruction. Urological intervention is not contraindicated but it is sensible to try patients on anticholinergic medication, preferably one without central effects, if symptoms of urgency or nocturia predominate.

Voiding cystometry is useful in cases where conservative measures have failed and demonstrate most commonly detrusor overactivity (67–75%) and/or obstructed voiding with hypotonic detrusor or detrusor sphincter dyssynergia being far less common (Pavlakis et al. 1983, Araki et al. 2000). Urodynamic studies are mandatory if prostate surgery is being considered.

Diabetes mellitus

Diabetes can result in a wide range of complications including incontinence, recurrent infections, decrease in sensation, and retention of urine. Cystopathy was once considered an uncommon complication, but the greater use of techniques for studying bladder function have shown that this is incorrect, although the condition is mostly asymptomatic and discovered incidentally. It develops gradually over several years with progressive loss of bladder sensation and impairment of bladder emptying, eventually culminating in chronic low-pressure urinary retention. Urodynamic studies demonstrate impaired detrusor contractility, reduction in the urinary flow rate, and increased post-micturition residual volume and reduction in bladder sensation. The sequence of pathophysiological events that result in diabetic neurocystopathy are uncertain, but it seems likely that there is involvement of both the vesical sensory afferent fibres, causing a reduced awareness of bladder filling, and involvement of parasympathetic efferent fibres to the detrusor, decreasing the ability of the bladder to contract. The bladder neck, which is principally innervated by sympathetic fibres, is competent in most cases of diabetic cystopathy, suggesting that, as in the cardiovascular system, sympathetic denervation is probably a late phenomenon.

Damage to the urothelium itself may result in alteration in the multiple receptors and ion channels that regulate the response to stretch and nociception. The detrusor smooth muscle itself is a target for damage resulting in reduced contractility.

Diabetics may have a reduced immune function and therefore greater susceptibility to infection. *Escherichia coli* with Type 1 fimbria adhere twice as well to diabetic epithelial cells compared with control cells (Geerlings et al. 2002).

Asymptomatic diabetics with cystopathy should be made aware of their disorders since having lost their normal desire to micturate, they may void infrequently. They should be advised to void at regular intervals and before going to bed at night. Symptomatic patients are best managed by CISC. Recurrent urinary tract infections may require prophylaxis with antibiotics especially if the residual volumes are high. The multi-system nature of diabetes affecting almost all body systems can make management very challenging.

References

Abrams, P. (1997). Urodynamics in Clinical Practice. In *Urodynamics* (P.Abrams (Ed)), pp. 148–72. Springer.

Abrams, P., Cardozo, L., Fall, M., *et al.* (2002). The standardisation of terminology of lower urinary tract function: report from the Standardisation Sub-committee of the International Continence Society. *Neurourol. Urodyn.* **21**, 167–78.

Araki, I., Kitahara, M., Oida, T., and Kuno, S. (2000). Voiding dysfunction and Parkinson's disease: urodynamic abnormalities and urinary symptoms. *J. Urol.* **164**, 1640–43.

Araki, I. and Kuno, S. (2000). Assessment of voiding dysfunction in Parkinson's disease by the international prostate symptom score. *JNNP* **68**, 429–33.

Beck, R. O., Betts, C. D., and Fowler, C. J. (1994). Genitourinary dysfunction in multiple system atrophy: clinical features and treatment in 62 cases. *J. Urol.* **151**, 1336–41.

Benarroch, E. E. (2003). Brainstem in multiple system atrophy: clinicopathological correlations. *Cell Mol. Neurobiol.* **23**, 519–26.

Campos-Sousa, R. N., Quagliato, E., da Silva, B. B., de, C. R., Jr., Ribeiro, S. C., and de Carvalho, D. F. (2003). Urinary symptoms in Parkinson's disease: prevalence and associated factors. *Arq Neuropsiquiatr.* **61**, 359–63.

Chandiramani, V. A., Palace, J., and Fowler, C. J. (1997). How to recognize patients with parkinsonism who should not have urological surgery. *Br. J. Urol.* **80**, 100–104.

Chess-Williams, R., Chapple, C. R., Yamanishi, T., Yasuda, K., and Sellers, D. J. (2001). The minor population of M₃-receptors mediate contraction of human detrusor muscle in vitro. *J. Auton. Pharmacol.* **21**, 243–48.

Christmas, T. J., Kempster, P. A., Chapple, C. R., Frankel, J. P., Lees, A. J., Stern, G. M., and Milroy, E. J. (1988). Role of subcutaneous apomorphine in parkinsonian voiding dysfunction. *Lancet* **2**, 1451–53.

Delodovici, M. L. and Fowler, C. J. (1995). Clinical value of the pudendal somatosensory evoked potential. *Electroencephalogr. Clin. Neurophysiol.* **96**, 509–515.

de Seze, M. P., Wiart, L., de Seze, M. P., *et al.* (2004). Intravesical capsaicin versus resiniferatoxin for the treatment of detrusor hyperreflexia in spinal cord injured patients: a double-blind, randomized, controlled study. *J Urol.* **171**, 251–55.

Eardley, I., Quinn, N. P., Fowler, C. J., Kirby, R. S., Parkhouse, H. F., Marsden, C. D., and Bannister, R. (1989). The value of urethral sphincter electromyography in the differential diagnosis of parkinsonism. *Br. J. Urol.* **64**, 360–62.

Ertekin, C., Colakoglu, Z., and Altay, B. (1995). Hand and genital sympathetic skin potentials in flaccid and erectile penile states in normal potent men and patients with premature ejaculation. *J. Urol.* **153**, 76–79.

Fowler, C. J. (1996). Investigation of the neurogenic bladder. *JNNP* **60**, 6–13.

Fowler, C. J. (2000). Intravesical treatment of overactive bladder. *Urology* **55**, 60–64.

Geerlings, S. E., Meiland, R., van Lith, E. C., Brouwer, E. C., Gaastra, W., and Hoepelman, A. I. (2002). Adherence of type 1-fimbriated Escherichia coli to uroepithelial cells: more in diabetic women than in control subjects. *Diabetes Care* **25**, 1405–1409.

Grosse, J., Kramer, G., and Stohrer, M. (2005). Success of Repeat Detrusor Injections of Botulinum A Toxin in Patients with Severe Neurogenic Detrusor Overactivity and Incontinence. *European Urology* **47**, 653–59.

Harper, M., Popat, R. B., Dasgupta, R., Fowler, C. J., and Dasgupta, P. (2003). A minimally invasive technique for outpatient local anaesthetic administration of intradetrusor botulinum toxin in intractable detrusor overactivity. *BJU. Int.* **92**, 325–26.

Khera, M., Somogyi, G. T., Kiss, S., Boone, T. B., and Smith, C. P. (2004). Botulinum toxin A inhibits ATP release from bladder urothelium after chronic spinal cord injury. *Neurochem. Int.* **45**, 987–93.

Kirchhof, K., Apostolidis, A. N., Mathias, C. J., and Fowler, C. J. (2003). Erectile and urinary dysfunction may be the presenting features in patients with multiple system atrophy: a retrospective study. *Int. J. Impot. Res.* **15**, 293–98.

Lang, A. E. and Obeso, J. A. (2004). Challenges in Parkinson's disease: restoration of the nigrostriatal dopamine system is not enough. *Lancet Neurol.* **3**, 309–316.

Lee, E. A., Kim, B. J., and Lee, W. Y. (2002). Diagnosing multiple system atrophy with greater accuracy: combined analysis of the clonidine-growth hormone test and external anal sphincter electromyography. *Mov Disord.* **17**, 1242–47.

Mannen, T., Iwata, M., Toyokura, Y., and Nagashima, K. (1982). The Onuf's nucleus and the external anal sphincter muscles in amyotrophic lateral sclerosis and Shy-Drager syndrome. *Acta Neuropathol.(Berl)* **58**, 255–60.

Mansfield, K. J., Liu, L., Mitchelson, F. J., Moore, K. H., Millard, R. J., and Burcher, E. (2005). Muscarinic receptor subtypes in human bladder detrusor and mucosa, studied by radioligand binding and quantitative competitive RT-PCR: changes in ageing. *Br. J. Pharmacol.* **144**, 1089–99.

Palace, J., Chandiramani, V. A., and Fowler, C. J. (1997). Value of sphincter electromyography in the diagnosis of multiple system atrophy. *Muscle Nerve* **20**, 1396–1403.

Pavlakis, A. J., Siroky, M. B., Goldstein, I., and Krane, R. J. (1983). Neurourologic findings in Parkinson's disease. *J. Urol.* **129**, 80–83.

Podnar, S. and Fowler, C. J. (2004). Sphincter electromyography in diagnosis of multiple system atrophy: technical issues. *Muscle Nerve* **29**, 151–56.

Pontari, M. A., Braverman, A. S., and Ruggieri, M. R., Sr. (2004). The M₂ muscarinic receptor mediates in vitro bladder contractions from patients with neurogenic bladder dysfunction. *Am. J. Physiol Regul. Integr. Comp Physiol* **286**, R874–80.

Popat, R. B., Apostolidis, A. N., Kalsi, V., and Fowler, C. J. (2005). A comparison between the response of patients with idiopathic detrusor overactivity (IDO) and neurogenic detrusor overactivity (NDO) to the first intradetrusor injection of botulinum A toxin. *J Urol.* **174**(3), 984–9.

Rapp, D. E., Lucioni, A., Katz, E. E., O'Connor, R. C., Gerber, G. S., and Bales, G. T. (2004). Use of botulinum-A toxin for the treatment of refractory overactive bladder symptoms: an initial experience. *Urology* **63**, 1071–75.

Reitz, A., Stohrer, M., Kramer, G., *et al.* (2004). European experience of 200 cases treated with botulinum-A toxin injections into the detrusor muscle for urinary incontinence due to neurogenic detrusor overactivity. *Eur. Urol.* **45**, 510–515.

Sakakibara, R., Hattori, T., Uchiyama, T., Kita, K., Asahina, M., Suzuki, A., and Yamanishi, T. (2000). Urinary dysfunction and orthostatic hypotension in multiple system atrophy: which is the more common and earlier manifestation? *J. Neurol. Neurosurg. Psychiatry* **68**, 65–69.

Sakakibara, R., Shinotoh, H., Uchiyama, T., Sakuma, M., Kashiwado, M., Yoshiyama, M., and Hattori, T. (2001). Questionnaire-based assessment of pelvic organ dysfunction in Parkinson's disease. *Auton. Neurosci.* **92**, 76–85.

Schick, E., Jolivet-Tremblay, M., Dupont, C., Bertrand, P. E., and Tessier, J. (2003). Frequency-volume chart: the minimum number of days required to obtain reliable results. *Neurourol. Urodyn.* **22**: 92–96.

Schurch, B., Stohrer, M., Kramer, G., Schmid, D. M., Gaul, G., and Hauri, D. (2000). Botulinum-A toxin for treating detrusor hyperreflexia in spinal cord injured patients: a new alternative to anticholinergic drugs? Preliminary results. *J. Urol.* **164**, 692–97.

Schurch, B. and de Seze, M. P. (2004). Botulinum Toxin A (Botox) in neurogenic urinary incontinence: results from a multicentre randomised, controlled trial. *Neurourol Urodyn* **23**, 609–10.

Sung, J. H., Mastri, A. R., and Segal, E. (1979). Pathology of Shy-Drager syndrome. *J. Neuropathol. Exp. Neurol.* **38**, 353–68.

Sussman, D. and Garely, A. (2002). Treatment of overactive bladder with once-daily extended-release tolterodine or oxybutynin: the antimuscarinic clinical effectiveness trial (ACET). *Curr. Med. Res. Opin.* **18**, 177–84.

Thor, K. B. and Katofiasc, M. A. (1995). Effects of duloxetine, a combined serotonin and norepinephrine reuptake inhibitor, on central neural control of lower urinary tract function in the chloralose-anesthetized female cat. *J. Pharmacol. Exp. Ther.* **274**, 1014–24.

Tison, F., Arne, P., Sourgen, C., Chrysostome, V., and Yeklef, F. (2000). The value of external anal sphincter electromyography for the diagnosis of multiple system atrophy. *Mov Disord.* **15**, 1148–57.

Uchiyama, T., Sakakibara, R., Hattori, T., and Yamanishi, T. (2003). Short-term effect of a single levodopa dose on micturition disturbance in Parkinson's disease patients with the wearing-off phenomenon. *Mov Disord.* **18**, 573–78.

Valldeoriola, F., Valls-Sole, J., Tolosa, E. S., and Marti, M. J. (1995). Striated anal sphincter denervation in patients with progressive supranuclear palsy. *Mov Disord.* **10**, 550–55.

Vodusek, D. B. (2001). Sphincter EMG and differential diagnosis of multiple system atrophy. *Mov Disord.* **16**, 600–607.

Wong, D. T., Bymaster, F. P., Mayle, D. A., Reid, L. R., Krushinski, J. H., and Robertson, D. W. (1993). LY248686, a new inhibitor of serotonin and norepinephrine uptake. *Neuropsychopharmacology* **8**, 23–33.

Zinner, N. R. (2005). Stress Urinary Incontinence in Women: Efficacy and Safety of Duloxetine. *European Urology Supplements* **4**, 29–37.

CHAPTER 38

Investigation and treatment of sexual dysfunction in autonomic diseases

Stacy Elliott

The area of sexuality illustrates one of the most integrated systems of the body. No other system of autonomic innervation demonstrates the mind–body connection as well as the emotionally connected one of sexual function.

This chapter will focus on the role and investigation of the autonomic nervous system (ANS) in both men and women during sexual arousal, ejaculation (in men) and orgasm. The primary functions of the ANS in sexual neurophysiology will be delineated at the central, spinal cord and local neurotransmitter level. Sexual dysfunction will be defined, and clinical examples of sexual changes in pertinent autonomic disease entities will be illustrated. Lastly, a brief overview of the available therapies will be mentioned.

Forty years ago, ground-breaking laboratory work of two researchers (Masters and Johnson 1966) resulted in a model of the physiological sexual response cycle. They proposed a four-phase 'sexual mountain' of rising and declining sexual arousal:

1 excitement

2 plateau [high arousal before orgasm]

3 orgasm

4 resolution [the reversal and/or dissipation of phase 1].

The excitement or arousal stage consists of pelvic vasocongestion and neuromuscular tension resulting in tumescence and/or erection of the erectile tissues in both men and women and additionally, in women, vaginal lubrication and accommodation (lengthening and uterine lifting). The plateau phase is clinically recognized as the 'pre-orgasmic' phase: typically men have maximal erection and rigidity, are undergoing seminal emission leading to ejaculatory inevitability (the 'point of no return'), and the outer third of the vagina forms an 'orgasmic platform' in women. Orgasm, a pleasant experience recognized in the genital area, brain or total body, is accompanied by rhythmic contractions of the pelvic floor muscles in both men and women, as well as smooth muscle contractions of internal and accessory organ structures (seminal vesicles, urethra prostate, etc). Orgasm and ejaculation, the process of antegrade seminal fluid expulsion in men, are neurologically independent but usually occur contemporaneously (Bhasin and Benson 2006).

The Masters and Johnson model has been criticized as being unrepresentative of the general population and too focused on pelvic physiology and not inclusive of the complexity of real life sexuality (i.e. subjective factors are generally overlooked) (Rosen and Rosen 2006). Recognizing the need to incorporate the cerebral aspects of sexuality, it was modified by Helen Singer Kaplan into three phases: desire, excitement, and orgasm (Kaplan 1974). Since then many more models have been published, the most recent being an 'alternate' model applicable to women (Basson 2001) and a clinically applicable model of human sexual response (Stevenson and Elliott 2007), both which envisage the biopsychosocial approach to sexuality. In a recent survey, the heterogeneity of female sexual response was emphasized when women subjects equally endorsed three varied models (Masters and Johnson, Kaplan, and Basson) as representing their own sexual experience (Sand and Fisher 2007). However, the original Masters and Johnson model, while not explaining the observed patterning of autonomic, somatic, and central concomitants of the sexual response at the time (Rosen and Rosen 2006), is still the most appropriate framework now to discuss *the role and investigation of the autonomic nervous system.* That said, it must be recognized that central factors obviously influence the neurophysiological outcome of the phases: contextual, emotional and hormonal interplay with the ANS account for the minute-to-minute variability in sexual response (Stevenson and Elliott 2007). Furthermore, ageing, disease, surgery, trauma, medications, and chemotherapy can cause endocrine, neural, and vascular components of sexual response to be altered, the details of which are beyond the scope of this chapter.

Complexity of neural pathways involved in sexual arousal

It is not fully understood how sexual desire, arousal, ejaculation and orgasm are mediated. It is known that the somatic and autonomic nervous systems, directed by the brain, affect spinal cord pathways and local spinal reflexes and peripheral nerves. The brain exerts supratentorial control over the spinal cord reflexes: a release of this 'inhibition' allows for the natural physiological unfolding of the sexual reflexes. The autonomic nerves connect the central nervous system (CNS) to the genitalia. In male rats, the anatomical site for the descending inhibitory action has been identified in the rostral pole of the paragigantocellular nucleus bilaterally located in the oblongata (Marson and McKenna 1990).

Brain initiated signals are the result of interpretation of imagery and fantasy, of visual, auditory and olfactory inputs (including the little known role of pheromones in man), and of ascending signals from somatic (usually tactile) stimulation. Ascending afferent pathways can initiate, reinforce or inhibit central sexual arousal, which will then have similar effects on a local sexual spinal reflex. While the traditional concept of sexual responses follows a 'hard wired' model with neural connections extending from the brain to the peripheral nerve receptors at the sexual end organs, there are neuroendocrine (Rowland 2006), other biological factors (Bancroft 2002) and possibly other non-CNS pathways that are significant. For example, there is growing evidence of a nociceptive vagal-solitary pathway from the vaginocervix region in women with complete spinal cord injuries (SCI) (so far not identified in men with SCI), consistent with pathways already described in basic rat studies (Hubscher 2006, Komisaruk and Wallman 1977), and confirmed by functional magnetic resonance imaging (fMRI) in the human female (Komisaruk et al. 2004, Komisaruk and Sansone 2003). Brain neuroplasticity can also play a role after sensory or motor injury (Dancause 2006), especially after SCI (Behrman et al. 2006): there are many anecdotal cases of renewed arousal and orgasm following stimulation of sensate non-sexual areas after SCI (Elliott 2002, Tepper 2001). Sensory substitution after SCI is also a new science (Bach-y-Rita 1999) and work in the area of sexual sensory substitution is currently ongoing (Borisoff et al. 2008).

The recent expansion in the knowledge about local genital physiological, biochemical, and genomic processes far outpace that of our knowledge of CNS control in man: correspondingly, most of our information on CNS control is from rat studies, the relevance of which, especially in the area of orgasm, will be understandably limited (De Tejada et al. 2004). However, in the autonomic area, animal models are what we have, excepting those human experimental studies of subjective and objective sexual responses and imaging. These various functional imaging modalities, including positron emission tomography (PET) and fMRI undertaken using human subjects experiencing sexual arousal, show activation of the higher cortex, the limbic and paralimbic cortex, and the limbic and other subcortical regions (Rees et al. 2007). These data infer that brain areas that integrate cognitive, motivational and autonomic components (Mouras et al. 2003), are also those responsible for sexual arousal. Most fMRI studies use visual exotic stimuli against controls (non-erotic stimuli), but olfactory stimuli has also been used (Huh et al. 2006), as well as cerebral correlates with volumetric plethysmography of the penis during arousal (Moulier V et al. 2006). There may even be gender differences in the brain imaging of sexual excitation and inhibition (Laan et al. 2006). Functional imaging of the brain in humans during sexual arousal and orgasm will advance the field far beyond basic animal studies in the next century.

Autonomic innervation of the genitalia

The CNS is connected to the genitalia by the autonomic nerves. Sympathetic preganglionic fibres arise from the intermediolateral gray cell column and dorsal commissure of the lower thoracic (T10) to upper lumbar (L2) segments of the spinal cord, and likely receive input from the descending supraspinal centres (Rehman

and Melman 2001). Preganglionic fibres leave the cord via the ventral roots of T10–L2 enroute to the paravertebral sympathetic chain, where they take one of two routes:

1 They descend to synapse with ganglia at the lower lumbar or sacral level (paravertebral pathway) enroute to the sacral pelvic or cavernosal nerves.

2 They pass through the corresponding chain ganglia without synapsing and enter the lumbar splanchnic nerves to synapse there (prevertebral pathway) or in the superior hypogastric plexus (Rehman and Melman 2001).

The superior hypogastric plexus sits in front of the promontory of the sacrum and divides inferiorly into the right and left hypogastric nerves, and contains additional branches of the 3rd and 4th lumbar sympathetic ganglia, as well as sacral parasympathetic and visceral afferent nerve fibres (Snell 2001).

Parasympathetic preganglionic input arises from the sacral (S2–S4) spinal cord, whose preganglionic neurons are situated in the intermediolateral cell column. The dendrites these preganglionic neurons receive input from are laminae V, VII, IX and X of the spinal cord (implying that these neurons receive afferent (sensory) information from both visceral and somatic structures) and they also project to descending axons from supraspinal centres to integrate and coordinate the ANS (i.e. hypothalamus, reticular formation and midbrain) (Rehman and Melman 2001). The axons of these sacral parasympathetic preganglionic neurons leaving through the ventral routes (similar to sympathetic preganglionic neurons) unite to form the pelvic splanchnic nerves (pelvic nerve) which, when joined by sympathetic fibres of the inferior hypogastric nerve to form the inferior hypogastric plexus (pelvic plexus). The pelvic plexus is therefore the main crossroad for genital autonomic nerves, consisting of parasympathetic fibres from the sacral roots (S2–S4) and sympathetic nerve fibres from the thoracolumbar sympathetic nerve roots (T11–L2) (Yang and Jiang 2009). However, not all axons conveyed by hypogastric or pelvic nerves synapse in the pelvic pexis (Rehman and Melman 2001). The inferior hypogastric plexus contains postganglionic sympathetic fibres, preganglionic and postganglionic parasympathetic fibres, and visceral afferent fibres (Snell 1992). In addition, somatic sensory information from the sacral region also provides information from the genitalia.

The pelvic sexual organs therefore receive innervation from the spinal cord in three ways:

- sacral parasympathetic (pelvic nerves and pelvic plexus)
- thoracolumbar sympathetic (hypogastric nerves and lumbar sympathetic chain)
- somatic (bilateral pudendal nerves) (Chuang and Steers 1999, Mathias and Frankel 1992).

Specific anatomical nerve distribution to the male and female internal and external genitalia can be found in current readings (Beck 1999a, Rehman and Melman 2001, Giuliano and Julia-Guilloteau 2006, Pauls et al. 2006), but in general, follow the major arteries of the abdomen and pelvis (Yang and Jiang 2009).

Autonomic nervous system pathways in the phases of sexual response

The sexual response can be thought of as a series of reflexes (i.e. involuntary events in response to a stimulus). The afferent arms of the reflex can include genital and extragenital erogenous touch, and special senses interpreted by the brain, including fantasy. The efferent reflex arm includes not only the induced genital changes, but systemic autonomic influences in heart rate, respiratory rate, skin vasomotor responses (flushing and perspiration), as well as emotional and sensory benefits (pleasure, reduction in pain, etc) (Yang and Jiang 2009). The highly coordinated autonomic and somatic functions, modulated by emotional and other factors, lead to variable perceptions of sexual response which can be different not only for each person but for every sexual situation.

Arousal

Arousal consists of penile erection in the male and engorgement of blood in the labia, vaginal wall (resulting in lubrication), and clitoral erectile tissue in the female. Anatomically, these responses involve the pelvic nerve (from the parasympathetic nucleus), the hypogastric and the lumbosacral chain sympathetic chain (which contain fibres originating from both the intermediolateral cell column and dorsal grey commissure of thoracolumbar levels (T12–L2) of the spinal cord), and the pudendal nerve, a somatic nerve whose cell body motoneurons are located in Onuf's nucleus (S2–S4) (Giuliano and Julia-Guilloteau 2006). Both somatic and autonomic afferent nerves form part of the general afferent segment of the entire nervous system and probably travel alongside or mixed together enroute to the brain via the spinal cord. Autonomic nerves will be activated by stretch or lack of oxygen verses touch, rather than by touch or temperature like the somatic nerves (Snell 2001), but both types of nerves appear critical to recognize stimuli as 'sexual'.

There are two neurological pathways for penile and clitoral erection: reflexogenic and psychogenic. The *reflexogenic pathway* is triggered by direct stimulation of the genital organs (usually via touch, pressure or friction) and conveyed to the pudendal nerve via the dorsal nerve. In this reflex, the afferent component is conveyed by the pudendal nerve to the S2–S4 segments of the spinal cord (Beck 1999a). The efferent component returns from the sacral parasympathetic centre, contributing fibres to the pelvic nerve and onto the cavernosal nerves at the genitalia. Pudendal afferent pathway interneurons in the dorsal commissure and medal dorsal horn not only activate the sacral preganglionic neurons to initiate reflex erection, but also send sensations to the brain. Complete spinal cord injury above the level of the sacral cord eliminates the central inhibitory brain control, enhancing the reflex mechanism initiated by touch (Rehman and Melman 2001).

The *psychogenic pathway* is of supraspinal origin (auditory, imaginative, visual etc.) with the thalamic (somatosensory and visual), rhinencephalon (olfactory), limbic (emotion, fantasy, and memory) afferent structures involved via the medial preoptic area (MPOA), paraventricular of hypothalamus (PVN) and reticular activating systems (the latter involved with nocturnal arousal during rapid eye movement [REM] sleep) (Rehman and Melman 2001). Efferent pathways from the MPOA enter the medial forebrain bundle (MFB), continue down through the midbrain segmental region near the lateral part of the substantia nigra, and, finally via the ventrolateral portion of the pons and medulla, to arrive at the spinal centres. The long efferent tracts of the CNS between cortex, cord, and ANS must be intact to elicit the sacral parasympathetic and thoracolumbar sympathetic pathways (Beck 1999a). The use of brain imaging techniques such as PET (Tiihonen et al. 1994) and fMRI have demonstrated areas in the brain associated

with imagery, visual sexual stimulation, arousal, and orgasm in both sexes (Goldstein et al. 2004, Meston et al. 2004).

While the psychogenic and reflexogenic pathways can act independently, they usually act synergistically to determine the erectile response via a final common pathway involving a sacral parasympathetic route (Chuang and Steers 1999). The sympathetic nervous system (SNS) maintains the male penile erection capacity after injury to parasympathetic pathways (Chuang and Steers 1999), has a role in the development of psychogenic erections (Sipski et al. 2007), and is instrumental in erectile detumescence (Beck 1999a).

Both men and women undergo measurable arousal during REM sleep (Gerdes 1997, Lundberg 1999) and in men, measurement of this erectile phenomenon has been used to differentiate 'organic' from 'psychogenic' erectile dysfunction (ED). However, measuring REM sleep erections, from simple home monitoring nocturnal penile tumescence (NPT) testing to more refined sleep-lab testing is used to objectively demonstrate the potential for full erections during sleep and thus provides a test that is relatively free from psychologically mediated events (Rosen et al. 2004). However, NPT testing has not proven that reliable in the differentiation of organic neurogenic ED, as the neurogenic pathways to initiate and maintain nocturnal erections are probably different from those involving psychogenic and reflexogenic pathways (Beck 1999b). This is illustrated in multiple sclerosis (Staerman et al. 1996), where nocturnal erections are preserved despite clear disturbance with daytime, erotic erections.

In men, vascular congestion results in tumescence of the erectile tissue. Interference with the neuronal messaging to allow vascular inflow from psychogenic or organic causes will result in lack of erection. Neurostimulation of the lumbar sympathetic trunk in dogs and monkeys antagonizes the relaxing action of papaverine on the cavernous smooth muscle and arterioles in papaverine induced erection (Diederichs et al. 1991). Once blood accumulates inside the corpora cavernosa (tumescence), a veno-occlusive mechanism (venule and emissary vein occlusion by the tunica albuginea) ensues, allowing for intracavernous pressure to increase to mean blood pressure (BP), resulting in a full erection state. Contraction of the ischiocavernosus muscle further increases intracavernosal pressure to the rigid state (Rehman and Melman 2001). Despite adequate arousal, men may have erection dysfunction secondary to poor arterial inflow from a vascular or neurogenic cause, from a venous leak due to inadequate compression of emissary veins as they pierce through the stretched tunica due to ageing or tunical scarring, or from excessive venous outflow through large abnormal veins draining the corpora. Conversely, priapism, a prolonged, unwanted, non-sexual erection, has been categorized into two clinically relevant subtypes: 'low flow' resulting from an abnormal veno-occlusive state leading to hypoxia in the cavernosal tissues, and 'high flow', caused by arterial trauma with normal venous flow and oxygenation. While both types require medical attention, 'low flow' is a medical emergency.

The neurological mechanisms of arousal in women are similar to those of men: the parasympathetic pathway is responsible for clitoral engorgement, vaginal congestion, lubrication, and lengthening of the vagina (Giuliano and Julia-Guilloteau 2006). An effective erection of the clitoris occurs with sexual stimulation, which may or may not be noticed by women in sexual encounters. Extensive pelvic vasocongestion (uterine, vaginal, urethral, labial, and pelvic ligaments) is also present in women. Clitoral erection may not occur simultaneously with vaginal lubrication, and often requires more intense stimulation (Lundberg 1999) than that required for lubrication. Vaginal venous drainage is probably also reduced at the same time blood flow is increased, leading to vasocongestion and genital engorgement, clitoral tumescence, and increased genital sensitivity (Wagner and Levin 1980). This veno-occlusive mechanism is less prominent in the female corporal bodies due to a less effectual tunica; however, priapism is possible in women (Lundberg 1999, Goldstein et al. 2004). Blood flow studies have looked indirectly at the role of the ANS on arousal and orgasm in women.

There is evidence for a facilitory role of peripheral adrenergic activation on sexual arousal in women: ephedrine (50 mg), an α- and β-agonist, facilitated vaginal photoplethysmography measures of sexual arousal, and clonidine, an α_2-adrenergic agonist that blocks peripheral sympathetic outflow, decreased this response (Meston and Gorzalka 1996). Intense acute exercise to induce SNS activity enhanced vaginal engorgement in women (Meston and Gorzalka 1996). It may be that there is a threshold for sympathetic stimulation to enhance arousal in women, and too much may cause reversal of arousal. This may have to do with the fact that sympathetic fibres in the hypogastric nerve pass through the ganglionic relay stations in the pelvic plexus and can produce vasodilation of vulva congestion as well as the opposite (de Groat 1999).

Secretory pathways are also under autonomic control. In males, autonomic (parasympathetic) stimulation results in mucus secretion from bulbourethral (Cowper's gland) and Littre's glands (de Groat and Booth 1980), which lubricates the urethra. In some men, Cowper's gland secretion can be quite noticeable in the plateau phase, just prior to ejaculation. Male internal accessory organ function is dependent on adequate testosterone levels. In women, the sexually aroused vagina becomes lubricated and elongated. At higher arousal levels, an orgasmic platform is formed at the distal outer third of the vaginal (Masters and Johnson 1996). Vaginal fluid, thought to be a plasma transudate from the blood circulating through the vessels of the vaginal epithelium and containing desquamated cervical and vaginal cells and cervical secretions, is increased during mental or physical sexual arousal. Normal lubrication depends on both intact innervation and on normal oestrogen levels (Lundberg 1999).

Muscles of the pelvic floor are also involved in sexual function and are innervated by the pudendal nerve. In men, the bulbocavernosus (BC) muscle invests the bulb of the urethra and the distal corpus spongiosum and increases turgor during erection beyond that attainable by arterial pressure alone: the ischiocavernosus (IC) muscle helps ejaculate semen (Shetty and Farah 1999). In women, passive dilation of the vagina results in a reflex contraction of both the BC and IC, indirectly affecting the clitoris and sensory perception of the clitoris (Shafik 1993).

Ejaculation

Ejaculation is a complex reflex that consist of two distinct phases: emission and expulsion (or propulsatile ejaculation). In contrast to genital arousal, where the parasympathetic nervous system (PNS) predominates, the SNS triggers ejaculation. Preganglionic sympathetic fibres leave the spinal cord from the first and second lumbar segments, then synapse with either the postganglionic neurons in their respective ganglia or in the lower lumbar or pelvic parts of the sympathetic trunks (Snell 2001). Postganglionic fibres

are then distributed to the vas deferens, the seminal vesicles and the prostate through the hypogastric nerves, where they stimulate contractions of the smooth muscle in the walls of these structures (Snell 2001).

Semen consists of combined secretions of the testes (including spermatozoa), vas deferens, seminal vesicles and prostate gland, and bulbourethral glands. Seminal emission, the first phase of ejaculation, is conducted by thoracolumbar sympathetic outflow from the presacral and hypogastric nerve (T10–L2). Seminal emission involves transport of semen into the prostatic urethra via the ejaculatory ducts in the prostate. Parasympathetic innervation allows for seminal vesicle and prostate secretions, which form most the volume of semen (Rehman and Melman 2001). The sympathetic hypogastric nerve (L1, 2) closes the bladder neck to prevent retrograde ejaculation.

Expulsion, the second phase of ejaculation, propels the seminal bolus distally out the urethral meatus in a rhythmic fashion (typically 10–15 contractions) (Yang and Jiang 2009) This phase is under combined parasympathetic and somatic control via the pelvic nerve at S2–4: the former is responsible for the spasmodic contraction of the seminal vesicles, prostate, and urethra, and the latter for rhythmic pelvic floor contractions of the BC and IC muscles and periurethral striated muscles.

Animal models have been primarily used to investigate the neural circuits and descending spinal pathways involved in ejaculation. Spinal ejaculatory circuits described include autonomic circuits at the thoracolumbar and lumbosacral levels mediating the emission phase, somatic circuits at the lumbosacral level responsible for the sequential, rhythmic contraction of the bulbospongiosus muscle involved in expulsion, and a proposed ejaculatory pattern generator in the lumbar cord (Johnson 2006). However, the ability of anaesthetized rats to exhibit ejaculatory behaviour following acute thoracic spinalization (Gravitt and Marson 2007), and humans with complete transaction of the spinal cord above the 10th thoracic segmental level to ejaculate with vibrostimulation (Elliott 2003), demonstrates that both emission and expulsion can occur despite the loss of connectivity with supraspinal structures. It appears that the most probable neural components responsible for the generation of ejaculation reside within the lumbosacral cord in an ejaculation centre or generator (McKenna 1999a). This centre was elucidated in male rats (Truitt and Coolen 2002), and appears to integrate the sensory inputs that are necessary to trigger ejaculation as well as coordinate the sympathetic, parasympathetic, and somatic outflow to induce the two phases of ejaculation described above. A population of interneurons in the lumbar spinal cord levels 3 and 4, which later came to be referred to as lumbar spinothalamic 'Lst cells', were discovered in male rats. The Lst cells appear to have supraspinal thalamic projections, as well as projections to the parasympathetic and sympathetic preganglionic neurons, the pudendal motoneurons, and are in the anatomical location to be able to receive sensory inputs through the pudendal nerve (Allard et al. 2005, Young et al. 2009). It has also been observed that Lst cell activation is exclusively associated with ejaculatory behaviour, as opposed to the sexual activity preceding (Young et al. 2009). Lesions of Lst cells completely ablate ejaculatory function (Allard et al. 2005). It has been proposed that the Lst cells operate through a glutamatergic N-methyl-D-aspartate (NMDA) driven mechanism of action (Young et al. 2009).

Orgasm

Orgasm, the pleasant physical and mental sensation of climax, is currently only partially understood neurologically. It appears to be relayed through both the somatic and autonomic systems (Goldstein et al. 2004). In men, it is often incorrectly assumed to be synonymous with ejaculation: while they usually occur together, they are separate neurological entities. Researchers have described orgasm as being primarily a localized, genitally based reflex triggered by internal and/or external genital stimulation, which can improve with reinforcement (Sipski et al. 2001). Orgasm, or components of orgasm, have also been described as the cerebral interpretation of either centrally generated afferents (de Groat and Booth 1980), those arriving from non-spinal pathways, such as the vagus nerve (Komisaruk and Whipple 1991, Hubscher and Berkeley 1994) or from non-genital erogenous zones (Bach-y-Rita 1999). It is assumed that the strength of the pelvic floor contractions (somatic), the degree of engorgement of the internal genitalia (autonomic), and duration and degree of central arousal are factors in the subjective intensity of orgasmic release. It appears that awareness of internal contractions of the uterus in women (Lundberg 1999) or urethral and intraprostatic pressures in men can also contribute to the subjective orgasmic experience, since hysterectomy or radical prostatectomy can, in some patients, affect the post-surgical quality of orgasm.

The role of the ANS during orgasm is poorly defined due to lack of investigative methodology and no universal definition of orgasm. The urogenital (UG) reflex, a reflex mimicking human orgasmic response seen after acute spinalization in anaesthetized rats, is being used as a model to examine the CNS control of genital reflexes. It is necessary to cut descending inhibitory inputs in order to observe the UG reflex (McKenna et al. 1991, Giuliano and Julia-Guilloteau 2006). Both the UG reflex in animal models and the observed pelvic changes during orgasmic release in humans seem to require coordinated autonomic and somatic neural mechanisms, and data suggest that intact sacral cord reflexes may be necessary (Goldstein et al. 2004). Brain neurons containing serotonin reuptake transporters seem to be involved in the tonic inhibition of the UG reflex (Gravitt and Marson 2007). Clinically in humans, once male orgasm is initiated, even if sexual stimulation is stopped, the completion is automatic: cessation of sexual stimulation in the middle of either clitoral or vaginally induced orgasm can result in the halting of the female orgasm (Sherfey 1972). Furthermore, men experience a refractory period after orgasm or ejaculation, a proposed central build-up of neuronal extracellular K^+ (Tuckwell 1989), such that a second orgasm is not possible until (presumably) steady state is reached. Unlike men, women do not have a physiological refractory period (Master and Johnson 1966), and have the capacity to have extended, repeated (multiple) or compounded orgasms. However, some men clearly claim to have the physiological capacity for multiple male orgasms prior to the cumulative ejaculation, usually without losing erection. This ability, or the potential to learn it, seems to be correlated to pelvic floor control (Chia and Arava 1996).

Neurologically, orgasm is the least understood of the sexual phases. It is probably a complicated combination of the proposed somatic spinal cord reflex with unquantifiable autonomic and cerebral influences, any of which could potentially dominate in any one orgasmic experience or be adequate within themselves to be considered an 'orgasm' by the individual. In both neurologically intact and spinal cord injured human brain imaging studies, the event of orgasm activates specific regions of the brain over and beyond those activated during arousal, where others are deactivated, likely reducing the inhibitory serotonergic tone descending to the lumbosacral cord (Rees et al. 2007). The cerebral component is further exemplified after disruption of pathways following nerve injury: cerebral afferents may dominate if perception of local somatic input is destroyed. For example, after SCI, perineal muscle contraction and genital sensation may be absent, but approximately 50% of women with various levels and completeness of SCI (Sipski et al. 2001) experience orgasm, and men with SCI who experience orgasm may or may not experience this with ejaculation (Sipski et al. 2006). Orgasm, particularly in women, can be reached purely through respiratory movements, by stimulation of the ear, neck, hands, or even by thought alone (Lundberg 1999), the latter being demonstrated by Tantric sex practices. This is fortunate for persons with altered genital sensation: for example, in some men and women with multiple sclerosis, SCI or cauda equina injury, they can, with time and often the use of either prolonged genital or non-genital stimulation, have what is described by them as orgasm, even if the orgasm is altered in terms of frequency, duration, and intensity: with SCI, this may or may not be a form of autonomic dysreflexia (AD) interpreted as sexual over time (Elliott 2002, Courtois et al. 2004).

Persons with SCI have provided invaluable information in elucidating the autonomic components on the perception of orgasm. Orgasmic ability in women with SCI appears not to be dependent on the remaining sensation at the T11–L2 or S2–S5 dermatomes (the respective origins for the sympathetic [hypogastric] and parasympathetic [pelvic] innervation of the genitals), nor is it solely dependent on completeness of injury, or whether upper or lower motor neuron injury affects their sacral cord segments. However, in one study, women with both complete and lower motor neuron injures (n = 6) were significantly less likely to report the ability to achieve orgasm following injury as compared with a grouped sample of women with all other levels of SCI (n = 56), but when placed in a laboratory setting, these differences did not appear, suggesting self-report was more reliable than laboratory based work in the area of orgasm (Sipski et al. 2001). It does appear that both men and women with a SCI that interferes with their sacral reflex arc are less likely to self-report or have laboratory based evidence of orgasmic response.

The perceived physiological and orgasmic sensations at ejaculation in men with SCI are also related to autonomic sensation, especially if the climacteric experience of ejaculation is related to autonomic dysreflexia (AD) (Courtois et al. 2008). While tetraplegic men are more likely to experience AD than paraplegic men, the latter seem more able to achieve ejaculation through natural (self or partner) stimulation than with the more powerful vibrostimulation (use of a high amplitude, high speed vibrator on the penis), which is so successful in tetraplegics. Tetraplegics did not differ from paraplegics sensitive to AD on perceived cardiovascular and muscular sensations, but perceived significantly more autonomic sensations, and generally more physiological sensations than those men with lower lesions who did not experience AD. The climactic experience of ejaculation seems related then to AD, with few sensations being reported when AD is not reached, pleasurable climactic sensation being reported when mild to moderate AD is reached, and unpleasant or painful sensation reported with severe AD (Courtois et al. 2008).

A neuroendocrine component is likely involved in the attainment and perception of orgasm. Low androgen levels make orgasm more difficult to reach in both men and women, but oestrogen does not seem to influence orgasmic potential (Meston et al. 2004, Rees et al. 2007). Oxytocin is known to rise inconsistently in humans during sexual arousal (Carmichael et al. 1994) and orgasm (Murphy et al. 1990) and may work synergistically with sex steroids to facilitate orgasm (Nappi et al. 2006). Increased prolactin is noted for about an hour following orgasm in both men and women (Goldstein et al. 2004), but the functional implications of these changes are not entirely understood (Bancroft 2005). Oxytocin plasma levels are highly correlated with the intensity of muscular contractions during orgasm in both men and women (Anderson-Hunt and Dennerstein 1995). Hyperprolactinaemia interferes with testosterone biosynthesis, effects the release of oxytocin, and may alter brain dopamine levels, resulting in an inhibitory action on sexual desire and reduced potency in men (Rehman and Melman 2001, Nappi et al. 2006).

Disconcerting urges or spontaneous orgasm may occur in patients with lesions in specific parts of the CNS (Lundberg 1999), either locally in the sacral cord (Kuhr et al. 1995) or centrally in the brain (Sandel 1997). Temporal lobe epilepsy can precipitate non-sexual, spontaneous orgasm, especially in women (Remillard et al. 1983, Reading and Will 1997). A newly described intrusive and unwanted entity where women become involuntarily aroused genitally for extended periods of time in the absence of subjective sexual desire, where the genital and clitoral arousal does not go away with one or more orgasm and the arousal is considered at least moderately distressing, is called persistent genital arousal disorder (PGAD) (Leiblum et al. 2007). There are vascular, pharmacological, idiopathic, hormonal, and psychological theories proposed for the aetiology of PGAD, including a CNS or peripheral nervous system disorder that may lead to persistent neurological stimulation or facilitation of the autonomic nerves regulating smooth muscle control of the clitoris, resulting in labial and/or vaginal engorgement from increased blood flow (Goldstein et al. 2006). Due to the reluctance of women to discuss such a condition, special attention must be given to questioning women with autonomic disorders about feelings of non-sexual genital arousal. Ultimately this may help elucidate this dysfunction.

Resolution

The SNS is responsible for detumescence (loss of erection), which is initiated either by ejaculation, orgasm, lack of arousal or other psychogenic factors (i.e. performance anxiety). In women, orgasm is presumed to cause the decreased release of several neuropeptides responsible for vasomotor and sensory nerve function and capillary permeability, and to enhance the release of adrenergic system transmitters, thus effectively decreasing the blood flow and production of vaginal lubrication (Meston et al. 2004). Similarly in men, detumescence occurs when the balance of neuropeptides dictates smooth muscle constrictor tone: this is primarily mediated by norepinephrine (noradrenaline), which actives the adrenergic receptors on the penile smooth muscle membrane (de Tejada et al. 2004). In men, it also appears that serotonin may have a significant role in the initiation of detumescence and maintenance of flaccidity (Uckert et al. 2003).

Autonomic control of local genital engorgement and erection

The pelvic autonomic nerve fibres release three important neurotransmitters: norepinephrine, also known as noradrenaline (from sympathetic fibres), acetylcholine (from parasympathetic fibres), and neuronal nitric oxide (NO) (from non-adrenergic, non-cholinergic [NANC] fibres). Parasympathetic stimulation causes vasodilatation of the arteries, increasing blood flow to the erectile tissue in the penis or clitoris/vulva. Vasodilatory preganglionic neurons (primarily parasympathetic) become activated, the activities of the vasoconstrictor preganglionic neurons (mainly sympathetic) become suppressed, and erectile tissue tumescence occurs (Chuang and Steers 1999).

Locally the release of NO and other facilitory neurotransmitters such as vasoactive intestinal peptide (VIP) supplying the arterioles of the corpora in males results in smooth muscle relaxation and erection and tumescence of clitoral tissue in women (Burnett et al. 1997, Beck 1999a): noradrenaline and neuropeptide Y (NPY) are the primary inhibitors of genital arousal response (Goldstein et al. 2004). Acetylcholine likely acts synergistically with other vasodilators released by nerves or contained within vascular structures in both men and women: sympathetic pathways may produce erection via a cholinergic mechanism (Chuang and Steers 1999). Calcitonin-gene-related peptide and substance P appear to have a role in afferent sensory input (Chuang and Steers 1999). Serotonin has variable effects (mainly inhibitory for erection and ejaculation) depending on the receptor sites (brain, raphe nucleus, spinal cord, and autonomic ganglia) (Abdo et al. 2004).

Two sources of NO exist: that released from nerve endings secondary to arousal, and NO released from healthy endothelial lining. During sexual activity, it is primarily the neuronal NO that diffuses into the smooth muscle cell, increasing the intracellular levels of cyclic guanosine monophosphate (cGMP). Hyperpolarization of the smooth muscle cell occurs through the opening of K^+ channels, decreasing intracellular calcium, and relaxing the smooth muscle (de Tajada et al. 2004). The process is terminated by the enzyme phosphodiesterase V (PDE5) that reduces cGMP and cyclic adenosine monophosphate (cAMP) levels in the smooth muscle in both men and women (D'Amati et al. 2002).

The female vagina is densely innervated by adrenergic nerves (sympathetic in origin) and parasympathetic nerves around blood vessels that control vaginal vasodilatation secretomotor function (Lundberg 1999). Paracervical ganglia contain nerve fibres that release NO, regulating uterine vascular tone (Lundberg 1999). Identification of autonomic nerve fibres in the human vagina show that there are significantly more fibres in the more distal than proximal area, and that the anterior wall (the most sensitive part of the vagina) displays a denser innervation than the posterior one (Goldstein et al. 2004).

Testosterone has an important role in normal male sexual function, and hypogonadal states result in reduced libido and sexual fantasies in young men but not in diminution of erectile responses to visual erotic stimulation (Burns-Cox and Gingell 1999). Testosterone levels are related to the frequency of NPT and to spontaneous erections, but there is no relationship between the levels of serum testosterone and the presence or absence of ED in community studies (Burns-Cox and Gingell 1999). However, the activity of neuronal nitric oxide synthase (nNOS), the enzyme response for NO production, is androgen dependant (de Tajada et al. 2004). Since testosterone is necessary for the functional maintenance of seminal vesicles, epididymis, and prostate, and for spermatogenesis, lowered levels can affect the amount of ejaculate and semen quality. As the serum levels of testosterone decline below normal, the first affect noticed is declining sexual drive, followed by a reduction in ejaculate volume (from lack of accessory organ hormonal support) and difficulty reaching orgasm (by raising the orgasmic threshold). Finally, loss of nocturnal erections, which are more androgen sensitive, will occur, and visually stimulated erections are the last to diminish (Kwan et al. 1983). This fact, as well as the multifactorial nature of ED, is why androgen replacement is relatively ineffective in reversing moderate to severe ED.

Testosterone is an important hormone for sexual desire and arousability in women, especially in relation to oestrogen levels. A minimal level of oestrogen appears to be necessary for the active neurogenic vasodilatation of clitoral cavernosal tissue and vaginal arterioles supplying the vaginal submucosal capillary plexus (Basson 2004). VIP also requires a minimum amount of oestrogen for its activity (Palle et al. 1991). Measurements of serum testosterone and sexual function in women is currently under investigation and debate, as the phenomenon of intracrinology (production of testosterone within the cell for its use from adrenal and ovarian precursors) (Labrie et al. 2006), the variability of hormone levels during menstrual cycles, premenopause and postmenopause, and the complexity of evaluating subjective versus objective sexual arousal in women makes the physiological study of female sexual function difficult.

The sexual dysfunctions and their relationship to autonomic function

Disruption or inhibition of the central control mechanism for the spinal cord reflexes results in sexual dysfunction, as also does the disruption of either the afferent or efferent arc of the local spinal cord reflex. Autonomic dysfunctions understandably affect sexual function. The complexity of the autonomic innervation to the sexual organs means that conditions that alter the ANS will be accompanied by some form of sexual dysfunction. These can be classified as arousal (difficulties with penile erection, clitoral engorgement, vaginal lubrication, and vaginal accommodation), ejaculation, and orgasmic problems. It should be remembered that a sexual dysfunction, like orthostatic hypotension, can actually be a symptom of autonomic problems (i.e. ED in a man with diabetes). ED can even be the presenting symptom, as it is in multiple system atrophy (MSA) (Kirchhof et al. 2003) where it can predate the onset of other neurological symptoms by several years (Beck et al. 1994), or be the sentinel symptom of cardiovascular autonomic neuropathy, as seen in alcoholics (Ravaglia et al. 2004).

Definitions of sexual dysfunction

The sexual dysfunctions are grouped as follows (Lewis et al. 2004).

 Sexual interest/desire dysfunction consists of diminished or absent feelings of sexual interest or desire, absent sexual thoughts or fantasies (spontaneous desire), and lack of responsive desire (that which appears after entering into sexual activity). Sexual desire problems can certainly be the sequela of other autonomic sexual dysfunctions or chronic illness conditions.

 Sexual aversion disorder is extreme anxiety or disgust at the anticipation of/or attempt to have any sexual activity.

Female
Female sexual arousal dysfunction

 Genital arousal dysfunction is a self-reported condition, where there is minimal vulvar swelling or vaginal lubrication from any type of sexual stimulation or reduced sexual feeling on the genitalia.

 Subjective sexual arousal dysfunction is the absence of or markedly diminished feelings of sexual arousal (sexual excitement or sexual pleasure) from any type of sexual stimulation even if vaginal lubrication or other signs of sexual response occur.

 Combined genital and subjective arousal dysfunction is the absence of any subjective or objective (genital) arousal.

 Persistent genital arousal disorder (newly coined PGAD) is a spontaneous, intrusive, and unwanted sexual arousal (tingling, throbbing, and pulsation) in the absence of sexual interest or desire, unrelieved by orgasm.

 Orgasmic dysfunction is a lack of orgasm, markedly diminished intensity of orgasmic sensations, or marked delay of orgasm from any kind of stimulation.

Dyspareunia (persistent pain from attempted or completed penile vaginal sexual intercourse) and vaginismus (persistent and recurrent difficulty for vaginal entry of any object due to involuntary spasm) are sexual pain issues for women.

Male

 Erection dysfunction is the consistent or recurrent inability of a man to attain and/or maintain an erection sufficient for the sexual activity.

 Early ejaculation is ejaculation that occurs sooner than desired, either before or after penetration over which the sufferer has no or minimal control.

 Delayed ejaculation is undue delay in reaching a climax during sexual activity.

 Male orgasmic dysfunction is inability to achieve an orgasm, markedly decreased intensity of orgasmic sensations, or marked delay of orgasm during conscious sexual activity.

 Anejaculation is the absence of ejaculation during orgasm (but can also refer to the condition of absence of the emission and expulsion phases of ejaculation and accompanying orgasm, such as in SCI).

There are other diagnoses more psychologically related (such as sexual aversion disorder) that are not as relevant to this chapter on autonomic dysfunctions.

Diagnosis and investigation of neurogenic sexual dysfunction
Sexual history

The single most effective tool in investigating sexual concerns is a complete sexual history. The onset and duration of the disorder can help delineate the probability of organicity. Differentiating the situations when adequate versus inadequate arousal is present assists in the investigation of the psychological component responsible for the CNS triggering of the neurotransmitter cascade. Men and women who experience sexual difficulties regardless of maximal psychosexual arousal presumably have an organic component requiring a form of medical treatment beyond psychologically based, talk-oriented sexual therapy. It is important to remember that the sexual history, medical history, and physical exam provide the basis for ordering any neurophysiological testing.

Physical examination

The diagnosis of neurogenic causes of sexual dysfunction requires a detailed history, neurological genital examination for discrepancies in light touch, pain and temperature, and the use of perineal reflex testing. The genital neurological exam is helpful in predicting sexual function after trauma or neurogenic disease. For example, in men, intact spinal sacral reflexes as demonstrated by positive bulbocavernosus reflex (BCR) and anal wink tested can assist in predicting whether reflex (versus psychogenic) arousal, erection and ejaculation to genital stimulation may be possible. However, the BCR does not test autonomic function. Anal tone may have an autonomic contribution. Testing for pinprick sensation on the glans penis or clitoral area defines the intact ascent of the spinothalamic tract to the brain, and ability to voluntarily contract the anal sphincter demonstrates intact descending corticospinal tracts: positive affirmation of these somatic two tests together predict the *neurological ability* to experience genitally derived orgasm (Szasz 1983). The presence of the BC and anal wink reflexes stemming from the S4–5 level further predicts the relative capacity for genital orgasm when there is some loss of genital sensation. Non-genitally induced orgasmic responses may be triggered by non-genital stimulation (such as breasts and ears), may be cerebrally induced (such as seen in sleep or Tantric sex practices), or may be alternate interpretations of other autonomic or somatic sensations, such as with milder to moderate forms of autonomic dysreflexia, as noted before.

Investigation of neurogenic and autonomic sexual dysfunction

Practically, investigations for neurogenic alterations to sexual function are reserved for a select group of patients in the few centres where such testing is available. A thorough sexual history, documented disturbances of the bladder and bowel, and genital neurological exam allow the practical *inference* of autonomic disturbance, but not proof. There is no current widely available 'neurogenic sexual function' test equivalent to bladder investigations like urodynamics: even if there was, only a neurological diagnosis and not a definitive autonomic problem could be established (Betts and Fowler 1992).

Assessment of suspected neurogenic sexual dysfunction relies almost exclusively on tests of the somatic nervous system. Commonly used investigational methods are limited because most are only designed to assess the pudendally mediated afferent component of the genital arousal reflex (Gerdes 1997). Conventional neurophysiological procedures like sacral reflex latencies, cortical somatosensory evoked potentials, pudendal evoked potentials (PEP), and sphincter electromyography (EMG) evaluate the function of rapidly conducting, thick myelinated nerve fibres which do not contribute to the diagnostic process of autonomic sexual difficulties. As such, neurophysiologic testing is becoming more sophisticated, since the evaluation of small nerve fibres is what is important (Hilz and Marthol 2003).

Individual tests for motor (somatic efferent), sensory (somatic afferent) and autonomic components of the neural network have been developed. Bulbocavernous EMG and reflex latency testing assesses the motor component (large myelinated fibres), and sensory methods include nerve conduction velocity, evoked potentials, biothesiometry, and thermal threshold testing. The somatic investigations test nerve conduction velocities and evoked potentials with well-known reproducibility and validity (Rosen et al. 2004). Autonomic testing is not well standardized and lacks reproducibility, validity, and comparability because it simultaneously measures a chain of events or reactions involving receptors, small fibres and target organ. Autonomic fibres are small diameter, poorly or non-myelinated, and conduct neural impulses relatively slowly (Yang and Jiang 2009). Each individual component may also be influenced by confounding factors (i.e. medication, temperature, alterations to fluid volume, receptor or target organ dysfunction), and the interaction between the parasympathetic and sympathetic nervous systems is complex in the pelvic plexus (Rosen et al. 2004). To use autonomic testing means tailoring the test to the small fibres or target organs and eliminating (if possible) confounding factors. Furthermore, the electrical stimuli necessary to depolarize the autonomic fibre is different and the recording signals are more difficult to consistently capture (Yang and Jiang 2009).

Most tests of the ANS assess physiological responses to parasympathetic or sympathetic stimulation to diagnose generalized autonomic function: it is difficult to measure specific autonomic nerve transmission to identify a local abnormality (Beck and Fowler 1999) as compared with responses to parasympathetic or sympathetic activation. Loss of variation of the cardiovascular reflex tests (heart rate variability and BP in response to deep breathing or sudden inspiration, changes in posture from lying to standing, cold stimuli, isometric exercise, or Valsalva manoeuvre) is indicative of autonomic dysfunction (Rosen et al. 2004, Beck and Fowler 1999). These and other tests for autonomic dysfunction suggest, but do not confirm, an autonomic component to the sexual dysfunction. However, in this regard these tests can be highly variable. For example, generalized parasympathetic impairment was demonstrated in 53% of men with ED (n = 30), as noted by abnormal heart rate variability found to both deep inspiration and standing tests (Kunesh et al. 1992), whereas cardiovascular reflex testing was not found to be accurate or predictive of identifying neuropathy in another study (Robinson et al. 1987).

There are methods to try and measure autonomic function within the genitalia themselves. Since the ANS plays such an important role in sexual response and assessment of autonomic pathways can bear critical importance in the evaluation of sexual dysfunction, tests such as corpus cavernosum EMG (CCEMG) and evoked cavernous activity (ECA) may be of some assistance. CCEMG and ECA primarily assess the sympathetic autonomic pathways (responsible for detumescence) to the penis, but it is felt that a technique that identifies sympathetic denervation would likely identify that which would also affect parasympathetic innervation (responsible for tumescence): as yet, there is no technology to discern neuropathy specific to parasympathetic fibres (Yang and Jiang 2009).

CCEMG attempts to measure direct penile autonomic function. Sympathetic skin responses (SSR) measures a sudomotor related potential (the change in voltage on the skin surface secondary to sweat gland activity in either the palms of the hands or soles of the foot) that is evoked in response to sympathetic activation (an electrical stimulus applied to the median nerve or posterior tibial nerve): it has also been attempted on the genitalia. ECA has also been explored on both men and women. These are addressed below and further examples are given with the individual chronic conditions.

CCEMG

Bioelectrical activity of the corpus cavernosum was found to be recordable using concentric needle electrodes with a method called CCEMG. The signals from the electrodes were thought to be sympathetic signals, since they declined when smooth muscle relaxation and erection occurred (Wagner et al. 1989). CCEMG readings were originally compressed by time, making analysis of individual electrodes difficult. An extended time base was initiated to allow better reading of the signals and was renamed SPACE (single potential analysis of cavernosal EMG) (Stief et al. 1992), but it soon became apparent that the reported bioelectric activity could not represent single cavernosal smooth muscle potentials, so the acronym SPACE was abandoned (Junemann et al. 1993). Since CCEMG readings were thought to be sympathetically mediated, both mental stimulation, pain, and stress associated with cavernosal needle insertion increased the frequency of potentials (Beck and Fowler 1999). CCEMG is still regarded as a relatively new, 'experimental' technique (Rosen et al. 2004), and lack of standardization or recording techniques and objective criteria to characterize the recorded signals (CC-potentials) hinder the clinical application of this method. However, an easier and more objective way to analyse the CCEMG for less experienced clinicians was suggested by applying digital signal processing techniques (Kellner et al. 2000, Stief et al. 1997).

While CCEMG has not been widely used to evaluate neurogenic ED due to its technical and practical difficulties, it is a significant improvement in the ability to assess the ANS involved in ED. Recently, a revised method of recording and interpretive methodology of the CCEMG was shown to discriminate patients with ED from those with conditions associated with cavernous smooth muscle degeneration and/or autonomic neuropathy from men with reported normal erectile function (Meuleman et al. 2007). It was also found to be reproducible under controlled conditions and under the influence of confounding factors (intake of caffeine, alcohol and smoking), except after ejaculation, where measurements were interfered with (Jiang et al. 2007). Currently, CCEMG is believed to be able to diagnose cavernous myopathy and neuropathy in patients caused by cavernosal smooth muscle degeneration, diabetes mellitus, and radical prostatectomy, helping to make the decision regarding appropriate therapies (Yang and Jiang 2009). It is likely that the CCEMG will be utilized more when software is introduced that can more easily analyse the signal traces.

Evoked cavernous activity

Concentric needle recording electrodes are placed into each CC, with frequency filters for recording set within 0.2 and 100 Hz, and stimulation of the median nerve occurs with a brief pulse to evoke a generalized sympathetic discharge. ECA is temporally associated with hand and foot SSR, which confirms the sympathetic nature of the ECA, as does the slow wave morphology, habituating nature, and induction of responses with startling stimulus. As with SSR, the most important aspect of the test is the presence or absence of the response, versus the latency and amplitude of measurements. The easy to perform ECA has not been widely validated, but has a waveform that can be interpreted (Yang and Jiang 2009).

Sympathetic skin responses

Similar to the ECA, the SSR is a test that measures conductance changes in the palmar and planar skin in response to a noxious stimulus. (Yang and Jiang 2009). With SSR, after medial nerve stimulation, resultant excitatory impulses from the brain descend through the spinal cord entering the sympathetic trunk at the level of T1–T4 and reach the palm via the brachial plexus (palmar SSR), or enter the sympathetic trunk at the level of T11–L3 and reach the sole via the sciatic nerve (plantar SSR). SSR is believed to be a multiple synapse potential with a long latency that requires supraspinal connections (Wang 1997), and the latency of SSR is not dependant on the types of stimuli (Elie 1990). Palmar and plantar SSR can therefore be used in numerous groups, including the detection of mixed neuronal neuropathies (Shahani 1984) and autonomic failure in patients with SCI (Curt et al. 1996). Palmar and plantar SSR has also been used to study erection and ejaculatory function in normal men and in those with erection and/or ejaculatory failure (Park et al. 1988).

SSR was first measured on the genital skin in 1987 (Ertekin et al. 1987) using various electrical stimuli to nerves at the wrist, knee, or directly to the dorsal nerve to the penis with the active electrode on the mons pubis and the reference electrode on the dorsum of the penis. SSR recorded from the genitalia was found to be present in normal individuals but not in some diabetic men with ED with and without previously diagnosed polyneuropathy (Opsomer et al. 1996). The penile sympathetic skin response (PSSR) has been characterized by shorter latency and higher amplitude in men with normal erections, but by longer latency and lower amplitude in those men with ED (Zhu and Shen 2001): it was felt these findings legitimized PSSR as an electrophysiological method in assisting the diagnosis of ED. There appears to be combined value of perineal SSR with other electrophysiological and urodynamic recordings: one group of SCI researchers concluded that the loss of BCR and detrusor areflexia implied loss of somatic and parasympathetic reflex activity and correlated with loss of reflex erection, whereas loss of psychogenic erections correlated with loss of perineal SSR (Schmid et al. 2003).

Interestingly, whether the PSSR and CCEMG are recording the same sympathetic potentials is under debate since CCEMG activity, but not SSR, is abolished after intracavernosal injection of prostaglandin E1 (PGE) (the same drug injected in penile vascular testing to relax penile smooth muscle leading to erection) (Beck and Fowler 1999, Derouet et al. 1995).

One study (Salinas et al. 2003) looked at the usefulness of CCEMG in the diagnosis of ED in men who also underwent neurophysiological studies, including BC muscle electromyography, S2–4 latency period, pudendal nerve somatosensory potentials and genital SSR before and after injection of PGE1. While there was no significant relationship between patients with peripheral neurological lesion and patients with inferior autonomic lesion on evoked EMG (EEMG), there was a significant relationship between patients with suprasacral neurological lesion and patients with superior autonomic lesion on CCEMG. The authors concluded that isolated application of pudendal nerve neurophysiological techniques for the diagnosis of ED was not enough, and that autonomic innervation studies should be included. However, there may be a correlation between CCEMG and the SSR: some potentials present only on the genital skin bear a striking resemblance to SSR, which raises the question of the origin of recording made with surface electrodes and (by inference) also those made by needle electrodes (Beck and Fowler 1999). However, these recordings seem to represent some form of autonomic activity on the genital skin. ECA also seemed to be more reliable for determining autonomic involvement in the pathophysiology of erectile dysfunction than the CCEMG or penile sympathetic skin responses due to false-negative results on the latter two (Yilmaz et al. 2002). Urethral evoked SSR and viscerosensory evoked potentials have also been used as diagnostic tools in patients with SCI to evaluate urogenital autonomic afferent innervation (Schmid et al. 2004).

Autonomic testing in women

Effective validated tools for investigation of female sexual dysfunction are lacking. Quantitative sensory testing (administration of temperature and vibration stimuli to determine thresholds) appears to have potential in assessment and ongoing evaluation of neurogenic sexual dysfunction in women (Vardi et al. 2006). Similar to ECA, direct evaluation of the autonomic innervation of the clitoris and bulb has been attempted: after placement of concentric needles into 22 healthy women, spontaneous activity recordings were obtained in 13 subjects (Yilmaz et al. 2004). Median nerve activation of the SNS evoked activity in the clitoris and bulb in 18 and 21 women, respectively. Hand SSRs were done and present in all subjects. Evoked genital response latencies were similar to hand SSR latency. Like CCEMG and ECA in men, this test may be helpful in the future with assessment of neurogenic sexual autonomic dysfunction in women.

Both left hand sympathetic skin responses and genital region SSR (g-SSR) were done in women with and without diabetes (Secil et al. 2005). While it was found to be more difficult to elicit g-SSR in diabetic women than in normal controls, mean amplitude was significantly decreased in the diabetic group.

Investigation of vascular causes of sexual dysfunction

Most organic problems with male arousal are vasculogenic versus neurogenic, and the number and sophistication of tests to assess erectile dysfunction are reflective of that. In males, the ability to obtain and maintain an adequate erection after neurological signalling requires adequate arterial inflow, effective veno- occlusion and relatively normal anatomy. Neurologically, the parasympathetic signals must be intact for the smooth muscle relaxation and vasodilatation to even occur. Indirectly then, the more common vascular investigations will give information about the neurogenic component, based on the theory that neurological impulses initiate a series of vascular changes associated with sexual function (Meston et al. 2004). For example, in women, vaginal photoplethysmography, a measure of vaginal blood flow (Prause and Janssen 2006) has been used as an indirect outcome measure of neurological integrity in women with incomplete SCI (Sipski et al. 1995), although the use in women with complete SCI is inconclusive (Meston et al. 2004). Thirty men with ED who underwent urological, angiological, and neurological examination with complementary

neurophysiological tests of somatosensory and autonomic function demonstrated a lack of correlation between vascular and general autonomic abnormalities, demonstrating that patients must be well screened for both before going for vascular operations (Kunesch et al. 1992).

In men, vascular tests involving penile injections of neurotransmitters to elicit smooth muscle relaxation effectively bypass the natural neurogenic input, thereby testing the potential of the vascular and veno-occlusive system. In men, subjective arousal (the man's recognition of the state of genital arousal) correlates well with objective arousal (i.e. penile tumescence measurements). Women are comparatively unaware of their genital sexual responses and tend to define sexual arousal in terms of their state of subjective feeling. This and other factors make the diagnosis of female sexual arousal disorder a complicated issue compared with male ED (Van Lunsen and Laan 2004). Currently vaginal pulse amplitude (VPA), which measures a change in amplitude with increased blood flow as assessed by photoplethysmography, is thought to reflect vascular events only in the genitalia, but it may reflect complex interactions between sympathetic and parasympathetic regulatory processes and between circulatory and vaginal BP (Levin 1998). Vaginal photoplethysmography is the most sensitive, specific, and reliable physiological measure of vaginal vasocongestion (Van Lunsen and Laan 2004) and neurological causes of sexual dysfunction, but pelvic MRI along with vaginal photoplethysmography is also being used to assess vaginal wall anatomy and response (Maravilla et al. 2003). Pulse wave Doppler ultrasonography can measure changes to vaginal and clitoral arteries, and duplex ultrasound can measure changes in blood flow velocity in the vagina, clitoris urethra, and labia. Laser Doppler velocimetry, vaginal pH measurements, vaginal compliance, and vaginal oxygen tension measurements and MRI appear promising but are currently insufficiently evaluated (Meston et al. 2004).

In males, investigative methods of arterial, vasculogenic erectile failure include the penile/brachial index, a measurement of penile systolic pressure compared with brachial pressure, the use of erectogenic intracavernosal injection agents to see if an erection ensues (intracavernosal injection test), and the use of colour duplex ultrasonography following intracavernosal injection to measure the increase in diameter of the cavernosal arteries post-injection and the increase in cavernosal volume. The more invasive, selective pudendal arteriography is only used prior to vascular surgery or reconstruction (Beck 1999b). Venous leak can also be investigated by colour Doppler ultrasonography studies, cavernosometry and cavernosography. Cavernosometry specifically assesses cavernosal venous outflow resistance by monitoring the rate of saline infused into the corpora cavernosa to create an erection (high perfusion rates and low intracavernosal pressure indicates venous insufficiency), whereas cavernosography involves infusion of contrast media to identify sites of venous leakage (Gerdes 1997).

Conditions of autonomic dysfunction and their expected sexual changes

Since autonomic dysfunction may be due to afferent, central or efferent 'disorders' (Bennett and Gardiner 1992), the medical conditions associated with autonomic sexual dysfunction would be too many to mention. Basic principles and frameworks to assess and manage the complex sexual changes with illness are helpful, and can be found in other works (Stevenson and Elliott 2007).

However, in any condition with autonomic dysfunction, *alterations in sexuality* can be categorized into five areas:

- direct involvement with the autonomic pathways (neurological) responsible for sexual functioning

- indirect neurological sequela, such as cognitive changes, sensory or motor alterations, bladder and bowel incontinence, spasticity, tremor

- sexual changes secondary to treatment of the condition (i.e. medications) or other non-neurogenic risk factors (i.e. cardio-vascular disease) for sexual dysfunction

- biopsychological factors associated with the condition, such as fatigue, depression or anxiety, impaired fertility, perceived loss of sexual attractiveness, altered sexual self-esteem, fertility issues

- relationship and societal issues, such as current sexual context, ability to work, perception of self, alteration in gender specific roles, partner or community sexual misconceptions.

Each of these five areas can, in turn, contribute to specific sexual dysfunctions. For example, a woman wheelchair bound with multiple sclerosis may have sexual disinterest, sexual arousal disorder, and anorgasmia based on both physical and psychosocial factors. She may have diminished genital sensation, adductor spasm making intercourse difficult, problems with positioning and weakness, concerns of incontinence with sexual activity, poor sexual self-image, reliance on caretakers (including her husband) for bladder, bowel and perineal hygiene that make her feel less independent and sexual, restricted social accessibility, overwhelming fatigue, and antidepressant use. However, despite these odds, she may wish the intimacy of partner connection and the physical pleasure of being sexual, and therefore pursue therapies to enhance arousal and orgasm. As another example, in a man with Parkinson's disease (PD), the changed appearance and flat affect, alteration in mood and sexual desire secondary to dopamine therapy, hand tremors made worse by intentional touch to a partner, awkward-ness of movement, and change of his gender role will affect his sexuality as much if not more than the neurotransmission related changes to erection dysfunction. That is why incorporating the context of the person is as critical as any medical intervention. In all these conditions, if there is a partner, they may have their own sexual issues or relationship questions, especially if they are in the care-giving role. The interrelationship feedback loop for both the person with the autonomic condition and their partner is complex and needs to be considered in sexual rehabilitation.

Clinical examples: specific autonomic conditions and their expected sexual changes

Multiple system atrophy and Parkinson's disease

An example of the type of sexual dysfunction found in primary autonomic failure would be that seen in MSA and PD. Both these conditions have severe loss of intermediolateral column cells, prob-ably through different pathological processes (Bannister and Mathias 1992). While little has been written about sexual problems in MSA, a striking feature is that ED is often the first symptom of MSA and usually predates the onset of other neurological symp-toms, including hypotension, by several years (Beck et al. 1994).

In contrast, ED often affects men only years after PD diagnosis is established (Chandiramani et al. 1997), although there can be an unfair increase in libido after treatment with L-dopa (Uitti et al. 1989). Since the ED is a separate complaint from hypotension, the underlying aetiology of ED may be centralized and possibly dopamine-dependant (Kirchhof et al. 2003). It has also been reported that women with MSA may also have reduced genital sensitivity (Oertel et al. 2003).

Studies of men with PD indicate that they suffer a higher incidence of libido problems, ED, and premature ejaculation than age-matched controls, with multifactorial causes (Chandiramani and Fowler 1999). Depression, drugs, changes in the dynamics of the dyadic relationship, and neurotransmitter modulation can affect primarily sexual drive in men with PD (Chandler 1999). While low desire is the most common complaint, high or height-ened drive has also been associated with the use of dopaminergic agents: this may be a result of improved general well-being, a spe-cific true increase in biological drive, or even sexual disinhibition seen in those patients who develop 'acute brain syndrome' with treatment (Bowers et al. 1971). The problem of ED often plagues men with PD, and can lead to ineffectual and frustrating pursuit of intercourse (Basson 1996).

Women with PD can also have difficulties, including spasm of perivaginal musculature. Difficulties with lubrication are not noted, suggesting a reserve of this arousal phase compared with men in the presence of autonomic neuropathy (Basson 1996). Age and gender do not dictate the level of dysfunction in men and women with PD. In one study of young people with PD (36–56 years of age), 70% of the women and 20% of the men had low drive (Wermuth and Stenager 1995). While it is clear that dopaminergic mechanisms have a role in both determination of desire and induc-tion of penile erection, it is not resolved whether there is a unique neurological genital dysfunction that is a feature of PD (Rees et al. 2007).

Multiple sclerosis

Autonomic dysfunction can cause significant disability in patients with MS, especially in the areas of micturition, arousal and orgas-mic disorders, sudomotor and gastrointestinal disturbance. Cardiovascular and sudomotor autonomic abnormalities in patients with MS are likely due to plaques distributed throughout the brainstem and spinal cord affecting the spinothalamic sensory and anatomically widespread autonomic regulatory areas and their connections (McDougall and McCleod 2003). The neurogenic sex-ual changes of 11 patients with MS and ED were analysed with penile injections and multiple neurological tests, including SPACE, SSR and cystometry, and the most frequent lesion was complete suprasacral and parasympathetic (upper motor neuron type), whereas peripheral autonomic lesions were less frequent (Salinas et al. 1998). Autonomic symptoms usually correlated with MS severity (McDougall and McLeod 2003) and sexual symptoms most often correlate with bladder and bowel dysfunction (Mattson et al. 1995). It is estimated that during the course of this chronic disease, more than 50% of women with MS and about 75% of men with MS experience some form of sexual dysfunction, including temporary or long-term disinterest in sex, sexual arousal disorders, inability to experience orgasm or altered orgasm, and difficulty with sexual positioning due to spasm, fatigue, and muscle weak-ness (Smeltzer and Kelley 1997). For men, ED can be partial and wane with MS remission until finally total failure of erectile function can occur. Men with MS can have preserved nocturnal and morning erections, with frustrating inability to attain daytime erotic erections (not of a psychogenic aetiology) (Kikeby et al. 1988). Loss of orgasmic capacity is the most dominant complaint for women with MS seeking treatment (Dasgupta et al. 2004), and orgasm capacity has been positively correlated with the presence of urge incontinence (Borello-France et al. 2004).

Congenital dopamine-beta-hydroxylase deficiency

The importance of the SNS in the physiological closure of the bladder neck and ejaculation is illustrated in the report of two men (siblings) with dopamine-beta-hydroxylase (DBH) deficiency (Mathias et al. 1990). DBH is an enzyme that converts dopamine into noradrenaline, so deficiency results in the absence of noradrenaline and adrenaline at the sympathetic nerve endings, with preservation of the neurotransmitters of parasympathetic nerve endings (Beck 1999a). These men had ejaculatory problems (one had retrograde ejaculation, the other delayed or absent ejaculation) but one also had erection difficulties.

Diabetes mellitus

Diabetic polyneuropathy suggests that small fibre sensory function is affected before that mediated by large myelinated fibres. Both onset of ED and diabetic cystopathy is insidious, with retrograde ejaculation more prevalent with diabetic cystopathy due to inadequate closure of the bladder neck (Dasgupta and Thomas 1999). Approximately 50% of men with diabetes mellitus (DM) will have ED from neurogenic, vascular, endothelial, smooth muscle factors, and psychogenic factors. Autonomic neuropathy of the pelvic nerves may promote increased oxidative stress, nerve hypoxia, and raised protein kinase C production, affecting smooth muscle contractility (Boulton et al. 2005), and is at least three to five times more prevalent in the diabetic population than among the general population (Tilton 1997). Interestingly, in the early stages of DM, ED may be brought on by poor glycaemic control, and reversed once metabolic control is reattained: it is thought that this temporary dysfunction is due to sorbitol and water accumulation in autonomic nerve fibres (Tilton 1997).

The strongest association with ED in diabetic men is the presence of autonomic neuropathy (Tilton 1997). The initial diabetic pathology in the small unmyelinated fibres leads to functional abnormalities, such as postural hypotension and disordered thermal sensation. The bulk of neurogenic evidence toward penile neurotransmitter depletion, specifically NO and VIP, is potentially at the receptor level. Once diabetic pathology has progressed to the large myelinated fibres (producing the classic 'glove and stocking' peripheral neuropathy), clinically it is observed that ED is almost always present, probably a result of permanent autonomic fibre changes.

Diabetic neuropathy provides a good example of the relevance of certain neurogenic tests evaluating sexual function. Since diabetic autonomic neuropathy primarily affects the small unmyelinated nerves and affects the larger fibres relatively late in the disease, a test like the BCR has little role in the diagnosis of neuropathic ED in diabetic men. CCEMG may provide better evidence in the future. PEP would also not be of assistance, since they do not demonstrate prolonged latencies in patients with peripheral neuropathy, only spinal cord dysfunction (Beck and Fowler 1999). With generalized autonomic function testing, single breath beat-to-beat

variation and orthostatic BP changes were noted in 20% of men with DM (Nisen et al. 1993), whereas investigators of another study found 55% of men with DM and ED showed abnormal cardiovascular responses to deep breathing, but 26% other men with DM and normal erection function also showed these abnormalities (Quadri et al. 1989)

Studies of loss of libido in men with DM suggest that it is a psychological reaction to loss of erectile function (Tilton 1997). Orgasm and functional ejaculation problems (i.e. premature ejaculation) are seen less often in men with DM than ED, probably because autonomic neuropathy has a more pronounced effect on the PNS than the SNS (Tilton 1997). However, as a result of the diabetic neuropathy, in some men the internal vesicle sphincter may not close properly during ejaculation, resulting in seminal expulsion into the bladder versus distally down the urethral meatus (retrograde ejaculation).

Women with DM also experience sexual dysfunction, especially libido issues. However, despite similar pathophysiology, arousal problems in women with DM (when compared with non-diabetic controls) are not as prevalent as in men with DM. However, women with DM do experience more vaginal infections and urinary tract infections, which can result in decreased sexual interest and decreased vaginal lubrication. Orgasm does not appear to be specifically affected (Tilton 1997). The most consistent finding in women with diabetes is a correlation between sexual dysfunction and depression (Bhasin et al. 2007).

In MS, both sexes have multifactorial sexual concerns, not the least of which is dealing with a chronic illness along with bladder, renal, bowel, mobility concerns, and depression and its treatment. Sexual satisfaction and frequency of activity often decreases (Tilton 1997).

Spinal cord injury

Of prime importance is the introduction of the development of international standards to document sexual and reproductive function after SCI (Sipski-Alexander 2007), part of an iniative to undertake a long-awaited and necessary document titled *International Standards to Document Remaining Autonomic Function after Spinal Cord Injury* (Alexander et al. 2009). This is an attempt to acknowlege the importance and clinical relevance of the ANS and the changes that occur to the sexual functioning of persons with SCI.

The level and completeness of SCI will affect the pathways of the ANS. Men and women with compete cervical SCI will have a dependence on the reflexogenic pathway, while injury of the lumbosacral cord will interfere with it, and arousal may be reliant on mental stimulation alone. For example, due to loss of tonic inhibitory control that reduces the sensory threshold and onset of erectile responses (McKenna 1999), men with SCI at the cervical level will have preserved, if not enhanced, reflex erection, especially if the lesion is complete (Chuang and Steers 1999). The ability to have reflex erections/vaginal lubrication is lost if the sacral spinal cord is injured or if the pudendal nerve or pelvic nerve is destroyed (Chuang and Steers 1999). Men with injuries to their sacral cord or lower are often dependent on intact psychogenic pathways to elicit an erection: they are also dependent on maintaining their mental sexual arousal, unlike those men dependent on reflex erections, in order to obtain and maintain their erection. The compensatory mechanism of the SNS maintaining erections after injury to parasympathetic pathways brings with it another potential clinical problem for the man dependant on psychogenic erections: while he struggles to maintain his erection through activation of sexually arousing mental thought, he is activating the sympathetic chain, and such adrenergic stimulation following SCI can bring about the first stage of ejaculation, seminal emission resulting in unwanted detumescence. Furthermore, although a spinal lesion between the two psychogenic and reflexogenic pathways should result in maintenance of good erectile function (Courtois et al. 1993), this specific lesion results in loss of spinal interplay between the two erection centres, and the loss of communication can clinically make the erection worse.

Approximately 40–50% (Alexander et al. 1993) of men with SCI are able to achieve orgasm, but may or may not have ejaculation (Sipski et al. 2006): ejaculatory dysfunction is very common following SCI and results in the necessity of sperm retrieval methodology for fertility (Elliott 2002).

Women with SCI presumably have similar reflex and psychogenic centres to men, but laboratory based studies have concluded more precisely that those women with SCI who have a higher ability to perceive a combination of light touch and pinprick sensation in the T11–L2 dermatomes were more likely to experience psychogenic lubrication, and that psychogenic control of female genital vasocongestion is dependent on sympathetic stimulation (Goldstein et al. 2004). This was also recently established with respect to erectile function in men with SCI (Sipski et al. 2007). Women with injury of the lower motor neurons and S2–S5 dermatomes are less likely to reach orgasm through direct genital stimulation compared with women with injury at or above T11 (Sipski et al. 1997, Sipski et al. 1995). However, loss of sacral reflexes did not completely preclude orgasm reporting, and overall, orgasm is possible in about 50% of women with SCI (Sipski et al. 1995, Sipski et al. 1997, Elliott 2003). Orgasmic genital potential may therefore differ from non-genital but reported orgasmic release.

In women with complete SCI, the vagus nerve appears to provide a spinal cord-bypass pathway for vaginal-cervical sensibility, and activation of this pathway can produce analgesia and orgasm (Komisaruk and Whipple 2005, Whipple et al. 1996). Whether this vagal pathway is an accessory to CNS functioning or becomes activated with CNS injury is not clear. In female rats, the vagus innervates the ovaries, oviduct, uterus, and cervix, and abdominal vagotomy disrupts the oestrous cycle, but whether or not the vagus innervates portions of the male urogenital tract is unknown (Hubscher 2006).

Of prime importance in men and women with SCI is the risk of AD with sexual activity, especially seen with ejaculation in men (Sheel et al. 2005). Besides the possible (and even lethal) consequences of severe hypertension, the symptoms of pounding headaches, nausea, flushing, and sweating are not conducive to continue sexual activity, or to even initiate it. Symptomatic control of AD and adaptation of AD from negative to possibly positive sexual interpretation can assist with this problem. However, AD can be 'silent' (asymptomatic) but the significant cardiovascular risks of AD associated with sexual activity in those vulnerable still remain (Claydon et al. 2006, Ekland et al. 2008). Malignant AD has also been described stemming from sexual practices (Elliott and Krassioukov 2006)

Lesions of the cauda equina or conus medullaris

Both somatic and parasympathetic fibres can be affected in cauda equina syndrome causing complete or incomplete saddle paraesthesias and various disruptions of bladder, bowel and sexual function. Unwelcomed spontaneous ejaculation has also been reported (Kuhr et al. 1995). Significant sexual impairment in men with lesions of the cauda equina or conus medullaris is poorly correlated with neurological and EMG findings (Podnar 2002). In general, sexual function changes in persons with these levels of lesions have received little attention. Clinically, men with this type of lesion who have ED unfortunately do not respond as well to the PDE5 inhibitors or intracavernosal injections.

Iatrogenic autonomic nerve damage

Autonomic nerve damage during surgery plays a critical role in the aetiology of sexual dysfunction, bladder dysfunction, and colorectal motility disorders. Surgeons are becoming more aware of the sexual benefits of nerve sparing procedures. While ED and ejaculatory disorders are seen following abdominal, bladder, bowel, and prostate surgery, attempts to spare the autonomic pathways during surgery do appear to result in some sexual benefits. This is especially true with radical prostatectomy (Smith and Christmas 1999) where the degree of sparing of the neurovascular bundle containing the autonomic nerves is critical to potency rates (Burnett 2006). Sural nerve grafting for sacrificed nerves holds mild promise (Sim et al. 2006). The ANS has also been implicated in post-surgical penile shortening. Early penile length changes may be related to sympathetic hypertonia in corporal smooth muscle and sympathetic hyperinnervation secondary to neural trauma, whereas late changes are likely due to denervation smooth muscle atrophy, apoptosis, and fibrosis (Fraiman et al. 1999, Savoie et al. 2003). Evaluating the autonomic innervation of the penis after nerve sparing radical prostatectomy may be possible using evoked cavernous activity (Yilmaz et al. 2006).

In operative treatment of rectal cancer, parasympathetic nerve sparing can result in preserved potency without undue risk of cancer recurrence (Enker 1992). Sexuality preserving cystectomy and neobladder construction (where the prostate is preserved) has improved outcomes for erectile function and continence (Nieuwenhuijzen et al. 2005).

While studies are limited in women, attempts are being made to be more proactive in nerve sparing in such procedures as hysterectomy (Maas et al. 2003) and pelvic suspension surgeries (Flynn et al. 2006) in the hope that arousal, lubrication and orgasmic potential will be preserved. Surgical preservation of the pelvic autonomic nerves in both laparoscopic and traditional radial hysterectomy may reduce the morbidity of impaired bladder function, defecation problems and sexual dysfunction (Bradford and Meston 2006). Preliminary results of sexuality preserving cystectomy and neobladder in women also look promising (Horenblas et al. 2001).

Treatments for sexual dysfunction

Effective treatments for male sexual dysfunction are now widely available. Men who are at risk for cardiovascular events should be assessed prior to recommendation for erection enhancement (Conti et al. 1999). For men, ED can be treated with direct, indirect and mechanical methods. The least invasive method should always be tried first. Mildly erectogenic drugs such as yohimbine have been replaced with the more recent and efficacious phosphodiesterase V inhibitors (PDE5i) including sildenafil (Viagra®), vardenafil (Levitra®), and tadalafil (Cialis®). Since the inhibition of the PDE5 enzyme results in the preservation of cGMP and prolongation of the smooth muscle relaxant effect in the penile tissues, it is an indirect way to enhance the natural erectile tumescence in men who have NO sources still available. In other words, those men with autonomic nerve damage interfering with the ability of the nerve to release NO (or who are simply not aroused) will not respond as well to the PDE5i drugs as those who do (or who also have excellent source of endothelial NO). The degree of 'end-organ' autonomic nerve involvement will dictate the efficacy (and ultimately the dose) of the PDE5i: for example, in men with SCI, the efficacy of sildenafil citrate depends on sparing of either sacral (S2–S4) or thoracolumbar (T10–L2) spinal segments (Schmid et al. 2000), sparing the reflex or psychogenic pathways respectively. Men with SCI who have higher injuries and no sacral nerve damage have ample end-organ NO sources, so often a smaller PDE5i dose is all that is needed. Men whose periprostatic nerves are injured during radical prostatectomy will not respond well to the PDE5i because of the lack of neurogenic NO; hopefully with the passage of time and nerve growth PDE5i therapy becomes more effective. Excessive endothelial damage (i.e. extensive endothelial damage from atherosclerosis, smoking, or chronic hypertension) will also interfere with the ability of the PDE5i due to the lack of endothelial NO. Men with peripheral nerve damage from trauma or surgery, or who have significant vascular issues will usually need higher doses of PDE5i due to the reduced sources of NO. Caution should be administered when giving PDE5i to those men with neurological disorders where hypotension is a risk. Since sildenafil has been shown to decrease systolic BP by approximately 8 mmHg and diastolic by 3–5 mmHg, men with hypotension secondary to quadriplegia should start with the lowest dose of a PDE5i (Sheel et al. 2005). Sildenafil did not have much effect on BP in men with ED and PD, but a significant postural BP fall occurred in those men with ED with MSA: lying and standing BP was advised prior to prescribing sildenafil (Hussain et al. 2002).

Direct methods to create an erection include the intracavernosal injection (ICI) of erection-inducing agents. These agents increase the level of intracellular cAMP in the smooth muscle causing relaxation similar to cGMP. These agents (notably prostaglandin E1 [PGE1], papaverine, and phentolamine) can be used singly or mixed together for better efficacy. Intracavernosal injection is the most efficacious and unsurpassed method for erection enhancement to date. PGE1 may have some early side effects of penile pain (30–50%) and prolonged erection (1%), which both diminish with time, and are more prevalent in the neurogenic population. The rare side-effect of hypotension usually occurs only with high doses. The latter effect is negligible with neurogenic ED since therapy requires only small doses of ICI (Hatzichristou 1999). Moxisylyte hydrochloride (Erectos®), an α-adrenergic blocking agent, is not as effective an ICI option as PGE1 but has a low incidence of local or systemic side-effects in patients with neurogenic ED (Linsenmeyer and Perkash 1991). The use of PGE1 in a pellet form administered into the urethra (MUSE®) is less efficacious since it must diffuse into the corpora cavernosa from the corpora spongiosum, but MUSE is also less invasive. MUSE, especially when contained in the penis by a penile ring at the base, claims to be a viable alternative following radical prostatectomy (Raina et al. 2005) but does not work well in the SCI population (Bodner et al. 1999). For patients with neurogenic ED, these direct forms of therapy (especially ICI) bypass the need for the NO/cGMP pathway and will often work in PDE5i failures.

One non-medicinal option for ED are mechanical aids such as vacuum pumps and/or erectile rings. A cylinder is placed over the penis and vacuum created with a pump, inducing primarily venous blood into the penis to create an erection. An erectile ring placed at the base of the penis maintains the erection, but should be removed after 30–45 minutes. Men with genital sensory deficits must be cautioned against leaving the ring on for more than the recommended time as pain will not be felt. The more invasive penile prosthesis implantation is reserved for failure of all the above reversible methods.

The choice of ED therapy is based on efficacy, safety, financial expense, and partner involvement. Practical issues will also determine use: a man with insulin-dependent diabetes mellitus and diabetic autonomic neuropathy will predictably have ED and even retrograde ejaculation, and, due to vision difficulties from retinal changes, poor hand function and possibly nitrate use for angina, be limited in his therapeutic options for ED. Furthermore, sensation and motor changes, decubitus ulcers, kidney failure and other problems associated with chronic illness will affect his sexuality in numerous ways.

Ejaculatory dysfunctions require various therapies depending on the aetiology and whether it is primarily a sexual or fertility concern (Elliott 2001, McMahon et al. 2004). For some men with SCI, the chance of ejaculation and/or orgasmic perception may be improved with the addition of oral midodrine, an α-stimulating drug (Courtois et al. 2008). Testosterone replacement for men with low normal and normal testosterone levels at baseline in various trials show that testosterone use in men is associated with small improvements in satisfaction with erectile function and moderate improvement in libido (Bolona et al. 2007). Often not mentioned in studies of this nature is the positive effect testosterone replacement has with orgasmic attainment, as men become hypogonadal with age and experience delayed ejaculation.

Therapies for female sexual dysfunction

There are currently no well-evaluated, available medicinal therapies for female sexual dysfunction. Testosterone replacement, effective in hypogonadal men, only assists sexual dysfunction in women (especially libido) in well-evaluated, testosterone deficient patients. Since the expression of PDE isoforms are found in the human clitoris, vagina, and labia minora (Mayer et al. 2005), sildenafil (Viagra®) has been tried and been shown to enhance vaginal engorgement during erotic stimulus in healthy women without sexual dysfunction, but there is not enough conclusive evidence that treatment with sildenafil is really effective therapeutically in women with sexual arousal disorders (Goldstein et al. 2004). Significant increases in subjective arousal were noted with sildenafil in women with SCI, although a borderline drug effect was noted by VPA (Sipski et al. 2000). Sildenafil has also shown some efficacy in selected sexual dysfunctions in women with MS (Dasgupta et al. 2004), which may be due to vasocongestion of the pelvis and temporarily improved sensation of the engorged clitoris. Topical prostaglandin preparations used to enhance genital arousal have not yet been tried in women with SCI.

Based on the theory that orgasm is a spinal cord reflex, studies examining the efficacy of either vibrostimulation or clitoral vacuum stimulation procedures are underway. For women, the use of vibrators has been helpful, and the site of effective stimulation may vary from around the area of injury, to the clitoris, inside the vagina, or on the cervix. Eros Therapy, a vacuum device inducing clitoral vascular engorgement, is the only US Food and Drug Administration cleared-to-market device available by prescription to treat female sexual dysfunction and may prove to be of benefit in increasing orgasmic responses in women with decreased sensation or SCI. Theoretically, by initiating the BCR and vasocongestion, this therapy may also improve sensory awareness in those women with some pelvic floor sensory preservation.

In all forms of genitally based therapy for men or women, it is as important to address the psychological aspects of sexual dysfunction, as well as the sexual context (the overall sexual relationships and current sexual frequency) within a partnered relationship. Sex therapy can have a vital independent or collaborative role in the management of any sexual dysfunction. The use of sexual counselling, the introduction of sexual aids, discussions around bladder and bowel continence, pain control, sexual positioning and sexual self-image and confidence are all part of the sexual rehabilitative process. It is important to maximize the physiological potential before addressing limitations, and to encourage a positive, open attitude for successful rehabilitation (Elliott 2003). Future specific therapies aimed at autonomic verses somatic nerve enhancement will serve to elucidate even further the role of the ANS in arousal, ejaculation and especially orgasm in men and women.

Acknowledgments

The author would like to express thanks to those who have educated and supported her in the field of sexuality and autonomic function (Dr Andrei Krassioukov, the Sexual Health Clinicians of GF Strong Rehabilitation Center, Dr John Steeves of ICORD, Mr Rick Hansen of the Man in Motion Foundation, Dr Ron Stevenson, Dr Chris Mathias, Dr Lynne Weaver, Dr George Szasz, Professor Emeritus) and to Maureen Piper for preparation of this chapter.

References

Abdo, C., Incrocci, L., Perelamn, M., et al. (2004). Disorders of orgasm and ejaculation in men. 21st ed. In TF Lue, R Basson, R Rosen, F Giuliano, S Khoury and F Montorsi, eds. Sexual dysfunctions in men and women, pp. 409–68. Health Publications, Paris.

Alexander, C. J., Sipski, M. L. and Findley, T. W. (1993). Sexual activities, desire, and satisfaction in males pre- and post-spinal cord injury. Archives of Sexual Behavior, 22 (3), 217–28.

Alexander, M. S., Biering-Sorensen, F., Bodner, D., et al. (2009). International standards to document remaining autonomic function after spinal cord injury. Spinal Cord. 47(1), 36–43.

Allard, J., Truitt, W. A., McKenna, K. E. and Coolen, L. M. (2005). Spinal cord control of ejaculation. World J Urol., 23(2), 119–26.

Anderson-Hunt, M., Dennerstein, L. (1995). Oxytocin and female sexuality. Gynecol. Obstet. Invest. 40, 217–21.

Bach-y-Rita, P. (1999). Theoretical aspects of sensory substitution and of neuro- transmission-related reorganization in spinal cord injury. Spinal Cord, 37, 465–74.

Bancroft, J. (2002). Biological factors in human sexuality. J Sex Res., 39, 15–21.

Bancroft, J. (2005). The endocrinology of sexual arousal. J Endocrinol., 186, 411–27.

Bannister, R. and Mathias, C. J. (1992). Introduction and classification of autonomic disorders. In R Bannister and C Mathias, eds. Autonomic failure, a textbook of clinical disorders of the autonomic nervous system, pp. 1–12. 3rd ed. Oxford University Press, Oxford.

Basson, R. (1996). Sexuality and Parkinson's disease. Parkinsons & Related Disorders, 2(4), 177–85.

Basson, R. (2001). Human Sex-Response Cycles. J Sex Marital. Ther., 27(1), 33–43.

Basson, R., Leiblum, S., Brotto, L., et al. (2004) Revised definitions of women's sexual dysfunction. J Sex. Med. 1(1), 40–48.

Beck, R. and Fowler, C. J. (1999). Neurological testing in erectile dysfunction. In C Carson, R Kirby and I Goldstein, eds. Textbook of erectile dysfunction, pp. 257–66. ISIS Medical Media, Oxford.

Beck, R. O., (1999b). Investigation of Male Erectile Dysfunction. In C Fowler, ed. Neurology of bladder, bowel and sexual dysfunction, pp. 145–60. Butterworth Heinemann, Boston.

Beck, R. O. (1999a). Physiology of Male sexual function and dysfunction in neurological disease. In C Fowler, ed. Neurology of bladder, bowel and sexual dysfunction, pp. 47–56. Butterworth Heinemann, Boston.

Beck, R. O., Betts, C. D. and Fowler, C. J. (1994). Genito-urinary dysfunction in multiple system atrophy: clinical features and treatment in 62 cases. J Urol., 151, 1336–41.

Behrman, A. L., Bowden, M. G. and Nair, P. M. (2006). Neuroplasticity after spinal cord injury and training: an emerging paradigm shift in rehabilitation and walking recovery. Physical Therapy, 86(10), 1406–25.

Bennett, T. and Gardiner, S. M. (1992). A commentary on clinical tests of autonomic function. In R Bannister and C Mathias, eds. Autonomic failure, a textbook of clinical disorders of the autonomic nervous system, pp. 391–412. 3rd ed. Oxford University Press, Oxford.

Betts, C. D. (1999). Bladder and sexual dysfunction in multiple sclerosis. In C Fowler, ed. Neurology of bladder, bowel and sexual dysfunction, pp. 289–308. Butterworth Heinemann, Boston.

Betts, C. D. and Fowler, C. J. (1992). Investigation and treatment of bladder and sexual dysfunction in diseases affecting the autonomic nervous system. In R Bannister and C Mathias, eds. Autonomic failure, a textbook of clinical disorders of the autonomic nervous system, pp. 462–78. 3rd ed. Oxford University Press, Oxford.

Bhasin, S., Enzlin, P., Coviello, A. and Basson, R. (2007). Sexual dysfunction in men and women with endocrine disorders. The Lancet, 369, 597–611.

Bhasin, S. and Benson, G. S. (2006). Male sexual dysfunction. In JD Neill, ed. Knobil and Neill's physiology of reproduction, pp. 1173–94. 3rd ed. Elsevier, Boston.

Bodner, D. R., Haas, C. A., Krueger, B., Seftel, A. D. (1999) Intraurethral alprostadil for treatment of erectile dysfunction in patients with spinal cord injury. Urology 53(1), 199–202.

Bolona, E. R., Uraga, M. V., Haddad, R. M., et al. (2007). Testosterone use in men with sexual dysfunction: a systematic review and meta-analysis of randomized placebo-controlled trials. Mayo Clin. Proc. 82(1), 20–28.

Borello-France, D., Leng, W., O'Leary, M., et al. (2004). Bladder and sexual function among women with multiple sclerosis. Multiple Sclerosis, 10(4), 455–61.

Borisoff, J. (2008). Personal communication on Proof of concept study of sensory substitution for the functional recovery of sexual sensation in individuals with chronic spinal cord injury (Birch G (PI), Borisoff J, Elliott SL.) Neil Squire Foundation and ICORD, Vancouver BC Canada

Boulton, A. J. M., Vinik, A. J., Arezzo, J. C., et al. (2005). Diabetic neuropathies. A statement by the American Diabetes Association. Diabetes Care, 28, 956–62.

Bowers, J. R., Woert, M. V. and Davis, L. (1971). Sexual behaviour during L-dopa treatment for parkinsonism. Am. J Psychiatry, 127, 127–29.

Bradford, A., Meson, C. Hysterectomy and alternative therapies. In I Goldstein, CM Meston, SR Davis and AM Traish, eds. Women's Sexual Function and Dysfunction, pp. 658–65. Taylor & Francis, New York.

Burnett, A. I., Calvin, T. C., Silver, R. I., et al. (1997). Immuno-chemical description of nitric oxide synthase isoforms in human clitoris. J Urol., 158, 278.

Burnett, A. L. (2006). Erectile function outcomes in the current era of anatomic nerve-sparing radical prostatectomy. *Rev. Urol.* **8**(2), 47–53.

Burns-Cox, N. and Gingell, J. C. (1999). Erectile dysfunction: endocrinological therapies, risks and benefits of treatment. In C Carson, R Kirby and I Goldstein, eds. *Textbook of Erectile Dysfunction*, pp. 327–44. ISIS Medical Media, Oxford.

Carmichael, M. S., Warburton, V. L., Dixen, J. and Davidson, J. M. (1994). Relationships among cardiovascular, muscular, and oxytocin responses during human sexual activity. *Archives of Sexual Behavior* **23**, 59–79.

Caruso, S., Intelisano, G., Lupo, L. and Agnello, C. (2001). Premenopausal women affected by sexual arousal disorder treated with sildenafil: A double-blind, cross-over, placebo-controlled study. *International Journal of Obstetrics and Gynecology*, **108**, 623–28.

Chandiramani, V. A., Palace, J. and Fowler, C. J. (1997). How to recognize patients with parkinsonism who should not have urological surgery? *Br. J Urol.*, **80**, 100–4.

Chandiramani, V. A. and Fowler, C. J. (1999). Urogenital disorders in Parkinson's disease and multiple system atrophy. In C Fowler, ed. *Neurology of bladder, bowel and sexual dysfunction*, pp. 245–54. Butterworth Heinemann, Boston.

Chandler, B. J. (1999). Impact of neurological disability on sex and relationships. In ML Sipski CJ and Alexander, eds. *Sexual function in people with disability and chronic illness*, pp. 69–93. Aspen Publication, Gaithersburg.

Chia, M. and Arvava, D. A. (1996). *The multiorgasmic man*. HarperCollins Publishers, New York

Chuang, A. T. and Steers, W. D. (1999). Neurophysiology of penile erection. In C Carson, R Kirby and I Goldstein, eds. *Textbook of erection dysfunction*, pp. 59–72. ISIS Medical Media Inc., Oxford.

Claydon, V. E., Elliott, S. L., Sheel, A. W., Krassioukov, A. (2006). Cardiovascular Responses to Vibrostimulation for Sperm Retrieval In Men with Spinal Cord Injury. *J Spinal Cord Med.* **29**, 207–16.

Conti, C. R., Pepine, C. J. and Sweeney, M. (1999). Efficacy and safety of sildenafil citrate in the treatment of erectile dysfunction in patients with ischemic heart disease. *Am. J Cardiol.*, **83**(5A), 28C–34C.

Courtois, F., Charvier, K., Leriche, A., *et al.* (2008). Perceived Physiological and Orgasmic sensations at Ejaculation in Spinal Cord Injured Men. *J Sex Med.* **5**, 2419–30

Courtois, F. J., Charvier, K. F., Leriche, A. and Raymond, D. P. (1993). Sexual function in spinal cord injured men. I. Assessing sexual capacity. *Paraplegia* **31**, 771–84.

Courtois, F. J., Geoffrion, R., Landry, E., Belanger, M. (2004). H-reflex and physiologic measures of ejaculation in men with spinal cord injury. *Arch. Phys. Med. Rehabil.* **85**(6), 910–18.

Dancause, N. (2006). Neurophysiological and anatomical plasticity in the adult sensorimotor cortex. *Reviews in Neuroscience* **17** (6), 561–80.

Dasgupta, P. and Thomas, P. K. (1999). Peripheral Neuropathy. In C Fowler, ed. *Neurology of bladder, bowel and sexual dysfunction*, pp. 339–52. Butterworth Heinemann, Boston.

Dasgupta, R., Wiseman, O. J., Kanabar, G., Fowler, C. J. and Mikol, D. D. (2004). Efficacy of sildenafil in the treatment of female sexual dysfunction due to multiple sclerosis. *J Urol.* **171**, 1189–93.

De Tejada, I. S., Angula, J., Cellek, S., *et al.* (2004). Physiology of erectile function and pathophysiology of erectile dysfunction. 21st ed. In TF Lue, R Basson, R Rosen, F Giuliano, S Khoury and F Montorsi, eds. *Sexual dysfunctions in men and women*, pp. 287–43. Health Publications, Paris.

de Groat, W. C. and Booth, A. M. (1980). Physiology of male sexual function. *Ann. Int. Med.* **2** (2), 329–33.

de Groat, W. C. (1999). Neural control of the urinary bladder and sexual organs. In JJ Mathias and R Bannister R, eds. *Autonomic failure 4th Edition. A textbook of clinical disorders of the autonomic nervous system* University Press, Oxford.

Derouet, H., Jost, W. H., Osterhage, J., *et al.* (1995). Penile sympathetic response in erectile dysfunction. *European Urology*, **28**, 314–19.

Diederichs, W., Stief, C. G., Lue, T. F., Tanagho, E. A. (1991). Sympathetic inhibition of papaverine induced erection. *J Urol.*, **146**(1), 195–8.

D'Amati, G., di Gioia, C. R., Bologna, M., *et al.* (2002). Type V phosphodiesterase expression in the human vagina. *Urology*, **60**, 191–202.

Ekland, M. B., Krassioukov, A. V., McBride, K. E., Elliott, S. L. (2008). Incidence of autonomic dysreflexia and silent autonomic dysreflexia in men with SCI undergoing sperm retrieval: implications for clinical practice. *J Spinal Cord Med.* **31**(1), 33–39.

Elie, B. and Guibeneue, P. (1990). Sympathetic skin response: normal results in different experimental conditions. *Electroencephalography and Clinical Neurophysiology* **76**, 258–67.

Elliott, S. (2001). Assessing orgasmic and ejaculatory problems in clinical practice. *Med Aspects of Human Sexuality*. pp. 26–30

Elliott, S. (2002). Ejaculation and orgasm: Sexuality in men with SCI. *Top. Spinal Cord Inj. Rehabil.* **8**(1), 1–15.

Elliott, S. (2003). Sexual dysfunction and infertility in men with spinal cord disorders. In V Lin, ed. *Spinal cord medicine: Principles and practice*, pp. 349–65. Demos Medical Publishing, New York.

Elliott S., Krassioukov, A. (2006). Malignant autonomic dysreflexia following ejaculation in spinal cord injured men. Epub 2005 Sep 27 *Spinal Cord*, Jun; 44(6):386–92.

Elliott, S. L. Problems of sexual function after spinal cord injury. (2006). In LC Weaver and C Polosa, eds. *Autonomic Dysfunction After Spinal Cord Injury, Prognosis in Brain Research*, pp. 387–99. Elsevier, Boston

Enker, W. E. (1992). Potency, cure and local control in the operative treatment of rectal cancer. *Arch. Surg.*, **127**(12), 1396–401.

Ertekin, C., Ertekin, N., Mutlu, S., *et al.* (1987). Skin potentials recorded from the extremities and genital regions in normal and impotent subjects. *Acta Neurologica Scandinavica* **76**, 28–36.

Flynn, M. K., Weidner, A. C. and Amundsen, C. L. (2006). Sensory nerve injury after uterosacral ligament suspension. *American Journal of Obstetricians and Gynecologists*, **195**(6), 1869–72.

Fraiman, M. C., Lepor, H., McCullough, A. R. (1999). Changes in Penile Morphometrics in Men with Erectile Dysfunction after Nerve-Sparing Radical Retropubic Prostatectomy. *Molecular Urology*, **3**(2), 109–15.

Gerdes, C. A. (1997). Psychophysiologic and laboratory testing. In ML Sipski and CJ Alexander, eds. *Sexual function in people with disability and chronic illness*, pp. 221–46. Aspen Publication, Gaithersburg.

Giuliano, F. and Julia-Guilloteau, V. (2006). Neurophysiology of female genital response. In I Goldstein, CM Meston, SR Davis and AM Traish. *Women's Sexual Function and Dysfunction*, pp. 168–73. Taylor & Francis, New York.

Goldstein, I., Elise, J. B. De and Johnson, J. A. (2006). Persistent arousal syndrome and clitoral priapism. In I Goldstein, CM Meston, SR Davis and AM Traish, eds. *Women's Sexual Function and Dysfunction*, pp. 674–85. Taylor & Francis, New York.

Goldstein, I., Giraldi, A., Kodigliu, A., *et al.* (2004). Physiology of female sexual function and pathophysiology of female sexual dysfunction in sexual medicine. 21st ed. In TF Lue, R Basson, R Rosen, F Giuliano, S Khoury and F Montorsi, eds. *Sexual dysfunctions in men and women*, pp. 685–747. Health Publications, Paris.

Gravitt, K., Marson, L. (2007). Effect of the destruction of cells containing the serotonin reuptake transporter on urethrogenital reflexes. *J Sex. Med.* **4**(2), 322–31.

Hatzichristou, D. M. (1999). Treatment of Sexual Dysfunction and Infertility in Patients with Neuroloical Diseases. In C Fowler, ed. *Neurology of bladder, bowel and sexual dysfunction*, pp. 209–25. Butterworth Heinemann, Boston.

Hilz, M. J. and Marthol, H. (2003). Erectile dysfunction—value of neurophysiologic diagnostic procedures. *Urologe A*, **42**(10), 1345–50.

Horenblas, S., Meinhardt, W., Ijzerman, W., Moonen, L. F. (2001). Sexuality preserving cystectomy and neobladder: initial results. *J Urol.* **166**(3), 837–40.

Hubscher, C. H. (2006). Ascending spinal pathways from sexual organs: effects of chronic spinal lesions. In LC Weaver and C Polosa, eds. Progress in Brain Research, 152—*Autonomic dysfunction after spinal cord injury*, pp. 401–14. Elsevier, Oxford.

Hubscher, C. H. and Berkeley, K. J. (1994). Responses of neurons in caudal solitary nucleus of female rats to stimulation of vagina, cervix, uterine horn and colon. *Brain Research* **664**, 1–8.

Huh, J., Park, K., Oh, K., Kim, H. J. and Jeong, G. W. (2006). Brain activation areas of olfactory sexual stimulation using functional MRI. *J Sex. Med.* **3**(S5), 435.

Hussain, I. F., Brady, C. M., Swinn, M. J., Mathias, C. J., and Fowler, C. J. (2002) Treatment of erectile dysfunction with sildenafil citrate (Viagra) in parkinsonism due to Parkinson's disease or multiple system atrophy with observations on orthostatic hypotension. *Journal of Neurology, Neurosurgery and Psychiatry* **72**(5), 371–74.

Jiang, X., Holsheimer, J., Wagner, G., Mulders, P., Wijkstra, H., Meuleman, E. (2007). A reproducibility study of corpus cavernosum electromyography in young healthy volunteers under controlled conditions. *J Sex. Med.* **4**, 183–90.

Johnson, R. D. (2006). Descending pathways modulating the spinal circuitry for ejaculation: effects of chronic spinal cord injury. In LC Weaver and C Polosa, eds. *Autonomic Dysfunction After Spinal Cord Injury. Progress in Brain Research*, **152**, 415–26. Elsevier, Boston.

Junemann, K. P., Burhle, C. P. and Stief, C. G. (1993). Current trends in corpus cavernosum EMG. *Int. J Impot. Res.* **5**, 105–8.

Kaplan, H. S. (1974). *The new sex therapy*. Brunner/Mazel, New York.

Kellner, B., Stief, C. G., Hinrichs, H., Hartung, C. (2000). Computerized classification of corpus cavernosum electromyogram signals by the use of discriminate analysis and artificial neural networks to support diagnosis of erectile dysfunction. *Urological Researc*, **28**, 6–13.

Kikeby, H. J., Poulsen, E. U., Peterson, T. and Dorup, J. (1988). Erectile dysfunction in multiple sclerosis. *Neurology* **38**, 1366–71.

Kirchhof, K., Apostolidis, A. N., Mathias, C. J. and Fowler, C. J. (2003). Erectile and urinary dysfunction may be the presenting features in patients with multiple system atrophy: a retrospective study. *Int. J Impot. Res* **15**(4), 293–98.

Komisaruk, B. R., Whipple, B., Crawford, A., Liu, W. C., Kalnin, A. and Mosier, K. (2004). Brain activation during vaginocervical self-stimulation and orgasm in women with complete spinal cord injury: fMRI evidence of mediation by the vagus nerves. *Brain Research* **1024** (1–2), 77–88.

Komisaruk, B. R. and Wallman, J. (1977). Antinociceptive effects of vaginal stimulation in rats: neurophysiological and behavioral studies. *Brain Research*, **137**, 85–107.

Komisaruk, B. R. and Whipple, B. (2005). Functional MRI of the brain during orgasm in women. *Ann. Rev. Sex Res.* **16**, 62–86.

Komisaruk, B. R., Whipple, B. (1991). Physiological and perceptual correlates of orgasm produced by genital or non-genital stimulation. In P Kothari, ed. *The Proceedings of the First International Conference on Orgasm*, pp. 69–73. VRP Publishers, Bombay.

Komisaruk, B. R. and Sansone, G. (2003). Neural pathways mediating vaginal function: the vagus nerves and spinal cord oxytocin. *Scandinavian Journal of Psychology.* **44**, 241–50.

Kuhr, C. S., Heiman, J., Cardenas, D., Bradley, W., Berger, R. E. (1995) Premature emission after spinal cord injury. *J Urol.* **153**, 429–31.

Kunesch, E., Reiners, K., Muller-Mathias, V., Strohmeyer, T., Ackermann, R., Freund, H. J. (1992). Neurological risk profile in organic erectile impotence. *Journal of Neurology, Neurosurgery and Psychiatry* **55**, 275–281.

Kwan, M., Greenleaf, W. J., Mann, J., Crapo, L., Davidson, J. M. (1983) The nature of androgen action on male sexuality: a combined laboratory— self-report study on hypogonadal men. *J Clin Endocrinol Metab* **57**, 557–62

Laan, E., van Stegeren, A. and Scholte, S. (2006). Brain imaging of gender differences in sexual excitation and inhibition. RT-2.2. *J Sex. Med.*, **3**(S5), 355.

Labrie, F., Belanger, A., Belanger, P. *et al.* (2006). Androgen glucuronides, instead of testosterone, as the new markers of androgenic activity in women. *J Steroid Biochem Mol Biol*, **99**, 182–88.

Leiblum, S., Seehus, M., Brown, C. (2007). Persistant Genital Arousal:Disorded or Normative Aspect of Female Sexual Response? *J Sex Med* **4**, 680–89.

Levin, R. J. (1998). Assessing human female sexual arousal by vaginal photoplethysmography—a critical examination. *Sexologies* **6**, 26–31.

Lewis, R. W., Fugl-Meyer, K. S., Bosch, R. *et al.* (2004). Definitions, Classification, and Epidemiology of Sexual Dysfunction. 21st ed. In TF Lue, R Basson, R Rosen, S Khoury and F Montorsi, eds. *Sexual dysfunctions in men and women*, pp. 39–72. Health Publications, Paris.

Lindsenmeyer, T. A. and Perkash, I. (1991). Infertility in men with spinal cord injury. *Arch. Phys. Med. Rehabil.* **72**, 747–54.

Lundberg, P. O. (1999). Physiology of female sexual function and effect of neurologic disease. In C Fowler, ed. *Neurology of bladder, bowel and sexual dysfunction*, pp. 33–46. Butterworth Heinemann, Boston.

Maas, C. P., Trimbos, J. B., DeRuiter, M. C., van de Velde, C. J. and Kenter, G. G. (2003). Nerve sparing radical hysterectomy: latest development and historical perspective. *Critical Review of Oncology and Hematology,* **48**(3), 271–79.

Maravilla, K. R., Heiman, J. R. and Garland, P. A. (2003). Imaging of the sexual arousal response in women. *Journal of Sex and Marital Therapy*, **20**(S1), 71–6.

Marson, L., McKenna, K. E. (1990).The identification of a brainstem site controlling the spinal sexual reflexes in male rats. *Brain Research* **515**, 303–308

Master, W. H. and Johnson, V. (1966). *Human Sexual Response*. Little, Brown and Co, Boston.

Mathias, C. J., Bannister, R. and Cortelli, R., *et al.* (1990). Clinical, autonomic and therapeutic observations in two siblings with postural hypotension and sympathetic failure due to an inability to synthesize noradrenalin from dopamine because of a deficiency of dopamine beta-hydrolyse. *Q J Med.* **75**, 617–33.

Mathias, C. J. and Frankel, H. L. (1992). Autonomic disturbances in spinal cord lesions. 3rd ed In R Bannister and C Mathias, eds. *Autonomic failure, a textbook of clinical disorders of the autonomic nervous system*, 839–81. Oxford University Press, Oxford.

Mattson, D. H. (1995). Sexual Function in Multiple Sclerosis. *Multiple Sclerosis: Clinical Issues* **2**(3), 1–13.

Mayer, M., Stief, C. G., Truss, M. C., Uckert, S. (2005). Phosphodiesterase inhibitors in female sexual dysfunction. *World Journal Urology*, **23**(6), 393–97.

McDougall, A. J. and McLeod, J. G. (2003). Autonomic nervous system functions in multiple sclerosis. *J Neurol. Sci.*, **215**(1–2), 79–85.

McKenna, K. (1999). The brain is the master organ in sexual function: central nervous system control of male and female sexual function. *Int. J Impot. Res.*, **11**(S1), S48–55.

McKenna, K. E. (1999a). Ejaculation: in: Knobil E, Neill J, eds. *Encyclopedia of Reproduction*. New York: Academic Press; 1999, 1002–8.

McKenna, K. E., Chung, S. K. and McVary, K. T. (1991). A model for the study of sexual function in anesthetised male and female rats. *Am. J Physiol.*, **261**(5 Pt 2), R1276–85.

McMahon, C. G., Abdo, C., Hull, E., *et al.* (2004). Disorders of Orgasm and Ejaculation in Men 21st ed. In TF Lue, R Basson, R Rosen, F Giuliano, S Khoury and F Montorsi, eds. *Sexual dysfunctions in men and women*, pp. 409–68. Health Publications, Paris.

Meston, C. M., Hull, E., Levin, R. J. and Sipski, M. (2004). Woman's orgasm chapter 21 in sexual medicine sexual dysfunctions in men and women. In TF Lue, R Basson, R Rosen, F Giuliano, S Khoury and F Montorsi, eds. *Sexual dysfunctions in men and women*, pp. 783–850. Health Publications, Paris.

Meston, C. M. and Gorzalka, B. B. (1996). Differential effects of sympathetic activation on sexual arousal in sexually dysfunctional and functional women. *J Abnorm. Psychol.* **105**, 582–91.

Meuleman, E., Jiang, X., Holsheimer, J., Wagner, G., Knipscheer, B., Wijkstra, H. (2007). Corpus cavernosum electromyography with revised methodology: an explorative study in patients with erectile dysfunction and men with reported normal erectile function. *J Sex. Med.* **4**, 191–98.

Moulier, V., Mouras, H., Pelegrini-Issac, M. *et al* (2006). Neuroanatomical correlates of penile erection evoked by photographic stimuli in human males. *Neuroimage* **33**(2), 689–99.

Mouras, H., Stoleru, S., Bittoun, J., *et al.* (2003). Brain processing of visual stimuli in healthy men: a functional magnetic resonance imaging study. *Neuroimage* **20**(2), 855–69.

Murphy, M. R., Checkley, S. A., Seckl, J. R. and Lightman, S. L. (1990). Naloxone inhibits oxytocin release at orgasm in man. *Journal of Clinical Endocrinology & Metabolism* **71**, 1056–58.

Nappi, R. E., Ferdeghini, F., Polatti, F. (2006). Mechanisms involved in desire and arousal dysfunction 203–209. In I. Goldstein, C. M. Meston, S. R. Davis and A. M. Traish, eds. *Women's Sexual Function and Dysfunction*, pp. 203–209. Taylor & Francis, New York.

Nieuwenhuijzen, J. A., Meinhardt, W., Horenblas, S. (2005). Clinical outcomes after sexuality preserving cystectomy and neobladder (prostate sparing cystectomy) in 44 patients. *J Urol.* **73**(4):1314–17.

Nisen, H. O., Larsen, A., Lindstrom, B. L., Ruutu, M. L., Virtanen, J. M., Alfthan, O. S. (1993). Cardiovascular reflexes in the neurological evaluation of impotence. *Br. J Urol,* **71**(2), 199–203

Oertel, W. H., Wachter, T., Quinn, N. P., Ulm, G. and Brandstadter, D. (2003). Reduced genital sensitivity in female patients with multiple system atrophy of parkinsonian type. *Movement Disorders* **18**(4), 430–2.

Opsomer, R. J., Boccasena, P., Traversa, R. and Rossini, P. M. (1996). Sympathetic skin responses from the limbs and genitalia: normative study and contribution to the revaluation of neuro-urological disorders. *Electroencephalography and Clinical Neurophysiology* **101**, 25–31.

Ottesen, B., Pedersen, B., Neilson, J., *et al* (1987). Vasoactive intestinal polypeptide (VIP) provokes vaginal lubrication in normal women. *Peptides* **8**, 797–800.

Palle, C., Bredkjaer, H. E., Fahrenkrug, J., *et al.* (1991). Vasoactive intestinal polypeptide loses its ability to increase vaginal blood flow after menopause. *Obstetrics and Gynecology* **161**, 556–8.

Park, Y. C., Esa, A., Sugiyama, T., Kaneko, S. and Kurita, T. (1988). Sympathetic skin response: a new test to diagnose ejaculation dysfunction. *J Urol.,* **139**, 539.

Pauls, R., Mutema, G., Segal, J., *et al.* (2006). A prospective study examining the anatomic distribution of nerve density in the human vagina. *J Sex. Med.* **3**(6), 979–87.

Podnar, S., Oblak, C., Vodusek, D. B. (2002). Sexual function in men with cauda equina lesions: a clinical and electormyographic study. *J Neurol. Neurosurg. Psychiatry.* **73**(6), 715–20.

Prause, N., Janssen, E. (2006). Blood flow: vaginal photoplethysmography. In I Goldstein, CM Meston, SR Davis and AM Traish, eds. *Women's Sexual Function and Dysfunction*, pp. 359–67. Taylor & Francis, New York.

Quadri, R.,Veglio, M., Flecchia, D., Tonda, L., De Lorenzo, F., Chiandussi, L., Fonzo, D. (1989). Autonomic neuropathy and sexual impotence in diabetic patients: analysis of cardiovascular reflexes. *Andrologia* **21**(4), 346–52.

Raina, R., Agarwal, A., Ausmundson, S., Mansour, D. and Zippe, C. D. (2005). Long-term efficay and compliance of MUSE for erectile dysfunction following radical prostatectomy: SHIM (IIEF-5) analysis. *International Journal of Impotence Research* **17** (1), 86–90.

Ravaglia, S., Marchioni, E., Costa, A., Maurelli, M. and Moglia, A. (2004). Erectile dysfunction as a sentinel symptom of cardiovascular autonomic neuropathy in heavy drinkers. *Journal of Peripheral Nervous System* **9**(4), 209–14.

Reading, P. J. and Will, R. G. (1997). Unwelcome orgasms: Case Report. *Lancet* **350**, 1946.

Rees, P. M., Fowler, C. J. and Maas, C. P. (2007). Sexual Function in men and women with neurological disorders. *Lancet* **369**, 512–25.

Rehman, J. and Melman, A. (2001). Normal anatomy and physiology in current clinical urology: In JJ Mulcahy, ed. *Male sexual function: A guide to Clinical Management*. pp. 1–46. Human Press Inc., Totowa.

Remillard, G. M., Andermann, F., Testa, G. F., *et al.* (1983). Sexual ictal manifestations predominate in women with temporal lobe epilepsy: a finding suggesting sexual dimorphism in the human brain. *Neurology* **33**, pp 323–30.

Robinson, L. Q., Woodcock, J. P., Stephenson, T. P. (1987) Results of investigation of impotence in patients with overt or probable neuropathy. *Br. J Urol.* **60**, 583–87.

Rosen, L. R. and Rosen, R. C. (2006). Fifty years of female sexual dysfunction research and concepts: from Kinsey to the present. In I Goldstein, CM Meston, SR Davis and AM Traish, eds. *Women's Sexual Function and Dysfunction*, pp. 3–10. Taylor & Francis, New York.

Rosen, R., Hatzichristou, D., Broderick, G., *et al.* (2004). Clinical evaluation and symptom Scales: sexual dysfunction assessment in men. 21st ed. In TF Lue, R Basson, R Rosen, F Giuliano, S Khoury and F Montorsi, eds. *Sexual dysfunctions in men and women,* pp. 175–241. Health Publications, Paris.

Rowland, D. L. (2006). Neurobiology of sexual response in men and women. *CNS Spectrums*, **11**:8(S9), 6–12.

Sakakibara, R. and Fowler, C. J. (1999). Vertebral control of bladder, bowel and sexual function and effects of brain disease. In C Fowler, ed. *Neurology of bladder, bowel and sexual dysfunction*, pp. 229–44. Butterworth Heinemann, Boston.

Salinas, C. J., Virseda, C. M., Saenz de Tejada, I., *et al.* (2003). New Contributions of the usefulness of electromyography of cavernous bodies in the diagnosis of erectile dysfunction. *Archivos españoles de urología*, **56**(1), 61–8.

Salinas, C. J.,Virseda, C. M., Samblas, G. R., *et al.* (1998). [Neurobiology of erectile dysfunction in multiple sclerosis]. *Archivos españoles de urología*, **51**(2), 167–70.

Sand, M., Fisher, W. (2007). Women's Endorsement of Models of Female Sexual Response: The Nurse's Sexuality Study. *J Sex Med* **4**, 708–719.

Sandel, M. E. (1997). Traumatic brain injury. In ML Sipski and CJ Alexander, eds. *Sexual function in people with disability and chronic illness*, pp. 221–46. Aspen Publication, Gaithersburg.

Savoie, M., Kim, S. S., Soloway, M. S. (2003). A prospective study measuring penile length in men treated with radical prostatectomy for prostate cancer. *J Urol.* **169**(4), 1462–64.

Schmid, D. M., Curt, A., Hauri, D. and Schurch, B. (2003). Clinical value of combined electrophysiological and urodynamic recording to assess sexual disorders in spinal cord injured men. *Neurourology and Urodynamics* **22**(4), 314–21.

Schmid, D. M., Reitz, A., Curt, A., Hauri, D., Schurch, B. (2004). Urethral evoked sympathetic skin responses and viscerosensory evoked potentials as diagnostic tools to evaluate urogenital autonomic afferent innervation in spinal cord injured patients. *J Urol.* **171**, 1156–60.

Schmid, D. M., Schurch, B. and Hauri, D. (2000). Sildenafil in the treatment of sexual dysfunction in spinal cord injured males. *European Urology* **38**(2), 184–93.

Secil, Y., Ozdedeli, K., Altay, B., Aydogdu, I., Yilmaz, C., Ertekin, C. (2005). Sympathetic skin response recorded from the genital region in normal and diabetic women. *Neurophysiol. Clin.* **35**(1):11–7.

Shafik, A. (1993). Vaginocavernosus reflex: clinical significance and role in the sexual act. *Gynecologic and Obstetric Invesigation* **35**, 114–17.

Shahani, B. T., Halperin, J. J., Boulu, P. and Cohen, J. (1984). Sympathetic skin response—a method of assessing unmyelinated axon dysfunction in peripheral neuropathies. *Journal of Neurology, Neurosurgery and Psychiatry* **47**, 536–42.

Sheel, A. W. and Krassioukov, A. V., Inglis, J. T. and Elliott, S. L. (2005). Autonomic dysreflexia during sperm retrieval in spinal cord injury: influence of lesion level and sildenafil citrate. *J Appl. Physiol.* **99**(1), 53–58.

Sherfey, M. J. (1972). *The Nature and Evolution of Female Sexuality.* Random House, New York.

Shetty, S. D. and Farah, R. N. (1999). Anatomy of erectile function. In C Carson, R Kirby, Irwin Goldstein, eds. *Textbook of erectile dysfunction,* pp. 25–29. Oxford, UK: ISIS Medical Media, Oxford.

Sim, H. G., Kilot, M., Lange, P. H., Ellis, W. J., Takayama, T. K. and Yang, C. C. (2006). Two-year outcome of unilateral nerve interposition graft after radical prostatectomy. *Urology* **68**(8), 1290–4.

Sipski, L., Rosen, R. C., Alexander, C. J., Hamer, R. M. (2000). Sildenafil effects on sexual and cardiovascular responses in women with spinal cord injury. *Urology* **55**(6), 812–5.

Sipski, M., Alexander, C., Gomez-Marin, O. and Spalding, J. (2007). The effects of spinal cord injury on psychogenic sexual arousal in males. *J Urol.,* **177**(1), 247–51.

Sipski, M., Alexander, C. J. and Gomez-Marin, O. (2006). Effects of level and degree of spinal cord injury on male orgasm. *Spinal Cord,* **44**(12),798–804.

Sipski, M. L., Alexander, C. J. and Rosen, R. (2001). Sexual arousal and orgasm in women: Effects of spinal cord injury. *Ann. Neurol.* **49**, 35–44.

Sipski, M. L., Alexander, C. J. and Rosen, R. C. (1995). Orgasm in women with spinal cord injuries: a laboratory based assessment. *Arch. Phys. Med. Rehabil.* **76**, 811–18.

Sipski, M. L., Craig, A. J., Rosen, R. C. (1997). Physiological parameters associated with sexual arousal in women with incomplete spinal cord injuries. *Arch. Phys. Med. Rehabil* **78**, 305–13.

Sipski-Alexander M., Bodner, D., Brackett, N., Elliott, S., Jackson, A., Sonksen, J. (2007b). The development of International Standards to Document Sexual and Reproductive Function after Spinal Cord Injury: A preliminary report. *J Rehab Res & Dev* **44**(1), 83–98.

Smeltzer, S. C. and Kelley, C. L. (1997). Multiple Sclerosis. In ML Sipski and CJ Alexander, eds. *Sexual function in people with disability and chronic illness,* pp. 177–88. Aspen Publication, Gaithersburg.

Smith, G. L. and Christmas, T. J. (1999). Potency preserving surgery. In C Carson, R Kirby and I Goldstein, eds. *Textbook of erectile dysfunction,* pp. 599–606. ISIS Medical Media, Oxford.

Snell, S. S. (2001). *Clinical neuroanatomy for medical students,* pp. 395–426. 5th ed. Lippincott Williams & Wilkins, Philadelphia.

Staerman, F., Guiraud, P., Coeurdacier, P., Menard, D., Edan, G. and Lobel, B. (1996). Value of nocturnal penile tumescence and rigidity (NPTR) recording in impotent patients with multiple sclerosis. *Int. J Impot.* **8**, 241–45.

Stevenson, R. W. D. S. and Elliott, S. L. (2007). Sexuality and Illness In S Leiblum, ed. 4th ed. *Principles and Practice of Sex Therapy,* pp. 313–49. Guilford Press, New York.

Stief, C. G., Kellner, B., Hartung, C., *et al.* (1997). Computer-assisted evaluation of smooth—muscle electromyogram of the corpora cavernosa by fast Fourier transformation *European Urology* **31**(3), 329–34.

Stief, C. G., Thon, W. F., Djamilian, M., *et al.* (1992). Transcutaneous registration of cavernous smooth muscle electrical activity: non-invasive diagnosis of neurogenic autonomic impotence. *J Urol.* **147**, 47–50.

Szasz, G. (1983). Sexual health care. In C Zejdlik, ed. *Management of the spinal cord injured,* pp. 25–152. Wadsworth Health Sciences Division, Monterey.

Tepper, M. (2001). *Personal Communication.* sexualhealth.com (owned and operated by the Sexual Health Network, Inc; Pennsylvania.

Tiihonen, J., Kuikka, J., Kupila, J., *et al.* (1994). Increasing cerebral blood flow of the prefrontal cortex in man during orgasm. *Neuroscience Letters* **170**, 241–3.

Tilton, M. C. (1997). Diabetes and amputation. In ML, Sipski CJ and Alexander, eds. *Sexual function in people with disability and chronic illness,* pp. 279–302. Aspen Publication, Gaithersburg.

Truitt, W. A. and Coolen, L. M. (2002). Identification of a potential ejaculation generator in the spinal cord. *Science* **297**, 1566–9.

Tuckwell, H. C. (1989). A neurophysiological theory of reproductive process. *Int. J Neurosci.* **44**, 143–8.

Uckert, S., Fuhlenriede, M. H., Becker, A. J., *et al.* (2003) *Urological Research* **31**(2), 55–60.

Uitti, R., Tanner, C., Rajput, A. *et al.* (1989). Hypersexuality with antiparkinsonism therapy. *Clinical Neuropharmacology* **5**, 375–83.

Van Lunsen, R. H. W. and Laan, E. L. (2004). Genital vascular responsiveness and sexual feelings in midlife women: psychophysiologic, brain and genital imaging studies. *Menopause* **11**(6), 441–748.

Vardi, Y., Gedalia, U. and Gruenwald, I. (2006). Neurological testing: quantified sensory testing. In I Goldstein, CM Meston, SR Davis and AM Traish, eds. *Women's Sexual Function and Dysfunction,* pp. 399–403. Taylor & Francis, New York.

Wagner, G., Gerstenberg, T. and Levin, R. J. (1989). Electrical activity of corpus cavernosum during flaccidity and erection of the human penis: a new diagnostic method? *J Urol.* **142**, 723–25.

Wagner, G. and Levin, R. J. (1980). Electrolytes in vaginal fluid during the menstrual cycle of coitally active and inactive women. *Journal of Reproductive Fertility* **60**, 17–27.

Wang, J. J. (1997). Analysis of sympathetic skin response of 83 normal subjects. *Journal of Clinical Electroencephalography* **6**, 201–3.

Wermuth, L. and Stenager, E. (1995). Sexual problems in young patients with Parkinson's disease. *Acta Neurologica Scandinavica* **91**, 453–5.

Whipple, B., Gerdes, C. A. and Komisaruk, B. R. (1996). Sexual response to self stimulation in women with complete spinal cord injury. *J Sex. Res.* **33**, 231–40.

Yang, C. C., Jiang, X. (2009). Clinical autonomic neurophysiology and the male sexual respsonse.An Overview. *J Sex. Med.,* **6**(suppl 3), 221–28.

Yarnitsky, D., Sprecher, E., Barilan, Y. and Vardi, Y. (1995). Corpus cavernosum electromyogram: spontaneous and evoked electrical activities. *J Urol.* **153**, 653–4.

Yilimaz, U., Ellis, W., lange, P., Yang, C. (2006). Evoked cavernous activity: measuring autonomic innervation following pelvic surgery. *Int. J Impot. Res.* **18**(3), 296–301.

Yilimaz, U., Soylu, A., Ozcan, C., Kutlu, R., Gunes, A. (2002). Evoked cavernous activity. *J Urol.* **167**(1), 188–91.

Yilmaz, U., Kromm, B. G. and Yang, C. C. (2004). Evaluation of the autonomic innervation of the clitoris and bulb. *J Urol.,* **172**(5 Pt 1), 1930–4.

Young, B., Coolen, L., McKenna, K. (2009). Neural regulation of ejaculation. *J Sex. Med.,* **6**(suppl 3), 229–33.

Zhu, G-Y, and Shen, Y. (2001). Sympathetic skin response: a new test to diagnose erectile dysfunction. *Asian J Androl.* **3**, 45–8.

PART IV

Primary Autonomic Failure: Clinical and Pathological Studies in Pure Autonomic Failure, Multiple System Atrophy, and Parkinson's Disease

CHAPTER 39

Clinical features and evaluation of the primary autonomic failure syndromes

Roger Bannister, Valeria Iodice, Ekawat Vichayanrat and Christopher J. Mathias

Classification

The clinical classification of primary autonomic failure adopted in this book (see Introduction) is:

1 Patients with pure autonomic failure (PAF), without associated neurological disorders, formerly known as 'idiopathic orthostatic hypotension'.

2 Patients with multiple system atrophy (MSA). MSA comprises a group of central neurological degenerations, often but not always including parkinsonism (Bannister and Oppenheimer 1972, Stefanova et al. 2009). The combination of autonomic failure (AF) and MSA was known as the Shy–Drager syndrome (Shy and Drager 1960, Smith et al. 1996). For brevity, in this chapter the use of the acronym MSA can be taken to mean MSA associated with AF. MSA in the form of striatonigral degeneration (SND) may occasionally occur without the symptoms of AF (Fearnley and Lees 1990).

3 Patients with Parkinson's disease (PD).

4 Patients with AF associated with progressive disabling cognitive impairment and parkinsonian features, known as Diffuse Lewy body disease or dementia with Lewy bodies (DLB) (Larner et al. 2000, McKeith et al. 2005).

Of these four primary autonomic disorders, MSA is the most common. Hughes et al. (1992), summarizing the results from the Parkinson's Disease Brain Bank at the Institute of Neurology, London, found that seven of the first 100 cases, supposed in life by the referring physicians to have PD, in fact had SND or MSA. This is consistent with further observations (Colosimo et al. 1995). MSA prevalence rates range from 1.9 to 4.4/100,000 (Chrysostome et al. 2004, Schrag et al. 1999) and the incidence has been estimated at 3/100,000 per year (Bower et al. 1997). The largest clinical series of MSA reported so far, 475 MSA cases recruited from 2001 by the European MSA Group shows that the disease presents uniformly across Europe (Köllensperger et al. 2010). MSA may have a prevalence rate as high as 10 per 100,000, by comparison with the prevalence rate of 100–150 per 100,000 for PD. PAF is much less common than MSA, and AF with PD rarer still.

In PD, the reported prevalence and incidence of orthostatic hypotension (OH), often used as an index of AF in PD, varies considerably. Some consider it to be rare (Colosimo et al. 1995). Others report modest orthostatic falls (Meco et al. 1991, Sandroni et al. 1991) that do not fulfill current definition criteria of orthostatic hypotension. This differs from a high prevalence, which consistently reported OH in more than 40% of patients with PD from other studies (Uono 1973, Senard et al.1997, Lipp et al. 2009). The disparity in prevalence estimated could be the result of differences in definition of OH and the methods used to measure the blood pressure changes. Whether this also reflects variations in the type of patient studied, the influence of the many factors that modify blood pressure control (such as increasing age, duration of the disorder, and drug therapy), is unclear (Van Dijk et al. 1993, Hillen et al.1996, Kujawa et al. 2000). Most previous studies were based on cohorts of patients recruited through hospital PD clinics, which may introduce bias and underestimate the phenomenon. OH was reported in 42 out of 89 patients with PD (47%) in a community-based population study (Allcock et al. 2004). A recent meta-analysis of 25 studies calculated an OH prevalence of 30% with large statistical heterogeneity between studies (Velseboer et al. 2011). Clearly, these findings, as well as other reports on autonomic function in PD (see p. 487, Chapter 45 and Asahina et al. 2012) indicate that autonomic dysfunction/failure can occur in PD and at any stage but it is more prevalent in later stages (Velseboer et al. 2011).

Prevalence of DLB in the general population differs among age groups and ethnicity. Approximately 5% of the population was reported in a population aged 75 years and older in Finland (Rahkonen et al. 2003, and this figure was 2% in a population aged 65 years in the UK (Stevens et al. 2002). From these studies, DLB accounts for 11–22% of all dementia patients, the second most common type of dementia in older people after Alzheimer's disease. Autonomic dysfunction in DLB is not uncommon and now features in the revised criteria for the clinical and pathologic diagnosis of DLB (McKeith et al. 2005). An earlier pathological study showed that most confirmed DLB patients had urinary incontinence and constipation as the most frequent symptoms, while

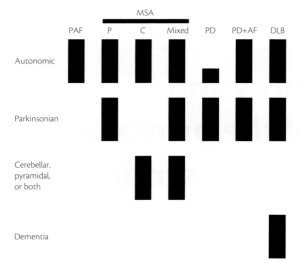

Fig. 39.1 Schematic representation of the major clinical features in some of the primary autonomic failure syndromes. These include, the three forms of Multiple System Atrophy (parkinsonian, MSA-P; cerebellar, MSA-C; and mixed, MSA-M), pure autonomic failure (PAF), Parkinson's disease (PD), Parkinson's disease with autonomic failure (PD+AF) and Dementia with Lewy Bodies (DLB). The partially filled histogram in PD is to indicate that there is evidence for localized but not generalized AF, unlike PD+AF. From Iodice et al. (2012).

almost one-third of these patients experienced episodic hypotension associated with syncopal episodes (Horimoto et al. 2003).

In 1996 a Consensus Panel of international experts (Schatz et al. 1996), defined MSA as 'a sporadic progressive adult onset disorder characterized by autonomic dysfunction, parkinsonism, and ataxia in any combination' (Fig. 39.1). The features of this disorder include:

- parkinsonism (bradykinesia with rigidity or tremor or both), usually with poor or unsustained motor response to chronic levodopa (L-3,4-dihydroxyphenylalanine [L -DOPA]) therapy
- cerebellar or corticospinal signs
- orthostatic (postural) hypotension, impotence, urinary incontinence or retention, usually preceding or within 2 years of the onset of motor symptoms.

A second Consensus Panel (Gilman et al. 2008) concluded that a diagnosis of possible MSA requires at least one feature suggesting autonomic dysfunction in addition to parkinsonism or a cerebellar syndrome, and at least one additional feature including findings on history, clinical examination, and results from either structural or functional imaging. Therefore the diagnosis of possible MSA can be made on both clinical and imaging results.

Characteristically, these features cannot be explained by medications or other disorders. Parkinsonism and cerebellar features quite commonly occur in combination. However, certain features may predominate. When parkinsonian features predominate, the term striatonigral degeneration is often used (Fearnley and Lees 1990). When cerebellar features predominate, the term olivopontocerebellar atrophy or degeneration is often used. When AF predominates, the term Shy–Drager syndrome is often used. These manifestations may occur in various combinations and evolve with time.

Clinical features of primary autonomic failure

The clinical features of AF can be described separately from the neurological features that are characteristic of MSA or PD.

The particular autonomic functions affected differ in degree from patient to patient but are remarkably similar in all three groups (Iodice et al. 2011). The patients are usually middle aged or elderly. In MSA, males are affected more often than females. In men, impotence and loss of libido are commonly the first symptoms. Patients living in hot climates may complain of inability to sweat, which could lead to hyperpyrexia and collapse in the tropics but rarely causes problems in temperate countries. The most dramatic symptom, however, and the most common reason for seeking medical advice, is postural dizziness, or even fainting, on standing erect, especially in the morning or after meals or exercise.

One curious symptom of AF, which presumably reflects a phase of denervation supersensitivity, is that in some patients, over a few weeks or months, an autonomic function may appear hyperactive before failure occurs. This may, in particular, be noted in salivation or sweating and in sexual function in the male in which more frequent spontaneous erection may precede erectile failure.

Postural hypotension

The postural attacks may be 'drop' attacks resembling sudden brainstem vascular dysfunction, but more commonly there is a gradual fading of consciousness over half a minute or so while the patient is standing or walking. A neck ache radiating to the occipital region of the skull and to the shoulders often precedes actual loss of consciousness. The neck ache may be due to ischaemia in continuously contracting postural muscles in the neck and back in a 'coathanger' distribution (Bleasdale-Barr and Mathias 1998), but the mechanism of this common and virtually unique symptom of postural hypotension is unknown. This ache may be associated with a progressive anterior cervical flexion—anterocollis.

Occasionally, patients may complain of other symptoms suggesting muscle ischaemia. For example, some have described the classic symptoms of angina on exercise and others have described leg symptoms that have features suggestive of 'claudication' affecting the cauda equina. Perhaps surprisingly, despite a very low systolic blood pressure of under 60 mmHg during exercise at the time anginal symptoms occur, the electrocardiogram usually fails to show T-wave inversion or other signs of ischaemia, although a prolonged QT time (although without changes in QT dispersion) has been documented in primary AF (Lo et al. 1996).

In the postural hypotensive attacks, usually after a visual disturbance or sensation of dizziness, the patient may then fall slowly to his knees; experience teaches him that, after lying flat, there will be recovery and loss of all symptoms, including the neck ache, within a few minutes. The recovery from such transient neurological symptoms is usually complete and occlusive cerebrovascular incidents are rare, possibly because many patients, after years of postural hypotension, have not only preserved but enhanced compensatory cerebral autoregulation (Thomas and Bannister 1980). The attacks of loss of consciousness also differ from normal fainting in that the patient usually does not sweat, and there is no vagally induced bradycardia (Chapter 56). In our units, pre-syncopal symptoms (light-headedness, dizziness, and visual disturbance) are generally the most common presenting symptoms followed by syncope (loss of consciousness, blackouts or fainting) among primary autonomic failure patients.

Symptoms are strikingly worse in the mornings, in hot weather, and also after meals and exercise, all of which cause an unfavourable redistribution of blood volume. The disease is likely to be progressive for several years before significant incapacity occurs, because autonomic compensatory mechanisms postpone overt failure. A few patients, if treated by bed rest for hypotensive symptoms, develop persistent recumbent hypertension, mainly due to loss of baroreflexes, of such severity that they may develop papilloedema with retinal haemorrhages.

Visual disturbances

Sometimes there are transient visual disturbances, scotomata, hallucinations, or tunnel vision, suggesting occipital-lobe ischaemia. The symptoms of visual disturbance may be particularly striking in some patients with AF. One observant patient was able to classify the disturbances into three kinds. First, there was a disturbance of primary colours, but particularly yellow and red, in which they became brilliant, and secondary colours, or pastel shades, appeared non-existent. Secondly, objects might appear in a photonegative form, that is dark shades being light and the light shades being dark, mostly in various shades of green. Finally, if he did not lie down promptly and had developed a severe neck ache and one of the previous disturbances of vision had been present for several minutes, he would then find that his central vision was blurred. On closing his eyes he would see a very clear oval orange or yellow shape filling the whole of the central field with a dark background outside it and in the very centre what appeared to be an irregularly shaped black hole. Once this particular disturbance had occurred it might take some 30 min to subside completely.

On occasion patients describe visual disturbances accompanied by neck and even lumbar aching, brought on by physical exertion while standing, particularly after a meal. The effects of arm exercise, such as washing up after meals or using an ironing board, appear, under conditions of critically reduced systolic blood pressure, to imitate the effects of the subclavian steal syndrome. This is similar to the visual disturbances described by Ross Russell and Page (1983) in patients with critical underperfusion of the brain and retina with extensive occlusive disease of the extracranial arteries. In patients with AF, however, such symptoms are relatively benign and patients quickly learn to use them as a warning sign that they must lie down quickly to restore an adequate perfusion pressure.

Defective sweating

Defective sweating (Fig. 39.2) causes the risk of hyperpyrexia and collapse in hot climate. Hypohidrosis was present in 59% of individuals with PAF in our Units. The testing of thermoregulatory sweating is described in Chapter 31.

Sexual function

Sexual function in the male is lost early. Failure of erection occurs first, though occasionally after an initial period with excessive erections, and later is followed by disturbance of ejaculation consistent with progressive parasympathetic and then sympathetic failure. Erectile dysfunction was reported in 73% of male PAF patients. As discussed in Chapter 38, complex techniques using pharmacological agents or electrical stimulation may enable some sexual function to be achieved for a time.

Urinary function

Nocturia is common in PAF patients and can be a presenting symptom in approximately 50% of these patients. Urinary symptoms in MSA-P are very common and usually severe compared with PD. A recent study showed that urinary symptoms occurred early and were reported in all MSA-P patients within 2 years after diagnosis (Swaminath et al. 2010). Furthermore, urinary symptoms in patients with MSA-P were not related to the severity of parkinsonian symptoms in contrast to patients with PD.

Gastrointestinal function

As the disease advances there may be difficulties with swallowing (Mathias 1996). In combination with laryngeal paresis this may increase the risk of pulmonary infection and even sudden death. Bowel control is sometimes affected, with constipation, intermittent diarrhoea, or rectal incontinence as symptoms. A few cases of MSA with predominant bowel disturbance and cholinergic dysfunction (including salivation) have been described (Khurana et al. 1980, Khurana 1994). A marked disturbance of bowel function with a predominance of diarrhoea and faecal incontinence suggests the possibility of amyloid.

Cognitive function

Cognitive profiles were recently evaluated in six patients with PAF who presented with cognitive impairment (Heims et al. 2006). Deficits of speed and attention were found to be the most common type of cognitive impairment following by frontal executive dysfunction. There was no direct relationship between cognitive function and white matter lesions on cerebral imaging.

Clinical motor features of multiple system atrophy

Three principal forms of motor disturbance occur in MSA:

◆ parkinsonian

◆ cerebellar

◆ pyramidal.

Parkinsonism

The term 'striatonigral degeneration' (SND) was first used by Adams et al. (1964) and later by Fearnley and Lees (1990), to describe patients with a parkinsonian syndrome with special pathological distinguishing features (Chapter 41). Often the disorder was clinically indistinguishable from PD and, with hindsight, these

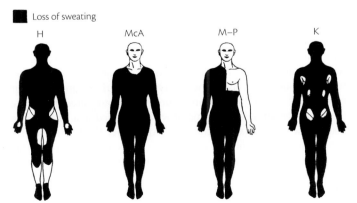

Fig. 39.2 Sweating response to 1°C rise in central body temperature in four patients with autonomic failure. From Bannister et al. 1967, with permission.

patients, especially if autonomic defects had been looked for and found, should probably now be classified as having MSA (MSA-P). In this disease there is a predominance of rigidity without much tremor, associated with progressive loss of facial expression and limb akinesis. The limbs show rigidity on examination, without the classical 'cog wheel' or 'lead pipe' rigidity of PD. Facial expression is often less affected than in PD. The patient has difficulty in standing, walking, or turning and has difficulty in feeding himself. Salivation is reduced. As a result of akinesis, the speech becomes faint and slurred. The patient's gait becomes slow and clumsy, superficially resembling PD, with an attitude of stooping and often extreme forward cervical flexion, which makes forward gaze difficult. In MSA, analysis of the dysarthria (Kluin et al. 1996) and of the motor disturbances, including ataxia and spasticity (Fetoni et al. 1997) have been reported.

Cerebellar

The cerebellar form of MSA (MSA-C) associated with olivopontocerebellar atrophy (OPCA) was not included in Shy and Drager's original clinical description of only two cases. In this form there is a prominent disturbance of gait with truncal ataxia which frequently makes it impossible for the patient to stand without support. In addition, marked slurring of speech with irregularity of speed of diction has the features describe above for SND. There may also be a mild or moderate intention tremor affecting the arms and legs. This form of MSA is to be distinguished from familial OPCA in which the associated clinical features may include optic atrophy, retinitis pigmentosa, chorea, cataracts, and areflexia (Harding 1981, Gilman and Quinn 1996) but without autonomic failure.

Pyramidal

In either the parkinsonian or cerebellar forms of degeneration there may be a pyramidal increase in tone, together with impaired rapid hand and foot movements and exaggerated deep-tendon jerks and bilateral extensor plantar responses. It is, of course, difficult to detect a pyramidal disturbance of tone in the presence of the extrapyramidal disturbance. Primitive reflexes such as the palmomental reflex may also be present.

Other clinical features in multiple system atrophy

Muscle wasting and neuropathy

Progressive muscle wasting not infrequently occurs although this is not nearly as marked as in motor neurone disease. Fasciculation occurs rarely, but on electromyographic examination there is usually some evidence of denervation with little evidence of any abnormality of peripheral nerve motor conduction. Rarely in PAF and uncommonly in MSA there is clinical and electrophysiological evidence of a mild distal sensorimotor neuropathy with the report of a mild reduction of myelinated fibre density (Cohen et al. 1987) and unmyelinated fibre density (Kanda et al. 1996).

Cognitive function

Dementia is no more common than might be expected on the basis of chance in patients of this age group, though more detailed testing of cognitive function has shown deficits in visuospatial organization and visuomotor ability, similar to those seen in PD (Testa et al. 1993; Pillon et al. 1995, Monza et al. 1998). It is surprising to observe preserved intellectual function in a patient who is almost totally incapacitated in terms of motor control, postural blood pressure regulation, and bladder disturbance. This is, of course, in striking contrast to the neuronal degeneration of presenile dementia (Alzheimer's disease) in which the predominant degeneration affects cortical cholinergic neurones. It is also in contrast to the intellectual impairment which is a feature of some cases of PD. Comprehensive neuropsychological tests and single photon emission computed tomography (SPECT) were compared between each subtype of MSA (Kawai et al. 2008). The results demonstrated that MSA-P patients were more likely to have severe involvement of visuospatial and constructional function, verbal fluency and executive function while patients with MSA-C showed only visuospatial and constructional function involvement compared to controls. MSA-P patients also tended to have a wide and severe impairment in cognitive function compared with MSA-C and the neuropsychological impairment was also significantly correlated with a decrease perfusion in prefrontal in SPECT which may suggest prefrontal involvement in MSA-P. A later study also suggested that cognitive impairment in MSA may correlate with prefrontal lobe atrophy and disease duration (Chang et al. 2009).

Affect

There is no evidence of a mood defect when allowance is made for the considerable physical disability of patients with MSA, as confirmed by detailed testing in patients with the parkinsonian forms that indicate an overall normal affective state (Pillon et al. 1995). This is surprising in view of the hypothesis that central catecholamine function plays a part in the preservation of normal mood and that patients with depression can be helped by augmenting central noradrenergic function.

Sensory function

In two cases out of a personal series of more than 150 patients with MSA, there was sensory loss in the legs, confirmed by loss of sural sensory action potentials in one and by post-mortem studies in the other (Bannister and Oppenheimer 1972). Nerve conduction studies in MSA confirm the presence of a mixed sensorimotor axonal neuropathy (Pramstaller et al. 1995).

Pupils

Abnormalities recorded in patients with MSA include Horner's syndrome, alternating anisocoria, and abnormal pupillary responses to drugs. Ponsford, Paul, and Bannister (unpublished observations) studied 16 patients with MSA and compared them with patients with PD and age-matched controls. There was alternating anisocoria in five patients. This was variable and different from the alternating resting anisocoria which was noted in a single case of acute pandysautonomia. It was concluded that in MSA the disturbance was due to a central lesion rather than to unilateral hypersensitivity to cholinergic drugs on one side and to adrenergic drugs on the contralateral side. Alternating anisocoria differs from the variable but consistently lateralized anisocoria in the patients with pandysautonomia and the pupillotonia of the Holmes–Adie syndrome which reflects the different hypersensitivity of the two pupils to circulating cholinergic drugs.

In more than half the patients with MSA or PD, with or without AF, there was an abnormal and excessive constrictor response to methacholine. The degree of constriction in the more sensitive pupils was in the same range as in the Holmes–Adie syndrome. More than half of the patients with AF, whether PAF, MSA or AF with PD, showed an abnormal sensitivity.

Pupillary response to eye-drop tests was recently proposed as a useful aid for distinguishing PD and MSA. However the pupillary measurement in these disorders need further study to confirm the usefulness of these tests for this purpose (Yamashita et al. 2010)

Ocular movements

There is frequently restriction of conjugate ocular movements in advanced MSA, but this is usually an upward rather than a downward restriction and is less severe than in progressive supranuclear palsy (PSP), in which the ocular movement disorder dominates the clinical picture. Nuchal rigidity and striatonigral features in PSP, superficially resembling MSA, may make the differential diagnosis difficult at an early stage. In due course the ocular movement disorder of PSP becomes more apparent and this, with the lack of autonomic symptoms and signs, will distinguish it from MSA.

Detailed testing of ocular movements by Dr T. J. Anderson of the National Hospital, London (personal communication) has shown that only a minority of patients with probable MSA have normal eye movements. Often the findings are similar to those of idiopathic PD, with hypometria of saccades, particularly upwards saccades. Prominent slowing of saccades is not normally seen and suggests familial OPCA or PSP. A supranuclear gaze paresis, seldom severe and usually affecting vertical more than horizontal gaze, is present in up to 20% of cases. Cerebellar eye signs—particularly gaze-evoked nystagmus, saccadic dysmetria, and poor smooth pursuit and vestibulo-ocular response suppression—are often present in patients with other features of cerebellar dysfunction, but may be found in the absence of cerebellar ataxia or limb dysmetria. Down-beat nystagmus (DBN) is present in up to a third of cases of MSA. In a minority of these, the DBN is noted in the head upright (i.e. sitting) position, but in most it is only elicited on positioning the patient with the head hanging (Dix–Hallpike or Barany manoeuvre) and may be of relatively short duration.

Oculomotor function in 30 probable MSA patients, which included 6 pathologically confirmed cases, were reviewed recently. The results indicated that excessive square wave jerks, mild-moderate hyhpometria of saccades, impaired vestibuloocular reflex (VOR) suppression, spontaneous nystagmus or positioning DBN were suggestive of MSA while the presence of slow saccades or moderate-to-severe gaze restriction suggested a diagnosis other than MSA (Anderson et al. 2008).

Olfactory dysfunction

Olfactory dysfunction has also been reported in MSA but the severity is less prominent than in PD, Alzheimer's disease and DLB. This study also demonstrated impaired olfaction in PAF with a similar severity to MSA (Silveira-Moriyama et al. 2009). A later study evaluated olfactory and autonomic function in 23 PD patients with different severity of smell dysfunction (Goldstein et al. 2010). Patients with PD were divided into two groups; 11 anosmia and 12 normal/moderate microsmia by the University of Pennsylvania Smell Inventory Test (UPSIT). Baroreflex-cardiovagal gain, baroreflex sympathoneural function, microdialysate levels of norepinephrine and dihydroxyphenylglycol (DHPG) from muscle during supine and tilting were used as markers for autonomic function. Cerebral 6-[^{18}F]fluorodopamine PET was also used as functional imaging and 6-[^{18}F]fluorodopamine-derived radioactivity in different organs (interventricular myocardial septum, free wall, liver, spleen, and renal cortex) for assessing cardiac/organ-selective extracardiac noradrenergic denervation. The results showed baroreflex-cardiovagal gain, baroreflex sympathoneural function, noradrenergic denervation in cardiac/extracardiac organ-selective were significantly lower in PD with anosmia compared to those with normal/moderate microsmia but there was no correlation between cerebral 6-[^{18}F]Fluorodopamine PET, Unified Parkinson's Disease Rating Scale (UPDRS) score, and olfactory dysfunction. These findings suggested the association between olfactory function, baroreflex failure and cardiac/extracardiac noradrenergic denervation were not correlated with parkinsonian symptoms and striatal dopaminergic denervation.

Disturbances of breathing

Rhythm and depth control

The disturbance of breathing may occur during the day, with involuntary inspiratory gasps (Bannister et al. 1967) or 'cluster' breathing, apparently normal breathing interspersed with regular apnoeic periods lasting about 20 seconds (Lockwood 1976), which appear to have a central origin. At night the patients may develop the sleep apnoea syndrome. The sleep apnoea may be 'central' with cessation of respiratory motor activity, or 'obstructive' in which there is a disturbance of the pharyngeal and laryngeal muscles. There is, in addition, evidence of an alteration of CO_2 sensitivity MSA, probably due to the brainstem lesion. The patient of Guilleminault et al. (1977) with MSA also had a reduced amount of rapid eye movement (REM) sleep and had disturbed non-REM sleep. This study showed that pulmonary arterial pressure rose progressively during sleep in direct association with each apnoeic episode and related hypoxaemia and hypocapnia, but without the extreme bradycardia which occurred in the REM sleep of patients who did not have AF.

Laryngeal function

At night, stridor with consequent hypoxia may secondarily cause disturbances of brainstem function and apnoea. The laryngeal stridor is due to a bilateral defect of the laryngeal abductors (Williams et al. 1979, Guindi et al. 1980, Harcourt et al. 1996) with changes of denervation on laryngeal electromyography (Guindi et al. 1981). At post-mortem, atrophy of the posterior cricoarytenoid muscles was found, due to an unusual form of denervation (Bannister et al. 1981). In the only case in which the laryngeal nerve was studied at post-mortem there appeared to be a reduced number of nerve fibres, although the nucleus ambiguus, thought to be the nucleus from which neurones innervating the laryngeal abductors arise, failed to show any selective neuronal loss. Once stridor and apnoea occur, continuous positive airway pressure (CPAP), nasal surgery, and arytenoidectomy can be considered, but usually tracheostomy cannot be long delayed. It is justified because such patients may manage well for several years before other symptoms become troublesome or incapacitating. However, sudden death during sleep remains a frequent cause of death in MSA (Munschauer et al. 1990).

Urinary function

Bladder symptoms are a combination of urgency, frequency, and nocturia due to uninhibited detrusor activity, or incontinence due to sphincter weakness, or, later, overflow incontinence due to an atonic bladder. During attempted evacuation there may be a weak or interrupted stream or incomplete evacuation, with residual urine. At its most severe there may be a complete inability to urinate. In MSA there may be various combinations of upper and lower motor neurone lesions affecting the detrusor and internal and external sphincter muscles.

As described in Chapter 38, degeneration of sacral autonomic neurons (Onuf's nucleus) leads to loss of both autonomic and somatic efferents as the nucleus has a status intermediate between ordinary somatic motoneurons and autonomic neurons. Anal and urethral sphincter impairment results from the loss of both innervations. Urinary incontinence, usually without retention, is the result. There is, in addition, detrusor instability with lack of the capacity to initiate micturition in MSA, which is probably the result of a lesion of the pontine centre for micturition. Very occasionally, reduction of the outflow resistance can be achieved surgically, although routine operations based on the common belief that the patient may have prostatism almost always make these patients worse. An appropriate operation, however, may postpone the need for the use of surgical drainage in the male. Ureteric sphincter implants are now available. In younger females with good co-ordination, intermittent self-catheterization may sometimes be an acceptable management instead of continuous drainage or the use of incontinence pads.

Autonomic cardiovascular and sudomotor investigations

As discussed in Chapter 22 the presence of orthostatic hypotension and abnormality of cardiovascular autonomic testing itself does not separate MSA from other parkinsonian syndromes (Mathias and Kimber 1999, Riley and Chelimsky 2003, Lipp et al. 2009, Iodice et al. 2011). Conversely, the distribution of anhidrosis and the anhidrosis percentage is significantly different between MSA and PD patients, as MSA patients have more widespread anhidrosis (Iodice et al. 2012). Furthermore, the distribution of anhidrosis confirmed the peripheral or ganglionic involvement in PD with AF and central-preganglionic involvement in MSA (Lipp et al. 2009).

Biochemical investigations

The most useful investigation is the measurement of plasma noradrenaline, taken under standard resting conditions, which is in the normal range in MSA but low in PAF (Mathias, 2009). In neither disorder does the level rise on tilting or standing, because of the impairment of baroreceptor pathways (Chapter 22). The low levels also help to separate the rare syndrome of dopamine-beta-hydroxylase deficiency (Chapter 49), which may not at first appear to differ from PAF, apart from its earlier age of onset. Low plasma noradrenaline levels without a rise on tilt can also been seen in patients with PD + AF and DLB (Oka et al. 2007) consistent with autonomic postganglionic impairment.

The growth hormone (GH) response to clonidine (Chapter 22) is normal in PAF patients where the lesion is localized in the peripheral autonomic pathway and abnormal in MSA patients, consistent with a predominant central lesion (Thomaides et al. 1992, Kimber et al. 1997).

Growth hormone secretion from the pituitary gland is stimulated by growth hormone releasing hormone (GHRH) and inhibited by somatostatin (Muller et al. 1999, Giustina et al. 1998). The growth hormone response to arginine, an amino acid that inhibits somatostatin release, is significantly reduced in patients with MSA compared with PD patients (Pellecchia et al. 2006, Zhang et al. 2010).

Neurophysiology investigations

Involvement of the peripheral nervous system (PNS) has been described in patients with MSA, and is relatively common in some neurodegenerative proteinopathies. Abnormal nerve conduction was present in MSA patients and was significantly more frequent in MSA-P compared with MSA-C (Abele M et al. 2000). Several studies have indicated that sphincter electromyography may be helpful in differentiating MSA from PD (Palace et al. 1997, Stocchi et al. 1997, Tison et al. 2000, Sakakibara et al. 2000, Winge et al. 2010). However, this has not been confirmed by other studies (Giladi et al. 2001, Giladi et al. 2000, Schwarz et al. 1997) and it is still matter for debate.

Skin vasomotor response

The skin vasomotor response (SkVR) is markedly reduced in patients with PAF have compared with MSA and normal controls, confirming the extensive postganglionic sympathetic denervation seen in PAF patients (Young et al. 2006). An attenuated SkVR is also present in patients with DLB and Parkinson disease with dementia (PDD) but not in PD patients (Akaogi et al. 2009).

Skin biopsy

In contrast to MSA, which is a preganglionic disorder, autonomic pathology in PD, DLB and PAF shows that these are postganglionic diseases. Autonomic and somatic innervation, as determined in skin biopsies also shows impairment in individual PD case reports (Donadio et al. 2005, Donadio et al. 2008, Dabby et al. 2006, Nolano et al. 2008). PAF patients showed marked postganglionic sympathetic denervation while MSA patients had preserved skin autonomic innervation (Donadio et al. 2010). Alpha-synuclein accumulation in skin nerve fibres revealed by skin biopsy has been described in patients with PAF, PD and DLB (Ikemura et al. 2008, Shishido et al. 2010, Miki et al. 2010).

Other investigations

See also Chapter 22.

Computerized tomography brain scanning

With the computerized tomography (CT) scan the enlargement of the cisterna ambiens associated with brainstem atrophy in MSA is visible along with atrophy of the pons and cerebral peduncles. In the cerebellar forms, atrophy of the vermis and cerebellar cortex is visible (Savoiardo et al. 1983, Huang and Plaitakis 1984).

Magnetic resonance imaging of the brain

The putaminal changes that are unique to MSA can be identified by T_1 weighted magnetic resonance imaging (MRI) (Pastakia et al. 1987). Brown et al. (1987) found that MRI changes ranked with the severity of the rigidity but not the other parkinsonian features of tremor or bradykinesia. The advances in MRI have increased the precision of diagnosis of MSA (Wenning et al. 2011). Fulham et al. (1991) showed that the most common MRI finding in MSA, present in 82% of their series, was cerebellar atrophy, which was seen in many patients whose symptoms were parkinsonian rather than cerebellar, e.g. Fig. 39.3. The second most common finding, present in more than half the patients in their series, was hypodensity in the posterolateral putaminal region, which matches exactly the region of cell loss found pathologically in MSA (Fig. 39.3a). Half the MSA patients have a specific further defect, anterior globose hyperintensity (Konagaya et al. 1994). In contrast, the MRI scans in patients with PAF were normal. Several studies also found other abnormalities including atrophy of putamen, lower brainstem, middle cerebellar peduncles (MCPs) and cerebellum (Bhattacharya et al. 2002). Hypersignal intensity in the pons and MCPs in MSA is not universal but may occasionally result in the 'hot-cross bun' sign (Fig. 39.3b). In other primary autonomic failure syndromes, extensive ischaemic damage in the deep cerebral white matter can be evident in pure autonomic failure (Fig. 39.3c) and generalized mild-moderate atrophy can be present in dementia with Lewy bodies (Fig. 39.3d).

An abnormal MRI scan provides a reliable method of diagnosing MSA even though the neurological signs of parkinsonism or cerebellar atrophy may be slight. Clearly, as with PD, the pathological

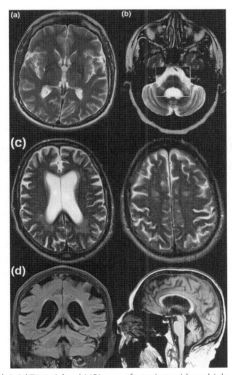

Fig. 39.3 (a) Axial T2-weighted MRI scan of a patient with multiple system atrophy demonstrating putaminal atrophy and marked putaminal hypointensity. (b) Axial T2-weighted MRI scan of a patient with multiple system atrophy demonstrating the cruciform abnormal signal within the pons (hot cross bun sign). (c) Axial T2-weighted MRI scan of a patient with pure autonomic failure demonstrating extensive ischaemic damage in the deep cerebral white matter. (d) Coronal and sagital T1-weighted MRI scan of a patient with dementia with Lewy bodies demonstrating generalized mild-moderate atrophy with more ventricular than sulcal dilatation..

changes in the brain in MSA may precede by some years the development of recognizable neurological clinical signs. In contrast, a normal MRI scan in a patient with severe orthostatic hypotension but without neurological symptoms strengthens the likelihood of the diagnosis of PAF. Though the MRI changes usually distinguish MSA from PD, at any rate in the late stages, MRI does not reliably distinguish between MSA and PSP (Savoiardo et al. 1994).

Quantitative MR using MRI volumetry (MRV) with a region-of-interest (ROI) approach was recently used to compare the volume loss of different individual brain structures. Significant volume reduction in striatum, brainstem, and cerebellum were commonly reported in MSA. This technique may help differentiate MSA from PD. More recently, there have been a few studies using voxel based morphometry (VBM) for the quantitative assessment of basal ganglia and infratentorial volume in MSA (Brenneis et al. 2006). One study was also showed more prominent infratentorial region abnormalities in MSA-C compared with MSA-P (Minnerop et al. 2007). Volume loss in several cortical regions was demonstrated in both MSA subtypes in these studies. Diffusion-weighted imaging (DWI) was an alternative quantitative MRI technique which has proved useful for discriminating PD and MSA. Increased diffusivity of putamen and MCP was consistently found in patients with MSA in different studies (Schocke et al. 2004, Seppi et al. 2006a). Although increased putaminal diffusivity was also reported in PSP but this abnormality in MCP was more likely to be seen in MSA-P compared with PSP (Nicoletti et al. 2006). A recent longitudinal study also suggested that DWI may be useful for monitoring disease progression in MSA patients (Seppi et al. 2006b).

Neuroimaging studies using radioligands

The use of positron emission tomography (PET) in defining the morphological and neurochemical characteristics of the cerebral lesions in MSA and PAF are described in Chapter 40. Allied investigations include the use of SPECT (Schulz et al. 1994, Pirker et al. 1997).

Presynaptic dopaminergic imaging studies (PET or SPECT) may help separate parkinsonian disorders from non-parkinsonian conditions but cannot distinguish MSA from other parkinsonian syndromes. In contrast the postsynaptic dopaminergic imaging using dopamine (D2) receptor binding using [123I]iodobenzamide (IBZM) SPECT was shown to be useful for differentiating MSA-P and PD. Although reduced putaminal D2 receptor binding was commonly seen in MSA while normal D2 availability was usually normal or elevated in PD, the overlapping ranges between MSA-P and PD partly explained the lower accuracy compared to DWI-MRI in separating these disorders.

18F-fluorodeoxyglucose (18F-FDG) PET was also helpful for detecting the difference between typical from atypical parkinsonian disorders, particularly when combined with computer-assisted statistical parametric mapping. Striatal, brainstem and cerebellar hypometabolism were commonly seen in MSA patients while increased metabolism in putamen and reduced frontotemporal metabolism were found in most patients with PD.

Cardiac 123I-meta-iodobenzyl guanidine (MIBG) imaging has been helpful for make a distinction between PD and MSA. A number of previous studies demonstrated that cardiac MIBG uptake is markedly reduced in Parkinson's disease even in the early stage of disease (Spiegel et al. 2005) which is resulting from postganglionic sympathetic dysfunction. This uptake was typically normal in MSA which can be explained by the preganglionic lesion in nature. Previous studies using MIBG to identify patients with PD from normal subjects showed that the sensitivity varies from 84.3% to 89.7%, and specificity ranged from 89.5% to 94.6% when using MIBG for discriminating between PD from MSA (Braune 2001, Sawada et al. 2009). According to these results, cardiac MIBG may provide an additional benefit for separating PD and MSA when using it as a further investigation. However, the considerable overlap in the reduction of cardiac reuptake between PD, MSA, DLB and PSP indicated that MIBG cannot entirely discriminate PD from these disorders.

Brainstem auditory evoked potentials

The usefulness of brainstem auditory evoked responses in providing an easier, non-invasive means of assessing the integrity of brainstem function in multiple sclerosis (Prasher and Gibson 1980) led us to investigate its use in patients with AF (Prasher and Bannister 1986). A group of patients with PAF and uncomplicated PD failed to show any abnormality. However, in nearly all patients with MSA there was a disruption of the brainstem responses in the pontomedullary region with delay or reduction of components of the response generated beyond this region (Fig. 39.4). The brainstem auditory evoked potentials, which are now widely available, may be helpful in distinguishing at an early stage the patients developing MSA from the patients with PAF, in whom the prognosis is so much better and the management easier. These findings have been confirmed by Vamatsu et al. (1987).

Cognitive events-related potentials

Cognitive event-related potentials provide a unique means of separating decision processes from motor involvement. The cerebral potentials are associated with information processing, especially the timing of sensory stimulus discrimination and categorization, together with the reaction time measures. These studies were undertaken in four patients with MSA at the National Hospital Human Movement and Balance Unit (D. K. Prasher, personal communication). They showed normal results by comparison with patients with PD, in whom they were all delayed. These findings are of interest in view of normal intellectual function in MSA.

Distinction between multiple system atrophy with striatonigral degeneration and olivopontocerebellar atrophy

Clearly, there are difficulties in distinguishing clinically the degree of SND and OPCA in patients with the features of both. In our experience careful attempts to elicit signs of striatonigral disease and cerebellar disease will usually give a correct diagnosis of MSA as judged by the only real criterion, the ultimate pathological verification. There may be only limited value in striving clinically to separate SND from OPCA, although we attempt to do so on the grounds of clinical signs at diagnosis. PET studies suggest that subclinical nigrostriatal involvement is present in most patients with the cerebellar form of MSA (Rinne et al. 1995) and the ultimate pathology usually shows the changes of both MSA and OPCA (Fearnley and Lees 1990) (Chapter 41), even though in life one form may predominate at first diagnosis and in the early stages. The association with AF, however, marks out the cerebellar form of MSA from the other progressive cerebellar syndromes, especially

predominantly inherited cases, which have little relationship with SND (Gilman and Quinn 1996).

Autonomic failure and Parkinson's disease

The question of whether, and to what degree, autonomic involvement occurs in PD has been discussed for many years (Obeso et al. 2010). The problem has been confused by the clinical description of supposed minor autonomic disturbances in PD, whose significance is difficult to assess, such as greasy skin or unequal pupils. Autonomic impairment, and in particular postural hypotension, in a patient with parkinsonism may be due to a variety of possibilities (Table 39.1), including unexpected effects of drugs, as has been described with selegiline (Churchyard et al. 1997). Autonomic involvement should be defined as measurable sympathetic or parasympathetic dysfunction, assessed by physiological or biochemical means (Mathias 2009). If a battery of tests of the kind described in Chapter 22 is undertaken, some parkinsonian patients can have AF according to defined autonomic criteria or localized AF, unlike PD+AF, which results in subtle or modest autonomic dysfunction. As alluded to earlier in the introduction, the exact prevalence of AF, and even localized AF, in PD is unclear with differences in reports due to various factors such as differences in definitions of AF, experimental methods and the type of patient studied, as well as other factors such as increasing age, disease duration and drug therapies. The AF syndrome associated with PD as defined by these tests is less common than the association of AF with MSA, particularly in the early stages of PD where autonomic disturbances may be modest or subtle (Asahina et al. 2012). The mechanisms for autonomic dysfunction/failure in PD may involve a variety of factors, including, lewy body accumulation and cell loss in key autonomic regulatory areas, such as the hypothalamus, medulla, locus coeruleus and raphe, dorsal vagal motor nuclei, intermediolateral cell column and autonomic ganglia, cardiac sympathetic denervation and alpha-synuclein pathology in the ventrolateral medulla and enteric plexus (Asahina et al. 2012).

Clinical distinction between multiple system atrophy and Parkinson's disease

The differential diagnosis clinically between MSA and PD can sometimes be difficult. There are, however, certain clinical features that should make the clinician suspicious that the true diagnosis is MSA, and not PD. Until the diagnosis becomes unequivocal clinically, which is usually within a year or so of presentation, it may sometimes be justified to preface the diagnosis with 'probable'. In this group a patient with the diagnosis of probable PD may well become a patient with probable MSA. The clinical features favouring a clinical diagnosis of MSA may be listed.

◆ *Marked orthostatic hypotension*—mild orthostatic hypotension occurs in PD and this effect is exaggerated by the action of levodopa used in its treatment. The hypotension may be worse on standing or after exercise and food.

◆ *Levodopa unresponsiveness*—it should be remembered, however, that about 30% of patients with MSA show a significant but short-lived improvement in their akinetic-rigid symptoms when taking levodopa (Chapter 46).

◆ *Erectile impotence* in males, some in their forties (Chapter 38) is unlikely to be prominent in PD, though, of course, it will be present if the AF syndrome is associated with PD.

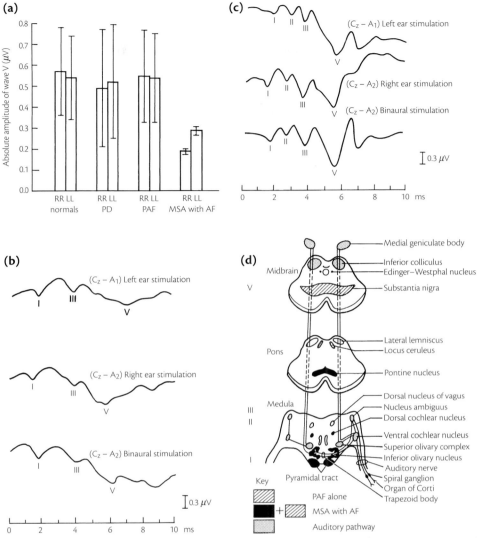

Fig. 39.4 **(a)** Mean and standard deviation of absolute amplitude of Wave V for the groups tested; PD, Parkinson's disease; PAF, pure autonomic failure; MSA with AF, multiple system atrophy with autonomic failure. Note the major reduction in the mean and variance of the amplitude of wave V in MSA. **(b)** Brainstem responses of MSA: bilateral abnormalities more severe on the left. **(c)** Brainstem responses of PAF: normal in amplitude and latency. **(d)** This diagram shows sites involved in PAF alone that clearly do not affect the brainstem auditory evoked potential. As these sites, which involve central autonomic control, are also affected in MSA it is necessary to exclude the site common to both syndrome. Therefore, by subtraction, the remaining sites in which degeneration is exclusive to the MSA component of the syndrome may be obtained. The auditory pathways are also shown with the Roman numerals indicating the generator sites of the brainstem potentials.

Table 39.1 Possible causes of postural hypotension and autonomic dysfunction in a patient with parkinsonian features

◆ Multiple system atrophy
◆ Parkinson's disease with autonomic failure
◆ Side-effects of anti-parkinsonian therapy including levodopa and selegiline
◆ Coincidental disease causing autonomic dysfunction such as diabetes mellitus
◆ Concomitant administration of drugs for an allied condition:
• antihypertensives (for hypertension)
• α-adrenoceptor blockers (for benign prostatic hyperplasia)

Adapted from Mathias 1996, with permission.

◆ *Urinary symptoms*, usually frequency, urgency, and a poor and intermittent stream (Chapter 37) raise the suspicion of MSA when they occur in younger males or in older males in the absence of prostatic hypertrophy, or in women in the absence of other causes such as pelvic trauma with multiple births.

◆ Mild pyramidal or cerebellar signs or both.

◆ A parkinsonian syndrome in which *rigidity and akinesis* are more marked than tremor.

◆ *Nocturnal stridor*, which may be inspiratory or expiratory and may be extraordinarily loud, sometimes likened to the braying of a donkey. The recent onset of snoring at night or sudden inspiratory gasps during the day may be a warning of more rapid progression of the disease.

It should be stressed that the diagnosis of MSA can be difficult but can only be based on clinical features and investigation. The most that can be expected is a probable diagnosis which may eventually be confirmed at post-mortem. The accuracy of diagnoses clinically at two stages, prior to death and histological confirmation, have confirmed previous impressions that MSA is underdiagnosed (Litvan et al. 1997).

Clinical distinction between pure autonomic failure and early multiple system atrophy

There is a second area in which diagnosis can be difficult. The wrong clinical diagnosis of PAF may be made in a patient who is in fact in the earliest stage of developing MSA or, much less commonly, PD. We made this error in a 68-year-old with severe postural hypotension but no other detectable signs of a neurological disorder. We thought she had PAF. We did, however, note that her plasma noradrenaline was in the normal range which should have made us suspicious that she might be developing MSA. In fact, 2 years after postural hypotension had been diagnosed, she developed a tremor of one hand. In the course of the next 18 months she developed all the signs of an akinetic-rigid syndrome with nocturnal stridor requiring a tracheostomy; in other words she had typical MSA. After this experience we have made the plasma noradrenaline value an essential part of the investigation of all our patients. The progression of symptoms was also useful to distinguish MSA and PAF. Sudomotor dysfunction is more likely to occur earlier in PAF. Respiratory dysfunction was not present in PAF in contrast to patients with MSA (Mabuchi et al. 2005).

Clinical course of primary autonomic failure

The clinical progression of patients with PAF is relatively benign since the hypotensive symptoms can usually be controlled (Chapter 47), so that life expectancy is only a little reduced; sphincter disturbance may be minimal. Occasionally, patients may survive from diagnosis for more than 20 years, raising the possibility that in some the lesion is non-progressive.

A recent study confirmed the rapid deterioration of conditions in MSA compared with patients with PAF, who had slower disease progression and better prognosis (Mabuchi et al. 2005).

Patients with AF and PD fare less well than patients with uncomplicated PD but, again, may survive for many years.

Patients with MSA face a distressing progression of their disability, unmitigated by any loss of insight, as their intelligence is almost always preserved. They often remain surprisingly cheerful, especially when attempts to help them with various drug regimens are pursued. The attempts are entirely justifiable since there is never any single drug regimen that can be applied automatically to patients with such a variety of sites and extents of their lesions. However, within a few years, some patients with MSA can barely move, due to the extrapyramidal and pyramidal weakness, and have a sphincter disturbance that may be helped but cannot be cured. Their survival is considerably poorer than for patients with PAF. The survival curves in various series indicate a mean of 7.5 years (Testa et al. 1996), 8.9 years (Schulz et al. 1994), and 9.3 years (Wenning et al. 1994), consistent with our earlier observations.

When the parkinsonian and cerebellar forms were compared, there did not appear to be a difference between the groups (Testa et al. 1996). Of clinical relevance is the individual survival, from 1 year to 15 years, again a wide range as we had noted previously. The pre-terminal development is often sleep apnoea or stridor.

Death in sleep may be due to stridor or apnoea causing hypoxia and may sometimes be a providential release. The denervation super-sensitivity of α- and β-adrenoceptors of the heart may render these patients more liable to cardiac arrhythmias from which they may die, as in patients with diabetic autonomic neuropathy (Page and Watkins 1978).

Despite all the physiological, biochemical, and pharmacological investigations in patients with AF, it must be stressed that the diagnosis remains a clinical one in individual cases. The final verification of the correctness of the diagnosis lies in the post-mortem examination (Chapter 41), but, from a practical point of view, the diagnosis in life is important because of the prognostic implications and the consideration of supportive and preventative aspects of care of the patient's acute and other disabilities. In order to help patients, their partners, relatives, and carers, support organizations have been formed; in the UK 'The Multiple System Atrophy Trust', currently focuses on MSA and the primary AF syndromes, and in the USA, the Shy–Drager Association has similar interests.

References

Abele, M., Schulz, J. B., Bürk, K., Topka, H., Dichgans, J., Klockgether, T. (2000). Nerve conduction studies in multiple system atrophy. *Eur Neurol.* **43**(4), 221–3.

Adams, R. D., van Bogaert, L., van der Eecken, H. (1964). Striato-nigral degeneration. *J. Neuropathol. Exp. Neurol.* **23**, 584–608.

Akaogi, Y., Asahina, M., Yamanaka, Y., Koyama, Y., Hattori, T. (2009). Sudomotor, skin vasomotor, and cardiovascular reflexes in 3 clinical forms of Lewy body disease. *Neurology.* **73**(1), 59–65.

Allcock, L.M., *et al.* (2004), Frequency of orthostatic hypotension in a community based cohort of patients with Parkinson's disease. *J Neurol Neurosurg Psychiatry.* **75**(10), 1470–1.

Anderson, T., *et al.* (2008). Oculomotor function in multiple system atrophy: clinical and laboratory features in 30 patients. *Mov Disord.* **23**(7), 977–84.

Asahina, M., Vichayanrat, E., Low, D. A., Iodice, V., and Mathias, C. J. (2012). Autonomic dysfunction in parkinsonian disorders: assessment and pathophysiology. *J Neurol. Neurosurg. Psychiatry.* [Epub ahead of print].

Bannister, R., Ardill, L., and Fentem, P. (1967). Defective autonomic control of blood vessels in idiopathic orthostatic hypotension. *Brain* **90**, 725–46.

Bannister, R., Gibson, W., Michaels, L., and Oppenheimer, D. R. (1981). Laryngeal abductor paralysis in multiple system atrophy. *Brain* **104**, 351–68.

Bannister, R. and Oppenheimer, D. R. (1972). Degenerative diseases of the nervous system associated with AF. *Brain* **95**, 457–74.

Bhattacharya, K., *et al.* (2002), Brain magnetic resonance imaging in multiple-system atrophy and Parkinson disease: a diagnostic algorithm. *Arch Neurol.* **59**(5), 835–42.

Bleasdale-Barr, K. M. and Mathias, C. J. (1998). Neck and other muscle pains in AF: their association with orthostatic hypotension. *J. Roy. Sci. Med.* 91, 355–9.

Bower, J. H., Maraganore, D. M., McDonnell, S. K., Rocca, W. A. (1997). Incidence of progressive supranuclear palsy and multiple system atrophy in Olmsted County, Minnesota, 1976 to 1990. *Neurology.* **49**, 1284–88.

Braune, S. (2001), The role of cardiac metaiodobenzylguanidine uptake in the differential diagnosis of parkinsonian syndromes. *Clin Auton Res.* **11**(6), 351–5.

Brenneis, C., *et al.* (2006), Cortical atrophy in the cerebellar variant of multiple system atrophy: a voxel-based morphometry study. *Mov Disord.* **21**(2), 159–65.

Brown, R. T., Polinsky, R. J., DiChiro, G., Pastakia, B., Wener, L., and Simmons, J. T. (1987). MRI in AF. *J. Neurol. Neurosurg. Psychiat.* **50**, 913–14.

Chang, C.C., *et al.* (2009), Cognitive deficits in multiple system atrophy correlate with frontal atrophy and disease duration. *Eur J Neurol.* **16**(10), 1144–50.

Chrysostome, V., Tison, F., Yekhlef, F., Sourgen, C., Baldi, I., Dartigues, J. F. (2004). Epidemiology of multiple system atrophy: a prevalence and pilot risk factor study in Aquitaine, France. *Neuroepidemiology.* **23**, 201–208.

Churchyard, A., Mathias, C. J., Boonkongchuen, P., and Lees, A. J. (1997). Autonomic effects of selegiline: possible cardiovascular toxicity in Parkinson's disease. *J. Neurol. Neurosurg. Psychiat.* **63**, 228–34.

Cohen, J., Low, P., Fealey, R., Sheps, S., and Jiang, N.-S. (1987). Somatic and autonomic function in progressive AF and multiple system atrophy. *Ann. Neurol.* **22**, 692–9.

Colosimo, C., Albanese, A., Hughes, A. J., De Bruin, V. M. S., and Lees, A. J. (1995). Some specific clinical features differentiate multiple system atrophy (striato-nigral variety) from Parkinson's disease. *Arch. Neurol.* **52**, 294–8.

Consensus statement (1996). Consensus statement on the definition of orthostatic hypotension, pure AF and multiple system atrophy. *Clin. Auton. Res.* **6**, 125–6.

Dabby, R., Djaldetti, R., Shahmurov, M., *et al.* (2006). Skin biopsy for assessment of autonomic denervation in Parkinson's disease. *J Neural Transm.* **113**(9), 1169–76. Epub 2006 Jul 13.

Donadio, V., Cortelli, P., Elam, M., *et al.* (2010) Autonomic innervation in multiple system atrophy and pure AF. *J Neurol. Neurosurg. Psychiatry.* **81**(12), 1327–35.

Donadio, V., Montagna, P., Nolano, M., *et al.* (2005). Generalised anhidrosis: different lesion sites demonstrated by microneurography and skin biopsy. *J Neurol. Neurosurg. Psychiatry.* **76**(4), 588–91.

Donadio, V., Nolano, M., Elam, M., *et al.* (2008). Anhidrosis in multiple system atrophy: a preganglionic sudomotor dysfunction? *Mov Disord.* **30**;23(6), 885–8.

Fearnley, J. M., Lees, A. J. (1990). Striatonigral degeneration: a clinico-pathological study. *Brain* **113**, 1823–42.

Fetoni, V., Genitrini, S., Monza, D. *et al.* (1997). Variations in axial, proximal and distal motor response to L-dopa in multisystem atrophy and Parkinson's disease. *Clin. Neuropharmacol.* **20**, 239–44.

Fulham, M. J., Dubinsky, R. M., Polinsky, R. J., *et al.* (1991). Computed tomography, magnetic resonance imaging and positron emission tomography with [18F] fluorodeoxyglucose in multiple system atrophy and pure AF. *Clin. Auton. Res.* **1**, 27–36.

Ghaemi, M., *et al.* (2002), Differentiating multiple system atrophy from Parkinson's disease: contribution of striatal and midbrain MRI volumetry and multi-tracer PET imaging. *J Neurol Neurosurg Psychiatry.* **73**(5), 517–23.

Giladi, N., Simon, E. S., Korczyn, A. D. *et al.* (2000). Anal sphincter EMG does not distinguish between multiple system atrophy and Parkinson's disease. *Muscle Nerve.* **23**, 731–4.

Giladi, R., Giladi, N., Korczyn, A. D., Gurevich, T., Sadeh, M. (2001). Quantitative anal sphincter EMG in multisystem atrophy and 100 controls. *J Neurol Neurosurg Psychiatry.* **71**, 596–9.

Gilman, S., Wenning, G. K., Low, P. A., *et al.* (2008). Second consensus statement on the diagnosis of multiple system atrophy. *Neurology.* **71**(9), 670–6.

Gilman, S. and Quinn, N. P. (1996). The relationship of MSA to sporadic olivopontocerebellar atrophy and other forms of late onset cerebellar atrophy. *Neurology* **46**, 1197–9.

Giustina, A., Veldhuis, J. D. (1998). Pathophysiology of the neuroregulation of growth hormone secretion in experimental animals and the human. *Endocr Rev.* **19**, 717–97.

Goldstein, D.S., Sewell, L, and Holmes, C. (2010). Association of anosmia with AF in Parkinson disease. *Neurology.* **74**(3), 245–51.

Guilleminault, C., Tilkian, A., Lehrman, K., Forno, L., and Dement, W. C. (1977). Sleep apnoea syndrome: states of sleep and autonomic dysfunction. *J. Neurol. Neurosurg. Psychiat.* **40**, 718–25.

Guindi, G. M., Bannister, R., Gibson, W., and Payne, J. K. (1981). Laryngeal electromyography in multiple system atrophy with AF. *J. Neurol. Neurosurg. Psychiat.* **44**, 49–53.

Guindi, G. M., Michaels, M., Bannister, R., and Gibson, W. (1980). Pathology of the intrinsic muscles of the larynx. *Clin. Otolaryngol.* **6**, 101–9.

Harcourt, J., Spraggs, P., Mathias, C., and Brookes, G. (1996). Sleep-related breathing disorders in the Shy-Drager syndrome. Observations on investigation and management. *Eur. J. Neurol.* **3**, 186–90.

Harding, A. E. (1981). Idiopathic late onset cerebellar ataxia. A clinical and genetic study of 36 cases. *J. Neurol. Sci.* **51**, 259–71.

Heims, H.C., *et al.*, (2006). Cognitive functioning in orthostatic hypotension due to pure AF. *Clin Auton Res.* **16**(2), 113–20.

Hillen, M.E., Wagner, M. L., and Sage, J. I. (1996). 'Subclinical' orthostatic hypotension is associated with dizziness in elderly patients with Parkinson disease. *Arch Phys Med Rehabil.* **77**(7), 710–2.

Horimoto, Y., *et al* (2003). Autonomic dysfunctions in dementia with Lewy bodies. *J Neurol.* **250**(5), 530–3

Huang, Y. O. and Plaitakis, A. (1984). Morphological changes of olivopontocerebellar atrophy in computed tomography and comments on its pathogenesis. *Adv. Neurol.* **41**, 39–85.

Hughes, A. J., Daniel, S. E., Kilford, L., and Lees, A. J. (1992). The accuracy of clinical diagnosis of idiopathic Parkinson's disease: a clinical pathological study of 100 cases. *J. Neurol. Neurosurg. Psychiat.* **55**, 181–2.

Ikemura, M., Saito, Y., Sengoku, R., *et al.* (2008). Lewy body pathology involves cutaneous nerves. *J Neuropathol Exp Neurol.* **67**(10), 945–53.

Iodice, V., Low, D. A., Vichayanrat E. and Mathias, C. J. (2011). Cardiovascular autonomic dysfunction in MSA and Parkinson's Disease: similarities and differences. *J Neurol. Sci.* **310**, 133–8.

Iodice, V., Low, D. A., Vichayanrat, E. and Mathias, C. J. (2012). Cardiovascular autonomic dysfunction in Parkinson's disease and Parkinsonian dyndromes. In *Parkinson's Disease.* (Eds. M. Ebadi, Z. K. Wszolek and R. F. Pfeiffer). pp 353–374. Florida: CRC Press.

Kanda, T., Tsukagoshi, H., Oda, M., Miyamoko, K., and Tanabe, H. (1996). Changes of unmyelinated fibres in sural nerve in ALS, PD and MSA. *Acta Neuropath. Berlin* **91**, 145–54.

Kawai, Y., *et al.* (2008). Cognitive impairments in multiple system atrophy: MSA-C vs MSA-P. *Neurology.* **70**(16 Pt 2), 1390–6.

Khurana, R. K. (1994). Cholinergic dysfunction in Shy–Drager syndrome: effect of the parasympathomimetic agent, bethanechol. *Clin. Auton. Res.* **4**, 5–13.

Khurana, R. K., Nelson, E., Azzarelli, B., and Garcia, J. H. (1980). Shy–Drager syndrome: diagnosis and treatment of cholinergic dysfunction. *Neurology, Minneapolis* **30**, 805–9.

Kluin, K. J., Gilman, S., Lohman, M., and Junck, L. (1996). Characteristics of dysarthria of multiple system atrophy. *Arch. Neurol.* **53**, 545–8.

Konagaya, Y., Konagaya, M., and Iida, M. (1994). Clinical and magnetic resonance imaging study of extrapyramidal syndromes in multiple system atrophy. *J. Neurol. Neurosurg. Psychiat.* **57**, 1528–31.

Kujawa, K., *et al.* (2000), Acute orthostatic hypotension when starting dopamine agonists in Parkinson's disease. *Arch Neurol.* **57**(10), 1461–3.

Köllensperger, M., Geser, F., Ndayisaba, J. P., *et al.*; EMSA-SG (2010). Presentation, diagnosis, and management of multiple system atrophy in Europe: final analysis of the European multiple system atrophy registry. *Mov Disord.*, **15**;25(15), 2604–12.

Larner, A. J., Mathias, C. J., and Rossor, M. N. (2000). AF preceding dementia with Lewy bodies. *J Neurol.* **247**(3), 229–31.

Lipp, A., Sandroni, P., Ahlskog, J. E., *et al.* (2009). Prospective differentiation of multiple system atrophy from Parkinson disease, with and without AF. *Arch Neurol.* **66**(6), 742–50.

Litvan, I., Goetz, C. G., Jankovic, J. *et al.* (1997). What is the accuracy of the clinical diagnosis of multiple system atrophy? *Arch. Neurol.* **54**, 937–44.

Lo, S. S., Mathias, C. J., St. John Sutton & M. (1996). QT interval and dispersion in primary AF. *Heart* **75**, (5), 498–501.

Lockwood, A. H. (1976). The Shy–Drager syndrome with abnormal respiration and antidiuretic hormone release. *Arch. Neurol., Chicago* **33**, 292–5.

Mabuchi, N., *et al.* (2005), Progression and prognosis in pure AF (PAF): comparison with multiple system atrophy. *J Neurol Neurosurg Psychiatry.* **76**(7), 947–52.

Mathias, C. J. (1996). Gastrointestinal dysfunction in multiple system atrophy. *Sem. Neurol.* **16**, 251–8.

Mathias, C. J. (1996). Disorders affecting autonomic function in parkinsonian patients. In: *Parkinson's Disease*, (ed. L. Battistin, G. Scarlato, T. Caraceni, and S. Ruggieri.) *Advances in Neurology*, **69**, pp. 383–91, Lippincott-Raven, Philadelphia.

Mathias, C. J. and Kimber, J. R. (1999). Postural hypotension: causes, clinical features, investigation, and management. *Annu Rev Med.* **50**, 317–36.

Mathias, C. J. (2009). Autonomic Dysfunction. In: Clarke, C., Howard, R., Rossor, M., and Shorvon, S. (eds). *Neurology: A Queen Square Textbook.* 1st Edition. Chichester: Wiley Blackwell. pp. 871–92.

McKeith, I. G., Dickson, D. W., Lowe, J., *et al.* (2005). Diagnosis and management of dementia with Lewy bodies: third report of the DLB Consortium. *Neurology.* **65**, 1863–72.

Meco, G., L. Pratesi, and V. Bonifati (1991), Cardiovascular reflexes and autonomic dysfunction in Parkinson's disease. *J Neurol.* **238**(4), 195–9.

Miki, Y., Tomiyama, M., Ueno, T., *et al.* (2010). Clinical availability of skin biopsy in the diagnosis of Parkinson's disease. *Neurosci Lett.* 2010 29;**469**(3), 357–9.

Minnerop, M. *et al.* (2007), Voxel-based morphometry and voxel-based relaxometry in multiple system atrophy-a comparison between clinical subtypes and correlations with clinical parameters. *Neuroimage.* **36**(4), 1086–95.

Monza, D., Soliveri, P., Radice, D. *et al.* (1998). Cognitive dysfunction and impaired organization of complex motility in degenerative parkinsonian syndromes. *Arch. Neurol.* **55**, 372–8.

Muller, E. E., Locatelli, V., Cocchi, D. (1999). Neuroendocrine control of growth hormone secretion. *Physiol. Rev.* **79**:511–607.

Munschauer, F., Loh, L., Bannister, R., and Newsom Davis, J. (1990). Abnormal respiration and sudden death during sleep in multiple system atrophy with AF. *Neurology* **40**, 677–9.

Nicoletti, G., *et al.* (2006), Apparent diffusion coefficient measurements of the middle cerebellar peduncle differentiate the Parkinson variant of MSA from Parkinson's disease and progressive supranuclear palsy. *Brain.* **129**(Pt 10), 2679–87.

Nolano, M., Provitera, V., Estraneo, A., *et al.* (2008) Sensory deficit in Parkinson's disease: evidence of a cutaneous denervation. *Brain*, **131** (Pt 7), 1903–11.

Obeso, J. A., *et al.* (2010). Missing pieces in the Parkinson's disease puzzle. *Nat. Med.* **16**(6), 653–61.

Oka, H., Morita, M., Onouchi, K., Yoshioka, M., Mochio, S., Inoue, K. (2007) Cardiovascular autonomic dysfunction in dementia with Lewy bodies and Parkinson's disease. *J Neurol Sci.* 15;**254**(1–2), 72–7.

Page, M. McB. and Watkins, P. J. (1978). Cardiorespiratory arrest and diabetic autonomic neuropathy. *Lancet* **i**, 14–16.

Palace J., Chandiramani V. A., Fowler C. J. (1997). Value of sphincter electromyography in the diagnosis of multiple system atrophy. *Muscle Nerve* **20**, 1396–403.

Pastakia, B., Polinsky, R., DiChiro, G., Simmons, J. T., Brown, R., and Wener, L. (1987). Multiple system atrophy (Shy–Drager syndrome) MR imaging. *Radiology* **159**, 499–502.

Pellecchia, M.T., *et al.* (2011). Progression of striatal and extrastriatal degeneration in multiple system atrophy: A longitudinal diffusion-weighted MR study. *Mov Disord.* (Early view online version).

Pellecchia, M. T., Longo, K., Pivonello, R., *et al.* (2006) Multiple system atrophy is distinguished from idiopathic Parkinson's disease by the arginine growth hormone stimulation test. *Ann Neurol.* **60**(5), 611–5.

Pillon, B., Gouider-Khouja, N., Deweer, B. *et al.* (1995). Neuropsychological pattern of striatonigral degeneration: comparison with Parkinson's disease and progressive supranuclear palsy. *J. Neurol. Neurosurg. Psychiat.* **58**, 174–9.

Pirker, W., Asenbaum, S., Wenger, S. *et al.* (1997). Iodine 123-Epidepride-SPECT: Studies in Parkinson's disease, multiple system atrophy and Huntington's disease. *J. Nucl. Med.,* **38**, 1711–17

Pramstaller, P. P., Wenning, G. K., Smith, S. J., Beck, R.O., Quinn, N. P., and Fowler, C. J. (1995). Nerve conduction studies, skeletal muscle EMG and sphincter EMG in multiple system atrophy. *J. Neurol. Neurosurg. Psychiat.* **58**, 618–21.

Prasher, D. K., Bannister, R. (1986). Brainstem auditory evoked potentials in patients with multiple system atrophy with progressive AF (Shy–Drager syndrome). *J. Neurol. Neurosurg. Psychiat.* **49**, 278–89.

Prasher, D. K. and Gibson, P. R. (1980). Brainstem auditory evoked potentials. A comparative study of monaural vs binaural stimulation in the detection of multiple sclerosis. *J. Clin. Neurophysiol.* **50**, 247–53.

Rahkonen, T.,*et al.* (2003). Dementia with Lewy bodies according to the consensus criteria in a general population aged 75 years or older. *J Neurol Neurosurg Psychiatry.* **74**(6), 720–4.

Riley, D. E. and Chelimsky, T. C. (2003). Autonomic nervous system testing may not distinguish multiple system atrophy from Parkinson's disease. *J Neurol. Neurosurg. Psychiatry.* **74**(1), 56–60.

Rinne, J. O., Burn, D. J., Mathias, C. J., Quinn, N. P., Marsden, D. C., and Brooks, D. J. (1995). Positron emission tomography studies on the dopaminergic system and striatal opiod binding in the olivopontocerebellar atrophy variant of multiple system atrophy. *Ann. Neurol.* **37**, 568–73.

Ross Russell, R. W. and Page, N. G. R. (1983). Critical perfusion of brain and retina. *Brain* **106**, 419–34.

Sakakibara, R., Hattori, T., Uchiyama, T. *et al.* (2000) Urinary dysfunction and orthostatic hypotension in multiple system atrophy: which is the more common and earlier manifestation? *J Neurol Neurosurg Psychiatry.* **68**, 65–9.

Sandroni, P., *et al.* (1991), Autonomic involvement in extrapyramidal and cerebellar disorders. *Clin Auton Res.* **1**(2), 147–55.

Savoiardo, J. W., Bracchi, M., Passerini, A., Visciani, A., DiDonato, S., and Cocchinni, F. (1983). Computed tomography of olivopontocerebellar atrophy. *Am. J. Neuroradiol.* **4**, 509–12.

Savoiardo, M. *et al.* (1994). Magnetic resonance imaging in progressive supranuclear palsy and other parkinsonian disorders. *J. Neurol. Transm.* Suppl. **42**, 93–110.

Sawada, H., *et al.* (2009), Diagnostic accuracy of cardiac metaiodobenzylguanidine scintigraphy in Parkinson disease. *Eur J Neurol.* **16**(2), 174–82.

Schatz, I. J. (1996), Consensus statement on the definition of orthostatic hypotension, pure autonomic failure and multiple system atrophy. *Neurology.* **46**, 1470.

Schocke, M.F., *et al.* (2004). Trace of diffusion tensor differentiates the Parkinson variant of multiple system atrophy and Parkinson's disease. *Neuroimage.* **21**(4), 1443–51.

Schrag,A., Ben Shlomo, Y., Quinn, N. P. (1999) Prevalence of progressive supranuclear palsy and multiple system atrophy: a cross-sectional study. *Lancet,* **354**, 1771–75.

Schulz, J. B., Klockgether, T., Petersen, D. et al. (1994). Multiple system atrophy: natural history, MRI morphology, and dopamine receptor imaging with [123]IBZM-SPECT. J. Neurol. Neurosurg. Psychiat. **57**, 1047–56.

Schwarz, J., Kornhuber, M., Bischoff, C., Straube, A. (1997) Electromyography of the external anal sphincter in patients with Parkinson's disease and multiple system atrophy: frequency of abnormal spontaneous activity and polyphasic motor unit potentials. Muscle Nerve. **20**, 1167–72.

Senard, J.M., et al. (1997) Prevalence of orthostatic hypotension in Parkinson's disease. J Neurol Neurosurg Psychiatry. **63**(5), 584–9.

Seppi, K., et al. (2006a). Topography of putaminal degeneration in multiple system atrophy: a diffusion magnetic resonance study. Mov Disord. **21**(6), 847–52.

Seppi, K., et al. (2006b). Progression of putaminal degeneration in multiple system atrophy: a serial diffusion MR study. Neuroimage. **15**, 240–5.

Shishido, T., Ikemura, M., Obi, T., et al. (2010) alpha-synuclein accumulation in skin nerve fibers revealed by skin biopsy in pure AF. Neurology. **16**;74(7), 608–10.

Silveira-Moriyama, L., Mathias, C. J., Lydia M., et al (2009), Hyposmia in pure autonomic failure. Neurology, **72**(19), 1677–81.

Smith, G. D., Watson, L. P., Mathias, C. J. (1996). Neurohumoral, peptidergic and biochemical responses to supine exercise in two groups with primary autonomic failure: Shy-Drager syndrome/multiple system atrophy and pure autonomic failure. Clin. Auton. Res. **6**, 255–62.

Spiegel, J., et al. (2005), FP-CIT and MIBG scintigraphy in early Parkinson's disease. Mov Disord. **20**(5), 552–61.

Stefanova, N., Bücke, P., Duerr, S., Wenning, G. K. (2009) Multiple system atrophy: an update. Lancet Neurol. **8**(12), 1172–8.

Stevens, T., et al. (2002), Islington study of dementia subtypes in the community. Br J Psychiatry. **180**, 270–6.

Stocchi, F., Carbone, A., Inghilleri, M. et al. (1997). Urodynamic and neurophysiological evaluation in Parkinson's disease and multiple system atrophy. J Neurol Neurosurg Psychiatry. **62**, 507–11.

Swaminath, P.V., et al. (2010), Urogenital symptoms in Parkinson's disease and multiple system atrophy-Parkinsonism: at onset and later. J Assoc. Physicians India, **58**, 86–90.

Testa, D., Fetoni, V., Soliveri, P., Musicco, M., Palazzini, E., and Girotti, F. (1993). Cognitive and motor performance in multiplesystem atrophy and Parkinson's disease compared. Neuropsychologia **31**, 207–10.

Testa, D., Filippini, G., Farinotti, M., Palazzini, E., and Caraceni, T. (1996). Survival in multiple system atrophy: a study of prognostic factors in 59 cases. J. Neurol. **243**, 401–4.

Thomaides, T. N., et al. (1992), Growth hormone response to clonidine in central and peripheral primary autonomic failure. Lancet **340**(8814), 263–6.

Thomas, D. J. and Bannister, R. (1980). Preservation of autoregulation of cerebral blood flow in AF. J. Neurol. Sci. **44**, 205–12.

Tison F., Arne P., Sourgen C., Chrysostome V., Yeklef F. (2000). The value of external anal sphincter electromyography for the diagnosis of multiple system atrophy. Mov Disord. **15**, 1148–57.

Turkka, J. (1986). Autonomic dysfunction in Parkinson's disease. Acta universitatis Ouluensis **D142**, 15–66.

Uono, Y. (1973). Parkinsonism and autonomic dysfunction. Auton Nerv Syst (Tokyo). (10), 163–70.

Vamatsu, D., Hamada, J., and Gotoh, F. (1987). Brainstem auditory evoked responses and CT findings in multiple system atrophy. J. Neurol. Sci. **77**, 161–71.

Van Dijk, J.G., et al. (1993), Autonomic nervous system dysfunction in Parkinson's disease: relationships with age, medication, duration, and severity. J Neurol Neurosurg Psychiatry. **56**(10), 1090–5.

Velseboer, D. C., de Haan, R. J., Wieling, W. et al. (2011). Prevalence of orthostatic hypotension in Parkinson's disease: a systematic review and meta-analysis. Parkinsonism Relat. Disord. **17**, 724–9.

Wenning, G. K., Ben Shlomo, Y., Magalhaes, M., Daniel, S. E., and Quinn, N. P. (1994). Clinical features and natural history of multiple system atrophy. An analysis of 100 cases. Brain **117**, 835–45.

Wenning, G. K., Krismer, F., and Poewe, W. (2011). New insights into atypical parkinsonism. Curr Opin Neurol. **24**(4), 331–8.

Williams, A., Hanson, D., and Calne, D. B. (1979). Vocal cord paralysis in the Shy–Drager syndrome. J. Neurol. Neurosurg. Psychiatr. **42**, 151–3.

Winge, K., Jennum, P., Lokkegaard, A., Werdelin, L. (2010) Anal sphincter EMG in the diagnosis of parkinsonian syndromes. Acta Neurol Scand. **121**(3), 198–203.

Yamashita, F., et al. (2010). Pupillary autonomic dysfunction in multiple system atrophy and Parkinson's disease: an assessment by eye-drop tests. Clin Auton Res. **20**(3), 191–7.

Young, T. M., Asahina, M., Nicotra, A., Mathias, C. J. (2006). Skin vasomotor reflex responses in two contrasting groups of AF: multiple system atrophy and pure AF. J Neurol. **253**(7), 846–50.

Zhang, K., Zeng, Y., Song, C., Fu, Y., Wan, Q. (2010). The comparison of clonidine, arginine and both combined: a growth hormone stimulation test to differentiate multiple system atrophy from idiopathic Parkinson's disease. J Neurol. **257**(9), 1486–91.

CHAPTER 40

Neuroimaging in autonomic failure syndromes

David J. Brooks

Introduction

Neurodegenerative conditions associated with autonomic failure include Parkinson's disease (PD), multiple system atrophy (MSA), and pure autonomic failure (PAF). The pathological hallmark of idiopathic late-onset PD is degeneration of pigmented and other brainstem nuclei (substantia nigra compacta, locus coeruleus, dorsal nuclei of the vagus, nucleus accumbens, and nucleus basalis of Meynert) associated with neuronal Lewy inclusion bodies. Interestingly, it has been reported that Lewy bodies in the dorsal nucleus of the vagus may precede involvement of the substantia nigal compacta (Braak et al. 2003). This raises the question as to why autonomic failure is a relatively late manifestation of typical sporadic PD. The Lewy body is an eosinophilic inclusion that contains aggregated alpha-synuclein, degenerating neurofilaments, and shows ubiquitin immunoreactivity. The loss of cells from the substantia nigra results in profound dopamine depletion in the striatum, ventral projections to putamen being more affected than dorsal projections to head of caudate (Fearnley and Lees 1991, Kish et al. 1988).

The pathology of MSA targets the substantia nigra and putamen, brainstem and cerebellar nuclei, and the intermediolateral columns of the cord. It is associated with argyrophilic neuronal and glial inclusions which contain alpha-synuclein (Papp and Lantos 1994, Wenning and Jellinger 2005). The loss of nigrostriatal dopaminergic projections is more uniform in MSA than in PD, leading to a relatively greater involvement of caudate dopamine projections (Fearnley and Lees 1990, Goto et al. 1989). In its early stages MSA may present as autonomic failure, an akinetic-rigid syndrome (MSA-P) or as progressive ataxia (MSA-C). Around 50% of patients with the akinetic-rigid variant show an initial response to levodopa making it difficult to distinguish them from PD on clinical criteria alone (Fearnley and Lees 1990). In a retrospective clinical pathological series Litvan and colleagues reported that only 25% of MSA cases were initially diagnosed correctly and this had only improved to 50% at endstage (Litvan et al. 1998). Conversely, around 10% of cases initially thought to have PD are later found to have MSA at autopsy (Quinn 1989).

Those PAF patients who have come to autopsy have shown either degeneration of the intermediolateral columns of the spinal cord similar to that found in MSA or Lewy bodies in the substantia nigra and sympathetic ganglia (Vanderhaegen et al. 1970). It can be seen, therefore, that the reported pathology of PAF has overlap features with both MSA and PD.

The syndrome of MSA includes striatonigral degeneration (SND), now termed MSA-P, and olivopontocerebellar atrophy (OPCA), now termed MSA-C, as part of the spectrum. Argyrophilic neuronal and glial inclusions characteristic of MSA have been reported in both isolated SND and OPCA (Papp and Lantos 1994). At post-mortem patients clinically diagnosed as SND usually have subclinical cerebellar degeneration while patients diagnosed as sporadic OPCA show subclinical striatonigral degeneration.

In addition to sporadic MSA, there is a large series of hereditary spinocerebellar ataxias (SCA) (Klockgether et al. 2000, Wullner 2003). Those which are associated with CAG repeat expansions in their causatives genes (e.g. SCA1, SCA2, SCA3, SCA7) can also manifest parkinsonism along with or in the absence of cerebellar ataxia and so can mimic MSA, though they tend to present at a younger age, and autonomic dysfunction is rarely a feature.

Magnetic resonance imaging

Conventional structural T1 and T2-weighted magnetic resonance imaging (MRI) is of limited value for differentiating neurodegenerative disorders associated with autonomic failure. Frequently MRI is normal in these syndromes but, occasionally, PD patients may show increased signal from the substantia nigra on T2-weighted MRI (Duguid et al. 1986). High field MRI, utilizing special grey and white matter signal suppressing inversion recovery sequences, is more sensitive for detecting abnormal signal from the substantia nigra compacta in patients with PD. In one series (Hutchinson and Raff 2000) all 6 cases with established PD showed altered nigral signal while in a second series (Hu et al. 2001) 7 out of 10 patients showed nigral MRI abnormalities. All 10 cases of PD in this second series had reduced putamen 6-[^{18}F]fluorodopamine (F-DOPA) uptake. The true sensitivity and specificity of this MRI approach for detecting nigral degeneration remains to be established.

While the striatum appears normal on T2-weighted MRI in PD, in MSA the lateral putamen can show reduced signal due to iron deposition and this may be bordered by a rim of increased signal due to gliosis (Schrag et al. 2000) (Fig. 40.1). If concomitant pontocerebellar degeneration is also present the lateral as well as longitudinal pontine fibres become evident as high signal on T2 MRI manifesting as the 'hot-cross bun' sign. Cerebellar and pontine

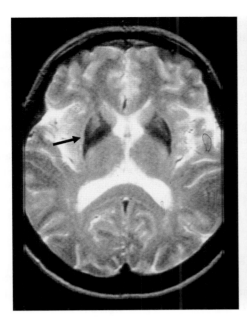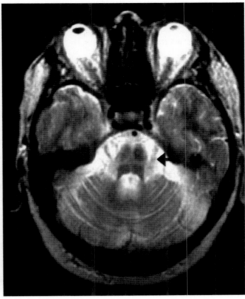

Fig. 40.1 T2-weighted magnetic resonance images showing low lateral putamen signal and the pontine 'hot-cross bun' sign in multiple system atrophy.

atrophy may be visually obvious with increased signal evident in the cerebellar peduncles (Savoiardo et al. 1990). These changes are usually only evident in patients with well established disease where putamen and brainstem atrophy can also be demonstrated with formal magnetic resonance volumetry.

More recently the use of diffusion-weighted imaging (DWI) and diffusion tensor MRI have been developed for discriminating atypical from typical parkinsonian syndromes. DWI reflects the movement of water molecules along fibre tracts in the brain—anisotropic diffusion. By applying static field gradients this anisotropy can be quantified as an apparent diffusion coefficient (ADC). In intact brain the central nervous system is organized in bundles of fibre tracts along which water molecules move. Degenerative disease removes restrictions to water molecule movement so reducing anisotropy and increasing the ADC. It has been reported that cases with clinically probable MSA-P can be discriminated from typical PD patients as they all show significantly higher regional ADC values in the putamen (Seppi et al. 2003). How sensitive this approach is for classifying grey parkinsonian cases is currently being determined.

Transcranial sonography

Transcranial sonography (TCS) allows the echogenicity of the midbrain and basal ganglia to be examined through temporal bone windows. In a series of 112 patients with clinically probable PD, TCS detected increased midbrain echogenicity in 103 of these subjects (Berg et al. 2001). This increased signal was most noticeable contralateral to the more clinically affected limbs and in patients with levodopa induced motor complications though did not correlate with disability rated with the Columbia University Rating Scale (CURS). Pathological studies have suggested that this nigral hyperechogenicity, when present, probably reflects the increased iron deposition present in parkinsonian nigra (Berg et al. 2002). However, in a 5-year follow up study of PD cases these workers reported that there was no significant change in TCS findings despite an increase in Unified Parkinson's Disease Rating Scale

(UPDRS) score from 26 to 45 (Berg et al. 2005). This suggests that midbrain hyperechogenicity may be a trait rather than state marker for susceptibility to PD.

A drawback from a diagnostic point of view is that 8.6% of elderly healthy individuals were also found to show midbrain hyperechogenicity (Berg et al. 1999). The presence of midbrain hyperechogenicity was associated with 'soft' signs of parkinsonism and, in half of these subjects, mildly but significantly reduced levels of striatal 6F-DOPA uptake. It remains to be seen how many of these TCS positive elderly individuals will convert to clinical PD.

TCS has been used to try and discriminate atypical from typical parkinsonian disorders. 16 MSA, 9 progressive supranuclear palsy (PSP), and 25 age-matched PD patients were prospectively studied and, whereas 24 of the 25 (96%) PD patients exhibited hyperechogenicity of the substantia nigra, only 2 of 23 (9%) atypical parkinsonian cases (1 MSA and 1 PSP) showed abnormal signal (p <0.001) (Walter et al. 2003). In contrast, lentiform nucleus hyperechogenicity was found in 17 out of 22 (77%) atypical parkinsonian patients but in only 5 of 22 (23%) IPD patients (p< 0.001). The PSP cases showed a widened third ventricle compared with the PD and MSA cases. These findings are of interest and suggest that TCS may have a role for discriminating MSA from PD. To date, only clinical probable cases have been studied and so it is not clear how well this technique would perform with early grey cases. A puzzling finding is the lack of midbrain hyperechogenicity in MSA as it is well established that nigral degeneration is present in these patients at post-mortem.

Functional imaging

Functional imaging provides a means of detecting and characterizing *in vivo* the regional changes in brain metabolism and receptor binding that characterize disorders of autonomic function. There are three main approaches to functional imaging:

◆ Positron emission tomography (PET) allows quantitative examination of regional cerebral blood flow (rCBF), glucose and oxygen metabolism (rCMRGlc, rCMRO$_2$), and brain pharmacology.

- Single photon emission computed tomography (SPECT) gives semi-quantitative estimates of rCBF and receptor binding.
- Proton magnetic resonance spectroscopy allows *in vivo* measurements of brain metabolism and pH.

Metabolic studies

[18]F-fluorodeoxyglucose (^{18}F-FDG) PET measurements of resting regional cerebral glucose metabolism (rCMRGlc) primarily reflect the metabolic activity of synaptic vesicles in nerve terminals. Consequently, levels of basal ganglia glucose metabolism provide a measure of metabolic activity of interneurons and afferent projections to those nuclei but not the activity of basal ganglia efferent projections. In levodopa (L-3,4-dihydroxyphenylalanine [L-DOPA]) responsive hemiparkinsonian patients with early disease, ^{18}F-FDG PET shows relatively increased lentiform nucleus glucose metabolism contralateral to the affected limbs (Miletich et al. 1988). PD patients with established bilateral disease have normal levels of striatal metabolism though covariance analysis reveals an abnormal metabolic pattern with relatively raised lentiform nucleus and reduced frontal rCMRGlc (Eidelberg et al. 1990).

^{18}F-FDG PET studies in patients with the full syndrome of sporadic MSA reveal reduced levels of striatal, cerebellar, and brainstem glucose metabolism (Gilman et al. 1994) (Fig. 40.2). In patients with clinically probable MSA-P (levodopa resistant parkinsonism without autonomic failure or ataxia) levels of striatal glucose metabolism have also been reported to be reduced (De Volder et al. 1989, Eidelberg et al. 1993, Otsuka et al. 1991). Eidelberg and co-workers also reported that akinetic-rigid patients with low levels of striatal glucose metabolism, irrespective of their levodopa response, showed little improvement after pallidotomy (Eidelberg et al. 1996). Overall, ^{18}F-FDG PET detects the presence of striatal degeneration in over 80% of early cases where atypical parkinsonism is suspected.

Fulham and colleagues reported patterns of brain ^{18}F-FDG uptake in seven MSA-C patients with autonomic failure and in eight pure autonomic failure patients (clinical disease duration 5–26 years) (Fulham et al. 1991). They found significantly reduced cerebellar and frontal glucose utilization in the MSA-C patients but normal levels of rCMRGlc in PAF. These findings suggest that

PET may provide a potential means of delineating whether patients presenting with isolated autonomic failure have PAF or a multisystem disturbance. Glucose utilization has also been examined in cases of sporadic and familial OPCA (Gilman et al. 1994, Rosenthal et al. 1988). The OPCA patients showed reduced cerebellar and brainstem glucose metabolism; individual levels correlating inversely with the level of ataxia present.

Proton magnetic resonance spectroscopy (MRS) also provides a potential means of discriminating MSA from PD. N-acetyl aspartate (NAA) is found in high concentrations in neurons and is believed to be a metabolic marker of neuronal integrity. Reduced NAA:creatine ratios in the proton MRS signal from the lentiform nucleus in 6 of 7 clinically probable MSA-P cases has been reported, whereas 8 of 9 probable PD cases showed normal levels of putamen NAA (Davie et al. 1995).

Dopaminergic dysfunction

F-DOPA PET is a marker of dopamine terminal dopa decarboxylase activity and dopamine storage capacity. ^{11}C-nomifensine binds to dopamine transporters (DAT) on nigrostriatal terminals as do tropane tracers such as ^{123}I-beta-CIT and ^{123}I-FP-CIT. and so also provide a measure of the functional integrity of nigrostriatal projections (Tedroff et al. 1990, Brooks et al., 1990b, Leenders et al. 1990).

In patients with clinically probable MSA-P the function of both the presynaptic and postsynaptic dopaminergic systems are impaired. As in PD, putamen 6F-DOPA uptake is reduced to around 50% of normal levels in established MSA-P and individual levels of putamen 6F-DOPA uptake correlate with locomotor status (Brooks et al. 1990a, Brooks et al. 1990b). In patients with the full syndrome of MSA, mean caudate 6F-DOPA uptake is significantly more depressed than in PD though the individual ranges overlap (Fig. 40.3). This finding suggests that the nigra is more extensively involved by the pathology of SND than PD and pathological studies corroborate this conclusion. However, the pattern of caudate and putamen 6F-DOPA uptake only discriminates MSA-P from PD with 70% specificity (Burn et al. 1994). Given this, ^{18}F-FDG PET and DWI MRI appear to provide more sensitive tools than 6F-DOPA PET for this purpose. When Pirker and colleagues examined ^{123}I-beta-CIT binding in 18 MSA patients these

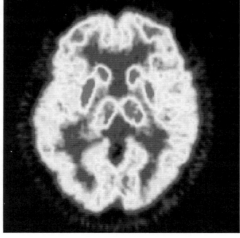
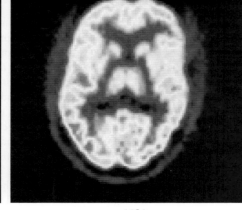

Fig. 40.2 ^{18}F-fluorodeoxyglucose positron emission tomography images of regional cerebral glucose metabolism. The multiple system atrophy (MSA) case shows reduced resting basal ganglia function. See also Plate 16.

Normal   MSA

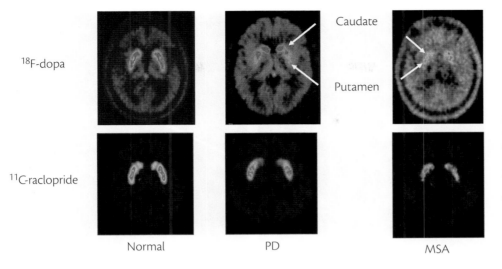

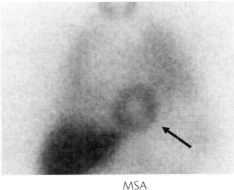

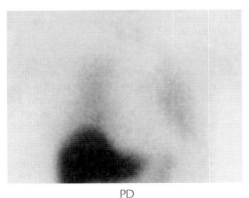

Fig. 40.3 F-DOPA and ^{11}C-raclopride positron emission tomography images of dopamine storage capacity and D2 receptor binding. The multiple system atrophy (MSA) case shows reduced caudate and putamen 6F-DOPA and ^{11}C-raclopride uptake. Caudate 6F-DOPA uptake and striatal ^{11}C-raclopride binding are preserved in Parkinson's disease (PD). See also Plate 17.

workers concluded that, while ^{123}I-beta-CIT SPECT reliably discriminated PD and MSA from normal, it could not reliably discern the two parkinsonian conditions (Pirker et al. 2000).

Striatal dopamine D1 and D2 receptor binding has been studied in MSA-P. ^{11}C-SCH23390 and ^{11}C-raclopride PET showed significant, though mild, reductions in mean putamen D1 and D2 binding, and an overlap between MSA-P, normal, and PD ranges was evident (Brooks 1993) (Fig. 40.3. Striatal D1 and D2 binding, therefore, does not appear to provide a sensitive discriminator of MSA-P from PD. In support of this viewpoint, in their series of probable MSA-P compared with PD cases Seppi and co-workers (Seppi et al. 2004) reported that the predictive value of ^{123}I-IBZM SPECT, a marker of D2 binding, was 75% versus 97% for DWI MRI. Schwarz and co-workers (Schwarz et al. 1992) found reduced striatal D2 binding with ^{123}I-IBZM SPECT in only 8 of 12 *de novo* parkinsonian patients who showed a negative apomorphine response. As a significant number of parkinsonian patients who respond poorly to levodopa retain normal levels of striatal D2 binding, it seems likely that degeneration of downstream brainstem and pallidal rather than striatal projections is responsible for their poor response to levodopa. Seppi and co-workers (Seppi et al. 2001) have used ^{123}I-IBZM SPECT to objectively longitudinally monitor striatal degeneration in a group of early MSA patients. They found an annual 10% loss of striatal D2 binding in their 18-month study and concluded that ^{123}I-IBZM SPECT provides a

valid future approach for testing the efficacy of putative neuroprotective agents in MSA.

^{123}I-MIBG SPECT has been used to study the functional integrity of cardiac sympathetic innervation in PD and MSA (Druschky et al. 2000, Nagayama et al. 2005) (Fig. 40.4). In PD there is a severe reduction in mediastinal ^{123}I-MIBG signal, even in cases where no clinical evidence of autonomic failure was present, while this is milder or absent in MSA. This finding suggests a greater involvement of postganglionic sympathetic innervation of the heart in PD compared with MSA though an overlap in ranges is seen. Having said that, normal cardiac ^{123}I-MIBG SPECT imaging effectively excludes a diagnosis of PD but not MSA.

Opioid dysfunction

The basal ganglia are rich in opioid peptides and their binding sites and these are differentially affected in SND and PD (Goto et al. 1990). ^{11}C-diprenorphine is a nonspecific opioid antagonist binding with equal affinity to μ, κ, and δ sites. In non-dyskinetic PD patients caudate and putamen ^{11}C-diprenorphine uptake is preserved whereas putamen uptake is significantly reduced in patients with MSA (Burn et al. 1995).

Overlap between PAF, OPCA, and SND

In order to determine the overlap between PAF, OPCA, and SND, groups of these patients have been studied with PET and proton MRS.

Fig. 40.4 Meta-iodobenzyl guanidine (MIBG) single photon emission computed tomography (SPECT) images in Parkinson's disease (PD) and multiple system atrophy (MSA). It can be seen that sympathetic innervation of the myocardium remains relatively intact in MSA. Reproduced from Braune S. et al. *Neurology* 1999; **53**: 1020–1025.

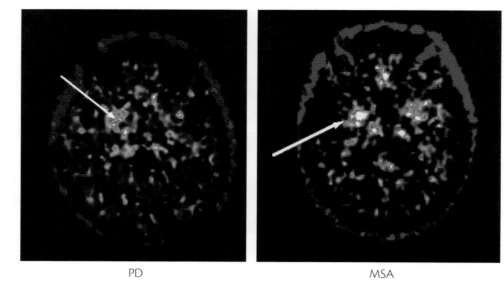

Fig. 40.5 ^{11}C-PK11195 positron emission tomography images of microglial activation in Parkinson's disease (PD) and multiple system atrophy (MSA). Both conditions show increased basal ganglia uptake but this is more extensive in MSA. See also Plate 18. Courtesy of A Gerhard.

PD   MSA

In one series of 7 PAF patients, putamen 6F-DOPA uptake was found to be abnormal in 2, suggesting that subclinical nigral dysfunction was present (Brooks et al. 1990b). One of these patients subsequently developed MSA. In a series of 10 sporadic OPCA patients with autonomic failure, 7 revealed reduced putamen 6F-DOPA uptake while 4 had reduced putamen ^{11}C-diprenorphine binding indicative of the presence of subclinical SND (Rinne et al. 1995). Reduced levels of striatal 6F-DOPA uptake (Otsuka et al. 1994), striatal glucose metabolism (Gilman et al. 1994), and lentiform NAA:creatine signal (Davie et al. 1995) have also been reported in other series of sporadic OPCA cases. It would seem, therefore, that most sporadic OPCA cases with autonomic failure show functional imaging evidence of subclinical striatonigral dysfunction.

Glial activation in multiple system atrophy

[11]C-PK11195 PET, an *in vivo* marker of microglial activation, has been used to study neuroinflammatory changes in MSA (Gerhard et al. 2003). Widespread subcortical increases in ^{11}C-PK11195 uptake were seen, particularly in nigra, putamen, pallidum, thalamus, and brainstem (Fig. 40.5). These changes were more extensive than those associated with PD but again there was significant overlap in the findings for these two conditions (Gerhard et al. 2001).

Conclusion

In summary, MRI reveals reduced lateral putamen signal in T2-weighted scans of MSA-P patients while DWI sensitively detects reduced anisotropy throughout the striatum. TCS does not detect the midbrain hyperechogenicity characteristic of PD but may show altered lentiform nucleus signal. 6F-DOPA PET sensitively reveals reduced striatal, cerebellar, and brainstem glucose metabolism, striatal dopamine storage, and opioid binding in MSA. The presence of reduced striatal metabolism can help distinguish MSA-P from PD in cases where clinical doubt exists. MIBG cardiac scintigraphy can also be helpful for this purpose, as sympathetic innervation is preserved in most cases of MSA but reduced in PD.

Sporadic MSA-C patients show reduced cerebellar and brainstem glucose metabolism and the majority also have evidence of subclinical nigral and striatal dysfunction as evidenced by reduced striatal 6F-DOPA and ^{11}C-diprenorphine uptake, glucose metabolism, and levels of NAA. This suggests that MSA-P and MSA-C are simply part of an MSA continuum, in line with pathological findings. Most patients with PAF have an intact nigrostriatal dopaminergic system, arguing against this condition being a variant of PD or MSA despite some pathological overlap. PET is capable, however, of detecting subclinical nigrostriatal dysfunction in occasional PAF patients when this is present.

References

Berg, D., Becker, G., Zeiler, B., *et al.* (1999). Vulnerability of the nigrostriatal system as detected by transcranial ultrasound. *Neurology* **53**, 1026–31.

Berg, D., Merz, B., Reiners, K., Naumann, M., Becker, G. (2005). Five-year follow-up study of hyperechogenicity of the substantia nigra in Parkinson's disease. *Movement Disorders* (in press).

Berg, D., Roggendorf, W., Schroder, U., *et al.* (2002). Echogenicity of the substantia nigra: association with increased iron content and marker for susceptibility to nigrostriatal injury. *Arch. Neurol.* **59**, 999–1005.

Berg, D., Siefker, C., Becker, G. (2001). Echogenicity of the substantia nigra in Parkinson's disease and its relation to clinical findings. *J Neurol.* **248**, 684–9.

Braak, H., Tredici, K. D., Rub, U., de Vos, R. A., Jansen Steur, E. N., Braak, E. (2003). Staging of brain pathology related to sporadic Parkinson's disease. *Neurobiol. Aging* **24**, 197–211.

Brooks, D. J. (1993). Functional imaging in relation to parkinsonian syndromes. *J. Neurol. Sci.* **115**, 1–17.

Brooks, D. J., Ibañez, V., Sawle, G. V., *et al.* (1990a). Differing patterns of striatal 18F-dopa uptake in Parkinson's disease, multiple system atrophy and progressive supranuclear palsy. *Ann. Neurol.* **28**, 547–55.

Brooks, D. J., Salmon, E. P., Mathias, C. J., *et al.* (1990b). The relationship between locomotor disability, autonomic dysfunction, and the integrity of the striatal dopaminergic system, in patients with multiple system atrophy, pure autonomic failure, and Parkinson's disease, studied with PET. *Brain* **113**, 1539–52.

Burn, D. J., Rinne, J. O., Quinn, N. P., Lees, A. J., Marsden, C. D., Brooks, D. J. (1995). Striatal opioid receptor binding in Parkinson's disease, striatonigral degeneration, and Steele-Richardson-Olszewski syndrome: An 11C-diprenorphine PET study. *Brain* **118**, 951–58.

Burn, D. J., Sawle, G. V., Brooks, D. J. (1994). The differential diagnosis of Parkinson's disease, multiple system atrophy, and Steele-Richardson-Olszewski syndrome: Discriminant analysis of striatal 18F-dopa PET data. *J. Neurol. Neurosurg. Psychiat.* **57**, 278–84.

Davie, C. A., Wenning, G. K., Barker, G. J., *et al.* (1995). Differentiation of multiple system atrophy from idiopathic Parkinson's disease using proton magnetic resonance spectroscopy. *Ann. Neurol.* **37**, 204–210.

De Volder, A. G., Francard, J., Laterre, C., *et al.* (1989). Decreased glucose utilisation in the striatum and frontal lobe in probable striatonigral degeneration. *Ann. Neurol.* **26**, 239–47.

Druschky, A., Hilz, M. J., Platsch, G., *et al.* (2000). Differentiation of Parkinson's disease and multiple system atrophy in early disease stages by means of I-123-MIBG-SPECT. *J Neurol. Sci.* **175**, 3–12.

Duguid, J. R., De La Paz, R., DeGroot, J. (1986). Magnetic resonance imaging of the midbrain in Parkinson's disease. *Ann. Neurol.* **20**, 744–47.

Eidelberg, D., Moeller, J. R., Dhawan, V., *et al.* (1990). The metabolic anatomy of Parkinson's disease: complementary [18F] fluorodeoxyglucose and [18F]fluorodopa positron emission tomographic studies. *Mov Disord* **5**, 203–13.

Eidelberg, D., Moeller, J. R., Ishikawa, T., *et al.* (1996). Regional metabolic correlates of surgical outcome following unilateral pallidotomy for Parkinson's disease. *Ann. Neurol.* **39**, 450–59.

Eidelberg, D., Takikawa, S., Moeller, J. R., *et al.* (1993). Striatal hypometabolism distinguishes striatonigral degeneration from Parkinson's disease. *Ann. Neurol.* **33**, 518–27.

Fearnley, J. M., Lees, A. J. (1990). Striatonigral degeneration: A clinicopathological study. *Brain* **113**, 1823–42.

Fearnley, J. M., Lees, A. J. (1991). Ageing and Parkinson's disease: Substantia nigra regional selectivity. *Brain* **114**, 2283–2301.

Fulham, M. J., Dubinsky, R. M., Polinsky, R. J., *et al.* (1991). Computed tomography, magnetic resonance imaging, and positron emission tomography with [18F]fluorodeoxyglucose in multiple system atrophy and pure autonomic failure. *Clin. Autonomic Res.* **1**, 27–36.

Gerhard, A., Banati, R. B., Cagnin, A., Brooks, D. J. (2001). In vivo imaging of activated microglia with [C-11]PK11195 positron emission tomography (PET) in idiopathic and atypical Parkinson's disease. *Neurology.* **56** Supp 3, A270.

Gerhard, A., Banati, R. B., Goerres, G. B., *et al.* (2003). [(11)C](R)-PK11195 PET imaging of microglial activation in multiple system atrophy. *Neurology* **61**, 686–9.

Gilman, S., Koeppe, R. A., Junck, L., Kluin, K. J., Lohman, M., St Laurent, R. T. (1994). Patterns of cerebral glucose metabolism detected with positron emission tomography differ in multiple system atrophy and olivopontocerebellar atrophy. *Ann. Neurol.* **36**, 166–75.

Goto, S., Hirano, A., Matsumoto, S. (1989). Subdivisional involvement of nigrostriatal loop in idiopathic Parkinson's disease and striatonigral degeneration. *Ann. Neurol.* **26**, 766–70.

Goto, S., Hirano, A., Matsumoto, S. (1990). Met-enkephalin immunoreactivity in the basal ganglia in Parkinson's disease and striatonigral degeneration. *Neurology* **40**, 1051–56.

Hu, M. T., White, S. J., Herlihy, A. H., Chaudhuri, K. R., Hajnal, J. V., Brooks, D. J. (2001). A comparison of (18)F-dopa PET and inversion recovery MRI in the diagnosis of Parkinson's disease. *Neurology* **56**, 1195–200.

Hutchinson, M., Raff, U. (2000). Structural changes of the substantia nigra in Parkinson's disease as revealed by MR imaging. *Am. J Neuroradiol.* **21**, 697–701.

Kish, S. J., Shannak, K., Hornykiewicz, O. (1988). Uneven pattern of dopamine loss in the striatum of patients with idiopathic Parkinson's disease. *N. Engl. J. Med.* **318**, 876–80.

Klockgether, T., Wullner, U., Spauschus, A., Evert, B. (2000). The molecular biology of the autosomal-dominant cerebellar ataxias. *Mov Disord* **15**, 604–12.

Litvan, I., Booth, V., Wenning, G. K., *et al.* (1998). Retrospective application of a set of clinical diagnostic criteria for the diagnosis of multiple system atrophy. *Journal of Neural Transmission* **105**, 217–27.

Miletich, R. S., Chan, T., Gillespie, M., Di Chiro, G., Stein, S. (1988). Contralateral basal ganglia metabolism is abnormal in hemiparkinsonian patients. An FDG-PET study. *Neurology.* **38**, S260.

Nagayama, H., Hamamoto, M., Ueda, M., Nagashima, J., Katayama, Y. (2005). Reliability of MIBG myocardial scintigraphy in the diagnosis of Parkinson's disease. *J Neurol. Neurosurg. Psychiatry* **76**, 249–51.

Otsuka, M., Ichiya, Y., Hosokawa, S., *et al.* (1991). Striatal blood flow, glucose metabolism, and 18F-dopa uptake: difference in Parkinson's disease and atypical parkinsonism. *J. Neurol. Neurosurg. Psychiat.* **54**, 898–904.

Otsuka, M., Ichiya, Y., Kuwabara, Y., *et al.* (1994). Striatal 18F-Dopa uptake and brain glucose metabolism by PET in patients with syndrome of progressive ataxia. *J. Neurol. Sci.* **124**, 198–203.

Papp, M. I., Lantos, P. L. (1994). Cellular pathology of multiple system atrophy: a review. *J. Neurol. Neurosurg. Psychiat.* **57**, 129–33.

Pirker, W., Asenbaum, S., Bencsits, G., *et al.* (2000). [I-123]beta-CIT SPECT in multiple system atrophy, progressive supranuclear palsy, and corticobasal degeneration. *Mov Disord* **15**, 1158–67.

Quinn, N. (1989). Multiple system atrophy—the nature of the beast. *J. Neurol. Neurosurg. Psychiatry.* **52**, 78–89.

Rinne, J. O., Burn, D. J., Mathias, C. J., Quinn, N. P., Marsden, C. D., Brooks, D. J. (1995). PET studies on the dopaminergic system and striatal opioid binding in the olivopontocerebellar atrophy variant of multiple system atrophy. *Ann. Neurol.* **37**, 568–73.

Rosenthal, G., Gilman, S., Koeppe, R. A., *et al.* (1988). Motor dysfunction in olivopontocerebellar atrophy is related to cerebral metabolic rate studied with positron emission tomography. *Ann. Neurol.* **24**, 414–19.

Savoiardo, M., Strada, L., Girotti, F., *et al.* (1990). Olivopontocerebellar atrophy: MR diagnosis and relationship to multisystem atrophy. *Radiology* **174**, 693–96.

Schrag, A., Good, C. D., Miszkiel, K., *et al.* (2000). Differentiation of atypical parkinsonian syndromes with routine MRI. *Neurology* **54**, 697–702.

Schwarz, J., Tatsch, K., Arnold, G., *et al.* (1992). 123I-iodobenzamide-SPECT predicts dopaminergic responsiveness in patients with de-novo parkinsonism. *Neurology* **42**, 556–61.

Seppi, K., Donnemiller, E., Riccabona, G., Poewe, W., Wenning, G. (2001). Disease progression in PD vs MSA: A SPECT study using 123-I IBZM. *Parkinsonism and related disorders.* Vol **7**, S24.

Seppi, K., Schocke, M. F., Donnemiller, E., *et al.* (2004). Comparison of diffusion-weighted imaging and [123I]IBZM-SPECT for the differentiation of patients with the Parkinson variant of multiple system atrophy from those with Parkinson's disease. *Mov Disord* **19**, 1438–45.

Seppi, K., Schocke, M. F., Esterhammer, R., *et al.* (2003). Diffusion-weighted imaging discriminates progressive supranuclear palsy from PD, but not from the parkinson variant of multiple system atrophy. *Neurology* **60**, 922–7.

Vanderhaegen, J. J., Perier, O., Sternon, J. E. (1970). Pathological findings in idiopathic orthostatic hypotension: its relationship with Parkinson's disease. *Arch. Neurol.* **22**, 207–214.

Walter, U., Niehaus, L., Probst, T., Benecke, R., Meyer, B. U., Dressler, D. (2003). Brain parenchyma sonography discriminates Parkinson's disease and atypical parkinsonian syndromes. *Neurology* **60**, 74–7.

Wenning, G. K., Jellinger, K. A. (2005). The role of alpha-synuclein in the pathogenesis of multiple system atrophy. *Acta Neuropathol (Berl)* **109**, 129–40.

Wullner, U. (2003). Genes implicated in the pathogenesis of spinocerebellar ataxias. *Drugs Today (Barc)* **39**, 927–37.

CHAPTER 41

Neuropathology of multiple system atrophy

Janice L. Holton and Tamas Revesz

Introduction

Multiple system atrophy (MSA) is now recognized as a sporadic adult onset disease of unknown aetiology with characteristic neuropathological features. Originally three separate disorders were described:

- olivopontocerebellar atrophy (OPCA) (Dejerine and Thomas 1900) in which patients manifest predominantly cerebellar symptoms
- striatonigral degeneration (SND) (Adams et al. 1961) with a largely parkinsonian presentation
- Shy–Drager syndrome in which the autonomic system is primarily affected (SDS) (Shy and Drager 1960).

The term MSA was first used in 1969 to encompass all three entities as it was realized that OPCA, SND, and SDS can be concurrent (Graham and Oppenheimer 1969). This grouping was justified with the recognition that the Papp-Lantos body or glial cytoplasmic inclusion (GCI) is the pathological hallmark of all clinical subtypes of the disease (Papp et al. 1989). Consensus clinical criteria for the diagnosis of MSA now recommend that patients are classified according to their predominant motor disorder; those with predominant parkinsonism are classified as MSA-P, replacing the term SND, while MSA-C, rather than OPCA, describes those with largely cerebellar features. The term SDS is no longer recommended for use (Gilman et al. 2008).

Macroscopic features

The brain weight may be within the normal range for age or be slightly diminished. In cases with marked cerebellar involvement the brainstem and cerebellum can contribute less than 10% of the total brain weight. On external examination the bulk of the inferior olivary nuclei may be reduced, and atrophy of the pons, which often has a wedge-shaped profile, may be evident. On slicing the brain a number of changes can be found, the distribution of changes often reflecting the predominant clinical features (Fig. 41.1). The putamen frequently shows macroscopic abnormalities most marked in the caudal and dorsolateral parts of the nucleus with reduction in width, flattening of the normally convex lateral border, and greyish discolouration. The substantia nigra and locus coeruleus show marked loss of pigmentation. In the cerebellum there may be obvious cortical atrophy with narrowing of the folia, and the white matter shows loss of bulk with grey discolouration. Sections through the pons may reveal reduction in size of the pontine base with decreased bulk of the transverse pontine fibres and the middle cerebellar peduncles. Examination of the

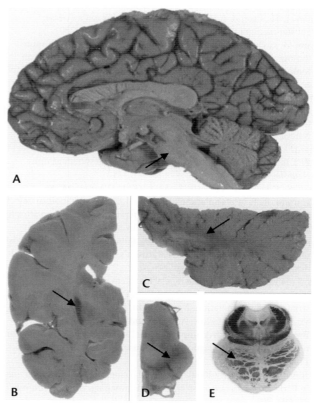

Fig. 41.1 Examination of the brain in multiple system atrophy shows reduction in size of the pontine base (**A**) (arrow). The putamen shows marked grey discolouration and reduction in width (**B**) (arrow). In the cerebellum there is mild atrophy of the cortex with reduction in width of the folia and also discolouration and diminution in bulk of the white matter (**C**) (arrow). The substantia nigra is pale (**D**) (arrow) and in the pons there is a decrease in the size of the pontine base due to loss of the transverse fibres (**E**) (arrow). Luxol fast blue stain.

medulla may show a decrease in size of the inferior olivary nucleus. Cortical atrophy affecting motor and premotor areas can sometimes be observed (Dickson et al. 1999a, Lantos and Quinn 2003, Lantos 1998).

Macroscopic features of multiple system atrophy

◆ Putamen atrophy and discolouration

◆ Pallor of the substantia nigra and locus coeruleus

◆ Atrophy of the pontine base

◆ Cerebellar cortical and white matter atrophy

◆ Atrophy of the inferior olive

Histological changes

Histological changes are widespread in MSA and in a large series of cases were not found to be restricted solely to striatonigral or olivopontocerebellar regions regardless of the clinical phenotype (Ozawa et al. 2004). The major features are widespread neuronal loss, gliosis and loss of myelin with specific glial and neuronal inclusions. Neuronal loss is most severe in the substantia nigra, putamen, pontine base, locus coeruleus, inferior olivary nucleus, cerebellar cortex, intermediolateral column of the spinal cord, and Onuf's nucleus, although many other regions may be affected to a lesser extent (Lantos and Quinn 2003, Ozawa et al. 2004).

The pathological hallmark of MSA has been accepted to be the GCI first described in 1989 (Fig. 41.2) (Papp et al. 1989). The first description of these inclusions was made in Gallyas silver impregnation preparations, in which oligodendroglial inclusions of varying size and shape including triangular, sickle, conical, oval and flame-shaped were observed often displacing the nucleus to one side of the cell. GCIs are widely distributed in the central nervous system and are most frequent in motor cortical regions, dorsolateral putamen, caudate nucleus, internal and external capsules, globus pallidus, pontine nuclei, reticular formation, middle cerebellar peduncle, and cerebellar white matter (Inoue et al. 1997, Papp et al. 1989). In addition to cytoplasmic inclusions oligodendrocytes may also possess rare rod-shaped intranuclear inclusions stained in silver impregnation preparations (Papp and

Lantos 1992). Argyrophilic neuronal cytoplasmic inclusions, which are round, oval or kidney-shaped, are also present most frequently in the pontine and inferior olivary nuclei (Kato and Nakamura 1990, Nishie et al. 2004b, Yokoyama et al. 2001). Fine argyrophilic thread-like inclusions often in the form of a loose basket-like network beneath the nuclear membrane may be found in neuronal nuclei most often in the pontine base but also in other areas. Argyrophilic neuronal processes or neuropil threads are also present, most commonly in regions containing neuronal or glial inclusions (Papp and Lantos 1992).

In addition to the argyrophilic properties of the glial and neuronal inclusions in MSA it was recognized that they could also be identified using ubiquitin immunohistochemistry (Papp et al. 1989, Papp and Lantos 1992, Kato and Nakamura 1990). More importantly it was subsequently demonstrated that one of the principal components of GCIs, neuronal cytoplasmic inclusions, glial and neuronal nuclear inclusions, and neuropil threads is alpha-synuclein, thus placing MSA in the group of alpha-synucleinopathies, which also includes idiopathic Parkinson's disease and dementia with Lewy bodies (Arima et al. 1998, Gai et al. 1998, Mezey et al. 1998, Spillantini et al. 1998, Wakabayashi et al. 1998).

Pathological changes also occur in the white matter in MSA. While changes leading to loss of myelin in areas such as the middle cerebellar peduncle and cerebellar white matter may be secondary to neuronal loss there is also evidence that myelin degradation may be a primary event. A study employing monoclonal antibodies that specifically recognize damaged myelin demonstrated widespread myelin damage in MSA even in areas that appeared normal using conventional stains for myelin and in those without GCIs, suggesting that myelin breakdown may be an early feature of MSA (Matsuo et al. 1998).

Alpha-synuclein immunoreactive structures in multiple system atrophy

◆ Glial cytoplasmic inclusions (oligodendroglial)

◆ Glial nuclear inclusions (oligodendroglial)

◆ Neuronal cytoplasmic inclusions

◆ Neuronal nuclear inclusions

◆ Neuropil threads

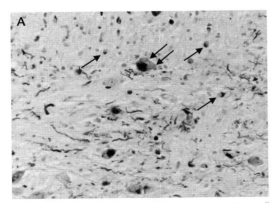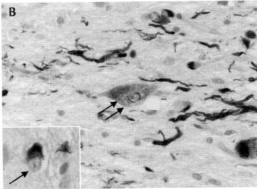

Fig. 41.2 Immunohistochemical staining for alpha-synuclein demonstrates intracellular inclusions in multiple system atrophy. In the pontine base there are numerous GCIs (arrows), and alpha-synuclein immunoreactive neuronal processes. Neuronal cytoplasmic inclusions (double arrow) are also found in this site **(A)**. At higher magnification a neuron containing both a cytoplasmic and a nuclear inclusion is demonstrated **(B)** (double arrow). Occasional oligodendrocytes contain alpha-synuclein-positive rod shaped nuclear inclusions **(B: inset)** (midbrain). Bar represents 50 μm in A, 25 μm in B and 17 μm in the inset in **B**.

Ultrastructure

Ultrastructural examination has shown that GCIs are composed of randomly arranged tubules, which are round or ovoid in cross-section, coated with granular material, and measuring 20–30 nm in diameter (Arima et al. 1992, Arima et al. 1998, Dickson et al. 1999a, Dickson et al. 1999b, Kato and Nakamura 1990, Nakazato et al. 1990, Papp, et al. 1989, Papp and Lantos 1992). Isolated filaments are of two types; the first, known as twisted filaments, are 5–18 nm in diameter with a periodicity of 70–90 nm, while the second are straight filaments 10 nm in diameter. Immunoelectron microscopy shows that both types of filament contain alpha-synuclein (Spillantini et al. 1998). Neuronal cytoplasmic inclusions are composed of tubular structures of similar diameter to that of GCIs with a variable number of associated ribosome-like granular particles (Papp and Lantos 1992, Yokoyama et al. 2001). Inclusions in neuronal processes comprise loosely arranged or more densely packed tubules with similar characteristics to those described in GCIs, with uncoated tubules 5–10 nm in diameter and those with a granular coating having diameters up to 40 nm (Dickson et al. 1999a, Papp and Lantos 1992). Neuronal and glial nuclear inclusions are composed of densely arranged tubules often forming bundles (Nishie et al. 2004b, Papp and Lantos 1992).

Distribution of pathology and clinicopathological correlations

In an early study examination of the relationship between the density of GCIs and the severity of neuronal loss showed no correlation in most anatomical sites (Papp and Lantos 1994). A further study of cases with either OPCA or SND showed a similar distribution of GCIs in all cases regardless of the pathological subtype or the severity of pathological changes. In cases without histological evidence of OPCA the cerebellar white matter contained many GCIs, which were increased in number in moderate OPCA. However, there was a decrease in the pathological load in severe OPCA suggesting that GCIs may have a role in the development of the disease process in this site. In other white matter areas, including the pyramidal tract and internal capsule, GCIs increased in number with increasing severity of both OPCA and SND. There was a positive correlation between putaminal GCI load and the severity of SND, but no similar relationship was evident for OPCA (Inoue et al. 1997). Biochemical investigation of the abundance of SDS-insoluble alpha-synuclein in a small series of cases showed no difference between OPCA and SND (Dickson et al. 1999b).

A recent comprehensive study has addressed a number of issues in a series of 100 MSA cases using semiquantitative analysis of neuronal loss, GCI density, neuronal cytoplasmic inclusion density, and gliosis in 24 brain areas chosen to include striatonigral (StrN) and olivopontocerebellar (OPC) regions. The authors examined the relationship between GCIs and neuronal loss, the prevalence of StrN-predominant and OPC-predominant pathological changes, and whether any correlations can be drawn between the distribution of pathology and clinical features. The study showed that all cases demonstrated both SND and OPCA and that this pathology was equivalent in almost half of the cases while in 34% SND was most severe and in 17% OPCA was the predominant finding. The number of GCIs was increased in StrN and OPC regions with disease duration and was also associated with increased neuronal loss

in both regions taken as a whole, although it was noted that neuronal loss in the substantia nigra predominated over GCI accumulation suggesting that in this site neuronal loss may be independent of GCIs. The distribution and frequency of neuronal cytoplasmic inclusions was similar in OPCA and SND indicating that these inclusions are not associated with subtypes of the disease. As might be expected cases with SND predominance had exhibited more severe bradykinesia in life than those with OPCA dominant pathology and the latter group had displayed more frequent cerebellar signs. Those patients with less severe involvement of the putamen were found to have shown greater responsiveness to L-DOPA in life. It was also of interest that relatively mild involvement of the substantia nigra was associated with parkinsonian features although the development of cerebellar signs required a greater degree of cerebellar pathology (Ozawa et al. 2004).

Pathological changes in components of the autonomic system are thought to give rise to clinical autonomic failure in MSA. There is evidence of a supraspinal contribution to autonomic failure as neuronal loss has been reported in a number of structures including the dorsal motor nucleus of the vagus (Sung et al. 1979, Benarroch et al. 2006) the catecholaminergic neurons of ventrolateral medulla (Benarroch et al. 1998), the serotonergic neurons of the nucleus raphé obscurus, nucleus raphé pallidus, nucleus raphé magnus and ventrolateral medulla (Benarroch et al. 2004), the Edinger–Westphal nucleus, the locus coeruleus (Wenning et al. 1997) and the posterior hypothalamus (Shy and Drager 1960) including the tuberomamillary nucleus (Nakamura et al. 1996). Most importantly, Papp and Lantos showed large numbers of GCIs in the brainstem pontomedullary reticular formation which is involved in cardiac regulation and the control of both respiration and micturition in addition to chemoreception and baroreception, thus providing a supraspinal histological counterpart for impaired visceral function (Papp and Lantos 1994). Neuronal loss in the ventrolateral nucleus ambiguus, a source of cardiac vagal innervation, is likely to contribute to cardiovagal failure in MSA (Benarroch et al. 2006).

Degeneration of sympathetic preganglionic neurons in the intermediolateral column of the thoracolumbar spinal cord is considered contributory to orthostatic hypotension (Bannister and Oppenheimer 1972, Wenning et al. 1997). Formal quantification of cell loss in this region has demonstrated that most cases of MSA with predominant pathology in either the StrN or OPC system show loss of intermediolateral cells. Cell counts in patients with autonomic failure were on average 25% of the controls, while in cases without autonomic failure there was around 50% depletion, with some overlap occurring between the two groups (Oppenheimer 1980). A subsequent study failed to correlate the severity of cell loss in the intermediolateral columns with the degree of autonomic failure suggesting a contribution from pathology in other sites (Gray et al. 1988).

Disordered bladder, rectal, and sexual function in SND and OPCA have been associated with cell loss in parasympathetic preganglionic nuclei of the spinal cord. These neurons are localized rostrally in Onuf's nucleus between sacral segments S2 and S3, and more caudally in the inferior intermediolateral nucleus chiefly in the S3 and S4 segments (Konno et al. 1986). Although neurons of Onuf's nucleus resemble somatic motor neurons morphologically, the sparing of this cell column in motor neurone disease and its involvement in MSA supports the view that it is part of the parasympathetic system concerned with innervation of the anal and urethral sphincters.

In the peripheral component of the autonomic nervous system, Bannister and Oppenheimer (1972) have described atrophy of the glossopharyngeal and vagus nerves. A recent study described alpha-synuclein positive inclusions in the sympathetic ganglia in 2 of 8 MSA cases, which were interpreted as representing neuronal cytoplasmic inclusions (Nishie et al. 2004a). However, this observation has been questioned by a further, larger study in which alpha-synuclein positive neuronal cytoplasmic inclusions in the sympathetic ganglia with features of Lewy bodies were found in 11 of 26 cases. The presence of such inclusions correlated with increased disease duration (Sone et al. 2005). This finding may be due to concomitant Lewy body pathology in MSA, which is known to occur in around 10% of cases (Ozawa et al. 2004). No alpha-synuclein positive inclusions have been observed in Schwann cells (Nishie et al. 2004a, Sone et al. 2005). No pathology has been reported in the visceral enteric plexuses or in the innervation of glands, blood vessels, or smooth muscle.

Diagnosis

A definite diagnosis of MSA relies on neuropathological examination (Trojanowski and Revesz 2007) and the finding of alpha-synuclein positive GCIs in the characteristic distribution as described above is required to make this diagnosis. Clinically MSA-P may be confused with other parkinsonian syndromes including idiopathic Parkinson's disease (IPD) and the sporadic tauopathies, progressive supranuclear palsy (PSP), in which involvement of the Onuf nucleus with sphincter disturbance can occur in late stages of the disease (Scaravilli et al. 2000), and corticobasal degeneration (CBD). Neuropathological examination can clearly distinguish MSA from both PSP and CBD. The macroscopic changes typically found in PSP include pallor of the substantia nigra and locus coeruleus, decreased bulk of the midbrain tegmentum and pontine tegmentum together with thinning of the superior cerebellar peduncle. The subthalamic nucleus is characteristically affected showing loss of bulk with dark discolouration and the cerebellar dentate nucleus is often discoloured and may appear indistinct. Histological examination of the brain confirms neuronal loss with gliosis in the affected nuclei. Immunohistochemical staining shows widespread accumulation of phosphorylated tau in the form of neurofibrillary tangles, neuropil threads and oligodendroglial coiled bodies, as well as the characteristic tufted astrocytes, which are most frequently found in the posterior frontal neocortex and in the striatum (Hauw and Agid (2003). In CBD the macroscopic findings most commonly described are frontal atrophy, which may be asymmetrical and more pronounced in a parasagittal distribution. Pallor of the substantia nigra and atrophy of the midbrain tegmentum are seen and there may be reduction in size of the caudate and thalamus. Histological examination is characterized by the presence of tau-immunopositive neurofibrillary tangles, neuropil threads, and coiled bodies similar to those found in PSP. Of note is that the astrocytic tau pathology in CBD differs from that of PSP in that the characteristic lesion is the astrocytic plaque and tufted astrocytes are not a feature. In both PSP and CBD the insoluble tau which accumulates is predominantly composed of four repeat tau isoforms (Dickson and Litvan 2003). The neuropathological features of IPD have been described elsewhere in this volume (Chapters 44 and 45).

MSA-C may have clinical similarities with hereditary spinocerebellar ataxias particularly SCA2 and SCA3 in which parkinsonian symptoms may be a prominent component. There are limited descriptions of the neuropathological findings in the spinocerebellar ataxias in the literature. The macroscopic abnormalities include cerebral, cerebellar and pontine atrophy, pallor of the substantia nigra, and decrease in size of the inferior olivary nucleus. Ubiquitin immunoreactive neuronal intranuclear inclusions are a feature of spinocerebellar ataxias associated with CAG repeat expansions in the coding sequence of the affected gene such as SCA1, SCA2 and SCA3 and these inclusions can also be identified using the antibody 1C2 which recognizes expanded polyglutamine tracts (Mizusawa et al. 2003). Careful neuropathological sampling to include neocortex, hippocampus, basal ganglia, midbrain, pons, medulla, cerebellum and spinal cord, and the use of immunohistochemical staining for alpha-synuclein, tau, amyloid-β and ubiquitin should facilitate an accurate neuropathological diagnosis in MSA. The occurrence of MSA with other neuropathological abnormalities should always be excluded. The most common pathology found in conjunction with MSA is the presence of Lewy bodies in around 10% of cases (Ozawa et al. 2004). There are rare reports in the literature of MSA in conjunction with pathological changes of progressive supranuclear palsy (Silveira-Moriyama et al. 2009). Concomitant Alzheimer pathology with Aβ plaques and neurofibrillary tangles pathology should be systematically documented in all cases.

Differential diagnosis

- Progressive supranuclear palsy (tauopathy)
- Corticobasal degeneration (tauopathy)
- Idiopathic Parkinson's disease (alpha-synucleinopathy)
- Spinocerebellar ataxias

Biochemistry

The protein composition of GCIs and the other cellular inclusions in MSA has been the subject of many immunohistochemical studies. The early studies demonstrated that GCIs contain ubiquitin together with α- and β-tubulin (Papp et al. 1989). The microtubule associated protein tau has also been demonstrated in GCIs and has been found to consist of normal adult tau rather than the hyperphosphorylated tau associated with neurofibrillary tangles in Alzheimer's disease (Cairns et al. 1997a). An important contribution to our understanding of MSA was made when it was discovered that GCIs and other cellular inclusions in MSA contain the presynaptic protein alpha-synuclein and that alpha-synuclein immunohistochemistry is a more sensitive and specific marker of these inclusions than ubiquitin immunohistochemistry (Spillantini et al. 1998, Gai et al. 1998, Wakabayashi et al. 1998). Other studies have identified many additional protein components of GCIs including synphilin-1 (Wakabayashi et al. 2002), 14–3-3 proteins (Komori et al. 2003), neurosin (Iwata et al. 2003), DJ-1 (Neumann et al. 2004), SUMO-1 (Pountney et al. 2005a), αB-crystallin (Pountney et al. 2005b) and dorfin (Hishikawa et al. 2003).

The normal cellular function of alpha-synuclein is still unknown, although it has been shown to localize close to synaptic vesicles (Clayton and George 1999, Goedert 2001). Biochemical protein fractionation studies in MSA have shown that there is an increase in the total amount of immunoreactive alpha-synuclein compared with controls and that this is largely due to an increase in the sodium dodecyl sulphate (SDS) soluble alpha-synuclein fraction compared with those fractions soluble in phosphate buffered saline or Triton X-100 (Dickson et al. 1999b). These authors also demonstrated that there is a significant amount of SDS-soluble alpha-synuclein in brain regions in which there are few GCIs, indicating that increased protein insolubility may be independent of inclusion formation. A further study confirmed the presence of an increase in SDS-soluble alpha-synuclein in MSA but also showed increased insolubility of alpha-synuclein in Lewy bodies when compared with that in MSA (Campbell et al. 2001). The intracellular accumulation of alpha-synuclein in MSA is unlikely to be caused by an increase in protein synthesis as the expression levels of alpha-synuclein messenger RNA (mRNA) were found to be no different to those of controls, indicating that transcriptional regulation of the alpha-synuclein gene is unlikely to be important in disease pathogenesis (Ozawa et al. 2001).

Immunohistochemical analysis of GCIs in MSA using antibodies recognizing a variety of alpha-synuclein epitopes has demonstrated that full length alpha-synuclein is present although antibodies raised against epitopes in the C-terminal region of the molecule stain more weakly suggesting that these epitopes may be hidden. In contrast, all of the antibodies stained cortical Lewy bodies with equal intensity indicating that there may be either conformational differences between alpha-synuclein in MSA and in Lewy bodies or that alpha-synuclein undergoes different protein interactions in GCIs and Lewy bodies (Duda et al. 2000b). Under physiological conditions alpha-synuclein is not phosphorylated however, post-translational modification with phosphorylation of serine residue 129 has been demonstrated in GCIs and other intracellular inclusions of MSA and also in Lewy bodies. Such phosphorylation of alpha-synuclein has also been shown to promote fibril formation *in vitro* (Fujiwara et al. 2002, Nishie et al. 2004a). Nitration of alpha-synuclein in GCIs and Lewy bodies has also been observed suggesting that oxidative damage leading to nitration may play a role in inclusion formation (Giasson et al. 2000, Duda et al. 2000a).

Biochemical features

◆ Alpha-synuclein is a major component of intracellular inclusions in MSA.

◆ A wide variety of other proteins is also present in GCIs.

◆ Accumulation of alpha-synuclein with increased insolubility occurs in MSA.

◆ Full length alpha-synuclein is present in GCIs.

◆ Alpha-synuclein undergoes phosphorylation and nitration in MSA

Genetics

Only rare familial examples of MSA have been described (Wullner et al. 2009). The alpha-synuclein gene (*SNCA*) has been a candidate gene in MSA as alpha-synuclein is a major component of GCIs and three different missense mutations in addition to duplication and triplication have been described in the gene for this protein in familial Parkinson's disease (Polymeropoulos et al. 1997, Kruger et al. 1998, Zarranz et al. 2004, Chartier-Harlin et al. 2004,

Singleton et al. 2003). Interestingly in affected members of the family with *SNCA* triplication not only were Lewy bodies, the characteristic hallmark of Parkinson's disease, found but there were also glial inclusions with features of GCIs. However, in MSA no mutations have been identified in *SNCA* (Ozawa et al. 1999). Common genetic variability in *SNCA* has been implicated in MSA (Scholz et al. 2009). No effect of genetic variability in the genes for ApoE, cytochrome P450-II D6, tau, UCHL-1, or synphillin has been demonstrated (Cairns et al. 1997b, Plante-Bordeneuve et al. 1995, Morris et al. 2000, Healy et al. 2005). No expansions in the genes for SCA1 and SCA3 have been identified in MSA thus excluding the possibility that MSA could represent a sporadic form of either disease (Bandmann et al. 1997). A genome wide association study for MSA is in progress.

◆ There are only very rare familial cases of MSA.

◆ No mutations in *SNCA* have been associated with MSA.

◆ *SNCA* triplication is associated with Lewy bodies and glial inclusions.

Animal models

A number of different approaches have been taken to produce animal models of MSA and have been reviewed recently (Stefanova et al. 2005b). As it is believed that GCIs may play an important role in the pathogenesis of MSA, several groups have sought to develop transgenic mouse models of the disease in which alpha-synuclein is expressed by oligodendrocytes. A model in which human alpha-synuclein was expressed in oligodendrocytes under the control of the oligodendroglial-specific proteolipid protein promoter resulted in mice with histological abnormalities but no overt motor phenotype. Oligodendroglial inclusions with morphological features similar to those of GCIs were found although these were not argyrophilic. These inclusions contained phosphorylated alpha-synuclein which, similar to MSA, showed increased detergent insolubility (Kahle et al. 2002). When these mice are exposed to the mitochondrial toxin 3-nitropropionic acid (3-NP) they develop more severe motor impairments than similarly treated wild-type controls and also more marked loss of Purkinje cells and neurons in the striatum, locus coeruleus and inferior olive (Stefanova et al. 2005a). Oligodendroglial expression of human alpha-synuclein under the control of the 2',3'-cyclic nucleotide 3'-phosphodiesterase (CNP) promoter also provides a mouse model of MSA. These mice have a normal lifespan but develop age-related motor deficits. There is reduction in brain weight and loss of oligodendrocytes and neurons, including anterior horn cells, although dopaminergic neurons are unaffected. GCI-like inclusions are present and there is age-dependent accumulation of insoluble alpha-synuclein. Ultrastructural examination demonstrates myelin breakdown and accumulation of alpha-synuclein filaments (Yazawa et al. 2005). A further transgenic mouse model using the myelin basic protein promoter to achieve over-expression of human alpha-synuclein in oligodendrocytes led to widespread oligodendroglial accumulation of phosphorylated fibrillar alpha-synuclein with reduced solubility. The degree of alpha-synuclein expression correlated with the severity of the neurological deficit with tremor, ataxia, seizures and early death occurring in animals with the highest expression levels and mild tremor in those with low levels of gene expression. Transgenic animals showed degeneration of white matter tracts, decreased cortical dendritic density and loss of dopaminergic fibres in the basal ganglia (Shults et al. 2005). These transgenic mouse models of MSA indicate that over-expression of alpha-synuclein by oligodendrocytes can lead to insoluble alpha-synuclein accumulation and consequent neurodegeneration.

Cell models

There are a number of cell models for Parkinson's disease in which alpha-synuclein is expressed in neurons. In MSA the major site in which alpha-synuclein accumulates is the oligodendroglial cytoplasm and therefore it is desirable to develop cell models to examine this process. Although alpha-synuclein is not usually expressed by adult oligodendrocytes expression has been observed in cultured rat oligodendrocytes during development with downregulation of expression relating to maturation. These findings raise the possibility that GCIs may result from altered oligodendroglial alpha-synuclein expression by oligodendrocytes (Richter-Landsberg et al. 2000). More recently it has been demonstrated that oligodendrocytes do not express alpha-synuclein mRNA in controls or MSA cases indicating that alpha-synuclein over-expression by oligodendrocytes is unlikely to be important in the pathogenesis of MSA (Miller et al. 2005). Cultured human astrocytoma cells and astrocytes also express alpha-synuclein mRNA and in the former this expression can be increased by stimulation using the inflammatory cytokine interleukin-1β (Tanji et al. 2001). Other studies have utilized astrocytoma cell lines transfected with alpha-synuclein to demonstrate cytoplasmic aggregation of alpha-synuclein. Such cells show increased susceptibility to oxidative stress and increased rates of apoptosis (Stefanova et al. 2001; Stefanova et al. 2002).

Conclusion

The neuropathological features of MSA are now clearly established enabling this disease to be distinguished from other syndromes with parkinsonian features or ataxia. Recent work has demonstrated that, at least at the time of death, there is pathological involvement of both StrN and OPC regions and that these areas are equally affected in around half of the cases. The relationship between a predominantly parkinsonian syndrome in life and more severe pathology in StrN regions and more prominent cerebellar ataxia with OPCA dominant pathology has been well established. The role of the Papp-Lantos body, or GCI, in the pathogenesis of the disease is a focus of study. Much is now known about the protein composition of these inclusions and their importance in disease progression has been emphasized by the findings that they increase in number with disease duration and that neuronal loss also increases with increased GCI load. The presence of alpha-synuclein as the most abundant component of the intracellular inclusions of MSA suggests that this protein is pivotal in the process of inclusion formation. Post-translational modification of alpha-synuclein has been identified in intracellular inclusions but there is no evidence that mutations in the gene for alpha-synuclein play a role in disease pathogenesis although gene triplication has been found to be associated with both Lewy bodies and glial inclusions resembling GCIs. The recent development of cell culture and animal models of MSA may provide further insight into the pathogenesis of MSA.

References

Adams, R. D., van Bogaert, L. and van der Eeken, H. (1961). Dégénérescences nigro-striées et cérébello-nigro-striées. *Psychiat Neurol*, **142**, 219–59.

Arima, K., Murayama, S., Mukoyama, M. and Inose, T. (1992). Immunocytochemical and ultrastructural studies of neuronal and oligodendroglial cytoplasmic inclusions in multiple system atrophy. 1. Neuronal cytoplasmic inclusions. *Acta Neuropathol.(Berl)*, **83**, 453–60.

Arima, K., Ueda, K., Sunohara, N., *et al.* (1998). NACP/alpha-synuclein immunoreactivity in fibrillary components of neuronal and oligodendroglial cytoplasmic inclusions in the pontine nuclei in multiple system atrophy. *Acta Neuropathol.(Berl)*, **96**, 439–44.

Bandmann, O., Sweeney, M. G., Daniel, S. E., *et al.* (1997). Multiple-system atrophy is genetically distinct from identified inherited causes of spinocerebellar degeneration. *Neurology*, **49**, 1598–1604.

Bannister, R. and Oppenheimer, D. R. (1972). Degenerative diseases of the nervous system associated with autonomic failure. *Brain*, **95**, 457–74.

Benarroch, E. E., Schmeichel, A. M., Low, P. A. and Parisi, J. E. (2004). Involvement of medullary serotonergic groups in multiple system atrophy. *Ann.Neurol.*, **55**, 418–22.

Benarroch, E. E., Schmeichel, A. M., Sandroni, P., Low, P. A. and Parisi, J. E. (2006). Involvement of vagal autonomic nuclei in multiple system atrophy and Lewy body disease. *Neurology*, **14**, 378–83.

Benarroch, E. E., Smithson, I. L., Low, P. A. and Parisi, J. E. (1998). Depletion of catecholaminergic neurons of the rostral ventrolateral medulla in multiple system atrophy with autonomic failure. *Ann. Neurol.*, **43**, 156–63.

Cairns, N. J., Atkinson, P. F., Hanger, D. P., Anderton, B. H., Daniel, S. E. and Lantos, P. L. (1997a). Tau protein in the glial cytoplasmic inclusions of multiple system atrophy can be distinguished from abnormal tau in Alzheimer's disease. *Neurosci.Lett.*, **230**, 49–52.

Cairns, N. J., Atkinson, P. F., Kovacs, T., Lees, A. J., Daniel, S. E. and Lantos, P. L. (1997b). Apolipoprotein E e4 allele frequency in patients with multiple system atrophy. *Neurosci.Lett.*, **221**, 161–64.

Campbell, B. C., McLean, C. A., Culvenor, J. G., *et al.* (2001). The solubility of alpha-synuclein in multiple system atrophy differs from that of dementia with Lewy bodies and Parkinson's disease. *J.Neurochem.*, **76**, 87–96.

Chartier-Harlin, M. C., Kachergus, J., Roumier, C., *et al.* (2004). Alpha-synuclein locus duplication as a cause of familial Parkinson's disease. *Lancet*, **364**, 1167–69.

Clayton, D. F. and George, J. M. (1999). Synucleins in synaptic plasticity and neurodegenerative disorders. *J.Neurosci.Res.*, **58**, 120–29.

Dejerine, J. and Thomas, A. A. (1900). L'atrophie olivo-ponto-cérébelleuse. *Nouv Iconogr Salpêtr*, **13**, 330–70.

Dickson, D. W., Lin, W., Liu, W. K. and Yen, S. H. (1999a). Multiple system atrophy: a sporadic synucleinopathy. *Brain Pathol.*, **9**, 721–32.

Dickson, D. W., Liu, W., Hardy, J., *et al.* (1999b). Widespread alterations of alpha-synuclein in multiple system atrophy. *Am.J.Pathol.*, **155**, 1241–51.

Dickson, D. W. and Litvan, I. (2003). Corticobasal degeneration. In D. W. Dickson, ed. *Neurodegeneration: the molecular pathology of dementia and movement disorders*, pp. 115–131. ISN Neuropath Press, Basel.

Duda, J. E., Giasson, B. I., Chen, Q., *et al.* (2000a), Widespread nitration of pathological inclusions in neurodegenerative synucleinopathies. *Am.J.Pathol.*, **157**, 1439–45.

Duda, J. E., Giasson, B. I., Gur, T. L., *et al.* (2000b). Immunohistochemical and biochemical studies demonstrate a distinct profile of alpha-synuclein permutations in multiple system atrophy. *J.Neuropathol.Exp. Neurol.*, **59**, 830–41.

Fujiwara, H., Hasegawa, M., Dohmae, N., *et al.* (2002). alpha-Synuclein is phosphorylated in synucleinopathy lesions. *Nat.Cell Biol.*, **4**, 160–64.

Gai, W. P., Power, J. H., Blumbergs, P. C. and Blessing, W. W. (1998). Multiple-system atrophy: a new alpha-synuclein disease? *Lancet*, **352**, 547–48.

Giasson, B. I., Duda, J. E., Murray, I. V., *et al.* (2000). Oxidative damage linked to neurodegeneration by selective alpha-synuclein nitration in synucleinopathy lesions. *Science*, **290**, 985–89.

Gilman, S., Wenning, G. K., Low, P. A., *et al.* (2008). Second consensus statement on the diagnosis of multiple system atrophy. *Neurology*, **71**, 670–6.

Goedert, M. (2001). Alpha-synuclein and neurodegenerative diseases. *Nat. Rev.Neurosci.*, **2**, 492–501.

Graham, J. G. and Oppenheimer, D. R. (1969). Orthostatic hypotension and nicotine sensitivity in a case of multiple system atrophy. *J Neurol Neurosurg Psychiatry*, **32**, 28–34.

Gray, F., Vincent, D. and Hauw, J. J. (1988). Quantitative study of lateral horn cells in 15 cases of multiple system atrophy. *Acta Neuropathol. (Berl)*, **75**, 513–18.

Hauw J. J., and Agid Y. (2003). Progressive supranuclear palsy (PSP) or Steele-Richardson-Olszewski disease. In D. W. Dickson, ed. *Neurodegeneration: the molecular pathology of dementia and movement disorders*, pp. 103–114. ISN Neuropath Press, Basel.

Healy, D. G., Abou-Sleiman, P. M., Quinn, N., *et al.* (2005). UCHL-1 gene in multiple system atrophy: a haplotype tagging approach. *Mov Disord.*, **20**, 1338–43.

Hishikawa, N., Niwa, J., Doyu, M., *et al.* (2003). Dorfin localizes to the ubiquitylated inclusions in Parkinson's disease, dementia with Lewy bodies, multiple system atrophy, and amyotrophic lateral sclerosis. *Am.J.Pathol.*, **163**, 609–619.

Inoue, M., Yagishita, S., Ryo, M., Hasegawa, K., Amano, N. and Matsushita, M. (1997). The distribution and dynamic density of oligodendroglial cytoplasmic inclusions (GCIs) in multiple system atrophy: a correlation between the density of GCIs and the degree of involvement of striatonigral and olivopontocerebellar systems. *Acta Neuropathol.(Berl)*, **93**, 585–91.

Iwata, A., Maruyama, M., Akagi, T., *et al.* (2003). Alpha-synuclein degradation by serine protease neurosin: implication for pathogenesis of synucleinopathies. *Hum.Mol.Genet.*, **12**, 2625–35.

Kahle, P. J., Neumann, M., Ozmen, L., *et al.* (2002). Hyperphosphorylation and insolubility of alpha-synuclein in transgenic mouse oligodendrocytes. *EMBO Rep.*, **3**, 583–88.

Kato, S. and Nakamura, H. (1990). Cytoplasmic argyrophilic inclusions in neurons of pontine nuclei in patients with olivopontocerebellar atrophy: immunohistochemical and ultrastructural studies. *Acta Neuropathol.(Berl)*, **79**, 584–94.

Komori, T., Ishizawa, K., Arai, N., Hirose, T., Mizutani, T. and Oda, M. (2003). Immunoexpression of 14–3-3 proteins in glial cytoplasmic inclusions of multiple system atrophy. *Acta Neuropathol.(Berl)*, **106**, 66–70.

Konno, H., Yamamoto, T., Iwasaki, Y. and Iizuka, H. (1986). Shy-Drager syndrome and amyotrophic lateral sclerosis. Cytoarchitectonic and morphometric studies of sacral autonomic neurons. *J Neurol Sci*, **73**, 193–204.

Kruger, R., Kuhn, W., Muller, T., *et al.* (1998). Ala30Pro mutation in the gene encoding alpha-synuclein in Parkinson's disease. *Nat.Genet.*, **18**, 106–108.

Lantos, P. L. (1998). The definition of multiple system atrophy: a review of recent developments. *J.Neuropathol.Exp.Neurol.*, **57**, 1099–1111.

Lantos, P. L. and Quinn, N. (2003). Multiple System Atrophy. In DW Dickson, ed. *Neurodegeneration: the molecular pathology of dementia and movement disorders*, pp. 203–214. ISN Neuropath Press, Basel.

Matsuo, A., Akiguchi, I., Lee, G. C., McGeer, E. G., McGeer, P. L. and Kimura, J. (1998). Myelin degeneration in multiple system atrophy detected by unique antibodies. *Am.J.Pathol.*, **153**, 735–44.

Mezey, E., Dehejia, A., Harta, G., Papp, M. I., Polymeropoulos, M. H. and Brownstein, M. J. (1998). Alpha synuclein in neurodegenerative disorders: Murderer or accomplice? *Nat Med*, **4**, 755–57.

Miller, D. W., Johnson, J. M., Solano, S. M., Hollingsworth, Z. R., Standaert, D. G. and Young, A. B. (2005). Absence of alpha-synuclein mRNA expression in normal and multiple system atrophy oligodendroglia. *J Neural Transm*, **112**, 1613–24.

Mizusawa, H., Clark, H. B. and Koeppen, A. H. (2003). Spinocerebeller ataxias. In D. W. Dickson, ed. *Neurodegeneration: the molecular pathology of dementia and movement disorders*, pp. 242–56. ISN Neuropath Press, Basel.

Morris, H. R., Vaughan, J. R., Datta, S. R., *et al.* (2000). Multiple system atrophy/progressive supranuclear palsy: alpha-Synuclein, synphilin, tau, and APOE. *Neurology*, **55**, 1918–20.

Nakamura, S., Ohnishi, K., Nishimura, M., *et al.* (1996). Large neurons in the tuberomammillary nucleus in patients with Parkinson's disease and multiple system atrophy. *Neurology*, **46**, 1693–96.

Nakazato, Y., Yamazaki, H., Hirato, J., Ishida, Y. and Yamaguchi, H. (1990). Oligodendroglial microtubular tangles in olivopontocerebellar atrophy. *J.Neuropathol.Exp.Neurol.*, **49**, 521–30.

Neumann, M., Muller, V., Gorner, K., Kretzschmar, H. A., Haass, C. and Kahle, P. J. (2004). Pathological properties of the Parkinson's disease-associated protein DJ-1 in alpha-synucleinopathies and tauopathies: relevance for multiple system atrophy and Pick's disease. *Acta Neuropathol.(Berl)*, **107**, 489–96.

Nishie, M., Mori, F., Fujiwara, H., *et al.* (2004a). Accumulation of phosphorylated alpha-synuclein in the brain and peripheral ganglia of patients with multiple system atrophy. *Acta Neuropathol.(Berl)*, **107**, 292–98.

Nishie, M., Mori, F., Yoshimoto, M., Takahashi, H. and Wakabayashi, K. (2004b). A quantitative investigation of neuronal cytoplasmic and intranuclear inclusions in the pontine and inferior olivary nuclei in multiple system atrophy. *Neuropathol.Appl.Neurobiol.*, **30**, 546–54.

Oppenheimer, D. R. (1980). Lateral horn cells in progressive autonomic failure. *J Neurol Sci*, **46**, 393–404.

Ozawa, T., Okuizumi, K., Ikeuchi, T., Wakabayashi, K., Takahashi, H. and Tsuji, S. (2001). Analysis of the expression level of alpha-synuclein mRNA using postmortem brain samples from pathologically confirmed cases of multiple system atrophy. *Acta Neuropathol (Berl).*, **102**, 188–90.

Ozawa, T., Paviour, D., Quinn, N. P., *et al.* (2004). The spectrum of pathological involvement of the striatonigral and olivopontocerebellar systems in multiple system atrophy: clinicopathological correlations. *Brain*, **127**, 2657–71.

Ozawa, T., Takano, H., Onodera, O., *et al.* (1999). No mutation in the entire coding region of the alpha-synuclein gene in pathologically confirmed cases of multiple system atrophy. *Neurosci.Lett.*, **270**, 110–112.

Papp, M. I., Kahn, J. E. and Lantos, P. L. (1989). Glial cytoplasmic inclusions in the CNS of patients with multiple system atrophy (striatonigral degeneration, olivopontocerebellar atrophy and Shy-Drager syndrome). *J.Neurol.Sci.*, **94**, 79–100.

Papp, M. I. and Lantos, P. L. (1992). Accumulation of tubular structures in oligodendroglial and neuronal cells as the basic alteration in multiple system atrophy. *J.Neurol.Sci.*, **107**, 172–82.

Papp, M. I. and Lantos, P. L. (1994). The distribution of oligodendroglial inclusions in multiple system atrophy and its relevance to clinical symptomatology. *Brain*, **117**, 235–43.

Plante-Bordeneuve, V., Bandmann, O., Wenning, G., Quinn, N. P., Daniel, S. E. and Harding, A. E. (1995). CYP2D6-debrisoquine hydroxylase gene polymorphism in multiple system atrophy. *Mov Disord.*, **10**, 277–78.

Polymeropoulos, M. H., Lavedan, C., Leroy, E., *et al.* (1997). Mutation in the alpha-synuclein gene identified in families with Parkinson's disease. *Science*, **276**, 2045–47.

Pountney, D. L., Chegini, F., Shen, X., Blumbergs, P. C. and Gai, W. P. (2005a). SUMO-1 marks subdomains within glial cytoplasmic inclusions of multiple system atrophy. *Neurosci.Lett.*, **381**, 74–79.

Pountney, D. L., Treweek, T. M., Chataway, T., *et al.* (2005b). Alpha B-crystallin is a major component of glial cytoplasmic inclusions in multiple system atrophy. *Neurotox.Res.*, **7**, 77–85.

Richter-Landsberg, C., Gorath, M., Trojanowski, J. Q. and Lee, V. M. (2000). Alpha-synuclein is developmentally expressed in cultured rat brain oligodendrocytes. *J.Neurosci.Res.*, **62**, 9–14.

Scaravilli, T., Pramstaller, P. P., Salerno, A., *et al.* (2000). Neuronal loss in Onuf's nucleus in three patients with progressive supranuclear palsy. *Ann. Neurol.*, **48**, 97–101.

Scholz, S. W., Houlden, H., Schulte, C., *et al.* (2009). SNCA variants are associated with increased risk for multiple system atrophy. *Ann. Neurol.*, **65**, 610–4.

Shults, C. W., Rockenstein, E., Crews, L., *et al.* (2005). Neurological and neurodegenerative alterations in a transgenic mouse model expressing human alpha-synuclein under oligodendrocyte promoter: implications for multiple system atrophy. *J Neurosci.* **25**, 10689–99.

Shy, G. M. and Drager, G. A. (1960). A neurologic syndrome associated with orthostatic hypotension. *Arch Neurol*, **2**, 511–27.

Silveira-Moriyama, L., Gonzalez, A. M., O'Sullivan, S. S., *et al.* (2009). Concomitant progressive supranuclear palsy and multiple system atrophy: more than a simple twist of fate? *Neurosci. Lett.*, **467**, 208–11.

Singleton, A. B., Farrer, M., Johnson, J., *et al.* (2003). Alpha-synuclein locus triplication causes Parkinson's disease. *Science*, **302**, 841.

Sone, M., Yoshida, M., Hashizume, Y., Hishikawa, N. and Sobue, G. (2005). Alpha-synuclein-immunoreactive structure formation is enhanced in sympathetic ganglia of patients with multiple system atrophy. *Acta Neuropathol.(Berl)*, **110**, 19–26.

Spillantini, M. G., Crowther, R. A., Jakes, R., Cairns, N. J., Lantos, P. L. and Goedert, M. (1998). Filamentous alpha-synuclein inclusions link multiple system atrophy with Parkinson's disease and dementia with Lewy bodies. *Neurosci.Lett.*, **251**, 205–208.

Stefanova, N., Emgard, M., Klimaschewski, L., Wenning, G. K. and Reindl, M. (2002). Ultrastructure of alpha-synuclein-positive aggregations in U373 astrocytoma and rat primary glial cells. *Neurosci. Lett.*, **323**, 37–40.

Stefanova, N., Klimaschewski, L., Poewe, W., Wenning, G. K. and Reindl, M. (2001). Glial cell death induced by overexpression of alpha-synuclein. *J.Neurosci.Res.*, **65**, 432–38.

Stefanova, N., Reindl, M., Neumann, M., *et al.* (2005a). Oxidative stress in transgenic mice with oligodendroglial alpha-synuclein overexpression replicates the characteristic neuropathology of multiple system atrophy. *Am.J.Pathol.*, **166**, 869–76.

Stefanova, N., Tison, F., Reindl, M., Poewe, W. and Wenning, G. K. (2005b). Animal models of multiple system atrophy. *Trends Neurosci.* **28**, 501–6.

Sung, J. H., Mastri, A. R. and Segal, E. (1979). Pathology of Shy-Drager syndrome. *J Neuropathol Exp Neurol*, **38**, 353–68.

Tanji, K., Imaizumi, T., Yoshida, H., *et al.* (2001). Expression of alpha-synuclein in a human glioma cell line and its up-regulation by interleukin-1beta. *Neuroreport*, **12**, 1909–1912.

Trojanowski, J. Q. and Revesz, T. (2001). Proposed neuropathological criteria for the post mortem diagnosis of multiple system atrophy. *Neuropathol. Appl. Neurobiol.*, **33**, 615–20.

Wakabayashi, K., Engelender, S., Tanaka, Y., *et al.* (2002). Immunocytochemical localization of synphilin-1, an alpha-synuclein-associated protein, in neurodegenerative disorders. *Acta Neuropathol. (Berl)*, **103**, 209–214.

Wakabayashi, K., Yoshimoto, M., Tsuji, S. and Takahashi, H (1998). Alpha-synuclein immunoreactivity in glial cytoplasmic inclusions in multiple system atrophy. *Neurosci.Lett.*, **249**, 18.0–82.

Wenning, G. K., Tison, F., Ben Shlomo, Y., Daniel, S. E. and Quinn, N. P. (1997). Multiple system atrophy: a review of 203 pathologically proven cases. *Mov Disord.*, **12**, 133–47.

Wullner, U., Schmitt, I., Kammal, M., *et al.* (2009). Definite multiple system atrophy in a German family. *J. Neurol. Neurosurg. Psychiatry*, **80**, 449–50.

Yazawa, I., Giasson, B. I., Sasaki, R., *et al.* (2005). Mouse model of multiple system atrophy alpha-synuclein expression in oligodendrocytes causes glial and neuronal degeneration. *Neuron*, 45, 847–59.

Yokoyama, T., Kusunoki, J. I., Hasegawa, K., Sakai, H. and Yagishita, S. (2001). Distribution and dynamic process of neuronal cytoplasmic inclusion (NCI) in MSA: correlation of the density of NCI and the degree of involvement of the pontine nuclei. *Neuropathology.*, **21**, 145–54.

Zarranz, J. J., Alegre, J., Gomez-Esteban, J. C., *et al.* (2004). The new mutation, E46K, of alpha-synuclein causes Parkinson and Lewy body dementia. *Ann.Neurol.*, **55**, 164–73.

CHAPTER 42

Autonomic ganglia and preganglionic neurons in autonomic failure

Margaret R. Matthews

Introduction: classes of autonomic failure

Autonomic failure (AF) may arise as a secondary consequence of more general disorders involving the nervous system, as in multiple sclerosis, or in toxic or diabetic peripheral neuropathy, described elsewhere in this volume, or it may arise as a specific feature of certain primary degenerative disorders of the nervous system. These include importantly multiple system atrophy (MSA), pure autonomic failure (PAF), and the autonomic failure that may occur in Parkinson's disease (PD with AF). The neuropathological and neurochemical changes associated with these conditions will be considered here.

As is outlined in the introduction to this volume, the neurons and pathways of the autonomic nervous system, in each of its divisions (sympathetic, parasympathetic and enteric), comprise the following hierarchy: ganglionic neurons and their postganglionic axons innervating effectors (cardiac muscle, smooth muscle and gland cells) in the periphery; innervation of the ganglia from preganglionic neurons in the brainstem (parasympathetic) or the spinal cord (sympathetic at thoracolumbar, parasympathetic at sacral levels); and higher levels of control mediated via the cerebral cortex, the limbic system including the amygdala and septal area, the hypothalamus, and nuclei of the brainstem reticular formation. AF may be associated with dysfunction or pathological changes at any of several levels in these pathways; thus, it may result from derangements of the postganglionic axons, as in peripheral neuropathies, or of ganglionic neurons, or of preganglionic neurons. Disorders of the central pathways involved in control of the preganglionic neurons may also lead, or contribute, to AF. More than one of these levels is often found to be involved on post-mortem examination in a particular case, even though the initial defect may have been more restricted, and the likely explanation for this is that secondary, transneuronal changes may become superimposed upon a primary lesion in this highly interdependent system. There is therefore a problem in establishing what may have been the first site or sites of the disorder.

Clinical studies come closest to revealing this, since they may be undertaken as soon as the diagnosis is suspected. Tests are available that explore differentially the integrity of postganglionic axons, the efficacy of preganglionic control, and the function of central pathways (Chapter 22). The evidence from clinical evaluation points to a primarily preganglionic and central lesion in MSA and a primarily postganglionic or ganglionic lesion in PAF. Thus, it is typical to find in patients showing orthostatic hypotension that the level of resting supine plasma noradrenaline is within normal limits in MSA but low in PAF, although in neither condition does it rise during head-up tilt; and the respective responses to injected tyramine and to the cholinomimetic edrophonium indicate integrity of peripheral noradrenergic nerve endings and of ganglionic neurons in MSA but not in PAF. In MSA, however, a selective deficit may develop in ganglionic sudomotor neurons (Kumazawa et al. 1989, Low and Fealey 1992). Clonidine demonstrates central involvement in MSA but not in PAF. In PD with AF, where the onset of AF tends to occur relatively late in the disease, both central and peripheral lesions may already coexist and may contribute in different ways to the AF, leading either to orthostatic hypotension via peripheral sympathetic neurocirculatory failure (Goldstein et al. 1997) or to urinary and gastrointestinal dysfunction, in which the respective roles of peripheral and central lesions are uncertain (Magaelhaes et al. 1995).

It has, in this way, become increasingly evident that there are important differences between the type of AF that occurs in MSA and that which occurs in PAF, or in PD with AF, and that these differences reflect differences in site of the primary lesion and therefore perhaps in aetiology. Neuropathological studies reinforce this distinction. Nonetheless, the identity of the primary cause or causes of the neuronal changes underlying the AF in either group of cases, as also in PD, still remains elusive. Genetic polymorphisms may be contributory factors (e.g. Infante et al. 2005).

Neuropathological changes in autonomic failure

Preganglionic neurons and central pathways

Neuropathological studies in AF, notably by Oppenheimer (1980), who also reviewed earlier work, have strongly supported the possibility of a primary lesion at sympathetic preganglionic level in

MSA, by showing that there is, in almost all cases of MSA with AF, considerable loss of thoracolumbar intermediolateral column (IML) neurons, amounting to 75% or more of control numbers. Cases of PD with AF, however, also showed severe loss of IML neurons, and moderate loss has been found in PD without AF. Oppenheimer's work has emphasized the importance of systematic counting of neurons in samples of adequate extent, with age-matched controls for comparison. More recent series have produced similar results (e.g. Gray et al. 1988, Low and Fealey 1992). It was already apparent that in the IML a loss of 50% of neurons may be overlooked if no adequate counts are made, and it is now confirmed that 50% or even more of IML neurons may be lost without overt AF. In PAF, however, a ganglionic lesion may coexist with a loss of up to 50% of IML neurons (Low and Fealey 1992, van Ingelghem et al. 1994).

Counts of preganglionic parasympathetic neurons at sacral spinal levels have likewise shown severe neuron loss in MSA (Konno et al. 1986). Consistent neuron loss is also present in Onuf's nucleus of the sacral cord, from which the external urethral and anal sphincter muscles are innervated, in cases of MSA with sphincter disturbances (Konno et al. 1986); and sphincter electromyography gives clear evidence of denervation and reinnervation in such patients (Beck et al. 1994), so consistently that an instance of abnormal sphincter EMG in a subject with PAF raises the suspicion that this presages the future development of MSA (Bajaj et al. 1996). Loss of neurons has also been reported in the dorsal motor nucleus of the vagus, both in MSA (Gray et al. 1988) and in PD with AF (Forno 1996); and in PD this nucleus consistently shows Lewy bodies, typical of the disease, in common with other pigmented nuclei of the brainstem (Hughes et al. 1993, Forno 1996). Similar Lewy bodies have sometimes been seen in the IML in PD, including the sacral IML (Oyanagi et al. 1990). Severe depletion of catecholaminergic C1 neurons in the ventrolateral medulla and of A2 neurons in the dorsomedial medulla (region of dorsal vagal nucleus) has been observed in MSA, and some depletion, but less severe, in PD (Gai et al. 1993, Kato et al. 1995). Medullary serotonergic neurons in raphe nuclei and the ventrolateral medulla also show severe depletion in MSA, but not in PD. These include neurons projecting to spinal preganglionic neurons (Benarroch et al. 2004). Other parasympathetic central nuclei are less consistently examined, but in MSA there have been occasional reports of neuron loss in the Edinger–Westphal nucleus, and loss of facial and glossopharyngeal central parasympathetic neurons has also been suspected. In PD, Lewy bodies have regularly been found in the Edinger–Westphal nucleus (Forno 1996).

In the nucleus ambiguus in MSA, apart from possible loss of its periambigual parasympathetic neurons (Chapter 2) there may be loss of neurons innervating the abductors of the vocal cords, the posterior crico-arytenoid muscles, seen in terms of neurogenic atrophy of the muscles and neuron loss and gliosis in the nucleus ambiguus (Hayoshi et al. 1997). This is the basis of the potentially life-threatening state of laryngeal stridor. Muscles of the palatopharyngeal isthmus may be similarly affected (Lapresle and Annabi 1979). Neither the nucleus ambiguus nor Onuf's nucleus shows involvement in PD. The neurons in these groups, which share vulnerability in MSA, innervate striated muscles regulating entry to and exit from the tracts derived developmentally from the endoderm (i.e. the laryngeal and oesophageal, and anal and urethral, orifices). The relevant neurons in the nucleus ambiguus are

branchiomotor neurons. It seems very possible that their common susceptibility in MSA might be founded in common factors in their development and, or, environment.

Although some of the same cell groups may show involvement in PD and in MSA, the regular occurrence of Lewy bodies in PD and their general absence in MSA assists in distinguishing the two conditions centrally. Some central neurons in MSA show cytoplasmic and, or, intranuclear inclusions (NCIs, NNIs), but these are relatively few and lack the characteristic, distinctively concentric features of Lewy bodies. A consistent positive discriminator in central nervous pathways in MSA is, however, an abundance of oligodendroglial cytoplasmic inclusions, which are argyrophilic and ubiquitinated, containing loosely arranged, granule-associated coarse filaments resembling microtubules. These are found in affected neuronal groups before the cell loss becomes severe, and also profusely in tracts of nerve fibres presynaptic to these (Papp and Lantos 1994). The filamentous elements both of Lewy bodies and of the GCIs, NCIs and NNIs of MSA have all been shown to be immunoreactive for alpha-synuclein, normally a presynaptic protein, and this accumulation precedes ubiquitination (e.g. Wakabayashi et al. 1998, Spillantini et al. 1998) (Chapter 41).

Ganglia and ganglionic neurons

Sympathetic ganglia have not often been examined in pathological studies of AF, and have seldom been described quantitatively. Enteric and parasympathetic ganglia have been studied in only a few instances. Here also, however, there emerges a distinction between two types of AF.

In MSA with AF (Table 32.1 of Matthews 1992a) it has been typical to report either no obvious abnormality in sympathetic ganglia, or some foci of gliosis and possible loss of neurons, or sometimes neuronophagia, not quantified. Spokes et al. (1979), in silver preparations, noted some depletion of nerve fibres, and argentophil debris. Gliosis could of itself indicate loss of nerve fibres and terminals, and not exclusively loss of neurons: gliosis may be seen in the globus pallidus in MSA in conjunction with severe loss of neurons from the putamen. Any morphological changes reported in sympathetic ganglionic neurons in MSA have tended to be nonspecific, falling within the normal age-related range of appearances, and published micrographs and counts have indicated at least a moderate density, and sometimes quite a high density, of surviving neurons. Four (27%) of the MSA cases reported by Gray et al. (1988), which had severe AF, are unusual in showing 'marked neuronal loss' in sympathetic ganglia.

In PAF, however, and in PD, it has been characteristic to find Lewy bodies (and often numerous Lewy body-like 'eosinophilic bodies' of bizarre, serpiginous form, now regarded as intraneuritic Lewy bodies) in the sympathetic ganglia, with or without obvious neuronal loss (Table 32.1 of Matthews 1992a), just as in the pigmented neurons of the brainstem in PD. Rajput and Rozdilsky (1976) found Lewy bodies in sympathetic ganglia in 5 of 6 PD cases, with 'axonal swellings' in the other, and reported (without formal counting) slight to severe loss and atrophy of the ganglionic neurons, roughly correlated with the degree of orthostatic hypotension, in the three cases of PD which also showed AF. The subject with severest AF and greatest loss of sympathetic neurons showed only 'minimal reduction' of neurons in the IML, whereas a subject with MSA and AF was judged to have moderate loss of IML neurons and no more than slight neuron loss in the sympathetic stellate ganglion.

Goldstein et al. (1997) found no demonstrable cardiac uptake of ^{18}F-6-fluorodopamine on thoracic PET scan, coupled with other indices of peripheral sympathetic cardiac denervation, in two PD patients with orthostatic hypotension. This observation has provided a basis for clinical discrimination between early PD and MSA (Braune et al. 1999, Druschky et al. 2000). Hague et al. (1997), in a subject with PAF of long standing, reported the presence of Lewy bodies both in central neurons (in substantia nigra, locus coeruleus, substantia innominata) and in sympathetic ganglionic neurons, including peripheral autonomic (presumptive sympathetic) axons at distal sites: in the epicardial fat, in peri-adrenal tissue, and in the muscularis of the urinary bladder. Such findings have suggested the possibility of a primary lesion in PD, and now also in PAF, affecting in common neurons of similar or related phenotypes. The disease process is, however, not restricted to catecholaminergic, or monoaminergic, neurons, either centrally, where the cholinergic nucleus basalis is regularly involved, or peripherally. Wakabayashi et al. (1993), while confirming the consistency of occurrence of Lewy bodies in sympathetic ganglia in cases of PD, reported in 12 such cases (and also in five non-parkinsonian subjects with many Lewy bodies in the central nervous system) an increased incidence of Lewy bodies in enteric neurons and in neurons of cardiac and pelvic plexuses, in comparison with an extensive control series. Takeda et al. (1993) found Lewy bodies, both intrasomatic and intraneuritic, in the submandibular ganglion as well as in myenteric ganglia in a case of PD. Thus, there may be widespread involvement of peripheral autonomic neurons, sympathetic, parasympathetic and enteric, by the pathological process which leads to the formation of Lewy bodies in PD and in diffuse Lewy body disease or the pre-parkinsonian state; and the latter may include PAF, since it is now reported that central as well as peripheral neurons may develop Lewy bodies in this condition also (Hague et al. 1997).

Since the autonomic ganglia appear to differ distinctively in these two forms of AF, it is clearly important to examine them carefully for any further evidence that may throw light on the pathological processes involved.

Why is it so difficult to be sure about the underlying changes? There are various reasons, some of which are common to all neuropathological studies while others are peculiar to the autonomic nervous system. First, the basic defect may be biochemical, metabolic, or regulatory, and may not express itself in gross structural terms. Secondly, the condition may be well advanced before it presents clinically. This is perhaps particularly true of the autonomic nervous system, which, unlike the somatic motor system, shows no clearly defined functional demarcation between an upper (higher centres) and a lower motor neuron (IML) lesion. In this context the fact that the earliest symptom in MSA is often sphincter disturbance from involvement of Onuf's nucleus, which innervates striated muscle, offers a valuable cue to immediate and follow-up evaluation of autonomic functions. There are both divergence and convergence of preganglionic neurons on to ganglionic neurons, and the latter may receive multiple inputs which have the characteristic that they are subthreshold, requiring coincidence of several inputs to bring the neuron to the threshold for firing. The peripheral effectors are smooth or cardiac muscle and gland cells; neuroeffector contacts are typically not close; and electrotonic coupling in the effector organ is frequent or invariable. The interstitial dropping-out of peripheral sympathetic nerve endings may be initially compensated by diffusion of transmitter, since fewer nerve endings mean less high-affinity reuptake, by increase in receptor density, and by electrotonic coupling, until the changes have become extreme. Moreover, collateral sprouting of residual preganglionic nerves in the ganglia (cf. Liestøl et al. 1986) and also of postganglionic nerves in the periphery is further able to compensate to a remarkable extent. A slowly progressive change may thus not become clinically evident until the underlying pathological changes are severe, as in the case of IML neuron loss in MSA with AF (Oppenheimer 1980).

By this time, secondary trophic and degenerative changes may well have occurred, involving not only neurons but also satellite or Schwann cells, supporting tissues, and vasculature. As far as the neurons are concerned, these secondary changes are likely to be transneuronal in character, but could be either anterograde or retrograde. Much knowledge has accrued latterly concerning retrograde trophic influences on neurons, and this has arisen largely from studies of autonomic and sensory ganglia, relating to nerve growth factor and, more recently, to brain-derived, ciliary, and other tissue-derived neurotrophic factors, which govern the development and maintenance of peripheral ganglion cells (Thoenen 1991). A similar control may be expected to apply in the case of the preganglionic neurons. Survival and phenotypic specification may be governed by different factors, and a neuron may be induced to change its phenotype by target-derived factor(s) after it has reached and innervated the target, as in the case of the sympathetic sudomotor neuron, which is initially adrenergic but undergoes a cholinergic transformation after it has innervated the sweat glands. Anterograde influences may also be important, as is well exemplified by the striated muscle fibre: trophic maintenance is influenced by activation, and in its absence shrinkage and a varying degree of dedifferentiation may occur. Whether in the long term denervation may lead to neuronal death is uncertain: it depends strongly on age, on the type of neuron, and the presence or absence of other inputs.

From the time of onset of AF a patient may survive for several or even many years. The availability of biopsy is strictly limited (e.g. to the peripheral autonomic terminals as seen in muscle or skin biopsies), since the removal of ganglia would be too destructive; and the possibility of early biopsy is virtually ruled out by the lateness of presentation. Post-mortem changes may preclude the finer aspects of the eventual analysis, and agonal changes, involving intense nervous discharges, may also have supervened, as the terminal event is often apparently asphyxial.

Desiderata for studying the ganglia post-mortem

These include early chilling of the body and early removal of tissues, to optimize tissue preservation; extensive sampling within the autonomic nervous system; the obtaining of adequate age-matched control material for comparison; and the use of appropriate fixation schedules: for example, buffered 4% formaldehyde followed by paraffin embedding for conventional histology, including neuron counting, or by cryostat or frozen sections for enzyme histochemistry and immunohistochemistry; buffered 3% glutaraldehyde followed by resin-embedding for electron microscopy and for light microscopy of 1 μm sections; or alternatively, especially where little tissue is obtainable, Bouin's fluid, or Zamboni's fixative (buffered 2% formaldehyde with 15% saturated picric acid), which is compatible with both immunohistochemistry and electron microscopy as well as conventional histology. In practice, for various reasons, it may only be possible to fulfil a limited number of these criteria.

Experimental observations

Matthews (1992a) reported a study of sympathetic ganglia from six subjects dying with MSA and AF, aged 46–77 years, two subjects dying with clinically pure AF, aged 58 years and 70 years, and ganglia from 10 subjects dying of other causes, aged 16–98 years.

Light microscopy

No Lewy bodies were found in any ganglia from the control or MSA subjects. The ganglia of subjects with MSA were well populated with neurons which resembled those of control ganglia in size, general cytology, and packing density. Almost all neurons had conspicuous aggregates of lipofuscin granules. Nissl material was, however, relatively scanty. In silver-stained preparations many neurons were seen to have well-preserved dendritic arborizations (Fig. 42.1). Some of these dendritic patterns were perhaps unusually complex and profuse, and some processes unusually stout, but no gross distortions were observed. Some of the smaller neurons showed no stainable arborizations; but failure to stain processes in this material cannot necessarily be taken to imply their absence.

Semi-quantitative cytological comparisons were made in 1-μm resin-embedded sections from comparable mid-ganglion levels (Fig. 42.2). In superior cervical ganglia (SCGs) of three control subjects (ages 16, 64, 98 years), the mean packing density of neurons in areas of neuropil averaged 7.1 nucleated neuronal profiles (NNP) in a standard reference area (range of means 5.6–8.3). In SCGs of three subjects with MSA (ages 59, 60, 77 years) the corresponding average was 8.9 NNP (range of means 6.8–10.4). This hardly suggests neuronal loss, but might indicate compaction consequent on reduction of other elements such as preganglionic nerve fibres and extent of dendritic trees. Schmidt et al. (1993) found no decrease of neuronal packing density with age in sympathetic ganglia of control, non-diabetic subjects.

In the control ganglia, a mean of 91% of NNP (range 84–95%) showed distinct Nissl granules. In all three MSA subjects, fewer NNP (37, 46, and 72%) showed distinct Nissl granules. Heavy clumps or masses of lipofuscin bodies were relatively few in the youngest control subject (35% of NNP) but their incidence differed little between the other two (87% and 84%) and the subjects with MSA (range 78–93%, mean 84%). The proportion of NNP

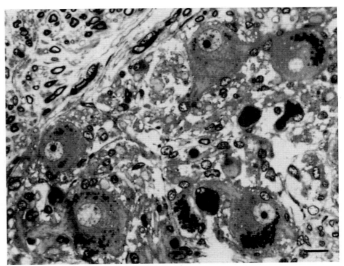

Fig. 42.2 1-μm section of an Araldite-embedded thoracic ganglion of a subject with multiple system atrophy, stained with methylene blue and Azur II. Most of the neurons have eccentric nuclei and contain arcs or masses of darkly stained lipofuscin bodies, but also contain some distinct Nissl material (intermediate grey clumps). Scale bar, 20 μm.

showing centrally situated, rather than eccentric, nuclei was similar in the two groups (control mean 15%, range 11–24%; MSA mean 13%, range 8–18%). The mean diameters of the five to eight largest and smallest neurons were compared, for two subjects from each group, and were not found to differ markedly.

Thus, in the MSA group of subjects with AF, the principal observed difference from the controls lay in the reduced incidence of distinct Nissl granules in the neuronal cell bodies. No consistent abnormalities were noted in the vasculature or in adventitious cells in the ganglia; but in one MSA subject there was some perivenular lymphocytic infiltration, part of a generalized distribution associated with a long-standing leukaemic condition (Waldeström macroglobulinaemia).

In sympathetic ganglia from the two subjects with PAF, the packing densities of NNP in the neuropil were strikingly reduced, to means of 3.4 and 2.2 per standard reference area, and there was similar heavy depopulation of neurons, with scattered evidence of neuronophagia, in all ganglia studied. Lewy bodies were seen in both subjects, with mean incidences of 1.1 and 1.25 per NNP; these were sometimes in neuronal somata and sometimes in enlarged neuronal processes. In the surviving neurons, however, the mean incidence of visible Nissl granules was high (92 and 93% of NNP), and the proportions of NNP which showed massed lipofuscin bodies (82% in each case) resembled those reported above for the MSA and control subjects. In these ganglia, therefore, the salient and distinctive features were the evidence of loss of neurons and the presence of Lewy bodies. In the younger PAF subject an entire SCG was available for neuron-counting in serial paraffin sections. Corrected counts of all neuronal nuclei in every fiftieth section, of 10 μm thickness, yielded an estimate of 214,002 neurons in the entire ganglion. When compared with the mean figure of approximately 937,000 (range 760,370–1,041,652) obtained from four ganglia of young adults by Ebbesson (1963), this suggests a loss of over 75% of neurons, which is much greater than might be expected to occur with age in normal subjects.

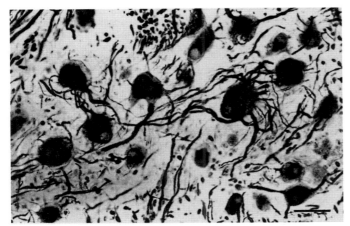

Fig. 42.1 Neurons of a thoracic sympathetic ganglion from a subject with multiple system atrophy. Silver preparation (Glees and Marsland). Scale bar, 50 μm.

Histochemistry, immunohistochemistry, *in situ* hybridization

In frozen sections of a thoracic ganglion from the younger PAF subject specific acetylcholinesterase activity was demonstrable, after prolonged incubation, with a normal distribution in the few surviving neuronal cell bodies and in parts of the surrounding neuropil, but not in nerve bundles.

Immunofluorescence histochemistry by the indirect method was performed on sections from ganglia of two subjects with MSA (males aged 56 and 77 years) and one with PAF (female, aged 58 years, from whom neuron counts were made in the SCG), in comparison with ganglia from three young (ages 17–27 years) and four older male control subjects (ages 57–85 years), with the following results.

Sensory nerve collaterals

In the control subjects prevertebral ganglia (coeliac–superior mesenteric; CSMG) contained perineuronal networks of finely varicose nerve fibres immunoreactive for substance P (SP), and likewise for calcitonin-gene-related peptide (CGRP), which surrounded individual neurons or clusters of neurons. Both these peptides are found in primary sensory neurons, in many of which they coexist, and the intraganglionic networks are attributable to collateral terminal branches of sensory nerve fibres from the viscera that traverse the prevertebral ganglia en route to the dorsal root ganglia and spinal cord (Matthews et al. 1987). In thoracic and lumbar paravertebral ganglia only occasional, solitary varicose trails were seen, which were immunoreactive for SP or CGRP. No obvious differences were found between the younger and older control subjects. Similar networks in a prevertebral ganglion, resembling those in the controls both in distribution and in density, and occasional solitary fibres in paravertebral ganglia, were found in one of the MSA subjects (Fig. 42.3b, c). (No prevertebral ganglion was available from the other MSA subject.) The coeliac ganglion of the subject with PAF showed localized baskets of SP- and CGRP-immunoreactive varicosities surrounding some of the residual neurons, but not those with Lewy bodies or dystrophic neurites. These findings suggest that such trophic interactions as may be required for the maintenance of these sensory collateral networks are still present and operative, not only in older control subjects equally with younger subjects, but also in MSA, and in relation to some surviving neurons in PAF.

Neuromedin B immunoreactivity in ganglia

In the CSMG of control subjects, neuromedin B (NMB) immunoreactivity was observed in finely varicose nerve fibres and pericellular networks surrounding many groups of neurons (Matthews et al. 1992b). Paravertebral ganglia showed only very occasional NMB-immunoreactive (-IR) fibres. A similar distribution of NMB-IR fibres was found in the MSA subjects, and some remnants of NMB networks also persisted in the CSMG of the PAF subject. Additionally, ileal myenteric ganglia of three control subjects were found to contain occasional NMB-IR neurons, and networks of NMB-IR fibres were observed surrounding some of the ganglionic neurons. In contrast, only scanty NMB-IR nerve fibre networks were found in spinal-cord sections, in superficial laminae of the dorsal horn. It cannot be excluded that the intraganglionic NMB-IR nerve networks in the CSMG are collateral branches of sensory nerve fibres, but it is also possible that they may originate from

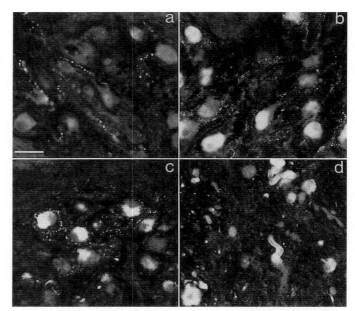

Fig. 42.3 Immunofluorescent staining for neuropeptides in the coeliac ganglion: **(a)** enkephalin, **(b)** substance P, **(c)** calcitonin-gene-related peptide, all from a case of multiple system atrophy; **(d)** neuropeptide Y in dystrophic neurites, from a case of pure autonomic failure. Scale bar, 50 μm. Some neurons in **(b)** and **(c)** show intensely autofluorescent lipofuscin masses.

neurons in the enteric nerve plexuses and that, like sensory nerve collaterals, they may persist in MSA and to some extent in PAF.

Enkephalin-immunoreactive elements

In the control prevertebral ganglia, equally in younger and older subjects, short trails and perineuronal arcs of coarse enkephalin-immunoreactive varicosities were scantily distributed from place to place. Similar enkephalin-immunoreactive nerve elements, similarly distributed, were found in the prevertebral ganglion of the MSA subject (Fig. 42.4a) and occasionally, near to some of the surviving neurons, in the PAF subject.

In the paravertebral ganglia of all the control subjects, profuse pericellular networks of finely varicose, slender, enkephalin-immunoreactive nerve fibres were seen, surrounding clusters of neurons from place to place throughout the ganglia (Fig. 42.4a). In the two MSA subjects, although the post-mortem intervals (10 hours, 13 hours) had been shorter than for any of the controls (21–48 hours, mean 31 hours), only slight and scanty enkephalin-immunoreactive networks were found in thoracic and lumbar paravertebral ganglia (Fig. 42.4b). In a thoracic ganglion of the PAF subject, no enkephalin-immunoreactive fibres or varicosities could be detected. This could have either of two causes:

- ante-mortem loss, through degeneration
- post-mortem degradation of these very fine nerve fibres, since in this case the post-mortem interval was long (84 hours), although cooling had been begun early.

The question must remain open.

The fine enkephalin-immunoreactive networks in the paravertebral ganglia are attributable to preganglionic nerve fibres. Clearly, these do not represent all the preganglionic nerve endings, since not all neurons are surrounded by them. In the rat, enkephalin and choline acetyltransferase, the acetylcholine-synthesizing enzyme,

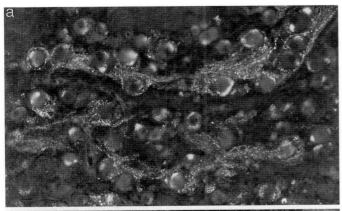

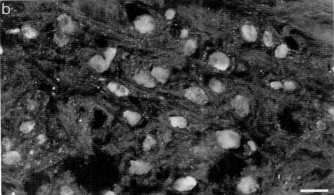

Fig. 42.4 Immunofluorescent staining for enkephalin in thoracic paravertebral ganglia: **(a)** from a young control subject, calcitonin-gene-related peptide from a case of multiple system atrophy. Very few trails of fine enkephalin-immunoreactive fibres are present in **(b)**. Most of the solitary bright points in this field represent lipofuscin autofluorescence. Scale bar, 50 μm.

have been shown to coexist in some of the preganglionic sympathetic neurons (Kondo et al. 1985). The severe depletion of enkephalin-immunoreactive networks in paravertebral ganglia in MSA suggests, first, that the corresponding IML neurons are heavily depleted, and secondly, that this loss has not been fully compensated by whatever intraganglionic sprouting may have occurred from the nerve endings of surviving enkephalin-immunoreactive neurons. The same could well also apply to the other, non-enkephalin-immunoreactive preganglionic neurons. In the PAF subject, absence of enkephalin-immunoreactive networks could indicate retrograde transneuronal loss of the preganglionic neurons from target deprivation, consequent upon the severe neuron depopulation of the ganglion. It is appropriate to consider whether death of preganglionic neurons from target deprivation could contribute to the loss of enkephalin-immunoreactive nerve networks in the MSA subjects, since there is evidence for selective loss of sudomotor ganglionic neurons in this condition (Low and Fealey 1992). Upon this point, however, the available evidence is conflicting, one study (Schmitt et al. 1988) suggesting that presumptive sudomotor neurons in human paravertebral sympathetic ganglia are not innervated by enkephalin-immunoreactive nerve fibres and another (Järvi and Pelto-Huikko 1990) indicating the contrary.

Neuropeptide Y immunoreactivity in ganglia

A proportion of sympathetic ganglionic neurons contains neuropeptide Y (NPY)-immunoreactive material in addition to noradrenaline.

These include vasoconstrictor neurons, and neurons innervating the heart and vas deferens, *inter alia*. In the young control subjects many ganglionic neurons showed moderate immunoreactivity for NPY, and a few short varicose trails and somewhat larger foci of more intense immunoreactivity were seen in the surrounding neuropil (Fig. 42.5a). In older subjects these additional foci of more intense immunoreactivity were more numerous and widespread, and the NPY immunoreactivity of the cell bodies also appeared more intense (Fig. 42.5c). In the ganglia of the MSA subjects this difference was at least as strongly marked, and possibly greater, placing them in sharp contrast with the ganglia of the younger subjects (Fig. 42.5b). The additional foci may represent NPY-rich short intracapsular dendrites or additional dendritic branches of the neurons, which increase with age, and might be particularly profusely developed, or strongly charged with NPY, in the MSA

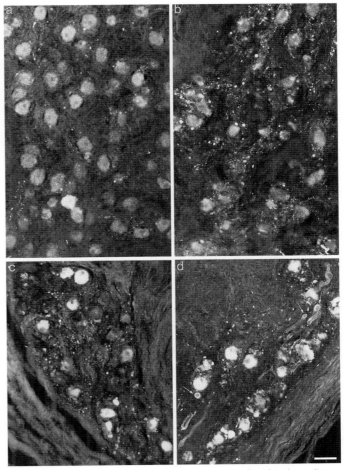

Fig. 42.5 Immunofluorescent staining for neuropeptide Y (NPY) in the coeliac ganglion. **(a)** From a young control subject, aged 17 years, **(b)** from a case of multiple system atrophy, subject aged 77 years, **(c)** from an old control subject, aged 85 years. NPY immunoreactivity is visible in most of the neurons in **(a)** and **(b)**, but in **(c)** is partly obscured by lipofuscin masses. Irregular varicose trails and larger foci of bright immunofluorescence are much more numerous in **(c)** than in **(a)** and are particularly conspicuous in **(b)**. Section **(d)** is from the case of pure autonomic failure illustrated also in Fig. 42.3d, and shows the prevalence of Lewy bodies and dystrophic neurites, some with strong peripheral NPY immunoreactivity (arrows), in a region unusually well populated with surviving neurons. Scale bar, 50 μm.

subjects, there perhaps reflecting low recruitment and engorgement with undischarged secretory material, and perhaps the formation of local collateral sprouts and synapses (cf. Ramsay and Matthews 1985). In the PAF subject, many of the Lewy bodies and dystrophic neurites showed NPY immunoreactivity in their peripheral zone, marginal to the halo (Fig. 42.5d).

Tyrosine hydroxylase immunoreactivity

Tyrosine hydroxylase (TH) is a cytoplasmic enzyme of the sympathetic neuron, which is of interest as being the rate-limiting enzyme in catecholamine synthesis. It is also subject to up-regulation via incoming nerve impulses. A low cytoplasmic level of immunofluorescent signal for TH, approximately $1.8 \times$ primary-antibody blank level, was demonstrable in neurons of a ganglion from a young control subject by image densitometry of film micrographs exposed for a standard interval. Similar measurements in the corresponding ganglion of an MSA subject gave a value of approximately $1.2 \times$ antibody blank level. These measurements were made with precautions to avoid deposits of lipofuscin in the neurons. They indicate that TH-like material and a presumptive catecholamine productive capacity may persist in sympathetic ganglionic neurons in MSA despite a severe degree of decentralization, which harmonizes with the observation of normal supine plasma noradrenaline levels in this condition.

In situ hybridization for tyrosine hydroxylase messenger RNA

Cryostat sections of ganglia of the same two MSA subjects and the PAF subject and ganglia from three younger and three older male control subjects, all from the above series, were examined by *in situ* hybridization for TH messenger RNA (mRNA) (Foster et al. 1990). Sections from MSA subjects and both older and younger controls showed similar levels of binding of the ^{35}S-labelled TH mRNA antisense oligonucleotide probe used (Fig. 42.6a, c; Fig. 42.6a). In contrast, sections from the PAF subject showed very low levels of probe binding over the few remaining neurons (Fig. 42.6b; Fig. 42.7b); neurons containing Lewy bodies did not differ noticeably from those without such inclusions. All the sections studied showed low levels of hybridization to a TH sense probe, employed to reflect nonspecific binding (Fig. 42.6d). Binding of this probe was localized almost exclusively to collections of lipofuscin in the ganglionic neurons. This study indicated that TH mRNA is detectable post-mortem in human sympathetic neurons by *in situ* hybridization. The finding that TH probe binding was similar in MSA and in control ganglia suggests that TH biosynthetic pathways may be functioning normally in the ganglionic neurons of MSA subjects, despite the deficiencies in preganglionic pathways. In the case of PAF studied, the low level of TH antisense probe binding did not differ appreciably from the level of non-specific binding indicated by the sense probe. Any conclusion that TH biosynthesis in surviving neurons was reduced in this case must, however, be tentative because of the long post-mortem delay of over 80 h, already noted.

Electron microscopy

Not all the material was sufficiently well preserved to be informative. Questions addressed included general neuronal cytology (Fig. 42.8), the presence and type of synapses, the completeness of satellite cell cover of the neurons, and the state of the preganglionic and postganglionic nerve fibres.

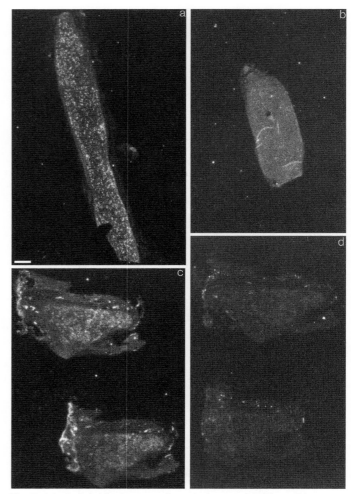

Fig. 42.6 *In situ* hybridization autoradiographs (reverse phase) from slide-mounted cryostat sections. **(a)** Paravertebral (lumbar) ganglion from a case of multiple system atrophy, **(b)** coeliac ganglion from a case of pure autonomic failure, **(c)** stellate ganglion from a control subject aged 66 years, all showing extent of binding of the antisense probe for tyrosine hydroxylase messenger RNA; **(d)** coeliac ganglion of the same control subject, adjacent section to that in **(c)**, showing low level of nonspecific binding of the sense probe. Scale bar, 1 mm.

In the youngest control subject, synapses were readily localizable with an incidence of approximately 6–10 per grid square of side 100 µm; they were of cholinergic preganglionic type (Fig. 42.9) (Matthews 1983) and were mostly axodendritic. In the subjects with MSA similar synapses were present (Fig. 42.10), occurring in clusters in areas of dendritic neuropil, but were much less frequent, and tended to be greatly expanded and depleted of vesicles. This appearance was not necessarily just a post-mortem artefact, since it appeared equally in ganglia fixed within 8 hours and over 36 hours post-mortem: it recalled the appearance of nerve endings heavily overstimulated by black widow spider venom, and could possibly have reflected intense sympathetic discharges in surviving preganglionic endings in the ante-mortem period. In addition, occasional synapses were seen containing tubular vesicles with a relatively electron-dense content (Fig. 42.11); these resemble a type of adrenergic nerve ending and could be intrinsic synapses, which can increase appreciably in incidence in denervated (and presumably in partly denervated) ganglia (Ramsay and Matthews 1985).

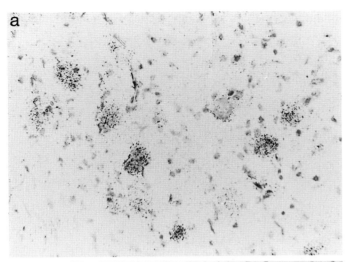

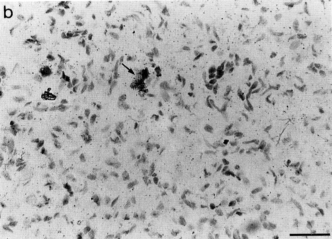

Fig. 42.7 *In situ* hybridization autoradiographs lightly counterstained with toluidine blue, light micrography. Scale bar, 50 µm. **(a)** Lumbar ganglion of a 66-year-old control subject, showing heavy binding of antisense probe for tyrosine hydroxylase messenger RNA over ganglionic neurons; **(b)** coeliac ganglion of the subject with pure autonomic failure showing some binding of the same probe over a neuron containing a Lewy body (arrow) but little or no binding elsewhere; the binding in this specimen did not differ appreciably from the nonspecific binding of the sense probe.

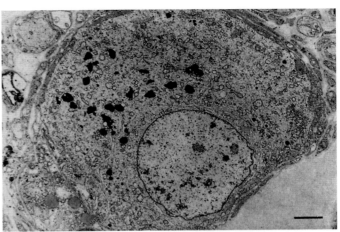

Fig. 42.8 Electron micrograph of a neuron from the superior cervical ganglia of a subject with multiple system atrophy. The nucleus is markedly eccentric. The cytoplasm shows numerous lipofuscin bodies and little rough endoplasmic reticulum (Nissl material). At the lower right, the satellite sheath of the neuron is very thin and in places deficient (cf. Fig. 42.12). Scale bar, 5 µm.

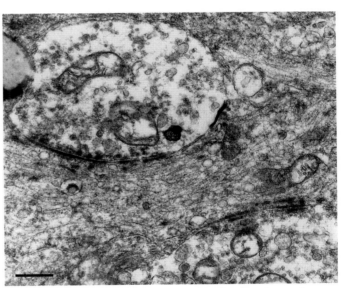

Fig. 42.9 Two synapses of cholinergic type on a dendrite from the superior cervical ganglia of a control subject aged 16 years. Scale bar, 0.5 µm.

Neuroneuronal attachment plaques were seen both in control and in MSA ganglia (Fig. 42.11).

Neuron–satellite relations did not seem to differ markedly between control and MSA ganglia. In both, neurons or their dendrites could show short, sometimes multiple, regions of their surfaces devoid of satellite cell cover (Fig. 42.12); these appeared to be at least as frequent in the MSA ganglia. There was possibly some tendency for the enveloping satellite cell processes to be thinner in the MSA ganglia; but further study, of material better matched as to age and preservation, would be required to clarify this question.

In one MSA subject the preganglionic and postganglionic nerve fibres were sufficiently well preserved for study. Among the preganglionic nerve fibres there was evidence of loss of axons, in the form of collagen-filled Schwann cell channels; myelinated fibres were few, and other Schwann–axon units contained each only one or two non-myelinated axons. The indications of fibre loss are consistent with the well-documented loss of IML neurons in MSA. Some of the non-myelinated axons were singly ensheathed and of relatively large diameter, up to 4 µm, which suggests possible demyelination, or hypertrophy without accompanying myelination. These axons were well populated with longitudinally oriented microtubules and neurofilaments, and did not appear to be pathologically swollen. Among the postganglionic fibres in the internal carotid trunk there was also some suggestion of fibre loss, in the form of collagen-filled channels in Schwann cells, and here also there was a wide range of diameters of non-myelinated axons, suggesting possible denervation atrophy of some neurons and hypertrophy of others. The number of fibres per Schwann unit was not unduly high, ranging mostly from 2 to 6; thus, there was little evidence of axon sprouting at this level.

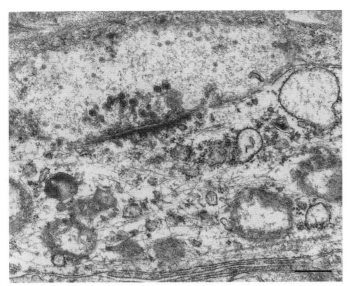

Fig. 42.10 Axodendritic synapse from the superior cervical ganglia of a subject with multiple system atrophy. The presynaptic profile is heavily depleted of synaptic vesicles and shows evidence of numerous coated vesicles, suggesting recent extensive liberation of transmitter. Scale bar, 0.5 μm.

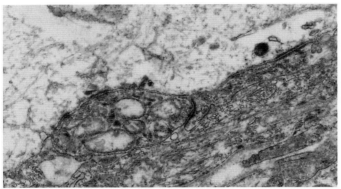

Fig. 42.11 Two synapses of possible adrenergic type from the same presynaptic profile, one axodendritic and the other probably axosomatic, from the superior cervical ganglia of a subject with multiple system atrophy (same ganglion as Fig. 42.10). On the right the dendrite is linked with the presumptive soma by an attachment plaque. ×21,000.

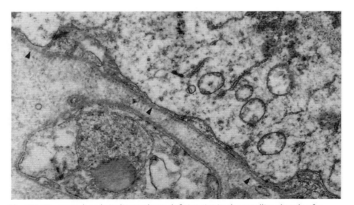

Fig. 42.12 Arrowheads indicate short deficiencies in the satellite sheath of a neuron, from the superior cervical ganglia of a subject with multiple system atrophy. ×13,000.

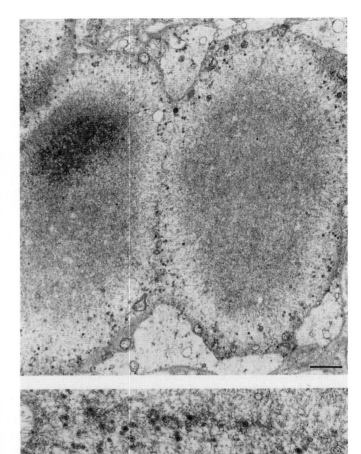

Fig. 42.13 Electron micrograph of two Lewy bodies filling adjacent parts of a neurite, possibly an axon, from the superior cervical ganglia of a subject with pure autonomic failure. Scale bar, 2 μm. Below is shown at higher magnification part of the periphery of the Lewy bodies, where dense-cored vesicles are associated with the margins of the fibrillary masses. Scale bar, 0.5 μm.

In the older subject with PAF, although preservation of the interneuronal neuropil was poor, information was obtained on the nature of the Lewy bodies in these sympathetic neurons (Fig. 42.13): a mass of densely fibrillar material with an amorphous denser core was surrounded by a rim of dense-cored vesicles, which were associated with radiating marginal filaments of the mass (cf. Forno and Norville 1976). Densely packed lysosomal bodies in addition to much lipofuscin were seen in some neurons; but otherwise the surviving neurons, apart from those containing Lewy bodies, did not look grossly abnormal.

Conclusion

This study in sympathetic ganglia has indicated a clear difference in ganglionic pathology, and hence presumably in underlying cause of the AF, between MSA and pure AF.

In MSA the neurons of sympathetic ganglia are not in general severely reduced in number and do not exhibit major abnormalities, apart from a relative lack of Nissl material which might indicate a partial denervation atrophy of long standing. There is confirmatory evidence of the loss of preganglionic nerve fibres, and there is evidence suggesting that, despite any regenerative sprouting from surviving fibres, by the time AF supervenes there is a severe deficiency of preganglionic nerve endings in the ganglia. The loss of preganglionic nerve endings appears to be selective, since other demonstrable fibre systems, for example sensory collateral nerve networks, seem at least as profuse as in normal subjects. It has not so far proved feasible to determine whether they may actually be increased in MSA ganglia, by some mechanism of sprouting in response to the partial denervation. It is possible however that NPY-immunoreactivity in neurons and their processes may be increased in these ganglia, by more than the increment with age which this study has revealed in control subjects. TH and its mRNA may still be demonstrable in these sympathetic neurons, in MSA with AF.

In PAF, on the other hand, the packing density of ganglionic neurons may be severely reduced; and counts in one complete SCG have indicated a neuronal loss of over 75%, which resembles the proportional loss of IML neurons at which AF becomes severe (Oppenheimer 1980). Some of the surviving ganglionic neurons show Lewy bodies, many display eosinophilic Lewy-like bodies in distorted, dystrophic neurites, and some show evidence of an intense lysosomal activity, but almost all of the remainder show well-defined Nissl granules and do not appear grossly abnormal for the age of the subject.

It therefore seems reasonable to assume, as a working hypothesis, that the prime determinants of these two forms of AF are, respectively, the loss of preganglionic and of ganglionic neurons. To this must be added, in MSA, the losses of branchiomotor neurons and of caudal sphincteric motoneurons (Onuf's nucleus) which underlie the development of laryngeal and sphincter problems; and in PD with AF, and possibly also in PAF (Hague et al. 1997), the as yet incompletely defined contribution of the involvement of central as well as peripheral neurons. The initial causes of these losses of neurons remain obscure, although they evidently differ: in both 'Lewy body disease' and MSA abnormal intraneuronal accumulations of filamentous material occur which in each case includes alpha-synuclein as an early constituent, but the different forms taken by these accumulations and their differential sensitivity for different classes of neurons suggest differences of origin. These might reside for example either in the primary abnormality that leads to the deposition of alpha-synuclein or in specific, possibly transmitter-related housekeeping functions of the cell which dictate the precise configuration and intracellular location of the accumulations. In each case the axonal transport system of the neuron and the proper functioning of its nerve terminals are presumably grossly disrupted. In both cases the material may become ubiquitinated, but this is a nonspecific sign of non-lysosomal protein degradation. It is not clear in either case whether the same abnormality which causes the accumulations also leads to neuronal death. Some families suffering early-onset PD show mutations of the alpha-synuclein gene, which might promote neurotoxicity. Neurons containing Lewy bodies may still, however, if catecholaminergic, exhibit tyrosine hydroxylase; and their nuclei and cytoplasmic organelles usually appear intact (Forno 1996). The apparently short-lived stage of intraneuronal granulofilamentous accumulations in MSA is possibly a more direct precursor of neuronal death, since few such accumulations are seen at stages when neuronal loss has become pronounced. It remains to be confirmed by counting to what extent there may be loss of ganglionic

neurons in the AF which can develop in Parkinson's disease; but it appears likely that PAF, PD, and PD with AF are different manifestations of the same disease process. The ramifications of the secondary consequences remain likewise to be unravelled. As Oppenheimer (1980) clearly showed, loss of IML neurons in PAF, or in AF with PD, can be quite as severe as that found in MSA. This could be a retrograde neuronal death, consequent upon target deprivation and related to the profundity and duration of the latter. Indeed, the loss of IML neurons in MSA might itself be due to disruption of a retrograde trophic influence from the ganglionic neurons, which might arise, for example, from inadequate production or release of essential neurotrophic factor(s), without overt morphological changes in the ganglionic neurons. The demonstration of apparently normal prevertebral sensory collateral nerve networks in MSA suggests, however, that any deficiency of trophic substance must be highly specific for the preganglionic neurons.

The observations reported here denote some advances to date but also present challenges for verification and questions for exploration. The wider range of approaches and techniques now available, including genetic studies, offers renewed hope of progress in resolving the basic problems of causation, and hence possibly of prevention, in these devastatingly disabling conditions of AF.

Acknowledgements

This work received MRC support. Thanks are due to Mr P. J. Belk and Mr M. Masih for technical assistance and to Mr B. Archer and Mr C. Beesley for photographic work. Generous gifts of primary antibodies from A. C. Cuello (SP, Enk, TH) and J. M. Polak (CGRP, NPY, NMB) are gratefully acknowledged. The author is indebted to the late Dr D.R. Oppenheimer, Professor M. M. Esiri, Drs J. R. Ponsford, M. Rossi, N. D. Francis and F. Scaravilli for assistance in obtaining ganglia, and to the late Professor L. W. Duchen for access to paraffin-embedded material.

References

Bajaj, N. P. S., Fowler, C. and Chaudhuri, K. R. (1996). Pure AF with abnormal sphincter electromyography: a case report. *Clin. Auton. Res.,* **6**, 279.

Beck, R. O., Bett, C. D., and Fowler, C. J. (1994). Genitourinary dysfunction in multiple system atrophy: clinical features and treatment in 62 cases. *J Urology,* **151**, 1336–41.

Benarroch, E. E., Schmeichel, A. M., Low, P. A. and Parisi, J. E. (2004). Involvement of medullary serotonergic groups in multiple system atrophy. *Ann. Neurol.,* **55**, 418–22.

Braune, S., Reinhardt, M., Schnitzer, R., Riedel, A. and Lucking, C. H. (1999). Cardiac uptake of [123I]MIBG separates Parkinson's disease from multiple system atrophy. *Neurology,* **54**, 1877–78.

Druschky, A., Hilz, M. J., Platsch, G. et al. (2000). Differentiation of Parkinson's disease and multiple system atrophy in early disease stages by means of I-123-MIBG-SPECT. *J Neurol Science,* **175**, 1–2.

Ebbesson, S. O. E. (1963). A quantitative study of human superior cervical sympathetic ganglia. *Anatomical Record,* **146**, 353–6.

Forno, L. S. (1996). Neuropathology of Parkinson's disease. *J Neuropathol. Exp. Neurol.,* **55**, 259–72.

Forno, L. S. and Norville, R. L. (1976). Ultrastructure of Lewy bodies in the stellate ganglion. *Acta neuropathologica, Berlin,* **34**, 183–97.

Foster, O. J. F., Matthews, M. R., Lightman, S. L. and Bannister, R. (1990). *In situ* hybridisation studies of sympathetic ganglia in multiple system atrophy and pure AF. *J Auton. Nerv. Syst.,* **31**, 171.

Gai, W. P., Geffen, L. B., Denoroy, L. and Blessing, W. W. (1993). Loss of C1 and C3 epinephrine-synthesizing neurons in the medulla oblongata in Parkinson's disease. *Ann. Neurol.*, **33**, 357–67.

Goldstein, D. S., Holmes, C., Cannon, R. O. III., Eisenhofer, G., and Kopin, I. J. .(1997). Sympathetic cardioneuropathy in dysautonomias. *New Engl. J Med.*, **336**, 696–702.

Gray, F., Vincent, D. and Hauw, J. J. (1988). Quantitative study of lateral horn cells in 15 cases of multiple system atrophy. *Acta neuropathologica, Berlin*, **75**, 513–18.

Hague, K., Lento, P., Morgello, S., Caro, S., and Kaufmann, H. (1997). The distribution of Lewy bodies in pure AF: autopsy findings and review of the literature. *Acta neuropathologica, Berlin*, **94**, 192–6.

Hayoshi, M., Isozaki, E., Oda, M., Tanabe, H. and Kimura, J. (1997). Loss of large myelinated fibres of the recurrent laryngeal nerve in patients with multiple system atrophy and vocal cord palsy. *Journal of Neurology, Neurosurgery and Psychiatry*, **62**, 234–48.

Hughes, A. J., Daniel, C. J., and Lees, A. J. (1993). A clinico-pathological study of 100 cases of Parkinson's disease. *Arch. Neurol.*, **50**, 140–8.

Infante, J., Llorca, J., Berciano, J. and Combarras, O. (2005). Interleukin-8, intercellular adhesion molecule-1 and tumour necrosis factor-alpha gene polymorphisms and the risk for multiple system atrophy. *J Neurol. Sci.*, **228**, 11–13.

Järvi, R. and Pelto-Huikko, M. (1990). Localization of neuropeptide Y in human sympathetic ganglia: correlation with met-enkephalin, tyrosine hydroxylase and acetylcholinesterase. *Histochemical Journal*, **22**, 87–94.

Kato, S., Oda, M., Hayashi, H. *et al.* (1995). Decrease of medullary catecholamine neurons in multiple system atrophy and Parkinson's disease and their preservation in amyotrophic lateral sclerosis. *J Neurol. Sci.*, **132**, 216–21.

Kondo, N., Kuramoto, H., Wainer, B. H. and Yanaihara, N. (1985). Evidence for the coexistence of acetylcholine and enkephalin in the sympathetic preganglionic neurons of rats. *Brain Research*, **335**, 309–14.

Konno, H., Yamamoto, T., Iwasaki, Y. and Iizuka, H. (1986). Shy–Drager syndrome and amyotrophic lateral sclerosis: cytoarchitectonic and morphometric studies of sacral autonomic neurons. *J Neurol. Sci.*, **73**, 193–204.

Kumazawa, K., Sobue, G., Nakao, N., and Mitsuma, T. (1989). Postganglionic sudomotor function in multiple system atrophy. *Rinsho Shinkeigaku, Japan* **29**, 1357–63. (English abstract).

Lapresle, J. and Annabi, A. (1979). Olivopontocerebellar atrophy with velopharyngolaryngeal paralysis: a contribution to the somatotopy of the nucleus ambiguus. *J Neuropathol. Exp. Neurol.*, **38**, 401–6.

Liestøl, K., Maehlen, J. and Njå, A. (1986). Selective synaptic connections: significance of recognition and competition in mature sympathetic ganglia. *Trends in Neuroscience*, **9**, 21–4.

Low, P. A. and Fealey, R. D. (1992). Pathological studies of the sympathetic neuron. In R. G. Bannister and C. J. Mathias, ed. *AF. A textbook of disorders of the autonomic nervous system*, (3rd edn.) pp. 586–92. Oxford University Press, Oxford.

Magaelhaes, M., Wenning, G. K., Daniel, S. E. and Quinn, N. P. (1995). Autonomic dysfunction in pathologically confirmed multiple system atrophy and idiopathic Parkinson's disease—a retrospective comparison. *Acta neurologica scandinavica*, **91**, 98–102.

Matthews, M. R. (1983). The ultrastructure of junctions in sympathetic ganglia of mammals. In L-G Elfvin, ed. *Autonomic ganglia*, pp. 27–66. John Wiley, Chichester.

Matthews, M. R. (1992a). Autonomic ganglia in multiple system atrophy and pure AF. In R. G. Bannister and C. J. Mathias, ed. *AF. A textbook of disorders of the autonomic nervous system*, (3rd edn.) pp. 593–621. Oxford University Press, Oxford.

Matthews, M. R. (1992b). Neuromedin B immunoreactive networks are present in human sympathetic ganglia and may persist in AF. *Clin. Auton. Res.*, **2**, 71.

Matthews, M. R., Connaughton, M. and Cuello, A. C. (1987). Ultrastructure and distribution of substance P. immunoreactive sensory collaterals in the guinea pig prevertebral sympathetic ganglia. *J Compar. Neurol.*, **258**, 28–51.

Oppenheimer, D. R. (1980). Lateral horn cells in progressive AF. *J Neurol. Sci.*, **46**, 393–404.

Oyanagi, K., Wakabayashi, K., Ohama, E. *et al.* (1990). Lewy bodies in the lower sacral parasympathetic neurons of a patient with Parkinson's disease. *Acta neuropathologica, Berlin*, **80**, 558–9.

Papp, P. L. and Lantos, M. I. (1994). The distribution of oligodendroglial inclusions in multiple system atrophy and its relevance to clinical symptomatology. *Brain*, **117**, 235–43.

Rajput, A. H. and Rozdilsky, B. (1976). Dysautonomia in Parkinsonism: a clinico-pathological study. *Journal of Neurology, Neurosurgery and Psychiatry*, **39**, 1092–100.

Ramsay, D. A. and Matthews, M. R. (1985). Denervation-induced formation of adrenergic synapses in the superior cervical sympathetic ganglion of the rat and the enhancement of this effect by postganglionic axotomy. *Neuroscience*, **16**, 997–1026.

Schmidt, R. E., Plurad, S. B., Parvin, S. A., and Roth, K. A. (1993). Effect of diabetes and aging on human sympathetic autonomic ganglia. *Am. J Pathol.*, **143**, 143–53.

Schmitt, M., Kummer, W., and Heym, C. (1988). Calcitonin gene-related peptide (CGRP)-immunoreactive neurons in the human cervico-thoracic paravertebral ganglia. *Journal of Chemical Neuroanatomy*, **1**, 287–92.

Spillantini, M. G., Crowther, R. A., Jakes, R., Cairns, N. J., Lantos, P. L. and Goedart, M. (1998). Filamentous alpha-synuclein inclusions link multiple system atrophy with Parkinson's disease and dementia with Lewy bodies. *Neuroscience Letters*, **251**, 205–208.

Spokes, E. G. S., Bannister, R. and Oppenheimer, D. (1979). Multiple system atrophy with AF—clinical, histological and neurochemical observations on four cases. *J Neurol. Sci.*, **43**, 59–82.

Takeda, S., Yamazaki, K., Miyakawa, T. and Arai, H. (1993). Parkinson's disease with involvement of the parasympathetic ganglia. *Acta neuropathologica, Berlin*, **86**, 397–8.

Thoenen, H. (1991). The changing scene of neurotrophic factors. *Trends in Neuroscience*, **14**, 165–70.

Wakabayashi, K., Hayashi, S., Kakita, A. *et al.* (1998). Accumulation of α-synuclein/NACP is a cytopathological feature common to Lewy body disease and multiple system atrophy. *Acta neuropathologica*, **96**, 445–52.

Wakabayashi, K., Takahashi, H., Ohama, E., Takeda, S. and Ikuta, F. (1993). Lewy bodies in the visceral autonomic nervous system in Parkinson's disease. *Advances in Neurology*, **60**, 609–12.

van Ingelghem, E., van Zandijcke, M. and Lammens, M. (1994). Pure AF: a new case with clinical, biochemical and autopsy data. *Journal of Neurology, Neurosurgery and Psychiatry* **57**, 745–7.

CHAPTER 43

Experimental models to define multiple system atrophy and autonomic failure

Nadia Stefanova and Gregor K. Wenning

Key points

- Multiple system atrophy (MSA) is an adult onset, sporadic neurodegenerative disorder that presents with autonomic failure in addition to motor impairment resulting from a combination of parkinsonism, cerebellar ataxia and, pyramidal signs.

- Animal models play an important role to study disease pathogenesis as well as test novel therapeutic strategies.

- Three approaches have been used to model key features of MSA with or without autonomic failure in experimental models: neurotoxin approach, transgenic approach, and combined approach.

- Neurotoxins that induce selective loss of dopaminergic nigral neurons and GABAergic medium spiny neurons in striatum have been applied to reproduce dual striatonigral degeneration in rats, mice and primates.

- The unilateral double-lesion rat model of MSA-P is a prominent tool to study neurotransplantation strategies for MSA to restore dopaminergic response.

- Transgenic models based on overexpression of alpha-synuclein in oligodendrocytes have indicated the role of glial cytoplasmic inclusions (GCIs) in the pathogenesis of MSA and their role to induce secondary degeneration related to endogenous alpha-synuclein aggregation in axons, mitochondrial impairment and microglial activation.

- Overexpression of α_{1B}-adrenergic receptor in mice causes an apoptotic multisystem neurodegeneration with a parkinsonian motor disorder and a grand mal seizure disorder accompanied by dysautonomia.

- Dysfunction of calcium channels may contribute to model pure autonomic dysfunction. Lack of the α_{1B} subunit of N-type calcium channels in knockout mice has induced autonomic failure with significant sympathetic nerve dysfunction, but no other apparent behavioural defects or neuroanatomical abnormalities

- The combined alpha-synuclein + 3-nitropropionic acid (αSYN + 3NP) mouse model of MSA reproduces cardinal features of MSA pathology and represents a novel test bed to study the pathogenesis of the disease.

Introduction

Progressive autonomic failure (PAF) occurs in Parkinson's disease (PD), MSA and dementia with Lewy bodies (DLB). These disorders are characterized by neuronal or oligodendroglial αSYN inclusions. Among the alpha-synucleinopathies PAF is most common in MSA, an adult onset, sporadic neurodegenerative disorder that also presents with motor impairment resulting from a combination of poorly levodopa-responsive parkinsonism, cerebellar ataxia, and pyramidal signs. The term MSA was first introduced in 1969 (Graham and Oppenheimer 1969); however, cases of the disease were previously described as striatonigral degeneration (SND), olivopontocerebellar atrophy (OPCA), Shy–Drager syndrome, or idiopathic orthostatic hypotension. SND is the predominant neuropathology in 80% of the MSA cases that manifest with parkinsonism (MSA-P). The remaining 20% develop predominant cerebellar ataxia (MSA-C) associated with OPCA. Autonomic dysfunction including urogenital failure and orthostatic hypotension is common in both motor presentations and reflects degenerative lesions of central autonomic pathways (Wenning et al. 2004). Most patients deteriorate rapidly and survival beyond 10 years of disease onset is unusual. Epidemiological studies suggest a prevalence of 1.9–4.9 per 100,000 people (Wenning et al. 2004) and an incidence of 3 patients per 100,000 population per year (Bower et al. 1997). Differential diagnosis of MSA-P versus PD may be difficult initially due to PD-like features in some MSA-P patients (Wenning et al. 2000a). There is a lack of effective therapies particularly for the motor features of MSA.

MSA brains reveal different degrees and combinations of neuronal loss in the striatum, substantia nigra pars compacta (SNc), cerebellum, pons, inferior olives, and the intermediolateral column of the spinal cord (Daniel 1999, Jellinger 2003). Glial pathology comprises astrogliosis (Schwarz et al. 1996), microglial activation

(Ishizawa et al. 2004), and argyrophilic (oligodendro)glial cytoplasmic inclusions (GCIs) (Papp et al. 1989). Since the discovery of αSYN as a principal component of GCIs (Spillantini et al. 1998, Wakabayashi et al. 1998) MSA has been classified as a member of the alpha-synucleinopathies family together with PD and DLB (Dickson et al. 1999). αSYN is a neuronal protein, which is not normally expressed in adult oligodendrocytes (Solano et al. 2000). In contrast to neuronal αSYN inclusions in PD and DLBD, MSA is characterized by oligodendroglial αSYN inclusion pathology suggesting a unique but poorly understood pathogenic mechanism that may ultimately lead to neuronal cell loss via disturbance of axonal function. The recent working hypothesis of MSA as a primary oligodendrogliopathy (Wenning et al. 2008) has been strengthened by the finding of early dysregulation in p25α/tubulin polymerization promoting protein (TPPP), recorded before any accumulation of GCIs (Orosz et al. 2004). In vitro experiments have demonstrated that p25α/TPPP is a potent stimulator of αSYN aggregation. (Lindersson et al. 2005) and in MSA brains, p25α/TPPP has been shown to strongly co-localize with oligodendroglial αSYN positive GCIs (Song et al. 2007, Jellinger 2005, Lindersson et al. 2005).

Animal models are an important tool to study the pathways underlying human neurodegenerative disorders. Further, they are essential to test and validate novel neuroprotective therapies that are necessary to modulate disease progression. In addition to the motor symptoms, however, modelling the full-blown pathology of MSA has proven to be a difficult task (Table 43.1). One major limitation in the development of experimental models of neurodegenerative disorders is the incomplete current knowledge on the aetiology and pathogenesis of the disorders as well as the failure to model the progressive course of the human pathology.

Three approaches have been used to model key features of MSA with or without autonomic failure in experimental models. The first approach has been based on the administration of available selective toxins in rodents to reproduce SND-like striatal and nigral neuronal loss (i.e. the pathology underlying MSA-P). Secondly, genetically modified mouse models (transgenic for αSYN, α_{1B}-adrenoceptor or knockouts for α_{1B}-subunit of N-type calcium channels) were developed to study candidate molecular pathways of glial and neuronal degeneration/dysfunction in MSA and autonomic failure. Finally, a combined approach to mimic the role of both genetic predisposition and environmental factors has been introduced.

Neurotoxin models

Neurotoxins have been widely used in modelling different neurodegenerative disorders due to their ability to selectively destroy certain neuronal populations. Neurotoxins that induce selective loss of dopaminergic nigral neurons and GABAergic medium spiny neurons in striatum have been applied to reproduce dual SND-like pathology. Dependent on the metabolism of the neurotoxins they are applied either systemically or locally (stereotaxically) into the brain. Further, to induce dual striatal and nigral lesions single or double toxin approaches may be applied.

Selective nigral toxins are classically used to model the dopaminergic neuronal loss in SNc of PD. 6-Hydroxydopamine (6-OHDA) is a hydroxylated analogue of the natural dopamine, which does not cross the blood–brain barrier. In experimental rodent models of PD, 6-OHDA is preferentially injected stereotaxically into striatum, SNc, or medial forebrain bundle (MFB), to destroy the nigral dopaminergic neurons and thus to reproduce the pathological features responsible for motor impairments in PD (Ungerstedt 1968, Ichitani et al. 1991, Sauer and Oertel 1994, Kirik et al. 1998). 1-methyl-4-phenyl-1,2,3,6-tetrahydropyridine (MPTP) induces PD-like symptoms in several species including mouse, dog, cat, and monkey (Burns et al. 1983, Heikkila et al. 1984, Langston et al. 1984, Schneider and Markham 1986, Wilson et al. 1987, Gerlach

Table 43.1 Experimental models of MSA

Species	Paradigm	Motor impairment	Autonomic failure	Atypical phenotype	SND	OPCA	CAD*	α-syn pathology
rat	Unilateral sequential 6-OHDA (mfb) and QA (striatum)	+	−	−	+	−	−	−
rat	Unilateral simultaneous 6-OHDA + QA (striatum)	+	−	−	+	−	−	−
rat	Unilateral 3-NP (striatum)	+	−	−	+	−	−	−
rat	Unilateral MPP+ (striatum)	+	−	−	+	−	−	−
mouse	Systemic, sequential MPTP (i.p.) + 3-NP (i.p.)	+	−	−	+	−	−	−
mouse	Systemic, simultaneous MPTP and 3-NP (i.p.)	+	−	−	+	−	−	−
mouse	Systemic 3-NP (i.p.)	+	−	−	+	−	−	−
primate	Systemic sequential MPTP (i.p.) + 3-NP (i.p.)	+	−	−	+	−	−	−
mouse	α-Synuclein transgenic with proteolipid protein (PLP) promoter	−	−	−	+	−	+	+
mouse	α-Synuclein transgenic with 2', 3'-cyclic nucleotide 3'-phosphodiesterase (CNP) promoter	+	?	−	+	−	+	+
mouse	α-Synuclein transgenic with myelin basic protein (MBP) promoter	+	?	−	−	−	+	+
mouse	α_{1B}-AR transgenic	+	+	+	+	−	+	+
mouse	α-Synuclein transgenic with proteolipid protein (PLP) promotor + systemic 3-NP	+	?	−	+	+	+	+

*central autonomic degeneration.

and Riederer 1996). When systematically administered to animals, MPTP crosses the blood–brain barrier and is converted, mainly in glial cells, into 1-methyl-4-phenylpyridinium ion (MPP$^+$). MPP$^+$ is a major inhibitor of mitochondrial complex I, triggering cell death of dopaminergic neurons (Blum et al. 2001).

Striatal neurotoxins have been first applied in experiments modelling the selective neuronal loss in Huntington's disease (HD), (Beal et al. 1986, Ferrante et al. 1993, Brouillet et al. 1999). Quinolinic acid (QA) is a well-known endogenous tryptophan metabolite at the kynurenine level. QA is a glutamate agonist with relative selectivity for the N-methyl-D-aspartate (NMDA) receptor (Stone 1993). It exerts its neurotoxic actions through mechanisms involving excitotoxicity, reactive oxygen species formation and oxidative stress (Foster et al. 1983, Behan et al. 1999, Santamaria et al. 2001). When injected into the striatum, QA produces a selective pattern of striatal neuronal degeneration with loss of GABAergic projecting medium spiny neurons and relative sparing of somatostatin/neuropeptide Y/NADPH-diaphorase containing interneurons (Figueredo-Cardenas et al. 1997, Figueredo-Cardenas et al. 1998). 3-Nitropropionic acid (3NP) is another neurotoxic compound that causes neuronal degeneration within the basal ganglia when injected systematically or directly into the striatum (Brouillet et al. 2005). 3NP is a mitochondrial toxin that inhibits both complex II-III of the respiratory chain and the tricarboxylic acid through inactivation of the succinate dehydrogenase (SDH) enzyme (Alston et al. 1977).

The first effort to model MSA in rodents was made in 1996. Wenning and co-workers (Wenning et al. 1996) based the idea on reproducing SND in rats by applying selective nigral and striatal neurotoxins, which had previously been used to mimic PD and HD in rats, respectively. 6-OHDA was administered into the left medial forebrain bundle, followed by intrastriatal injection of QA into the ipsilateral striatum. The unilateral 6-OHDA lesion resulted in ipsilateral rotation to amphetamine-induced dopamine release and contralateral rotation to apomorphine (dopamine receptor agonist). Following the subsequent striatal lesion, amphetamine-induced ipsilateral rotation persisted, but apomorphine-induced contralateral rotation was reduced or abolished. The unilateral double-lesion rat model was further characterized by Scherfler and co-workers (Scherfler et al. 2000) who evaluated motor deficits reflecting limb akinesia and deficits of complex motor function in rats subjected to a unilateral double lesion of the nigrostriatal and striatonigral projection. Both behavioural and histopathological studies demonstrated a complex interaction of nigral and striatal lesions depending on the lesion sequence. The study raised the issue whether loss of dopaminergic neurons might protect against the striatal disease process occurring in MSA-P. A modified partial unilateral model of early-stage SND based on simultaneous low dose QA and 6-OHDA injections into the lateral striatum was proposed subsequently (Ghorayeb et al. 2001). This strategy was designed to induce simultaneous and anatomically related striatal and nigral degeneration closely reflecting the human disease process and to avoid reduction of QA striatal toxicity by prior dopamine depletion. However, it remains unknown whether the disease process of MSA-P starts at a nigral or striatal level or both and what is the contribution of nigral and striatal pathology to parkinsonism in MSA (Wenning et al. 2002).

Further, the stereotaxic double-lesion rat model of MSA-P was shown to reproduce the typical levodopa-unresponsive motor disability accompanied by levodopa-induced dyskinesia with orolingual predominance (Stefanova et al. 2004a) in contrast to the 6-OHDA rat model. Comparative pulsatile levodopa treatment in MSA-P and PD rats demonstrated that the combination of striatal and nigral lesion in MSA-P rats leads to loss of levodopa responsiveness of the spontaneous motor activity, probably related to the loss of striatal dopamine receptors in contrast to PD rats. However, dyskinesias were preserved and striatal FosB/ΔFosB up-regulation in MSA-P and PD rats correlated with the severity of levodopa-induced dyskinesias. The MSA-P double lesion rat model therefore supports the idea that different pathophysiological mechanisms underlie dyskinesia and motor response to levodopa therapy (Mouradian et al. 1989, Hughes et al. 1992).

The unilateral double lesion rat model has been widely used to test neuroprotective (Stefanova et al. 2004b, Mantoan et al. 2005, Scherfler et al. 2005) and neurorestorative (Wenning et al. 1996, Schocke et al. 2000, Puschban et al. 2000a, Puschban et al. 2000b, Wenning et al. 2000b, Waldner et al. 2001) strategies for MSA-P. Most of the neuroprotective studies failed to demonstrate significant effects, probably reflecting the complexity of the double lesion paradigm that is required to reproduce SND pathology. In contrast, several agents have been shown to protect striatum and/or substantia nigra in single lesion models of HD or PD. Riluzole, an anti-glutamatergic drug, showed striatal, but not nigral protection in the double-lesion rat model of MSA-P (Scherfler et al. 2005). Minocycline, which had a significant neuroprotective effect in PD and HD models (Chen et al. 2000, Wu et al. 2002, Wang et al. 2003), was ineffective in the MSA-P rat model both at striatal and nigral level despite efficient suppression of microglial and astroglial activation (Stefanova et al. 2004b). Finally, caspase inhibition failed to exert neuroprotection in the MSA-P rat model (Mantoan et al. 2005). Grafting in the double-lesion rat model has shown that embryonic allografts of mesencephalic and striatal origin survive the transplantation in SND with, however, poor dopaminergic reinnervation of the lesioned striatum. Yet, striatal grafts could restore the apomorphine-induced contralateral rotation (Wenning et al. 1996) suggesting a possibility to restore the dopamine response in the lesioned striatum of SND.

The simplified 'single toxin-double lesion' approach was developed to avoid neurotoxins interactions based on the use of a single toxin able to elicit degeneration in both the striatum and the SNc to reproduce MSA-P/SND-like pathology. Intrastriatal 3NP injections were first applied to model advanced MSA-P/SND and to assess the effects of embryonic allografts upon drug-induced rotation asymmetries and complex-motor behavioural deficits measured by paw reaching tests (Waldner et al. 2001). Unfortunately, significant dopamine depletion (−45%) was achieved only at the expense of complete destruction of the lesioned striatum. The severity of the striatal lesion precluded functional effects of the embryonic grafts upon amphetamine- and apomorphine-induced rotations and forelimb use. In addition to 3NP, MPP$^+$, the active metabolite of the MPTP, was also used to generate a double lesion model of MSA-P/SND. Intrastriatal administration of MPP$^+$ caused retrograde and irreversible damage to the dopaminergic system and produced marked excitotoxic lesions of the striatum therefore providing an alternative 'single toxin-double lesion' approach for modelling MSA-P/SND (Ghorayeb et al. 2002). MPP$^+$ administration resulted in loss of the amphetamine-induced ipsilateral bias observed also in the 6-OHDA group and of the apomorphine-induced ipsilateral bias like that observed in the QA group. The 'single toxin-double lesion' paradigm may thus advantageously replace or complement these earlier models, particularly in regard to the better lesion size control obtained with a single toxin.

In an attempt to reproduce the bilateral lesion pattern in MSA-P, selective neurotoxins have been used to develop systemic models of MSA-P where striatal and nigral lesions are bilateral. 3NP and MPTP were intraperitoneally injected in mice in various sequence and dose paradigms (Stefanova et al. 2003, Fernagut et al. 2004, Diguet et al. 2005). In general, the observations in the systemic mouse model confirmed those from the unilateral double-lesion rat model. 3NP-treated mice displayed altered gait patterns, impaired motor performance and activity parameters correlating with the severe neuropathology in striatum and SNc (Fernagut et al. 2004). Studies of the systemic double toxin double lesion mouse model revealed that MPTP-induced nigral lesions attenuate 3NP striatal toxicity and, reciprocally, that 3NP-induced striatal lesions reduce MPTP toxicity (Stefanova et al. 2003). The experiments confirmed the complex integrative mechanisms that are likely to regulate the vulnerability of the striatum and SNc to cell death in MSA-P. Again, neuroprotective studies had limited success with riluzole providing limited 'neuronal rescue' with a subtle motor improvement in the systemic MSA-P mouse model (Diguet et al. 2005).

The same paradigm of MPTP and 3NP intoxication has been transferred to non-human primates to reproduce the SND pathology of MSA-P (Ghorayeb et al. 2000, Ghorayeb et al. 2002). levodopa-responsive parkinsonian features emerged after MPTP injections. Subsequent chronic 3NP administration aggravated the motor symptoms and abolished the levodopa response. In vivo magnetic resonance imaging revealed striatal damage that correlated with the onset of poor levodopa response. Histopathology confirmed striatal degeneration and severe dopaminergic cell loss in the SNc. The model therefore reproduced levodopa-unresponsive parkinsonism and SND-like pathologic changes characteristic of MSA-P. However, the ethical limitations of this model restrict its use in larger studies.

In conclusion, the neurotoxin models, either stereotaxic or systemic, reproduce neuronal cell loss in striatum and SNc, therefore modelling the SND pathology of MSA-P. These models may serve to study basic aspects of dopaminergic dysfunction in MSA-P as well as functional and structural effects of neuroprotection and regeneration therapies targeting the nigro-striato-nigral pathway. Yet, the neurotoxin models are limited to reproducing SND without specifically affecting the olivopontocerebellar system or inducing autonomic dysfunction, which are the other two cardinal clinical presentations of MSA. Further, the specific oligodendroglial αSYN pathology of MSA is lacking in these models.

Transgenic models

Alpha-synuclein transgenic models

The transgenic models of MSA have been generally created to reproduce the GCI pathology of the disease and to study the role of αSYN in its pathogenesis. Principally, all the models use specific oligodendroglial promotors to target the overexpression of human αSYN in oligodendrocytes.

The first transgenic mouse with oligodendroglial expression of human αSYN was developed by using the proteolipid protein (PLP) promotor (Kahle et al. 2002). Marked insolubility of the transgenic αSYN and hyperphosphorylation at serine 129 were observed like in the human disease. The GCI-like pathology in these mice triggered microgliosis, which was demonstrated to contribute to the neurodegeneration (Stefanova et al. 2007). There was mild loss of dopaminergic neurons in SNc that was correlated with shortened stride length in aged transgenic mice (Stefanova et al. 2005). Recent analysis identified in addition progressive neuronal loss in cholinergic brain stem nuclei as well as neurodegeneration of the Onuf's nucleus analogue in (PLP)-αSYN transgenic mice (Stemberger et al. 2010). However, full-blown pathology of MSA was not replicated in these mice.

Parallel efforts were made to create transgenic mice with oligodendroglial expression of human αSYN by applying the 2′, 3′-cyclic nucleotide 3′-phosphodiesterase (CNP) promotor (Yazawa et al. 2005). These experiments showed that oligodendroglial αSYN pathology induces axonal degeneration combined with accumulation of endogenous αSYN. However, selective neuropathology of the human disease was not reproduced. The motor phenotype correlated with neurodegeneration in the spinal cord, while the motor disability (parkinsonism and ataxia) in MSA patients is due to SND and OPCA both of which were absent in the transgenic model.

Finally, a third transgenic model of GCI-like pathology was developed by using the myelin basic protein (MBP) promotor to overexpress human αSYN in oligodendrocytes (Shults et al. 2005). The mice developed progressive accumulation of detergent insoluble, hyperphosphorylated αSYN in oligodendrocytes along the axonal tracts in the brainstem, basal ganglia, cerebellum, corpus callosum, and neocortex. The white matter tracts displayed intense astrogliosis, myelin pallor, and decreased neurofilament immunostaining. The GCI-like pathology induced decreased dendritic density in the neocortex and loss of dopaminergic fibres in the basal ganglia. The oligodendrocytic alpha-synucleinopathy was accompanied by mitochondrial alterations and disruption of the myelin lamina in the axons.

In summary, transgenic mice with oligodendroglial αSYN overexpression reproduce the GCI pathology of MSA. These models indicated that GCIs play a crucial role in the pathogenesis of the disease and may trigger neurodegenerative changes. However, although isolated neurodegeneration was observed in cortical, brainstem, and spinal cord regions, the transgenic mice failed to reproduce the characteristic neuronal multisystem dysfunction observed in the human disease MSA. Autonomic functions have not been tested in the transgenic mice with oligodendroglial αSYN overexpression, however preliminary observations suggest changed heart rate variability in (PLP)-αSYN transgenic mice (unpublished data).

α$_{1B}$-Adrenergic receptor transgenic model

An alternative way to reproduce MSA-like pathology in rodents was discovered inadvertently in functional studies of the α$_{1B}$-adrenergic receptor in the central nervous system. Overexpression of α$_{1B}$-adrenergic receptor in mice caused an apoptotic multisystem neurodegeneration with a levodopa-responsive parkinsonian motor disorder and dopaminergic neuronal loss in SNc and a grand mal seizure disorder accompanied by neurodegeneration of the cerebral cortex. (Zuscik et al. 2000). αSYN inclusion formation was reported in these transgenic mice (Papay et al. 2002); however, the protein was nitrated but not phosphorylated in contrast to the human disease. Further, autonomic failure was observed comprising reduced catecholamine levels together with basal hypotension, bradycardia, reproductive problems, and weight loss (Zuscik et al. 2001). α_{1B}-Adrenoceptor transgenic mice displayed an increased heart to body weight ratio indicative of cardiac hypertrophy. Functional deficits included an increased isovolumetric relaxation time, a decreased heart rate, and cardiac output. Transgenic mice were hypotensive (Fig. 43.1) and exhibited a decreased pressor response as well as loss of sympathetic nerve activity (Fig. 43.2).

Taken together, the scarce information on the expression of adrenergic receptors in MSA as well as the major shortcomings of the α_{1B}-adrenoreceptor transgenic mouse (i.e. recurrent grand mal seizures and a generalized pattern of brain damage, (Seppi et al. 2001)) make it difficult to correlate the disease pathogenesis with the mouse model overexpressing α_{1B}-adrenergic receptors and limits its future applications.

Deficiency of α_{1B} subunit of N-type calcium channels

Further studies on central autonomic function have lead to studies of the N-type voltage-dependent Ca^{2+} channels which are considered to play essential role in neurotransmitter release at sympathetic nerve terminals. Lack of the α_{1B} subunit of N-type calcium channels in knockout mice has induced autonomic failure with reduction of baroreflex response and dramatic decrease of the positive inotropic responses to electrical sympathetic neuronal stimulation (Ino et al. 2001). Although this model has significant sympathetic nerve dysfunction, no other apparent behavioural defects or neuroanatomical abnormalities have been detected. These studies demonstrated that dysfunction of calcium channels may contribute to model pure autonomic dysfunction without further neurodegeneration.

A novel optimized two factor design

Genetic (Ozawa et al. 2001, Infante et al. 2005, Miller et al. 2005) and environmental factors (Nee et al. 1991, Hanna et al. 1999, Chrysostome et al. 2004, Vanacore et al. 2005) are likely to contribute to the etiopathogenesis of MSA. In order to generate an optimized model of MSA and to avoid the shortcomings of isolated neurotoxin or genetic models we have combined these approaches in a novel strategy. 3NP was systemically applied to transgenically modified mice with oligodendroglial αSYN overexpression (Stefanova et al. 2005). As a result there was a striking replication of human MSA neuropathology in this novel mouse model. It included severe SND with loss of striatal GABAergic medium spiny neurons, loss of dopaminergic neurons in the SNc and loss of dopaminergic nigrostriatal fibres (Fig. 43.3). 3NP exposure of

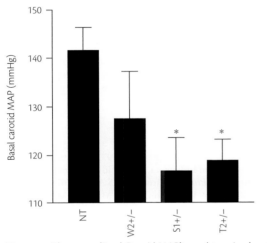

Fig. 43.1 Mean carotid pressure (Basal Carotid MAP) was determined under basal conditions in conscious mice via an in-dwelling catheter. The asterisks indicate the significance from the NT group (p = 0.05). NT, non-transgenic; W, wild type α_{1B}AR transgenic; S, single mutant α_{1B}AR transgenic; T, triple mutant α_{1B}AR transgenic. With permission from Zuscik MJ, Chalothorn D, Hellard D et al. (2001). *J Biol. Chem.*, **276**, 13738–43.

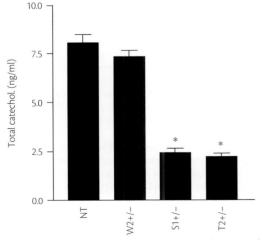

Fig. 43.2 Total plasma epinephrine and norepinephrine levels in mice. The asterisks in each part of the figure indicate the significance from the NT group (p = 0.05). NT, non-transgenic; W, wild type α_{1B}AR transgenic; S, single mutant α_{1B}AR transgenic; T, triple mutant α_{1B}AR transgenic. With permission from Zuscik MJ, Chalothorn D, Hellard D et al. (2001). *J Biol. Chem.*, **276**, 13738–43.

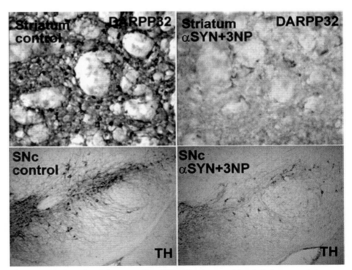

Fig. 43.3 Striatonigral degeneration (SND) in the combined alpha-synuclein + 3-nitropropionic acid (αSYN + 3NP) model of multiple system atrophy demonstrated by loss of striatal DARPP32-immunopositive neurons in striatum and loss of tyrosine hydroxylase (TH)-immunopositive neurons in substantia nigra pars compacta (SNc). Reprinted from Am. J. Pathol. 2005 166: 869–876 with permission from the American Society for Investigative Pathology.

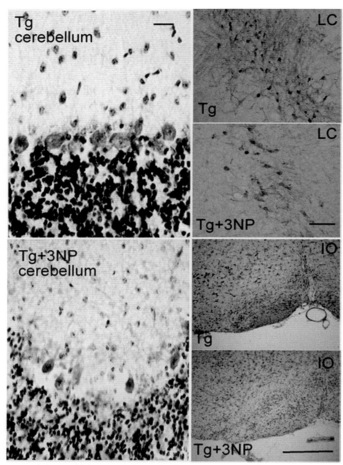

Fig. 43.4 Olivopontocerebellar atrophy (OPCA) in the combined alpha-synuclein + 3-nitropropionic acid (αSYN + 3NP) model of multiple system atrophy demonstrated by loss of Purkinje cells in the cerebellum (cresyl violet), loss of tyrosine hydroxylase (TH)-immunopositive neurons in locus coeruleus (LC), and loss of neurons in the inferior olive (IO, cresyl violet). Reprinted from Am. J. Pathol. 2005 166: 869–876 with permission from the American Society for Investigative Pathology.

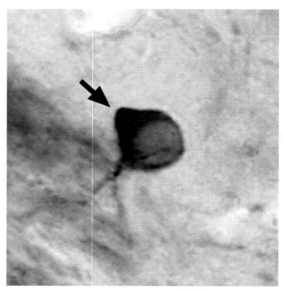

Fig. 43.5 GCI-like alpha-synuclein-immunopositive oligodendroglial inclusion (arrow) in the combined αSYN + 3NP model of multiple system atrophy. Reprinted from Am. J. Pathol. 2005 166: 869–876 with permission from the American Society for Investigative Pathology.

References

Alston, T. A., Mela, L., and Bright, H. J. (1977). 3-Nitropropionate, the toxic substance of Indigofera, is a suicide inactivator of succinate dehydrogenase. *Proc.Natl.Acad.Sci.U.S.A*, **74**, 3767–71.

Beal, M. F., Kowall, N. W., Ellison, D. W., Mazurek, M. F., Swartz, K. J., and Martin, J. B. (1986). Replication of the neurochemical characteristics of Huntington's disease by quinolinic acid. *Nature*, **321**, 168–71.

Behan, W. M., McDonald, M., Darlington, L. G., and Stone, T. W. (1999). Oxidative stress as a mechanism for quinolinic acid-induced hippocampal damage: protection by melatonin and deprenyl. *British Journal of Pharmacology*, **128**, 1754–60.

Blum, D., Torch, S., Lambeng, N., *et al.* (2001). Molecular pathways involved in the neurotoxicity of 6-OHDA, dopamine and MPTP: contribution to the apoptotic theory in Parkinson's disease. *Prog. Neurobiol.*, **65**, 135–72.

Bower, J. H., Maraganore, D. M., McDonnell, S. K., and Rocca, W.A. (1997). Incidence of progressive supranuclear palsy and multiple system atrophy in Olmsted County, Minnesota, 1976 to 1990. *Neurology*, **49**, 1284–8.

Brouillet, E., Conde, F., Beal, M. F., and Hantraye, P. (1999). Replicating Huntington's disease phenotype in experimental animals. *Prog. Neurobiol.*, **59**, 427–68.

Brouillet, E., Jacquard, C., Bizat, N., and Blum, D. (2005). 3-Nitropropionic acid: a mitochondrial toxin to uncover physiopathological mechanisms underlying striatal degeneration in Huntington's disease. *J Neurochem.*, **95**, 1521–40.

Burns, R. S., Chiueh, C. C., Markey, S. P., Ebert, M. H., Jacobowitz, D. M., and Kopin, I. J. (1983). A primate model of parkinsonism: selective destruction of dopaminergic neurons in the pars compacta of the substantia nigra by N-methyl-4-phenyl-1,2,3,6-tetrahydropyridine. *Proc.Natl.Acad.Sci.U.S.A*, **80**, 4546–50.

Chen, M., Ona, V. O., Li, M., *et al.* (2000). Minocycline inhibits caspase-1 and caspase-3 expression and delays mortality in a transgenic mouse model of Huntington disease. *Nat.Med.*, **6**, 797–801.

Chrysostome, V., Tison, F., Yekhlef, F., Sourgen, C., Baldi, I., and Dartigues, J. F. (2004). Epidemiology of multiple system atrophy: a prevalence and pilot risk factor study in Aquitaine, France. *Neuroepidemiology*, **23**, 201–8.

(PLP)- αSYN transgenic mice induced degeneration of the cerebellar Purkinje cells, pons and inferior olives replicating human OPCA (Fig. 43.4). Further, αSYN overexpression exacerbated astrogliosis and microglial activation in the degenerating areas following 3NP exposure. The MSA-like neuropathology in the combined αSYN + 3NP mouse model caused severe motor impairment comprising hindlimb and truncal dystonia, decreased horizontal and vertical locomotor activity, poor pole test performance demonstrating disturbed balance and cerebellar dysfunction, and shortening of the stride length.

The combined αSYN + 3NP mouse model of MSA represents a novel test bed to study the pathogenesis of the disease. It is the first model to replicate selective SND and OPCA in the presence of GCI-like structures (Fig. 43.5), neurodegeneration in medullary and spinal autonomic centers, microgliosis and astrogliosis, all typical of MSA. Finally, it provides an invaluable test-bed to study new therapeutic approaches for this severely disabling and rapidly progressive neurodegenerative disorder.

Daniel, S. (1999), The neuropathology and neurochemistry of multiple system atrophy. In: *Autonomic failure*, C. J. Mathias & R. Bannister, eds., Oxford University Press, Oxford.

Dickson, D. W., Lin, W., Liu, W. K., and Yen, S. H. (1999). Multiple system atrophy: a sporadic synucleinopathy. *Brain Pathology*, **9**, 721–32.

Diguet, E., Fernagut, P. O., Scherfler, C., Wenning, G., and Tison, F. (2005). Effects of riluzole on combined MPTP + 3-nitropropionic acid-induced mild to moderate striatonigral degeneration in mice. *J Neural Transm.*, **112**, 613–31.

Fernagut, P. O., Diguet, E., Bioulac, B., and Tison, F. (2004). MPTP potentiates 3-nitropropionic acid-induced striatal damage in mice: reference to striatonigral degeneration. *Exp.Neurol.*, **185**, 47–62.

Ferrante, R. J., Kowall, N. W., Cipolloni, P. B., Storey, E., and Beal, M. F. (1993). Excitotoxin lesions in primates as a model for Huntington's disease: histopathologic and neurochemical characterization. *Exp. Neurol.*, **119**, 46–71.

Figueredo-Cardenas, G., Chen, Q., and Reiner, A. (1997). Age-dependent differences in survival of striatal somatostatin-NPY-NADPH-diaphorase-containing interneurons versus striatal projection neurons after intrastriatal injection of quinolinic acid in rats. *Exp.Neurol.*, **146**, 444–57.

Figueredo-Cardenas, G., Harris, C. L., Anderson, K. D., and Reiner, A. (1998). Relative resistance of striatal neurons containing calbindin or parvalbumin to quinolinic acid-mediated excitotoxicity compared to other striatal neuron types. *Exp.Neurol.*, **149**, 356–72.

Foster, A. C., Collins, J. F., and Schwarcz, R. (1983). On the excitotoxic properties of quinolinic acid, 2,3-piperidine dicarboxylic acids and structurally related compounds. *Neuropharmacology*, **22**, 1331–42.

Gerlach, M. and Riederer, P. (1996). Animal models of Parkinson's disease: an empirical comparison with the phenomenology of the disease in man. *J Neural Transm.*, **103**, 987–1041.

Ghorayeb, I., Fernagut, P. O., Aubert, I., *et al.* (2000). Toward a primate model of L-dopa-unresponsive parkinsonism mimicking striatonigral degeneration. *Mov Disord.*, **15**, 531–6.

Ghorayeb, I., Fernagut, P. O., Stefanova, N., Wenning, G. K., Bioulac, B., and Tison, F. (2002). Dystonia is predictive of subsequent altered dopaminergic responsiveness in a chronic 1-methyl-4-phenyl-1,2,3,6-tetrahydropyridine + 3-nitropropionic acid model of striatonigral degeneration in monkeys. *Neurosci.Lett.*, **335**, 34–8.

Ghorayeb, I., Puschban, Z., Fernagut, P. O. and others (2001). Simultaneous intrastriatal 6-hydroxydopamine and quinolinic acid injection: a model of early-stage striatonigral degeneration. *Exp. Neurol.*, **167**, 133–47.

Graham, J. G. and Oppenheimer, D. R. (1969). Orthostatic hypotension and nicotine sensitivity in a case of multiple system atrophy. *J Neurol. Neurosurg.Psychiatry*, **32**, 28–34.

Hanna, P. A., Jankovic, J., and Kirkpatrick, J. B. (1999). Multiple system atrophy: the putative causative role of environmental toxins. *Archives of Neurology*, **56**, 90–4.

Heikkila, R. E., Hess, A., and Duvoisin, R. C. (1984). Dopaminergic neurotoxicity of 1-methyl-4-phenyl-1,2,5,6-tetrahydropyridine in mice. *Science*, **224**, 1451–3.

Hughes, A. J., Colosimo, C., Kleedorfer, B., Daniel, S. E., and Lees, A. J. (1992). The dopaminergic response in multiple system atrophy. *J Neurol.Neurosurg.Psychiatry*, **55**, 1009–13.

Ichitani, Y., Okamura, H., Matsumoto, Y., Nagatsu, I., and Ibata, Y. (1991). Degeneration of the nigral dopamine neurons after 6-hydroxydopamine injection into the rat striatum. *Brain Research*, **549**, 350–3.

Infante, J., Llorca, J., Berciano, J., and Combarros, O. (2005). Interleukin-8, intercellular adhesion molecule-1 and tumour necrosis factor-alpha gene polymorphisms and the risk for multiple system atrophy. *J Neurol.Sci.*, **228**, 11–3.

Ino, M., Yoshinaga, T., Wakamori, M., *et al.* (2001). Functional disorders of the sympathetic nervous system in mice lacking the alpha 1B subunit (Cav 2.2) of N-type calcium channels. *Proc.Natl.Acad.Sci.U.S.A*, **98**, 5323–8.

Ishizawa, K., Komori, T., Sasaki, S., Arai, N., Mizutani, T., and Hirose, T. (2004). Microglial activation parallels system degeneration in multiple system atrophy. *J Neuropathol.Exp.Neurol.*, **63**, 43–52.

Jellinger, K. A. (2003). Neuropathological spectrum of synucleinopathies. *Mov Disord.*, **18** Suppl 6, S2–12.

Jellinger, K. A. (2006) P. 25alpha immunoreactivity in multiple system atrophy and Parkinson disease. *Acta Neuropathol,* **112**, 112.

Kahle, P. J., Neumann, M., Ozmen, L., *et al.* (2002). Hyperphosphorylation and insolubility of alpha-synuclein in transgenic mouse oligodendrocytes. *EMBO Rep.*, **3**, 583–8.

Kirik, D., Rosenblad, C., and Bjorklund, A. (1998). Characterization of behavioral and neurodegenerative changes following partial lesions of the nigrostriatal dopamine system induced by intrastriatal 6-hydroxydopamine in the rat. *Exp.Neurol.*, **152**, 259–77.

Langston, J. W., Forno, L. S., Rebert, C. S., and Irwin, I. (1984). Selective nigral toxicity after systemic administration of 1-methyl-4-phenyl-1,2,5,6-tetrahydropyrine (MPTP) in the squirrel monkey. *Brain Research*, **292**, 390–4.

Lindersson, E., Lundvig, D., Petersen, C., *et al.* (2005). p. 25 alpha Stimulates alpha-synuclein aggregation and is co-localized with aggregated alpha-synuclein in alpha-synucleinopathies. *J Biol Chem*, **280**, 5703–5715.

Mantoan, L., Stefanova, N., Egger, K. E., Jellinger, K. A., Poewe, W., and Wenning, G. K. (2005). Failure of caspase inhibition in the double-lesion rat model of striatonigral degeneration (multiple system atrophy). *Acta Neuropathol.(Berl)*, **109**, 191–7.

Miller, D. W., Johnson, J. M., Solano, S. M., Hollingsworth, Z. R., Standaert, D. G., and Young, A. B. (2005). Absence of alpha-synuclein mRNA expression in normal and multiple system atrophy oligodendroglia. *J.Neural Transm.*, **112**, 1613–24.

Mouradian, M. M., Heuser, I. J., Baronti, F., Fabbrini, G., Juncos, J. L., and Chase, T. N. (1989). Pathogenesis of dyskinesias in Parkinson's disease. *Annals of Neurology*, **25**, 523–6.

Nee, L. E., Gomez, M. R., Dambrosia J., Bale S., Eldridge R., and Polinsky, R. J. (1991). Environmental-occupational risk factors and familial associations in multiple system atrophy: a preliminary investigation. *Clin Auton.Res.*, **1**, 9–13.

Orosz, F., Kovacs, G. G., Lehotzky, A., *et al.* (2004) TPPP/p. 25: from unfolded protein to misfolding disease: prediction and experiments. *Biol.Cell*, **96**, 701–711.

Ozawa, T., Okuizumi, K., Ikeuchi, T., Wakabayashi, K., Takahashi, H., and Tsuji, S. (2001). Analysis of the expression level of alpha-synuclein mRNA using postmortem brain samples from pathologically confirmed cases of multiple system atrophy. *Acta Neuropathol.(Berl)*, **102**, 188–90.

Papay, R., Zuscik, M. J., Ross, S. A., *et al.* (2002). Mice expressing the alpha(1B)-adrenergic receptor induces a synucleinopathy with excessive tyrosine nitration but decreased phosphorylation. *J Neurochem.*, **83**, 623–34.

Papp, M. I., Kahn, J. E., and Lantos, P. L. (1989). Glial cytoplasmic inclusions in the CNS of patients with multiple system atrophy (striatonigral degeneration, olivopontocerebellar atrophy and Shy-Drager syndrome). *J Neurol.Sci.*, **94**, 79–100.

Puschban, Z., Scherfler, C., Granata, R., *et al.* (2000a). Autoradiographic study of striatal dopamine re-uptake sites and dopamine D1 and D2 receptors in a 6-hydroxydopamine and quinolinic acid double-lesion rat model of striatonigral degeneration (multiple system atrophy) and effects of embryonic ventral mesencephalic, striatal or co-grafts. *Neuroscience*, **95**, 377–88.

Puschban, Z., Waldner, R., Seppi, K. *et al.* (2000b). Failure of neuroprotection by embryonic striatal grafts in a double lesion rat model of striatonigral degeneration (multiple system atrophy). *Exp. Neurol.*, **164**, 166–75.

Santamaria, A., Jimenez-Capdeville, M. E., Camacho, A., Rodriguez-Martinez, E., Flores, A., and Galvan-Arzate, S. (2001). In vivo hydroxyl radical formation after quinolinic acid infusion into rat corpus striatum. *Neuroreport*, **12**, 2693–6.

Sauer, H. and Oertel, W. H. (1994). Progressive degeneration of nigrostriatal dopamine neurons following intrastriatal terminal lesions with 6-hydroxydopamine: a combined retrograde tracing and immunocytochemical study in the rat. *Neuroscience*, **59**, 401–15.

Scherfler, C., Puschban, Z., Ghorayeb, I., *et al.* (2000). Complex motor disturbances in a sequential double lesion rat model of striatonigral degeneration (multiple system atrophy). *Neuroscience*, **99**, 43–54.

Scherfler, C., Sather, T., Diguet, E. *et al.* (2005). Riluzole improves motor deficits and attenuates loss of striatal neurons in a sequential double lesion rat model of striatonigral degeneration (parkinson variant of multiple system atrophy). *J Neural Transm.*, **112**, 1025–33.

Schneider, J. S. and Markham, C. H. (1986). Neurotoxic effects of N-methyl-4-phenyl-1,2,3,6-tetrahydropyridine (MPTP) in the cat. Tyrosine hydroxylase immunohistochemistry. *Brain Research*, **373**, 258–67.

Schocke, M. F., Waldner, R., Puschban, Z., *et al.* (2000). In vivo magnetic resonance imaging of embryonic neural grafts in a rat model of striatonigral degeneration (multiple system atrophy). *Neuroimage.*, **12**, 209–18.

Schwarz, J., Weis, S., Kraft, E., *et al.* (1996). Signal changes on MRI and increases in reactive microgliosis, astrogliosis, and iron in the putamen of two patients with multiple system atrophy. *J Neurol.Neurosurg. Psychiatry*, **60**, 98–101.

Seppi, K., Puschban, Z., Stefanova, N., *et al.* (2001). Overstimulation of the alpha1B-adrenergic receptor causes a 'seizure plus' syndrome. *Nat. Med*, 7, p. 132.

Shults, C. W., Rockenstein, E., Crews, L., *et al.* (2005). Neurological and neurodegenerative alterations in a transgenic mouse model expressing human alpha-synuclein under oligodendrocyte promoter: implications for multiple system atrophy. *J Neurosci.*, **25**, 10689–99.

Solano, S. M., Miller, D. W., Augood, S. J., Young, A. B., and Penney, J. B., Jr. (2000). Expression of alpha-synuclein, parkin, and ubiquitin carboxy-terminal hydrolase L1 mRNA in human brain: genes associated with familial Parkinson's disease. *Annals of Neurology* 47, 201–10.

Song, Y. J., Lundvig, D. M., Huang, Y., *et al.* (2007) p. 25alpha relocalizes in oligodendroglia from myelin to cytoplasmic inclusions in multiple system atrophy. *Am J Pathol,* **171**, 1291–1303.

Spillantini, M. G., Crowther, R. A., Jakes, R., Cairns, N. J., Lantos, P. L., and Goedert, M. (1998). Filamentous alpha-synuclein inclusions link multiple system atrophy with Parkinson's disease and dementia with Lewy bodies. *Neurosci.Lett.*, **251**, 205–8.

Stefanova, N., Lundblad, M., Tison, F., Poewe, W., Cenci, M. A., and Wenning, G. K. (2004a). Effects of pulsatile L-DOPA treatment in the double lesion rat model of striatonigral degeneration (multiple system atrophy). *Neurobiol.Dis.*, **15**, 630–9.

Stefanova, N., Mitschnigg, M., Ghorayeb, I., *et al.* (2004b). Failure of neuronal protection by inhibition of glial activation in a rat model of striatonigral degeneration. *J Neurosci.Res.*, **78**, 87–91.

Stefanova, N., Puschban, Z., Fernagut, P. O., *et al.* (2003). Neuropathological and behavioral changes induced by various treatment paradigms with MPTP and 3-nitropropionic acid in mice: towards a model of striatonigral degeneration (multiple system atrophy). *Acta Neuropathol.(Berl)*, 106, 157–66.

Stefanova, N., Reindl, M., Neumann, M., Kahle, P. J., Poewe, W., and Wenning, G. K. (2007). Microglial activation mediates neurodegeneration related to oligodendroglial alpha-synucleinopathy: Implications for multiple system atrophy. *Mov Disord.*

Stefanova, N., Reindl, M., Neumann, M., *et al.* (2005). Oxidative stress in transgenic mice with oligodendroglial alpha-synuclein overexpression replicates the characteristic neuropathology of multiple system atrophy. *American Journal of Pathology*, 166, 869–76.

Stemberger, S., Poewe, W., Wenning, G. K., and Stefanova, N. (2010). Targeted overexpression of human alpha-synuclein in oligodendroglia induces lesions linked to MSA-like progressive autonomic failure. *Experimental Neurology*, **224**, 459–64.

Stone, T. W. (1993). Neuropharmacology of quinolinic and kynurenic acids. *Pharmacol.Rev.*, **45**, 309–79.

Ungerstedt, U. (1968). 6-Hydroxy-dopamine induced degeneration of central monoamine neurons. *Eur.J Pharmacol.*, **5**, 107–10.

Vanacore, N., Bonifati, V., Fabbrini, G., *et al.* (2005). Case-control study of multiple system atrophy. *Mov Disord.*, **20**, 158–63.

Wakabayashi, K., Yoshimoto, M., Tsuji, S., and Takahashi, H. (1998). Alpha-synuclein immunoreactivity in glial cytoplasmic inclusions in multiple system atrophy. *Neurosci.Lett.*, **249**, 180–2.

Waldner, R., Puschban, Z., Scherfler, C., *et al.* (2001). No functional effects of embryonic neuronal grafts on motor deficits in a 3-nitropropionic acid rat model of advanced striatonigral degeneration (multiple system atrophy). *Neuroscience*, **102**, 581–92.

Wang, X., Zhu, S., Drozda, M., *et al.* (2003). Minocycline inhibits caspase-independent and -dependent mitochondrial cell death pathways in models of Huntington's disease. *Proc.Natl.Acad.Sci.U.S.A*, **100**, 10483–7.

Wenning, G. K., Ben Shlomo, Y., Hughes, A., Daniel, S. E., Lees, A., and Quinn, N. P. (2000a). What clinical features are most useful to distinguish definite multiple system atrophy from Parkinson's disease? *J Neurol.Neurosurg.Psychiatry*, **68**, 434–40.

Wenning, G. K., Colosimo, C., Geser, F., and Poewe, W. (2004). Multiple system atrophy. *Lancet Neurol.*, **3**, 93–103.

Wenning, G. K., Granata, R., Laboyrie, P. M., Quinn, N. P., Jenner, P., and Marsden, C. D. (1996). Reversal of behavioural abnormalities by fetal allografts in a novel rat model of striatonigral degeneration. *Mov Disord.*, **11**, 522–32.

Wenning, G. K., Seppi, K., Tison, F., and Jellinger, K. (2002). A novel grading scale for striatonigral degeneration (multiple system atrophy). *J Neural Transm.*, **109**, 307–20.

Wenning, G. K., Stefanova, N., Jellinger, K. A., *et al.* (2008) Multiple system atrophy: a primary oligodendrogliopathy. *Ann Neurol,* in press

Wenning, G. K., Tison, F., Scherfler, C., *et al.* (2000b). Towards neurotransplantation in multiple system atrophy: clinical rationale, pathophysiological basis, and preliminary experimental evidence. *Cell Transplant.*, **9**, 279–88.

Wilson, J. S., Turner, B. H., Morrow, G. D., and Hartman, P. J. (1987). MPTP produces a mosaic-like pattern of terminal degeneration in the caudate nucleus of dog. *Brain Research*, **423**, 329–32.

Wu, D. C., Jackson-Lewis, V., Vila, M., *et al.* (2002). Blockade of microglial activation is neuroprotective in the 1-methyl-4-phenyl-1,2,3,6-tetrahydropyridine mouse model of Parkinson disease. *J.Neurosci.*, **22**, 1763–71.

Yazawa, I., Giasson, B. I., Sasaki, R., *et al.* (2005). Mouse model of multiple system atrophy alpha-synuclein expression in oligodendrocytes causes glial and neuronal degeneration. *Neuron*, **45**, 847–59.

Zuscik, M. J., Chalothorn, D., Hellard, D., *et al.* (2001). Hypotension, autonomic failure, and cardiac hypertrophy in transgenic mice overexpressing the alpha 1B-adrenergic receptor. *J Biol.Chem.*, **276**, 13738–43.

Zuscik, M. J., Sands, S., Ross, S. A., *et al.* (2000). Overexpression of the alpha1B-adrenergic receptor causes apoptotic neurodegeneration: multiple system atrophy. *Nat.Med*, **6**, 1388–94.

CHAPTER 44

Development of Parkinson's disease-related pathology in the enteric and central nervous systems

Heiko Braak and Kelly Del Tredici-Braak

Distinction between parkinsonism and Parkinson's disease

The syndrome parkinsonism includes bradykinesia or hypokinesia, cogwheel rigidity, postural instability, and resting tremor. These motor dysfunctions are common in individuals with a significant reduction of dopamine in the central nervous system and can be induced by a variety of causes, such as intoxication (substance abuse), traumata, vascular alterations, infections, genetically based familial forms of parkinsonism, or degenerative diseases, including the tauopathies progressive supranuclear palsy (PSP) and Alzheimer's disease (AD), and the synucleinopathies multiple system atrophy (MSA) and Lewy body disease (LBD). LBD encompasses three related subentities: pure autonomic failure (PAF), sporadic Parkinson's disease (PD), and the clinical entity referred to as diffuse Lewy body disease (DLBD) (McKeith et al. 1996, 2005, Hague et al. 1997, Arai et al. 2000, Fahn 2003, Litvan et al. 2003, Geser et al. 2005, Galvin et al. 2006, Kaufmann and Goldstein 2010).

In LBD, the underlying pathological process is linked to the formation of aberrant proteinaceous inclusion bodies in a limited number of neuronal types distributed throughout the peripheral, enteric, and central portions of the nervous system (PNS/ENS/CNS) (Jellinger 1991, McKeith et al. 1996, 2005, Takahashi and Wakabayashi 2001, 2005, Jellinger and Mizuno 2003, Braak and Del Tredici 2008, 2009, Braak et al. 2004, 2007, Langston 2006, Cersósimo and Benarroch 2008). Because the intraneuronal inclusions do not routinely accompany ageing—they do not appear in 'controls,' not even in the very old (Saito et al. 2004, Chu and Kordower 2007)—they can be regarded as pathological, and assessment of their presence is a prerequisite for the post-mortem diagnosis of LBD (Dickson 1998, Dickson et al. 2009, Iwanaga et al. 1999). Individuals with parkinsonism but lacking these lesions should be classified with the above-mentioned heterogeneous group of motor disorders outside of LBD (Galvin et al. 2001, Pankratz and Foroud 2004, Attems et al. 2007). The present chapter chiefly refers to the pathology underlying sporadic (idiopathic) PD,

the most widespread form of parkinsonism (Parkinson 1817, Lavedan 1998, Trojanowski and Lee 2003, Eriksen et al. 2005, Hardy and Lees 2005, de Lau and Breteler, 2006, Dorsey et al. 2007).

Sporadic Parkinson's disease is a protein misfolding disorder and a synucleinopathy: alpha-synuclein aggregation, Lewy neurites, pale bodies, and Lewy bodies

A process of misfolding, abnormal aggregation, as well as overexpression and/or inefficient elimination of the neuronal protein alpha-synuclein underlies the formation of the hallmark inclusion bodies (Kopito 2000, McNaught et al. 2002, Ciechanover and Brundin 2003, Eriksen et al. 2003, 2005, Olanow et al. 2004, Berg et al. 2005, Lundvig et al. 2005, Olanow and McNaught, 2006, Chu and Kordower 2007, Pan et al. 2008). Affected nerve cells can survive for an as yet unknown period of time, possibly decades, but most probably forfeit much of their functional integrity long before they die. The consequences of the lesions are disrupted neurotransmitter production (Dugger and Dickson 2010), dysfunctional axonal transport, and premature neuronal loss at multiple sites (German et al. 1992, Henderson et al. 2000, Zarow et al. 2003, Orimo et al. 2005), which in all likelihood not only induce but also sustain the development of the PD-associated clinical picture, including both motor dysfunctions and a variety of non-motor symptoms.

The natively unfolded alpha-synuclein molecule is soluble in the cytosol and, in mature nerve cells, it preferentially occurs in the axon, particularly in presynaptic boutons (Spillantini et al. 1997, Trojanowski and Lee 1998, 2000, Dickson 1999, Golbe 1999, Duda et al. 2000, Goedert 2001). The protein exists in many, although not all, neuronal types and, as such, nerve cells require a sufficient supply of the physiological alpha-synuclein to become involved at all in the aberrant protein metabolism associated with LBD (Braak et al. 2001). In affected neurons, part of the alpha-synuclein molecule adopts a β-pleated sheet configuration and in this misfolded form the molecule shows a marked tendency to aggregate with additional alpha-synuclein molecules and other proteins (Trojanowski and Lee 1998, 2000, Dickson 1999, Duda et al. 2000, Goedert 2001, Walker and LeVine 2001, Jellinger 2003a, Norris et al. 2004, Tofaris and Spillantini 2005, 2007, Schulz-Schaeffer 2010). Intrinsic and extrinsic factors that contribute to the induction and maintenance of the aggregation process are as yet unknown (Fortin et al. 2005, McAllister et al. 2005). The aggregated material forms spindle- or thread-like and, in part, arborizing Lewy neurites (LNs) (Fig. 44.1a,b,c) within the dendrites and axons of involved nerve cells (Braak et al. 1994) and punctate structures (Fig. 44.1c,e) or smoothly contoured pale bodies and Lewy bodies (LBs) (Fig 44.1b,d,f) within nerve cell somata (Lewy 1912, Lowe 1994, Takahashi and Wakabayashi 2001, 2005, Apaydin et al. 2002, Kuusisto et al. 2003, Saito et al. 2003, Wakabayashi et al. 2007). It has been proposed that pale bodies represent forerunners of LBs (Dale et al. 1992, Del Tredici and Braak 2004, Wakabayashi et al. 2007).

Differences in axon length and/or the degree to which the involved axons have undergone myelination may predispose some neurons to harsher fates than others (Hill 1987, Braak and Del Tredici 2004, 2009, Braak et al. 2004). In PD, only projection neurons with a long and thin unmyelinated or poorly myelinated axon are prone to develop LNs and LBs (Braak and Del Tredici 2008, Braak et al. 2006c). By contrast, all short-axoned local circuit neurons and all projection cells with a short axon or a long axon insulated by a thick-calibre myelin sheath remain intact.

The Parkinson's disease-related pathological process includes 'incidental' disease in the prodromal phase and, later, a manifest symptomatic phase with no signs of remission

Because LNs and LBs can be seen at autopsy in the nervous system of individuals who did not manifest PD-associated motor signs or dysfunctions during their lifetime, many authors subdivide PD into a prodromal (i.e., premotor) and a symptomatic phase (Forno 1969, 1996, Koller et al. 1991, Jenner 1993, Sawle 1993, Morrish et al. 1998, Wolters et al. 2000, Berendse et al. 2001, Tissingh et al. 2001, Langston 2006, Wolters and Braak 2006, Hawkes 2008, Hawkes et al. 2010, Claassen et al. 2010, Savica et al. 2010). The designations "prodromal" or "presymptomatic" phase, however, also implies that even when mild intraneuronal alpha-synuclein-containing inclusion body pathology is present in persons without the classic PD motor symptoms, such 'incidental' LNs/LBs represent incipient PD and are the harbingers of the symptomatic phase (Gibb and Lees 1988, Wakabayashi et al. 1993b, Lang and Lozano 1998, Lang and Obeso 2004, Del Tredici et al. 2002, Mikolaenko et al. 2005, Bloch et al. 2006, Klos et al. 2006, Ross et al. 2006, Abbott et al. 2007, Beach et al. 2008, Dickson et al. 2008, Fujishiro et al. 2008, Markesbery et al. 2009) (Fig. 44.2).

Once initiated, the pathological process associated with PD progresses without remission and can take years to reach its full extent, provided it is not terminated prematurely by the individual's death (Hely et al. 2008, Kempster et al. 2010). At the same time, the lesions increase in topographic extent, apparently according to a predictable sequence, so that additional brain regions and portions of the nervous system become drawn into the disease process. In fact, its predictable caudo-rostral advance in the brain is one of the major

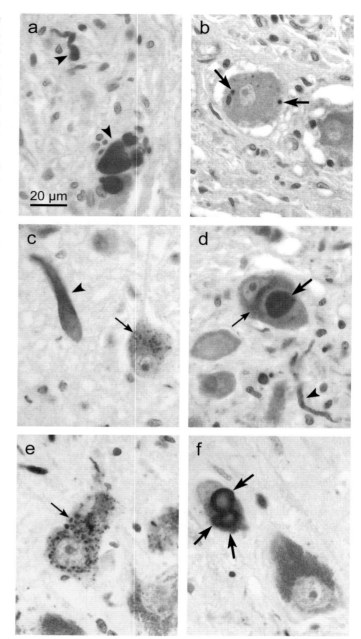

Fig. 44.1 Inclusion bodies in idiopathic Parkinson's disease. (Syn-1 [Transduction Laboratories] immunoreactions in 6 µm paraffin sections). **(a)** Lewy neurites (arrowheads) and **(b)** Lewy bodies (arrows) in the myenteric plexus of the esophagus. **(c)** Club-shaped Lewy neurite (arrowhead) and abnormal particulate alpha-synuclein (arrow) in a cholinergic neuron of the dorsal motor vagal nucleus. With time, the immunolabelled punctate material aggregates to form a Lewy body or bodies (see **d**). **(d)** Mature Lewy body (large arrow) crowned by lipofuscin pigment (small arrow) in a cholinergic nerve cell of the dorsal motor vagal nucleus. Arrowhead points to a thread-like Lewy neurite. **(e)** Abnormal particulate alpha-synuclein (arrow) in a dopaminergic melanized neuron of the substantia nigra pars compacta. **(f)** Three Lewy bodies (arrows) fill out a nigral neuron containing neuromelanin. Compare the normal (still uninvolved) melanized neuron to the right. Scale bar in **a** is valid for **b–f**. Reproduced in part with kind permission from Springer Science+Business Media: *Cell and Tissue Research*, Stages in the development of Parkinson's disease-related pathology, **318**, 2004, 121–34, Braak, H., et al.

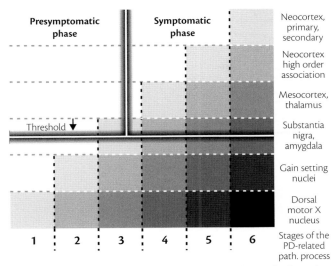

Fig. 44.2 Presymptomatic (prodromal) and symptomatic phases of Parkinson's disease. Incidental Lewy neurites and Lewy bodies are detectable in the brain of asymptomatic individuals. In the symptomatic phase, an individual neuropathological threshold is presumably exceeded (arrow). The gradually increasing slope and intensity of the blocks below the diagonal are intended to show the increasing severity of the pathology and growing number of involved brain regions. With permission from Braak, H., et al. (2006c), *Movement Disorders*, Wiley.

attributes of the pathological process in PD (Braak and Del Tredici 2008, 2009, Braak et al. 2003a, Dickson et al. 2010) (Fig. 44.3).

Where does Parkinson's disease begin in the human nervous system?

In sporadic PD, the earliest LNs and LBs in the brain appear to occur at predisposed sites and to advance from there in a predictable manner throughout other vulnerable regions (Fig. 44.3) (Braak and Del Tredici 2008, 2009, Braak et al. 2003a, Jellinger 2003b, 2004, Neumann et al. 2004, Müller et al. 2005, Halliday et al. 2006, 2008, Ushikado et al. 2006, Dickson et al. 2010). In so doing, the PD-related pathological process leaves a distinctive lesional pattern in its wake. Despite the imperfect state of knowledge regarding the pathogenesis of PD, preliminary data may support the hypothesis that the process may begin in the olfactory system and ENS, then gain access to the CNS via the vagal nerve, and ascend from lower brainstem nuclei until it reaches the cerebral cortex (Braak et al. 2003b, 2006a, Hawkes et al. 2007). Initial attempts to explore the first affected sites *outside* of the CNS rest upon the outcome of extended post-mortem screening procedures that include non-symptomatic cases with incidental LBD pathology (Del Tredici et al. 2002, 2010, Bloch et al. 2006, Fumimura et al. 2007, Minguez-Castellanos et al. 2007, Beach et al. 2010). The task presents a challenge insofar as the profiles of some of the potentially earliest involved nerve cell types in the not readily accessible PNS and ENS are still unknown.

Some of the earliest Parkinson's disease-related lesions occur in the autonomic nervous system

With few exceptions, detailed information about the progressive involvement of the sympathetic nervous system in PD is still meagre (Forno and Norville, 1976, Forno et al. 1986, Wakabayashi and Takahashi 1997a, Iwanaga et al. 1999, Orimo et al. 2005, 2007, 2008, Minguez-Castellanos et al. 2007, Fumimura et al. 2007, Orimo et al. 2008, Ghebremedhin et al. 2009, Del Tredici et al. 2010, Miki et al. 2009). As regards the ENS and part of the para-sympathetic system within the CNS, preliminary observations point to affection early in the disease process (Braak et al. 2006a). Recent reports also point out that the peripheral vagal nerve becomes involved during the prodromal phase (Bloch et al. 2006, Del Tredici et al. 2010) (Fig. 44.4d). It has long been known that ENS lesions occur in symptomatic cases (Jager et al. 1960, Qualman et al. 1984, Wakabayashi and Takahashi 1997b, Wakabayashi et al. 1988, 1990, 1991, 1993a, Matthews 1999) but there is also evidence for their existence in the pre-symptomatic disease phase (Braak et al. 2006a, 2006b, Abbott et al. 2007, Beach et al. 2010). This phenomenon of early ENS involvement is, in cases observed up to now, always accompanied by mild CNS lesions. It remains to be seen whether LNs and LBs consistently appear in the peripheral autonomic nervous system even in the absence of CNS lesions.

Symptomatic and pre-symptomatic cases with lesions in peripheral organs notably exhibit LNs in the submandibular gland (Fig. 44.4a), sympathetic autonomic ganglia (Fig. 44.4b), and in the wall of the distal esophagus (Fig. 44.4c), gastric cardia, fundus, and pylorus regions. Only a few of the many cell types within the ENS (Bishop and Polak 1999, Costa et al. 2000, Furness 2000, Timmermans et al. 2001, Anlauf et al. 2003) are prone to develop the lesions, for instance the inhibitory nitrergic vasoactive intestinal polypeptide (VIP) neurons in both the myenteric and submucous plexuses (Wakabayashi et al. 1990, 1993). Whereas punctate aggregations of alpha-synuclein presumably represent an early somatic change in PD, cells with more advanced pathology exhibit globose LBs that can fill large portions of the cell body (Fig. 44.4c). ENS neurites contain aggregates of varying size and shape. Axons with thread-like aggregations are found within the fibre strands that interconnect the ganglia but also in terminal branches of visceromotor neurons that profusely arborise between the smooth muscles.

Of particular interest are axons given off from the submucous plexus (Fig. 44.5b). Some extend into the muscle layer of the mucosa where they split up into terminal ramifications (Fig. 44.5e). Others, however, even reach the lamina propria of the mucosa (Fig. 44.5c) and take an upward course aligned parallel to the gastric glands (Figs. 44.5a,b,d). These axons protrude into and ramify within the mucosa where they are only micrometers away from the body's innermost environment (Braak et al. 2006a).

Here, it is important to emphasise that uninterrupted axonal connectivities exist linking the ENS with the CNS as well as all of the presently known sites within the brain that are susceptible to PD. The successive involvement of these sites prompts the question whether an as yet unknown environmental neurotropic pathogen may induce the protein misfolding and aggregation process in the nerve plexuses of the gastrointestinal tract and progress by way of retrograde axonal transport and transsynaptic/transneuronal transmission (Pearson et al. 1985, Saper et al. 1987, DeLacoste and White 1993, Pearson 1996, McBride et al. 2001, Li et al. 2008, Angot and Brundin 2009, Desplats et al. 2009) into the CNS, thereby providing the most straightforward explanation for the caudo-rostral disease propagation that characterizes PD neuropathologically (Braak et al. 2003b) (Fig. 44.6a).

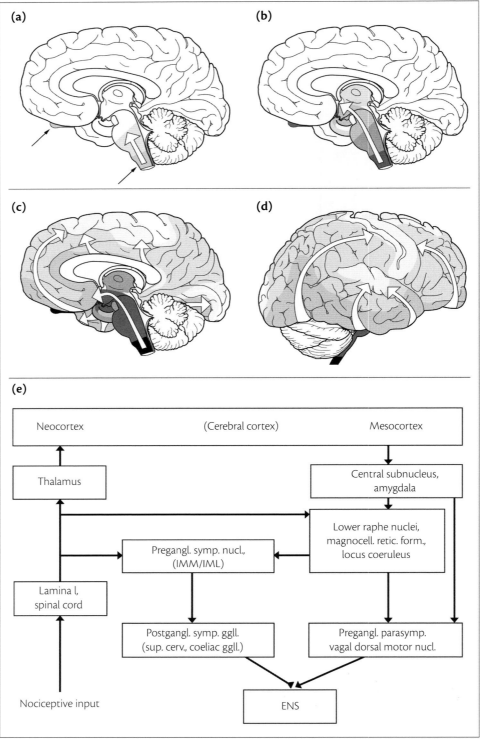

Fig. 44.3 Distribution and progression of Parkinson's disease-related pathology in the brain. The earliest lesions develop in the dorsal motor vagal nucleus and often in the anterior olfactory nucleus (see black arrows in **a**). Thereafter, the pathology takes an essentially ascending course from the lower brainstem through basal portions of the midbrain and forebrain until it reaches the cerebral cortex (see white arrows in **a–d**). The cortical affection begins in the anteromedial temporal mesocortex and proceeds through high order sensory association and prefrontal areas into first order sensory association and pre-motor areas, as well as primary sensory and motor fields of the neocortex. **a–d**. The variation in shading represents the sequential topographic advance, distribution pattern, and severity of the Lewy pathology in six neuropathological stages. Reprinted from *Neurobiology of Aging*, **24**, Braak, H., Del Tredici, K., Rüb, U., de Vos, R.A.I., Jansen Steur, E.N.H., and Braak, E., Staging of brain pathology related to sporadic Parkinson's disease. 197–211 Copyright (2003), with permission from Elsevier. **e**. Diagram summarizing known anatomical connectivities between the enteric nervous system (ENS) and autonomic relay nuclei of the peripheral nervous system and lower brainstem/spinal cord, and between layer I of the spinal dorsal horn and sympathetic relay nuclei of the spinal cord. Nociceptive input can activate sympathetic outflow via the sympathetic preganglionic neurons of the intermediomedial and intermediolateral nuclei (IMM / IML) of the spinal cord. **Abbreviations**: magnocell. retic. form. – magnocellular reticular formation, postgangl. symp. ggll. – postganglionic sympathetic ganglia, pregangl. symp. nucl. – preganglionic sympathetic nuclei, vagal dorsal motor nucl. – dorsal motor nucleus of the vagal nerve.

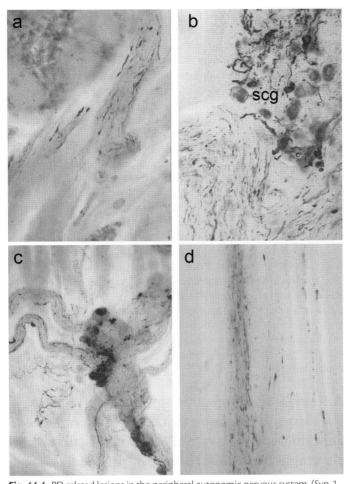

Fig. 44.4 PD-related lesions in the peripheral autonomic nervous system. (Syn-1 [Transduction Laboratories] immunoreactions in 100 μm PEG-embedded tissue sections). **a.** Lewy neurites in nerve fibres within the connective tissue of the submandibular gland from a PD patient with stage 6 brain pathology (female, 86 years of age). Lewy pathology in the submandibular gland can occur early (i.e., in incidental cases with stage 2 brain pathology) and, in symptomatic PD, may be related to reduced salivary secretion. **b.** Superior cervical ganglion (scg) and attached sympathetic trunk with Lewy pathology in a symptomatic case with stage 4 brain pathology (male, 75 years of age). The paravertebral and prevertebral sympathetic ganglia represent the "final neuron" directly before the end organs which they innervate. **c.** Tangentially cut section through the vagally influenced distal esophagus (Auerbach plexus) showing Lewy bodies and Lewy neurites in a patient with PD stage 5 brain pathology (male, 61 years of age). Note also the circular and longitudinal muscle layers visible in the background. Problems with swallowing and with sialopenia are not relieved by dopamine replacement therapy. **d.** Peripheral vagal nerve (mediastinum) from a symptomatic individual (female, 71 years of age) with stage 6 brain pathology. Reproduced in part with permission of Springer from Del Tredici, K., et al. (2008). Acta Neuropathologica **115**, 379–84.

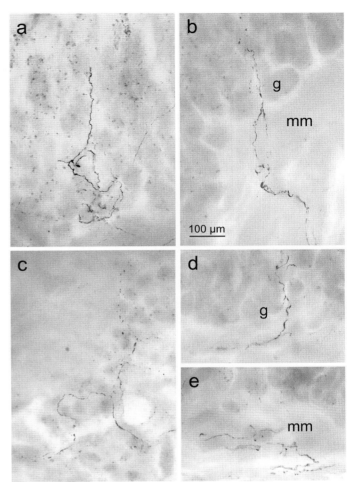

Fig. 44.5 Aggregated intra-axonal alpha-synuclein in the gastric submucous plexus. (Syn-1 [Transduction Laboratories] immunoreactions in 150 mm cryosections). **a,b,d,e** display details of immunoreactive axonal fibres filled with abnormal-synuclein aggregates generated by the gastric Meissner plexus from a PD patient with stage 4 brain pathology (female, 69 years of age), whereas **c** is from a non-symptomatic individual (male, 65 years of age) at stage 3. **a–e** show terminal branches of pathologically altered axons that reach the lamina propria of the gastric mucosa. **a**, **b**, and **d** show ramifications that ascend through the muscularis mucosa (mm) and run parallel to the gastric glands (g). **e.** Abnormally altered axons penetrate the muscularis mucosa (mm) and ramify within this layer. Scale bar in **b** is valid for **a–e**. Reprinted from Neuroscience Letters, **396**, Braak, H., de Vos, R.A.I., Bohl, J., and Del Tredici, K., Gastric a-synuclein immunoreactive inclusions in Meissner's and Auerbach's plexuses in cases staged for Parkinson's disease-related brain pathology, 67–72, Copyright 2006, with permission from Elsevier.

Uptake of exogenous substances is known to occur preferably at synapses and, from there, such substances are transferred to the cell body via retrograde axonal transport (Saper et al. 1987, Sotelo and Triller 1997). Neuroactive substances, including neurotropic viruses, unconventional pathogens with prion-like properties, or slow neurotoxins are taken up in this manner—frequently by receptor-mediated endocytosis (Strack et al. 1989, Card 1998, Helke et al. 1998, Prusiner 1998, Mufson et al. 1999, Wadsworth et al. 1999, Rinaman et al. 2000, Brown 2001, Murer et al. 2001, Nicotera 2001, Gosh 2002, Palka-Santini et al. 2003). The myelin sheath serves as a barrier to viruses attempting to pass from the surroundings into the axon (Hill 1987). The reverse, however, is also true: the absence of a myelin sheath around axons generated by postganglionic visceromotor neurons and preganglionic neurons of the dorsal motor vagal nucleus not only facilitates but also virtually invites entrance by viruses or neurotropic pathogens

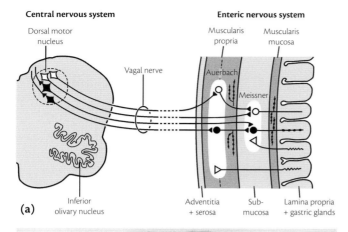

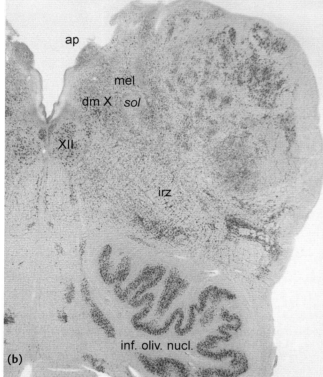

Fig. 44.6 **(a)** Diagram showing the interconnections between the enteric nervous system (ENS) and the dorsal motor vagal nucleus. A neurotropic agent capable of passing through the mucosal epithelial barrier of the gastrointestinal tract could enter terminal axons of postganglionic VIPergic neurons (black, rounded cell bodies) in the submucous plexus and, via retrograde axonal and transneuronal transport either directly or indirectly by way of cell bodies in the myenteric plexus, reach the preganglionic cholinergic neurons (black, diamond-shaped cell bodies) of the dorsal motor nucleus of the vagal nerve. Two triangular-shaped cells (white) represent uninvolved primary viscerosensory neurons in the enteric nervous system. Two rounded cells there (white) indicate cholinergic excitatory visceromotor neurons. Reprinted from *Neuroscience Letters*, **396**, Braak, H., de Vos, R.A.I., Bohl, J., and Del Tredici, K., Gastric a-synuclein immunoreactive inclusions in Meissner's and Auerbach's plexuses in cases staged for Parkinson's disease-related brain pathology, 67–72, Copyright 2006, with permission from Elsevier. VIP, vasoactive intestinal peptide. **(b)** Tissue section at the level of the dorsal motor vagal nucleus through the medulla oblongata of a control case (male, 56 years of age, 400 μm PEG-embedded section, stained with aldehyde fuchsin for lipofuscin pigment and Darrow red for basophilic material). Sections of 100–400 μm thickness facilitate topographical orientation based on the nerve cell shapes, sizes, and pigmentation patterns, and serve here to demonstrate the normal anatomy. ap, area postrema; dm X, dorsal motor vagal nucleus; inf. oliv. nucl., inferior olivary nucleus; irz, intermediate reticular zone; mel, melanized neurons (A2 group) in the dorsal motor vagus areal; *sol*, solitary tract; XII, hypoglossus nucleus (twelfth cranial nerve); PEG, polyethylene glycol.

(Morrison et al. 1991, Card 1998, Rinaman et al. 2000, Matsuda et al. 2004, Jang et al. 2009).

Most of the neuronal types located within the CNS are protected against uptake of substances from the extracellular milieu beyond the CNS by the blood–brain barrier. Only axons of nerve cells that project outside of the CNS (such as those given off from preganglionic neurons of the dorsal motor vagal nucleus) lack such protection. For example, an intravenous injection of horseradish peroxidase results in retrograde labelling of the dorsal motor vagal nucleus (Broadwell and Brightman 1976). Provided the putative pathogen could penetrate the esophageal, gastric, or intestinal (jejunum, colon) mucosal barrier, it could be incorporated into terminal axons of susceptible postganglionic visceromotor neurons (Phillips et al. 2008). From there, it could pass transsynaptically directly into unmyelinated preganglionic fibres of the vagus nerve or indirectly via nerve cells of the myenteric plexus. In this manner, the pathogen could overcome the distance from the gastrointestinal mucosa to the CNS via retrograde axonal transport (Fig. 44.6a). The mucosa of the gastrointestinal tract appears to be susceptible to an assault because it is innervated by the dorsal motor vagal nucleus (Richards and Sugarbaker 1995, Hopkins et al. 1996, Cersósimo and Benarroch 2008). Moreover, the thin epithelial lining of the gut is susceptible to microbleeding and chronic infection (Strang 1965, Altschuler 1996, Dobbs et al. 2000, Palka-Santini et al. 2003).

A neuropathological staging system of the Parkinson's disease-related lesions in the central nervous system (brain) postulates six stages based on the topographical distribution pattern and extent of the lesions

Within the brain, the first LNs usually develop at two sites more or less simultaneously, namely, the dorsal motor nucleus of the vagal nerve together with the adjoining intermediate reticular zone and/or the olfactory bulb with the related anterior olfactory nucleus (Del Tredici et al. 2002; Braak and Del Tredici 2009, Braak et al. 2003a) (Fig. 44.2). Its cellular islands are dispersed throughout the olfactory tract. These islands and the retrobulbar-olfactory portion of the anterior olfactory nucleus develop a network of LNs (Daniel and Hawkes 1992, Pearce et al. 1995, Mesholam et al. 1998, Hawkes et al. 1999, Berendse et al. 2001, Doty 2001, Doty et al. 1992, Tissingh et al. 2001, Hawkes 2003, Ponsen et al. 2004, Price 2004, Stiasny-Kolster et al. 2005, Hubbard et al. 2007). In subsequent disease stages, the lesions appear in more remote olfactory sites (piriform and periamygdalear regions) without advancing into the medial nucleus of the amygdala and into non-olfactory structures (Braak et al. 2003a, 2003b, Hubbard et al. 2007). From the dorsal motor vagal nucleus of the medulla oblongata the main disease process takes an essentially upward route through lower and upper brainstem nuclei until it reaches the neocortex (Fig. 44.2).

Neuropathological stages 1–2: Pathology in the medulla oblongata and pontine tegmentum

The dorsal motor vagal nucleus is almost always involved in stage 1 (Fig. 44.6b). In addition to the LNs there (Fig. 44.7), LNs may be seen in the adjoining intermediate reticular zone (Fig. 44.6b).

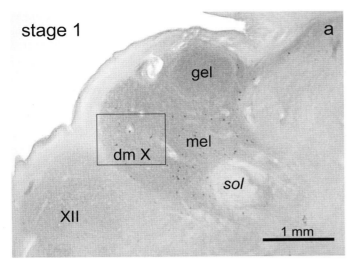

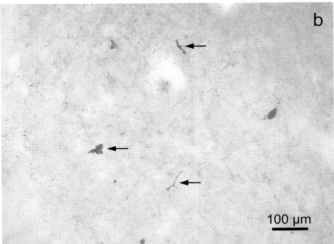

Fig. 44.7 (a) Dorsal motor vagal nucleus from a non-symptomatic neuropathological stage 1 case (male, 71 years of age), Syn-1 [Transduction Laboratories] immunoreaction in 100 μm PEG-embedded tissue section. **(b)** Detail micrograph from **a** showing incidental Lewy body pathology (arrows point to Lewy neurites). In the majority of cases and regions examined, the appearance of Lewy neurites precedes that of pale bodies and/or Lewy bodies. dm X, dorsal motor vagal nucleus; gel, gelatinosus nucleus; mel, melanoneurons; *sol*, solitary tract; XII, motor nucleus of the hypoglossus nerve (twelfth cranial nerve); PEG, polyethylene glycol.

The hypothesis regarding invasion by an environmental or prion-like pathogen rests, in part, upon the fact that the earliest brain lesions consistently develop in the dorsal motor vagal nucleus and that a pathogenic transfer apparently does not take place at sites where little or no opportunity exists for transneuronal contact between the CNS and ENS (Braak and Del Tredici 2009).

The preganglionic projection neurons of the dorsal motor vagal nucleus generate long and unmyelinated fibres that connect the CNS with the postganglionic neurons of the ENS (Fig. 44.6a) (Huang et al. 1993, Hopkins et al. 1996). The myelinated viscerosensory fibres of the vagus nerve terminate in the small-celled nuclei that accompany the solitary tract. These viscerosensory nuclei as well as the gelatinosus subnucleus remain virtually uninvolved in PD (Del Tredici et al. 2002, Braak and Del Tredici 2009). The sturdily myelinated visceromotor projections that originate from the second motor vagal nucleus, the ambiguus nucleus, directly

innervate (among others) the striated muscles of the upper gastrointestinal tract but do not establish connections to the ENS (Fig. 44.8). The ambiguus nucleus does not become affected at any point during the course of the disease (Braak et al. 2003a,b).

The catecholaminergic melanized neurons (Figs. 44.6b, 44.7a) within the dorsal vagus area (A2 group) and intermediate reticular zone (A1 group) give off ascending projections to higher levels of the CNS (Saper et al. 1991, Huang et al. 1993, Hopkins et al. 1996) and those located more rostrally in the ventrolateral medulla (A5 group) provide descending input to preganglionic sympathetic neurons in the intermediolateral cell column of the spinal cord (Strack et al. 1989). In the early pre(motor)symptomatic stages, these catecholaminergic melanized neurons (A1, A2, A5 groups) show no signs of involvement (Halliday et al. 1990, Del Tredici et al. 2002, Benarroch et al. 2005).

In stage 2, the disease process goes beyond the limits of the medullary dorsal motor nucleus to include the lower raphe nuclei and magnocellular portions of the reticular formation, in particular the gigantocellular reticular nucleus (Fig. 44.8). LNs also appear within the coeruleus-subcoeruleus complex (German et al. 1992, Zweig et al. 1993, Braak et al. 2000, Boeve et al. 2007). All of these nuclei form a functional adaptive gain or level setting system (Benarroch 2009). Their sparingly myelinated descending fibre tracts comprise a pain control system that partially inhibits the spinal and medullary relay nuclei for somatosensory and viscerosensory input. In addition, they function as a motor control system by modulating the excitability level of medullary and spinal premotor and motor neurons. This system is capable of limiting the conduction of incoming

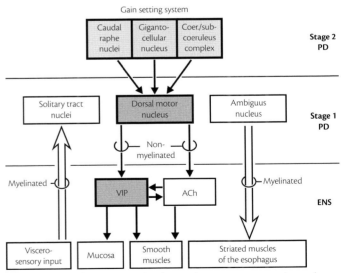

Fig. 44.8 Fibre pathways connecting the enteric nervous system and central nervous systems by way of the vagal nerve. Myelinated visceroafferent fibres terminate in the small-celled nuclei that surround the solitary tract. Myelinated visceroefferent fibres from the ambiguus nucleus innervate the striated muscles of the upper esophagus. Unmyelinated preganglionic fibres from the dorsal motor vagal nucleus contact ganglion cells of the enteric plexuses. Affected nuclei and nerve cell types in early non-symptomatic stages are indicated by boldface framing. Well-myelinated viscerosensory and visceromotor fibres (thick white arrows) do not develop alpha-synuclein immunoreactive aggregates. In stage 2 cases, the gain (level) setting nuclei become involved and supplement the affection of the dorsal motor vagal nucleus. ACh, cholinergic neurons in the enteric nervous system; coer./subcoeruleus complex, coeruleus-subcoeruleus complex; VIP, vasoactive intestinal peptide nitrergic neurons in the enteric nervous system.

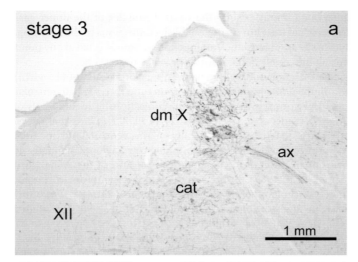

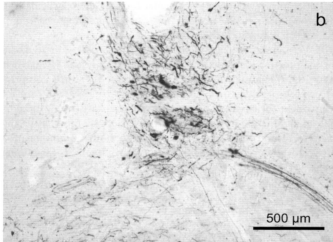

Fig. 44.9 **(a)** Dorsal motor vagal nucleus from a non-symptomatic individual (male, 65 years of age) with stage 3 pathology, Syn-1 [Transduction Laboratories] immunoreaction in a 100 μm PEG-embedded tissue section. The dorsal motor vagal nucleus (dm X) shows a clear increase of involvement (compare Fig. 44.7 with Fig. 44.9). All other subnuclei of the dorsal vagal area as well as the adjoining motor nucleus of the hypoglossal nerve (XII) notably remain virtually unaffected. Thread-like aggregations within axons indicate the intramedullary course of bundles of the vagal nerve (ax). Frequently, the catecholaminergic tract (cat) can likewise be followed because of the presence of α-synuclein aggregates within its axons. **(b)** Detail micrograph from **a**. **PEG,** polyethylene glycol.

pain signals in a given situation and placing motor neurons in a heightened state of preparedness for action (Braak et al. 2000, Koutcherov et al. 2004). It also plays a central role in the modulation of cognitive functions (Benarroch et al. 2007, Sara 2009). The fact that the gain/level setting nuclei, and only these, become simultaneously affected in stage 2 is in keeping with the hypothesis that retrograde axonal and transneuronal transport via pre-existing pathways may play a key role in the progress of the pathology (Fig. 44.8).

Neuropathological stages 3–4: Pathology in the mesecephalic tegmentum, basal forebrain, meso- and allocortex

Cases with stage 3 pathology show increasingly severe involvement of the dorsal motor vagal areal, including intensely

immunopositive LNs in both intramedullary and extramedullary portions of the vagus nerve (Fig. 44.9). In stage 3, the ascending disease process enters the basal midbrain and forebrain (Braak et al. 2003a, Braak and Del Tredici 2009). It first encroaches on the central subnucleus of the amygdala (Fig. 44.10a) and thereafter involves the amygdalar basolateral nuclei. In unconventionally thick (100 μm), polyethylene glycol-embedded hemisphere sections,

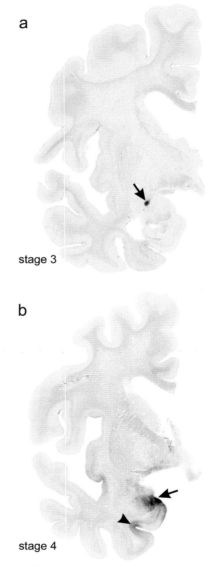

Fig. 44.10 Pathological changes associated with neuropathological stages 3 and 4 of sporadic Parkinson's disease (PD) in 100 μm hemisphere sections immunostained for alpha-synuclein (Syn-1, Transduction Laboratories). The darkened tissue areas indicate the presence of PD-related lesions that can be recognized macroscopically from stage 3 onwards in hemisphere sections. **(a)** Hemisphere section of a non-symptomatic individual (female, 86 years of age) at stage 3. The arrow points to a single darkened spot showing the central subnucleus of the amygdala. Allocortical, mesocortical, and neocortical areas are uninvolved at this stage. **(b)** Hemisphere section of a symptomatic individual (female, 90 years of age) at stage 4. More severe involvement of the amygdala (arrow) is accompanied by beginning affection of the anteromedial temporal mesocortex (arrowhead). Note that neocortical areas are not immunolabelled. With permission from Braak, H., et al. (2006c). *Movement Disorders*, Wiley.

a network of LNs fills the central subnucleus, distinctly setting it off from surrounding regions (Fig. 44.10a). Additional lesions evolve in the pedunculopontine tegmental nucleus (Hirsch et al. 1987, Jellinger 1988, Zweig et al. 1989, Pahapill and Lozano 2000), the oral raphe nuclei, magnocellular nuclei of the basal forebrain (medial septal nucleus, interstitial nucleus of the diagonal band, basal nucleus of Meynert), and hypothalamic tuberomamillary nucleus.

The central subnucleus of the amygdala generates a descending and poorly myelinated fibre tract that exerts superordinate 'limbic' influence on both the gain setting nuclei and the dorsal motor vagal nucleus (Bohus et al. 1996, Liubashima et al. 2000) (Fig. 44.13). That the earliest PD-related pathology in the amygdala develops within this subnucleus also speaks for the working hypothesis that a postulated pathogen may utilize either the group of adaptive gain setting nuclei or the medullary dorsal motor vagal nucleus to reach the amygdalar central subnucleus and, from there, the substantia nigra, basalolateral nuclei of the amygdala, and magnocellular nuclei of the basal forebrain (Fig. 44.13).

The pars compacta of the substantia nigra becomes involved in stage 3. LNs appear first, followed by punctate aggregations, pale bodies, and LBs in dopaminergic melanized neurons (A9 group) that generate thin and sparsely myelinated axons (Braak and Braak 1986, Braak et al. 2003a, Del Tredici and Braak 2004) (Fig. 44.13).

At stage 4, a specific portion of the cerebral cortex, namely the transition zone between allocortex and neocortex, i.e. the poorly myelinated anteromedial temporal mesocortex, is drawn into the disease process (Braak 1980, Braak and Braak 1992, Braak et al. 2003a, Braak and Del Tredici 2009) (Fig. 44.10b). A network of LNs develops in the superficial layers of this phylogenetically late-evolving and ontogenetically late-maturing region, whereas projection neurons in the deeper layers develop LBs. The anteromedial temporal mesocortex sends reciprocal (bidirectional) projections to the entorhinal region, hippocampal formation, and amygdala (Fig. 44.11). To understand the functional consequences of

the increasingly severe lesions that develop in this region, it is important to realise that it is involved in the transfer of data from sensory association areas to the prefrontal cortex (cross-hatched arrow in Fig. 44.11). As if through a bottleneck or eye of a needle, all vital information coming from neocortical high-order sensory association areas is siphoned through the anteromedial temporal mesocortex to the amygdala, entorhinal region, and hippocampal formation before heading for the prefrontal neocortex. Bilateral impairment of this important data-stream opens the way for memory dysfunction and cognitive decline. Decreased limbic input to the prefrontal cortex can also lead to loss of initiative and other forms of hypofrontality (Braak et al. 2005).

To the extent that the amygdala—in particular its basolateral subnuclei—receive strong input from the anteromedial temporal mesocortex (Fig. 44.11), a neurotropic pathogen might well be able to reach this cortical region by means of axonal and transneuronal (transsynaptic) transport. At some point during stages 3 and 4, the pre-symptomatic phase usually gives way to the clinically manifest (i.e. somatomotor) phase of PD (Braak and Del Tredici 2008, 2009, Braak et al. 2003a).

Neuropathological stages 5–6: Pathology in the neocortex

In stages 5 and 6, the pathological process attains its greatest topographic extent (Fig. 44.12). Most of the remaining projection neurons in the most important parasympathetic centre of the lower brainstem, the dorsal motor vagal nucleus, are involved (Fig. 44.12). With the temporal mesocortex as its starting point (Figs. 44.10b,44.13a), the inclusion body pathology gradually occupies the neocortex (Fig. 44.13b). Lesions appear initially in the prefrontal and high-order sensory association areas of the neocortex (stage 5) (Fig. 44.13a), next within the reaches of premotor and first order sensory association areas, and, finally, in the primary fields of the neocortex (stage 6) (Fig. 44.13b)

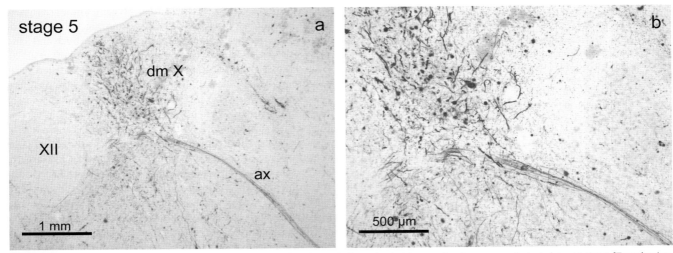

Fig. 44.11 Dorsal motor vagal nucleus from a symptomatic patient with Parkinson's disease (male, 76 years of age) at neuropathological stage 5, Syn-1 [Transduction Laboratories] immunoreaction in a 100 μm PEG (polyethylene glycol)-embedded tissue section. In comparison to Fig. 44.9, again a remarkable increase in the severity of involvement can be observed. At this stage, most of the remaining projection neurons in the dorsal motor vagal nucleus (dm X) show intraneuronal inclusion bodies and their axons (ax) often can be followed throughout the entire medulla oblongata and even beyond into the peripheral portions of the vagal nerve. Note that at this advanced stage the motor nucleus of the hypoglossal nerve (XII) still remains uninvolved. **(b)** Detail micrograph from **a**.

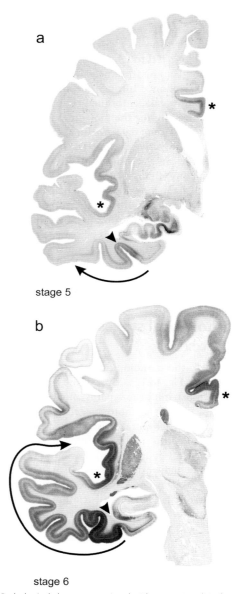

stage 5

stage 6

Fig. 44.12 Pathological changes associated with stages 5 and 6 of sporadic PD in 100 m hemisphere sections immunostained for -synuclein (Syn-1, [Transduction Laboratories] immunoreaction. **a. Section from a PD patient at neuropathological stage 5** (male, 80 years of age). A dense network of Lewy neurites and Lewy bodies-containing projection neurons emerges in the anteromedial temporal mesocortex (arrowhead). The disease process encroaches upon the related insular and cingulate mesocortex (asterisks). From the mesocortex, the pathology progresses into the high order association fields of the neocortex. The immunoreactivity gradually tapers off the closer it gets to the secondary and primary fields of the temporal neocortex (arrow). Note that the gyrus of Heschl along the superior temporal convolution is still unaffected. **b. Section from a PD patient at neuropathological stage 6** (female, 78 years of age). Cortical involvement gains additional momentum. Areas of the insular, cingulate (asterisks), and temporal mesocortex (arrowhead) continue to show strong immunoreactivity. The cortical changes increase both in severity and extent. The disease process reaches even the secondary and, in advanced stage 6 cases, primary neocortical fields, as seen here from the mild affection of the primary auditory field in Heschl's gyrus (arrow). Reproduced with permission of John Wiley & Sons from Braak, H., et al. (2006c). *Movement Disorders* **21**, 2042–51.

(Braak and Del Tredici 2005, 2008, 2009, Braak et al. 2003a, Del Tredici and Braak 2004). Patients in these neuropathological stages manifest the full range of disease-related symptoms. Damage to the olfactory, autonomic, limbic, and somatomotor systems can become compounded by supervening deficits in the cerebral cortex (Mesulam 1998, Hurtig et al. 2000, Jellinger 2000, Korczyn 2001, Aarsland et al. 2003, Braak et al. 2005). Once again, existing fibre interconnectivities between cortical areas are in concert with the proposed hypothesis of the systematic advance of a pathogenic agent.

Future prospects: More than dopamine replacement

PD is by no means a monosystemic disorder of the human nervous system. To be sure, the majority of the dopaminergic melanized neurons in the substantia nigra perish in the course of the disease process, and it is indisputable that this nigral neuronal loss causes somatomotor dysfunctions, e.g. akinesia, hypokinesia. Nevertheless, parallel and even prior to the pathological developments in the substantia nigra, considerable damage occurs in projection neurons of extranigral structures that belong to diverse functional and transmitter systems. Some of the very earliest lesions that can be seen light microscopically occur within the autonomic nervous system—outside the CNS (Bloch et al. 2006, Braak et al. 2006a, Minguez-Castellanos et al. 2007, Miki et al. 2009, Del Tredici et al. 2010). These findings have their counterparts in the fact that during the course of PD non-motor and motor symptoms arise that cannot be accounted for by a reduction of dopamine in the striatum and/or do not respond to dopamine replacement therapy (Quinn et al. 1987, Doty et al. 1988, , Hely et al. 2008, Lang and Obeso 2004, Adler 2005, Ahlskog 2005, Verbaan et al. 2007, Sethi 2008, Olanow et al. 2010). Olfactory and autonomic dysfunctions, for instance, have long been known to contribute to the symptomatology of PD (Rajput and Rozdilsky 1976, Korczyn 1990, Magalhaes et al. 1995, Martignoni et al. 1995, Quigley 1996, Siddiqui et al. 2002, Jost 2003, Micieli et al. 2003, Ahlskog 2005, Magerkurth et al. 2005, Lee et al. 2006, Martinez et al. 2007, Verbaan et al. 2007, Sethi 2008, Evatt et al. 2009, Pfeiffer 2010). Recent studies designed to detect such signs have shown that autonomic failure has to be counted among the early phenomena in PD (Awerbuch and Sandyk 1994, Hishikawa et al. 2000, Larner et al. 2000, Abbott et al. 2001, 2007, Pfeiffer 2003, Kaufmann et al. 2004). The postulated systematic progression of the pathological process opens up a prospective for clinicians who want to follow the disease dynamic and shifts of symptomatology. It is hoped that it may help them reconcile these changes with the devolution of the pathological process.

In closing, it appears necessary to reconsider carefully whether it is appropriate to continue to base the diagnosis of PD largely on the presence of somatomotor symptoms alone. Particularly for the recognition of the *early* phase of the disorder, the non-motor symptoms have to be taken into consideration as well (Chaudhuri et al. 2006, Ross et al. 2006, Abbott et al. 2007, Haehner et al. 2007, Olanow et al. 2010). Such efforts could lead to a shift away from the current emphasis on motor symptoms which, relatively speaking, appear late in the disease course, and away from the one-sided focus on dopamine replacement toward an early assessment of PD as well as early onset therapeutic strategies with the goal of forcing the pathological process into remission.

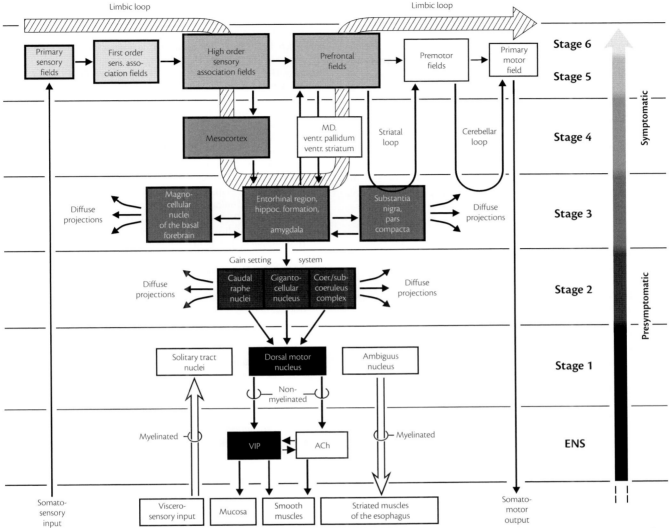

Fig. 44.13 Schematic diagram showing the gradual ascent and expansion progression of the neuropathological process underlying PD. The greater the intensity of the shading, the more severe the pathology in the regions or structures involved (symbolized by graded shading of the ascending arrow at right hand margin). White indicates non-involvement or very minimal affection. Affected subcortical nuclei and cortical areas are indicated by boldface framing. The enteric nervous system (ENS) is connected via the vagal nerve with the brainstem. Unmyelinated preganglionic fibres from the dorsal motor vagal nucleus contact ganglion cells of the enteric nervous system. This fibre pathway is susceptible to the PD-related lesions (**stage 1**). In contrast to unmyelinated fibers, the well-myelinated viscerosensory input and the visceromotor fibers from the ambiguus nucleus resist the pathology (see Fig. 8). Thereafter, the gain setting nuclei of the brainstem become involved and supplement the affection of the dorsal motor vagal nucleus (**stage 2**). The central nucleus of the amygdala, the pedunculopontine tegmental nucleus, and substantia nigra, as well as the magnocellular nuclei of the basal forebrain follow suit and become the focus of initially subtle and, then, more severe changes (**stage 3**). The sparsely myelinated, descending projections that originate in the central nucleus of the amygdala influence both the gain/level setting nuclei and the dorsal motor vagal nucleus. The anteromedial temporal mesocortex develops the first lesions within the cerebral cortex (**stage 4**). The diagram includes the chief components of the limbic loop/circuit, e.g. the entorhinal region, hippocampal formation, and amygdala. Observe the insertion of the anteromedial temporal mesocortex into the afferent trunk of the limbic loop and that of the ventral striatum, ventral pallidum, and mediodorsal thalamic nuclei into the efferent trunk (thick hatched arrow). Normal functions of the limbic loop/circuit depend on the structural integrity of the anteromedial temporal mesocortex. Severe involvement of the mesocortex thus leads to a marked reduction of the data-transfer from the sensory neocortex via entorhinal region, hippocampal formation, and amygdala to the prefrontal cortex. Thereafter, the lesions advance into the neocortex, initially making inroads into the extended prefrontal and high order sensory association areas (**stage 5**), followed by incursions into premotor and first order sensory association areas, and eventually affecting primary fields (**stage 6**). The gradual involvement of the cerebral cortex can pave the way for cognitive impairment. The dysfunctions of the visceromotor and somatomotor systems become supplemented by deterioration of cortically-controlled cognitive executive functions.
Abbreviations: ACh—cholinergic neurons in the enteric nervous system; coer./subcoeruleus complex—coeruleus-subcoeruleus complex; hippoc. formation—hippocampal formation; MD—mediodorsal nuclei of the thalamus; ventr. pallidum—ventral pallidum; ventr. striatum—ventral striatum; VIP—vasoactive intestinal peptide nitrergic neurons in the enteric nervous system. Reproduced in part with kind permission from Springer Science+Business Media: *Cell and Tissue Research*, Stages in the development of Parkinson's disease-related pathology, **318**, 2004, 121–34, Braak, H., et al.

Acknowledgements

Funding for this project was made possible by the German Research Council (Deutsche Forschungsgemeinschaft), the Hilde Ulrichs Foundation (Florstadt-Staden, Germany), and the Michael J. Fox Foundation for Parkinson's Disease Research. We wish to express our thanks to Jürgen R.E. Bohl, M.D. (Department of Neuropathology, Johannes Gutenberg University, Mainz), Hansjürgen Bratzke M.D. (Institute for Forensic Medicine, Goethe University, Frankfurt am Main), and Rob A.I. de Vos, M.D. (Laboratorium Pathologie Oost Nederland, Enschede) for autopsy material, as well as to Mr Mohamed Bouzrou, Ms Birgit Meseck-Selchow, Ms. Siegried Baumann (tissue preparations and immunohistochemistry), Ms I. Szász-Jacobi and Mr. Stephan Mayer (graphics) for their adept technical support.

References

Aarsland, D., Andersen, K., Larsen, J. P., Lolk, A., and Kragh-Sorensen, P. (2003). Prevalence and characteristics of dementia in Parkinson disease. An 8-year prospective study. *Archives of Neurology* **60**, 387–92.

Abbott, R. D., Petrovitch, H., White, L. R., *et al.* (2001). Frequency of bowel movements and the future risk of Parkinson's disease. *Neurology* **57**, 456–62.

Abbott, R. D., Ross, G. W., Petrovitch, H., *et al.* (2007). Bowel movement frequency in late-life and incidental Lewy bodies. *Movement Disorders* (May 21; Epub ahead of print).

Adler, C. H. (2005) Nonmotor complications in Parkinson's disease. *Movement Disorders* **20** (Suppl 11), 23–29.

Ahlskog, J. E. (2005). Challenging conventional wisdom: the etiologic role of dopamine oxidative stress in Parkinson's disease. *Movement Disorders* **20**, 271–82.

Altschuler, E. (1996). Gastric helicobacter pylori infection as a cause of idiopathic Parkinson disease and non-arteric anterior optic ischemic neuropathy. *Medical Hypotheses* **47**, 413–414.

Angot, E. and Brundin, P. (2009). Dissecting the potential molecular mechanisms underlying alpha-synuclein cell-to-cell transfer in Parkinson's disease. *Parkinsonism and Related Disorders* **15**(Suppl 3), S143–S147.

Anlauf, M., Schäfer, M. K. H., Eiden, L., and Weihe, E. (2003). Chemical coding of the human gastrointestinal nervous system: cholinergic, VIPergic, and catecholaminergic phenotypes. *Journal of Comparative Neurology* **459**, 90–111.

Apaydin, H., Ahlskog, J. E., Parisi, J. E., Boeve, B. F., and Dickson, D. W. (2002). Parkinson disease neuropathology: later-developing dementia and loss of the levodopa response. *Archives of Neurology* **59**, 102–112.

Arai, K., Kato, N., Kashiwado, K., and Hattori, T. (2000). Pure autonomic failure in association with human alpha-synucleinopathy. *Neuroscience Letters* **296**, 171–73.

Attems, J., Quass, M., and Jellinger, K. A. (2007). Tau and α-synuclein brainstem pathology in Alzheimer disease: relation with extrapyramidal signs. *Acta Neuropathologica* **113**, 53–62.

Awerbuch, G. I. and Sandyk, R. (1994). Autonomic functions in the early stages of Parkinson's disease. *International Journal of Neuroscience* **74**, 9–16.

Beach, T. G., Adler, C. H., Sue, L. L., *et al.* (2008). Reduced striatal tyrosine hydroxylase in incidental Lewy body disease. *Acta Neuropathologica* **115**, 445–51.

Beach, T. G., White, C. L. 3rd, Hladik, C. L., *et al.*, Arizona Parkinson's Disease Consortium. (2008). Olfactory bulb alpha-synucleinopathy has high specificity and sensitivity for Lewy body disorders. *Acta Neuropathologica* **117**, 169–174.

Beach, T. G., Adler, C. H., Sue, L. L., *et al.*, and Arizona Parkinson's Disease Consortium. (2010). Multi-organ distribution of phosphorylated a-synuclein histopathology in subjects with Lewy body disorders. *Acta Neuropathologica* **119**, 689–702.

Benarroch, E. E., Schmeichel, A. M., Low, P. A., Boeve, B. F., Sandroni, P., and Parisi, J. (2005). Involvement of medullary regions controlling sympathetic output in Lewy body disease. *Brain* **128**, 338–44.

Benarroch, E. E. (2009). The locus coeruleus norepinephrine system. *Neurology* **73**, 1699–1704.

Berendse, H. C., Booij, J., Francot, C. M. J. E., Bergmans, P. L. M., Hijman, R., Stoof, J. C., and Wolters, E. C. (2001). Subclinical dopaminergic dysfunction in asymptomatic Parkinson's disease patients' relatives with a decreased sense of smell. *Annals of Neurology* **50**, 34–41.

Berg, D., Niwar, M., Maass, S., *et al.* (2005). Alpha-synuclein and Parkinson's disease: Implications from the screening of more than 1,900 patients. *Movement Disorders* **20**, 1191–94.

Bishop, A. E. and Polak, J. M. (1999). The gut and the autonomic nervous system. In: C.J. Mathias and Sir R. Bannister, eds. *Autonomic Failure: A Textbook of Clinical Disorders of the Autonomic Nervous System*, (4th edn.), pp. 117–25. Oxford and New York: Oxford University Press.

Bloch, A., Probst, A., Bissig, H., Adams, H., and Tolnay, M. (2006). α-Synuclein pathology of the spinal and peripheral autonomic nervous system in neurologically unimpaired elderly subjects. *Neuropathology and Applied Neurobiology* **12**, 284–95.

Boeve, B. F., Silber, M. H., Saper, C. B., *et al.* (2007). Pathophysiology of REM sleep behavior disorder and relevance to neurodegenerative disease. *Brain* **129**, 3103–114.

Bohus, B., Koolhaas, J. M., Luiten, P. G. M., Korte, S. M., Roozendaal, B., and Wiersma, A. (1996). The neurobiology of the central nuleus of the amygdala in relation to neuroendocrine and autonomic outflow. *Progress in Brain Research* **107**, 447–60.

Braak, H. (1980). *Architectonics of the Human Telencephalic Cortex*. Berlin: Springer.

Braak, H., Braak, E., Yilmazer, D., de Vos, R. A. I., Jansen, E. N. H., Bohl, J., and Jellinger, K. (1994). Amygdala pathology in Parkinson's disease. *Acta Neuropathologica* **88**, 493–500.

Braak, H., Del Tredici, K., Gai, W. P., and Braak, E. (2001). Alpha-synuclein is not a requisite component of synaptic boutons in the adult human central nervous system. *Journal of Chemical Neuroanatomy* **20**, 245–52.

Braak, H., Del Tredici, K., Rüb, U., de Vos, R. A. I., Jansen Steur, E. N. H., and Braak, E. (2003a). Staging of brain pathology related to sporadic Parkinson's disease. *Neurobiology of Aging* **24**, 197–211.

Braak, H., Ghebremedhin, E., Rüb, U., Bratzke, H., and Del Tredici, K. (2004). Stages in the development of Parkinson's disease-related pathology. *Cell and Tissue Research* **318**, 121–34.

Braak, H., Müller, C. M., Bohl, J. R., Rüb, U., de Vos, R. A. I., and Del Tredici, K. (2006c). Stanley Fahn Lecture 2005: the staging procedure for the inclusion body pathology associated with sporadic Parkinson disease reconsidered. *Movement Disorders* **21**, 2042–51.

Braak, H., Müller, C. M., Rüb, U., Ackermann, H., Bratzke, H., de Vos, R. A. I., and Del Tredici, K. (2006b). Pathology associated with sporadic Parkinson's disease—where does it end? *Journal of Neural Transmission Supplements* **70**, 89–97.

Braak, H., Rüb, U., Gai, W. P., and Del Tredici, K. (2003b). Idiopathic Parkinson's disease: possible routes by which vulnerable neuronal types may be subject to neuroinvasion by an unknown pathogen. *Journal of Neural Transmission* **110**, 517–36.

Braak, H., Rüb, U., Jansen Steur, E. N. H., Del Tredici, K. and de Vos, R. A. I. (2005). Cognitive status correlates with neuropathological stage in Parkinson disease, *Neurology* **64**, 1404–1410.

Braak, H., Rüb, U., Sandmann-Keil, D., Gai, W. P., de Vos, R. A. I., Jansen Steur, E. N. H., Arai, K., and Braak, E. (2000). Parkinson's disease: affection of brain stem nuclei controlling premotor and motor neurons of the somatomotor system. *Acta Neuropathologica* **99**, 489–95.

Braak, H., Sastre, M., Bohl, J. R. E., de Vos, R. A. I., and Del Tredici, K. (2007). Parkinson's disease: lesions in dorsal horn layer I, involvement of parasympathetic and sympathetic pre- and postganglionic neurons. *Acta Neuropathologica* **113**, 421–29.

Braak, H. and Braak, E. (1986). Nuclear configuration and neuronal types of the nucleus niger in the brain of the human adult. *Human Neurobiology* 5, 71–82.

Braak, H. and Braak, E. (1992). The human entorhinal cortex: normal morphology and lamina-specific pathology in various diseases. *Neuroscience Research* 15, 6–31.

Braak, H. and Del Tredici, K. (2004). Poor and protracted myelination as a contributory factor to neurodegenerative disorders. *Neurobiology of Aging* 25, 19–23.

Braak, H. and Del Tredici, K. (2008). Nervous system pathology in sporadic Parkinson's disease. *Neurology* 70, 1916–25.

Braak, H. and Del Tredici, K. (2009). Neuroanatomy and pathology of sporadic Parkinson's disease. *Advances in Anatomy, Embryology and Cell Biology* 201, 1–119.

Braak, H., de Vos, R. A. I., Bohl, J., and Del Tredici, K. (2006a). Gastric α-synuclein immunoreactive inclusions in Meissner's and Auerbach's plexuses in cases staged for Parkinson's disease-related brain pathology. *Neuroscience Letters* 396, 67–72.

Broadwell, R. D. and Brightman, M. V. (1976). Entry of peroxidase into neurons of the central and peripheral nervous systems from extracerebral and cerebral blood. *Journal of Comparative Neurology* 166, 257–84.

Brown, P. (2001). The pathogenesis of transmissible spongiform encephalopathy: routes to the brain and the erection of therapeutic barricades. *Cellular and Molecular Life Sciences* 58, 259–65.

Card, J. P. (1998). Exploring brain circuitry with neurotropic viruses: new horizons in neuroanatomy. *Anatomical Record* 253, 176–85.

Castillo, P. R., Del Tredici, K., and Braak, H. (2007). Pathophysiology of REM sleep behavior disorder and relevance to neurodegenerative disease. *Brain* 129, 3103–14.

Cersósimo, M. G., Benarroch, E. E. (2008). Neural control of the gastrointestinal tract: implications for Parkinson disease. *Movement Disorders* 23, 1065–75.

Chaudhuri, K. R., Healy, D. G., and Schapira, A. H. (2006). Non-motor symptoms of Parkinson's disease: diagnosis and management. *Lancet Neurology* 5; 235–45.

Chu, Y. and Kordower, J. H. (2007). Age-associated increases of a-synuclein in monkeys and humans are associated with nigrostriatal dopamine depletion: is this the target for Parkinson's disease? *Neurobiology of Disease* 25, 134–49.

Ciechanover, A. and Brundin, P. (2003). The ubiquitin proteasome system in neurodegenerative diseases: sometimes the chicken, sometimes the egg. *Neuron* 40, 427–46.

Claassen, D. O., Josephs, K. A., Ahlskog, J. E., Silber, M. H., Tippman-Peikert, M., and Boeve, B. F. (2010). REM sleep behaviour disorder preceding other aspects of synucleinopathies by up to a half a century. *Neurology* 75, 494–9.

Costa, M., Brookes, S. J. H., and Hennig, G. W. (2000). Anatomy and physiology of the enteric nervous system. *Gut* (Suppl. 4) 47, iv15–19.

Dale, G. E., Probst, A., Luthert, P., Martin, J., Anderton, B. H., and Leigh, P. N. (1992). Relationship between Lewy bodies and pale bodies in Parkinson's disease. *Acta Neuropathologica* 83, 525–29.

Daniel, S. E. and Hawkes, C. H. (1992). Preliminary diagnosis of Parkinson's disease by olfactory bulb pathology. *The Lancet* 340, 186.

DeLacoste, M. C. and White, C. L. (1993). The role of cortical connectivity in Alzheimer's disease pathogenesis: a review and model system. *Neurobiology of Aging* 14, 1–16.

Del Tredici, K., Rüb, U., de Vos, R. A. I., Bohl, J. R. E., and Braak, H. (2002). Where does Parkinson disease pathology begin in the brain? *Journal of Neuropathology and Experimental Neurology* 61, 413–26.

Del Tredici, K. and Braak, H. (2004). Idiopathic Parkinson's disease: Staging an α-synucleinopathy with a predictable pathoanatomy. In: P. Kahle, and C. Haass, eds. *Molecular Mechanisms in Parkinson's Disease*, pp. 1–32. Georgetown, Texas: Landes Bioscience.

Del Tredici, K. and Braak, H. (2008). A not entirely benign procedure: progression of Parkinson's disease. *Acta Neuropathologica* 115, 379–84.

Del Tredici, K., Hawkes, C. H., Ghebremedhin, E., and Braak, H. (2010). Lewy pathology in the submandibular gland of individuals with incidental Lewy body disease and sporadic Parkinson's disease. *Acta Neuropathologica* 119, 703–13.

Desplats, P., Lee, H. J., Bae, E. J., et al. (2009). Inclusion formation and neuronal cell death through neuron-to-neuron transmission of alpha-synuclein. *Proceedings of the National Academy of Science USA* 106, 13010–5.

Dickson, D. W. (1998). Aging in the central nervous system. In: M. R. Markesbery, ed. *Neuropathology of Dementing Disorders*, pp. 56–88. London and New York: Arnold.

Dickson, D. W. (1999). Tau and synuclein and their role in neuropathology. *Brain Pathology* 9, 657–61.

Dickson, D. W., Fujishiro, H., DelleDonne, A., et al. (2008). Evidence that incidental Lewy body disease is presymptomatic Parkinson's disease. *Acta Neuropathologica* 115, 437–44.

Dickson, D. W., Braak, H., Duda, J. E., et al. (2009). Diagnostic criteria for the neuropathological assessment of Parkinson disease. *Lancet Neurology* 8, 1150–7.

Dickson, S. W., Uchikado, H., Fujishiro, H., and Tsuboi,, Y. (2010). Evidence in favor of Braak staging of Parkinson's disease. *Movement Disorders* 25(Suppl. 1), S78–S82.

Dobbs, S. M., Dobbs, R. J., Weller, C., and Charlett, A. (2000). Link between Helicobacter pylori infection and idiopathic parkinsonism. *Medical Hypotheses* 55, 93–98.

Dorsey, E. R., Constantinescu, R., Thompson, J. P., et al. (2007). Projected numbers of people with Parkinson's disease in the most populous nations. 2005 through 2030. *Neurology* 68, 284–386.

Doty, R. L. (2001). Olfaction. *Annual Review of Psychology* 52, 423–52.

Doty, R. L., Deems, D. A., and Steller, S. (1988). Olfactory dysfunction in parkinsonism: a general deficit unrelated to neurologic signs, disease stage, or disease duration. *Neurology* 38, 1237–44.

Doty, R. L., Stern, M. B., Pfeiffer, C., Gollomp, S. M., and Hurtig, H. I. (1992). Bilateral olfactory dysfunction in early stage treated and untreated idiopathic Parkinson's disease. *Journal of Neurology, Neurosurgery, and Psychiatry* 55, 138–142.

Duda, J. E., Lee, V. M. Y., and Trojanowski, J. Q. (2000). Neuropathology of synuclein aggregates: new insights into mechanism of neurodegenerative diseases. *Journal of Neuroscience Research* 61, 121–27.

Dugger, B. N. and Dickson, D. W. (2010). Cell type specific sequestration of choline acetyltransferase and tyrosine hydroxyalase within Lewy bodies. *Acta Neuropathologica* doi.10.1007/s00401-010-0739-1.

Eriksen, J. L., Dawson, T. M., Dickson, D. W., and Petrucelli, L. (2003). Caught in the act: α-synuclein is the culprit in Parkinson's disease. *Neuron* 40, 453–56.

Eriksen, J. L., Zbigniew, W., and Petrucelli, L. (2005). Molecular pathogenesis of Parkinson disease. *Archives of Neurology* 62, 353–57.

Evatt, M. L., Chaudhuri, K. R., Chou, K. L., et al. (2009). Dysautonomia rating scales in Parkinson's disease: sialorrhea, dysphagia, and constipation – critique and recommendations by Movement Disorders Task Force on Rating Scales for Parkinson's disease. *Movement Disorders* 24, 635–46.

Fahn, S. (2003). Description of Parkinson's disease as a clinical syndrome. *Annals of the New York Academy of Sciences* 991, 1–14.

Forno, L. S. (1969). Concentric hyaline intraneuronal inclusions of Lewy body type in the brain of elderly persons (50 incidental cases): Relationship to parkinsonism. *Journal of the American Geriatrics Society* 17, 557–75.

Forno, L. S. (1996). Neuropathology of Parkinson's disease. *Journal of Neuropathology and Experimental Neurology* 55, 259–72.

Forno, L. S., Sternberger, L. A., Sternberger, N. H., Strefling, A. M., Swanson, K., and Eng, L. F. (1986). Reaction of Lewy bodies with antibodies to phosphorylated and non-phosphorylated neurofilaments. *Neuroscience Letters* 64, 253–58.

Forno, L. S. and Norville, R. L. (1976). Ultrastructure of Lewy bodies in the stellate ganglion. *Acta Neuropathologica* **34**, 183–97.

Fortin, D. L., Nemani, V. M., Voglmaier, S. M., Anthony, M. D., Ryan, T. A., and Edwards, R. H. (2005). Neural activity controls the synaptic accumulation of a-Synuclein. *Neurobiology of Disease* **25**, 10913–21.

Fujishiro, H., Frigerior, R., Burnett, M., *et al.* (2008). Cardiac sympathetic denervation correlates with clinical and pathologic stages of Parkinson's disease. *Movement Disorders* **23**, 1085–92.

Fumimura, Y., Ikemura, M., Saito, Y., *et al.* (2007). Analysis of the adrenal gland is useful for evaluating pathology of the peripheral autonomic nervous system in Lewy body disease. *Journal of Neuropathology and Experimental Neurology* **66**, 354–62.

Furness, J. B. (2000). Types of neurons in the enteric nervous system. *Journal of the Autonomic Nervous System* **81**, 87–96.

Galvin, J. E., Lee, V. M. Y., and Trojanowski, J. Q. (2001). Synucleinopathies. Clinical and pathological implications. *Archives of Neurology* **58**, 186–90.

Galvin, J. E., Pollack, J., and Morris, J. C. (2006). Clinical phenotype of Parkinson disease dementia. *Neurology* **67**, 1605–611.

German, D. C., Manaye, K. F., and White, C. L. 3rd. (1992). Disease-specific patterns of locus coeruleus cell loss. *Annals of Neurology* **32**, 667–76.

Geser, F., Wenning, G. K., Poewe, W., and McKeith, I. (2005). How to diagnose dementia with Lewy bodies: state of the art. *Movement Disorders Suppl.12* **20**, 11–20.

Ghebremedhin, E., Del Tredici, K., Langston, J. W., and Braak, H. (2009). Diminished tyrosine hydroxylase immunoreactivity in the cardiac conduction system and myocardium in Parkinson's disease. *Acta Neuropathologica* **118**, 777–84.

Gibb, W. R. and Lees, A.J. (1988). The relevance of the Lewy body to the pathogenesis of idiopathic Parkinson's disease. *Journal of Neurology, Neurosurgery, and Psychiatry* **51**, 745–52.

Goedert, M. (2001). The significance of tau and α-synuclein inclusions in neurodegenerative diseases. *Current Opinion in Genetics & Development* **11**, 343–51.

Golbe, L. I. (1999). Alpha synuclein and Parkinson's disease. *Movement Disorders* **14**, 6–9.

Gosh, S. (2002). Intestinal entry of prions. *Zeitschrift für Gastroenterologie* **40**, 37–39.

Haehner, A., Hummel, T., Hummel, C., Sommer, U., Junghanns, S., and Reichmann, H. (2007). Olfactory loss may be a first sign of idiopathic Parkinson's disease. *Movement Disorders* **22**, 839–42.

Hague, K., Lento, P., Morgello, S., Caro, S., and Kaufmann, H. (1997). The distribution of Lewy bodies in pure autonomic failure: autopsy findings and review of the literature. *Acta Neuropathologica* **94**, 92–96.

Halliday, G., Del Tredici, K., and Braak, H. (2006). Critical appraisal of the Braak staging of brain pathology related to sporadic Parkinson's disease. *Journal of Neural Transmission Supplements* **70**, 99–103.

Halliday, G. M., Hely, M., Reid, W., and Morris, J. (2008). The progression of pathology in longitudinally followed patients with Parkinson's disease. *Acta Neuropathologica* **115**, 409–415.

Halliday, G. M., Lee, Y. V., Bloombergs, P. C., *et al.* (1990). Neuropathology of immunohistochemically identified brainstem neurons in Parkinson's disease. *Annals of Neurology* **72**, 373–85.

Hardy, J. and Lees, A. J. (2005). Parkinson's disease: a broken nosology. *Movement Disorders* 20 (Suppl. 12) **20**, S2–S4.

Hawkes, C. H. (2003). Olfaction in neurodegenerative disorder. *Movement Disorders* **18**, 364–72.

Hawkes, C. H. (2008). Parkinson's disease and aging: same or different process? *Movement Disorders* **23**, 47–53.

Hawkes, C. H., Del Tredici, K., and Braak, H. (2007). Parkinson's disease: A dual hit hypothesis. *Neuropathology and Applied Neurobiology* **33**, 599–614.

Hawkes, C. H., Del Tredici, K., and Braak, H. (2010). A timeline for Parkinson's disease. *Parkinsonism and Related Disorders* **16**, 79–84.

Hawkes, C. H., Shephard, B. C., and Daniel, S. E. (1999). Is Parkinson's disease a primary olfactory disorder? *Quarterly Journal of Medicine* **92**, 473–80.

Helke, C. J., Adryan, K. M., Fedorowicz, J., *et al.* (1998). Axonal transport of neurotrophins by visceral afferent and efferent neurons of the vagus nerve of the rat. *Journal of Comparative Neurology* **393**, 102–117.

Hely, M. A., Reid, W. G., Adena, M. A., Halliday, G. M., and Morris, J. G. (2008). The Sydney multicenter study of Parkinson's disease: the inevitability of dementia at 20 years. *Movement Disorders* **23**, 837–44.

Henderson, J. M., Carpenter, K., Cartwright, H., and Halliday, G. H. (2000). Loss of thalamic intralaminar nuclei in progressive supranuclear palsy and Parkinson's disease: clinical and therapeutic implications. *Brain* **123**, 1410–21.

Hill, T. J. (1987). Ocular pathogenicity of herpes simplex virus. *Current Eye Research* **6**, 1–7.

Hirsch, E. C., Graybill, A. M., Duyckaerts, C., and Javoy-Agid, F. (1987). Neuronal loss in the pedunculopontine tegmental nucleus in Parkinson disease and in progressive supranuclear palsy. *Proceedings of the National Academy of Sciences USA* **84**, 5976–80.

Hishikawa, N., Hashizume, Y., Hirayama, M., *et al.* (2000). Brainstem-type Lewy body disease presenting with progressive autonomic failure and lethargy. *Clinical Autonomic Research* **10**, 139–43.

Hopkins, D. A., Bieger, D., de Vente, J., and Steinbusch, H. W. M. (1996). Vagal efferent projections: viscerotopy, neurochemistry and effects of vagotomy. *Progress in Brain Research* **107**, 79–96.

Huang, X. F., Törk, I., and Paxinos, G. (1993). Dorsal motor nucleus of the vagus nerve: a cyto- and chemoarchitectonic study in the human. *Journal of Comparative Neurology* **330**, 158–82.

Hubbard, P. S., Esiri, M. M., Reading, M., McShane, R., Nagy, Z. (2007). Alpha-synuclein pathology in the olfactory pathways of dementia patients. *Journal of Anatomy* **211**, 117–24.

Hurtig, H. I., Trojanowski, J. Q., Galvin, J., *et al.* (2000) Alpha-synuclein cortical Lewy bodies correlate with dementia in Parkinson's disease. *Neurology* **54**, 1916–21.

Iwanaga, K., Wakabayashi, K., Yoshimoto, M., *et al.* (1999). Lewy body-type degeneration in cardiac plexus in Parkinson's and incidental Lewy body diseases. *Neurology* **52**, 1269–71.

Jager, W., den Hartog, W. A., and Bethlem. J. (1960). The distribution of Lewy bodies in the central and autonomic nervous system in idiopathic paralysis agitans. *Journal of Neurology, Neurosurgery, and Psychiatry* **23**, 283–90.

Jang, H., Boltz, D. A., Webster, R. G., and Smeyne, R. J. (2009). Viral Parkinsonism. *Biochimica et Biophysica Acta* **1892**, 714–21.

Jellinger, K. (1988). The pedunculopontine nucleus in Parkinson's disease, progressive supranuclear palsy and Alzheimer's disease. *Journal of Neurology, Neurosurgery, and Psychiatry* **51**, 540–43.

Jellinger, K. (1991). Pathology of Parkinson's disease. Changes other than the nigrostriatal pathway. *Molecular and Chemical Neuropathology* **14**, 153–97.

Jellinger, K. A. (2000). Morphological substrates of mental dysfunction in Lewy body disease: an update. *Journal of Neural Transmission Supplements* **59**, 185–212.

Jellinger, K. A. (2003a). Neuropathological spectrum of synucleinopathies. *Movement Disorders (Suppl. 6)* **18**, 2–12.

Jellinger, K. A. (2003b). Alpha-synuclein pathology in Parkinson's and Alzheimer's disease brain: incidence and topographic distribution—a pilot study. *Acta Neuropathologica* **106**, 191–201.

Jellinger, K. A. (2004) Lewy body-related α-synucleinopathy in the aged human brain. *Journal of Neural Transmission* **111**, 1219–35.

Jellinger, K. A. and Mizuno, Y. (2003). Parkinson's disease. In: D. W. Dickson, ed. *Neurodegeneration: The Molecular Pathology of Dementia and Movement Disorders*, pp. 159–87. Basel: ISN Neuropath Press.

Jenner, P. (1993). Presymptomatic detection of Parkinson's disease. *Journal of Neural Transmission Supplements* **40**, 23–36.

Jost, W. H. (2003). Autonomic dysfunctions in idiopathic Parkinson's disease. *Journal of Neurology* **250** (Suppl. 1), 28–30.

Kaufmann, H., Nahm, K., Purohit, D., and Wolfe, D. (2004). Autonomic failure as the initial manifestation of Parkinson's disease and dementia with Lewy bodies. *Neurology* **63**, 1093–95.

Kaufmann, H., and Goldstein, D. S. (2010). Pure autonomic failure: a restricted Lewy body synucleinopathy or early Parkinson disease? *Neurology* **74**, 536–7.

Kempster, P. A., O'Sullivan, S. S., Holton, J. L., Revesz, T., and Lees, A. J. (2010). Relationships between age and late progression of Parkinson's disease: a clinico-pathological study. *Brain* **133**, 1755–62.

Klos, K. J., Ahlskog, J. E., Josephs, K. A., *et al.* (2006). α-Synuclein pathology in the spinal cord of neurologically asymptomatic aged individuals. *Neurology* **66**, 1100–1102.

Koller, W. C., Langston, J. W., Hubble, J. P., *et al.* (1991). Does a long preclinical period occur in Parkinson's disease? *Neurology* (Suppl. *2*) **41**, 8–13.

Kopito, R. R. (2000). Aggresomes, inclusion bodies and protein aggregation. *Trends in Cellular Biology* **10**, 524–30.

Korczyn, A. D. (1990). Autonomic nervous system disturbances in Parkinson's disease. *Advances in Neurology* **53**, 463–68.

Korczyn, A. D. (2001). Dementia in Parkinson's disease. *Journal of Neurology* (Suppl. *3*) **248**, 1–4.

Koutcherov, Y., Huang, X. F., Halliday, G., and Paxinos, G. (2004). Organization of human brain stem nuclei. In: G. Paxinos and J.K. Mai, eds. *The Human Nervous System*, (2nd edn.), pp. 273–321. San Diego and London: Elsevier Academic Press.

Kuusisto, E., Parkkinen, L., and Alafuzoff, I. (2003). Morphogenesis of Lewy bodies: dissimilar incorporation of α-synuclein, ubiquitin, and p. 62. *Journal of Neuropathology and Experimental Neurology* **62**, 1241–53.

Lang, A. E. and Lozano, A. M. (1998). Parkinson's disease: first of two parts. *The New England Journal of Medicine* **339**, 1044–53.

Lang, A. E. and Obeso, J. A. (2004). Challenges in Parkinson's disease: restoration of the nigrostriatal dopamine system is not enough. *The Lancet Neurology* **3**, 309–316.

Langston, J. W. (2006). The Parkinson's complex: parkinsonism is just the tip of the iceberg. *Annals of Neurology* **59**, 591–96.

Lantos, P. L. and Quinn, N. (2003). Multiple system atrophy. In: D. W. Dickson, ed. *Neurodegeneration: The Molecular Pathology of Dementia and Movement Disorders*, pp. 203–214. Basel: ISN Neuropath Press.

Larner, A. J., Mathias, C. J., and Rossor, M. N. (2000). Autonomic failure preceding dementia with Lewy bodies. *Journal of Neurology* **247**, 229–31.

Lavedan, C. (1998). The synuclein family. *Genetic Research* **8**, 871–80.

Lee, P. H., Yeo, S. H., Kim, H. J., and Youm, H. Y. (2006). Correlation between cardiac ^{123}I-MIBG and odor identification in patients with Parkinson's disease and multiple system atrophy. *Movement Disorders* **21**, 1975–77.

Lewandowski, ed. *Handbuch der Neurologie*, Bd. 3, pp. 920–933. Berlin: Springer.

Lewy, F. H. (1912). Paralysis agitans. I. Pathologische Anatomie. In: M. Lewandowski, ed. *Handbuch der Neurologie*, Bd. 3, pp. 920–33. Berlin: Springer.

Li, J. Y., Englund, E., Holton, J. L., *et al.* (2008). Lewy bodies in grafted neurons in people with Parkinson's disease suggest host-to-graft disease propagation. *Nature Medicine* **14**, 501–3.

Litvan, I., Bhatia, K. P., Burn, D. J., *et al.* (2003). SIC Task force appraisal of clinical diagnostic criteria for Parkinsonian disorders. *Movement Disorders* **18**, 467–86.

Liubashima, O., Jolkkonen, E., and Pitkänen, A. (2000). Projections from the central nucleus of the amygdala to the gastric related area of the dorsal vagal complex: a Phaseolus vulgaris leucoagglutinin study in rat. *Neuroscience Lettters* **291**, 85–88.

Lowe, J. (1994). Lewy bodies. In: D. P. Calne, ed. *Neurodegenerative Diseases*, pp. 51–69. Philadelphia: Saunders.

Lundvig, D., Lindersson, E., and Jensen, P. H. (2005). Pathogenic effects of α-synuclein aggregation. *Molecular Brain Research* **134**, 3–17.

Magalhaes, M., Wenning, G. K., Daniel, S. E., and Quinn, N. P. (1995). Autonomic dysfunction in pathologically confirmed multiple system atrophy and idiopathic Parkinson's disease—a retrospective comparison. *Acta Neurologica Scandinavica* **91**, 98–102.

Magerkurth, C., Schnitzer, R., and Braune, S. (2005). Symptoms of autonomic failure in Parkinson's disease: prevalence and impact on daily life. *Clinical Autonomic Research* **15**, 76–82.

Markesbery, W. R., Jicha, G. A., Liu, H., and Schmitt, F. A. (2009). Lewy body pathology in normal elderly subjects. *Journal of Neuropathology and Experimental Neurology* **68**, 816–22.

Martignoni, E., Pacchetti, C., Godi, L., Micieli, G., and Nappi, G. (1995). Autonomic disorders in Parkinson's disease. *Journal of Neural Transmission Supplements* **45**, 11–19.

Matsuda, K., Park, C.H., Synden, Y., Kimura, T., Ochiai, K., Kida, H., and Umemura, T. (2004). The vagus nerve is one route of transneural invasion for intranasally inocculated influenza A virus in mice. *Veterinary Pathology* **41**, 101–107.

Matthews, M. R. (1999). Autonomic ganglia and preganglionic neurones in autonomic failure. In: C.J. Mathias and Sir R. Bannister, eds. *Autonomic Failure: A Textbook of Clinical Disorders of the Autonomic Nervous System*, (4th edn.), pp. 329–39. Oxford and New York: Oxford University Press.

McAllister, C., Karymov, M. A., Kawano, Y., Lushnikov, A. Y., Mikheikin, A., Uversky, V. N., and Lyubchenko, Y. L. (2005). Protein interactions and misfolding analyzed by AFM force spectroscopy. *Journal of Molecular Biology* **354**, 1028–42.

McBride, P. A., Schulz-Schaeffer, W. J., Donaldson, M., *et al.* (2001). Early spread of scrapie from the gastrointestinal tract to the central nervous system involves autonomic fibers of the splanchnic and vagus nerves. *Journal of Virology* **75**, 9320–7.

McKeith, I. G., Dickson, D. W., Lowe, J., *et al.* (2005). Diagnosis and management of dementia with Lewy bodies: third report of the DLB consortium. *Neurology* **65**, 1863–72.

McKeith, I. G., Galasko, D., Kosaka, K., *et al.* (1996). Consensus guidelines for the clinical and pathological diagnosis of dementia with Lewy bodies (DLB): Report of the consortium on DLB international workshop. *Neurology* **47**, 1113–24.

McNaught, K. S. T. P., Shashidharan, P., Perl, D. P., Jenner, P., and Olanow, C. W. (2002). Aggresome-related biogenesis of Lewy bodies. *European Journal of Neuroscience* **16**, 2136–48.

Mesholam, R. L., Moberg, P. J., Mahr, R. N., and Doty, R. L. (1998). Olfaction in neurodegerative disease. A meta-analysis of olfactory functioning in Alzheimer's and Parkinson's diseases. *Archives of Neurology* **55**, 84–90.

Mesulam, M. M. (1998). From sensation to cognition. *Brain* **121**, 1013–52.

Micieli, G., Tosi, P., Marcheselli, S., and Cavallini, A. (2003). Autonomic dysfunction in Parkinson's disease. *Neurological Sciences* **24**, 32–34.

Miki, Y., Mori, F., Wakabayashi, K., Kuroda, N., and Orimo, S. (2009). Incidental Lewy body disease restricted to the heart and stellate ganglion. *Movement Disorders* **24**, 2299–301.

Mikolaenko, I., Pletnikova, O., Kawas, C. H., O'Brien, R., Resnick, S. M., Crain, B., and Troncoso, J. C. (2005). Alpha-synuclein lesions in normal aging, Parkinson disease, and Alzheimer disease: evidence from the Baltimore Longitudinal Study of Aging (BLSA). *Journal of Neuropathology and Experimental Neurology* **64**, 156–62.

Minguez-Castellanos, A., Chamorro, C. E., Escamilla-Sevilla, F., *et al.* (2007). Do α-synuclein aggregates in autonomic plexuses predate Lewy body disorders? A cohort study. *Neurology* **68**, 2012–2028.

Morrish, P. K., Rakashi, J. S., Bailey, D. L., Sawle, G. V., and Brooks, D. J. (1998). Measuring the rate of progression and estimating the preclinical period of Parkinson's disease with (18F)dopa PET. *Journal of Neurology, Neurosurgery, and Psychiatry* **64**, 314–319.

Morrison, L. A., Sidman, R. L., and Fields, B. N. (1991). Direct spread of reovirus from the intestinal lumen to the central nervous system through vagal autonomic nerve fibers. *Proceedings of the National Academy of Sciences USA.* **88**, 3852–56.

Mufson, E. J., Kroin, J. S., Sendera, T. J., and Sobreviela, T. (1999). Distribution and retrograde transport of trophic factors in the central nervous system: Functional implications for the treatment of neurodegenerative diseases. *Progress in Neurobiology* **57**, 451–84.

Murer, M. G., Yan, Q., and Raisman-Vozari, R. (2001). Brain-derived neurotrophic factor in the control human brain, and in Alzheimer's disease and Parkinson's disease. *Progress in Neurobiology* **63**, 71–124.

Müller, C. M., de Vos, R. A. I., Maurage, C. A., Thal, D. R., Tolnay, M., and Braak, H. (2005). Staging of sporadic Parkinson disease-related alpha-synuclein pathology: inter- and intra-rater reliability. *Journal of Neuropathology and Experimental Neurology* **64**, 623–28.

Neumann, M., Müller, V., Kretzschmar, H. A., Haass, C., and Kahle, P.J. (2004). Regional distribution of proteinase-K-resistant α-synuclein correlates with Lewy body disease stage. *Neuropathology and Experimental Neurology* **63**, 1225–35.

Nicotera, P. (2001). A route for prion neuroinvasion. *Neuron* **31**, 345–48.

Norris, E. H., Giasson, B. I., and Lee, V. M. (2004). α-Synuclein: normal function and role in neurodegenerative diseases. *Current Topics in Developmental Biololgy* **60**, 17–54.

Olanow, C. W., Perl, D. P., DeMartin, G. N., and McNaught K. St. P. (2004). Lewy-body formation is an aggresome-related process: a hypothesis. *The Lancet Neurology* **3**, 496–503.

Olanow, C. W. and McNaught, K. St. P. (2006). Ubiquitin-Proteasome system and Parkinson's disease. *Movement Disorders* **21**, 1806–23.

Olanow, C. W., Stocchi, F., and Lang, A. E. (2010). *The Non-Dopaminergic Features of Parkinson's Disease.* Oxford: Blackwell (in press).

Orimo, S., Amino, T., Itoh, Y., *et al.* (2005). Cardiac sympathetic denervation precedes neuronal loss in the sympathetic ganglia in Lewy body disease, *Acta Neuropathologica* **109**, 583–88.

Orimo, S., Takahashi, A., Uchihara, T., Mori, F., Kakita, A., Wakabayashi, K., and Takahashi, H. (2007). Degeneration of cardiac sympathetic nerve begins in the early disease process of Parkinson's disease. *Brain Pathololgy* **17**, 24–30.

Orimo, S., Uchihara, T., Nakamura, A., Mori, F., Kakita, A., Wakabayashi, K., and Takahashi, H. (2008). Axonal alpha-synuclein aggregates herald centripetal degeneration of cardiac sympathetic nerve in Parkinson's disease. *Brain* **131**, 642–50.

Pahapill, P. A. and Lozano, A. M. (2000). The pedunculopontine nucleus and Parkinson's disease. *Brain* **123**, 1767–83.

Palka-Santini, M., Schwarz-Henke, B., Hösel, M., Renz, D., Auerochs, S., Brondke, H., and Doerfler, W. (2003). The gastrointestinal tract as the portal of entry for foreign macromolecules: Fate of DANN and proteins. *Molecular Genetics and Genomics* **270**, 201–215.

Pan, T., Kondo, S., Le, W., and Jankovic J. (2008). The role of autophagy-lysosome pathway in neurodegeneration associated with Parkinson's disease. *Brain* **131**, 1969–78.

Pankratz, N. and Foroud, T. (2004). Genetics of Parkinson disease. *NeuroRx* **2**, 235–42.

Parkinson, J. (1817). *An essay on the shaking palsy.* London: Whittingham and Rowland.

Pearce, R. K., Hawkes, C. H., and Daniel, S. E. (1995). The anterior olfactory nucleus in Parkinson's disease. *Movement Disorders* **10**, 283–87.

Pearson, R. C. A. (1996). Cortical connections and the pathology of Alzheimer's disease. *Neurodegeneration* **5**, 429–34.

Pearson, R. C. A., Esiri, M. M., Hiorns, R. W., Wilcock, G. K., and Powell, T. P. S. (1985). Anatomical correlates of the distribution of the pathological changes in the neocortex in Alzheimer's disease. *Proceedings of the National Academy of Sciences USA* **82**, 4531–34.

Pfeiffer, R. F. (2003). Gastrointestinal dysfunction in Parkinson's disease. *The Lancet Neurology* **2**, 107–116.

Pfeiffer, R. F. (2010). Gastrointestinal, urological, and sexual dysfunction in Parkinson's disease. *Movement Disorders* **25**(*Suppl.* 1), S94–S97.

Phillips, R. J., Walter, G. C., Wilder, S. L., Baronowski, E. A., and Powley, T. L. (2008). Alpha-synuclein immunopositive myenteric neurons and vagal preganglionic terminals: autonomic pathway implicated in Parkinson's disease? *Neuroscience* **153**, 733–50.

Ponsen, M. M., Stoffers, D., Booij, J., van Eck-Smit, B. L., Wolters, E. C., and Berendse, H. W. (2004). Idiopathic hyposmia as a preclinical sign of Parkinson's disease. *Annals of Neurology* **56**, 173–81.

Price, J. L. (2004). Olfaction. In *The Human Nervous System,* (2nd edn.), (ed. G. Paxinos and J.M. Mai), pp. 1198–1212. Elsevier Academic Press, San Diego and London.

Prusiner, S. B. (1998). Prions. *Proceedings of the National Academy of Sciences USA* **95**, 13363–83.

Qualman, S. J., Haupt, H. M., Yang, P., and Hamilton, S. R. (1984). Esophageal Lewy bodies associated with ganglion cell loss in achalasia. Similarity to Parkinson's disease. *Gastroenterology* **87**, 848–56.

Quigley, E. M. (1996). Gastrointestinal dysfunction in Parkinson's disease. *Seminars in Neurology* **16**, 245–50.

Quinn, N. P., Rossor, M. N., and Marsden, C. D. (1987). Olfactory threshold in Parkinson's disease. *Journal of Neurology, Neurosurgery, and Psychiatry* **50**, 88–89.

Rajput, A. H. and Rozdilsky, B. (1976). Dysautonomia in Parkinsonism: a clinicopathological study. *Journal of Neurology, Neurosurgery, and Psychiatry* **39**, 1092–100.

Richards, W. G. and Sugarbaker, D. J. (1997). Neuronal control of esophageal functions. *Chest Surgery Clinics of North America* **5**, 157–71.

Rinaman, L., Levitt, P., and Card, J. P. (2000). Progressive postnatal assembly of limbic-autonomic circuits revealed by central transneuronal transport of pseudorabies virus. *Journal of Neuroscience* **20**, 2731–41.

Ross, G. W., Abbott, R. D., Petrovitch, H., *et al.* (2006). Association of olfactory dysfunction with incidental Lewy bodies. *Movement Disorders* **21**, 2062–67.

Saito, Y., Kawashima, A., Ruberu, N. N., *et al.* (2003). Accumulation of phosphorylated α-synuclein in aging human brain. *Journal of Neuropathology and Experimental Neurology* **62**, 644–54.

Saito, Y., Ruberu, N. N., Sawabe, M., *et al.* (2004). Lewy body-related α-synucleinopathy in aging. *Journal of Neuropathology and Experimental Neurology* **63**, 742–49.

Saper, C. B., Sorrentino, D. M., German, D. C., and de Lacalle, S. (1991). Medullary catecholaminergic neurons in the normal human brain and in Parkinson's disease. *Annals of Neurology* **29**, 577–84.

Saper, C. B., Wainer, B. H., and German, D. C. (1987). Axonal and transneuronal transport in the transmission of neurological disease: potential role in system degenerations, including Alzheimer's disease. *Neuroscience* **23**, 389–98.

Sara, J. S. (2009). The locus coeruleus and noradrenergic modulation of cognition. *Nature Reviews Neuroscience* **10**, 211–23.

Savica, R., Rocca, W. A., and Ahlskog, J. E. (2010). When does Parkinson disease start? *Archives of Neurology* **67**, 798–801.

Sawle, G. V. (1993). The detection of preclinical Parkinson's disease: what is the role of positron emission tomography? *Movement Disorders* **8**, 271–77.

Schulz-Schaeffer, W. J. (2010). The synaptic pathology of a-synuclein aggregation in dementia with Lewy bodies, Parkinson's disease and Parkinson's disease dementia. *Acta Neuropathologica* **120**, 131–43.

Sethi, K. (2008). Levodopa unresponsive symptoms in Parkinson's disease. *Movement Disorders* **23** (Suppl. 3), S521–33.

Siddiqui, M. F., Rast, S., Lynn, M. J., Auchus, A. P., and Pfeiffer, R. F. (2002). Autonomic dysfunction in Parkinson's disease: a comprehensive symptom survey. *Parkinsonism and Related Disorders* **8**, 277–84.

Sotelo, C. and Triller, A. (1997). The central neuron. Inv: D.I. Graham and P.L. Lantos, eds. *Greenfield's Neuropathology*, (6th edn.), pp. 3–62. London: Arnold.

Spillantini, M. G., Schmidt, M. L., Lee, V. M. Y., Trojanowski, J. Q., Jakes, R., and Goedert, M. (1997). α-synuclein in Lewy bodies. *Nature* **388**, 839–40.

Stiasny-Kolster, K., Doerr, Y., Möller, J. C. Hoffken, H., Behr, T. M., Oertel, W. H., and Mayer, G. (2005). Combination of 'idiopathic' REM sleep behaviour disorder and olfactory dysfunction as possible indicator for α-synucleinopathy demonstrated by dopamine transporter FP-CIT-SPECT. *Brain* **128**, 126–37.

Strack, A. M., Sawyer, W. B., Hughes, J. H., Platt, K. B., and Loewy, A. D. (1989). A general pattern of CNS innervation of the sympathetic outflow demonstrated by transneuronal pseudorabies viral infections. *Brain Research* **491**, 156–62.

Strang, R. R. (1965). The association of gastro-duodenal ulceration with Parkinson's disease. *Medical Journal of Australia* **52**, 842–43.

Takahashi, H., and Wakabayashi, K. (2001). The cellular pathology of Parkinson's disease. *Neuropathology* **21**, 315–22.

Takahashi, H. and Wakabayashi, K. (2005). Controversy: Is Parkinson's disease a single disease entity? Yes. *Parkinsonism and Related Disorders* **11**, 31–37.

Timmermans, J. P., Hens, J., and Adriaensen, D. (2001). Outer submucous plexus: an intrinsic nerve network involved in both secretory and motility processes in the intestine of large mammals and humans. *Anatomical Record* **262**, 71–78.

Tissingh, G., Berendse, H. W., Bergmanns, P., De Waard, R., Drukarch, B., Stoof, J. C., and Wolters, E. C. (2001). Loss of olfaction in *de novo* and treated Parkinson's disease: possible implication for early diagnosis. *Movement Disorders* **16**, 41–46.

Tofaris, G. K. and Spillantini, M. G. (2005). Alpha-synuclein dysfunction in Lewy body diseases. *Movement Disorders* **20**, 37–44.

Tofaris, G. K. and Spillantini, M. G. (2007). Physiological and pathological properties of α-synuclein. *Cellular and Molecular Life Sciences* **64**, 2194–2201.

Trojanowski, J.Q. and Lee, V.M. (2003). Meeting summary—cell biology of Parkinson's disease and related neurodegenerative disorders. *Science of Aging Knowledge Environment* **13**, 23.

Trojanowski, J. Q. and Lee, V. M. Y. (1998). Aggregation of neurofilament and α-synuclein proteins in Lewy bodies—implications for the pathogenesis of Parkinson-disease and Lewy body dementia. *Archives of Neurology* **55**, 151–52.

Trojanowski, J. Q. and Lee, V. M. Y. (2000). 'Fatal attractions' of proteins. A comprehensive hypothetical mechanism underlying Alzheimer's disease and other neurodegenerative disorders. *Annals of the New York Academy of Sciences* **924**, 62–67.

Ushikado, H., Lin, W. L., DeLucia, M. W., and Dickson, D. W. (2006). Alzheimer disease with amgydala Lewy bodies: a distinct form of alpha-synucleinopathy. *Journal of Neuropathology and Experimental Neurology* **65**, 685–97.

Verbaan, D., Marinus, J., Visser, M., van Rooden, S. M., Stiggelbout, A. M., and van Hilten, J.J. (2007). Patient-reported autonomic symptoms in Parkinson disease. *Neurology* **69**, 333–41.

Wadsworth, J. D. F., Jackson, G. S., Hill, A. F., and Collinge, J. (1999). Molecular biology of prion propagation. *Current Opinion in Genetics & Development* **9**, 338–45.

Wakabayashi, K., Takahashi, H., Ohama, E., Takeda, S., and Ikuta, F. (1991). Lewy bodies in the visceral autonomic nervous system in Parkinson's disease. In: F. Ikuta, ed. *Neuropathology in brain research*, pp. 133–41. Amsterdam, London and New York, Tokyo: Excerpta Medica.

Wakabayashi, K., Takahashi, H., Ohama, E., Takeda, S., and Ikuta. F. (1993a). Lewy bodies in the visceral autonomic nervous system in Parkinson's disease. *Advances in Neurology* **60**, 609–612.

Wakabayashi, K., Takahashi, H., Ohama, E., and Ikuta, F. (1990). Parkinson's disease: an immunohistochemical study of Lewy body-containing neurons in the enteric nervous system. *Acta Neuropathologica* **79**, 581–83.

Wakabayashi, K., Takahashi, H., Oyanagi, K., and Ikuta, F. (1993b). Incidental occurrence of Lewy bodies in the brain of elderly patients—the relevance to aging and Parkinson's disease. *No To Shinkei* **45**, 1033–38.

Wakabayashi, K., Takahashi, H., Takeda, S., Ohama, E., and Ikuta, F. (1988). Parkinson's disease: the presence of Lewy bodies in Auerbach's and Meissner's plexuses. *Acta Neuropathologica* **76**, 217–21.

Wakabayashi, K., Tanji, K., Mori, F., and Takahashi, H. (2007), The Lewy body in Parkinson's disease: molecules implicated in the formation and degradation of alpha-synuclein aggregates. *Neuropathology* **27**, 494–506.

Wakabayashi, K. and Takahashi, H. (1997a). The intermediolateral nucleus and Clarke's column in Parkinson's disease. *Acta Neuropathologica* **94**, 287–89.

Wakabayashi, K. and Takahashi, H. (1997b). Neuropathology of autonomic nervous system in Parkinson's disease. *European Neurology* (Suppl. 2) **38**, 2–7.

Walker, L. C. and LeVine, H. (2001). The cerebral proteopathies. Neurodegenerative disorders of protein conformation and assembly. *Molecular Neurobiology* **21**, 83–95.

Wolters, E. C., Francot, C., Bergmans, P., Winogrodzka, A., Booij, J., Berendse, H. W., and Stoof, J. C. (2000). Preclinical (premotor) Parkinson's disease. *Journal of Neurology* (Suppl. 2) **247**, 103–109.

Wolters, E. C. and Braak H. (2006). Parkinson's disease: premotor clinico-pathological correlations. *Journal of Neural Transmission Supplements* **70**:309–319.

Zarow, C., Lyness, S. A., Mortimer, J. A., and Chui, H. C. (2003). Neuronal loss is greater in the locus coeruleus than nucleus basalis and substantia nigra in Alzheimer and Parkinson diseases. *Archives of Neurology* **60**, 337–41.

Zweig, R. M., Cardillo, J. E., Cohen, M., Giere, S., and Hedreen, J. C. (1993). The locus ceruleus and dementia in Parkinson's disease. *Neurology* **43**, 986–9891.

Zweig, R. M., Jankel, W. R., Hedreen, J. C., Mayeux, R., and Price, D. L. (1989). The pedunculopontine nucleus in Parkinson's disease. *Annals of Neurology* **26**, 41–46.

de Lau, L. M. L. and Breteler, M. M. B. (2006). Epidemiology of Parkinson's disease. *Lancet Neurology* **5**, 525–35.

CHAPTER 45

Parkinson's disease and autonomic failure

Pietro Cortelli and Christopher J. Mathias

Introduction

Parkinson's disease (PD) is a neurodegenerative disorder characterized by motor symptoms, such as stiffness, tremor, bradykinesia and non-motor symptoms (NMS) represented by loss of smell, sleep and mood disorders, autonomic symptoms (AS) that may be the earliest manifestations of the disease (Tolosa et al. 2007). Autonomic dysfunction in PD patients has been recognized since the first description of the disease by James Parkinson in 1817 (Parkinson 1817). The clinical manifestations may be various and are represented by gastrointestinal, urogenital, cardiovascular, sudomotor and thermoregulatory symptoms, pupillary abnormalities, and sleep and respiratory disorders (Siddiqui et al. 2002, Magerkurth et al. 2005, Wüllner et al. 2007, Iodice et al. 2012).

In the past years more importance has been given to diagnosis, management, and the impact on quality of life for patients with PD of NMS.

A self-reported questionnaire for NMS has been developed and validated (Chaudhuri et al. 2007). It assesses the presence of 30 common symptoms regarding sleep, mood and cognition, hallucinations, olfaction and AS (cardiovascular, gastrointestinal, urinary, sexual, sweating and weight disturbances) and it's designed to provide a rapid screen for NMS to aid clinical management. The relationship between dysautonomia and disease-related variables such as age at onset, disease duration and severity, concomitant medications is still not clear (Singer et al. 1992, Mathias 2003, Chaudhuri and Hu 2000). This topic of debate is particularly important because autonomic dysfunction is considered an important clinical marker for the diagnosis of multiple system atrophy (MSA) in which parkinsonism is a feature, but prognosis and neuropathology are different from PD (Iodice et al. 2011). Moreover, new medications and surgical options for treating PD which are ineffective in MSA (Lezcano et al. 2004) emphasizes the need for diagnostic modalities such as an appropriate evaluation of ANS functions to distinguish PD from other neurodegenerative diseases. This chapter will review the various aspects of autonomic dysfunction in PD.

Definitions and diagnosis

PD is characterized clinically by slowly progressive symptoms and pathologically by degeneration of the pigmented neuromelanin bearing cells of the zona compacta of the substantia nigra. The term Parkinson syndrome may be preferable, as the disorder may not be a single clinicopathological entity. The presence of Lewy bodies (LB) is a pathological hallmark of PD. However, these may be absent in some inherited forms of parkinsonism that are clinically indistinguishable in some cases from PD.

The clinical diagnosis of PD based on the cardinal features akinesia, muscular rigidity and resting tremor, may seem to be simple but several clinicopathological studies have shown a significant false positive rate of diagnosis. In spite of recent advances in structural and functional neuroimaging, the diagnosis of the disease still remains clinical. In the absence of a biological marker, misdiagnosis is high during the early stages of the illness even amongst movement disorder specialists. This has an impact on studies not only of epidemiology in the general population but also early clinical trials studying symptomatic and neuroprotective therapies in PD. In the absence of a biomarker, diagnosis depends on certain clinical diagnostic criteria. Assessment of the clinical features suggests that an accuracy of 90% may be the highest that can be expected using current diagnostic criteria (Hughes et al. 2001).

Involvement of the autonomic nervous system in Parkinson's disease

Severe dysautonomia is common in the advanced stage of PD because of the neuropathological progression of the disease and the effect of treatment (Tolosa et al. 2007). Several studies have shown that AS may precede motor symptoms for many years and this could be explained by the earliest involvement of peripheral ganglia.

The first studies investigating dysautonomia in idiopathic PD were particularly focused on OH (Appenzeller and Goss 1971, Gross et al. 1972). The authors documented a substantial fall in blood pressure (BP) during head-up tilting and they suggested that OH may be the result of a central defect above the level of the medulla. Since then several authors reported abnormalities of the autonomic nervous system (ANS) on cardiovascular (Goetz et al. 1986, Turkka et al. 1987, Meco et al. 1996, van Dijk et al. 1993), sudomotor, gastrointestinal, and bladder function (Chaudhuri 2001, Siddiqui et al. 2002, Visser et al. 2004), and the pathogenesis of these dysfunctions in PD has been linked to neuronal damage in central areas of autonomic regulation. LB, the pathological hallmark of idiopathic PD, and cell loss are detected in:

- autonomic regulatory areas such as the hypothalamus, parabrachial nucleus, intermediate reticular zone of the medulla, locus coeruleus, and raphe
- preganglionic parasympathetic region such as the Edinger–Westphal nucleus and dorsal vagal motor nuclei
- preganglionic sympathetic neurons in the intermediolateral cell column
- neurons in paravertebral and prevertebral autonomic ganglia (Gibb 1988).

These findings, however, may not necessarily correlate with clinical autonomic dysfunction. The most consistent pathological substrate of autonomic failure in PD is significant cell loss in the intermediolateral cell columns, although to a lesser degree than in MSA (Bannister and Oppenheimer 1972, Oppenheimer 1980).

A novel neuropathological view of PD has been proposed by Braak and colleagues after a systematic mapping with alpha-synuclein immunocytochemistry of 41 PD brains, 69 brains with incidental LB pathology and 58 control brains (Braak et al. 2003). The results of these studies show that LB pathology evolves in six consecutive stages affecting multiple neuronal systems. Lesions initially occur in the medulla oblongata, namely the dorsal motor nucleus of the glossopharyngeal and vagal nerves, and in the anterior olfactory nucleus (stage 1). In stage 2, monoaminergic nuclei of the brainstem (raphe nuclei, locus coeruleus) are involved, whereas the substantia nigra becomes affected only at stage 3. In subsequent stages, the pathological alterations take an ascending course with increasing involvement of the cerebral cortex, beginning with the anteromedial temporal mesocortex followed by neocortical areas. Spinal cords and sympathetic ganglia were not studied and therefore, whether the disease process in PD regularly involves sympathetic ganglia remains unsettled.

This view of PD as a multisystemic disorder starting in the medulla oblongata, the anterior olfactory nucleus and probably in peripheral ganglia correspond to the recognition that NMS including autonomic disturbances are a frequent, if not inevitable, feature of PD.

The relationship between AS and other NMS is not clear. Studies have found an association between impaired autonomic cardiovascular function and visual hallucinations (Oka et al. 2007a) while no significant correlation was found between orthostatic hypotension (OH), postprandial hypotension (PPH) and cognitive impairment (Idiaquez et al. 2007). Anosmia has been found associated with baroreflex failure and cardiac noradrenergic denervation, independently of parkinsonism or striatal dopaminergic denervation (Goldstein et al. 2010).

Prevalence of self-reported AS in 3414 PD patients and correlation with sex, age, and disease duration has been assessed by means of the German PD Database (Wüllner et al. 2007). A significant correlation of OH and urinary incontinence with age and disease duration was found while sexual dysfunction and sleep disturbances were related only to age and disease duration respectively.

The prevalence of autonomic impairment in patients with PD varies greatly among studies (14–80%) and the correlation between its severity and disease-related variables in not well documented.

Magerkurth et al. evaluated AS and impact on daily life in 141 PD patients and 50 healthy controls (Magerkurth et al. 2005). Patients with PD were subjected to standard laboratory evaluation of autonomic functioning and divided in subjects with normal and abnormal functioning. In patients prevalence of orthostatic dizziness, bladder dysfunction, erectile dysfunction, and hyperhidrosis was significantly higher than in controls. Impaired cardiovascular function was found in 32% of PD patients in which orthostatic dizziness, bladder dysfunction, erectile dysfunction, and constipation were significantly higher than in PD patients with normal autonomic functioning. Bladder dysfunction, orthostatic dizziness, and constipation were the most disturbing AS in PD patients compared with controls.

The occurrence of AS has been assessed in a controlled cohort of 420 patients with PD by SCOPA-AUT questionnaire (Verbaan et al. 2007). The results of this study showed a greater complaint of AS in PD patients than in controls with a more pronounced difference is in the gastrointestinal and urinary domains. Age, disease severity and medication use resulted to be related to more AS.

In summary, AS seem to be very common in PD patients even in the earliest stages of the disease or even before motor symptoms appear (the so called 'pre-motor phase'). This could be explained by the early neuropathological involvement of the autonomic peripheral ganglia. The relationship between dysautonomia and disease-related features is still subject to debate. The impact of concomitant medications (L-dihydroxyphenylalanine [L-DOPA]) on autonomic failure is still equivocal, and some authors have found no correlation (Goldstein et al. 2005).

Clinical features

Cardiovascular system

Hypotension or hypertension may result from disruption of autonomic control. As organ function is dependent upon an adequate perfusion pressure, the symptoms arising from hypotension (such as syncope with head-up postural change) often are more prominent than those resulting from hypertension.

Cardiovascular dysregulation may be present in PD patients but the role of medications or of deep brain stimulation (DBS) of subthalamic nucleus is still unclear (Stemper et al. 2006, Holmberg et al. 2005).

Orthostatic hypotension

A cardinal feature of failure of the sympathetic nervous system is OH (see Chapter 22). It is defined as a fall in systolic BP of 20 mm Hg or more, or in diastolic BP of 10 mm Hg or more, on either standing or head-up tilt to at least 60° (Schatz 1996). OH reduces perfusion of organs. Hypoperfusion of the brain can result in dizziness, visual disturbances and impaired cognition that often precede loss of consciousness. These symptoms occur on assuming the upright posture, especially when getting out of bed in the morning, when patients often are at their worst. Many recognize the association between postural change and symptoms of cerebral hypoperfusion and either sit down or lie flat; some even assume curious postures such as squatting or stooping that now are recognized as reducing hypotension (Wieling et al. 1993). With time symptoms may diminish for reasons that include improved cerebrovascular autoregulation. However, a transcranial Doppler study evidenced an impaired cerebral autoregulation in PD patients, independently of dopaminergic treatment (Vokatch et al. 2007). Occasionally the BP falls precipitously and syncope may occur rapidly, similar to a drop attack. Falls are more common in elderly and frail patients and may be the cause of serious morbidity with subsequent loss of independence. Orthostatic hypotension (OH) and postprandial hypotension (PPH) have an increased prevalence in the elderly and are well-recognized risk factors for falls. In parkinsonian patients these features, in association with their movement disorder enhances the propensity to falls. There is a variety of non-cerebral symptoms associated with OH that result from underperfusion of various organs (Mathias et al. 1999). Measurement of BP should be an integral component of the clinical evaluation of all parkinsonian patients (Asahina et al. 2012). This should be performed both supine and standing, or sitting if it is difficult for the patient to stand. Laboratory testing using a tilt table is advisable, as this enables accurate evaluation of OH if present and provides a baseline, ideally prior to initiation of drug therapy. In the laboratory, tilt table testing should be combined with autonomic screening tests to determine if OH is present, and if so whether it is the consequence of failure of the ANS or the result of non-neurogenic factors (Table 45.1). As recently reported, in some patients with PD, the blood pressure may fall later when upright, after 10 min of standing, which is of importance in evaluating the cause of falls, especially as some PD patients may remain relatively still and frozen when upright (Jamnadas-Khoda et al. 2009; see Figure 45.1). As previously emphasized, the presence of OH and such testing itself does not separate MSA from other parkinsonian syndromes or disorders where autonomic dysfunction occurs (Mathias 1996, Mathias and Kimber 1999, Riley and Chelimsky 2003), which is the reason for the range of tests described in the different disorders. A prospective ongoing study of MSA and PD showed that the severity, distribution, and pattern of autonomic deficits at study entry can distinguish MSA from PD, and MSA from PD with autonomic

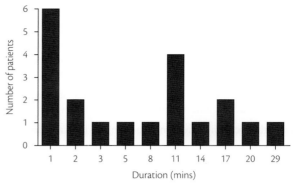

Fig. 45.1 Frequency of orthostatic hypotension (OH) with time after head-up tilting. OH occurs frequently after 3 min (the recommended duration for recording OH). From Jamnadas-Khoda et al. (2009).

failure, and that these differences are increased at follow-up (Lipp et al. 2009).

Twenty-four hour non-invasive BP and heart rate (HR) monitoring, which can be obtained in the home environment, often provides valuable information (Fig 45.2), including on the effects of treatment (Senard et al. 1992, Alam et al. 1993, Alam et al. 1995, Cortelli et al. 1996). There have been varying levels of resting BP reported in PD. These include low basal levels (Yahr 1970, Barbeau et al. 1971), which was not confirmed in a large study in PD patients not on dopaminergic agents (Aminoff et al. 1975). Various factors, ranging from age, stage of disease, drug treatment and associated disorders may contribute to these differences. In PD, the reported prevalence and incidence of OH varies considerably. Some consider it to be rare (Colosimo et al. 1995). Others report a modest orthostatic fall (systolic mean fall of 11mm Hg in 20 patients [Meco et al 1991], and 10 mm Hg in 35 patients [Sandroni et al. 1991]) that do not fulfil current definition criteria of OH. This differs from a high prevalence reported in other studies (43% of 80) (Uono 1973) and 58% of 91 patients (Senard et al. 1997). Whether this reflects variations in the type of patient studied, the influence of the many factors that modify BP control (such as increasing age, duration of the disorder, and drug therapy), or differences in methods to evaluate OH, is unclear (van Dijk et al. 1993, Orskov et al. 1987, Piha et al. 1988, Mesec et al. 1993, Hillen et al. 1996, Kujawa et al. 2000). Impaired mobility itself and motor fluctuations may contribute to autonomic dysfunction, as is known to occur, especially in elderly bed-bound patients (Kihara et al. 1998, Pursiainen et al. 2007a). Post-mortem studies have emphasized the difficulties of *in vivo* diagnosis and in separating PD from non-PD disorders such as MSA that inadvertently and erroneously may have been included as PD patients (Rajput et al. 1990, Hughes et al. 1992, Litvan et al. 1997). However, this alone is unlikely to account for the considerably higher prevalence in some studies. In the PD study by Senard and co-workers (Senard et al. 1997), of the 58% with OH, 38.5% were symptomatic. However, there may be dissociation between symptoms suggestive of cerebral hypoperfusion and OH; in a study by Turkka (1987), 12 out of 15 PD patients complained of dizziness, but OH was present in only 4 suggesting that other factors were contributing.

Recently in order to overcome the limitations of the previous studies (concomitant medications and lack of follow-up to confirm a clinical diagnosis) 60 *de novo* PD underwent autonomic

Table 45.1 Possible causes of orthostatic hypotension and autonomic dysfunction in a patient with parkinsonian features

Side-effects of anti-parkinsonian therapy, including:
◆ L-DOPA, bromocriptine, pergolide
◆ The combination of L-DOPA and catechol-*O*-methyltransferase inhibitors (tolcapone)
◆ The monoamine oxidase 'B' inhibitor, selegiline
Coincidental disease causing autonomic dysfunction (e.g. diabetes mellitus)
Coincidental administration of drugs for an allied condition
◆ Antihypertensives
◆ α-adrenoceptor blockers (for benign prostatic hypertrophy)
◆ Vasodilators (for ischaemic heart disease)
◆ Diuretics (for cardiac failure)
◆ Sildenafil (for erectile failure)
Multiple system atrophy (Shy–Drager syndrome)
Parkinson's disease with autonomic failure
Diffuse Lewy body disease

Adapted from Mathias 1996, Mathias and Kimber 1999.

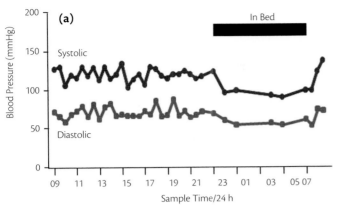

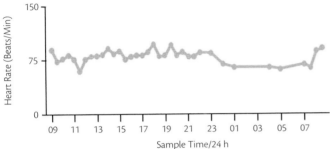

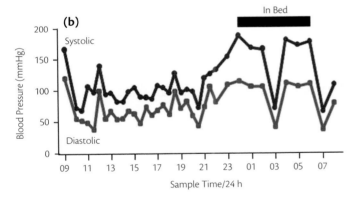

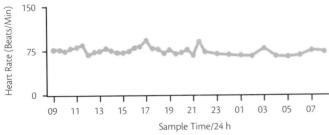

Fig. 45.2 24-hour non-invasive ambulatory blood pressure profile, showing systolic and diastolic blood pressure and heart rate at intervals through the day and night. **(a)** The changes in a normal subject with no postural fall in blood pressure; there was a fall in blood pressure at night while asleep, with a rise in blood pressure on wakening. **(b)** The marked fluctuations in blood pressure in a patient with pure autonomic failure. The marked falls in blood pressure are usually the result of postural changes, either sitting or standing. Supine blood pressure, particularly at night, is elevated. Getting up to micturate causes a marked fall in blood pressure (at 03:00 hours). There is a reversal of the diurnal changes in blood pressure. There are relatively small changes in heart rate, considering the marked changes in blood pressure. From Mathias 1996a, with permission.

cardiovascular function evaluation and then they were followed up at least 7 years (Bonuccelli et al. 2003). The diagnosis of idiopathic PD was confirmed in 51 subjects who showed a quite high prevalence of sympathetic and parasympathetic failure at the onset of the disease. When using a decrease of 20 mmHg in systolic BP, 14% of the PD patients had a OH at the onset of the disease discrediting the myth that OH is the hallmark of MSA, especially when occur early in the course of the disease. Data from retrospective studies show differences in the frequency and severity of autonomic dysfunction between MSA and PD (Wenning et al. 1999, Magalhaes et al. 1995): symptomatic OH within 1 year of disease onset predicted MSA in 75% patients (Wenning et al. 1999) and pathological autonomic reactions were found at an older age and after a longer disease duration in patients with PD than in MSA (Holmberg et al. 2001). However, in another retrospective study of ANS testing, no difference was found between PD and MSA suggesting that current clinical criteria for PD and MSA based on the presence of dysautonomia may be inappropriate (Riley and Chelimsky 2003). In clinical practice the rule that the presence of symptomatic OH in a patient with parkinsonism should lead to consideration of MSA, especially when there are additional non-cardiovascular features of autonomic failure, is still well grounded but it should not lead to erroneous avoiding of dopaminergic treatment.

Goldstein evaluated 35 cases of PD with OH to assess whether OH may be an early finding. He found that 60% of patients were affected by OH before or within a year after onset of symptomatic motor symptoms (Goldstein 2006).

A clinical study found that 50% of PD patients are affected by OH that correlates with age, male sex, and use of dopaminergic medications (Allcock et al. 2006). No correlation with disease severity and duration was found.

In PD, the mechanisms responsible for OH warrant discussion. Some studies exclude generalized autonomic failure, and speculate on central lesions in the upper brainstem, that affect postural control of BP but spare other reflexes, such as the Valsalva manoeuvre (Appenzeller and Goss 1971, Gross et al. 1972, Aminoff and Wilcox 1971, Kuno 1989). Other studies suggest that autonomic failure in PD, is similar to that observed in pure autonomic failure (PAF). In PD with autonomic failure there are subnormal levels of basal plasma noradrenaline, and an impaired plasma noradrenaline response to head-up postural challenge (Turkka et al. 1986, Senard et al. 1990, Durrieu et al. 1990). This may explain why such patients do not respond to certain drugs used to treat OH, such as yohimbine, whose benefits are dependent on intact post-ganglionic sympathetic pathways (Senard et al. 1993). In PD with autonomic failure, drugs that act on α-adrenoceptors, such as midodrine and its metabolite, are more likely to be effective. Supine hypertension may occur in patients with PD with autonomic failure as in MSA (Alam et al. 1995, Goldstein et al. 2003a). This may be a problem at night if such patients lie supine and horizontal, as demonstrated on the 24-hour ambulatory BP profiles (Fig. 45.2b). The probable mechanisms for supine hypertension include inappropriate sympathetic tone, the movement of intra- and extravascular fluid from the peripheral to the central vascular compartment, impaired baroreflexes, and supersensitivity even to small amounts of circulating catecholamines or to pressor agents used for therapy (Alam et al. 1995, Shannon et al. 2010). Patients may report a fullness of the head or a throbbing headache while lying flat. It is unclear to what extent supine hypertension contributes to morbidity and mortality in such patients. Debate continues on the 'safe' upper limits of supine hypertension and the use of anti-hypertensive drugs at night. However, even short-acting anti-hypertensives are likely to enhance OH, and increase vulnerability to falls of patients who need to get up at night to micturate, because of nocturia and urinary bladder dysfunction. The use of head-up tilt at night, together with a small nocturnal meal or alcoholic beverage (thus beneficially utilizing the hypotensive effects of food and alcohol) may transiently diminish supine hypertension.

In one of the early post-mortem reports on PD with OH, it was noted that the sympathetic ganglia were involved (Fichefet et al. 1965). LB have been observed in the autonomic ganglia of PD (Wakabayashi et al. 1993, Wakabayashi et al. 1997) and also in PD with OH (Rajput and Rozdilsky 1976), and may indicate peripheral involvement of the ANS. This differs from MSA, where sympathomimetic drugs that act through residual postganglionic sympathetic pathways, such as ephedrine, often are effective (Mathias and Kimber 1999). The mechanisms and pathophysiological basis of OH in the different parkinsonian disorders thus are of relevance for diagnosis and importantly for determining which drugs are more likely to provide effective benefit. The association between PD, OH and LB density in the posterior left insular cortex has been shown in a neuropathological study, underlying the role of central autonomic network in the genesis of OH (Papapetropoulos and Mash 2007).

Postprandial hypotension

In normal individuals food ingestion does not change systemic BP, but there are a number of changes in gastrointestinal and pancreatic hormones accompanied by compensatory cardiac and regional haemodynamic responses (see Chapter 28).

PPH has been recognized as an independent predictor of all-cause mortality in older low-level-care residents (Fisher et al. 2005).

In PD, there are varying reports on the extent of PPH. In PD patients not on drug therapy, a small postprandial fall in BP while supine was reported without exacerbation of OH post-meal (Thomaides et al. 1993); these observations differ from those reported previously by Micieli et al. (1987) who noted a greater incidence and degree of hypotension. In elderly parkinsonian patients PPH is more frequent (82% compared with 41% in controls) than OH (13% vs 6% in controls); the combination of levodopa (L-DOPA) (125 mg) and benserazide did not significantly aggravate either (Mehagnoul-Schipper et al. 2001). In PD the lowering of BP by food ingestion may account for worsening motor control after a meal, especially in patients on antiparkinsonian drugs that may contribute to vasodilatation (Chaudhuri et al. 1997). In PD, exercise causes minimal or no fall in BP and does not appear to unmask OH.

Drug-induced hypotension

Drugs may induce hypotension may be caused either by causing autonomic dysfunction or because of their cardiovascular side effects of drugs (Chapter 71). This applies to treatment with antiparkinsonian drugs (Table 45.2). In PD, there is variability in the ability of dopaminergic drugs to lower BP. Some may cause OH (Calne et al. 1970, Quinn et al. 1981, Tanner et al. 1982, Johns et al. 1984, Piha et al. 1988, Camerlingo et al. 1990), although other reports conclude that there has been no alteration of cardiovascular reflexes or enhancement of OH (Goetz et al. 1986, Kujawa et al. 2000,

Table 45.2 Overview of gastrointestinal dysfunction in Parkinson's disease

Mouth
◆ Pooling of saliva
◆ Jaw tremors
Salivary glands
◆ Reduced saliva production
◆ Low swallowing frequency causes drooling
Pharinx
◆ Oropharyngeal dysphagia
Oesophagus
◆ Slow oesophageal transit
◆ Segmental oesophageal spasm
◆ Gastro-oesophageal influx
Stomach
◆ Gastroparesis
◆ Early satiety
◆ Weight loss
Small intestine
◆ Dilatation
Colon
◆ Dismotility
◆ Constipation, megacolon, volvulus, bowel perforation
Rectum
◆ Difficulty in defecation

Ballantyne 1973, Sachs et al. 1985). The tendency to hypotension is likely to increase in patients who are older, have cardiovascular disease, and have either occult or evident AF, as part of MSA or PD with AF. Hypotension with dopaminergic drugs may result from vasodilatation induced by dopaminergic receptor stimulation. Thus peripheral dopa-decarboxylase inhibitors may reduce the hypotensive effects of l-dopa, although the central effects of l-dopa or other dopaminergic agents may contribute (Calne et al. 1973, Montastruc et al. 1985). Selegiline in PD may cause OH by mechanisms that are unclear; they include the central effects of its metabolite methylamphetamine and interactions with L-DOPA and ergoline derivatives (Karoum et al. 1982, Churchyard et al. 1997, Turkka et al. 1997, Churchyard et al. 1999, Pursiainen et al. 2007b). The induction of marked hypotension following L-DOPA challenge in a parkinsonian patient should necessitate consideration of autonomic failure and MSA (Mathias 2000) (Fig. 45.3).

Treatment of orthostatic, postprandial, exercise-induced and drug-associated hypotension

See Chapters 28, 30, 47, 61, and 71.

Heart rate control

Patients with PD usually are older and some may be predisposed to cardiac dysrhythmias, especially when on antiparkinsonian drugs with cardiovascular effects. There also may be an intrinsic

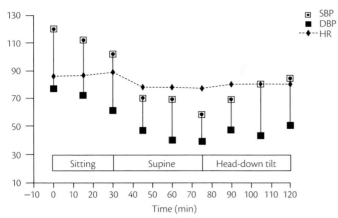

Fig. 45.3 Systolic and diastolic blood pressure in a patient with parkinsonian features before and after a standard L-DOPA challenge (250 mg of L-DOPA, with 25 mg carbidopa). The patient was initially seated but blood pressure fell and was so low that he needed to be laid supine and horizontal, and then head down. On further investigation, the final diagnosis in this patient was autonomic failure and the parkinsonian form of multiple system atrophy. From Mathias 2000, with permission.

propensity to the development of arrhythmias in PD with impaired who have cardiac sympathetic innervation; the mechanisms may include denervation supersensitivity. The QT interval is the electrocardiographic description of ventricular depolarization and repolarization, and if abnormal may identify patients at risk of developing ventricular fibrillation and sudden cardiac death.

Patients with PD show blunted HR changes to various stimuli. HR variability (HRV) and HR response have been evaluated by means of 24 hours recording and head-up tilt test. A reduced HR variability in the time and frequency domains were found during tilt test in PD without AS comparing with controls (Barbic et al. 2007). These findings may suggest that initial alteration in cardiac autonomic activity may precede the appearing of a symptomatic OH.

In PD, atrial and ventricular arrhythmias initially were reported with L-DOPA (Barbeau 1969, McDowell et al. 1970), but this was not confirmed in later studies (Hunter et al. 1971, Jenkins et al. 1972, Tanner et al. 1987). Tremor artefacts on the electrocardiogram may result in an erroneous diagnosis of dysrhythmias as in PD (Pallis et al. 1970, Freemon 1971, Saint-Pierre 1973). Hypotension may induce a tachycardia and thus could increase the dysrhythmic potential. The introduction of dopa-decarboxylase inhibitors (such as carbidopa) was considered a means of avoiding potential dysrhythmogenic effects (Mars and Krall 1971, Desjacques et al. 1973) by reducing hypotension secondary to increasing dopamine levels. There is no clear evidence that dopaminergic agents, such as pergolide increase the tendency to dysrhythmias (Lieberman et al. 1982, Tanner et al. 1985). Whether certain drugs predispose susceptible individuals (such as those with sympathetic cardiac denervation) to dysrhythmias is not known.

Investigation of cardiac sympathetic innervation

Control of HR exerted by the sympathetic nervous system is difficult to assess. An alternative, although this does not provide functional evaluation, is the use of imaging techniques that determine the integrity of cardiac sympathetic innervation. The physiological analogue of noradrenaline, meta-iodobenzyl guanidine (MIBG) is

actively transported into sympathetic nerve terminals by a noradrenaline transporter; its iodinated form ^{123}I-MIBG can be readily detected by myocardial scintigraphy.

In MSA, consistent with a preganglionic lesion, noradrenaline transport is preserved, as in normal subjects (Orimo et al. 1999, Braune et al. 1999). In peripheral autonomic disorders, such as diabetes mellitus with a cardiac autonomic neuropathy, uptake is diminished (Claus et al. 2002). In central disorders with spinocerebellar atrophy, such as Machado–Joseph disease, reduced MIBG uptake also occurs (Kazuta et al. 2000) and one explanation is peripheral denervation secondary to central and trans-synaptic degeneration. In PD there is impaired uptake, suggesting cardiac sympathetic denervation (Orimo et al. 1999, Kazuta et al. 2000, Hakusui et al. 1994, Kanzaki et al. 1998, Braune et al. 1998, Yoshita 1998, Satoh et al. 1999, Reinhardt et al. 2000, Druschky et al. 2000, Ohmura 2000, Courbon et al. 2003, Oka et al. 2007b). This occurs even in the absence of clinical features suggesting autonomic failure at an early stage of PD (Courbon et al. 2003, Takatsu et al. 2000). Uptake in PD does not appear to be affected by dopaminergic drug therapy, and the results differ from vascular parkinsonism (Orimo et al. 1999) and progressive supranuclear palsy (PSP) (Yoshita et al. 1998). It has been suggested that the defect is exclusive to PD but this needs further evaluation, as limited uptake also occurs in Machado–Joseph disease (Kazuta et al. 2000). In the study by Orimo et al. (1999), HRV was impaired only in a small proportion of PD (11%). The dissociation of functional autonomic testing with reduced cardiac MIBG uptake is consistent with the suggestion that autonomic screening tests predominantly assess parasympathetic, and not sympathetic, cardiac activity. However, among patients with neurogenic OH those with cardiac sympathetic denervation was demonstrated an impaired inotropic response to tyromine and an exaggerated response to isoproterenol suggesting a decreased ability to release norepinephrine from sympathetic nerves with supersensitivity of cardiac β-adrenoceptors (Imrich et al. 2009). Sympathetic cardiac innervation also has been assessed with ^{18}F-fluorodeoxyglucose (^{18}F-FDG) and positron emission tomography (Goldstein et al. 1997, Goldstein et al. 2000) with similar results to those obtained from MIBG scanning; uptake in MSA is similar to normal subjects, with minimal uptake in PD with autonomic failure. Cardiac uptake, using this technique, as was described with MIBG scanning also is impaired in PD without OH and diminishes with time (Goldstein et al. 2002, Li et al. 2002).

One study failed to find a relationship between cardiac sympathetic denervation assessed by myocardial MIBG uptake and disease-related features (duration of the disease, stage and treatment) except for bladder symptoms (Matsui et al. 2006). Another study found a correlation between cardiac sympathetic denervation and the phenotype of PD with a less impaired myocardial MIBG uptake in tremor dominant type than in akinetic rigid type or mixed type at the same stage of the disease (Spiegel et al. 2007).

Peripheral sympathetic denervation in the majority of PD, albeit only to the heart, appears surprising, considering that the manifestations of PD are central in origin. The combined MIBG and 18F FD cardiac scanning data in PAF and MSA, taken in conjunction with neuroendocrine and function neuroimaging mapping, is consistent with sparing of brain autonomic centres and intracerebral sympathetic pathways in PAF and PD, and their involvement in MSA (Thomaides et al. 1992, Kaufmann et al. 1992, Kimber et al. 1997, Kimber and Mathias 1999, Critchley et al. 2001,

Critchley et al. 2002). Confirmation that MIBG and ¹⁸F-FDG scanning provide a true indication of cardiac sympathetic denervation has been obtained from post-mortem studies in a few patients with PD and MSA; in heart muscle of PD patients, in comparison with controls and MSA, there is diminished tyrosine hydroxylase activity (Orimo et al. 2001, Orimo et al. 2002). Furthermore, in PD with autonomic failure, other organs, such as the adrenal medulla appear spared, as levels of adrenaline and its metabolite, metanephrine, are within the normal range (Goldstein et al. 2003b). It remains unclear why selective cardiac sympathetic denervation should occur in PD even at a relatively early stage of the disease.

Orimo et al. (2005) in two patients with PARK2, assessed cardiac sympathetic innervation *in vivo* with MIBG myocardial scintigraphy and post-mortem with myocardial tissue immunohistochemistry with antibodies against tyrosine hydroxylase; they did not find abnormalities in this genetic form of PD and the authors suggest that MIBG could represent a useful tool to distinguish PD from familiar forms of parkinsonism. Moreover, Orimo et al. examined immunohistochemically the cardiac tissue, sympathetic ganglia and medulla oblongata at the level of dorsal vagal nucleus in 20 patients with incidental LB disease that is thought to be the presymptomatic stage of PD (Orimo et al. 2007). They found various degrees of cardiac sympathetic nerve involvement in these patients, suggesting that cardiac sympathetic nerve degeneration begins in the early disease process of PD and it occurs before neuronal cell loss in the dorsal vagal nucleus.

Gastrointestinal function

The most commonly seen non-motor feature of PD is gastrointestinal dysfunction (Pfeiffer 2003) (Table 45.2). Abnormalities include impaired motility of the oesophagus, impaired emptying of the stomach, and disorders of intestinal function, most notably constipation. Up to 25–30% of PD patients below the age of 55–60 years, and up to 75% of patients over 60 years of age complain of constipation (Oertel et al. 1996). An epidemiological study of 6790 men followed prospectively in the Honolulu Heart Program showed that men with less than one bowel movement per day had a 4.5-fold excess risk of developing PD versus men with more than two bowel movements per day. These observations are compatible with the view that constipation is part of an early PD.

Another study assessed constipation in 156 PD patients and 148 controls over 65 years by means of a simple questionnaire based on the Rome criterion (Kaye et al. 2006). They found that constipation is three times more frequent in PD patients than in control (59% vs 21%). Stomach and intestinal functions are controlled largely by the autonomic and enteric nervous systems. The bulk of parasympathetic innervation of the gastrointestinal tract is derived from the dorsal motor nucleus of the vagus nerve, which supplies the stomach, small intestine, and proximal colon. Parasympathetic supply to the middle and distal colon is via sacral nerves. Sympathetic supply to the entire gastrointestinal tract arises from cells of the intermediolateral column of the spinal cord at T5–L3 levels. Information is passed by both parasympathetic and sympathetic sources to the enteric nervous system, where cholinergic neurons in the myenteric plexus can either stimulate contraction of smooth muscle cells in the gut wall or excite surface epithelial cells to absorb or secrete fluid and electrolytes (Camilleri and Bharucha 1996). In general terms, parasympathetic signals act

as the 'accelerator' to the gastrointestinal tract and stimulate its function, whereas sympathetic fibres serve as the 'brake' (Camilleri and Bharucha 1996). In PD the involvement of the dorsal motor nucleus of the vagus nerve is well documented, but involvement of other centres, such as the median raphe nucleus of the pons, has also been described (Gai et al. 1995, Halliday et al. 1990).

The presence of α-synuclein aggregates in abdomino-pelvic autonomic plexuses in the general population maybe a risk factor for the development of LB disorders. In a recent study abdominal surgical specimens of 100 subjects have been immunohistochemically evaluated to assess the presence of alpha-synuclein. They found that alpha-synuclein was present in 9% of subjects and that 16 alpha-synuclein positive subjects showed a reduced myocardial MIBG uptake (Minguez-Castellano et al. 2007).

Although these changes in parasympathetic autonomic supply to the gut could certainly account for the impairment of gastrointestinal function in PD, abnormalities in the enteric nervous system within the gut itself have also been identified, including both LB formation and loss of dopaminergic neurons (Kupsky et al. 1987, Wakabayashi et al. 1990, Singaram et al. 1995) Clinically this results in apparently slowed transit time of stool secondary to impaired colonic muscle contraction (Jost and Schimrigk 1993). A second syndrome, resulting in a primary abnormality of defecation, (straining, incomplete evacuation) may also occur irrespective of colonic transit time and may reflect involvement of the pelvic floor musculature. This distinction may have therapeutic implications, a dopaminergic agonist may improve rather worsen defecatory dysfunction in these patients, and injections of botulinum toxin into the puborectalis muscle have been used successfully to relax a dystonic process (Albanese et al. 1997). Other abnormalities associated with the gastrointestinal tract in PD include megacolon and sigmoid volvulus.

Sialorrhoea and dysphagia

Sialorrhoea and dysphagia are common symptoms in PD with a relevant impact on quality of life and morbidity. Evaluation scales have been developed and validated (Perez Lloret et al. 2007, Yael Manor et al. 2007) to provide a clinical tool for detection of these disturbances.

Sialorrhoea occurs frequently in PD and may be a manifestation of pharyngeal akinesia and swallowing difficulties. The production of saliva appears to be impaired in about 50% of parkinsonian patients in comparison with controls (Oertel et al. 1996). However, the overabundance of saliva is not the result of excessive saliva formation, but the consequence of inefficient and infrequent swallowing. In fact, saliva production in PD is typically diminished (Bagheri et al. 1999, Bateson et al. 1973, Eadie 1963). Swallowing may also be directly regulated by central pattern generators in the medial reticular formation of the rostral medulla and the reticulum adjacent to the solitary nucleus, which project to the nucleus ambiguus and dorsal motor nucleus of the vagus nerve (Hunter et al. 1997, Hamdy et al. 1999, Miller 1986). These generators contain the neural programmes that direct the sequential movements of the many oral, pharyngeal, and oesophageal muscles used in normal swallowing. In PD, the nucleus ambiguus is spared, but the pedunculopontine tegmental nucleus and the dorsal motor nucleus of the vagus nerve are not (Jellinger 1987). Thus, dysphagia in PD can result from defective coordination of the oral, pharyngeal, and oesophageal musculature, owing to the combination of dysfunction in the medullary central pattern generators and increased inhibitory outflow from the pallidum to the pedunculopontine tegmental nucleus (Hunter et al. 1997). Within the oesophageal myenteric plexus, however, Lewy bodies have been identified; this finding suggests that at least some part of parkinsonian dysphagia results from direct damage to the enteric nervous system (Qualman et al. 1984). This is supported by the fact that dysphagia appears to be dominant when the patient undergoes fluctuation in motor performance and is in the 'off' state (Koller et al. 1994). Disabilities may include abnormal lingual control and the inability to propel a bolus of food into the pharynx. This may lead to silent aspiration with repetitive reflux of food. Retention of food and medication in the valleculum may also contribute to erratic levodopa response later in the course of the disease. Dysmotility of oesophagus has been reported in up to 70% of patients with PD (Edwards et al. 1994). Bradykinetic swallowing EMG abnormalities have been described in PD, even in asymptomatic patients (Alfonsi et al. 2007).

Urinary and bladder dysfunction

Nervous bladder control depends on the functioning of almost all parts of the ANS such as suprapontine and pontine structures, spinal connections and peripheral nerves (Winge and Fowler 2006). However, urinary difficulties in PD may arise from central neuroanatomical involvement of the detrusor motor area in the frontal lobes which is connected to a similar functional area in the ponto-mesencephalic reticular formation (Koller et al. 1994, Stocchi et al. 1997).

Up to 75% of PD patients may develop forms of urinary difficulties. In men, prostatic hypertrophy and in women consequences of traumatic childbirth need to be considered as possible contributory factors to urinary difficulties.

The misdiagnosis with MSA could also have influenced the results of previous epidemiological studies and some authors suggest that urinary symptoms prevalence in PD patients diagnosed with modern criteria is between 27% and 39% (Winge and Fowler 2006).

Clinically, it appears that detrusor hyperreflexia and the resultant detrusor hyperactivity seem to affect patients with PD preferentially. Detrusor hyperactivity leads to urinary urgency, nocturia, frequency, and dribbling.

Night-time urinary frequency is the most common urinary symptom complained by PD patients (>60%) and may cause great difficulty with sleep and often is followed by increased voiding frequency (16–36%); other disturbances can be urgency (33–54%) (Winge and Fowler 2006), and incontinence of urine that occurs much less commonly in PD and is often secondary to akinesia as a late feature. Approximately 20% of patients have incomplete voiding, due to unsustained detrusor contraction or external sphincter dysfunction, with prostatic obstruction possibly superimposed in men (Sotolongo 1988). The most common pattern found during urodynamic studies is detrusor hyperreflexia, manifested by inability to suppress detrusor contraction during the filling phase, resulting in involuntary voiding. In addition, patient with PD may have external sphincter bradykinesia and pseudosynergy that contribute to obstruction and increased bladder pressure. Unlike MSA, detrusor areflexia is relatively rare (8–10%) and the external urinary sphincter is only occasionally

dysfunctional in PD. The effect of dopaminergic treatment on bladder control and urodynamic parameters are unpredictable in the individual patient, thought most patients experience significant changes (Winge et al. 2004) whereas subthalamic deep brain stimulation seems to have a significant effect leading to a normalization of pathologically increased bladder sensitivity (Seif et al. 2004) (Herzog et al. 2006, Winge et al. 2007). Some authors found a correlation between urinary disturbances and PD stage, suggesting a possible relationship between dopaminergic degeneration and bladder dysfunction but this is still matter of debate (Winge and Fowler 2006).

Male sexual function

Sexual dysfunction is more frequently reported by PD patients than by age-matched controls. The most common sexual dysfunctions are erectile dysfunction and loss of ejaculation control in male and 'non-sensuality' in female (Papatsoris et al. 2006).

Disturbances of male sexual function may occur in PD either secondary to drugs (tricyclic antidepressants, beta-blockers, anticholinergics) or spontaneously, particularly in some patients below 50 years of age (Oertel et al. 1996). Women reported difficulties with arousal (87.5%), with reaching orgasm (75.0%), with low sexual desire (46.9%), and with sexual dissatisfaction (37.5%) (Bronner et al. 2004). Men reported erectile dysfunction (68.4%), sexual dissatisfaction (65.1%), premature ejaculation (40.6%), and difficulties reaching orgasm (39.5%) (Bronner et al. 2004). Premorbid sexual dysfunction may contribute to cessation of sexual activity during the course of the disease (among 23.3% men and 21.9% women). Associated illnesses, use of medications, and advanced stage of PD contributed to sexual dysfunction. The profound impairment in the dimensions of sexual arousal, behaviour, orgasm, and drive, has been confirmed in PD patients (Yu et al. 2004). In contrast, the same study reveals an increase in sexual fantasy with greater PD duration, suggesting that patients with advancing disease remain interested in sex and that sexual dysfunction in PD is clinically relevant in this. The prevalence of low testosterone level in a PD registry resulted considerably higher than that in the general male population over 60 years of age suggesting a possible cause of sexual dysfunction in PD (Okun et al. 2002).

Sildenafil citrate (50 mg) is efficacious in the treatment of erectile dysfunction in PD; however, it may unmask or exacerbate hypotension and measurement of lying and standing BP before prescribing sildenafil to men with parkinsonism is strongly recommended (Hussain et al. 2001). Other treatment options are dopaminergic agonists or intracavernously injected prostaglandin (Papatsoris et al. 2006).

A clear-cut history of impotence may point more towards a diagnosis of MSA.

Skin changes and seborrhoea

Seborrhoea (seborrhoea oleosa) and hyperhidrosis are common problems in patients with PD. The phenomenon of increased sebum production was first described in the 1920s (Cohn 1920) and appears to be particularly severe in postencephalitic PD. However, a number of investigations have also shown seborrhoea in idiopathic PD (Baas and Fischer 1984, Burton and Shuster 1970, Burton et al. 1973, Kohn et al. 1973, Martignoni et al. 1997, Pochi et al. 1962). The prevalence of seborrhoea in PD varies from

18.6% up to 52% (Baas and Fischer 1984). The cause of seborrhoea in PD is still unclear. However, the significant correlation between sebum values at the different parts of the body indicates that the physiological distribution pattern of sebum production (forehead, sternum, extremities) is maintained in PD. This suggests a systemically effective stimulation of the sebaceous glands. α-melanocyte stimulating hormone, a neuropeptide derivative of pro-opiomelanocortin has often been suggested as the stimulant (Baas and Fischer 1984, Villares and Carlini 1989, Wintzen and Gilchrest 1996). If systemic stimulation of the sebaceous glands is taking place, the lack of correlation between the laterality of the neurological symptoms and sebum production can be explained. This has also been found in other investigations (Baas and Fischer 1984; Burton et al. 1973). This overexcretion of sebum can also be attributed to hyperactivity of the parasympathetic component of the autonomic nervous system. Male PD subjects had the highest excretion rate, suggesting a possible role for androgens, but iatrogenic influences and the effect of ageing (Fischer et al. 2001) should be taken into account.

Thermoregulation

It has been estimated that sweating disturbance occurs in 30–50% of patients with PD, and hypohidrosis is more frequent than hyperhidrosis. Sweating may also be modified by motor fluctuations (Pursiainen et al. 2007c). Prognosis of dyshidrosis is not clear and pathogenesis involves central and postganglionic abnormalities (Hirayama 2006).

The hypothalamus plays an important role in the maintenance of normal core body temperature; other central neural systems important in the regulation of body temperature are found in the cerebral cortex, thalamus, brainstem, and spinal cord. Peripheral sweat gland function is regulated by the sympathetic nervous system. PD patients show abnormal sympathetic skin responses (SSR) and this abnormalities are more marked in subjects complaining of sweating disturbances (Schestatsky et al. 2006). Patients with PD often complain about increased sweating on their face, neck, arms, and back, and seborrhea on face and head (Mano et al. 1994). Clinical reports in idiopathic PD have shown abnormal thermoregulation, which consists of heat intolerance and hypothermia (Appenzeller and Goss 1971, Gubbay and Barwick 1966) and it was attributed to dysfunction of the ANS. The underlying basis were defective thermoregulatory mechanism in PD patients, such as reduced or absent sweating response when their core temperature was increased or peripheral vasodilatation reflex impairment when the skin was heated (Appenzeller and Goss 1971, Fischer et al. 2001). The SSR, a sweating reflex associated with thermoregulation, was also found to be abnormal. Its latency was prolonged and its amplitude reduced. On the basis of these clinical findings, it has been postulated an inappropriate activation of the sympathetic nervous system as the cause of the thermoregulation disability in PD patients (Fischer et al. 2001, Djaldetti et al. 2001)

Nevertheless, there are no data on experimental studies in animals about the possible role of the basal ganglia on thermoregulatory functions. The circadian rhythm of body core temperature and the analysis of mean degrees changes during the different sleep phases are normal in PD suggesting that the coupling between the mechanisms of sleep and the normally associated withdrawal of the sympathetic tone which mainly involve neurons of the median preoptic anterior hypothalamic regions is not altered in PD (Pierangeli et al. 2001).

Weight loss

Unintended weight loss it is a common feature of PD and disease severity, advanced age, visual hallucinations in the advanced stage and possibly dementia may predict weight loss (Uc et al. 2006). The reason for progressive, weight loss in PD is not clear, although many hypotheses have been advanced. Weight loss can be the result of either reduced energy intake or increased energy expenditure. Reduced energy intake can result from either decreased food intake or impaired food absorption. When dietary intake in PD patients has been assessed, however, no significant differences from controls have been uncovered (Abbott et al. 1992, Beyer et al. 1995, Durrieu et al. 1992, Wszolek and Markopoulou 1998, Toth et al. 1997). The idea that dysphagia might cause reduced caloric intake and weight loss has been put forward by some investigators (Nozaki et al. 1999) but discounted by others (Jankovic et al. 1992). A more direct role for dopamine in parkinsonian weight loss can be postulated. Dopamine modulates reward systems (including appetite) in the brain, and obese individuals show decreased striatal dopamine D2 receptor availability (Wang et al. 2001). Furthermore, dopamine antagonist medications and stereotactic surgery for treatment of motor PD symptoms can induce significant weight gain. Therefore the basis for unintended weight loss in PD is largely unexplained but considering that PD symptoms and decreased cognitive function were more severe in patients with weight loss this could be an expression of a more severe neurodegeneration (Lorefalt et al. 2004). Mean body mass index (BMI) in 100 cases of idiopathic PD was found to be 9% reduced in comparison to that in patients with either essential tremor or no neurologic disease. A similar reduction in BMI was also discovered among the 24 cases of PD in whom retrospective BMI data were available from their presymptomatic years suggesting that alterations in nutrient intake or metabolism could reflect early changes in the central autonomic network preceding the emergence of classical extrapyramidal manifestation of PD (Cheshire and Wszolek 2005).

Pupillary changes

The size and reactivity of the pupils are controlled by the sympathetic and parasympathetic components of the ANS. Constriction of the pupils is mediated via the parasympathetic fibres of the third cranial nerve that arise from the Edinger–Westphal nucleus of the midbrain. Pupillary dilatation is mediated via the sympathetic pathways. Micieli et al. (1991) found abnormally slow pupillary responses to light and pain in patients with PD. Application of pharmacological agents to the eye demonstrated the peripheral ANS to be intact in these PD patients; papillary abnormalities resulted from central autonomic dysfunction centred in the parasympathetic Edinger–Westphal nucleus of the midbrain.

Autonomic aspects of pharmacological therapy in Parkinson's disease

Virtually all antiparkinsonian treatment can lead to exacerbation of pre-existing mild dysautonomia and, in particular, enhance or aggravate OH. L-DOPA, the gold standard of treatment in PD, can worsen OH but also may have significant interaction with meal times and occasionally result in worsening of PPH (Chaudhuri et al. 1997). Dopamine agonists, particularly bromocriptine, pergolide and apomorphine injections, can cause cardiovascular dysautonomia, in particular OH. Caution should therefore be exercised in patients undergoing L-DOPA or apomorphine challenge tests as such patients are particularly prone to develop OH and even syncope. The syndrome of akinetic crisis or malignant L-DOPA withdrawal can be associated with significant dysautonomia. In akinetic crisis patients may develop gastrointestinal dysautonomia leading to dysphagia and faecal retention. In both akinetic crisis and malignant L-DOPA withdrawal, thermoregulatory dysautonomia may lead to hyperthermia, similar to neuroleptic malignant syndrome, associated with other features of peripheral dysautonomia such as tachypnoea, tachycardia and sweating disorders. Use of psychoactive drugs such as amantadine and selegiline, particularly in the evening, can cause significant difficulties with sleep pattern and lead to rapid eye movement (REM) behaviour disorders (RBDs) or even agitation at night, again associated with tachycardia and/or sweating. Considerable concern has arisen over the use of selegiline in older patients due to an unexplained increased mortality seen in these patients when selegiline is used in conjunction with L-DOPA in comparison to patients on levodopa alone (Ben Shlomo et al. 1998). Two studies have shown that selegiline may indeed diminish autonomic responsiveness and increase the risk of OH in PD (Churchyard et al. 1997, Turkka et al. 1997). However, the study reported by the Parkinson's Disease Research Group of the UK provides limited support for the hypothesis that the autonomic side-effects of selegiline are responsible for the increased death rate seen in patients treated with a combination of selegiline and L-DOPA. Hyperhidrosis and abdominal pain have been reported with long-term administration of tolcapone, which also appears to cause diarrhoea in some patients (Rajaput et al. 1997). The nature of this diarrhoea is similar to diarrhoea seen in diabetic patients with autonomic failure.

Treatments effective for autonomic symptoms in Parkinson's disease

Although common, autonomic symptoms of PD are underdiagnosed and undertreated.

There is a paucity of research concerning treatment of autonomic symptoms in PD and a concerted and multidisciplinary effort needs to be made for fulfilling this urgent unmet need.

There are few dedicated controlled trials of drugs to treat autonomic symptoms in PD that were recently reviewed by the Quality Standards Subcommittee of the American Academy of Neurology (Zesiewicz et al. 2010).

Conclusions

◆ Parkinson's disease (PD) has mainly been characterized in terms of motor impairments.

◆ The clinical spectrum of PD is more extensive, including cognitive, mood, sleep, and a broad spectrum of autonomic features involving gastrointestinal, urinary, sexual, cardiovascular, thermoregulatory, respiratory, and pupillomotor functions.

◆ The overall prevalence of autonomic features varies considerably from 2% for urinary incontinence to 72% for constipation and

in part, they have been related with disease duration, disease severity, or use of antiparkinsonian drugs.

◆ Autonomic dysfunction in patients with PD is a serious problem; it is associated with depression and impacts on daily functioning and quality of life.

◆ Subtle autonomic disturbances that can at least partly be related to the degeneration of the vagal nerve are an early and frequent sign of PD. For several autonomic symptoms, including gastrointestinal and urinary problems, orthostatic hypotension, and erectile dysfunction, therapeutic interventions have become available.

◆ Investigation of cardiovascular autonomic dysfunction in parkinsonism is important for a variety of reasons that include determining the precise diagnosis and in predicting prognosis.

◆ In parkinsonian disorders, understanding the pathophysiological basis of the autonomic abnormality aids targeting of therapy, improves management strategies, and should benefit such patients.

References

Abbott, R. A., Cox, M., Markus, H., Tomkins, A. (1992). Diet, body size and micronutrient status in Parkinson's disease. *Eur. J Clin. Nutrition* **46**, 879–84.

Alam, M., Pavitt, D. V., Mathias, C. J. (1993). Cumulative sums of 24 hour blood pressure profiles in patients with sympathetic denervation. *J Hypertension.* **11**(suppl 5), s286–287.

Alam, M., Smith, G. D. P., Bleasdale-Barr, K., Pavitt, D. V., Mathias, C. J. (1995). Effects of the peptide release inhibitor, Octreotide, on daytime hypotension and on nocturnal hypertension in primary autonomic failure. *J Hypertension* **13**, 1664–69.

Albanese, A., Maria, G., Bentivoglio, A., Brisinda, G., Cassetta, E., Tonali, P. (1997). Severe constipation in Parkinson's disease relieved by botulinum toxin. *Mov. Disord.* **12**, 764–66.

Alfonsi, E., Versino, M., Merlo, I. M. *et al.* (2007). Electrophysiologic patterns of oral-pharyngeal swallowing in parkinsonian syndromes. *Neurology* **68**, 583–90.

Allcock, L. M., Kenny, R. A., Burn, D. J. (2006). Clinical phenotype of subjects with Parkinson's disease and orthostatic hypotension: autonomic symtom and demographic comparison. *Mov. Disord.* **21**, 1851–55.

Aminoff, M. J., Gross, M., Laatz, B., Vakil, S. D., Petrie, A., Calne, D. B. (1975). Arterial blood pressure in patients with Parkinson's disease. *JNNP* **38**, 73–77.

Aminoff, M. J., Wilcox, C. S. (1971). Assessment of autonomic function in patients with a parkinsonian syndrome. *BMJ* **4**, 80–84.

Appenzeller, O., Goss, J. E. (1971). Autonomic deficits in Parkinson's syndrome. *Arch. Neurol.* **24**(1), 50–57.

Asahina, M., Vichayanrat, E., Low, D. A., Iodice, V., Mathias, C. J. (2012). Autonomic dysfunction in parkinsonian disorders: assessment and pathophysiology. *J Neurol. Neurosurg. Psychiatry.* [Epub ahead of print].

Baas, H. and Fischer, P. A. (1984). Salbengesicht. Zentrale Dysregulation der Talgsekretion beim Parkinson-Syndrom. In: Fischer, P. A. (Hrsg), ed. *Vegetativstörungen beim Parkinson-Syndrom.* Editiones Roche, Basel, p. 221–23;

Bagheri, H., Damase-Michel, C., Lapeyre-Mestre, M., *et al.* (1999). A study of salivary secretion in Parkinson's disease. *Clin. Neuropharmacol.* **22**(4), 213–15.

Ballantyne, J. P. (1973). Early and late effects of levodopa on the cardiovascular system in Parkinson's disease. *J Neurol. Sci,* **19**, 97–103.

Bannister, R., Oppenheimer, D. R. (1972). Degenerative disease of the nervous system associated with autonomic failure. *Brain* **95**, 457–74.

Barbeau, A. (1969). L-dopa therapy in Parkinson's disease: nine years experience. *Can. Med. Assoc. J* **101**, 791–96.

Barbeau, A., Mars, H., Gillo-Joffroy. (1971). Adverse clinical side effects of levodopa therapy. In: Markham, C. H., ed. *Recent Advances in Parkinson's Disease*. Blackwell, Oxford, p. 203–37;

Barbic, F., Perego, F., Canesi, M. *et al.* (2007). Early abnormalities of vascular and cardiac autonomic control in Parkinson's disease without orthostatic hypotension. *Hypertension* **49**, 120–26.

Bateson, M. C., Gibberd, F. B., Wilson, R. S. E. (1973). Salivary symptoms in Parkinson's disease. *Arch. Neurol.* **29**, 274–75.

Ben Shlomo, Y., Churchyard, A., Head, J., *et al.* (1998). Investigations by Parkinson's Disease Research Group of the united Kingdom into excess mortality seen with combined levodopa and selegiline treatment in patients with early, mild Parkinson's Disease: further result of randomised trial and confidential enquiry. *BMJ* **316**, 1191–95.

Beyer, P. L., Palarino, M. Y., Michalek, D., Busenbark, K., Koller, W. C. (1995). Weight change and body composition in patients with Parkinson's disease. *J Am. Diet Assoc.* **95**, 979–83.

Bonuccelli, U., Lucetti, C., Del Dotto, P., *et al.* (2003). Orthostatic hypotension in de novo Parkinson disease. *Arch. Neurol.*, **60**(10), 1400–1404.

Braak, H., Del Tredici, K., Rub, U., Vos, R. A. de, Jansen Steur, E. N., Braak, E. (2003). Staging of brain pathology related to sporadic Parkinson's disease. *Neurobiology of Aging* **24**, 197–211.

Braune, S., Reinhardt, M., Bathmann, J., Krause, T., Lehmann, M., Lucking, C. H. (1998). Impaired cardiac uptake of meta-[123]-iodobenzylguanidine in Parkinson's disease with autonomic failure. *Acta Neurologica Scandinavica* **97**, 307–14.

Braune, S., Reinhardt, M., Schnitzer, R., Riedel, A., Lucking, C. H. (1999). Cardiac uptake of [123i]MIBG separates Parkinson's disease from multiple system atrophy. *Neurology* **53**, 1020–26.

Bronner, G., Royter, V., Korczyn, A. D., Giladi, N. (2004). Sexual dysfunction in Parkinson's disease. *J Sexual Marital Therapy* **30**(2), 95–105.

Burton, J. L., Cartlidge, M., Cartlidge, N. E. F., Shuster, S. (1973). Sebum excretion in Parkinsonism. *Br J Dermatol.* **88**, 263–66.

Burton, J. L., Shuster, S. (1970). Effect of L-dopa on seborrhoea of Parkinsonism. *Lancet* **ii**, 19–20.

Calne, D. B., Brennan, A. S., Spiers, D., Stern, G. M. (1970). Hypotension caused by l-dopa. *BMJ* **1**, 474–75.

Calne, D. B., Reid, J. L., Vakil, S. D., George, C. F., Rao, S. (1973). Effects of carbidopa-levodopa on blood pressure in man. In: M. D. Yahr, ed. *Advances in Neurology* Vol 2. *Treatment of Parkinsonism*. Raven Press, New York, p. 149–59;

Camerlingo, M., Ferrar, B., Gazzaniga, G. C., Casto, L., Cesana, B. M., Mamoli, A. (1990). Cardiovascular reflexes in Parkinson's disease: long-term effects of levodopa treatment on de novo patients. *Acta Neurologica Scandinavica* **81**, 346–48.

Camilleri, M., Bharucha, A. E. (1996). Gastrointestinal dysfunction in neurologic disease. *Seminars in Neurology* **16**, 203–216.

Chaudhuri, K. R. (2001). Autonomic dysfunction in movement disorders. *Curr. Opin. Neurol.* **14**, 505–511.

Chaudhuri, K. R., Love-Jones, S., Ellis, C. M. *et al.* (1997). Postprandial hypotension and parkinsonian state in Parkinson's disease. *Mov. Disord.* **12**, 877–84.

Chaudhuri, K. R., Hu, M. (2000). Central autonomic dysfunction. In *Handbook of clinical neurology*, Vol 75 (31): The autonomic nervous system. Part II. Dysfunctions O. Appenzeller ed. Elseviere Science, 161–202;

Chaudhuri, K. R., Martinez-Martin, P., Brown, R. G. *et al.* (2007). The metric properties of a novel non-motor symptoms scale for Parkinson's disease: results from an international pilot study. *Mov. Disord.* **22**(13), 1901–911.

Cheshire, W. P. Jr, Wszolek, Z. K. (2005). Body mass index is reduced early in Parkinson's disease. *Parkinsonism Related Disorders* **11**(1), 35–38.

Churchyard, A., Mathias, C. J., Lees, A. J. (1997). Autonomic effects of selegiline: possible cardiovascular toxicity in Parkinson's disease. *JNNP* **63**, 228–34.

Churchyard, A., Mathias, C. J., Lees, A. J. (1999). Selegiline-induced postural hypotension in Parkinson's disease: a longitudinal study on the effects of drug withdrawal. *Mov. Disord.* **2**, 246–51.

Claus, D., Meudt, O., Rozeik, C., Engelmann-Kempe, K., Huppert, P. E., Wietholtz. (2002). Prospective investigation of autonomic cardiac neuropathy in diabetes mellitus. *Clin Auton Res.* **12**, 373–78.

Cohn, T. (1920). Encephalitis ohne Lethargie bei der Grippeepidemie. *Zentr. Bl. Neurol.* **38**, 260–64.

Colosimo, C., Albanese, A., Hughes, A. J., de Bruin, V. M. S., Lees, A. J. (1995). Some specific clinical features differentiate multiple system atrophy (striatonigral variety) from Parkinson's disease. *Arch. Neurol.* **52**, 294–98.

Cortelli, P., Pierangeli, G., Provini, F., Plazzi, G., Lugaresi, E. (1996). Blood pressure rhythms in sleep disorders and dysautonomia. *Ann. N Y Acad. Sci.* **783**, 204–21.

Courbon, F., Brefel-Courbon, C., Thalamas, C., *et al.* (2003). Cardiac MIBG scintigraphy is a sensitive tool for detecting cardiac sympathetic denervation in Parkinson's disease. *Mov. Disord.* **18**, 890–97.

Critchley, H. D., Mathias, C. J., Dolan, R. J. (2001). Neuroanatomical basis for first-and second order representations of bodily states. *Nature Neuroscience* **4**, 207–212.

Critchley, H. D., Mathias, C. J., Dolan, R. J. (2002). Fear conditioning in humans: the influence of awareness and autonomic arousal on functional neuroanatomy. *Neuron* **33**, 653–63.

Desjacques, P., Moret, P., Gauthier, G. (1973). Effect cardiovasculaires de las L-dopa et de l'inhibiteur de la decarboxylase chez les malades atteints de la maladie de Parkinson. *Schweizerische medizinische Wochenschrift* **103**, 1783–85.

Djaldetti, R., Melamed, E., and Gadoth, N. 2001. Abnormal skin wrinkling in the less affected side in hemiparkinsonism: A possible test for sympathetic dysfunctions in Parkinson's disease. *Biomedicine & Pharmacotherapy* **55**, 474–78.

Druschky, A., Hilz, M. J., Platsch, G. *et al.* (2000). Differentiation of Parkinson's disease and multiple system atrophy in early disease stages by means of I-123-MIBG-SPECT. *J Neurol. Sci.* **175**, 3–12.

Durrieu, G., Llau, M. E., Rascol, O., Senard, J. M., Rascol, A., Montastruc, J. L. (1992). Parkinson's disease and weight loss: a study with anthropometric and nutritional assessment. *Clin. Auton. Res.* **2**, 153–57.

Durrieu, G., Senard, J. M., Rascol, O., Tran, M. A., Lataste, X., Rascol, A., Montastruc, J. L. (1990). Blood pressure and plasma catecholamines in never-treated parkinsonian patients: effect of a D1 agonist (CY 208–243). *Clin. Neuropharmacol.* **16**, 70–76.

Eadie, M. J. (1963). Gastric secretion in parkinsonism. *Australasian Annals of Medicine* **12**, 346–50.

Edwards, L. L., Quigley, E. M., Harned, R. K., Hofman, R., Pfeiffer, R. F. (1994). Characterization of swallowing and defecation in Parkinson's disease. *Am. J Gastroenterol.* **89**(1), 15–25.

Fichefet, J. P., Sternon, J. E., Franken, L., Demanet, J. C., Vanderhaeghen, J. J. (1965). Etude anatomo-clinique d'un cas d'hypotension orthostatique 'idiopathique'. Considerations pathogeniques. *Acta Cardiologia* **20**, 332–48.

Fischer, M. Gemende, I., Marsch, W. C., Fischer, P. A. (2001). Skin function and skin disorders in Parkinson's disease. *Journal of Neural Transmission* **108**(2), 205–213.

Fisher, A. A., Davis, M. W., Srikusalanukul, W., Budge, M. M. (2005). Post-prandial hypotension predicts all-cause mortality in older, low-level care residents. *Journal of American Geriatric Society* **53**, 1313–20.

Freemon, F. R. (1971). Parkinsonism and cardiac arrhythmias. *Lancet* **2**, 83–84.

Gai, W. P., Blessing, W. W., Blumbergs, P. C. (1995). Ubiquitinpositive degenerating neurites in the brainstem in Parkinson's disease. *Brain* **118**, 1447–59.

Gibb, W. R. G. (1988). The Lewy body and Autonomic failure. In: Bannister, R., ed. *Autonomic failure; A textbook of clinical disorders of the Autonomic Nervous System*. 2nd ed Oxford: Oxford University press, pp. 484–97;

Goetz, C. G., Luteg, W. and Tanner, C. M. (1986). Autonomic dysfunction in Parkinson's disease. *Neurology* **6**, 72–75.

Goldstein, D. S. (2006). Orthostatic hypotension as an early finding in Parkinson's disease. *Clin. Auton. Res.* **16**, 46–54.

Goldstein, D. S., Eldadah, B. A., Holmes, C. et al. (2005). Neurocirculatory abnormalities in Parkinson disease with orthostatic hypotension: indipendence from levodopa treatment. *Hypertension* **46**, 1333–39.

Goldstein, D. S., Holmes, C., Cannon, R. O. III, Eisenhofer, G., Kopin, I. J. (1997). Sympathetic cardioneuropathy in dysautonomias. *N Engl. J Med.* **336**, 696–702.

Goldstein, D. S., Holmes, C., Dendi, R., Bruce, S., Li, S-T. (2002). Orthostatic hypotension from sympathetic denervation in Parkinson's disease. *Neurology* **58**, 1247–55.

Goldstein, D. S., Holmes, C., Li, S. T., Bruce, S., Metman, L. V., Cannon, R. O. (2000). Cardiac sympathetic denervation in Parkinson disease. *Ann. Int. Med.* **133**, 338–47.

Goldstein, D. S., Pechnik, S., Holmes, C., Eldadah, B., Sharabi, Y. (2003a). Association between supine hypertension and orthostatic hypotension in autonomic failure. *Hypertension* **42**, 136–42.

Goldstein, D. S., Holmes, C., Sharabi, Y., Brentzel, S., Eisenhofer, G. (2003b). Plasma levels of catechols and metanephrines in neurogenic orthostatic hypotension. *Neurology* **60**, 1327–32.

Goldstein, D. S., Sewell, L., Holmes, C. (2010). Association of anosmia with autonomic failure in Parkinson disease. *Neurology* **74**, 245–51.

Gross, M., Bannister, R., Godwin-Austen, R. (1972). Orthostatic hypotension in Parkinson's disease. *Lancet* **1**(7743), 174–76.

Gubbay, S. S. and Barwick, D. D. (1966). Two cases of accidental hypotermia in Parkinson's disease with unusual EEEG findings. *JNNP* **29**, 459–66.

Hakusui, S., Yasuda, T., Yanagi, T. et al. (1994). A radiological analysis of heart sympathetic functions with with meta-[123I] iodobenzylguanadine in neurological patients with autonomic failure. *J Auton. Nerv. Syst.* **49**, 81–84.

Halliday, G. M., Blumbergs, P. C., Cotton, R. G., Blessing, W. W., Geffen, L. B. (1990). Loss of brainstem serotonin- and substance P-containing neurons in Parkinson's disease. *Brain Research* **510**, 104–107.

Hamdy, S., Rothwell, J. C., Brooks, D. J., Bailey, D., Aziz, Q., Thompson, D. G. (1999). Identification of the cerebral loci processing human swallowing with H2 15O PET activation. *J Neurophysiol.* **81**, 1917–26.

Herzog, J., Weiss, P. H., Assmus, A. et al. (2006). Subthalamic stimulation modulates cortical control of urinary bladder in Parkinson's disease. *Brain* **129**, 336–75.

Hillen, M. E., Wagner, M. L., Sage, J. I. (1996). 'Subclinical' orthostatic hypotension is associated with dizziness in elderly patients with Parkinson disease. *Archives of Physical Medicine and Rehabilitation* **77**, 710–712.

Hirayama, M. (2006). Sweating dysfunction in Parkinson's disease. *J Neurol.* **253**(S7), 42–47.

Holmberg, B., Corneliusson, O., Elam, M. (2005). Bilateral stimulation of nucleus subthalamicus in advanced Parkinson's disease: no efffects on, and of, autonomic dysfunction. *Mov. Disord.* **20**(8), 976–81.

Holmberg, B., Kallio, M., Johnels, B., Elam, M. (2001). Cardiovascular reflex testing contributes to clinical evaluation and differential diagnosis of Parkinsonian syndromes. *Mov. Disord.* **16**(2), 217–25.

Hughes, A. J., Daniel, S. E., Kilford, L., Less, A. J. (1992). Accuracy of clinical diagnosis of idiopathic Parkinson's disease: a clinicopathological study of 100 cases. *JNNP* **55**, 181–84.

Hughes, A. J., Daniel, S. E., Lees, A. J. (2001). Improved accuracy of clinical diagnosis of Lewy body Parkinson's disease. *Neurology*, **57**,1497–99.

Hunter, K. R., Hollman, A., Laurence, D. R., Stern, G. M. (1971). Levodopa in parkinsonian patients with heart disease. *Lancet* **1**, 932–34.

Hunter, P. C., Crameri, J., Austin, S., Woodward, M. C., Hughes, A. J. (1997). Response of parkinsonian swallowing dysfunction to dopaminergic stimulation. *JNNP* **63**, 579–83.

Hussain, I. F., Brady, C. M., Swinn, M. J., Mathias, C. J., Fowler, C. J. (2001). Treatment of erectile dysfunction with sildenafil citrate (Viagra) in parkinsonism due to Parkinson's disease or multiple system atrophy with observations on orthostatic hypotension. *JNNP* **71**, 371–74.

Idiaquez, J., Benarroch, E. E., Rosales, H., Milla, P., Rìos, L. (2007). Autonomic and cognitive dysfunction in Parkinson's disease. *Clin. Auton. Res.* **17**, 93–98.

Imrich, R., Eldadah, B. A., Bentho, O., et al. (2009). Functional effects of cardiac sympathetic denervation in neurogenic orthostatic hypotension. *Parkinsonism Relat. Disord.* **15**, 122–27.

Iodice, V., Low, D. A., Vichayanrat E. and Mathias, C. J. (2011). Cardiovascular autonomic dysfunction in MSA and Parkinson's disease: similarities and differences. *J Neurol. Sci.* **310**, 133–8.

Iodice, V., Low, D. A., Vichayanrat, E. and Mathias, C. J. (2012). Cardiovascular autonomic dysfunction in Parkinson's disease and Parkinsonian dyndromes. In *Parkinson's Disease*. (Eds. M. Ebadi, Z.K. Wszolek and R.F. Pfeiffer). pp 353–74. Florida: CRC Press.

Jamnadas-Khoda, J., Koshy, S., Mathias, C. J., Muthane, U. B., Ragothaman, M., Dodaballapur, S. K. (2009). Are current recommendations to diagnose orthostatic hypotension in Parkinson's disease satisfactory? *Mov. Disord.* **24**(12), 1747–51.

Jankovic, J., Wooten, M., Van der Linden, C., Jansson, B. (1992). Low body weight in Parkinson's disease. *Southern Medical Journal* **85**, 351–54.

Jellinger, K. (1987). Overview of morphological changes in Parkinson's disease. In: Yahr, M. D., Bergmann, K. J., eds. *Advances in Neurology*, volume 45: Parkinson's disease. New York: Raven Press, 1–18.

Jenkins, R. B., Mendelson, S. H., Lamid, S., Klawans, H. L. (1972). Levodopa therapy of patients with parkinsonism and heart disease. *Br. Med. J* **3**, 512–514.

Johns, D. W., Ayers, C. R., Carey, R. M. (1984). The dopamine agonist bromocriptine induces hypotension by venous and arteriolar dilatation. *Journal of Cardiovascular Pharmacology* **6**, 582–87.

Jost, W. H., Schimrigk, K. (1993). Cisapride treatment of constipation in Parkinson's disease. *Mov. Disord.* **8**(3), 339–43.

Kanzaki, N., Sato, K., Jayabara, T. (1998). Improved cardiac iodine-123 metaiodobenzyleguanidine accumulation after drug therapy in a patient with Parkinson's disease. *Nuclear Medicine Communications* **22**, 697–99.

Karoum, F., Chuang, L. W., Eisler, T. et al. (1982). Metabolism of (-) deprenyl to amphetamine and metamphetamine may be responsible for deprenyl's therapeutic benefit: a biochemical assessment. *Annali of Neurology* **32**, 503–509.

Kaufmann, H., Oribe, E., Miller, M., Knott, P., Wiltshire-Clement, M., Yahr, M. D. (1992). Hypotension-induced vasopressin release distinguishes between pure autonomic failure and multiple system atrophy with autonomic failure. *Neurology* **42**, 590–93.

Kaye, J., Gage, H., Kimber, A., Storey, L., Trend, P. (2006). Excess burden of constipation in Parkinson's disease: a pilot study. *Mov. Disord.* **21**(8), 1270–73.

Kazuta, T., Hayashi, M., Shimizu, T., Iwasaki, A., Nakamura, S., Hirai, S. (2000). Autonomic dysfunction in Machado-Joseph disease assessed by iodine123-labeled metaiodobenzylguanidine myocardial scintigraphy. *Clin. Auton. Res.* **10**, 111–115.

Kihara, M., Takahashi, M., Nishimoto, K. et al. (1998). Autonomic dysfunction in elderly bedfast patients. *Age Ageing* **27**, 551–55.

Kimber, J. R., Watson, L., Mathias, C. J. (1997). Distinction of idiopathic Parkinson's disease from multiple system atrophy by stimulation of growth hormone release with clonidine. *Lancet* **349**, 1877–81.

Kimber, J. R. and Mathias, C. J. (1999). Neuroendocrine responses to Levodopa in multiple system atrophy (MSA). *Mov. Disord.* **14**, 981–87.

Kohn, S. R., Pochi, P. E., Strauss, J. S., Sax, D. S., Feldman, R. G., Timberlake, W. H. (1973). Sebaceous gland secretion in Parkinson's disease during L-dopa treatment. *The Journal of Investigative Dermatology* **60**, 134–36.

Koller, W. C., Silver, D. S., Leiberman, A. (1994). An algorithm for the management of Parkinson's disease. *Neurology* **44** (S10), S9–S52.

Kujawa, K., Leurgans, S., Raman, R., Blasucci, L., Goetz, C. G. (2000). Acute orthostatic hypotension when starting dopamine agonists in Parkinson's disease. *Arch. Neurol.* **57**, 1461–63.

Kuno, S. (1989). Parkinson's disease and its autonomic disorders. *Mod Physician (Tokyo)* **9**, 1214–1219.

Kupsky, W. J., Grimes, M. M., Sweeting, J., Bertsch, R., Cote, L. J. (1987). Parkinson's disease and megacolon: concentric hyaline inclusions (Lewy bodies) in enteric ganglion cells. *Neurology* **37**, 1253–55.

Lezcano, E., Gomez-Esteban, J. C., Zarranz, J. J. et al. (2004). Parkinson's disease-like presentation of multiple system atrophy with poor response to STN stimulation: a clinicopathological case report. *Mov. Disord.* **19**(8), 973–77.

Li, S. T., Dendi, R., Holmes, C., Goldstein, D. S. (2002). Progressive loss of cardiac sympathetic innervation in Parkinson's disease. *Annali of Neurology* **52**, 220–23.

Lieberman, A. N., Goldstein, M., Gopinathan, G. et al. (1982). Further studies with pergolide in Parkinson disease. *Neurology* **32**, 1181–84.

Lipp, A., Sandroni, P., Ahlskog, J. E., et al. (2009). Prospective differentiation of multiple system atrophy from Parkinson disease, with and without autonomic failure. *Arch. Neurol.* **66**, 742–50.

Litvan, I., Goetz, C. G., Jankovic, J. et al. (1997). What is the accuracy of the clinical diagnosis of multiple system atrophy? *Arch. Neurol.* **54**, 937–44.

Lorefalt, B., Ganowiak, W., Palhagen, S., Toss, G., Unosson, M., Granerus, A. K. (2004). Factors of importance for weight loss in elderly patients with Parkinson's disease. *Acta Neurologica Scandinavica* **110**(3), 180–87.

Magalhaes, M., Wenning, G. K., Daniel, S. E., Quinn, N. P. (1995). Autonomic dysfunction in pathologically confirmed multiple system atrophy and idiopathic Parkinson's disease—a retrospective comparison. *Acta Neurologica Scandinavica* **91**(2), 98–102.

Magerkurth, C., Schnitzer, R., Braune, S. (2005). Symptoms of autonomic failure in Parkinson's disease: prevalence and impact on daily life. *Clin. Auton. Res.* **15**, 76–82.

Mano, Y., Nakamuro, T., Takayanagi, T. et al. (1994). Sweat function in Parkinson's disease. *J Neurol.* **241**, 573–76.

Mars and Krall. (1971). L-dopa and cardiac arrhythmias. *N Engl. J Med.* **285**, 1437.

Martignoni, E., Godi, E., Pacchetti, C. et al. (1997). Is seborrhea a sign of autonomic impairment in Parkinson's disease? *Journal of Neural Transmission* **104**, 1295–1304.

Mathias, C. J. (1996a). Disorders of the autonomic nervous system in childhood. In *Principles of Child Neurology.* (Ed. B Berg). pp. 413–36. New York: McGraw-Hill.

Mathias C. J. (1996). Disorders affecting autonomic function in Parkinsonian patients. In: *Parkinson's Disease.* Eds. Battistini, L., Scarlato, G., Caraceni, T., Ruggieri, S. Raven Press, New York, pp. 383–91.

Mathias, C. J. (2000). Autonomic dysfunction. In: *Oxford Textbook of Geriatric Medicine.* Second Edition. Ed. J Grimley-Evans. Oxford University Press, Oxford, pp. 833–52.

Mathias, C. J. (2003). Autonomic diseases: clinical features and laboratory evaluation. *JNNP* **74** (S3), s31–41.

Mathias, C. J., Mallipeddi, R., Bleasdale-Barr, K. (1999). Symptoms associated with orthostatic hypotension in pure autonomic failure and multiple system atrophy. *J Neurol.* **246**, 893–98.

Mathias, C. J. and Kimber, J. R. (1999). Postural hypotension—causes, clinical features, investigation and management. *Ann. Rev. Med* **50**, 317–36.

Matsui, H., Nishinaka, K., Oda, M., Komatsu, K., Kubori, T., Udaka, F. (2006). Does cardiac MIBG uptake in Parkinson's disease correlate with major autonomic symptoms? *Parkinsonism and Related Disorders* **12**, 284–88.

McDowell, F. H., Lee, J. E., Swift, T., Sweet, R. D., Ogsburg, J. S., Kessler, J. T. (1970). Treatment of Parkinson's syndrome with L-dihydroxyphenalalinine (levo-dopa). *Annali of Internal Medicine* **72**, 29–35.

Meco, G., Gasparini, M. and Doricchi, F. (1996). Attentional functions in multiple system atrophy and Parkinson's disease. *JNNP;* **60**, 393–98.

Meco, G., Pratesi, L., Bonifati, V. (1991). Cardiovascular reflexes and autonomic dysfunction in Parkinson's disease. *J Neurol.* **238**, 195–99.

Mehagnoul-Schipper, J., Boerman, R. H., Hoefnagels, W. H. L., Jansen, R. W. M. M. (2001). Effect of levodopa on orthostatic and post-prandial hypotension in elderly parkinsonian patients. *The Journals of Gerontology. Series A, Biological sciences and medical sciences* **56A**, M749–55.

Mesec, A., Sega, S., Kiauta, T. (1993). The influence of the type, duration, severity and levodopa treatment of Parkinson's disease on cardiovascular autonomic responses. *Clin. Auton. Res.* **3**, 339–44.

Micieli, G., Martignoni, E., Cavallini, A., Sandrini, G., Nappi, G. (1987). Postprandial and orthostatic hypotension in Parkinson's disease. *Neurology* **37**, 383–93.

Micieli, G., Tassorelli, C., Martignoni, E. et al. (1991). Disordered pupil reactivity in Parkinson's disease. *Clin. Auton. Res.* **1**, 55–58.

Miller, A. J. (1986). Neurophysiological basis of swallowing. *Dysphagia* **1**, 91–100.

Minquez-Castellanos, A., Chamorro, C. E., Escamilla-Sevilla, F. et al. (2007). Do α-synuclein aggregates in autonomic plexuses predate Lewy body disorders? *Neurology* **68**, 2012–2018.

Montastruc, J. L., Chamontin, B., Rascol, A. (1985). Parkinson's disease and hypertension: Chronic bromocriptine treatment. *Neurology* **35**, 1644–7.

Nozaki, S., Saito, T., Matsumura, T., Miyai, I., Kang, J. (1999). Relationship between weight loss and dysphagia in patients with Parkinson's disease. *Rinsho Shinkeigaku* **39**, 1010–1014.

Oertel, W. H., Quinn, N. P. (1996). Parkinsonism. In: T. Brandt, L. R. Kaplan, J. Dicaghans, H. C. Diener, C. Kennard (Eds) *Neurological Disorders. Cause and Treatment,* 64. San FDiego, CA, Academic Press, 715–72.

Ohmura, M. (2000). Loss of 123I-MIBG uptake by the heart in Parkinson's disease: assessment of cardiac sympathetic denervation and diagnostic value. *Journal of Nuclear Medicine* **41**, 1594–95.

Oka, H., Yoshioka, M., Onouchi, K. et al. (2007a). Impaired cardiovascular autonomic function in Parkinson's disease with visual hallucinations. *Mov. Disord.* **22**(10), 1510–1514.

Oka, H., Yoshioka, M., Morita, M. et al. (2007b). Reduced cardiac 123I-MIBG uptake reflects cardiac sympathetic dysfunction in Lewy body disease. *Neurology* **69**, 1460–65.

Okun, M. S., McDonald, W. M., DeLong, M. R. (2002). Refractory nonmotor symptoms in male patients with Parkinson disease due to testosterone deficiency: a common unrecognized comorbidity. *Arch. Neurol.* **59**(5), 807–811.

Oppenheimer, D. R. (1980). Lateral horn cells in progressive autonomic failure. *Journal of Neurological Sciences* **46**, 393–404.

Orimo, S., Amino, T., Yokochi, M. et al. (2005). Preserved cardiac sympathetic nerve accounts for normal cardiacuptake of MIBG in PARK2. *Mov. Disord.* **20**(10), 1350–53.

Orimo, S., Oka, T., Miura, H., et al. (2002). Sympathetic cardiac denervation in Parkinson's disease and pure autonomic failure but not in multiple system atrophy. *JNNP* **73**, 776–78.

Orimo, S., Ozawa, E., Nakade, S., Sugimoto, T., Mizusawa, H. (1999). 123I-metaiodobenzylguanidine myocardial scintigraphy in Parkinson's disease. *JNNP* **67**, 189–94.

Orimo, S., Ozawa, E., Oka, T. *et al.* (2001). Different histopathology accounting for a decrease in myocardial MIBG uptake in PD and MSA. *Neurology* 57, 1140–41.

Orimo, S., Takahashi, A., Uchihara, T. *et al.* (2007). Degeneration of cardiac sympathetic nerve begins in the early disease process of Parkinson's disease. *Brain Pathology* 17, 24–30.

Orskov, I., Jakobsen, J., Dupont, E., de Fine Olivarius, B., Christensen, N. J. (1987). Autonomic function in parkinsonian patients relates to duration of disease. *Neurology* 37, 1173–78.

Pallis, C. A., Calne, D. B. (1970). A case of 'atrial flutter' due to tremor artifacts. *Lancet* 2, 1313.

Papapetropoulos, S. and Mash, D. C. (2007). Insular pathology in Parkinson's disease patients with orthostatic hypotension. *Parkinsonism and Related Disorders* 13, 308–311.

Papatsoris, A. G., Deliveliotis, C., Singer, C., Papapetropoulos, S. (2006). Erectile dysfunction in Parkinson's disease. *Urology* 67, 447–51.

Parkinson, J. (1817). *An essay on the shaking palsy*. London: Sherwood, Neely and Jones;

Perez Lloret, S., Piràn Arce, G., Rossi, M., Caivano Nemet, M. L., Salsamendi, P., Merello, M. (2007). Validation of a new scale for the evaluation of sialorrhea in patients with Parkinson's disease. *Mov. Disord.* 22 (1), 107–111.

Pfeiffer, R. F. (2003). Gastrointestinal dysfunction in Parkinson's disease. *Lancet Neurology* 2(2), 107–116.

Pierangeli, G., Provini, F., Maltoni, P. *et al.* (2001). Nocturnal body core temperature falls in Parkinson's disease but not in Multiple-System Atrophy. *Mov. Disord.* 16(2), 226–32.

Piha, S. J., Rinne, J. O., Rinne, J. O., Seppanen, A. (1988). Autonomic dysfunction in recent onset and advanced Parkinson's disease. *Clinical Neurology and Neurosurgery* 90, 221–26.

Pochi, P. E., Strauss, J. S., Mescon, H. (1962). Sebum production and fractional 17-ketosteroid excretion in Parkinsonism. *The Journal of Investigative Dermatology*, 38, 45–51.

Pursiainen, V., Korpelainen, T. J., Haapaniemi, H. T., Sotaniemi, A. K., Myllylä, V. V. (2007a). Blood pressure and heart rate in parkinsonian patients with and without wearing-off. *Eur. J Neurol.* 14, 373–78.

Pursiainen, V., Korpelainen, T. J., Haapaniemi, H. T., Sotaniemi, A. K., Myllylä, V. V. (2007b). Selegiline and blood pressure in patients with Parkinson's disease. *Acta Neurologica Scandinavica* 115, 104–108.

Pursiainen, V., Haapaniemi, H. T., Korpelainen, T. J., Sotaniemi, A. K., Myllylä, V. V. (2007c). Sweating in parkinsonian patients with wearing-off. *Mov. Disord.* 22 (6), 828–32.

Qualman, S. J., Haupt, H. M., Yang, P., Hamilton, S. R. (1984). Esophageal Lewy bodies associated with ganglion cell loss in achalasia: similarity to Parkinson's disease. *Gastroenterology* 87, 848–56.

Quinn, N., Illas, A., Lermitte, F., Agid, Y. (1981). Bromocriptine in Parkinson's disease: a study of cardiovascular effects. *JNNP*; 44, 426–29.

Rajput, A. H., Martin, W., St Hilaire, M. H., Dorflinger, E., Peddar, S. (1997). Tolcapone improves motor function in parkinsonian patients with the wearing 'off' phenomenon: a double blind, placebo controlled multicentre trial. *Neurology* 49, 1066–71.

Rajput, A. H., Rozdilsky, B., Rajput, A., Ang, L. (1990). Levodopa therapy and pathological basis of Parkinson's syndrome. *Clinical Neuropharmacology* 13, 553–58.

Rajput, A. H. and Rozdilsky, B. (1976). Dysautonomia in parkinsonism: a clinicopathological study. *JNNP* 39, 1092–1100.

Reinhardt, M. J., Jungling, F. D., Krause, T. M., Braune, S. (2000). Scintigraphic differentiation between two forms of primary dysautonomia early after onset of autonomic dysfunction; value of cardiac and pulmonary iodine-123 MIBG uptake. *European Journal of Nuclear Medicine* 27, 595–600.

Riley, D. E., Chelimsky, T. C. (2003). Autonomic nervous system testing may not distinguish multiple system atrophy from Parkinson's disease. *JNNP* 74, 56–60.

Sachs, C., Bergland, B., Kajser, L. (1985). Autonomic cardiovascular responses in parkinsonism: effect of levodopa with dopa-decarboxylase inhibition. *Acta Neurologica Scandinavica* 71, 37–42.

Saint-Pierre, A. (1973). ECG artifacts simulating atrial flutter. *JAMA* 224, 1534.

Sandroni, P., Ahiskog, E., Fealey, R. D., Low, P. A. (1991). Autonomic involvement in extrapyramidal and cerebellar disorders. *Clin. Auton. Res.* 1, 147–55.

Satoh, A., Serita, T., Seto, M. *et al.* (1999). Loss of 123I-MIBG uptake by the heart in Parkinson's disease: assessment of cardiac sympathetic denervation and diagnostic value. *Journal of Nuclear Medicine* 40, 371–75.

Schatz, I. J., Bannister, R., Freeman, R. L. *et al.* (1996). Consensus Statement on the definition of orthostatic hypotension, pure autonomic failure and multiple system atrophy. *Clin. Auton. Res.* 6, 125–26.

Schestatsky, P., Valls-Solé, J., Ehlers, J. A., Rieder, C. R. M., Gomes, I. (2006). Hyperhidrosis in Parkinson's disease. *Mov. Disord.* 21 (10), 1744–48.

Seif, C., Herzog, J., van der Horst, C. *et al.* (2004). Effect of subthalamic deep brain stimulation on the function of the urinary bladder. *Annali of Neurology* 55(1), 118–20.

Senard, J. M., Chamentin, B., Rascol, A., Montastruc, J. L. (1992). Ambulatory blood pressure in patients with Parkinson's disease without and with orthostatic hypotension. *Clin. Auton. Res.* 2, 99–104.

Senard, J. M., Rai, S., Lapeyre-Mestre, M. *et al.* (1997). Prevalence of orthostatic hypotension in Parkinson's disease. *JNNP* 63, 578–89.

Senard, J. M., Rascol, O., Durrieu, G. *et al.* (1993). Effects of Yohimbine on plasma catecholamine levels in orthostatic hypotension related to Parkinson's disease or multiple system atrophy. *Clinical Neuropharmacology* 16, 70–76.

Senard, J. M., Valet, P., Durrieu, G. *et al.* (1990). Adrenergic supersensitivity in parkinsonians with orthostatic hypotension. *European Journal of Clinical Investigation* 20, 613–619.

Shannon, J. R., Jordan, J., Diedrich, A. *et al.* (2010). Sympathetically mediated hypertension in autonomic failure. *Circulation* 101(23), 2710–5.

Siddiqui, M. F., Rast, S., Lynn, M. J., Auchus, A. P., Pfeiffer, R. F. (2002). Autonomic dysfunction in Parkinson's disease: a comprehensive symptom survey. *Parkinsonism Related Disorders* 8(4), 277–84.

Singaram, C., Ashraf, W., Gaumnitz, E. A., *et al.* (1995). Dopaminergic defect of enteric nervous system in Parkinson's disease patients with chronic constipation. *Lancet* 346, 861–64.

Singer, C., Weiner, W. J., Sanchez-Ramos, J. R. (1992). Autonomic dysfunction in men with Parkinson's disease. *European Neurology* 32(3), 134–40.

Sotolongo, J. R. (1988). Voiding dysfunction in Parkinson's disease. *Seminars in Neurology* 8(2), 166–69.

Spiegel, J., Hellwig, D., Farmakis, G. *et al.* (2007). Myocardial sympathetic degeneration correlates with clinical phenotype of Parkinson's disease. *Mov. Disord.* 22 (7), 1004–1008.

Stemper, B., Beric, A., Welsch, G., Haendl, T., Sterio, D., Hilz, M. J. (2006). Deep brain stimulation improves orthostatic regulation of patients with Parkinson disease. *Neurology* 67, 1781–85.

Stocchi, F., Carbone, A., Inghilleri, M. *et al.* (1997). Urodynamic and neurophysiological evaluation in Parkinson's disease and multiple system atrophy. *JNNP* 62(5), 507–511.

Takatsu, H., Nishida, H., Matsuo, H. *et al.* (2000). Cardiac sympathetic denervation from the early state of Parkinson's disease: clinical and experimental studies with radiolabeled MIBG. *Journal of Nuclear Medicine* 41, 71–77.

Tanner, C. M., Chhablani, R., Goetz, C. G., Klawans, H. L. (1985). Pergolide mesylate: lack of cardiac toxicity in patients with cardiac disease. *Neurology* 35, 918–21.

Tanner, C. M., Goetz, C. G., Glantz, R. H., Glatt, S. L., Klawans, H. L. (1982). Pergolide mesylate and idiopathic Parkinson disease. *Neurology* **32**, 1175–79.

Tanner, C. M., Goetz, C. G., Klawans, H. L. (1987). Autonomic nervous system disorders. In: Koller, W. C. ed. *Handbook of Parkinson's Disease*. Marcel Dekker, pp. 145–70.

Thomaides, T., Bleasdale-Barr, K., Chaudhuri, K. R., Pavitt, D. V., Marsden, C. D., Mathias, C. J. (1993). Cardiovascular and hormonal responses to liquid food challenge in idiopathic Parkinson's disease, multiple system atrophy and pure autonomic failure. *Neurology* **43**, 900–904.

Thomaides, T., Chaudhuri, K. R., Maule, S., Watson, L., Marsden, C. D., Mathias, C. J. (1992). The growth hormone response to clonidine in central and peripheral primary autonomic failure. *Lancet*, **340**, 263–66.

Tolosa, E., Compta, Y., Gaig, C. (2007). The premotor phase of Parkinson's disease. *Parkinsonism and Related Disorders* **13**, S2–S7.

Toth, M. J., Fishman, P. S., Poehlman, E. T. (1997). Free-living daily energy expenditure in patients with Parkinson's disease. *Neurology* **48**, 88–91.

Turkka, J., Suominen, K., Tolonen, U., Sotaniemi, K., Myllyla, V. V. (1997). Selegiline diminishes cardiovascular autonomic responses in Parkinson's disease. *Neurology* **48**, 662–67.

Turkka, J. T. (1987). Correlation of the severity of autonomic dysfunction to cardiovascular reflexes and to plasma noradrenaline levels in Parkinson's disease. *European Neurology* **26**, 203–210.

Turkka, J. T., Juujarvi, K. K., Lapinlampi, T. O., Myllyla, V. V. (1986). Serum noradrenaline response to standing up in patients with Parkinson's disease. *European Neurology* **25**, 355–61.

Turkka, J. T., Tolonen, U., Myllylav, V. (1987). Cardiovascular reflexes in Parkinson's disease. *European Neurology* **26**, 104–112.

Uc, E. Y., Struck, L. K., Rodnitzky, R. L., Zimmerman, B., Dobson, J., Evans, W. J. (2006). Predictors of weight loss in Parkinson's disease. *Mov. Disord.* **21** (7), 930–36.

Uono, Y. (1973). Parkinsonism and autonomic dysfunction. *Auton Nerv Syst (Tokyo)* **10**, 163–70.

Van Dijk, J. G., Haan, J., Zwinderman, K., Kremer, B., Van Hilten, B. J. and Roos, R. A. C. (1993). Autonomic nervous system dysfunction in Parkinson's disease: relationships with age, medication, duration and severity. *JNNP* **56**, 1090–95.

Verbaan, D., Marinus, J., Visser, M., van Rooden, S. M., Stiggelbout, A. M., van Hilten, J. J. (2007). Patient-reported autonomic symptoms in Parkinson disease. *Neurology* **69**, 333–41.

Villares, J. C. B., Carlini, E. A. (1989). Sebum secretion in idiopathic Parkinson's disease: effect of anticholinergic and dopaminergic drugs. *Acta Neurologica Scandiavica* **80**, 57–63.

Visser, M., Marinus, J., Stiggelbout, A. M., Van Hilten, J. J. (2004). Assessment of autonomic dysfunction in Parkinson's disease: the SCOPA-AUT. *Mov. Disord.* **19**(11), 1306–1312.

Vokatch, N., Grötzsch, H., Mermillod, B., Burkhard, P. R., Sztajzel, R. (2007). Is cerebral autoregulation impaired in Parkinson's disease? A transcranial Doppler study. *Journal of Neurological Sciences* **245**, 49–53.

Wakabayashi, K., Takahashi, H. (1997). Neuropathology of autonomic nervous system in Parkinson's disease. *European Neurology* **38**, 2–7.

Wakabayashi, K., Takahashi, H., Ohama, E., Ikuta, F. (1990). Parkinson's disease: an immunohistochemical study of Lewy-body containing neurons in the enteric nervous system. *Acta Neuropathologica* **79**, 581–83.

Wakabayashi, K., Takahashi, H., Ohama, E., Takeda, S., Ikuta, F. (1993). Lewy bodies in the visceral autonomic nervous system in Parkinson's disease. *Advances in Neurology* **60**, 609–612.

Wang, G. J., Volkow, N. D., Logan, J., *et al.* (2001). Brain dopamine and obesity. *Lancet* **357**, 354–57.

Wenning, G. K., Scherfler, C., Granata, R. *et al.* (1999). Time course of symptomatic orthostatic hypotension and urinary incontinence in patients with postmortem confirmed parkinsonian syndromes: a clinicopathological study. *JNNP* **67**(5), 620–23.

Wieling, W., van Lieshout, J. J., van Leeuwen, A. M. (1993). Physical manoeuvres that reduce postural hypotension. *Clin. Auton. Res.* **3**, 57–65.

Winge, K., Fowler, C. J. (2006). Bladder dysfunction in Parkinsonism: mechanism, prevalence, symptoms and management. *Mov. Disord.* **21**(6), 737–45.

Winge, K., Krøyer Nielsen, K., Stimpel, H., Lokkegaard, A., Rusborg Jensen, S., Werdelin, L. (2007). Lower urinary tract symptoms and bladder control in advanced Parkinson's disease: effect of deep brain stimulation in the subthalamic nucleus. *Mov. Disord.* **22** (2), 220–25.

Winge, K., Werdelin, L. M., Nielsen, K. K., Stimpel, H. (2004). Effects of dopaminergic treatment on bladder function in Parkinson's disease. *Neurourology and Urodynamics* **23**(7), 689–96.

Wintzen, M., Gilchrest, B. A. (1996). Proopiomelanocortin, its derived peptides, and the skin. *The Journal of Investigative Dermatology* **106**, 3–10.

Wszolek, Z. K. and Markopoulou, K. (1998). Olfactory dysfunction in Parkinson's disease. *Clin. Neurosci.* **5**, 94–101.

Wüllner, U., Schmitz-Hübsch, T., Antony, G. *et al.* (2007). Autonomic dysfunction in 3414 Parkinson's disease patients enrolled in the German Network on Parkinson's disease (KNP e.V.). *European Journal of Neurology*; Epub ahead of print;

Yael Manor, M. A., Giladi, N., Cohen, A., Fliss, D. M., Cohen, J. T. (2007). Validation of a swallowing disturbance questionnaire for detecting dysphagia in patients with Parkinson's disease. *Mov. Disord.* **22** (13), 1917–21.

Yahr, M. D. (1970). General discussion on clinical effects of l-dopa upon blood pressure. In: Barbeau A, McDowell FH eds. *L-dopa and parkinsonism*. Philadelphia, FA Davis, pp. 266–8;

Yoshita, M. (1998). Differentiation of idiopathic Parkinson's disease from striatonigral degeneration and progressive supranuclear palsy using iodine-123 and metaiodobenzylguanadine myocardial scintigraphy. *Journal of Neurological Science* **155**, 60–66.

Yoshita, M., Hayashi, M., Hirai, S. (1998). Decreased myocardial accumulation of 123I-metaiodobenzylguanidine in Parkinson's disease. *Nuclear Medicine Communications* **19**, 137–42.

Yu, M., Roane, D. M., Miner, C. R., Fleming, M., Rogers, J. D. (2004). Dimensions of sexual dysfunction in Parkinson disease. *American Journal of Geriatric Psychiatry* **12**(2), 221–26.

Zesiewicz, T. A., Sullivan, K. L., Arnulf, I., *et al.* (2010). Quality Standards Subcommittee of the American Academy of Neurology. Practice Parameter: treatment of nonmotor symptoms of Parkinson disease: report of the Quality Standards Subcommittee of the American Academy of Neurology. *Neurology* **74**, 924–31.

CHAPTER 46

Treatment of the motor disorders of multiple system atrophy

Uday Muthane and Andrew J. Lees

Introduction

Clinicopathological studies at the UK Parkinson's Disease Society Brain Research Centre at the Institute of Neurology, Queen Square, London have defined the clinical criteria of multiple system atrophy (MSA) (Ben Shlomo et al. 1995) and have improved the accuracy of diagnosing MSA during life (Gilman et al. 1998a). MSA presents as either autonomic failure, a motor disorder manifesting as parkinsonism, cerebellar ataxia or both. Studies from the UK suggest predominance of the parkinsonian phenotype (MSA-P) (Wenning et al. 1994) while studies from Japan report predominance of the cerebellar variety (MSA-C) (Watanabe et al. 2002).

At the bedside, the parkinsonian phenotype of MSA (MSA-P) resembles Parkinson's disease (PD) and distinguishing them clinically can be difficult (Wenning et al. 1994). Of the 370 brains of patients dying with a parkinsonian syndrome seen at the UK Parkinson's Disease Society Brain Research Centre up to 1992, 35 (9.5%) showed pathological changes of MSA. Twelve of these cases remained misdiagnosed as PD until their death and even retrospectively reviewing the case material it was impossible in 10 of these to diagnose MSA (Ben Shlomo et al. 1995). The clinical diagnosis of MSA is based on clinical criteria established using neuropathologically examined cases from the Queen Square Brain Bank for Neurological Disorders. A study comparing these two published criteria showed that application of either of the criteria was superior to the actual clinical diagnosis at the initial visit but there was little difference by the last visit (Osaki et al. 2002).

Clinical features suggesting an early diagnosis of MSA are: rigidity, autonomic dysfunction, and a poor initial response to L-dihydroxyphenylalanine (L-DOPA) with early motor fluctuations (Wenning et al. 2000). When at least two of these features occur, MSA can be diagnosed with a reasonable sensitivity (87%) and specificity (70.5%). The predictive value improves close to death when clinical features like speech or bulbar dysfunction, dysautonomia, poor response to L-DOPA, absence of L-DOPA induced confusion and falls are present. These features help diagnose MSA with high sensitivity (90.3%) and specificity (92.6%) MSA (Wenning et al. 2000). Treatment of MSA is mainly symptomatic and treating the motor disorder plays a key role in improving the patient's quality of life.

Treatment of the parkinsonian syndrome in multiple system atrophy

Most patients with MSA present with parkinsonism and are, therefore, frequently treated with L-DOPA. It is incorrect to believe that all MSA patients do not respond to L-DOPA. Early in the illness, some patients with MSA-P respond excellently to L-DOPA and, therefore, can be confused with PD (Wenning et al. 1994). The initial response to L-DOPA being poor is common in MSA-P (72%) compared with PD (12%) (Wenning et al. 2000). Acute challenge with oral L-DOPA or subcutaneous apomorphine is used in research and, occasionally, in a clinical setting to assess their dopaminergic responsiveness. This testing is also recommended as part of pre-surgical evaluation for PD (Langston et al. 1992) to exclude conditions like MSA where the response is often poor.

Acute challenges with oral L-DOPA or subcutaneous apomorphine to assess dopaminergic responsiveness

Acute dopaminergic challenge improves motor functions in pathologically confirmed and clinically suspected MSA patients (Hughes et al. 1992). A recent consensus statement (Albanese et al. 2001) reiterates the value of acute dopaminergic challenge using L-DOPA or apomorphine in the diagnosis and therapy of parkinsonian disorders and is incorporated in the guidelines for experimental studies on parkinsonian patients.

Assessing dopaminergic responsiveness in MSA is of limited diagnostic value but it is helpful to know the chances of improvement on long-term L-DOPA treatment.

In the apomorphine test, the peripheral dopamine receptor antagonist drug, domperidone, is given in a dose of 30 mg three times a day for at least 24 hours before apomorphine is given subcutaneously in a fasting state serially in doses of 1.5, 3.0, 4.5, and 7.0 mg. The test is continued until an unequivocal response occurs, intolerable side-effects are experienced, or the maximum dose is reached.

An acute challenge using apomorphine and L-DOPA improves nearly 25% of clinically definite MSA patients and, subsequently, these patients have a sustained improvement on L-DOPA therapy. Few patients had negative responses to acute challenges and failed to benefit from L-DOPA therapy. A further 8 patients with possible MSA were tested, 5 of whom had negative responses to the challenges and failed to respond to L-DOPA therapy. One had positive responses to both apomorphine and the L-DOPA test and responded well to chronic L-DOPA, and a further 2 patients had equivocal responses to both apomorphine and L-DOPA and subsequently responded to long-term L-DOPA therapy (Hughes et al. 1990). In contrast, Oertel and colleagues (1989) did not observe any clinical benefit following apomorphine administration in five clinically definite MSA patients. In another study evaluating the apomorphine and oral L-DOPA tests in 45 previously untreated patients with PD, 9 cases failed to respond either to an acute challenge or long-term L-DOPA therapy and one of them developed pyramidal signs and autonomic dysfunction in the 12 months of follow-up, suggesting a diagnosis of MSA. Parati et al. gave acute L-DOPA challenges to 8 clinically probable MSA cases and only 4 (50%) had a positive response (Parati et al. 1993). It has been our subjective impression that patients who turn out to have MSA tend to have more adverse events when challenged with L-DOPA or subcutaneous apomorphine in the early stages, and a profound drop of blood pressure with orthostatic symptoms is particularly suggestive of early MSA.

Hughes performed a meta-analysis of 340 parkinsonian patients who had undergone apomorphine test and suggests that this test has a greater role in assessing dopaminergic responsiveness than in improving the diagnosis. The test has 80% sensitivity and 96% positive predictive value to predict an L-DOPA response in *de novo* patients. However, the false-negative rate of 20% indicates that all newly diagnosed parkinsonian patients should undergo an adequate trial with levodopa (Hughes 1999).

The diagnostic accuracy of apomorphine test to differentiate PD (n = 83) was better than non-PD (MSA: 28, unclassified parkinsonism: 17) following acute challenges with oral L-DOPA/carbidopa (250/25 mg) and subcutaneous apomorphine (1.5, 3 and 4.5 mg). L-DOPA improved motor functions better than apomorphine and at least 18% improvement suggests the patient has PD rather than MSA. Apomorphine at 4.5 mg had the best degree of improvement. A good agreement exists between acute challenges with L-DOPA/carbidopa and apomorphine, using both tests improves the reliability to differentiate PD from MSA and has a good predictive value for subsequent improvement to chronic L-DOPA therapy (Rossi et al. 2000).

Acute L-DOPA challenge

Patient does not take dopaminergic drugs for 12 hours (practical 'off') and their motor response is assessed using timed tapping and walking tests at 15 minute intervals and four-point scales for tremor and dyskinesia after taking a single dose of L-DOPA/DOPA decarboxylase inhibitor (250/25 mg) in a fasting state (Langston et al. 1992). The motor benefit before and after taking L-DOPA is assessed using the Unified Parkinson's Disease Rating Scale (UPDRS).

While performing acute L-DOPA challenge to categorize a cohort of parkinsonian patients into PD and MSA-P and evaluate their motor response some patients develop symptomatic orthostatic hypotension (OH). Anecdotal cases are reported when a challenge with apomorphine (Bowron 2004) and the first dose of dopamine agonists cause OH in PD. However, a single parkinsonian patient with profound fall in blood pressure following an acute L-DOPA

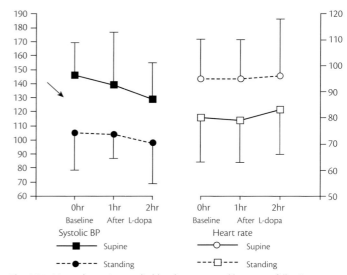

Fig. 46.1 Mean change in systolic blood pressure and heart rate following acute challenge with L-dihydroxyphenylalanine (L-DOPA) in the parkinsonian type of multiple system atrophy. The magnitude of baseline orthostatic hypotension is greater in MSA-P than in Parkinson's disease. Fall in systolic blood pressure occurs after an hour and lasts for more than 2 hours.

challenge actually had MSA-P (Mathias 2000). Merello et al. reported a sensitivity and specificity of acute L-DOPA challenge to predict clinical diagnosis of PD as 70.9% and 81.4%, respectively; positive predictive ratio was 88.6%. Their study indicates that a positive result of initial acute L-DOPA challenge predicts chronic L-DOPA responsiveness as major criterion of PD in all patients (Merello et al. 2002).

Acute L-DOPA challenge causes hypotension in lying position (PD: 28%, MSA-P: 26%) and in MSA this lasts for more than 2 hours (Fig. 46.1). Fall in supine blood pressure was more frequent in MSA-P (26%) than in PD (4.7%) and lasted for 3 hours in 4 patients. Acute L-DOPA challenge precipitated OH in 3 (10%) MSA patients and worsened pre-existing OH in 8 (26%) of them (Sarangmath et al. 2004).

Chronic treatment with dopaminergic drugs

Improving parkinsonian symptoms is the mainstay of treating the motor disorder of MSA.

L-DOPA

L-DOPA improves parkinsonian features in MSA. An initial significant improvement occurs with L-DOPA in 29% (Wenning et al. 1994) to 84% (Goetz et al. 1984) of MSA patients. This improvement, in some, lasts for nearly 10 years (Goetz et al. 1984). In 203 pathologically proven cases of MSA, L-DOPA administration resulted in a good or excellent response in 28% of patients and 27% developed dyskinesia (Wenning et al. 1997). This improvement occurs in younger patients (< 49 years of age) and is maintained in 13% of patients (Wenning et al. 1994). L-DOPA induced dyskinesia appear after 3.5+/-1.8 yrs (Goetz, Tanner, & Klawans 1984) and motor fluctuations (Lang et al. 1986).

L-DOPA-induced dyskinesia, in PD, commonly begins in the limbs; it is frequently choreiform and eventually spreads to become generalized. Contrary to this in MSA, these dyskinesia are dystonic and involve the face and neck region (Wenning et al. 1994). Unilateral facial dystonic spasms are particularly suggestive of MSA (Quinn 2006, Wenning et al. 1996) and can improve with botulinum toxin injections. In a recent review of therapeutic strategies in MSA, chronic L-DOPA treatment results in motor fluctuations in 14.8–60.6% and dyskinesia in 15–55% (Table 46.1). A prompt and marked improvement with L-DOPA is therefore infrequent in MSA, but could occur early in the illness. Even if L-DOPA improves parkinsonian signs in the initial stages, eventually as the disease progresses, the response is poor (Quinn 1994, Wenning et al. 1994, 1995).

All patients with MSA should receive an adequate trial of L-DOPA (with a DOPA-decarboxylase inhibitor) by gradually increasing doses of at least 1 g/day of L-DOPA for a period of 3 months to determine if they improve (Gilman et al. 1998b). High doses of levodopa were not neurotoxic in a transgenic MSA mouse model with oligodendroglial alpha-synuclein inclusions, behavioural and neuropathological indices (Stefanova et al. 2007). Starting one pill of carbidopa/L-DOPA (25/100) and gradually increasing it once in 3 days, depending on the patient's tolerance, eventually to 2 pills three times a day helps reaching the required dose. Optimization of parkinsonian symptoms in MSA is crucial as they are disabling, but this is limited by L-DOPA precipitating and worsening pre-existing postural hypotension in 39% of patients (Wenning et al. 1994). Nevertheless, it is worth trying to treat OH by using different strategies and medications while attempting to verify if L-DOPA is helpful.

Treating with L-DOPA often induces sleepiness in MSA compared with PD. L-DOPA causes excessive daytime drowsiness, including sleep episodes while driving. The exact cause for this is not known but is believed this is due to more widespread pathology in the pedunculopontine nucleus, locus coeruleus and dorsal raphe nucleus in MSA compared with PD (Seppi et al. 2006).

Amantadine

Open-label use of amantadine had caused improvement in MSA patients, thus Wenning et al. (2005) conducted a double-blind, placebo-controlled crossover trial of amantadine in 8 patients with MSA. Amantadine did not produce a clinically significant antiparkinsonian effect, but as this study had few patients it is difficult to make firm conclusions (Wenning 2005). It is possible that amantadine does have a mild antiparkinsonian effect in MSA.

Dopamine agonists

Results with the dopamine agonists have been even more disappointing. Goetz and colleagues using doses of 10–80 mg daily of bromocriptine, reported benefit in 5 patients who had responded to L-DOPA and 1 patient who had failed to respond to L-DOPA (Goetz et al. 1984). Williams et al. (1979) also reported temporary benefit in an occasional patient; others, however, have had more disappointing results (Williams et al. 1979). Gautier and Durand (1977) in a controlled trial with lisuride (mean dose 2.4 mg daily), found that only 1 of 7 patients with MSA and autonomic failure had improvement in parkinsonian features and another, who had been deriving considerable benefit from L-DOPA before the study began, failed to respond at all to large doses of lisuride (Gautier and Durand 1977). Severe psychiatric side-effects occurred in 6 patients on lisuride, with nightmares, isolated visual hallucinations, and toxic confusional states (Lees and Bannister 1981). Wenning et al. (1994) reported a response to oral dopamine agonists in 4 of 46 patients. None of 30 patients receiving bromocriptine improved, but 3 of 10 who received pergolide had some benefit.

Table 46.1 Therapeutic effects of L-DOPA in parkinsonian type of multiple system atrophy

Reference	Treated cases (n)	P/M confirmed (n)	Mean L-DOPA dose (mg/day)	Motor benefit n (%)*	Motor fluctuations (%)	Dyskinesias (%)	Adverse effects (n)
Goetz et al. (1984)	19	1	NA (up to 3000)	16 (84)	NA	52	12 (SD, 7; H, 5)
Fearnley and Lees (1990)	10	10	NA (range: 341–924)	4 (40)	20	40	4 (OH, 2; NV, 1; H, 1)
Rajput et al. (1990)	6	6	NA (at least 1500)	2 (33)	NA	NA	NA
Staal et al. (1990)	27	2	NA	8 (30)	14.8	NA	4 (AP)
Hughes et al. (1992)	20	20	580	15 (75)	55	55	NA
Wenning et al. (1994)	78	14	300–600	30 (40)	NA	21.7	34 (OH, 29; C, 5)
Albanese et al. (2001)	20	NA	750 or 800	12 (60)	NA	NA	NA
Colosimo et al. (1995)	16	16	NA (>800)	11 (67)	NA	NA	NA
Gouider-Khouja et al. (1995)	18	NA	>750	0 (0)	NA	44.5	NA
Wenning et al. (1995)	33	33	NA	15 (45)	60.6	51.5	7 (C, 3; H, 2; N, 2)
Wenning et al. (1997)	NA	all	NA	NA	NA	NA	NA
Testa et al. (2001)	67	NA	NA	53 (79)	NA	NA	NA
Boesch et al. (2002)	24	5	NA (up to 1200)	15 (63)	20.8	50	NA
EMSA-SG, unpublished data (Wenning et al. 2005)	216	NA	686	89 (41)	19.4	15.2	NA

Only reports/studies with a more than or equal to 6 patients are considered; acute L-DOPA challenge tests are excluded.
* Benefit: at least moderate response.
AP, acute psychosis; C, confusion; EMSA-SG, European MSA-Study Group; H, hallucinations; L-DOPA, L-3,4-dihydroxyphenylalanine; n, number; N, nightmares; NA, not available; NV, nausea or vomiting; OH, orthostatic hypotension; P/M, post-mortem; SD, sleep disruption.
(Modified from Wenning 2005, Wenning et al. 2005)

Of the l-DOPA responders, 22% (2 of 9) had good or excellent response to at least one orally active dopamine agonist (Wenning et al. 1994).

Serotonergic drugs

Friess et al. evaluated the role of paroxetine, a selective serotonin reuptake inhibitor, on the motor symptoms in a small number of MSA patients who were randomly assigned to either paroxetine (n = 11) or placebo (n = 9) on the basis that serotonin modulates dopaminergic transmission in the basal ganglia. Paroxetine marginally improved limb agility and speech but the cerebellar signs did not improve. This study shows the possible role of modulating non-dopaminergic systems in improving motor deficits in MSA (Friess et al. 2006).

Treatment of focal dystonia

Boesch (2002) reported dystonia in 46% of l-DOPA naive MSA patients at the first neurological visit (Boesch et al. 2002). Antecollis was present in 6 patients (25%) and unilateral limb dystonia in 5 patients (21%). l-DOPA initially improved this in MSA-P patients but not in MSA-C. MSA-P patients developed l-DOPA-induced dyskinesias after 2.3 years (range 0.5–4) and in most the dystonia was craniocervical dystonia, although some developed limb or generalized dystonia. Bruxism in a patient with MSA improved with low doses of l-DOPA/carbidopa (Wali 2004). Botulinum toxin can be used to treat antecollis and orofacial dystonia with lower lip retraction associated with MSA (Muller et al. 2002). However, injections of botulinum toxin to treat cervical dystonia in MSA should be used cautiously as one patient developed prolonged dysphagia lasting for nearly 4 months (Thobois et al. 2001). Laryngeal stridor in MSA is due to dystonia, and injections of botulinum toxin into the vocalis muscle can improve this disabling symptom (Merlo et al. 2002). Injections of botulinum toxin can be used to treat cricopharyngeal dystonia that causes dysphagia in MSA patients.

Restless leg syndrome

Recently, rapid eye movement (REM)-induced sleep behaviour disorder (RBD) is considered as the prodrome of MSA (Montplaisir 2004). MSA patients commonly have sleep disorders and Vetrugno et al. (2004) in a series of 19 patients reported that all snored, 42% had stridor, and 37% had an obstructive sleep apnoea syndrome. The oxygen saturation varies considerably in MSA patients while they are asleep. All these patients had RBD, and 88% had periodic limb movements during sleep (PLMS) (Wetter et al. 2000). These sleep disorders are also present in untreated PD patients and could be due to dopaminergic deficiency rather than due to dopaminergic treatment (Vetrugno et al. 2004). RLS and RBD improve with ropinirole or l-DOPA given at bedtime, and using drugs before going to sleep might improve difficulty in turning in bed (Trenkwalder et al. 2005, Bogan et al. 2006).

Treatment of cerebellar symptoms

Patients with MSA can present as sporadic ataxia; this clinical presentation is the most common in the Japanese (Watanabe et al. 2002). Within the large group of 'idiopathic' late-onset cerebellar ataxia are patients with sporadic olivopontocerebellar atrophy who have striking cerebellar signs as their major disability. Some of these patients—but by no means all—go on to develop autonomic failure and mild parkinsonism.

Treatment of cerebellar signs remains disappointing and as yet there is no effective management of cerebellar ataxia in MSA. Adding clonazepam, 0.5 mg at bedtime, increasing to 1 mg may improve action tremor (Wenning et al. 2005).

Functional surgery in multiple system atrophy

Preoperative evaluation of parkinsonian patients before lesioning or deep brain stimulation (DBS) involves re-confirming the clinical diagnosis is PD. This is crucial as results are best in patients with PD. Posteroventral pallidotomy in three MSA patients had marginal or little benefit (Pereira et al. 2004). Neuronal firing in the globus pallidum interna (GPi) is low in MSA-P but high in PD, and this could be a reason for a poor therapeutic response in MSA-P. However, GPi firing rate alone might not be a determinant of a good response to surgery in parkinsonian patients with PD (Dostrovsky et al. 2003).

Another patient diagnosed as MSA as she had early falls, rapid progression, stridor, and cortical myoclonus together with magnetic resonance imaging (MRI) showing mild cerebellar and brainstem atrophy, underwent bilateral pallidal DBS as she was l-DOPA responsive and had severe generalized peak-dose dyskinesia. Pallidal stimulation in this patient reduced rigidity and l-DOPA-induced dyskinesia lasting for 15 months. Bilateral pallidal stimulation resulted in improvement of dystonia involving the neck, trunk, eyes, and larynx in a patient with MSA but resulted in worsening his slowness and anarthria (Santens et al. 2006).

Few l-DOPA-responsive MSA patients underwent subthalamic nucleus (STN) DBS and the diagnosis of MSA was known only at follow-up or autopsy. An important reason for poor or suboptimal responses to DBS is MSA being misdiagnosed as PD due to a good response to l-DOPA. When 41 patients reporting suboptimal responses following DBS from two movement disorder centres were retrospectively analysed, there were two MSA patients who were misdiagnosed as PD despite being screened by movement disorder specialists (Okun et al. 2005). Thus, even l-DOPA-responsive MSA patients might not improve with DBS (Chou et al. 2004, Huang et al. 2005).

Nevertheless, STN DBS has helped improve motor symptoms in l-DOPA-responsive MSA patients. Tarsy et al. (2003) reported improvement of l-DOPA-responsive upper extremity slowness but worsening of speech, swallowing, and gait following bilateral STN DBS. This symptomatic improvement can last for short periods (Lezcano et al. 2004, Visser-Vandewalle et al. 2003), and long-term in an occasional patient (Visser-Vandewalle et al. 2003).

The poor results of pallidotomy and DBS in MSA patients suggest that motor symptoms of MSA possibly involve different parts than in PD. A recent review of DBS in MSA reports that almost all authors report functionally limiting dysphagia, dysarthria, postural instability, and death from respiratory failure within 7 months of surgery (Shih and Tarsy 2007). Thus, DBS is best avoided in patients with MSA, but can be used to treat the few patients who improve with l-DOPA and develop disabling l-DOPA dyskinesia.

Neural transplantation

Neural transplantation aims to improve functional deficits by replacing lost nigral neurons and possibly effecting a change in the striatal circuitry. Wenning et al. (2000) suggest that embryonic mesencephalic grafts alone or in combination with striatal grafts can partially reverse drug-induced rotation asymmetries without improving deficits of complex motor function in animal studies (Wenning et al. 2000d). Shocke et al. (2000) produced lesions in the striatum and nigra by injecting 3-nitropropionic acid in a rat model. They showed that in these animals, the sensitivity of detecting mesencephalic and striatal grafts was 100% on T1- and T2-weighted MRI. Puschban et al. (2000b) showed that embryonic striatal grafts failed to protect against striatal quinolinic acid (QA)-induced excitotoxicity in a previously established double lesion rat model of striatonigral degeneration. These authors show that striatal grafts implanted into host striatum before lesions are made using excitotoxins were unable to protect in the presence of severe dopaminergic denervation. These studies show that neural transplantation in experimental models of MSA has little promise, and further studies are required before they can be used in humans. Recently, Puschban et al. (2000a) reported survival of embryonic mesencephalic grafts in an experimental model. The surviving dopaminergic neurons had re-innervated the adult striatum and improved rotation behaviour in the graft group. This study suggests a possibility that embryonic transplantation might be a therapeutic intervention in patients with early MSA having mild parkinsonism (Puschban et al. 2000a). However, in light of the results of fetal nigral transplants in two human PD studies, it is necessary to be cautious and use a systematic approach to study their role in MSA.

Recently, Lee et al. (2007) injected mesenchymal stem cells intra-arterially in 11 MSA patients. This resulted in improvement of the Unified MSA rating scale scores as compared with control, non-injected MSA patients lasting for at least 12 months. Patients injected with stem cells had significantly reduced orthostasis and cerebellar dysfunction. This clinical improvement was also accompanied by improvement on serial positron emission tomography scan in the cerebellum and frontal white matter in the group treated with mesenchymal stem cells. None of the patients had any serious adverse effects. This preliminary study shows that mesenchymal stem cell therapy is safe and delayed the progression of neurological deficits with achievement of functional improvement in the follow-up period in patients with MSA (Lee et al. 2007). It will be important to compare results of injecting stem cells with effects of fetal transplantation to determine if stem cells provide a better option in treating this disease.

References

Albanese A., Bonuccelli U., Christine B. K., Chaudhuri R., Colosimo C., Tobias E., Melamed E., Pierre P., Teus V. L., Zappia M. (2001). Consensus statement on the role of acute dopaminergic challenge in Parkinson's disease. *Movement Disorders* 16: 197–201.

Ben Shlomo, Y., Magalhaes, M., Daniel, S. E., Quinn, N. P. (1995). Clinicopathological study of 35 cases of multiple system atrophy. *J. Neurol. Neurosurg. Psychiat* 58 (160): 166.

Boesch, S. M., Wenning, G. K., Ransmayr, G., Poewe, W. (2002). Dystonia in multiple system atrophy. *J Neurol Neurosurg. Psychiatry.* 72(3): 300–303.

Bogan, R. K., Fry, J. M., Schmidt, M. H., Carson, S. W., Ritchie, S. Y. (2006). Ropinirole in the treatment of patients with restless legs syndrome: a US-based randomized, double-blind, placebo-controlled clinical trial. *Mayo Clin Proc.* 81 (1): 17–27.

Bowron, A. (2004). Practical considerations in the use of apomorphine injectable, *Neurology* 62(6) Suppl 4, S32–36.

Chou, K. L., Forman, M. S., Trojanowski, J. Q., Hurtig, H. I., & Baltuch, G. H. (2004). 'Subthalamic nucleus deep brain stimulation in a patient with levodopa-responsive multiple system atrophy. Case report', *J Neurosurg.* 100(3), 553–56.

Colosimo, C., Albanese, A., Hughes, A. J., de Bruin, V. M., & Lees, A. J. (1995), Some specific clinical features differentiate multiple system atrophy (striatonigral variety) from Parkinson's disease', *Arch Neurol* 52(3), 294–98.

Dostrovsky, J. O., Tang, J., Lozano, A. M., & Hutchison, W. D. (2003). *Altered pattern of neuronal firing in pallidal neurons in Huntington's and Parkinson's disease patients.* Society for Neuroscience; 2003.Washington, DC. (Abstract)

Fearnley, J. M. & Lees, A. J. (1990). Striatonigral degeneration. A clinicopathological study. *Brain*, 113, 1823–42.

Friess, E., Kuempfel, T., Modell, S., Winkelmann, J., Holsboer, F., Ising, M., & Trenkwalder, C. (2006). Paroxetine treatment improves motor symptoms in patients with multiple system atrophy. *Parkinsonism. Relat Disord.*, 12(7), 432–37.

Gautier, J.-C. & Durand, J. P. (1977), Traitement des syndromes parkinsonien par la bromocriptine, *Nouv. Presse Med.*, 6(3), 171–74.

Gilman, S., Low, P., Quinn, N., *et al.* (1998). Consensus statement on the diagnosis of multiple system atrophy. American Autonomic Society and American Academy of Neurology. *Clin Auton. Res.*, 8(6), 359–62.

Goetz, C. G., Tanner, C. M., & Klawans, H. L. (1984). The pharmacology of olivopontocerebellar atrophy. *Adv. Neurol.*, 41, 143–8.

Gouider-Khouja, N., Vidailhet, M., Bonnet, A. M., Pichon, J., & Agid, Y. (1995). "Pure" striatonigral degeneration and Parkinson's disease: a comparative clinical study. *Mov Disord.*, 10(3), 288–94.

Huang, Y., Garrick, R., Cook, R., O'Sullivan, D., Morris, J., & Halliday, G. M. 2005, Pallidal stimulation reduces treatment-induced dyskinesias in "minimal-change" multiple system atrophy, *Mov Disord.* 20(8), 1042–47.

Hughes, A. J. (1999). Apomorphine test in the assessment of parkinsonian patients: a meta-analysis. *Adv.Neurol.*, 80, 363–8.

Hughes, A. J., Lees, A. J., & Stern, G. M. (1990). Apomorphine test to predict dopaminergic responsiveness in Parkinsonian syndrome. *Lancet*, 335(32).

Hughes, A. J., Colosimo, C., Kleedorfer, B., Daniel, S. E., and Lees, A. J. (1992). The dopaminergic response in multiple system atrophy., *JNNP*, 55, 1009–1013.

Lang, A. E., Birnbaum, A., Blair, R. D., & Kierans, C. (1986). Levodopa dose-related fluctuations in presumed olivopontocerebellar atrophy. *Mov Disord.*, 1(2), 93–102.

Langston, J. W., Widner, H., Goetz, C. G., Brooks, D. J., Fahn, S., & Watts, R. (1992). Core assesment program for intracerebral transplantations (CAPITT). *Movement Disorders.*, 7, 2–13.

Lee, P. H., Kim, J. W., Bang, O. Y., Ahn, Y. H., Joo, I. S., & Huh, K. (2007). Autologous mesenchymal stem cell therapy delays the progression of neurological deficits in patients with multiple system atrophy', *Clin Pharmacol.Ther.*, vol.

Lees, A. J. & Bannister, R. (1981). The use of lisuride in the treatment of multiple system atrophy with autonomic failure (Shy-Drager syndrome). *J Neurol Neurosurg.Psychiatry.*, 44(4), 347–51.

Lezcano, E., Gomez-Esteban, J. C., Zarranz, J. J., *et al.* (2004). 'Parkinson's disease-like presentation of multiple system atrophy with poor response to STN stimulation: a clinicopathological case report', *Mov Disord.*, 19(8), 973–77.

Mathias, C. J. (2000). Autonomic dysfunction and the elderly. In: *Oxford Textbook of Geriatric medicine*, 2nd edn, Sir John Grimley Evans, ed., Oxford University Press, Oxford, pp. 833–52.

Merello, M., Nouzeilles, M. I., Arce, G. P., & Leiguarda, R. (2002). Accuracy of acute levodopa challenge for clinical prediction of sustained long-term levodopa response as a major criterion for idiopathic Parkinson's disease diagnosis. *Mov Disord.*, 17(4), 795–98.

Merlo, I. M., Occhini, A., Pacchetti, C., & Alfonsi, E. (2002). Not paralysis, but dystonia causes stridor in multiple system atrophy. *Neurology.*, 58(4), 649–52.

Montplaisir, J. (2004). Abnormal motor behavior during sleep. *Sleep Med.*, 5 Suppl 1:S31–4.

Muller, J., Wenning, G. K., Wissel, J., Seppi, K., & Poewe, W. (2002). Botulinum toxin treatment in atypical parkinsonian disorders associated with disabling focal dystonia. *J Neurol.*, 249(3), 300–304.

Oertel, W. H., Gasser, T., Ippisch, R., Trenkwalder, C., & Poewe, W. (1989). Apomorphine test for dopaminergic responsiveness. *Lancet*, ii, 1261–62.

Okun, M. S., Tagliati, M., Pourfar, M., Fernandez, H. H., Rodriguez, R. L., Alterman, R. L., & Foote, K. D. (2005). Management of referred deep brain stimulation failures: a retrospective analysis from 2 movement disorders centers. *Archives of Neurology*, 62(8), 1250–55.

Osaki, Y., Ben-Shlomo, Y., Wenning, G. K., et al. (2002). Do published criteria improve clinical diagnostic accuracy in multiple system atrophy? *Neurology*, 59(1486), 1491.

Parati, E. A., Fetoni, V., Geminiani, G. C., et al. (1993), Response to L-DOPA in multiple system atrophy. *Clin. Neuropharmacol.*, 16(2), 139–44.

Pereira, L. C., Palter, V. N., Lang, A. E., Hutchison, W. D., Lozano, A. M., & Dostrovsky, J. O. 2004, 'Neuronal activity in the globus pallidus of multiple system atrophy patients', *Mov Disord.*, 19(12), 1485–92.

Puschban, Z., Scherfler, C., Granata, R., et al. (2000a). Autoradiographic study of striatal dopamine re-uptake sites and dopamine D1 and D2 receptors in a 6-hydroxydopamine and quinolinic acid double-lesion rat model of striatonigral degeneration (multiple system atrophy) and effects of embryonic ventral mesencephalic, striatal or co-grafts. *Neuroscience.*, 95(2), 377–88.

Puschban, Z., Waldner, R., Seppi, K., et al. (2000b). Failure of neuroprotection by embryonic striatal grafts in a double lesion rat model of striatonigral degeneration (multiple system atrophy). *Exp. Neurol.*, 164(1), 166–75.

Quinn, N. (1994). Multiple system atrophy. In: *Movement Disorders*, 3rd edn, C. D. Marsden & S. Fahn, eds, Butterworth-Heinemann, London, pp. 262–81.

Quinn, N. (2006). Unilateral facial dystonia in multiple system atrophy. *Mov Disord* 7 (Suppl. 1), 79. 2006. (Abstract)

Rajput, A. H., Rozdilsky, B., Rajput, A., & Ang, L. (1990). Levodopa efficacy and pathological basis of Parkinson syndrome. *Clin Neuropharmacol.*, 13(6), 553–58.

Rossi, P., Colosimo, C., Moro, E., Tonali, P., & Albanese, A. (2000). Acute challenge with apomorphine and levodopa in Parkinsonism', *Eur. Neurol.*, 43(2), 95–101.

Santens, P., Vonck, K., De Letter, M., et al. (2006). Deep brain stimulation of the internal pallidum in multiple system atrophy. *Parkinsonism.Relat Disord.*, 12(3), 181–83.

Sarangmath, N., Dodaballapur, S. K., Mathias, C. J., & Muthane, U. B. (2004). Levodopa-induced hypotensionin multiple system atrophy and Parkinson's disease: Characteristics and factors that predict its occurrence. *Movement Disorders* 19[Suppl. 9], S334. (Abstract)

Schocke, M. F., Waldner, R., Puschban, Z., et al. (2000). In vivo magnetic resonance imaging of embryonic neural grafts in a rat model of striatonigral degeneration (multiple system atrophy). *Neuroimage.*, 12(2), 209–218.

Seppi, K., Hogl, B., Diem, A., Peralta, C., Wenning, G. K., & Poewe, W. (2006). Levodopa-induced sleepiness in the Parkinson variant of multiple system atrophy. *Mov Disord.*, 21(8), 1281–83.

Shih, L. C. & Tarsy, D. (2007). Deep brain stimulation for the treatment of atypical parkinsonism. *Mov Disord*, in press.

Staal, A., Meerwaldt, J. D., van Dongen, K. J., Mulder, P. G., & Busch, H. F. (1990). Non-familial degenerative disease and atrophy of brainstem and cerebellum. Clinical and CT data in 47 patients. *J Neurol Sci.*, 95(3), 259–69.

Stefanova, N., Kollensperger, M., Hainzer, M., Cenci, A., Poewe, W., & Wenning, G. K. (2007). High dose levodopa therapy is not toxic in multiple system atrophy: experimental evidence. *Mov Disord.*, 22(7), 969–73.

Testa, D., Monza, D., Ferrarini, M., Soliveri, P., Girotti, F., & Filippini, G. (2001). Comparison of natural histories of progressive supranuclear palsy and multiple system atrophy. *Neurol Sci.*, 22(3), 247–51.

Thobois, S., Broussolle, E., Toureille, L., & Vial, C. (2001). 'Severe dysphagia after botulinum toxin injection for cervical dystonia in multiple system atrophy', *Mov Disord.*, 16(4), 764–65.

Trenkwalder, C., Paulus, W., & Walters, A. S. (2005). The restless legs syndrome. *Lancet Neurol.*, 4(8), 465–75.

Vetrugno, R., Provini, F., Cortelli, P., et al. (2004). Sleep disorders in multiple system atrophy: a correlative video-polysomnographic study. *Sleep Med.*, 5(1), 21–30.

Visser-Vandewalle, V., Temel, Y., Colle, H., & van der, L. C. (2003). Bilateral high-frequency stimulation of the subthalamic nucleus in patients with multiple system atrophy—parkinsonism. Report of four cases. *J Neurosurg.*, 98(4), 882–87.

Wali, G. M. (2004). Asymmetrical awake bruxism associated with multiple system atrophy. *Mov Disord.*, 19(3), 352–55.

Watanabe, H., Saito, Y., Terao, S., et al. (2002). Progression and prognosis in multiple system atrophy: an analysis of 230 Japanese patients, *Brain*, 125(5), 1070–83.

Wenning, G. K. (2005). Placebo-controlled trial of amantadine in multiple-system atrophy. *Clin Neuropharmacol.*, 28(5), 225–27.

Wenning, G. K., Ben Shlomo, Y., Hughes, A., Daniel, S. E., Lees, A., & Quinn, N. P. (2000). What clinical features are most useful to distinguish definite multiple system atrophy from Parkinson's disease? *J Neurol Neurosurg.Psychiatry*, 68(4), 434–40.

Wenning, G. K., Ben Shlomo, Y., Magalhaes, M., Daniel, S. E., & Quinn, N. P. (1994). Clinical features and natural history of multiple system atrophy: An analysis of 100 cases. *Brain*, 117(835), 845.

Wenning, G. K., Ben Shlomo, Y., Magalhaes, M., Daniel, S. E., & Quinn, N. P. (1995). Clinicopathological study of 35 cases of multiple system atrophy. *J. Neurol. Neurosurg. Psychiatry*, 58(2), 160–66.

Wenning, G. K., Geser, F., & Poewe, W. (2005). Therapeutic strategies in multiple system atrophy. *Mov Disord.*, 20 Suppl 12:S67–76.

Wenning, G. K., Quinn, N. P., Daniel, S. E., Garratt, H., & Marsden, C. D. (1996). Facial dystonia in pathologically proven multiple system atrophy: a video report. *Mov Disord.*, 11(1), 107–109.

Wenning, G. K., Tison, F., Ben Shlomo, Y., Daniel, S. E., & Quinn, N. P. (1997). Multiple system atrophy: a review of 203 pathologically proven cases. *Mov Disord.*, 12(2), 133–47.

Wenning, G. K., Tison, F., Scherfler, C., et al. (2000d). Towards neurotransplantation in multiple system atrophy: clinical rationale, pathophysiological basis, and preliminary experimental evidence. *Cell Transplant.*, 9(2), 279–88.

Wetter, T. C., Collado-Seidel, V., Pollmacher, T., Yassouridis, A., & Trenkwalder, C. (2000). Sleep and periodic leg movement patterns in drug-free patients with Parkinson's disease and multiple system atrophy. *Sleep.*, 23(3), 361–67.

Williams, A. C., Nutt, J., & Lakes, C. R. (1979). Actions of bromocriptine in the Shy–Drager and Steele–Richardson–Olszewski syndromes. In: *Dopaminergic ergots and motor control*, K. Fuxe & D. B. Calne, eds, Pergamon Press, Oxford, pp. 271–83.

CHAPTER 47

Treatment of orthostatic hypotension

Christopher J. Mathias, Valeria Iodice,
David A. Low and Roger Bannister

General principles

The treatment of postural (orthostatic) hypotension due to autonomic failure is fraught with difficulties, many caused by inaccurate localization of the sites of the lesions. Treatment requires targeting; as Ehrlich commented on chemotherapy, 'we must learn to aim and aim in a chemical sense'. In autonomic failure, treatment has to be directed to overcoming precisely identified defects. This chapter focuses on the management of orthostatic hypotension (OH) due to primary autonomic failure, but many of the principles outlined here are applicable to postural hypotension due to other causes.

In secondary autonomic failure there may be special factors, which are covered in other chapters. Some examples of these include:

◆ insulin affecting postural hypotension in diabetes (Chapter 53)

◆ difficulties in managing postural hypotension in tetraplegics, as pressor drugs can lead to severe hypertension (Chapter 66)

◆ the aggravating effects of hypoalbuminaemia due to protein loss in amyloidosis, making treatment with fludrocortisone very difficult

◆ the successful treatment of postural hypotension in dopamine-beta-hydroxylase deficiency, with the replacement prodrug, dihydroxyphenylserine (Chapter 49).

Some principles of management are common to all patients.

Cerebral blood flow

It is important not to be over concerned about a low standing blood pressure if the patient is without symptoms. Some patients can tolerate a standing systolic blood pressure (SBP) as low as 70 mmHg without dizziness or syncope, probably because cerebral blood flow is maintained at an adequate level because of the capacity of the cerebral circulation for autoregulation. Several studies have attempted to clarify whether in autonomic failure there is a reduced fall of cerebral blood flow for a standard fall of mean arterial pressure. In five patients with multiple system atrophy (MSA), autoregulation was preserved down to a SBP close to 60 mmHg which is well below the 80 mmHg at which autoregulation fails in

normal subjects (Thomas and Bannister 1980). Results in a further three patients with pure autonomic failure (PAF) showed a similar trend. A shift of autoregulation to the left in autonomic failure almost certainly occurs and the reason some have failed to record it is probably that, when cerebral blood flow was measured during tilt, the arterial pressure may have been transiently much lower than the recorded pressure. There was evidence of this in one patient with autonomic failure who developed symptoms of cerebral ischaemia when his systolic pressure fell transiently to 40 mmHg and the clearance curve changed (Fig. 47.1), implying a transient fall in flow (Thomas and Bannister 1980). The change in autoregulation may be the result of prolonged exposure to lower than normal arterial pressure, causing some changes in the response of normally innervated vessels, or because cerebral vessels are partially or completely sympathectomized in autonomic failure. It has been suggested that the major sympathetic innervation is to the extraparenchymal vessels, the intraparenchymal vessels being under myogenic and metabolic control. If this is so, the sympathetic innervation at the lower level of autoregulation may normally reduce cerebral blood flow by constricting extraparenchymal vessels. Whatever the explanation, it is certain that patients with autonomic failure have a remarkable tolerance to low blood pressure without developing postural hypotensive symptoms. Studies of the cerebral circulation with continuous measurements using the non-invasive technique of near-infrared (NIR) spectroscopy have provided further information. Patients with MSA and presyncopal symptoms have marked ScO_2 (an index of arterial O_2 saturation) reduction during tilting, whereas those without presyncopal symptoms did not, and cerebral autoregulation was preserved (Asahina et al. 2006, Pavy-Le Traon et al. 2006, Hunt et al. 2006). There was a marked reduction in cerebral oxygenation when BP fell below the lower limit of cerebral autoregulation (SBP <80 mmHg). These observations suggest that prominent ScO_2 reductions are related to orthostatic symptoms and ScO_2 monitoring may be useful to detect cerebral hypoperfusion in autonomic failure (Suzuki et al. 2008). NIR spectroscopy confirms impaired cardiovascular and cerebrovascular responses to postural change in PAF patients and provides a template for investigating the rate of change of systemic blood pressure, cerebral oxygenation and

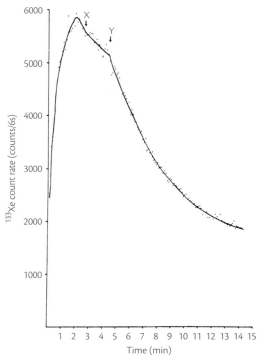

Fig. 47.1 Cerebral ^{133}Xe count rates/6 seconds in patient G. K. with pure autonomic failure tilted to 45°. At point X, the blood pressure fell suddenly to a systolic pressure of 40 mmHg. The rate of ^{133}Xe clearance decreased and the patient developed symptoms of cerebral ischaemia. At point Y, the tilt table was lowered, blood pressure rose, and the rate of clearance increased. From Thomas and Bannister 1980, with permission.

haemodynamics in response to head-up tilt in such patients (Tachtsidis et al. 2005).

Recumbent (supine) hypertension

A second principle that has to be considered in treatment is the tendency of patients with autonomic failure to develop recumbent hypertension owing principally to defective baroreceptor reflexes, supersensitivity, and treatment with drugs such as fludrocortisone. Clearly, this may result in a reactive increase of cerebrovascular resistance, leading to the likelihood of cerebral ischaemic symptoms when such patients stand suddenly. Some patients, if nursed lying flat, may develop severe hypertension and run the risk of developing complications such as papilloedema, other features of hypertensive retinopathy, and cerebral haemorrhage. Supine hypertension in PAF has been associated with left ventricular hypertrophy (Vagaonescu et al. 2000, Maule et al. 2006) and end-organ damage in the kidney associated with anaemia and low plasma renin activity (Garland et al. 2009).

There is concern about using antihypotensive agents in such patients. Nocturnal antihypertensive therapy has been suggested but this has potential dangers in patients who often have nocturia and thus run undue risks from hypotension if they need to arise from bed to empty their bladder at night. Clonidine appears to reduce blood pressure and nocturnal natriuresis in patients with supine hypertension and autonomic failure (Shibao et al. 2006). There is no improvement in orthostatic tolerance in the morning raising the possibility of residual hypotensive effects even in the morning.

Yohimbine in the morning to counteract any residual effect of clonidine has been suggested (Shibao et al. 2006).

More information on the effects of the treatment will emerge from 24-hour blood pressure monitoring, as in the case of the peptide release inhibitor octreotide that reduces postprandial and postural hypotension but does not increase nocturnal hypertension (Alam et al. 1995). The hypotensive effects of food could be utilized to reduce supine hypertension in autonomic failure as noted in a subject with gastrostomy feeding (Young and Mathias 2008)

Control of blood volume

A third principle is that, although loss of baroreflexes determines the immediate response of blood pressure to standing, control of blood volume is the long-term and more important adjustment to postural hypotension in autonomic failure. Blood volume is influenced by various factors, including low-pressure receptors, the kidney and various hormones such as antidiuretic hormone, atrial natriuretic peptides, and the renin–angiotensin–aldosterone system.

Limitations of treatment

All methods of treatment, directly or indirectly, aim either at reducing the vascular volume into which pooling occurs on standing, or increasing the volume of blood available for pooling. A reduction of the volume into which the blood may pool by pressor drugs has its limitations. Unless the drugs increase the responsiveness of vessels to small amounts of noradrenaline that still can be liberated, they will aggravate the tendency to recumbent hypertension. An increase in blood volume runs the risk of overloading the circulation, thus leading to cardiac failure and peripheral oedema. Many patients with autonomic failure have defects of renal preservation of sodium when recumbent and are sensitive to sodium depletion, which leads to a reduction of intravascular and extracellular fluid volume. Though we are aware that many patients continue to receive a variety of treatments in different medical centres, it is probable that any treatment with pressor drugs that temporarily enables a patient to become more mobile will improve the patient's other homeostatic responses to standing. Hence, an improvement, even if sustained, may be erroneously attributed to a particular form of treatment when it might, under controlled conditions, be possible to withdraw or replace it with a safer method.

Testing of drugs

There has been a series of reports of treatment with many different drugs, usually given empirically for a short uncontrolled trial, often in patients with an imprecise diagnosis of autonomic failure. It may reasonably be asked whether any pressor drug is effective if so many different treatments have been proposed. It is also reasonable to question whether the effect of drugs can be monitored, when the lack of baroreceptor reflexes in autonomic failure leads to marked fluctuations with changes of posture and other events, such as food ingestion, over the course of 24 hours, so that adequate maintenance of blood pressure is as difficult as targeting in a video space game. In any attempt to measure the benefit of a drug in autonomic failure, the recumbent and standing blood pressure must be taken under standard conditions, preferably four times a day by trained staff. A number of factors, in addition to postural change, can influence blood pressure, including food ingestion and even moderate exercise (Alam et al. 1995); these need to be both considered and incorporated into the assessment protocols. There is increasing use of non-invasive, 24-hour ambulatory blood pressure and heart rate recorders, and some are reliable at low blood pressures, thus providing useful information for therapeutic studies (Chapter 23). As blood pressure of patients with autonomic failure usually continues to fall when they stand; the duration of standing has to be recorded. Ideally, the blood pressure should be recorded 2 minutes after the onset of standing, because intra-arterial recordings have shown that by then any fall in pressure will be clearly apparent. Another approach is to record the duration of standing (standing time), but this may not be practical especially in those with additional neurological deficits, and other disabilities in whom there may be further reasons for difficulties in standing and mobility. In a recent study delayed OH (after 3 minutes of tilting) occurred in 20% of patients with Parkinson's disease (PD); in PD tilting for longer than the recommended 3 minutes appears to be needed (Jamnadas-Khoda J et al. 2009).

Prior to drug treatment it is advisable to have an equilibrium period of a week on a standard daily sodium diet of 150 mmol with monitoring of position and physical activity during the day and consistent head-up tilt at night. The ideal would be to measure the haematocrit, plasma protein, urea, creatinine, and electrolytes every 3 days, weigh the patient on accurate scales twice daily, measure day and night fluid balance and urinary sodium and potassium excretion, and measure blood pressure at least four times a day while lying and standing before meals and exercise.

Drug combinations

Since patients with autonomic failure often have lesions at more than one site, it should always be considered whether a combination of drugs may be more effective than a single drug. For example, drugs with central, ganglionic, and postganglionic effects may have synergistic actions. At the sympathetic terminals, drugs that increase noradrenaline release may be combined with drugs that reduce re-uptake of the transmitter or increase the sensitivity of receptors. Similarly, drugs that affect intravascular and extracellular fluid volume (such as fludrocortisone and desmopressin), release of vasodilatatory hormones (such as octreotide), or other factors influencing blood pressure, may be of value in combination (Mathias, 2009).

Approaches to treatment

Advice on factors that influence blood pressure

A number of factors have now been defined, which can considerably lower blood pressure and thus enhance the postural fall and therefore the symptoms accompanying postural hypotension (Mathias, 2010). The pathophysiological mechanisms accounting for a number of these have been worked out, and in a number of situations avoidance measures can be instituted. Therefore, patients should be advised on these factors.

Diurnal changes in blood pressure

The supine blood pressure in patients with autonomic failure is lowest in the morning and rises gradually during the day. This has been confirmed by non-invasive measurements and also by using continuous ambulatory intra-arterial blood pressure recordings (Fig. 47.2). The circadian changes in blood pressure are the reverse of those in normal subjects, in whom the blood pressure falls during sleep and rises prior to awakening. The low level of blood pressure in the morning appears to be the result of nocturnal polyuria and natriuresis,

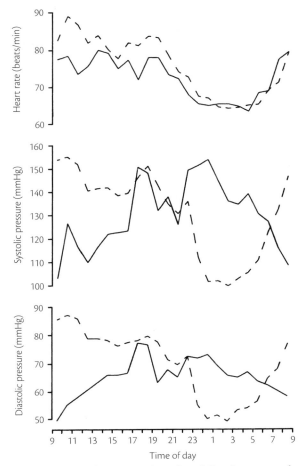

Fig. 47.2 Overall trend in heart rate and systolic and diastolic pressures of six subjects with autonomic failure (—) compared with those derived from a matched group of six subjects with normal or elevated blood pressure (—). Lines join pooled hourly means. With permission from Mann, S., Altman, D. G., Raftery, E. B., and Bannister, R., Circadian variation of blood pressure in autonomic failure. *Circulation* **68**, 477–83 (1983).

which can result in a substantial overnight weight loss, at times over 1 kg (Mathias et al. 1986, Omboni et al. 2001). The reduction in extracellular fluid volume is likely to contribute to the low blood pressure as it is improved by administration of desmopressin. The low supine blood pressure aggravates the symptoms of postural hypotension in the morning, and some patients find it extremely difficult to conduct their normal activities for a few hours after waking. Methods of preventing morning postural hypotension are described below.

Straining during micturition and defaecation

A number of patients suffer from either urinary bladder problems or from constipation. Straining might result in a Valsalva manoeuvre being performed; this can result in a substantial reduction in blood pressure without the recovery mechanisms that normally come into play. Episodes of hypotension in some situations may be particularly dangerous, for example when patients lose consciousness while propped against a lavatory wall and may not fall to the ground and thus automatically correct their low blood pressure.

Exposure to a warm environment

Patients exposed to tropical or subtropical temperatures tend to have greater symptoms for a variety of reasons. They often lack the ability to sweat, and their core temperature therefore can rise. Uncompensated vasodilatation often ensues and the blood pressure may fall. Adequate precautions therefore should be taken by patients travelling to warm countries or in tropical areas, who should be aware of the possible worsening of postural hypotension. Patients should be warned of the probability of deterioration after a hot bath, especially if prolonged.

Effect of food and alcohol

The majority of patients with autonomic failure have substantial postprandial hypotension (Chapter 28). This occurs soon after food ingestion and may last for up to 3 hours after a standard meal. The supine blood pressure can be lowered to levels of 80/50 mmHg even in the supine position and therefore these patients often exhibit increased symptoms of postural hypotension. Carbohydrate appears to be the major component causing the hypotension, and this may be linked to the release of insulin and other gastrointestinal hormones which have vasodilatatory properties. Vasodilatation in the gut, not compensated for by defective sympathetic reflexes, is the probable cause of the reduction in pressure. Food ingestion enhances postural hypotension in PAF and MSA (Mathias et al. 1991). The pathophysiology and management of postprandial hypotension is described in Chapter 28. Alcohol has the potential to cause mesenteric vasodilatation and will lower blood pressure in these patients.

Effect of exercise

It is now recognized that most patients with autonomic failure have exercise-induced hypotension (Smith et al. 1995a); the fall in blood pressure may occur even during relatively mild forms of exertion, such as walking upstairs or even while on level ground. The symptoms and circumstances vary between individual patients (Chapter 30). Exercise-induced hypotension occurs even while supine, and can compound the hypotensive effects of postural change during and even after the cessation of exercise (Smith and Mathias 1995). The hypotension is presumably due to vasodilatation in exercising muscle that is not accompanied by adequate compensatory changes in different vascular regions as occur normally (Puvi-Rajasingham et al. 1997).

Effect of drugs with vasoactive properties

Both the patient and the physician should be aware that drugs with vasoactive properties, even if only a minor action of the agent, may result in substantial vascular and blood pressure changes because of supersensitivity. The responses to pressor agents and particularly sympathomimetics, have already been described (Chapter 22). Vasopressor responses may occur to a variety of agents acting on receptors other than adrenoceptors. An example is the drug Saralasin, which has an immediate pressor response because of its initial agonist activity on angiotensin II receptors (Mathias et al. 1984), despite being an angiotensin II antagonist. Even drugs administered via the intra-ocular or intranasal route may have clinically important effects; an example is the use of β-adrenoceptor blockers for glaucoma which occasionally can cause bradycardia and lower blood pressure (Vahidassr et al. 1997). Drugs used for non-autonomic features also may unmask or enhance postural hypotension and an example is hypotension induced by L-dopa in certain parkinsonian patients; its hypotensive effects may at times draw attention to underlying autonomic failure and the diagnosis of MSA. Antidepressants and particularly tricyclic agents, may also

increase the postural blood pressure fall (Freeman et al. 2011). Marked hypotension may also occur with drugs which have vasodilatory properties. An example is glyceryl trinitrate, which routinely is used sublingually in patients with angina pectoris; when given to patients with autonomic impairment even in the supine position, it can result in severe hypotension. Medication which can enhance postural hypotension include neuroleptics, and drugs used for prostatism (Prazosin, Terazosin), for erectile dysfunction (Sildenafil), that induce autonomic neuropathy (amiodarone, vincristine, cisplatin) and also Insulin.

Head-up tilt at night

The first line of treatment in a patient with autonomic failure is to attempt to increase the patient's blood volume by the use of head-up tilt at night. Fig. 47.3 shows the change in lying and standing blood pressure and body weight in a patient placed in the head-up position at night (Bannister et al. 1969). The increase of 2.6 kg in body weight points to a progressive increase in extracellular fluid volume, which was reversed on the one night when the patient slept flat. The effect of this procedure was studied further in one patient followed on a 90 mmol per day sodium diet in whom water and sodium balance was monitored. As shown in Fig. 47.4, the patient was losing more sodium and water during the night than during the day for each of 5 days until head-up tilt at night was introduced, when the nocturnal loss of sodium and water was reversed over the subsequent 5 days. Head-up body tilt at night is likely to operate by reducing renal arterial pressure and promoting renin release with consequent angiotensin II formation, leading to aldosterone release, and thus increasing blood volume for patients with autonomic failure who can still release renin (Bannister et al. 1977). Patients with autonomic failure have complex defects of renal sodium conservation (Chapter 39) that can result in excessive nocturnal polyuria. Some patients with PAF, with incapacitating postural hypotension until the introduction of head-up tilt, have been maintained satisfactorily for years solely by this form of treatment.

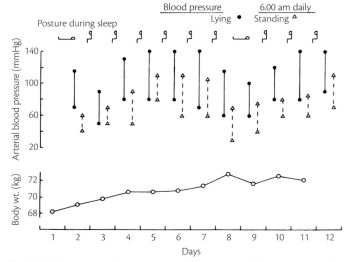

Fig. 47.3 The change in the early morning blood pressure (lying and standing) in a patient (H) with autonomic failure and multiple system atrophy studied when he slept in the sitting position for 10 days with one interruption. The changes in blood volume and body weight are also shown. From Bannister et al. 1969, with permission.

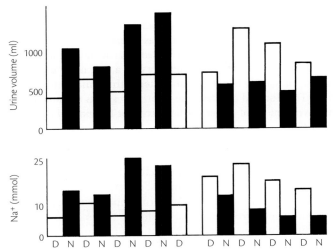

Fig. 47.4 Diurnal changes in water and sodium excretion in a patient with autonomic failure and multiple system atrophy during 5 days lying flat at night and 5 days of head-up tilt at night. D, day; N, night.

Water ingestion

Drinking 250–500 ml of water raises blood pressure substantially in various autonomic failure syndromes, improving hypotensive symptoms and improving orthostatic tolerance (Young and Mathias 2004). The pressor effect of water also ameliorates exercise induced hypotension (Humm et al. 2008). The pressor effect is in part due to an increase in systemic vascular resistance (Cariga and Mathias 2001) and some studies suggest may in part be noradrenaline mediated (Jordan et al. 2000, Shannon et al. 2002). Local changes in osmolality induced by water drinking may elicit a pressor response through activation of vanniloid 4 (Trpv4) receptors located on peripheral osmoreceptors; it is speculated that osmo-sensors in the liver and portal vasculature may induce the pressor response (May and Jordan 2011). Further details of the pressor effect of water and the mechanisms suggested are in Chapter 34.

Positions and manoeuvres to raise blood pressure

A number of positions and manoeuvres have been increasingly recognized as being helpful to patients with severe OH. The beat-by-beat recording of blood pressure with the Finapres (now Finometer) and the Portapres has enabled evaluation of the magnitude of rise induced by many of these manoeuvres (Wieling et al. 1993). The term 'physical countermeasures' has been used, and these include crossing the legs while standing, squatting, abdominal compression, bending forward, placing one foot on a chair and stooping as if to tie shoe laces (Fig. 47.5). They appear to raise blood pressure either by raising vascular resistance or by increasing venous return. The effect of leg muscle pumping and tensing (Ten Harkel et al. 1994) may be of particular value in subjects with exercise-induced hypotension, who are at their worst on ceasing exercise, presumably because of lower limb pooling (Chapter 30).

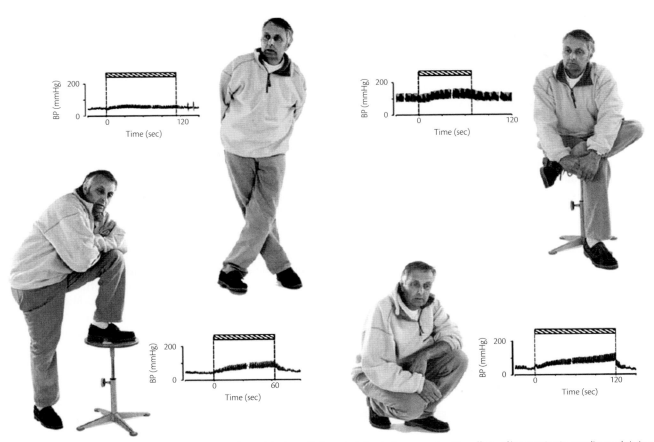

Fig. 47.5 Physical countermaneuvres using isometric contractions of the lower limbs and abdominal compression. The effects of leg crossing in standing and sitting positions, placing a foot on a chair and squatting on blood pressure in a 54 year old male patient with PAF and incapiciating OH. The patient was standing (sitting) quietly prior to the maneuvres. Bars indicate the duration of the maneuvres. From Wieling et al. (2004).

Leg crossing improves cerebral perfusion and oxygenation in patients with sympathetic failure (Harms et al. 2010). Squatting, bending forward and abdominal compression improve blood pressure control in familial dysautonomia (Tutaj et al. 2006).

External support to prevent pooling

The application of graduated pressure to the lower half of the body and legs reduces the amount of blood pooling in the legs on standing and so temporarily improves central blood volume and left ventricular filling. However, there must be concern that this treatment is in danger of reducing the intrinsic myogenic reaction of smooth muscle in response to stretch caused by increased intravascular pressure on standing, in addition to preventing other compensatory hormone and other responses to a low blood pressure. Thus the patient with OH is more vulnerable than ever when *not* wearing the support garment. In practice, a support garment may be necessary temporarily in order to achieve mobility in a patient who has been recumbent as a result of severe postural hypotension for some time, or because of an intercurrent illness. Then, as the effect of head-up tilt and drugs such as fludrocortisone produce a benefit, a counterpressure garment may be abandoned.

Originally, antigravity suits devised for aviators were used; these were certainly effective (Fig. 47.6), but were uncomfortable. The graded counterpressure support garments of the Jobst type (Sheps 1976) are more comfortable. Elastic pressure stockings are often recommended but are often not patient-acceptable, and do not appear to provide the value they should. The use of abdominal binders may provide benefit; this may be in the form of a corset, or an inflatable abdominal band, as has been demonstrated in children (Tanaka et al. 1997).

Cardiac pacing

There have been reports of benefit obtained by implantation of a cardiac pacemaker and elevation of heart rate during postural change. The benefit noted by Moss et al. (1980) occurred in a patient who apparently had an incomplete autonomic lesion, and therefore had the potential to vasoconstrict at times. In patients with more severe lesions, in whom there are low plasma noradrenaline levels at rest and in response to tilt, there appears to be no benefit. Beneficial effects of tachypacing are unlikely in patients who have maximal arteriolar and venous dilatation, as cardiac output is dependent upon venous return which is often considerably reduced in such patients. Occasionally, cardiac pacing may be needed to prevent excessive bradycardia in response to elevation of blood pressure by drugs, as described in a patient in whom atrial demand pacing was needed to protect against vagal overactivity in the presence of a severe sympathetic autonomic neuropathy

(Bannister et al. 1986). In this patient administration of drugs to raise blood pressure resulted in severe bradycardia and consequent dysrhythmias (Fig. 47.7). Assessment was initially made with atropine, which raised the heart rate but resulted in unacceptable side-effects. Atrial pacing was performed, initially with a temporary pacemaker, which was clearly beneficial, and later with permanent implantation. This enabled effective use of pressor agents without the fear of development of either cardiac arrest or a serious dysrhythmia (Fig. 47.8).

There have been further studies on the efficacy of atrial tachypacing, as observed in five patients with severe OH who were resistant to multiple interventions that included non-pharmacological measures, sympathomimetic amines, mineralocorticoids, selective serotonin reuptake inhibitors, and droxidopa. Neither syncope nor presyncope occurred in any patient for up to 3 months of follow-up when combined with implantation of a cardiac pacemaker (Kohno et al. 2007). It may be that advances in pacemaker technology may benefit some patients.

Noradrenaline infusion devices

One potential future advance may be the utilization of devices which are closely linked to blood pressure control and postural change and which administer short-acting pressor agents. One such device was described by Polinsky et al. (1983). They used an electromechanical device, utilizing the arterial transducer to record blood pressure from one arm while controlling the rate of an intravenous infusion of noradrenaline into the opposite arm (Fig. 47.9). There do not appear to have been further developments, although advances in drug administration, using either implantable devices or mini-infusion pumps, linked to the ability to non-invasively measure blood pressure on a beat-by-beat basis, should lead to further advances. This will be of especial benefit to severely impaired patients in whom multiple drug therapy has failed.

In Table 47.1 an attempt has been made to classify these agents on the basis of their main actions in helping postural hypotension.

Plasma volume expansion and reduction of natriuresis
Fludrocortisone

Fludrocortisone is the most commonly used drug treatment and has multiple pharmacological effects (Chobanian et al. 1979). In an initial dose of 0.1 mg at night, in some patients with autonomic failure, fludrocortisone approaches most closely to the ideal of a drug which increases effective vasoconstriction on standing, by augmenting the action of noradrenaline released by some remaining normal sympathetic efferent activity but without aggravating recumbent hypertension. In normal subjects, fludrocortisone also sensitizes vascular receptors to pressor amines (Schmidt et al. 1966).

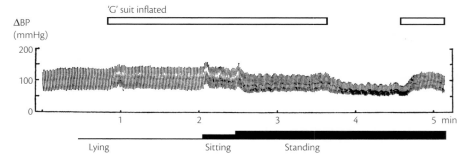

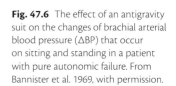

Fig. 47.6 The effect of an antigravity suit on the changes of brachial arterial blood pressure (ΔBP) that occur on sitting and standing in a patient with pure autonomic failure. From Bannister et al. 1969, with permission.

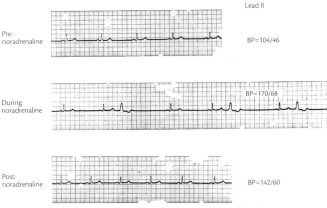

Fig. 47.7 Electrocardiographic tracings before, during and after intravenous infusion of noradrenaline. Sinus bradycardia and coupled beats occur when the blood pressure is elevated to 170/68 mmHg. This is reversed when the blood pressure returns to normal. From Bannister et al. 1986, with permission.

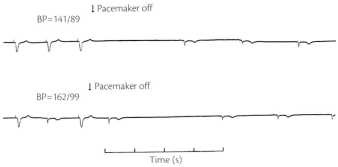

Fig. 47.8 Electrocardiographic (ECG) tracings, initially with pacemaker off, on upper trace. There are pacemaker triggered complexes followed by a pause and then sinus bradycardia. During noradrenaline infusion (lower trace) with the blood pressure elevated, there are alternating pacemaker-induced and intrinsic complexes. Following exclusion of the pacemaker there is a longer pause before endogenous rhythm takes over. The elevation in blood pressure appears to enhance sinus node suppression. From Bannister et al. 1986, with permission.

Fludrocortisone may also increase the fluid content of vessel walls, so increasing their resistance to stretching (Tobian and Redleaf 1958).

In a study of MSA, 0.1 mg of fludrocortisone daily did not increase body weight but caused a shift to the left of the noradrenaline infusion sensitivity curve and a significant rise in standing blood pressure (Davies et al. 1979). This effect may be less apparent in patients with PAF (Chobanian et al. 1979). It was speculated that fludrocortisone might increase the number of α-adrenoceptors, change their structure, or decrease the clearance rate by the uptake-2 mechanism by smooth muscle of blood vessels. There is an increase in the α-adrenoceptors of platelets and β-adrenoceptors of lymphocytes in autonomic failure and these changes are increased further after treatment with fludrocortisone (Bannister et al. 1981, Davies et al. 1982). In autonomic failure there also is an increase in the pressor response to angiotensin II which is not affected by fludrocortisone, indicating a probable change in angiotensin vascular receptors as well as α-adrenoceptors (Davies et al. 1979).

In higher doses with careful supervision, fludrocortisone can expand the blood volume, improve cardiac output, and so reduce postural hypotension. Patients with autonomic failure have a normal or slightly low plasma volume when supine but this does not, as in normal subjects, fall on standing owing to the lack of vasoconstriction, probably because the lowered arterial pressure compensates for the raised hydrostatic pressure in the legs on standing. Patients with autonomic failure lose twice as much body weight as control subjects when on a low-sodium diet, with a corresponding increase in their postural hypotension. The resting plasma renin activity in autonomic failure is usually low, with a reduced rise on standing, though this is increased by sodium restriction or by dopamine infusion. This suggests that renin synthesis and storage are intact but release may be defective. Aldosterone secretion may be reduced in autonomic failure but it is unclear whether the defect is the result of a chronic reduction of angiotensin stimulation of aldosterone secretion rather than an adrenal defect. The dose of fludrocortisone likely to increase the blood volume by replacing aldosterone levels without overloading the circulation requires delicate and continuous adjustment probably because of the baroreflex defect, in contrast to the situation in a patient with Addison's disease. As with other forms of treatment, each patient shows variations in response which are the result of the different types of lesion present in each patient. The combination of fludrocortisone (0.1 mg) with head-up tilt at night and a high salt diet (150–200 mmol sodium/day) is an effective means of improving postural hypotension (Ten Harkel et al. 1992), and symptoms are reduced with only minimal side-effects (such as ankle oedema) and without the causation of hypokalaemia.

Desmopressin

Desmopressin (DDAVP) is a vasopressin analogue which acts specifically upon the V_2 receptors on the renal tubules, which are responsible for the antidiuretic effects of vasopressin (antidiuretic hormone). It has virtually no activity on the V_1 receptor, which is responsible for the vasoconstriction induced by vasopressin. In patients with autonomic failure, nocturnal polyuria, overnight weight loss, and the subsequent reduction in extracellular fluid volume and intravascular volume, account for the low morning blood pressures and for the increased severity of symptoms from postural hypotension. Intramuscular DDAVP prevents nocturnal polyuria and reduces overnight weight loss, and raises the supine blood pressure in the morning, thus improving symptoms resulting from postural change (Mathias et al. 1986) (Fig. 47.10). Because of the lack of direct vascular effects of DDAVP an increased tendency to supine hypertension is not present. Studies with intranasal DDAVP indicate that it is equally effective in the short term and also in the long term; doses between 5 μg and 40 μg given at bedtime as a single dose are of benefit both in relation to preventing nocturia (which can also be a problem especially in those with bladder involvement) and also in morning postural hypotension. An oral form of DDAVP is available and should have advantages over the intranasal form. Tablets of 200 μg have been used successfully in adolescents and adults with nocturnal enuresis (Janknegt et al. 1997); 400 μg tablets are also available.

However, DDAVP has the potential to cause side-effects. Some patients, and in particular those with PAF, may be exquisitely sensitive to its action and hyponatraemia can readily ensue (Mathias et al. 1986). In these patients, low starting doses of intranasal DDAVP should be administered under careful supervision to ensure that hyponatraemia does not occur, before stabilization. In some patients, natriuresis continues as before and occasionally is in excess and DDAVP needs to be combined with fludrocortisone and sodium supplements to ensure that the patient remains in

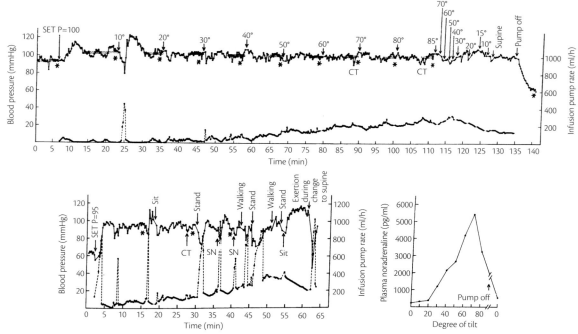

Fig. 47.9 Mean blood pressure (upper trace in each record), noradrenaline infusion rate (lower trace in each record), and plasma noradrenaline levels during clinical trial of a sympathetic neural prosthesis. The * indicates points at which blood samples were obtained. CT, clear throat; SN, sneeze. Reprinted from *The Lancet*, **i**, Polinsky, R. J., Samaras, G. M., and Kopin, I. J., Sympathetic neural prosthesis for managing orthostatic hypertension, 901–4, Copyright (1983), with permission from Elsevier.

Table 47.1 Drugs used in the treatment of postural hypotension

Site of action	Drugs	Predominant action
Plasma volume: expansion	◆ Fludrocortisone	◆ Mineralocorticoid effects—increased plasma volume
		◆ Sensitization of α-adrenoceptors
Kidney: reducing diuresis	◆ Desmopression	◆ Vasopressin$_2$-receptors on renal tubules
Vessels: vasoconstriction (adrenoceptor-mediated)	◆ Ephedrine	◆ Indirectly acting sympathomimetic
Resistance vessels	◆ Midodrine*, phenylephrine, methylphenidate	◆ Directly acting sympathomimetics
Capacitance vessels	◆ Tyramine	◆ Release of noradrenaline
	◆ Clonidine	◆ Postsynaptic α_2-adrenoceptor agonist
	◆ Yohimbine	◆ Presynaptic α_2-adrenoceptor antagonist
	◆ DL-DOPS and L-DOPS	◆ Pro-drug resulting in formation of noradrenaline
	◆ Dihydroergotamine	◆ Direct action on α-adrenoceptors
Vessels: vasoconstriction (non-adrenoceptor mediated)	◆ Triglycyl-lysine-vasopressin (glypressin)	◆ Vasopressin$_1$-receptors on blood vessels
Vessels: prevention of vasodilatation	◆ Propranolol	◆ Blockade of β_2-adrenoceptors
	◆ Indomethacin	◆ Prevents prostaglandin synthesis
	◆ Metoclopramide	◆ Blockade of dopamine receptors
Vessels: prevention of postprandial hypotension	◆ Caffeine	◆ Blockade of adenosine receptors
	◆ Octreotide	◆ Inhibits release of vasodilator gut/pancreatic peptides
	◆ Acarbose, Voglibose	◆ Intestinal α-glucosidase inhibitors
Enhancing sympathetic ganglionic transmission	◆ Pyridostigmine	◆ Inhibition of acetylcholinesterase
Heart: stimulation	◆ Pindolol, xamoterol	◆ Intrinsic sympathomimetic action
Red cell mass: increase	◆ Erythropoietin	◆ Stimulates red cell production

*Through its active metabolite.
DOPS, dihydroxyphenylserine.

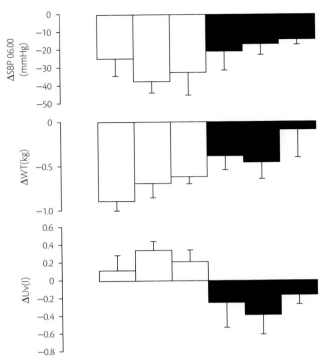

Fig. 47.10 Desmopressin (DDAVP) in the treatment of autonomic failure. From above, morning postural hypotension, difference between sitting and lying systolic pressure (ΔSBP), change in body weight overnight (ΔWt), and change in urine volume between night and day (ΔUv). The open rectangles show the changes during a 3-day control period and the closed rectangles the changes after 2 µg of intramuscular DDAVP each evening for 3 days. The mean results in five patients with autonomic failure show after DDAVP a reduction in postural hypotension and a gain in extracellular and intravascular fluid volume as measured by the reduction in nocturnal weight loss and nocturnal urinary volume.

sodium balance. The long-term efficacy and safety of nocturnal intranasal desmopressin in reducing nocturnal polyuria and nocturia has been confirmed in MSA (Sakakibara et al. 2003).

We have treated patients with intranasal DDAVP for many years with regular monitoring of plasma osmolality or plasma sodium levels and with no long-term side-effects. (Mathias and Young 2003, Mathias 2001).

Drugs causing vasoconstriction

Drugs acting as vasoconstrictors can be divided broadly into those working through the sympathetic nervous system and/or its receptors and those with actions on non-adrenergic receptors. Examples of the latter include vasopressin and its analogue, glycopressin, acting on V$_1$ receptors. Most of these drugs act on resistance vessels and will be described below, along with dihydroergotamine, which acts predominantly on capacitance vessels.

Directly acting agents

A variety of agents have been used which act directly on α-adrenoceptors. These include agents such as phenylephrine, phenylpropanolamine, methylphenidate, and midodrine. A factor to be kept in mind is the potential of these agents to cause severe constriction in peripheral vessels. This might be a disadvantage, especially in the elderly who are more likely to have peripheral vascular abnormalities.

Of the sympathomimetic vasoconstrictor agents, midodrine has been studied extensively (Kaufmann et al. 1988, Jankovic et al. 1993, Fouad-Tarazi et al. 1995, Low et al. 1997). Midodrine is a prodrug that is metabolized to the active form, desglymidodrine, which acts on α$_1$-adrenoceptors to cause constriction of both arterial resistance and venous capacitance vessels. It is absorbed fairly rapidly, with peak concentrations within 20–40 minutes and with a short half-life, in the region of 30 minutes. It is administered in doses of 2.5–10 mg given three times daily. Its side-effects include goose skin (cutis anserina), tingling of the skin and pruritus, especially of the scalp; the pruritus can be severe in some patients. Impaired urine flow, hesitancy, and urinary retention may occur, especially in the male, presumably because of its adrenoceptor agonist effects on the internal sphincter. It may be of particular value in patients with severe postural hypotension and in those with peripheral lesions, as in PAF. Surprisingly, some patients on midodrine become worse, for reasons that are unclear; in these patients there may be a reduction in intra- and extravascular fluid volume, as manifested by weight loss (Kaufmann et al. 1988).

Indirectly acting agents

Ephedrine acts by both releasing noradrenaline and also by acting directly on adrenoceptors. This drug may have a role in patients with central lesions (such as in MSA) and in patients with incomplete lesions, where a combination of its direct effects and the release of noradrenaline may be of benefit. As with other agents, there is the potential to cause supine hypertension. The value of the drug in patients with severe sympathetic lesions is probably minimal. The starting dose is 15 mg three times daily. With larger doses of ephedrine (in excess of 30 mg, three times daily), side-effects such as tachycardia, insomnia, decreased appetite and tremulousness may occur, in part due to central stimulation.

Drugs predominantly releasing noradrenaline

Tyramine is an agent that raises blood pressure by the release of noradrenaline from the sympathetic nerve endings. In some patients with autonomic failure there may be sufficient sparing of nerve endings for this to be achieved, and the effects of tyramine can be potentiated by the concurrent administration of a monoamine oxidase inhibitor. This applies even to the newer selective monoamine oxidase inhibitors, as has been reported in a case treated with moclobemide (Karet et al. 1994). A number of foods, especially certain cheeses and Bovril, contain *p*-tyramine and this may have been partially responsible for the erratic blood responses, except that these were also obtained using chemically pure *p*-tyramine when studied in combination with phenelzine (Fig. 47.11) (Davies et al. 1978); in these studies the marked fluctuation of blood pressure that occurred along with pronounced supine hypertension made such treatment potentially hazardous. The improvement in postural hypotension caused by this combination appears to be less effective than that caused by midodrine or ephedrine, and its use largely has been abandoned.

α$_2$-Adrenoceptor agonists

Clonidine is an α$_2$-adrenoceptor agonist, which is highly lipophilic and has actions both centrally and peripherally. Its central actions, which result in withdrawal of sympathetic tone, are responsible for the fall in supine blood pressure in both normal subjects and hypertensive patients. In tetraplegics, therefore, with a decentralized

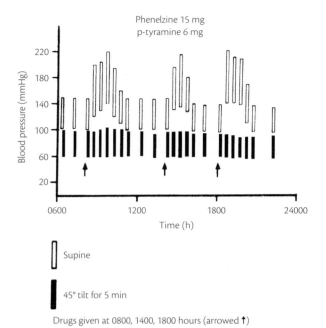

Phenelzine 15 mg
p-tyramine 6 mg

□ Supine

■ 45° tilt for 5 min

Drugs given at 0800, 1400, 1800 hours (arrowed ↑)

Fig. 47.11 Blood pressure and heart rate before and after treatment of a patient with pure autonomic failure with phenelzine and p-tyramine. Reprinted from *The Lancet*, **i**, Davies, B., Bannister, R., and Sever, P., Pressor amines and monoamine oxidase inhibitors for treatment of postural hypotension in progressive autonomic failure. Limitations and hazards, 172–5, Copyright (1978), with permission from Elsevier.

sympathetic nervous system, clonidine does not lower resting blood pressure (Mathias et al. 1979); however, it is capable of attenuating the pressor response to urinary bladder stimulation, indicating that it may have effects either on spinal sympathetic neurones or on presynaptic α_2-adrenoceptors in the periphery (Chapter 66). When given intravenously to tetraplegics there is an initial pressor response (Mathias and Frankel, unpublished observations) which results from its normally transient peripheral postsynaptic effects causing vasoconstriction. These are probably a combination of both postsynaptic α_1- and α_2-adrenoceptor effects. These effects are probably the basis for the observations of the benefit of clonidine in some patients with autonomic failure. Our own experience with the use of clonidine in the management of postural hypotension in autonomic failure patients has not been favourable, and it may be that the drug is only of benefit in those with complete lesions involving postganglionic fibres where there is extreme pressor sensitivity to α-adrenoceptor agents. This is consistent with the observations of Thomaides et al. (1992) who studied the systemic and regional haemodynamic responses to intravenous clonidine (2 µg/kg body weight) in MSA and PAF; blood pressure fell in MSA but rose in PAF. Clonidine may be of benefit in reducing supine hypertension in autonomic failure patients (Shibao et al. 2006)

Presynaptic α_2-adrenoceptor antagonists

Yohimbine is an α_2-adrenoceptor antagonist which can act both centrally and peripherally. The blockade of presynaptic α_2-adrenoceptors may facilitate the release of noradrenaline at nerve terminals. The drug has been used in single doses with benefit in autonomic failure with probable partial lesions, thus resulting in accentuation of noradrenaline release (Onrot et al. 1987). The drug may have a role in patients with autonomic failure with

central lesions, as reported in MSA (Senard et al. 1993a); it does not appear to be effective in parkinsonian patients with autonomic failure of presumed peripheral origin (Senard et al. 1993b). It has not been evaluated in the long term and it is not known whether it has advantages over ephedrine and midodrine. Combined use of yohimbine and pyridostigmine (cholinesterase inhibitor) showed no significant synergistic effect on standing blood pressure; however, the patients had severe autonomic failure with minimal residual sympathetic function which may have accounted for the lack of effect (Shibao et al. 2010).

Enhancement of ganglionic neurotransmission

Pyridostigmine inhibits the enzyme acetylcholinesterase and increases the transmission of impulses from cholinergic neurons across the synaptic cleft. It does not cross the blood–brain barrier and its effects result from enhancement of ganglionic neurotransmission and not due to stimulation of the central cholinergic system. The facilitatory effect on sympathetic ganglionic neurotransmission results in increased vascular adrenergic tone during orthostasis without enhancement of sympathetic tone while supine (Singer W et al. 2003). The effect of pyridostigmine on standing blood pressure has been tested in an open label study and then in a double-blind, randomized 4-way crossover study alone or in combination with midodrine. Pyridostigmine improves blood pressure during standing although it appears to be of benefit mainly in patients with mild OH. Further studies, however, have not confirmed these results especially in patients with severe autonomic failure (Shibao et al. 2010).

Increased production of noradrenaline

The prodrug, dihydroxyphenylserine (DOPS) in the laevo form (L) or racemic mixture (DL), raises levels of plasma noradrenaline when decarboxylated, as described in the management of postural hypotension in dopamine-beta-hydroxylase deficiency (Chapter 49). Since 1980, DOPS has been used, often with success, in hypotension associated with a variety of disorders, including, familial amyloidosis (Carvalho et al. 1997), spinal cord injury (Muneta et al. 1992), children with orthostatic intolerance (Tanaka et al. 1996), Parkinson's disease (Mathias et al. 2001), PAF and MSA (Kaufmann et al. 1991, Mathias et al. 2001) and autoimmune autonomic neuropathy (Gibbons et al. 2005). It has been used in doses of 250–500 mg twice daily. The mechanisms by which DL- and L-DOPS raise blood pressure in autonomic failure are unclear. This may be through the rise in plasma noradrenaline levels and thus direct stimulation of peripheral postsynaptic adrenoceptors. If so, it could be more effective in patients with PAF (who have a greater degree of pressor supersensitivity), than patients with MSA, although this has not been the observation in two separate studies (Hoeldtke et al. 1984, Kaufmann et al. 1991), albeit in a small number of patients. The administration of DOPS has been shown, using microneurographic techniques, to increase sympathetic nerve activity in a patient with MSA (Kachi et al. 1988) and also in normal subjects (Iwase et al. 1992). DOPS has the ability to enter the central nervous system, and enhancing sympathoneural activity may be a factor in raising blood pressure, especially in patients with MSA who usually have preserved postganglionic sympathetic pathways. The value of L-DOPS in the management of OH in PAF, MSA and PD has been evaluated in pan-European multicentre trials (Mathias et al. 2001). Concomitant use of dopa-decarboxylase inhibitors in the doses used to treat patients with PD does not appear to blunt the efficacy of L-dihydroxyphenylserine (L-DOPS) in PD (Mathias et al. 2008).

Dopaminergic agents

A dopaminergic prodrug, ibopamine, that also has weak α- and β-adrenoceptor agonist activity, has been studied in three patients with pure autonomic failure (Rensma et al. 1993). Within 10–30 minutes after administration there was substantial improvement in orthostatic tolerance, that lasted for 20–50 minutes. These effects were reversed by the α-adrenoceptor blocker phentolamine, favouring a predominant effect on these receptors. The pharmacokinetic profile was highly variable, and in one patient there was severe hypertension and tachycardia. There have been no further reports on the use of this agent.

Predominantly venoconstrictor agents with direct action on α-adrenoceptors

Dihydroergotamine has a long history in treatment of postural hypotension since reports by Nordenfelt and Mellander (1972). It acts as a direct α-adrenoceptor agonist, stimulating venous capacity vessels although resistance vessels may even show slight dilatation when normally innervated. It increases central blood volume by about 120 ml with only a slight rise in venous pressure. Nordenfelt and Mellander (1972) studied patients with intact sympathetic function but liable to syncope (so-called 'sympathotonic' OH) and their results are not directly applicable to autonomic failure. When there is sympathetic denervation as in autonomic failure, dihydroergotamine almost certainly causes constriction of resistance vessels (Bevegard et al. 1974). It is highly effective after venous injection and abolishes postural hypotension almost completely for half an hour even in severe cases of autonomic failure, sometimes temporarily improving the Valsalva response, these benefits being obtained at the price of severe recumbent hypertension. The effectiveness of intravenous dihydroergotamine was confirmed by Jennings et al. (1979) in two patients with PAF and two with MSA. They showed reduction of the excessive fall of central blood volume on standing. An oral dose of 30 mg daily was needed in three out of four patients to improve their postural hypotension, and the addition of fludrocortisone resulted in further improvement.

The major disadvantage of dihydroergotamine is its poor bioavailability. One approach has been to combine it with oral glyceryl trinitrate, which was reported to increase its bioavailability and thus increase its efficacy. However, studies in our unit, using such a combination in our patients with autonomic failure, did not provide any evidence of beneficial effect when dihydroergotamine with placebo was compared with dihydroergotamine in combination with 0.5 mg of glyceryl trinitrate. In some patients there may even have been a fall in blood pressure, presumably because of the vasodilator effects of glyceryl trinitrate. Increasing the daily oral dose of dihydroergotamine may be of benefit in some patients, keeping in mind the potential complication of peripheral vasoconstriction. Dihydroergotamine can also be given parenterally, either subcutaneously or intramuscularly, as in the prevention of thromboembolic complications. It has been used with benefit intramuscularly in autonomic failure resulting from alcoholism and diabetes. Other ergot derivatives have also been assessed in patients with autonomic failure; ergotamine tartrate can be given orally, and has been used in doses of 2–5 mg daily with some benefit.

Vasopressin₁-receptor agonists

Stimulation of V_1-receptors in blood vessels results in constriction. The drug triglycyl-lysine-vasopressin (glypressin), an analogue of vasopressin with predominant V_1 effects, results in constriction of arteries, mainly in the splanchnic and skin circulation, and may reduce postural hypotension (Rittig et al. 1991). Further studies using this approach are awaited.

Prevention of vasodilatation

A variety of drugs has been used on the premise that blood pressure control can be improved by preventing vasodilatatory mechanisms.

β-Adrenoceptor blockade

Propranolol was introduced in the treatment of autonomic failure on the grounds, despite the obvious α-adrenoceptor defect, that α-adrenoceptor agonist induced vasodilatation might also contribute to the OH and should be reversed by the β-adrenoceptor blocking properties of propranolol. It may also act on presynaptic β-adrenoceptors and so reduce the release of noradrenaline. Chobanian et al. (1977) reported beneficial effects in four patients with PAF on oral propranolol in doses of 40–240 mg daily but, as they were already taking 0.3–0.5 mg fludrocortisone daily and had an excessive salt intake, no clear conclusion can be drawn. They later withdrew propranolol in one patient because it caused severe recumbent hypertension, and they reported that in two patients episodes of 'syncope' still occurred in the early morning when orthostatic intolerance was most severe. In practice propranolol has not proved sufficiently encouraging for other trials to be reported.

Other forms of postural intolerance and hypotension have been treated with propranolol. Some patients do not appear to have autonomic failure, but have orthostatic tachycardia or a hyperadrenergic orthostatic response leading to postural hypotension, partially due to a decreased cardiac output. The tachycardia is probably emotionally determined and is accompanied by a mounting sense of anxiety when standing, associated with over-breathing, and then sometimes, paradoxically, increasing bouts of vagally induced bradycardia, which may eventually lead to syncope. Propranolol reduces the initial tachycardia and may benefit such patients. Some patients with autonomic failure or diabetes mellitus, and in whom there is sparing of cardiac sympathetic efferents but impaired sympathetic tone to the vascular bed, have a compensatory tachycardia and deteriorate if this compensatory mechanism is blocked by propranolol.

Prostaglandin synthetase inhibitors

Indomethacin was first proposed on the theoretical basis that some prostaglandins are potent vasodilators and their effect may be inhibited by indomethacin, which also may have several other effects that modify pressor responses. Improvement with indomethacin was reported in four patients with postural hypotension (Kochar and Itskovitz 1978). However, the diagnosis was uncertain in one of them, in that the standing blood pressure was within the normal range for her age and, in all, the diagnosis of autonomic failure and MSA was based on clinical features without the benefit of physiological tests. Oral indomethacin (50 mg three times daily) increased sensitivity to infused noradrenaline and angiotensin II in four patients with MSA but the pressor effect was only significant on recumbent blood pressure, probably because the hydrostatic stresses on standing require compensatory constriction of different blood vessels in different vascular beds (Davies et al. 1980). Inhibition of prostaglandin synthesis may be a factor because urinary prostaglandin excretion was greater than in normal subjects and was decreased by indomethacin. The lack of improvement in the standing blood pressure might also have been due to a decrease in plasma renin activity due to indomethacin. Benefit has been reported from the combined effect of fludrocortisone and flurbiprofen in PAF (Watt et al. 1981). Since both prostaglandin inhibitors and fludrocortisone have pressor effects, we have decided, in some cases failing to respond to fludrocortisone alone, to add indomethacin because both substances appear to increase smooth muscle sensitivity to noradrenaline and, in larger doses, may increase blood volume. Drugs such as indomethacin have side-effects, including gastric–duodenal ulceration.

Dopamine antagonists

Metoclopramide, a dopamine antagonist, has been used on the basis that it blocks the vasodilator effects of dopamine. In a single patient with postural hypotension after an extensive sympathectomy, Kuchel et al. (1980) reported an improvement in postural hypotension. They postulated that this was the result of the drug inhibiting the vasodilator and natriuretic effects of the excess dopamine released. In four patients with PAF, in whom plasma dopamine levels were similar to those of normal subjects, intravenous metoclopramide (10 µg) caused a small but significant fall in blood pressure. A similar dose given to patients with dopamine-beta-hydroxylase deficiency, in whom plasma dopamine levels were elevated, lowered blood pressure substantially (Chapter 49). These observations do not favour a role for these drugs in the treatment of postural hypotension, except in situations where concurrent drug therapy (such as with L-dopa or apomorphine) elevates peripheral dopamine levels and stimulates vasodilatatory dopaminergic receptors. However, caution is necessary in patients with supersensitivity of central dopamine receptors who may be vulnerable to the extrapyramidal side-effects, and antagonists with mainly peripheral effects, such as domperidone, may be preferable.

Drugs preventing postprandial hypotension

Dilatation within the splanchnic circulation following a meal is probably the cause of the marked postprandial fall in blood pressure in patients with autonomic failure. Splanchnic vasodilatation may result from the release of vasodilatatory neuropeptides. Drugs such as dihydroergotamine seem to have minimal effects in preventing postprandial hypotension. The beneficial use of other agents, and particular octreotide, is discussed in Chapter 28. It should be noted that octreotide also reduces postural hypotension (Armstrong and Mathias 1991) and may provide some benefit in exercise-induced hypotension (Smith et al. 1995b). Long acting preparations of somatostatin analogues may be of value in some (Hoeldtke et al. 2007, Colao et al. 2010).

Acarbose (100 mg 20 minutes before food) and Voglibose (200 µg 10 minutes before food) inhibit intestinal α-glucosidase activity, and thus delay glucose absorption, decrease the breakdown of complex carbohydrate. These actions have been shown to decrease the release of vasodilatatory gastrointestinal hormones including insulin, and thus reduce postprandial hypotension in autonomic disorders (Maruta et al. 2006, Shibao et al. 2007, Jian and Zhou 2008).

Drugs acting on the heart

Pindolol

Pindolol has additional partial β-adrenoceptor agonist activity (so-called intrinsic sympathomimetic activity) which should cause less reduction in resting heart rate than a pure beta-blocker might be expected to cause. The initial encouraging report was by Frewin et al. (1980) on two patients with diabetic autonomic neuropathy who probably had supersensitivity to noradrenaline. It was followed by Man in't Veld and Schalekamp (1981), who showed benefits in three patients with autonomic failure, two of whom had amyloidosis and one following acute autonomic neuropathy. They argued that, when receptor occupancy is low as is assumed in the postganglionic lesion of autonomic failure, there was a strong possibility that even a partial β-agonist would act as a full agonist and its agonist effect would be enhanced by denervation hypersensitivity and lack of baroreflexes. They also raised the possibility that pindolol might have an effect on β-adrenoceptors in veins and, like dihydroergotamine, might increase venous tone. They showed that the improvement in postural hypotension was due to an improvement in cardiac output but vascular resistance was unchanged. Their patients had an increase in cardiac rate. However, this enthusiasm was premature. Davies et al. (1981) reported briefly on five patients studied under standard conditions after a control period. Pindolol was given in an adequate dose, gauged by the heart rate response to intravenous isoprenaline, but did not increase blood pressure or cause symptomatic benefit at any dose level. The trend was towards a decrease in lying and standing pressure. Pindolol did not have a chronotropic action and there was instead a tendency for the pulse rate to decrease with increasing doses of pindolol. Two patients had raised jugular venous pressure after 3 days on 15 mg daily and frank cardiac failure after 45 mg daily for 3 days. Pindolol causes a rightward shift of the isoprenaline dose–response curve so that, although in theory pindolol acts more as a sympathetic agonist than a competitive antagonist, its β-blocking action was still pronounced. In our patients there was evidence of increased receptor numbers and denervation super-sensitivity to noradrenaline. Therefore, the view put forward by Man in't Veld and Schalekamp (1981), that their patients responded because of the partial agonist effect of pindolol may not be the only explanation.

Prenalterol and xamoterol

Two other beta-blockers with α_1-adrenoceptor partial agonist effects have been assessed in autonomic failure. Prenalterol was found to be effective (Goovaerts et al. 1984). Xamoterol has also been shown in a number of patients to benefit postural hypotension (Mehlsen and Trap-Jensen 1985, Mathias et al. 1990). However, xamoterol, like pindolol, has the potential to cause cardiac failure and has been withdrawn.

Erythropoietin

Erythropoietin is a polypeptide that is produced mainly in the kidney. It stimulates red blood cell production. The level of oxygen to the kidney is a key factor in its synthesis as stimuli such as hypoxia, blood loss, or chronic anaemia increase erythropoietin levels. The role of the sympathetic nervous system in erythropoietin synthesis is unclear; previously we had noted low haemoglobin levels, with normocytic, normochromic anaemia, mainly in pure autonomic failure patients. Further studies indicate that in autonomic failure the anaemia is not associated with an appropriate increase in erythropoietin levels, as otherwise would be expected (Biaggioni et al. 1994).

Erythropoietin is now produced using recombinant techniques, and it was first used in postural hypotension by Hoeldtke and Streeten (1993), in a dose of 50 units/kg body weight, three times a week for 6–8 weeks. It raised haemoglobin levels and red cell volume, but it had no effect on plasma volume in eight patients with postural hypotension, of whom four had diabetic autonomic neuropathy, three PAF, and one sympathotonic OH. Following erythropoietin, there was a rise in both systolic and diastolic blood pressure with an improvement in postural hypotension and symptoms. Erythropoietin in primary chronic autonomic failure has since been used successfully by other groups (Biaggioni et al. 1994, and Perera et al. 1995). It may be of particular value in autonomic failure where anaemia may be a complication, as in diabetic autonomic neuropathy with renal failure and amyloidosis patients (Kawakami et al. 2003) (Chapters 50, 53). It is not known whether erythropoietin will be effective in reducing postural hypotension in the large number of patients with autonomic failure who are not anaemic.

Summary of management approaches

The management of postural hypotension entails consideration of a large number of factors (Mathias and Kimber, 1998). Some of these include the marked lability of blood pressure (at times with supine hypertension), the variability of symptoms despite a similar blood pressure fall, and the effects of activities in daily life that can worsen postural hypotension substantially. The patient must be made aware that the treatment, even with a combination of drugs, is unlikely to be a substitute for the rapid and complex responses of the autonomic nervous system. The physician, and in many situations the patient also, should be aware that various non-neurogenic factors that lower blood pressure can worsen postural hypotension; an example is even modest fluid loss induced by vomiting or diarrhoea. The management, therefore, is dependent upon an integrated approach, with education of the patient of particular importance. A summary is provided in Table 47.2, outlining the non-pharmacological and pharmacological approaches that we use.

The non-pharmacological approaches are an important component of the patient's contribution to management (Mathias et al. 2012). Awareness of the various factors that worsen hypotension is important, together with the means to avoid these. Some are readily definable, while others, such as exercise, need to be related specifically to the individual as the severity of exertion causing symptomatic hypotension will vary. The patient, often with the help of the partner or carers, will need to implement measures to reduce postural hypotension. Some, such as increasing salt intake either by the liberal addition of salt at meals or salt tablets, often may need explanation, as the risks of high salt intake have been so well publicized that a low intake is often erroneously adhered to. Exercise is needed to maintain an adequate muscle mass and improve circulatory control. The type of, and even position during, exercise will need to be modified, depending upon the degree of hypotension and associated neurological and musculoskeletal disabilities. Thus, in some patients it may need to be performed while lying flat. There may be advantages in swimming, because the subject is semi-supine with the supportive external pressure of water. An important component is the utilization of various

Table 47.2 Outline of non-pharmacological and pharmacological measures used in the management of postural hypotension due to neurogenic failure

Non-pharmacological measures
To be avoided
◆ Sudden head-up postural change (especially on waking)
◆ Prolonged recumbency
◆ Straining during micturition and defaecation
◆ High environmental temperature (including hot baths)
◆ 'Severe' exertion
◆ Large meals (especially with refined carbohydrate)
◆ Alcohol
◆ Drugs with vasodepressor properties
To be introduced
◆ Head-up tilt during sleep
◆ Small, frequent meals
◆ High salt intake
◆ Judicious exercise (including swimming)
◆ Body positions and manoeuvres
To be considered
◆ Water ingestion
◆ Elastic stockings
◆ Abdominal binders
Pharmacological measures
◆ Starter drug: fludrocortisone
◆ Sympathomimetics: ephedrine, midodrine, L-DOPS
◆ Specific targeting: octreotide, desmopressin, erythropoietin
◆ Ganglionic nicotinic receptor stimulation: pyridostigmine

It should be emphasized that non-neurogenic factors, such as fluid loss due to vomiting or diarrhoea, may substantially worsen neurogenic postural hypotension and will need to be rectified.
Adapted from Mathias et al. 2012, with permission.

positions and manoeuvres to raise blood pressure in different circumstances, that again need to be tailored to the patient's associated disabilities.

Drugs should be used when it is clear that non-pharmacological approaches alone are not beneficial. A valuable starter drug with minimal side-effects is low-dose fludrocortisone. This can be followed by the sympathomimetic drugs, ephedrine (especially in those with central or incomplete lesions) or midodrine (in those with peripheral lesions). If the combination of fludrocortisone and sympathomimetics does not produce the desired effects, then selective targeting is needed, depending upon the pathophysiological disturbances. Thus, octreotide may be of value in those with postprandial hypotension, desmopressin in those with nocturnal polyuria, and erythropoietin in those with associated anaemia. The drug treatment, therefore, needs to be individually tailored.

Finally, the management of postural hypotension in each patient will need to be linked to non-autonomic features and any other medical disorder, and must be relevant to their life style. Thus the treatment of parkinsonism and introduction of L-DOPA may necessitate changes in dosage or frequency of drugs to control hypotension. In the cerebellar form of MSA there may be marked truncal ataxia, and exercise and walking programmes will need to be modified; such patients may, in due course, be safer in a wheelchair to reduce the risk of falling and trauma. The laboratory evaluation of postural hypotension also needs consideration, as blood pressure measurements are made usually with passive change (such as head-up tilt) or while standing still, precisely the measures that we encourage our patients to avoid. The evaluation of standing time, advocated by some, is often irrelevant in practice, as this will be influenced by many factors that worsen postural hypotension in daily life, and also by the additional neurological disabilities, as in patients with MSA. However, measurements of blood pressure are necessary for evaluation, and have their value, although in the individual patient symptoms and the ability to function independently are the crucial factors. The increasing availability of home blood pressure monitors should, in general, be discouraged, as unfortunately there are many patients shackled to monitors that inadvisably have been recommended; these are not even a poor second to the patient's symptoms! The key aims, therefore, in the management of postural hypotension are to ensure that the patient is appropriately mobile and functional, is on low-risk therapy that prevents falls and associated trauma, and is able to maintain a suitable quality of life. The same principles of pharmacological treatment of postural hypotension could generally be used in patients with orthostatic intolerance (eg. PoTS) but some exceptions would need to be applied, such as, cardioselective β-blockers may be useful in some patients with PoTS, alternatively, ephedrine may have beneficial effects in patients with autonomic failure but not in PoTS.

References

Alam, M., Smith, G. D. P., Bleasdale-Barr, K., Pavitt, D. V., and Mathias, C. J. (1995). Effects of the peptide release inhibitor, Octreotide, on daytime hypotension and on nocturnal hypertension in primary autonomic failure. *J. Hypertension.* 13, 1664–9.

Armstrong, E. and Mathias, C. J. (1991). The effects of the somatostatin analogue, octreotide, on postural hypotension, before and after food ingestion in primary autonomic failure. *Clin. Auton. Res.* 2, 135–40.

Asahina, M., Sato, J., Tachibana, M., Hattori, T. (2006). Cerebral blood flow and oxygenation during head-up tilt in patients with multiple system atrophy and healthy control subjects. *Parkinsonism Relat Disord*, 12, 472–7.

Bannister, R., Ardill, L., and Fentem, P. (1969). An assessment of various methods of treatment of idiopathic OH. *Q. J. Med.* 38, 377–95.

Bannister, R., Boylston, A. W., Davies, I. B., Mathias, C. J., Sever, P. S., and Sudera, D. (1981). Beta-receptor numbers and thermodynamics in denervation supersensitivity. *J. Physiol. London* 319, 369–77.

Bannister, R., Da Costa, D. F., Hendry, W. G., Jacobs, J., and Mathias, C. J. (1986). Atrial demand pacing to protect against vagal overactivity in sympathetic autonomic neuropathy. *Brain* 109, 345–56.

Bannister, R., Sever, P., and Gross, M. (1977). Cardiovascular reflexes and biochemical responses in progressive autonomic failure. *Brain* 100, 327–44.

Bevegard, S., Castenfors, J., and Lindblad, L.-E. (1974). Haemodynamic effects of dihydroergotamine in patients with postural hypotension. *Acta Med. Scand.* 196, 473–7.

Biaggioni, I., Robertson, D., Krantz, D. S., Jones, M., and Hale, V. (1994). The anaemia of primary autonomic failure and its reversal with recombinant erythropoietin. *Ann. Int. Med.* 121, 181–6.

Cariga, P., Mathias, C. J. (2001). Haemodynamics of the pressor effect of oral water in human sympathetic denervation due to autonomic failure. *Clin Sci.* 101, 313–319.

Carvalho, M. J., van den Meirackers, A. H., Boomsma, F. *et al.* (1997). Improved orthostatic tolerance in familial amyloidotic polyneuropathy with unnatural noradrenaline precursor L-threo-3,4,-dihydroxyphenylserine. *J. Autonom. Nerv. Syst.* 62, 63–71.

Chobanian, A. V., Volicer, L., Liang, C. S., Kershaw, G., and Tifft, C. (1977). Use of propranolol in the treatment of idiopathic OH. *Trans. Ass. Am. Physcns.* 90, 324–34.

Chobanian, A. V., Volicer, L., Tifft, C., Gavras, H., Liang, C., and Faxon, D. (1979). Mineralocorticoid-induced hypotension in patients with OH. *New Engl. J. Med.* 301, 68–73.

Colao, A., Faggiano, A., and Pivonello, R. (2010). Somatostatin analogues: treatment of pituitary and neuroendocrine tumors. *Prog Brain Res* 182, 281–94.

Davies, B., Bannister, R., Hensby, C., and Sever, P. (1980). The pressor actions of noradrenaline, angiotensin 11 in chronic autonomic failure treated with indomethacin. *Br. J. Clin. Pharmacol.* 10, 223–9.

Davies, B., Bannister, R., Mathias, C. J., and Sever, P. (1981). Pindolol in postural hypotension; the case for caution. *Lancet* i, 982–3.

Davies, B., Bannister, R., Sever, P., and Wilcox, C. S. (1979). The pressor actions of noradrenaline, angiotensin 11 and saralasin in chronic autonomic failure treated with fludrocortisone. *Br. J. Clin. Pharmacol.* 8, 253–60.

Davies, B., Bannister, R., and Sever, P. (1978). Pressor amines and monoamine oxidase inhibitors for treatment of postural hypotension in progressive autonomic failure. Limitations and hazards. *Lancet* i, 172–5.

Davies, B., Sudera, D., SagneHa, E. *et al.* (1982). Increased numbers of alpha-receptors in sympathetic denervation supersensitivity in man. *J. Clin. Invest.* 69, 779–84.

Fouad-Tarazi, F. M., Okabe, M., and Goran, H. (1995). α-sympathomimetic treatment of autonomic insufficiency with OH. *Am. J. Med.* 99, 604–10.

Freeman, R., Wieling, W., Axelrod, F. B., *et al.* (2011). Consensus statement on the definition of OH, neurally mediated syncope and the postural tachycardia syndrome. *Clin. Auton. Res.* 21, 69–72.

Frewin, D. B., Leonello, P. P., Pentall, R. K., Hughes, L., and Harding, P. E. (1980). Pindolol in OH: possible therapy? *Med. J. Aust.* 1, 128.

Garland, E. M., Gamboa, A., Okamoto, L., *et al.* (2009) Renal impairment of pure autonomic failure. *Hypertension.* 54, 1057–61.

Gibbons, C. H., Vernino, S. A., Kaufmann, H., Freeman, R. (2005). L-DOPS therapy for refractory OH in autoimmune autonomic neuropathy. *Neurology.* 65, 1104–6

Goovaerts, J., Ver faillie, C., Fagard, R., and Knochaert, D. (1984). Effect of prenalterol on OH in the Shy–Drager syndrome. *BMJ.* 288, 817–18.

Harms, M. P., Wieling, W., Colier, W. N., Lenders, J. W., Secher, N. H., van Lieshout, J. J. (2010). Central and cerebrovascular effects of leg crossing in humans with sympathetic failure. *Clin Sci (Lond).* 118, 573–81.

Hoeldtke, R. D., Cilmi, K. M., and Mattis-Graves, K. (1984). DL-Threo-3, 4-dihydroxyphenylserine does not exert a pressor effect in OH. *Clin. Pharmacol. Ther.* 36, 302–6.

Hoeldtke, R. D., and Streeten, D. H. P. (1993). Treatment of OH with erythropoietin. *New Engl. J. Med.* 329, 611–15.

Hoeldtke, R. D., Bryner, K. D., Hoeldtke, M. E., Hobbs, G. (2007). Treatment of autonomic neuropathy, postural tachycardia and orthostatic syncope with octreotide LAR. *Clin Auton Res.* 217:334–40.

Humm, A. M., Mason, L. M., Mathias, C. J. (2008). Effects of water drinking on cardiovascular responses to supine exercise and on OH after exercise in pure autonomic failure. *J Neurol Neurosurg Psychiatry.* 79, 1160–4.

Hunt, K., Tachtsidis, I., Bleasdale-Barr, K., Elwell, C., Mathias, C., Smith, M. (2006). Changes in cerebral oxygenation and haemodynamics during postural blood pressure changes in patients with autonomic failure. *Physiol Meas.* 27, 777–85.

Iwase, S., Mano, T., Kunimoto, M., and Saito, M. (1992). Effect of L-threo-3, 4,-dihydroxyphenylserine on muscle sympathetic nerve activity in humans. *J. Autonom. Nerv. Syst.* 39, 159–67.

Jamnadas-Khoda, J., Koshy, S., Mathias, C. J., Muthane, U. B., Ragothaman, M., Dodaballapur, S. K. (2009). Are current recommendations to diagnose OH in Parkinson's disease satisfactory? *Mov Disord.* 24, 1747–51.

Janknegt, R. A., Zweers, H. M. M., Delaere, K. P.J., Kloet, A. G., Khoe, S. G. S., and Arendsen, H. J. (1997). Oral desmopressin as a new treatment modality for primary nocturnal enuresis in adolescents and adults: a double-blind, randomized, multicenter study. *J. Urol.* **157**, 513–17.

Jankovic, J., Gilden, J. L. D., Heine, B. C., *et al.* (1993). Neurogenic OH: a double blind, placebo controlled study with midodrine. *Am. J. Med.* **95**, 38–48.

Jennings, G., Esler, M., and Holmes, R. (1979). Treatment of OH with dihydroergotamine. *BMJ.* **ii**, 307–8.

Jian, Z. J. and Zhou, B. Y. (2008). Efficacy and safety of acarbose in the treatment of elderly patients with postprandial hypotension. *Chin. Med. J. (Engl).* **121**(20), 2054–9.

Jordan, J., Shannon, J. R., Black, B. K., Ali, Y., Farley, M., Costa, F., Diedrich, A., Robertson, R. M., Biaggioni, I., Robertson, D. (2000). The pressor response to water drinking in humans: a sympathetic reflex? *Circulation.* **101**, 504–9.

Kachi, T., Iwase, S., Mano, T., Saito, M., Kunimoto, M., and Sobue, I. (1988). Effect of L-threo-3,4-dihydroxyphenylserine on muscle sympathetic nerve activity in Shy–Drager syndrome. *Neurology* **38**, 1091–4.

Karet, F. E., Dickerson, J. E. C., Brown, J., and Brown, M. J. (1994). Bovril and moclobemide: a novel therapeutic strategy for central autonomic failure. *Lancet* **344**, 1263–5.

Kaufmann, H., Brannan, T., Krakoff, L., Yahr, M. D., and Mandeli, J. (1988). Treatment of OH due to autonomic failure with a peripheral α-adrenergic agonist (midodrine). *Neurology* **38**, 951–6.

Kaufmann, H., Oribe, E., and Yahr, M. D. (1991). Differential effect L-threo-3,4-dihydroxyphenylserine in pure autonomic failure and multiple system atrophy with autonomic failure. *J. Neurol. Transm.* **3**, 143–8.

Kawakami, K., Abe, H., Harayama, N., Nakashima, Y. (2003). Successful treatment of severe OH with erythropoietin. *Pacing Clin Electrophysiol.* **26**, 105–7.

Kochar, M. S. and Itskovitz, H. D. (1978). Treatment of idiopathic OH (Shy–Drager syndrome) with indomethacin. *Lancet* **i**, 1011–14.

Kohno, R., Abe, H., Oginosawa, Y., Nagatomo, T., Otsuji, Y. (2007). Effects of atrial tachypacing on symptoms and blood pressure in severe OH. *Pacing Clin Electrophysiol.* **30**, 203–6.

Kuchel, O., Bun, N. T., Gutkowska, J., and Genest, J. (1980). Treatment of severe OH by metoclopramide. *Ann. Int. Med.* **93**, 841–3.

Low, P. A., Gilden, J. L., Freeman, R., Sheng, K.-N., and McElligott, M. A. (1997). Efficacy of midodrine vs placebo in neurogenic OH. A randomized, double-blind multicenter study. *J. Am. Med. Ass.* **277**, 1046–51.

Man in't Veld, A. J. and Schalekamp, M. A. D. H. (1981). Pindolol acts as betaadrenoceptor agonist in OH: therapeutic implications. *BMJ.* **282**, 929–31.

Mann, S., Altman, D. G., Raftery, E. B., and Bannister, R. (1983). Circadian variation of blood pressure in autonomic failure. *Circulation* **68**, 477–83.

Maruta, T., Komai, K., Takamori, M., and Yamada, M. (2006). Voglibose inhibits postprandial hypotension in neurologic disorders and elderly people. *Neurology* **66**(9), 1432–4.

Mathias, C. J. (2001). A sound night's rest may do no good in autonomic failure! *Clin Sci.* **10**, 619–20

Mathias, C. J. (2008). L-dihydroxyphenylserine (Droxidopa) in the treatment of OH: the European experience. *Clin Auton Res.* **18**, 25–9.

Mathias, C. J. (2009). Autonomic Dysfunction. In: Clarke, C., Howard, R., Rossor, M., Shorvon, S. (eds). *Neurology: A Queen Square Textbook.* 1st Edition. Chichester: Wiley Blackwell. p. 871–92.

Mathias, C. J. (2010). Disorders of the Autonomic Nervous System. In: Warrell, D. A., Cox, T. M., Firth, J. D. (eds). *Oxford Textbook of Medicine.* 5th Edition. Oxford: Oxford University Press.

Mathias, C. J., Fosbraey, P., de Costa, D. F., Thorley, A., and Bannister, R. (1986). Desmopressin reduces nocturnal polyuria, reverses overnight weight loss and improves morning postural hypotension in autonomic failure. *BMJ.* **293**, 353–4.

Mathias, C. J., Holly, E., Armstrong, E., Shareef, M., and Bannister, R. (1991). The influence of food on postural hypotension in three groups with chronic autonomic failure: clinical and therapeutic implications. *J. Neurol. Neurosurg. Psychiat.* **54**, 726–30.

Mathias, C. J., Iodice, V. and Low, D. A. (2012). Autonomic Dysfunction—Recognition, Diagnosis, Investigation and Management. In: Barnes, M. P. and Good, D. C. *Handbook of Clinical Neurology. Neurological Rehabilitation.* Vol 110. 3rd Series. Amsterdam: Elsevier.

Mathias, C. J., O'kuchu, M., Raimbach, S. J., Watson, L., and Bannister, R. (1990). Xamoterol reduces postural hypotension in both pure autonomic failure and multiple system atrophy. *J. Neurol.* **237**, (Suppl. 1): s24.

Mathias, C. J., Reid, J. L., Wing, L. M. H., Frankel, H. L., and Christensen, N. J. (1979). Antihypertensive effects of clonidine in tetraplegic subjects devoid of central sympathetic control. *Clin. Sci.* **57**, 425–6.

Mathias, C. J., Senard, J. M., Braune, S., Watson, L., Aragishi, A., Keeling, J. E., Taylor, M. D. (2001). L-threo-dihydroxyphenylserine (L-threo-DOPS; droxidopa) in the management of neurogenic orthostatic hypotension: a multi-national, multi-center, dose-ranging study in multiple system atrophy and pure autonomic failure. *Clin. Auton. Res.* **11**(4), 235–42.

Mathias, C. J., Unwin, R. J., Pike, F. A., Frankel, H. L., Sever, P. S. and Peart, W. S. (1984). The immediate pressor response to saralarin in man: evidence against sympathetic activation and for intrinsic angiotensin I-like myotropism. *Clin. Sci.* **66**, 517–24.

Mathias, C. J., Young TM. (2003) Plugging the leak—benefits of the vasopressin-2 agonist, desmopressin in autonomic failure. *Clin. Auton. Res.* **13**, 85–7.

Mathias, C. J. and Alam, M. (1995). The influence of certain daily activities on 24 hour ambulatory blood pressure in hypotensive, normotensive and hypertensive subjects. *Clin. Auton. Res.* **5**, 321.

Mathias, C. J. and Kimber, J. R. (1998). Treatment of postural hypotension. *J. Neurol. Neurosurg. Psychiat.* **65**, 285–9.

Maule, S., Milan, A., Grosso, T., Veglio, F. (2006). Left ventricular hypertrophy in patients with autonomic failure. *Am J Hypertens.* **19**, 1049–54.

May, M., Jordan, J. (2011). The osmopressor response to water drinking. *Am. J. Physiol. Regul. Integr. Comp. Physiol.* **300**, R40–6.

Mehlsen, J., and Trap-Jensen, J. (1985). Use of xamoterol, a new selective betaadrenoreceptor partial agonist, in the treatment of postural hypotension. *Proceedings of the International Symposium on Cardiovascular Pharmacotherapy, Geneva,* Abstract **73**.

Moss, A. J., Glaser, W., and Topol E. (1980). Atrial tachypacing in the treatment of a patient with primary OH. *New Engl. J. Med.* **302**, 1456–7.

Muneta, S., Iwata, T., Hiwada, K., Murakami, E., Sato, Y., and Imamura, Y. (1992). Effect of L-threo-3,4,-dihydroxyphenylserine on OH in a patient with spinal cord injury. *Jap. Circ. J.* **56**, 243–7.

Nordenfelt, I., and Mellander, S. (1972). Central haemodynamic effects of dihydroergotamine in patients with OH. *Acta Med. Scand.* **191**, 115–20.

Omboni, S., Smit, A. A., van Lieshout, J. J., Settels, J. J., Langewouters, G. J., Wieling, W. (2001). Mechanisms underlying the impairment in orthostatic tolerance after nocturnal recumbency in patients with autonomic failure. *Clin Sci.* **101**, 609–18.

Onrot, J., Goldberg, M. R., Biaggioni, I., Wiley, R. G., Hollister, A. S., and Robertson, D. (1987). Oral yohimbine in human autonomic failure. *Neurology* **37**, 215–20.

Pavy-Le Traon, A., Hughson, R.L., Thalamas, C., Galitsky, M., Fabre, N., Rascol, O., Senard, J.M., (2006). Cerebral autoregulation is preserved in multiple system atrophy: A transcranial Doppler study. *Mov Disord.* **21**. 2122–6.

Perera, R., Isola, L., and Kaufmann, H. (1995). Effect of recombinant erythropoietin on anemia and OH in primary autonomic failure. *Clin. Auton. Res.* **5**, 211–14.

Polinsky, R. J., Samaras, G. M., and Kopin, I. J. (1983). Sympathetic neural prosthesis for managing orthostatic hypertension. *Lancet* **i**, 901–4.

Puvi-Rajasingham, S., Smith, G. D. P., Akinola, A., and Mathias, C. J. (1997). Abnormal regional blood flow responses during and after exercise in human sympathetic denervation. *J. Physiol.* **505**, 481–9.

Rensma, P. L., van den Meiracker, A. H., Boomsma, F., Man in't Veld, A. J., and Schalekamp, M. A. (1993). Effects of ibopamine on postural hypotension in pure autonomic failure. *J. Cardiol. Pharmacol.* **21**, 863–8.

Rittig, S., Arentsen, J., Sorensen, K., Matthiesen, T., and Dupont, E. (1991). The hemodynamic effects of triglycyl-lysine-vasopressin (glypressin) in patients with parkinsonism and OH. *Movement Disorders* **6**, 21–8.

Sakakibara, R., Matsuda, S., Uchiyama, T., Yoshiyama, M., Yamanishi, T., Hattori, T. (2003). The effect of intranasal desmopressin on nocturnal waking and urination in multiple system atrophy patients with nocturnal polyuria. *Clin. Aut. Res.* **13**, 106–8.

Schmidt, P. G., Eckstein, J. W., and Abboud, F. M. (1966). Effect of 9-alpha-fluorohydrocortisone on forearm vascular responses to norepinephrine. *Circulation* **34**, 620–6.

Senard, J. M., Rascol, O., Durrieu, G., *et al.* (1993a). Effects of yohimbine on plasma catecholamine levels in OH related to Parkinson disease or multiple system atrophy. *Clin. Neuropharmacol.* **1**, 70–6.

Senard, J. M., Rascol, O., Rascol, A., and Montastruc, J. L. (1993b). Lack of yohimbine effect on ambulatory blood pressure recoding: a double-blind cross-over trial in parkinsonians with OH. *Fund. Clin. Pharmacol.* **7**, 465–70.

Shannon, J. R., Diedrich, A., Biaggioni, I., Tank, J., Robertson, R. M., Robertson, D., Jordan, J. (2002). Water drinking as a treatment for orthostatic syndromes. *Am J Med.* **112**, 355–60.

Sheps, S. G. (1976). The use of an elastic garment in the treatment of idiopathic OH. *Cardiology* **62**, (Suppl. 1), 271–9.

Shibao, C., Gamboa, A., Abraham, R., *et al.* (2006). Clonidine for the treatment of supine hypertension and pressure natriuresis in autonomic failure. *Hypertension.* **47**, 522–6.

Shibao, C., Gamboa, A., Diedrich, A., Dossett, C., Choi, L., Farley, G., Biaggioni, I. (2007). Acarbose, an alpha-glucosidase inhibitor, attenuates postprandial hypotension in autonomic failure. *Hypertension* **50**(1), 54–61.

Shibao, C., Okamoto, L. E., Gamboa, A., *et al.*, (2010). Comparative efficacy of yohimbine against pyridostigmine for the treatment of OH in autonomic failure. *Hypertension.* **56**, 847–51.

Singer, W., Opfer-Gehrking, T. L., McPhee, B. R., Hilz, M. J., Bharucha, A. E., Low, P. A. (2003). Acetylcholinesterase inhibition: a novel approach in the treatment of neurogenic OH. *J. Neurol Neurosurg. Psychiatry.* **74**, 1294–8.

Smith, G. D. P., Alam, M., Watson, L. P., and Mathias, C. J. (1995b). Effects of the somatostatin analogue, octreotide, on exercise induced hypotension in human subjects with chronic sympathetic failure. *Clin. Sci.* **89**, 367–73.

Smith, G. D. P., Watson, L. P., Pavitt, D. V., and Mathias, C. J. (1995a). Abnormal cardiovascular and catecholamine responses to supine exercise in human subjects with sympathetic dysfunction. *J. Physiol. London,* **485**, 255–65.

Smith, G. D. P., and Mathias, C. J. (1995). Postural hypotension enhanced by exercise in patients with chronic autonomic failure. *Q. J. Med.* **88**, 251–6.

Suzuki, K., Asahina, M., Suzuki, A., Hattori, T. (2008). Cerebral oxygenation monitoring for detecting critical cerebral hypoperfusion in patients with multiple system atrophy during the head-up tilt test. *Intern Med.* **47**, 1681–7.

Tachtsidis, I., Elwell, C. E., Leung, T. S., *et al.*, (2005). Rate of change in cerebral oxygenation and blood pressure in response to passive changes in posture: a comparison between pure autonomic failure patients and controls. *Adv Exp Med Biol.* **566**, 187–93.

Tanaka, H., Yamaguchi, H., and Tamaih, H. (1997). Treatment of orthostatic intolerance with inflatable abdominal band. *Lancet* **349**, 175.

Ten Harkel, A. D. J., van Lieshout, J. J., and Weiling, W. (1994). Effect of leg muscle pumping and in tensing on orthostatic arterial pressure; a study in normal subjects and in patients with autonomic failure. *Clin. Sci.* **87**, 533–58.

Ten Harkel, A. D. J., van Lieshout, J. J., and Wieling, W. (1992). Treatment of OH with sleeping in the head-up tilt position and in combination with fludrocortisone. *J. Intern. Med.* **232**, 139–45.

Thomaides, T. N., Chaudhuri, K. R., Maule, S., and Mathias, C. J. (1992). Differential responses in superior mesenteric artery blood flow may explain the variant pressor responses to clonidine in two groups with sympathetic denervation. *Clin. Sci.* **83**, 59–64,

Thomas, D. J., and Bannister, R. (1980). Preservation of autoregulation of cerebral blood flow in autonomic failure. *J. Neurol. Sci.* **44**, 205–12.

Tobian, L. and Redleaf, P. D. (1958). Ionic composition of the aorta in renal and adrenal hypertension. *Am. J. Physiol.* **192**, 325–30.

Tutaj, M., Marthol, H., Berlin, D., Brown, C. M., Axelrod, F. B., Hilz, M. J. (2006). Effect of physical countermaneuvers on OH in familial dysautonomia. *J Neurol.* **253**, 65–72.

Vagaonescu, T. D., Saadia, D., Tuhrim, S., Phillips, R. A., Kaufmann, H. (2000). Hypertensive cardiovascular damage in patients with primary autonomic failure. *Lancet.* **355**, 725–6.

Vahidassr, M. D., Foy, C. J., O'Malley, T., and Passmore, A. P. (1997). Eye drops and lethargy. *J. R. Soc. Med.* **90**, 155.

Watt, S. J., Tooke, J. E., Perkins, C. M., and Lee, M. (1981). The treatment of idiopathic OH: a combined fludrocortisone– flurbiprofen regime. *Q. J. Med.* **50**, 205–212.

Wieling, W., van Lieshout J. J., and van Leeuwen A. M. (1993). Physical manoeuvres that reduce postural hypotension. *Clin. Ant. Res.* **3**, 57–65.

Wieling, W., Colman, N., Krediet, C. T., and Freeman, R. (2004). Nonpharmacological treatment of reflex syncope. *Clin. Auton. Res.* **14** Suppl 1, 62–70.

Young, T. M., and Mathias, C. J. (2004). The effects of water ingestion on orthostatic hypotension in two groups of chronic autonomic failure: multiple system atrophy and pure autonomic failure. *J. Neurol. Neurosurg. Psychiatry* **75**(12), 1737–41.

Young, T. M., Mathias, C. J. (2008). Treatment of supine hypertension in autonomic failure with gastrostomy feeding at night. *Auton Neurosci.* **5**, 77–8.

PART V

Peripheral Autonomic Neuropathies

CHAPTER 48

Familial dysautonomia

Felicia B. Axelrod

Key points

- Familial dysautonomia is one of the hereditary sensory and autonomic neuropathy disorders that affects neuronal development and survival and results in sensory and autonomic dysfunction.

- DNA diagnosis and general population screening is now possible.

- Although absence of emotional tearing is a consistent feature, there is considerable variation in expression of other systemic symptoms including gastrointestinal dysmotility, vomiting crises, and small fibre sensory dysfunction.

- Cardiovascular perturbations include orthostatic hypotension and episodic hypertension, as well as bradyarrhythmia.

- The disease is progressive but supportive treatments can decrease morbidity and mortality.

Introduction

Familial dysautonomia (FD), originally termed the Riley–Day syndrome (Riley et al. 1949), is an autosomal recessive disorder with extensive central and peripheral autonomic perturbations. It is now appreciated that FD is one example of a group of rare disorders termed hereditary sensory and autonomic neuropathies (HSAN) (Axelrod 2002, Axelrod 2004, Axelrod and Hilz 2003). Within this classification FD is termed HSAN type 2. The HSANs can be thought of broadly as entities in which normal migration and maturation of neural-crest-derived cells has been impeded, especially those destined to evolve into the sensory and autonomic populations. The genetic defect affects prenatal neuronal development so that symptoms are present from birth, although individual expression varies widely. Because the entire autonomic nervous system is affected, there is a pervasive effect on the functioning of other systems. However, with supportive treatments of the various manifestations, the prognosis for affected individuals has improved and a growing number of individuals affected with FD are surviving into adulthood (Axelrod et al. 2002). Because the FD population is largely genetically homogeneous, it serves as an excellent model with which to understand autonomic dysfunction caused by depleted unmyelinated neurons. Now that the gene for FD has been discovered we anticipate that we will gain further insight into the interrelationship of neuropathological lesions and the biochemical and physiological factors controlling the autonomic nervous system.

Genetics

FD results from a recessive genetic defect with a remarkably high carrier frequency in individuals of Ashkenazi Jewish extraction. In this population, the carrier rate has been estimated to be 1 in 30, with a disease frequency of 1 in 3600 live births (Maayan et al. 1987). In 1993 the FD gene was localized to the long arm of chromosome 9 (9q31) with a single major haplotype accounting for >99.5% of all FD chromosomes in the Ashkenazi Jewish population, which strongly suggested a founder mutation (Blumenfeld et al. 1993). In January 2001 it was reported that a unique non-coding splicing mutation in the *IKBKAP* gene is involved in all cases of FD described to date (Anderson et al. 2001, Slaugenhaupt et al. 2001). This major FD mutation is a T to C change located at base pair 6 of intron 20 (IVS20 + 6 T>C) of the gene *IKBKAP* that resides on the distal long arm of chromosome 9 (q31). The mutation causes a splicing alteration that leads to variable skipping of exon 20 in the *IKBKAP* message. Examination of multiple cell types from autopsied tissue revealed that the mutation causes a tissue specific decrease in the efficiency of splicing (Slaugenhaupt et al. 2001). Consistent with, and perhaps contributing to, the neurodegenerative phenotype of FD, neuronal tissues show the greatest reduction in correctly spliced *IKBKAP* transcripts. The other, less common, Ashkenazi Jewish mutation is a missense on exon 19 date (Anderson et al. 2001, Slaugenhaupt et al. 2001). A third mutation, also a missense mutation, was found in one patient whose mother was not of Jewish background (Leyne et al. 2003).

The other HSANs do not have the same ethnic bias as FD and are presumed to have unique genotypes accounting for their subtle phenotypic differences. Because all of the HSANs affect neuronal development, possible candidates are genes that encode neurotrophins, their receptors, or any proteins that might participate in a neurotrophin-related signal transduction pathway. In fact HSAN type 4 has been shown to result from mutations in the gene that encodes a neurotrophin receptor, NTRK1, which is located on chromosome 1 (Axelrod 2002, Axelrod and Hilz 2003, Indo et al. 1996).

Neuropathology

Although clinical manifestations suggest both central and peripheral nervous system involvement, consistent neuropathological lesions have only been described for the peripheral nervous system. Pathological findings indicate that within the peripheral sensory and autonomic systems individuals affected with FD suffer from incomplete neuronal development as well as progressive neuronal degeneration. Investigations are yet to be performed to see whether similar lesions are present in the central autonomic tracts.

Sensory nervous system

Intrauterine development and postnatal maintenance of dorsal root ganglion neurons are abnormal. The dorsal root ganglia are grossly reduced in size due to decreased neuronal population. Within the spinal cord, lateral root entry zones and Lissauer's tracts are severely depleted of axons (Pearson and Pytel 1978a). With increasing age, the numbers of neurons in dorsal root ganglia decrease more than one would expect as part of normal ageing and there is an abnormal increase in the number of residual nodules of Nageotte. In addition, loss of dorsal column myelinated axons becomes evident in older patients. Neuronal depletion in dorsal root ganglia and spinal cord is consistent with reports of decreased size of the sural nerve in FD patients (Pearson et al. 1975). The sural nerve is reduced in area and contains markedly diminished numbers of non-myelinated axons, as well as diminished numbers of small-diameter myelinated axons. Even in the youngest subject, extensive pathology has been evident, as might be expected from the fact that this is a developmental disorder. The sural nerve findings are sufficiently characteristic for familial dysautonomia to differentiate it from other sensory neuropathies (Axelrod 2002, Axelrod and Hilz 2003).

Autonomic nervous system

Consistent with an actual decrease in neuronal numbers, the mean volume of superior cervical sympathetic ganglia is reduced to 34% of the normal size (Pearson and Pytel 1978a) (Fig. 48.1), yet staining for tyrosine hydroxylase is enhanced in the neurons that are present in the sympathetic ganglia (Pearson et al. 1979). Decreased numbers of neurons in the intermediolateral grey columns of the spinal cord suggests involvement of preganglionic neurons (Pearson and Pytel 1978a). Furthermore, autonomic nerve terminals cannot be demonstrated on peripheral blood vessels (Grover-Johnson and Pearson 1979). Lack of innervation is consistent with postural hypotension, as well as exaggerated responses to sympathomimetic and parasympathomimetic agents (Smith et al. 1965, Bickel et al. 2002). Other than the sphenopalatine ganglia, which are consistently reduced in size with low total neuronal counts, other parasympathetic ganglia, such as the ciliary ganglia, do not seem to be affected (Pearson and Pytel 1978b). The paucity of neurons in the sphenopalatine ganglion would explain the supersensitivity of the lachrymal gland to infused methacholine (Smith et al. 1965).

Neurophysiology

Chemoreceptor and baroreceptor dysfunction

Denervation extending to chemoreceptors and baroreceptors has never been demonstrated pathologically but is strongly suggested by physiological studies (Stemper et al. 2004). During hypoxia (12% O_2), patients with FD initially increase ventilation but with continued hypoxia, ventilation decreases (Stemper et al. 2004, Edelman et al. 1970, Bernardi et al. 2002, Maayan et al. 1992). These observations suggest that patients with FD have normal peripheral chemoreceptors but an inordinate central depression of

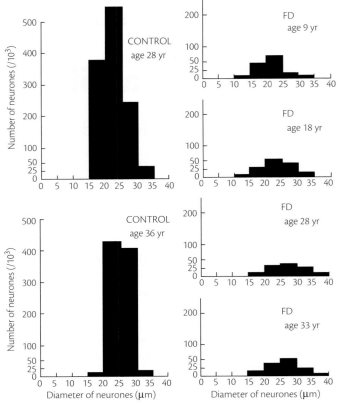

Fig. 48.1 Histograms of neuron distribution in sympathetic ganglia in patients with familial dysautonomia and controls. Reprinted from *J. Neurol. Sci.*, **39**, Pearson J, Pytel B., Quantitative studies of sympathetic ganglia and spinal cord intermedio-lateral gray columns in familial dysautonomia, 47–59, copyright 1978, with permission from Elsevier.

ventilation by hypoxia. Furthermore, hypoxia induces profound circulatory responses consistent with sympathetic denervation (Edelman et al. 1970, Bernardi et al. 2002). In contrast to controls, when FD subjects are exposed to hypoxia during rebreathing, there is a marked decrease in heart rate and systemic blood pressure (Fig. 48.2).

Studies of blood flow have described inappropriate arteriolar and venous tone responses to both upright positioning and cold stimuli (Mason et al. 1966, Hilz et al. 1997, Hilz et al. 2002, Brown et al. 2003). In individuals with FD, vascular resistance did not increase with either stimulus. In addition organ hypoperfusion coexists during hyperfusion of terminal vessels (Stemper et al. 2003). It is also now well recognized that individuals with FD consistently manifest orthostatic hypotension without compensatory tachycardia (Stemper et al. 2004, Ziegler et al. 1976, Axelrod et al. 1993).

Catecholamine metabolism

On measurement of urinary catecholamine metabolites, FD patients were found to have elevated levels of homovanillic acid (HVA) and normal to low levels of vanillylmandelic acid (VMA), resulting in elevated HVA:VMA ratios (Smith et al. 1963) These findings are consistent with the later neuropathological descriptions of a decreased sympathetic neuronal population. Although supine plasma levels of noradrenaline are normal or elevated, FD patients, like most other patients with neurogenic orthostatic

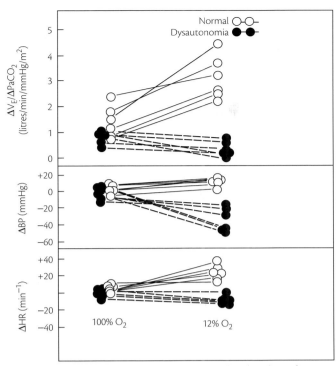

Fig. 48.2 Ventilatory and cardiovascular responses to the rebreathing of 100% and 12% oxygen by six dysautonomic and six normal subjects. Left-hand points: 100% O_2, right-hand points: 12% O_2. Upper panel: ventilatory response to CO_2 expressed as increase in ventilation per mmHg increase in $PaCO_2$ normalized for body surface area. Middle panel: each point represents the change in mean systemic blood pressure from the beginning to the end of a rebreathing period. Lower panel: each point represents the change in heart rate from the beginning to the end of a rebreathing period. In contrast to control subjects, rebreathing 12% O_2 by dysautonomia subjects resulted in a lower ventilatory response to CO_2 than during 100% rebreathing, bradycardia, and a substantial fall in systemic blood pressure. With permission from Edelman NH, Cherniack NS, Lahiri S, Richards E, Fishman AP (1970). *J. Clin. Invest* **49**, 1153–65.

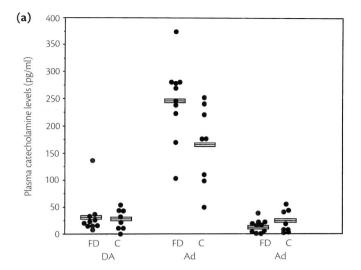

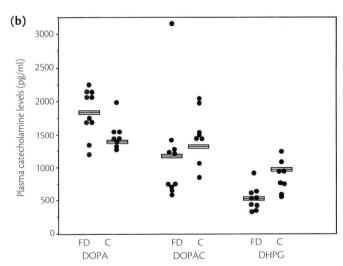

Fig. 48.3 Supine catechol values for 10 patients with familial dysautonomia (FD) and 8 control subjects. FD values are averages from two to three testing sessions. Control values are absolute values. Horizontal bars are means. **(a)** Catecholamine: DA, dopamine; Ad, adrenaline; **(b)** catechol metabolites: DOPA, dihydroxyphenylalanine; DOPAC, dihydroxyphenylacetic acid; DHPG, dihydroxyphenylglycol. From Axelrod et al. 1996, with permission.

hypotension, do not have an appropriate increase in plasma levels of noradrenaline and dopamine-beta-hydroxylase (DBH) with standing (Ziegler et al. 1976, Axelrod et al. 1996, Axelrod et al. 1994). In addition, FD patients appear to have a distinctive pattern of plasma levels of catechols (Axelrod et al. 1996, Fig. 48.3). Regardless of posture, plasma levels of DOPA are disproportionately high and plasma levels of dihydroxyphenylglycol (DHPG) are low resulting in elevated plasma DOPA:DHPG ratios (Fig. 48.4) which are not seen in other disorders associated with neurogenic orthostatic hypotension. The low levels of DHPG could be a consequence of either decreased availability of axoplasmic noradrenaline or decreased sequential activity of monoamine oxidase (MAO) and aldehydic reductase on noradrenaline. The high plasma dopa levels are consistent with FD subjects having an increased proportion of tyrosine hydroxylase in superior cervical ganglia (Pearson et al. 1979).

When FD subjects are supine, there is a strong correlation between mean blood pressure and plasma levels of noradrenaline, but when they are upright, the correlation is seen only with plasma dopamine levels (Fig. 48.5) suggesting that in FD patients dopamine may serve to maintain upright blood pressure. During emotional crises, plasma noradrenaline and dopamine levels are markedly elevated

and vomiting usually coincides with the high dopamine levels. The elevation of plasma Noradrenaline is attributed to peripheral conversion of dopamine by DBH. Diazepam sedates patients in crises and relieves vomiting, possibly by enhancing γ-aminobutyric acid (GABA) and damping the release of dopamine.

Other vascular modulators

Supine early morning plasma renin activity is elevated in FD subjects and the release of renin and aldosterone is not co-ordinated (Rabinowitz et al. 1974). In FD individuals with supine hypertension, an increase in plasma atrial natriuretic peptide (ANP) has also been demonstrated (Axelrod et al. 1994). The combination of these factors may serve to explain the exaggerated nocturnal urine volume and increased excretion of salt in some FD individuals, especially during stress and hypertension.

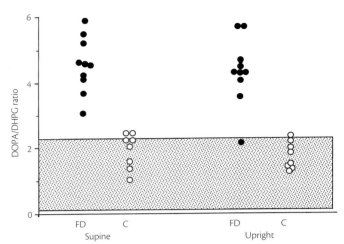

Fig. 48.4 Ratio of dihydroxyphenylalanine to dihydroxyphenylglycol (DOPA:DHPG) for 10 patients with familial dysautonomia (FD) and 8 control subjects. FD values (●) are averages from two to three testing sessions. Control values (o) are absolute values. The grey area indicates the normal range of this ratio in plasma (0.13–2.28). From Axelrod et al. 1996, with permission.

Clinical features and management

Diagnostic criteria

Although genetic diagnosis is available, initial evaluation utilizes clinical criteria that are based upon the ethnic bias for this disorder as well as a constellation of signs attributed to sensory and autonomic dysfunctions (Axelrod 2002, Axelrod 2004, Axelrod and Hilz 2003). This is primarily a neurological disorder, but the clinical features are pervasive and involve many other systems (Table 48.1). The diagnosis should be suspected by history and physical examination, which can provide much of the essential information. Clinical confirmation is then obtained by ascertaining the presence of five 'cardinal' criteria (i.e. absence of overflow emotional tears, absent lingual fungiform papillae (Fig. 48.6), depressed patellar reflexes, lack of an axon flare following intradermal histamine (Fig. 48.7), and documentation of Ashkenazi Jewish extraction) (Axelrod 2002, Axelrod 2004, Axelrod and Hilz 2003). Further supportive evidence is provided by findings of decreased response to pain and temperature, orthostatic hypotension, periodical erythematous blotching of the skin, and increased sweating. In addition, cine-oesophagrams may reveal delay in cricopharyngeal closure, tertiary contractions of the oesophagus, gastro-oesophageal reflux, and delayed gastric emptying.

Because individuals affected with the other HSANs will also fail to produce an axon flare after intradermal histamine and because there can be extreme variability in expression, clinical criteria are not always sufficient. For a definitive diagnosis, sural nerve biopsy has now been replaced by DNA molecular testing that can identify the FD *IKBKAP* mutations.

Sensory system

In the younger patient, sensory abnormalities appear to be limited to the unmyelinated neuronal population, but in the older patient there is progressive involvement of myelinated neurons of the dorsal column tracts (Axelrod et al. 1981). Although pain sensation is decreased, it is not completely absent and there is usually sparing of palms, soles of feet, neck, and genital areas, with these areas

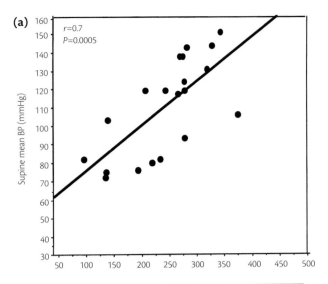

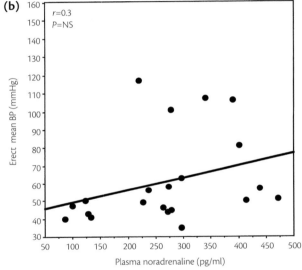

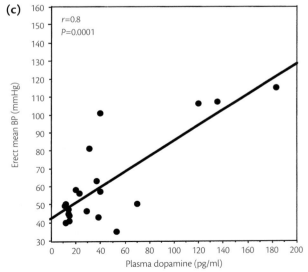

Fig. 48.5 (a) Correlation of mean blood pressure and plasma level of noradrenaline in patients with dysautonomia (FD) when supine and erect. **(b)** Correlation of mean blood pressure and plasma level of dopamine in FD subjects when erect.

Table 48.1 Clinical features of familial dysautonomia

System	Common symptoms	Frequency (%)
Ocular	◆ Decreased tears	>60
	◆ Corneal analgesia	>60
Gastrointestinal dysfunction	◆ Dysphagia	>60
	◆ Oesophageal and gastric dysmotility	>60
	◆ Gastro-oesophageal reflux	67
	◆ Vomiting crises	40
Pulmonary	◆ Aspirations	NA
	◆ Insensitivity to hypoxia	NA
	◆ Restrictive lung disease	NA
Orthopaedic	◆ Spinal curvature	90
	◆ Aseptic necrosis	15
Vasomotor	◆ Postural hypotension	100
	◆ Blotching	99
	◆ Excessive sweating	99
	◆ Hypertensive crises	>60
Neurological	◆ Decreased deep tendon reflexes	95
	◆ Dysarthria	NA
	◆ Decreased pain sensation	NA
	◆ Decreased temperature sensation	NA
	◆ Decreased vibration (after 13 years)	NA
	◆ Progressive ataxia (in adult years)	NA
	◆ Less than average IQ	38

NA, percentages not available.

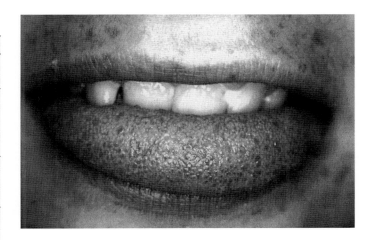

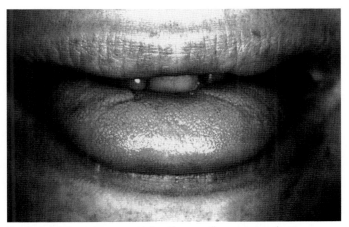

Fig. 48.6 (a) Normal tongue with fungiform papillae present on the tip, **(b)** dysautonomic tongue.

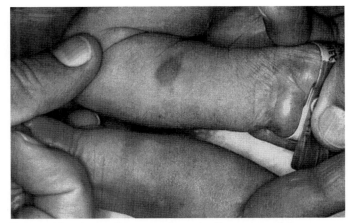

Fig. 48.7 Histamine test. Dysautonomic reaction (forearm on top) demonstrates a narrow areola surrounding the wheal. Normal reaction (lower forearm) displays diffuse axon flare around a central wheal.

often being exquisitely sensitive. Temperature appreciation, as documented by sympathetic skin responses and Thermotest readings to both hot and cold stimuli, is also affected (Hilz et al. 1999, Hilz and Axelrod 2000). With both pain and temperature perceptions, the trunk and lower extremities are more affected and older individuals have greater losses than younger (Axelrod et al. 1981). In the older individual, vibration sense, and occasionally joint position, becomes abnormal and Rombergism may be noted suggesting the development of spinocerebellar atrophy. Visceral sensation is intact so patients are able to perceive discomfort with pleuritic or peritoneal irritation.

Peripheral sensory deprivation makes the FD patient prone to self-injury. In addition to inadvertent trauma to joints and long bones, causing Charcot joints, aseptic necrosis, and unrecognized fractures, some patients will self-mutilate by picking at their fingers to the point of bleeding. Spinal curvature, which can be early and pernicious in its course, requires extreme care in fitting of braces to avoid development of pressure decubiti on insensitive skin.

Central sensory deficits include decreased pain perception along the branches of the trigeminal nerve, diminished corneal reflexes, and decreased taste perception, especially in recognition of sweet flavour, which corresponds to the absence of fungiform papillae on the tip of the tongue.

Although the motor system is spared, the young child with FD is frequently hypotonic, which may be due to a combination of central deficits and decreased tone of stretch receptors. Older patients develop a broad-based and mildly ataxic gait, with special difficulties

in performing rapid movements or turning. Gait abnormalities can be severe enough to require the use of walkers or wheelchairs.

Autonomic dysfunction

Pervasive autonomic dysfunction results in protean functional abnormalities affecting other systems and yielding a myriad of clinical manifestations. As the disorder has variable expression, there are individual variations. Some of these manifestations are apparent at birth and others become more prominent and problematic as a function of age.

Gastrointestinal system

Oropharyngeal incoordination is one of the earliest signs of FD. Poor sucking or discoordinated swallowing is observed in 60% of infants in the neonatal period. Oral incoordination can persist in the older patient and be manifested as a tendency to drool. Cine-radiographic swallowing studies, using various food consistencies, are used to assess function and provide guidelines for therapy. Liquids are more apt to be aspirated. If dysphagia impedes maintenance of nutrition, or if respiratory problems persist, then gastrostomy is recommended (Axelrod and Maayan 2002).

The most prominent manifestation of abnormal gastrointestinal dysmotility in FD individuals is the propensity to vomit. Vomiting can occur intermittently as part of a systemic reaction to physical or emotional stress or it can occur daily in response to the stress of arousal. Because vomiting is often associated with hypertension, tachycardia, diffuse sweating, and even personality change, this constellation of signs has been termed the dysautonomic crisis (Axelrod 2002, Axelrod and Hilz 2003, Axelrod and Maayan 2002). Diazepam is considered to be the most effective anti-emetic for the dysautonomic crisis and can be administered orally, intravenously, or rectally at 0.1–0.2 mg/kg/dose (Axelrod 2005, Axelrod and Maayan 2002). Subsequent doses of diazepam are repeated at 3-hour intervals until the crisis resolves. If diastolic hypertension persists (>90 mm Hg) after giving diazepam, then either chloral hydrate or clonidine (0.004 mg/kg/dose) is suggested. Clonidine can be repeated at 3–6-hour intervals. The crisis usually resolves abruptly and is marked by return of personality to normal and return of appetite.

Gastro-oesophageal reflux (GER) is another common problem and should be considered in FD individuals with frequent vomiting (Sundaram and Axelrod 2005). If GER is identified, medical management, including prokinetic agents and H_2 antagonists, should be tried. However, if pneumonia, haematemesis, or apnoea occur, then surgical intervention (fundoplication) is recommended (Axelrod 2005, Axelrod and Maayan 2002). After surgery, dysautonomic crises may continue but retching will be substituted for vomiting (Sundaram and Axelrod 2005).

Respiratory system

Aspiration is the major cause of lung infections. Most of the lung damage occurs during infancy and early childhood when oral incoordination is extremely poor and the diet contains mostly liquids. If gastro-oesophageal reflux is present, the risk for aspiration increases (Axelrod and Maayan 2002, Axelrod and Maayan 1998).

The ventilatory response to lung infection is often altered due to insensitivity to hypoxia and hypercapnia (Edelman et al. 1970, Bernardi et al. 2002, Maayan et al. 1992). Low oxygen saturations do not cause tachypnoea and can cause syncope as hypoxia induces both hypotension and bradycardia. Dysautonomic patients must be cautious in settings where the partial pressure of oxygen is decreased, such as at high altitudes or during aeroplane travel. When the aeroplane's altitude exceeds 39,000 feet ($\simeq$ 12,000 m), the cabin pressure will be equivalent to more than 6000 feet ($\simeq$ 2000 m), and supplemental oxygen probably will be necessary. Diving and underwater swimming can be potential hazards.

Cardiovascular irregularities

Consistent with sympathetic dysfunction, patients exhibit rapid and severe orthostatic decreases in blood pressure, without appropriate compensatory increases in heart rate. Clinical manifestations of postural hypotension include episodes of light-headedness or dizzy spells. Some patients complain of 'weak legs'. On occasion, there may be syncope. Symptoms tend to be worse in the morning, in hot or humid weather, when the bladder is full, before a large bowel movement, after a long car ride, coming out of a movie theatre, or with fatigue. Symptoms referable to hypotension become more prominent in the adult years and can limit function and mobility. Postural hypotension is treated by maintaining adequate hydration and encouraging lower-extremity to increase muscle tone and promote venous return (Axelrod and Maayan 2002). In a retrospective study fludrocortisone was shown to have clinical efficacy (Axelrod et al. 2005). Fludrocortisone significantly increased mean blood pressures and decreased dizziness and leg cramping. In addition cumulative survival was significantly higher in fludrocortisone-treated patients than in non-treated patients during the first decade. In subsequent decades, the addition of midodrine, an α-adrenergic agonist, improved cumulative survival (Fig. 48.8). In a previous study of the clinical efficacy of midodrine, it was shown that an average dose of 0.25 mg/kg/day produced clinical improvement (Axelrod et al. 1995).

General anaesthesia has the potential for inducing severe hypotension. With greater attention to stabilization of the vascular bed by hydrating the patient before surgery and titrating the anaesthetic to continuously monitored arterial blood pressure, anaesthetic risk has been greatly reduced.

In the older patients, supine hypertension can become prominent despite the retention of severe responses to orthostatic challenge.

Hypertension can also occur intermittently in response to emotional stress or visceral pain, or as part of the crisis constellation. The hypertension will respond to the same medications recommended for crisis management. Hypertension can also exist without

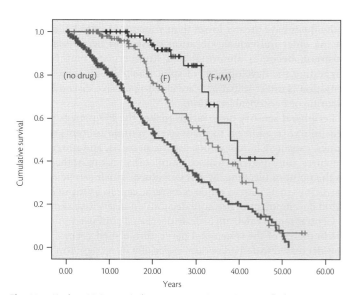

Fig. 48.8 Kaplan–Meier survival curves comparing patients on fludrocortisone alone (F), patients on both fludrocortisone and midodrine (F + M), and patients not treated with either of these two drugs (No drug) over the entire study period. Modified from Axelrod et al. 2005, with permission.

any other symptoms. Because blood pressure is so labile in individuals with FD, asymptomatic hypertension is not usually treated as the hypertension is usually transitory and appears to be better tolerated than hypotension.

Although FD subjects consistently exhibit orthostatic instability, they have variable electrocardiographic findings. As part of the progressive nature of FD, there is worsening of sympathetic dysfunction and development of parasympathetic dysfunction. Heart rate variability studies, using power spectral analysis, indicate that with exertion there is inappropriate persistence of parasympathetic activity and failure to enhance sympathetic activity (Maayan et al. 1987). Prolongation of the QTc and JTc occurs in some patients and may be an ominous sign (Glickstein et al. 1993, Axelrod et al. 1997, Glickstein et al. 1999). In a retrospective review of FD patients, it was noted that 3.7% had pacemakers placed and that asystole was the most frequent electrocardiographic finding (85%), other electrocardiographic abnormalities included bradycardia, AV block, prolonged QTc and prolonged JTc (Gold-von Simson et al. 2005). Data from this review suggested that pacemaker placement might protect FD patients from fatal bradyarrhythmia.

Renal problems

Azotaemia is frequently prerenal in origin. Although clinical signs of dehydration may not be present, blood urea nitrogen values often can be reduced by simple hydration. Renal function appears to deteriorate with advancing age and patients with FD are more likely to develop chronic renal disease than the general population (Matalon et al. 2006). According to the findings of Matalon et al., 19% of patients who remained alive at 25 years of age eventually required dialysis. Renal biopsies performed on individuals with uncorrectable azotaemia revealed significant ischaemic-type glomerulosclerosis and deficient vascular innervation (Pearson et al. 1980). Renal hypoperfusion secondary to cardiovascular instability or inadequate hydration has been suggested as the cause of the progressive renal disease. Patients with FD who eventually required dialysis showed a greater degree of orthostatic hypotension and were less likely to have had a feeding gastrostomy tube placed for hydration before 15 years of age (Matalon et al. 2006). In further support of the cardiovascular instability hypothesis are the studies utilizing the technique of renal artery Doppler blood velocity waveform analysis (Axelrod et al. 1993). In contrast to controls, when FD patients assumed the erect position and exercised, renal systolic velocity decreased as reflected in an increased A/B ratio, the ratio of the peak systolic velocity (point A) to the end diastolic velocity (point B). An increase in A/B ratio can be interpreted as consistent with a decrease in the end diastolic flow (Fig. 48.9). Thus, aggressive treatment of postural hypotension, including assuring adequate hydration, appears to be justified.

Ophthalmological manifestations

Individuals with FD do not cry with overflow tears. Corneal hypaesthesia compounds the ocular status, as it results in decreased blink frequency and indifference to corneal trauma. Epithelial erosions of the exposed cornea and conjunctiva are the hallmarks of dry-eye states. These lesions may become confluent, leading to patchy areas of de-epithelialization. Early treatment of corneal epithelial erosions includes increased frequency of tear substitutes, attention to the general state of hydration, and the search for precipitating systemic factors that might have disturbed the patient's

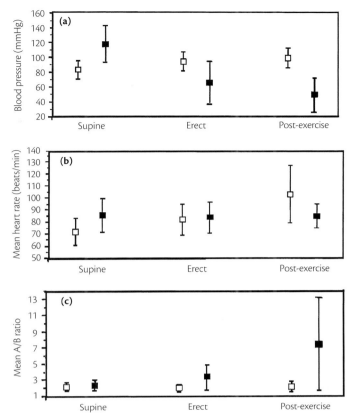

Fig. 48.9 Haemodynamic response to change in position and exercise in controls (□) and patients with familial dysautonomia (FD) (■). **(a)** Mean blood pressures with 1 SD bars, p = 0.0001, **(b)** mean heart rates with 1 SD bars, p = 0.0002, **(c)** mean A/B ratios with 1 SD bars, p = 0.005. From Axelrod et al. 1993, with permission.

fragile catecholamine homeostasis (Axelrod and D'Amico 1995). Persistent erosions or ulcerations may require a therapeutic soft contact lens, occlusion of the lachrymal puncta or small lateral tarsorrhaphies that limit the area exposed to surface evaporation. Corneal grafts generally have not been successful as the dry anaesthetic cornea is an unfavourable environment for a corneal graft. The importance of restoring the patient's homeostasis when treating ocular complications in familial dysautonomia cannot be overemphasized. Failure to correct dehydration or even a low-grade systemic infection can thwart the most heroic efforts at ocular therapy.

Other ophthalmological features include hyperreactivity to sympathetic and parasympathetic agents as well as tendency to myopia, optic pallor, and strabismus.

Central nervous system features (intelligence/emotion/seizures)

Emotional lability has been considered one of the prominent features of FD and was stressed in its original description (Riley et al. 1949). It is now appreciated that the behavioural abnormalities tend to be part of the crisis constellation and may be secondary to periodic catecholamine imbalance. The prompt normalization of personality in response to benzodiazepines supports this hypothesis (Axelrod and Maayan 1998).

Most affected individuals are of normal intelligence. In one study, 38% of FD patients had less than average intelligence (Welton et al. 1979) but correlation with other systemic problems was not available. Individuals with FD usually perform well on the Similarities subtest of the WISC (Wechsler Intelligence Scale for Children), which suggests that verbal intellect is relatively spared.

About 25% of FD patients have abnormal EEGs but less than 10% actually have a true seizure disorder. In the population of FD patients who have had a seizure, the incidence of an abnormal EEG rises to 65%. Anticonvulsant therapy should be used in these cases.

Prolonged breath-holding with crying can be severe enough to result in cyanosis, syncope, and decerebrate posturing and has been thought to represent a type of seizure activity. Breath-holding is frequent in the early years, occurring at least one time in 63% of patients. This phenomenon probably is a manifestation of insensitivity to hypoxia and hypercapnia. It can become a manipulative manoeuvre with some children. In our experience, the episodes are self-limited, cease by 6 years of age, and have never been fatal. However, hypoxia due to an infection can produce seizures with a more severe outcome.

Metabolic seizures, induced by hyponatraemia, have been observed during extremely hot weather when fluid and salt intake have failed to compensate for the excessive sweating manifested by these patients. Hyponatraemic seizures have also occurred with severe infections or protracted crises.

Progressive features (peripheral and central problems)

As survival has improved for the FD population (Axelrod et al. 2002), an adult FD population has evolved which has confirmed the progressive nature of the disorder. Slow progressive peripheral degeneration is appreciated clinically, as the older patients exhibit further worsening of sensory loss (Axelrod et al. 1981) and neuropathologically, as the number of neurons in dorsal root ganglia diminish and residual nodules of Nageotte increase abnormally with age (Pearson and Pytel 1978a). Adult FD patients do not appear to appreciate the decline in their sensory abilities but they frequently complain of poor balance, unsteady gait, and difficulty concentrating. They are prone to depression, anxieties, and even phobias. With increasing age, sympathovagal balance becomes more precarious with worsening of orthostatic hypotension, development of supine hypertension, and even occasional bradyarrhythmias (Axelrod et al. 1997, Gold-von Simson et al. 2005). In addition the cardiovascular instability appears to lead to chronic kidney disease in the adult population (Matalon et al. 2006)

Prognosis

With greater understanding of the disorder and development of treatment programmes, survival statistics have markedly improved so that increasing numbers of patients are reaching adulthood. Survival statistics prior to 1960 reveal that 50% of patients died before 5 years of age. Current survival statistics indicate that a newborn with FD has a 50% probability of reaching 40 years of age (Axelrod et al. 2002). Many FD adults have been able to achieve independent function. Both men and women with FD have married and reproduced. All offspring have been phenotypically normal despite their obligatory heterozygote state. Although pregnancies were tolerated well, at time of delivery blood pressures were labile.

Causes of death are less often related to pulmonary complications, indicating that aggressive treatment of aspirations has been beneficial. Of recent concern have been the patients who have succumbed to unexplained deaths, which may have been the result of unopposed vagal stimulation or a sleep abnormality. A few adult patients have died of renal failure.

Future goals

The FD genetic mutation does not cause complete loss of function. Instead, it results in a tissue-specific decrease in splicing efficiency of the *IKBKAP* transcript, cells from patients retain some capacity to produce normal mRNA and IKAP protein (Slaugenhaupt et al. 2001). It has been speculated that by raising the amount of the normal or wild type IKAP protein, the progression of the disease will be slowed and that the clinical symptoms of FD may be reduced (Anderson et al. 2003a). Anderson et al. (2003a) state that tocotrienols, unsaturated vitamin E, in cell culture generally increase IKAP levels. They have proposed this as a treatment for FD patients and suggest using 50–200 mg a day (Anderson et al. 2003a). Only one clinical trial is presently underway and there have been favourable anecdotal reports, especially in regard to increasing baseline eye moisture.

Another approach to therapy would be to alter splicing patterns of mammalian messenger RNA. Two agents appear to have this effect, EGCG (epigallocatechin gallate) and kinetin, a plant cytokinin (Anderson et al. 2003b, Slaugenhaupt et al. 2004)). Objective assessment of efficacy for these treatments still awaits verification by clinical trials.

Discovery of the genetic defect in FD should also yield valuable insight into the processes involved in normal development and maintenance of the sensory and autonomic nervous systems. This information may serve to aid us in providing more definitive treatments to individuals affected with FD and may foster innovative treatment approaches for other adult-onset or acquired autonomic disorders.

References

Anderson, S. L., Coli, R., Daly, I. W., *et al.* (2001). Familial dysautonomia is caused by mutations of the IKAP gene. *Am. J. Hum. Genet.* 68, 753–8.

Anderson, S. L., Qiu, J., Rubin, B. Y. (2003a). Tocotrienols induce IKBKAP expression: a possible therapy for familial dysautonomia. *Biochem. Biophys. Res. Commun.* **306**, 303–9.

Anderson, S. L., Qiu, J., Rubin, B. Y. (2003b). EGCG corrects aberrant splicing of IKAP mRNA in cells from patients with familial dysautonomia. *Biochem. Biophys. Res. Commun.* **310**(2), 627–33.

Axelrod, F. B. (2002). Hereditary Sensory and Autonomic Neuropathies: Familial Dysautonomia and other HSANs. *Clin. Auton. Res.* **12** Supplement 1, 2–14.

Axelrod, F. B. (2004). Familial Dysautonomia (Invited Review). *Muscle and Nerve* **29**, 352–63.

Axelrod, F. B. (2005). Familial dysautonomia: A review of the current pharmacological treatments. *Expert Opin. Pharmocother* **6**, 561–67.

Axelrod, F. B., D'Amico, R. (1995). Familial dysautonomia. In: Fraunfelder, F. T., Hampton Roy F., eds. *Current Ocular Therapy*, 4th edition. pp. 413–415. WB Saunders, Philadelphia.

Axelrod, F. B., Glickstein, J. S., Weider, J., Gluck, M. C., Friedman, D. (1993). The effects of postural change and exercise on renal haemodynamics in familial dysautonomia. *Clin. Auton. Res.* **3**, 195–200.

Axelrod, F. B., Goldberg, J. D., Rolnitzky, L., *et al.* (2005). Fludrocortisone in Patients with Familial Dysautonomia: Assessing Effect on Clinical Parameters and Gene Expression. *Clin. Auton. Res.* **15**, 284–91.

Axelrod, F. B., Goldberg, J. D., Ye, X. Y., Maayan, C. (2002). Survival in familial dysautonomia: Impact of early intervention. *J Pediatr.* **141**, 518–23.

Axelrod, F. B., Goldstein, D. S., Holmes, C., Berlin, D., Kopin, I. (1996). Pattern of plasma catechols in familial dysautonomia. *Clin. Auton. Res.* **6**, 205–9.

Axelrod, F. B., Hilz, M. J. (2003). Inherited Autonomic Neuropathies. *Seminars in Neurology* **23**, 381–90.

Axelrod, F. B., Iyer, K., Fish, I., Pearson, J., Sein, M. E., Spielholz, N. (1981). Progressive sensory loss in familial dysautonomia. *Pediatrics* **65**, 517–22.

Axelrod, F. B., Krey, L., Glickstein, J. S., Weider-Allison, J., Friedman, D. (1995). Preliminary observations on the use of midodrine in treating orthostatic hypotension in familial dysautonomia. *J Auton. Nerv. Syst.* **55**, 29–35.

Axelrod, F. B., Krey, L., Glickstein, J. S., *et al.* (1994). Atrial natriuretic peptide and catecholamine response to orthostatic hypotension and treatments in familial dysautonomia. *Clin. Auton. Res.* **4**, 311–18.

Axelrod, F. B., Maayan Ch (1998). Familial dysautonomia. In: Chernick, V., Boat, T. F., eds. *Kendig's Disorders of the Respiratory Tract in Children*, 6th edition, pp. 1103–1106. WB Saunders, Philadelphia.

Axelrod, F. B., Maayan Ch (2002). Familial dysautonomia. In: Burg, F. D., Ingelfinger, J. R., Polin, R. A., Gershon, A. A., eds. *Gellis and Kagen's Current Pediatric Therapy*,17th edition, pp. 437–41. WB Saunders, Philadelphia.

Axelrod, F. B., Putman, D., Berlin, D., Rutkowski, M. (1997). Electrocardiographic measures and heart rate variability in patients with familial dysautonomia. *Cardiology* **88**, 133–40.

Bernardi, L., Hilz, M., Stemper, B., Passino, C., Welsch, G., Axelrod, F. B. (2002). Respiratory and cerebrovascular responses to hypoxia and hypercapnia in familial dysautonomia. *Am. J Respir. Crit. Care. Med.* **167**, 141–9.

Bickel, A., Axelrod, F. B., Schmetz, M., Marthal, H., Hilz, M. J. (2002) Dermal microdialysis provides evidence for hypersensitivity to noradrenaline in patients with familial dysautonomia. *J Neurol. Neurosurg. Psychiatry* **73**, 299–302.

Blumenfeld, A., Slaugenhaupt, S. A., Axelrod, F. B., *et al.* (1993). Localization of the gene for familial dysautonomia on Chromosome 9 and definition of DNA markers for genetic diagnosis. *Nature. Genet.* **4**, 160–4.

Brown, C. M., Stemper, B., Welsch, G., Brys, M., Axelrod, F. B., Hilz, M. J. (2003). Orthostatic challenge reveals impaired vascular resistance control but normal venous pooling and capillary filtration in familial dysautonomia. *Clinical Science* **104**, 163–9.

Edelman, N. H., Cherniack, N. S., Lahiri, S., Richards, E., Fishman, A. P. (1970). The effects of abnormal sympathetic nervous function upon the ventilatory response to hypoxia. *J. Clin. Invest* **49**, 1153–65.

Glickstein, J. S., Axelrod, F. B., Friedman, D. (1999). Electrocardiographic repolarization abnormalities in familial dysautonomia: an indicator of cardiac autonomic dysfunction. *Clin. Auton. Res.* **9**, 109–12.

Glickstein, J. S., Schwartzman, D., Friedman, D., Rutkowski, M., Axelrod, F. B. (1993). Abnormalities of the corrected QT interval in familial dysautonomia: an indicator of autonomic dysfunction. *J Pediatrics* **122**, 925–8.

Gold-von Simson, G., Rutkowski, M., Berlin, D., Axelrod, F. B. (2005). Review of pacemaker experience in patients with familial dysautonomia. *Clin. Auton. Res.* (accepted for publication)

Grover-Johnson, N., Pearson, J. (1976). Deficient vascular innervation in familial dysautonomia, an explanation for vasomotor instability. *Neuropath. Appl. Neurobiol.* **2**, 217–24.

Hilz, M. J., Axelrod, F.B. (2000) Quantitative sensory testing of thermal and vibratory perception in familial dysautonomia. *Clin. Aut. Res.* **10**, 177–83.

Hilz, M. J., Axelrod, F. B., Braeske, K., Stemper, B. (2002). Cold pressor test demonstrates residual sympathetic cardiovascular activation in familial dysautonomia. *J Neurol. Sci.* **196**, 81–9.

Hilz, M. J., Axelrod, F. B., Sauer, P., Hagler, A., Russo, H., Neundorfer, B. (1997). Cold face stimulation demonstrates parasympathetic dysfunction in familial dysautonomia. *J Auton. Nerv. Sys.* **65**, 111.

Hilz, M. J., Axelrod, F. B., Schweibold, G., Kolodny, E. H. (1999) Sympathetic skin response following thermal, electrical, acoustic and inspiratory gasp stimulation in familial dysautonomia patients and healthy persons. *Clin. Aut. Res.* **9**,165–77.

Indo, Y., Tsuruta, M., Hayashida, Y., *et al.* (1996). Mutations in the NTRKA/NGF receptor gene in patients with congenital insensitivity to pain with anhidrosis. *Nature Genet.,* **13**, 485–8.

Leyne, M., Mull, J., Gill, S. P., *et al.* (2003). Identification of the first non-Jewish mutation in Familial Dysautonomia. *Am. J of Med. Genet.* **118A**, 305–8.

Maayan Ch, Axelrod, F. B., Akselrod, S., Carley, D. W., Shannon, C. D. (1987). Evaluation of autonomic dysfunction in familial dysautonomia by power spectral analysis. *J Autonom. Nerv. Syst.* **21**, 51–8.

Maayan Ch, Carley, D. W., Axelrod, F. B., Grimes, J., Shannon, D. C. (1992). Respiratory system stability and abnormal carbon dioxide homeostasis. *J Appl. Physiol.* **72** (3), 1186–93.

Maayan Ch, Kaplan, E., Shachar Sh, Peleg, O., Godfrey, S. (1987). Incidence of familial dysautonomia in Israel 1977–1981. *Clin. Genet.* **32**, 106–8.

Mason, D. T., Kopin, I. J., Braunwald, E. (1966). Abnormalities in reflex control of the circulation in familial dysautonomia. *Am. J Med.* **41**, 898–909.

Matalon, A., Elkay, L., Tseng, C. H., Axelrod, F. B. (2006). The Prevalence and Severity of Renal Disease in Familial Dysautonomia. *American Journal of Kidney Diseases* **48**, 780–86.

Pearson, J., Brandeis, L., Goldstein, M. (1979). Tyrosine hydroxylase immunohistoreactivity in familial dysautonomia. *Science* **206**, 71–2.

Pearson, J., Dancis, J., Axelrod, F. B., Grover-Johnson, N. (1975) The sural nerve in familial dysautonomia. *J Neuropathol. Exp. Neurol.* **34**, 413–24.

Pearson, J., Gallo, G., Gluck, M., Axelrod, F. B. (1980). Renal disease in familial dysautonomia. *Kidney Int.* **17**, 102–12.

Pearson, J., Pytel, B. (1978a). Quantitative studies of sympathetic ganglia and spinal cord intermedio-lateral gray columns in familial dysautonomia. *J. Neurol. Sci.* **39**, 47–59.

Pearson, J., Pytel, B. (1978b). Quantitative studies of ciliary and sphenopalatine ganglia in familial dysautonomia. *J Neurol. Sci.* **39**, 123–30.

Rabinowitz, D., Landau, H., Rosler, A., Moses, S. W., Rotem, Y., Freier, S. (1974). Plasma renin activity and aldosterone in familial dysautonomia. *Metabolism* **23**, 1–5.

Riley, C. M., Day, R. L., McL Greeley, D., Langford, W. S. (1949). Central autonomic dysfunction with defective lacrimation. Report of 5 cases. *Pediatrics* **3**, 468–77.

Slaugenhaupt, S. A., Blumenfeld, A., Gill, S. P., *et al.* (2001). Tissue-specific expression of a splicing mutation in the IKBKAP gene causes familial dysautonomia. *Am. J Hum. Genet.* **68**, 598–604.

Slaugenhaupt, S. A., Mull, J., Leyne, M., *et al.* (2004). Rescue of a human mRNA splicing defect by the plant cytokinin kinetin. *Hum. Mol. Genet* **13**, 429–36.

Smith, A. A., Hirsch, J. I., Dancis, J. (1965). Responses to infused methacholine in familial dysautonomia. *Pediatrics* **36**, 225–30.

Smith, A. A., Taylor, T., Wortis, S. B. (1963). Abnormal catecholamine metabolism in familial dysautonomia. *New Engl. J Med.* **268**, 705–7.

Stemper, B., Axelrod, F., Marthol, H., Brown, C., Brys, M., Welsch, G., Hilz, M. J. (2003). Terminal vessel hyperperfusion despite organ hypoperfusion in familial dysautonomia, *Clinical Science* **105**(3): 295–301.

Stemper, B., Bernardi, L., Axelrod, F. B., Welsch, G., Passino, C., Hilz, M. J. (2004). Sympathetic and parasympathetic baroreflex dysfunction in familial dysautonomia. *Neurology* **63**, 1427–31.

Sundaram, V., Axelrod, F. B. (2005). Gastroesophageal reflux in familial dysautonomia:Correlation with crisis frequency and sensory dysfunction. *J Ped. Gastroenterol. and Nutrition* **40**, 429–33.

Welton, W., Clayson, D., Axelrod, F. B., Levine, D. B. (1979). Intellectual development and familial dysautonomia. *Pediatrics* **63**, 708–12.

Ziegler, M. G., Lake, R. C., Kopin, I. J. (1976). Deficient sympathetic nervous system response in familial dysautonomia, *New Engl. J Med.* **294**, 630–3.

CHAPTER 49

Dopamine-beta-hydroxylase deficiency—with a note on other genetically determined causes of autonomic failure

Christopher J. Mathias and Roger Bannister

Introduction

Dopamine-beta-hydroxylase (DBH) is the enzyme that converts dopamine into noradrenaline (Fig. 49.1). It is present within vesicles in sympathetic nerve endings and within the adrenal medulla and is released stoichiometrically with noradrenaline during sympathetic stimulation. It can be measured readily in plasma, and studies in both animals and man indicate that the major contribution to circulating levels is from sympathetic nerve endings. It was once thought that it might serve as a better indicator of sympathetic nervous activity than noradrenaline. Further studies, however, have indicated that there are marked differences within normal subjects and that plasma levels are largely genetically predetermined. Its half-life is probably in the region of about 30 minutes and is considerably longer than that of noradrenaline. This can be a disadvantage with short-lived sympathetic stimuli. Furthermore, it has a much larger molecular weight (290 kDa compared with 169 kDa for noradrenaline) and it reaches the circulation predominantly by lymphatic channels rather than through diffusion. Studies from a variety of sources indicate that in man it is not as sensitive an indicator of short-term or long-term changes in sympathetic activity as is noradrenaline (Mathias et al. 1976, Weinshilboum 1978).

Interest in DBH in autonomic disorders was stimulated by the lower plasma levels observed in familial dysautonomia (Weinshilboum and Axelrod 1971) and later in familial amyloid polyneuropathy (Suzuki et al. 1980). In the latter group, further evidence of a functional DBH deficit was provided by successful treatment of their hypotension with the agent DL-dihydroxyphenylserine (DOPS), which bypassed the deficient enzymatic component (Fig. 49.2). There was a resurgence of interest in the late 1980s with the description of two patients with a congenital deficiency of DBH resulting in severe postural hypotension due to sympathetic adrenergic failure (Robertson et al. 1986, Man in't Veld et al. 1987a). Since then five further cases have been described, two of whom are siblings (see Table 49.1).

The clinical features, autonomic deficits, results of routine and specialized investigations, together with the management of DBH deficiency are described. There will also be a short discussion on differences from other genetically determined causes of autonomic failure and orthostatic hypotension.

Clinical features

Presentation

Of the 12 patients, 8 are female (Table 49.1). All were diagnosed after 20 years of age (except the most recent at 16 years), although in most patients their history was suggestive of autonomic failure from birth or early childhood. In patients 2, 3 and 9 there were other complicating features (hypoglycaemia and probably incorrectly diagnosed epilepsy). In all, the reason for investigation and subsequent diagnosis was directly related to symptoms and signs of postural hypotension. This was recognized only in their teens or later. Patient 8 was a 31-year-old woman with long-standing orthostatic hypotension, treated unsuccessfully for anaemia (Gomes et al. 2003) who also developed diarrhoea. No details of clinical examinations are provided, with the assumption that there were no specific additional clinical features. Patient 12 was diagnosed at 73 years, although he had symptoms since early childhood (Despas et al. 2010).

Family history

In none of the cases was there a history of a similar problem in previous generations. Patient 7 had a maternal grandfather who died at an early age (less than 30 years) of a blood pressure problem, but details were not available. There was no evidence of consanguinity. The patients were of white Caucasian stock; of Scottish, Irish, Dutch, and northern English descent except for patient 2 who also had Cherokee Indian lineage. There was a history of miscarriages in some of their parents. The brother and sister in the UK (patients 5 and 6) were the only siblings in the family.

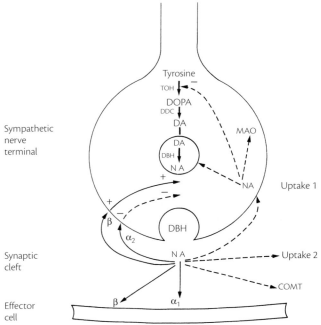

Fig. 49.1 Schema of some pathways in the formation, release, and metabolism of noradrenaline from sympathetic nerve terminals. Tyrosine is converted into dihydroxyphenylalanine (DOPA) by tyrosine hydroxylase (TOH). DOPA is converted into dopamine (DA) by dopa-decarboxylase (DDC). In the vesicles, DA is converted into noradrenaline (NA) by dopamine β-hydroxylase (DBH). Nerve impulses release both DBH and NA into the synaptic cleft by exocytosis. NA acts predominantly on α_1-adrenoceptors but has actions on β-adrenoceptors on the effector cell of target organs. It also has presynaptic adrenoceptor effects. Those acting on α_2-adrenoceptors inhibit NA release while those acting on β-adrenoceptors stimulate NA release. NA may be taken up by a neuronal (uptake 1) process into the cytosol, where it may inhibit further formation of DOPA through the rate-limiting enzyme TOH. NA may be taken into vesicles or metabolized by monoamine oxidase (MAO) in the mitochondria. NA may be taken up by a higher-capacity but lower-affinity extraneuronal process (uptake 2) into peripheral tissues such as vascular and cardiac muscle, and certain glands. NA is also metabolized by catechol-*o*-methyl transferase (COMT). NA measured in plasma is thus the overspill which is not affected by these numerous processes. From Mathias 1996.

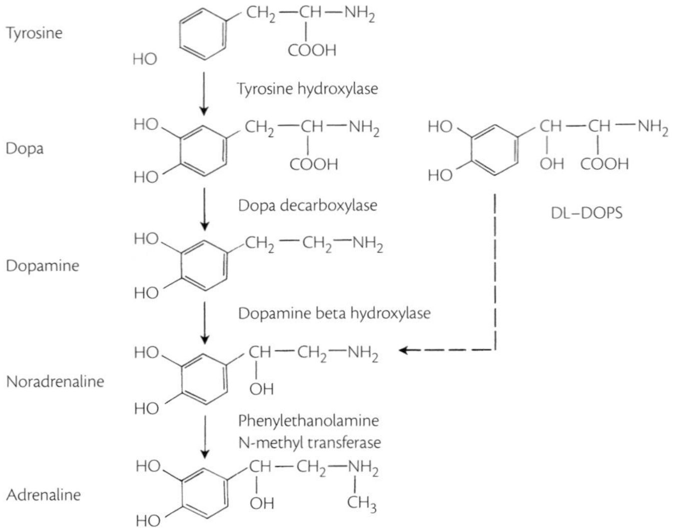

Evaluations of the parents of patients 5 and 6 confirmed normal autonomic function and catecholamine levels.

In a mouse model where gene targeting resulted in absence of DBH, most homozygous embryos died *in utero* (Thomas et al. 1995). Death of the embryos was due to cardiovascular failure. Treatment with DOPS prevented fetal loss; this was reversed by the addition of a dopa decarboxylase inhibitor, carbidopa. It was thought that the survival of the embryos was dependent upon catecholamine transfer across the placenta, as all the embryos of homozygous mothers died *in utero*. The high fetal loss in these studies may explain the rarity of human DBH deficiency.

Pre-adult manifestations

All, except for patient 5 and 8, were unwell from early childhood. Patient 7 was 4 weeks premature. There was a strong association between their symptoms, syncope, and exercise which was avoided especially in patients 3 and 6. In patient 7, dizziness was more frequent and severe in a warm environment. As a child, patient 6 had difficulty in walking, which her mother attributed to her not trying.

Fig. 49.2 Biosynthetic pathway in the formation of noradrenaline and adrenaline. The structure of DL-DOPS is indicated on the right. It is converted directly to noradrenaline by dopa decarboxylase, thus bypassing dopamine β-hydroxylase.

Epilepsy was considered in patients 2 and 3 who were unsuccessfully tried on anti-epileptic medication. At birth patient 3 had episodes of hypoglycaemia and hypothermia. Physical growth in all appeared to be normal, and sexual maturation was not delayed. Symptoms, however, became more apparent in their teens; in patient 5, however, this only emerged at 13 years. The mother of patient 7 was mainly concerned that she did not have the energy of a normal 14-year-old girl.

Patient 9 had decreased development of the central face, brachydactyly, a high palate, micrognathia, hypotonia and ataxia. Patient 11 had bilateral iris coloboma, short hands and high arched feet presumed to be separate from DBH deficiency. Whether the clinical manifestations in their teens were associated with greater activity, worsening of their condition, or sharpening of their ability to associate symptoms with specific events is not clear.

Clinical manifestations at diagnosis

Autonomic function

Symptoms pointed to postural hypotension, with blurring of vision, dizziness, and at times syncope (Table 49.2). This was often worse in the morning, during exercise, and during hot weather. Postural symptoms were not worse after food ingestion except in patient 2. Patient 5 occasionally had aching in the back of the neck and shoulders after meals. In patient 6, food often reduced postural symptoms but there was no evidence of hypoglycaemia. In patients 5 and 6, precordial pain occasionally occurred during exertion, and was reproduced during exercise testing with electrocardiography (ECG), but without concomitant evidence of ischaemia on the ECG. They both also had weakness and paraesthesiae in the legs during exertion, suggestive of ischaemia to the spinal cord. On formal testing immediately post-exercise, no objective evidence of a neurological or vascular deficit in the periphery was obtained.

Patients 1–4, 7 and 9 had bilateral partial ptosis, presumably related to the lack of sympathetic tone to Muller's muscle in the upper lid. Patient 1 had nasal stuffiness probably due to vasodilatation secondary to lack of sympathetic vasoconstriction, as seen in

Table 49.1 Details of twelve patients with dopamine-beta-hydroxylase deficiency

Reference	Robertson et al. (1986)	Biaggioni et al. (1990)	Man in't Veld et al. (1987a)	Man in't Veld et al. (1988)	Mathias et al. (1990)	Mathias et al. (1990)	Thompson et al. (1995)	Gomes et al. (2003)	Cheshire et al. (2006)	Robertson et al. (2005)	Erez et al. (2010)	Despas et al. (2010)
Sex	F	M	F	F	M	F	F	F	M	F	F	M
Patient	1	2	3	4	5[a]	6[a]	7	8	9	10	11	12
Origin	Scotch-Irish	Dutch, Scotch-Irish, Cherokee	Dutch[b]	Dutch[b]	English	English	English	Dutch	American	Irish/Scottish	USA	French
Consanguinity	—	—	None	—	None	None	None	—	—	—	—	—
Siblings	1 brother	—	1 brother, 1 sister	—	1 sister	1 brother	1 brother	?	?	?	?	?
Family affected	No	No	No	—	Yes (sister)	Yes (brother)	No[c]	No	No	No	No	No
Age when postural hypotension recognized (years)	25	33	21	20	29	21	14	31	24	22	16	73

[a]Patients 5 and 6 are siblings. No details provided.
[b]Presumed, as no details provided.
[c]See text.

acute tetraplegia (Guttmann's sign) and after α-adrenoceptor blockers such as phenoxybenzamine. It is recorded that patients 2, 5, and 6 were aware of their ability to sweat. There were no abnormalities in relation to lacrimation or salivation. There was normal gut and large bowel function, except for intermittent diarrhoea in patients 1 and 2. Urinary bladder function was normal in all. Patient 6 had nocturia. Patient 10 had primary enuresis. In patient 5, erection was preserved but ejaculation took a prolonged time to achieve, or was absent. Patient 2 was originally described as impotent (Biaggioni and Robertson 1987) but was later reported to have difficulty in maintaining an erection and to have retrograde ejaculation (Biaggioni et al. 1990).

On Patient 8, 10 and 11 no other clinical features were described; in Patient 11 sweating and thermoregulation were preserved; he had normal pupillary reactions with no mention of ptosis.

Neurological and mental function

There were no major neurological abnormalities. Mild ptosis was present in patients 1–4. Patient 2 had reduced deep tendon reflexes. Muscle hypotonia, weakness of the facial musculature, and sluggish deep tendon reflexes were reported in patients 3 and 4. No neurological deficits were recorded in patients 5 and 6. There was no evidence of impairment of mental function and detailed psychometric examinations in patients 5 and 6 were normal.

Miscellaneous

Patients 2 and 6 had renal impairment with an elevated creatinine level (220 and 150 mmol/l, respectively). In patient 6 this was due to an episode of glomerulonephritis which had been treated successfully with steroids when she was 21 years, but which left her with an elevated but stable creatinine level; she had remained mildly anaemic (Hb I0g/dl). Patients 3 and 4 had brachydactyly and a high palate. Patient 2 had atrial fibrillation and patient 3 had negative or flat T waves in the precordial leads of the ECG.

Patient 8 was initially found to have low erythropoietin levels prior to the diagnosis of DBH deficiency. She had a low haemoglobin that responded to subcutaneous erythropoietin. This increased her haemoglobin concentration but her postural dizziness remained. She was then started on oral L-DOPS, and within a few weeks her dizziness had improved. Her haemoglobin remained stable even after stopping erythropoietin.

Autonomic investigations

Physiological

Cardiovascular

The investigations indicated sympathetic adrenergic failure (Table 49.3). All had severe postural hypotension, and in those who underwent detailed autonomic testing an abnormal Valsalva manoeuvre, but with an adequate rise in heart rate when the blood pressure fell, showing preserved baroreceptor afferent and vagal efferent pathways. In patients 1, 5, and 6 there was a small rise in blood pressure and heart rate during some of the pressor tests; patient 7 was reported as having a suppressed blood pressure rise during the cold pressor test. The responses, in the absence of noradrenaline, suggested the presence of alternative although less effective mechanisms which raise blood pressure. These include vagal withdrawal, which can raise heart rate and cardiac output, and pressor effects exerted through dopamine, neuropeptides (such as neuropeptide Y), or purines (such as adenosine triphosphate) released from otherwise intact sympathetic nerve terminals. Heart rate responses to deep breathing and hyperventilation were present indicating functional cardiac vagus nerves.

The responses to food ingestion were tested in patients 5 and 6. In neither was there a fall in supine blood pressure or an accentuation of postural hypotension after food (Mathias et al. 1990); this differs from observations in patients with primary chronic autonomic

Table 49.2 Clinical symptoms and signs in twelve patients[a] with dopamine-beta-hydroxylase deficiency

Reference	Robertson et al. (1986)	Biaggioni et al. (1990)	Man in't Veld et al. (1987a)	Man in't Veld et al. (1988)	Mathias et al. (1990)	Mathias et al. (1990)	Thompson et al. (1995)	Gomes et al. (2003)	Cheshire et al. (2006)	Robertson et al. (2005)	Erez et al. (2010)	Despas et al. (2010)
Symptoms and signs	Patient 1	Patient 2	Patient 3	Patient 4	Patient 5	Patient 6	Patient 7	Patient 8	Patient 9	Patient 10	Patient 11	Patient 12
Autonomic												
Postural symptoms	+	+	+	+	+	+	+	+	+	+	+	+
Postural hypotension	+	+	+	+	+	+	+	+	+	+	+	+
Postural rise in heart rate	+	+	+	+	+	+	+	+	+	NR	NR	+
Sweating	+	+	+	+	+	+	+			NR	NR	
Bowels	ID	ID	N	N	N	N	N	Diarrhoea		NR	NR	+
Urinary bladder	N	N	N	N	N	N	N			NR	NR	+
Sexual												
Maturation (or menarche)	N	N	N	N	N	N	N			NR	NR	N
Erection		Impaired			N					NR	NR	N
Ejaculation		Retrograde			Delayed or absent							N
Partial ptosis	+	+	+	+	-	-	+					N
Neurological	N	Reduced deep tendon reflexes	Hypotonia, facial weakness, sluggish deep tendon reflexes		N	N				NR	NR	
Higher function	N	N	N	N	N	N	N			NR	NR	
Miscellaneous		Hyper-extensible joints	Brachydactyly, high palate									

N, normal; +, symptom or sign present; –, symptom or sign absent; ID, intermittent diarrhoea.
[a] Patient details in Table 49.1

failure due to pure autonomic failure and multiple system atrophy (Fig. 49.3). Possible mechanisms for this difference indicate their ability to influence cardiac output and to release vasoactive neurotransmitters other than noradrenaline (Chapter 24). Neither patient 5 nor 6 had a fall in supine blood pressure with bicycle exercise, and this differed again from the patients with pure autonomic failure (PAF) and multiple system atrophy (MSA); their blood pressure did not go up with exercise as occurs normally, consistent with their inability to increase circulating noradrenaline and adrenaline levels (Smith et al. 1995) (Fig. 49.4). However, when patients 5 and 6 stood up after exercise there was a marked fall in blood pressure that was considerably greater than pre-exercise (Smith and Mathias 1995). It is likely that the absence of exercise-induced hypotension while supine was due to similar mechanisms that prevented the fall in blood pressure during food ingestion in these patients. The enhanced postural hypotension after exercise presumably reflects the limitations of these secondary mechanisms, and indicates the importance of neurally mediated vasoconstriction as exerted through noradrenaline.

Spectral analysis of heart rate variability was performed in Patient 7 (Fig. 49.5). At rest the high frequency, respiratory-related variability (0.2–0.3 Hz) linked to parasympathetic activity was preserved, while the low frequency heart rate variability (0.1 Hz) that reflects sympathetic activation was not present; with head-up tilt there was a marked reduction in high frequency heart rate variability suggesting vagal withdrawal.

Patient 12 had a meta-iodobenzyl guanidine (MIBG) scan with a wash-out rate above the normal laboratory rate indicating that cardiac sympathetic nerves cardiac sympathetic nerves could take up and store catecholamines, and favouring a normal density, thus separating DBH deficiency from PAF. The higher wash out rate was considered to be due to elevated sympathetic nerve traffic, as had been demonstrated using microneurography.

Sweating

Sweating was preserved in all patients. The thermoregulatory sweating response was tested in patients 3–6 and was present, although in patients 5 and 6 this was patchy when compared with

Table 49.3 Summary of physiological autonomic investigations in twelve patients[a] with DBH deficiency

Reference	Robertson et al. (1986)	Biaggioni et al. (1990)	Man in't Veld et al. (1987a)	Man in't Veld et al. (1988)	Mathias et al. (1990)	Mathias et al. (1990)	Thompson et al. (1995)	Gomes et al. (2003)	Cheshire et al. (2006)	Robertson et al. (2005)	Erez et al. (2010)	Despas et al. (2010)
Physiological investigations	Patient 1	Patient 2	Patient 3	Patient 4	Patient 5	Patient 6	Patient 7	Patient 8	Patient 9	Patient 10	Patient 11	Patient 12
Sympathetic adrenergic								A	A			
Head-up postural change-BP	↓	↓	↓	↓	↓	↓	↓	A	A	A	A	A
Valsalva manoeuvre												
-BP	A	A	A	A	A	A	A					
-Phase IV-HR	A	A	A	A	A	A	A					
Pressor tests	A	A	A	A	A	A	A					
Sympathetic cholinergic												N
Sweating	N	N	N	N	P	P	N		N (post-ganglionic)			N
Parasympathetic									N			N
Sinus arrhythmia	+	+	+	+	+	+	+					N
Hyperventilation-HR	↑	↑	↑	↑	↑	↑						
Head-up postural change-HR	↑	↑	↑	↑	↑	↑	↑		↑			
Valsalva manoeuvre Phase II-HR	↑	↑	↑	↑	↑	↑	↑					
Schirmer's test					N	N						
Miscellaneous												
Food on BP					↔	↔						
Exercise on BP					↔	↔						
Nocturnal polyuria					+	+						
Nocturnal natriuresis					+	+						

BP, blood pressure; HR, heart rate; A, abnormal; N, normal; P, preserved but patchy; ↓, fall; ↑, rise; ↔, no change; +, symptom present; no symbol, not described.
[a] Patient details in Table 49.1.

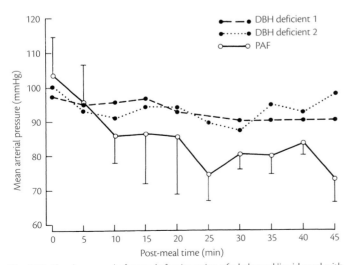

Fig. 49.3 Blood pressure before and after ingestion of a balanced liquid meal with measurements in the supine position, in five patients with pure autonomic failure (PAF) and in patients 5 and 6 with dopamine beta hydroxylase (DBH) deficiency. (1 and 2, respectively, in figure). From Mathias et al. 1990.

normal individuals. Patient 3 sweated profusely when hypoglycaemia was induced by insulin.

Lacrimation and salivation

There were no symptoms to suggest xerostomia. Schirmer's test was normal in patients 5 and 6.

Pupillary studies

Detailed studies in patients 5 and 6 have been made while on and off L-DOPS (Bremner and Smith 2006). They had bilateral Horner's syndrome and the physiological studies indicated normal light and near reflexes with normal amplitude but with redilatation lag. Pharmacological studies with phenylephrine showed supersensitivity. Stopping L-DOPS did not affect the findings.

Nocturnal polyuria and natriuresis

This was recorded in patients 5 and 6. Both had nocturnal polyuria and excreted large amounts of sodium (Fig. 49.6). In patient 3, sodium output was reported as high but details were not provided.

Electrophysiological studies

Sympathetic microneurography was performed in patient 2 (Rea et al. 1990) and 7. This demonstrated a rise in muscle sympathetic

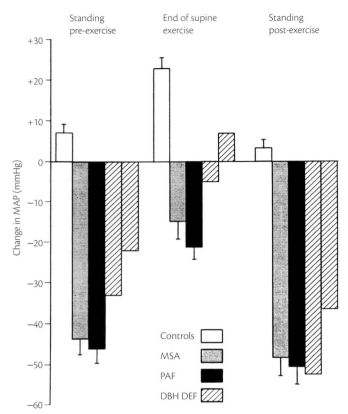

Fig. 49.4 Change in mean arterial blood pressure (MAP) at the end of 9 minutes of supine exercise on a bicycle, and on standing before exercise and after exercise in normal subjects (controls), and patients with multiple system atrophy (MSA), pure autonomic failure (PAF) and patients 5 and 6. Exercise raises supine blood pressure in normal subjects and lowers blood pressure in MSA and PAF, but with little change in patients 5 and 6. After exercise, however, blood pressure on standing falls further in both patients. From Smith and Mathias 1995, with permission.

nerve activity with pressor stimuli (despite no change in blood pressure) and a fall in nerve discharge with phenylephrine, both consistent with functional preservation of sympathetic nerve activity (Fig. 49.7a,b and Fig. 49.5).

Biochemical investigations

Plasma catecholamines

The key findings were the virtual absence of circulating levels of noradrenaline and adrenaline, with abnormally elevated levels of dopamine (Fig. 49.8a). Patient 1 was reported to have detectable plasma adrenaline levels but this was later retracted (Biaggioni et al. 1990) on the basis that the levels observed were probably due to cross-reactivity with high levels of dopamine. The evidence of an inability to convert dopamine to noradrenaline suggested a lack of DBH activity which was confirmed (Fig. 49.8b). In patients 2–4 the precursor substance to dopamine, dihydroxyphenylalanine, was also elevated in plasma. The high levels of dopamine suggested lack of inhibition of tyrosine hydroxylase, the rate-limiting enzyme, which is normally inhibited by intraneuronal noradrenaline. Despite these high basal levels, definite elevations in plasma dopamine levels were associated with physiological and/or pharmacological stimulation in all patients (Fig. 49.9). Neither intravenous tyramine (patients 1–4), nor insulin-induced hypoglycaemia

(patients 3 and 4) caused an elevation in noradrenaline or adrenaline levels (respectively), as they normally do.

Cerebrospinal fluid catecholamines

In patients 2 and 3, noradrenaline and adrenaline were not detectable in cerebrospinal fluid, while dopamine and its metabolites were elevated (Fig. 49.10). These observations are consistent with undetectable DBH immunoreactivity in cerebrospinal fluid in such patients (O'Connor et al. 1994). Post-mortem findings in patient 9 at 28 years of age showed no central involvement except for lack of DBH immunoreactivity in the rostral ventrolateral medulla (Cheshire et al. 2006).

Urinary catecholamine measurements

The urinary metabolites of dopamine (homovanillic acid and 3-methoxytyramine) were normal or elevated while those of noradrenaline (normetanephrine) and adrenaline (metanephrine) were either extremely low or undetectable (Fig. 49.11). This was consistent with the observations in plasma.

Noradrenaline and adrenaline kinetics

In patient 7, total body noradrenaline and adrenaline spillover to plasma was measured using radiotracer methods, (Thompson et al. 1995) (Fig. 49.5). At rest, total body noradrenaline spillover was very low (38 ng/minute) compared with normal individuals (519 ± 43 ng/minute) and patients with PAF (251 ± 22 ng/minute). Adrenaline secretion was almost undetectable. During head-up tilt in patient 7, total body noradrenaline spillover fell to 27 ng/minute, with a minimal fall in adrenaline clearance (from 1.9 ng/minute to 1.7 ng/minute). This contrasts with normal subjects during head-up tilt, when noradrenaline spillover increases (to 677 ± 8 ng/minute).

Tissue studies

Electron microscopy was performed on axillary and gluteal skin in patients 5 and 6 and did not show any structural abnormalities of sympathetic nerve terminals. In these patients, immunohistochemical staining indicated the presence of tyrosine hydroxylase but not DBH. In patient 3, immunohistochemistry of skin biopsy material was negative for DBH and noradrenaline and positive for dopamine, but no details of methodology were provided. Immunofluorescence to vasoactive intestinal polypeptide, neuropeptide Y, substance P, and calcitonin-gene related peptide was present in patients 5 and 6, similar to that in normal subjects.

Pharmacological

A series of investigations further emphasized the enzymatic deficiency and the associated autonomic abnormalities (Table 49.4). There was pressor supersensitivity to both noradrenaline and to clonidine, emphasizing α-adrenoceptor up-regulation (Figs 49.12a and 49.13). There was a depressor response to isoprenaline with an exaggerated heart rate response, probably due to a combination of a-adrenoceptor supersensitivity and also vagal withdrawal in response to the fall in blood pressure (Fig. 49.12b,c). Tyramine did not raise levels of plasma noradrenaline in patients 1–4 (Fig. 49.14); edrophonium administration in patients 3 and 4 had no effect, but raised levels of plasma dopamine. The functional role of high circulating levels of dopamine varied: in patients 1 and 2 there was no response to oral metoclopramide, in patients 3 and 4 intravenous metoclopramide raised blood pressure, while an identical dose in patients 5 and 6 lowered blood pressure (Fig. 49.15). The reasons for these differences are not known.

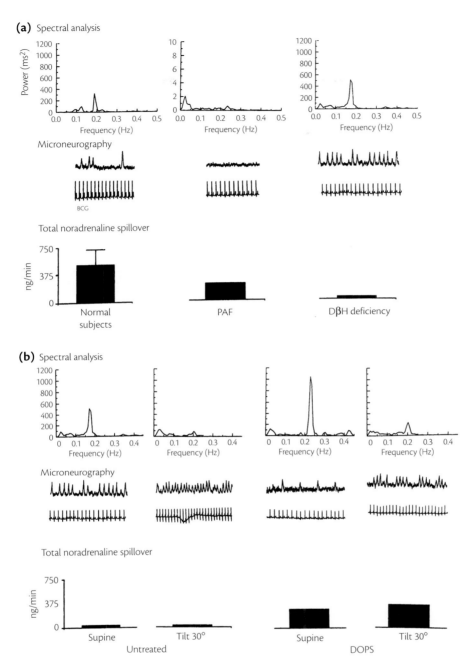

Fig. 49.5 Heart rate spectral analysis, muscle sympathetic nerve activity (microneurography) and total noradrenaline spillover in normal subjects, patients with pure autonomic failure (PAF), and patient 7 with dopamine-beta-hydroxylase deficiency. From Thompson et al. 1995, with permission. In **(a)**, at rest, only high frequency respiratory-related variability (0.2 to 0.3 Hz; representing parasympathetic activity) was present without the low frequency heart rate variability (0.01 Hz; that reflects sympathetic activity); muscle sympathetic nerve activity was greater than in normal individuals, while noradrenaline spillover was extremely low. In **(b)**, data in patient 7 alone is provided, while supine and during head-up tilt to 30° while untreated and after L- dihydroxyphenylserine (L-DOPS). With L-DOPS there was an increase in the high frequency peak, but the low frequency variability remained undetectable; muscle sympathetic nerve activity fell to within the normal range. There was an increase in noradrenaline spillover while supine but a lower than expected rise with head-up tilt.

Genetic studies

Genetic studies have been performed in a number of the DBH patients and extensively in normal healthy subjects. In four families there was truncating, splice site or missense mutation in the DBH gene (Deinum et al. 2004). Despite some family members described having absent plasma concentrations of DBH there was no evidence of orthostatic hypotension. To explain this dissociation it was noted that they were heterozygous for the mutations, suggesting a reduction of DBH but not enough to impair the synthesis of noradrenaline needed to prevent orthostatic hypotension. A locus in the 5' flanking region of the DBH gene is likely to be responsible for absent plasma DBH, which is present in 4% of the normal population who do not have orthostatic symptoms.

Thus both plasma concentrations and the DBH genotype need to be considered in understanding DBH deficiency.

In patient 11, there were additional clinical features and a mosaic cytogenetic abnormality.

Other familial and hereditary autonomic disorders

The presence of the disorder at birth and the recognition of siblings with DBH deficiency places this condition among other familial and hereditary autonomic disorders, some of which are described briefly below. In most of these disorders there are associated neurological deficits, which immediately separate them

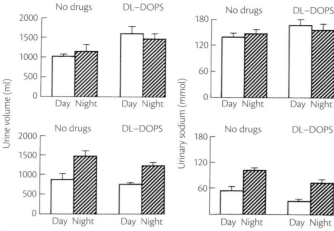

Fig. 49.6 Day (open histograms) and night (hatched histograms) urine volumes (left panels) and urinary sodium excretion (right panels) in patient 5 (upper panels) and patient 6 (lower panels) with DBH deficiency, before and after drug therapy with DL-DOPS. From Mathias et al. 1990.

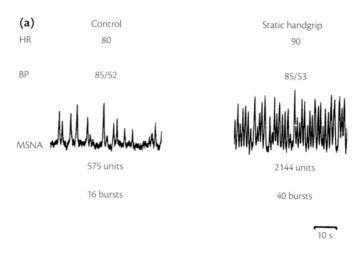

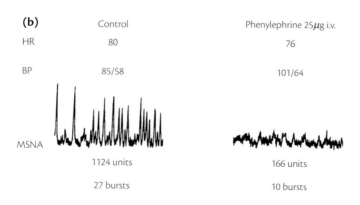

Fig. 49.7 Heart rate (HR), blood pressure (BP), and muscle sympathetic nerve activity (MSNA) recorded from the peroneal nerve in a patient with DBH deficiency (patient 2): (a) before and during isometric exercise (static handgrip); and (b) during injection of phenylephrine. Isometric exercise increases MSNA and phenylephrine decreases MSNA indicating that baroreflex pathways are intact. With permission from Rea R, Biaggioni I, Robertson RM, Haile V, Robertson D. (1990). Reflex control of sympathetic nerve activity in dopamine-beta-hydroxylase deficiency. *Hypertension* **15**, 107–12.

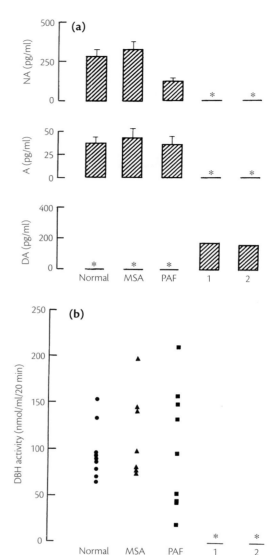

Fig. 49.8 (a) Mean levels (± SEM) of plasma noradrenaline (NA), adrenaline (A), and dopamine (DA) in 10 normal subjects, 12 patients with multiple system atrophy (MSA), and 8 patients with pure autonomic failure (PAF). Individual values on the first occasion in patients 5 and 6 (1 and 2, respectively, in figure) with DBH deficiency are indicated. The asterisk indicates undetectable levels, which were below 5 pg/ml for NA and A and 20 pg/ml for DA. (b) Scattergram showing DBH activity in 10 normal subjects, 7 MSA, and 9 PAF patients. In patients 5 and 6 (1 and 2, respectively, in figure) activity was undetectable. From Mathias et al. 1990.

from congenital DBH deficiency. In two of the disorders (familial hyperbradykinism and adrenoleukodystrophy) there are no autonomic deficits, but there are overlapping features, such as postural hypotension.

Riley–Day syndrome (familial dysautonomia)

Riley–Day syndrome is an autosomal recessive disorder with autonomic abnormalities often present from birth and is described in Chapter 48.

Familial 'Shy–Drager' like syndrome

There have been two reports of a familial syndrome with postural hypotension, sphincter involvement, and multiple neurological deficits. The age of onset, however, was the late thirties or early

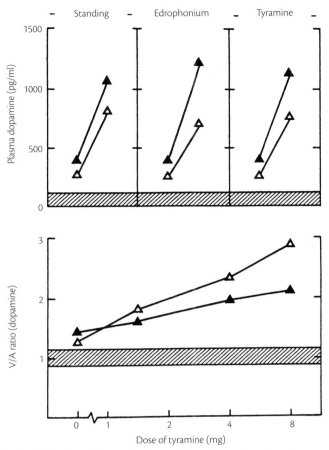

Fig. 49.9 Effect of standing, edrophonium and tyramine or plasma dopamine and the venous/arterial (V/A) ratio for dopamine in two patients (3 and 4) with congenital DBH deficiency. (Filled triangles, patient 3; open triangles, patient 4; hatched area, 95 per cent confidence intervals in normals). Reprinted by permission from Macmillan Publishers Ltd: *Am. J. Hypertens.* Man in't Veld AJ et al, copyright (1988).

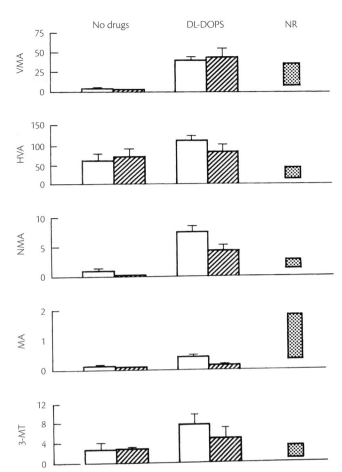

Fig. 49.11 Twenty-four hour urinary secretion of catecholamine metabolites in patient 5 (open histograms) and patient 6 (filled histograms) with DBH deficiency, before and after treatment with DL-DOPS. Bars indicate ± SEM and relate to collections over 3 consecutive days. VMA, vanillylmandelic acid; HVA, homovanillic acid; 3-MT, 3-methoxy-tyramine; MA, metadrenaline; NMA, normetadrenaline. Normal range (NR) indicated by stippled histogram on right. HVA and 3-MT are metabolites of dopamine. From Mathias et al. 1990.

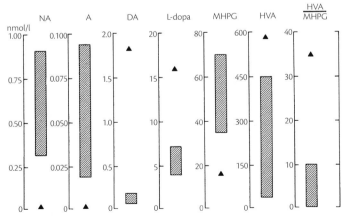

Fig. 49.10 Plasma catecholamine concentrations, 3-methoxy-4-hydroxyphenyl ethylene glycol (MHPG) and homovanillic acid (HVA) in cerebrospinal fluid (CSF) of patient 3 with DBH deficiency. NA, noradrenaline; A, adrenaline, DA, dopamine, L-dopa = L-dihydroxyphenylalanine. Reprinted from *The Lancet*, **i**, Man in't Veld AJ, Boomsma F, Moleman P, Schalekamp MADH. Congenital dopamine beta-hydroxylase deficiency. A novel orthostatic syndrome, 183–7, Copyright 1987, with permission from Elsevier.

forties in the first family (Lewis 1964) and even later in the second (Ilson et al. 1982). Details of the autonomic disorder in these patients are limited.

Familial amyloidosis (familial amyloid polyneuropathy)

Familial amyloidosis is characterized by abnormal deposition of fibrillar amyloid protein predominantly into peripheral and autonomic nerves, and is described in Chapter 50.

Other hereditary peripheral neuropathies

Other hereditary peripheral neuropathies are described in Chapter 51, and include porphyria (the acute intermittent, variegate, and copro-porphyria forms), where the inheritance is autosomal dominant. Widespread autonomic involvement may occur including tachycardia and hypertension, which is thought to be related to baroreceptor denervation, in addition to other factors. There are a number of hereditary sensory and autonomic neuropathies (Thomas 1992) where the key feature is the sensory neuropathy. The autonomic abnormalities often include the urinary bladder and sweat glands.

Table 49.4 Summary of pharmacological investigations in twelve patients[a] with DBH deficiency. Responses relate to blood pressure unless otherwise stated

Reference	Robertson et al. (1986)	Biaggioni et al. (1990)	Man in't Veld et al. (1987a)	Man in't Veld et al. (1988)	Mathias et al. (1990)	Mathias et al. (1990)	Thompson et al. (1995)	Gomes et al. (2003)	Cheshire et al. (2006)	Robertson et al. (2005)	Erez et al. (2010)	Despas et al. (2010)
Pharmacological investigations	Patient 1	Patient 2	Patient 3	Patient 4	Patient 5	Patient 6	Patient 7	Patient 8	Patient 9	Patient 10	Patient 11	Patient 12
Noradrenaline	↑++	↑++	↑++	↑++	↑++	↑++						
Isoprenaline (BP)	↓++	↓++	↓++	↓++	↓++	↓++						
HR response	↑++	↑++	↑++	↑++	↑++	↑++						
Tyramine	↔b	↔b	↔b	↔b								
Clonidine	↑++	↑++	↑++	↑++	↑++	↑++						
Edrophonium					↔b	↔b						
Atropine (HR)	N	N	N	N	N	N	N					
Metoclopramide	↔	↔	↑	↑	↓	↓						
DL-DOPS	↑	↑	↑	↑	↑	↑						
L-DOPS					↑	↑	↑	↑	↑	↑		↑
L-DOPS + carbidopa					↔	↔						

BP, blood pressure; HR, heart rate; N, normal; ↑, rise; ↓, fall; ↔, no response; ++, excessive response; no symbol, not described.
[a] Patient details described in Table 49.1.
[b] Includes plasma noradrenaline response.

Fabry–Anderson disease

Fabry–Anderson disease is an X-linked glycolipid lysosomal storage disease (Iannacone and Rosenberg 1996). It results from mutation of the α-galactosidase genes situated on the X chromosome and there are a number of variants. The enzymatic deficiency results in accumulation of its main natural substrate, ceramide trihexoside being deposited in connective tissues. Globoside, a tetrahexoside which is its major precursor, is also found in red blood cells, blood vessels, and the kidney. A characteristic of the disease is skin deposits resulting in angiokeratoma, hence the alternative name angiokeratoma corporis diffusum. In addition, the peripheral and autonomic nervous systems, the kidney, the gastrointestinal tract, and the blood vessels themselves are affected. Vascular dilatation and constriction may be impaired directly or through autonomic involvement. In a detailed study of 10 males (Cable et al. 1982), lacrimal and salivary secretion and abnormal pupillary responses to pilocarpine were found in half the cases. The responses to postural change and the plasma noradrenaline levels were normal in all. Impaired sweating was found in all 10 cases. Detailed studies in a single case suggest that both skin sympathetic nerve activity and sweat gland dysfunction may contribute to anhidrosis (Yamamoto et al. 1996). Long-term enzyme therapy with Agalsidase alpha or beta may halt disease progression and should be used with adjunctive therapies; the effects on autonomic features is not known (Germain 2010).

Allgrove's syndrome

Allgrove's syndrome is a paediatric disorder in which there is alacrima, achalasia and adrenocortical insufficiency due to insensitivity to corticotrophin (Allgrove et al. 1978). It is also known as Triple A syndrome and is a rare genetic disorder caused by mutations in the achalasia-addisonianism-alacrima syndrome (*AAAS*) gene, which encodes a tryptophan aspartic acid (WD) repeat-containing protein named alacrima-achalasia-adrenal insufficiency neurological disorder (ALADIN) (Cho et al. 2009). An autonomic neuropathy may be present, as described in four children tested between 6 years and 8 years of age (Gazarian et al. 1995) and two Hispanic adolescents (Chu et al. 1996); orthostatic hypotension, with decreased heart rate variability and impaired responses to deep breathing was reported. The features appear to result from progressive degeneration of cholinergic neurones, although the observations on orthostatic hypotension suggest additional involvement. The relationship between early onset achalasia and the *ALADIN* gene remains unclear (Jung et al. 2011).

Mitochondrial encephalomyopathy

Mitochondrial encephalomyopathy are disorders in which there are structural or biochemical defects in mitochondria, thus impairing oxidative phosphorylation, and affecting a number of systems (Iannaccone and Rosenberg 1996). Abnormalities vary in different subgroups. In Leigh syndrome, there is vomiting and gastrointestinal abnormalities, similar to the patients with myoneural gastrointestinal encephalopathy. In Kearns–Sayre syndrome there is cardiac involvement. In mitochondrial encephalomyopathy with lactic acidosis and stroke-like episodes (MELAS) there is both gastrointestinal and cardiac involvement. Whether the abnormalities result from involvement of the autonomic nervous system is unclear. In a recent report of three children with a mitochondrial encephalomyopathy, there was gastrointestinal dysmotility, cardiac arrhythmias, decreased lacrimation, supersensitivity to methacholine, altered sweating, postural hypotension and apnoea; some of these features were attributed to autonomic dysfunction (Zelnik et al. 1996). The clinical course in these patients was variable, and differed from other groups with mitochondrial encephalomyopathy.

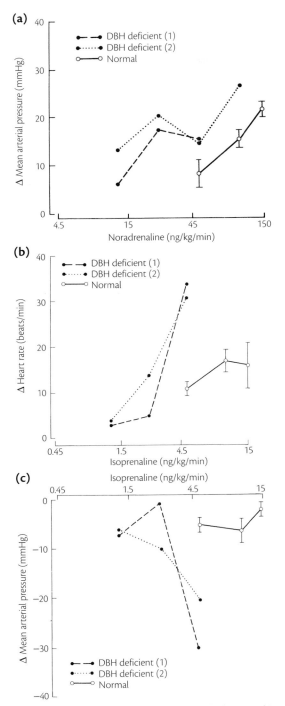

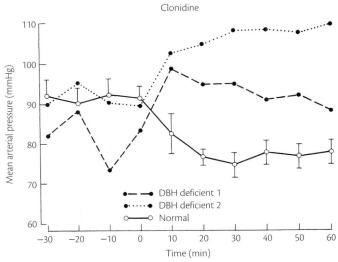

Fig. 49.13 Blood pressure changes following intravenous clonidine given at time 0 (2 μg/kg infused over 10 min) in six normal subjects and in patients 5 and 6 (1 and 2, respectively, in figure) with DBH deficiency. In the normal subjects there is a substantial and significant fall in blood pressure after clonidine. From Mathias et al. 1990.

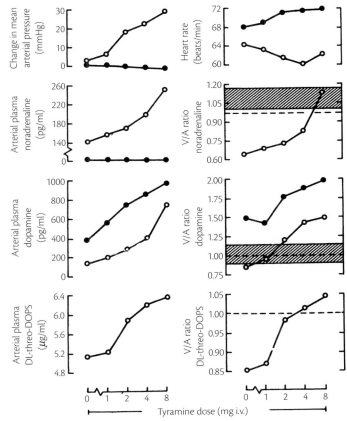

Fig. 49.12 (a) Change in mean blood pressure in normal subjects and in patients 5 and 6 (1 and 2, respectively, in figure) with DBH deficiency after incremental intravenous infusion of noradrenaline. In patient 5 the pulse rate fell to 40 beats/min after the third dose infusion and no further doses were administered. (b) and (c) Rise in heart rate (b) and fall in mean blood pressure (c) in normal subjects and in patients 5 and 6 (1 and 2, respectively, in figure) after incremental intravenous infusion of isoprenaline. From Mathias et al. 1990.

Fig. 49.14 Effects of tyramine before (●–––●) and after (○–––○) treatment with DOPS in patient 3. V/A venous/arterial. Hatched areas indicate 95 per cent confidence interval of V/A ratios for noradrenaline and dopamine in 30 untreated patients with borderline hypertension under basal conditions. Prior to treatment with DL-DOPS, tyramine has no effects on blood pressure and plasma noradrenaline levels. This is changed after treatment with DOPS. From Man in't Veld et al. 1987b.

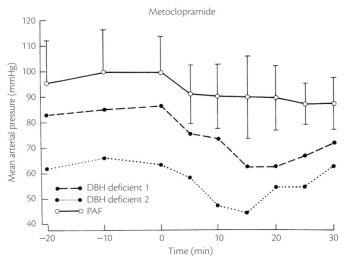

Fig. 49.15 Blood pressure changes before and after the dopamine antagonist metoclopramide (10 mg given as 2.5 mg i.v. every 2.5 minutes from time 0) in four patients with pure autonomic failure (PAF) and patients 5 and 6 (1 and 2 in figure, respectively) with DBH deficiency. From Mathias et al. 1990.

Tyrosine hydroxylase, DBH, and sensory neuropeptide deficiency

A patient with sympathetic adrenergic failure, who had preserved sweating and parasympathetic function, and thus with findings similar to those in DBH deficiency has been described (Anand et al. 1991). In addition, she had undetectable plasma dopamine levels, with immunohistochemical evidence of absent neuronal tyrosine hydroxylase, DBH and the sensory neuropeptides, substance P and calcitonin-gene-related peptide. Dopa decarboxylase activity was present and she could convert oral L-3, 4-dihydroxyphenylalanine (L-DOPA) into dopamine and L-DOPS to noradrenaline. There was an impaired histamine response on skin testing. Nerve growth factor (NGF) levels in skin were subnormal. The combined autonomic and sensory neuropeptide deficit appeared related to a reduction in NGF. Thus, there were marked differences from isolated DBH deficiency.

In experimental studies using gene targeting, inactivation of tyrosine hydroxylase, when performed in mid-gestation *in utero*, results in death of 90% of mutant embryos probably as a result of cardiovascular failure; this can be prevented by the administration of L-DOPA (dihydroxyphenylalanine), indicating the importance of catecholamines for mouse foetal development and post-natal survival (Zhou et al. 1995). This may be of relevance to this particular patient and raises the possibility that the pathological process accounting for her syndrome (that included tyrosine hydroxylase deficiency) was likely to have occurred either in the later stages of pregnancy, or post-partum.

Aromatic L-amino acid decarboxylase deficiency

Three children (including monozygotic twins) with aromatic L-amino acid decarboxylase (AADC) deficiency have been described (Hyland et al. 1992). The twins (1 year old) had reduced plasma dopamine, noradrenaline, and adrenaline levels, along with absent DBH in plasma. Whole blood serotonin levels were low. Cerebrospinal fluid levels of dopamine and serotonin metabolites were reduced. AADC was not present in liver tissue and was reduced in plasma. The previous sibling had died soon after birth

and limited information suggested a similar disorder. The autonomic abnormalities included temperature and blood pressure instability, excessive sweating, miosis, and ptosis. Heart rate variation was preserved. The neurological features (oculogyric crises and abnormal movements) were consistent with a cerebral deficiency of dopamine and responded to dopamine agonists (bromocriptine) and monoamine oxidase inhibitors. The parents appeared normal, except for plasma AADC levels that were <20% of controls. They were first cousins. The inheritance of the disorder appears to be autosomal recessive.

Fatal familial insomnia

Fatal familial insomnia is an autosomal dominant condition characterized by selective degeneration of the anterior and dorso-medial thalamic nuclei. It is an inherited prion disease. It presents in the third or fourth decade with progressive insomnia, ataxia, dysarthria, and myoclonus along with hypertension, tachycardia, and sweating. The autonomic investigations suggest preserved parasympathetic but higher background and stimulated sympathetic activity (Cortelli et al. 1991). Recent positron emission tomography scanning studies confirm hypometabolism of the thalamus and cingulate cortex although there is variable involvement of other brain regions (Cortelli et al. 1997).

Menkes' kinky hair disease (trichopoliodystrophy)

Menkes' kinky hair disease (MD) is a focal degenerative disorder of grey matter in which there is a maldistribution of body copper with low serum copper and caeruloplasmin levels (Menkes 1995). MD is inherited as an X-linked recessive trait due to mutations in the *ATP7A* gene; the majority of *ATP7A* mutations are intragenic mutations or partial gene deletions. ATP7A is an energy-dependent transmembrane protein, which is involved in the delivery of copper to the secreted copper enzymes and in the export of surplus copper from cells. Variants have been described (Proud et al. 1996). There is reduced activity of DBH, which is dependent on copper as a cofactor. This results in impaired conversion of dopamine to noradrenaline. MD presents in infancy with vomiting, hypothermia, and neurological abnormalities such as hypotonia and poor head control. An important pointer to the diagnosis is the appearance of the hair which is colourless and friable. Most infants have delayed growth and development, and the mean age at death is 19 months, although survival to 13 years of age has been recorded. Early copper-histidine replacement may be beneficial (Kaler et al. 1996).

Familial hyperbradykininism

Patients with familial hyperbradykininism have symptoms suggestive of postural hypotension (Streeten et al. 1972). During head-up postural change the systolic (but not necessarily the diastolic) blood pressure, usually fails and there is a marked rise in heart rate. Associated signs include cutaneous dilatation in the face and the lower limbs, which may turn purple. There are no neurological deficits. The findings have been attributed to excessive bradykinin levels. The postural hypotension, therefore, is not due to autonomic failure. These patients appear to benefit from propranolol, fludrocortisone, and the serotonin antagonist, cyproheptadine.

Adrenoleukodystrophy

Adrenoleukodystrophy (ALD) is a peroxisomal disorder that is related to the deposition of very long-chain fatty acids (VLCFA) such as hexocosanoate C26 :0) in cerebral white matter and in the adrenal cortex. It is thought to be due to an enzymatic defect in degradation of long-chain fatty acids, (Iannacone and Rosenberg 1996). X-linked adrenoleukodystrophy (X-ALD) confers a life-long risk for neurological deterioration (Moser et al. 2000 and Moser et al. 2001). In adulthood male phenotypes from adrenomyeloneuropathy (AMN), a spastic paraparesis that is due to a chronic axonopathy of the spinal cord (van Geel et al. 1999), to adult cerebral ALD (ACALD), a rapidly progressive brain disorder involving inflammatory demyelination; in females heterozygous for X-ALD, neurological symptoms are also frequent and incapacitating (van Geel et al. 1999, 2001). Abnormally high levels of plasma VLCFA are diagnostic for X-ALD but unfortunately do not correlate with symptom severity or predict the pathology of the phenotype (van Geel et al. 1999, 2001). Conventional imaging reveals distinct lesion patterns in demyelinating and axonopathic phenotypes, but is poorly sensitive, resulting in delays in diagnosis and treatment.

There are three forms, which result in adrenocortical failure (Addison's disease) and therefore may cause a low supine blood pressure and also postural hypotension; thus, the latter, is not the result of autonomic failure. In the childhood form, with presentation between 4 years and 8 years of age, there may be deafness, dementia, cortical blindness, and tetraparesis. In the adult form, the presentation is usually between 20 years and 30 years of age, with a longer life expectancy. In this form spastic paraparesis and polyneuropathy are common. A mixed form has been described. The symptomatic heterozygote form, which may occur in females, does not appear to involve the adrenal cortex.

Like hyperbradykininism, there is no evidence of autonomic failure accounting for the postural hypotension, and deficiency of cortisol and aldosterone is responsible.

Management of DBH deficiency

The main problem in patients with DBH deficiency is postural hypotension, which responds unsatisfactorily to conventional approaches and drugs (Chapter 47). In patients 1–4 details of drug combinations used were not provided. Patient 5 improved on fludrocortisone alone but did not benefit from desmopressin at night despite having nocturnal polyuria; patient 6 needed a combination of fludrocortisone, dihydroergotamine, and desmopressin at night, that helped partially.

Metyrosine is a drug that inhibits the rate-limiting enzyme tyrosine hydroxylase and is used in patients with malignant phaeochromocytoma to prevent the formation of noradrenaline. In patient 1 it was used successfully to raise supine blood pressure and improve postural hypotension. This was thought to be due to reducing the formation of dopamine (Biaggioni et al. 1987). However, in this same patient the dopamine antagonist, metoclopramide, had no effect on blood pressure. The reasons for this difference are not clear.

The drug that has been particularly beneficial in all patients with DBH deficiency is dihydroxyphenylserine (DOPS). It is similar in structure to noradrenaline (Fig. 49.2), except that it has a carboxyl group as in DOPA. Therefore it is acted upon by dopa-decarboxylase, which is present both intraneurally and in a number of extraneuronal tissues including the kidney and liver, and is converted directly into noradrenaline, thus bypassing the DBH enzymatic step. The drug crosses the blood–brain barrier, as has been demonstrated in

animal studies (Kato et al. 1987). Its effects on reducing postural hypotension were described initially by Suzuki et al. (1980), in patients with familial amyloidosis. It is available either as the racemic mixture (DL-DOPS) or in the laevo form (L-DOPS). The L form is thought to be the active form, based on both animal studies and on observations in patients with familial amyloidosis, where it was effective in half the dosage of the DL form (Suzuki et al. 1982).

In each of the patients, DL-DOPS had remarkable effects. There were definite improvements, with an elevation of supine blood pressure and more importantly, a reduction in postural hypotension (Fig. 49.16). There were no mood changes in patients 1 and 2. In patients 3, 5 and 6 the description indicated that use of the drug effectively changed their lives. Patient 3 could cycle, climb stairs and sit in the sun without feeling faint; she could not do this previously. Patients 5 and 6 were less tired and fatigued, especially in the morning. In patient 5, the symptoms of postural hypotension were virtually eliminated, and in patient 6 they were considerably improved. They both became far more active physically and noted perspiration to a greater extent on exertion, especially around the axillae and groins. Both noted cutis anserina (goose pimples) over the forearms and thighs, that they had not seen previously. In patient 7, symptoms of orthostatic intolerance disappeared. Patient 10 completed a marathon as a result of the beneficial effects of L-DOPS (Robertson et al. 2005)

The change in patient 6 improved a strained marital relationship. She was at times slightly more aggressive than previously and even challenged her mother-in-law for the first time, having previously wished to do so but having been too timid. Neither patient 5 or 6 had difficulty in sleeping, which is consistent with observations in patients 3 and 4. After DOPS, patient 5 may have had an increase in the number of nightmares, which she had suffered from for many years. There was little doubt, however, that initially on DL-DOPS and later with L-DOPS, Patients 5 and 6 were symptomatically far better than when their blood pressure was raised to an equivalent degree on the conventional therapy described above (i.e. fludrocortisone in patient 5 and fludrocortisone, dihydroergotamine, and desmopressin in patient 6). The treatment with DL-DOPS had no effect on nocturia in patient 6, and in both patients the nocturnal diuresis and natriuresis continued (Fig. 49.6). Whether the overall improvement was related to the effects of the drug (including central effects) or nonspecifically to the rise in blood pressure and reduction in postural hypotension was not entirely clear.

An additional advantage of DL- and L-DOPS in patient 5 was the improvement in sexual function, as he was able to achieve ejaculation, which had been difficult or impossible previously. The effect of DOPS on sexual function in the other male (patient 2), was not described.

Levels of plasma noradrenaline rose in each of the patients to whom DL-DOPS was administered; there was also a rise in patients 5, 6 and 7 who were also given L-DOPS. In patients 1–3 there was a further increase in plasma noradrenaline levels with postural challenge (Fig. 49.17), as occurred in patient 7. This was not consistently observed in patients 5 and 6 (Fig. 49.16a, b) when given either DL-DOPS or L-DOPS. In patients 5 and 6 this may imply inadequate intraneuronal replacement. In patient 3 the ability of tyramine to release noradrenaline after DL-DOPS was provided as evidence of intraneuronal replacement. However, noradrenaline formed extraneuronally (dopa decarboxylase is extensively distributed, especially in liver and kidneys) would have been incorporated

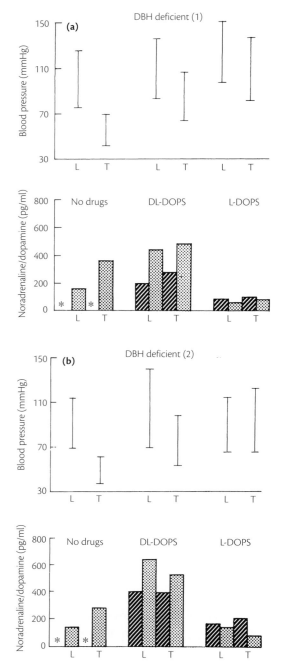

Fig. 49.16 Blood pressure (systolic and diastolic) while lying (L) and during head-up tilt (T) in (a) patient 5 and (b) patient 6 (b) with DBH deficiency (1 and 2, respectively, in figures), before and during treatment with DL-DOPS and L-DOPS. Plasma noradrenaline (hatched histogram) and dopamine (stippled histogram) levels are indicated before and during tilt. Plasma noradrenaline was undetectable (* = <5pg/ml) in both while off drugs. From Mathias et al. 1990.

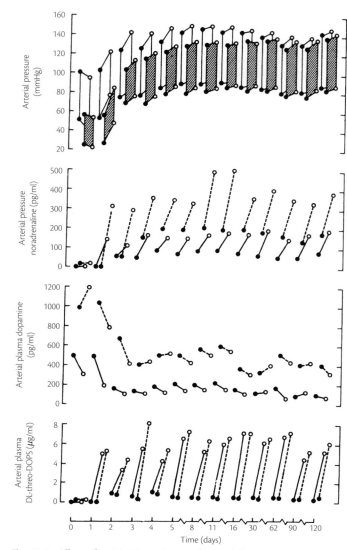

Fig. 49.17 Effects of DL-DOPS in patient 3 with DBH deficiency. Open columns and solid lines indicate values with the patient supine, hatched columns and broken lines with the patient standing. (Filled circle) 12 h after dosing: (open circle) 2 h after dosing. Reprinted from *The Lancet*, **ii**, Man in't Veld AJ, Van den Meiracker AH, Boomsma F, Schalekamp MADH. Effect of unnatural noradrenaline precursor on sympathetic control and orthostatic hypotension in dopamine beta-hydroxylase deficiency, 1172–5, Copyright 1987 with permission from Elsevier.

by uptake mechanisms into the cytosol and this could have been released by tyramine, not necessarily indicating intraneuronal conversion of DL-DOPS to noradrenaline and release of noradrenaline by neuronal impulses. The data in patients 5 and 6 suggest that extraneuronal formation of noradrenaline may have played a more important role in them. In patient 7, the noradrenaline spillover at rest was extremely low and rose to within the normal range during

treatment with L-DOPS. During head-up tilt, however, the noradrenaline spillover, although initially increased by L-DOPS, remained below the normal range. Another explanation provided was that the replacement dose, although clinically satisfactory, may have not provided adequate biochemical replacement of noradrenaline. In patient 7 there was a marked increase in plasma concentration of dihydroxyphenylethylene glycol (DHPG) the intraneuronal metabolite of noradrenaline, providing evidence of noradrenaline synthesis within sympathetic nerves.

In patients 5 and 6, adrenaline remained undetectable in plasma and the metabolites of adrenaline in urine (metadrenaline) did not change (Fig. 49.11) until after 3 months of therapy. This raised the question of abnormalities in the conversion of noradrenaline to adrenaline, either because of an atrophic adrenal medulla or because of the absence of the enzyme phenylethanolamine N-methyl transferase (PNMT). A similar conclusion, based on barely detectable changes in adrenaline secretion after L-DOPS, was reported in patient 7. Further evidence of the inability to form adrenaline was obtained in patients 5 and 6 in whom insulin hypoglycaemia was induced while they were on treatment with L-DOPS. During hypoglycaemia, there was no rise in plasma adrenaline levels, and a small rise in plasma noradrenaline levels. The absence of a rise of metadrenaline excretion in urine was also noticed in patients with familial amyloidosis who were given L-DOPS (Suzuki et al. 1982).

In patients 5 and 6, the question of whether DOPS had direct pressor effects was tested by pretreating them with the dopa-decarboxylase inhibitor carbidopa, in a dose sufficient to prevent peripheral decarboxylation. L-DOPS was then administered and, unlike in previous studies, it had no beneficial effect either on blood pressure or on their ability to stand. This was consistent with a lack of its conversion to noradrenaline, which could not be detected in plasma. Thus L-DOPS alone, even in patients with known adrenoceptor supersensitivity, has no direct pressor effects.

Another point of interest is the question of the central effects of DOPS. This has been partially discussed in relation to behavioural and mood changes and may also be relevant to the blood pressure responses. Animal studies indicate that DL- and L-DOPS enter the brain (Kato et al. 1987). In patients 5 and 6, L-DOPS in the same dose as DL-DOPS was equally effective; theoretically it should have been doubly effective. One possibility is greater formation of noradrenaline within the central nervous system, as has been clearly demonstrated in animal studies, that reduces centrally induced sympathetic discharge and would thus have negated the peripheral effects of the drug (Araki et al. 1981). This would be consistent with the lower levels of plasma dopamine observed after L-DOPS, as compared with levels after L-DOPS (Fig. 49.1a, b). There may also have been other effects including a central reduction of dopamine levels. Both patients 5 and 6 felt that DL-DOPS was 'better' than L-DOPS, though this has not been quantified. In repeat studies after 25 years of treatment with L-DOPS in patients 5 and 6, there was no evidence of any neurological or behavioural impairment and they continue to benefit considerably from the drug.

References

Allgrove, J., Clayden, G. S., Grant, D. B. (1978). Familial glucocorticoid deficiency with achalasia of the cardia and deficient tear production. *Lancet* **1**, 1284–6.

Anand P., Rudge P., Mathias, C. J. et al. (1991). New autonomic and sensory neuropathy with loss of adrenergic sympathetic functions and sensory neuropeptides. *Lancet* **337**, 1253–4.

Araki, H., Tanaka, C., Fujiwara, H., Nakamura, Ohmura, I. (1981). Pressor effect of L-threo-3, 4-dihydroxyphenylserine in rats. *J. Pharm. Pharmacol.* **33**, 772–7.

Biaggioni, I., Goldstein, D. S., Atkinson, T., Robertson, D. (1990). Dopamine beta-hydroxylase deficiency in humans. *Neurology* **40**, 370–3.

Biaggioni, I., Robertson, D. (1987). Endogenous restoration of noradrenaline by precursor therapy in dopamine beta-hydroxylase deficiency. *Lancet* **ii**, 1170–2.

Birkmeyer, W., Birkmeyer, G., Lechner, Riederer, P. (1983). DL-3, 4-threo-DOPS in Parkinson's disease: effects on orthostatic hypotension and dizziness. *J Neurol Transmission* **58**, 305–13.

Bremner, F. D., Smith, S. E. (2006). Pupil Abnormalities in Selected Autonomic Neuropathies. *Journal of Neuro-Ophthalmology.* **26**, 209–19.

Cable, W. J. L., Kolodny, E. H., Adams, R. D. (1982). Fabry disease: impaired autonomic function. *Neurology* **32**, 498–502.

Chen, Y., Wen, G., Rao, F., et al. (2010). Human dopamine beta-hydroxylase (DBH) regulatory polymorphism that influences enzymatic activity, autonomic function and blood pressure. *J Hypertens.* **28**, 76–86.

Cheshire, W. P., Jr., Dickson, D. W., Nahm, K. F., Kaufmann, H. C., Benarroch, E. E., (2006). Dopamine-hydroxylase deficiency involves the central autonomic network. *Acta. Neuropathol.* **112**, 227–9.

Cho, A. R., Yang, K. J., Bae, Y., et al. (2009). Tissue-specific expression and subcellular localization of ALADIN, the absence of which causes human triple A syndrome. *Exp. Mol. Med.* **41**, 381–6.

Chu, M. L., Berlin, D., Axelrod, F. B. (1996). Allgrove syndrome: documenting cholinergic dysfunction by autonomic tests. *J. Pediatr.* **129**, 156–9.

Cortelli P., Parchi P., Contin, M., et al. (1991). Cardiovascular dysautonomia in fatal familial insomnia. *Clin. Aut. Res.*, 15–122.

Cortelli P., Perani, D., Parchi P., et al. (1997). Cerebral metabolism in fatal familial insomnia: Relation to duration, neuropathology, and distribution of protease-resistant prion protein. *Neurology* **49**, 126–33.

Deinum, J., Steenbergen-Spanjers, G. C. H., Jansen, M., et al (2004). DBH gene variants that cause low plasma dopamine β hydroxylase with or without a severe orthostatic syndrome. *J Med Genet* **41**, 38.

Despas, F., Pathak, A., Berry M., et al. (2010) DBH deficiency in an elderly patient: efficacy and safety of chronic droxidopa. *Clin Auton Res.* **20**, 205–7

Erez, A., Li, J., Geraghty, M. T., et al. (2010). Mosaic deletion 11p. 13 in a child with dopamine beta-hydroxylase deficiency—Case report and review of the literature. *Am. J Med. Genet. Part A.* **152**, 732–6.

Gazarian, M., Cowell, C. T., Bonney, M., Grigo, W. G. (1995). The '4A' syndrome: adrenocorticol insufficiency associated with achalasia, alacrima, autonomic and other neurological abnormalities. *Eur. J. Pediatr.* **154**, 18–23.

Germain, D. P. (2010). Fabry disease. *Orphanet J Rare Dis.* **5**, 30.

Goldstein, D. S., Holmes, C., and Axelrod, B. (2008) Plasma catechols in familial dysautonomia long-term follow-up study. *Neruochem. Res.* **33**, 1839–93.

Gomes, M., Deinum, J., Timmers, H. J., Jacques, W. M., Lenders, J.W. M.,(2003). Occam's razor; anaemia and orthostatic hypotension. *Lancet.* **18**, 1282

Hyland, K., Surtees, R. A., Rodeck, A. H., Clayton, T. (1992). Autonomic effects of Aromatic L-amino acid decarboxylase deficiency: Clinical features, diagnosis and treatment of a new inborn error of neurotransmitter amine synthesis. *Neurology* **42**, 1980–88.

Iannaccone, S. T., Rosenberg, R. N. (1996). Principles of molecular genetics and neurologic diseases. In: *Principles of Child Neurology*. Ed. B. Berg. McGraw-Hill, New York, pp. 461–606.

Ilson, J., Parrish, M., Fahn, S., Cote, L. J. (1982). Familial Shy-Drager syndrome: clinical, biochemical and pathological findings. *Neurology* **32**, A160.

Jung, K. W., Yoon, I. J., Kim do, H., et al. (2011). Genetic Evaluation of ALADIN Gene in Early-Onset Achalasia and Alacrima Patients. *J Neurogastroenterol Motil.* **17**, 169–73.

Kaler, S. G., Das, S., Levinson, B., et al. (1996). Successful early copper therapy in Menkes disease associated with a mutant transcript containing a small In-frame deletion. *Biochem. Mol. Med.* **57**, 37–46.

Kato, T., Karai, N., Katsuyama, M., Nakamura, M., Katsube, J. (1987). Studies on the activity of L-threo-3, 4-dihydroxyphenylserine (L-DOPS) as a catecholamine precursor in the brain: Comparison with that of L-DOPA. *Biochem. Pharmacol.* **36**, 3051–7.

Kim, C. H., Zabetian, C. P., Cubells, J. F., et al. (2002). Mutations in the dopamine beta-hydroxylase gene are associated with human norepinephrine deficiency. *Am. J Med. Genet.* **108**, 140–7.

Kim, K. S., Kim, C. H., Koˇhnke, M. D., Kranzler, H. R., Gelernter. J., Cubells, J. F. (2003) A revised allele frequency estimate and haplotype analysis of the DBH deficiency mutation IVS1 + 2T.C in African- and European-Americans. *Am. J Med. Genet.* **123**, 190–2.

Lewis, P. (1964). Familial orthostatic hypotension. *Brain* **87**, 719–28.

Man in't Veld, A.J., Boomsma, F., Lenders, J., *et al.* (1988). Patients with congenital dopamine beta-hydroxylase deficiency. A lesson in catecholamine physiology. *Am. J. Hypertens.* **1**, 231–8.

Man in't Veld, A. J., Boomsma, F., Moleman, P., Schalekamp, M. A. D. H. (1987a). Congenital dopamine beta-hydroxylase deficiency. A novel orthostatic syndrome. *Lancet* **i**, 183–7.

Man in't Veld, A. J., Van den Meiracker, A. H., Boomsma, F., Schalekamp, M. A. D. H. (1987b). Effect of unnatural noradrenaline precursor on sympathetic control and orthostatic hypotension in dopamine beta-hydroxylase deficiency. *Lancet* **ii**, 1172–5.

Mathias, C. J. (1996). Disorders of the autonomic nervous system. In: *Neurology in Clinical Practice.* 2nd edition. Eds. W. G. Bradley, R. B. Daroff, G. M. Fenichel, C. D. Marsden. Butterworth-Heinemann, Boston, USA, 82: pp. 1953–81.

Mathias, C. J., Bannister, R., Cortelli, P. *et al.* (1990). Clinical autonomic and therapeutic observations in two siblings with postural hypotension and sympathetic failure due to an inability to synthesize noradrenaline from dopamine because of a deficiency of dopamine beta-hydroxylase. *Q. J. Med.* **75**, 617–33.

Mathias, C. J., Smith, A. D., Frankel, H. L., Spalding, J. K. M. (1976). Dopamine beta-hydroxylase release during hypertension from sympathetic nervous overactivity in main. *Cardiovasc. Res.* **10**, 176–81.

Menkes, J. H. (1995). Metabolic diseases of the nervous system. In: *Textbook of Child Neurology* (ed. JH Menkes). Williams & Wilkins Baltimore, Maryland. pp. 29–151.

Moser, H. W., Loes, D. J., Melhem, E. R., *et al.* (2000). X-Linked adrenoleukodystrophy: overview and prognosis as a function of age and brain magnetic resonance imaging abnormality. A study involving 372 patients. *Neuropediatrics* **31**, 227–39.

Moser, H., Smith, K. & Watkins, P. (2001). X-linked adrenoleukodystrophy. In: Scriver, C. & Sly, W. S. (eds). *The Metabolic and Molecular Bases of Inherited Disease.* pp. 3257–301. McGraw Hill, New York, NY.

O'Connor, D. T., Cervenka, J. H., Stone, R. A., *et al.* (1994). Dopamine beta-hydroxylase immunoreactivity in human cerebrospinal fluid: properties, relationship to central noradrenergic neuronal activity and variation in Parkinson's disease and dopamine beta-hydroxylase deficiency. *Clin. Sci.* **86**, 149–58.

Proud, V. K., Mussell, H. G., Kaler, S. G., Young, D. W., Percy, A. K. (1996). Distinctive Menkes disease variant with occipital horns: delineation of natural history and clinical phenotype. *Am. J. Med. Genet.* **65**, 44–51.

Rea, R., Biaggioni, I., Robertson, R. M., Haile, V., Robertson, D. (1990). Reflex control of sympathetic nerve activity in dopamine-beta-hydroxylase deficiency. *Hypertension* **15**, 107–12.

Robertson, D., Garland, E. M., Raj, S. R., Demartinis, N. (2005). Case report. Marathon runner with severe autonomic failure. *Lancet* **366**, 513.

Robertson, D., Goldberg, M. R., Onrot, J., Hollister, A. S., Wiley, R., Thompson, J. G., Robertson, R. M. (1986). Isolated failure of autonomic noradrenergic neurotransmission. Evidence for impaired beta-hydroxylation of dopamine. *New Engl. J. Med.* **314**, 1494–7.

Smith, G. D. P., Mathias, C. J. (1995). Postural hypotension enhanced by exercise in patients with chronic autonomic failure. *Q. J. Med.,* **88**, 251–6.

Smith, G. D. P., Watson, L. P., Pavitt, D. V., Mathias, C. J. (1995). Abnormal cardiovascular and catecholamine responses to supine exercise in human subjects with sympathetic dysfunction. *J. Physiol.* (London), **485**, 255–65.

Suzuki, S., Higa, S., Sakoda, S., *et al.* (1982). Pharmacokinetic studies of oral L-threo-3, 4-dihydroxyphenylserine in normal subjects and patients with familial amyloid polyneuropathy. *Eur. J. Clin. Pharmacol.* **23**, 463–8.

Suzuki, S., Higa, S., Tsuga, I., *et al.* (1980). Effects of infused L-threo-3, 4-dihydroxyphenylserine in patients with familial amyloid polyneuropathy. *Eur. J. Clin. Pharmacol.* **17**, 429–35.

Thomas, P. K. (1992). Autonomic involvement in inherited neuropathies. *Clin. Aut. Res.* 2, 51–6.

Thomas, S. A., Matsumoto, A. M., Palmiter, R. D. (1995). Noradrenaline is essential for mouse fetal development. *Nature* **374**, 643–6.

Thompson, J. M., O'Callaghan, C. J., Kingwell, B. A., Lambert, G. W., Jennings, G. L., Esler, M. D. (1995). Total norepinephrine spillover, muscle sympathetic nerve activity and heart-rate spectral analysis in a patient with dopamine b-hydroxylase deficiency. *J. Aut. Nerv. System* **55**, 198–206.

Tulen, J. H., Man in't Veld, A. J., Mechelse, K., and Boomsma, F. (1990). Sleep patterns in congenital dopamine beta-hydroxylase deficiency. *J Neurol.* **237**, 98–102.

van Geel, B. M., Assies, J., Haverkort, E. B., *et al.* (1999). Progression of abnormalities in adrenomyeloneuropathy and neurologically asymptomatic X-linked adrenoleukodystrophy despite treatment with 'Lorenzo's oil' *J Neurol. Neurosurg. Psychiatry.* **67**, 290–9.

van Geel, B. M., Bezman, L., Loes, D. J., *et al.* (2001). Evolution of phenotypes in adult male patients with X, linked adrenoleukodystrophy. *Ann. Neurol.* **49**, 186–94.

Weinshilboum, R. M. (1978). Serum dopamine beta-hydroxylase. *Pharmacol. Rev.* **30**, 133–66.

Weinshilboum, R., and Axelrod, J. (1971). Serum dopamine-beta-hydroxylase activity. *Circ. Res.* **28**, 307–15.

Yamamoto, K., Sobue, G., Iwase, S., Kumazawa, K., Mitsuma, T., Mano, T. (1996). Possible mechanism of anhidrosis in a symptomatic female carrier of Fabry's disease: an assessment by skin sympathetic nerve activity and sympathetic skin response. *Clin. Aut. Res.* **6**, 107–10.

Zabetian, C. P., Romero, R., Robertson, D., *et al.* (2003). A revised allele frequency estimate and haplotype analysis of the DBH deficiency mutation IVS1 + 2T—> C in African- and European-Americans. *Am J Med Genet A.* 1, 190–2.

Zelnik, N., Axelrod, F. B., Leshinsky, E., Griebel, M. L., Kolodny, E. H. (1996). Mitochondrial encephalomyopathies presenting with features of autonomic and visceral dysfunction. *Pediatric Neurology* **14**, 251–4.

Zhou, Q-Z., Quaife, C. J., Palmiter, R. D. (1995). Targeted disruption of the tyrosine hydroxylase gene reveals that catecholamines are required for mouse fetal development. *Nature* **374**, 640–3.

CHAPTER 50

Hereditary amyloid neuropathy

Sinéad M. Murphy and Mary M. Reilly

Introduction

The hereditary amyloid neuropathies, more commonly known as the familial amyloid polyneuropathies (FAP), are a heterogeneous group of autosomal dominant disorders originally described by Andrade in Portuguese patients in 1952 (Andrade 1952). FAP is one of a group of conditions called the amyloidoses that are characterized by deposition of a fibrillar protein with abundant beta pleated structure in the extracellular space (Benson 1989). The staining of amyloid with congo red dye and the subsequent viewing of it microscopically under crossed polarized light gives a characteristic apple green birefringence. Many different proteins have been described to form amyloid and it is the individual constituent protein that defines the various types of amyloidosis (Reilly and King 1993). Amyloidosis is usually either systemic or localized. The most common systemic forms are primary light chain amyloidosis (constituent protein kappa or lambda light chains), secondary or reactive amyloidosis (constituent protein serum amyloid A) and familial amyloid polyneuropathy (constituent proteins transthyretin, apolipoprotein A-1 or gelsolin). There are also many localized forms of amyloidosis including some that affect the nervous system (e.g. Alzheimer's disease).

Amyloid neuropathy, classically seen in FAP, can also be a feature of primary light chain amyloidosis and dialysis related amyloidosis (constituent protein β_2-microglobulin) (Reilly and Staunton 1996). In primary light chain amyloidosis, two types of neuropathy are described, a compression neuropathy such as carpal tunnel syndrome and a generalized neuropathy with autonomic involvement (Kyle 1992). In patients on long-term dialysis, carpal tunnel syndrome, due to β_2-microglobulin amyloid, may be found.

In FAP, the most common fibril protein deposited as amyloid is a variant form of transthyretin (TTR, formerly known as pre-albumin) (Costa et al. 1978) but FAP can also occur secondary to apolipoprotein A-1 deposition (Nichols et al. 1988) and to gelsolin deposition (Ghiso et al. 1990). Although there are now over 100 amyloidogenic point mutations and one trinucleotide deletion in the *TTR* gene (Connors et al. 2003), the first described mutation, methionine 30 (Met 30), originally described in Portuguese patients with TTR-related FAP (Dwulet and Benson 1983), is still the most common worldwide. Clinically the neuropathy in TTR-related FAP starts as a small fibre neuropathy and progresses to a more generalized sensory motor neuropathy commonly associated with autonomic dysfunction, a cardiomyopathy and vitreous involvement. In the past two decades major progress has been made in the understanding of FAP, particularly TTR-related FAP, and in the treatment of TTR-related FAP with liver transplantation.

History

In 1842, Rokitansky described a specific condition giving rise to an enlarged liver and spleen associated with certain chronic diseases, later known as amyloidosis. The term amyloid was originally coined in 1853 by Virchow following his studies on isomers of starch in humans and his observation of the cellulose like nature of the sago grains in the sago spleens described by Chistensen (Virchow 1853). The earliest descriptions of amyloid clearly refer to secondary amyloidosis, that is amyloid associated with chronic infections such as tuberculosis and osteomyelitis. The association of multiple myeloma and amyloid (primary light chain amyloid) was noted in 1867 and in the first part of the 20th century the association of Bence Jones protein with amyloid formation and the finding of increased bone marrow cells in primary amyloidosis was recorded (Cohen 1992). The modern method of staining for amyloid with the congo red dye was introduced by Bennhold in 1922 and shortly afterwards it was found that all amyloid had positive green birefringence after congo red staining. By 1959, Cohen had shown that amyloid could be clearly visualized, isolated and characterized as a fibrous protein (Cohen and Calkins 1959).

The first description of amyloidosis clinically and pathologically affecting the peripheral nerves was by Königstein in 1925 (Königstein 1925). He noted that the clinical involvement of the peripheral nerves seemed to be much greater that the histological involvement, a finding now well recognized in FAP. In 1938, Navasquez and Treble described a case of polyneuropathy secondary to amyloidosis with associated autonomic features. Hereditary amyloid neuropathy was first described by Andrade in 1952 (Andrade 1952). His original description of FAP was of 'a peculiar form of peripheral neuropathy' known for generations among the local people as 'mal dos pesinhos' (foot disease). He gave a detailed description of 74 patients with a disease which started insidiously in the second or third decade of life and was characterized by a 'progressive lowering of the general state of health, gastrointestinal disturbances, premature impotence, and a syndrome of involvement of the peripheral neurone starting and predominating in the lower extremities' (Andrade 1952). He demonstrated that the disease was often familial and that the average duration of the illness was seven to ten years. The size of the problem in Portugal has gradually come to light with over 500 kindreds now known to be affected. The suggestion that the fibril protein in FAP was immunologically related to TTR was made in 1978 (Costa et al. 1978) and the first point mutation (Met 30) in the TTR gene associated with FAP and accounting for the original Portuguese cases was described in 1983 (Dwulet and Benson 1983). There have been more than 100 amyloidogenic TTR point mutations subsequently described but TTR Met 30 associated with FAP is still the most common and best characterized.

In 1969 Van Allen described an Iowan kindred with a typical clinical picture of FAP (Van Allen et al. 1969), in which the constituent amyloid protein has subsequently been shown to be a variant of apolipoprotein A-1 with an arginine for glycine substitution at position 26 (Nichols et al. 1990).

The third form of FAP was originally described by Meretoja in a Finnish kindred in 1969 (Meretoja 1969). Clinically this is different from classical FAP and is characterized by corneal lattice dystrophy and a progressive cranial neuropathy. The fibril protein in this disease is an abnormal fragment of gelsolin, usually associated with a substitution of asparagine for aspartic acid at position 15 (Levy et al. 1990).

Classification

In the past FAP has been classified into four different types based on clinical presentation although this classification has now been replaced by a classification based on the nature of the constituent amyloidogenic protein. The four types of FAP in the original classification were: type I (lower limb onset) originally and mainly described in Portuguese (Andrade 1952), Japanese (Araki et al. 1968) and Swedish (Andersson 1970) kinships; type II (upper limb onset) originally described in the Indiana/Swiss (Mahloudji et al. 1969) and in the German/Maryland (Nichols et al. 1989) kinships; type III (lower limb neuropathy, nephropathy and gastric ulcers) originally described in an Iowa kinship (Van Allen et al. 1969) and type IV (cranial nerve involvement with corneal lattice dystrophy) originally described in a Finnish kindred (Meretoja 1969).

In the more modern classification FAP is divided into three types, transthyretin-related FAP, apolipoprotein A-1 related FAP and gelsolin-related FAP. Transthyretin-related FAP (TTR-related FAP) is so named as TTR is the constituent amyloid protein. This encompasses types I and II of the original classification, both of which are secondary to TTR deposition. Apolipoprotein A-1 related FAP (apolipoprotein A-1 related FAP) secondary to apolipoprotein A-1 deposition encompasses type III of the original classification. Gelsolin-related FAP secondary to gelsolin deposition, is the same as type IV in the original classification. In TTR-related amyloidosis and apolipoprotein A-1 related amyloidosis, a neuropathy is not always present so in this chapter the three different forms of hereditary amyloidosis that can be associated with a neuropathy will be referred to as TTR amyloidosis, apolipoprotein A-1 amyloidosis and gelsolin amyloidosis.

There are now over 100 pathogenic TTR point mutations described, most of which are associated with hereditary amyloid neuropathy, and it is clear with the ever increasing number of different mutations being described that there are overlapping clinical syndromes between specific mutations. Nevertheless in an individual patient the ethnic origin, or in some cases the presenting clinical feature, may alert the clinician to suspect a particular mutation.

Transthyretin amyloidosis

TTR amyloidosis is the most common cause of inherited amyloid neuropathy, and since the recognition that the fibril protein in this type of amyloidosis was immunologically related to TTR was made in 1978 (Costa et al. 1978), TTR amyloidosis has been recognized throughout the world. The cardinal clinical features in TTR amyloidosis associated with a neuropathy are of a sensory motor peripheral neuropathy usually with autonomic involvement, a cardiomyopathy and to a lesser extent vitreous and renal involvement (Reilly and King 1993). Many other systems can be involved as described below. The first point mutation in the TTR gene to be described in TTR amyloidosis was the methionine 30 (Met 30) point mutation in 1983 (Dwulet and Benson 1983). This has subsequently been shown to be by far the most common point mutation in TTR amyloidosis and this type of amyloidosis is a major cause of morbidity and mortality in areas where this type of amyloidosis is endemic, such as the Oporto region of Portugal.

Clinical features of transthyretin amyloidosis
Transthyretin amyloidosis methionine 30
TTR amyloidosis Met 30 is the best characterized of all the amyloidosis associated TTR point mutations as it occurs most commonly. The detailed original description of this type of amyloidosis by Andrade in 74 patients (Andrade 1952) fits well with the subsequent description of further cases. As well as describing a peripheral and autonomic neuropathy starting in the second or third decade of life, he noted that the disease was often familial and that the average duration of the disease was 7–10 years, with patients usually succumbing to cachexia, intercurrent infection or cardiovascular collapse. In his series patients usually presented with sensory symptoms including hypo- or analgesia, painless injuries, burns, paraesthesia or pain in the lower limbs. Pain was often a significant feature especially secondary to slight cutaneous stimuli. From these presentations he concluded that there was a pattern to the sensory loss, starting with the loss of thermal sensibility and progressively involving pain, touch, and deep sensibility. He described the motor system becoming involved later with the lower limbs again being involved first. As the disease progressed the reflexes were gradually lost. He noted anisocoria, gastrointestinal disturbances including constipation, diarrhoea, abdominal distension and progressive weight loss and genitourinary disturbances especially impotence. Post mortem studies were carried out in two of these cases where amyloid was found deposited in the peripheral nerves, kidneys, heart, pancreas, skin, lungs, and stomach. In the peripheral nerves amyloid was deposited within the nerve bundles and in spinal roots and ganglia.

Subsequent descriptions of this type of amyloidosis, particularly in the Portuguese cases, are very similar. The cardinal feature remains a length dependent sensory and motor neuropathy that usually starts in the lower limbs with symptoms of small fibre involvement predominating initially. This gives rise to the classical examination findings of a dissociated sensory loss more pronounced for pain and temperature than for light touch (Adams 2001). Eventually all sensory modalities are involved which can lead to complications secondary to painless injury to the feet including ulcers, cellulitis, osteomyelitis and Charcot joints (Reilly and King 1993). Motor involvement typically occurs later in the course of the disease initially with wasting and weakness in the lower limbs but gradually progressing to upper limbs accompanied by a progressive loss of tendon reflexes. The neuropathy can be very severe and disabling in the latter stages of the disease. Carpal tunnel syndrome can occur in TTR amyloidosis Met 30 but is not usually the presenting feature (Benson 1991) unlike in other forms of TTR amyloidosis as described below.

Neurophysiological studies confirm an axonal neuropathy. In the early stages the only abnormalities detected may be in small fibre function such as abnormal thermal thresholds. Later the sensory action potentials become progressively reduced and eventually absent, initially in the lower limbs but eventually in the upper limbs. The sensory conduction velocities are usually normal or close to normal. The motor amplitudes are normal at first but become progressively reduced and eventually are often absent especially in the lower limbs. Motor conduction velocities are usually normal or close to normal.

As Andrade suggested in his original description autonomic involvement can be early and can be severe. Symptomatically this usually manifests with orthostatic hypotension, alternating constipation and diarrhoea, severe gastric distension and retention and genitourinary problems including sexual impotence and urinary disturbances (Reilly and King 1993). The gastrointestinal symptoms can be very troublesome and can include diarrhoea triggered by meals, explosive diarrhoea and nocturnal diarrhoea. Recurrent vomiting can more rarely be a prominent symptom (Adams 2001). Examination findings include scalloped pupils, postural hypotension, an abnormal Valsalva response and a fixed pulse rate. Pupillography and formal autonomic testing is usually abnormal especially as the disease progresses demonstrating both sympathetic and parasympathetic involvement. The autonomic neuropathy can be very debilitating and in the terminal stages of the disease patients can be bedbound due to a combination of a severe peripheral and autonomic neuropathy.

The other frequently involved system in TTR amyloidosis Met 30 is the heart. Although pathological involvement of the heart was shown in Andrade's original cases, subsequent studies have confirmed the importance of cardiac involvement in the overall clinical picture. One Portuguese study of 60 cases showed that all patients had cardiac involvement in advanced disease (Fonseca et al. 1991). Clinically the cardiac involvement usually presents with an arrhythmia, heart block or heart failure. Electrocardiography abnormalities include widespread T-wave and Q-wave repolarization changes and various conduction disturbances. Echocardiography is abnormal in cardiac amyloidosis showing a restrictive cardiomyopathy with thickened interventricular septum and thickened ventricular walls with greatly refractile echoes (termed a granular sparkling appearance) (Hungo and Ikeda 1986). Preserved wall motion at the left ventricular apex with basal and midsection hypokinesis is a characteristic finding (Belkin et al. 2010). [123]Iodine-labelled serum amyloid protein (SAP) scans are also used but do not detect cardiac amyloid reliably (Hazenberg et al. 2006). More recently, bone scintigraphy has been demonstrated to be useful for detecting cardiac amyloid deposition (Puille et al. 2002, Wechalekar et al. 2007).

Vitreous amyloid deposits are well recognized in TTR amyloidosis Met 30 and are often the presenting feature in Swedish patients (Sousa et al. 1993). Other systems including the central nervous system may be involved in TTR amyloidosis Met 30 but they are less common and are discussed below (see 'Other system involvement in TTR amyloidosis').

TTR amyloidosis Met 30 is most commonly seen in patients of Portuguese and Swedish origin (Planté-Bordeneuve and Said 2000) but is now recognized worldwide (Reilly and Staunton 1996). It had been postulated that all patients with TTR Met 30 were Portuguese in origin with a common founder but haplotype studies have clearly shown many founders for this mutation (Ii and Sommer 1993, Reilly et al. 1995a, Yoshioka et al. 1989). There is marked clinical heterogeneity in cases of TTR amyloidosis Met 30 with some consistency in each major cluster of the disease, in relation to both age of onset and the nature of the initial presentation. Portuguese patients and patients of Portuguese descent tend to present in a classical manner with a lower limb sensory neuropathy in their twenties and thirties whereas Swedish patients with the same mutation and surprisingly the same haplotype, usually present in their late fifties with vitreous involvement (Sousa et al. 1993). In Japan, the TTR Met 30 cases in the two main endemic areas of Arao city and Ogawa village present early like the Portuguese cases but the other patients presenting outside these areas often present later (46–80 years) with a slightly different phenotype including less autonomic involvement (Ikeda et al. 2002). Worldwide variations in both age of onset and clinical presentation is well documented with TTR amyloidosis Met 30.

Other transthyretin amyloidosis point mutations

A similar clinical picture to that seen with TTR amyloidosis Met 30 is described with many other TTR point mutations. No specific clinical picture predicts a specific mutation but there are a few mutations that deserve further comment.

TTR amyloidosis Tyr 77 is the second commonest TTR point mutation associated with TTR amyloidosis which has been shown to have multiple founders (Reilly et al. 1995a). This mutation was originally described in a German kindred from Illinois but has since been described in families from many countries including France, UK, USA, and Spain (Reilly et al. 1995b). Disease onset is usually later than TTR amyloidosis Met 30, often in the fifties. The clinical features are otherwise similar to TTR amyloidosis Met 30 except for a high incidence of carpal tunnel syndrome (which can be the presenting feature) and the absence of vitreous involvement.

Other TTR amyloidosis mutations that classically present in the upper limbs and often with carpal tunnel syndrome are Ser 84 (Dwulet and Benson 1986) and His 58 (Nichols et al. 1989). This type of TTR amyloidosis (FAP type II in the original classification) was originally described in two kindreds, an Indiana family of Swiss origin (Ser 84) and a Maryland family of German origin (His 58). The clinical presentation is of a generalized neuropathy starting in the upper limbs often with associated autonomic failure and occasionally with cardiomyopathy. This type of upper limb presentation has now been described with many TTR mutations (Reilly and Staunton 1996).

TTR amyloidosis Ala 60 has been found in the US, Ireland, UK and Australia and to date all patients that have had haplotype studies done have been shown to have a common founder in northwest Ireland (Reilly et al. 1995c). TTR amyloidosis Ala 60 has also been described in Japan but no haplotype data is available (Kotani et al. 2002). The TTR amyloidosis Ala 60 families therefore represent the second largest group of families with a common mutation presenting in different areas to be traced to a common founder, the largest being those of known Portuguese origin with TTR amyloidosis Met 30. TTR amyloidosis Ala 60 typically presents late in the sixth or seventh decade and both large fibre sensory loss and motor involvement are more prominent than in TTR amyloidosis Met 30. Cardiomyopathy is often a major feature and is commonly the presenting feature.

A more aggressive and rapid disease course is described in TTR amyloidosis with some mutations including TTR Pro 55 (Jacobson et al. 1992), TTR Lys 54 (Togashi et al. 1999) and TTR Ser 25 (Yazaki et al. 2000).

Central nervous system involvement in transthyretin amyloidosis

Until recently, involvement of the central nervous system (CNS) in TTR amyloidosis was considered to be very rare although postmortem studies had shown leptomeningeal amyloid deposition that usually was asymptomatic. In 1980, Goren first described the rare syndrome of oculoleptomeningeal amyloidosis (OLMA) (Goren et al. 1980) and subsequently this has been shown to be associated with TTR point mutations (Brett et al. 1999). The clinical features vary even within a kindred and include vitreous opacities, progressive dementia, stroke, subarachnoid haemorrhage, ataxia, hydrocephalous, seizures, spasticity, and episodes of fluctuating consciousness often with focal neurological signs (Brett et al. 1999). Magnetic resonance imaging (MRI) may show meningeal enhancement in the brain and spinal cord and the cerebrospinal fluid (CSF) protein can be raised. The other typical TTR amyloidosis features, including peripheral neuropathy and cardiomyopathy, are usually mild although one patient with a TTR Pro 12 mutation was described with a severe peripheral neuropathy and prominent central manifestations (Brett et al. 1999). OLMA has been described in association with 9 TTR point mutations, Gly 30, Met 30, Gly 18, Pro 12, Ser 64, Pro 36, Glu 53, Cys 114 and His 69 (Blevins et al. 2003) and as it has been described with the common Met 30 mutation, OLMA should be considered a rare part of the TTR amyloidosis syndrome.

Other system involvement in transthyretin amyloidosis

In post-mortem studies amyloid is often found to be widely distributed in TTR amyloidosis and yet many systems are only rarely symptomatic. Kidney involvement can occur but is often asymptomatic and may only be picked up when patients are being considered for liver transplantation. Gastrointestinal involvement can occur independently from the gastrointestinal symptoms secondary to autonomic involvement and includes a protein losing enteropathy (Reilly and King 1993). Rarely, symptomatic muscle, bone and pulmonary involvement occur.

Course

TTR amyloidosis is a slowly progressive illness in most patients except for the more aggressive forms described above. The course is best described for TTR amyloidosis Met 30 and has been divided into three stages (Coutinho et al. 1980). Stage 1 is characterized by a mainly sensory neuropathy in the lower limbs where the patient is still independently ambulant. In stage 2, after a mean interval of 5.6 years there is a more generalized sensory motor neuropathy affecting gait (may need walking aids) and beginning to affect the upper limbs. In stage 3, which occurs after a mean of 10.4 years, the patient is either confined to a wheelchair or bedridden. Death usually occurs after an interval of about 10 years with TTR amyloidosis Met 30 and is usually due to infections, cachexia, cardiac

or autonomic complications (Adams 2001). The course of the disease varies somewhat for other TTR mutations.

Pathology of transthyretin amyloidosis

All types of amyloid found in the peripheral nervous system occur as extracellular, amorphous, eosinophilic deposits (Reilly and King 1993). The most widely used technique to demonstrate amyloid is a combination of alkaline congo red (Fig. 50.1a) and polarizing filters to demonstrate the characteristic apple-green birefringence (Fig. 50.1b). It is important to identify the constituent fibril protein in amyloid, particularly to distinguish between TTR amyloidosis and AL (light chain) amyloidosis as they can present with a very similar clinical picture. Immunohistochemical studies using monoclonal antibodies for TTR (Fig. 50.1c) and kappa or lambda light chains are used for this purpose but are not always reliable (Adams 2001). A negative study from immunostaining for TTR does not exclude TTR amyloidosis. More recently, liquid chromatography tandem mass spectrometry with laser dissection (LMD/MS) of amyloid plaques has been demonstrated to reliably differentiate between different types of amyloid deposits in nerve biopsies (Klein et al. 2011). TTR amyloidosis Met 30 is the best characterized pathologically as it is the most common type of TTR amyloidosis.

Amyloid deposits can be found in any part of the peripheral nervous system, including the nerve trunks, plexuses and sensory and autonomic ganglia. In the ganglia, they often form deposits around the small ganglion cells. In the peripheral nerves, amyloid deposits occur extracellularly in the epi-, peri-, or endoneurium (Fig. 50.2). The size and number of deposits vary, with both large and small deposits described. The deposits are often found around blood vessels where they may form a symmetrical annulate cuff. Larger deposits can be seen unrelated to blood vessels with a globular form surrounding collagen fibrils. One study of both post-mortem nerves and sural nerve biopsies from patients with varying stages of TTR amyloidosis has demonstrated that amyloid deposition in the endoneurium starts angiocentrically in the small vessel walls and surrounding tissue (Araki and Shigehira 2000). The same study showed that in more advanced cases, deposits were also seen in the subperineurial and/or epineurial regions. Electron microscopy (EM) demonstrates that amyloid is composed of fibrils with a characteristic ultrastructural appearance. The fibrils are straight nonbranching tubules with a diameter of 8 nanometres (Fig. 50.3), which in cross-section have a very dense, hard-edged profile. A study of the ultrastructure of amyloid fibrils in TTR amyloidosis Met 30 showed that the amyloid fibrils were composed of two protofilaments twisted at 180 degrees to the right and left alternatively with a periodicity of 125–135 nm (Katsuragi et al. 2000). The fibrils may form disorganized mats or radiating arrays and they are often closely related to the basal lamina, both of Schwann cells and perineurial cells.

In TTR amyloidosis it is well recognized that the neuropathy is due to progressive axonal loss characterized by fibres undergoing Wallerian degeneration. The axonal loss initially affects unmyelinated and small myelinated fibres and later affects the larger myelinated fibres (Dyck and Lambert 1969, Thomas and King 1974). The loss of unmyelinated axons is indicated by the occurrence of flat sheets of Schwann cell processes. Although occasionally recent Wallerian type degeneration and macrophage infiltration is seen in affected nerves it is more usual not to demonstrate active pathology.

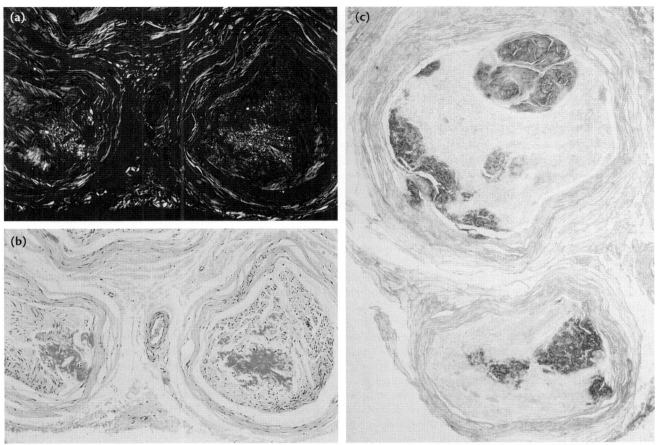

Fig. 50.1 Endoneurial amyloid deposits visualized by Congo red staining **(a)** and, again after Congo red staining but viewed by polarization optics **(b)** showing the green birefringence displayed by the deposit. **(c)** Demonstrates positive immunostaining of the endoneurial amyloid deposits for transthyretin. ×100.

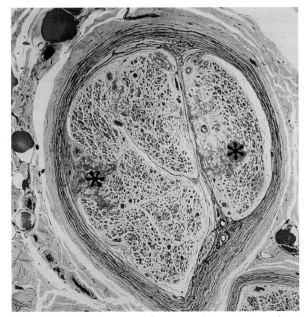

Fig. 50.2 Semithin transverse section of sural nerve biopsy specimen, showing severe loss of myelinated nerve fibres and the presence of endoneurial amyloid deposits (asterisks). Thionin and acridine orange stain; ×100.

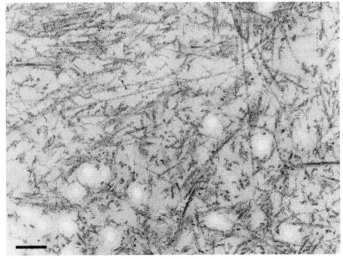

Fig. 50.3 Electron micrograph of amyloid fibrils showing the straight, unbranched, 'rigid' appearance. Bar = 0.1 μm.

Teased fibre studies have shown that there may also be segmental demyelination and remyelination (Dyck and Lambert 1969). This could result from demyelination secondary to Schwann cell dysfunction or demyelination secondary to axonal atrophy. There is usually little evidence of axonal regeneration. As the disease progresses the number of remaining nerve fibres declines with the gradual replacement of the endoneurial contents by amyloid.

Genetics/epidemiology of transthyretin amyloidosis

The original suggestion that the fibril protein in TTR amyloidosis was immunologically related to TTR was made by Costa et al. (1978). The three-dimensional structure of plasma TTR is known. TTR is a tetramer (55 kDa) composed of four identical monomer subunits. Each monomer shows extensive β-pleated structure with eight β-pleated sheets arranged in two parallel plates. Two monomers combine to form a dimer and the two dimers bond non-covalently to form the tetramer (Benson 1991). Over 90% of TTR is produced in the liver with the remainder produced in the choroid plexus and retina. The mature protein has two known functions; it is responsible for about 20% of plasma thyroxine binding and it also binds with retinal binding proteins.

TTR is the product of a single copy gene on chromosome 18 (18q11.2—q12.1) (Wallace et al. 1995). This gene has four exons which code for a 127 amino acid mature protein and an 18 residue signal peptide. The protein is mainly encoded by exons 2, 3 and 4 whereas exon 1 encodes a signal peptide and the first three amino acids of the mature protein. There have been more than 100 point mutations reported in TTR (Connors et al. 2003), all in exons 2, 3 and 4 and most of these are pathogenic, usually presenting with the clinical features of TTR amyloidosis neuropathy and more rarely with just a cardiomyopathy (Planté-Bordeneuve and Said 2000). A case of TTR amyloidosis has been reported secondary to a trinucleotide deletion in exon 4 (Uemichi et al. 1997). Several non-pathogenic point mutations have been described including Thr 109, associated with euthyroid hyperthyroxinaemia (Moses et al. 1986) and neutral polymorphisms detected in healthy people including Met 119 and Ser 6.

The various point mutations in the TTR gene described in TTR amyloidosis usually exist in the heterozygous state and are inherited in an autosomal dominant manner. The TTR Met 30 mutation is the commonest worldwide and therefore has been studied most extensively. As stated above, haplotype studies have shown multiple founders for this mutation which may be partially explained by the occurrence of the mutation in a CpG dinucleotide hotspot (Yoshioka et al. 1989). Homozygosity for the TTR Met 30 mutation has now been described in at least 18 people and is not associated with either earlier onset or more aggressive disease than the heterozygotes (Ikeda et al. 2002), unlike most autosomal dominant conditions where homozygotes are more severely affected than heterozygotes. Patients homozygous for the TTR Met 30 mutation have been reported to have later onset disease and a higher incidence of vitreous deposits (Sandgren et al. 1990). Some TTR Met 30 homozygotes have been documented to be asymptomatic up to the age of 70 years. These observations could be due to other genetic factors. The description of a discordant phenotype of TTR amyloidosis Met 30 in monozygotic twins suggests that acquired factors are also likely to affect the phenotype in TTR amyloidosis (Holmgren et al. 1997). Compound heterozygosity has been described for non-pathogenic and pathogenic TTR point mutations

usually occurring on different alleles (Saraiva 2001b). The Ser 6 polymorphism has been described in association with many pathogenic TTR point mutations but it does not seem to influence the clinical course of the disease (Alves et al. 1996). Conversely, if either of the two TTR polymorphisms, Met 119 or His 104, occur with Met 30 they provide a protective effect as demonstrated by a more benign disease course (Coelho 1996; Terazaki et al. 1999). The mechanism behind this has been shown to be increased tetramer stability conferred by the non-pathogenic mutations as discussed below (Alves et al. 1997).

The penetrance for TTR amyloidosis varies even for patients with the same mutation. Epidemiological studies in northern Portugal found a TTR amyloidosis prevalence rate of 1/1000 and a gene carrier frequency of 1/538. In this group the mean age of onset is 33 with almost complete penetrance (Sousa et al. 1995). In Japan the patients with TTR Met 30 from the two endemic foci who have early onset disease are similar to the Portuguese patients and have a higher rate of penetrance than the patients from the non-endemic foci, who also present later with a different disease course as described above (Ikeda et al. 2002). The penetrance rates for other mutations vary but reduced penetrance has been reported with TTR Ala 60 (Reilly et al. 1995c). TTR amyloidosis patients have been described with unaffected parents but nearly all TTR mutations seem to be inherited, with reduced penetrance accounting for the unaffected parents. There was probable evidence for a de novo mutation in a patient with the Arg 47 TTR mutation as neither parent carried the mutation (Murakami et al. 1992). There is also a report of a family with TTR Ser 25 which originated in a paternal germline mosaicism (Yazaki et al. 2000). There are other interesting epidemiological observations in patients with TTR Met 30, which have yet to be fully understood. Anticipation has been described in Portuguese, Swedish and early onset Japanese TTR Met 30 patients (Planté-Bordeneuve and Said 2000) but unlike other neurodegenerative diseases demonstrating anticipation, the anticipation in TTR Met 30, at least in the Portuguese families, has been shown not to be due to triplet repeat expansions (Soares et al. 1999). Portuguese and Swedish families with TTR Met 30 both show more affected men than women with women having a slightly later age of onset (Sousa et al. 1993). These families also show an earlier age of onset when the disease is inherited from an affected mother (Hellman et al. 2008). It has been suggested that mitochondrial DNA polymorphisms may, at least in part, explain the parent-of-origin effect in FAP (Bonaiti et al. 2010). Similarly, in late onset TTR Met 30 in French patients (Planté-Bordeneuve and Said 2000) and also in late onset TTR Met 30 in Japanese patients, there is an unusually high male to female ratio with asymptomatic carriers usually being females detected late in life (Ikeda et al. 2002). In the French patients the TTR Met 119 polymorphism has been excluded as a genetic modifier in these patients. All of these observations suggest strongly that there are other genetic and environmental factors affecting the phenotype in TTR amyloidosis which have yet to be identified.

Pathogenesis of transthyretin amyloidosis

TTR amyloid is composed of protein fibrils and non-fibrillary constituents such as serum amyloid P and glycosaminoglycans present in all types of amyloid. As stated above, these fibrils exist in a β-pleated structure with eight β-pleated sheets arranged in two parallel plates, a structure allowing possible infinite self aggregation

(Hund et al. 2001). The amyloidogenic potential of TTR is presumed to be partially due to its extensive β-pleated structure. Further evidence for this is seen in senile systemic amyloidosis, a condition affecting approximately 20% of people over 80 years of age (Pitkanen et al. 1984), in which normal transthyretin is deposited in the heart as amyloid (Westermark et al. 1990). More recently it has also been observed that the TTR deposited in the heart in TTR amyloidosis is composed of both mutated TTR and normal TTR (Yazaki et al. 2000).

X-ray crystallography studies of TTR secondary to various mutations have been carried out to investigate if conformational changes caused by the various mutations could account for the increased amyloidogenicity of mutant TTR. The results show that generally TTR amyloidosis point mutations do not alter the native TTR folded structure significantly except for the Pro 55 TTR mutation (Saraiva 2001b), which is associated with a particularly aggressive form of TTR amyloidosis. The solved structure of other mutant TTRs points towards a destabilization of the tetrameric structure of the protein suggesting that these mutations increase the amyloidogenicity of TTR by reducing formation of the physiological soluble tetramer and increasing the formation of the pro-amyloidogenic monomer (Hund et al. 2001). The importance of the TTR tetramer stability is further demonstrated in studies of patients who are compound heterozygotes for the TTR Met 30 and the TTR Met 119 mutations. As stated above it has been noted that these compound heterozygotic patients have a more benign disease course than FAP patients heterozygous for the TTR Met 30 mutation. Studies, by semi-denaturing isoelectric focusing, have shown that the TTR Met 30 has a higher tendency for dissociation of the tetramer into monomers than wild type TTR. Conversely, TTR Met 119 showed higher resistance to dissociation into monomers than wild type TTR. When TTR from compound heterozygotes Met 30/Met 119 were studied they showed the same resistance to dissociation as wild type TTR (Alves et al. 1997). Thus the TTR Met 119 mutation appears to have a protective effect by counteracting the weaker subunit interactions of the Met 30 tetramers (Saraiva 2001a).

Many clinical and epidemiological observations, including the variations in phenotypes and age of onset in patients with the same mutation, are difficult to explain by limiting pathogenetic studies to TTR amyloidogenesis. Other genetic factors, including perhaps polymorphisms of the non-fibrillary amyloid constituents, and environmental factors that might modify the phenotype have yet to be described.

Despite the advances in the understanding of the pathogenesis of TTR amyloidosis many questions remain particularly regarding the cause of the neuropathy in TTR amyloidosis. The initial hypothesis was that the neuropathy was due to ischaemia, based on the finding of amyloid deposits in the walls of vasa nervorum. This is now thought to be unlikely because ischaemia would be expected to cause the loss of large myelinated fibres first, unlike in amyloid neuropathy where the small myelinated and unmyelinated fibres are affected first and are known to be less sensitive to ischaemia. The second hypothesis suggests that localized compression of the Schwann cells in the endoneurium could lead to the neuropathy. It is already known that carpal tunnel syndrome seen in many types of TTR amyloidosis is probably due to a compression neuropathy secondary to amyloid deposition in the closed space of the carpal tunnel. Against the compression hypothesis for the neuropathy

generally is the fact that the unmyelinated fibres which are primarily affected in TTR amyloidosis are more resistant to compression than myelinated fibres. The third and more likely hypothesis speculates as to whether amyloid deposits could have a toxic or metabolic effect on the endoneurium. A study suggested that TTR fibrils may bind to the receptor for advanced glycation end products (RAGE) on specific cell targets and induce a stress response which may result in peripheral nerve dysfunction (Sousa et al. 2001b). TTR deposition has been shown to occur in peripheral nerve years before amyloid fibril formation (Sousa et al. 2001a). There is also evidence that the toxicity may be related to early stages of fibril formation whereas the mature full-length fibrils may represent an inert end stage (Andersson et al. 2002). Transgenic mice studies have been used to try to understand the pathogenesis of the neuropathy in TTR amyloidosis further but transgenic mice, whether expressing the human TTR Met 30 or other mutations or the human TTR Met 30 mutation and various regulatory regions have not yet shown amyloid deposition in the peripheral nerves. The pattern of amyloid deposition in these mice is otherwise similar to that seen in autopsy cases of human TTR amyloidosis (Takaoka et al. 1997). Further research is obviously needed to elucidate the exact mechanisms underlying the neuropathy in TTR amyloidosis.

Differential diagnosis of transthyretin amyloidosis

The characteristic combination of a predominantly small fibre neuropathy with autonomic involvement and cardiac disease should always raise the suspicion of hereditary amyloid neuropathy, especially if there is a family history. Diagnostic difficulties arise early in the disease when the patient may just present with a sensory neuropathy mainly involving the small fibres and no apparent family history. The main differentials for this type of neuropathy are diabetes mellitus, leprosy, HIV infection, toxic neuropathy due to neurotoxic drugs, occasionally vasculitic neuropathy and idiopathic small fibre neuropathy. Amyloid becomes much more likely when there is a significant autonomic component but diabetes is still a possibility as are hereditary sensory and autonomic neuropathy, Fabry's disease and Tangier disease if the history is long. Most of the above differentials are easily excluded but the differentiation between the various types of amyloid neuropathy, especially AL amyloidosis and TTR amyloidosis, can be difficult without immunohistochemical staining and molecular diagnosis.

Diagnosis of transthyretin amyloidosis

The evaluation of a patient with TTR amyloidosis is initially concerned with establishing the diagnosis and then evaluating the extent and stage of the disease.

The diagnosis of TTR amyloidosis requires the diagnosis of amyloidosis first and then the characterization of the nature of the constituent amyloid fibril protein. The diagnosis requires a high level of clinical suspicion. It should always be considered in patients with a neuropathy and a known family history of TTR amyloidosis and in patients with a known family history of TTR amyloidosis who do not have a neuropathy but who present with a cardiomyopathy, carpal tunnel syndrome or vitreous deposits. The diagnosis should also be kept in mind in patients with an unexplained small fibre neuropathy especially with autonomic involvement or a cardiomyopathy regardless of family history. Once the clinical suspicion is present the diagnosis of amyloid can be made by direct examination of biopsy material from rectum, peripheral nerve, heart, subcutaneous fat or other tissue. The actual tissue biopsied will depend on the clinical presentation but in practice a rectal biopsy is often the initial choice if amyloid is suspected followed if necessary by a peripheral nerve biopsy. Rectal biopsy is considered more sensitive than nerve biopsy presumably because the patchy nature of amyloid deposits may make the diagnosis more difficult in a limited nerve biopsy. The sensitivity of gastrointestinal biopsies is approximately 85% (Hund et al. 2001). The most widely used technique for diagnosis is a combination of alkaline congo red and polarizing filters to demonstrate the characteristic apple green birefringence (Reilly and Staunton 1996). The nature of the amyloid fibril protein is characterized by immunohistochemistry using the indirect immunoperoxidase method where monoclonal antibodies are used which are directed against γ and κ light chain derived amyloid, amyloid A and TTR. The method is not completely reliable as there may not be sufficient amyloid present and the antibodies, especially the light chain antibodies, may lack specificity (Adams 2001). More recently LMD/MS has been demonstrated to accurately identify specific amyloid protein in nerve biopsies where immunostaining was unable to subtype the amyloid (Klein et al. 2011). If AL amyloid is suspected and the antibodies to TTR are negative it may be worth pursuing immunofixation and electrophoresis of serum and urine even if the light chain antibodies were also negative. However, one study found that approximately 10% of patients thought to have AL amyloid actually had FAP; therefore, genetic testing for TTR should be considered even in the presence of a paraprotein (Lachmann et al. 2002).

If TTR amyloid is confirmed or if there is no definite diagnosis of AL amyloidosis, the next step is to search for variant TTR. In practice this usually means proceeding to direct sequencing of the TTR gene but other methods can be initially used. In heterozygotic patients with TTR amyloidosis, both normal and variant TTR circulate in the blood. Variant TTR can be detected by a variety of means including isoelectric focusing in urea gradients (Altland et al. 1987), immunoassay using specific monoclonal antibodies (Goldsteins et al. 1999) and electrospray ionization mass spectrometry after immunoprecipitation with polyclonal TTR antibodies (Ando et al. 1996b). Direct sequencing of the TTR gene is used to characterize new mutations although other methods to screen for the presence of a TTR mutation may be used initially. These methods are continuously being updated and include single strand conformation polymorphism analysis (Orita et al. 1989), denaturing gradient gel electrophoresis and chemical cleavage of mismatch method (Cotton 1989). TTR point mutations in a family with a known mutation can be detected using the polymerase chain reaction (PCR) with subsequent digestion with an appropriate restriction enzyme. The above molecular genetic methods can be used not only for diagnostic testing but also for pre-symptomatic and pre-natal testing in families with known mutations. Both require pre-test and post-test genetic counselling. One of the difficulties in counselling for presymptomatic testing especially in the rarer TTR mutations is the lack of accurate information for penetrance.

Once the diagnosis has been made the extent and stage of the disease needs to be accurately assessed, especially if liver transplantation is being considered. The extent of systemic amyloid deposition can be assessed using scintigraphic studies with ^{123}iodine-labelled SAP, as SAP is deposited in all types of amyloidosis (Holmgren et al. 1993) (Fig. 50.4). SAP scanning can also

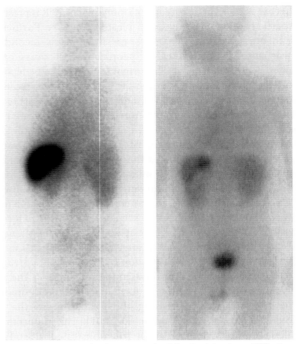

Fig. 50.4 Posterior whole-body scintigraphy following injection of ^{123}iodine-labelled serum amyloid protein component in a patient with transthyretin methionine 30 associated familial amyloid polyneuropathy, before (left) and 2 years after liver transplantation (right). The amyloid deposits in the spleen, kidneys, and adrenal glands have regressed between the two studies. (Figure kindly supplied by Dr P. N. Hawkins.)

occasionally be used diagnostically but it is not widely available. The main limitation of this technique is that it does not detect amyloid deposition in the peripheral nerves or CNS and is not completely reliable at detecting amyloid in the heart (Hazenberg et al. 2006). Peripheral nerve involvement can be assessed clinically, with nerve conduction studies, electromyography and occasionally nerve biopsy. Detailed autonomic testing is especially important in pre-liver transplant patients. CNS involvement if present can be studied by MRI imaging with gadolinium and CSF analysis. An ophthalmologic assessment is necessary to look for vitreous deposits. Cardiac assessment is important and requires at the least an electrocardiogram (ECG), an echocardiogram and sometimes a 24 hour ECG. N-terminal pro-brain natriuretic peptide (NT-proBNP) and troponin are used to screen for cardiac involvement (Dispenzieri et al. 2004). More recently, bone scintigraphy demonstrating cardiac uptake has been shown to have high specificity for cardiac amyloid deposition, but endomyocardial biopsy remains the gold standard (Wechalekar et al. 2007). Renal involvement although not usually symptomatic needs to be assessed. The patient's general health, mobility and nutritional status are also important.

Treatment of transthyretin amyloidosis

Until the 1990s the treatment of TTR amyloidosis was limited to rehabilitative measures and symptomatic therapies. These measures remain important in the overall management of the patient. Neuropathic pain can be very troublesome especially early on in the disease and is treated with the usual agents that are used for this type of pain including various anticonvulsants and antidepressants. The autonomic neuropathy often requires treatment including pharmacological treatment of the postural hypotension with drugs such as fludrocortisone and midodrine (Adams 2001). The known cardiac complications may need addressing including the insertion of a pacemaker for cardiac conduction disturbances. Other non-neurological manifestations including the gastrointestinal, vitreous and renal disturbances may need addressing.

Since the early 1990s liver transplantation has been used in the treatment of TTR amyloidosis. Liver transplantation was first suggested as a potential treatment for TTR amyloidosis because approximately 90% of TTR is produced in the liver. The first liver transplants for TTR amyloidosis were performed in two Swedish patients in 1990 (Holmgren et al. 1991). As predicted, the biochemical effect of liver transplantation is good as demonstrated by a dramatic reduction in variant TTR in plasma (Holmgren et al. 1993). A SAP scintigraphy study has also demonstrated a diminished amyloid load postoperatively (Fig. 50.2) with 50% of TTR Met 30 patients who had a liver transplant showing a decrease in activity indicating diminished amyloid load (Rydh et al. 1998). There have now been almost 1800 liver transplants done worldwide for TTR amyloidosis according to the Familial Amyloidotic Polyneuropathy World Transplant Registry (FAPWTR) (http://www.fapwtr.org). This register is based in Sweden and the purpose of the register is to monitor the international results of liver transplantation for TTR amyloidosis. The figure of 1800 is an underestimate as not all transplants are reported to the register. The transplanted liver is usually taken from a cadaver but both living donor transplants and domino transplants have been used. A number of Japanese TTR amyloidosis patients have had living donor transplants as full cadaver liver transplantation is uncommon in Japan because brain death has not been widely accepted as a definition of death (Ikeda et al. 2002). Domino liver transplantation arose because liver amyloid deposition in TTR amyloidosis is minimal (Shaz et al. 2000). In this procedure, after a TTR amyloidosis patient has been transplanted with a new liver, the liver from the TTR amyloidosis patient is then transplanted into a non-amyloidotic patient who needs a new liver usually for palliative reasons, such as a liver neoplasm (Hund et al. 2001). Initial follow-up of patients who received liver transplants from TTR amyloidosis patients showed no evidence of development of early amyloidosis (Bittencourt et al. 2002). However, longer follow-up of TTR liver recipients have demonstrated that systemic amyloid deposition occurs not uncommonly (Sousa et al. 2004, Takei et al. 2007) and symptomatic amyloidosis may occur (Conceicao et al. 2010, Llado et al. 2010). Despite this, domino liver transplant is still considered justified in selected patients. There have now been over 900 domino liver transplants done with TTR amyloidosis livers reflecting the overall shortage of livers for transplantation (http://www.fapwtr.org).

Although there is now a consensus of opinion that liver transplantation halts or slows the progression of TTR amyloidosis in most Met 30 patients, it is clear that better data is needed to establish efficacy. Prospective controlled trials have not been done. Most of the information is available for TTR Met 30 patients, as these account for 93% of patients transplanted in the worldwide register (http://www.fapwtr.org). There is some suggestion that the patients with mutations other than Met 30 do not do as well, especially from the cardiac point of view, but as the numbers for patients transplanted with differing (non-Met 30) mutations are small, this suggestion has to be interpreted with caution. General well being, gastrointestinal symptoms and nutritional state are the most frequent indices reported to improve (Coelho 1996).

If the transplant is done at a relatively early stage in the disease, when patients have only a moderate neuropathy, there is clinical and electrophysiological stability in the neuropathy in 76% of transplanted patients according to one series (Adams et al. 2000). The same study showed a marked reduction in axonal loss by a histometric comparative study between 7 transplanted patients and 4 control non-transplanted TTR amyloidosis patients. In other studies the results of the response of the peripheral neuropathy to transplantation varied from lack of neuropathy progression post-transplantation to some improvement post-transplant (Suhr et al. 2000). One study demonstrated continued deposition of wildtype amyloid in the nerve of a patient following liver transplantation (Liepnieks et al. 2010). The conclusion to date is that a moderate improvement in the peripheral neuropathy is seen in some patients particularly if transplanted early in the disease course.

Early reports suggested that the symptoms of autonomic neuropathy improved post transplant although this has not been confirmed in patients with short or long follow-up by non-invasive autonomic testing (Adams et al. 2000, Hornsten et al. 2008). Despite this, some studies do report an improvement in some of the autonomic symptoms (Adams et al. 2000, Bergethon et al. 1996).

Most TTR Met 30 patients seem to have unchanged cardiac amyloid deposition post transplant and indeed improvement has been noted in some patients. Many patients require pacemakers preoperatively. There have been a number of worrying reports of progression of cardiac disease post transplantation in patients with other TTR point mutations if there was echocardiographic evidence of ventricular wall or valve thickening preoperatively (Pomfret et al. 1998, Stangou et al. 1998, Okamoto et al. 2008). This is thought to be due to wildtype TTR being deposited as amyloid on existing amyloid deposits (Yazaki et al. 2000). It may be necessary to consider combined liver and heart transplants in these patients. Recent reports have also described cardiac progression postoperatively in TTR Met 30 patients (Okamoto et al. 2008, Olofsson et al. 2002).

The global mortality from liver transplantation is about 22% with a five year survival of 77% (Herlenius et al. 2004). The surgery is usually technically straightforward but perioperative circulatory instability secondary to autonomic dysfunction can be problematical. Arrhythmias can also occur perioperatively and as stated above pacemakers are often fitted preoperatively. Death is most common in the first 6 months postoperatively, usually due to infections or cardiocirculatory problems. Mortality has been related to the length of the disease and nutritional status preoperatively. Although symptomatic renal disease is not common preoperatively, renal dysfunction can be a major postoperative problem so detailed preoperative renal assessment is mandatory. Because of the high mortality and the shortage of liver donors, liver transplantation should probably be directed more at the young and rapidly worsening cases than at the old and slowly advancing cases.

There was a concern that as some TTR is produced in the choroid plexus CNS TTR syndromes may be seen post transplant, and this has been documented in TTR Cys 114 (Ando et al. 2004). In addition, *de novo* vitreous amyloid deposits have been documented post-transplant presumably due to local TTR synthesis in the retina (Ando et al. 1996a).

Liver transplantation has emerged as a treatment that should be considered in TTR amyloidosis patients. The important prognostic factors are modified body mass index, disease duration and the presence of a non-Met 30 TTR mutation (Herlenius et al. 2004). Survival after transplantation appears to be closely related to nutritional status pre transplant, having a disease duration of less than seven years and whether autonomic involvement is present (Herlenius et al. 2004). There probably is not yet enough information about transplants on non-Met 30 TTR mutations to say that having one is a definite bad prognostic factor. Older patients may also not do as well if they have other medical problems. The optimum time for liver transplantation has yet to be determined but the evidence suggests that it should be considered early (Suhr et al. 2000). This is particularly important in younger patients who are otherwise healthy. In older patients the duration and severity of the disease, the coexistence of other medical disorders and the mortality of the procedure need all to be considered before a transplant is recommended.

Although liver transplantation is the first treatment for TTR amyloidosis and should be considered in affected patients, it is associated with a significant mortality and other safer and more effective treatments are being researched. Both plasmaphoresis and immunoadsorption have been tried with the aim of reducing the high blood levels of variant TTR but neither treatment has been shown to be useful in the long term. A gene therapy approach using ribozymes to degrade variant and native TTR messenger RNA and thus suppress TTR production has been successful *in vitro* and this approach may be a potential treatment for TTR amyloidosis (Tanaka et al. 2001). Currently various chemotherapeutic approaches for the treatment of TTR amyloidosis are being researched and look promising. Several non-steroidal anti-inflammatory drugs including flufenamic acid, diclofenac, flurbiprofen and resveratrol, and other structurally similar compounds have been shown to inhibit the formation of amyloid fibrils *in vitro* (Klabunde et al. 2000). One such non-steroidal agent, diflunisal, is in clinical use in patients not considered suitable for liver transplant. Diflunisal stabilizes amyloid precursor protein; evidence of efficacy is awaited. A derivative of diflunisal, iododiflunisal is now being evaluated in experimental studies (Gillmore and Hawkins 2006). Another drug has been developed, R-1-[6-[R-2-carboxy-pyrrolidin-1-yl]-6-oxo-hexanoyl]-pyrrolidine-2-carboxylic acid (CPHPC) that both inhibits SAP binding to amyloid fibrils and leads to the rapid clearance of SAP by the liver with re-distribution of SAP from the tissues to the plasma (Kolstoe and Wood 2010; Pepys et al. 2002). As SAP binds to fibrils in all types of amyloidosis and is known to protect amyloid fibrils from degradation this approach is potentially very useful. Preliminary pilot studies in systemic amyloidosis including some patients with TTR amyloidosis have confirmed the rapid clearance of SAP from the blood following an infusion of this drug. Halogenated biarylamine compounds have been demonstrated to stabilize the tetrameric form of TTR, preventing dissociation and aggregation (Johnson et al. 2008); fx-1006a (tafamidis) has recently completed phase II clinical trials (publication awaited) (http://clinicaltrials.gov/ct2/show/NCT00694161). These compounds need further evaluation but these developments raise the possibility of alternative treatments to liver transplantation for TTR amyloidosis in the future.

Prognosis of transthyretin amyloidosis

The average life expectancy for patients with untreated TTR amyloidosis associated with neuropathy is about 10 years as discussed above. There are ethnic differences in survival in patients with the same mutation with Swedish Met 30 patients having an average life expectancy of 14 years and French patients with Met 30 of less than 10 years (Planté-Bordeneuve et al. 1998). Some less common TTR point mutations have a more aggressive course as described above. The five-year survival for patients with TTR amyloidosis who have had a liver transplant is 77% (Herlenius et al. 2004). This figure is likely to improve further as the optimum conditions and timing for liver transplantation are determined and as newer genetic and chemotherapeutic treatments are developed.

Apolipoprotein A-1 amyloidosis

In 1969 Van Allen described a kindred in Iowa with familial amyloid polyneuropathy associated with a high incidence of gastric ulcers and renal failure (Van Allen et al. 1969). The age of onset of the Iowa type of amyloidosis is in the thirties and the neuropathy is similar to TTR amyloidosis beginning in the lower limbs with small fibre symptoms and progressing to the upper limbs with motor involvement occurring later than sensory involvement. Autonomic neuropathy is not prominent. In the original family there were two distinguishing features from TTR amyloidosis which is why this type of amyloidosis was classified separately as FAP type III; there is a high incidence of both gastric ulcers and renal failure reported. Post mortem studies confirm amyloid deposition throughout the peripheral nervous system including nerves, roots and dorsal root ganglia (Van Allen et al. 1969).

Apolipoprotein A-1 amyloidosis was termed FAP type III in the old FAP classification. Apolipoprotein A-1, the gene for which is on chromosome 11, was found to be the constituent fibril protein in 1988 (Nichols et al. 1988) and in 1990 an arginine for glycine substitution at position 26 of the protein was reported as the causative mutation of this autosomal dominant condition. Apolipoprotein A-1 is the major protein constituent of high density lipoprotein and the constituent amyloid protein in apolipoprotein A-1 amyloidosis is the amino terminal 83 residues of the mature 243 amino acid long apolipoprotein A-1 with the Gly26Arg mutation (Nichols et al. 1990). It is of interest that although apolipoprotein A-1 itself is not predicted to have extensive β-pleated structure, the first 55 residues of the 83 amino terminal fragment referred to above is predicted to have mostly β-pleated structure. This phenotype has only been described with the Gly26Arg mutation, but there are now 12 different apolipoprotein A-1 mutations associated with systemic non-neuropathic amyloidosis (Gillmore et al. 2006, Gillmore et al. 2001) usually with marked major organ involvement including liver, renal and cardiac. The Gly26Arg apolipoprotein A-1 mutation has also been described in non-neuropathic systemic amyloidosis.

The diagnosis is established by demonstrating amyloid on an appropriate tissue biopsy with subsequent immunohistochemical staining for apolipoprotein A-1. Sequencing of the apolipoprotein A-1 gene reveals a guanine to cysteine mutation giving rise to the Gly26Arg substitution.

Symptomatic treatment (e.g. for painful neuropathy) is important as described for TTR amyloidosis but most patients eventually develop renal failure requiring dialysis. Although apolipoprotein

A-1 is partially produced in the liver, liver transplantation to reduce the production of the abnormal precursor protein has only rarely been used for this type of amyloid neuropathy (Testro et al. 2007). In apolipoprotein A-1 non-neuropathic systemic amyloidosis organ transplantation is recommended for severe organ (e.g. liver or kidney) failure. A report of hepatorenal transplantation in a patient with hereditary non-neuropathic systemic amyloidosis and the apolipoprotein A-1 Gly26Arg mutation (with severe renal and hepatic involvement) is of interest as the plasma levels of variant apolipoprotein A-1 decreased by 50% post transplant and there was evidence of amyloid regression in the heart and spleen postoperatively as quantified by [123]iodine SAP scanning (Gillmore et al. 2001). This raises the question that liver transplantation may be a future treatment for apolipoprotein A-1 amyloidosis.

Gelsolin amyloidosis

Gelsolin amyloidosis was first described in a Finnish kindred by Meretoja in 1969 (Meretoja 1969). Clinically this type of amyloidosis usually presents in the thirties with corneal lattice dystrophy which may be asymptomatic. This is due to amyloid deposition in the corneal branches of the trigeminal nerve (Mendell 2001). This is followed by a progressive cranial neuropathy. The facial nerve is the commonest cranial nerve involved with the upper fibres as manifested by forehead muscle weakness initially being affected. Other cranial nerves may also be affected including the vestibulo-cochlear, hypoglossal and trigeminal with varying clinical manifestations (Reilly and Staunton 1996). Peripheral nerve involvement does occur but is usually a mild sensory neuropathy. There also may be mild autonomic involvement. Neurophysiological tests show a higher incidence of carpal tunnel syndrome than is suspected clinically. The neuropathy is predominantly axonal but slow nerve conduction velocities, prolonged distal motor latencies, and conduction block all point towards an additional demyelinating element (Kiuru and Seppalainen 1994). The facial skin is involved at first appearing thickened but becoming lax with time. Minor neuropsychological, MRI and evoked potential abnormalities have been described suggesting mild CNS involvement (Kiuru et al. 1995). A post-mortem study has shown widespread spinal, cerebral and meningeal amyloid angiopathy associated with deposition of gelsolin amyloid (Kiuru et al. 1999). Cardiac involvement is rare clinically but cardiac involvement has been shown in autopsy studies (Kiuru et al. 1994).

The fibril protein in this type of amyloidosis is an abnormal fragment of a plasma protein, gelsolin, a calcium binding protein that fragments actin filaments (Yin et al. 1984). Gelsolin is mainly derived from muscle. The gene for gelsolin is located on chromosome 9 and codes for two separate proteins, one intracellular and one extracellular with an additional 25 amino acid residues, by starting at two different transcriptional sites. There have been two mutations described in the gelsolin gene associated with this type of amyloidosis. The first is a substitution of asparagine for aspartic acid at residue 187 (position 15 of the amyloid protein) (Levy et al. 1990). This has been described in over 200 Finnish kindreds and also in patients of Dutch (de le Chapelle et al. 1992), Japanese (Sunada et al. 1993), and US origin (Ghiso et al. 1990). We have seen a family with this mutation of Russian ancestry (personal observation). Two homozygotes for this mutation have been described, both more severely affected than heterozygotes. The second mutation involves the same codon, a tyrosine for aspartic acid at residue 187 and has been reported in a Danish family and a Czech family (de le Chapelle et al. 1992). The amyloid fibrils in this type of amyloidosis are composed of the internal degradation products of an abnormal fragment of gelsolin which begins at position 173 of the plasma protein. An abnormal 65 kD gelsolin species has been shown to be the circulating precursor of tissue amyloid in this type of amyloidosis. Residue 187 is thought to be a critical site where a substitution of an amino acid with an uncharged (asparagine) or hydrophobic side chain (tyrosine or valine) creates a conformation that is highly amyloidogenic (Maury et al. 1994). It has been discovered that the protease furin is responsible for gelsolin protein proteolysis-induced amyloidosis in familial amyloidosis, Finnish type (Chen et al. 2001). The two described mutations prevent calcium from binding to domain 2 and allow gelsolin to misfold, allowing furin access to a site not normally exposed in the wildtype protein (Sacchettini and Kelly 2002).

The diagnosis is established by biopsy with amyloid being demonstrated as described above. The gene can be sequenced to look for causative mutations. There is no specific treatment other than symptomatic treatment. Liver transplantation is not an option as gelsolin is not produced in the liver. There is interest in developing furin inhibitors as a therapeutic strategy (Sacchettini and Kelly 2002).

Acknowledgements

Dr Michael Groves is kindly acknowledged for help in producing Figs 50.1a,b,c,d and e. Professor Philip Hawkins is kindly acknowledged for supplying Fig. 50.2.

MMR is grateful to the Medical Research Council (MRC) and the Muscular Dystrophy Campaign, and SMM and MMR are grateful to the NINDS/ORD (1U54NS065712–01) for their support.

References

Adams, D. (2001). Hereditary and acquired amyloid neuropathies. *J Neurol.* **248**, 647–57.

Adams, D., Samuel, D., Goulon-Goeau, C. *et al.*, (2000). The course and prognostic factors of familial amyloid polyneuropathy after liver transplantation. *Brain.* **123**, 1495–1504.

Altland, K., Becker, P. and Banzhoff, A., (1987). Paraffin oil protected high resolution hybrid isoelectric focusing for the demonstration of substitutions of neutral amino acids in denatured proteins: the case of four human transthyretin (prealbumin) variants associated with familial amylodotic polyneuropathy. *Electrophoresis.* **8**, 293–97.

Alves, I. L., Hays, M. T. and Saraiva, M. J. M., (1997). Comparative stability and clearance of [Met30] transhyretin and [met119] transthyretin. *European Journal of Biochemistry.* **249**, 662–68.

Alves, I. L., Jacobson, D. R., Torres, M. F., Holmgren, G., Buxbaum, J. and Saraiva, M. J. M., (1996). Transthyretin Ser 6 as a natural polymorphism in familial amyloidotic polyneuropathy. *Amyloid.* **3**, 242–44.

Andersson, K., Olofsson, A., Nielsen, E. H., Svehag, S. E. and Lundgren, E., (2002). Only amyloidogenic intermediates of transthyretin induce apoptosis. *Biochemical and Biophysical Research Communications.* **294**, 309–314.

Andersson, R., (1970). Hereditary amyloidosis with polyneuropathy. *Acta Medica Scandinavica.* **188**, 85–94.

Ando, Y., Ando, E., Tanaka, Y. *et al.*, (1996a). De novo amyloid synthesis in ocular tissue in familial amyloidotic polyneuropathy after liver transplantation. *Transplantation.* **62**, 1037–38.

Ando, Y., Ohlsson, P. I., Suhr, O. *et al.*, (1996b). A new simple and rapid screening method for variant transthyretin (TTR) related amyloidosis. *Biochemical and Biophysical Research Communications.* **228**, 480–83.

Ando, Y., Terazaki, H., Nakamura, M. *et al.*, (2004). A different amyloid formation mechanism: de novo oculoleptomeningeal amyloid deposits after liver transplantation. *Transplantation.* **77**, 345–49.

Andrade, C., (1952). A peculiar form of peripheral neuropathy: Familial atypical generalized amyloidosis with special involvement of the peripheral nervous system. *Brain.* **75**, 408–27.

Araki, S., Mawatari, S., Ohta, M., Nakajima, A. and Kuroiwa, Y., (1968). Polyneuritic amyloidosis in a Japanese family. *Arch. Neurol.* **18**, 593–602.

Araki, S. and Shigehira, Y., (2000). Pathology of familial amyloidotic polyneuropathy with TTR Met 30 in Kumamoto, Japan. *Neuropathology.* **20**, S47–51.

Belkin, R. N., Kupersmith, A. C., Khalique, O. *et al.*, (2010). A novel two-dimensional echocardiographic finding in cardiac amyloidosis. *Echocardiography.* **27**, 1171–76.

Benson, M. D., (1989). Familial amyloid polyneuropathy. *Trends in Neurosciences.* **12**, 88–92.

Benson, M. D., (1991). Inherited amyloidosis. *Journal of Medical Genetics.* **28**, 73–78.

Bergethon, P. R., D., S. T., Lewis, D., Simms, R. W., Cohen, A. S. and Skinner, M., (1996). Improvement in the polyneuropathy associated with familial amyloid polyneuropathy after liver transplantation. *Neurology.* **47**, 944–51.

Bittencourt, P. L., Couto, C. A., Leitao, R. M. *et al.*, (2002). No evidence of de novo amyloidosis in recipients of domino liver transplantation: 12 to 40 months (mean 24) month follow-up. *Amyloid.* **9**, 194–96.

Blevins, G., Macaulay, R., Harder, S. *et al.*, (2003). Oculoleptomeningeal amyloidosis in a large kindred with a new transthyretin variant Tyr69His. *Neurology.* **60**, 1625–30.

Bonaiti, B., Olsson, M., Hellman, U., Suhr, O., Bonaiti-Pellie, C. and Plante-Bordeneuve, V., (2010). TTR familial amyloid polyneuropathy: does a mitochondrial polymorphism entirely explain the parent-of-origin difference in penetrance? *European Journal of Human Genetics.* **18**, 948–52.

Brett, M., Persey, M. R., Reilly, M. M. *et al.*, (1999). Transthyretin Leu12Pro is associated with systemic, neuropathic and leptomeningeal amyloidosis. *Brain.* **122**, 183–90.

de le Chapelle, A., Tolvanen, R., Boysen, G. *et al.*, (1992). Gelsolin derived familial amyloidosis caused by asparagine or tyrosine substitution for aspartic acid at residue 187. *Nature Genetics.* **2**, 157–60.

Chen, C. D., Huff, M. E., Matteson, J. *et al.*, (2001). Furin initiates gelsolin familial amyloidosis in the Golgi through a defect in CA^{2+} stabilization. *The EMBO Journal.* **20**, 6277–87.

Coelho, T., (1996). Familial amyloid polyneuropathy: new developments in genetics and treatment. *Current Opinions in Neurology.* **9**, 355–59.

Cohen, A. S., (1992). History of amyloidosis. *Journal of Internal Medicine.* **232**, 509–510.

Cohen, A. S. and Calkins, E., (1959). Electron microscopic observations on a fibrous component of amyloid of diverse origins. *Nature.* **183**, 1202–1203.

Conceicao, I., Evangelista, T., Castro, J. *et al.*, (2010). Acquired amyloid neuropathy in a Portuguese patient after domino liver transplantation. *Muscle & Nerve.* **42**, 836–39.

Connors, L. H., Lim, A., Prokaeva, T., Roskens, V. A. and Costello, C. E., (2003). Tabulation of human transthyretin (TTR) variants, 2003. *Amyloid.* **10**, 160–84.

Costa, P., Figueira, A. S. and Bravo, R. R., (1978). Amyloid fibril protein related to pre-albumin in familial amyloidotic polyneuropathy. *Proceedings of the National Acadamy of Sciences.* **75**, 4499–4503.

Cotton, R. G. H., (1989). Detection of single base changes in nucleic acids. *The Biochemical Journal.* **263**, 1–10.

Coutinho, P., Martins Da Silva, A., Lopes Lima, J. and Resende Barbosa, A. (1980). Forty years of experience with type 1 amyloid neuropathy. Review of 483 cases. In *Amyloid and Amyloidosis*, (ed. Glenner, G. G., Pinho, P., Costa, E. and Falcao De Freitas, A., pp. 88–98. Excerpta Medica, Amsterdam.

Dispenzieri, A., Gertz, M. A., Kyle, R. A. *et al.*, (2004). Serum cardiac troponins and N-terminal pro-brain natriuretic peptide: a staging system for primary systemic amyloidosis. *Journal of Clinical Oncology.* **22**, 3751–57.

Dwulet, F. E. and Benson, M. D., (1983). Polymorphism of human plasma thyroxine binding prealbumin. *Biochemical and Biophysical Research Communications.* **114**, 657–62.

Dwulet, F. E. and Benson, M. D., (1986). Characterization of a transthyretin (pre-albumin) variant associated with familial amyloidotic polyneuropathy, type II (Indiana/Swiss). *The Journal of Clinical Investigation.* **78**, 880–86.

Dyck, P. J. and Lambert, E. H., (1969). Dissociated sensation in amyloidosis. *Arch. Neurol.* **20**, 490–507.

Fonseca, C., Ceia, F., Nogueira, J. S. *et al.*, (1991). Myocardiopathy caused by Portuguese-type familial amyloidotic polyneuropathy. Sequential morphological and functional study of 60 cases. *Revista Portuguesa de Cardiologica.* **10**, 909–916.

Ghiso, J., Haltia, M., Prelli, F., Novello, J. and Frangione, B., (1990). Gelsolin variant (ASN 187) in familial amyloidosis, Finnish type. *The Biochemical Journal.* **272**, 827–30.

Gillmore, J. D., Stangou, A. J., Lachmann, H. J. *et al.*, (2006). Organ transplantation in hereditary Apolipoprotein AI amyloidosis. *American Journal of Transplantation.* **6**, 2342–47.

Gillmore, J. D., Stangou, A. J., Tennent, G. A. *et al.*, (2001). Clinical and biochemical outcome of hepatorenal transplantation for hereditary systemic amyloidosis associated with apolipoprotein AI Gly26Arg. *Transplantation.* **71**, 986–92.

Gillmore, J. D. and Hawkins, P. N., (2006). Drug insight: emerging therapies for amyloidosis. *Nature Clinical Practice Nephrology.* **2**, 263–70.

Goldsteins, S. G., Persson, H., Andersson, K. *et al.*, (1999). Exposure of cryptic epitopes on transthyretin only in amyloid and in amyloidogenic mutants. *Proceedings of the National Acadamy of Sciences.* **96**, 3108–3113.

Goren, H., Steinberg, M. C. and Farboody, G. H., (1980). Familial oculoleptomeningeal amyloidosis. *Brain.* **103**, 473–95.

Hazenberg, B. P. C., van Rijswijk, M. H., Piers, D. A. *et al.*, (2006). Diagnostic performance of 123I-labeled serum amyloid P. component scintigraphy in patients with amyloidosis. *Am. J Med.*, **119**, 355.e315–324.

Hellman, U., Alarcon, F., Lundgren, H.-E., Suhr, O. B., Bonaiti-Pellie, C. and Plante-Bordeneuve, V., (2008). Heterogeneity of penetrance in familial amyloid polyneuropathy, ATTR Val30Met, in the Swedish population. *Amyloid.* **15**, 181–86.

Herlenius, G., Wilczek, H. E., Larsson, M. and Ericzon, B.-G., (2004). Ten years of international experience with liver transplantation for familial amyloidotic polyneuropathy: results from the familial amyloidotic polyneuropathy world transplant registry. *Transplantation.* **77**, 64–71.

Holmgren, G., Ando, Y. and Wikström, L., (1997). Discordant symptoms in monozygotic twins with familial amyloidotic polyneuropathy (FAP TTR met30) amyloid. *International Journal of Experimental and Clinical Investigation.* **4**, 178–80.

Holmgren, G., Ericzon, B.-G., Groth, C.-G. *et al.*, (1993). Clinical improvement and amyloid regression after liver transplantation in hereditary transthyretin amyloidosis. *The Lancet.* **341**, 1113–1116.

Holmgren, G., Steen, L., Ekstedt, J. *et al.*, (1991). Biochemical effect of liver transplantation in two Swedish patients with familial amyloidotic polyneuropathy (FAP-met^{30}). *Clinical Genetics.* **40**, 242–46.

Hornsten, R., Suhr, O., Jensen, S. M. and Wiklund, U., (2008). Outcome of heart rate variability and ventricular late potentials after liver transplantation for familial amyloidotic polyneuropathy. *Amyloid.* **15**, 187–95.

Hund, E., Linke, R. P., Willig, F. and Grau, A., (2001). Transthyretin-associated neuropathic amyloidosis. *Neurology.* **56**, 431–35.

Hungo, M. and Ikeda, S., (1986). Echocardiographic assessment of the evolution of amyloid heart disease: a study with familial amyloid polyneuropathy. *Circulation.* **73**, 249–56.

Ii, S. and Sommer, S. S., (1993). The high frequency of TTR Met 30 in familial amyloidotic polyneuropathy is not due to a founder effect. *Human Molecular Genetics.* **2**, 1303–1305.

Ikeda, S., Nakazato, M., Ando, Y. and Sobue, G., (2002). Familial transthyretin-type amyloid polyneuropathy in Japan. *Neurology.* **58**, 1001–1007.

Jacobson, D. R., McFarlin, D. E., Kane, I. and Buxbaum, J. N., (1992). Transthyretin Pro55, a variant associated with early-onset, aggressive, diffuse amyloidosis with cardiac and neurologic involvement. *Human Genetics.* **89**, 353–56.

Johnson, S. M., Connelly, S., Wilson, I. A. and Kelly, J. W., (2008). Biochemical and structural evaluation of highly selective 2-arylbenzoxazole-based transthyretin amyloidogenesis inhibitors. *Journal of Medicinal Chemistry.* **51**, 260–70.

Katsuragi, S., Miyakawa, T., Ando, Y. and Terazaki, H., (2000). High-resolution ultrastructure of amyloid fibrils in familial amyloid polyneuropathy. *Journal of Electron Microscopy (Tokoyo).* **49**, 579–81.

Kiuru, S., Matikainen, E., Kupari, M., Haltia, M. and Palo, J., (1994). Autonomic nervous system and cardiac involvement in familial amyloidosis, Finnish type (FAF). *J Neurol. Sci.* **126**, 40–48.

Kiuru, S., Salonen, O. and Haltia, M., (1999). Gelsolin-related spinal and cerebral amyloid angiopathy. *Ann. Neurol.* **45**, 305–311.

Kiuru, S., Seppalainen, A.-M., Salonen, O., Hokkanen, L., Somer, H. and Palo, J., (1995). CNS abnormalities in patients with familial amyloidosis of the Finnish type (FAF). *Amyloid.* **2**, 22–30.

Kiuru, S. and Seppalainen, A. M., (1994). Neuropathy in familial amyloidosis, Finnish type (FAF): electrophysiological studies. *Muscle & Nerve.* **17**, 299–304.

Klabunde, T., Petrassi, H. M., Oza, V. B., Raman, P., Kelly, J. W. and Sacchettini, J. C., (2000). Rational design of potent human transthyretin amyloid disease inhibitors. *Nature Structural Biology.* **7**, 312–20.

Klein, C. J., Vrana, J. A., Theis, J. D. *et al.*, (2011). Mass spectrometric-based proteomic analysis of amyloid neuropathy type in nerve tissue. *Arch. Neurol.* **68**, 195–99.

Königstein, H., (1925). Über Amyloidose der haut. *Archives of Dermatology and Syphilology.* **148**, 330–83.

Kotani, N., Hatori, T., Yamagata, S. *et al.*, (2002). Transthyretin Thr60Ala Appalachian-type mutation in a Japanese family with familial amyloidotic polyneuropathy. *Amyloid.* **9**, 31–34.

Kolstoe, S. E. and Wood, S. P., (2010). Drug targets for amyloidosis. *Biochemical Society Transactions.* **38**, 466–70.

Kyle, R. A., (1992). Amyloidosis. *Journal of Internal Medicine.* **232**, 507–508.

Lachmann, H. J., Booth, D. R., Booth, S. E. *et al.*, (2002). Misdiagnosis of hereditary amyloidosis as AL (primary) amyloidosis. *N Engl. J Med.* **346**, 1786–91.

Levy, E., Haltia, M., Fernandez-Madrid, I. *et al.*, (1990). Mutation in gelsolin gene in Finnish hereditary amyloidosis. *The Journal of Experimental Medicine.* **172**, 1865–67.

Liepnieks, J. J., Zhang, L. Q. and Benson, M. D., (2010). Progression of transthyretin amyloid neuropathy after liver transplantation. *Neurology.* **75**, 324–27.

Llado, L., Baliellas, C., Casasnovas, C. *et al.*, (2010). Risk of transmission of systemic transthyretin amyloidosis after domino liver transplantation. *Liver Transplantation.* **16**, 1386–92.

Mahloudji, M., Teasdall, R. D., Adamkiewics, J. J., Hartmann, W. H., Lambird, P. A. and McKusick, V. A., (1969). The genetic amyloidoses with particular reference to hereditary neuropathic amyloidosis, Type II (Indiana or Rukavina type). *Medicine.* **48**, 1–37.

Maury, C. P., Nurmiaho-Lassila, E. L. and Rossi, H., (1994). Amyloid fibril formation in gelsolin derived amyloidosis. Definition of the amyloidogenic region and evidence of accelerated amyloid formation of mutant Asn-187 and Tyr-187 gelsolin peptides. *Laboratory Investigation.* **70**, 558–64.

Mendell, J. R. (2001). Familial amyloid polyneuropathies. In *Diagnosis and management of peripheral nerve disorders*, (ed. Mendell, J. R., Kissel, J. T. and Cornblath, D. R., pp. 477–91. Oxford University Press, New York.

Meretoja, J., (1969). Familial systemic paramyloidosis with lattice dystrophy of the cornea, progressive cranial neuropathy, skin changes and various internal symptoms. *Annals of Clinical Research.* **1**, 314–24.

Moses, A. C., Rosen, H. N., Moller, D. E. *et al.*, (1986). A point mutation in transthyretin increases affinity for thyroxine and produces euthyroid hyperthyroxinemia. *The Journal of Clinical Investigation.* **86**, 2025–33.

Murakami, T., Maeda, S., Yi, S. *et al.*, (1992). A novel transthyretin mutation associated with familial amyloidotic polyneuropathy. *Biochemical and Biophysical Research Communications.* **182**, 520–26.

Nichols, W. C., Dwulet, F. E., Liepnieks, J. and Benson, M. D., (1988). Variant apolipoprotein A-1 as a major constituent of a human hereditary amyloid. *Biochemical and Biophysical Research Communications.* **156**, 762–68.

Nichols, W. C., Gregg, R. E., Brewer, H. B. J. and Benson, M. D., (1990). A mutation in apolipoprotein A-1 in the Iowa type of familial amyloidotic polyneuropathy. *Genomics.* **8**, 318–23.

Nichols, W. C., Liepnieks, J. J., McKusick, V. A. and Benson, M. D., (1989). Direct sequencing of the gene for Maryland/German familial amyloidotic polyneuropathy type II and genotyping by allele-specific enzymatic amplification. *Genomics.* **5**, 535–40.

Okamoto, S., Yamashita, T., Ando, Y. *et al.*, (2008). Evaluation of myocardial changes in familial amyloid polyneuropathy after liver transplantation. *Internal Medicine.* **47**, 2133–37.

Olofsson, B.-E., Backman, C., Karp, K. and Suhr, O. B., (2002). Progression of cardiomyopathy after liver transplantation in patients with familial amyloidotic polyneuropathy, Portuguese type 1. *Transplantation.* **73**, 745–51.

Orita, M., Iwahana, H. and Sekiya, T., (1989). Detection of polymorphisms of human DNA by gel electrophoresis as single-strand conformation polymorphisms. *Proceedings of the National Acadamy of Sciences.* **86**, 2766–70.

Pepys, M. B., Herbert, J., Hutchinson, W. L. *et al.*, (2002). Targeted pharmacological depletion of serum amyloid P. component for treatment of human amyloidosis. *Nature.* **417**, 254–59.

Pitkanen, P., Westermark, P. and Cornwell III, G. G., (1984). Senile systemic amyloidosis. *American Journal of Pathology.* **117**, 391–99.

Planté-Bordeneuve, V., Lalu, T., Misrahi, M. *et al.*, (1998). Genotypic-phenotypic variations in a series of 65 patients with familial amyloid ployneuropathy. *Neurology.* **51**, 708–714.

Planté-Bordeneuve, V. and Said, G., (2000). Transthyretin related familial amyloidotic polyneuropathy. *Current Opinions in Neurology.* **13**, 569–73.

Pomfret, E. A., Lewis, W. D., Jenkins, R. L. *et al.*, (1998). Effect of orthoptic liver transplantation on the progression of familial amyloidotic polyneuropathy. *Transplantation.* **65**, 918–25.

Puille, M., Altland, K., Linke, R. P. *et al.*, (2002). 99mTc-DPD scintigraphy in transthyretin-related familial amyloidotic polyneuropathy. *European Journal of Nuclear Medicine and Molecular Imaging.* **29**, 376–79.

Reilly, M., Adams, D., Davis, M. B., Said, G. and Harding, A. E., (1995a). Haplotype analysis of French, British and other European patients with familial amyloid polyneuropathy (Met 30 and Tyr 77). *J Neurol.* **242**, 664–68.

Reilly, M. M. and Staunton, H., (1996). Peripheral nerve amyloidosis. *Brain Pathology.* **6**, 163–77.

Reilly, M. M., Adams, D., Booth, D. R. *et al.*, (1995b). Transthyretin gene analysis in European patients with suspected familial amyloid polyneuropathy. *Brain.* **118**, 849–56.

Reilly, M. M. and King, R. H. M., (1993). Familial amyloid polyneuropathy. *Brain Pathology.* **3**, 165–76.

Reilly, M. M., Staunton, H. and Harding, A. E., (1995c). Familial amyloid polyneuropathy (TTR ala 60) in north west Ireland: a clinical, genetic, and epidemiological study. *JNNP.* **59**, 45–49.

Rydh, A., Suhr, O., Hietala, S.-O., Ahlstrom, K. R., Pepys, M. B. and Hawkins, P. N., (1998). Serum amyloid P. scintigraphy in familial amyloid polyneuropathy: Regression of visceral amyloid following liver transplantation. *European Journal of Nuclear Medicine*. **25**, 709–713.

Sacchettini, J. C. and Kelly, J. W., (2002). Therapeutic strategies for human amyloid diseases. *Nature Reviews*. **1**, 267–75.

Sandgren, O., Holmgren, G. and Lundgren, E., (1990). Vitreous amyloidosis associated with homozygosity for the transthyretin methionine-30 gene. *Archives of Ophthalmology*. **108**, 1584–86.

Saraiva, M. J. M., (2001a). Transthyretin amyloidosis: a tale of weak interactions. *FEBS Letters*. **498**, 201–203.

Saraiva, M. J. M., (2001b). Transthyretin mutartions in hyperthyroxinemia and amyloid disease. *Human Mutation*. **17**, 493–503.

Shaz, B. H., Gordon, F., Lewis, W. D., Jenkins, R. L., Skinner, M. and Khettry, U., (2000). Orthotopic liver transplantation for familial amyloidotic polyneuropathy: a pathological study. *Humand Pathology*. **31**, 40–44.

Soares, M., Buxbaum, J., Sirugo, G. *et al.*, (1999). Genetic anticipation in Portuguese kindreds with familial amyloidotic polyneuropathy is unlikely to be caused by triplet repeat expansions. *Human Genetics*. **104**, 480–85.

Sousa, A., Andersson, R., Drugge, U., Holmgren, G. and Sandgren, O., (1993). Familial amyloidotic polyneuropathy in Sweden: Geographical distribution, age of onset, and prevalence. *Human Heredity*. **43**, 288–94.

Sousa, A., Coehlo, T., Barros, J. and Sequeiros, J., (1995). Genetic epidemiology of familial amyloidotic polyneuropathy (FAP)-type 1 in Povoa do Varzim and Vila do Conde (north of Portugal). *American Journal of Human Genetics*. **60**, 512–21.

Sousa, M. M., Cardoso, I., Fernandes, R., Guimaraes, A. and Saraiva, M. J. M., (2001a). Deposition of transthyretin in early stages of familial amyloidotic polyneuropathy, Evidence for toxicity of nonfibrillar aggregates. *American Journal of Pathology*. **159**, 1993–2000.

Sousa, M. M., Du Yan, S., Fernandes, R., Guimaraes, A., Stern, D. and Saraiva, M. J. M., (2001b). Familial amyloid polyneuropathy: receptor for advanced glycation end products-dependent triggering of neuronal inflammatory and apoptotic pathways. *The Journal of Neuroscience*. **21**, 7576–86.

Sousa, M. M., Ferrao, J., Fernandes, R. *et al.*, (2004). Deposition and passage of transthyretin through the blood-nerve barrier in recipients of familial amyloid polyneuropathy livers. *Laboratory Investigation*. **84**, 865–73.

Stangou, A. J., Hawkins, P. N., Heaton, N. D. *et al.*, (1998). Progressive cardiac amyloidosis following liver transplantation for familial amyloid polyneuropathy. *Transplantation*. **66**, 229–33.

Suhr, O. B., Herlinius, G., Friman, S. and Ericzon, B.-G., (2000). Liver transplantation for hereditary transthyretin amyloidosis. *Liver Transplantation*. **6**, 263–76.

Sunada, Y., Shimizu, T., Nakase, H. *et al.*, (1993). Inherited amyloid polyneuropathy type IV (gelsolin variant) in a Japanese family. *Ann. Neurol*. **33**, 57–62.

Takaoka, Y., Tashiro, F., Yi, S. *et al.*, (1997). Comparison of amyloid deposition in two lines of transgenic mouse that model familial amyloidotic polyneuropathy, type 1. *Transgenic Research*. **6**, 261–69.

Takei, Y., Gono, T., Yazaki, M. *et al.*, (2007). Transthyretin-derived amyloid deposition on the gastric mucosa in domino recipients of familial amyloid polyneuropathy livers. *Liver Transplantation*. **13**, 215–218.

Tanaka, K., Yamada, T., Ohyagi, Y., Asahara, H., Horiuchi, I. and Kira, J., (2001). Suppression of transthyretin expression by ribozymes: a possible therapy for familial amyloidotic polyneuropathy. *Journal of the Neurological Sciences*. **183**, 79–84.

Terazaki, H., Ando, Y., Misumi, S. *et al.*, (1999). A novel compound heterozygote (FAP ATTR Arg104His/Val30Met) with high serum transthyretin (TTR) and retinal binding protein (RBP) levels. *Biochemical and Biophysical Research Communications*. **264**, 365–70.

Testro, A. G., Brennan, S. O., Macdonell, R. A. L., Hawkins, P. N. and Angus, P. W., (2007). Hereditary amyloidosis with progressive peripheral neuropathy associated with Apolipoprotein AI Gly26Arg: outcome of hepatorenal transplantation. *Liver Transplantation*. **13**, 1028–31.

The effects of FX-1006a on transthyretin stabilization and clinical outcome measures in patients with V122I or wild-type TTR amyloid cardiomyopathy. http://clinicaltrials.gov/ct2/show/NCT00694161. Accessed March 2011.

Thomas, P. K. and King, R. H. M., (1974). Peripheral nerve changes in amyloid neuropathy. *Brain*. **97**, 395–406.

Togashi, S., Watanabe, H., Nagasaka, T. *et al.*, (1999). An aggressive familial amyloidotic polyneuropathy caused by a new variant transthyretin Lys 54. *Neurology*. **53**, 637–39.

Uemichi, T., Liepnieks, J. J. and Benson, M. D., (1997). A trinucleotide deletion in the transthyretin gene (delta V 122) in a kindred with familial amyloidotic polyneuropathy. *Neurology*. **48**, 1667–70.

Van Allen, M. W., Frohlich, J. A. and Davis, J. R., (1969). Inherited predisposition to generalized amyloidosis. Clinical and pathological study of a family with neuropathy, nephropathy and peptic ulcer. *Neurology*. **19**, 10–25.

Virchow, R., (1853). Découverte d'une substance qui donne lieu au mêmes reactions chimiques que la cellulose vegetable, dans le corps human. *Comptes rendus de l'Academie des Sciences*. **37**, 492–93.

Wallace, M. R., Naylor, S. L., Kluve-Beckerman, B. *et al.*, (1995). Localization of the pre-albumin gene to chromosome 18. *Biochemical and Biophysical Research Communications*. **129**, 753–58.

Wechalekar, K., Ng, F. S., Poole-Wilson, P. A. *et al.*, (2007). Cardiac amyloidosis diagnosed incidentally by bone scintigraphy. *Journal of Nuclear Cardiology*. **14**, 750–53.

Westermark, P., Sletten, K., Johansson, B. and Cornwell III, G. G., (1990). Fibril in senile systemic amyloidosis derived from normal transthyretin. *Proceedings of the National Acadamy of Sciences*. **87**, 2843–45.

Yazaki, M., Tokuda, T., Nakamura, A. *et al.*, (2000). Cardiac amyloid in patients with familial amyloid polyneuropathy consists of abundant wild-type transthyretin. *Biochemical and Biophysical Research Communications*. **274**, 702–706.

Yin, H. L., Kwaitkowski, D. J., Mole, J. E. and Cole, F. S., (1984). Structure and biosynthesis of cytoplasmic and secreted variants of gelsolin. *The Journal of Biological Chemistry*. **259**, 5271–76.

Yoshioka, K., Furuya, H., Sasaki, H. *et al.*, (1989). Haplotype analysis of familial amyloidotic polyneuropathy. Evidence for multiple origins of the Val-Met mutation most common to the disease. *Human Genetics*. **82**, 9–13.

CHAPTER 51

Autonomic dysfunction in peripheral nerve disease

Michael Donaghy

Many peripheral neuropathies have the potential to cause autonomic dysfunction. Usually this autonomic involvement is clinically mild, or remains subclinical. Clinically prominent involvement of small-diameter myelinated and unmyelinated nerve fibres particularly occurs in diabetes, amyloid neuropathy, hereditary sensory and autonomic neuropathies, and some infections, particularly Chagas' disease. Because of their ubiquitous distribution throughout the body, peripheral nerve dysfunction can affect blood pressure and heart rate control, gastrointestinal motility, micturition, sexual functioning, temperature control, sweating, and pupil control. In routine practice, autonomic manifestations of polyneuropathies most frequently produce loss of distal sweating, and postural hypotension. In particular, loss of sweating in the hands and feet is often under-recognized in its importance in contributing to symptomatology. Lack of secretion of sweat oils contributes to hard skin, and fissures that may provide the nidus for ulceration. Loss of sweating on the finger pulp deprives the skin of that moist adhesive quality necessary to perform fine manipulations, such as sorting papers, and thereby contributes to difficulties with manipulation.

This chapter addresses those peripheral nerve disorders in which autonomic abnormalities may be a clinically significant component of the overall symptomatology (Table 51.1). Some important autonomic peripheral neuropathies are addressed separately elsewhere: diabetic autonomic failure (Chapter 53), paraneoplastic autonomic neuropathy (Chapter 52), familial dysautonomia (Chapter 48), and amyloid neuropathy (Chapter 50).

Structure of the autonomic nervous system

Both the sympathetic and parasympathetic components of the peripheral nervous system contain both unmyelinated and myelinated axons (McLeod 1980, McLeod 1999). Unmyelinated fibres predominate, forming about 80% of the nerve fibres in the cervical vagus nerve of humans. Most myelinated nerve fibres are 2–6 μm in diameter. There are a few larger diameter fibres (12–16 μm) many of which are afferents. Morphometric analysis of myelinated sympathetic nerve fibres has shown shorter internodal lengths in relation to overall fibre diameter than in the peripheral somatic nervous system (Fig. 51.1) (McLeod 1999).

Clinical features and investigation of autonomic dysfunction in peripheral neuropathy

Loss of sweating from the feet and hands is a common early symptom. Patients may note that their socks no longer become sweaty, that their fingertips are slippery and have no grip when handling paper, or that their hand and foot skin 'seems dry all the time'. Loss of sweating probably results from impaired postganglionic sympathetic cholinergic functioning in the fibres which travel within peripheral nerve trunks to innervate sweat glands. Given that most peripheral neuropathies are length-dependent disorders, malfunction of this postganglionic neuron is more likely than degeneration or demyelination of the preganglionic sympathetic efferent fibres. Informal clinical assessment may reveal that the foot or finger skin is dry to touch. Formal demonstration of sympathetic cholinergic function may be undertaken by thermoregulatory sweat testing using an indicator powder mixture and controlled heating. More technically complicated assessments can be made by the quantitative sudomotor-axon-reflex test, sympathetic skin responses, or sweat imprint methods (Chapter 31). Hyperhidrosis, usually patchy, may occur in the autonomic instability and the acute phase of Guillain–Barré syndrome, in incomplete peripheral nerve injuries associated with causalgic pain (complex regional pain syndrome) and occasionally in toxic or infiltrative neuropathies. When there is significant loss of sweating from hands and legs, compensatory hyperhidrosis may be evident on the face and trunk.

Postural hypotension, causing faintness on standing, or syncope, is the aspect of autonomic peripheral nerve function most easily quantifiable in the clinic by comparing lying and standing blood pressures. It represents abnormal sympathetic adrenergic function and reflects damage to the small myelinated and the unmyelinated nerve fibres in the baroreflex pathways and in the splanchnic outflow. Most typically it is seen in diabetic and amyloid peripheral neuropathy, in which the small nerve fibres degenerate. By contrast, surges of hypertension may occur in acute Guillain-Barré syndrome.

Impaired heart rate control due to cardiac parasympathetic-nervous-system dysfunction is not commonly symptomatic. However, it is another aspect of peripheral autonomic fibre function which is easily assessable in the clinic, by electrocardiographic

Table 51.1 Clinically important autonomic peripheral neuropathy

		Other neuropathies causing autonomic dysfunction
1.	Diabetic (Chapter 53)	
2.	Amyloid deposition (Chapter 50)	◆ Primary amyloidosis
		◆ Familial amyloidosis
3.	Hereditary sensory and autonomic neuropathy	◆ Autosomal dominant sensory neuropathy (HSAN type I)
		◆ Autosomal recessive sensory neuropathy (HSAN type II)
		◆ Anderson–Fabry's disease
		◆ Multiple symmetric lipomatosis
		◆ Porphyria
		◆ Familial dysautonomia (HSAN type III) (Riley–Day syndrome) (Chapter 48)
		◆ Anhidrotic sensory neuropathy (HSAN type IV)
		◆ Small myelinated fibre deficiency (HSAN type v)
4.	Idiopathic polyneuritis	◆ Guillain–Barré syndrome
5.	Paraneoplastic (Chapter 52)	
6.	Toxic	◆ Alcohol
		◆ Vincristine
		◆ Cisplatin
		◆ Taxol
		◆ Amiodarone
		◆ Perhexiline
		◆ Vacor
		◆ Seafood toxicity (Ciguatoxin)
		◆ Heavy metals
7.	Infections	◆ *Trypanosoma cruzi* (Chagas' disease)
		◆ Leprosy
		◆ Botulism
		◆ HIV
		◆ Diphtheria

measurement of the respiratory sinus arrhythmia, or the heart rate responses to the Valsalva manoeuvre, or to standing. This abnormality of vagal cardiac control is particularly detectable in diabetic neuropathy.

The other visceral and ocular symptoms of peripheral autonomic nerve dysfunction are less easy to quantify in clinical practice. Abnormal micturition, erectile impotence, and loss of vaginal lubrication are typical symptoms of autonomic peripheral neuropathy, most frequently encountered in diabetes and amyloidosis. Altered amplitudes of pupil and motor responses, or mild degrees of ptosis are rarely symptomatic. Autonomic disorders of the gastrointestinal tract may cause vomiting due to gastroparesis or nocturnal diarrhoeal episodes in diabetes, while a paralytic ileus may be a presenting feature of acute idiopathic autonomias, which masquerade as acute surgical emergencies. Standard clinical and neurophysiological testing for a peripheral neuropathy is poorly

sensitive to involvement of the small axons of the autonomic nervous system. For instance, the tendon reflexes, and motor and sensory nerve conduction studies reflect the function of large myelinated nerve fibres. Most peripheral neuropathies causing autonomic dysfunction will also show evidence of reduced pinprick and thermal sensations distally. In evaluating small axon integrity in peripheral neuropathy patients, it may be informative to compare lying and standing blood pressure, and measure the sinus arrhythmia response to deep breathing. The unmyelinated fibres of peripheral nerves can be assessed through the neurogenic flare reaction (also known as the axon reflex flare reaction) occurring 5–15 minutes after iontophoresis of histamine dichloride into the skin (Bickel et al. 2002).

Biopsy is relatively uninformative in investigating autonomic peripheral neuropathy. Extensive morphometric studies on unmyelinated fibre, and small myelinated fibre populations in sural nerve biopsies are laborious to undertake, and rarely yield diagnostic informative unobtainable more simply by the above methods. Although skin biopsies may demonstrate a reduction in the number of sweat glands, and allow quantification of skin neural innervation (Facer et al. 1998) this assessment is rarely used in routine diagnostic clinical practice. Rectal or peripheral nerve biopsy can be critical in detecting amyloid deposition, particularly in primary amyloidosis where molecular genetic testing will not be informative.

Diabetes

Abnormal autonomic function is detectable in a sixth of all patients with insulin-dependent diabetes although symptoms of autonomic peripheral neuropathy only occur in relatively fewer (O'Brian et al. 1986). The autonomic neuropathy usually coexists with a small fibre sensory peripheral neuropathy and the main symptoms are abnormal sweating or diarrhoea. Less frequently, patients suffer postural hypotension, vomiting from gastroparesis, micturition difficulties, bladder infection due to antony, sexual impotence and retrograde ejaculation. Diabetic autonomic neuropathy is considered in detail in Chapter 53.

Amyloid neuropathy

Autonomic features are a prominent component of the polyneuropathy due to primary amyloidosis, and some forms of familial amyloidosis. These are considered in Chapter 50.

Hereditary sensory and autonomic neuropathies

The hereditary sensory and autonomic neuropathies (HSAN) reflect failure of development, or degeneration, of subpopulations of peripheral sensory and autonomic neurons. Impaired appreciation of pain leads to a mutilating acropathy as a result of lack of self protection. Skin ulceration and fissuring, long bone fractures, Charcot joints and digit autoamputation are the principle features. Various classifications have been posed for the HSANs including descriptive/genetic classifications (Donaghy et al. 1987), and a closely contiguous numerical classification into types I to V (Dyck et al. 1983). Increasingly, such phenotypic classification is being replaced by, and further subdivided by, characterization of the molecular genetic abnormality (Axelrod 2002).

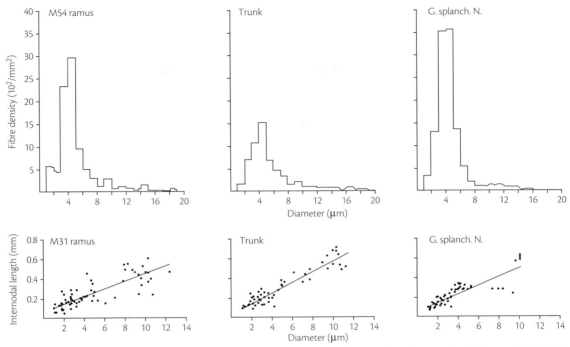

Fig. 51.1 Control subjects. (Above) diameter distribution of myelinated fibres in white ramus, sympathetic trunk, and greater splanchnic nerve. (Below) relationship between internodal length and diameter of myelinated fibres in white ramus, trunk and greater splanchnic nerve. With permission from McLeod J.G. Copyright Elsevier (1980).

Within this group of disorders, those most likely to have significant autonomic features are the autosomal recessive disorder familial dysautonomia (Riley–Day syndrome) and the autosomal recessive selective deficiency of unmyelinated (HSAN IV) or small myelinated (HSAN V) sensory nerve fibres.

Familial dysautonomia (HSAN type III)

This autosomal recessive disorder principally occurs in Ashkenazi Jews involving mutation of the *IKBKAP* gene on chromosome 9 with resultant depletion in the numbers of unmyelinated sensory and autonomic neurons. Affected infants vomit, have impaired thermal regulation, sweat excessively, develop patchy skin blotching, have impaired tear formation and are prone to pulmonary infection. The tongue is characteristically bare of fungiform papillae. This disorder is discussed in detail elsewhere (Chapter 48) (Axelrod 2004).

Hereditary anhidrotic sensory neuropathy (HSAN type IV)

Patients with this autosomal recessive neuropathy suffer from congenital insensitivity to pain. Presentation is in infancy with pyrexial episodes, failure to thrive, retarded development, failure to respond to painful stimuli, anhidrosis, and mild mental retardation. Peripheral nerves show a severely diminished unmyelinated fibre population, and small dorsal root ganglion neurones are largely absent (Swanson et al. 1965). This rare condition often leads to premature death, often around the time of unexplained fever. It is this form of HSAN in which anhidrosis is particularly widespread and severe, probably contributing to thickening and callous formation of the skin, dystrophic nails, and scalp hair loss. Skin biopsies show that sweat glands and blood vessels are completely devoid of nerve fibres, pointing to a developmental disorder, rather than

a degeneration affecting peripheral nerves (Axelrod 2004, Verze et al. 2000). The disorder is due to various mutations affecting the *TRKA* gene on chromosome 1, encoding a receptor tyrosine kinase that autophosphorylates in response to nerve growth factor (Indo 2002). It is hypothesized that the resulting defect in nerve growth factor signal transduction at its receptor leads to developmental apoptosis of neurons dependent upon nerve growth factor. At least 25 frameshift, non-sense, missense and spice mutations of the *TRKA* gene have been identified (Indo 2002). Correspondingly, it has emerged that the clinical spectrum of this disorder is wider than the initially identified uniformly fatal infantile syndrome. Studies of these older surviving children have documented the breadth of the autonomic and sensory peripheral nerve dysfunction, and highlighted associated neuroendocrine disturbances affecting thermal control and circadian rhythms (Ohto et al. 2004, Loewenthal et al. 2005). The treatment of this disorder is symptomatic, with prompt control of hyperthermia, prevention of self-mutilation and awareness of impaired ability to cope with stresses such as thirst or surgery (Axelrod 2002, Loewenthal et al. 2005).

Deficiency of small myelinated sensory fibres (HSAN type V)

Kinships have been described with autosomal recessive inheritance of a severe mutilating acropathy with or without corneal opacification due to neurotrophic keratitis (Donaghy et al. 1987, Dyck et al. 1983). Pain and temperature sensation are completely absent from the limbs. Motor function, tendon reflexes and kinaesthetic sensations are normal, as are motor and sensory nerve conduction. Sural nerve biopsies show selective reduction of the smaller myelinated fibre population. Patients show patchy anhidrosis (Donaghy et al. 1987, Low et al. 1978). In keeping with the variable phenotype of this condition, the genetic basis is heterogeneous. In one patient a novel *TRKA* gene mutation suggested that HSAN V was not truly distinct from HSAN IV, but simply represented a different manifestation of *TRKA* gene mutations (Houlden et al. 2001). However, another patient with the HSAN V phenotype has shown no mutation on sequencing the *TRKA* gene (Toscano et al. 2002). A further problem with classification in this area includes patients with congenital indifference to pain, only one family of which has been described with normal morphometric examination of peripheral nerve (Landrieu et al. 1990). This disorder, which was described on an autosomal dominant basis, has been considered part of the spectrum of HSAN V (Houlden et al. 2001, Toscano et al. 2002). In particular, the question of an abnormality of transmitter function, or of the central pain pathways in the face of an apparently normal unmyelinated fibre population has been hypothesized to explain the apparent normality of the unmyelinated fibre population in peripheral nerves in congenital indifference to pain, and HSAN V (Houlden et al. 2001).

HSAN types I and II

These hereditary sensory neuropathies, autosomal dominant and recessive respectively, involve various patterns of sensory loss. A pan-sensory disorder also involving proprioceptive function is typical of HSAN II; more selective pain and temperature sensory loss is more typical of HSAN I. A severe acromutilating neuropathy occurs in both, with a mild degree of anhidrosis predominantly in the regions of impaired sensation. Classic neuropathic signs such as tendon areflexia are usual, and both neuropathies seem to progressively worsen through life (Denny-Brown 1951, Nukada et al. 1982). Similar forms of HSAN have been inherited as an X-linked recessive (Jestico et al. 1985) and an autosomal recessive form has been associated with spastic paraplegia (Cavanagh et al. 1979). The molecular genetic abnormality in HSAN I involves a mutation in the SPTLC 1 (serine palmitoyltransferase, long-chain base subunit 1) on chromosome 9 (Dawkins et al. 2001). Three geographically widespread missense mutations have been reported (Geraldes et al. 2004). Serine palmitoyltransferase is the rate-limiting enzyme synthesizing ceramide and sphingomyeline. HSAN II has been associated with mutations in a chromosome 12 gene, known as HSN II, particularly identified in French Canadians (Roddier et al. 2005, Lafreniere et al. 2004).

Familial distal dysautonomia

A family has been described with probable autosomal dominant inheritance of peripheral dysautonomia, represented by dry hands and feet with variable vasomotor symptoms, but without sensory loss (Robinson et al. 1989).

Other inherited sensory and autonomic neuropathies

Adult onset of anosmia, followed by anhidrosis and sensory loss, but without acromutilation, with probable autosomal recessive inheritance, has been described (Sakae et al. 2001). A triple A (Allgrove) syndrome of **A**chalasia, **A**lacrima, **A**drenal abnormalities is also associated with sexual impotence, orthostatic hypotension and varying progressive neurological disorders; in keeping with the heterogeneous nature of the condition it is associated with varying mutations of the triple A gene, ALADIN (**A**lacrima, **A**chalasia, **A**drenal Insufficiency, **N**eurological disorder) (Houlden et al. 2002).

Multiple symmetric lipomatosis; Madelung's disease

These patients develop multiple subcutaneous lipomata over the upper trunk and proximal arms, associated with an axonal peripheral neuropathy, usually sensory motor but occasionally with autonomic features. Generally patients present in middle age and there may be a background of excessive consumption (Enzi et al. 1985), or a familial basis (Chalk et al. 1990). Multiple symmetric lipomatosis is a heterogeneous disorder, caused in some patients by mitochondrial DNA deletions (Klopstock et al. 1994). While a largely alcoholic population showed hyperhidrosis, impotence, and abnormal cardiovascular reflexes (Enzi et al. 1985), autonomic symptoms were not noted in a group of non-alcoholic familial cases (Chalk et al. 1990).

Anderson–Fabry disease

This X-linked disorder is also known as angiokeratoma corporis diffusum, and is due to α-galactosidase deficiency. Boys present in childhood or early adult life with burning pain and paraesthesiae distally in the limbs. Episodes of pain may be provoked by heat or exercise and can prevent walking. Excess lysosomal storage of glycosphingolipids occurs in blood vessel walls in selected neuronal populations, including ganglia (deVeber et al. 1992). Anhidrosis, and dry mouth or eyes may occur, with disordered intestinal mobility in older patients (Cable et al. 1982), although cardiovascular autonomic function seems normal (Morgan et al. 1990). It is not known whether the anhidrosis is due to the demonstrated reduction in intra-epidermal small nerve fibres (Scott et al. 1999) or is primary due to a sweat gland abnormality (Kang et al. 1987).

Porphyric neuropathy

A distinctive pattern of neuropathy can occur in attacks of acute hepatic porphyria. Typically such attacks, which may be precipitated by drug administration, start with abdominal pain, with subsequent psychiatric problems and other neurological symptoms. The peripheral neuropathy, if it occurs, usually involves autonomic symptoms. Indeed the abdominal pain at the onset of an attack presumably indicates an autonomic neuropathy with constipation, pseudo-obstruction and other evidence of reduced gastrointestinal motility (Albers and Fink 2004). Abnormalities of autonomic function may be demonstrable during attacks, and may even occur alone (Laiwah et al. 1985, Stewart and Hensley 1981). The neuropathy usually follows the abdominal pain by a few weeks, progressing over subsequent weeks, and can cause severe paralysis reminiscent of Guillain–Barré syndrome. Episodic hypertension or tachycardia may also be reminiscent of Guillain–Barré syndrome.

Acute polyneuritis

Guillain-Barré syndrome

This condition produces severe ascending paralysis due to acute and diffuse demyelination or conduction block affecting spinal roots and peripheral nerves. It is usually post-infective and recovers spontaneously. The severity may be attenuated, and the speed of recovery hastened by early treatment with intravenous immunoglobulin or plasma exchange (Plasma Exchange/Sandoglobulin Guillain–Barré Syndrome Trial Group 1997). The crude average annual incidence rate varies in different countries from 0.6 to 1.9 per 100,000 people (Ropper et al. 1991). The condition is usually post infectious, with preceding cytomegalovirus, campylobacter jejune and Epstein–Barr virus infections being most frequently identified. Inflammatory cell infiltrates, with associated demyelination are found in peripheral nerves. It should be noted that spinal nerve roots may be particularly affected.

Autonomic dysfunction occurs in over 60% of patients with Guillain–Barré syndrome (Zochodne 1994). It particularly contributes to the cardiac arrhythmias which are a leading cause of death, particularly in elderly patients (Dalos et al. 1988). Systolic hypertension and reduced R-R interval variation were particularly noted in those patients developing serious arrhythmias (Winer and Hughes 1988). Indeed, such arrhythmias occur in over 10% of patients and caused or contributed to death in 7% in a general hospital setting. The likelihood of autonomic neuropathy cannot be predicted from the severity of the motor and sensory nerve abnormalities. Both over- and under-activity of the sympathetic or parasympathetic nervous systems may occur with wide fluctuations in blood pressure and heart rate, episodes of facial flushing, pupil abnormalities, patchy anhidrosis, excessive sweating, paralytic ileus, or urinary retention. Paroxysms of increased autonomic activity, causing hypertension, tachycardia or facial flushing are of poor portent, and can be the antecedents of sudden cardiac death (Winer and Hughes 1988, Lichtenfeld 1971). The pathophysiological basis of these varied autonomic manifestations is not known. Lymphocytic infiltrations of autonomic ganglia have been described (Panegyres and Mastaglia 1989) raising the possibility that autoimmune attack upon the autonomic nervous system is part of the pathology. Alternatively, the acute oedema and infiltration of nerve roots in Guillain–Barré syndrome could affect the autonomic outflow.

Given that autonomic dysfunction plays a major part in the morbidity and mortality of Guillain–Barré syndrome, its management is of importance. There is no consensus about the use of pharmacological agents to prevent fluctuations in blood pressure and cardiac rate. Generally, intense vigilance with electrocardiographic and blood pressure monitoring is advised, proceeding to drug or pacemaker treatment of significant abnormalities as they arise.

Idiopathic autonomic neuropathy

Two relatively unusual pure clinical profiles of idiopathic autonomic neuropathy have been defined. A subacute form of rapid onset, sometimes preceded by an infectious illness has been called by the various syndromic terms of acute pan-autonomic neuropathy, idiopathic autonomic neuropathy and acute pan-dysautonomia. Those cases of gradual onset and slow progression have been referred to as pure autonomic failure. About a quarter of such patients have ganglionic acetylcholine receptor antibodies (Sandroni et al. 2004). Such seropositivity was markedly more likely if there were pupil abnormalities and associated Sjögren's syndrome, and the seropositive group are more likely to have a subacute onset. Presenting symptoms are most commonly orthostatic hypotension and gastrointestinal abnormalities, sweating disorders and micturition disorders (Sakakibara et al. 2004). Apart from the association with Sjögren's disease (Wright et al. 1999), subacute autonomic neuropathy has occurred in systemic lupus erythematosus (Hoyle et al. 1985). The subacute form usually follows a monophasic course, but the recovery is usually incomplete. There are reports of individual patients responding well to treatment with intravenous immunoglobulin (Heafield et al. 1996, Smit et al. 1997, Mericle and Triggs 1997).

Idiopathic sensory neuropathy

The syndrome of acute idiopathic sensory neuropathy (Windebank et al. 1990) is sometimes associated with pan-dysautonomia (Yokota et al. 1994). Both preganglionic and postganglionic autonomic neurons may be involved (Tohgi et al. 1989), and T-lymphocytic infiltration of autonomic ganglia occurs (Hainfellner et al. 1996). It seems likely that the disorder including sensory disturbance is related to pure idiopathic autonomic neuropathy, and the same approach to management of their acute polyneuritis should be undertaken. Patients with the chronic painful feet syndrome, associated with reduced numbers of intra-epidermal nerve fibres on skin biopsy, also have predominantly cholinergic autonomic symptoms, including skin vasomotor disturbances, hypertension and impotence, but do not have generalized autonomic failure with postural hypotension (Novak et al. 2001).

Adie's pupil and the Ross syndrome

Adie's tonic pupil is an idiopathic condition thought to result from loss of post-ganglionic cholinergic parasympathetic innervation of the iris sphincter by the ciliary ganglion. Hyporeflexia, particularly of the ankle jerks, has been a long-recognized association of Adie's tonic pupil. The Ross syndrome describes the triad of tonic pupil, tendon hyporeflexia and segmental anhidrosis. Adie's pupil and the Ross syndrome are probably part of the same idiopathic clinical spectrum. The disorder not progressive usually, and the symptoms generally consist of a noted a pupil asymmetry, and segmental anhidrosis sometimes with heat intolerance (Weller et al. 1992).

Lambert–Eaton myasthenic syndrome

Lambert–Eaton myasthenic syndrome causes weakness due to autoimmune mediated decrease in acetylcholine release from the presynaptic terminal at the neuromuscular junction. There is a corresponding diminution in acetylcholine release in the autonomic nervous system. This produces autonomic abnormalities in over 90% of patients, with significant autonomic failure in 20% (O'Suilleabhain et al. 1998). Autonomic failure is most marked in older patients with cancer. Common autonomic symptoms are reduced sweating and salivation, cardiovagal reflexes are often abnormal on measuring sinus arrhythmia, but a wide range of autonomic symptoms and signs may occur, with impotence common in men. The immunopharmacological basis for autonomic involvement remains uncertain since seropositivity for N-type CAT + channel antibodies does not correlate closely with the autonomic features (O'Suilleabhain et al. 1998).

Paraneoplastic autonomic neuropathy

The clinical presentation of this disorder is the same as that of idiopathic autonomic neuropathy. Gastrointestinal symptoms such as pseudo-obstruction, constipation or gastroparesis are particularly common and may occur as isolated features. Most patients have small-cell lung carcinoma and associated anti-Hu antineuronal antibody. This condition is considered in detail in Chapter 52.

Toxin-induced autonomic neuropathy

Although not individually commonly encountered, a wide range of neurotoxins can produce autonomic symptoms.

Alcohol

Axonal degeneration polyneuropathy, predominantly affecting sensory axons, occurs in chronic alcoholism (Behse and Buchthal 1977). In practice, neuropathy is unlikely until a lifetime alcohol consumption of 15 kg of ethanol per kilogram bodyweight is reached (Monforte et al. 1995). Autonomic neuropathy occurs and associates with increased risk of cardiovascular death (Johnson and Robinson 1988). Significant autonomic neuropathy is present in about a third of patients with alcoholic polyneuropathy, and is symptomatic in roughly half of these (Ravaglia et al. 2004). Damage to the parasympathetic system seems to predominate, with erectile dysfunction a particularly common autonomic symptom, often occurring in isolation (Ravaglia et al. 2004).

Autonomic neuropathy also occurs in patients with non-alcoholic hepatic cirrhosis (Bajaj et al. 2003, McDougall et al. 2003). Although autonomic function may improve in individual patients after hepatic transplantation, in the majority autonomic features remain relatively unchanged (McDougall et al. 2003).

Drugs

Symptomatic autonomic neuropathy most usually follows administration of oncological drugs. **Vincristine** can produce postural hypotension, constipation, abdominal pain, paralytic ileus and urinary retention starting within days of commencement of therapy. Abdominal discomfort is the usual first symptom, and can be sudden and severe mimicking an acute abdomen (Donaghy 1996). These symptoms are usually associated with symptoms of a somatic peripheral neuropathy such as sensory disturbance in hands and feet and loss of the ankle reflexes. Usually vincristine-induced autonomic symptoms resolve slowly from about 2 weeks after stopping the drug. **Taxol** can cause a severe autonomic neuropathy, with postural hypotension in addition to the well-recognized sensory polyneuropathy (Jerian et al. 1993). Autonomic neuropathy, usually mild, occurs in association with the sensory polyneuropathy induced by **cisplatin** treatment (Rosenfeld and Broder 1984, Boogerd et al. 1990).

Prolonged administration of the cardiac anti-arrhythmic drugs **amiodarone** and **perhexiline** can cause polyneuropathy, with associated postural hypotension (Manolis et al. 1987, Fraser et al. 1977).

Industrial and agricultural toxins

Poisoning with a number of heavy metals causes peripheral neuropathy. There is associated tachycardia and hypotension in the acute paralysis of **thallium** poisoning, and this may be of delayed onset (Davis et al. 1981, Nordentoft et al. 1998). Abnormalities of cardiovascular autonomic reflexes have been attributed to chronic **lead** toxicity in workers exposed to multiple metals (Murata and Araki 1991). Abnormal cardiovascular reflexes have been noted in workers chronically exposed to **organic solvents**; this abnormality was most marked in those also showing signs of peripheral neuropathy (Matikainen and Juntunen 1985). Ingestion of the rodenticide **vacor** (N-3-pyridylmethyl-N'-*p*-nitrophenyl urea) produces severe autonomic disturbance involving both sympathetic and parasympathetic function, with postural hypotension as an early feature and associated with peripheral neuropathy (LeWitt 1980).

Seafood toxins

Ciguatera poisoning occurs after consumption of large fish which have eaten the toxin-containing dinoflagellate *Gambierdiscus toxicus* which has entered the seafood chain when consumed by smaller fish. More than three quarters of cases of poisoning have primary neurological features: paraesthesiae, dysaesthesiae, and heightened pain perception. Weakness and cerebellar dysfunction are less frequent. In severe cases autonomic involvement may cause brady-cardia or hypotension (Pearn 2001, Allsop et al. 1986). Ciguatoxin binds to and activates the voltage sensitive sodium channel.

Infections

Leprosy

Hypohidrosis classically accompanies the loss of nociception in the territories of nerves affected by leprosy. This hypohidrosis can result either from mycobacterial damage to the unmyelinated fibres innervating sweat glands, or from loss of the sweat glands as a result of skin damage (Facer et al. 1998). In addition to this focal anhidrosis, patients with the more generalized lepromatous form of leprosy have demonstrable dysautonomia affecting cardiovascular reflexes, and syncope, gustatory sweating and impotence are reported by some (Shah et al. 1990). Parasympathetic cardiovascular reflexes are commonly and earlier affected than the sympathetic reflexes. There has been some interest in assessing vasomotor reflexes as an indicator of early nerve damage (Beck et al. 1991) and an ultrasound Doppler method for detecting muscle vasomotor reflexes may have more utility than the detection of skin reflexes using laser Doppler flow velocimetry (Wilder-Smith et al. 2000).

Human immunodeficiency virus

As for the small fibre sensory neuropathy, autonomic dysfunction is most common and severe by the AIDS stage of the disease, but can be observed earlier (Gluck et al. 2000, Freeman et al. 1990, Ruttimann et al. 1991). Syncope, diminished sweating, diarrhoea, micturition abnormalities and impotence are symptomatic in a subgroup of those with demonstrably abnormal autonomic function. Autonomic neuropathy is frequently asymptomatic (Villa et al. 1992). Autonomic abnormalities of pupil control are noteworthy. Sometimes autonomic abnormalities in HIV infection may reflect central nervous system disease.

Chagas' disease

Infection with the protozoal parasite *Trypanosoma cruzi* causes Chagas' disease in at least twenty million people of the population in Latin America (Fernandez et al. 1992). Gastrointestinal motility abnormalities are common causing achalasia, mega-oesophagus, aperistalsis, dysphagia, constipation, intestinal volvulus and mega-colon (Santos et al. 2000). These changes reflect damage to the neurones of the submucosal and myenteric plexuses.

Cardiovascular autonomic involvement leads to cardiac arrhythmias, cardiac failure, sudden death and postural hypotension. Both vagal and sympathetic abnormalities are demonstrable in many asymptomatic patients (Junqueira and Soares 2002, Iosa et al. 1990, Oliveira et al. 2002, Ribeiro et al. 2001, Villar et al. 2004). *T. cruzi* DNA is demonstrable in oesophageal tissue of patients without mega-oesophagus and it has been proposed that the emergence of Chagas' disease in the 30–40% of infected individuals reflects variation in host immune response (Tarleton 2003, Vago et al. 2003).

Diphtheria

Paralysis, descending from the palate, occurs in about 15% of patients with palatal diphtheria infection. Of those developing palatal paralysis, a generalized sensory polyneuropathy affecting the limbs occurs roughly three weeks later (Logina and Donaghy 1999). Autonomic disturbances are detectable in all patients with severe diphtheritic polyneuropathy (Piradov et al. 2001). Paralysis of accommodation due to ciliary muscle involvement produces blurred vision for near objects. The pupillary reactions to light and on convergence are unimpaired. Thirty% of patients develop impaired bladder control. Abnormalities of vagal cardiovascular reflexes are well recognized. Blood pressure swings or cardiac arrhythmia can reflect either autonomic neuropathy or cardiomyopathy (Logina and Donaghy 1999). There are different views about whether postural hypotension due to sympathetic involvement is common; it may reflect differences in severity and the timing of testing (Piradov et al. 2001, Idiaquez 1992). The combination of paralysed accommodation, yet with sparing of the light reflex is a distinguishing feature between diphtheritic and botulism-related pupillary changes (Freeman 2005).

Botulism

The toxins of *Clostridium botulinum* bind to the 'snare' proteins of cholinergic presynaptic nerve terminals, preventing fusion of synaptic vesicles and reducing exocytosis of acetylcholine. The main clinical manifestations of botulism are a descending paralysis starting in the extraocular and bulbar muscles. The blockade of cholinergic autonomic synapses lead to a dry mouth, dry eyes, urinary retention, blurred vision and constipation. Impaired pupillary responses to both light and accommodation are typical. Impaired blood pressure responses to standing occur (Vita et al. 1987). Occasionally, autonomic dysfunction may be the leading symptom of botulism (Merz et al. 2003).

Treatment of autonomic neuropathy

In some, the underlying causative disorder may be treated in its own right. The general principles of treating autonomic neuropathy follow those for treating other autonomic manifestations (Vita et al. 1987). Threatened syncope due to orthostatic hypotension is helped by fluid and salt repletion, mineralocorticoid administration, and sympathomimetic pressor agents. Gastroparesis may respond to dietary modification or metoclopramide, domperidone or erythromycin. Intermittent self-catheterization may be required for urinary retention. Focal hyperhidrosis can be relieved by botulinum toxin injection intracutaneously. The dry cracked skin of hypohidrosis may lead to foot ulceration and daily use of skin oils may reduce the risk. Phosphodiesterase inhibitors such as sildenafil can be effective in erectile impotence, but may exacerbate orthostatic hypotension (Vita et al. 1987). Lubricants may compensate for failure of vaginal secretions.

References

Albers, J. W., Fink, J. K. (2004). Porphyric neuropathy. *Muscle 30 Nerve*, 410–22.

Allsop, J. L., Martini, L., Lebris, H., Pollard, J., Walsh, J., Hodgkinson, S. (1986). [Neurologic manifestations of ciguatera. 3 cases with a neurophysiologic study and examination of one nerve biopsy]. *Rev. Neurol. (Paris)*, **142**, 590–7.

Axelrod, F. B. (2002). Hereditary sensory and autonomic neuropathies. Familial dysautonomia and other HSANs. *Clin. Auton. Res.*, **12** Suppl 1, I2–14.

Axelrod, F. B. (2004). Familial dysautonomia. *Muscle Nerve*, **29**, 352–63.

Bajaj, B. K., Agarwal, M. P., Ram, B. K. (2003). Autonomic neuropathy in patients with hepatic cirrhosis. *Postgrad Med J*, **79**, 408–11.

Beck, J. S., Abbot, N. C., Samson, P. D., *et al.* (1991). Impairment of vasomotor reflexes in the fingertips of leprosy patients. *J Neurol. Neurosurg. Psychiatry*, **54**, 965–71.

Behse, F. Buchthal, F. (1977). Alcoholic neuropathy: clnical, electrophysiological, and biopsy findings. *Ann. Neurol*, **2**, 95–110.

Bickel, A., Kramer, H. H., Hilz, M. J., Birklein, F., Neundorfer, B., Schmelz, M. (2002). Assessment of the neurogenic flare reaction in small-fiber neuropathies. *Neurology*, **59**, 917–9.

Boogerd, W., ten Bokkel Huinink, W. W., Dalesio, O., Hoppenbrouwers, W. J., van der Sande, J. J. (1990). Cisplatin induced neuropathy: central, peripheral and autonomic nerve involvement. *J Neurooncol.*, **9**, 255–63.

Cable, W. J., Kolodny, E. H., Adams, R. D. (1982). Fabry disease: impaired autonomic function. *Neurology*, **32**, 498–502.

Cavanagh, N. P., Eames, R. A., Galvin, R. J., Brett, E. M., Kelly, R. E. (1979). Hereditary sensory neuropathy with spastic paraplegia. *Brain*, **102**, 79–94.

Chalk, C. H., Mills, K. R., Jacobs, J. M., Donaghy, M. (1990). Familial multiple symmetric lipomatosis with peripheral neuropathy. *Neurology*, **40**, 1246–50.

Dalos, N. P., Borel, C., Hanley, D. F. (1988). Cardiovascular autonomic dysfunction in Guillain-Barre syndrome. Therapeutic implications of Swan-Ganz monitoring. *Arch. Neurol.*, **45**, 115–7.

Davis, L. E., Standefer, J. C., Kornfeld, M., Abercrombie, D. M., Butler, C. (1981). Acute thallium poisoning: toxicological and morphological studies of the nervous system. *Ann. Neurol.*, **10**, 38–44.

Dawkins, J. L., Hulme, D. J., Brahmbhatt, S. B., Auer-Grumbach, M., Nicholson, G. A. (2001). Mutations in SPTLC1, encoding serine palmitoyltransferase, long chain base subunit-1, cause hereditary sensory neuropathy type I. *Nat. Genet.*, **27**, 309–12.

Denny-Brown, D. (1951). Hereditary sensory radicular neuropathy. *J Neurochem.*, **14**, 237–52.

deVeber, G. A., Schwarting, G. A., Kolodny, E. H., Kowall, N. W. (1992). Fabry disease: immunocytochemical characterization of neuronal involvement. *Ann. Neurol.*, **31**, 409–15.

Donaghy, M. (1996). Vincristine and neuropathies. *Prescriber's J*, **36**, 116–19.

Donaghy, M., Hakin, R. N., Bamford, J. M., *et al.* (1987). Hereditary sensory neuropathy with neurotrophic keratitis. Description of an autosomal recessive disorder with a selective reduction of small myelinated nerve fibres and a discussion of the classification of the hereditary sensory neuropathies. *Brain*, **110** (Pt 3), 563–83.

Dyck, P. J., Mellinger, J. F., Reagan, T. J., *et al.* (1983). Not 'indifference to pain' but varieties of hereditary sensory and autonomic neuropathy. *Brain* **106** (Pt 2), 373–90.

Enzi, G., Angelini, C., Negrin, P., Armani, M., Pierobon, S., Fedele, D. (1985). Sensory, motor, and autonomic neuropathy in patients with multiple symmetric lipomatosis. *Medicine (Baltimore)*, **64**, 388–93.

Facer, P., Mathur, R., Pandya, S. S., Ladiwala, U., Singhal, B. S., Anand, P. (1998). Correlation of quantitative tests of nerve and target organ dysfunction with skin immunohistology in leprosy. *Brain*, **121** (Pt 12), 2239–47.

Fernandez, A., Hontebeyrie, M., Said, G. (1992). Autonomic neuropathy and immunological abnormalities in Chagas' disease. *Clin. Auton. Res.*, **2**, 409–12.

Fraser, D. M., Campbell, I. W., Miller, H. C. (1977). Peripheral and autonomic neuropathy after treatment with perhexiline maleate. *Br. Med. J*, **2**, 675–6.

Freeman, R. (2005). Autonomic peripheral neuropathy. *Lancet*, **365**, 1259–70.

Freeman, R., Roberts, M. S., Friedman, L. S., Broadbridge, C. (1990). Autonomic function and human immunodeficiency virus infection. *Neurology*, **40**, 575–80.

Geraldes, R., de Carvalho, M., Santos-Bento, M., Nicholson, G. (2004). Hereditary sensory neuropathy type 1 in a Portuguese family-electrodiagnostic and autonomic nervous system studies. *J Neurol. Sci*, **227**, 35–8.

Gluck, T., Degenhardt, E., Scholmerich, J., Lang, B., Grossmann, J., Straub, R. H. (2000). Autonomic neuropathy in patients with HIV: course, impact of disease stage, and medication. *Clin. Auton. Res.*, **10**, 17–22.

Hainfellner, J. A., Kristoferitsch, W., Lassmann, H., *et al.* (1996). T-cell-mediated ganglionitis associated with acute sensory neuronopathy. *Ann. Neurol.*, **39**, 543–7.

Heafield, M. T., Gammage, M. D., Nightingale, S., Williams, A. C. (1996). Idiopathic dysautonomia treated with intravenous gammaglobulin. *Lancet*, **347**, 28–9.

Houlden, H., King, R. H., Hashemi-Nejad, A., *et al.* (2001). A novel TRK A (NTRK1) mutation associated with hereditary sensory and autonomic neuropathy type V. *Ann. Neurol.*, **49**, 521–5.

Houlden, H., Smith, S., De Carvalho, M., *et al.* (2002). Clinical and genetic characterization of families with triple A (Allgrove) syndrome. *Brain*, **125**, 2681–90.

Hoyle, C., Ewing, D. J., Parker, A. C. (1985). Acute autonomic neuropathy in association with systemic lupus erythematosus. *Ann. Rheum. Dis.*, **44**, 420–4.

Idiaquez, J. (1992). Autonomic dysfunction in diphtheritic neuropathy. *J Neurol. Neurosurg. Psychiatry*, **55**, 159–61.

Indo, Y. (2002). Genetics of congenital insensitivity to pain with anhidrosis (CIPA) or hereditary sensory and autonomic neuropathy type IV. Clinical, biological and molecular aspects of mutations in TRKA(NTRK1) gene encoding the receptor tyrosine kinase for nerve growth factor. *Clin. Auton. Res*, **12** Suppl 1, I20–32.

Iosa, D., Dequattro, V., Lee, D. D., Elkayam, U., Caeiro, T., Palmero, H. (1990). Pathogenesis of cardiac neuro-myopathy in Chagas' disease and the role of the autonomic nervous system. *J Auton. Nerv. Syst*, **30** Suppl, S83–7.

Jerian, S. M., Sarosy, G. A., Link, C. J., Jr., Fingert, H. J., Reed, E., Kohn, E. C. (1993). Incapacitating autonomic neuropathy precipitated by taxol. *Gynecol. Oncol.*, **51**, 277–80.

Jestico, J. V., Urry, P. A., Efphimiou, J. (1985). An hereditary sensory and autonomic neuropathy transmitted as an X-linked recessive trait. *J Neurol. Neurosurg. Psychiatry*, **48**, 1259–64.

Johnson, R., Robinson, B. (1988). Mortality in alcoholics with autonomic neuropathy. *J Neurol. Neurosurg. Psychiatry*, **51**, 476–80.

Junqueira, L. F., Jr., Soares, J. D. (2002). Impaired autonomic control of heart interval changes to Valsalva manoeuvre in Chagas' disease without overt manifestation. *Auton. Neurosci.*, **97**, 59–67.

Kang, W. H., Chun, S. I., Lee, S. (1987). Generalized anhidrosis associated with Fabry's disease. *J Am. Acad. Dermatol.*, **17**, 883–7.

Klopstock, T., Naumann, M., Schalke, B., *et al.* (1994). Multiple symmetric lipomatosis: abnormalities in complex IV and multiple deletions in mitochondrial DNA. *Neurology*, **44**, 862–6.

Lafreniere, R. G., MacDonald, M. L., Dube, M. P., *et al.* (2004). Identification of a novel gene (HSN2) causing hereditary sensory and autonomic neuropathy type II through the Study of Canadian Genetic Isolates. *Am. J Hum. Genet.*, **74**, 1064–73.

Laiwah, A. C., Macphee, G. J., Boyle, P., Moore, M. R., Goldberg, A. (1985). Autonomic neuropathy in acute intermittent porphyria. *J Neurol. Neurosurg. Psychiatry*, **48**, 1025–30.

Landrieu, P., Said, G., Allaire, C. (1990). Dominantly transmitted congenital indifference to pain. *Ann. Neurol.*, **27**, 574–8.

LeWitt, P. A. (1980). The neurotoxicity of the rat poison vacor. A clinical study of 12 cases. *N Engl. J Med.*, **302**, 73–7.

Lichtenfeld, P. (1971). Autonomic dysfunction in the Guillain-Barre syndrome. *Am. J Med.*, **50**, 772–80.

Loewenthal, N., Levy, J., Schreiber, R., *et al.* (2005). Nerve growth factor-tyrosine kinase A pathway is involved in thermoregulation and adaptation to stress: studies on patients with hereditary sensory and autonomic neuropathy type IV. *Pediatr. Res.*, **57**, 587–90.

Logina, I., Donaghy, M. (1999). Diphtheritic polyneuropathy: a clinical study and comparison with Guillain-Barre syndrome. *J Neurol. Neurosurg. Psychiatry*, **67**, 433–8.

Low, P. A., Burke, W. J., McLeod, J. G. (1978). Congenital sensory neuropathy with selective loss of small myelinated fibers. *Ann. Neurol.*, **3**, 179–82.

Manolis, A. S., Tordjman, T., Mack, K. D., Estes, N. A., 3rd. (1987). Atypical pulmonary and neurologic complications of amiodarone in the same patient. Report of a case and review of the literature. *Arch. Intern. Med.*, **147**, 1805–9.

Matikainen, E., Juntunen, J. (1985). Autonomic nervous system dysfunction in workers exposed to organic solvents. *J Neurol. Neurosurg. Psychiatry*, **48**, 1021–4.

McDougall, A. J., Davies, L., McCaughan, G. W. (2003). Autonomic and peripheral neuropathy in endstage liver disease and following liver transplantation. *Muscle Nerve*, **28**, 595–600.

McLeod, J. (1980). Autonomic nervous system. In *The physiology of peripheral nerve disease*, Sumner, A. (ed) pp. 432–83. Saunders: Philadelphia.

McLeod, J. (1999). Autonomic dysfunction in peripheral nerve disease. In *Autonomic failure: a textbook of clinical disorders of the autonomic nervous system*, Mathias, C. & Bannister, R. (eds) pp. 367–77. Oxford University Press: Oxford.

Mericle, R. A., Triggs, W. J. (1997). Treatment of acute pandysautonomia with intravenous immunoglobulin. *J Neurol. Neurosurg Psychiatry*, **62**, 529–31.

Merz, B., Bigalke, H., Stoll, G., Naumann, M. (2003). Botulism type B presenting as pure autonomic dysfunction. *Clin. Auton. Res*, **13**, 337–8.

Monforte, R., Estruch, R., Valls-Sole, J., Nicolas, J., Villalta, J., Urbano-Marquez, A. (1995). Autonomic and peripheral neuropathies in patients with chronic alcoholism. A dose-related toxic effect of alcohol. *Arch. Neurol.*, **52**, 45–51.

Morgan, S. H., Rudge, P., Smith, S. J., *et al.* (1990). The neurological complications of Anderson-Fabry disease (alpha-galactosidase A deficiency)—investigation of symptomatic and presymptomatic patients. *Q J Med*, **75**, 491–507.

Murata, K., Araki, S. (1991). Autonomic nervous system dysfunction in workers exposed to lead, zinc, and copper in relation to peripheral nerve conduction: a study of R-R interval variability. *Am. J Ind. Med.*, **20**, 663–71.

Nordentoft, T., Andersen, E. B., Mogensen, P. H. (1998). Initial sensorimotor and delayed autonomic neuropathy in acute thallium poisoning. *Neurotoxicology*, **19**, 421–6.

Novak, V., Freimer, M. L., Kissel, J. T., *et al.* (2001). Autonomic impairment in painful neuropathy. *Neurology*, **56**, 861–8.

Nukada, H., Pollock, M., Haas, L. F. (1982). The clinical spectrum and morphology of type II hereditary sensory neuropathy. *Brain*, **105** (Pt 4), 647–65.

O'Brien, I. A., O'Hare, J. P., Lewin, I. G., Corrall, R. J. (1986). The prevalence of autonomic neuropathy in insulin-dependent diabetes mellitus: a controlled study based on heart rate variability. *Q J Med*, **61**, 957–67.

O'Suilleabhain, P., Low, P. A., Lennon, V. A. (1998). Autonomic dysfunction in the Lambert-Eaton myasthenic syndrome: serologic and clinical correlates. *Neurology*, **50**, 88–93.

Ohto, T., Iwasaki, N., Fujiwara, J., *et al.* (2004). The evaluation of autonomic nervous function in a patient with hereditary sensory and autonomic neuropathy type IV with novel mutations of the TRKA gene. *Neuropediatrics*, **35**, 274–8.

Oliveira, E., Ribeiro, A. L., Assis Silva, F., Torres, R. M. Rocha, M. O. (2002). The Valsalva maneuver in Chagas disease patients without cardiopathy. *Int. J Cardiol.*, **82**, 49–54.

Panegyres, P. K., Mastaglia, F. L. (1989). Guillain-Barre syndrome with involvement of the central and autonomic nervous systems. *Med. J Aust.*, **150**, 655–9.

Pearn, J. (2001). Neurology of ciguatera. *J Neurol. Neurosurg. Psychiatry*, **70**, 4–8.

Piradov, M. A., Pirogov, V. N., Popova, L. M., Avdunina, I. A. (2001). Diphtheritic polyneuropathy: clinical analysis of severe forms. *Arch. Neurol.*, **58**, 1438–42.

Plasma Exchange/Sandoglobulin Guillain-Barre Syndrome Trial Group (1997). Randomised trial of plasma exchange, intravenous immunoglobulin, and combined treatments in Guillain-Barre syndrome. Plasma Exchange/Sandoglobulin Guillain-Barre Syndrome Trial Group. *Lancet*, **349**, 225–30.

Ravaglia, S., Marchioni, E., Costa, A., Maurelli, M., Moglia, A. (2004). Erectile dysfunction as a sentinel symptom of cardiovascular autonomic neuropathy in heavy drinkers. *J Peripher. Nerv. Syst.*, **9**, 209–14.

Ribeiro, A. L., Moraes, R. S., Ribeiro, J. P., *et al.* (2001). Parasympathetic dysautonomia precedes left ventricular systolic dysfunction in Chagas disease. *Am. Heart J*, **141**, 260–5.

Robinson, B., Johnson, R., Abernethy, D., Holloway, L. (1989). Familial distal dysautonomia. *J Neurol. Neurosurg. Psychiatry*, **52**, 1281–5.

Roddier, K., Thomas, T., Marleau, G., *et al.* (2005). Two mutations in the HSN2 gene explain the high prevalence of HSAN2 in French Canadians. *Neurology*, **64**, 1762–7.

Ropper, A., Wijdicks, E., Truax, B. (1991). *Guillain-Barre syndrome.* F A Davis: Philadelphia.

Rosenfeld, C. S., Broder, L. E. (1984). Cisplatin-induced autonomic neuropathy. *Cancer Treat. Rep.*, **68**, 659–60.

Ruttimann, S., Hilti, P., Spinas, G. A., Dubach, U. C. (1991). High frequency of human immunodeficiency virus-associated autonomic neuropathy and more severe involvement in advanced stages of human immunodeficiency virus disease. *Arch. Intern. Med.*, **151**, 2441–3.

Sakae, N., Yamada, T., Arakawa, K., *et al.* (2001). Adult-onset hereditary sensory and autonomic neuropathy accompanied by anosmia but without skin ulceration. *Acta Neurol Scand*, **104**, 316–9.

Sakakibara, R., Uchiyama, T., Asahina, M., Suzuki, A., Yamanishi, T., Hattori, T. (2004). Micturition disturbance in acute idiopathic autonomic neuropathy. *J Neurol. Neurosurg. Psychiatry*, **75**, 287–91.

Sandroni, P., Vernino, S., Klein, C. M., *et al.* (2004). Idiopathic autonomic neuropathy: comparison of cases seropositive and seronegative for ganglionic acetylcholine receptor antibody. *Arch. Neurol.*, **61**, 44–8.

Santos, S. L., Barcelos, I. K., Mesquita, M. A. (2000). Total and segmental colonic transit time in constipated patients with Chagas' disease without megaesophagus or megacolon. *Braz. J Med. Biol. Res.*, **33**, 43–9.

Scott, L. J., Griffin, J. W., Luciano, C., *et al.* (1999). Quantitative analysis of epidermal innervation in Fabry disease. *Neurology*, **52**, 1249–54.

Shah, P. K., Malhotra, Y. K., Lakhotia, M., Kothari, A., Jain, S. K., Mehta, S. (1990). Cardiovascular dysautonomia in patients with lepromatous leprosy. *Indian J Lepr.*, **62**, 91–7.

Smit, A. A., Vermeulen, M., Koelman, J. H., Wieling, W. (1997). Unusual recovery from acute panautonomic neuropathy after immunoglobulin therapy. *Mayo Clin. Proc.*, **72**, 333–5.

Stewart, P. M., Hensley, W. J. (1981). An acute attack of variegate porphyria complicated by severe autonomic neuropathy. *Aust. N Z J Med.*, **11**, 82–3.

Swanson, A. G., Buchan, G. C., Alvord, E. C, Jr. (1965). Anatomic changes in congenital insensitivity to pain. Absence of small primary sensory neurons in ganglia, roots, and Lissauer's tract. *Arch. Neurol.*, **12**, 12–8.

Tarleton, R. L. (2003). Chagas disease: a role for autoimmunity? *Trends Parasitol.*, **19**, 447–51.

Tohgi, H., Sano, M., Sasaki, K., *et al.* (1989). Acute autonomic and sensory neuropathy: report of an autopsy case. *Acta Neuropathol. (Berl)*, **77**, 659–63.

Toscano, E., Simonati, A., Indo, Y., Andria, G. (2002). No mutation in the TRKA (NTRK1) gene encoding a receptor tyrosine kinase for nerve growth factor in a patient with hereditary sensory and autonomic neuropathy type V. *Ann. Neurol.*, **52**, 224–7.

Vago, A. R., Silva, D. M., Adad, S. J., Correa-Oliveira, R., d'Avila Reis, D. (2003). Chronic Chagas disease: presence of parasite DNA in the oesophagus of patients without megaoesophagus. *Trans. R Soc. Trop. Med. Hyg.*, **97**, 308–9.

Verze, L., Viglietti-Panzica, C., Plumari, L., *et al.* (2000). Cutaneous innervation in hereditary sensory and autonomic neuropathy type IV. *Neurology*, **55**, 126–8.

Villa, A., Foresti, V., Confalonieri, F. (1992). Autonomic nervous system dysfunction associated with HIV infection in intravenous heroin users. *Aids*, **6**, 85–9.

Villar, J. C., Leon, H., Morillo, C. A. (2004). Cardiovascular autonomic function testing in asymptomatic T. cruzi carriers: a sensitive method to identify subclinical Chagas' disease. *Int. J Cardiol.*, **93**, 189–95.

Vita, G., Girlanda, P., Puglisi, R. M., Marabello, L., Messina, C. (1987). Cardiovascular-reflex testing and single-fiber electromyography in botulism. A longitudinal study. *Arch. Neurol.*, **44**, 202–6.

Weller, M., Wilhelm, H., Sommer, N., Dichgans, J., Wietholter, H. (1992). Tonic pupil, areflexia, and segmental anhidrosis: two additional cases of Ross syndrome and review of the literature. *J Neurol.*, **239**, 231–4.

Wilder-Smith, E. P., Wilder-Smith, A. J., Nirkko, A. C. (2000). Skin and muscle vasomotor reflexes in detecting autonomic dysfunction in leprosy. *Muscle Nerve*, **23**, 1105–12.

Windebank, A. J., Blexrud, M. D., Dyck, P. J., Daube, J. R., Karnes, J. L. (1990). The syndrome of acute sensory neuropathy: clinical features and electrophysiologic and pathologic changes. *Neurology*, **40**, 584–91.

Winer, J. B. Hughes, R. A. (1988). Identification of patients at risk of arrhythmia in the Guillain-Barre syndrome. *Q J Med.*, **68**, 735–9.

Wright, R. A., Grant, I. A., Low, P. A. (1999). Autonomic neuropathy associated with sicca complex. *J Auton. Nerv. Syst.*, **75**, 70–6.

Yokota, T., Hayashi, M., Hirashima, F., Mitani, M., Tanabe, H., Tsukagoshi, H. (1994). Dysautonomia with acute sensory motor neuropathy. A new classification of acute autonomic neuropathy. *Arch. Neurol.*, **51**, 1022–31.

Zochodne, D. W. (1994). Autonomic involvement in Guillain-Barre syndrome: a review. *Muscle Nerve*, **17**, 1145–55.

CHAPTER 52

Autoimmune and paraneoplastic autonomic neuropathies

Steven Vernino and Angela Vincent

Key points

- Cancer patients may have autonomic dysfunction due to direct effects of the malignancy or due to remote effects mediated by the immune system.

- Acute or subacute autonomic failure can result from an autoimmune 'paraneoplastic' response to tumour antigens that cross reacts with autonomic ganglia or nerves.

- Paraneoplastic autonomic neuropathy can present as widespread autonomic failure or as isolated severe gastrointestinal dysmotility.

- Autonomic failure can also occur as a non-paraneoplastic idiopathic autoimmune disorder specifically targeting autonomic nerves or ganglia.

- Autonomic dysfunction is also commonly seen in patients with Lambert–Eaton myasthenic syndrome, autoimmune neuromyotonia or Morvan's syndrome both with and without tumours.

- Patients with autoimmune or paraneoplastic autonomic neuropathy may have specific serum autoantibodies.

- Some cases of autoimmune autonomic neuropathy are caused by antibodies specific for ganglionic nicotinic acetylcholine receptors.

- Experimental autoimmune animal models of autonomic neuropathy have been described.

Introduction

Acute or subacute autonomic failure can be caused by certain drugs and toxins or in association with systemic disorders that affect the nerves more diffusely (e.g. diabetes, amyloidosis). Once these causes are excluded, many cases of acute or subacute autonomic failure may be attributed to autoimmunity targeting the autonomic nerves and/or ganglia. In addition to the time course of the symptoms, several clinical observations support this concept. Subacute autonomic failure may occur in association with known autoimmune neuromuscular disorders, such as myasthenia gravis, Lambert–Eaton myasthenic syndrome or acquired neuromyotonia, or may be associated with occult cancer (paraneoplastic autonomic neuropathy).

When subacute autonomic neuropathy occurs in isolation, the syndrome often follows a viral prodrome, has a monophasic course, and can be associated with elevated cerebrospinal fluid protein and neuron-specific autoantibodies. Until recently, subacute idiopathic autonomic neuropathy was considered to be a pure autonomic variant of the Guillain–Barré syndrome, but recent evidence suggests that some cases, at least, may be due to a specific immune response to the α3-type neuronal nicotinic acetylcholine receptor (AChR) in autonomic ganglia. Indeed, an animal model of autonomic failure has been induced by immunization against α3-type neuronal nicotinic AChR. The manifestations of autoimmune forms of peripheral autonomic failure are reviewed in this chapter with special consideration of autonomic dysfunction in cancer patients and the emerging experimental and laboratory evidence for specific autoantibodies in both cancer and non-cancer cases.

Autonomic dysfunction in cancer patients

Tumours may occasionally affect the autonomic nervous system directly. Brainstem tumours, even in the absence of increased intracranial pressure, can cause alterations in blood pressure (including orthostatic hypotension or paroxysmal hypertension) or gastrointestinal motor dysfunction (notably intractable vomiting) if medullary autonomic centres are affected (Finestone and Teasell 1993). Tumours in the frontal lobes can cause urinary or bowel dysfunction (Andrew and Nathan 1964). Brain tumours, however, rarely cause an autonomic syndrome in isolation.

Systemic cancers can occasionally impinge directly on peripheral autonomic structures. A variety of tumours originating in the lung apex, mediastinum or cervical vertebral column may extend into the area of the cervical sympathetic chain. Bulky metastases to the cervical chain lymph nodes can also affect these structures. Damage to the preganglionic sympathetic fibres classically results in Horner's syndrome (unilateral miosis, ptosis, and facial anhidrosis).

Patients with cancer outside the nervous system can, and often do, experience autonomic dysfunction even in the absence of direct involvement of autonomic structures by tumour. Symptoms like orthostatic hypotension may be readily explained in the context of anorexia, weight loss and hypovolaemia in the cancer patient.

Peripheral autonomic neuropathy may also occur secondary to the neurotoxic effects of chemotherapy agents (Hancock and Naysmith 1975). Less commonly, a patient with cancer will develop a more specific severe panautonomic or enteric neuropathy caused by an immunological response to the cancer that remotely damages autonomic nerves (paraneoplastic autonomic neuropathy) (Lucchinetti et al. 1998).

Paraneoplastic disorders—general concepts

Neurological paraneoplastic syndromes represent rare, but severe neuroimmunological complications of malignancy. The tumours most commonly associated with these syndromes are small-cell lung carcinoma (SCLC), ovarian carcinoma, breast carcinoma, lymphoma, and thymoma. In general, paraneoplastic neurological disorders have a subacute onset and relentlessly progressive clinical course. Typically, the neurological presentation antedates the diagnosis of malignancy; and the cancer, when found, tends to be localized and responsive to treatment. Clinical neurological manifestations, by contrast, can be varied and multifocal. Several distinct clinical syndromes are easily recognized including sensory neuronopathy (PSN), cerebellar degeneration, limbic encephalitis, Lambert–Eaton myasthenic syndrome (LEMS), and opsoclonus-myoclonus, but it should be appreciated that these characteristic syndromes can also occur in patients without cancer. Paraneoplastic disorders of the peripheral nerves or ganglia most commonly manifest as sensorimotor neuropathy, polyradiculoneuropathy, or sensory neuronopathy. Dysautonomia can occur in combination with any of the recognized paraneoplastic syndromes (notably with Lambert–Eaton syndrome) or can be the sole manifestation of paraneoplastic autoimmunity. Peripheral autonomic failure can be present in patients whose major symptoms involve the central nervous system (especially in combination with limbic encephalitis and SCLC). Thus, many patients have a combination of symptoms that do not fit neatly into a single syndromic classification. Certain tumours, particularly SCLC and thymoma, are often associated with highly mixed clinical syndromes. Moreover, it can sometimes be difficult to decide whether a particular neurological condition should be classified as paraneoplastic or not. A review has highlighted some of these issues and suggested criteria for defining paraneoplastic disorders as definite or probable (Graus et al. 2004).

Antibody tests

Antibodies in paraneoplastic conditions fall into two categories. Firstly, one of the main indications of a paraneoplastic condition is the presence of a serum autoantibody to a paraneoplastic or 'onconeural' antigen. There are a growing number of reported antibodies that can be detected routinely in academic or commercial clinical laboratories as well as less common antibodies which have been reported in only a small number of cases. The antigens are generally cytoplasmic or nuclear proteins and the antibodies can be detected by a combination of immunohistochemistry and western blotting. Many of the well-recognized onconeural antibodies are listed in Table 52.1, and Table 52.2 highlights those autoantibodies which may be associated with the autonomic syndromes discussed in this chapter. In general, a particular antibody correlates more closely with a particular type of malignancy than with a single clinical syndrome. Some patients may simultaneously produce two or more different antibodies (Pittock et al. 2004). Seropositivity for any one of the onconeural antibodies should prompt further consideration of an underlying malignancy, even if routine imaging studies and other cancer screening tests are negative. Importantly, there is increasing evidence that positron emission tomography (PET) imaging of the body is more sensitive than computed tomography for detecting small tumour foci (Rees et al. 2001). Nevertheless, some patients, around 30%, with typical neurological diseases and associated tumours do not have any of the recognized onconeural antibodies, while other patients have a well-recognized antibody but no detectable tumour. (Graus et al. 2004, Candler et al. 2004).

Secondly, there are a group of ion channel autoantibodies that can be found in patients with both paraneoplastic and non-paraneoplastic disorders. These antibodies are considered to be pathogenic since they bind to ion channels or associated proteins that are involved in synaptic transmission, the patients tend to improve clinically after plasma exchange or other immunotherapies, and the conditions can be transferred to experimental animals by injection of patients' immunoglobulin G (Vernino et al. 2004a, Lambert and Lennon 1988, Vincent 2002). The antigens include the voltage-gated calcium channels that are responsible for neurotransmitter release at the neuromuscular junction and at ganglionic synapses in the autonomic nervous system, voltage gated potassium channels that are responsible for the repolarization of the nerve terminals after each nerve impulse, and nicotinic acetylcholine receptors (both muscle and neuronal ganglionic types). Until very recently, these antibodies have been detected by immunoprecipitation of the ion channel target that has been pre-tagged with a highly specific and radiolabelled antigen. Other techniques are being developed as will be described below. These new tests for antibodies to cell surface antigens and more about the antibodies and the associated diseases are reviewed in Vincent et al. 2011.

Paraneoplastic autonomic neuropathy

Paraneoplastic autonomic neuropathy typically presents as a subacute panautonomic neuropathy (indistinguishable from non-paraneoplastic autoimmune autonomic neuropathy, discussed below). Limited presentations may also occur, most notably severe gastrointestinal dysmotility without other autonomic features (paraneoplastic enteric neuropathy). As with other paraneoplastic disorders, the symptoms usually precede the diagnosis of cancer, and the tumours, when found, are limited in stage or only locally metastatic (regional lymph nodes) (Maddison et al. 1999). Hence, since the patient has no symptoms directly referable to their tumour, the autonomic symptoms cannot be attributed to direct effects of the tumour, non-specific consequences of chronic illness or to chemotherapy-induced neuropathy.

The time course of paraneoplastic panautonomic neuropathy varies from acute autonomic failure to a more insidious onset over several months. Orthostatic hypotension and anhidrosis (dry skin and/or heat intolerance) reflect sympathetic failure. Resting and orthostatic plasma catecholamine levels may be reduced. Parasympathetic failure manifests as impaired cardiovagal function (tachycardia and impaired heart rate response to deep breathing, Valsalva and upright tilt), erectile dysfunction, dry eyes and mouth, and/or dilated and poorly reactive pupils. Patients may have bladder dysfunction although there is no consistent pattern to the

Table 52.1 Neuronal paraneoplastic autoantibodies

Antibody name *	Antigen(s)	Tumour	Associated syndromes
Neuronal nuclear and cytoplasmic antibodies*			
Anti-Hu ANNA-1	*HuD, HuC, Hel-N1*	SCLC	Encephalomyelitis, sensory neuronopathy, autonomic and sensorimotor neuropathies, ataxia
CRMP-5 anti-CV2	*CRMP-5*	SCLC or thymoma	Encephalomyelitis, chorea, neuropathy, optic neuritis
anti-Yo PCA-1	*CDR34 and CDR62*	Ovarian or breast cancer	Paraneoplastic cerebellar degeneration
Anti-Ma	*Ma1 and Ma2*	Lung, breast or testicular	Limbic and brainstem encephalitis
Anti-amphiphysin	*Amphiphysin*	Lung or breast cancer	Encephalomyelitis, neuropathy, 'stiff-person syndrome'
PCA-2	Unknown (280kD)	SCLC	Encephalomyelitis
anti-Ri ANNA-2	*Nova*	Lung or breast cancer	Ataxia, opsoclonus-myoclonus, neuropathy
anti-Tr	Unknown	Hodgkin lymphoma	Paraneoplastic cerebellar degeneration
ANNA-3	Unknown (170kD)	SCLC	Encephalomyelitis
Recoverin	*Recoverin*	SCLC	Cancer-associated retinopathy
Ion channel antibodies†			
P/Q-type VGCC	Neuronal Ca++ channels	SCLC (~50%)	Lambert-Eaton syndrome
Muscle AChR	Muscle AChR	Thymoma (~15%)	Myasthenia gravis
Ganglionic (α3-type) AChR	Neuronal ganglionic AChR	SCLC (≤ 15%)	Autonomic neuropathy
VGKC-complex	Proteins associated with neuronal K+ channels	Thymoma (<20%) or SCLC (<5%)	Neuromyotonia; limbic encephalitis

* When alternate nomenclature exists, both are given. The neuronal and cytoplasmic antibodies are listed in approximate order of decreasing frequency.

† The ion channel antibodies are more commonly found in a non-paraneoplastic context.

AChR, (nicotinic) acetylcholine receptor; ANNA, antineuronal nuclear antibody; PCA, Purkinje-cell antibody, SCLC, small-cell lung carcinoma; VGCC, voltage-gated calcium channel; VGKC, voltage-gated potassium channel; VGKC complex, voltage-gated potassium channel complex.

urinary complaints. Gastrointestinal complaints are very common, usually severe constipation, gastroparesis or intestinal pseudo-obstruction. Even if the time course in unclear, the presence of pupillary abnormalities and prominent gastrointestinal symptoms help distinguish autoimmune and paraneoplastic autonomic neuropathies from the more chronic degenerative autonomic disorders

Table 52.2 Antibodies associated with prominent autonomic syndromes

Clinical syndrome	Associated antibodies	Tumours
Diffuse autonomic neuropathy	ANNA-1 CRMP-5	SCLC or thymoma (≥ 80%)
Diffuse autonomic neuropathy	Ganglionic AChR	Usually not paraneoplastic Sometimes SCLC (≤ 10%)
Enteric neuropathy	ANNA-1, CRMP-5	SCLC or thymoma
Enteric neuropathy	Ganglionic AChR, VGKC	Usually not paraneoplastic Thymoma or SCLC (≤ 10%)
LEMS	VGCC, ANNA-1	SCLC (~50%)
Neuromyotonia/ Morvan's syndrome	VGKC-complex, CRMP-5	Usually not paraneoplastic Up to 50% have thymoma, rarely SCLC

AChR, acetylcholine receptor; ANNA, antineuronal nuclear antibody; CRMP-5, collapsin response-mediated protein 5; LEMS, Lambert–Eaton myasthenic syndrome; SCLC, small-cell lung carcinoma; VGCC, voltage-gated calcium channel; VGKC, voltage-gated potassium channel.

(Klein et al. 2003). Standard autonomic testing demonstrates the autonomic deficits but does not usually differentiate paraneoplastic autonomic neuropathy from other causes of severe pandysautonomia.

Paraneoplastic disorders often present as multifocal neurological disorders. When subacute autonomic failure develops in combination with another peripheral or central neurological syndrome, paraneoplastic disease should rise to the top of the differential diagnosis. A common example is autonomic or enteric neuropathy in combination with limbic encephalitis (memory loss, seizures and behavioral changes); SCLC is the most common tumour association. Another recognized scenario is autonomic neuropathy in combination with sensory ganglionopathy (pure sensory neuropathy) also associated with SCLC. Paraneoplastic dysautonomia also commonly occurs in the setting of paraneoplastic ataxia or brainstem encephalitis, Lambert–Eaton syndrome or Morvan's syndrome (discussed later in this chapter).

The autoantibody most commonly associated with paraneoplastic autonomic neuropathy is anti-Hu, also known as antineuronal nuclear antibody type 1 (ANNA-1). SCLC is found in more than 80% of patients who are seropositive for ANNA-1 (Lucchinetti et al. 1998). This antibody recognizes a family of 35–40 kDa neuronal nuclear RNA-binding proteins and labels the nuclei (and to a lesser extent, the cytoplasm) of all neurons. Characteristically, ANNA-1 also binds to peripheral neurons in autonomic ganglia and in the myenteric plexus (Fig. 52.1).

Treatment of paraneoplastic autonomic neuropathy generally consists of supportive symptomatic treatments to alleviate the most

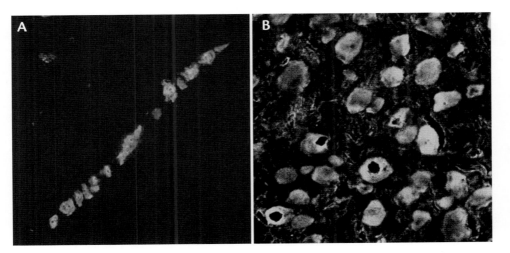

Fig. 52.1 Binding of antineuronal nuclear antibody type 1 (ANNA-1) antibodies to autonomic ganglia neurons. Human ANNA-1 antibodies bound to rabbit autonomic tissues were detected by indirect immunofluorescence. ANNA-1 binds to the nuclei and cytoplasm of **(A)** enteric neurons in myenteric plexus and **(B)** sympathetic neurons in superior cervical ganglia. See also Plate 19.

problematic symptoms, orthostatic hypotension and gastrointestinal dysmotility. Every effort should be made to locate and treat the underlying malignancy. In some cases, autonomic function improves once the malignancy is effectively treated (Vernino et al. 2000, Park et al. 1972). Plasma exchange or intravenous immunoglobulin have also been effective in individual reports (Bohnen et al. 1997). Patients with paraneoplastic neurological disorders seem to achieve prolonged cancer remission more often than patients with similar tumours (Maddison et al. 1999, Keime-Guibert et al. 1999). This may reflect the effects of the vigorous immune response against the cancer in these patients, but it is also possible that this observation is due to earlier diagnosis in cases that present with neurological symptoms (Maddison et al. 1999). Nevertheless, even with prompt diagnosis and appropriate treatment, many patients are left with some degree of residual autonomic deficits.

Although SCLC is the most commonly associated cancer, dysautonomia may also be encountered with thymoma, with or without associated symptoms of myasthenia gravis (Vernino and Lennon 2004, Viallard et al. 2005). Subtle pupillary abnormalities have been noted in patients with myasthenia gravis, but overt subacute autonomic dysfunction has been reported in only 13 cases of myasthenia gravis, most in association with thymoma (Rakocevic et al. 2003, Vernino et al. 2001). Similar to lung cancer-related paraneoplastic autonomic neuropathy, symptoms ranged from isolated gastroparesis to severe panautonomic failure. Intestinal pseudo-obstruction was a common feature. Patients with myasthenic and prominent autonomic dysfunction must be carefully evaluated for the alternative diagnosis of LEMS and for underlying thymoma or lung carcinoma, and antibodies against ganglionic AChR should be looked for in patients with myasthenia gravis who have significant autonomic failure.

Paraneoplastic enteric neuropathy

Gastrointestinal hypomotility is a common and disabling feature of paraneoplastic autonomic neuropathy. Quite often, the paraneoplastic syndrome can be limited to the gut and is better classified as a paraneoplastic enteric neuropathy. This syndrome can occur in patients with known malignancy but more typically precedes the diagnosis of cancer (Chinn and Schuffler 1988, Lhermitte et al.

1980, Condom et al. 1993, Lucchinetti et al. 1998). Features vary from severe gastroparesis, intestinal pseudo-obstruction, severe constipation, or a combination of these. Oesophageal dysmotility (including achalasia) has also been reported (Liu et al. 2002, Lucchinetti et al. 1998, Vernino and Lennon 2004). Patients present with nausea, early satiety, bloating, abdominal pain, constipation and resultant weight loss. Patients may regurgitate undigested food many hours after eating. In severe cases, even fluid intake may be compromised leading to dehydration. Imaging studies show dilated loops of bowel, and motility studies reveal delayed gastric emptying, diffuse intestinal hypomotility, and absent or uncoordinated motor complexes. Such patients are often presumed to have bowel obstruction, but endoscopy and exploratory laparotomy fail to identify an obstruction.

Gastrointestinal dysmotility is usually refractory to treatment with motility-enhancing agents or surgical decompression. To survive, many patients need to have supplemental nutrition supplied through jejunostomy feeding tubes or intravenously. Gastrostomy feeding is usually not tolerated because of gastroparesis and vomiting. There have been several cases of improvement following cancer chemotherapy (Sodhi et al. 1989) or with plasma exchange and immunosuppression (Vernino et al. 2004b).

Pathologically, paraneoplastic dysmotility has been associated with inflammatory destructive process affecting myenteric ganglia of the gut. In post-mortem or surgical samples of the oesophagus, stomach, small bowel, and colon, every area shows abnormalities in the myenteric plexus with reduction in neurons and axons, and lymphocytoplasmic infiltration (Fig. 52.2) (Jun et al. 2005, Chinn and Schuffler 1988). Pathological examination in another case showed intact myenteric plexus and a prominent loss of interstitial cells of Cajal (Pardi et al. 2002).

Neuron-specific autoantibodies may play a role both diagnostically and pathophysiologically. Among patients with ANNA-1 (anti-Hu) antibodies, more than 10% had a paraneoplastic syndrome limited to gastrointestinal dysmotility (Lucchinetti et al. 1998). ANNA-1 antibodies bind to the nuclei of neurons throughout the nervous system and characteristically bind to neurons in the myenteric plexus ganglia (Fig. 52.1). Other patients with paraneoplastic dysmotility related to SCLC have IgG antibodies specifically reactive with neurons of the myenteric and submucosal plexuses of jejunum and stomach (Lennon et al. 1991), although the target of

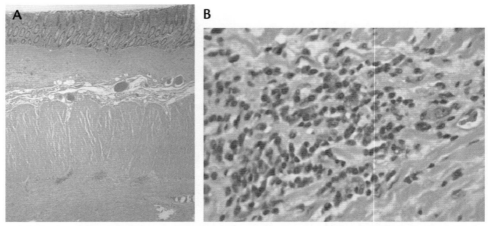

Fig. 52.2 Lymphoplasmacytic infiltration of myenteric plexus ganglia in a bowel section from a patient with paraneoplastic enteric neuropathy. **A:** A full thickness view of the colon shows normal mucosa and submucosa. There is a chronic inflammatory infiltrate between the longitudinal and circular layers of the muscularis propria. (H&E, 20x). **B:** A dense lymphoplasmacytic infiltrate is noted in the location of the myenteric plexus. Ganglion cells can be seen surrounded by inflammation (H&E, 400x). See also Plate 20. With permission from Jun, S., Dimyan, M., Jones, K. D. and Ladabaum, U. (2005), *Neurogastroenterology & Motility*, Wiley.

these antibodies is not yet clear. At least one case of thymoma-associated gastric pseudo-obstruction was associated with antibodies to voltage-gated potassium channel complex (VGKC) (and associated neuromyotonia) (Viallard et al. 2005). VGKC antibodies can also be associated with gastric motility defects in non-tumour cases (Knowles et al. 2002).

Investigators have shown that antibodies from patients with paraneoplastic dysmotility can induce cell death in cultured myenteric neurons (De Giorgio et al. 2003, Schafer et al. 2000), but most evidence suggests that the ganglionitis is caused primarily by cell-mediated immunity rather than a direct antibody effect.

Lambert–Eaton myasthenic syndrome

LEMS is an acquired, antibody-mediated disorder of neuromuscular junction transmission. Antibodies against P/Q-type voltage-gated calcium channels cause an impairment in presynaptic calcium influx and a reduction in the release of acetylcholine (Lambert and Lennon 1988, Vincent et al. 1989). Around 50–60% of adult LEMS patients have a malignancy, most commonly SCLC.

Weakness and fatigue are the usual presenting complaints, but autonomic symptoms are present in about 75% of patients. Often the autonomic symptoms are mild, and patients do not volunteer them unless specifically asked. Dry mouth and impotence (in men) are extremely common. Other cholinergic autonomic symptoms may be present, including dry eyes, reduced sweating, abnormal pupillary function, and constipation (O'Neill et al. 1988). Adrenergic symptoms like postural hypotension and ptosis are less common.

Examination shows symmetrical proximal weakness, reduced or absent reflexes and normal sensation. While autonomic complaints are relatively few, autonomic tests show widespread autonomic abnormalities. Calcium-channel antibodies, detected by immuno-precipitation of P/Q-type calcium channels, are found in nearly 100% of patients with LEMS (Lennon et al. 1995, Motomura et al. 1995), but they do not distinguish between paraneoplastic and non-paraneoplastic forms of the disease, and they can sometimes be associated with other autoimmune neurological disorders, such as cerebellar ataxia with lung cancer (Voltz et al. 1999, Graus et al. 2002).

To try to exclude the presence of a SCLC in LEMS cases at risk, anti-Hu and collapsin response-mediated protein 5 (CRMP-5) antibodies, in particular, should also be investigated (Table 52.1).

Neuromyotonia and Morvan's syndrome

Several other autoimmune neuromuscular disorders are associated with autonomic dysfunction. Acquired neuromyotonia (or Isaacs syndrome) is an autoimmune disorder characterized by peripheral nerve hyperexcitability. Electromyography shows spontaneous firing of motor units in multiplet discharges at irregular intervals with a high intraburst frequency. These discharges are often characterized as myokymia or neuromyotonia. Clinical features include muscle stiffness, cramps, myokymia, hyperhidrosis, and hypersalivation (Hart et al. 2002, Newsom-Davis and Mills 1993). Serum from about 40% of patients contains antibodies (IgG) that precipitate ^{125}I-dendrotoxin-VGKC of the Kv1.1, 1.2 and 1.6 subtypes (Shillito et al. 1995, Vernino and Lennon 2002), although it is now clear that the antibodies are often directed against proteins complexed with these Kv1 subtypes, such as contactin-2 associated protein, contactin-2 itself or leucine-rich, glioma inactivated 1 protein rather than the Kv1 subtypes themselves (Irani et al. 2010).

A proportion of patients with neuromyotonia, report some disturbance of the central nervous system such as sleep problems, anxiety, personality change (Vernino and Lennon 2002, Hart et al. 2002). The French physician Augustin Marie Morvan first used the term 'la chorée fibrillaire' in 1870 to describe a syndrome characterized by peripheral nerve hyperexcitability, dysautonomia, insomnia, and fluctuating delirium (Morvan, 1890). Recently, a number of cases have been reported in the English literature and the autoimmune pathogenesis of this disorder established (Madrid et al. 1996, Liguori et al. 2001, Lee et al. 1998, Barber et al. 2000, Irani et al 2010). Typical presentation of Morvan's syndrome includes muscle twitching, hyperhidrosis, insomnia, fluctuating cognition, and limb paraesthesia. Patients complain of burning pain in skin, joints, or muscles. Needle electromyography (EMG) typically reveals spontaneous muscle fibre activity with fasciculations, multiplets, and myokymic and neuromyotonic discharges. Dysautonomia is a prominent feature of Morvan's syndrome.

Excessive autonomic activity is suggested by new onset hypertension, piloerection, vasomotor instability in the hands and feet, tachycardia, extrasystoles (Liguori et al. 2001, Lee et al. 1998, Josephs et al. 2004, Spinazzi et al. 2008) and increased urinary or serum catecholamines. Paroxysms of sweating, piloerection and salivation can occur, and one case had hyperlacrimation.

In addition to autonomic hyperactivity, patients with autoimmune neuromyotonia (Isaacs or Morvan's syndrome) may also experience autonomic failure including constipation, intestinal pseudo-obstruction (Viallard et al. 2005) orthostatic hypotension and cardiovagal failure (Josephs et al. 2004). Both neuromyotonia and Morvan's syndrome can be associated with thymoma, and less commonly, SCLC. It appears that the incidence of VGKC antibodies is higher in those cases with a tumour (Hart et al. 2002), but even so many cases are VGKC antibody negative. A thorough search for other autoantibodies or onconeural antibodies in these patients has not yet been systematically performed. Antibodies to Contactin-2 associated protein, which is tightly complexed with the VGKC Kv1 subunits, are relatively frequent in patients with Morvan's syndrome or isolated neuromyotonia, particularly in those with thymomas. These antibodies are detected by measuring by indirect immunofluorescence binding of IgG to the surface of cells that have been transfected with cDNAs encoding these proteins (see Irani et al. 2010).

Autoimmune autonomic ganglionopathy

Pure acute dysautonomia was first described as a discrete clinical entity by Young et al. in 1969 (Young et al. 1969, Young et al. 1975). This disorder was characterized by subacute onset, monophasic course with partial recovery, sympathetic and parasympathetic failure, and no significant evidence of somatic peripheral neuropathy. Clinical and laboratory data from larger groups of these cases suggested an immunological basis (Suarez et al. 1994, Hart and Kanter 1990). More recently, specific antibodies directed against the neuronal AChR in autonomic ganglia have been found in many patients with this disorder (Vernino et al. 2000). Based on this finding, the term autoimmune autonomic ganglionopathy (AAG) was proposed to highlight the nature of the disorder.

The clinical features of AAG (also known as acute panautonomic neuropathy, idiopathic autonomic neuropathy, acute pandysautonomia) are essentially indistinguishable from paraneoplastic autonomic neuropathy. The distinction may not be possible until cancer is diagnosed or another neurological syndrome becomes evident. As with the paraneoplastic form, the symptoms of AAG reflect involvement of parasympathetic, sympathetic and enteric nervous systems. Less common patterns are those of selective cholinergic failure, selective adrenergic neuropathy, or isolated gastrointestinal dysmotility. The typical presentation is highly characteristic; severe pandysautonomia affecting a previously healthy individual (Suarez et al. 1994). Common presenting symptoms are orthostatic hypotension and gastrointestinal dysfunction; each of these symptoms occurring in more than 70% of patients (Suarez et al. 1994). Parasympathetic failure is also prominent with dry eyes, dry mouth, impaired pupillary light reflex, and disturbances of bladder and bowel function. A presumed antecedent viral infection may be reported in about 60% of cases, with a flu-like illness or upper respiratory infection being the most frequent association (Suarez et al. 1994). Specific preceding viral infections

have been reported, with Epstein–Barr virus being the most common association (Yahr and Frontera 1975). The spinal fluid protein is often elevated (Suarez et al. 1994, Hart and Kanter 1990).

The acute or subacute onset of autonomic failure occurs with relative or complete sparing of somatic nerve fibres. Neuropathic symptoms, such as tingling in the distal extremities, occur in approximately 25% of patients, but these symptoms are not accompanied by objective signs or electrophysiological evidence of somatic neuropathy. When significant sensory neuropathy is present, a diagnosis of acute sensory and autonomic neuropathy is more appropriate.

The main differential diagnoses are paraneoplastic autonomic neuropathy and Guillain–Barré syndrome. Patients with a paraneoplastic autonomic neuropathy may be clinically indistinguishable until a cancer, usually SCLC, is detected. In Guillain–Barré syndrome, the brunt of the process affects the somatic nerves, causing diffuse muscle weakness and areflexia, which provides a clear distinction from autonomic neuropathy. The temporal profile helps distinguish autoimmune autonomic neuropathies from the chronic ones, but if the time course of symptoms is unclear, chronic forms of dysautonomia (including pure autonomic failure, diabetes or amyloidosis) must also be considered.

About 50% of patients with the typical clinical features of AAG have high titers of autoantibodies directed against the ganglionic AChR (Vernino et al. 2000). This receptor is a pentameric transmembrane complex consisting of two AChR α3 subunits in combination with AChR β subunits. The α3-type ganglionic AChR mediates fast synaptic transmission in all peripheral autonomic ganglia and is homologous but genetically and immunologically distinct from the AChR at the neuromuscular junction. Serum ganglionic AChR antibody levels in AAG cases correlate with the severity of autonomic failure clinically and with the severity on laboratory testing (Vernino et al. 2000, Klein et al. 2003). Although the finding of high levels of ganglionic AChR antibody is specific for the diagnosis of AAG, a negative antibody test does not rule out the diagnosis. Ganglionic AChR antibodies can also be found in patients with lung cancer-related and thymoma-related autonomic neuropathy, so a positive test does not exclude a paraneoplastic cause (Vernino et al. 2000, Vernino and Lennon 2004). Clinically, patients with ganglionic AChR antibodies more often have a subacute onset and generally show more prominent cholinergic dysautonomia (sicca complex, pupillary abnormalities, and gastrointestinal tract symptoms) compared with seronegative autonomic neuropathy patients (Sandroni et al. 2004).

Recognition of ganglionic AChR antibodies has allowed for the serological detection of autoimmune autonomic neuropathy and led to a better appreciation of the spectrum of this disorder, including the observation that some cases are characterized by insidious symptom onset, without antecedent event, and gradual progression (Klein et al. 2003, Goldstein et al. 2002). Such chronic cases may initially be indistinguishable from degenerative forms of autonomic failure. Often, laboratory autonomic function testing shows diffuse abnormalities, which suggest a postganglionic autonomic neuropathy. However, in some cases, the pattern of laboratory findings is more selective and suggests a problem at the level of the autonomic ganglia. Low plasma catecholamine levels may be associated with evidence of robust cardiac sympathetic innervation by fluorodopamine PET imaging (Goldstein et al. 2009). Anhidrosis with preserved postganglionic sudomotor nerve function may also be seen (Fig. 52.3).

These clinical laboratory patterns may initially be attributed to preganglionic autonomic failure rather than ganglionic impairment.

The clinical course of AAG is typically monophasic and patients often show spontaneous stabilization or recovery. Recurrences are uncommon. However, the recovery is typically incomplete (Suarez et al. 1994, Hart and Kanter 1990, Feldman et al. 1991, Yahr and Frontera 1975). Only one patient in three shows a major functional improvement. The mainstay of treatment is symptomatic management of autonomic failure including blood pressure support, bowel management, and supplemental moisture for dry eyes and mouth. Acetylcholinesterase inhibitors have been used to alleviate neurogenic orthostatic hypotension (Singer et al. 2003), and this class of drugs might be particularly appropriate to treat AAG where the pathophysiology is presumed to be impaired ganglionic cholinergic synaptic transmission.

There is no proven specific treatment for AAG, but it is reasonable to consider immunomodulatory therapies including plasma exchange, intravenous immunoglobulin, steroids or immunosuppressant drugs especially as an early therapeutic intervention (within 8 weeks of onset) for patients with marked autonomic failure. There are numerous reports of beneficial responses to intravenous immunoglobulin, plasma exchange, or immunosuppression (Iodice et al. 2009). The recovery of autonomic function after plasma exchange can be dramatic but short-lived, so combination immunotherapy is often required (Fig. 52.4) (Gibbons et al. 2008, Schroeder et al. 2005). Because of the expense and potential risks of immune therapy, it is critical to quantitate autonomic deficits before and after treatment to determine efficacy.

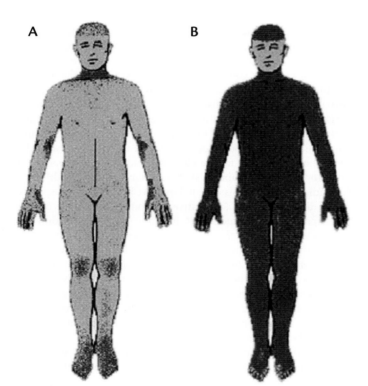

Fig. 52.3 Sweating abnormalities in a patient with autoimmune autonomic ganglionopathy. This 63-year-old man presented with the acute onset of gastroparesis, orthostatic light-headedness and dry skin. **A:** At presentation, thermoregulatory sweat test (TST) showed total body anhidrosis (91% loss of sweating). However, the quantitative sudomotor axon reflex test (QSART) responses were entirely normal at three sites in the lower extremity and in the arm. Ganglionic acetylcholine receptor antibodies were found in the patient's serum (0.4 nmol/L; normal < 0.05). Without treatment, the patient spontaneously improved. He became completely asymptomatic. **B:** Nine months later, the TST showed nearly normal heat-induced sweating (2% anhidrosis). Anhidrosis with normal QSART responses can be seen in disorders affecting preganglionic sympathetic autonomic neurons or with blockade of autonomic ganglia. The rapid spontaneous recovery in this patient supports the latter explanation. Adapted from Vernino S., Low, P.A., Fealey, R. D., Stewart, J. D., Farrugia, G. & Lennon, V. A. (2000).

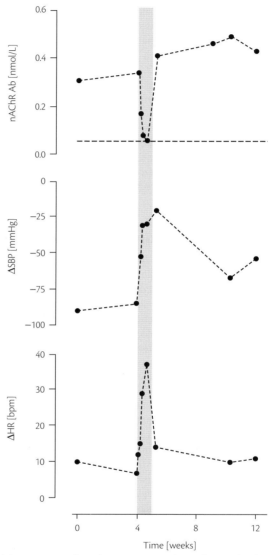

Fig. 52.4 Improvement of autoimmune autonomic ganglionopathy after plasma exchange (PLEX). A 43-year-old man presented with a long history (more than 10 years) of autonomic failure. Symptoms included orthostatic syncope, dry mouth, loss of sweating, dilated pupils, constipation, and early satiety. He had not responded to trials of symptomatic medications. Ganglionic acetylcholine receptor (AChR) antibodies were detected in his serum (7 times the upper limit of normal). PLEX was performed daily for 5 days. The upper graph shows the immediate, but transient, decrease in ganglionic AChR antibody levels during PLEX. Orthostatic blood pressure and heart rate changes are shown in the lower two graphs. With PLEX, the orthostatic blood pressure drop improved from 80 mmHg to 20 mmHg and the patient became able to stand without symptoms. With treatment, an appropriate reflex orthostatic heart rate increment appeared. Adapted from Schroeder et al. (2005).

Experimental models of autoimmune autonomic neuropathy

Several animal models of autoimmune or antibody mediated autonomic neuropathy have been developed, and these have proved insights into autonomic pathophysiology in humans.

Forty years ago, Appenzeller et al. reported an active immunization model of sympathetic failure. Rabbits immunized with extracts of sympathetic ganglia showed impaired vasomotor function (Appenzeller et al. 1965). While the autonomic and histological lesions were mild, the vasomotor abnormalities (namely failure of heat-induced reflex vasodilation in the ear) were only seen in animals that produced antibodies specific for sympathetic ganglia. The investigators ultimately decided that their model had limited value in understanding human acute autonomic neuropathy. However, it did show that autonomic tissues contained antigens that could be specifically targeted by the immune system.

Severe selective sympathectomy can be induced by treating newborn rats with antiserum against nerve growth factor (Brody 1964). Rats that survive show diffuse sympathetic failure including ptosis, miosis, and vasoconstrictor hypersensitivity to catecholamines. Ganglionic sympathetic neurons fail to develop normally. Adult rats treated with monoclonal antibodies against acetylcholinesterase also develop severe sympathetic failure (Brimijoin and Lennon 1990). The acetylcholinesterase antibodies appear to cause a permanent immunological destruction of preganglionic sympathetic nerves.

Animal models of autoimmune disorders associated with ion channel antibodies depend on either active or passive immunization. The sine quo non of antibody-mediated diseases is the ability to transfer the disease to a healthy animal by administering antibody (passive transfer). Patient IgG (or plasma) is injected intraperitoneally into mice or rats to achieve circulating antibody levels of 20–80% of those in the donor patients. The animals may not show overt signs of the disorder, but physiological investigations, either *in vivo* or on tissue preparations *in vitro*, demonstrate the appropriate abnormalities. For instance, mice treated repeatedly with IgG from patients with LEMS did not show obvious muscle weakness but had a marked reduction in the calcium channel dependent release of acetylcholine at the motor nerve terminals (Lang et al. 1981). In addition, parasympathetic transmission in the bladder and sympathetic cholinergic synaptic transmission in the vas deferens were subtly altered (Waterman et al. 1997). The lack of clinical autonomic involvement in the animals is likely due to the fact that other calcium ion channels can be upregulated to compensate for the loss of the P/Q-type channels, both at the neuromuscular junction and at autonomic synapses (e.g. Waterman et al. 1997).

Autoimmune autonomic ganglionopathy can be induced in mice by passive transfer of IgG from affected rabbits or humans (Vernino et al. 2004a). These mice show electrophysiological evidence of impaired ganglionic synaptic transmission due to a postsynaptic deficit (Wang et al. 2010). An animal model of experimental autoimmune autonomic ganglionopathy (EAAG) can also be induced in rabbits by immunization with the ganglionic acetylcholine receptor. Rabbits with EAAG manifest symptoms of chronic autonomic failure similar to those seen in AAG patients. Histological and electrophysiological studies of EAAG indicate that this autoimmune form of autonomic neuropathy is caused by an immune-mediated loss of ganglionic AChR and impairment in ganglionic synaptic transmission (Vernino et al. 2003, Lennon et al. 2003, Wang et al. 2007). EAAG recapitulates the clinical phenotype of human autoimmune autonomic neuropathy, including gastrointestinal dysmotility, dilated and poorly responsive pupils, decreased lacrimation, reduced heart rate variability, dilated bladder, reduced levels of plasma catecholamines, and hypotension (Vernino et al. 2003). As in patients with AAG, more severe autonomic dysfunction correlates with higher antibody levels (Vernino et al. 2003).

Summary

Autonomic dysfunction in patients with cancer is fairly common. Clinicians should be aware that peripheral autonomic neuropathy (especially enteric neuropathy) can occur as an autoimmune paraneoplastic phenomenon either in isolation or in combination with other syndromes. We now know that the autonomic nervous system can be the target of autoimmunity even in the absence of cancer. Autoimmune autonomic neuropathy (and its animal model) is an example of a severe, but potentially treatable, form of autonomic failure.

References

Andrew, T. and Nathan, P. (1964) Lesions of the anterior frontal lobes and disturbances of micturition and defecation. *Brain*, 233–262. **87**

Appenzeller, O., Arnason, B., Adams, R. (1965) Experimental autonomic neuropathy: An immunologically induced disorder of reflex vasomotor function. *JNNP*, **28**, 510–515.

Barber, P. A., Anderson, N. E., Vincent, A. (2000) Morvan's syndrome associated with voltage-gated K + channel antibodies. *Neurology*, **54**, 771–772.

Bohnen, N., Cheshire, W., Lennon, V., Berg, C. V. D. (1997) Plasma exchange improves function in a patient with ANNA-1 seropositive paraneoplastic autonomic neuropathy. *Neurology*, **48**, A131.

Brimijoin, S. & Lennon, V. A. (1990) Autoimmune preganglionic sympathectomy induced by acetylcholinesterase antibodies. *Proc. Nat. Acad. Sci.*, **87**, 9630–9634.

Brody, M. (1964) Cardiovascular responses following immunological sympathectomy. *Circ. Res.*, **15**, 161–167.

Candler, P. M., Hart, P. E., Barnett, M., Weil, R. & Rees, J. H. (2004) A follow up study of patients with paraneoplastic neurological disease in the United Kingdom. *JNNP*, **75**, 1411–5.

Chinn, J. S. & Schuffler, M. D. (1988) Paraneoplastic visceral neuropathy as a cause of severe gastrointestinal motor dysfunction. *Gastroenterology*, **95**, 1279–1286.

Condom, E., Vidal, A., Rota, R., Graus, F., Dalmau, J. & Ferrer, I. (1993) Paraneoplastic intestinal pseudo-obstruction associated with high titres of Hu autoantibodies. *Virchows Arch. A Pathol. Anat. Histopathol.*, **423**, 507–511.

De Giorgio, R., Bovara, M., Barbara, G., *et al.* (2003) Anti-HuD-induced neuronal apoptosis underlying paraneoplastic gut dysmotility. *Gastroenterology*, **125**, 70–9.

Feldman, E. L., Bromberg, M. B., Blaivas, M. & Junck, L. (1991) Acute pandysautonomic neuropathy. *Neurology*, **41**, 746–8.

Finestone, H. M. & Teasell, R. W. (1993) Autonomic dysreflexia after brainstem tumor resection. A case report. *Am J. Phys. Med. Rehab.*, **72**, 395–7.

Gibbons, C. H., Vernino, S. A. & Freeman, R. (2008) Combined immunomodulatory therapy in autoimmune autonomic ganglionopathy. *Arch. Neurol.*, **65**, 213–7.

Goldstein, D., Holmes, C., Dendi, R., Li, S.-T., Brentzel, S. & Vernino, S. (2002) Pandysautonomia associated with impaired ganglionic neurotransmission and circulating antibody to the neuronal nicotinic receptor. *Clin. Auton. Res.*, **12**, 281–285.

Goldstein, D. S., Holmes, C. & Imrich, R. (2009) Clinical laboratory evaluation of autoimmune autonomic ganglionopathy: Preliminary observations. *Autonomic Neuroscience-Basic & Clinical*, **146**, 18–21.

Graus, F., Delattre, J. Y., Antoine, J. C. (2004) Recommended diagnostic criteria for paraneoplastic neurological syndromes. *JNNP*, **75**, 1135–40.

Graus, F., Lang, B., Pozo-Rosich, P., Saiz, A., Casamitjana, R. & Vincent, A. (2002) P./Q type calcium-channel antibodies in paraneoplastic cerebellar degeneration with lung cancer. *Neurology.*, **59**, 764–6.

Hancock, B. W. & Naysmith, A. (1975) Vincristine-induced autonomic neuropathy. *Br. Med. J*, **3**, 207.

Hart, I. K., Maddison, P., Newsom-Davis, J., Vincent, A. & Mills, K. R. (2002) Phenotypic variants of autoimmune peripheral nerve hyperexcitability. *Brain.*, **125**, 1887–95.

Hart, R. G. & Kanter, M. C. (1990) Acute autonomic neuropathy. Two cases and a clinical review. *Arch. Int. Med.*, **150**, 2373–6.

Iodice, V., Kimpinski, K., Vernino, S., Sandroni, P. & Low, P. A. (2009) Immunotherapy for autoimmune autonomic ganglionopathy. *Autonomic Neuroscience-Basic & Clinical*, **146**, 22–5.

Irani, S. R., Alexander S., Waters P., *et al.* (2010) Antibodies to Kv1 potassium channel-complex proteins Leucine-rich, glioma inactivated 1 protein and Contactin-2-associated protein in limbic encephalitis, Morvan's syndrome and acquired neuromyotonia *Brain* in press

Josephs, K. A., Silber, M. H., Fealey, R. D., Nippoldt, T. B., Auger, R. G. & Vernino, S. (2004) Neurophysiologic studies in Morvan syndrome. *J Clin. Neurophysiol.*, **21**, 440–5.

Jun, S., Dimyan, M., Jones, K. D. & Ladabaum, U. (2005) Obstipation as a paraneoplastic presentation of small cell lung cancer: case report and literature review. *Neurogastroenterology & Motility*, **17**, 16–22.

Keime-Guibert, F., Graus, F., Broet, P., Rene, R., Molinuevo, J. L., Ascaso, C. & Delattre, J. Y. (1999) Clinical outcome of patients with anti-Hu-associated encephalomyelitis after treatment of the tumor. *Neurology.*, **53**, 1719–23.

Klein, C. M., Vernino, S., Lennon, V. A., *et al.* (2003) The spectrum of autoimmune autonomic neuropathies. *Ann. Neurol.*, **53**, 752–758.

Knowles, C. H., Lang, B., Clover, L., Scott, S. M., Gotti, C., Vincent, A. & Martin, J. E. (2002) A role for autoantibodies in some cases of acquired non-paraneoplastic gut dysmotility. *Scand. J Gastroenterol.*, **37**, 166–170.

Lambert, E. H. & Lennon, V. A. (1988) Selected IgG rapidly induces Lambert-Eaton myasthenic syndrome in mice: complement independence and EMG abnormalities. *Muscle and Nerve,* **11**, 1133–1145.

Lang, B., Newsom-Davis, J., Wray, D., Vincent, A. & Murray, N. (1981) Autoimmune aetiology for myasthenic (Eaton-Lambert) syndrome. *Lancet*, **2**, 224–226.

Lee, E. K., Maselli, R. A., Ellis, W. G. & Agius, M. A. (1998) Morvan's fibrillary chorea: a paraneoplastic manifestation of thymoma. *J Neurol. Neurosurg. Psychiatry*, **65**, 857–862.

Lennon, V. A., Ermilov, L. G., Szurszewski, J. H. & Vernino, S. (2003) Immunization with neuronal nicotinic acetylcholine receptor induces neurological autoimmune disease. *J Clin. Invest.*, **111**, 907–13.

Lennon, V. A., Kryzer, T. J., Griesmann, G. E., *et al.* (1995) Calcium-channel antibodies in the Lambert-Eaton syndrome and other paraneoplastic syndromes. *New Engl. J Med.*, **332**, 1467–1474.

Lennon, V. A., Sas, D. F., Busk, M. F., Scheithauer, B., Malagelada, J. R., Camilleri, M. & Miller, L. J. (1991) Enteric neuronal autoantibodies in pseudoobstruction with small-cell lung carcinoma. *Gastroenterology*, **100**, 137–142.

Lhermitte, F., Gray, F., Lyon-Caen, O., Pertuiset, B. F. & Bernard, P. (1980) [Paralysis of digestive tract with lesions of myenteric plexuses. A new paraneoplastic syndrome (author's transl)]. *Revue Neurologique*, **136**, 825–36.

Liguori, R., Vincent, A., Clover, L., *et al.* (2001) Morvan's syndrome: peripheral and central nervous system and cardiac involvement with antibodies to voltage-gated potassium channels. *Brain*, **124**, 2417–2426.

Liu, W., Fackler, W., Rice, T. W., Richter, J. E., Achkar, E. & Goldblum, J. R. (2002) The pathogenesis of pseudoachalasia: a clinicopathologic study of 13 cases of a rare entity. *American Journal of Surgical Pathology*, **26**, 784–8.

Lucchinetti, C. F., Kimmel, D. W. & Lennon, V. A. (1998) Paraneoplastic and oncologic profiles of patients seropositive for type 1 antineuronal nuclear autoantibodies. *Neurology.*, **50**, 652–7.

Maddison, P., Newsom-Davis, J., Mills, K. R. & Souhami, R. L. (1999) Favourable prognosis in Lambert-Eaton myasthenic syndrome and small-cell lung carcinoma. *Lancet*, **353**, 117–8.

Madrid, A., Gil-Peralta, A., Gil-Neciga, E., Gonzalez, J. R. & Jarrin, S. (1996) Morvan's fibrillary chorea: remission after plasmapheresis. *Journal of Neurology*, **243**, 350–3. 27

Morvan, A. (1890) De la choree fibrillaire. *Gazette hebdomadaire de médecine et de chirurgie*, 173–176.

Motomura, M., Johnston, I., Lang, B., Vincent, A., Newsom-Davis, J. (1995) An improved diagnostic assay for Lambert-Eaton myasthenic syndrome. *J Neurol. Neurosurg. Psychiatry.* **58**, 85–7

Newsom-Davis, J. & Mills, K. R. (1993) Immunological associations of acquired neuromyotonia (Isaacs' syndrome) Report of five cases and literature review. *Brain*, **116**, 453–469.

O'Neill, J. H., Murray, N. M. & Newsom-Davis, J. (1988) The Lambert-Eaton myasthenic syndrome. A review of 50 cases. *Brain*, **111**, 577–96.

Pardi, D. S., Miller, S. M., Miller, D. L., Burgart, L. J., Szurszewski, J. H., Lennon, V. A. & Farrugia, G. (2002) Paraneoplastic dysmotility: loss of interstitial cells of Cajal. *American Journal of Gastroenterology*, **97**, 1828–33.

Park, D. M., Johnson, R. H., Crean, G. P. & Robinson, J. F. (1972) Orthostatic hypotension in bronchial carcinoma. *Br. Med. J*, **3**, 510–1.

Pittock, S. J., Kryzer, T. J. & Lennon, V. A. (2004) Paraneoplastic antibodies coexist and predict cancer, not neurological syndrome. *Ann. Neurol.*, **56**, 715–9.

Rakocevic, G., Barohn, R., Mcvey, A. L., Damjanov, I., Vernino, S. & Lennon, V. (2003) Myasthenia gravis, thymoma, and intestinal pseudo-obstruction: a case report and review. *J Clin. Neuromusc. Dis.*, **5**, 93–95.

Rees, J. H., Hain, S. F., Johnson, M. R., *et al.* (2001) The role of [18F] fluoro-2-deoxyglucose-PET scanning in the diagnosis of paraneoplastic neurological disorders. *Brain*, **124**, 2223–31.

Sandroni, P., Vernino, S., Klein, C. M., Lennon, V. A., Benrud-Larson, L., Sletten, D. & Low, P. A. (2004) Idiopathic autonomic neuropathy: comparison of cases seropositive and seronegative for ganglionic acetylcholine receptor antibody. *Arch. Neurol.*, **61**, 44–8.

Schafer, K. H., Klotz, M., Mergner, D., Mestres, P., Schimrigk, K. & Blaes, F. (2000) IgG-mediated cytotoxicity to myenteric plexus cultures in patients with paraneoplastic neurological syndromes. *Journal of Autoimmunity*, **15**, 479–84.

Schroeder, C., Vernino, S., Birkenfeld, A. L., *et al.* (2005) Plasma exchange for primary autoimmune autonomic failure. *N Engl. J Med.*, **353**, 1585–90.

Shillito, P., Molenaar, P. C., Vincent, A., *et al.* (1995) Acquired neuromyotonia: evidence for autoantibodies directed against K + channels of peripheral nerves. *Ann. Neurol.*, **38**, 714–722.

Singer, W., Opfer-Gehrking, T. L., Mcphee, B. R., Hilz, M. J., Bharucha, A. E. & Low, P. A. (2003) Acetylcholinesterase inhibition: a novel approach in the treatment of neurogenic orthostatic hypotension. *JNNP*, **74**, 1294–8.

Sodhi, N., Camilleri, M., Camoriano, J. K., Low, P. A., Fealey, R. D. & Perry, M. C. (1989) Autonomic function and motility in intestinal pseudoobstruction caused by paraneoplastic syndrome. *Digestive Diseases & Sciences*, **34**, 1937–42.

Suarez, G. A., Fealey, R. D., Camilleri, M. & Low, P. A. (1994) Idiopathic autonomic neuropathy: Clinical, neurophysiologic, and follow-up studies on 27 patients. *Neurology*, **44**, 1675–1682.

Spinazzi, M., Argentiero, V., Zuliani, L., Palmieri, A., Tavolato, B., Vincent, A. (2008) Immunotherapy-reversed compulsive, monoaminergic, circadian rhythm disorder in Morvan syndrome. *Neurology.* **71**, 2008–10.

Vernino, S. & Lennon, V. A. (2002) Ion channel and striational antibodies define a continuum of autoimmune neuromuscular hyperexcitability. *Muscle and Nerve,* **26**, 702–707.

Vernino, S. & Lennon, V. A. (2004) Autoantibody profiles and neurological correlations of thymoma. *Clinical Cancer Research,* **10**, 7270–7275.

Vernino, S., Cheshire, W. P. & Lennon, V. A. (2001) Myasthenia gravis with autoimmune autonomic neuropathy. *Autonomic Neuroscience-Basic & Clinical,* **88**, 187–92.

Vernino, S., Ermilov, L. G., Sha, L., Szurszewski, J. H., Low, P. A. & Lennon, V. A. (2004a) Passive transfer of autoimmune autonomic neuropathy to mice. *J Neurosci.,* **24**, 7037–42.

Vernino, S., Low, P. A. & Lennon, V. A. (2003) Experimental autoimmune autonomic neuropathy. *J Neurophysiol.,* **90**, 2053–9.

Vernino, S., Low, P. A., Fealey, R. D., Stewart, J. D., Farrugia, G. & Lennon, V. A. (2000) Autoantibodies to ganglionic acetylcholine receptors in autoimmune autonomic neuropathies. *N Engl. J Med.,* **343**, 847–855.

Vernino, S., O'Neill, B. P., Marks, R. S., O'Fallon, J. R. & Kimmel, D. W. (2004b) Immunomodulatory Treatment Trial for Paraneoplastic Neurological Disorders. *Neuro-Oncology,* **6**, 55–62.

Viallard, J.-F., Vincent, A., Moreau, J.-F., Parrens, M., Pellegrin, J.-L. & Ellie, E. (2005) Thymoma-associated neuromyotonia with antibodies against voltage-gated potassium channels presenting as chronic intestinal pseudo-obstruction. *European Neurology,* **53**, 60–63.

Vincent, A. (2002) Unravelling the pathogenesis of myasthenia gravis. *Nature Reviews Immunology,* **2**, 797–804.

Vincent, A., Lang, B. & Newsom-Davis, J. (1989) Autoimmunity to the voltage-gated calcium channel underlies the Lambert-Eaton myasthenic syndrome, a paraneoplastic disorder. *Trends in Neurosciences,* 496–502.

Vincent, A., Bien, B. G., Irani, S. R., Waters, P. (2011) Autoantibodies associated with diseases of the CNS: new developments and future challenges. *Lancet Neurol.,* **10**(8), 759–72. Review.

Voltz, R., Carpentier, A. F., Rosenfeld, M. R., Posner, J. B. & Dalmau, J. (1999) P./Q-type voltage-gated calcium channel antibodies in paraneoplastic disorders of the central nervous system. *Muscle & Nerve,* **22**, 119–22.

Wang, Z., Low, P. A. & Vernino, S. (2010) Antibody-mediated impairment and homeostatic plasticity of autonomic ganglionic synaptic transmission. *Experimental Neurology,* **222**, 114–9.

Wang, Z., Low, P. A., Jordan, J., *et al.* (2007) Autoimmune autonomic ganglionopathy: IgG effects on ganglionic acetylcholine receptor current. *Neurology,* **68**, 1917–21.

Waterman, S., Lang, B. & Newsom-Davis, J. (1997) Effect of Lambert-Eaton myasthenic syndrome antibodies on autonomic neurons in the mouse. *Ann. Neurol.,* **42**, 147–156.

Yahr, M. D. & Frontera, A. T. (1975) Acute autonomic neuropathy. Its occurrence in infectious mononucleosis. *Arch. Neurol.,* **32**, 132–3.

Young, R., Asbury, A., Adams, R. & Corbett, J. (1969) Pure pandysautonomia with recovery. *Trans. Am. Neurol. Ass.,* **94**, 355–357.

Young, R. R., Asbury, A. K., Corbett, J. L. & Adams, R. D. (1975) Pure pan-dysautonomia with recovery. *Brain,* **98**, 613–636.

CHAPTER 53

Autonomic failure in diabetes

Michael Edmonds

Introduction

Autonomic neuropathy is an important complication of diabetes resulting in increased morbidity and mortality. Autonomic dysfunction is common although symptomatic autonomic neuropathy is rare. Thus diabetic autonomic neuropathy can take two forms: subclinical neuropathy, which is diagnosed by the presence of abnormal autonomic function tests, and symptomatic or clinical neuropathy, which presents with the classic signs and symptoms. Autonomic neuropathy can involve many systems, including cardiovascular, gastrointestinal, genitourinary, and respiratory systems. Autonomic neuropathy may also result in haemodynamic and structural abnormalities in the arterial system. Cardiovascular autonomic neuropathy represents the most serious complication. Although symptomatic autonomic neuropathy is rare, many patients with abnormal autonomic tests do not respond appropriately to cardiovascular stresses because of impaired autonomic reflexes and this leads to an approximately five-fold risk of mortality.

This chapter will be divided into the following sections:

- Epidemiology
- Pathogenesis
- Cardiovascular autonomic neuropathy
- Circulatory changes in neuropathy (peripheral vascular system and cerebrovascular system)
- Gastrointestinal autonomic neuropathy
- Genitourinary autonomic neuropathy
- Respiratory responses and arrests
- Sweating abnormalities
- Abnormalities of pupils
- Abnormal responses to hypoglycaemia
- Clinical associations of autonomic neuropathy
- Erythropoetin depletion in autonomic neuropathy
- Natural history and prognosis
- Management

Epidemiology

Prevalence data for diabetic autonomic neuropathy varies considerably from 1.6% to 90% depending on type of autonomic function tests used, populations examined, and type and stage of disease (Boulton et al. 2005). A prospective study has shown the prevalence of autonomic neuropathy in the EURODIAB IDDM Complications Study to be 36% when autonomic neuropathy was defined as an abnormality of at least one of two tests of autonomic function (changes in heart rate and blood pressure [BP] from lying to standing) (Kempler et al. 2002). The prevalence of impaired autonomic function tests was 54% in Type 1 and 73% in Type 2 diabetic patients who were drawn from the population-based Rochester Diabetic Neuropathy Study (Low et al. 2004). Rates of autonomic neuropathy as assessed by pupillary tests in adolescents were also similar in Type 2 compared with Type 1 (61% in Type 1 diabetes vs 57% in Type 2 diabetes) (Eppens et al. 2006). Although these studies indicate that autonomic impairment as assessed by autonomic function tests are common, symptomatic autonomic neuropathy is a rare but nevertheless devastating complication of diabetes mellitus, especially in Type 1 diabetic patients.

A distinct syndrome exists in young insulin dependent diabetic subjects in their twenties and thirties, often women, who develop symptomatic autonomic neuropathy often associated with Charcot joints and foot ulceration, and associated with grossly abnormal autonomic function tests, serious loss of thermal sensation, and increased peripheral blood flow (Fig. 53.1A and 53.1B). They demonstrate medial calcification of the arteries of the feet despite their youth, yet do not experience numbness of their feet, retaining normal light touch and near-normal vibration perception (Fig 53.2). The clinical manifestations are almost solely due to small nerve fibre damage. This striking syndrome is not rare, is highly destructive, and is clearly different from the commoner problem of numb, ulcerated feet (Winkler et al. 2000).

Pathogenesis

The cause of autonomic neuropathy is not fully understood. There may be multiple causative mechanisms including metabolic insult to nerve fibres, reduced blood supply, growth factor deficiency and autoimmune damage leading to the differing presentations of autonomic injury in diabetes (Schmidt 2002).

Exposure to hyperglycaemia remains the principle metabolic insult and an important risk factor for autonomic neuropathy. Studies have also stressed role of vascular factors in the pathogenesis of autonomic neuropathy. The EURODIAB IDDM Complications Study has shown a strong relationship between autonomic neuropathy and the presence of cardiovascular disease risk factors including cigarette smoking, total cholesterol:high-density lipoprotein (HDL)-cholesterol ratio, fasting triglyceride,

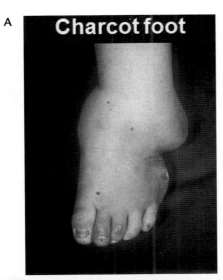

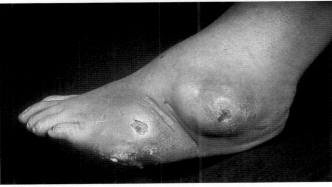

Fig. 53.1 Charcot foot showing deformity and ulceration.

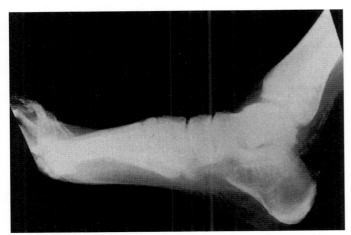

Fig. 53.2 Medial calcification in the arteries of a young, severely neuropathic, insulin-dependent diabetic.

diastolic BP and low HDL-cholesterol as well as confirming significant correlations between autonomic neuropathy and age, duration of diabetes and HbA1c. As a key finding, autonomic neuropathy was related to the presence of cardiovascular disease (Kempler et al. 2002). In the prospective part of the study, measurements were available for 956 participants who did not have evidence of cardiac

autonomic neuropathy at baseline. On follow-up, hyperglycaemia, hypertension, distal symmetric polyneuropathy and retinopathy, predicted the risk of autonomic neuropathy which developed in 163 (17%) subjects yielding an incidence of 23.4 per 1000 person-years.

Studies have suggested that loss of the neurotrophic effects of insulin and/or insulin-like growth factor-I (IGF-I) on sympathetic neurons rather than hyperglycaemia per se, may be crucial in the development of autonomic neuropathy (Schmidt et al. 2004). The sympathetic neuropathology developing in rat models of hypoinsulinaemic type 1 diabetes was compared with that in a hyperglycaemic and hyperinsulinaemic type 2 diabetes rat model. The hyperinsulinaemic rats developed neuroaxonal dystrophy (NAD), a distinctive distal axonopathy involving terminal axons and synapses, which represents the neuropathologic hallmark of diabetic sympathetic autonomic neuropathy. However, the hypoinsulinaemic rat, in comparison, failed to develop NAD in excess of that of age-matched controls. This argues that hyperglycemia alone is not sufficient to produce sympathetic ganglionic NAD, but rather that it may be the diabetes-induced superimposed loss of trophic support, likely of IGF-I, insulin, or C-peptide, that ultimately causes NAD.

Autoimmune factors may also be important. In an autopsy study of patients with symptoms of autonomic neuropathy, Duchen and colleagues found infiltration of lymphocytes, macrophages and plasma cells in and about autonomic nerve bundles and ganglia (Duchen et al. 1980). Immunological mechanisms might underlie symptomatic autonomic neuropathy. An association of severe autonomic deficit with iritis was initially described (Guy et al. 1984). Autoantibodies to autonomic nervous tissue structures including vagus nerve, cervical ganglion and adrenal medulla are a feature of patients with symptomatic diabetic autonomic neuropathy (Ejskjaer et al. 1998). Furthermore such antibodies have been shown to persist and in studies 2 years apart, there is a high degree of concordance of both positive and negative results (Cachia et al. 1997). Autoantibodies against sympathetic and parasympathetic nervous tissues are relatively specific for Type 1 diabetes. Indeed, autoantibodies against sympathetic nervous tissue in cardiac autonomic denervation have been described in Type 1 diabetes (Schsnell et al. 1996). However, in Type 2 diabetes, autoantibodies against autonomic nervous tissues showed no association with cardiac autonomic dysfunction (Schnell et al. 2000).

Further evidence to support the importance of autoimmunity has come from a long term 14 year study of autonomic function and the presence of auto antibodies in 41 patients with autonomic neuropathy (Granberg et al. 2005). A total of 56% of patients had antibodies to the autonomic nervous system including sympathetic ganglion, vagus nerve, or adrenal medulla. An index of autonomic neuropathy was 7.5 times more likely to become abnormal in patients who were autoantibody positive compared to those who were autoantibody negative. A further study investigated autonomic nervous function and the presence of autoantibodies to sympathetic and parasympathetic nervous structures, to glutamic acid decarboxylase (GAD) and tyrosine phosphatase (IA-2/ICA512) in 85 adolescents with insulin-dependent diabetes mellitus but no autonomic symptoms (Zanone et al. 1998). Only 7 patients (8%) had anti-vagus nerve autoantibodies, 7 other patients (8%) had anti-cervical ganglia autoantibodies, while all controls were negative (p < 0.05). Anti-adrenal medulla antibodies were detected in 16 patients (19%) and in 2 control subjects (p <0.02).

However, patients positive for one or more autoantibody showed a trend for lower values of deep breathing test and the 30:15 ratio test on standing, compared with healthy control subjects, which failed to reach conventional significance values (p = 0.17 and p = 0.07, respectively) There was no association between autoimmunity to nervous tissue structures and presence of GAD and IA-2/ICA512, and no correlation between these two autoantibodies and values of cardiovascular tests. Thus, it is not established whether antibodies to the autonomic nervous system are innocent bystanders or neurotoxins and whether they cause, contribute to or simply reflect nervous tissue damage (Vinik et al. 2005).

Cardiovascular autonomic neuropathy

Cardiac denervation

Heart rate variability

Resting tachycardia is an early sign of autonomic neuropathy. Depression of heart rate variability has been observed in autonomic neuropathy, heart transplantation, congestive heart failure, myocardial infarction myocardial ischaemia, and other cardiac and non-cardiac diseases. However, the clinical implication of heart rate variability analysis has been clearly recognized specifically in two clinical conditions (Tesfaye et al. 2010):

◆ as a predictor of risk of arrhythmic events or sudden cardiac death after acute myocardial ischaemia

◆ as a clinical marker of evolving diabetic neuropathy.

The demonstration of loss of heart rate variability during deep breathing indicates the presence of vagal denervation of the heart, which becomes increasingly common with the lengthening duration of diabetes. In population studies, decreased heart rate variability has had predictive value for mortality among healthy adults. It is a well-established risk factor for arrhythmic events and mortality among post-myocardial-infarction patients but has only moderate sensitivity and specificity (Stein and Kleiger 1999). It is thought that decreased parasympathetic innervation exposes the heart to unopposed stimulation by sympathetic nerves (Gorman and Sloan 2000).

Sympathetic and parasympathetic abnormalities

Cardiac denervation involves both parasympathetic and sympathetic fibres. Resting tachycardia due to parasympathetic damage may represent one of the earlier signs. Sympathetic denervation was thought to develop after parasympathetic changes had occurred, but newer techniques suggest that sympathetic changes might occur very early in the course of diabetes. The progress of diabetic cardiac parasympathetic dysfunction as reflected by loss of heart rate variability may parallel the impairment of sympathetic function as measured by of the uptake of radiolabeled analogues of noradrenaline, by the sympathetic nerve terminals of the heart (Stevens 2001). Quantitative scintigraphic assessment of the cardiac sympathetic innervation of the heart is possible with either iodine-123-meta-iodobenzyl guanidine (^{123}I-MIBG) and single photon emission computed tomography (SPECT) or carbon-11 hydroxyephedrine (^{11}C-HED) and positron emission tomography (PET). Deficits of left ventricular ^{123}I-MIBG and ^{11}C-HED retention have been identified in diabetic subjects without abnormalities on cardiovascular reflex testing indicating an increased sensitivity to detect cardiac autonomic neuropathy.

Several studies have shown an early sympathetic involvement before evidence of vagal neuropathy and ^{123}I-MIBG myocardial scintigraphy appears to be a useful diagnostic tool in the early detection and evaluation of the progression of myocardial sympathetic nerve dysfunction (Flotats and Carrió 2009). The finding of a higher than expected prevalence of MIBG regional abnormalities in patients without signs or symptoms of autonomic neuropathy suggests that cardiac autonomic nerve damage occurs earlier than previously thought in diabetic patients whose cardiovascular tests are still completely normal (Giordano et al. 2000). Deficits begin distally in the left ventricle and may extend proximally. Since this abnormality occurs in the inferior segment, an inferior-to-anterior count ratio, an index of regional MIBG uptake may be suitable for the evaluation of this condition (Hattori et al. 1996). However, the clinical significance and subsequent fate of small regional defects has not been fully established (Stevens et al. 1999). Impaired myocardial MIBG uptake correlates with altered left ventricle diastolic filling and myocardial electrophysiological deficits and is predictive of sudden death and recently MIBG myocardial scintigraphy has been shown to be useful for predicting cardiac events and long-term mortality in Type 2 diabetes (Nagamachi et al. 2006). However, it is not used routinely in the assessment of autonomic function (Scott and Kench 2004).

Left ventricular dysfunction

There is evidence of left ventricular (LV) dysfunction in particular diastolic dysfunction in patients with autonomic neuropathy (Willenheimer et al. 1998). LV diastolic dysfunction may be detected early in Type1 diabetic patients. Parasympathetic impairment and nocturnal elevations in BP could be the link between autonomic neuropathy and diastolic ventricular dysfunction (Monteagudo et al. 2000). Diastolic function is usually impaired first followed by systolic dysfunction (Irace et al. 1996). Type 1 diabetic patients with autonomic neuropathy have impaired LV filling pattern at rest, slightly increased LV systolic function, and a higher LV working load, in comparison to patients without autonomic neuropathy (Didangelos et al. 2003). Diabetic patients with autonomic neuropathy also have left ventricular hypertrophy (LVH) (Nishimura et al. 2004). Impaired parasympathetic activity, which indicates cardiovascular autonomic neuropathy, was also associated with the presence of LVH in diabetic patients on haemodialysis. The co-existence of cardiovascular autonomic neuropathy and LVH may be one of the key factors for the high incidence of cardiovascular events in these patients (Nishimura et al. 2004).

Decreased myocardial reserve

Diabetic autonomic neuropathy is also associated with an impaired vasodilator response of coronary resistance vessels to increased sympathetic stimulation, which is related to the degree of sympathetic neuropathy (Di Carli et al. 1999). There was a significant correlation between BP response to dipyridamole and myocardial perfusion reserve index. Type 1 diabetic patients with autonomic neuropathy have a decreased myocardial perfusion reserve capacity when challenged with a vasodilatator. The underlying mechanism may be defective myocardial sympathetic vasodilatation or a lack of ability to maintain BP during vasodilatation, or both (Taskiran et al. 2002). Patients with diabetic autonomic neuropathy do not have a normal hemodynamic response to exercise even in the absence of ischaemic heart disease. The responses of heart rate, BP and cardiac output to exercise are significantly impaired in diabetic patients with neuropathy (Vinik and Ziegler 2007).

Autonomic neuropathy and coronary heart disease risk

There is an association between autonomic neuropathy and increased coronary heart disease risk (Ziegler 1999). Tachycardia increases the risk of atherosclerosis (Beer et al. 1984). Additionally, distensibility of the vascular wall is reduced by tachycardia (Mangoni et al. 1996). Reduced heart rate variability is associated with increased progression of coronary atherosclerosis (Huikuri et al. 1999). In the EURODIAB Complications Study, autonomic neuropathy was related to the development of coronary artery disease in men (Soedamah-Muthu et al. 2004).

Indeed cardiovascular autonomic neuropathy may be a component of the metabolic syndrome. Autonomic neuropathy 5 years after diagnosis of Type 2 diabetes is associated with an unfavourable metabolic risk profile and parasympathetic neuropathy in Type 2 diabetic patients is associated with features of the insulin resistance syndrome (Gottsater et al. 1999). However, in a further study, autonomic neuropathy was associated with BP levels, but not with dyslipidaemia, smoking, or obesity (Spallone et al. 1997). Nevertheless, a high insulin level seems to have a predictive role in the development of parasympathetic autonomic neuropathy irrespective of obesity and glycaemia (Toyry et al. 1996b). Insulin resistance may be associated with altered balance between parasympathetic and sympathetic pathways (Lindmark et al. 2003). There may also be a link between hepatic parasympathetic denervation and insulin resistance (Takayama et al. 2000). Recently insulin resistance has been shown to be associated with both peripheral and autonomic neuropathy (Lee et al. 2012). Cardiovascular autonomic neuropathy is associated with platelet activation in Type 1 diabetes mellitus and this may reflect an increased prothrombotic state in diabetic cardiovascular autonomic dysfunction (Rauch et al. 1999). Furthermore, cardiovascular autonomic neuropathy is related to increased plasminogen activator inhibitor (Szelag et al. 1999).

Silent myocardial ischaemia

Asymptomatic coronary artery disease and myocardial infarctions are common in diabetic subjects. It is assumed that autonomic neuropathy is responsible for painless myocardial ischaemia and silent acute myocardial infarction but this is not proven and the association between autonomic neuropathy and silent myocardial ischaemia remains controversial. The increased incidence of asymptomatic myocardial infarctions and coronary artery disease in diabetic patients may reflect accelerated coronary atherosclerosis and the proportion of silent disease relative to symptomatic disease or episodes may not be increased in diabetes (Airaksinen 2001).

However, patients with silent myocardial ischaemia have a higher prevalence of autonomic neuropathy, hypertension, dyslipidemia and microalbuminuria than those without. In the Detection of Ischemia in Asymptomatic Diabetics (DIAD) study, silent myocardial ischemia occurred in greater than one in five asymptomatic patients with Type 2 diabetes and cardiac autonomic dysfunction was a strong predictor of ischaemia. Overall, 1123 patients with Type 2 diabetes, aged 50–75 years, with no known or suspected coronary artery disease were studied and a total of 113 patients (22%) had silent ischemia, including 83 with regional myocardial perfusion abnormalities and 30 with normal perfusion but other abnormalities (i.e. adenosine-induced ST-segment depression, ventricular dilation, or rest ventricular dysfunction). Moderate or large perfusion defects were present in 33 patients. The strongest predictors for abnormal tests were abnormal Valsalva (odds ratio [OR] 5.6), male sex (2.5), and diabetes duration (5.2). However, on follow-up over a 4.8-year period, the cardiac event rates were low and were not significantly reduced by screening for myocardial ischemia (Young et al. 2009).

Thus Type 1 and Type 2 diabetic patients with autonomic neuropathy and other cardiovascular risk factors may be at increased risk for silent myocardial ischemia. On a practical basis, autonomic neuropathy is independently associated with asymptomatic coronary artery disease. Thus patients may experience equivalents of angina such as breathlessness or fatigue. Silent myocardial ischaemia should be suspected in patients presenting with acute left ventricular failure, collapse, vomiting and ketoacidosis.

Cardiovascular morbidity and mortality

Autonomic neuropathy as assessed by decreased heart rate variability is an independent risk factor for mortality in diabetic patients (Pop-Busui et al. 2010). This may be due to autonomic neuropathy per se or associated co-morbidities. An evaluation of the independent contribution of cardiac autonomic dysfunction to mortality risk in a population-based sample of 487 individuals with Type 1 diabetes showed a four-fold higher mortality rate in those with cardiac autonomic neuropathy at baseline versus those without. (Orchard et al. 1996). However, after adjusting for baseline differences between the patients with and without neuropathy in markers related to nephropathy, coronary heart disease, duration of diabetes, and hypertension, the relative risk decreased from 4.03 to 1.37 and was no longer statistically significant.

However, in the Horn study of a glucose tolerance-stratified sample from a general population subjects with diabetes, impaired autonomic function was associated with an approximately doubled risk of mortality. The elevated risk was not observed in subjects without diabetes, hypertension, or prevalent cardiovascular disease (Gerritsen et al. 2001). The associations between autonomic neuropathy, and the risk of sudden cardiac death were studied among 462 diabetic patients (151 Type 1) enrolled in the Rochester Diabetic Neuropathy Study, and 21 cases of sudden cardiac death were identified over 15 years of follow-up (Suarez et al. 2005). Sudden cardiac death was correlated with atherosclerotic heart disease and nephropathy, and to a lesser degree with autonomic neuropathy and HDL cholesterol. Although autonomic neuropathy was associated with sudden cardiac death, it was thought unlikely to be its primary cause. However, autonomic neuropathy may contribute to excess mortality in patients after acute myocardial infarction (Whang and Bigger 2003).

The presence of heart rate variability is an independent risk factor for cardiovascular morbidity and mortality in Type 1 diabetic patients with nephropathy (Astrup et al. 2006). In patients with nephropathy, this was significantly associated with fatal and nonfatal cardiovascular disease after adjustment for cardiovascular risk factors. A meta-analysis of published data demonstrated that reduced cardiovascular autonomic function, as measured by heart rate variability, was strongly (i.e. relative risk is doubled) associated with increased risk of myocardial ischemia and mortality. The pooled relative risk for studies that defined cardiac autonomic neuropathy with the presence of two or more abnormalities was

3.45 (95% confidence interval [CI] 2.66–4.47; p < 0.001) compared with 1.20 (1.02–1.41; p = 0.03) for studies that used one measure (Vinik et al. 2003).

In asymptomatic diabetic patients, cardiac autonomic neuropathy appears to be a better predictor of major cardiac events than silent myocardial ischaemia. The risk linked to cardiac autonomic neuropathy appears to be independent of silent myocardial ischaemia but is highest when it is associated with silent myocardial ischaemia (Cosson et al. 2005). Furthermore, when the prognostic value of cardiac autonomic neuropathy was examined in relation to perfusion defects in diabetic patients with suspected coronary artery disease it remained a significant predictor of death and cardiac events after adjustment for perfusion defects (both p <0.02), and provided prognostic information incremental to that offered by perfusion defects alone (p <0.003 and p <0.006, respectively) (Lee et al. 2003). The actual mode of death is not fully established. Often they are sudden. Arrhythmias have been suggested as the heterogeneity of sympathetic innervation in response to injury is highly arrhythmogenic.

Blood pressure abnormalities

BP abnormalities include loss of circadian rhythm, postural hypotension, postprandial hypotension, and hypotension during anaesthesia.

Loss of circadian rhythm

Patients with autonomic neuropathy have disturbed circadian rhythms of BP (Spallone et al. 2003). They lose the normal diurnal BP variation in which night time BP is overall lower than that in the daytime, suggesting that there is a relative sympathetic overdrive due to predominantly parasympathetic impairment of cardiovascular innervation. This occurs both in both normotensive and hypertensive Type 2 patients with asymptomatic autonomic neuropathy. Monitoring BP over 24 hours confirms this flattening in nocturnal BP reduction at night and shows increased BP values (Ikeda et al. 1993). This may cause cardiac hypertrophy and is postulated as one possible cause of increased mortality (Jermendy et al. 1996). Patients in whom BP decreases during the night incur less damage to the brain, kidneys, heart, and blood vessels than people with elevated nocturnal BP (Izzedine et al. 2006).

Postural hypotension
Presentation
Maintenance of BP on standing depends on afferent impulses from baroreceptors (namely in the carotid sinus and aortic arch and on efferent sympathetic impulses to the heart and blood vessels.) Postural hypotension, that is a fall in systolic pressure of more 30 mm Hg on standing, occurs in diabetic subjects with advanced neuropathy, although symptoms are infrequent. Disabling hypotension when systolic pressure falls below 70 mmHg on standing is rare.

Blood flow studies show that the reduction in foot blood flow on standing observed in normal subjects is diminished in diabetic patients with postural hypotension, although significant vasoconstriction still occurs (Flynn et al. 1988). Another important mechanism is the failure of the splanchnic bed to vasoconstrict on standing. However, this was no worse than in diabetics without hypotension so that the importance of this mechanism in diabetic autonomic neuropathy remains uncertain (Watkins and Edmonds 1999).

Failure of cardiac acceleration and reduced cardiac output both contribute to the problems. Noradrenaline levels are generally reduced in diabetics with postural hypotension. An excess of noradrenaline is found in some patients with hypotension due to reduced intravascular volume rather than autonomic neuropathy. Failure of renin responses on standing, though probably not responsible for acute postural hypotension, may or may not be present. Anaemia may also contribute to postural hypotension as treatment with erythropoetin has been shown to improve the anaemia and postural hypotension.

Insulin is known to have cardiovascular effects (Yki and Utriainent 1998). It causes a reduction in plasma volume, an increase of peripheral blood flow from vasodilatation and an increase in heart rate. In patients with autonomic neuropathy, insulin may cause or exacerbate postural hypotension to the point of fainting whether it is given intravenously or subcutaneously, and occasionally a blackout may occur from hypotension and this may be confused with hypoglycaemia (Fig. 53.3). These effects of insulin are likely to be due to the insulin itself and not to changes in blood glucose concentration.

Both hypotension and its symptoms fluctuate spontaneously to a remarkable degree and may persist for many years without necessarily deteriorating (Sampson et al. 1990). The explanation is unclear although insulin itself may partly be responsible for exacerbating the condition and fluid retention may improve it (Zoccali 2000).

Management
Few patients develop symptoms sufficiently severe to need treatment. When they do, it is first essential to stop any drugs that exacerbate hypotension notably diuretics, tranquillizers and antidepressants. Simple treatment should always be tried and include raising the head of the bed and wearing full length elastic stockings but the benefits are slight. Mild symptoms may respond to raising the head of the bed about 10 cm, which helps to maintain postural vascular tone. Observations on insulin dependent diabetic patients established that while food causes a large increase in mesenteric blood flow the latter does not coincide with an exacerbation of their hypotension (Purewal and Watkins 1995).

Measures that increase plasma volume are the most effective, although oedema is a troublesome side-effect that renders the treatment unacceptable. A high salt uptake or fludrocortisone

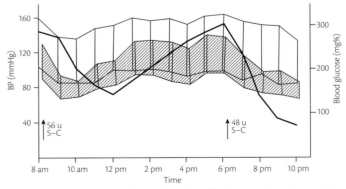

Fig. 53.3 Diurnal variation of lying and standing blood pressure in a 48-year-old man with severe autonomic neuropathy. Insulin was given subcutaneously (S–C) at times shown by the vertical arrows. The unhatched area shows supine blood pressure, the hatched area the standing blood pressure, and the continuous line the blood glucose.

sometimes in high doses up to 0.4 mg daily can be effective. It acts by increasing peripheral vascular tone and extracellular fluid and blood volume.

The use of an orally active adrenergic agonist midodrine can help and can be given in addition to fludrocortisone. It has an exclusively peripheral pressor effect on arterial and venous capacitance vessels. The dose should be titrated from 2.5 mg to 10.0 mg three times a day to reduce the risk of an exaggerated pressor response due to denervation supersensitivity (Freeman 2005). In a small number of patients octreotide is of value in the treatment of postural hypotension in diabetic autonomic neuropathy

Intranasal administration of an antidiuretic agent such as desmopressin (DDAVP) can improve symptomatic postural hypotension by reducing nocturnal diuresis. Recombinant human erythropoietin administered subcutaneously to anaemic autonomic neuropathy patients increases standing BP (Winkler et al. 2001). However, in a recent pharmacosurveillance study, the most common therapy was midodrine followed by a combination of midodrine and fludrocortisone (Pathak et al. 2005).

Many other treatments have been suggested. Their effectiveness is inconsistent. Some regimes are hazardous and supine hypertension is a common sequel and these treatments include beta blockers with partial agonist activity such as pindolol and the use of caffeine, non-steroidal anti-inflammatory drugs, clonidine and metoclopramide. Ergotamine may be considered in refractory cases of postural hypotension. In a recent case report, a patient who failed to respond to non-pharmacological measures, fludrocortisone, midodrine, octreotide, erythropoietin and increased caffeine intake was eventually commenced on half a Cafergot suppository (giving him a dose of ergotamine 1 mg and caffeine 50 mg). This resulted in dramatic clinical improvement (Toh et al. 2006).

Postprandial hypotension

In diabetic patients with autonomic neuropathy, postprandial hypotension may also occur and there is a concordance of postprandial hypotension with cardio-vascular autonomic neuropathy (Trofimiuk et al. 2003). The fall in BP is attenuated when gastric emptying and small intestinal carbohydrate absorption are slowed by dietary (e.g. guar) or pharmacological (e.g. acarbose) means (Gentilcore et al. 2006).

Hypotension during anaesthesia

In diabetes, severe hyopotension can occur during anaesthesia as a consequence of cardiovascular autonomic neuropathy. There is a significant relationship between heart rate variability preoperatively and BP stability during anaesthesia induction (Knüttgen et al. 2005). Diabetic patients may require more intra-operative BP support by vasosupressor drugs. (Bruckner et al. 2005). Cardiorespiratory arrests have been reported perioperatively in diabetic subjects and there is increased intraoperative morbidity in diabetic patients with autonomic neuropathy (Burgos et al. 1989).

Cardiovascular autonomic function tests

Bedside cardiovascular tests have been developed which indicate the presence or absence of autonomic neuropathy (Table 53.1). Their use to exclude the condition is at least as important as its confirmation; the tests are extremely sensitive, and as many as one-fifth of all diabetic patients have one or more abnormalities, while only rarely suffering from symptomatic autonomic neuropathy.

When symptoms such as diarrhoea or gastroparesis occur, autonomic tests must be abnormal, and other conditions excluded, before they can be attributed to diabetic autonomic neuropathy. It has been suggested that patients should be screened for cardiac autonomic neuropathy either at time of diagnosis in type 2 diabetes or within 5 years after diagnosis of type 1 diabetes (unless an individual has symptoms suggestive of autonomic dysfunction earlier). Early measurement of heart rate variation can serve as a baseline from which interval tests can be compared (Manzella and Paolisso 2005).

The tests fall into 4 groups:

- simple non-invasive cardiovascular reflex tests
- spectral analysis of heart rate variation
- measurement of baroreflex sensitivity
- measurement of QT interval.

Simple non-invasive cardiovascular reflex tests

Beat-to-beat variation of heart rate has been used to assess dysfunction of the vagal nerve for many years. The most commonly used battery of non-invasive tests includes heart rate response to deep breathing, heart rate response to standing and Valsalva manoeuvre and BP fall on standing. A further test was designed to evaluate BP changes during sustained hand grip.

These tests form the core of diagnosis of cardiac autonomic neuropathy. They are validated, reliable and reproducible. They correlate with each other and with tests of peripheral somatic nerve function. Computerized systems are available to make the performance of the tests easier and to improve the analysis of results during tests on the changes of heart rate. The computer programme measures the length of individual R-R intervals with immediate display of the results. Age-specific and sex-specific reference values for a wide range of different autonomic function measures in an elderly population are also available (Gerritsen et al. 2003).

Spectral analysis of heart rate variability

The development of power-spectrum analysis has facilitated the diagnosis of autonomic neuropathy. Heart rate variation can be assessed in the time domain (by statistical analysis of R-R intervals) and the frequency domain (by spectral analysis of a series of successive R-R intervals). ECG recordings are made for at least 5 minutes to allow spectral analysis to be carried out. However, the optimum duration of the tracing is 10 minutes. Where there are

Table 53.1 Normal values for autonomic function

Test	Normal	Borderline	Abnormal
Heart rate variation on deep breathing (beats/minute)	> 15	11–14	< 10
Heart rate increase on standing, at 15 seconds (beats/minute)	> 15	13–14	< 12
Heart rate increase on standing, 30:15 ratio	>1.04	1.01–1.03	< 1.00
Valsalva ratio	> 1.21	-	<1.20
Postural systolic pressure fall at 2 minutes (mmHg)	< 10	11–29	> 30

These tests decline with age. The figures given here generally apply in those less than 60 years of age.

slow fluctuations in heart rate a prolonged 24-hour recording is necessary (Kempler 2002).

In the time domain, the simplest parameter is the standard deviation of R-R intervals, whereas the most commonly used indices are the mean calculated from the differences of consecutive R-R intervals and the number of R-R intervals recorded over a period where the difference of consecutive R-R intervals exceeds 50 ms. Heart rate variation can also be measured in the frequency domain. Plotting the length of the R-R interval against time produces a periodic curve which can be broken down in to different wave components. These are characterized by their frequency (range) and amplitude representing a given power. Three frequency components are usually measured:

◆ a high frequency (HF) component, which is a reflection of respiratory sinus arrhythmia and is an index of vagal activity

◆ a low frequency (LF) component reflecting vasomotor activity and is dependent on both sympathetic and vagal tone

◆ a very low frequency (VLF) band representing the influence of the peripheral vasomotor and renin-angiotensin system (Stein and Kleiger 1999).

Diabetic autonomic neuropathy is associated with a reduction of heart rate variation. Both the LF and HF components diminish before the onset of clinical neuropathy. This suggests similar damage to both sympathetic and parasympathetic pathways of the heart. Heart rate variation in long-term diabetes using 24-hour ambulatory recordings is abnormal and reproducible over a 12-month interval with very little variation in all heart rate variation parameters, especially in those of parasympathetic activity (Burger et al. 1997).

Twenty four hour assessments of heart, including spectral analysis, compare favourably with conventional tests (Takase et al. 2002). In a study that performed four cardiovascular tests of autonomic function (deep breathing, lying to standing, Valsalva manoeuvre, postural hypotension) and simultaneous 24-hour recordings of BP and electrocardiography (ECG), the significant correlation of day–night pattern of BP and sympathovagal activity to standard cardiovascular reflex tests, supported the usefulness of 24-hour BP monitoring and spectral analysis of heart rate variability in diabetic neuropathy (Spallone et al. 1996).

In conclusion, spectral analysis of heart rate variation appears a convenient method to assess various degrees of diabetic autonomic dysfunction: it appears easy to perform, while giving results similar to traditional methods, with greater sensibility (Spallone et al. 2011).

Measurement of baroreflex sensitivity

The arterial baroreflex maintains the stability of BP. Changes in BP lead to stimulation of the baroreceptors which activates cardiac vagal fibres and sympathetic outflow to the heart and the peripheral blood vessels. Vagal tone is maintained by reflex mechanisms which are activated by continuous input from baroreceptors. Thus baroreflex sensitivity can be measured from the reflex heart rate response to changes in BP. A change in BP can be induced pharmacologically or the spontaneous fluctuations of BP in steady state conditions may be used (Jermendy et al. 1996).

Thus, short non-invasive recording of the BP and R-R interval signals are taken in the supine patient, i.e. under conditions suitable for routine outpatient evaluation. The baroreflex sensitivity is

determined by the regression analysis of changes induced in the length of R-R interval by spontaneous fluctuations in BP.

Baroreflex sensitivity is impaired in diabetes and its measurement is helpful in the early detection of cardiac autonomic neuropathy (Frattola et al. 1997). After myocardial infarction the analysis of baroreflex sensitivity has a significant prognostic value independent of left ventricular ejection fraction and ventricular arrhythmias, and it significantly adds to the prognostic value of heart rate variation.

In conclusion, these estimates of baroreceptor function may provide a powerful tool for assessing cardiovascular autonomic neuropathy at any stage, including the early stage, which is not detected by conventional tests (Ziegler et al. 2001).

Measurement of the QT interval

The length of the QT interval is influenced by autonomic nervous tone. A long QT interval may reflect imbalance between right and left heart sympathetic nerve activity. Electric instability reflected by abnormally long QT intervals increases the risk of severe abnormal rhythms and sudden death. This was first described with the long QT syndrome. A prolonged QT interval due to autonomic neuropathy can be seen in a proportion of patients with Type I diabetes. The length of the QT interval (QTc) is dependent on heart rate. Therefore a corrected QT interval must be obtained by dividing the QT length measured in seconds with the square root of the length R-R interval. QTc values above 440ms are considered abnormal. QTc prolongation is associated with major degrees of autonomic neuropathy (Tentolouris et al. 1997). In a cohort-based prospective study, QTc prolongation was predictive of increased mortality in Type 1 diabetic patients (Veglio et al. 2000).

The usefulness of the QTc interval is under debate. A meta-analysis concluded that QTc prolongation is a specific albeit insensitive indicator of autonomic failure (Whitsel et al. 2000). Other data suggest that in Type 1 diabetic patients, QT abnormalities can occur independently of autonomic dysfunction or myocardial ischaemia and may be related to the processes which increase urinary albumin leakage (Earle et al. 2000). Experimental hypoglycaemia in adults with Type 1 diabetes causes an abnormal ECG, with increases in QT interval (Heller 2002). When cardiac repolarization was studied during clamped hypoglycaemia in patients with Type 1 diabetes, with and without autonomic neuropathy, there was lengthening of QTc during hypoglycaemia in all groups with no significant differences between the groups, suggesting that autonomic dysfunction did not contribute to hypoglycaemia-induced QTc lengthening in Type 1 diabetes (Lee et al. 2004).

QT dispersion (QTd) may be more important than the measurement of QT interval length (Kumhar et al. 2000). QT dispersion is the difference between the longest and shortest QT intervals recorded by the 12-lead ECG. Increasing QT dispersion reflects electrical instability of the left ventricular musculature. In normoalbuminuric Type 1 diabetic patients, increased QTc dispersion was associated with reduced nocturnal fall in BP and an altered sympathovagal balance (Poulsen et al. 2001). However, in EURODIAB IDDM STUDY, prevalence of QTd prolongation was associated with ischaemic heart disease and diastolic BP but not neuropathy. Although QTd was statistically related to duration of QTc, increased QTd and increased QTc identified different patients (Veglio et al. 2002). Age-adjusted QTd interval was not different between patients with Types 1 and 2 diabetes. Cardiac autonomic neuropathy was not associated with QTd interval in both types of diabetes. Furthermore, microalbuminuria was found to be the strongest predictor of QTd in patients with Type 2 diabetes (Psallas et al. 2006).

A further study in type 2 diabetes, assessed the cardiac autonomic influences on QT indices using the measurements of baroreflex sensitivity, heart rate variability, and cardiac ^{123}I-meta-iodobenzyl guanidine scintigraphic findings and showed that baroreflex sensitivity negatively correlated with the maximum and minimum QTc intervals as well as QT/QTc dispersion (Takahashi et al. 2004). However, the high-frequency power and the ratio of low-frequency power to high-frequency power of heart rate variability did not correlate with any QT indices. The percentage washout rate of ^{123}I- meta-iodobenzyl guanidine positively correlated with QT/QTc dispersion, but not with maximum and minimum QTc intervals. This indicated that cardiac vagal dysfunction was related to QT interval prolongation while both sympathetic and vagal dysfunctions were related to increased QT dispersion in Type 2 diabetic patients.

Circulatory changes in neuropathy

Blood flow and vascular responses

Sympathetic denervation causes loss of vasoconstricter tone and peripheral vasodilatation, associated with opening of arteriovenous shunts. Skin blood flow increases substantially and this can occur in the absence of other clinical evidence of neuropathy. These blood flow changes explain some of the clinical features of the neuropathic foot notably the excessively warm skin, bounding pulses and marked venous distension. The venous PO2 is increased because of arteriovenous shunting. Capillary pressure is increased and may contribute to neuropathic oedema, which can occasionally be severe and sometimes reversed by administration of ephedrine. However, nutritive capillary blood flow is not compromised by shunting and has been shown directly by television microscopy to be normal or even increased (Korzon-Burakowska and Edmonds 2006).

Blood flow responses to various stimulae are also abnormal. Sympathetic stimulation by coughing or standing normally induces peripheral vasoconstriction. Neuropathic patients show blunting of these responses. Maximal vasodilatation in response to heating is reduced. Although this defect is partly attributable to the effects of hyperglycaemia on the microvasculature, failure of nitric oxide dependent smooth muscle vasodilatation in neuropathy has been described in diabetic foot patients (Pitei et al. 1997).

Increased blood flow in the neuropathic foot may sometimes be related to the presence of pain and a reduction of blood flow can be associated with diminution of pain in these cases. Bone blood flow is also elevated in these patients and this is thought to contribute to the osteopenia that predisposes to the development of Charcot joints particularly in Type 1 diabetic patients (Petrova et al. 2005).

Structural changes

Sympathetic denervation of the peripheral arterial system may occur quite early in the evolution of neuropathy and has major effects on blood flow and vascular responses and causes structural changes in the arterial wall (Edmonds 2004). Vascular sympathetic denervation can lead to degeneration of the smooth muscle of arteries leading to medial arterial calcification and stiffening

of the arteries. (Fig. 53.2) This calcification may assume the histological characteristics of bone.

Unilateral lumbar sympathectomy in humans, both in diabetics and non-diabetics, has been shown to result in medial wall calcification on the ipsilateral side (Goebel and Fuessl 1983). Unilateral sympathectomy in animals leads to excess deposition of cholesterol on the operated side and the occurrence of cholesterol sclerosis in the rabbit's aorta was accelerated by removal of the coeliac ganglion (Harrison 1938). Furthermore, in animal models, denervation of smooth muscle leads to striking pathological changes, including atrophy of muscle fibres with foci of degeneration (Kerper and Collier 1926). Arterial calcification is initiated within senescent atrophic smooth muscle (Morgan 1980).

Medial arterial calcification in the Pima Indians is significantly associated with an increased prevalence of cardiovascular mortality (Everhart et al. 1988). Medial calcification may be an important factor in the development of peripheral vascular disease, which in diabetes shows a predilection for the distal arteries below the knee and is unexplained. Chantelau reported an association of below knee atherosclerosis to medial arterial calcification (Chantelau et al. 1995).

Type 2 diabetes is associated with a significant reduction in the elastic properties of the aorta and duration of diabetes and presence of cardiac autonomic neuropathy were the main predictors of aortic distensibility (Tentolouris et al. 2003). In women, with Type 1 diabetes there is a correlation between increased aortic stiffness and parasympathetic dysfunction and increased arterial stiffness may be of importance in the increased susceptibility to cardiovascular complications in diabetic women (Ahlgren et al. 1999). In Type 1 diabetes, one third of patients have coronary artery calcification which is linked to both cardiac autonomic neuropathy and retinopathy (Thilo et al. 2004).

Thus autonomic neuropathy by causing sympathetic denervation can lead to calcification and stiffening of the arteries. This can predispose to loss of arterial elasticity and abnormal flow, which results in injury to the endothelium and predisposes to atherosclerosis. The influence of peripheral autonomic neuropathy in predisposing to stiffening of the peripheral arteries may provide an explanation for the distal distribution of the atherosclerosis.

Cerebrovascular diseases

Diabetic patients are at increased risk for cerebrovascular disease when compared to non-diabetic patients. Strokes are a significant source of morbidity and mortality and autonomic neuropathy is a significant independent risk factor for the occurrence of stroke. This may occur due to accelerated cerebral vascular damage and alterations in the regulation of cerebral blood flow in diabetic patients with autonomic neuropathy (Cohen et al. 2003). In Type 2 diabetic patients, autonomic neuropathy predicts the development of stroke in patients with non-insulin-dependent diabetes mellitus (Toyry et al. 1996a). Patients with cardiovascular autonomic neuropathy and orthostatic hypotension show instability in cerebral blood flow upon standing (Mankovsky et al. 2003) and autonomic neuropathy is associated with impairment of dynamic cerebral autoregulation in type 1 diabetes (Nasr et al. 2011).

Although autonomic neuropathy is recognized as an independent risk factor for stroke in diabetes, the mechanism by which autonomic nerves are involved in this pathology is unknown. Perivascular nitrergic nerves around the cerebral arteries degenerate in two phases in streptozotocin-induced diabetic rats. In the first phase, perivascular nitrergic nerve fibers remain intact while they lose their neuronal nitric oxide synthase content. This phase is reversible with insulin treatment. In the second phase, nitrergic cell bodies in the ganglia are lost via apoptosis in an irreversible manner. Throughout the two phases, irreversible thickening of the smooth muscle layer of cerebral arteries is observed. Thus nitrergic degeneration in diabetic cerebral arteries may be the link between diabetic autonomic neuropathy and stroke (Cellek et al. 2005).

Cardiovascular autonomic neuropathy is associated with atherosclerosis and narrowing of the carotid artery (Gottsater 2003). To clarify the associations between cardiovascular autonomic neuropathy and the progression of carotid artery atherosclerosis in Type 2 diabetic patients, cardiovascular autonomic nerve function and carotid artery ultrasound were carried out in 61 Type 2 diabetic patients, 5 years and 8 years after the diagnosis of diabetes. Cardiovascular autonomic neuropathy was linked with the degree of carotid atherosclerosis, which, in the carotid bulb, might affect baroreceptor function with the progression of Type 2 diabetes (Gottsater et al. 2005). In a follow-up study, autonomic dysfunction as measured by heart rate variation was associated with the extent and progression of carotid atherosclerosis in Type 2 diabetes (Gottsater et al. 2006).

Gastrointestinal autonomic neuropathy

Oesophageal problems

Abnormal oesophageal motility has been described but no definite symptoms have been attributed to this functional abnormality as autonomic damage to the upper gastrointestinal tract is often asymptomatic.

Gastroparesis

Pathogenesis

The pathogenesis of abnormal upper gastrointestinal sensory-motor function in diabetes is not fully understood and is likely to be multifactorial in origin. Diabetic autonomic neuropathy as well as hyperglycaemia has been shown to impair motor and sensory function. Morphological and biomechanical remodeling of the gastrointestinal wall occurs throughout the duration of diabetes, and may contribute to motor and sensory dysfunction (Zhao et al. 2006). Slow emptying and increased distal retention have been shown to be significantly associated with autonomic neuropathy (Stacher et al. 2003).

There is also evidence of smooth muscle degeneration, characterized by subtotal smooth muscle cell atrophy in the muscularis propria associated with transformed smooth muscle cells undergoing a form of necrobiosis, appearing as highly distinctive, homogeneous, round eosinophilic bodies. Since vagal degeneration does not normally cause gut smooth muscle degeneration these changes might represent an independent gastromyopathic process as the cause of gastroparesis (Watkins 1998). The molecular pathophysiology of diabetic gastroparesis is unknown, limiting the development of rational therapies. Animal studies point to a defect in the enteric nervous system as a major molecular cause of abnormal gastric motility in diabetes. This defect is characterized by a loss of nitric oxide signals from nerves to muscles in the gut resulting in delayed gastric emptying (Smith and Ferris 2003).

Presentation

Gastric emptying can be normal, accelerated or retarded in patients with diabetes (Phillips et al. 2006, Zhao et al. 2006), although gastric stasis is a feature of autonomic neuropathy (Stacher 2001). This sometimes, though rather surprisingly not always, causes vomiting (Watkins 1998) although radionuclide studies to measure gastric emptying indicate delay in 30–50% of outpatients with long-standing Type 1 (Ziegler et al. 1996) or Type 2 diabetes (O'Donovan et al. 2003). Symptomatic gastroparesis is a rare diabetic complication. The vomiting may be due to vagal denervation of the stomach. Studies have demonstrated the loss of myelinated and unmyelinated fibres in the vagus nerve.

Investigation

The diagnosis is difficult to establish and three approaches are needed. First, other obstructive causes should be excluded by endoscopic and barium studies, secondly the presence of gastric stasis needs to be established to detect decreased or absent peristalsis and thirdly, the presence of abnormal autonomic function should be demonstrated. Most patients with this complication suffer from other symptoms of autonomic neuropathy.

Gastric stasis must be confirmed by radio isotopic studies, using anterior and posterior cameras to exclude artefacts from stomach movements during the test. Liquids, solids and indigestible solids are emptied by the stomach at different rates and by different mechanisms. Radioisotope studies in diabetics with autonomic neuropathy have variously shown normal solid emptying, impairment of the usual differentiation between solid and liquid emptying, abnormal liquid emptying and abnormal solid and liquid emptying. Abnormal liquid emptying probably represents advanced disease. The 13C-octanoic acid breath test may be used to measure disordered gastric emptying in diabetics due to its highly significant positive correlation to scintigraphy (Zahn et al. 2003). Diabetic subjects complicated with cardiovascular autonomic neuropathy and dyspepsia may be at high risk of *Helicobacter pylori* infection and should be investigated and considered for eradication therapy (Gulcelik et al. 2005), although a previous report concluded that *H. pylori* infection was not associated with delayed gastric emptying or upper gastrointestinal symptoms in diabetes (Jones et al. 2002).

Management

Glycaemic control should be optimized as hyperglycaemia per se can delay gastric emptying. Prokinetic agents such as dopamine antagonists (metoclopramide and domperidone) enhance gastric tone and emptying. They may accelerate gastric emptying in diabetic autonomic neuropathy. Intravenous erythromycin (3 mg/kg every 8 hours) causes a substantial acceleration of gastric emptying. Oral administration may be used but is less effective in alleviating symptoms. Anti-emetic agents may also be used such as the serotonin (5-HT3) receptor antagonist (e.g. ondansetron). The very rare cases of intractable vomiting from gastroparesis may require more invasive treatment. Vomiting should be sufficiently severe to cause recurrent hospital admissions over a considerable period of time, since occasionally it may remit spontaneously even after an interval of as long as 2 years (Dowling et al. 1985).

The introduction of percutaneous endosocopic jejunostomy may benefit patients in the short term. This may alleviate the problem until a natural remission of vomiting occurs even after protracted periods of time. Sometimes a more definitive procedure is required and a two-thirds gastrectomy with Roux-en-Y loop anastomosed 60 mm from the gastric stump has proved to be successful (Ejskjaer et al. 1999). Gastric electrical stimulation otherwise known as gastric pacing has recently emerged as an effective strategy in the management of these patients as has the use of botulinum toxin to control symptoms of gastroparesis (Tang and Friedenberg 2011). The long-term outlook for patients, who have symptomatic gastroparesis and who have generally suffer multiple diabetic complications is poor (Watkins et al. 2003). However, patients with abnormal gastric emptying tests but not necessarily symptoms have a better prognosis (Kong et al. 1999).

Diabetic diarrhoea

Presentation

Diarrhoea is a very disagreeable symptom of autonomic neuropathy. Borborygmi and discomfort precede attacks of watery diarrhoea without pain or bleeding and usually without malabsorption. Faecal incontinence is common, especially at night, when exacerbations seem to be worse. Symptoms last from a few hours to a few days and then remit, with normal bowel action or even constipation (sometimes induced by treatment in between attacks).

Intermittent attacks of diabetic diarrhoea tend to persist over many years and rarely remit completely. Very few patients suffer almost continuous diarrhoea for which no other cause is discovered and they are very difficult to treat. The underlying cause of diabetic diarrhoea is not established. Gut denervation probably alters gut motility and bacterial overgrowth has been demonstrated in these cases. Thus gastroparesis might result in maldigestion of disaccharides and result in malabsorption of bile acids which may in turn cause diarrhoea. Neuromuscular dysfunction might cause a shortened transit time and there may be a secretory diarrhoea.

Investigation

Full investigation of diarrhoea in a diabetic patient is crucial in order not to overlook easily treatable causes such as coeliac disease which may be increased in Type I patients, pancreatic malabsorption or other rarer causes. Autonomic function tests should be abnormal otherwise autonomic diarrhoea is very unlikely and normal tests virtually exclude this as a cause. Nevertheless the presence of abnormal autonomic function is not alone sufficient to lead to a diagnosis of diabetic diarrhoea and may thus be very deceptive. The diagnosis is most likely to be correct in long-standing Type I patients with other autonomic symptoms such as gustatory sweating and postural hypotension.

Treatment

Tetracycline offers effective treatment in approximately half the patients and is given in one or two doses of 250mg at the onset of the attack, which is abruptly aborted. If this fails, a range of the anti-diarrhoea remedies could be tried, notably codeine phosphate, lomotil or loperamide. Clonidine reduces propulsive contractions and restores sympathetic tone and the long acting somatostatin analogue octreotide, which suppresses gastrointestinal mobility, may be useful in intractable diarrhoea

Various methods have been used to treat faecal incontinence ranging from relaxation, biofeedback techniques to surgical reconstruction of the anal sphincter. They are only partially successful. Control of associated diarrhoea often helps.

Gallbladder

Enlargement of the gallbladder, probably due to poor contraction, may be a feature of diabetes related to autonomic neuropathy. Studies by ultrasonography have not confirmed the enlargement of the gallbladder, but do suggest impaired muscular contraction. There are no known clinical effects from this.

Genitourinary autonomic neuropathy

Bladder dysfunction

Presentation

Autonomic neuropathy affecting the sacral nerves causes bladder dysfunction (Stief and Ziegler 2003). Bladder function tests are commonly abnormal in neuropathic diabetic patients but symptoms from neurogenic bladder in diabetes are relatively rare, usually occurring in diabetic patients who already have advanced complications. Most men with neurogenic bladder are also impotent.

Impairment of bladder function is chiefly the results of neurogenic detrusor muscle abnormality, while pudendal innervation of perineal and peri-urethral striated muscle is usually unaffected in diabetic neuropathy. Afferent damage results in impaired sensation of bladder filling and leads to detrusor areflexia. Thus the bladder pressure during cystometrography fails to increase as the bladder is filled. In advanced cases, bladder emptying is reduced because of impaired detrusor activity and possibly failure of the internal sphincter to open adequately. Measurements of urine flow show that the peak flow rate is reduced and that duration of flow is increased.

There are no symptoms in the early stages but later patients experience hesitancy during micturition, develop the need to strain, a feeble stream and a tendency to dribble. Micturition is sometimes in short, interrupted spurts which result from straining. Patients may be aware of lengthening intervals between micturition and also experience a sensation of inadequate bladder emptying. Gradually residual urine volume increases and in severe cases, gross bladder retention occurs with abdominal swelling and sometimes overflow incontinence as well. Bladder capacity may exceed one litre.

Investigation

Diagnosis of neurogenic bladder is usually possible especially in those patients with clinical evidence of severe neuropathy. It is important, however, to exclude bladder neck obstruction and especially prostatic obstruction in men. Ultrasound examination before and after emptying should be performed and cystoscopy is usually needed. Rarely diabetic neurogenic bladder causes hydroureter and hydronephrosis. Occasionally more sophisticated bladder function tests are needed. These include cystograms, cystometrography and urine flow rate measurements.

Treatment

The principles of treatment are to compensate for a deficient bladder sensation and thus prevent the development of a high residual urine volume. For those diabetic patients who have symptoms of cystopathy, education is important and may suffice. In particular the patient should be told to void every three hours during the daytime. Manual suprapubic pressure can increase the efficiency of bladder emptying. With more severe symptoms more active measures are needed. Pharmacotherapy has a limited place in treating detrusor areflexia. Bethanechol may be helpful in chronic states of of detrusor atony. An alpha I adrenoceptor blocker may help by reducing urethral resistance. Self-catherization three times daily is the recommended treatment for patients with chronic retention. Recurrent urinary tract infections are often troublesome in those patients and protracted courses of antibiotics changing monthly may be needed to prevent this problem.

Impotence

Presentation

The cause of impotence is probably multifactorial. Autonomic neuropathy is important (Carson et al. 2004). However, impotence in diabetes may be primarily due to endothelial dysfunction. It may also be due to vascular occlusions of the branches of internal pudendal artery. Furthermore in rare cases, erectile failure may be caused by Leriche syndrome.

Erectile dysfunction is often associated with atherosclerotic diseases, such as coronary heart disease, stroke, peripheral vascular disease. An association between erectile dysfunction and asymptomatic coronary artery disease angiographically verified has been shown in diabetic patients (Koppiker et al. 2003).

Several pathophysiological mechanisms may explain the relationship between erectile dysfunction and atherosclerosis including a common pattern of cardiovascular risk factors, the presence of autonomic neuropathy and endothelial dysfunction. Thus erectile dysfunction may be a marker of silent or early atherosclerotic diseases.

Neuropathic impotence is due to erectile failure resulting from damage to both parasympathetic and sympathetic innervation of the corpora cavernosa. VIPergic nerves are also important in the vasodilatation of erection and the concentration of vasoactive intestinal peptide (VIP) is low in the penile corpora in diabetics with autonomic neuropathy. Failure to achieve erection may also be the result of a concomitant sensory deficit in the dorsal nerve of the penis. The onset of neuropathic impotence is usually gradual, progressing slowly over months, but complete erectile failure is usually present within 2 years of the onset of symptoms. This history contrasts with psychogenic impotence, which begins suddenly and in which nocturnal erections are present.

The diagnosis of neuropathic impotence is diabetes is difficult. The use of intracavernosal injections of prostaglandin E1 (PGE1) is to some extent helpful in distinguishing neurogenic from vasculogenic impotence—it causes an erection in the former and fails to do so in the latter. This is helpful both in terms of diagnosis and in giving guidance in the choice of treatment. For centres with particular interest, other techniques are available. Thus it is possible to record nocturnal penile tumescence and rigidity during sleep. The absence of tumescence and rigidity over three successive nights is a strong indication of an organic cause of impotence. Vasculogenic impotence can be confirmed by a measurement of penile BP and by comparing it with the brachial systolic pressure thereby achieving a penile-brachial. When the ratio of penile to brachial pressure is 0.75 or less the diagnosis of penile vascular disease can be considered. Autonomic function tests give some guidance as the presence of autonomic neuropathy but they do not establish conclusively in an individual that it is the cause of impotence. A neuropathic cause can be more exactly defined by electophysiological testing of reflex

sexual pathways. Conduction velocity is reduced in the dorsal nerve of the penis in diabetic impotent patients and latency of the bulbocavernosus reflex is prolonged.

Treatment
Early intervention
Despite the availability of many treatments for impotence, early intervention and prevention by improved glycemic control and general reduction of associated risk factors should be stressed because many of the diabetes-related complications leading to impotence are irreversible (Koppiker et al. 2003).

Stop medications causing impotence
Medications associated with erectile dysfunction should be stopped if possible. These include anti-hypertensive drugs, diuretics, vasodilators, beta-blockers, angiotensin-converting enzyme (ACE) inhibitors and calcium-channel blockers, and antidepressants—both tricyclics and monoamine oxidase inhibitors.

Counselling
If the history reveals a psychological component, then the patient and his partner may be helped by appropriate discussion and advice. Counselling is always needed, especially if the impotence is psychogenic in origin. Neuropathic impotence is, however, permanent and there is no cure. This needs to be understood to eliminate suspicion and mistrust. Proper explanation often suffices and many seek no further treatment. Androgen treatment is contraindicated unless there is evidence of its deficiency because it merely serves to increase libido without restoring potency.

Oral pharmacological agents
The introduction of sildenafil (Viagra) has revolutionized the treatment of erectile dysfunction (Goldstein et al. 1998). Sildenafil produces a natural erectile response to sexual stimulation by enhancing the relaxant effect of nitric oxide on the corpora cavernosa. Nitric oxide is the pivotal neurotransmitter involved in the relaxation of the corpus cavernosal smooth muscle. It acts through a second messenger system involving guanylate cyclase. This enzyme converts guanosine triphosphate (GTP) into intracellular cyclic guanosine monophosphate (cGMP), a potent second messenger for smooth muscle relaxation. Detumescence is caused by sympathetic vasoconstrictor activity and the enzyme breakdown of cGMP by phosphodiesterase type 5 (PDE 5), which exists principally in the corpora cavernosa (Rendell et al. 1999).

Sildenafil is a selective inhibitor of GMP-specific PDE5 and therefore enhances the normal vasodilatory erectile mechanisms. The therapeutic window is up to 4 hours after administration of the single dose. Recommended dose is 50 mg taken approximately 60 minutes before sexual activity. It should be taken no more than once daily. The dose may be increased to 100 mg or reduced to 25 mg depending on its effect.

Sildenafil has peripheral vasodilatory properties and this results in modest decreases in BP in some patients, which is consistent with its known effects on the nitric oxide cGMP pathway. Sildenafil is contraindicated in patients using nitrates such as glyceryl trinitrate or nitric oxide donors such as sodium nitroprusside. It is contraindicated in patients with significant cardiac disease (Jackson et al. 1999).

Other phosphodiesterase inhibitor drugs available include tadalafil and vardenafil. For patients taking tadalafil, the duration of the therapeutic window of effectiveness is at least 24 hours in 80% of men. It has a rapid tissue distribution but a half-life of 17.5 hours. These characteristics potentially reduce the need for planning associated with most other treatments for erectile dysfunction but they are contraindicated in those taking nitrates. A study has also investigated the effect of a p38 MAPK inhibitor on penile neurovascular function in streptozotocin-induced diabetic mice; p38 MAPK inhibition corrected nitric oxide-dependent indices of diabetic erectile autonomic neuropathy and vasculopathy, and this therapeutic approach may result in further treatments for impotence (Nangle et al. 2006).

Vacuum devices

Erection can be induced by application of a partial vacuum to the penis after venous occlusion. This is applied with a specially designed reusable condom with a vacuum pump attached (Bosshardt et al. 1995). It is non-invasive, but the apparatus is cumbersome and relatively expensive. A vacuum is applied to the penis for a few minutes, causing tumescence and rigidity, which are sustained using a constricting ring at the base of the penis, but trabecular smooth muscle relaxation does not occur. By this mechanism, blood is simply trapped in both the intracorporal and extracorporal compartments of the penis. Many different devices are now manufactured. They all have three common components; a vacuum chamber, a pump and a constriction band that is applied to the base of the penis once an erection is achieved.

Intrcavernosal therapy

Direct injection of a vasodilator into the corpus cavernosum is a satisfactory treatment. Papavarine is a powerful direct smooth muscle relaxant that acts on both the trabecular muscle of the erectile tissue and the vascular tone inducing an erection that lasts for several hours. When vasoactive drugs were introduced papavarine was initially the most widely used agent for intracorporal self-injection. If papavarine alone fails, then combination therapy with phentolamine and papavarine may be beneficial. Phentolamine acts directly on the α-adrenoceptors of the vascular smooth muscle and potentiates the effects of papavarine.

However, prostaglandin E_1 (as alprostadil) is the most widely used agent and has become the drug of choice for intracavernous pharmacotherapy. PGE1 plays a natural role as a neurotransmitter in the natural erectile mechanism and alprostadil is as least as effective in treating erectile dysfunction as combination therapy with papavarine and phentolamine and has fewer side-effects. The recommended starting dose is 1.25 μg for patients with neurogenic impotence. The skin is drawn taught and the needle and syringe held at right angles. The injection is given near to the base of the penis on either side and avoiding any visible veins. Injection sites should be varied. After starting with a small dose the patient should titrate this upwards under medical supervision until a satisfactory erection lasting not more than 1 hour is achieved. The chief hazard is from a sustained erection (i.e. lasting more than 4 hours), which can lead to permanent damage if it is not treated promptly. Patients must be given written instructions: if vigorous exercise fails to reduce the erection, they should receive emergency treatment consisting of aspiration of blood and phenylephrine injection, which leads to prompt detumescence. Failure to achieve detumescence after 6–8 hours can cause irreversible ischaemic damage to the corpora cavernosa with subsequent fibrotic damage and permanent loss of erectile function. Other long-term problems are sepsis and

penile fibrosis, but these occur infrequently. Papavarine, phentolamine and alprostadil have a low rate of leakage into the systemic circulation.

Intraurethral therapy

Alprostadil has been developed for insertion into the urethra as a pellet through a specific polypropylene applicator. Once delivered, the pellet dissolves into the urethral mucosa and from there it enters the corpora. In a comparative study of intracavernosal and intraurethral application of alprostadil, the intracavernosal administration was shown to be more effective though there was a slightly higher incidence of local side-effects than with the intraurethral route of administration (Linet and Ogring 1996). It would seem that while the intraurethral route of administraton is associated with a lower overall success rate, the improved side-effect profile and acceptability to patients makes it a preferred option for some patients.

Surgical treatment

Surgical treatment of erectile dysfunction is usually reserved for patients in whom more conservative therapy has failed or for whom conservative therapy is contraindicated. Most of these patients will have significant arterial or venous disease. Surgically implantable penile prostheses are classified as either semi-rigid or inflatable. The simplest technique is the insertion of a malleable silastic rod which is often effective especially when ejaculation is retained. Semi-rigid rod devices were the first prostheses designed to restore erectile function and are used extensively More elaborate inflatable prostheses can be inserted but the apparatus is more complex, prone to failure and very expensive. Although the incidence of postoperative complications has decreased markedly, mechanical malfunction can still occur with any of the penile prosthetic devices. Another potential complication is infection (Carson 1999).

Respiratory responses and arrests

Autonomic neuropathy may be responsible for spontaneous respiratory arrest and unexplained sudden death. In most of these episodes there was some interference with respiration either by anaesthesia, drugs or bronchopneumonia. These episodes are transient and while temporary ventilation may be needed recovery to normal health is expected. Anaesthetists need to be forewarned of this possibility when patients with symptomatic autonomic neuropathy require even minor surgery.

These observations have led to further investigation of the respiratory system of diabetics with autonomic neuropathy and this falls into three parts.

- Control of ventilation in response to hypoxia with hypocapnia
- Pattern of respiration during sleep
- Bronchial reactivity to chemical and physical agents.

Control of ventilation in response to hypoxia with hypocapnia

The integrity of the ventilatory responses in autonomic neuropathy has been studied by measuring responses to hypoxia and hypercapnia in diabetic patients with and without neuropathy. Most studies have found a defective response to hypoxia in autonomic neuropathy (Scionti and Bottini 2003). The results regarding responses to hypercapnia have been conflicting in that both normal, ventilatory and reduced responses have been detected. Thus the true importance of abnormal ventilatory responses as a cause of respiratory arrest has yet to be established.

Pattern of respiration during sleep

Sleep apnoea has been reported in Type I diabetes, occasionally in association with autonomic neuropathy. (Rees et al. 1981). Heart rate responses to apnoeic episodes may be abnormal. Uncertainty still exists however, and in the study of Catterall et al. (1984) there was no evidence for sleep apnoea in diabetics with autonomic neuropathy. However, in a large group of diabetic patients of patients suffering from autonomic neuropathy 26% had obstructive sleep apnoea and none of the patients without autonomic neuropathy showed any breathing abnormalties (Ficker et al. 1998).

Bronchial reactivity to chemical and physical agents

The third area of study has assessed the integrity of respiratory reflexes, which affect bronchomotor tone. Airway tone is mainly under vagal control and is reduced in diabetics with autonomic neuropathy leading to diminished bronchodilatation in response to anticholinergic agents. Diabetics with autonomic neuropathy also show a degree of bronchoconstriction during inhalation of cold air and even more strikingly a diminished or even absent cough reflex in response to an inhaled irritant such as citric acid (Vianna et al. 1988) (Fig. 53.4). These deficits are due to neuropathic denervation and not to any intrinsic abnormality in bronchial smooth muscle which responds normally to direct stimulation by inhaled histamine. The perception of respiratory sensations in diabetic patients has also been measured in patients breathing through a tube manifold apparatus with resistance to airflow that was randomly varied. Diminished perception or respiratory resistance loads occurred in diabetics with neuropathy and this may render the patient prone to subclinical episodes of respiratory illness. Neuroadrenergic bronchopulmonary denervation may occur in diabetic patients with autonomic neuropathy despite normal clinical and respiratory function findings (Antonelli et al. 2002).

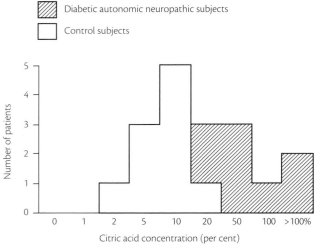

Fig. 53.4 Cough responses to inhaled citric acid in normal subjects and diabetics with severe autonomic neuropathy. The response may be impaired or even absent in autonomic neuropathy.

Sweating abnormalities

Peripheral

The sweat gland is an important structure with a complex peptidergic as well cholinergic innervation. Neuropeptide immunoreactivity especially of vasoactive intestinal polypeptide is low in diabetic sudomotor nerves (Levy et al. 1989). Measurement of sweating in the periphery is one of the few quantitative methods for assessing cholinergic nerve function.

There are various methods for studying sweat responses. The thermoregulatory sweat test involves whole body heating and sweating is detected by the application of alizarin red powder. This method assesses peripheral sympathetic function both preganglionic and postganglionic. The quantitative sudomotor axon reflex test (QSART) stimulates sweating by iontophoresis of acetylcholine and assesses postganglionic sympathetic function by the axon reflex. Direct stimulation of sweat glands either by iontophoresis of pilocarpine and counting sweat droplets on a silastic imprint, or by acetylcholine injection and counting iodine starch sweat spots assesses postganglionic sweat gland denervation. The sympathetic skin response (SSR) is a potential generated by a change in the electrical resistance of the skin, caused by activity of the sweat glands innervated by sympathetic sudomotor fibres. The potential difference between electrode plates placed on opposite surfaces of the foot is measured (Nazhel et al. 2001).

Studies of sympathetic peripheral neuropathy suggest that QSART can evaluate early diabetic neuropathy more precisely than SSR (Shimada et al. 2001). More important than differences in sensitivity is the specificity of QSART, which evaluates the postganglionic axon (instead of polysynaptic pathways in SSR) and provides quantitative data on the severity and pattern of autonomic deficit. Peripheral sympathetic adrenergic and cholinergic fibres simultaneously undergo early alterations in diabetic patients, even when there is no clinical neuropathy (Cacciatori et al. 1997). There is a close relationship between sudomotor and vagal cardiac neuropathy. This may reflect a C-fibre directed selectivity of the pathological process in autonomic diabetic neuropathy (Spitzer et al. 1997).

The most common sweating abnormality in diabetic neuropathy is in the feet, in the classic stocking distribution. Loss of sweating causes dryness of the feet and cracked skin, which might serve as a portal of entry for infection as a part of the pathogenesis of diabetic foot problems. Patients with diabetic neuropathy typically have decreased sweating in the feet but excessive sweating in the upper body. Redistribution of sudomotor responses is an early sign of sympathetic dysfunction with decreased sweating in the feet and increased sweating in the upper body (Hoeldtke et al. 2001).

Gustatory sweating

Gustatory sweating is a highly characteristic and not uncommon symptom of diabetic autonomic neuropathy. Sweating begins soon after starting to chew tasty food, especially cheese. It starts on the forehead, and spreads to involve the face, scalp, and neck, and sometimes the shoulders and upper part of the chest, compelling patients to keep a towel at the dinner table. Distribution of the sweating is in the territory of the superior cervical ganglion. It may be of sudden onset; its cause is unknown, although aberrant nerve regeneration has been suggested. It is occasionally sufficiently severe to need treatment. Gustatory sweating, once established, generally persists over many years although there can be remarkable and unexplained remission after renal transplantation.

Gustatory sweating is occasionally sufficiently severe to need treatment. (Fig. 53.5) Anticholinergic drugs are highly effective although side-effects may limit their use. Poldine methylsulphate is the best agent, and propantheline bromide can also be used. They are given half an hour before meals, but may also be effective if given before single meals at social occasions. The use of glycopyrrolate cream has been described made from glycopyrrolate powder and made into a cream using a standing cream base called Cetamacrogol normally at 0.5%, but 1% or 2% may be more effective. The cream is applied on alternate days to the areas affected by sweating, avoiding contact with the mouth, nose and eyes. The area must not be washed for 4 hours after application. The only contraindication known is narrow angle glaucoma which might be exacerbated if the eye is accidentally contaminated.

Some neuropathic patients complain of drenching night sweats requiring a change of clothes and bed clothes, and not precipitated by hypoglycaemia. This symptom is unexplained and rare.

Abnormalities of pupils

The pupil receives a substantial sympathetic and parasympathetic innervation and has been extensively studied as a visible mirror of autonomic denervation (Smith and Smith 1999). Pupillary autonomic neuropathy is an early sign of the development of systemic autonomic neuropathy and can be detected before the onset of cardiac autonomic neuropathy (Pittasch et al. 2002).

In diabetic neuropathy, various abnormalities have been reported. These include a decrease in pupil size, greater than

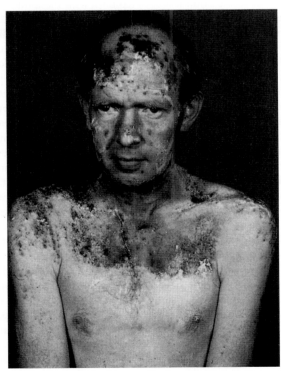

Fig. 53.5 Severe facial and shoulder sweating (gustatory sweating) seen a few minutes after eating cheese. The area of sweating is clearly delineated by the application of quinazarine powder which turns blue when moist.

expected for age; slowness to redilate after constricting to light; and a diminished light reflex amplitude. Hippus (i.e. the natural oscillatory movement of the pupil), is reduced in patients with neuropathy (Hreidarsson 1992). Finally, there is evidence of denervation hypersensitivity in the exaggerated response to directly acting sympathomimetic agents. Most of these observations require sophisticated apparatus with which to measure them, and they have not generally been adapted for bedside tests.

Abnormal responses to hypoglycaemia

Hypoglycaemia is a powerful stimulus of autonomic function causing sweating, tremor, tachycardia and an increase of pulse pressure with a notable rise of systolic BP. There are also major circulatory and endocrine changes in response to hypoglycaemia. Glucagon, adrenaline, noradrenaline, pancreatic polypeptide, somatostatin, adrenocorticotropic hormone (ACTH), growth hormone, and corticosteroids all increase in response to hypoglycaemia. The presence of autonomic neuropathy prevents the stimulated increase of pancreatic polypeptide and possibly of somatostatin while responses of the remaining hormones are unaffected beyond the diminished responses which occur anyway in long-term Type 1 diabetes regardless of the presence of neuropathy, notably for glucagon and adrenaline.

Loss of warning of hypoglycaemia has been attributed to autonomic neuropathy and in long-standing diabetes with duration over 20 years, autonomic neuropathy has been associated with an irreversible loss of adrenaline response to hypoglycaemia and impairment of autonomic symptoms (Bottini et al. 1997). However, studies in Type I patients of more than 15 years with and without loss of warnings of hypoglycaemia showed equal proportions of autonomic damage in the two groups. Furthermore patients with established autonomic neuropathy have similar autonomic and neuroglycopaenic symptoms to those without autonomic neuropathy (Hepburn et al. 1990, Frier 1993). The Diabetes Control and Complications (DCCT) study also showed a lack of relationship between loss of warning in those with tight control and the presence of autonomic neuropathy. (The Diabetes Control and Complications Trial Research Group 1993). The concept however that diminished autonomic symptoms and counter-regulatory changes may occur as a result of reduced central nervous system responses to hypoglycaemia has gained substantial support but these changes are independent of the presence or absence of autonomic neuropathy itself.

Although loss of warning of hypoglycaemia has been attributed to autonomic neuropathy, the phenomenon occurs chiefly in those subjected to repeated hypoglycaemia and can be reversed (Cranston et al. 1994). In this so-called hypoglycemia-associated autonomic failure, recent hypoglycaemia can lead to defective glucose counterregulation by reducing the adrenaline response to subsequent hypoglycemia in the background of an absent glucagon response and hypoglycemic unawareness by reducing the autonomic sympathetic neural and adrenomedullary response and therefore the neurogenic symptom responses to subsequent hypoglycaemia (Cryer 2002).

This leads to a vicious cycle of recurrent iatrogenic hypoglycaemia. Avoidance of iatrogenic hypoglycemia reverses hypoglycemia unawareness and improves the reduced adrenaline component of defective glucose counterregulation in most affected patients. The main factor regulating the magnitude of hypoglycemia associated autonomic failure is antecedent duration and frequency of hypoglycemia, but prior episodes of exercise, and autonomic neuropathy may also be important (Diedrich et al. 2002). Autonomic responses to hypoglycemia are further reduced during sleep in patients with type 1 diabetes and because of their reduced sympathoadrenal responses, these patients are substantially less likely to be awakened by hypoglycemia (Banarer and Cryer 2003).

The use of beta-blockers can, however, cause abrupt loss of warning of hypoglycaemia in delayed metabolic recovery. This occurs infrequently, perhaps in as few as one in 50 patients on beta-blockers, yet when it occurs it is dramatic and potentially dangerous and patients should always be warned of this hazard.

Clinical associations of autonomic neuropathy

Nephropathy

There is evidence of a link between autonomic neuropathy and nephropathy in that there is an association of 24-hour cardiac par-asympathetic activity and degree of nephropathy and the urinary albumin in Type 1 patients (Molgaard et al. 1992). The urinary albumin excretion rate is independently related to subclinical auto-nomic neuropathy in Type 2 diabetes (Wirta et al. 1999). Cardiovascular autonomic neuropathy and higher resting BP are both associated with microalbuminuria in older patients with Type 2 diabetes in agreement with the hypothesis that cardiovascular autonomic neuropathy and BP are linked to microalbuminuria by different biological pathways (Moran et al. 2004). In prospective studies, autonomic neuropathy and abnormal postural diastolic BP falls at baseline were associated with future renal complications (Forsen et al. 2004). Marked abnormalities in heart rate variability are significantly associated with and predictive of progressive renal deterioration at 1 year (Burger et al. 2002). The remarkable co-variation of degree of neuropathy and nephropathy has suggested a common pathogenetic mechanism. Furthermore, the reduced 24-hour vagal activity, even in the early stages of nephropathy, could be an important risk factor for cardiac death in insulin-dependent diabetic patients.

Retinopathy

In a study of risk factors for early onset proliferative retinopathy in insulin dependent diabetes, a striking relationship with cardiovas-cular autonomic neuropathy was found (Krolewski et al. 1992). In a further study of Type 1 diabetic patients with proteinuria, cardiac autonomic neuropathy was notably demonstrated in patients suf-fering from proliferative retinopathy (Zander et al. 1992). Cardiac autonomic neuropathy is thus significantly associated with the presence of retinopathy: an impairment of autonomic peripheral blood flow control might be a contributing factor in the formation of microvascular lesions (Valensi et al. 1997).

Erythropoietin depletion in autonomic neuropathy

Renal erythropoietin production is stimulated chiefly by the presence of anaemia and hypoxia. However, sympathetic innnervation of the kidney appears to have a modulating influence and renal den-ervation leads to a reduction of stimulated erythropoiesis due to a decreased reduction of erythropoietin. Studies of human auto-nomic neuropathy with postural hypotension including some patients with diabetes have demonstrated erythropoietin depletion.

Diabetic autonomic neuropathy may cause both anaemia and diminished erythropoietin production in patients without renal impairment (Winkler et al. 1999). Certainly, an erythropoietin-deficient anaemia is recognized in Type 1 diabetic patients with early nephropathy and symptomatic autonomic neuropathy. Diabetic patients with autonomic neuropathy have inappropriately low erythropoietin levels for the severity of their anaemia but they can mount an appropriate erythropoietin response to moderate hypoxia (Bosman et al. 2002). Recently, an early abnormality of erythropoietin regulation in Type 2 diabetes has been described before clinical nephropathy and this points to a contributory role of autonomic neuropathy in erythropoietin dysregulation (Spallone et al. 2004). The mechanism underlying the erythropoietin-deficient anaemia present in some diabetic patients remains unclear. The high incidence of low-production anaemia found in diabetic patients with autonomic neuropathy provides a rationale for the use of recombinant erythropoietin as a therapeutic trial for those in whom impaired erythropoietin production is documented. The goal is not only to reverse the anaemia, which is usually mild, but also to treat orthostatic hypotension (Jacob et al. 2003). Administration of erythropoietin may improve symptomatic postural hypotension.

Natural history and prognosis

Autonomic function tests have been used to detect early changes in the natural history and abnormalities can be detected in children Studies in diabetic children have shown that heart rate variation analysis can detect early subclinical alterations of the autonomic nervous system in asymptomatic patients with Type 1 diabetes, which seem to consist mainly of a parasympathetic impairment. Autonomic dysfunction is associated both with the duration and an inadequate metabolic control of the disease (Chessa et al. 2002). Neurological abnormalities were also demonstrable in a small pro-portion of diabetic children, who were younger than the rest of the population at the time of onset of their disease (Karavanaki and Baum 1999).

Autonomic function declines with age but in diabetes it deterio-rates on average faster than in normal subjects. Thus heart rate variation which normally decreases at approximately one beat per minute per 3 years declines three times faster in diabetic patients although there is substantial variation. Most patients who develop abnormal autonomic function do not become symptomatic. Established symptoms of autonomic neuropathy including diarrhoea, vomiting from gastroparesis and postural hypotension run a very protracted though intermitting course and rarely become disabling even over the 10–15 years during which these patients have been seen. Postural hypotension fluctuates substantially with corresponding variation in intensity of symptoms. Type 2 dia-betic patients with abnormal autonomic function tests have increased mortality, and patients with both abnormal autonomic tests and postural hypotension have higher mortality than those without (Chen et al. 2001). Gustatory sweating also tends to persist without remission although many patients describe disappearance of this symptom after renal transplantation.

Mortality of asymptomatic patients with autonomic dysfunction may be increased but the prognosis is generally good with 90% of patients (all under 50 years old) still alive 10 years later (O'Brien et al. 1991). (Fig. 53.6). In contrast, the outcome for those with

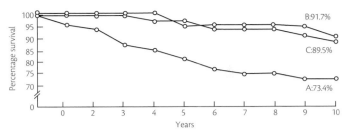

Fig. 53.6 Calculated 10-year survival (per cent) in groups A (symptomatic autonomic neuropathy; *n* = 49), B (abnormal heart rate variation; *n* = 24), and C (asymptomatic normal heart rate variation; *n* = 38). (From Sampson et al. (1990).)

symptomatic autonomic neuropathy is not as good, although even in this group 73% were still alive after a decade. Ewing and Clark described a poorer prognosis although patient selection was different (Ewing and Clarke 1986). The patients were older and some had renal damage. Those with postural hypotension appeared to have the highest mortality perhaps because of a premature development of left ventricular hypertrophy. Most deaths of these patients were from renal failure or myocardial infarction.

Although autonomic neuropathy is clearly associated with increased mortality, this may be explained by associations with complications (e.g. nephropathy) and increased cardiovascular risk factors (e.g. hypertension) (Orchard et al. 1996). In a study that investigated the incidence rate and potential predictors for cardiovascular autonomic neuropathy in a cohort of childhood-onset type 1 diabetic patients (subjects from the Epidemiology of Diabetes Complications Study), nephropathy was a significant risk factor for cardiac autonomic neuropathy and this association may explain some of the increased mortality (Stella et al. 2000).

As well as increased mortality, autonomic neuropathy may be responsible for spontaneous respiratory arrest and unexplained sudden death (Rathmann et al. 1993). Possible causes and mechanisms of sudden death include silent myocardial ischaemia/infarction, ventricular arrhythmias: prolongation of the QT interval, impaired respiratory reflexes to hypoxia and sleep apnoea syndrome and deficient haemodynamic response to cardiovascular stresses such as surgery, infection, and anaesthesia (Freeman 2005).

Management

Near normoglycaemia is now generally accepted as the primary approach to the prevention of diabetic neuropathy but is not achievable in most patients. The natural history of neuropathy is governed by the degree of glycaemic control. The deleterious effect of long-term poor glycaemic control on the development and progression of autonomic neuropathy is now accepted in the light of evidence from prospective large scale studies including the DCCT and the UK Prospective Diabetes Study. In diabetic subjects with early cardiovascular denervation, institution of good glycaemic control may prevent the development of further myocardial sympathetic nerve damage and enhanced cardiac risk. There is scintigraphic evidence that insulin improves cardiac autonomic innervation in diabetic patients (Schnell et al. 2004). A target-driven, long-term, intensified intervention aimed at multiple risk factors in patients with Type 2 diabetes and microalbuminuria reduced the risk of cardiovascular and microvascular events by about 50% including a significant reduction in autonomic neuropathy (Gaede et al. 2003).

As to specific treatment of the neuropathy, clinical experience with aldose reductase inhibitors has been disappointing Treatment of autonomic neuropathy with alpha lipoic acid, has been promising. This is a powerful free radical scavenger that improves nerve blood flow, and reduces nerve oxygen and lipid peroxidation and oxidative stress. Improvement of cardiac autonomic function as assessed by heart rate was demonstrated in the Deutsche Kardiale Autonome Neuropathie (DEKAN) study (Ziegler et al. 1997). Quinapril significantly increased parasympathetic activity in patients with autonomic neuropathy 3 months after treatment initiation and sustains this effect until the 6th month (Kontopoulos et al. 1997).

Conclusion

This chapter has focused on autonomic denervation in diabetic patients. Autonomic neuropathy as defined by abnormal autonomic tests is common but symptoms are rare. However, when present they can be devastating. The unfavourable connection between autonomic neuropathy and cardiovascular disease leads to considerable cardiovascular morbidity and mortality.

References

Ahlgren, A. R., Sundkvist, G., Wollmer, P., Sonesson, B., Lanne, T. (1999). Increased aortic stiffness in women with type 1 diabetes mellitus is associated with diabetes duration and autonomic nerve function. *Diabetic Medicine* **16**(4), 291–7.

Airaksinen, K. E. (2001). Silent coronary artery disease in diabetes—a feature of autonomic neuropathy or accelerated atherosclerosis? *Diabetologia* **44**(2), 259–66.

Antonelli, I., Fuso, L., Giordano, A., *et al.* (2002). Neuroadrenergic denervation of the lung in type I diabetes mellitus complicated by autonomic neuropathy. *Chest* **121**(2), 443.

Astrup, A. S., Tarnow, L., Rossing, P., Hansen, B. V., Hilsted, J., Parving, H. H. (2006). Cardiac autonomic neuropathy predicts cardiovascular morbidity and mortality in type 1 diabetic patients with diabetic nephropathy. *Diabetes Care* **29**(2), 334–9.

Banarer, S., Cryer, P. E. (2003). Sleep-related hypoglycemia-associated autonomic failure in Type 1 diabetes—reduced awakening from sleep during hypoglycemia. *Diabetes* **52**, 1195–1203.

Beer, P. A., Glagor, S., Zariu, C. K. (1984). Retarding effect of lowered heart rate on coronary atherosclerosis. *Science* **226**, 180– 82.

Bosman, D. R., Osborne, C. A., Marsden, J. T., Macdougall, I. C., Gardner, W. N., Watkins, P. J. (2002). Erythropoietin response to hypoxia in patients with diabetic autonomic neuropathy and non-diabetic chronic renal failure. *Diabet. Med.* **19**(1), 65–9.

Bosshardt, R. J., Farwerk, R., Sikora, R. *et al.* (1995). Objective measurement of the effectiveness, therapeutic success and dynamic mechanisms of vacuum device. *Br. J Urol.* **75**, 786–91.

Bottini, P., Boschetti, E., Pampanelli, S., *et al.* (1997). Contribution of autonomic neuropathy to reduced plasma adrenaline responses to hypoglycemia in IDDM: evidence for a nonselective defect. *Diabetes* **46**(5), 814–23.

Boulton, A. J. M., Vinik, A. I., Arezzo, J. C., *et al.* (2005). Diabetic Neuropathies: A statement by the American Diabetes Association. *Diabetes Care* **28**(4), 956.

Bruckner, I. M., Vlaiculescu, N. V., Negrila, A. N. (2005). The involvement of autonomic neuropathy in cardiovascular function in diabetes mellitus. In: Cheeta, D. (Ed.) *Vascular Involvement in Diabetes.* Karger: Basil, pp. 321–38.

Burger, A. J., Charlamb, M., Weinrauch, L. A., D'Elia, J. A. (1997). Short- and long-term reproducibility of heart rate variability in patients with long-standing type I diabetes mellitus. *Am. J Cardiol.* **80**(9), 1198–202.

Burger, A. J., D'Elia, J. A., Weinrauch, L. A., Lerman, I., Gaur, A. (2002). Marked abnormalities in heart rate variability are associated with progressive deterioration of renal function in type I diabetic patients with overt nephropathy. *Int. J. Cardiol.* **86**(2–3), 281–7.

Burgos, L. G., Ebert, T. J., Asiddao, C., et al. (1989). Increased intraoperative cardiovascular morbidity in diabetics with autonomic neuropathy. *Anesthesiology* **70**, 591–97.

Cacciatori, V., Dellera, A., Bellavere, F., Bongiovanni, L. G., Teatini, F., Gemma, M. L., Muggeo, M. (1997). Comparative assessment of peripheral sympathetic function by postural vasoconstriction arteriolar reflex and sympathetic skin response in NIDDM patients. *Am. J Med.* **102**(4), 365–70.

Cachia, M. J. Peakman, M., Zanone, M., Watkins, P. J., Vergani, D. (1997). Reproducibility and persistence of neural and adrenal autoantibodies in diabetic autonomic neuropathy. *Diabetic Medicine* **14**(6), 461–5.

Carson, C. C. (1999). Penile prostheses. In: Carson, C. C., Kirby, R. S., Goldstein, I. (Eds.) *Textbook of Erectile Dysfunction.* Oxford: Isis Medical Media.

Carson, C., Holmes, S., Kirby, R. S. (2004). *Fast facts: Erectile dysfunction.* Oxford: Health Press.

Catterall, J. R. et al. (1984). Breathing, sleep and diabetic autonomic neuropathy. *Diabetes* **33**, 1025–27.

Cellek, S., Anderson, P. N., Foxwell, N. A. (2005). Nitrergic neurodegeneration in cerebral arteries of streptozotocin-induced diabetic rats: a new insight into diabetic stroke. *Diabetes* **54**(1):212–9.

Chantelau, E., Lee, K. M., Jungblut, R. (1995). Association of below knee athrosclerosis to medial arterial calcification in diabetes mellitus. *Diab. Res. Clin. Prac.* **29**, 169–72.

Chen, H. S., Hwu, C. M., Kuo, B. I., et al. (2001). Abnormal cardiovascular reflex tests are predictors of mortality in Type 2 diabetes mellitus. *Diabet. Med.* **18**(4), 268–73.

Chessa, M., Butera, G., Lanza, G. A., et al. (2002). Role of heart rate variability in the early diagnosis of diabetic autonomic neuropathy in children. *Herz* **27**(8), 785–90.

Cohen, J. A., Estacio, R. O., Lundgren, R. A., Esler, A. L., Schrier, R. W. (2003). Diabetic autonomic neuropathy is associated with an increased incidence of strokes. *Auton Neurosci* **108**(1–2), 73–8.

Cosson, E., Attali, J. R., Valensi, P. (2005). Markers for silent myocardial ischemia in diabetes. Are they helpful? *Diabetes Metab.* **31**(2), 205–13.

Cranston et al. (1994). Restoration of hypoglycaemia unawareness in patients with long-duration insulin-dependent diabetes. *Lancet* **344**, 283–87.

Cryer, P. E. (2002). Hypoglycaemia: The limiting factor in the glycaemic management of type I and type II diabetes. *Diabetologia* **45**, 937–48.

Di Carli, M. F., Bianco-Batlles, D., Landa, M. E., Kazmers, A., Groehn, H., Muzik, O., Grunberger G. (1999). Effects of autonomic neuropathy on coronary blood flow in patients with diabetes mellitus. *Circulation* **100**(8), 813–9.

Didangelos, T. P., Arsos, G. A., Karamitsos, D. T., Athyros, V. G., Karatzas, N. D. (2003). Left ventricular systolic and diastolic function in normotensive type 1 diabetic patients with or without autonomic neuropathy: a radionuclide ventriculography study. *Diabetes Care* **26**(7), 1955–60.

Diedrich, L., Sandoval, D., Davis, S. N. (2002). Hypoglycemia associated autonomic failure. *Clin. Auton. Res.* **12**(5), 358.

Dowling, C. J., Kumar, S., Boulton, A. J. M., et al. (1985). Severe gastroperisis diabeticorum in a young patient with insulin dependent diabetes. *Br. Med. J* **310**, 308–311.

Duchen, L. W., Anjorin, A., Watkins, P. J., MacKay, J. D. (1980). Pathology of autonomic neuropathy in diabetes mellitus. *Ann. Intern. Med.* **92**, 301–303.

Earle, K. A., Mishra, B., Morocutti, A., Barnes, D., Chambers, J., Viberti, G. C. (2000). QT dispersion in microalbuminuric Type 1 diabetic patients without myocardial ischemia. *Journal of Diabetes & its Complications* **14**(5), 277–80.

Edmonds, M. E. (2004). Autonomic neuropathy. In: *International Textbook of Diabetes Mellitus.* DeFronzo, R. A., Ferrannini, E., Kenn, H., Zimmet, P. (Eds). John Wiley & Sons: Chichester, pp. 1263–81.

Ejskjaer, N. T., Zanone, M. M., Peakman, M. (1998). Autoimmunity in diabetic autonomic neuropathy: does the immune system get on your nerves? [Review] *Diabet. Med.* **15**(9), 723–9.

Ejskjaer, N., Bradley, J. L., Buxton-Thomas, M. S., et al. (1999). Novel surgical treatment and gastric pathology in diabetic gastroperisis. *Diabet. Med.* **16**, 488–95.

Eppens, M. C., Craig, M. E., Cusumano J, et al. (2006). Prevalence of Diabetes Complications in Adolescents With Type 2 Compared With Type 1 Diabetes. *Diabetes Care* **29**(6), 1300.

Everhart, J. E., Pettitt, D. J., Knowler, W. C., Rose, F. A., Bennett, P. H. (1988). Medial arterial calcification and its association with mortality and complications of diabetes. *Diabetologia* **31**, 16–33.

Ewing, D. J., Clarke, B. F. (1986). Autonomic neuropathy: its diagonosis and prognosis. In: *Clinics in Endocrinology & Metabalism.* Edt. Watkins, PJ. London: Saunders. pp 855–88.

Ficker, J. H., Dertinger, S. H., Siegfried, W., et al. (1998). Obstructive sleep apnoea and diabetes mellitus: the role of cardiovascular autonomic neuropathy. *Eur. Respir. J* **11**(1), 14–9.

Flotats, A., Carrió, I. (2009). The role of nuclear medicine technique in evaluating electrophysiology in diabetic hearts especially with 123I-MIBG cardiac SPECT imaging. *Minerva Endocrinol.* **34**(3), 263–71.

Flynn, ME, et al. (1988). Direct measurement of capillary blood flow in the Diabetic neuropathic foot. *Diabetologia* **31**, 652–56.

Forsen, A., Kangro, M., Sterner, G., Norrgren, K., Thorsson, O., Wollmer, P., Sundkvist, G. (2004). A 14-year prospective study of autonomic nerve function in Type 1 diabetic patients: association with nephropathy. *Diabet. Med.* **21**(8), 852–8.

Frattola, A., Parati, G., Gamba, P., et al. (1997). Time and frequency domain estimates of spontaneous baroreflex sensitivity provide early detection of autonomic dysfunction in diabetes mellitus. *Diabetologia* **40**(12), 1470–5.

Freeman, R. (2005). Autonomic peripheral neuropathy. *Lancet* **365**(9466), 1259–70.

Frier, B. M. (1993). *Hypoglycaemia unawareness in hypoglycaemia and diabetes.* Frier, B. M., Fisher, M. (Eds). London: Edward Arnold, pp 291–93.

Gaede, P., Vedel, P., Larsen, N., Jensen, G. V., Parving, H. H., Pedersen, O. (2003). Multifactorial intervention and cardiovascular disease in patients with type 2 diabetes. *N Engl. J Med.* **348**(5), 383–93.

Gentilcore, D., Jones, K. L., O'Donovan, D. G., Horowitz, M. (2006). Postprandial hypotension—novel insights into pathophysiology and therapeutic implications. *Curr. Vasc. Pharmacol.* **4**(2), 161–71.

Gerritsen, J., Dekker, J. M., TenVoorde, B. J., et al. (2001). Impaired autonomic function is associated with increased mortality, especially in subjects with diabetes, hypertension, or a history of cardiovascular disease: The Hoorn Study. *Diabetes Care* **24**(10), 1793.

Gerritsen, J., TenVoorde, B. J., Dekker, J. M., et al. (2003). Measures of cardiovascular autonomic nervous function: agreement, reproducibility, and reference values in middle age and elderly subjects. *Diabetologia* **46**(3), 330–8.

Giordano, A., Calcagni, M. L., Verrillo, A., Pellegrinotti, M., Frontoni, S., Spallone, V., Gambardella, S. (2000). Assessment of sympathetic innervation of the heart in diabetes mellitus using 123I-MIBG. *Diabetes, Nutrition & Metabolism—Clinical & Experimental* **13**(6), 350–5.

Goebel, F-D., Fuessl, H. S. (1983). Monckeberg's sclerosis after sympathetic denervation in diabetic and non diabetic subjects. *Diabetologia* **24**, 347–50.

Goldstein, I., Lue, T. F., Padma-Nathan, H. et al. (1998). Oral sildenafil in the treatment of erectile dysfunction. *N Engl. J Med.* **338**, 1397–1404.

Gorman, J. M., Sloan, R. P. (2000). Heart rate variability in depressive and anxiety disorders. *Am. Heart J.* **140**(4 Suppl), 77–83.

Gottsater, A., Ryden-Ahlgren, A., Szelag, B., *et al.* (2003). Cardiovascular autonomic neuropathy associated with carotid atherosclerosis in Type 2 diabetic patients. *Diabetic Medicine* **20**, 495–99.

Gottsater, A., Ahmed, M., Fernlund, P., Sundkvist, G. (1999). Autonomic neuropathy in Type 2 diabetic patients is associated with hyperinsulinaemia and hypertriglyceridaemia. *Diabetic Medicine* **16**(1), 49–54.

Gottsater, A., Szelag, B., Berglund, G., Wroblewski, M., Sundkvist, G. (2005). Changing associations between progressive cardiovascular autonomic neuropathy and carotid atherosclerosis with increasing duration of type 2 diabetes mellitus. *J Diabetes Complications* **19**(4), 212–7.

Gottsater, A., Ahlgren, A. R., Taimour, S., Sundkvist, G. (2006). Decreased heart rate variability may predict the progression of carotid atherosclerosis in type 2 diabetes. *Clin. Auton. Res.* **16**(3), 228–34.

Granberg, V., Ejskjaer, E., Peakman, M., Sundkvist, G. (2005). Autoantibodies to autonomic nerves associated with cardiac and peripheral autonomic neuropathy. *Diabetes Care* **28**, 1959–64.

Gulcelik, N. E., Kaya, E., Demirbas, B., *et al.* (2005). Helicobacter pylori prevalence in diabetic patients and its relationship with dyspepsia and autonomic neuropathy. *J Endocrinol. Invest.* **28**(3), 214–7.

Guy, R. J. C., Richards, F., Edmonds, M. E., Watkins, P. J. (1984). Diabetic autonomic neuropathy and iritis: an association suggesting an immunological cause. *Br. Med. J* **789**, 343–45.

Harrison, C. V. (1938). The effect of sympathectomy on the development of experimental arterial disease. *J Pathol.* **616**, 353–60.

Hattori, N., Tamaki, N., Hayashi, T., *et al.* (1996). Regional abnormality of iodine-123-MIBG in diabetic hearts. *Journal of Nuclear Medicine.* **37**(12), 1985–90.

Heller, S. R. (2002). Abnormalities of the electrocardiogram during hypoglycaemia: the cause of the dead in bed syndrome? *Int. J Clin. Pract.* **129**(Suppl), 27–32.

Hepburn, D. A. *et al.* (1990). Unawareness of hypoglycaemia in insulin trated diabetic patients: prevalence and relationship to autonomic neuropathy. *Diabet. Med.* **7**, 711–717.

Hoeldtke, R. D., Bryner, K. D., Horvath, G. G., Phares, R. W., Broy, L. F., Hobbs, G. R. (2001). Redistribution of sudomotor responses is an early sign of sympathetic dysfunction in type 1 diabetes. *Diabetes* **50**(2), 436–43.

Hreidarsson, A. B. (1992). The pupil of the eye in diabetes mellitus, an indicator of autonomic nervous dysfunction. *Dan. Med. Bull.* **39**, 400–408.

Huikuri, H. V., Jokinen, V., Syvanne, M., *et al.* (1999). Heart rate variability and progression of coronary atherosclerosis. *Arterioscler. Thromb. Vasc. Biol.* **19**(8), 1979–85.

Ikeda, T., Matsubara, T., Sato, Y., Sakamoto, N. (1993). Circadian BP variation in diabetic patients with autonomic neuropathy. *J Hypertens.* **11**(5), 581–7.

Irace, L., Iarussi, D., Guadagno, I., *et al.* (1996). Left ventricular performance and autonomic dysfunction in patients with long-term insulin-dependent diabetes mellitus. *Acta Diabetologica* **33**(4), 269–73.

Izzedine, H., Launay-Vacher, V., Deray, G. (2006). Abnormal BP circadian rhythm: a target organ damage? *Int. J Cardiol.* **107**(3), 343–9.

Jackson, G., Betteridge, J., Dean, J. *et al.* (1999). A systematic approach to ED in the cardiovascular patient: a consensus statement. *Int. J Clin. Pract.* **53**, 445–51.

Jacob, G., Costa, F., Biaggioni, I. (2003). Spectrum of autonomic cardiovascular neuropathy in diabetes. *Diabetes Care* **26**(7), 2174–80.

Jermendy, G., Ferenczi, J., Hernandez, E., Farkas, K., Nadas, J. (1996). Day-night BP variation in normotensive and hypertensive NIDDM patients with asymptomatic autonomic neuropathy. *Diabetes Research & Clinical Practice* **34**(2), 107–14.

Jones, K. L., Wishart, J. M., Berry, M., Russo, A., Xia, H. H. X., Talley, N. J., Horowitz, M. (2002). Helicobacter pylori infection is not associated with delayed gastric emptying or upper gastrointestinal symptoms in diabetes mellitus. *Dig. Dis. Sci.* **47**, 704–9.

Karavanaki, K., Baum, J. D. (1999). Prevalence of microvascular and neurologic abnormalities in a population of diabetic children. *Journal of Pediatric Endocrinology & Metabolism* **12**(3), 411–22.

Kempler, P. K. (Ed). (2002). *Clinical features, diagnosis and therapy of autonomic neuropathy in neuropathies.* Budapest: Springer Scientific. pp 79–141.

Kempler, P., Tesfaye, S., Chaturvedi, N., *et al.* (2002). Autonomic neuropathy is associated with increased cardiovascular risk factors: the EURODIAB IDDM Complications Study Group. *Diabet. Med.* **19**(11), 900–9.

Kerper, H. A., Collier, W. D. (1926). Pathological changes in arteries following partial denervation. *Proc. Soc. Exp. Biol. Med.* **24**, 493–94.

Knüttgen, D., Trojan, S., Weber, M., Wolf, M., Wappler, F. (2005). Präoperative Bestimmung der Herzfrequenzvariabilität bei Diabetikern zur Einschätzung des Blutdruckverhaltens während der Anästhesieeinleitung. *Anaesthesist* **54**(5), 442–9.

Kong, M. F., Horowitz, M., Jones, K. L., Wishart, J. M., Harding, P. E. (1999). Natural history of diabetic gastroparesis. *Diabetes Care* **22**(3), 503–7.

Kontopoulos, A. G., Athyros, V. G., Didangelos, T. P., Papageorgiou, A. A., Avramidis, M. J., Mayroudi, M. C., Karamitsos, D. T. (1997). Effect of chronic quinapril administration on heart rate variability in patients with diabetic autonomic neuropathy. *Diabetes Care* **20**(3), 355–61.

Koppiker, N., Boolell, M., Price, D. (2003). Recent advances in the treatment of erectile dysfunction in patients with diabetes mellitus. *Endocrine practice: official journal of the American College of Endocrinology and the American Association of Clinical Endocrinologists* **9**(1), 52–63.

Korzon-Burakowska, A., Edmonds, M. (2006). Role of the microcirculation in diabetic foot ulceration. *Int. J Low. Extrem. Wounds.* **5**(3), 144–8.

Krolewski, A. S., Barzilay, J., Warram, J. H., Martin, B. C., Pfeifer, M., Rand, L. I. (1992). Risk of early onset proliferative retinopathy in IDDM is closely related to cardiovascular autonomic neuropathy. *Diabetes* **41**, 430–37.

Kumhar, M. R., Agarwal, T. D., Singh, V. B., Kochar, D. K., Chadda, V. S. (2000). Cardiac autonomic neuropathy and its correlation with QTc dispersion in type 2 diabetes. *Indian Heart J* **52**(4), 421–6.

Lee, K. H., Jang, H. J., Kim, Y. H., *et al.* (2003). Prognostic value of cardiac autonomic neuropathy independent and incremental to perfusion defects in patients with diabetes and suspected coronary artery disease. *Am. J Cardiol.* **92**(12), 1458–61.

Lee, S. P., Yeoh, L., Harris, N. D., *et al.* (2004). Influence of autonomic neuropathy on QTc interval lengthening during hypoglycemia in type 1 diabetes. *Diabetes* **53**(6), 1535–42.

Lee, K. O., Nam, J. S., Ahn, C. W., *et al.* (2012). Insulin resistance is independently associated with peripheral and autonomic neuropathy in Korean type 2 diabetic patients. *Acta Diabetol* **49**(2), 97–103.

Levy, D. M. *et al.* (1989). Depletion of cutaneous nerves and neuropeptides in diabetes mellitus: an immunocyrochemical study. *Diabetologia* **32**, 427–33.

Lindmark, S., Wiklund, U., Bjerle, P., Eriksson, J. W. (2003). Does the autonomic nervous system play a role in the development of insulin resistance? A study on heart rate variabilty in first-degree relatives of Type 2 diabetes patients, and control subjects. *Diabetic Medicine* **20**, 399–405.

Linet, O. I, Ogring, F. G. (1996). Efficacy and safety of intracavernosal Alprostadil in men with erectile dysfunction. *N Engl. J Med.* **334**, 873–77.

Low, P. A., Benrud-Larson, L. M., Sletten, D. M., *et al.* (2004). Autonomic symptoms and diabetic neuropathy: a population-based study. *Diabetes Care* **27**(12), 2942–7.

Mangoni, A. A., Mircoli, L., Giannattasio, C., Ferrari, A. U., Mancia, G. (1996). Heart rate-dependence of arterial distensibilty in vivo. *J Hypertens.* **14**, 897–902.

Mankovsky, B. N., Piolot, R., Mankovsky, O. L., Ziegler, D. (2003). Impairment of cerebral autoregulation in diabetic patients with cardiovascular autonomic neuropathy and orthostatic hypotension. *Diabet. Med.* **20**(2), 119–26.

Manzella, D., Paolisso, G. (2005). Cardiac autonomic activity and Type II diabetes mellitus. *Clin. Sci. (Lond)* **108**(2), 93–9.

Molgaard, H., Christensen, P. D., Sorensen, K. E., Christensen, C. K., Mogensen, C. E. (1992). Association of 24-h cardiac parasympathetic activity and degree of nephropathy in IDDM patients. *Diabetes* **41**(7), 812–7.

Monteagudo, P. T., Moises, V. A., Kohlmann, O. Jr., Ribeiro, A. B., Lima, V. C., Zanella, M. T. Department of Medicine, Escola Paulista de Medicina, UNIFESP, Sao Paulo, Brazil. (2000). Influence of autonomic neuropathy upon left ventricular dysfunction in insulin-dependent diabetic patients. *Clinical Cardiology* **23**(5), 371–5.

Moran, A., Palmas, W., Field, L., *et al.* (2004). Cardiovascular autonomic neuropathy is associated with microalbuminuria in older patients with type 2 diabetes. *Diabetes Care* **27**(4), 972.

Morgan, A. J. (1980). Mineralised deposits in the thoracic aorta of aged rats: ultrastructural and electron probe x-ray microanalysis study. *Ext. Geront.* **15**, 563–73.

Nagamachi, S., Fujita, S., Nishii, R., *et al.* (2006). Prognostic value of cardiac I-123 metaiodobenzylguanidine imaging in patients with non-insulin-dependent diabetes mellitus. *Journal of Nuclear Cardiology* **13**(1), 34–42.

Nangle, M. R., Cotter, M. A., Cameron, N. E. (2006). Correction of nitrergic neurovascular dysfunction in diabetic mouse corpus cavernosum by p. 38 mitogen-activated protein kinase inhibition. *Int. J Impot. Res.* **3**, 258–63.

Nasr, N., Czosnyka, M., Arevalo, F., Hanaire, H., Guidolin, B., Larrue, V. (2011). Autonomic neuropathy is associated with impairment of dynamic cerebral autoregulation in type 1 diabetes. *Auton. Neurosci.* **160**(1–2), 59–63.

Nazhel, B., Yetkin, I., Irkec, C., Kocer, B. (2001). Sympathetic skin response in diabetic neuropathy. *Auton. Neurosci.* **92**(1–2), 72–5

Nishimura, M., Hashimoto, T., Kobayashi, H., *et al.* (2004). Association between cardiovascular autonomic neuropathy and left ventricular hypertrophy in diabetic haemodialysis patients. *Nephrology dialysis transplantation: official publication of the European Dialysis and Transplant Association—European Renal Association* **19**(10), 2532–8.

O'Brien, I. A., McFadden, J. P., Corrall, R. J. (1991). The influence of autonomic neuropathy on mortality in insulin-dependent diabetes. *Q J Med.* **79**(290), 495–502.

O'Donovan, D., Samson, M., Feinle, Cjones K.L., Horowitz, M. (2003). Gastrointestinal Tract In: *Textbook of Diabetic Neuropathy.* Eds Gries, R., Cameron, N., Low, P., Ziegler, D. Georg Thieme verlag Stuttgart G. pp 246–62.

Orchard, T. J., Lloyd, C. E., Maser, R. E., Kuller, L. H. (1996). Why does diabetic autonomic neuropathy predict IDDM mortality? An analysis from the Pittsburgh Epidemiology of Diabetes Complications Study. *Diabetes Res. Clin. Pract.* **34** (Suppl.), S165–71.

Pathak, A., Raoul, V., Montastruc, J. L., Senard, J. M. (2005). Adverse drug reactions related to drugs used in orthostatic hypotension: a prospective and systematic pharmacovigilance study in France. *European Journal of Clinical Pharmacology* **61** (5–6), 471.

Petrova, N. L., Foster, A. V., Edmonds, M. E. (2005). Calcaneal bone mineral density in patients with Charcot neuropathic osteoarthropathy: differences between Type 1 and Type 2 diabetes. *Diabet. Med.* **22**(6), 756–61.

Phillips, L. K., Rayner, C. K., Jones, K. L., Horowitz, M. (2006). An update on autonomic neuropathy affecting the gastrointestinal tract. *Curr. Diab. Rep.* **6**, 417–23.

Pitei, D. L., Watkins, P. J., Edmonds, M. E. (1997). NO-Dependent smooth muscle vasodilatation is reduced in the NIDDM patients with peripheral sensory neuropathy. *Diab. Med.* **14**, 284–90.

Pittasch, D., Lobmann, R., Behrens, B. W., Lehnert, H. (2002). Pupil signs of sympathetic autonomic neuropathy in patients with type 1 diabetes. *Diabetes Care* **25**(9), 1545–50.

Pop-Busui, R. (2010). Cardiac autonomic neuropathy in diabetes: a clinical perspective. *Diabetes Care* **33**(2), 434–41.

Poulsen, P. L., Ebbehoj, E., Arildsen, H., *et al.* (2001). Increased QTc dispersion is related to blunted circadian BP variation in normoalbuminuric type 1 diabetic patients. *Diabetes* **50**(4), 837–42.

Psallas, M., Tentolouris, N., Papadogiannis, D., Doulgerakis, D., Kokkinos, A., Cokkinos, D. V., Katsilambros, N. (2006). QT dispersion: comparison between participants with Type 1 and 2 diabetes and association with microalbuminuria in diabetes. *J Diabetes Complications* **20**(2), 88–97.

Purewal, T. S., Watkins, P. J. (1995). Postural-hypotension in diabetic autonomic neuropathy: a review. *Diab. Med.* **12**, 192–200.

Rathmann, W., Ziegler, D., Jahnke, M., Haastert, B., Gries, F. A. (1993). Mortality in diabetic patients with cardiovascular autonomic neuropathy. *Diabet. Med.* **10**(9), 820–4.

Rauch, U., Ziegler, D., Piolot, R., Schwippert, B., Benthake, H., Schultheiss, H. P., Tschoepe, D. (1999). Platelet activation in diabetic cardiovascular autonomic neuropathy. *Diabet. Med.* **16**(10), 848–52.

Rees, P. J. *et al.* (1981). Sleep apnoea in diabetic patients with autonomic neuropathy. *J R Soc. Med.* **74**, 192–95.

Rendell, M., Ragfer, J., Wicker, P. A. (1999). Sidenafil for treatment of ED in men with diabetes. *JAMA* **281**, 421–26.

Sampson, M. J. *et al.* (1990). Progression of diabetic autonomic neuropathy over a decade in insulin dependent diabetics. *Q. J. Med.* **75**, 635–46.

Schmidt, R. E., Dorsey, D. A., Beaudet, L. N., Parvin, C. A., Zhang, W., Sima, A. A. F. (2004). Experimental rat models of types 1 and 2 diabetes differ in sympathetic neuroaxonal dystrophy. *J Neuropathol. Exp. Neurol.* **63**(5), 450–60.

Schmidt, R. E. (2002). Neuropathology and pathogenesis of diabetic autonomic neuropathy. *Int. Rev. Neurobiol.* **50**, 257–92

Schnell, O., Muhr, D., Dresel, S., Tatsch, K., Ziegler, A. G., Haslbeck, M., Standl, E. (1996). Autoantibodies against sympathetic ganglia and evidence of cardiac sympathetic dysinnervation in newly diagnosed and long-term IDDM patients. *Diabetologia* **39**(8), 970–5.

Schnell, O., Schwarz, A., Muhr-Becker, D., Standl, E. (2000). Autoantibodies against autonomic nervous tissues in type 2 diabetes mellitus: no association with cardiac autonomic dysfunction. *Exp. Clin. Endocrinol. Diabetes* **108**(3), 181–6.

Schnell, O., Kilinc, S., Rambeck, A., Standl, E. (2004). [Insulin therapy improves cardiac autonomic function in type 2 diabetic patients] *Herz* **29**(5), 519.

Scionti, L., Bottini, P. (2003). Respiratory Tract. In: *Textbook of Diabetic Neuropathy.* Gries, R., Cameron, N., Low, P., Ziegler, D. Georg (Eds). Thieme verlag Stuttgart G, pp 242–45.

Scott, L. A., Kench, P. L. (2004). Cardiac autonomic neuropathy in the diabetic patient: Does ^{123}I-MIBG imaging have a role to play in early diagnosis? *Journal of Nuclear Medicine Technology* **32**(2), 66.

Shimada, H., Kihara, M., Kosaka, S., Ikeda, H., Kawabata, K., Tsutada, T., Miki, T. (2001). Peripheral sympathetic neuropathy. Comparison of SSR and QSART in early diabetic neuropathy—the value of length-dependent pattern in QSART. *Auton. Neurosci.* **92**(1–2), 72–5.

Smith, D. S., Ferris, C. D. (2003). Current Concepts in Diabetic Gastroparesis. *Drugs, Adis Internationa* 63(13):1339–58.

Smith SA, Smith SE. (1999). Pupil function: tests and disorders. In: Mathias, C. J. Bannister, R. (eds) *Autonomic Failure.* Oxford: Oxford Medical Publications, pp. 245–53.

Soedamah-Muthu, S. S., Chaturvedi, N., Toeller, M., *et al.* (2004). Risk factors for coronary heart disease in type 1 diabetic patients in Europe. *Diabetes Care* **27**(2), 530–7.

Spallone, V., Bernardi, L., Maiello, M. R., Cicconetti, E., Ricordi, L., Fratino, P., Menzinger, G. (1996). Twenty-four-hour pattern of BP and spectral analysis of heart rate variability in diabetic patients with various degrees of autonomic neuropathy. Comparison to standard cardiovascular tests. *Clinical Science* **91**(Suppl.), 105–7.

Spallone, V., Maiello, M. R., Cicconetti, E., Menzinger, G. (1997). Autonomic neuropathy and cardiovascular risk factors in insulin-dependent and non insulin-dependent diabetes. *Diabetes Research & Clinical Practice* **34**(3), 169–79.

Spallone, V., Menzinger, G., Ziegler, D. (2003). Diabetic autonomic neuropathy Cardiovascular System In: *Textbook of Diabetic Neuropathy*. Gries, R., Cameron, N., Low, P., Ziegler, D. Georg (Eds) Thieme verlag Stuttgart G, pp 225–40.

Spallone, V., Maiello, M. R., Kurukulasuriya, N., *et al.* (2004). Does autonomic neuropathy play a role in erythropoietin regulation in non-proteinuric Type 2 diabetic patients? *Diabet. Med.* **21**(11), 1174–80.

Spallone, V., Bellavere, F., Scionti, L., *et al.* (2011). Diabetic Neuropathy Study Group of the Italian Society of Diabetology. Recommendations for the use of cardiovascular tests in diagnosing diabetic autonomic neuropathy. *Nutr. Metab. Cardiovasc. Dis.* **21**(1), 69–78.

Spitzer, A., Lang, E., Birklein, F., Claus, D. (1997). Cardiac autonomic involvement and peripheral nerve function in patients with diabetic neuropathy. *Neundorfer. Funct. Neurol.* **12**(3–4), 115–22.

Stacher, G. (2001). Gastric stasis is a feature of autonomic neuropathy. Diabetes mellitus and the stomach. *Diabetologia* **44**(9), 1080–93. Review.

Stacher, G., Lenglinger, J., Bergmann, H., *et al.* (2003). Impaired gastric emptying and altered intragastric meal distribution in diabetes mellitus related to autonomic neuropathy? *Dig. Dis. Sci.* **48**(6), 1027–34.

Stein, P. K., Kleiger, R. E. (1999). Insights from the study of heart rate variability. *Annual Review of Medicine* **50**, 249–61.

Stella, P. *et al.* (2000). Cardiovascular autonomic neuropathy (expiration and inspiration ratio) in type 1 diabetes. Incidence and predictors. *J Diabetes Complications* **14**(1), 1–6.

Stevens, M. J. (2001). New imaging techniques for cardiovascular autonomic neuropathy: a window on the heart. *Diabetes Technol. Ther.* **3**(1), 9–22.

Stevens, M. J., Raffel, D. M., Allman, K. C., Schwaiger, M., Wieland, D. M. (1999). Regression and progression of cardiac sympathetic dysinnervation complicating diabetes: an assessment by C-11 hydroxyephedrine and positron emission tomography. *Metabolism: Clinical & Experimental* **48**(1), 92–101.

Stief, C. G., Ziegler, D. (2003). Urogenital System. In *Textbook of Diabetic Neuropathy*. Gries, R., Cameron, N., Low, P., Ziegler, D. (Eds). Georg Thieme verlag Stuttgart G, pp. 262–274.

Suarez, G. A., Clark, V. M., Norell, J. E., *et al.* (2005). Sudden cardiac death in diabetes mellitus: risk factors in the Rochester diabetic neuropathy study. *J Neurol. Neurosurg. Psychiatry* **76**(2), 240–5.

Szelag, B., Wroblewski, M., Castenfors, J., Henricsson, M., Berntorp, K., Fernlund, P., Sundkvist, G. (1999). Obesity, microalbuminuria, hyperinsulinemia, and increased plasminogen activator inhibitor 1 activity associated with parasympathetic neuropathy in type 2 diabetes [Letter]. *Diabetes Care* **22**, 1907–1908.

Takahashi, N., Nakagawa, M., Saikawa, T., *et al.* (2004). Regulation of QT indices mediated by autonomic nervous function in patients with type 2 diabetes. *Int. J Cardiol.* **96**(3), 375–79.

Takase, B., Kitamura, H., Noritake, M., Nagase, T., Kurita, A., Ohsuzu, F., Matsuoka, T. (2002). Assessment of diabetic autonomic neuropathy using twenty-four-hour spectral analysis of heart rate variability: a comparison with the findings of the Ewing battery. *Japanese Heart Journal* **43**(2), 127–35.

Takayama, S., Legare, D. J., Lautt, W. W. (2000). Dose-related atropine-induced insulin resistence: comparing intra-portal vs. intravenus administration. *Proc. West Pharmacol. Soc.* **43**, 33–34.

Tang, D. M., Friedenberg, F. K. (2011). Gastroparesis: approach, diagnostic evaluation, and management. *Dis. Mon.* **57**(2), 74–101.

Taskiran, M., Fritz-Hansen, T., Rasmussen, V., Larsson, H. B., Hilsted, J. (2002). Decreased myocardial perfusion reserve in diabetic autonomic neuropathy. *J Diabetes* **51**(11), 3306–10.

Taskiran, M., Rasmussen, V., Rasmussen, T., Fritz-Hansen, T., Larsson, H. B., Jensen, G. B., Hilsted, J. (2004). Left ventricular dysfunction in normotensive Type 1 diabetic patients: the impact of autonomic neuropathy. *Diabet. Med.* **21**(6), 524–30.

Tentolouris, N., Katsilambros, N., Papazachos, G., Papadogiannis, D., Linos A., Stamboulis, E., Papageorgiou, K. (1997). Corrected QT interval in relation to the severity of diabetic autonomic neuropathy. *European Journal of Clinical Investigation* **27**(12), 1049–54.

Tentolouris, N., Liatis, S., Moyssakis, I., *et al.* (2003). Aortic distensibility is reduced in subjects with type 2 diabetes and cardiac autonomic neuropathy. *Eur. J Clin. Invest.* **33**(12), 1075–83.

Tesfaye, S., Boulton, A. J., Dyck, P. J., *et al*, (2010). Diabetic neuropathies: update on definitions, diagnostic criteria, estimation of severity, and treatments. *Diabetes Care* **33**(10), 2285–93.

The Diabetes Control and Complications Trial Research Group. (1993). The effect of intensive treatment of diabetes on the development and progression of long-term complications in insulin-dependent diabetes mellitus. *N Engl. J Med.* **329**(14), 977–86.

Thilo, C., Standl, E., Knez, A., Reiser, M., Steinbeck, G., Haberl, R., Schnell, O. (2004). Coronary calcification in long-term type 1 diabetic patients—a study with multi slice spiral computed tomography. *Exp. Clin. Endocrinol. Diabetes* **112**(10), 561–5.

Toh, V., Duncan, E., Lewis, N., Fichter, L., Matthews, D. R. (2006). Ergotamine use in severe diabetic autonomic neuropathy. *Diabet. Med.* **23**(5), 574–6.

Toyry, J. P., Niskanen, L. K., Lansimies, E. A., Partanen, K. P., Uusitupa, M. I. (1996a). Uusitupa myocardial ischaemia. Autonomic neuropathy predicts the development of stroke in patients with non-insulin-dependent diabetes mellitus. *Stroke* **27**(8), 1316–8.

Toyry, J. P., Niskanen, L. K., Mantysaari, M. J., Lansimies, E. A. (1996b). Occurrence, predictors, and clinical significance of autonomic neuropathy in NIDDM. Ten-year follow-up from the diagnosis. *Diabetes* **45**(3), 308–15.

Trofimiuk, M., Huszno, B., Golkowski, F., Szybinski, Z. (2003). Postprandial hypotension and autonomic neuropathy in diabetic patients. *Folia-Med-Cracov* **44**(1–2), 117–28.

Valensi, P., Huard, J. P., Giroux, C., Attali, J. R. (1997). Factors involved in cardiac autonomic neuropathy in diabetic patients. *J Diabetes Complications* **11**(3), 180–7.

Veglio, M., Sivieri, R., Chinaglia, A., Scaglione, L., Cavallo-Perin, P. (2000). QT interval prolongation and mortality in type 1 diabetic patients: a 5-year cohort prospective study. Neuropathy Study Group of the Italian Society of the Study of Diabetes, Piemonte Affiliate. *Diabetes Care* **23**(9), 1381–3.

Veglio, M., Giunti, S., Stevens, L. K., Fuller, J. H., Perin, P. C. (2002). Prevalence of Q-T Interval Dispersion in Type 1 Diabetes and Its Relation With Cardiac Ischemia: The EURODIAB IDDM Complications Study Group. *Diabetes Care* **25**(4):702.

Vianna, L. G., Gilbey, S. G., Barnes, N. C., Guy, R. J., Gray, B. J. (1988). Cough threshold to citric acid in diabetic patients with and without autonomic neuropathy. *Thorax* **43**(7), 569–71.

Vinik, A. I., Maser, R. E., Mitchell, B. D., Freeman, R, (2003). Diabetic autonomic neuropathy (Technical Review). *Diabetes Care* **26**, 1553–79.

Vinik, A. I., Dharshan, A., Jagdeesh, U. (2005). Antibodies to Neuronal Structures: Innocent bystanders or neurotoxins? *Diabetes Care* **28**(8), 2067–72.

Vinik, A. I. and Ziegler, D. (2007). Diabetic cardiovascular autonomic neuropathy *Circulation* **115**(3), 387–97.

Watkins, P. J. (1998). The enigma of autonomic failure in diabetes. *Journal of the Royal College of Physicians of London* **32**, 360–365.

Watkins, P. J., Edmonds, M. E. (1999). Diabetic Autonomic Failure. In: *Autonomic Failure* 4th Edn. Oxford: Oxford University Press, pp 378–86.

Watkins, P. J., Buxton-Thomas, M. S., Howard, E. R. (2003). Long-term outcome after gastrectomy for intractable diabetic gastroparesis. *Diabet. Med.* **20**(1), 58–63.

Whang, W., Bigger, J. T. (2003). Comparison of the prognostic value of RR-interval variability after acute myocardial infarction in patients with versus those without diabetes mellitus. *Am. J Cardiology* **92**(3), 247–51.

Whitsel, E. A., Boyko, E. J., Siscovick, D. S. (2000). Reassessing the role of QTc in the diagnosis of autonomic failure among patients with diabetes: a meta-analysis. *Diabetes Care* **23**(2), 241–7.

Willenheimer, R. B., Erhardt, L. R., Nilsson, H., Lilja, B., Juul-Moller, S., Sundkvist, G. (1998). Parasympathetic neuropathy associated with left ventricular diastolic dysfunction in patients with insulin-dependent diabetes mellitus. *Scandinavian Cardiovascular Journal* **32**(1), 17–22.

Winkler, A. S., Marsden, J., Chaudhuri, K. R., Hambley, H., Watkins, P. J. (1999). Erythropoietin depletion and anaemia in diabetes mellitus. *Diabet. Med.* **16**(10), 813–9.

Winkler, A. S., Ejskjaer, N., Edmonds, M., Watkins, P. J. (2000). Dissociated sensory loss in diabetic autonomic neuropathy. *Diabet. Med.* **17**(6), 457–62.

Winkler, A. S., Landau, S., Watkins, P. J. (2001). Erythropoietin treatment of postural hypotension in anemic type 1 diabetic patients with autonomic neuropathy: a case study of four patients. *Diabetes Care* **24**(6), 1121–3.

Wirta, O. R., Pasternack, A. I., Mustonen, J. T., Laippala, P. J., Reinikainen, P. M. (1999). Urinary albumin excretion rate (UAER) is independently related to subclinical autonomic neuropathy in type 2 diabetes. *J Intern. Med.* **245**(4), 329–35.

Yki, J. H., Utriainent, T. (1998). Insulin-induced vasodilatation: physiology or pharmacology? *Diabetologia* **41**, 369–79.

Young, L. H., Wackers, F. J., Chyun, D. A., *et al.* (2009). DIAD Investigators.Cardiac outcomes after screening for asymptomatic coronary artery disease in patients with type 2 diabetes: the DIAD study: a randomized controlled trial. *JAMA* **301**(15), 1547–55.

Zahn A., Langhans, C. D., Hoffner, S., *et al.* (2003). Measurement of gastric emptying by 13C-octanoic acid breath test versus scintigraphy in diabetics. *Zeitschrift für Gastroenterologie* **41**, 383–90.

Zander, E., Seidlein, I., Herfurth, S., *et al.* (1992). Increased prevalence of proliferative retinopathy and cardiovascular autonomic dysfunction in IDDM patients with protein urea. *Exp. Clin. Endcrinol.* **99**, 102–107.

Zanone, M. M., Burchio, S., Quadri, R., *et al.* (1998). Autonomic function and autoantibodies to autonomic nervous structures, glutamic acid decarboxylase and islet tyrosine phosphatase in adolescent patients with IDDM. *J Neuroimmunol.* **87**(1–2), 1–10.

Zhao, J., Frøkjaer, J. B., Drewes, A. M., Ejskjaer, N. (2006). Upper gastrointestinal sensory-motor dysfunction in diabetes mellitus. *World J Gastroenterol.* **12**(18), 2846–57.

Ziegler, D., Schadewaldt, P., Pour Mirza, A., *et al.* (1996). [13C] octanoic acid breath test for non-invasive assessment of gastric emptying in diabetic patients: validation and relationship to gastric symptoms and cardiovascular autonomic function. *Diabetologia* **39**(7), 823–30.

Ziegler, D., Schatz, H., Conrad, F., Gries, F. A., Ulrich, H., Reichel, G. (1997). Effects of treatment with the antioxidant alpha-lipoic acid on cardiac autonomic neuropathy in NIDDM patients. A 4-month randomized controlled multicenter trial (DEKAN Study). Deutsche Kardiale Autonome Neuropathie. *Diabetes Care* **20**(3), 369–73.

Ziegler, D., Laude, D., Akila, F., Elghozi, J. L. (2001). Time- and frequency-domain estimation of early diabetic cardiovascular autonomic neuropathy. *Clin. Auton. Res.* **11**(6), 369–76.

Ziegler, D. (1999). Cardiovascular autonomic neuropathy:clinical manifestations and measurement. *Diab. Rev.* **7**, 342–57.

Zoccali, C. (2000). Cardiovascular risk in uraemic patients: is it fully explained by classicalclassic risk factors? *Nephrol. Dial. Transplant* **15**, 454–57.

PART VI

Other Disorders Associated with Autonomic Dysfunction

CHAPTER 54

Introduction to neurocardiology

Martin A. Samuels

In 1942, Walter Bradford Cannon published a remarkable paper entitled 'Voodoo' Death (Cannon 1942), in which he recounted anecdotal experiences, largely from the anthropology literature, of death from fright. These events, drawn from widely disparate parts of the world, had several features in common. They were all induced by an absolute belief that an external force, such as a wizard or medicine man, could, at will, cause demise and that the victim himself had no power to alter this course. This perceived lack of control over a powerful external force is the *sine qua non* for all the cases recounted by Cannon, who postulated that death was caused 'by a lasting and intense action of the sympathicoadrenal system.' Cannon believed that this phenomenon was limited to societies in which the people were 'so superstitious, so ignorant, that they feel themselves bewildered strangers in a hostile world. Instead of knowledge, they have fertile and unrestricted imaginations which fill their environment with all manner of evil spirits capable of affecting their lives disastrously.' Over the years since Cannon's observations, evidence has accumulated to support his concept that 'Voodoo' death is, in fact, a real phenomenon, but far from being limited to ancient peoples, may be a basic biological principal that provides an important clue to understanding the phenomenon of sudden death in modern society as well as providing a window into the world of neurovisceral disease. George Engel collected 160 accounts from the lay press of sudden death that were attributed to disruptive life events (Engel 1971). He found that such events could be divided into eight categories:

1 the impact of the collapse or death of a close person

2 during acute grief

3 on threat of loss of a close person

4 during mourning or on an anniversary

5 on loss of status or self-esteem

6 personal danger or threat of injury

7 after danger is over

8 reunion, triumph, or happy ending.

Common to all is that they involve events impossible for the victim to ignore and to which their response is overwhelming excitation, giving up, or both.

In 1957, Carl Richter, reported on a series of experiments aimed at elucidating the mechanism of Cannon's 'Voodoo' death (Richter 1957). Richter studied the length of time domesticated rats could swim at various water temperatures and found that at a water temperature of 93° these rats could swim for 60–80 minutes. However, if the animal's whiskers were trimmed, it would invariably drown within a few minutes. When carrying out similar experiments with fierce, wild rats, he noted that a number of factors contributed to the tendency for sudden death, the most important of which were restraint involving holding the animals and confinement in the glass swimming jar with no chance of escape. Trimming the rats' whiskers, which destroys possibly their most important proprioceptive mechanism, contributed to the tendency for early demise. In the case of the calm domesticated animals in which restraint and confinement were apparently not significant stressors, shaving the whiskers rendered these animals as fearful as wild rats with a corresponding tendency for sudden death. Electrocardiograms taken during the process showed a bradycardia developing prior to death and adrenalectomy did not protect the animals. Furthermore, atropine protected some of the animals and cholinergic drugs lead to an even more rapid demise. All this was taken as evidence that overactivity of the sympathetic nervous system was not the cause of the death but rather it was caused by increased vagal tone.

We now know that the apparently opposite conclusions of Cannon and Richter are not mutually exclusive, but rather that a generalized autonomic storm, occurring as a result of a life-threatening stressor will have both sympathetic and parasympathetic effects. The apparent predominance of one over the other depends on the parameter measured (e.g. heart rate, blood pressure) and the timing of the observations in relation to the stressor (e.g. early events tend to be dominated by sympathetic effects whereas late events tend to be dominated by parasympathetic effects).

In human beings, one of the easily accessible windows into autonomic activity is the electrocardiogram (ECG). Edwin Byer and colleagues reported six patients whose ECGs showed large upright T-waves and long QT intervals (Byer 1947). Two of these patients had hypertensive encephalopathy, one had a brainstem stroke with neurogenic pulmonary oedema, one had an intracerebral haemorrhage, one had a postpartum ischaemic stroke possibly related to toxaemia and one had no history except a blood pressure of 210/110. Based on experimental results of cooling or warming the endocardial surface of the dog's left ventricle, Byer concluded that these ECG changes were due to subendocardial ischaemia.

Levine reported on several disorders, other than ischaemic heart disease, which could produce ECG changes reminiscent of coronary disease (Levine 1953). Among these was a 69-year-old woman who was admitted and remained in coma. Her admission ECG showed deeply inverted T-waves in the anterior and lateral precordial leads. Two days later, it showed ST segment elevation with less deeply inverted T-waves, a pattern suggestive of myocardial infarction. However, at autopsy a ruptured berry aneurysm was found and no evidence of myocardial infarction or pericarditis was noted. Levine did not propose a specific mechanism but referred to experimental work on the production of cardiac arrhythmias by basal ganglia stimulation and ST and T-wave changes induced by injecting caffeine into the cerebral ventricle.

Burch et al. (1954) reported on 17 patients who were said to have 'cerebrovascular accidents' (i.e. strokes). In 14 of the 17, haemorrhage was demonstrated by lumbar puncture. It is not possible to determine which of these patients had haemorrhagic infarction, intracerebral haemorrhage and subarachnoid haemorrhage, and no data about the territory of the strokes is available. The essential features of the ECG abnormalities were:

◆ long QT intervals in all patients

◆ large, usually, inverted T-waves, in all patients

◆ U-waves in 11 of the 17 patients.

Cropp et al. (1960) reported on the details of the ECG abnormalities in 29 patients with subarachnoid haemorrhage. Of the 29, 22 patients survived; 2 of those who died had no post-mortem examination, leaving 5 in whom autopsies confirmed the presence of a ruptured cerebral aneurysm. In 3 of these 5, the heart and coronary arteries were said to be normal, but the details of the pathological examination are not revealed. The point is made that ECG changes seen in the context of neurological disease do not represent ischaemic heart disease but are merely a manifestation of autonomic dysregulation, possibly emanating from a lesion affecting the cortical representation of the autonomic nervous system. The authors argued that Brodman area 13 on the orbital surface of the frontal lobe and area 24 on the anterior cingulate gyrus were the cortical centres for cardiovascular control.

In contrast to this rather inconclusive clinical data, there is clear evidence that cardiac lesions can be produced as the result of nervous system disease. The concept of visceral organ dysfunction occurring as a result of neurological stimuli can be traced to Pavlov, who may have introduced the concept of a neurogenic dystrophy. Selye, a student of Pavlov, described the electrolyte-steroid-cardiopathy with necroses (ESCN) (Selye 1958). His view was that this cardiac lesion was common and often described using different names in the world's literature. He argued that this lesion was distinct from the coagulation necrosis that occurred as a result of ischaemic disease, but could exist in the same heart. Selye felt that certain steroids and other hormones created a predisposition for the development of ESCN, but that other factors needed were required for ESCN to develop. The most effective conditioning steroid was 2 alpha-methyl-9 alpha chlorocortisol. Among the factors that lead to ESCN in steroid sensitized animals were certain electrolytes (e.g. NaH_2PO_4), various hormones (e.g. vasopressin, adrenalin, insulin, thyroxin), certain vitamins (e.g. dihydrotachysterol), cardiac glycosides, surgical interventions (e.g. cardiac reperfusion after ischaemia), and psychic or nervous stimuli (e.g. restraint, fright). The cardiac lesions could not be prevented

with adrenalectomy, suggesting that the process, if related to autonomic hyperactivity, must exert its influence by direct neural connection to the heart rather than by a blood-borne route.

Cardiac lesions may be produced in rats by pretreating with either 2-alpha-methyl-9-alpha-flourohydrocortisone (flourocortisol), dihydrotachysterol (calciferol) or thyroxine (Synthroid) and then restraining the animals on a board for 15 hours or by using cold stress (Raab 1961). Agents that act by inhibition of the catecholamine-mobilizing reflex arc at the hypothalamic level (e.g. chlorpromazine) or by blockade of only the circulating, but not the neurogenic intramyocardial catecholamines (e.g. dibenamine) were the least effective in protecting cardiac muscle whereas those drugs that act by ganglionic blockade (e.g. mecamylamine) or by direct intramyocardial catecholamine-depletion (e.g. reserpine) were the most effective. Furthermore, it is clear that blood catecholamine levels are often normal but that identical ECG findings are seen with high systemic catecholamines. This clinical and pharmacological data support the concept that the cardiac necrosis is due to catecholamine toxicity and that catecholamines released directly into the heart via neural connections are much more toxic than those reaching the heart via the blood stream, though clearly the two routes could be additive in the intact, non-adrenalectomized animal. Intracoronary infusions of epinephrine reproduce the characteristic ECG pattern of neurocardiac disease which are reminiscent of subendocardial ischaemia, though no ischaemic lesion can be found in the hearts of dogs sacrificed after several months of infusions (Barger 1961). In the years that followed numerous reports emanated from around the world documenting the production of cardiac repolarization abnormalities in the context of various neurological catastrophes and proposing that this was due to an autonomic storm. It seemed likely that the connection between neuropsychiatric illness and the visceral organs would be provided by the autonomic nervous system.

Melville et al. (1963) produced ECG changes and myocardial necrosis by stimulating the hypothalamus of cats. With anterior hypothalamic stimulation, parasympathetic responses occurred with bradycardia predominating. Lateral hypothalamic stimulation produced tachycardia and ST segment depressions. With intense bilateral and repeated lateral stimulation, persistent, irreversible ECG changes occurred and post-mortem examination revealed a stereotyped cardiac lesion characterized by intense cytoplasmic eosinophilia with loss of cross striations and some haemorrhage. The coronary arteries were normal without occlusion. Although Melville referred to this lesion as 'infarction,' it is probably best to reserve that term for coagulative necrosis caused by ischaemia. This lesion is probably identical to Selye's ESCN and would now be called coagulative myocytolysis, myofibrillar degeneration or contraction band necrosis. More recently Oppenheimer has mapped the chronotropic organizational structure in the rat insular cortex, demonstrating that sympathetic innervation arises from a more rostral part of the posterior insula then does parasympathetic innervation (Oppenheimer 1990).

Despite the fact that myocardial damage could definitely be produced in animals, until the mid-1960s there was little recognition that this actually occurred in human beings with acute neurological or psychiatric illness until Koskelo et al. reported on three patients with ECG changes due to subarachnoid haemorrhage who were noted on post-mortem examination to have several small subendocardial petechial haemorrhages (Koskelo 1964).

Connor reported focal myocytolysis in 8% of 231 autopsies, with the highest incidence seen in patients dying of intracranial haemorrhages. The lesion reported by Connor conforms to the descriptions of Selye's ESCN or what might now be called myofibrillar degeneration, coagulative myocytolysis or contraction band necrosis. Connor pointed out that previous pathological reports probably overlooked the lesion because of the fact that it was multifocal with each individual focus being quite small requiring extensive tissue sampling. It is clear now that even Connor underestimated the prevalence of the lesion and that serial sections are required to rigorously exclude its presence (Connor, 1969).

Greenshoot and Reichenbach reported on 3 new patients with subarachnoid haemorrhage and a review of 6 prior patients from the same medical centre (Greenshoot 1969). All 9 of these patients had cardiac lesions of varying degrees of severity ranging from eosinophilia with preservation of cross striations to transformation of the myocardial cell cytoplasm into dense eosinophilic transverse bands with intervening granularity, sometimes with endocardial haemorrhages. Both the ECG abnormalities and the cardiac pathology could be reproduced in cats given mesencephalic reticular formation stimulation. Adrenalectomy did not protect the hearts, supporting the contention that the ECG changes and cardiac lesion are due to direct intracardiac release of catecholamines.

Hawkins and Clower injected blood intracranially into mice and thereby producing the characteristic myocardial lesions (Hawkins 1971). The number of lesions could be reduced but not obliterated by pretreatment with adrenalectomy and the use of either atropine or reserpine, which suggested that the cause of the lesions was in part due to sympathetic overactivity (humorally reaching the myocardium from the adrenal and by direct release into the muscle by intracardiac nerves) and in part due to parasympathetic overactivity. This supports the concept that the cause is an autonomic storm with both divisions contributing to the pathogenesis.

Jacob et al. (1972) experimentally produced subarachnoid haemorrhage in dogs and carefully studied the sequential haemodynamic and ultrastructural changes which occurred. The haemodynamic changes occurred in four stages and directly paralleled the effects seen with intravenous norepinephrine injections. These stages were:

1 dramatic rise in systemic blood pressure

2 extreme sinus tachycardia with various arrhythmias (e.g. nodal or ventricular tachycardia, bradycardia, atrioventricular block, ventricular premature beats, ventricular tachycardia, ventricular fibrillation with sudden death), all of which could be suppressed by bilateral vagotomy or orbital frontal resection

3 rise in left ventricular pressure parallel to rise in systemic pressure

4 up to twofold increase in coronary blood flow.

Ultrastructurally, a series of three stereotyped events occurred, which could be imitated exactly with norepinephrine injections. These were:

1 migration of intramitochondrial granules containing Ca++ to the periphery of the mitochondria,

2 disappearance of these granules

3 myofilament disintegration at the I bands while the density of the I-band was increased in the intact sarcomeres (Jacob 1972).

Partially successful efforts to modify the development of neuro-cardiac lesions were made by using reserpine pretreatment in mice subjected to simulated intracranial haemorrhage (McNair 1970) and by Hunt and Gore who pretreated a group of rats with propranolol and then attempted to produce cardiac lesions with intracranial blood injections. No lesions were found in the control animals, in 21 of the 46 untreated rats and in only 4 of the 22 treated rats (Hunt 1972). This suggested that neurological influences via catecholamines may be partly responsible for cardiac cell death due to ischaemic causes.

The phenomenology of the various types of myocardial cell death was finally clarified by Baroldi, who pointed out that there were three main patterns of myocardial necrosis:

1 coagulation necrosis, the fundamental lesion of infarction in which the cell loses its capacity to contract and dies in the atonic state with no myofibillar damage

2 colliquative myocytolysis, in which oedematous vacuolization with dissolution of myofibrils without hypercontraction occurs in the low-output syndromes

3 coagulative myocytolysis in which the cell dies in a hypercontracted state, with early myofibrillar damage, and anomalous irregular cross-band formations (Baroldi 1975).

Coagulative myocytolysis is seen in reperfused areas around regions of coagulation necrosis in transplanted hearts, in 'stone hearts', in sudden unexpected and accidental death, and in hearts exposed to toxic levels of catecholamines such as in patients with phaeochromocytoma. This is probably the major lesion described by Selye as ESCN and is clearly the lesion seen in animals and people suffering acute neurological or psychiatric catastrophes. Although coagulative myocytolysis is probably the preferred term, the terms myofibrillar degeneration and contraction band necrosis are commonly used in the literature. This lesion tends to calcify early and to have a multifocal subendocardial predisposition.

It is likely that the subcellular mechanisms underlying the development of coagulative myocytolysis involve calcium entry. Zimmerman and Hulsmann reported that the perfusion of rat hearts with calcium free media for short periods of time creates a situation such that upon readmission of calcium, there is a massive contracture followed by necrosis and enzyme release (Zimmerman 1966). This phenomenon, known as the calcium paradox, can be imitated almost exactly with reoxygenation followed by hypoxaemia and reperfusion following ischaemia. The latter called the oxygen paradox, has been linked to the calcium paradox by pathological calcium entry (Hearse 1978). This major ionic shift is probably the cause of the dramatic ECG changes seen in the context of neurological catastrophe, a fact that could explain the phenomenon of sudden unexpected death (SUD) in multiple contexts.

Although SUD is now recognized as a medical problem of major epidemiological importance, it has generally been assumed that neurological disease rarely results in SUD. In fact, it has been traditionally taught that neurological illnesses almost never cause sudden demise, with the only exceptions being the occasional patient who dies during an epileptic convulsion or rapidly in the context of a subarachnoid haemorrhage. Further, it has been assumed that the various SUD syndromes (e.g. sudden death in middle-aged men, sudden infant death syndrome [SIDS], sudden unexpected nocturnal death syndrome [SUNDS], frightened to death [a.k.a. 'Voodoo' death], sudden death during a seizure, sudden death during natural catastrophe, sudden death associated with drug abuse, sudden death in wild and domestic animals, sudden death during asthma attacks, sudden death during the alcohol withdrawal syndrome, sudden death during grief after a major loss, sudden death during panic attacks, sudden death from mental stress, and sudden death during war) are entirely separate and have no unifying mechanism. For example, it is generally accepted that sudden death in middle aged men is usually caused by a cardiac arrhythmia (i.e. ventricular fibrillation) that results in functional cardiac arrest, while most work on SIDS focuses on respiratory failure.

However, the connection between the nervous system and the cardiopulmonary system provides the unifying link that allows a coherent explanation for most, if not all, of the forms of SUD. Powerful evidence from multiple disparate disciplines allows for a neurological explanation for SUD (Samuels 1993).

Neurogenic heart disease

Definition of neurogenic electrocardiographic changes

A wide variety of changes in the ECG is seen in the context of neurological disease. Two major categories of change are regularly noted:

- arrhythmias
- repolarization changes.

It is likely that the increased tendency for life-threatening arrhythmias found in patients with acute neurological disease is due to the repolarization change, which increases the vulnerable period during which an extrasystole would be likely to result in ventricular tachycardia and/or ventricular fibrillation. Thus, the essential and potentially most lethal features of the ECG, which are known to change in the context of neurologic disease, are the ST segment and T-wave, reflecting abnormalities in repolarization. Most often, the changes are seen best in the anterolateral or inferolateral leads. If the ECG is read by pattern recognition by someone who is not aware of the clinical history, it will often be said to present subendocardial infarction or anterolateral ischemia. The electrocardiographic abnormalities usually improve, often dramatically with death by brain criteria.

The phenomenon is not rare. In a series of 100 consecutive stroke patients, 90% showed abnormalities on the ECG, compared with 50% of a control population of 100 patients admitted for carcinoma of the colon (Dimant 1977). This, of course, does not mean that 90% of stroke patients have neurogenic electrocardiographic changes. Obviously, stroke and coronary artery disease have common risk factors, so that many electrocardiographic abnormalities in stroke patients represent concomitant atherosclerotic coronary disease. Nonetheless, a significant number of stroke patients have authentic neurogenic electrocardiographic changes.

Mechanism of the production of neurogenic heart disease

Catecholamine infusion

Josué first showed that epinephrine infusions could cause cardiac hypertophy (Josué 1907). This observation has been reproduced on many occasions, documenting the fact that systemically administered catecholamines are not only associated with electrocardiographic changes reminiscent of widespread ischaemia but with a characteristic pathological picture in the cardiac muscle that is distinct from myocardial infarction. An identical picture may be found in human beings with chronically elevated catecholamines as is seen with phaeochromocytoma. Patients with stroke often have elevated systemic catecholamine levels, a fact which may, in part, account for the high incidence of cardiac arrhythmias and ECG changes seen in these patients. On light microscopy, these changes range from increased eosinophilic staining with preservation of cross-striations to total transformation of the myocardial cell cytoplasm into dense eosinophilic transverse bands with intervening granularity. In severely injured areas, infiltration of the necrotic debris by mononuclear cells is often noted, sometimes with haemorrhage. Ultrastructurally, the changes in cardiac muscle are even more widespread than they appear to be in light microscopy. Nearly every muscle cell shows some pathologic alteration, ranging from a granular appearance of the myofibrils to profound disruption of the cell architecture with relative preservation of ribosomes and mitochondria. Intracardiac nerves can be seen, identified by their external lamina, microtubules, neurofibrils, and the presence of intracytoplasmic vesicles. These nerves can sometimes be seen immediately adjacent to an area of myocardial cell damage. The pathological changes in the cardiac muscle are usually less at a distance from the nerve, often returning completely to normal by a distance of 2–4 um away from the nerve ending (Jacob 1972).

Myofibrillar degeneration (also known as coagulative myocytolysis and contraction band necrosis) is an easily recognizable form of cardiac injury distinct in several major respects from coagulation necrosis, the major lesion of myocardial infarction (Baroldi 1975, Karch 1986). In coagulation necrosis, the cells die in a relaxed state without prominent contraction bands. This is not visible by any method for many hours or even days. Calcification occurs only late and the lesion elicits a polymorphonuclear cell response. In stark contrast, in myofibrillary degeneration the cells die in a hypercontracted state with prominent contraction bands (Fig. 54.1). The lesion is visible early, perhaps within minutes of its onset. It elicits a mononuclear cell response and may calcify almost immediately (Rona 1985, Karch 1986).

Stress plus or minus steroids

A similar, if not identical, cardiac lesion can be produced using various models of 'stress.' This concept was applied to the heart when Selye published his monograph *The Chemical Prevention of Cardiac Necrosis* in 1958 (Selye 1958). He found that cardiac lesions probably identical to those described above could be regularly produced in animals that were pretreated with certain steroids, particularly 2-alpha-methyl-9-alpha-fluorohydrocortisone (fluorocortisol), and then subjected to various types of stress. Other hormones, such as dihydrotachysterol (calciferol) and thyroxine, could also sensitize animals for stress-induced mycardial lesions, but less potently than fluorocortisol. This so-called stress could be of multiple types, including restraint, surgery, bacteraemia, vagotomy, toxins, and others. He believed that the 'first mediator' in translating these widely disparate stimuli into a sterotyped cardiac lesion was the hypothalamus and that it, by its control over the autonomic nervous system, caused the release of certain agents that were toxic to the myocardial cell. Since Selye's original work, similar experiments have been repeated in many different types of laboratory animals with comparable results. Although the

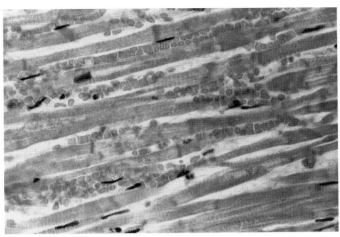

Fig. 54.1 Contaction band necrosis.

administration of exogenous steroids facilitates the production of cardiac lesions, it is clear that stress alone can result in the production of morphologically identical lesions.

Whether a similar pathophysiology could ever be operable in human beings is, of course, of great interest. Many investigators have speculated on the role of 'stress' in the pathogenesis of human cardiovascular disease and, in particular, on its relationship to the phenomenon of sudden unexpected death. A few autopsies on patients who experienced sudden death have shown myofibrillar degeneration. Cebelin and Hirsch reported on a careful retrospective analysis of the hearts of 15 victims of physical assault who died

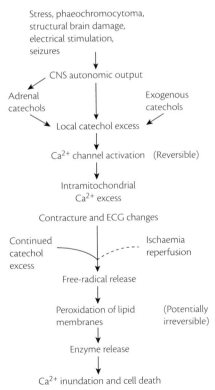

Fig. 54.2 Proposed cascade leading to neurogenic heart disease.

as a direct result of the assault, but without sustaining internal injuries. Eleven of the 15 individuals showed myofibrillar degeneration. Age and cardiac disease-matched controls showed little or no evidence of this change. This appears to represent a human stress cardiomyopathy (Cebelin 1980). Whether or not such assaults can be considered murder has become an interesting legal correlate of the problem.

Since the myofibrillar degeneration is predominantly subendocardial, it may involve the cardiac conducting system, thus predisposing to cardiac arrhythmias. This lesion, combined with the propensity of catecholamines to produce arrhythmias even in a normal heart may well raise the risk of a serious arrhythmia. This may be the major immediate mechanism of sudden death in many neurological circumstances, such as subarachnoid haemorrhage, stroke, epilepsy, head trauma, psychological stress, and increased intracranial pressure. Even the arrhythmogenic nature of digitalis may be largely mediated by the central nervous system. Further evidence for this is the antiarrhythmic effect of sympathetic denervation of the heart for cardiac arrhythmias of many types.

Furthermore, it is known that the stress-induced myocardial lesions can be prevented by sympathetic blockade using many different classes of anti-adrenergic agents, most notably, ganglionic blockers such as mecamylamine and catecholamine-depleting agents such as reserpine (Raab 1961). This suggests that catecholamines, either released directly into the heart by sympathetic nerve terminals or reaching the heart through the bloodstream after release from the adrenal medulla, may be excitotoxic to myocardial cells.

Reversible left ventricular dysfunction affecting the apex out of proportion to the base is known to occur in human beings (predominantly older women) after emotional stress (Ako 2006). This so-called myocardial stunning may present with chest pain, electrocardiographic abnormalities or frank heart failure (pulmonary oedema) and is usually associated with a modest myocardial enzyme (troponin) leak. Endocardial biopsies show contraction bands and plasma catecholamines are usually found to be elevated (Wittstein 2005). The characteristic appearance of the four chamber view of the echocardiogram or the ventriculogram shows a dilated apex and relatively uninvolved base producing an appearance that is reminiscent of the Japanese octopus trapping pot (takotsubo), a fact that has led to the naming of this phenomenon as the takotsubo-like cardiomyopathy (Kawai 2000). Takotsubo-like cardiomyopathy is known to increase in frequency around the time of large-scale stressors, such as earthquakes (Watanabe 2005). It is likely that the takotsubo-like cardiomyopathy represents the tip of an iceberg, below which lurks a much larger problem of neurally induced visceral organ damage, of which severe left ventricular apical ballooning is only one small, albeit dramatic, component.

Nervous system stimulation

Nervous system stimulation produces cardiac lesions histologically indistinguishable from those just described for stress, and catecholamine-induced cardiac damage. It has been known for a long while that stimulation of the hypothalamus can lead to autonomic cardiovascular disturbances, and many years ago, lesions in the heart and gastrointestinal tract had been produced using hypothalamic stimulation. It has been clearly demonstrated that stimulation of the lateral hypothalamus produces hypertension or ECG changes reminiscent of those seen in patients with central nervous system damage of various types. Furthermore, this effect on the blood pressure and ECG can be completely prevented by C2 spinal section and stellate ganglionectomy, but not by vagotomy, suggesting that the mechanism of the electrocardiographic changes is sympathetic rather than parasympathetic or humoral. Stimulation of the anterior hypothalamus produces bradycardia, an effect that can be blocked by vagotomy. Unilateral hypothalamic stimulation does not result in histological evidence of myocardial damage by light microscopy, but bilateral prolonged stimulation regularly produces myofibrillar degeneration indistinguishable from that produced by catecholamine injections and stress, as previously described (Melville 1963).

Other methods of producing cardiac lesions of this type include stimulation of the limbic cortex, the mesencephalic reticular formation, the stellate ganglion, and regions known to elicit cardiac reflexes such as the aortic arch. Experimental intracerebral and subarachnoid haemorrhages can also result in cardiac contraction band lesions. These neurogenic cardiac lesions will occur even in an adrenalectomized animal, although they will be somewhat less pronounced (Hawkins 1971). This evidence argues strongly against an exclusively humoral mechanism in the intact organism. High levels of circulating catecholamines exaggerate the electrocardiographic findings and myocardial lesions, but high circulating catecholamine levels are not required for the production of pathologic changes. These electrocardiographic abnormalities and cardiac lesions are stereotyped and identical to those found in the stress and catecholamine models already outlined. They are not affected by vagotomy and are blocked by manoeuvres that interfere with the action of the sympathetic limb of the autonomic nervous system, such as C2 spinal section, stellate ganglion blockade, and administration of anti-adrenergic drugs such as propranolol.

It seems clear that the insula is the region of the cerebral cortex that most directly affects cardiac structure and function. There is a great deal of clinical evidence that insular diseases are the most likely to produce neurally induced cardiac changes, though the issue of lateral dominance of one insula over the other has not yet been completely settled (Laowattana 2006, Ay 2006, Oppenheimer 2006, Cechetto 1987, Tokgozoglu 1999).

The histological changes in the myocardium range from normal muscle on light microscopy to severely necrotic (but not ischaemic) lesions with secondary mononuclear cell infiltration. The findings on ultrastructural examination are invariably more widespread, often involving nearly every muscle cell, even when the light microscopic appearance is unimpressive. The electrocardiographic findings undoubtedly reflect the total amount of muscle membrane affected by the pathophysiological process. Thus, the ECG may be normal when the lesion is early and demonstrable only by electron microscopy. Conversely, the ECG may be grossly abnormal when only minimal findings are present by light microscopy, since the cardiac membrane abnormality responsible for the electrocardiographic changes may be reversible. Cardiac arrhythmias of many types may also be elicited by nervous system stimulation along the outflow of the sympathetic nervous system.

Reperfusion

The fourth, and last, model for the production of myofibrillar degeneration is reperfusion, as is commonly seen in patients dying after a period of time on a left ventricular assist pump for cardiac surgery. Similar lesions are seen in hearts that were reperfused using angioplasty or fibrinolytic therapy. The mechanism by which reperfusion of ischaemic cardiac muscle produces myofibrillar degeneration involves entry of calcium after a period of relative deprivation (Braunwald 1985).

Sudden calcium influx by one of several possible mechanism (e.g. a period of calcium deficiency with loss of intracellular calcium, a period of anoxia followed by reoxygenation of the electron transport system, a period of ischemia followed by reperfusion, or opening of the receptor-operated calcium channels by excessive amounts of locally released norepinephrine) may be the final common pathway by which the irreversible contractures occur, leading to myofibrillar degeneration. Thus reperfusion induced myocardial cell death may be a form of apoptosis (programmed cell death) analogous to that seen in the central nervous system wherein excitotoxicity with glutamate results in a similar, if not identical, series of events (Gottlieb 1994).

The precise cellular mechanism for the electrocardiographic change and the histological lesion may well reflect the effects of large volumes of norepinephrine released into the myocardium from sympathetic nerve terminals (Eliot 1979). The fact that the cardiac necrosis is greatest near the nerve terminals in the endocardium and is progressively less severe as one samples muscle approaching the epicardium provides further evidence that catecholamine toxicity produces the lesion (Greenhoot 1969). This locally released norepinephrine is known to stimulate synthesis of adenosine 3',5'-cyclic phosphate, which in turn results in the opening of the calcium channel with influx of calcium and efflux of potassium. This efflux of potassium could explain the peaked T-waves (a hyperkalaemic pattern) often seen early in the evolution of neurogenic electrocardiographic changes (Jacob 1972). The actin and myosin filaments interact under the influence of calcium but do not relax unless the calcium channel closes. Continuously high levels of norepinephrine in the region may result in failure of the calcium channel to close, leading to cell death, and finally to leakage of enzymes out of the myocardial cell. Free radicals released as a result of reperfusion after ischemia or by the metabolism of catecholamines to the known toxic metabolite adrenochrome may contribute to cell membrane destruction, leading to leakage of cardiac enzymes into the blood (Meerson 1983, Singal 1982). Thus, the cardiac toxicity of locally released norepinephrine would represent a continuum ranging from a brief reversible burst of electrocardiographic abnormalities to a pattern resembling hyperkalaemia and then, finally, to an irreversible failure of the muscle cell with permanent repolarization abnormalities, or even the occurrence of transmural cardiac necrosis with Q waves seen on the ECG.

Histological changes would also represent a continuum ranging from complete reversibility in a normal heart through mild changes seen best with electron microscopy to severe myocardial cell necrosis with mononuclear cell infiltration and even haemorrhages. The level of cardiac enzymes released and the electrocardiographic changes would roughly correlate with the severity and extent of the pathologic process. This explanation, summarized in Fig. 54.2, would tie together all the observations in the catecholamine infusion, stress plus or minus steroid, nervous system stimulation, and reperfusion models.

In conclusion, there is powerful evidence suggesting that overactivity of the sympathetic limb of the autonomic nervous system is the common phenomenon that links the major cardiac and

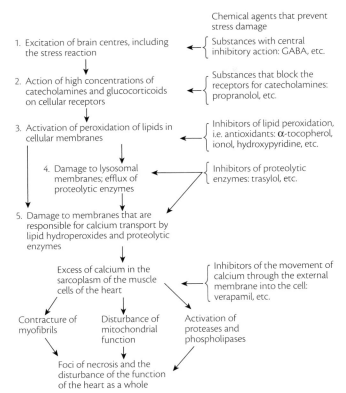

1. Excitation of brain centres, including the stress reaction ← { Chemical agents that prevent stress damage. Substances with central inhibitory action: GABA, etc.

2. Action of high concentrations of catecholamines and glucocorticoids on cellular receptors ← { Substances that block the receptors for catecholamines: propranolol, etc.

3. Activation of peroxidation of lipids in cellular membranes ← { Inhibitors of lipid peroxidation, i.e. antioxidants: α-tocopherol, ionol, hydroxypyridine, etc.

4. Damage to lysosomal membranes; efflux of proteolytic enzymes ← { Inhibitors of proteolytic enzymes: trasylol, etc.

5. Damage to membranes that are responsible for calcium transport by lipid hydroperoxides and proteolytic enzymes

Excess of calcium in the sarcoplasm of the muscle cells of the heart ← { Inhibitors of the movement of calcium through the external membrane into the cell: verapamil, etc.

Contracture of myofibrils

Disturbance of mitochondrial function

Activation of proteases and phospholipases

Foci of necrosis and the disturbance of the function of the heart as a whole

Fig. 54.3 Potential preventions and treatments of neurogenic heart disease.

pulmonary pathologies seen in neurological catastrophes. These profound effects on the heart and lungs may contribute in a major way to the mortality rates of many primarily neurologic conditions such as subarachnoid haemorrhage, status epilepticus, and head trauma. These phenomena may also be important in the pathogenesis of sudden unexpected death in adults, sudden infant death, sudden death during asthma attacks, cocaine and amphetamine related deaths, and sudden death during the alcohol withdrawal syndrome, all of which may be linked by stress and catecholamine toxicity (Fig. 54.2).

Investigations aimed at altering the natural history of these events using catecholamine receptor blockade, calcium-channel blockers, free radical scavengers, and antioxidants are ongoing in many centres around the world (Fig. 54.3).

References

Ako, J., Krishnankutty, S., Farouque, O., Honda, Y., Fitzgerald, P. J. (2006). Transient left ventricular dysfunction under severe stress: brain-heart relationship revisited. *Am J Med* **119**, 10–17.

Barger, A. C., Herd, J. A., Liebowitz, M. R. (1961). Chronic catherization of coronary artery induction of ECG pattern of myocardial ischemia by intracoronary epinephrine. *Proc Soc Experimental Biology and Medicine* **107**, 474–77.

Baroldi, F. (1975). Different morphological types of myocardial cell death in man. In Fleckstein A, Rona G, eds. *Recent Advances in Studies in Cardiac Structure and metabolism. Pathophysiology and Morphology of Myocardial Cell Alteration.* University Park Press, Baltimore, Vol 6, pp. 385–97.

Braunwald, E., Kloner, R. A. (1985). Myocardial reperfusion: a double-edged sword? *J. Clin Invest* **76**, 1713–1719.

Burch, G. E., Myers, R. Adildskov, J. A. (1954). A new electrocardiographic pattern observed in cerebrovascular accidents. *Circulation* **9**, 719–26.

Byer, E. Ashman, R., Toth, L. A. (1947). Electrocardiogram with large upright T wave and long Q-T intervals. *Am Heart J* **33**, 796–801.

Cannon, W. B. (1942). 'Voodoo' death. American Anthropologist.

Cebelin, M., Hirsch, C. S. (1980). Human stress cardiomyopathy. *Hum Pathol* **ll**, 123–32.

Cechetto, D. F., Saper, C. B. (1987). Evidence for a viscerotopic sensory representation in the cortex and thalamus in the rat. *J Comp Neurol*, **262**, 27–45.

Connor, R. C. R. (1969): Myocardial damage secondary to brain lesions. *Am Heart J.* **78**, 145–48.

Cropp, C. F., Manning, G. W. (1960). *Electrocardiographic change simulating myocardial ischemia and infarction associated with spontaneous intracranial haemorrhage.*

Dimant, J., Grob, D. (1977). Electrocardiographic changes and myocardial damage in patients with acute cerebrovascular accidents. *Stroke* **8**, 448–55.

Eliot, R. S., Todd, G. L., Pieper, G. M., Clayton, F. C. (1979). Pathophysiology of catecholamine-mediated myocardial damage. *J. S.Carolina Med. Assoc* **75**, 513–518.

Engel, G. (1971). Sudden and rapid death during psychological stress. *Ann Intern Med* **74**, 771–82.

Gottlieb, R., Burleson, K. O., Kloner, R. A., *et al* (1994). Reperfusion injury induces apoptosis in rabbit cardiomyocytes. *J Clin Invest* **94**, 1621–28.

Greenhoot, J. H., Reichenbach, D. D. (1969). Cardiac injury and subarachnoid haemorrhage. *J Neurosurg* **30**, 521–31.

Hawkins, W. E., Clower, B. R. (1971). Myocardial damage after head trauma and simulated intracranial haemorrhage in mice: the role of the autonomic nervous system. *Cardiovascular Res* **5**, 524–29.

Hearse, D. J., Humphrey, S. M., Bullock, G. R. (1978). The oxygen paradox and the calcium paradox:two facets of the same problem? *J Molecular Cellular Cardiol* **10**, 641–68.

Jacob, W. A., Van Bogaert, A., DeGroot-Lasseel, M. H. A. (1972). Myocardial ultrastructural and haemodynamic reactions during experimental subarachnoid haemorrhage. J *Molecular Cellular Cardiol* **4**, 287–98.

Josue, O. (1907). Hypertrophie cardiaque causee par l'adrenaline et la toxine typhique. *C R Soc Biol (Paris)* **63**, 285–87.

Karch, S. B., Billingham, M. E. (1986). Myocardial contraction bands revisited. *Human Path* **17**, 9–13.

Koskelo, P., Punsar, S., Sipila, W. (1964). Subendocardial haemorrhage and ECG changes in intracranial bleeding. *Brit Med J* **1**, 1479–83.

Laowattana, S., Zeger, S. L., Lima, J. A. C., Goodman, S. N., Wittstein, I. S., Oppenheimer, S. M. (2006). Left insular stroke is associated with adverse cardiac outcome. *Neurology* **66**, 477–483.

Levine, H. D. (1953). Non-specificity of the electrocardiogram associated with coronary heart disease. *Am J Med* **15**, 344–50.

McNair, J. L., Clower, B. R., Sanford, R. A. (1970). The effect of reserpine pretreatment on myocardial damage associated with simulated intracranial haemorrhage in mice. *Eur. J. Pharmacol* **9**, 1–6.

Meerson, F. Z. (1983). Pathogenesis and prophylaxis of cardiac lesions in stress. *Advances in Myocardiology* **4**, 3–21.

Melville, K. I., Blum, B., Shister, H. E., *et al.* (1963). Cardiac ischaemic changes and arrhythmias induced by hypothalamic stimulation. *Am J Cardiol*, **12**, 781–91.

Oppenheimer, S. M. (2006). Cerebrogenic cardiac arrhythmias: cortical lateralization and clinical significance. *Clin Auton Res*; **16**, 6–11.

Oppenheimer, S. M., Cechetto, D. F. (1990). Cardiac chronotropic organization of the rate insular cortex. *Brain Research* **533**, 66–72.

Raab, W., Stark, E., MacMillan, W. H., *et al.* (1961). Sympathogenic oriin and anti-adrenergic prevention of stress-induced myocardial lesions. *Am J Cardiol* **8**, 203–211.

Richter, C. P. (1957). On the phenomenon of sudden death in animals and man. *Psychosomatic Medicine* **19**, 191–98.

Rona, G. (1985). Catecholamine cardiotixicity. *J Molecular Cellular Cardiol* **17**, 291–306.

Samuels, M. A. (1993). Neurally induced cardiac damage. *Neurologic Clinics* **11**, 273–92.

Selye, H. (1958). *The Chemical Prevention of Cardiac Necrosis*. New York, Ronald Press.

Singal, P. K., Kapur, N., Dhillon, K. S., Beamish, R. E., Dhalla, N. A. (1982). Role of free radicals in catecholamine-induced cardiomyocaphy. *Can J Physiol Pharmacol* **60**, 1390–97.

Tokgozoglu, S. L., Batur, M. K., Topcuoglu, M. A., Saribas, O., Kes, S., Oto, A. (1999). Effects of stroke localization on cardiac autonomic balance and sudden death. *Stroke* **30**, 1307–1311.

Wittstein, I. S., Thiemann, D. R., Lima, J. A. C., *et al.* (2005). Neurohuymoral features of myocardial stunning due to sudden emotional stress. *N Engl J Med* **352**, 539–548.

Zimmerman, A. N. A., Hulsmann, W. C. (1966). Paradoxical influence of calcium ions on the permeability of the cell membranes of the isolated rate heart. *Nature* **211**, 616–47.

CHAPTER 55

Transient loss of consciousness

J. Gert van Dijk

Introduction

Attacks of 'transient loss of consciousness' (TLOC) are a frequently occurring medical problem. Syncope, the most frequent form of TLOC, accounts for up to 5% of emergency room visits and up to 3% of hospital admissions. TLOC may be due to a large variety of causes, including the 'common faint', epileptic seizures, autonomic failure, cardiac arrhythmias and functional disorders. In addition some disorders only rarely cause TLOC, such as vertebrobasilar transient ischaemic attacks (TIAs), and some may merely mimic TLOC, such as sleep attacks and cataplexy. TLOC is associated with two types of risks: the first concerns the consequences of loss of consciousness, such as falling, drowning or traffic accidents; these risks are largely independent of the cause of TLOC. The second type of risk is associated with the cause of TLOC, and differs strongly between causes: the prospects for quality of life, morbidity and mortality after a first TLOC episode are excellent for a 16-year-old with a vasovagal faint, but poor for a 70-year-old with an abnormal electrocardiogram (ECG) and antecedent heart disease.

Any disorder that is both common and carries significant risks deserves a correct diagnosis. Unfortunately, diagnostic mistakes appear to be uncomfortably common. Epidemiological surveys of syncope usually contain a category 'unexplained syncope' making up 10–20% of all cases. Estimates of the proportions of cases of presumed epilepsy in which the diagnosis was later shown to be something else vary, reaching a staggering 30% in some settings. There are several probable reasons for such high rates of misdiagnosis of TLOC.

The first is a combination of the wide range of causes of TLOC and medical specialization, ensuring that specialists have gaps in their knowledge. While neurologists are trained in epilepsy, they commonly receive little training in syncope. Loss of consciousness associated with myoclonic jerks is still often regarded as conclusive of an epileptic seizure; jerks are common enough in syncope to state that the fact of their presence should count for much less than details about their nature and duration. Similar knowledge gaps probably occur in other fields. 'Functional' or 'psychogenic' attacks pose problems for many specialists, including psychiatrists. Pseudo-epileptic attacks often take years to be diagnosed correctly; how often pseudo-syncope occurs is not even reliably known. The communication gap may be at its widest here: somatic specialists use the label 'functional' frequently, both when dealing with patients and in the scientific literature, but the term does not occur in the DSM-IV. Oddly, 'conversion' in the DSM-IV is limited to symptoms of a seemingly motor and sensory nature: as consciousness is not mentioned, pseudo-syncope cannot formally be categorized as such.

The second reason for misdiagnoses may be a lack of training in vasovagal syncope, an entity not claimed by any specialty as its own. While the diagnosis is easy in the vast majority of cases, the rare difficult cases, such as those occurring after physical exercise, during sleep or without any apparent trigger, cause confusion. 'Rare' is a relative term here: supposing that difficult presentations make up only 1% of all vasovagal attacks, the fact that vasovagal syncope affects about one third of the population means that the number of difficult cases is not that different from the numbers of people with epileptic seizures or cardiac syncope.

Thirdly and finally, there is no universally accepted system of labelling and classifying such disorders. The European Society of Cardiology has evolved a system starting in 2000, focusing mostly on syncope (Brignole et al. 2001, Brignole et al. 2004, ESC 2009, Van Dijk et al. 2009). A key problem in papers on syncope is an often occurring lack of clarity regarding its definition, causing confusion between a 'wide' interpretation, following which syncope might include epileptic seizures and concussion, and a 'narrow' one, limiting syncope to TLOC caused by cerebral hypoperfusion. The lack of clarity may be compounded by a failure of authors to follow their own definitions strictly: in many cases the given definition is of the wide type, but the lack of epileptic seizures or psychogenic attacks or other disorders in the results of such papers show that the concept used was not the one as defined. There are some other terminological problems as well: 'seizures' may imply an epileptic mechanism to many readers, but may only mean a type of 'attack' to others, who will use it to describe syncopal attacks as readily as epileptic ones.

The lack of a common ground is detrimental for patient care, with as a result high rates of incorrect diagnoses and inconsequential, inefficient and costly investigations. Medical education will suffer as it is difficult for students or residents to acquire an overview of the field. Finally, research suffers because results cannot be generalised confidently in view of unknown differences between study populations.

The present chapter provides a common ground for TLOC. Its primary purpose is to present an overview of the field through a classification designed to aid differential diagnosis. The classification is broadly based on pathophysiology, but does not adhere to pathophysiological lines painstakingly. In fact, pathophysiological details are overlooked at times to avoid clinical confusion. Examples are the sudden collapse of the circulation in syncope associated with physical exertion in structural cardiac disease. There is evidence that a reflex is involved, but this cause of syncope is categorized as 'cardiac' rather than as 'reflex syncope'. The result should be of use to medical students, residents, general practitioners, emergency room physicians, and specialists wishing to broaden their understanding of forms outside their specialty. As such, it touches on many disorders that do not or not directly involve the autonomic nervous system.

Meaning of 'consciousness' in the context of TLOC

According to the *Compact Oxford Dictionary* (online edition), 'conscious' means *'aware of and responding to one's surroundings'*, and 'unconscious' accordingly adds *'not'* to that statement. Plum and Posner, in their textbook on the diagnosis of stupor and coma (Posner 2007), distinguish between the arousal and content aspects of consciousness. 'Arousal' describes a state that ranges from being fully awake to unconsciousness in the sense of looking asleep but without the ability of being woken. 'Content' describes more complex phenomena such as self-awareness. Others may recognize these two aspects as 'quantitative' and 'qualitative' aspects of consciousness.

If consciousness can be used in two ways, it seems logical to do the same for 'loss of consciousness'. Following this reasoning examples of unconsciousness affecting arousal are disorders that cause patients to lie unresponsively on the floor, such as syncope. The question whether there still is content in these disorders may hold some interest, but is clinically irrelevant: for practical purposes a complete loss of 'arousal' also involves a loss of 'content'. Examples of unconsciousness affecting 'content' exclusively are epileptic seizures of the absence and complex partial types, in which patients show no or limited responsiveness, but sit or stand upright, look awake, and may be responsive to some degree. While this state is indeed labelled as 'unconscious' by some, this use does not conform to how 'unconscious' is interpreted by the common public, including the vast majority of physicians. For them active standing or sitting is not compatible with 'unconscious'. This distinction makes sense from a diagnostic point of view: a state in which a patient can remain standing or sitting suggests a different set of diagnoses than do states in which patients lose postural control. For this reason 'loss of consciousness' concerns the arousal aspect, implying a loss of postural control. Consciousness in states such as complex partial seizures and absence seizures can be labelled as 'altered' rather than lost.

'Loss of consciousness' as defined can be established after the fact through history taking from patients as well as eye witnesses. Three items are crucial: during the attack there should be a lack of normal responsiveness to external stimuli and an absence of voluntary motor control. The latter can be apparent as either stiffness or flaccidity, with or without muscle jerking. The third item is amnesia for the attack, established afterwards. Note that the reliance on history taking means that the presence of these items should strictly be preceded by 'apparent', as appearances can be misleading.

This approach recognizes functional disorders such as pseudo-epilepsy and pseudo-syncope as TLOC. In such states it is unclear to which extent patients are aware of themselves, their role in the attack or their surroundings. What is clear is that there are no gross abnormalities of cerebral function as evidenced by an EEG, definitely present in all other causes. Such thorny issues might suggest that these conditions have no place in a classification of TLOC. In fact, in the first version of the ESC classification they were considered as mimics rather than as TLOC (Brignole et al. 2001). The main reason to consider them as forms of TLOC is clinical utility. The triple presence of amnesia, abnormal responsiveness and absent voluntary motor control holds as much for these disorders as it does for generalized epileptic seizures or syncope, meaning they all belong together in the same differential diagnostic list. In this chapter not all forms receive equal attention. While syncope is described globally, its various forms are not described in full, as these are discussed in other chapters. A full description of all aspects of epileptic seizures has no place in a textbook on autonomic failure; the rare causes receive perhaps more attention than is warranted; the reason to include them in some detail is that they are rarely discussed together.

Transient loss of consciousness

TLOC concerns the state described above, further characterized by an onset lasting seconds to minutes, a duration also lasting seconds to minutes, and a spontaneous recovery. The wide range of time is necessary to accommodate all forms of TLOC. Note that 'recovery' here refers only to a restoration of consciousness itself. After generalized epileptic seizures patients may be drowsy and suffer from impaired cognitive function for many minutes, while restoration of cognitive function in syncope usually only takes a few seconds. Associated symptoms such as fatigue, nausea or sleepiness in syncope may last much longer, up to hours.

It may be fruitful to place TLOC in a wider context. Fig. 55.1 provides two decision nodes separating TLOC from other conditions: the first concerns the question whether or not consciousness appeared lost or not. If it did not, the differential diagnosis may include falls or states of altered consciousness, depending on the presentation. The second node concerns the four features that set TLOC aside from other forms of loss of consciousness. If these are not all met, the differential diagnosis is that of longer-lasting loss of consciousness. Whereas 'coma' is usually reserved for long-lasting forms. there is no common name for disorders with a duration of unconsciousness intermediate between TLOC and coma. Examples are metabolic derangements such as hypoglycaemia and various intoxications.

Introduction to the main categories of TLOC

The first level of division of TLOC is into traumatic and non-traumatic forms. Head trauma causing loss of consciousness occurs frequently. As the presence of a trauma is usually abundantly clear there is limited chance of diagnostic confusion, so this form will not be extensively discussed. Problems arise when head trauma may result from another form of TLOC, so more than one category may be involved at the same time. In such cases the symptoms of traumatic TLOC may overshadow those of the cause of the fall. In some cases it may not be possible to detect the presence of the reason for a fall, as for instance may be the case when someone is found with evidence of cranial trauma at the bottom of the stairs.

The second level of division concerns the four major groups forms of non-traumatic TLOC. Syncope is the first group, based

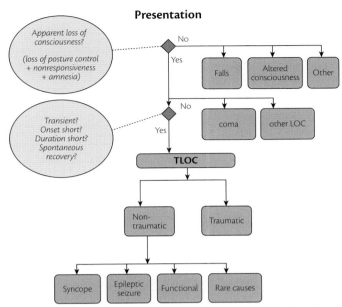

Presentation

Fig. 55.1 Transient loss of consciousness in a wider framework. Developed in collaboration with European Heart Rhythm Association (EHRA); Heart Failure Association (HFA); Heart Rhythm Society (HRS), Moya A, Sutton R, Ammirati F, Blanc JJ, Brignole M, Dahm JB, Deharo JC, Gajek J, Gjesdal K, Krahn A, Massin M, Pepi M, Pezawas T, Ruiz Granell R, Sarasin F, Ungar A, van Dijk JG, Walma EP, Wieling W., Guidelines for the diagnosis and management of syncope (version 2009): Task Force for the Diagnosis and Management of Syncope; European Society of Cardiology (ESC), *Eur Heart J.* 2009 **30**(21):2631–71, by permission of Oxford University Press.

on its frequency of occurrence. It is defined as TLOC due to global cerebral hypoperfusion. The underlying cause is almost always an insufficiency of the systemic circulation, expressed as low cardiac output and low blood pressure.

Epileptic seizures form the second largest group. In many countries, particularly ones in which English is not the first language, the English word 'seizure' is interpreted as synonymous with 'epileptic attack', but this use is not universal: the word can also be used to describe a syncopal attack. As this usage carries the risk of increasing confusing between epilepsy and syncope, 'epileptic seizure' will be used instead of the shorter 'seizure'.

'Functional' or 'psychogenic' attacks from the third group. Note that the word 'psychogenic' may be interpreted as offensive by some. Here it is not meant to denote anything else than that the attack has a presumed psychological origin, and concerns an expression of behaviour more than of a gross disturbance of brain function.

The category 'rare disorders and mimics' bundles miscellaneous disorders on purpose. A strict division along pathophysiological principles would elevate many of the disorders to the same level as syncope or epilepsy, with the implication that they may be regarded as equally important from a clinical diagnostic point of view. The reasons to consider the disorders in this category as being of secondary importance was that they feature fairly rarely in the differential diagnosis of TLOC. The disorders in question may be rare, as holds for cataplexy and a clinically relevant subclavian steal phenomenon, or rarely cause a loss of consciousness resembling other forms of TLOC (vertebrobasilar TIAs). For some disorders their presentation usually does not resemble other forms of TLOC

much, as is the case for excessive daytime sleepiness and cataplexy. Table 55.1 provides a more exhaustive classification of TLOC.

Syncope

Definition

Syncope can be defined as TLOC due to cerebral hypoperfusion.

Terminological remarks

TLOC and syncope were introduced as different entities on two hierarchical levels in 2001 (Brignole et al. 2001). Papers on syncope not adhering to this definition, either before or later, may be about other patient groups than implied in the present definition. The noun 'presyncope' is often used to describe a state resembling the prodromal phase of syncope but which is not followed by loss of consciousness. As such it may concern an aborted syncope but may also concern a different disorder. The adjective 'presyncopal' is used in a more literal sense, to describe the phase preceding unconsciousness.

As explained above, the classification of syncope represents a mixture of pathophysiological causes and clinical presentation patterns. 'Reflex syncope' contains forms in which mechanical factors such as straining are much more important than an autonomically mediated reflex (Table 55.1). Likewise, a reflex may well be involved in cardiac syncope during exercise due to structural cardiac disease; these are bundled as 'cardiac syncope' rather than as 'reflex syncope' to underline where attention should be paid: the heart.

Clinical description

Clinical nature of syncope

Syncope has a wide range of clinical presentations with differences in trigger patterns, prodromal symptoms and signs, speed of onset, ictal phenomena and postictal events. All these depend not only on the cause of syncope, but also on age and various other factors that affect the clinical presentation. Ultimately syncope depends on a failure of the circulation to perfuse the brain, so any factor affecting the circulation may affect whether or not syncope occurs. Such factors may operate through hypovolaemia (vomiting, diarrhoea, blood loss), skin vasodilatation (external heat, fever, alcohol use) or through impaired venous return (straining, prolonged coughing). A vertical body position (standing or sitting) increases the chances of syncope for nearly all forms, except for those that cause a virtual standstill of the circulation usually through severe bradycardia or asystole; those can occur in any position, including lying down. Given all these differences it is not wise to regard syncope as a condition with a single stereotypical clinical expression. The pathophysiology of the different forms does cause clinical patterns to emerge that greatly help differential diagnosis: a very sudden loss of consciousness without any warning accompanied by an equally sudden recovery in a lying subject should suggest a sudden cardiac standstill, while a very slow decrease in orthostatic blood pressure leaving someone standing without the clarity of mind to sit down, almost only occurs in severe autonomic failure. Such groupwise differences between presentations cardiac and vasovagal syncope have been tabulated (Sheldon et al. 2006). Unfortunately for clinical teaching, even within a single cause symptoms and signs can differ markedly between patients and even between episodes. A pattern must be sought building a narrative history from as many attacks as can be examined using history and

Table 55.1 Forms of non-traumatic transient loss of consciousness (TLOC)

This table provides a more detailed classification of TLOC (Van Dijk et al. 2009). Many forms are not discussed in the text. Forms particular to childhood have been left out. The group of 'mainly mechanical/hydraulic factors' concerns forms of syncope in which gravitational stress and increased intrathoracic pressure cause a temporary reduction in cardiac output.

Syncope

◆ Reflex (neurally mediated) syncope
  - Vasovagal
    ○ Pain, fear, instrumentation
    ○ Standing
  - Situational
    ○ Coughing, sneezing
    ○ Micturition/post-micturition
    ○ Gastrointestinal stimulation (swallowing, defecation, visceral pain)
  - Carotid sinus syncope
  - Mainly mechanical/hydraulic factors
    ○ Mess trick
    ○ Wind instruments, straining
◆ Syncope due to orthostatic hypotension
  - Primary autonomic failure
  - Secondary autonomic failure
  - Drug-induced autonomic failure
  - Volume depletion
◆ Cardiac syncope
  - Arrhythmias as primary cause
    ○ Bradycardia
      Sinus node dysfunction, atrioventricular node dysfunction
      Pacemaker/ICD malfunction
      Drug-induced
    ○ Tachycardia
      Supraventricular
      Ventricular
  - Structural diseases
    ○ Cardiac (valvular disease, infarction/ischaemia, hypertrophic cardiomyopathy,
      Cardiac masses, pericardial disease/tamponade
      Congenital anomalies of coronary arteries
    ○ Others (pulmonary embolus, acute aortic dissection, pulmonary hypertension)

Epileptic seizures

◆ Primary generalized
  - Tonic, clonic, tonic-clonic
  - Atonic
◆ Secondary generalized

Table 55.1 (*Continued*)

Functional TLOC

◆ Functional TLOC mimicking epileptic seizures ('pseudoseizures')
◆ Functional TLOC mimicking syncope ('pseudosyncope')

Miscellaneous and mimics

◆ Vertebrobasilar transient ischaemic attacks and stroke
◆ Subclavian steal syndrome
◆ Cataplexy
◆ Excessive daytime sleepiness
◆ Metabolic disorders (hypoglycaemia)
◆ 'Drop attacks'

eyewitness accounts (Gastaut 1974, Stephenson 1990, Colman et al. 2004, Thijs et al. 2008). The diagnosis often rests on a combination of clues rather than on one or two elements (Thijs et al. 2008).

Understanding symptoms and signs

The symptoms and signs of syncope may be divided into three ways. The first division is by order of appearance, distinguishing the presyncopal phase, also called the prodromal phase (i.e. before consciousness is lost), ictal and postictal events (Van Dijk et al. 2009, Wieling et al. 2009).

The second division is by cause, resulting in two subgroups. The first is related to the cause of syncope, meaning that these symptoms are extremely important for differential diagnosis. These symptoms mostly concern the presyncopal and postictal phases. Some examples follow: 'autonomic activation' (i.e. nausea, pallor and sweating) are typical for vasovagal syncope; palpitations or chest pain point towards cardiac syncope, and 'coat hanger pain' suggests orthostatic hypotension in the context of autonomic failure. Prodromal symptoms are often not reported by elderly subjects; putative reasons for this are a greater susceptibility to retrograde amnesia, a lesser degree of autonomic activation, or diminished sensitivity to the sometimes subtle symptoms (Kenny et al. 1991, Benke et al. 1997). Prodromal symptoms usually last for 30–60 seconds, but their duration is notoriously variable (Newman and Graves 2001, Alboni et al. 2002; del Rosso 2005).

The second subgroup by cause reflects the effects of hypoperfusion on the retina and brain. These are in principle independent of the course of syncope, and are ictal in nature or occur just before consciousness is lost. Light-headedness may fall into this group. While this is no doubt related to cerebral hypoperfusion, it is unclear what its pathophysiology is. There are after all no sensory nerve endings in the brain itself, and it is unclear whether the sensation can be regarded as a loss of a cerebral function. It may occur before changes are observed on the electroencephalogram [EEG]) Prodromal manifestations in this group include visual symptoms such as loss of colour vision, a darkening of vision, seeing white or a loss of peripheral vision. Auditory symptoms include the sensation that sounds come from a distance or the hearing of buzzing. Difficulty in thinking may also be observed, but usually only when the onset of syncope is slow enough to allow a level of self reflection to occur. One of the last symptoms before unconsciousness is only infrequently encountered: this concerns an inability to act while subjects are still aware of themselves (Rossen et al. 1943). In clinical practice this is only reported by those with very slow onset of syncope, as in some cases of autonomic failure.

Loss of consciousness usually lasts less than 20 seconds in syncope (Lempert et al. 1994, Stephenson 1990) but may last longer in subjects kept upright. Some subjects lie still while taking time to collect themselves, which may appear as prolonged unconsciousness. Unconsciousness is invariably accompanied by a loss of normal voluntary motor control, meaning subjects will fall if upright. Falls are often flaccid but may be stiff (Lempert et al. 1994) and there may be opisthotonus (Stephenson 1990). During unconsciousness the eyes are usually open, even if closed before, and are directed upwards or straight ahead (Rossen et al. 1943, Lempert et al. 1996, Stephenson 1990). A downbeat nystagmus has been described (Lempert et al. 1996, Stephenson 1990). Jerks of the limbs may occur, lasting only a few seconds. These jerks are usually small in amplitude, do not cause pronounced bending of the knees or elbows, are not rhythmic and not synchronous. Estimates of their rate of occurrence vary: they were reported in 12% of blood donors who had fainted in a retrospective study (Lin et al. 1982), but a prospective study in blood donors noted them in 42–46% (Newman and Graves 2001). Jerks occurred in 90% of subjects in whom syncope was induced using the fainting lark, a form of syncope with an almost instantaneous fall in blood pressure (Lempert 1994). Tilt-table testing of subjects with vasovagal syncope suggests that a few minor jerks are almost always present. It seems likely that the differing rates of myoclonic jerking in syncope are due to the level of attention: many small and non-recurring jerks are missed, and only more obvious jerks are noted by eyewitnesses. In short, the presence of such jerks does not differentiate syncope from epileptic seizures, but their nature does (see the section on epilepsy). Urinary incontinence occurs in about one quarter of syncope cases (Stephenson 1990, Hoefnagels et al. 1991, Romme et al. 2008) and so does not reliably differentiate between syncope and epilepsy either. Tongue biting is extremely rare in syncope (Stephenson 1990, Romme et al. 2008). If it occurs, it usually involves the tip of the tongue, not the side as in epilepsy (Benbadis 1995).

Consciousness is typically regained promptly in syncope, without confusion or later amnesia for the postictal stage. Patients may be amazed at what happened to them, however. The postictal stage may to some extent reflect the cause of the syncope: autonomic activation in reflex syncope may well continue after the attack. A pronounced red colour of the face during recovery has been noted as indicating arrhythmic syncope, but may also occur in reflex syncope, as it does not depend on the cause of syncope but on the rapidity of its onset and offset (Wieling et al. 2006). Fatigue and sleepiness after syncope may last several hours, particularly in children.

The third division of symptoms is by rate of occurrence: rapid or slow. If the rate of onset is very high, events may unfold too quickly for patients to recognize and report them later; the fact that their attention is diverted will probably contribute to this (Kenny et al. 1991, Sutton 1999). The most rapid onset is probably found in syncope associated with a sudden asystole; this may occur in arrhythmias, notably complete AV-block, or in cardioinhibitory forms of reflex syncope. Examples of the latter are syncope induced by carotid sinus massage (Kenny et al. 1991) and, in children, by eyeball pressure (Stephenson 1990). The time between asystole and loss of consciousness is counted in seconds: in children, after

eyeball pressure, the EEG flattened after about 9 seconds of asystole (Stephenson 1990). A few seconds may probably be subtracted from this to obtain the latency to unconsciousness, as this usually, at least in adults, occurs during the slow phase of the EEG, several seconds before the EEG flattens. When the arterial circulation in the neck is suddenly mechanically blocked, adult men lost consciousness in 5–6 seconds (Rossen et al. 1943). When cerebral hypoperfusion becomes impaired gradually, patients may have time to perceive and recollect more symptoms. An example of this condition is the -pure- vasodepressor type of reflex syncope, but the slowest onset of syncope is probably found in patients with primary autonomic failure. In such patients blood pressure can decrease so slowly, or become stable at such a low level, that patients may remain standing by themselves, but their cognitive processes are affected to such a degree that they cannot act of their own accord, so they do not reply and do not sit down.

As said, recognizing patterns in both the nature and rapidity of the various prodromal and ictal signs and symptoms contains crucial clues to the cause of syncope.

Pathophysiology

Retinal and cerebral hypoperfusion

The symptoms and signs of retinal and cerebral hypoperfusion are partly understood. Although the retina is perfused through the cerebral arterial system, retinal symptoms may be noticed before consciousness is lost. The explanation for this resides in intraocular pressure. This is normally about 18 mmHg (Whinnery and Shender 1993) and provides an impediment to perfusion not present in the brain itself. Studies from various sources indicate that arterial pressure at the level of the brain has to drop to 20–40 mmHg at the onset of syncope (Wieling et al. 2009). Note that, in the upright position, arterial pressure at the level of the heart will be 15–20 mm Hg higher than at brain level (Van Dijk 2003). Studies on induced syncope with EEG measurements showed that the EEG in syncope shows either temporary slowing or a slow-flat-slow pattern when cerebral perfusion lasts longer and/or is more pronounced. A flat phase, indicating profound cortical dysfunction, has most often been described for asystole (Stephenson 1990, Gastaut 1957, Breningstall 1996), but can occur without it (Sheldon et al. 1998). There is a minimum duration of asystole before the EEG flattens. This has been studied in detail in children mostly undergoing eyeball pressure to evoke syncope. The 'threshold' duration was 7–14 seconds in children 5 or 6 years of age, and rose to about 12 seconds of asystole for 12-year-olds. There is a larger reserve in older than in younger children (Stephenson 1990), but its nature is not entirely understood. Loss of muscle control and of reactivity starts in the slow phase; if there is a slow-flat-slow pattern consciousness is lost in the first slow phase and regained in the second. The flat phase of the EEG is invariably associated with loss of consciousness; stiffness has been noted as probably universal in children in this phase (Stephenson 1990). Clinical observations show that this is not the case in adults, however, in whom flaccidity predominates. Not all brain activity is lost during syncope, not even when the EEG is flat: breathing may continue, either shallow or with snoring (Newman and Graves 2001). The continuation of breathing during the flat phase of the EEG shows that the brainstem is still functioning. Persisting asystole in cardioinhibitory reflex syncope must also point to a functional brainstem, as it is the product of an increased vagal drive (it is tempting to think that asystole in reflex syncope must ultimately cause its own cessation through anoxia of the vagal nucleus). It has been suggested on clinical grounds that the presence of myoclonic jerks indicates either a prolonged or a severe cerebral hypoperfusion, but whether this is true or not is imperfectly known. Such jerks seem to occur preferentially during the beginning and end of syncopal episodes when there is slow activity in the EEG (author's observations). They are hypothetically due to a lack of inhibition from the cortex (Gastaut 1974).

Other symptoms and signs

The manifestations of 'autonomic activation' in vasovagal syncope are various, and include facial pallor, sweating, nausea with or without vomiting, wide pupils, increased peristalsis, an urge to void urine or to defecate, but not necessarily all at once. While their autonomic origin seems clear, their purpose is not.

Palpitations in cardiac syncope in principle point to a disturbed rhythm, but a sinus rhythm with strong beats or a high frequency may also be perceived and reported by patients as 'palpitations'. Chest pain suggests myocardial ischemia.

'Coat hanger pain' in autonomic failure is due to ischaemia of shoulder and neck muscles. It typically occurs in the vertical position and subsides quickly on lying down (Bleasdale-Barr and Mathias 1999, Robertson et al. 1994). Infrequently other organs may also suffer from orthostatic hypotension; pain in the lower back, the buttocks, and the chest has been described. Exercise-related precordial pain without coronary artery disease might also be due to systemic hypotension (Asahina et al. 2006). Symptoms typically develop in minutes or after longer periods of standing or walking and resolve on lying down (Robertson et al. 1994, Bleasdale-Barr and Mathias 1999, Mathias et al. 1999).

Epileptic seizures

Definition

An epileptic seizure is a transient occurrence of signs and/or symptoms due to abnormal excessive or synchronous activity in the brain (Fisher et al. 2005, Engel 2006). Note that the presence of an 'epileptic seizure' does not always equate with the presence of 'epilepsy', which is generally regarded as an abnormal tendency for epileptic seizures to recur (Fisher et al. 2005); in practice this holds mostly for attacks induced by fever, sleep and/or alcohol deprivation.

Terminological remarks

The international classification of epilepsy and epileptic seizures by the International League Against Epilepsy (ILAE) was obviously not designed to differentiate epilepsy from other causes of TLOC. As explained in the introduction, the TLOC point of view requires a distinction between disorders that leave a patient unconscious on the floor (i.e. TLOC), and those that leave the subject actively upright. Table 55.2 shows a shortened classification of seizure types (Engel 2006, Berg et al. 2010) highlighting types which types do and which do not fall under the TLOC heading. Only tonic, clonic, tonic-clonic and atonic epileptic seizures fall under the TLOC heading (Brignole et al. 2001, Brignole et al. 2004, Thijs et al. 2004, ESC 2009, Van Dijk et al. 2009). Note that the 'dyscognitive seizures', with or without automatisms largely conform to 'complex partial seizures'.

Table 55.2 Epileptic seizures and transient loss of consciousness (TLOC)

The first column shows the classification of seizure types of the International League Against Epilepsy (Engel 2006). The classification is abridged; where the ILAE classification is more extensive, this has been indicated by appending '...' to a seizure type. The distinction which forms do and which do not fall under the TLOC heading hinges on whether consciousness is lost causing a loss of normal motor control over the entire body, usually resulting in a fall.

ILAE Classification	Consciousness	
	Lost, with loss of motor control	Impaired, no loss of motor control
Self-limited epileptic seizures		
I. Generalized onset		
A. Tonic and/or clonic manifestations		
1. Tonic-clonic seizures	TLOC	
2. Clonic seizures	TLOC	
3. Tonic seizures	TLOC	
B. Absences ...		yes
C. Myoclonic seizure types ...		
D. Epileptic spasms		
E. Atonic seizures	TLOC	
II. Focal onset (partial)		
A. Local ...		
B. With ipsilateral propagation ...		
C. With contralateral spread		
1. Neocortical		
2. Limbic areas		
(dyscognitive seizures)		yes
D. Secondarily generalized		
1. Tonic-clonic seizures	TLOC	
2. Absence seizures		yes
3. Epileptic spasms ...		
III. Neonatal seizures		
Status epilepticus ...		

Note that the word 'seizure' on its own does not imply 'epileptic seizure' in all cases. The most notable exception is 'reflex anoxic seizures', sometimes used to describe a form of syncope in children (Stephenson 1990).

Clinical description

Most generalized tonic-clonic epileptic seizures are reported reliably by eyewitnesses as such. Problems arise when eyewitness accounts are lacking, or when eyewitnesses mistake limited myoclonic syncopal jerks for clonic movements and physicians fail to distinguish between eyewitness' observations from interpretations. The atonic and tonic epileptic seizure types resemble syncopal attacks more than tonic clonic seizures; luckily for differential diagnosis, both seizure types are rare and mostly affect people with known neurological problems or learning disabilities (So 1995).

Epileptic seizures are rarely triggered, in contrast to syncope. The key question in syncope is therefore 'what were you doing at the time', a question that most often does not yield any pattern in epilepsy. Triggering occurs in 'reflex epilepsies'; the best-known triggers are flashing lights (Trenité 2006). One of the very few triggers that can evoke syncope as well as epilepsy is startling, (Bakker et al. 2006) as it can evoke startle epilepsy (Tibussek et al. 2006) and syncope in the hereditary prolonged QT-syndrome (Levine et al. 2008).

Convulsive seizures may start with a focal onset, important for differential diagnosis: while the TLOC episode itself may be difficult to diagnose as syncope or seizure, signs of symptoms beforehand may help settle the question: attacks beginning with automatisms, smacking, mumbling, purposeless acts or with jerks of one extremity while the person is upright, strongly suggest an epileptic nature. The classical aura with a rising sensation in the abdomen or an unpleasant smell is not very common; however, aura patterns tend to repeat themselves in patients, who learn to recognise them as such (Van Donselaar et al. 1990).

Epileptic seizures usually last about one minute or more, longer than syncopal ones. Although eyewitnesses often overestimate the duration of any attack, the difference is still useful for diagnosis. In epilepsy, but not in syncope, jerks can begin unilaterally and before the fall. The jerks are coarse, and may involve pronounced bending of the knees and elbows. They are symmetric and rhythmic. Physicians should realise that eyewitnesses have no preconceptions about when to think that jerks were 'coarse' or 'subtle', so their answers may mean little unless checked. Mimicking the movements to eyewitnesses can help them recognize the nature of the jerks (Hoefnagels et al. 1991). The eyes are usually open, as in syncope, but there is a stronger tendency for gaze to be directed to one side. A blue facial colour can occur in epileptic seizures and in cardiac syncope but is not likely in reflex syncope (Sheldon et al. 2006, Colman et al. 2004). Other important clues are a lateral tongue bite, (Sheldon et al. 2006) a pronounced head deviation, (Sheldon 2002) or a cry at the beginning of an attack. Recovery after an epileptic seizure can be slow and be associated with disorientation and confusion for many minutes or longer (Hoefnagels et al. 1991). This should be distinguished from sleepiness and fatigue after syncope. Syncope patients can usually provide an uninterrupted account of events from the moment they regained consciousness, while patients after seizures may not recall events after the seizure clearly.

Pathophysiology

An epileptic seizure is characterized by abnormal patterns of excitability and synchrony among neurons in select brain areas (Engel 2006). 'Epilepsy', in the sense of a proven propensity for seizures to recur, requires an enduring alteration in the brain that increases the likelihood of future seizures (Fisher et al. 2005).

Functional transient loss of consciousness

Definition

'Functional' here concerns those forms of TLOC in which no somatic explanation can be given for the apparent loss of consciousness, and for which a psychological mechanism is surmised.

Terminological remarks

Note that the definition is based on a concept rather than on falsifiable criteria, and that it mainly relies on an absence of something

(somatic findings) rather than on positive criteria for what it does represent. This ambiguity is inherent in the somatoform disorders of the DSM-IV (Noyes et al. 2008), the group of disorders to which 'functional TLOC' belongs. Within this group, the best-fitting category is 'conversion disorder': part of the criteria for conversion disorder are unexplained symptoms or deficits affecting voluntary motor or sensory function that suggest a neurological or other general-medical condition, and that psychological factors are judged to be associated with the symptoms or deficits (Kroenke et al. 2007, Kroenke and Rosmalen 2006). Oddly, disorders of consciousness are not listed in the definition, which from the point of view of TLOC is an omission. In the International Classification of Diseases (ICD) conversion is classified as a dissociative disorder (Strassnig et al. 2006, LaFrance et al. 2006). Unfortunately, neither of these systems is used much in the literature to describe the disorders in question. A systematic search over 5 years yielded no studies even identifying the prevalence or incidence of conversion disorder (Strassnig et al. 2006). Of 26 papers on 'pseudoseizures' none defined them as conversion disorder (Strassnig et al. 2006). The latter finding illustrates the stark contrast between the hardly-used concept 'conversion disorder' and the proliferating research into 'functional' medical syndromes (Strassnig et al. 2006, Benbadis 2005).

Outside of psychiatry a variety of names may be encountered, including 'hysterical', 'psychosomatic', medically unexplained', 'unexplained', 'psychogenic', 'pseudo-syncope', 'pseudo-seizures' and 'pseudo-epilepsy'. The last two terms are used to describe attacks that resemble syncope or epileptic seizures respectively. Examples of the tendency to define disorders based on an absence of something are the phrases 'non-epileptic attack disorder (NEAD)' and 'non-epileptic seizures (NES)', used to distinguish such attacks from true epilepsy. The phrase 'psychogenic non-epileptic seizures' (PNES) is more clear in this respect.

A problem with the terminology is the reluctance of patients to accept a psychological explanation of their putative somatic problems, along with the interpretation that they are personally responsible for the condition as a direct result of it being psychological in nature (Kroenke et al. 2007). The term 'functional' has the advantages of stressing abnormality of a function rather than of a somatic structure, and avoiding stigmatization. It is also not likely to offend patients (Stone 2003).

Clinical notes

Note that the diagnosis of functional TLOC can often be made with near certainty (Benbadis 2005, Benbadis and Chichkova 2006, LaFrance 2008). This is in stark contrast to other functional disorders such as movement abnormalities or pain where certainty is very difficult to achieve (Reuber et al. 2005). Functional disorders are prone to suggestion, meaning attacks can often be documented. Provocation in functional TLOC mimicking epileptic seizures involved infusion of placebo or alcohol-soaked pads (Ribaï et al. 2006, Zaidi et al. 1999). The diagnosis commonly rests on combined video-EEG monitoring (Zaidi et al. 1999, LaFrance 2008). For most types of epilepsy a seizure cannot co-exist with a normal EEG; the few forms that can, such as frontal lobe epilepsy, are among the most difficult to diagnose (LaFrance 2008), but they do not resemble syncope. Tilt testing in syncope is expressly carried out to provoke an attack of syncope, so the procedure also lends itself well to provoking functional TLOC mimicking syncope; it has also been used to provoke PNES to good effect (Zaidi et al. 1999).

In principle a normal EEG during an attack of apparent loss of voluntary motor control and reactivity is sufficient to exclude syncope, but adding recordings of normal or elevated blood pressure and heart rate during periods of apparent responsiveness help to exclude syncope.

If patients can be investigated during attacks of functional TLOC, there should be no neurological abnormalities such as extensor plantar responses (unless previously existent) nor circulatory changes as in syncope.

Functional disorders are commonly associated with psychiatric comorbidity.

Pathophysiology

The nature of the mental or physiological cerebral process giving rise to functional TLOC is essentially unknown. A subtle neurological disorder cannot be excluded. Current investigations show abnormalities on tests such as functional magnetic resonance imaging, but whether these represent the cause or consequence of the condition is unknown. Functional attacks are believed not be intentionally produced by patients (Reuber et al. 2005), but, as intention cannot be proven, the involuntary nature of the attacks is unfalsifiable. Regardless of this it is wise to regard and explain them as wholly involuntary. Patients treat them as such, and subscribing to this point of view not only avoids counterproductive clashes, but provides a therapeutic opening (Reuber et al. 2005).

Rare causes and mimics

This group is bundled because the disorders described here occur relatively infrequently, not because they share a common aetiology or clinical presentation. Hence, descriptions are provided for the separate entities only.

Cataplexy

Cataplexy is not TLOC but may be mistaken for it. It concerns a bilateral loss of muscle tone with preserved awareness, usually evoked by emotions. In very rare cases cataplexy can occur as a symptom of a structural brainstem disorder (brain lesions, Niemann–Pick type C disease, Norrie disease, Prader–Willi syndrome and Coffin–Lowry syndrome). In practice cataplexy almost always points to narcolepsy. In fact, establishing that a patient with excessive daytime sleepiness has cataplexy is enough to diagnose 'narcolepsy with cataplexy' (the other main way is to show a lack of hypocretin in the cerebrospinal fluid) (AASM 2005).

Cataplexy concerns a flaccid paralysis of striated muscles. The precise pathophysiology is unknown. It is regarded as similar to rapid eye movement (REM) sleep atonia, a physiological phenomenon in which muscle tone drops during REM-sleep, presumably to prevent dreams being acted out (Overeem et al. 2001). Attacks may be partial, mostly concerning buckling of the knees and weakness of the neck, jaw, and facial muscles (AASM 2005, Overeem et al. 2001). Complete attacks affect most striated muscles except for those involved in respiration; those are unaffected, causing patients to slump to the floor. Although attacks commence suddenly, they usually take seconds to develop fully, allowing patients to break their fall with their hands. In the beginning of the attacks the paralysis is not continuous, causing jerking movements, particularly of the jaws and face. Attacks last several seconds to, rarely, minutes. Common triggers are laughing out loud, unexpectedly meeting strangers, trying to tell a joke, and the expectation of hitting a winning stroke in sports. During longer-lasting attacks patients may directly proceed from cataplexy to REM sleep. If so, there may be no memory of the final phase of the attack, but there is always recollection of the beginning, as patients are then fully aware: consciousness is normal.

This latter feature, the absence of amnesia, is crucial to recognize cataplexy as such. The presence of other characteristics of narcolepsy helps making a diagnosis: excessive daytime sleepiness, hypnagogic hallucinations, sleep onset paralysis, automatic behaviour and disturbed nocturnal sleep. Excessive daytime sleepiness is usually present, but cataplexy may precede it in some patients. The other telltale clue is the nature of the triggers, which do not or extremely rarely feature in TLOC. Laughter can also occur as an expression of epilepsy: gelastic epilepsy, occurring in children, is associated with hypothalamic hamartoma. Unlike cataplexy, laughter is then not appropriate for the circumstances and not accompanied by mirth (Harvey and Freedman 2007, Pearce 2004). Cataplexy can be mistaken for complex partial seizures as well as for tonic-clonic seizures (Macleod et al. 2005, Zeman et al. 2001). The role of emotions as a trigger and the flaccidity upon falling can cause confusion with neurally mediated syncope (Calabrò et al. 2007).

Excessive daytime sleepiness

Daytime sleepiness is defined as the inability to stay awake and alert during the major waking episodes of the day, resulting in unintended lapses into drowsiness or sleep (AASM 2005). As sleepiness involves the waking state confusion with TLOC should be uncommon. Some common causes of daytime sleepiness are sleep related breathing disorders, periodic limb movements in sleep and narcolepsy (AASM 2005). Attacks of unwanted sleep can cause such confusion however. Sleep is not normally considered a form of unconsciousness, so such attacks are a TLOC mimic rather a form of TLOC themselves. In most cases the resulting sleep during the day is recognized as sleep by both patients and bystanders, so diagnostic problems arise only rarely. In narcolepsy, 'automatic behaviour' results in patients continuing activities in semiautomatic fashion (AASM 2005), such as writing or working with a computer. However, the work done is usually meaningless, and patients have no recollection of having done anything during such a period. These states may cause confusion with complex partial seizures (Mihaescu and Malow 2003).

Transient ischaemic attacks

TIA concerns events of focal neurological dysfunction that resolve with a duration ranging from minutes to hours, up to 24 hours by definition.

TIAs of the cerebral areas supplied by the carotid arteries can affect many neurological functions, but consciousness is not among them, because not enough of the cortex is affected to cause unconsciousness. The only exception is when multiple large arteries are stenotic or occluded, because then an additional problem of a remaining supplying vessel may affect a large portion of the brain. Even then, however, the clinical presentation does not commonly concern loss of consciousness without any focal neurological signs. While such presentations have been reported (Stark and Wodak 1983), their paucity warns against ready acceptance of TIA as the diagnosis for this presentation. In patients with occlusion of multiple large vessels orthostatic TIAs are more likely: TIAs then occur only in the standing position, often when there is also orthostatic hypotension (Melgar and Weinand 2003, Dobkin 1989, Somerville 1984, Jardine 2007).

TIAs of the vertebrobasilar system are theoretically more likely to cause loss of consciousness because they can affect the function of the reticular ascending system. Even if consciousness is affected, there are always signs indicating focal dysfunction. The most common signs are limb weakness, gait and limb ataxia, oculomotor palsies, and oropharyngeal dysfunction (Savitz and Caplan 2005). Fewer than 1% of patients had a single presenting symptom (Savitz and Caplan 2005). Light-headedness is rare in vertebrobasilar TIAs (75% of patients), and this complaint never occurred as an isolated symptom. Although the word 'syncope' can be found in the literature as one of the clinical manifestations of vertebrobasilar TIAs, it is usually unclear how the word should be interpreted. Reliable descriptions of a TIA manifesting itself as isolated loss of consciousness have not been found. For practical purposes the following adage may be used: a TIA concerns a focal deficit without loss of consciousness, and syncope represents loss of consciousness without a focal deficit. This clinical difference parallels the key difference in the pathophysiology (i.e. regional hypoperfusion in TIAs and global hypoperfusion in syncope), which difference is not reflected in the phrase 'transient ischaemic attacks' (if taken literally this phrase would fit syncope perfectly).

Subclavian steal syndrome

The 'subclavian steal syndrome' refers to the symptoms and signs of insufficient vertebrobasilar blood flow as the result of occlusion or severe stenosis of the subclavian artery. In principle the words 'subclavian steal' merely refer to rerouting of blood flow when there is a stenosis or occlusion of the subclavian artery regardless of whether this causes symptoms or signs, but 'steal' and 'steal syndrome' are often used interchangeably.

Steal more often affects the left than the right side; blood reaches the brachial artery distal of a stenosis through the vertebral artery, in which it flows downward instead of upwards (Taylor et al. 2002). In turn, the vertebral artery receives its blood supply through Willis' circle, fed by the other vertebral artery and the carotid arteries. The majority of cases (64%) in which flow abnormalities consistent with subclavian steal were detected with ultrasound were asymptomatic (Hennerici et al. 1988). Of cases with symptoms, these concerned carotid artery flow areas in 31%, and vertebrobasilar symptoms in only 5% (Hennerici et al. 1988). In most patients there are multiple cerebral vascular abnormalities, affecting the other vertebral artery and/or the carotid arteries (Hennerici et al. 1988, Taylor et al. 2002). Clinical clues towards the presence of subclavian steal are pronounced blood pressure differences between the two arms, and the fact that symptoms can appear after exercise of the arm, most often the left one.

Loss of consciousness can be found in case reports as 'syncope', but, as for TIAs, it often remains unclear how the word should be interpreted. An isolated loss of consciousness is probably rare if it exists at all.

Clues for history taking

As stated in the introduction, TLOC concerns many causes belonging to various specialties. Most cases presumably end up being classified and interpreted correctly. Still, TLOC, and particularly syncope, is so common that a small proportion of uncertain diagnoses results in a sizable number of patients.

Experts agree that the diagnosis largely rests on history taking. The guidelines for syncope of the European Society of Cardiology stress a tiered approach, in which the first step consists of history taking, a physical examination and an ECG (ESC 2009). Specific investigations such as carotid compression or tilt table testing are requested based on the likelihood of underlying conditions emerging from this initial investigation. In this way, a shotgun approach (Landau 1996) ordering tests for just about any condition featuring in Table 55.1 is avoided. When the initial evaluation does not yield sufficient evidence, further analysis on based on risks, which for syncope boils down to underlying life-threatening cardiac disease. This model can be used for TLOC as a whole, with slight modifications: when the history suggests strongly suggests an epileptic seizure, an EEG becomes more attractive than an ECG.

How best to approach a patient may be influenced by the setting; in an emergency room establishing whether there is an immediate risk may take preference over subtleties of diagnosis, that do matter in a tertiary referral centre.

Weighing the evidence from the history should be done with an eye on the patient's epidemiological background: age, sex, and the previous medical history play a role in determining the a priori chance of any condition. Consider attacks of unconsciousness just after exercise; in a 75-year-old in whom they occur when resting at the top of the stairs these are likely to reflect post-exercise hypotension in a context of orthostatic hypotension and autonomic failure; when they occur on a sport field in a 30-year-old trained athlete, they suggest a much more benign form of syncope instead. The result of this is that items in the history rarely stand on their own; the diagnosis of TLOC often rests on a combination of clues rather than on one or two elements (Thijs et al. 2008). Ideally, the various elements should fit together similar to entries in a cross-word puzzle.

There have been attempts to use lists of items to derive rules for diagnosis (Sheldon et al. 2002, Sheldon et al. 2006). While these are very useful to unearth which items carry more weight than others, it is doubtful that they can reflect the process of weighing data that goes on inside an experienced clinician's mind. Whether this weighing process can be taught to others in a practical and quick manner or whether this requires extensive patient contacts over several years, may be a key problem in medical education. The items in Table 55.3 should be seen in this light; they are derived from multiple sources. Their relative importance for the various diagnoses almost certainly differs, but there is no evidence to order them according to their diagnostic impact. They are sorted by their time relation to the attack, and are provided in random order within each group. The list is not meant as something to be laboured through in its entirety; it may suggest questions for further enquiry. The best question to start with, particularly in syncope, probably is 'What were you doing at the time?'.

Acknowledgement

This chapter is based in part on: 'Dijk JG van, Thijs RD, Benditt DG, Wieling W. A guide to disorders causing transient loss of consciousness: focus on syncope. *Nat Rev Neurol* 2009; **5**: 438–448.

Table 55.3 Items in the history in cases of transient loss of consciousness

A. Prior to the attack	
◆ Lying	Epilepsy, cardiac syncope, functional attacks. Reflex syncope very rare (cardioinhibitory syncope due to instrumentation is possible, as is vasovagal syncope during sleep), orthostatic hypotension impossible
◆ Standing	All possible causes
◆ Standing or after standing up	Orthostatic hypotension, vasovagal syncope
◆ Micturition, defecation	Reflex syncope (situational form)
◆ Prolonged coughing	Reflex syncope (situational form)
◆ Swallowing	Reflex syncope (situational form), also carotid sinus hypersensitivity
◆ Laughing out loud, telling joke, unexpected meeting acquaintance	Cataplexy
◆ After a meal	Postprandial hypotension
◆ Head movements, pressure on the neck, shaving	Carotid sinus hypersensitivity, symptomatic form
◆ Fear, pain, stress	Reflex syncope (classic vasovagal form)
◆ During physical exercise	Cardiac: structural cardiopulmonary disease, less often orthostatic hypotension
◆ Directly after cessation of physical exercise	Post-exercise hypotension: in the elderly autonomic failure, in athletes vasovagal
◆ During exercise of the arms	Subclavian steal syndrome
◆ Palpitations	Cardiac: arrhythmia
◆ Startling (e.g. alarm clock)	Hereditary prolonged QT syndrome, startle epilepsy (very rarely)
◆ Flashing light	Epilepsy with photosensitivity
◆ Sleep deprivation	Epilepsy
◆ Heat	Reflex syncope, autonomic failure
B. At the onset of the attack	
◆ Nausea, sweating, pallor	'Autonomic activation': reflex syncope
◆ Pain in shoulders, neck ('coathanger pattern')	Ischaemia of local muscles: autonomic failure
◆ Rising sensation from abdomen, unpleasant smell or taste, or other phenomena specific to subject but recurring over attacks	Epileptic aura
◆ Shout at onset of attack	Epileptic seizure
C. During the attack (eyewitness account)	
◆ Fall:	
• Keeling over, stiff	Tonic phase epilepsy, rarely syncope
• Flaccid collapse	Syncope (all variants)
◆ Movements:*	
• Beginning before the fall	Epileptic seizure
• Beginning after the fall	Epileptic seizure, syncope
• Symmetric, synchronous	Epileptic seizure
• Asymmetric, asynchronous	Syncope, may be epileptic seizure
• Beginning at onset of unconsciousness	Epileptic seizure, syncope
• Beginning after onset unconsciousness	Syncope
• Lasting less than about 15 seconds	Syncope more likely than epileptic seizure
• Lasting for minutes	Epileptic seizure
• Restricted to one limb or one side	Epileptic seizure, rarely syncope
• Pelvic thrusting	Functional (pseudo-seizure)
• Movements with repeated waxing and waning in intensity or nature	Functional (pseudo-seizure)

Table 55.3 (*Continued*)

C. During the attack (eyewitness account)	
◆ Other aspects:	
• Automatisms (chewing, smacking, blinking)	Epileptic seizure
• Cyanosis of the face	Epileptic seizure, cardiac syncope
• Eyes open	Epilepsy as likely as syncope; argues against psychogenic
• Eyes closed (during nonresponsive state)	When consistent: psychogenic
• Tongue bitten	Much more often in epilepsy (lateral side of tongue) than in syncope (tip of the tongue)
• Urinary incontinence	Epileptic seizure as likely as syncope
• Paresis, ataxia, brain stem signs	Vertebrobasilar TIA, steal syndrome
• Motionless loss of consciousness lasts 10–30 minutes	Functional (pseudo-syncope)
• Foaming at the mouth	Epileptic seizure
• Bruises and other injuries	All causes, including functional
D. After the attack	
◆ Nausea, sweating, pallor	Autonomic activation: reflex syncope
◆ Clearheaded immediately on regaining consciousness	Syncope, may occur in epileptic seizure
◆ Confused with memory problems for many minutes after regaining consciousness	Epileptic seizure
◆ Sleepy after attack	Epileptic seizure as well as reflex syncope (particularly children)
◆ Aching muscles (not due to a fall)	Epileptic seizure
◆ Palpitations	Cardiac: arrhythmia
◆ Chest pain	Cardiac: ischemia
◆ Crying	Psychogenic attacks
E. Antecedent disorders	
◆ History of heart disease	Cardiac: arrhythmia or structural cardiac disease
◆ Hypertension	Orthostatic hypotension due to medication
◆ Parkinsonism	Orthostatic hypotension (autonomic failure)
◆ History of epilepsy	Epileptic seizure
◆ Structural brain damage	Epileptic seizure
◆ Psychiatric history	Functional, orthostatic hypotension due to medication
◆ Sudden death in family members	Arrhythmia, specifically prolonged QT syndrome
◆ Diabetes mellitus	Cardiac syncope, orthostatic hypotension, LOC due to hypoglycaemia
◆ Vasovagal syncope before 35 years of age	Vasovagal syncope (not strongly)
◆ No syncope before 35 years of age	Vasovagal syncope less likely
◆ Family history of vasovagal syncope	Vasovagal syncope more likely

* The word 'clonic' is in everyday use restricted to epilepsy, while the word 'myoclonus' is used for the movements in syncope as well as for certain types of epilepsy and to describe postanoxic movements. The word 'convulsions' is probably best reserved for epilepsy. 'Myoclonic jerks' has little connotation with a specific cause, and is preferable to avoid jumping to conclusions.

References

Alboni, P., Dinelli, M., *et al.* (2002). Haemodynamic changes early in prodromal symptoms of vasovagal syncope. *Europace* 2, 333–38.

American Academy of Sleep Medicine, (2005). *The international classification of sleep disorders. Diagnostic and coding manual*, second edition. Westchester, Illinois: American Academy of Sleep Medicine.

Asahina, M., Hiraga, A., Hayashi, Y., Mizobuchi, K., Sakakibara, R., Lee, K., Hattori, T. (2006). Ischemic electrocardiographic change induced by exercise in a patient with chronic autonomic failure. *Clin. Auton. Res.* 16, 72–75

Bakker, M. J., van Dijk, J. G., van den Maagdenberg, A. M., Tijssen, M. A. Startle syndromes. *Lancet Neurol.* 5, 513–524.

Benbadis, S. R. (2005). The problem of psychogenic symptoms: is the psychiatric community in denial? *Epilepsy & Behavior* 6, 9–14

Benbadis, S. R., Chichkova, R. (2006). Psychogenic pseudosyncope: an underestimated and provable diagnosis. *Epilepsy & Behavior* 9, 106–110.

Benbadis, S. R., Wolgamuth, B. R., Goren, H., Brener, S., Fouad-Tarazi, F. (1995). Value of tongue biting in the diagnosis of seizures. *Arch. Intern. Med.* 155, 2346–2349.

Benke, Th, Hochleitner, M., Bauer, G. (1997). Aura phenomena during syncope. *Eur. Neurol* 37, 28–32.

Berg, A. T., Berkovic, S. F., Brodie, M. J. *et al.* (2010). Revised terminology and concepts for organization of seizures and epilepsies: Report of the ILAE Commission on Classification and Terminology, 2005–2009. *Epilepsia* **51**, 676–685.

Bleasdale–Barr, K. M., Mathias, C. J. (1999). Neck and other muscle pains in autonomic failure; their association with orthostatic hypotension. *J R Soc. Med.* **91**, 2355–2359.

Breningstall, G. N. (1996). Breath-holding spells. *Pediatr. Neurol.* **14**, 91–97.

Brignole, M., Alboni, P., Benditt, D., *et al.* (2001). Task Force on Syncope, European Society of Cardiology. Guidelines on management (diagnosis and treatment) of syncope. *Eur. Heart. J.* **22**, 1256–306.

Brignole, M. *et al.* Task Force on Syncope, European Society of Cardiology. (2004). Guidelines on management (diagnosis and treatment) of syncope—update 2004. *Europace* **6**, 467–537.

Calabrò, R. S., Savica, R., Laganà, A., *et al.* (2007). Status cataplecticus misdiagnosed as recurrent syncope. *Neurol. Sci.* **28**, 336–338.

Colman, N., Nahm, K., van Dijk, J. G., Reitsma, J. B., Wieling, W., Kaufmann, H. (2004). Diagnostic value of history taking in reflex syncope. *Clin. Auton. Res.* **14** Suppl 1, 37–44.

Del Rosso, A., Alboni, P., Brignole, M., Menozzi, C., Raviele, A. (2005). Relation of clinical presentation of syncope to the age of patients. *Am. J Cardiol.* **96**, 1431–1435.

Dobkin, B. H. (1989). Orthostatic hypotension as a risk factor fir symptomatic occlusive cerebrovascular disease. *Neurology* **39**, 30–34.

Engel, J. (2006). Report of the ILAE Classification Core Group. *Epilepsia* **47**, 1558–1568.

European Society of Cardiology. (2009). Guidelines for the diagnosis and management of syncope (version 2009): the Task Force for the Diagnosis and Management of Syncope of the European Society of Cardiology (ESC). *Eur. Heart J* **30**, 2631–2671.

Fisher, R. S., van Emde, Boas, W., Blume, W., *et al.* (2005). Epileptic seizures and epilepsy. Definitions proposed by the International League against Epilepsy (ILAE) and the International Bureau for Epilepsy (IBE). *Epilepsia* **46**, 470–472.

Gastaut, H. (1974). Syncopes: generalized anoxic cerebral seizures. In: Magnus, O., Haas, A. M. editors. *Handbook of clinical neurology.* Vol 15. Chapter 42. Amsterdam: North Holland; pp. 815–36.

Gastaut, H., Fischer-Williams, M. (1957). Electro-encephalographic study of syncope: its difference from epilepsy. *Lancet* **2**, 1018–1025.

Harvey, A. S., Freeman, J. L. (2007). Epilepsy in hypothalamic hamartoma: clinical and EEG features. *Semin. Pediatr. Neurol.* **14**, 60–64.

Hennerici, M., Klemm, C., Rautenberg, W. (1988). The subclavian steal phenomenon: a common vascular disorder with rare neurologic deficits. *Neurology* **38**, 669–673.

Hoefnagels, W. A. J., Padberg, G. W., Overweg, J., van der Velde, E. A., Roos, R. A. C. (1991). Transient loss of consciousness: the value of the history for distinguishing seizure from syncope. *J Neurol.* **238**, 39–43.

Jardine, D. L., Hurrell, M. A., Fink, J. (2007). Tit-test diagnosis of hypotensive transient ischemic attacks. *Intern. Med. J* **37**, 498–501.

Kenny, R. A., Traynor, G. (1991). Carotid sinus syndrome—clinical characteristics in elderly patients. *Age Ageing* **20**, 449–454.

Kroenke, K., Rosmalen, J. G. M. (2006). Symptoms, syndromes, and the value of psychiatric diagnostics in patients who have functional somatic disorders. *Med. Clin. N Am.* **90**, 603–626.

Kroenke, K., Sharpe, M., Sykes, R. (2007). Revising the classification of somatoform disorders: key questions aand preliminary recommendations. *Psychosomatics* **48**, 277–285.

LaFrance, W. C. (2008). Psychogenic nonepileptic seizures. *Curr. Opin. Neurol.* **21**, 195–201.

LaFrance, W. C., Alper, K., Babcock, D., *et al.* (2006). Nonepileptic seizures treatment workshop summary. *Epilepsy & Behavior* **8**, 451–461.

Landau, W. M., Nelson, D. A. (1996). Clinical neuromythology XV. Feinting science: Neurocardiogenic syncope and collateral vasovagal confusion. *Neurology* **46**, 609–618.

Lempert, T., Bauer, M., Schmidt, D. (1994). Syncope: a videometric analysis of 56 episodes of transient cerebral hypoxia. *Ann. Neurol.* **36**, 233–237.

Lempert, T., von Brevern, M. (1996). The eye movements of syncope. *Neurology* **46**, 1086–1088.

Levine, E., Rosero, S. Z., Budzikowski, A. S., Moss, A. J., Zareba, W., Daubert, J. P. (2008). Congenital long QT syndrome: considerations for primary care physicians. *Cleve. Clin. J Med.* **75**, 591–600.

Lin, J. T. J., Ziegler, D. K., Lai, C. W., Bayer, W. (1982). Convulsive syncope in blood donors. *Ann. Neurol.* **11**, 525–528.

Macleod, S., Ferrie, C., Zuberi, S M. (2005). Symptoms of narcolepsy in children misinterpreted as epilepsy. *Epileptic Disord.* **7**, 13–17.

Mathias, C. J., Mallipeddi, R., Bleasdale-Barr, K. (1999). Symptoms associated with orthostatic hypotension in pure autonomic failure and multiple system atrophy. *J Neurol.* **246**, 893–898.

Melgar, M. A., Weinand, M. E. (2003). Thyrocervical trunk-external carotid artery bypass for positional cerebral ischemia dur to common carotid artery occlusion. Report of three cases. *Neurosurg. Focus* **14**, e7.

Mihaescu, M., Malow, B. A. (2003). Sleep disorders: a sometimes forgotten cause of nonepileptic spells. *Epilepsy & Behavior* **4**, 784–787.

Newman, B. H., Graves, S. (2001). A study of 178 consecutive vasovagal syncopal reactions from the perspective of safety. *Transfusion* **41**, 1475–1479.

Noyes, R., Stuart, S. P., Watson, D. B. A reconceptualization of the somatoform disorders. *Psychosomatics* **49**, 14–22.

Overeem, S., Mignot, E., van Dijk, J. G., Lammers, G. J. (2001). Narcolepsy: clinical features, new pathophysiological insights, and future perspectives. *J Clin. Neurophysiol.* **18**, 78–105.

Pearce, J. M. (2004). A note on gelastic epilepsy. *Eur. Neurol.* **52**, 172–174.

Posner, J. B., Saper, C. B., Schiff, N., Plum, F. (Eds). (2007). *Plum and Posner's Diagnosis of Stupor and Coma.* Oxford University Press, Oxford.

Reuber, M., Mitchell, A. J., Howlett, S. J., Crimlisk, Grünewald, R. A. (2005). Functional symptoms in neurology: questions and answers. *JNNP* **76**, 307–314.

Ribaï, P., Tugendhaft, P., Legros, B. (2006). Usefulness of prolonged video-EEG monitoring and provocative procedure with saline injection for the diagnosis of nonepileptic seizures of psychogenic origin. *J Neurol.* **253**, 328–332.

Robertson, D., Wade Kincaid, D., Halle, V., Robertson, R. M. (1994). The head and neck discomfort of autonomic failure: an unrecognized aetiology of headache. *Clin. Auton. Res.* **4**, 99–103.

Romme, J. J. *et al.* (2008). Influence of age and gender on the occurrence and presentation of reflex syncope. *Clin. Auton. Res.* **18**, 127–133.

Rossen, R., Kabat, H., Anderson, J. P. (1943). Acute arrest of cerebral circulation in man. *Arch. Neurol. Psychiatry* **50**, 510–518.

Savitz, S. I., Caplan, L. R. (2005). Vertebrobasilar disease. *NEJM* **352**, 2618–2626.

Sheldon, R., Rose, S., Connolly, S., Ritchie, D., Koshman, M. L., Frenneaux, M. (2006). Diagnostic criteria for vasovagal syncope based on a quantitative history. *Eur. Heart J.* **27**, 344–50.

Sheldon, R., Rose, S., Ritchie, D., *et al.* (2002). Historical criteria that distinguish syncope from seizures. *J Am. Coll. Cardiol.* **40**, 142–148.

Sheldon, R. S., Koshman, M. L., Murphy, W. F. (1998). Electroencephalographic findings during presyncope and syncope induced by tilt table testing. *Can. J Cardiol.* **14**, 811–816.

So, N. K. (1995). Atonic phenomena and partial seizures. A reappraisal. *Adv. Neurol.* **67**, 29–39.

Somerville, E. R. (1984). Orthostatic transient ischemic attacks: a symptom of large vessel occlusion. *Stroke* **15**, 1066–1067.

Stark, R. J., Wodak, J. (1983). Primary orthostatic cerebral ischaemia. *JNNP* **46**, 883–891.

Stephenson, J. B. P. (1990). *Fits and faints.* London: MAC Keith Press.

Stone, J., Campbell, K., Sharma, N., Carson, A., Warlow, C. P., Sharpe, M. (2003). What should we call pseudoseizures? The patient's perspective. *Seizure* **12**, 568–572.

Strassnig, M., Stowell, K. R., First, M. B., Pincus, H. A. (2006). General medical and psychiatric perspectives on somatoform disorders: separated by an uncommon language. *Curr. Opin. Psychiatry* **19**, 194–200.

Sutton, R. (1999). Vasovagal syncope: prevalence and presentation. An algorithm of management in the aviation environment. *Europ. Heart J Suppl.* **1**, D109–D113.

Taylor, C. L., Selman, W. R., Ratchson, R. A. (2002). Steal affecting the cntral nervous system. *Neurosurgery* **50**, 679–689.

Thijs, R. D., Wagenaar, W. A., Middelkoop, H. A., Wieling, W., van Dijk, J. G. (2008). Transient loss of consciousness through the eyes of a witness. *Neurology* **71**, 1713–1718.

Thijs, R. D., Wieling, W., Kaufmann, H., van Dijk, J. G. (2004). Defining and classifying syncope. *Clin. Auton. Res.* **14** Suppl 1, 4-8.

Tibussek, D., Wohlrab, G., Boltshauser, E., Schmitt, B. (2006). Proven startle-provoked epileptic seizures in childhood: semiologic and electrophysiologic variability. *Epilepsia* **47**, 1050–1058.

Trenité, D. G. (2006). Photosensitivity, visually sensitive seizures and epilepsies. *Epilepsy Res.* **70** Suppl 1, S269–279.

Van Dijk, J. G. (2003). Fainting in animals. *Clin. Auton. Res.* **13**, 247–255.

Webster, M. W., Downs, L., Yonas, H., Makaroun, M. S., Steed, D. L. (1994). The effect of arm exercise on regional cerebral blood flow in the subclavian steal syndrome. *Am. J Surg.* **168**, 91–93.

Whinnery, J. A., Shender, B S. (1993). The opticographic nerve: eye-level anatomic relationships within the central nervous system. *Aviat. Space Environm. Med.* **64**, 952–954.

Wieling, W., Krediet, C. T., Wilde, A. A. (2006). Flush after syncope: not always an arrhythmia. *J Cardiovasc. Electrophysiol.* **17**, 804–805.

Wieling, W., Thijs, R. D., van Dijk, N., Wilde, A. A. M., Benditt, D. G., van Dijk, J. G. (2009). Symptoms and signs of syncope. A review of the link between physiology and clinical clues. *Brain* **132**, 2630–2642.

Zaidi, A., Crampton, S., Clough, P., Fitzpatrick, A., Scheepers, B. (1999). Head-up tilting is a useful provocative test for psychogenic non-epeilptic seizures. *Seizure* **8**, 353–355.

Zeman, A., Douglas, N., Aylward, R. (2001). Narcolepsy mistaken for epilepsy. *BMJ* **322**, 216–218.

van Dijk, J. G., Thijs, R. D., Benditt, D. G., Wieling, W. (2009). A guide to disorders causing transient loss of consciousness: focus on syncope. *Nat. Rev. Neurol.* **5**, 438–448.

van Donselaar, C. A., Geerts, A. T., Schimsheimer, R. J. (1990). Usefulness of an aura for classification of a first generalized seizure. *Epilepsia* **31**, 529–535.

CHAPTER 56

Syncope and fainting: classification and pathophysiological basis

Roger Hainsworth and Victoria E. Claydon

Introduction

Syncope, or fainting, refers to a transient loss of consciousness usually resulting from temporarily inadequate cerebral blood flow. A syncopal attack is frequently preceded by sweating, pallor, blurring of vision, dizziness, and nausea. It is uncommon in supine subjects and usually when subjects become supine as the result of syncope they rapidly recover consciousness. There is a wide variation in the susceptibility of individuals to syncope. The fainting of pregnant women or soldiers standing motionless on hot parade grounds is well known. On the other hand, patients in heart failure rarely, if ever, faint. Syncope does not necessarily point to organic disease, although it is clearly important to exclude diseases such as epilepsy, autonomic neuropathies, cerebrovascular disease, as well as cardiac and endocrine disorders. Most healthy individuals can precipitate at least presyncopal symptoms if, particularly in a warm environment (causing skin vasodilatation), they hyperventilate (to constrict cerebral blood vessels) and, after having been in a crouching position, suddenly stand (to allow abdominal blood vessels to fill with blood and to increase the height to which blood must be pumped to the brain).

The onset of syncope can be gradual with ample warning signs, or it may be quite abrupt. Usually preceding the faint there is increased activity of the sympathetic nervous system, leading to a maintained or sometimes increased blood pressure accompanied by increases in heart rate and vascular resistance. Then there is a profound fall in arterial blood pressure, inadequate cerebral perfusion, and loss of consciousness. Often the syncopal attack is accompanied by vasodilatation and bradycardia. This is the vasovagal attack, a term introduced in 1932 by Sir Thomas Lewis.

In this chapter, the main causes of syncope are first categorized. The control of cerebral blood flow and its inadequacy in causing loss of consciousness is then discussed, followed by discussion of the factors leading to vasodilatation and to bradycardia and the consequences of these for the maintenance of blood pressure. Cardiac and neurological causes of syncope are described in Chapter 57. This chapter concentrates on fainting due to unexplained hypotension and, in particular, on vasovagal syncope. Possible trigger mechanisms for initiating vasovagal syncope, and a number of factors thought to predispose individuals to syncopal attacks, such as emotional stress, small plasma or blood volume, changes in cerebral function and the importance of skeletal muscle pumping activity are discussed.

Causes of syncope

Syncope is a transient loss of consciousness resulting from cerebral dysfunction due usually to cerebral hypoperfusion, although sometimes to metabolic disorders. Cerebral hypoperfusion results from either abnormally high cerebral vascular resistance or inadequate cerebral perfusion pressure. In some cases the cause of syncope may be identified as being secondary to some recognizable clinical condition, such as a cardiac arrhythmia or autonomic failure. However, in many cases the cause is not immediately apparent, but it occurs when in the upright position, often accompanied by vasodilatation and sometimes bradycardia. These faints are often referred to as vasovagal attacks or neurocardiogenic syncope.

The causes of syncope have been listed in Table 56.1 and have been classified on a pathophysiological basis. Cerebral hypoperfusion may result from systemic hypotension. Since blood pressure is dependent on cardiac output and total peripheral vascular resistance, any factor that decreases either variable must decrease blood pressure.

The most important physiological factor determining cardiac output is venous filling, since the heart can never pump out more blood than flows in. Therefore, excessive pooling of blood in dependent veins when upright, or a small blood volume, predisposes to syncope. Occasionally cardiac output may be impaired due to bradyarrhythmias, tachyarrhythmias, or valvular disease. These disorders are discussed in Chapter 57. Rarely, cardiac output may be reduced due to vagally-induced bradycardia in vasovagal syncope or 'carotid sinus syncope'. These are discussed later in this chapter.

Widespread and excessive vasodilatation causes blood pressure to fall; this is the main reason for the sudden fall in blood pressure in the vasovagal attack. Vasodilatation also occurs during thermal stress and in response to some reflex stimuli, as well as when vasoactive drugs are given. Normal vasoconstrictor responses are impaired in autonomic neuropathies.

Table 56.1 Causes of syncope

Low arterial blood pressure

◆ Low cardiac output

- Inadequate venous return—due either to excessive venous pooling or to low blood volume

- Cardiac causes—tachyarrhythmias, bradyarrhythmias, valvular disease, bradycardia

◆ Low total peripheral vascular resistance

- Vasovagal attacks

- Widespread cutaneous vasodilatation in thermal stress

- Reflex (autonomic) causes—vasovagal attacks, 'carotid sinus syndrome', visceral pain reflexes (may cause vasodilatation or vasoconstriction), decreased stimulation of visceral stretch receptors (e.g. voiding distended bladder)

- Vasodilator drugs

- Autonomic neuropathies

Increased resistance to cerebral blood flow

◆ Cerebral vasoconstriction

- Low $PaCO_2$, due to hyperventilation

- Cerebral vasospasm (?)

◆ Vascular disease—either extracranial or intracranial arteries

Other causes of cerebral dysfunction

◆ Epilepsy—may confuse with simple faints

◆ Metabolic and endocrine disorders—hypoglycaemia, Addison's disease, hypopituitarism

◆ Electrolyte disorders—may be associated with hypovolaemia or predispose to cardiac arrhythmias

Cerebral blood flow may be reduced as the result of cerebral vasoconstriction due to low blood levels of carbon dioxide caused by hyperventilation. This is often a manifestation of psychological stress and it also commonly occurs during orthostatic stress. Vascular disease involving extracranial and/or intracranial arteries may impede cerebral blood flow and predispose to syncope.

Syncope may result from cerebral dysfunction due to causes other than hypoperfusion. An obvious cause to consider is epilepsy, which may be misdiagnosed in cases of vasovagal attacks because of the tonic clonic movements that are sometimes seen. Metabolic disorders, notably hypoglycaemia, can also lead to loss of consciousness. Syncope may also occur in various other endocrine disorders, particularly Addison's disease and hypopituitarism, probably mainly due to low blood volume. Severe electrolyte disturbances may cause impaired consciousness or predispose to syncope from low blood volume or cardiac dysrhythmias.

Cerebral blood flow

The blood flow to the human brain normally remains relatively constant. Unlike tissues such as muscle or glands, in which changes in metabolic activity result in large changes in blood flow, changes in cerebral activity result in changes in flow that are usually too localized and, overall, too small to be apparent in estimates of total flow. Typical values of cerebral blood flow are 50–60 ml/minute per 100 g brain tissue, or about 15% of the resting cardiac output.

The brain cannot withstand more than a few seconds of total interruption of flow without loss of consciousness; interruption for longer periods results in irreversible damage.

Regulation of cerebral blood flow

Cerebral blood flow shows marked autoregulation. That means that cerebral blood flow remains almost constant over a wide range of perfusion pressures. Two mechanisms are postulated for causing relaxation of arteriolar smooth muscle to maintain a constant flow to a region when perfusion pressure decreases: relaxation in response to decreased stretch (the myogenic theory), and relaxation in response to an increase in local concentrations of vasodilator metabolites following a transient decrease in flow (the metabolic theory). There may also be a role for neurogenic autoregulation by the autonomic nervous system, although the significance of this is debated.

Changes in the level of carbon dioxide in the arterial blood are particularly effective in causing changes in cerebral blood flow. At normal levels of arterial pressure, an increase in PCO_2 from 5.3 to 7 kPa (40–52 mmHg) approximately doubles cerebral flow, whereas a decrease to 4 kPa (30 mmHg) halves it. The level of CO_2 in the perfusing blood also influences the autoregulation of cerebral blood flow. Autoregulation is abolished during hypercapnia; during hypocapnia cerebral blood flow is low at all perfusion pressures (Fig. 56.1).

Cerebral blood vessels are innervated to some extent by sympathetic vasoconstrictor nerves. These are thought to be relatively unimportant in most circumstances. There have been reports of a 'paradoxical' cerebral vasoconstriction which precedes the onset of syncope. However, this is now thought not to be due to active vasoconstriction but rather to the critical closing pressure of the vessels being reached, caused by the combination of hypotension and hypocapnic vasoconstriction (Carey et al. 2001).

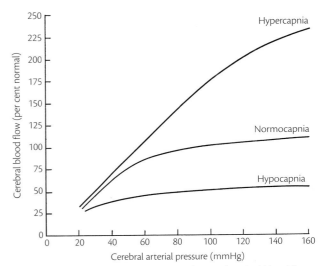

Fig. 56.1 Schematic diagram showing autoregulation of cerebral blood flow. The flow at normal cerebral perfusion pressure and normal arterial PCO_2 is taken as 100%. Cerebral perfusion pressure (cerebral arterial pressure minus intracranial pressure) is 5–10 mmHg less than cerebral arterial pressure. Above a pressure of about 60 mmHg the flow is largely independent of pressure. During hypercapnia the autoregulation is largely lost. During hypocapnia blood flow is only about 50% of the normal value, at all levels of CO_2.

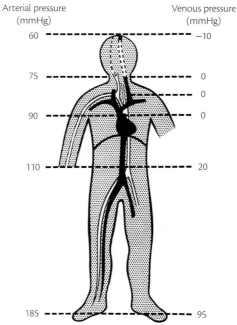

Arterial pressure (mmHg)   Venous pressure (mmHg)

Fig. 56.2 Effects of gravity on arterial and venous blood pressures in an erect, motionless man. Arterial and venous pressures in the lower part of the body are increased and in the upper part of the body decreased. Note that cerebral arterial pressure is about 15 mmHg lower than aortic root pressure. Because the brain is enclosed by rigid skull, the venous pressures may be below atmospheric. This results in a relatively constant arterial-venous pressure difference in different parts of the brain. With permission from Hainsworth, R. Copyright Elsevier (1985).

Cerebral blood flow during hypotension

It must first be appreciated that in the upright position cerebral arterial pressure is 15–30 mm Hg lower than that in the aortic arch and the difference is even greater compared with that in a dependent arm (Fig. 56.2). Consciousness starts to be lost when cerebral blood flow falls below about 25 ml/min/100g, half the normal flow. This level can be reached by severe hypocapnia (Pco_2 less than 4 kPa) achieved by hyperventilation, or by cerebral arterial pressure falling below about 40 mmHg (Fig. 56.1). In the upright position the critical level of cerebral arterial pressure would correspond to a mean brachial arterial pressure of about 70 mmHg; for example 90/60 mmHg (mean pressure is approximately diastolic plus 1/3 pulse pressure). Note, however, that flow is actually determined by cerebral perfusion pressure (i.e. arterial–venous) (or cerebrospinal fluid pressure) and, in the upright position, pressure in the cerebral venous sinuses is sub-atmospheric, which would reduce the gravitational effect on perfusion pressure. Syncope is much less likely to occur when subjects are supine, partly because cerebral arterial pressure is then the same as aortic pressure and partly because there is less pooling of blood in dependent veins.

Vasodilatation

Poiseuille's equation states that flow through a tube is proportional to pressure and the fourth power of the radius. By rearranging Poiseuille's equation, arterial pressure, P, can be seen to be dependent on cardiac output ($\dot{Q}$), and a term r, relating to the radius of resistance vessels:

$$P \propto \dot{Q}/r^4$$

Thus, the effect of vasodilatation on blood pressure depends on whether the change in r^4 is greater than the change in $\dot{Q}$. Vasodilatation can be particularly pronounced in skeletal muscle during exercise. At rest in a comfortable environment, the cardiac output (typically about 5.5 litres/minute) is distributed so that less than 20% of it perfuses skeletal muscle, even though muscle comprises nearly half the tissue mass. During severe exercise total muscle blood flow may increase from 1 to 20 litres/minute and it then forms the major part of the cardiac output. This intense vasodilatation, however, is usually associated with an increase rather than a decrease in blood pressure. The main reason for this is that the contracting muscles and increased respiratory activity return blood rapidly back to the heart, and this, together with an increased activity in cardiac sympathetic nerves, increases cardiac output. The same effect does not occur when there is vasodilatation in the absence of increased muscular activity. Thus administration of vasodilator drugs, such as sodium nitroprusside, or blocking sympathetic vasoconstrictor activity pharmacologically, results in vasodilatation with relatively little accompanying increase in cardiac output, so that the change in r^4 is greater than the change in $\dot{Q}$, and this results in a decrease in blood pressure.

Blood flow in the skin has been estimated to lie between as little as 20 ml/minute for the entire skin during cooling of both skin and body core, to as much as 3 litres/minute during severe heat load. Thermally induced vasodilatation results in a decrease in total vascular resistance and an increased volume of blood in cutaneous veins, and this may decrease blood pressure and predispose to fainting.

Mechanisms of vasodilatation

The diameter of blood vessels can change in response to neural, chemical and mechanical influences.

Sympathetic vasoconstrictor (noradrenergic) nerves increase the contraction of smooth muscle in both arterioles and veins. Resting discharge rate is quite low (<1 Hz) but this may increase up to about 10 Hz during severe stresses or baroreceptor unloading. Capacitance vessels have been shown to be more sensitive to low levels of sympathetic activity (Hainsworth 1986) (Fig. 56.3) and moderate levels of hypotension result in baroreceptor-mediated responses which maintain blood pressure more by capacitance vessel constriction than by increases in vascular resistance.

Blood flow to most regions of the body is regulated so that it is appropriate for the level of metabolic activity. This is achieved through the formation of metabolic products which dilate resistance vessels. Flow is thus determined by the balance between neurally mediated vasoconstriction and metabolically mediated vasodilatation. In circumstances, such as orthostatic stress, in which the degree of sympathetic activity is high, flow is reduced and metabolic products consequently accumulate. Abrupt removal of the normal vasoconstrictor activity would therefore result in an abrupt fall in vascular resistance and a consequent fall in blood pressure. This is illustrated in Fig. 56.4 in which it can be seen that during constant pressure perfusion of a dog's hindlimb, stimulation of the efferent sympathetic nerves decreased the blood flow. Immediately after switching off the stimulator, blood flow

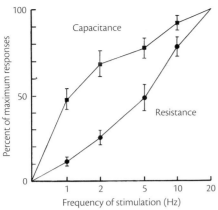

Fig. 56.3 Capacitance and resistance responses in abdominal circulation of anaesthetized dogs to stimulation of splanchnic nerves at various frequencies. Responses expressed as percentages of the changes at 20 Hz. Values are means ± SE from 14 dogs. Note that at 1 Hz the capacitance response was nearly 50% of maximal, whereas the resistance response was only about 10% maximal. Above 2 Hz there was little further response of capacitance but larger responses of resistance. Karim, F. and Hainsworth, R. (1976). *Am. J. Physiol.*, Am Physiol Soc, used with permission.

increased transiently to well above the steady-state value seen before stimulation.

Is flow also controlled by vasodilator nerves?

The importance of sympathetic adrenergic nerves in the control of blood pressure is undisputed. However, it has also been proposed that blood flow, particularly to skeletal muscle, is under the influence of sympathetic cholinergic vasodilator nerves. The importance of these nerves was thought to lie not only with their supposed ability to increase flow at the onset of exercise, but also that they might mediate the vasodilatation that precedes syncope.

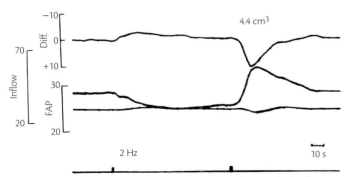

Fig. 56.4 Reactive hyperaemia in response to cessation of sympathetic efferent activity. A dog's hindlimb was perfused at constant pressure, and efferent sympathetic nerves to the limb were stimulated at 2 Hz for 90 seconds. Traces from above down are of the electronically subtracted difference between outflow of blood from the limb and inflow in ml/minute (an upward deflection indicates that outflow exceeds inflow and so the volume decreases), inflow in ml/minute, and femoral arterial perfusion pressure in kPa (1 kPa = 7.5 mmHg). Stimulation of sympathetic nerves caused a decrease in flow to the limb and a decrease in the volume of blood in the limb. After cessation of the stimulus, the flow increased and was initially much greater than the steady-state value in absence of stimulation. The increase in flow also resulted in the retention of blood within the limb. With permission from Hainsworth, R. et al. (1983), Hind-limb vascular-capacitance responses in anaesthetized dogs. *J. Physiol.* Wiley.

The evidence in support of cholinergic vasodilator responses in humans comes from experiments of fainting in which there was seen to be an increase in limb blood flow just before the onset of syncope and which was prevented by sympathetic block (Barcroft and Edholm 1945) and reduced by intra-arterial atropine (Blair et al. 1959). There is, however, considerable evidence against the existence of a cholinergic vasodilator supply to muscle in man. First, Uvnas (1966) looked for these nerves in many animals and found them only in some sub-primate species and not in any of several primates studied; their existence in humans therefore seems unlikely. Secondly, the observation that flow in an innervated limb increases transiently to become greater than that in a sympathect-omized limb is not evidence for active vasodilatation because it is likely that there would have been reactive hyperaemia following abrupt withdrawal of sympathetic tone (e.g. Fig. 56.4). The evidence in support of cholinergic vasodilatation provided by the administration of atropine is also not conclusive because, although atropine blocks the bradycardia occurring during a vasovagal attack, the fall in blood pressure is not prevented (Lewis 1932). Any small effect of atropine in human limbs may be an effect on the cutaneous circulation since thermally induced vasodilatation may be a cholinergic response associated with sweating. Further evidence against active muscle vasodilatation was provided by Wallin and Sundlof (1982) who recorded activity in efferent sympathetic nerves in humans during vasovagal fainting. They observed an abrupt cessation of nervous activity with the onset of the hypotension, but there was no suggestion of any increase in other nervous activity which might have been expected if vasodilator nerves had become active.

Is there are role for carbon dioxide in peripheral vasodilatation?

Hypocapnia is well known to cause constriction of cerebral vessels. However, hypocapnia has the opposite effect on the peripheral circulation, resulting in vasodilatation (Norcliffe et al. 2002a). During orthostatic stress there is a tendency to hyperventilate, and thus reduce arterial carbon dioxide levels. This may contribute to the peripheral vasodilatation that is seen immediately prior to a syncopal event. Interestingly, the sensitivity of the peripheral circulation to changes in carbon dioxide is greater in individuals prone to syncopal events compared to more orthostatically tolerant controls (Norcliffe et al. 2002a; Norcliffe-Kaufmann et al. 2008) and this could contribute to their poor orthostatic blood pressure control.

Cardiac output

By far the most important determinant of cardiac output is venous return. The heart clearly cannot pump out more blood that it receives. Changes in rate and force of cardiac contraction facilitate the ejection of the venous inflow, and failure of these responses to occur would limit the outflow when filling is high as, for example during severe exercise. However, they are unlikely to be of importance when filling is low as during orthostatic stress.

Effect of heart rate on cardiac output

Cardiac output is equal to the product of heart rate and stroke volume. Although this relationship is mathematically unarguable, it can be misleading because stroke volume is not independent of heart rate. Fig. 56.5 illustrates the effect of changes in heart rate

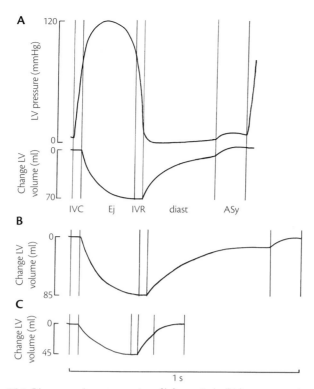

Fig. 56.5 Diagrammatic representation of left ventricular (LV) pressures and volumes during the cardiac cycle and the influence of heart rate. IVC, isovolumic contraction phase; Ej, ejection phase; IVR, isovolumic relaxation phase; diast, ventricular and atrial diastole; ASy, atrial systole. **A:** Pressure and volume changes at heart rate of 80 beats/minute (cycle length 0.75 seconds). Note the rapid ventricular filling during early diastole and the small contribution of atrial systole. Stroke volume is 70 ml and cardiac output is 5.6 litres/minute. **B:** Volume changes at a heart rate of 60 beats/minute (cycle length 1.0 seconds). Diastole is prolonged and there is a period of diastasis during which ventricular filling virtually ceases. Stroke volume increases to 85 ml and cardiac output is only slightly reduced at 5.1 litres/minute. **C:** Volume changes at a heart rate of 120 beats/minutes (cycle length 0.5 seconds). The shortening is mainly at the expense of diastole, which is greatly reduced. Atrial systole now makes a major contribution to ventricular filling. Stroke volume decreases to 45 ml and cardiac output again remains almost unchanged at 5.4 litres/minute.

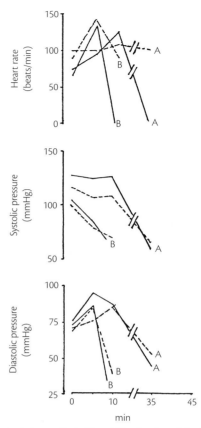

Fig. 56.6 Responses in two patients (A and B) to head-up tilting before (continuous lines) and after (interrupted lines) implantation of atrioventricular pacemakers. The pacemakers successfully prevented the asystole, but had no effect on the blood pressure change or on the time to onset of syncope. From El-Bedawi et al. 1994, with permission

when venous filling of the heart is not enhanced. A moderate decrease in heart rate, say to 60 beats/minute, results in longer time for cardiac filling so that the effect of the bradycardia is offset by an increase in stroke volume. Abnormal tachycardia would seriously reduce filling time and output would be impaired. Very severe bradycardia or asystole would be expected to decrease output, although preventing this in syncope patients has little effect on the symptoms or on the frequency of the attacks, as has been demonstrated in studies of the effects of cardiac pacemakers (El-Bedawi et al. 1994). Fig. 56.6 shows the effects of head-up tilting in two patients before and after implanting atrioventricular pacemakers. The pacemakers successfully prevented bradycardia but had no effect on the hypotension or on the time at which it occurred.

The effect of a change in heart rate on cardiac output depends on the rate of venous filling and also on whether it is accompanied by a change in the inotropic state. During exercise, an increase in heart rate is accompanied by a positive inotropic change which reduces the duration of systole and so preserves diastolic filling time. Venous filling pressure is high and this results in a large increase in output. Under these circumstances failure adequately to increase rate and force would be likely to limit the response. This is quite different from orthostatic stress when venous filling pressure would be low and changes in heart rate would then have little effect on cardiac output.

Importance of skeletal muscle pumping activity

Apart from when resting in the supine position, we can regard the circulation as being driven by three pumps in series: left heart, right heart and peripheral pumps. The peripheral pumps comprise the skeletal muscle-venous pump and the thoracoabdominal respiratory pump. When upright, it is the peripheral pumps that limit the venous pooling and the consequent fluid transudation that may lead to syncope (Brown and Hainsworth 1999). The main difference between walking, and even standing, and being passively tilted is the action of the muscle pump. It has been demonstrated that voluntary contractions of the lower limb musculature during orthostasis, using techniques such as leg crossing or buttock clenching, are effective methods of improving blood pressure in individuals prone to syncope (Krediet et al. 2002), presumably working at least partly through activation of the skeletal muscle pump. This would be likely to increase venous return and help to prevent or delay a syncopal event. We (Claydon and Hainsworth 2005) showed that involuntary skeletal muscle contractions associated with postural sway may also be important in the prevention of syncope.

Asymptomatic volunteers who show early presyncope during orthostatic stress testing, and yet never normally faint, demonstrate enhanced postural sway during normal standing. This would be likely to enhance venous return and, at least partly, explain why they remain asymptomatic despite their poor test results. Indeed, patients with recurrent syncope do not exhibit this enhancement of postural sway (Claydon and Hainsworth 2006).

Vasovagal syncope

Lewis (1932) described fainting attacks as being vasovagal because they were accompanied by hypotension and bradycardia. He considered that bradycardia usually was not the main cause of the faint, since heart rate rarely fell to very low levels (less than 40 beats/minute) and the hypotension was little affected by the administration of atropine which prevented the bradycardia.

Barcroft et al. (1944) performed an illuminating study in which they induced fainting in healthy subjects by bleeding and application of tourniquets to the legs. They observed that, before the onset of the faint, heart rate increased and there was also an increase in vascular resistance shown by blood pressure being relatively little changed despite the large decrease in cardiac output. Just before the faint, blood pressure decreased abruptly, and this was accompanied by decreases in heart rate and vascular resistance, but no further fall and perhaps even a small increase in cardiac output. Subsequent investigators have also made similar observations, of a fall in vascular resistance but no further fall in cardiac output during fainting.

Barcroft and Edholm (1945) reported an increase in forearm blood flow during fainting (Fig. 56.7) and suggested that the hypotension was due mainly to dilatation of vessels in skeletal muscle. Subsequently, based on animal work, Morita and Vatner (1985) suggested that vasodilatation in hypotensive haemorrhage may be more widespread.

Emotional stress leads to increases in heart rate and blood pressure with little change in total vascular resistance. However, if a vasovagal faint occurs, blood pressure, heart rate and forearm vascular resistance decrease abruptly.

Julu et al. (2003) described four phases of the cardiovascular responses leading up to syncope. In the first, blood pressure is well maintained with a large increase in vascular resistance but relatively little change in heart rate. In the second phase there is a progressive increase in heart rate. Phase 3 is characterized by instability with large oscillations of blood pressure and often heart rate. The final phase is presyncope with sudden decreases in blood pressure and heart rate, and symptoms of presyncope. The durations of the phases are quite variable but all can be recognized to some extent.

Thus, a vasovagal attack is usually preceded by evidence of increased sympathetic and decreased vagal activity. The main cause of the hypotension is vasodilatation due to inhibition of sympathetic vasoconstrictor activity. The bradycardia is usually relatively unimportant because heart rate is seldom greatly slowed and cardiac output does not usually decrease with the onset of the faint. Furthermore, prevention of bradycardia by pacing the heart does not necessarily prevent or even delay syncope (Fig. 56.6).

Patients with histories suggestive of fainting attacks are frequently investigated by determining the effects of head-up tilting, either alone or accompanied by administration of a vasodilator drug such as isoprenaline. We use a stress that combines head-up tilting with application of progressive lower-body suction

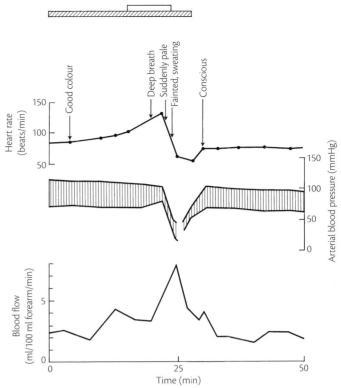

Fig. 56.7 Heart rate, arterial blood pressure, and forearm blood flow in a human subject during a haemorrhagic faint. Shaded bar: venous return impeded by application of tourniquets to both thighs; open bar: venesection. Note that initially blood pressure was relatively well maintained but that heart rate was increased. Then heart rate slowed and blood pressure fell. This was accompanied by an increase in forearm blood flow. With permission from Barcroft, H. and Edholm, O.G. (1945). On the vasodilatation in human skeletal muscle during post-haemorrhagic fainting. *J. Physiol.* Wiley.

(El-Bedawi and Hainsworth 1994) and have been able to induce syncope in almost all volunteer subjects tested if the stress is great enough. Fig. 56.8 shows responses obtained in a volunteer subject during the combined test. Head-up tilt alone did not induce hypotension but during the combined stress there were decreases in blood pressure and heart rate with symptoms of presyncope. It is important to note that vasovagal syncope is not necessarily an abnormal response. It is just that some people are more susceptible than others. The amounts of stress that are required to induce presyncope in volunteer subjects and in patients with suspected orthostatic intolerance are compared in Fig. 56.9. It can be noted that tilting with lower-body suction at −40 mmHg induces syncope in most subjects but that at −20 mmHg syncope is much more likely in the patients than in volunteers.

Many factors may be involved in the initiation of syncope and these are listed earlier in this chapter. The cardiac and neurological disorders leading to syncope are dealt with elsewhere. Most other fainting attacks seem to be associated with either a reduction in the return of blood to the heart and/or peripheral vasodilatation. Thus, when patients faint they are almost invariably standing or sitting up and often warm, and this results in dependent veins becoming distended with blood. The effects of posture are enhanced by performing the Valsalva manoeuvre. In this, intrathoracic and intra-abdominal pressures are increased by expiring against a resistance

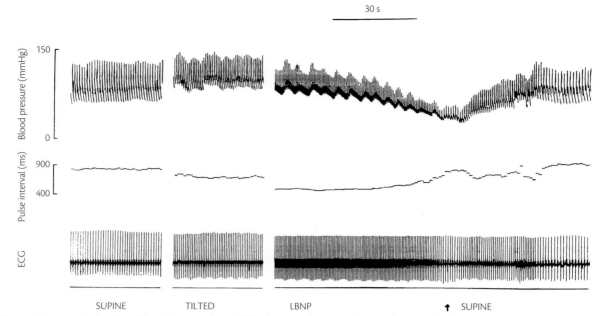

Fig. 56.8 Vasovagal syncope in a healthy subject. Traces are of arterial blood pressure (Finapres—finger at heart level), pulse interval, and ECG. Head-up tilting alone for 20 minutes caused an increase in diastolic pressure and a decrease in pulse interval. Addition of lower body negative pressure (LBNP) while still tilted caused a further decrease in pulse interval accompanied by a decrease in blood pressure, particularly systolic. Subsequently, blood pressure fell, with a small pulse pressure and an increase in pulse interval. The subject experienced symptoms of pre-syncope. From El-Bedawi and Hainsworth 1994, with permission.

or a closed glottis. Initially, the Valsalva results in an increase in arterial blood pressure as the thoracic and abdominal arteries are compressed. After a few seconds, owing to a decreased venous return into the abdomen and thorax due to the high pressures, cardiac output and blood pressure fall, possibly resulting in syncope. Two clinical manifestations of this are cough syncope and micturition syncope.

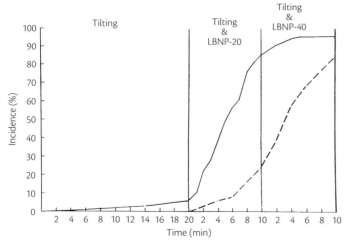

Fig. 56.9 Cumulative incidence of presyncope in volunteers (interrupted line) and patients with attacks of unexplained syncope (continuous line) to an orthostatic stress test of 20 minutes of 60° head-up tilt, followed while still tilted by lower body suction at −20 and −40 mmHg for 10 minutes at each. Note that tilting alone did not induce syncope in many subjects of either group, and that before the end of the test most subjects had developed syncope. The best discrimination between the groups was at the end of the first level of suction, when 85% of patients but only 20% of volunteers had developed symptoms. From Hainsworth and El-Bedawi 1994, with permission.

Paroxysms of coughing are effectively a Valsalva manoeuvre, but in addition, there may be reflex vasodilatation from stimulation of lung receptors (Daly et al. 1967). If sufficiently intense or prolonged, syncope may result.

Micturition syncope is particularly interesting as many diverse mechanisms seem to operate. Usually the problem occurs when a man stands to micturate after leaving a warm bed. His cutaneous circulation is dilated and therefore peripheral vascular resistance is low. He stands motionless so the muscle pump mechanism does not operate and the dependent capacitance vessels become distended leading to a decrease in venous return. He may have an enlarged prostate and have to perform a Valsalva type of strain. Relief of bladder distension may also result in reflex vasodilatation as the result of a reduced stimulus to bladder stretch receptors (Mary 1989).

What is the trigger for vasovagal syncope?

Although there have been several analyses of the haemodynamic changes that occur before and during the faint, the mechanism responsible for suddenly switching the apparently appropriate responses of vasoconstriction and tachycardia to the inappropriate ones of vasodilatation and bradycardia remains a matter for speculation. A number of possibilities have been suggested.

An abnormal baroreceptor reflex?

It has been suggested that vasovagal syncope might be triggered by stimulation of baroreceptors. In emotional syncope the faint is usually preceded by an increase in blood pressure. This, however, does not usually happen in orthostatic syncope. Furthermore, baroreceptors normally function as a stabilizing negative feedback system and would not be expected to induce sufficient vasodilatation to lower blood pressure abnormally.

In the so-called carotid sinus syndrome, syncope is thought to be caused by an exaggerated baroreceptor reflex. The original classical case was attributed to pressure on the sinus by a stiff winged collar, although the stimulus in most present cases is uncertain. The condition is most frequently diagnosed in older patients (Kenny and Richardson 2001). It is usually seen as an excessive bradycardia or an abnormal fall in blood pressure in response to carotid sinus massage. However, when we have studied such patients using a neck chamber to apply controlled carotid baroreceptor stimulation we have never seen syncope or abnormal hypotension. Part of the explanation for this apparent anomaly may be that some patients who are susceptible to orthostatically induced syncope have brisk baroreceptor responses (Wahbha et al. 1989, El-Sayed and Hainsworth 1995). Thus, many of the patients diagnosed as having carotid sinus syndrome may actually have poor orthostatic tolerance associated with brisk baroreceptor responses. It is interesting to note that patients who were treated successfully so that orthostatic tolerance improved also consistently showed decreases in baroreceptor sensitivity (El-Sayed and Hainsworth 1996).

Stimulation of cardiac receptors?

Another theory, which was popular for several years, is that the vasodilatation and bradycardia were responses to the Bezold–Jarisch reflex and resulted from abnormal stimulation of cardiac ventricular receptors (for references see Hainsworth 1991). The postulated mechanism was that, following haemorrhage or orthostasis, the ventricle would be contracting powerfully at a small volume and this would strongly stimulate ventricular mechanoreceptors. The basis for this was the observation by Oberg and Thoren (1972) that some ventricular non-myelinated afferents in the cat became excited under these conditions. The possible cardiac origin of syncope forms the rationale for infusing isoprenaline to subjects during orthostatic tests and for the use of beta-blocking drugs in treatment. However, it is very unlikely that stimulation of ventricular afferents has any significant part to play. First, in the original report of discharge in ventricular afferent nerves, only a few of them were actually excited under these conditions; in most the activity decreased. Secondly, other animal studies, in which the sympathetic nerves were stimulated and the heart bypassed, failed to show either vasodilatation or bradycardia (Al-Timman and Hainsworth, 1992, Drinkhill et al. 2001). Thirdly, studies carried out on humans with transplanted, and therefore denervated, ventricles have shown that orthostatic stress could still cause vasodilatation, hypotension, and syncope (Fitzpatrick et al. 1993). Finally, echocardiographic studies of patients at syncope have indicated that the heart is not necessarily near-empty (Novak et al. 1996), nor powerfully contracting (Liu et al. 2000). Furthermore, the Bezold–Jarisch reflex is not a response to mechanical stimulation; it is a response to chemical stimulation of cardiac receptors. The effect of isoprenaline infusion is probably related to some other property of the drug, possibly its action as a β_2-vasodilator. Furthermore, it is almost as effective in inducing syncope in normal subjects as in patients susceptible to fainting attacks (Kapoor and Brant 1992).

A defence mechanism?

Animal studies have defined a region in the hypothalamus which, when activated either by electrical stimulation or exposure of the animal to prey or predator, initiates a response called the 'defence reaction'. This response may include vasodilatation, particularly in muscle, and bradycardia. It may also be related to the 'playing dead' response seen in some animals. It is has also been suggested that emotionally induced fainting in humans may be comparable to activation of the hypothalamic defence area in animals. However, the mechanisms inducing vasodilatation seem to be different and there is no evidence for defence area involvement in human syncope.

A cerebral trigger?

Although the precipitating factors are not known, there is evidence that some central nervous mechanisms are involved. Opioids, probably of the delta subtype, may be implicated in the initiation of vasodilatation. Administration of naloxone has been shown to prevent the vasodilatation in rabbits, dogs, and rats (Morita and Vatner 1985), although it has not yet been shown to have the same effect in people. This may be because far greater doses were given to the animals. It has also been suggested that serotonergic mechanisms may also be involved (Chapter 53).

There are other hormonal influences on the brain that may be implicated in the initiation of vasovagal syncope. Vasopressin is suddenly and dramatically increased immediately before syncope (Davies et al. 1976). This would be expected to cause vasoconstriction. However, indirectly it increases the sensitivity of reflexes, including baroreflexes (Bishop and Hayworth 1991). Increased baroreceptor sensitivity would be likely to promote the inhibition of sympathetic control, and may also explain why, when patients are returned to supine after syncope induced by tilt testing, a single pressure pulse sometimes induces further vasodilatation and bradycardia (Hainsworth 2004).

Mercader et al. (2002) provided further support for the existence of a cerebral trigger for syncope. They demonstrated that, in patients with vasovagal syncope, during tilt testing with electroencephalographic (EEG) monitoring there was increased slow wave delta activity lateralized to the left side of the brain immediately prior to syncope. Furthermore, subjects who did not develop a vasovagal attack, including those who had a gradual and progressive fall in blood pressure due to autonomic failure, did not show this characteristic slowing of the EEG activity. Since these changes in the brain occurred prior to the onset of the vasovagal attack, in brain regions known to modulate cardiovascular control, it is tempting to suggest cause and effect. At this stage, however, there is insufficient evidence to draw firm conclusions, although this remains an exciting possibility in terms of identifying the trigger for syncope. Furthermore, subsequent research has highlighted EEG differences in patients suffering from syncope that can be identified between attacks (Mecarelli et al. 2004). They identified non-specific and diffuse slowing of baseline rhythms, particularly in the alpha rhythm, in syncope patients compared to controls at rest and during hyperventilation. They were able to identify EEG abnormalities (none of which were epileptiform in nature) in 79% of patients with vasovagal syncope (and only 31% of controls), again suggesting that there may be some cerebral trigger to the onset of syncope.

When one examines the time course of events leading to syncope, there is also some further evidence to suggest a central trigger. Research by Dan et al. (2002) showed that both presyncopal symptoms and reductions in cerebral blood flow velocity occurred prior to the fall in blood pressure in patients with orthostatic vasovagal syncope, highlighting the possible role of the cerebral circulation in initiating syncope.

These data suggest that, although the trigger for the switch to bradycardia and vasodilatation immediately prior to syncope remains elusive, we should continue examining the brain, rather than the heart, in order to solve this mystery.

Factors predisposing to vasovagal syncope

As mentioned previously, there are a number of external factors that are likely to increase an individual's susceptibility to syncope, such as prolonged orthostasis, heat stress and vasodilator agents. We have already noted that almost anyone can experience a vasovagal response given a sufficiently severe orthostatic challenge. However, why is it that some individuals, with no apparent pathology, are much more prone to vasovagal syncope than others? There are a number of factors that may predispose a person to vasovagal attacks.

Emotional stress

Many people faint at the sight of blood or the feel or sight of an intravenous needle. Also, and of particular relevance to orthostatic stress testing, people faint much earlier during head-up tilt if any intravascular instrumentation is employed (Stevens 1966). The mechanism for inducing vasodilatation and bradycardia during emotional stress is unknown.

Magnitude of vasoconstriction

The main mechanism by which blood pressure is maintained during orthostatic stress is via peripheral vasoconstriction. Individuals who are prone to vasovagal syncope have smaller vascular resistance responses to orthostatic stress (Sneddon et al. 1993, Brown and Hainsworth 2000). Furthermore, some measures known to increase orthostatic tolerance such as salt loading (Claydon and Hainsworth 2004) and water drinking (Schroeder et al. 2002) were associated with increased peripheral vasoconstriction during orthostasis. These findings suggest that an individual's susceptibility to syncope is related to the magnitude of peripheral vasoconstriction. This response is mediated mainly through baroreflexes, and vascular responses to baroreceptor stimulation are known to be enhanced during orthostatic stress (Cooper and Hainsworth

2001). The degree to which baroreceptor sensitivity is increased when upright is less in individuals prone to syncope (Cooper and Hainsworth 2002a), and this could explain their smaller vascular resistance response to orthostasis. The mechanism underlying the enhancement of baroreceptor sensitivity during orthostasis is uncertain, but one possibility is that it may be related to stimulation of subdiaphragmatic venous receptors (Doe et al. 1996).

Relation to plasma and blood volumes

Orthostatic stress results in a decrease in return of blood to the heart and a consequent decrease in cardiac output. This effect is enhanced by the loss of fluid from the plasma to the tissues in dependent regions (Brown and Hainsworth 1999). When cardiac output falls to below about half the supine value, syncope becomes very likely (El-Bedawi and Hainsworth 1994). This raises the possibility that a person's susceptibility to syncope might be related to his plasma or blood volume, and this indeed was shown to be the case (El-Sayed and Hainsworth 1995). The role of plasma volume has been further examined in patients by interventions designed to increase plasma volume. Several of these may be effective, including salt loading (El-Sayed and Hainsworth 1996; Cooper and Hainsworth 2002b), exercise training (Mtinangi and Hainsworth 1998) and sleeping head-up at 10° (Cooper and Hainsworth 2008). Results have shown that *changes* in plasma volume were correlated with changes in orthostatic tolerance (Fig. 56.10). As a result of these findings, many individuals who are liable to fainting have been advised to increase their salt and water intake, to expand plasma volume, and this usually ameliorates their symptoms. We examined the effect of water drinking alone, and found that drinking 500 ml water significantly increased orthostatic tolerance (Schroeder et al. 2002; Claydon et al. 2006). The mechanism underlying this effect is unknown. It is possible that it is mediated through an increase in plasma volume, although any effect on this is thought to be small (Jordan et al. 2000). It may be related to the increase in sympathetic efferent activity that has been reported to occur following water ingestion, although how this is mediated is not known.

It is possible, however, that the link between plasma volume and orthostatic tolerance may not necessarily be related to plasma volume per se, but rather to blood volume. Recent studies of high altitude dwellers who are polycythaemic from the high altitude

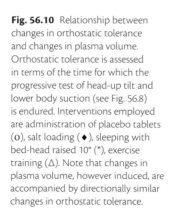

Fig. 56.10 Relationship between changes in orthostatic tolerance and changes in plasma volume. Orthostatic tolerance is assessed in terms of the time for which the progressive test of head-up tilt and lower body suction (see Fig. 56.8) is endured. Interventions employed are administration of placebo tablets (o), salt loading (♦), sleeping with bed-head raised 10° (*), exercise training (Δ). Note that changes in plasma volume, however induced, are accompanied by directionally similar changes in orthostatic tolerance.

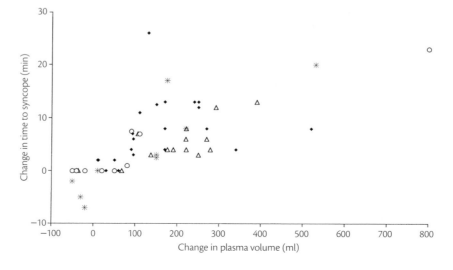

hypoxia to which they are exposed suggest that blood volume is the more important factor. These individuals have large packed cell and blood volumes, but normal plasma volumes, and have exceptionally good orthostatic tolerance (Claydon et al. 2004).

Autoregulation of cerebral blood flow

The ultimate cause of syncope, as mentioned previously, is a lack of blood flow to the brain. Since cerebral blood flow normally shows marked autoregulation, the question arises as to whether autoregulation is impaired in syncope patients. If autoregulation is effective, any decrease in cerebral perfusion pressure due to orthostasis should be buffered by a decrease in cerebrovascular resistance so that flow is constant. By examining the relationship between flow and pressure, using transcranial Doppler estimates of cerebral blood velocity, we have shown impaired cerebral autoregulation in patients with syncope (Claydon and Hainsworth 2003). The extent of impairment of autoregulation was found to be correlated with the impairment of orthostatic tolerance. The exact role of impaired autoregulation in predisposing to syncope is disputed and it has been suggested that this may be due to the heterogeneity of subjects studied and techniques used (see Edwards and Schondorf 2003).

Autoregulation is impaired during hypocapnia, and orthostasis is commonly associated with some degree of hyperventilation, which would lead to hypocapnia and cerebral vasoconstriction. Indeed, the combined stimulus of hypocapnia and hypotension is likely to play a fundamental role in the induction of syncope. We have reported that, in those individuals who are prone to syncope, hypocapnia causes a greater constriction of the cerebral vessels than in subjects who are resistance to syncopal attacks during tilt testing (Norcliffe et al. 2002b; Norcliffe-Kaufmann et al. 2008).

Summary

Vasovagal syncope is a transient loss of consciousness, due to temporarily inadequate cerebral blood flow, followed by a full recovery. Syncope usually occurs when the subject is upright and blood 'pools' in dependent vessels and gravity causes cerebral perfusion pressure to be lower than elsewhere. Most of the time, orthostatic stress does not result in hypotension because of the effects of reflexes, particularly baroreceptors, and cerebrovascular autoregulation. However, if the stress becomes too great, and this may occur earlier in particularly susceptible individuals, the normal sympathetic activity ceases and blood pressure falls. The hypotension is usually associated with a slowing of the heart rate, although this is rarely sufficient to make an important contribution to the syncope.

Several factors may predispose to syncope. Straining manoeuvres that impede venous return may initiate an attack and this, together with standing still with a warm dilated cutaneous circulation, may explain micturition syncope. Hypovolaemia also seems to be an important factor and increases in blood volume, whether from expansion of plasma volume or increased haematocrit, are of benefit in increasing orthostatic tolerance and preventing fainting. Susceptibility to syncope is also related to the magnitude of peripheral vasoconstriction and extent of utilization of skeletal muscle pumps. Alterations in cerebrovascular control are likely to be important in determining orthostatic tolerance.

The actual trigger mechanism which turns off sympathetic activity remains unknown. There have been suggestions that it is caused by inappropriate stimulation of baroreceptors or ventricular receptors. However, this is very unlikely and the responsible mechanism remains one of the continuing mysteries in cardiovascular physiology.

References

Al-Timman, J. K. A. and Hainsworth, R. (1992). Reflex vascular responses to changes in left ventricular pressures, heart rate and inotropic state in dogs. *Exp. Physiol.* **77**, 455–69.

Barcroft, H., McMichael, J. and Sharpey-Schafer, E.P. (1944). Post haemorrhagic fainting. Study by cardiac output and forearm flow. *Lancet* **i**, 289–91.

Barcroft, H. and Edholm, O.G. (1945). On the vasodilatation in human skeletal muscle during post-haemorrhagic fainting. *J. Physiol.* **104**, 161–75.

Bishop, V.S. and Hayworth, J.R. (1991). Hormonal control of cardiovascular reflexes. In: *Reflex control of the circulation,* (eds. I.H. Zucker and J.P. Gilmore), pp. 253–71. CRC Press, Boca Raton.

Blair, D. A., Glover, W. E., Greenfield, A. D. M. and Roddie, I. S. (1959). Excitation of cholinergic vasodilator nerves to human skeletal muscles during emotional stress *J. Physiol.* **148**, 633–47.

Brown, C. M. and Hainsworth, R. (1999). Assessment of capillary fluid shifts during orthostatic stress in normal subjects and subjects with orthostatic intolerance. *Clin. Auton. Res.* **9**, 69–73.

Brown, C.M. and Hainsworth, R. (2000). Forearm vascular responses during orthostatic stress in control subjects and patients with posturally related syncope. *Clin. Auton. Res.* **10**, 57–61.

Carey, B.J., Eames, P.J., Panerai, R.B. and Potter, J.F. (2001). Carbon dioxide, critical closing pressure and cerebral haemodynamics prior to vasovagal syncope in humans. *Clin. Sci.* **101**, 351–58.

Claydon, V.E., Norcliffe, L.J., Moore, J.P., Rivera-Ch, M., Leon-Velarde, F., Appenzeller, O., and Hainsworth, R. (2004). Orthostatic tolerance and blood volumes in Andean high altitude dwellers. *Exp. Physiol.* **89**, 565–71.

Claydon, V.E., Schroeder, C., Norcliffe, L.J., Jordan, J. and Hainsworth, R. (2006). Water drinking improves orthostatic tolerance in patients with posturally related syncope. *Clin. Sci.* **110**, 343–52.

Claydon, V.E. and Hainsworth, R. (2003). Cerebral autoregulation during orthostatic stress in healthy controls and in patients with posturally related syncope. *Clin. Auton. Res.* **13**, 321–29.

Claydon, V.E. and Hainsworth, R. (2004). Salt supplementation improves orthostatic cerebral and peripheral vascular control in patients with syncope. *Hypertension* **43**, 1–5.

Claydon, V.E. and Hainsworth, R. (2005). Increased postural sway in control subjects with poor orthostatic tolerance. *J. Am. Coll. Cardiol.* **46**, 1309–13.

Claydon, V.E. and Hainsworth, R. (2006). Postural sway in patients with syncope and poor orthostatic tolerance. *Heart* **92**, 1688–9.

Cooper, V.L. and Hainsworth, R. (2001). Carotid baroreceptor reflexes in humans during orthostatic stress. *Exp. Physiol.* **86**, 677–81.

Cooper, V.L. and Hainsworth, R. (2002a). Effects of head-up tilting on baroreceptor control in subjects with different tolerances to orthostatic stress. *Clin. Sci.* **103**, 221–26.

Cooper, V.L. and Hainsworth R. (2002b). Effects of dietary salt on orthostatic tolerance, blood pressure and baroreceptor sensitivity in patients with syncope. *Clin. Auton. Res.* **12**, 236–41.

Cooper, V.L. and Hainsworth R. (2008). Head-up sleeping improves orthostatic tolerance in patients with syncope. *Clin. Auton. Res.* **18**, 318–24.

Daly, M. de. B., Hazzledine, J. L. and Ungar, A. (1967). The reflex effects of alterations in lung volume on systemic vascular resistance in the dog. *J. Physiol.* **188**, 331–51.

Dan, D., Hoag, J.B., Ellenbogen, K.A., Wood, M.A., Eckberg, D.L., and Gilligan, D.M. (2002). Cerebral blood flow velocity declines before arterial pressure in patients with orthostatic vasovagal presyncope. *J. Am. Coll. Cardiol.* **39**, 1039–0145.

Davies, R., Slater, J.D., Forsling, M.L. and Payne N. (1976). The response of arginine vasopressin and plasma renin to postural change in normal man, with observations on syncope. *Clin. Sci. Mol. Med.* **51**, 267–74.

Doe, C.P.A., Drinkhill, M.J., Myers. D.S., Self, D.A. and Hainsworth, R. (1996). Reflex vascular responses to abdominal venous distension in anesthetized dogs. *Am. J. Physiol.* **271**, H1049–56.

Drinkhill, M.J., Wright, C.I. and Hainsworth, R. (2001). Reflex vascular responses to independent changes in left ventricular end-diastolic and peak systolic pressures and inotropic state in anaesthetised dogs. *J. Physiol.* **532**, 549–61.

Edwards, M.R. and Schondorf, R. (2003) Is cerebrovascular autoregulation impaired during neurally-mediated syncope? *Clin. Auton. Res.* **13**, 306–309.

El-Bedawi, K. M. Wahbha, M. M. A. E. and Hainsworth, R. (1994). Cardiac pacing does not improve orthostatic tolerance in patients with vasovagal syncope. *Clin. Auton. Res.* **4**, 233–7.

El-Bedawi, K. M. and Hainsworth, R. (1994). Combined head-up tilt and lower body suction: a test of orthostatic tolerance. *Clin. Auton. Res.* **4**, 41–7.

El-Sayed, H. and Hainsworth, R. (1995). Relationship between plasma volume, carotid baroreceptor sensitivity and orthostatic tolerance. *Clin. Sci.* **88**, 463–70.

El-Sayed, H. and Hainsworth, R. (1996). Salt supplement increases plasma volume and orthostatic tolerance in patients with unexplained syncope. *Heart* **75**, 134–40.

Fitzpatrick, A. P., Banner, N., Cheng, A., Yacoub, M. and Sutton, R. (1993). Vasovagal reactions may occur after orthotopic heart transplantation. *J. Am. Coll. Cardiol.* **21**, 1132–7.

Hainsworth, R. (1985). Arterial blood pressure. In *Hypotensive anaesthesia*, (ed. G. E. H. Enderby), pp. 3–29. Churchill Livingstone, Edinburgh.

Hainsworth, R. (1986). Vascular capacitance: its control and importance. *Rev. Physiol. Biochem. Pharmacol.* **105**, 101–73.

Hainsworth, R. (1991). Reflexes from the heart. *Physiol. Rev.* **71**, 617–58.

Hainsworth, R. (2004). Pathophysiology of syncope. *Clin. Auton. Res.* **14**, I18–24.

Hainsworth, R., Karim, F., McGregor, K. H. and Wood, L. M. (1983). Hind-limb vascular-capacitance responses in anaesthetized dogs. *J. Physiol.* **337**, 417–28.

Hainsworth, R. and El-Bedawi, K. M. (1994). Orthostatic tolerance in patients with unexplained syncope. *Clin. Auton. Res.* **4**, 239–44.

Jordan, J., Shannon, J.R. and Black, B.K. (2000). The pressor response to water drinking in humans: a sympathetic reflex? *Circulation* **101**, 504–509.

Julu, P.O., Cooper, V.L., Hansen, S., Hainsworth, R. (2003). Cardiovascular regulation in the period preceding vasovagal syncope in conscious humans. *J. Physiol.* **549**, 299–311.

Kapoor, W. N. and Brant, N. (1992). Evaluation of syncope by upright tilt testing with isoproterenol, a nonspecific test. *Ann. Int. Med.* **116**, 358–63.

Karim, F. and Hainsworth, R. (1976). Responses of abdominal vascular capacitance to stimulation of splanchnic nerves. *Am. J. Physiol.* **231**, 434–40.

Kenny, R.A., and Richardson, D.A. (2001). Carotid sinus syndrome and falls in older adults. *Am. J. Geriatr. Cardiol.* **10**, 97–99.

Krediet C.T., van Dijk, N., Linzer, M., van Lieshout, J.J., and Wieling, W. (2002). Management of vasovagal syncope: controlling or aborting faints by leg crossing and muscle tensing. *Circulation* **106**, 1684–89.

Lewis, T. (1932). Vasovagal syncope and the carotid sinus mechanism. *BMJ* **1**, 873–6.

Liu, J.E., Hahn, R.T., Stein, K.M., Markowitz, S.M., Okin, P.M., Devereux, R.B., and Lerman, B.B. (2000). Left ventricular geometry and function preceding neurally mediated syncope. *Circulation* **101**, 777–83.

Mary, D. A. S. G. (1989). The urinary bladder and cardiovascular reflexes. *Int. J. Cardiol.* **23**, 11–17.

Mecarelli, O., Pulitano, P., Vicenzini, E., Vanacore, N., Accornero, N. and De Marinis, M. (2004). Observations on EEG patterns in neurally-mediated syncope: an inspective and quantitative study. *Neurophysiol. Clin.* **34**, 203–207.

Mercader, M.A., Varghese, P.J., Potolicchio, S.J. Venkatraman, G.K. and Lee, S.W. (2002). New insights into the mechanism of neurally mediated syncope. *Heart* **88**, 217–55.

Morita, H. and Vatner, S. F. (1985). Effects of haemorrhage on renal nerve activity in conscious dog. *Circ. Res.* **57**, 788–93.

Mtinangi, B. L. and Hainsworth, R. (1998). Increased orthostatic tolerance following moderate exercise training in patients with unexplained syncope. *Heart* **80**, 596–600.

Norcliffe, L.J., Bush, V.E. and Hainsworth R. (2002a). The role of hypocapnia in the development of syncope during orthostatic stress. *J. Physiol.* **544P**, 84P.

Norcliffe, L.J., Bush, V.E. and Hainsworth R. (2002b). Patients with posturally related syncope have increased responsiveness of the cerebral circulation to carbon dioxide. *Clin. Auton. Res.* **12**, 316.

Norcliffe-Kaufmann, L.J., Kaufmann, H. and Hainsworth R. (2008). Enhanced vascular responses to hypocapnia in neurally mediated syncope. *Ann. Neurol.* **63**, 288–94.

Novak, V., Honos, G., and Schondorf, R. (1996). Is the heart "empty' at syncope? *J. Auton. Nerv. Syst.* **60**, 83–92.

Oberg, B. and Thoren, P. (1972). Increased activity in left ventricular receptors during haemorrhage or occlusion of the caval veins in the cat. A possible cause of vasovagal reaction. *Acta Physiol. Scand.* **85**, 164–73.

Schroeder, C., Bush, V.E., Norcliffe, L.J., Luft, F.C., Tank, J., Jordan, J. and Hainsworth, R. (2002). Water drinking acutely improves orthostatic tolerance in healthy subjects. *Circulation* **106**, 2806–2811.

Sneddon, J.F., Counihan, P.J., Bashir, Y., Haywood, G.A., Ward, D.E. and Camm, A.J. (1993). Impaired immediate vasoconstrictor responses in patients with recurrent neurally mediated syncope. *Am. J. Cardiol.* **71**, 72–76.

Stevens, P. M. (1966). Cardiovascular dynamics during orthostasis and influence of intravascular instrumentation. *Am. J. Cardiol.* **17**, 211–18.

Uvnas, B. (1966). Cholinergic vasodilator nerves. *Fed. Proc.* **25**, 1618–22.

Wahbha, M. M. A. E., Morley, C. A., Al-Shamma, Y. M. H. and Hainsworth, R. (1989). Cardiovascular reflex responses in patients with unexplained syncope. *Clin. Sci.* **77**, 547–53.

Wallin, B. G. and Sundlof, G. (1982). Sympathetic outflow to muscle during vasovagal syncope. *J. Auton. Nerv. System.* **6**, 287–91.

CHAPTER 57

Cardiac causes of syncope

Abhay Bajpai and A. John Camm

Introduction

Syncope from cardiac causes results from disorders of either cardiac rhythm or cardiac structure. Several potentially fatal cardiac diseases may present with syncope as their first premonitory symptom. Neural reflex mechanisms also operate in many cardiac conditions, but neurocardiogenic syncope is discussed in full details in Chapter 56.

The proportion of cardiac causes increases with advancing age (Table 57.1) (Olshansky 2005). Disturbances of cardiac rhythm comprise the second most common cause of syncope, the first being reflex neurocardiogenic syncope. In a review of 7814 participants in the Framingham Heart Study, cardiac causes of syncope were identified in about 10% of cases during an average follow-up period of 17 years (Soteriades 2002). Following an episode of syncope, it is the presence of underlying cardiac disease that determines the overall prognosis. Large population-based studies have previously shown that patients with cardiac syncope have high mortality rates (10% at 6 months and 18–33% at 1 year) in comparison with those with a non-cardiogenic cause (Kapoor 1983, Lempert 1994, Martin 1984), more recent studies have linked this higher mortality to the underlying structural heart disease (Middlekauff 1993, Kapoor 1996, Getchell 1999, Sarasin 2001). The risk of ventricular arrhythmias and sudden death increases with the severity of ventricular dysfunction. Thus, the presence of syncope may be a marker of the fatal underlying cardiac disease, but has not been shown per se to influence mortality.

Pathophysiology

Syncope from cardiac causes usually results from sudden reduction in cardiac output and cerebral blood flow, sufficient enough to cause transient global impairment of cerebral function. In addition, neural reflex mechanisms, degree of peripheral vasodilation, extent of hypoxia and use of medications which affect preload or afterload can simultaneously alter cerebral blood flow. Pathophysiological mechanisms are summarized in Fig. 57.1 and are discussed in greater details in Chapter 56.

Table 57.1 Common causes of syncope

Young (< 35 years)	Middle-age (35–65 years)	Elderly (> 65 years)
◆ Neurocardiogenic	◆ Neurocardiogenic	◆ Multifactorial
◆ Situational	◆ *Cardiac:*	◆ *Cardiac:*
◆ Psychiatric	• *Arrhythmic*	• *Arrhythmic*
◆ Less common, but life-threatening causes:	• *Mechanical/ obstructive*	• *Mechanical/ obstructive*
• Undiagnosed seizures		◆ Orthostatic
◆ *Cardiac:*		◆ Drug induced
• *LQTS/SVT/W-P-W syndrome/HCM*		◆ Neurocardiogenic

LQTS, long QT syndrome; SVT, supraventricular tachycardia; W-P-W, Wolff–Parkinson–White syndrome; HCM, hypertrophic cardiomyopathy. Causes discussed in this chapter are shown in italics. Adapted from Olshansky B (2005). Syncope: overview and approach to management. In: Grubb BP, Olshansky B, eds. *Syncope: Mechanisms and management*, Wiley.

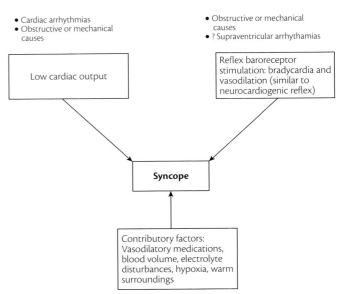

Fig. 57.1 Mechanisms of cardiogenic syncope.

Cardiac arrhythmias as cause of syncope

Cardiac arrhythmias can result in sudden fall in cardiac output and syncope without much warning. Arrhythmias commonly associated with syncope are bradyarrhythmias accompanying sinus node dysfunction ('sick sinus syndrome'), atrioventricular blocks or tachycardias of ventricular origin (Table 57.2). These usually occur in patients with structural heart disease.

Although cardiac arrhythmias can directly cause syncope, they can also be a part of complicated reflex response as in the case of neurocardiogenic syncope (bradyarrhythmias).

Bradyarrhythmias

Sinus node dysfunction

Also termed 'sick sinus syndrome' or sinoatrial disease, sinus node dysfunction comprises an array of sinus node and atrial arrhythmias that result in persistent or intermittent periods of inappropriately slow or fast heart rates (sinus bradycardia, sinus pauses, atrial tachycardia, atrial flutter and atrial fibrillation). Sinus node dysfunction is found in all age groups, but the prevalence increases with advancing age. Sinus node dysfunction can be intrinsic or extrinsic in nature (Table 57.3). Intrinsic sinus node dysfunction is usually the result of structural changes and replacement of sinoatrial cells by fibrous tissue. It must be emphasized that these same intrinsic or extrinsic factors may also simultaneously affect the function of the atrioventricular node and the remaining conduction system.

Intrinsic sinus node dysfunction is an important cause of bradycardia associated symptoms with a prevalence of syncope or dizziness ranging from 40% to 92% (Benditt and Sutton 2005).

Sinus node dysfunction can be divided into three subgroups: sinus bradycardia, sinus arrest, and bradycardia/tachycardia syndrome.

Sinus bradycardia is common in young, healthy individuals especially during the night due to high vagal tone. Heart rates above 35–40 beats/minute do not usually result in syncope and in most cases sinus bradycardia does not produce any symptoms. If symptoms occur, they are generally fatigue, lethargy, and light-headedness, especially during exercise. Sinus bradycardia in itself should not be considered as a cause of syncope unless demonstrated during a syncopal attack.

Sinus pause and sinus arrest (Fig. 57.2a) result from impaired automaticity of the sinus node or impaired conduction from the sinus node to the right atrium. The two cannot be distinguished

Table 57.2 Cardiac arrhythmias primarily associated with syncope

◆ Sinus node dysfunction (including bradycardia/tachycardia syndrome)
◆ Atrioventricular conduction system disease
◆ Ventricular tachycardias
◆ Paroxysmal supraventricular tachycardias
◆ Implanted device malfunction (pacemaker, ICD)
◆ Inherited syndromes (e.g. long QT syndrome, Brugada syndrome)
◆ Drug-induced proarrhythmias

ICD, implantable cardioverter defibrillator

Table 57.3 Causes of sinus node dysfunction

Intrinsic sinus node dysfunction	Extrinsic sinus node dysfunction
◆ Idiopathic degenerative disease	◆ Drugs: class I and III antiarrhythmic, propranolol, nadolol, α-methyldopa, reserpine, diltiazem, verapamil, carbamazepine, phenytoin, lithium and cardiac glycosides
◆ Ischaemic heart disease	◆ Hyperkalaemia
◆ Infiltrative disorders: tumours, amyloid	◆ Hypothyroidism
◆ Inflammatory conditions: pericarditis, myocarditis	◆ Neurally mediated response: carotid sinus syndrome, vasovagal, post-micturition, cough syncope
◆ Musculoskeletal problems: muscular dystrophies, Friedreich's ataxia	◆ Intracranial hypertension
◆ Collagen vascular diseases	◆ Obstructive jaundice
◆ Postoperative: mustard procedure for transposition of great arteries, atrial septal defect repair	

from each other from surface electrocardiographic (ECG) recording. Asymptomatic sinus pauses of up to 3 seconds in duration are a relatively common finding in ambulatory ECG recordings occurring in 6% of healthy subjects and do not pose any adverse prognostic risks (Crawford et al.1999). They are even more common in trained athletes due to high vagal tone (37%) (Viitasalo et al. 1982, Mazuz and Friedman 1983, Fagard 2003). Pauses in excess of 3 seconds may vary in their clinical presentation and demand further assessment to detect symptomatic correlations (Hilgard et al. 1985, Ector et al. 1983). Caution is recommended when interpreting sinus arrest as a cause of symptoms without demonstrating concomitant syncope.

Bradycardia-tachycardia syndrome is a form of sinus node dysfunction when atrial tachycardias (usually atrial fibrillation or atrial flutter) coexist with periods of bradyarrhythmias (Fig. 57.2b) Benditt et al.1995, Kaplan et al. 1973).

Syncope may occur due to fast or slow heart rates. A prolonged pause immediately following the termination of an atrial tachyarrhythmia (Fig. 57.2b) is one of the most frequent causes of presyncopal or syncopal symptoms in patients with sinus node disease. It must also be emphasized that presence bradycardia can also increase the susceptibility to tachycardia (e.g. rapid atrial fibrillation) or even ventricular tachyarrhythmias, particularly if the patient is being treated with antiarrhythmic drugs. Thus, implantation of a pacemaker will not only prevent bradycardic syncope, but also reduce the incidence of tachyarrhythmic episodes.

Atrioventricular conduction defects

Atrioventricular (AV) blocks can be congenital or acquired and present as first-degree, second-degree and third-degree (complete) AV blocks. Intermittent second-degree or complete heart block can lead to dizziness and syncope. When transient, these can be difficult to diagnose and in one study on patients with unexplained syncope, only 3% had high-degree AV block that could be demonstrated at the time of syncope (Kapoor et al. 1987). The long-term outcome of AV conduction defects, even if high-degree, depends

(a)

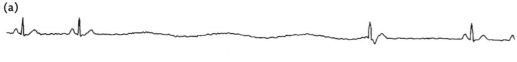

(b)

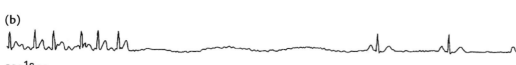

- - -1s - -

Fig. 57.2 Sinus node dysfunction. **(a)** Sinus arrest. There is a long asystolic pause. The third beat is a junctional escape beat. **(b)** Bradycardia-tachycardia syndrome.

significantly on the underlying disease process (e.g. occurrence during the course of a large anterior myocardial infarction and risk of sudden death from ventricular arrhythmias). The site of conduction defect can be located within the AV node, the bundle of His or the infra-His structures.

As a solitary finding first-degree AV block is generally of benign significance and does not require any treatment. It may be a more frequent finding among pilots (3.5%) but the long-term outcomes do not differ from that observed in the general population (Mathewson et al. 1976). However, if the PR interval is markedly prolonged (300–500 ms), atrial contraction may occur against the closed AV valves. This functional AV dissociation can occasionally manifest with hypotension, dizziness and even syncope resulting from a range of factors including loss of atrial contribution to cardiac output, excessive stretch of atrial walls triggering neuro-hormonal influences and retrograde ejection of blood into systemic and pulmonary veins. In these cases, restoration of AV synchrony by the use of a permanent dual-chamber pacemaker should be considered.

A prolonged PR interval associated with bifascicular block (left or right bundle branch block plus left anterior or posterior hemiblock) indicates greater involvement of the conduction system and can predict progression to higher-grade AV block (Kaul et al. 1988).

In second-degree block AV impulse transmission is intermittent (Fig. 57.3). Wenckebach (type I) AV block can be precipitated in almost all individuals by rapid atrial pacing. The presence of Wenckebach phenomenon during rapid atrial tachyarrhythmias can be protective and prevent development of rapid ventricular rates. It is also a common finding in trained young athletes as a result of high vagal tone, particularly during rest and sleep. It is unlikely to produce syncope and does not merit pacemaker therapy, even in the setting of acute myocardial infarction unless there is other evidence of diffuse conduction system disease.

Presence of type II second-degree AV block indicates more severe involvement of the infranodal conduction system and generally carries a worse prognosis. Patients are often symptomatic with recurrent syncope which is due to intermittent progression to complete AV block. Cardiac pacing is recommended in type II AV blocks.

Third-degree AV block may be high grade (when multiple consecutive P waves are blocked) or complete (Fig. 57.3c). There is no impulse transmission from the atria to the ventricles. The block can occur in the AV node or the infranodal conduction system and the cardiac rhythm depends on subsidiary pacemakers. Congenital complete heart block is a typical example of third-degree block located within the AV node. The subsidiary pacemaker is usually in the bundle of His, which being proximal results in an escape rhythm of 40–60 beats/minute with narrow QRS complexes. Congenital heart block is usually responsive to alterations in autonomic tone and drugs influencing the AV node function. Thus, syncope is rarely a presenting symptom in these patients. The acquired form on the other hand, is symptomatic and is most often secondary to coronary artery disease, degenerative processes, or drug toxicity. In the acquired form, the block is usually located in the bundle of His or infra-His conduction system, resulting in a slow distal ventricular escape rhythm with wide QRS complexes. Syncope is thus a common symptom in this setting. The block is usually unresponsive to autonomic tone and drugs (atropine, isoprenaline). Permanent pacemaker therapy is mandatory in these patients.

Tachyarrhythmias

About 25% of cases of syncope result from tachyarrhythmias. Of these, 85% are due to ventricular tachycardia (VT) and the remaining 15% result from supraventricular tachycardia (SVT) (Krol et al. 1987).

Supraventricular tachyarrhythmias

SVTs are common arrhythmias and can be present in 3% of population. Arrhythmias originating in the atria include atrial fibrillation, atrial flutter and atrial tachycardia. The incidence of atrial

(a)

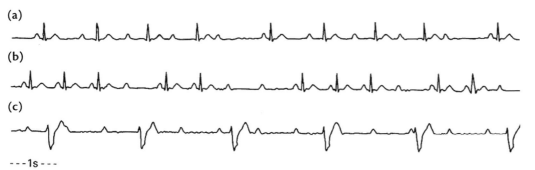

(b)

(c)

- - -1s - - -

Fig. 57.3 Atrioventricular conduction defect. **(a)** Mobitz Type I (Wenckebach type) second-degree AV block; **(b)** Mobitz Type II second-degree AV block; **(c)** third-degree AV block.

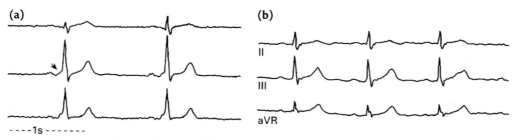

Fig. 57.4 (a) A patient with Wolff–Parkinson–White syndrome caused by an accessory pathway between left atrium and left ventricle. Due to inhomogeneous ventricular depolarization, the QRS complexes are pre-excited and have a delta wave (arrow). **(b)** Same patient after radiofrequency ablation of the accessory pathway. The delta wave is no longer seen.

fibrillation increases with age and is the most common arrhythmia requiring hospital admission. Atrial fibrillation and flutter are usually uncommon causes of syncope, except when they occur in the presence of an extranodal accessory pathway.

In young patients, SVT usually results from a re-entrant circuit that involves the AV node. The most common form is atrioventricular nodal re-entrant tachycardia (AVNRT) in which the re-entrant circuit is caused by splitting of the electrical connection between the right atrium and AV node, into two pathways communicating with each other via the AV node. In others, the re-entrant circuit is due to one or multiple accessory pathways between the atria and the ventricles (e.g. Wolff–Parkinson–White syndrome) giving rise to atrioventricular re-entrant tachycardia (AVRT). If the electrical impulse from the atria to the ventricles conducts through the accessory pathway, the ventricles become pre-excited and the characteristic delta wave is seen at the beginning of QRS complex (Fig. 57.4). These accessory pathways lack the normal restrictive properties of the AV node and can support the frequent conduction of impulses originating in the atria (atrial fibrillation or flutter) to cause extremely rapid ventricular rates leading to syncope or even sudden death from ventricular fibrillation (Fig. 57.5).

Most commonly, supraventricular arrhythmias are accompanied by mild symptoms such as palpitations and dizziness, but only rarely with syncope. If syncope develops, there is often concomitant sinus node dysfunction when syncope can occur during a long period of sinus pause at the moment when tachycardia terminates

SVTs are often paroxysmal and infrequent. Thus, they may be difficult to demonstrate on ambulatory ECG recordings and implantable loop recorders or electrophysiological testing may be needed. Treatment should be focused on treating the underlying arrhythmia since catheter-based ablation of re-entrant or accessory pathways can offer permanent cure from the arrhythmia.

Ventricular tachyarrhythmias

Ventricular tachyarrhythmias are the most common arrhythmias responsible for syncope. These include sustained (more than 30 s

duration) or non-sustained ventricular tachycardia (VT) and ventricular fibrillation (Fig. 57.6).

About 30% of patients with sustained VT experience syncope or near-syncope.

Risk factors for ventricular tachyarrhythmias include presence of underlying structural disease, ventricular hypertrophy or dilatation, conduction system disease, long QT syndromes and use of medications with proarrhythmic effects. The most common cause is coronary artery disease, especially following myocardial infarction leading to ischaemic cardiomyopathy. In this setting the tachycardia is usually due to development of areas of fibrosis and scarring which are arrhythmogenic in nature. Typical clinical manifestation is a monomorphic VT where QRS complexes have similar appearances. About 70–80% of patients with monomorphic VT have coronary artery disease. Reduced left ventricular systolic function, spontaneous non-sustained ventricular arrhythmias, late potentials on signal-averaged ECG, and reduced heart rate variability may predict ventricular tachyarrhythmias in patients following myocardial infarction (Hartikainen et al. 1996).

Ventricular arrhythmias are also found in patients with congenital heart disease (especially after repair of tetralogy of Fallot), valvular heart disease, arrhythmogenic right ventricular dysplasia (fibro-fatty infiltration of right ventricular myocardium (Fig. 57.7) (Frances 2005), and electrolyte disturbances, but they can occur in patients without any apparent structural abnormality of the heart. Idiopathic VT seems to arise from the right ventricular outflow tract in 80–90% of cases with no structural abnormality, but typically causes palpitations rather than syncope.

A particular type of polymorphic VT characterized by beat-to-beat variability of amplitude and polarity of the QRS complexes is termed torsade de pointes (Fig. 57.8). It is often self-terminating but occasionally degenerates into ventricular fibrillation. Torsade de pointes is usually associated with prolongation of QT interval which can be congenital or acquired. Congenital long QT syndrome (LQTS) has an incidence of 1 in 7000 and is caused by mutations in genes encoding cardiac ion channels, resulting in

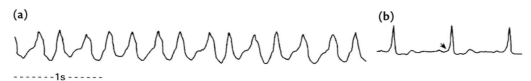

Fig. 57.5 (a) Rapid atrial fibrillation (220 beats/minute) in a patient with Wolff–Parkinson–White syndrome. **(b)** ECG of the same patient during sinus rhythm reveals delta waves (arrow).

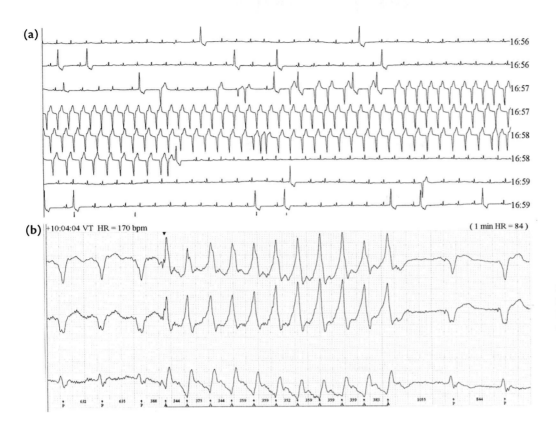

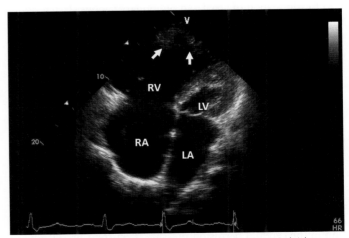

Fig. 57.6 **(a)** Holter recording revealing ventricular tachycardia. The patient experienced severe dizziness during the period of tachycardia. **(b)** Another example of ventricular tachycardia recorded during Holter monitoring. The tachycardia is of short duration, non-sustained and was an incidental finding in this patient with syncope from a different cause.

delayed depolarization and a prolonged QT interval (Keating et al. 1991, Jiang et al. 1994, Schott et al. 1995). Congenital LQTS is associated with increased mortality in the presence of syncope (Vincent 2000). The onset of torsade de pointes can follow two patterns. In the bradycardia-dependent type, slowing of heart rate (e.g. sleep, pauses following premature ventricular beats) results in marked QT prolongation, rendering the patients susceptible to tachycardia. In the second type, QT prolongation is associated with sympathetic activation and tachycardia is typically initiated during emotional or physical stress. Presence of syncope or aborted sudden death in the patient or a close relative can be predictive of increased risk of sudden death and implantable cardioverter defibrillator (ICD) should be considered (Zareba W et al. 2003).

The acquired type of LQTS is more common and is usually the result of drugs which prolong the QT interval (Table 57.4); other causes are bradycardia (complete heart block, sick sinus syndrome), hypothermia, metabolic disorders (hypokalaemia, hypomagnesaemia, and hypocalcaemia), myocardial ischaemia, myocarditis, or abnormal nutritional status (e.g. anorexia nervosa or intense weight reduction that involves the use of liquid protein diet) (Camm et al. 2004).

Brugada syndrome is a genetic disorder with autosomal dominant transmission and results from disorder of sodium channels. It is associated with characteristic changes on surface ECG which shows ST segment elevation in precordial leads V$_1$–V$_3$ with QRS morphology resembling a right bundle branch block. However, the ECG may be completely normal in some patients and intravenous infusion of sodium channel blocking agent (procainamide or ajmaline) will bring out the typical ECG changes and help establish a diagnosis (Fig. 57.9). Patients with Brugada syndrome are at risk of developing episodes of polymorphic VT causing syncope, or

ventricular fibrillation and sudden death. Inducibility of arrhythmia during electrophysiological studies is considered a strong predictor of outcome in these patients. Since no antiarrhythmic agent has been shown to be effective, high-risk patients should be considered for ICD therapy.

Ventricular fibrillation is often triggered by myocardial ischaemia. Electrolyte imbalances such as hypokalaemia and hypomagnesaemia, in the presence of ischaemia or myocardial dysfunction are common factors which predispose to ventricular fibrillation.

Fig. 57.7 Four-chamber view on 2D-echocardiogram showing apical right ventricular dysplasia with fibro-fatty infiltration of the myocardium (arrows). There is gross dilation of the right ventricle. This is an important cause of sudden arrhythmic death, often exertional, affecting young individuals and athletes. RV, right ventricle; RA, right atrium; LV, left ventricle; LA, left atrium.

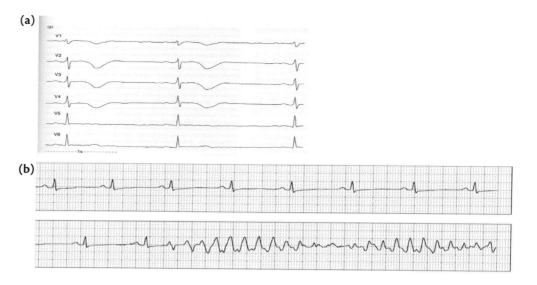

Fig. 57.8 (a) A patient with acquired long QT syndrome caused by thioridazine overdosing. The electrocardiogram (ECG) shows markedly prolonged QT interval of 0.70 seconds. **(b)** ECG from a different patient showing polymorphic ventricular tachycardia highly suggestive of torsade de pointes due to changing morphology and axis of QRS complexes. Previous recordings taken few hours before the arrhythmia had clearly shown prolongation of QT interval.

It can also result from abrupt changes in autonomic tone or degeneration of rapid monomorphic or polymorphic VT into fibrillation. Once ventricular fibrillation develops it is fatal and results in sudden death. Most patients sustaining out-of-hospital cardiac arrest due to ventricular fibrillation die before seeking medical advice.

Syncope related to pacemaker malfunction

In general, pacemaker generators are reliable and only rarely are problems encountered. Nevertheless, as with any other mechanical device, a pacemaker may malfunction to the extent of complete pacing failure. Syncope occurring in a patient with a permanent pacemaker should lead to suspicion of system failure or a new tachyarrhythmia. Most pacemaker malfunctions (e.g. diminishing battery life) can be detected early in time during regular pacing interrogations in follow-up clinics. Common pacemaker problems are shown in Table 57.5 and Fig. 57.10.

Use of ventricular pacing results in loss of AV synchrony, which may lead to atrial contraction against closed AV valves. This may lead to stimulation of atrial and pulmonary venous stretch receptors causing reflex peripheral vasodilation, hypotension and syncope, a clinical status referred to as pacemaker syndrome. Pacemaker syndrome can be prevented by assuming AV synchrony with dual-chamber pacemaker. The neurocardiogenic reflex is the most common cause of syncope in paced patients.

Obstructive and mechanical causes of syncope

Conditions that restrict the emptying or filling of the heart can cause syncope. As a result of obstruction, cardiac output is more or less fixed and does not rise during periods of increased demands such as exercise. Moreover, exercise causes arterial vasodilation and decreases peripheral vascular resistance adding to the reduction in the cerebral perfusion pressure. Recurrent presyncope or syncope induced by effort should lead to a suspicion of obstructive cardiac cause.

Cardiac disorders commonly resulting in obstructive syncope are listed in Table 57.6.

Aortic stenosis

Aortic stenosis (AS) is a common cause for obstructive cardiogenic syncope (Fig. 57.11). While rheumatic fever remains an important cause of AS in developing countries, congenital malformations (bicuspid aortic valve) and senile degenerative AS are common in the developed world.

Syncope may be a presenting symptom in nearly 40% of patients with severe AS (Grech and Ramsdale 1991). Typically, syncope occurs during physical effort. The possible mechanisms of syncope in AS are:

♦ systemic hypotension brought on by posture change or vasodilation from exercise in the presence of a fixed cardiac output

♦ high intracardiac pressures leading to stimulation of baroreceptors wit resultant bradycardia and vasodilation (similar to that seen in neurocardiogenic syncope)

Table 57.4 Drugs associated with prolongation of QT interval and torsade de pointes

Antiarrhythmic drugs	Antimicrobial drugs
♦ Quinidine	♦ Erythromycin
♦ Disopyramide	♦ Chloroquine
♦ Procainamide	♦ Halofantrine
♦ Ajmaline	♦ Sparfloxacin
♦ Flecainide	♦ Grepafloxacin
♦ Sotalol	♦ Fluconazole
♦ Amiodarone (relatively low risk)	♦ Ketoconazole
	♦ Pentamidine
	♦ Amantadine
Psychiatric drugs	**Other agents**
♦ Chlorpromazine	♦ Astemizole
♦ Thioridazine	♦ Terfenadine
♦ Haloperidol	♦ Cisapride
♦ Amitriptyline	♦ Organophosphates
♦ Lithium	♦ Cocaine

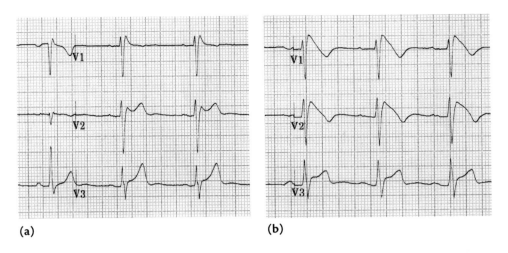

(a) **(b)**

Fig. 57.9 The Brugada syndrome. **(a)** Suspected diagnosis of Brugada syndrome on a baseline electrocardiogram. **(b)** Typical diagnostic changes of ST elevation in V1–V3 with a QRS morphology resembling right bundle branch block are seen after intravenous ajmaline challenge. Ajmaline is a sodium-channel blocking agent.

◆ development of AV block from extension of the calcific process

◆ ventricular and supraventricular tachyarrhythmias resulting from AS.

Patients with moderate to severe aortic stenosis often have left ventricular hypertrophy. A hypertrophied left ventricle is stiff and diastolic filling of the ventricle is critical for proper systolic function. A decrease in preload caused by vasodilator drugs (e.g. nitrates) may result in inadequate diastolic filling, further fall in cardiac output and syncope.

Syncope has prognostic significance in patients with aortic stenosis. Without valve replacement, the mean survival after syncope is 2–3 years (Ross and Braunwald 1968).

Hypertrophic cardiomyopathy

Hypertrophic cardiomyopathy (HCM) is an autosomal dominant disorder which manifests as pathological thickening of left ventricular wall that may be patchy, concentric or asymmetrical (Nishimura and Holmes 2004). Asymmetric hypertrophy of the interventricular septum produces subvalvular obstruction of the outflow tract between the upper septum and the mitral apparatus (Fig. 57.12). There is also abnormal motion of the anterior mitral leaflet towards the hypertrophied septum during the latter part of

systole which further obliterates the outflow tract. This dynamic obstruction of the ventricular outflow tract can be intermittent and depends on the catecholamine level, degree of contractility, state of hydration and ventricular volume. The smaller the ventricular volume, the greater is the degree of obstruction. Hypertrophied abnormal fibres are short, fragmented and there is usually fibrosis. This abnormal arrangement of muscle fibres makes the heart vulnerable to fatal ventricular tachyarrhythmias.

Syncope has been reported in up to 20% of patients with HCM. Patients with HCM may die suddenly with an annual mortality of 2.5% for adults and up to 6% for children and adolescents. HCM is the most common cause of sudden cardiac death (SCD) among athletes, found in 36% of those who die suddenly, but it is not known whether cardiomyopathy in athletes is genetically transmitted or represents undesirable consequences of high intensity training (Maron et al. 2003). The physiological mechanisms of syncope and sudden death in HCM are similar to those in valvular aortic stenosis with additional factors being—catecholamine sensitive

Table 57.5 Common causes of pacemaker malfunction

◆ Wire displacement

◆ Lead fracture and insulation defect

◆ Exit block: failure to cause depolarization due to raised threshold (e.g. tissue reaction around lead tip; poor contact; antiarrhythmic drugs)

◆ Battery failure

◆ Sensing failure

◆ False inhibition (oversensing): inhibition of ventricular pacing secondary to inappropriate sensing of skeletal muscle EMG potentials, spurious signals from electrode fracture, large T-wave voltage and electromagnetic interference (less with newer systems)

◆ Pacemaker mediated tachycardia

EMG, electromyography

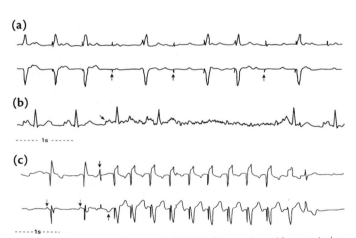

Fig. 57.10 Pacemaker malfunction. **(a)** Exit block in a patient with a ventricular pacemaker (VVI). Some pacing spikes (arrows) are not followed by ventricular capture. **(b)** Myopotential interference in a patient with an atrial pacemaker. The pacemaker interprets noise caused by muscular activity as spontaneous cardiac activity, resulting in pacemaker inhibition. An atrial pacing spike is denoted with an arrow. **(c)** Pacemaker-mediated tachycardia. Two first P waves are sensed correctly and they trigger ventricular pacing. A ventricular ectopic beat (arrows pointing down) is conducted

Table 57.6 Cardiac disorders associated with obstructive syncope

- ◆ Aortic stenosis
- ◆ Hypertrophic cardiomyopathy
- ◆ Prosthetic valve malfunction
- ◆ Cardiac tumors
- ◆ Pulmonary hypertension
- ◆ Pulmonary embolism
- ◆ Cardiac tamponade
- ◆ Right-to-left shunts
- ◆ Aortic dissection

outflow obstruction (effort or excitement), association of HCM with Wolff–Parkinson–White (W-P-W) syndrome (rapid AV conduction via the accessory pathway) and increased risk of massive myocardial infarction (high demand and external compression of coronary arteries).

The treatment of HCM includes use of negatively inotropic drugs such as beta-blockers, calcium-channel blockers, and antiarrhythmic agents amiodarone and disopyramide. Beta-blockers can reduce the subvalvular outflow tract obstruction by lowering the left ventricular end-diastolic pressure and increasing the end-diastolic volume. Dual-chamber pacing has been reported to decrease the obstructive gradient and may be helpful in symptomatic patients, especially those with significant outflow tract obstruction (Gregoratos and Abrams et al. 2002). Invasive procedures include alcohol ablation and surgical myomectomy of septal muscle. Patients with high risk of sudden death (Box 57.1) should be implanted with an implantable cardioverter defibrillator (ICD) (Frenneaux et al 1990, Maron et al 2000).

Prosthetic valve obstruction

Prosthetic valves are commonly implanted in aortic or mitral positions, obstruction of which can cause syncope. Usually the obstruction is caused by a large organized thrombus, and a tilting-disc type of valve appears to be more prone to thrombus formation when compared to bio-prosthetic valves. Patients may also present with features of heart failure, shock or peripheral embolism

Atrial masses

These can be due to primary malignancies, metastatic deposits or thrombus formation. Myxoma is the most common benign tumour of the heart. While myxomas can occur in any chamber, 75% are located in the left atrium. Myxomas are frequently pedunculated and may prolapse through the mitral (or tricuspid) valve causing obstruction and reduced ventricular filling. Syncope often occurs when patient changes position (Raynen 1995). Similarly, large mobile thrombi in the atria may also cause symptoms of heart failure and syncope (Fig. 57.13). Patients with severe mitral stenosis have an increased tendency toward left atrial thrombus formation and syncope can result from occlusion of an already stenotic valve by the thrombus.

Pulmonary hypertension

Pulmonary hypertension can be primary or secondary. Most cases of pulmonary hypertension are secondary to chronic cardiac (left ventricular dysfunction, increased pulmonary flow in left-to-right shunts) or pulmonary diseases (e.g. diffuse fibrosis, chronic obstructive airway diseases, sleep apnoea syndrome). In both primary and secondary forms, high pulmonary resistance compromises the cardiac output during periods of increased demand and causes syncope, which may be seen in up to 30% of patients (Fuster et al. 1984).

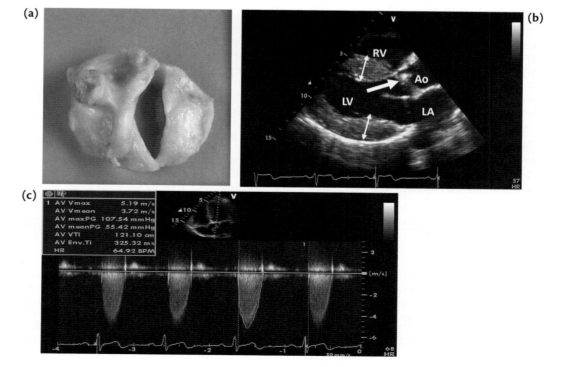

Fig. 57.11 Aortic stenosis. **(a)** A thickened, calcified and stenosed aortic valve with fusion of cusps. **(b)** 2D-echocardiogram showing calcific and poorly mobile aortic valve (bold arrow). There is also concentric ventricular hypertrophy (double arrows). **(b)** Continuous-wave Doppler recording revealed a high peak velocity of flow through the aortic valve (5.19 m/s) which corresponds to a mean pressure gradient of 55.4 mmHg across the aortic valve. LV, left ventricle, LA, left atrium, Ao, aorta.

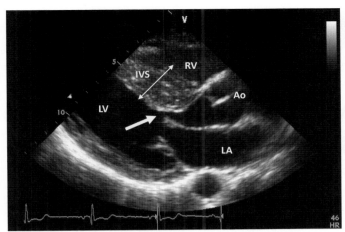

Fig. 57.12 Hypertrophic obstructive cardiomyopathy. The interventricular septum is 3 cm in thickness (double arrow). There is also anterior movement of the mitral valve leaflet towards the septum during systole, which further deteriorates the outflow obstruction (bold arrow). LV, left ventricle; IVS, interventricular septum; LA, left atrium; Ao, aorta.

Right-to-left shunts

In patients with large communications between the left and right sides of the heart (ventricular septal defect, tetralogy of Fallot etc.), right ventricular pressure tends to increase and can equal or exceed the pressure in the left ventricle and aorta. This reverses the left-to-right shunt (Eisenmenger's syndrome). A decrease in systemic vascular resistance (e.g. exercise, pyrexia) increases the right-to-left shunt. As a result, systemic oxygen saturation falls worsening the systemic hypoxaemia associated with these diseases and may precipitate a syncopal episode.

Pulmonary embolism

Syncope may be the first presenting symptom affecting 10–15% of patients with acute pulmonary embolism (Thames et al. 1969). The usual mechanism of syncope is sudden reduction of cardiac output (Fig. 57.14), but syncope can also result from a marked vagal response secondary to right ventricular overload and baroreceptor activation. In the long term, recurrent pulmonary embolism eventually results in secondary pulmonary hypertension (and cor pulmonale) giving rise to exercise or effort induced syncope. Associated arterial hypoxia and secondary hypocapnia also worsen the tendency to syncope (Wilk et al. 1995).

Cardiac tamponade

Acute cardiac tamponade decreases cardiac output by restricting the dilation of cardiac chambers during diastole to the extent that

---

Box 57.1 Risk factors for sudden cardiac death in hypertrophic cardiomyopathy

- ◆ Young age
- ◆ Family history of sudden infant death
- ◆ Extreme hypertrophy (septal thickness > 30 mm)
- ◆ Ventricular tachycardia
- ◆ Exercise induced hypotension

---

there may be a total collapse of the relatively thin walled right atrium and the ventricle from external compression. Acute tamponade may result from blunt or penetrating chest trauma, myocardial rupture secondary to infarction, acute aortic dissection or as a complication of invasive cardiac procedures. Pericardial diseases, including viral infections and malignant deposits, usually present with subacute effusion, but a large volume of fluid may eventually cause tamponade. Syncope results from acute reduction of cardiac output, bradycardia and hypotension from a neurocardiogenic reflex and associated factors such as blood loss, effect of medications and arrhythmias (Desanctis et al. 1987, Reddy et al. 1978).

Aortic dissection

Aortic dissection is commonly seen in men aged 50–70 years. It is more common in Afro-Caribbean than Caucasians. Predisposing factors include hypertension, pregnancy, coarctation of aorta, bicuspid or unicommissural aortic valves, Marfan's syndrome and other connective tissue disorders (e.g. systemic lupus erythematosus, giant cell arteritis, Ehlers–Danlos syndrome). Aortic dissection usually presents with acute, intense or tearing pain over the anterior chest or interscapular region and is commonly associated with syncope. Syncope may result either from the acute pain or from the dissection tracking back causing reduction of flow in the cerebral and coronary vessels, or leaking into the pericardium causing tamponade. Most patients have normal or elevated blood pressure which requires rapid control. Diagnosis is confirmed by transoesophageal echocardiography, computed tomography or cardiac magnetic resonance imaging (Crawford 1990).

Evaluation of a patient with suspected cardiac causes

The initial evaluation of a patient presenting with syncope consists of a detailed history, physical examination, postural blood pressure measurements and a standard 12-lead electrocardiogram. Careful history taking can provide vital clues towards a diagnosis. Important points in the patient's history and features on a standard electrocardiogram which increase the suspicion of a cardiogenic cause are summarized in Box 57.2 (Brignole et al. 2004, Moya et al. 2009).

Further investigations are needed if the initial work-up suggests a cardiac cause. Screening for electrolyte disorders and serum drug levels (e.g. digoxin, amiodarone) is essential. Specific cardiac investigations comprise echocardiography, exercise stress testing, prolonged ambulatory ECG monitoring (Holter recording, external or implantable loop-recorders) and invasive electrophysiological testing.

Echocardiography is useful in assessing structural abnormalities such as ventricular dysfunction, hypertrophy or valve defects. The diagnostic yield however, is low in the absence of a convincing cardiac history, physical signs and ECG abnormalities.

Exercise stress testing is recommended for patients presenting with effort induced syncope, chest pain or palpitations to assess for any cardiac ischaemia. Patients with exertion related syncope should also have a transthoracic echocardiogram in order to identify obstructive lesions, e.g. aortic stenosis. Exercise may also induce supraventricular or VT in those with ischaemia or high myocardial sensitivity to catecholamines. In patients with bradycardia and conduction system disease, exercise testing may reveal chronotropic incompetence, i.e. failure of heart rate to increase with exercise.

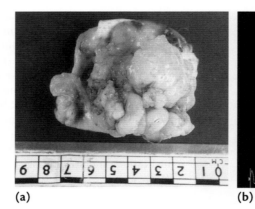

Fig. 57.13 (a) Post-surgical specimen of left atrial myxoma. **(b)** A large left atrial thrombus seen on trans-oesophageal echocardiogram.

(a)   **(b)**

Prolonged ambulatory ECG monitoring can be performed by various means. *Holter monitoring*, which is usually 24–48 hours of continuous ECG recording, is useful only if there are frequent episodes of syncope, since for the test to be diagnostic the arrhythmic episode needs to occur during the period of recording. Even so, many studies have shown poor correlation between rhythm abnormalities revealed during Holter recording and symptoms. As a result asymptomatic arrhythmias (e.g. non-sustained VT) may be misdiagnosed as cause of syncope (Gibson and Heitzman 1984, Lacroix 1991). Endless loop-recorders have emerged as useful devices to assess potential arrhythmic causes. The *external loop-recorders* can be attached for weeks or months and continuously record the ECG so that if a patient experiences symptoms or syncope, the data up to a fixed period preceding the episode can be saved by the patient manually activating the device upon awakening. The main disadvantage is that it requires patient input and knowledge of how and when to use. Infrequent events and inaccurate activation can reduce diagnostic accuracy (Schuchert et al. 2003). *Implantable loop-recorders* are devices which can be placed subcutaneously under local anaesthesia. These devices can record ECG continuously in their loop memory and have a battery life of up to 36 months. The device can either be triggered by the patient upon recovery or can automatically detect and save abnormal rhythms (Figs 57.15 and 57.16). They are useful when syncope is

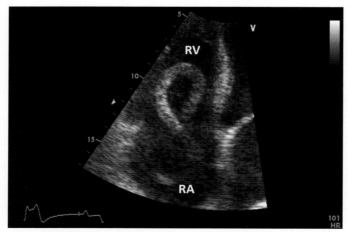

Fig. 57.14 2D image showing apical four-chamber view. There is a long, coiled thrombus seen entering into the right ventricle through the tricuspid valve. RA, right atrium; RV, right ventricle.

Box 57.2 History and electrocardiographic features suggestive of a cardiac cause

History

- Abrupt onset
- Absence of premonitory symptoms (unpleasant sight, smell, hearing, pain)
- Associated palpitations or chest pain following effort or exertion
- Syncope in supine position
- Presence of structural heart disease (e.g. aortic stenosis, ischaemic cardiomyopathy)
- Family history of sudden death
- Drug-related arrhythmia (e.g. antiarrhythmics, neuroleptics, digoxin, beta-blockers, cocaine)

12-lead ECG

- Evidence of acute ischaemia or infarction
- Sinus bradycardia, sinus pause > 3 seconds
- High degree AV blocks (second-degree type 2 and complete heart block)
- Alternating LBBB and RBBB; trifascicular block or bifascicular AV blocks (suggestive of diffuse conductive system disease)
- Broad QRS complex > 0.12 seconds
- Accessory pathway: short P-R interval; delta wave
- Prolonged corrected Q-T interval
- Non-sustained VT
- Pauses despite pacemaker (pacemaker malfunction)
- RBBB pattern with down-sloping ST segment elevation in leads V1–V3 (Brugada syndrome)
- Negative T waves in V1–V3, broad QRS in V1–V3, presence of epsilon waves or late potentials (ARVC)

AV, atrioventricular; LBBB and RBBB, left and right bundle branch blocks; VT, ventricular tachycardia; ARVC, arrhythmogenic right ventricular cardiomyopathy

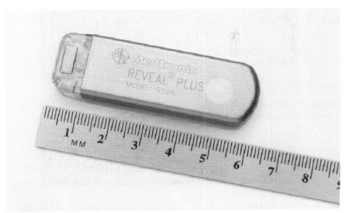

Fig. 57.15 An implantable loop recorder. Photo courtesy of Medtronic Inc.

infrequent or the cause remains unclear even after full evaluation (Krahn et al. 2003). There is increasing evidence that use of implantable loop-recorders during the initial evaluation is more likely to provide a diagnosis than conventional testing (Krahn et al. 2001, Parry 2010). Loop recorders have been also been found to be helpful in establishing symptom-ECG correlation in several other clinical settings such as patients with—suspected epilepsy where treatment has been ineffective; bundle branch block with high degree of suspicion of AV block but negative electrophysiological evaluation; those with structural heart disease or non-sustained VT where electrophysiological studied have been negative (Moya et al. 2009).

The *signal-averaged electrocardiogram* (SAECG) is a computer-processed surface ECG to detect low-amplitude potentials at the end of the QRS complex. The test consists of averaging several hundred QRS complexes by digital means. The presence of late potentials represents slow conduction in the viable strands of myocardium traversing fibrous scar tissue, thereby creating the substrate and conditions necessary for re-entrant ventricular arrhythmias. Presence of late potentials can be useful in identifying those at risk of ventricular arrhythmias following myocardial infarction. Absence of late potentials on the other hand, predicts

non-inducibility of monomorphic VT during invasive electrophysiological study (Winters et al. 1987), but the test is of poor predictive value in assessing the risk of arrhythmias with non re-entrant mechanisms or when the left ventricular ejection fraction is less than 40%.

Electrophysiological studies and ablation

Electrophysiological testing is an invasive procedure that involves measurements of electrical potentials and conduction times between different intracardiac sites by means of electrode-tipped catheters. It is indicated when initial evaluation suggests a high probability of a cardiac cause. The main aim is to induce a clinically important arrhythmia by stimulating various sites within the atria or the ventricles. Various supraventricular, junctional and ventricular arrhythmias can be identified, but sensitivity is low in bradyarrhythmias arising from sinus or AV nodal disease. The main use in patients with syncope is to induce monomorphic VT, responsible for syncope. The lower the ejection fraction, the higher is the likelihood of inducing VT. Rhythms such as non-sustained VT, polymorphic VT and ventricular fibrillation can be induced even in normal individuals. A negative test does not exclude ventricular arrhythmia as the cause of symptoms.

Once identified, the abnormal substrate or an accessory pathway (e.g. W-P-W syndrome; AV nodal re-entrant tachycardia) can be ablated by means of radiofrequency heat coagulation or cryo-ablation to offer a permanent cure from the arrhythmia.

Electrophysiological testing is highly recommended for all patients with a history of syncope and organic heart disease even if the non-invasive tests remain negative.

Sudden cardiac death and role of implantable cardioverter-defibrillators

ICD therapy has made possible the successful prevention of SCD. These are devices which can now be implanted in a similar fashion to permanent pacemakers and can abort a ventricular arrhythmia either by means of anti-tachycardia pacing or by direct defibrillation (Fig. 57.17). They also have a back-up function of single or dual chamber pacing for bradycardia.

Previously ICDs were implanted for secondary prevention after an episode of aborted sudden death, but subsequent to the evidence from recent trials are increasingly used for primary prevention in high risk individuals. The MADIT II trial demonstrated mortality reduction from prophylactic ICD implantation in post-myocardial infarction patients with a poor ejection fraction of ≤ 30% even without requiring inducibility at electrophysiological testing (Moss 2002). The recently completed Sudden Cardiac Death in Heart Failure (SCD-HeFT) trial shows significant mortality benefit in patients with heart failure and reduced left ventricular function (LVEF ≤ 35%) regardless of aetiology or additional risk factors (Bardy et al. 2005). Current guidelines recommend ICD therapy for individuals with syncope of unexplained origin in whom clinically relevant VT/VF is induced at electrophysiological study when antiarrhythmic therapy has been ineffective or discontinued due to intolerance or lack of compliance (Epstein et al. 2008). Prophylactic ICD therapy is also useful in patients with primary electrical defects, for example congenital long QT, Brugada syndrome and hypertrophic cardiomyopathy with syncope or a family history of SCD. A significant proportion of patients with

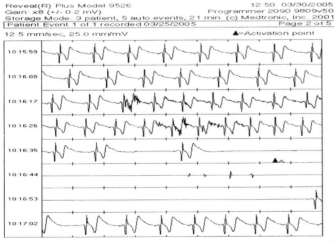

Fig. 57.16 Recordings from implantable loop recorder device revealing a period of long asystolic pause.

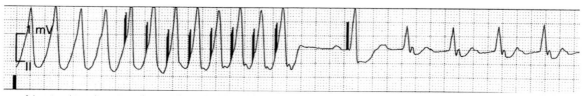

Fig. 57.17 Successful anti-tachycardia pacing of ventricular tachycardia (VT) by the implantable cardioverter defibrillator (ICD). The VT is relatively slow (150/minute) and is overdriven by a train of rapidly paced beats at 188/minute. ICDs are usually programmed to provide initial anti-tachycardia pacing followed by direct current shocks if overdrive pacing fails.

SCD, however, have normal ventricular function with no predisposing risk factors, and we as yet do not know how to identify these individuals.

Acknowledgements

Dr C Corbishley, Consultant Cellular Pathologist and Department of Echocardiography, St George's Hospital, London.

References

Bardy, G. H., Lee, K. L., Mark, D. B., *et al.* (2005); Sudden Cardiac Death in Heart Failure Trial (SCD-HeFT) Investigators. Amiodarone or an implantable cardioverter-defibrillator for congestive heart failure. *N Engl. J Med.* **352**(3), 225–37.

Benditt, D. G., Sakaguchi, S., Goldstein, M. A., *et al.* (1995). Sinus node dysfunction: Pathophysiology, clinical features, evaluation and treatment. In: Zipes, D. P., Jalife, J. eds. *Cardiac Electrophysiology: From Cell to Bedside*, pp. 1215–46. W B Saunders, Philadelphia.

Benditt, D. G. and Sutton, R. (2005). Bradyarrhythmias and syncope. In Grubb, B., Olshansky, B., eds. *Syncope: mechanisms and management*, pp. 92–120 Blackwell Futura, Massachusetts.

Brignole, M., Alboni, P., Benditt, D. G. *et al.* (2004). Guidelines on Management (Diagnosis and Treatment) of Syncope-Update 2004. The Task Force on Syncope, European Society of Cardiology. *Europace* **6**, 467–537.

Camm, A. J., Malik, M. and Yap, Y. G. (2004). *Acquired Long QT Syndrome.* Blackwell Futura, Oxford.

Crawford, E. S. (1990). The diagnosis and management of aortic dissection. *JAMA* **264**, 2537–41

Crawford, M. H., Bernstein, S. J., Deedwania, P. C. *et al.* (1999). ACC/AHA/ESC Guidelines for ambulatory electrocardiography. *J Am. Coll. Cardio.*, **34**, 912–48

DeSanctis, R. W., Doroghazi, R. M., Austen, W. G. and Buckley, M. J. (1987). Aortic dissection. *New Engl. J Med.* **317**, 1060–7.

Ector, H., Rolies, L., and De Geest, H. (1983). Dynamic electrocardiography and ventricular pauses of 3 seconds and more: etiology and therapeutic implications. *PACE* **6**, 548–51.

Epstein, A. E., DiMarco, J. P., Ellenbogen, K. A., *et al.* (2008). ACC/AHA/HRS 2008 guidelines for device-based therapy of cardiac rhythm abnormalities. A report of the American College of Cardiology/American Heart Association Task Force on Practice Guidelines. *Circulation* **117**; e350–408.

Fagard, R. (2003). Athlete's heart. *Heart*, **89**, 1455–61.

Frances, R. J. (2005). Arrhythmogenic right ventricular dysplasia/cardiomyopathy. A review and update *Int. J. Cardiol,* full article available online via Pubmed ahead of publication.

Frenneaux, M. P., Counihan, P. J., Caforio, A. L. P., Chikamori, T. and McKenna, W. J. (1990). Abnormal blood pressure response during exercise in hypertrophic cardiomyopathy. *Circulation* **82**, 1995–2002.

Fuster, V., Steele, P. M., Edwards, W. D., Gersh, B. J., McGoon, M. D., and Frye, R. L. (1984). Primary pulmonary hypertension: Natural history and the importance of thrombosis. *Circulation* **70**, 580–7.

Getchell, W. S., Larsen, G. C., Morris, C. D. and McAnulty, J. H. (1999). Epidemiology of syncope in hospitalized patients. *J Gen. Intern. Med.*, **14**, 677–87

Gibson, J. C. and Heitzman, M. R. (1984). Diagnostic efficacy of 24–hour electrocardiographic monitoring for syncope. *Am. J. Cardiol.* **53**, 1013–17.

Grech, E. D., and Ramsdale, D. R. (1991). Exertional syncope in aortic stenosis. *Am. Heart J.* **121**, 603–6.

Gregoratos, G., Abrams, J., Epstein, A. E., *et al.* (2002). ACC/AHA/NASPE 2002 guideline update for implantation of cardiac pacemakers and antiarrhythmia devices: summary article. A report of the American College of Cardiology/American Heart Association Task Force on Practice Guidelines (ACC/AHA/NASPE committee to update the 1998 pacemaker guidelines). *Circulation* **106**, 2145–61

Hartikainen, J. E., Malik, M., Staunton, A., Poloniecki, J. and Camm, A. J. (1996). Distinction between arrhythmic and nonarrhythmic death after acute myocardial infarction based on heart rate variability, signal-averaged electrocardiogram, ventricular arrhythmias and left ventricular ejection fraction. *J. Am. Coll. Cardiol.* **28**, 296–304.

Hilgard, J., Ezri, M. D. and Denes, P. (1985). Significance of ventricular pauses of three seconds or more detected on twenty-four hour Holter recordings. *Am. J. Cardiol.* **55**, 1005–8.

Jiang, C., Atkinson, D., Towbin, J. A., *et al.* (1994). Two long QT syndrome loci map to chromosomes 3 and 7 with the evidence for further heterogeneity. *Nature Genet.* **8**, 141–7.

Kaplan, B. M., Langendorf, R., Lev, M., Pick, A. (1973). Tachycardia-bradycardia syndrome (so called 'sick sinus syndrome'), *Am. J Cardiol.*, **26**, 497–508

Kapoor, W. N., Cha, R., Peterson, J. R., Wieand, H. S., and Karpf, M. (1987). Prolonged electrocardiographic monitoring in patients with syncope. *Am.J. Med.* **82**, 20–8.

Kapoor, W. N., Karpf, M., Wilband, H. S., Peterson, J. and Levey, G. (1983). A prospective evaluation and follow-up of patients with syncope. *New Engl. J. Med.* **309**, 197–204.

Kapoor, W. N. and Hanusa, B. (1996). Is syncope a risk factor for poor outcomes? Comparison of patients with and without syncope. *Am. J Med.*, **100**, 646–55.

Kaul, U., Dev, V., Narula, J., Malhotra, A. K., Talwar, K. K. and Bahatia, M. L. (1988). Evaluation of patients with bundle branch block and 'unexplained' syncope: A study based on comprehensive electrophysiologic testing and ajmaline stress. *PACE*, **11**, 289–97.

Keating, M. T., Atkinson, D., Dunn, C., Timothy, K., Vincent, G. M., and Leppert, M. (1991). Linkage of a cardiac arrhythmia, the long QT syndrome, and the Harvey ras-1 gene. *Science* **252**, 704–6.

Krahn, A. D., Kein, G. J., Yee, R. I. *et al.* (2001). Randomized Assessment of Syncope Trial: conventional diagnostic testing versus a prolonged monitoring strategy. *Circulation*, **104**, 46–51.

Krahn, A. D., Kein, G. J. and Skanes, A. C. (2003). Use of implantable loop recorders in evaluation of patients with unexplained syncope. *J Cardiovas. Electrophysiol.* **14**, S70–3.

Krol, R. B., Morady, F., Flaker, G. C. *et al.*(1987). Electrophysiologic testing in patients with unexplained syncope: clinical and non-invasive predictors of outcome. *J Am. Coll. Cardiol.* **10**, 358–63,

Lacriox, D., Dubuc, M., Kus, T. and Savard, P. (1991). Evaluation of arrhythmic causes of syncope: correlation between Holter monitoring, electrophysiologic testing and body surface mapping. *Am. Heart J,* **122**, 1346–54

Lempert, T., Bauer, M. and Schmidt, D. (1994). Syncope: a videometric analysis of 56 episodes of transient cerebral hypoxia. *Ann. Neurol.,* **36**, 233–37

Linzer, M., Yang, E. H., Estes, N. A. M., Wang, P., Vorperian, V. R. and Kapoor, W. N. (1997). Diagnosing syncope: Part II. Unexplained syncope. *Ann. Intern. Med.,* 127, 76–86

Maron, B. J. (2003). Sudden death in young athletes. *N Engl J Med.* **349**, 1064–75

Maron, B. J., Shen, W. K., Link, M. S., *et al.* (2000). Efficacy of implantable cardioverter-defibrillators for the prevention of sudden death in patients with hypertrophic cardiomyopathy. *N Engl J Med.* **342**, 365–73

Martin, G. J., Adams, S. L., Martin, H. G., Mathews, J., Zull, D. and Scanlon, P. J. (1984). Prospective evaluation of syncope. *Ann. Emer. Med.,* **13**, 499–504

Mathewson, F. A., Rabkin, S. W. and Hsu, P. H. (1976). Atrioventricular heart block: 27 year follow-up experience. *Trans. Assoc. Life Ins. Med. Dir. Am.,* **60**, 110–30.

Mazuz, M. and Friedman, H. S. (1983). Significance of prolonged electrocardiographic pauses in sinoatrial disease: Sick sinus syndrome. *Am. J. Cardiol.* **52**, 485–9.

Middlekauff, H., Stevenson, W., Stevenson, L. and Saxon, L. A. (1993). Syncope in advanced heart failure: high risk of sydden death regardless of origin of syncope. *J Am. Coll. Cardiol.,* **21**, 110–116

Moss, A. J., Zareba, W., Hall, W. J. *et al.* (2002). Prophylactic implantation of a defibrillator in patients with myocardial infarction and reduced ejection fraction. *N Engl J Med.* **346**, 877–83

Moya, A., Sutton, R., Ammirati, F., *et al.* (2009). Guidelines for the diagnosis and management of syncope (version 2009). *Eur. Heart J* **30**, 2631–71

Nishimura, R. A. and Holmes, D. R. Jr. (2004) Hypertrophic cardiomyopathy. *N Engl J Med.* **350**(13), 1320–7.

Olshansky, B. (2005). Syncope: overview and approach to management. In: Grubb BP, Olshansky B, eds. *Syncope: Mechanisms and management,* pp. 1–46. Blackwell Futura, Massachusetts.

Parry, S. W. and Matthews, I. G. (2010). Implantable loop-recorders in the investigation of unexplained syncope: a state of the art review. *Heart* **96**, 1611–16

Raynen, K. (1995). Cardiac myxomas. *New Engl. J. Med.* **333**, 1610–17.

Reddy, P. S., Curtis, E. I., O'Toole, S. D. and Shaver, J. A. (1978). Cardiac tamponade: haemodynamic observations in man. *Circulation* **58**, 265–72.

Ross, J. Jr and Braunwald, E. (1968). Aortic stenosis. *Circulation* **38**, (Suppl. 5), 61–7.

Sarasin, F. P., Louis-Simonet, M. and Carballo, D. (2001). Prospective evaluation of patients with syncope: a population based study. *Am. J Med.,* **111**, 177–84

Schott, J. J., Charpentier, F., Peltier, S. *et al.* (1995). Mapping of a gene for long QT syndrome to chromosome 4q25–27. *Am. J. Hum. Genet.* **57**, 1114–22.

Schuchert, A., Maas, R., Kretzschmar, C. *et al* (2003). Diagnostic yield of external ECG loop recorders in patients with recurrent syncope and negative tilt table testing. *PACE,* **26**(18), 37–40.

Soteriades, E. S., Evans, J. C., Larson, M. G., *et al.* (2002). Incidence and prognosis of syncope. *N Engl J Med.,* **347**(12), 878–85.

Thames, M., Alpert, J. and Dalen, J. (1969). Syncope in patients with pulmonary embolism. *JAMA* **238**, 2509–11.

Viitasalo, M. T., Kala, R. and Eisalo, A. (1982). Ambulatory electrocardiographic recording in endurance athletes. *Br. Heart J.* **47**, 213–20.

Vincent, G. M. (2000). Long QT syndrome. *Cardiol Clin* **18**, 309–25.

Wilk, J., Nardone, A., Jennings, C., *et al.* (1995) Unexplained syncope: when to expect pulmonary embolism. *Geriatrics* **50**(10), 46–50.

Winters, S. L., Steward, D. and Gones, J. A. (1987). Signal averaging of the surface QRS complex predicts inducibility of ventricular tachycardia in patients with syncope of unknown origin: a prospective study. *J. Am. Coll. Cardiol* **10**, 775–81.

Zareba, W., Moss, A. J., Daubert, J. P. *et al.* (2003). Implantable cardioverter defibrillator in high-risk long QT syndrome patients. *J Cardiovasc. Electrophysio.* **14**, 337–41.

CHAPTER 58

Paediatric aspects of neurally (autonomic) mediated syncope

John B.P. Stephenson

Introduction

Syncope is common in childhood, especially in infants and toddlers. This chapter will concentrate on that age group, referred to as early childhood.

Syncope is the most common paroxysmal event of early childhood, far outnumbering the better known epilepsies (Hindley et al. 2006). These usually are neurally (autonomic) mediated, but the varying terminology may be a bar to understanding and this therefore is dealt with initially.

Terminology

The terms used for the episodes to be discussed vary with the age and stage of development of the child and between doctors of different specialties and geographical origin, both within the English-speaking world and between other cultures and linguistic groups. Doubtless some of this multiplicity of terms results from uncertainty about what are the mechanisms involved. Another reason may be the constraints on the vocabulary used by paediatricians when speaking to parents about their children's attacks.

Syncope definition

It may seem surprising, but there is not even agreement as to the definition of the term syncope when applied to the very young. Those who deal with adults and particularly adult cardiologists would like to restrict the definition of syncope to the result of cerebral hypoperfusion due to failure of the systemic circulation. Particularly they would say that syncope is a transient loss of consciousness due to impaired blood flow to the brain.

Definition of syncope in early childhood

There are several reasons why the above definition cannot be applied to early childhood. The first reason is that the mechanism or mechanisms of what we call syncope in the very young is in the main speculative. This is because only rarely has it been possible to measure all the important variables in a spontaneous episode. The second reason is that in the most common of these syncopes, the so-called cyanotic breath-holding spell, what evidence there is points to anoxic anoxia (hypoxic hypoxia) as the mechanism, without necessarily any impairment of cerebral circulation at all. The Gastaut definition of syncope (Gastaut 1974), as an abrupt cutting off of energy substrates to the cerebral cortex, is preferred. It is implicit here that deficiency of glucose (as in hypoglycaemia) is excluded from the definition, so that in the simplest terms syncope is the state resulting from an insufficient supply of oxygen to the brain (Hainsworth 2004, Martin et al. 2010).

Syncope versus asphyxia

Some have argued that if the mechanism of acute loss of cerebral activity is hypoxia without impaired cerebral perfusion, then that is asphyxia and not syncope. Once again, this distinction is not possible in early childhood, for three reasons. First, in any individual case the pathophysiology is usually speculative. Secondly, when the mechanism has been determined, it has been found that a young child may have some episodes brought about by hypoxic hypoxia and others through circulatory collapse. Thirdly, when ictal recordings have been made, it is often the case that there is both an asphyxic element (hypoxic hypoxia) and an ischaemic element (circulatory failure) in the same episode of loss of cerebral activity.

Anoxic seizures

Gastaut (1974) called syncopes 'generalized anoxic cerebral seizures'. Since then the term anoxic seizure has been widely used for the predominantly motor seizure that is the visible manifestation of any severe syncope. Anoxic seizures, brought about through abrupt loss of cerebral activity, have only a superficial resemblance to epileptic seizures, in which by contrast there is an abrupt increase in cerebral activity.

Clinical recognition of childhood syncope

Although this chapter focuses on syncope in infants and young children, many of the features described may be observed or elicited in older individuals, as summarized by Lempert (1996).

Settings, situations, provocations, precipitants, stimuli and triggers

The tautologies in the subtitle emphasize the major clinical point that the history of what happened beforehand is the key to what transpired afterwards. Most syncopes occur in certain situations and most have provocations. If a bump on the head precedes the event in a toddler then what follows is a syncope with a high probability. If hair grooming precedes the event in an older child the same inference applies. This is the most important phase in which 'history is all' (Stephenson 1990).

Prodrome

When syncope is infrequent parents may recognize that the child's behaviour changes for hours or even days before an episode (Stephenson 2001). During this prodromal period the child may appear emotional, withdrawn, quiet, and pale, and complain of excessive noise. Stimuli that are at other times ineffective may easily induce an episode.

Aura or warning

It is well known that fading of vision and of hearing are premonitory symptoms in the older individual. Sometimes the pre-syncopal aura is more complex, including hallucinations and something akin to an out-of-body-experience.

Colour changes

Although pallor is frequent at the onset or at the conclusion of a syncopal episode, children with most so-called breath-holding spells (BHS) are cyanosed instead. In some episodes of syncope no colour change is recognized. In those with vagal mediated cardiac stand-still, a beetroot red flush may signal the re-starting of the heart.

Falls

Falls might seem to be an inevitable component of syncope but obviously is not so when the patient is already on the bed or on the floor, or too young to be upright. Falls may be stiff as well as limp.

Convulsions

Some sort of convulsive movements are the rule in syncopes. The most prominent is a tonic extension, commonly to opisthotonus, with clenching of the jaw and fisting of the hands. More after than before this hypertonia are random irregular jerks. These are better called spasms (they have some resemblance to epileptic infantile spasms) and may be repeated more than once. They may be asymmetrical, especially if the head is turned to one side. In the absence of anoxic-epileptic seizures (Stephenson et al. 2004), syncopal convulsions never involve prolonged regular rhythmic jerking.

Eye movements

The eyes may deviate up, or to either side; down-beat nystagmus is frequent, albeit it may not be easily noticeable.

Vocalizations

Various noises that have been described as growling, moaning, cackling, barking, grunting, snorting, gurgling, and groaning are not uncommon during the unconscious phase.

Tongue biting

Lateral tongue biting is only very rarely seen.

Urinary incontinence

In early childhood before bladder control is attained, urinary incontinence is seldom noticed, though active emptying of the bladder during a severe syncope may be seen as early as in the neonatal period. In later childhood, wetting is common in syncope, and embarrassing long before adolescence.

Automatisms

Complex movements during a syncope are not infrequent. They are usually very short, but occasionally may be prolonged for minutes.

Hallucinations and out-of-body experiences

In early childhood these strange perceptions are not volunteered, but certainly are a feature of the 'coming-to' (recovery) phase of syncopes well before school age. Elaborate distortions of perception are reported in later school age and in adolescence.

Recovery phase

In early childhood, sleep may follow immediately after the syncope, or the child may first wake up and then drift off to sleep soon after. Crying and general misery is common. Confusion in those old enough to determine this is said to last less than 30 seconds, but this is not always so. Those old enough to verbalize their feelings may describe great fatigue, pains, difficulty with any task, and an experience that other people are rushing about and talking too fast. Such feelings may last for hours or even days (Stephenson 2001). Parasomnias in the form of night terrors may occur in the days following a severe syncope.

Neurally medicated syncope in early childhood: vasovagal variants

The more common early childhood neurally mediated syncopes may be classified predominantly into three groups, with more classical vasovagal syncope making up a fourth.

Reflex anoxic seizures/reflex asystolic syncope

Most easy to understand is syncope in which there is a short latency pain-induced reflex arrest of the heart, the so-called reflex anoxic seizures (RAS) or reflex asystolic syncope (Whitehouse et al. 2002).

The terms used for RAS in the literature are legion. Examples include type II hypoxic crisis (Maulsby and Kellaway 1964), pallid infantile syncope (Lombroso and Lerman 1967), pallid syncopal attacks (Laxdal et al. 1969), white breath-holding (Stephenson 1978), vagal attacks (Stephenson 1978), vagal hypertonia (Lucet et al. 1984), vago-cardiac syncope and vagal cardio-inhibitory fainting fit (Stephenson 1990), infantile vasovagal syncope (Hannon 1997), infantile neurocardiogenic syncope (Hannon 1997), neurally mediated syncope with reflex anoxic seizures McLeod et al. 1999), pallid BHS (DiMario 2001), and BHS associated with significant bradycardia (Kelly et al. 2001).

The original description (Stephenson 1978) is as follows—'In a typical case an unsteady toddler on his own trips and falls. His mother hears the bump but no succeeding cry and hurries to him. She finds her child lying deathly still with eyes fixed upwards, lips dusky. As she lifts him, he abruptly stiffens into rigid extension with jaw clenched and hands fisted, gives a few jerks, and after what seems an age (but in fact is less than half a minute) relaxes limply with an absent far-away look. Then he opens his eyes, at once recognizes his mother, cries a little, and drifts off to sleep, his face distinctly pale.' This was written before video-recordings or monitoring studies were available, and has stood the test of time.

The best known and perhaps the most common stimulus to RAS is an accidental bump to the head or to the face, but an unpleasant knock to any part of the body may provoke RAS especially if the injury—however minor—is unexpected. There is nothing absolutely specific about the semiology but syncopes tend to be abrupt and violent, in keeping with the sudden arrest of cerebral circulation. Certain features are usual. The latency between the stimulus and the syncopal onset tends to be very short, maybe less than 10 seconds, during which time most children will cry out. Almost all have a colour change being described as white or grey (sometimes yellow or green), with blue lips (Lobban et al. 2002); rarely there is no colour change, and rarely there is a red flush at the conclusion. Stiffening of the trunk is usual, with waving or jerking of the extended limbs. The majority have been incontinent of urine in an episode, and most experience at least an hour of post-ictal sleep. Hallucinations, sometimes with features resembling near-death experiences, including out-of-body experiences, are reportedly not rare in RAS (Blackmore 1998).

The evidence supporting reflex vagal-mediated cardiac asystole as the mechanism comes from several sources. In early studies it was found that ocular compression would induce instant asystole and reproduce the natural syncope precisely (Stephenson 1978). Direct evidence for asystole came with the first ambulatory recordings in a boy with RAS in 1981 (Stephenson 1990, case 9.29, pp 102–3). In that and other studies it was found that the duration of EEG flattening was closely linked to the duration of asystole, and that additional factors were not needed to explain the syncope (Stephenson 1990, Fig. 7.9, p54) (Fig. 58.1). The effect of atropine in preventing RAS (Stephenson 1979, McWilliam and Stephenson 1984) added support for the proposed cardio-vagal mechanism. Numerous ECG traces during RAS have confirmed pure asystole

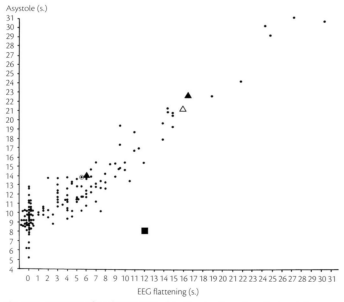

Fig. 58.1 Duration of isoelectric EEG related to duration of cardiac asystole. Each symbol represents one observation. Small filled circles: 144 children who had motor anoxic seizures induced by ocular compression when supine. Double circle: ocular compression result in child whose spontaneous reflex anoxic seizures induced by head bumps are shown as solid triangles (Stephenson 1990: case 9.29, p102–3). Open triangle: needle-induced asystole. Solid square: prolonged expiratory apnoea as shown in Fig. 58.3 (Stephenson 1990: Fig 7.8 p53 and 1991). Reprinted with permission from Stephenson JBP (1990). *Fits and Faints*. Copyright Mac Keith Press and Cambridge University Press.

(Fig. 58.2). Finally, several authors reported anecdotally elimination of such syncopes by cardiac pacing (Sreeram and Whitehouse 1996, Villain et al. 2000, Kelly et al. 2001, Legge et al. 2002). That this did not reflect the natural course was established by a blinded within-patient cross-over study of cardiac pacing in RAS (McLeod et al. 1999).

When children with RAS are paced and become free of syncope they may still experience very brief reflex events that are called by the parents 'near-misses' (McLeod and Stephenson 1999). Instead of syncope there is a gasp, draining of colour and eyes starting to roll, duration about two seconds, after a hurt (Stephenson and McLeod 2000, case 7, p12). The pathophysiology of these near-miss episodes has not been studied.

It is disturbing that RAS are still not well known to doctors, as a parent's anecdote illustrates (Warrington 2004).

Cyanotic breath-holding/cyanotic infantile syncope/ prolonged expiratory apnoea

More common but less well understood than RAS are cyanotic breath-holding spells (CBHS) (DiMario 1992, Breningstall 1996), otherwise called type I hypoxic crises (Maulsby and Kellaway 1964), cyanotic infantile syncope (Lombroso and Lerman 1967 or prolonged expiratory apnoea (PEA) (Southall et al. 1985). Simply known as BHS, these have been known and written about for centuries.

A detailed clinical analysis of severe BHS (of this cyanotic type) in 20 recruited children was made at the Hospital for Sick Children, Toronto, Canada (Gauk et al. 1963). They found that the initial history from the parents was of limited value: invariably the breath was said to be held in inspiration, and periods of apnoea up to 20 minutes were reported. After reassurance the parents were sent home and requested to make careful observations. At the next clinic visit all had observed that the apnoea was expiratory and the maximum duration was one minute. A remarkably consistent pattern emerged from the parental and clinical observations. There were four phases in all cases: provocation, apnoea, rigidity, and stupor. The provocation was usually a frustrating experience, but occasionally pain or a startle. A very brief period of crying, less than 15 seconds, preceded the apnoea. Sometimes there was no cry. Complete expiration was followed by apnoea with progressively deepening cyanosis and retained awareness for 10–15 seconds. Marked restlessness appeared after about 25 seconds and the child slowly twisted into opisthotonus with arms and legs violently extended, incontinent of urine and deeply cyanosed. Twitching was described but 'not convulsive movements'. At the conclusion the child gasped, colour promptly returned, but stupor or drowsiness lasted from minutes to several hours. Asystole was never observed.

Despite such CBHS being extremely common, very few affected individuals have been studied with monitoring equipment to determine the pathophysiology. Peiper (1939) was the first to show that the apnoea was *expiratory* and that during it the high diaphragm moved periodically. He studied one eight-month girl who consistently suffered apnoeic episodes when offered hated bananas.

The Toronto group (Gauk et al. 1963) were able to provoke a spell in two children from their series while a number of physiological modalities were monitored. The most interesting finding to this author was the arterial *hypertension* that accompanied the

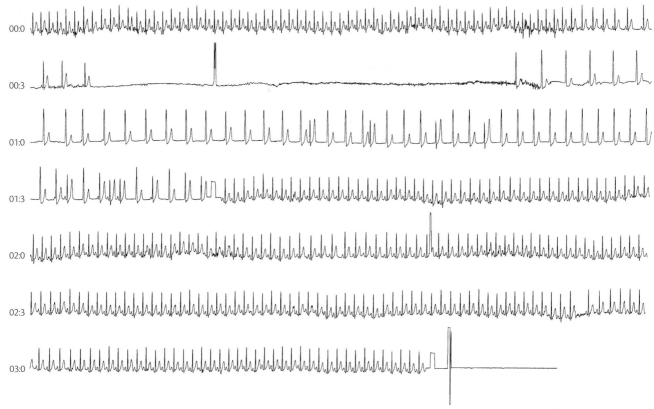

Fig. 58.2 Typical appearance of the electrocardiogram in reflex anoxic seizures as recorded on a cardiac loop recorder. Each line is 30 seconds. After bradycardia for a maximum of about 4 seconds there is asystole for 20.5 seconds. Tonic EMG is seen on the baseline from soon after the event marker that is shown as a high amplitude upward deflection. The trigger was a minor injury.

hypoxic syncope. The explanation for the hypoxia was postulated to be rapid oxygen utilization. In a later study (Gauk et al. 1966), the same authors showed that such BHS could occur without glottal closure, excluding the Valsalva manoeuvre as a mechanism.

Southall et al. (1985) studied 10 infants with what they called prolonged expiratory apnoea. They confirmed arterial hypertension in those episodes studied, and showed that continued expiratory activity continued to occur at low lung volumes with or without glottic closure. In five of their patients episodes continued after tracheostomy or the placement of a nasotracheal tube. They inferred that the very rapid fall in arterial PO_2 (to below 20 mm Hg within 20 seconds.) was due to lack of ventilation at maximum expiratory position in the presence of a rapid circulation time. They also postulated that this mechanism was a cause of neurodevelopmental damage and sudden death in young children, a proposition with which I disagreed (Stephenson 1985). The same authors (Southall et al. 1990) increased their patient number to 51, 28 of whom had physiological monitoring during cyanotic breath-holding attacks. Hypoxaemia occurred far more rapidly than could be explained by upper airways obstruction (Southall et al. 1987). On the basis of krypton-81m scans in seven of these patients the authors concluded that intrapulmonary shunting played a part in the rapid onset hypoxaemia, but this study has not so far as I know been replicated. Once again, I disputed the proposition that such episodes were an important cause of childhood mortality (Stephenson 1991).

Early childhood syncope/breath-holding with mixed or changing or indeterminate mechanism

Although RAS and CBHS/PEA have been described in the previous two sections as distinct entities, in practice there are many blurrings of the margins or boundaries.

In a population of children with so-called BHS, the majority will have only blue spells (CBHS/PEA), fewer will have only white spells (RAS), and a substantial proportion will have *both* types of spell (Maulsby and Kellaway 1964, Lombroso and Lerman 1967, Laxdal and Gomez 1969, Stephenson 1990, DiMario 2001).

Maulsby and Kellaway (1964) attempted to explain how both what they called type I (CBHS) and type II hypoxic crises (RAS) could occur in the same individual. Their clue lay in this observation: 'If one monitors respiration during ocular compression, a characteristic pattern is almost invariably observed. This consists of prolonged expiration, usually with an initial audible cry or "whine". This forced expiratory effort is usually begun simultaneously with cardiac arrest, and it is maintained during cardiac arrest into the phase of EEG hypersynchrony and iso-electric phase during which the child is otherwise unconscious, limp or convulsing— thus suggesting that this "breath-holding" is an involuntary, subcortical component of the reaction to ocular compression. The first inspiratory gasp, or relaxation of expiratory effort, usually occurs *after* EEG recovery has begun. . . .The electromyographic pattern of the abdominal expiratory muscles is quite similar during spontaneous breath-holding spells.' Maulsby and Kellaway (1964) went on 'An hypothesis. Although fragmentary, these data suggest a common mechanism which might relate the two types of hypoxic crises: The cardiac arrest (seen during ocular compression and during Type II hypoxic crises) and the respiratory response (seen during ocular compression, but most prominent in Type I hypoxic crises or breath-holding spell) could be simply two variably associated responses which are elicitable by emotional or painful stimuli and are mediated by a common brainstem reflex pathway. In this concept, one or other response pattern may predominate in any given situation. The respiratory response, prolonged forceful expiratory effort, appears to be the most common expression of the "reflex". The cardiac response may or may not occur; when it does consciousness is more quickly lost, as is evident from the description of Type II attacks. The end result is the same in both cases—syncope due to cerebral hypoxia.'

The author is of the opinion that all these varieties of early childhood syncopes are vasovagal variants, although syncope in any particular child seems more consistent than has been suggested in the literature. There is no disagreement that a young child may have syncopes that sometimes look blue and sometimes white, but the few multiple recordings available show a similar ECG or EEG/ECG pattern on each occasion. For example, the child with unequivocal CBHS, agreed to have PEA by Southall, had 15 spells recorded (Stephenson 1991). In each syncope a short cardiac asystole occurred immediately before the first hypoxic EEG change, the duration of asystole varying from 2 seconds to 8 seconds, and not a contributor to the cerebral hypoxia which was respiratory in origin (Fig. 58.1, 58.3) (Stephenson 1991).

To add to the complexity, some children may have both cardiac asystole and either expiratory apnoea or prolonged expiratory grunting at the same time (Stephenson 1990,1991, Sreeram and Whitehouse 1996, Stephenson and McLeod 2000). Fig. 58.4 demonstrates this. It is pertinent to note that the expiratory grunting that accompanies asystole continues into the phase of diffuse hypoxic EEG slowing.

Vasovagal syncope of classical or mature type

Several authors have noted that classical vasovagal syncope may be a sequel to what the author has called early childhood vasovagal variants. It is not surprising that classical vasovagal syncope (including blood-illness-injury phobia) may evolve step-by-step from infantile RAS (Stephenson et al. 2004, p7), but it is in keeping with the unitary view of this form of syncope that—in the long-term study from the Mayo Clinic (Laxdal et al. 1969)—four patients who originally had *cyanotic* syncopes (CBHS) in response to anger or frustration, had recurrent vasovagal syncope at 16–21 years of age.

Genetic data also support a relationship. In a case control study RAS co-segregated with vasovagal syncopes (Whitehouse et al. 2002). Faints, including needle/injury faints and pregnancy faints, were reported significantly more in parents and grandparents (Lobban et al. 2002).

Conclusions on common neurally mediated syncope

Childhood neurally mediated syncope and in particular the varieties of early childhood neurally mediated syncope are common but poorly understood conditions that give rise to considerable distress and suffering. Although there are obvious difficulties in pursuing research in this area, much remains to be learnt with respect to pathophysiology, genetics, and epidemiology. Such may allow some clarification of the nomenclature and in due course evidence-based treatment.

Rare monogenic neurally mediated syncope

In two single gene channelopathies affecting the nervous system, severe syncope may be a feature in the neonatal period and early infancy, sometimes with bathing an apparent trigger (Nechay and Stephenson 2009).

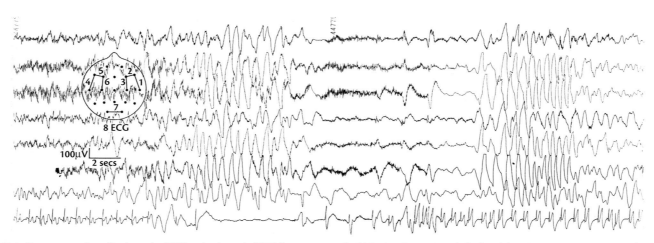

Fig. 58.3 Cassette recording of 7 channels of EEG and 1 channel of ECG from a 15-month girl. During the 40 seconds displayed there is a spontaneous cyanotic breath-holding spell with prolonged expiratory apnoea. Expiratory grunts lead to rapid cyanosis and decerebrate posturing (as shown in video 2, Stephenson 1991). The 8 second asystole is much too short to account for the 12 seconds of EEG flattening, as shown in Fig. 58.1. Reprinted with permission from Stephenson JBP (1990). *Fits and Faints.* Copyright Mac Keith Press and Cambridge University Press.

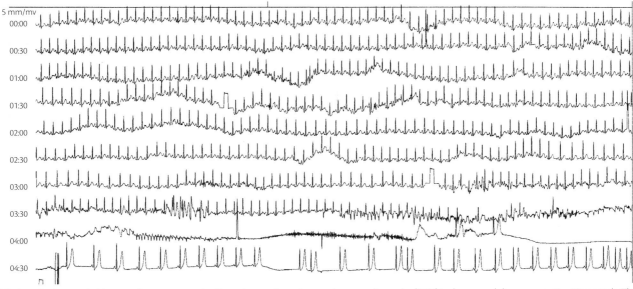

Fig. 58.4 An episode recorded by a cardiac event recorder. Five minutes of continuous electrocardiography (ECG) is shown, each line representing 30 seconds. The ECG shows, in the second half of the 8th line, tachycardia, then bradycardia, then complete asystole for 24 seconds, then two escape beats and further asystole (the total asystole being 40 seconds), then prolonged bradycardia, in part with absent P waves. The additional 'artefacts' are interesting and instructive. Towards the end of the 8th line there is not only an electromyographic (EMG) signal but a notched appearance to the baseline, which becomes more obvious during the asystolic period at the beginning of the 9th line. This represents rapid expiratory grunting at about 5 grunts/second. At the end of this run of expiratory grunts of diminishing amplitude is a tall sharp vertical deflection that represents the pressing of the event button by the mother. After this there is a black 'fuzz' on the baseline which is excessive EMG during the tonic phase of the (non-epileptic) anoxic seizure that is manifest as opisthotonus. The steady baseline in the 10th line probably reflects apnoea.

This episode was typical of the child's usual episodes or as the mother put it a 'normal' attack. She wanted a video to be put in: she had it in her hand, standing up. Having been insistently asking she went quiet. You could see the silent cry, no sound. Her colour was red, her lips darker, but not deep blue. Her head went back and her hands splayed palms upwards and her back arched completely rigid. Then it was as if all the air was out of her body and she gave a snort and went completely limp like a dish-towel, then absolutely white. She was incontinent, wetting herself (and later very upset about this). She came out of it in about half a minute and then went to sleep. Her mother pressed the event button of the cardiac event recorder as she was beginning to go stiff.

Hyperekplexia

In neonatal hyperekplexia (stiff-startle disorder with non-habituating head retraction on tapping the tip of the nose) profound apnoeic syncopes are a dangerous feature (Thomas et al. 2010), often treatable by the Vigevano manoeuvre (Vigevano et al. 1989) and preventable by oral clonazepam (Nigro and Lim 1992).

Hyperekplexia is a ligand-gated chloride channelopathy usually caused by mutations in either *GLRA1* (the gene for the alpha-subunit of the strychnine-sensitive glycine receptor) or *SLC6A5* (the gene for the presynaptic glycine transporter type 2 or Gly2) (Harvey et al. 2008). The ictal polygraphic pattern of these apnoeic syncopes is in my view pathognomonic of hyperekplexia, there being a combination of EEG flattening, junctional bradycardia and high voltage repetitive compound muscle action potentials (EMG 'spikes') on both EEG channels and on the ECG trace as in Fig. 58.5 (see also McMaster et al. 1999).

Paroxysmal extreme pain disorder

Neonatal—or even prenatal—severe syncope (that may include cardiac asystole and resemble reflex anoxic seizures) are a feature of paroxysmal extreme pain disorder (PEPD) that used to be called familial rectal pain and is now known to be a sodium channelopathy with mutations in *SCN9A* (Fertleman et al. 2007). Harlequin phenomena especially flushing of half of the face are

characteristic, and perineal stimulation ('wiping the bottom') a typical precipitation; carbamazepine usually helps (Fertleman et al. 2007).

Conclusions on rare neurally mediated syncope

Very severe syncopes in the neonatal period may reflect hyperekplexia or PEPD. Both may be difficult to diagnose without expert paediatric neurological advice but both are treatable and have genetic implications.

Key points

♦ Neurally mediated syncopes are common in early childhood.

♦ Terminology is confusing, both as to what is syncope in the very young and with respect to the nomenclature of the syncopes encountered.

♦ Clinical recognition depends on adequate history, especially in relation to setting and provocation.

♦ Three variants of immature vasovagal syncope are described.

♦ Reflex anoxic seizures are most easily understood as a short-latency pain-triggered reflex arrest of the heart, that is, reflex asystolic syncope.

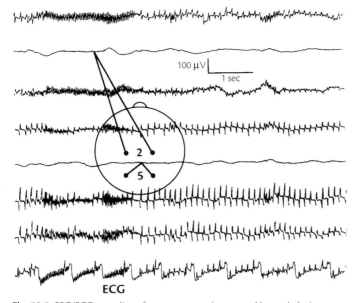

Fig. 58.5 EEG/ECG recording of severe syncope in neonatal hyperekplexia.

10s segment of cassette EEG/ECG during a severe non-epileptic convulsive syncope in a neonate with hyperekplexia due to a dominant negative mutation in the GlyT2 gene *SLC6A5*. Note that 'spikes', whether very rapidly recurring ('tonic') or at around 8 per second ('clonic'), are confined to scalp areas overlying muscle and so are absent at the vertex (channels 2 and 5, arrowed); similar activity is seen on the ECG channel. These 'spikes' represent repetitive muscle action potentials, whereas the EEG is virtually isoelectric. The underlying ECG also demonstrates severe bradycardia with junctional escape rhythm. With permission from Mary D. King, John B. P. Stephenson, *A Handbook of Neurological Investigations in Children*, Wiley.

♦ Cyanotic breath-holding spells are a more complex involuntary response to emotional stimuli with prolonged expiratory apnoea and profound oxygen desaturation.

♦ Mixed syncopes form a third group, including combinations of asystole and expiratory apnoea or expiratory grunting.

♦ Vasovagal syncope in its mature form may evolve from each of these three variants, suggesting common genetic mechanisms.

♦ Rare genetic forms of neurally mediated syncope peculiar to early infancy are seen in hyperekplexia and paroxysmal extreme pain disorder.

Acknowledgements

I thank Trudie Lobban for information and for the support she has given to patients and their families (http://www.stars.org.uk).

References

Blackmore, S. (1998). Experiences of anoxia: do reflex anoxic seizures resemble near-death experiences? *Journal of Near-Death Studies* 17, 111–20.

Breningstall, G. N. (1996). Breath-holding spells. *Pediatric Neurology* 14, 91–7.

DiMario, F. J. Jr (1992). Breath-holding spells in childhood. *American Journal of Diseases in Childhood* 146, 125–31.

DiMario, F. J. Jr (2001). Prospective study of children with cyanotic and pallid breath-holding spells. *Pediatrics* 107, 265–9.

Fertleman, C. R., Ferrie, C. D., Aicardi, J., *et al.* (2007). Paroxysmal extreme pain disorder (previously familial rectal pain syndrome). *Neurology* 69, 586–595.

Gastaut, H. (1974). Syncopes: generalised anoxic cerebral seizures. In: Vinken P. J., Bruyn G. W., eds *Handbook of Clinical Neurology Volume 15: The Epilepsies*, pp. 815–35. North-Holland, Amsterdam.

Gauk, E. W., Kidd, L., Prichard, J. S. (1963). Mechanism of seizures associated with breath-holding spells. *New England Journal of Medicine* **268**, 1436–41.

Gauk, E. W., Kidd, L., Prichard, J. S. (1966). Aglottic breath-holding spells. *New England Journal of Medicine* **275**, 1361–2.

Hainsworth, R. (2004). Pathophysiology of syncope. *Clinical Autonomic Research* **14** Suppl 1: i18–24.

Hannon, D. W. (1997). Breath-holding spells: waiting to inhale, waiting for systole, or waiting for iron therapy? *Journal of Pediatrics*, **130**, 510–2.

Harvey, R. J., Topf, M., Harvey, K., Rees, M. I. (2008). The genetics of hyperekplexia: more than startle! *Trends in Genetics* **24**, 439–47.

Hindley, D., Ali, A., Robson, C. (2006). Diagnoses made in a secondary care 'fits, faints, and funny turns' clinic. *Archives of Disease in Childhood* **91**, 206–209.

Kelly, A. M., Porter, C. J., McGoon, M. D., Espinosa, R. E., Osborn, M. J., Hayes, D. L. (2001). Breath-holding spells associated with significant bradycardia: successful treatment with permanent pacemaker implantation. *Pediatrics* **108**, 698–702.

Laxdal, T., Gomez, M. R., Reiher, J. (1969). Cyanotic and pallid syncopal attacks in children (breath-holding spells). *Developmental Medicine and Child Neurology*, **11**, 755–63

Legge, L. M., Kantoch, M. J., Seshia, S. S., Soni, R. (2002). A pacemaker for asystole in breath-holding spells. *Paediatrics & Child Health* 7, 251–4.

Lempert, T. (1996). Recognizing syncope: pitfalls and surprises. *Journal of the Royal Society of Medicine* **89**, 372–75.

Lobban, T., Bates, G., Curran, P., Collier, J., Whitehouse, W. P. (2002). Reflex Asystolic Syncope: a case controlled study of family history. *Clinical Autonomic Research* 13, 383.

Lombroso, C. T., Lerman, P. (1967). Breath-holding spells (cyanotic and pallid infantile syncope). *Pediatrics* **39**, 563–81.

Lucet, V., Toumieux, M. C., Pajot, N., Monod, N. (1984). Hypertonie vagale paroxystique dunourrisson. Apropos 14 cases. *Archives Francaises de Pediatrie*, **41**, 527–31.

Martin, K., Bates, G., Whitehouse, W. P. (2010) Transient loss of consciousness and *syncope* in children and young people: what you need to know. *Arch Dis Child Educ Pract Ed*, **95**, 66–72.

Maulsby, R., Kellaway, P. (1964) Transient hypoxic crises in children. In: Kellaway, P. Petersen, I., eds. *Neurological and electroencephalographic correlative studies in infancy*, pp. 349–60. Grune & Stratton, New York.

McLeod, K. A., Wilson, N., Hewitt, J., Norrie, J., Stephenson, J. B. P. (1999). Cardiac pacing for severe childhood neurally mediated syncope with reflex anoxic seizures. *Heart* **82**, 721–5.

McMaster, P., Cadzow, S., Vince, J. Appleton, J. (1999). Hyperekplexia: a rare differential of neonatal fits described in a developing country. *Annals of Tropical Paediatrics* **19b**, 345–48.

McWilliam, R. C., Stephenson, J. B. P. (1984). Atropine treatment of reflex anoxic seizures. *Archives of Disease in Childhood* 59, 473–5.

Nigro, M. A., Lim, H. C. (1992). Hyperekplexia and sudden neonatal death. *Pediatric Neurology* 8, 221–225.

Peiper, A. (1939). Das 'Wegbleiben'. *Monatschrift für Kinderheilkunde* **79**, 236–40.

Southall, D. P., Johnson, P., Morley, C. J. *et al.* (1985). Prolonged expiratory apnoea: a disorder resulting in episodes of severe arterial hypoxaemia in infants and young children. *Lancet* **ii**, 571–7.

Southall, D. P., Samuels, M. P., Talbert, D. G. (1990). Recurrent cyanotic episodes with severe arterial hypoxaemia and intrapulmonary shunting: a mechanism for sudden death. *Archives of Disease in Childhood* **65**, 953–61.

Southall D. P., Stebbens, V. A., Rees, S. V., Lang, M. H., Warner, J. O., Shinebourne, E. A. (1987). Apnoeic episodes induced by smothering: two cases identified by covert video surveillance. *British Medical Journal (Clinical Research Ed)* **294**(6588), 1637–41.

Sreeram, N., Whitehouse, W. (1996). Permanent cardiac pacing for reflex anoxic seizure. *Arch Dis Child* **75**, 462.

Stephenson, J., Breningstall, G., Steer, C. *et al.* (2004). Anoxic-epileptic seizures: home video recordings of epileptic seizures induced by syncopes. *Epileptic Disorders* **6**, 15–9.

Stephenson, J. B. P. (1978). Reflex anoxic seizures ('white breath-holding'): nonepileptic vagal attacks. *Archives of Disease in Childhood* **53**, 193–200.

Stephenson, J. B. P. (1979). Atropine methonitrate in management of near-fatal reflex anoxic seizures. *Lancet* **2**(8149), 955

Stephenson, J. B. P. (1985). Prolonged expiratory apnoea in children. *Lancet* **2**(8461), 953.

Stephenson, J. B. P. (1990). *Fits and Faints*. Mac Keith Press and Cambridge University Press, Cambridge and New York.

Stephenson, J. B. P. (1991). Blue breath-holding is benign. *Archives of Disease in Childhood* **66**, 255–7.

Stephenson, J. B. P. (2001). Anoxic seizures: self-terminating syncopes. *Epileptic Disorders* **3**, 3–6.

Stephenson, J. B. P., McLeod, K. A. (2000). Reflex Anoxic Seizures. In: David, T. J., ed. *Recent Advances in Paediatrics 18*. Churchill Livingstone, Edinburgh.

Stephenson, J. B. P., Whitehouse, W., Zuberi, S. M. (2004). Paroxysmal non-epileptic disorders: differential diagnosis of epilepsy. In Wallace, S. J., Farrell K., eds. *Epilepsy in Children*, p. 7. Arnold, London.

Thomas, R. H., Stephenson, J. B. P., Harvey, R. J., Rees, M. I. (2010). Hyperekplexia: stiffness, startle and syncope. *Journal of Pediatric Neurology* **8**, 11–14.

Vigevano, F., Di Capua, M., Dalla Bernardina, B. (1989). Startle disease: an avoidable cause of sudden infant death. *Lancet* **1**(8631), 216.

Villain, E., Lucet, V., Do Ngoc, D., Bonnet, D., Fraisse, A., Kachaner, J. (2000). Stimulation cardiaque dans les spasms du sanglot. *Archives des Maladies du Coeur et des Vaisseaux* **93**, 547–52.

Warrington, M. (2004). Living with reflex anoxic seizure. *Archives of Disease in Childhood* **89**, 682.

Whitehouse, W., Lobban, T., Gayatri, R., Collier, J., Bates, G. (2002). Reflex asystolic syncope: associated features, impact and family history. *Clinical Autonomic Research* **12**, 138.

CHAPTER 59

Syncope in the elderly

Rose Anne Kenny and Blair Grubb

Introduction

'Syncope' is derived from the Greek words '*syn*' (meaning 'together') and '*koptein*' (meaning 'cut'). It is a syndrome consisting of a relatively short period of temporary and self-limited loss of blood flow to the brain, which is most often the result of systemic hypotension (Brignole et al. 2001, Brignole et al. 2004). Syncope is more common in older persons than in any other age group due to a combination of age-related physiological and pathological changes, and its consequences reflect age-related factors pertinent to quality of life, confidence, independence and psychological and physical comorbidity. These elements combine to create potential difficulties in making a diagnosis, which has implications for the subsequent investigation and management of these patients. Causes of syncope are multifactorial, primarily due to increased co-morbidity and polypharmacy in this population, and there may be more than one attributable diagnosis. In addition, the history may be unreliable and events commonly unwitnessed. Furthermore, the consequences of syncope in older persons are greater compared to younger individuals, through the higher risk of serious injury, the increased rate of hospitalization, the consequent loss of confidence, reduction in independence, and the greater risk of death.

Therefore, syncope in the older person poses a challenge for investigation, diagnosis and management.

Falls

Syncope and falls are often considered as separate entities with different aetiologies. However, an overlap between the two has become increasingly evident and this is particularly so for neurally mediated syncope (Lipsitz et al. 1985, Davies and Kenny 1996, Parry et al. 2005). A 'fall' is defined as an event whereby an individual comes to rest on the ground or on another level with or without loss of consciousness. It may be categorized as 'extrinsic' (where the cause is environmental), or as 'intrinsic' (caused by age-related physiological and/or pathological changes). However, most falls, particularly in the very elderly, are attributable to a combination of the two. Falls can be further classified according to their clinical characteristics: clear recall of a trip or a slip is defined as 'accidental', but an episode with/without loss of consciousness *for no apparent reason* is 'unexplained' or 'non-accidental'.

Determination of a fall versus syncope relies on an accurate account of the event either from the patient or an eyewitness. If the patient has cognitive impairment or dementia, the details of the event may be incorrect, and in particular a fall or syncopal episode may not be witnessed or not reported. The estimated annual incidence of falls in this group is as high as 80% (van Dijk et al. 1993). This is compounded further by many syncopal episodes going unwitnessed in older persons—up to 60% (McIntosh et al. 1993a, McIntosh et al. 1993b). Another aspect is amnesia for loss of consciousness. This has been observed in particular in patients with CS syndrome (CSS) who present with unexplained falls and deny loss of consciousness (Parry et al. 2005); however, it is even the case in cognitively normal elderly subjects who fail to recall documented falls 3 months after the event (Cummings et al. 1988). This phenomenon is not confined to the elderly—there has been a similar observation in young adults where syncope was induced through a sequence of hyperventilation, orthostasis, and Valsalva manoeuvre (Lempert et al. 1994), and in older adults with postprandial hypotension and orthostatic hypotension (OH) (Aronow and Ahn 1994, Ward and Kenny 1996). This suggests that the phenomenon is generalized for cardiovascular syncope. Thus, amnesia for loss of consciousness and/or loss of postural stability during episodes of hypotension may explain why some patients report falls rather than syncope.

Age-related physiology and pathology

Older persons are more likely to have age-related physiological impairments of heart rate, blood pressure, and cerebral blood flow. For example, baroreflex sensitivity is blunted by ageing, manifesting as a reduction in heart rate response to hypotensive stimuli (Lipsitz et al. 1985, Lipsitz 1989, Ogawa et al. 1992). The elderly are also prone to reduced blood volume due to excessive salt wasting by the kidneys, diminished renin-aldosterone activity, a rise in atrial natriuretic peptide, and concurrent diuretic therapy-all contributing to hypotension and syncope. Low blood volume, together with age-related diastolic dysfunction, causes low cardiac output and increases susceptibility to OH and neurally mediated syncope (Chimenti et al. 2003). Furthermore, cerebral autoregulation, which maintains a constant cerebral perfusion pressure over a wide range of systemic blood pressure changes, is altered in the presence of hypertension and possibly by ageing. As a result, sudden mild to moderate declines in blood pressure that would not cause any embarrassment of cerebral perfusion in younger individuals can markedly affect perfusion pressures in older adults and leave them vulnerable to syncope.

With advancing age many organ systems will be affected by disease processes (overt or covert) with direct and indirect implications for syncope. The most common of these processes is atherosclerosis; related diseases include ischaemic heart disease, cerebrovascular disease, and renovascular disease. Each of these progresses with age, leading to a reduction in functional reserve of the organ and development of underlying organ dysfunction to varying degrees. In this situation any insult on the organ that increases demand will further compromise organ function, making it more likely to fail. In the context of syncope, this increases both the risk of events and the severity of the sequelae.

Polypharmacy is increasing (Kaufman et al. 2002), particularly in light of more aggressive treatment of cardiovascular disorders such as hypertension (present in 60% of persons over 70 years), and due to the presence of multiple diagnoses. One third of persons over 65 years are taking three or more prescribed medications. The impact of polypharmacy in the elderly is through the increased risk of adverse events per se, to which older persons are more susceptible; the increased risk of drug interactions; the altered metabolism of drugs, particularly with underlying renal and hepatic dysfunction; and the altered bioavailability due to altering substrate for the volume of distribution.

Thus, a combination of age related physiological and pathological factors combine to increase the prevalence and consequences of syncope in older persons. The commonest causes of syncope in the elderly are CSS, vasovagal syncope, OH, and cardiac arrhythmias (McIntosh et al. 1993a). CSS will be discussed in detail in this chapter. The other pertinent causes of syncope are dealt with in Chapters 56, 57 and 60.

CS hypersensitivity/CS syndrome

CS hypersensitivity (CSH) is defined by exaggerated heart rate and blood pressure responses to CS stimulation. The exaggerated heart rate response is referred to as 'cardioinhibition' and represents 3 seconds or more of asystole during CS stimulation. The exaggerated blood pressure response is referred to as 'vasodepression' and represents a drop in systolic blood pressure of 50 mmHg or more during CS stimulation. CSS is present when the exaggerated haemodynamic responses are the attributable cause of syncope. When both cardioinhibitory and vasodepressor responses are present they are referred to as 'mixed CSH'. These responses have been defined during 5–10 seconds of CS stimulation by longitudinal massage over the sinus.

Anatomy

The CS is located at the bifurcation of the internal and external carotid arteries, level with the thyroid cartilage. The sinus is a mechanoreceptor which responds to stretch stimulation and together with the aortic arch baroreceptors is the key regulator of heart rate and blood pressure activity during resting and dynamic activities.

The nerve fibres from the sinus join the Herring Brewer nerve for a short course before joining the glossopharyngeal nerve to the brainstem. The afferent input from the sinus is modulated in the brainstem. Efferent fibres from the brainstem travel via the vagus nerve and the sympathetic ganglia to the heart and peripheral vasculature. In patients with mixed CSH, CS massage rapidly inhibits sympathetic nerve activity (as measured by intraneural recording of sympathetic nerve traffic) and reduces heart rate (Luck et al. 1996).

Pathophysiology

The exact pathophysiology of CSH is unknown, in particular it is unknown whether it is a central or peripheral disorder. Baroreflex gain, as measured by heart rate and blood pressure responses to nitroprusside and phenylephrine, is significantly deceased in CSH and may play a role in pathophysiology (Morillo et al. 1999). To determine whether CSH is a central or local lesion Tea et al. (1996) conducted an investigation of central activity using brainstem auditory evoked potentials, somatosensory evoked potentials, blink reflexes and sympathetic skin responses. In 17 CSH and 17 age and sex-matched controls the response to 'central' tests were similar for patients and controls but tests of peripheral innervation of the sternocleidomastoid muscle differed between groups—76% of CSH patients had a pathological response compared with 24% of controls. Furthermore, the abnormality was bilateral in 53% of patients and in none of controls. The authors concluded that the neuromuscular structures surrounding the CS mechanoreceptors are denervated in CSH. In a follow-up study, Blanc et al. (1997) showed that both CSH and chronic denervation were common confounders in older persons. It may be that both represent age related neurodegeneration and studies of electromyographic (EMG) activity in other muscle groups are necessary before attributing a pathophysiological relationship for CSH and sternocleidomastoid activity.

In a neuropathological series, Miller et al. (2004) showed that the density of neurodegenerative hyperphosphorylated Tau protein was higher in CSH than case controls without CSH. The pathology was specifically increased in nuclei which regulate cardiovascular activity—the cardioreflex arc, the nucleus ambiguus and dorsal sensory nucleus of vagus nerve. The density of Tau deposition did not reflect the degree of Braak staging for Alzheimer pathology—suggesting a selective deposition in brainstem cardiovascular nuclei. Furthermore, the numbers of catecholaminergic neurons were depleted in the rostral ventrolateral medulla—particularly in the nucleus ambiguus.

In 1995 it was hypothesized that CSH was secondary to enhanced regulation of α_2-adrenoceptors due to atherosclerosis related to a reduction in carotid artery and sinus compliance and consequent deafferentation of the baroreflex (O'Mahony 1995). However, in a more recent study, administration of Yohimbine—an α_2-receptor antagonist—did not attenuate the heart rate or blood pressure response to patients with CSH/CSS (Parry et al. 2005). So, although the exact pathophysiology is unknown, recent data supports the contribution of central degeneration as at least one causal component.

Epidemiology

CSH rarely occurs in adults under 50 years, and increases in prevalence with advancing years. Reported prevalence rates vary according to the health status and age of the population studied (Table 59.1). In a recent community-based series Kerr et al. (2005) reported CSH in one third of asymptomatic persons over 65 years of age. There was no significant correlation between the presence of CSH and symptoms of presyncope, syncope or falls. The only variables which predicted an abnormal response were male sex and advancing age. The relevance of this high prevalence of abnormal

Table 59.1 Prevalence of carotid sinus hypersensitivity in non-syncopal subjects

Reference	No, Age (years) (mean ± SD/range)	Setting	Population characteristics	Technique CSM (duration) Definition of CSH	CSH	CI	VD	Mixed	Symptoms with CSH
Nathanson 1956	115 (30–81)	Unclear	71 had no prior symptoms	Right CSM (up to 30 s) / Asystole of 5s	?	115 (100)	?	?	
Smiddy et al. 1972	58 (all male)	Hospital inpatients	No cardiovascular disease, hypertension or cardioactive medication			5 (20% of those with an abnormal ECG)			5 syncope
Mankikar and Clark 1975	386 (60–104)	Nursing home		Supine asystole > 2 s	?	9	?	?	0
Hudson et al. 1985	333 (>50)	ECG Dept		5 s CSM (supine only) / Asystole of ≥3 s	?	14 (4)	?	?	10 (71) syncope
Volkmann et al. 1990	163 (58 ± 13)	Hospital. Source of patients?	All in sinus rhythm	Supine only (5–10 s) / Asystole > 3 s	?	32 (20)	?	?	?
Brignole et al. 1991	25 (60 ± 17; 16–84)	Hospital. Source of controls?	No evidence of organic disease: normal ECG and ECHO	Supine and upright (10 s) / Asystole ≥ 3 s	4(16)	2(8)	2(8)	0	1 (25)
Wentink et al. 1993	69 (23–91)	Community-dwellers (newspaper recruitment)	No IHD, cerebrovascular disease, Parkinson's disease, IDDM, weak pulsations or carotid bruits	Supine (5–10 s) / Asystole ≥ 3 s / SBP drop ≥ 50 mmHg	10 (14)	5 (7)	0	5 (7)	1 (10)
McIntosh et al. 1994	25 (61–87)	Outpatient	No intercurrent illness; no medication	Supine and upright (5 s) / Asystole ≥ 3 s / SBP drop ≥ 50 mmHg mixed	3 (12)	0	3 (12)	0	?
Jeffreys et al. 1996	95 (≥65)	GP practices	No previous MI/CVA	Supine only (5 s) / Sinus arrest ≥ 3 s	?	4 (4.2)	?	?	2 (50) dizziness
Ward et al. 1994	31 EH (74 ±7) 30 AI (79 ± 7) 35 CF (82 ± 8)	Inpatient/outpatient		Supine and upright (5s) / Asystole ≥3 s / SBP ≥ 50 mmHg drop	0 / 13 / 17	?	?	?	?
Morillo et al. 1999	30 (65 ± 14; 40–89)			Supine and upright (5 s) / Cannulated / SBP drop ≥ 50 mmHg/HR ≥ 40 bpm ± asystole ≥ 3 s / Asystole ≥ 3 s / No preceding significant SBP drop / SBP fall ≥ 50 mmHg and HR decrease <10% / SBP drop ≥ 50 mmHg and HR ≥ 40 bpm / Provocation of syncope or presyncope	2 (6.6)	0	0	2 (6.6)	2 (6.6)

Study	n (age)	Setting	Medications	Protocol					
Tsioufs et al. 2002	210 (34–78)	Coronary angiography patients	Cardiovascular medications stopped	Supine (5 to 10s) Vent asystole > 3s SBP drop ≥ 50 mmHg/30 mmHg with neuro symptoms Mixed	40 (26.6)	19(9)	5(2.4)	6 (2.9)	3
McGlinchey et al. 2002	32 (60–80)	University register		Supine and upright (5 s) Asystole > 3 s SBP fall ≥ 50 mmHg Mixed	4 (13)	2(50)	2(50)	0	?
Kumar et al. 2003	44 (> 60)	Hospital GP register		Supine and upright (5 s) Asystole ≥ 3 s SBP drop ≥ 50 mmHg Mixed	0	0	0	0	
Kerr et al. 2005	(a) 298 (b) X	(a) Community (b) Community-	(a) Unselected (b) No symptoms, no culprit medications	(a) and (b) Supine and upright (5s) Asystole ≥ 3s SBP drop ≥ 50 mmHg Mixed	X (X)				

CSM, carotid sinus massage; CSH, carotid sinus hypersensitivity; CI, cardioinhibitory; ECG, electrocardiogram; ECHO, echocardiography; HR, heart rate; IHD, ischaemic heart disease; SBP, systolic blood pressure; SD, standard deviation; VD, vasodepressor.

Table 59.2 Prevalence of cardioinhibitory and vasodepressor carotid sinus hypersensitivity/carotid sinus syndrome in symptomatic patients

Author	Year	Symptoms	N	Mean age	CI/Mixed	VD
Richardson[41]	2000	Falls and Syncope	1000	69	16%	13%
Puggioni[40]	2002	Syncope	1719	63	46%	43%
Kumar[38]	2003	Falls and Syncope	266	79	22%	43%
McIntosh[8]	1993	Falls and Syncope	65	78	19%	26%
O'Mahony[42]	1998	Falls and Syncope	54	76	2%	
Allcock[43]	2000	Falls and Syncope	120	78	22%	15%
Eltrafi[44]	2000	Falls and Syncope	139	74	24.4%	11.5%
Youde[45]	2000	Syncope	76	75 median (range 60–94)	12%	5%

CI, cardioinhibitory; VD, vasodepressor.

responses in asymptomatic older persons is unknown but raises the important question of what factors discriminate between asymptomatic and symptomatic CSH possibly lead to conversion to a symptomatic status. Long-term follow-up of this cohort, which is underway, may resolve some of these questions.

Conversely, CSH is a common and well-recognized cause of symptoms of falls and syncope in symptomatic older persons. CSH is the attributable cause of symptoms in 30% of older persons with unexplained falls or 'drop attacks' and a quarter of older persons with syncope (Parry and Kenny 2005) (Table 59.2).

Work from Puggioni et al. (2002) emphasizes the age-related prevalence of CSS as an attributable cause of symptoms in a large series of 1719 patients referred for investigation of syncope. In 41% of those over 80 years, CSS was the attributable cause of symptoms compared with only 4% of those under 40 years as detailed in the figure.

Symptomatic older persons with CSH are at a particularly high risk of injurious episodes. In one series, where CSH was the attributable cause of syncope or falls, 25% of persons had sustained a fracture (McIntosh et al. 1993a). In a further series, 40% of persons who had unexplained falls due to CSH had had at least one previous fracture (Kenny et al. 2001, McIntosh et al. 1993b). In one case controlled series, reproducible CSH was present in 36% of fracture neck of femur, none of elective surgery patients, 13% of acutely ill controls and 17% of outpatients (Ward et al. 1994). In one nursing home study, patients with CSH had a two fold increase in lacerations, a three-fold increase in fracture rates and a tenfold increase in the incidence of syncope compared with non-CSH patients, but the incidence of 'simple falls' was similar for CSH negative and CSH positive cohorts (Murphy et al. 1986).

The prevalence of CSH is particularly high in older persons attending the Accident and Emergency department with recurrent falls and syncope. In one UK series, 40% of attendees over 50 years presented with a fall or syncopal episode. Of these, 12% had unexplained falls or syncope and 73% of these had CSH, of whom a quarter had the cardioinhibitory type and benefited from cardiac pacing intervention (Richardson et al. 1997, Davies and Kenny 1998, Kenny and Richardson 2001).

Diagnosis

CSH is defined by the heart rate and blood pressure responses to CS massage (CSM). CSM is carried out over the CS, usually the point of maximum pulsation in the area of bifurcation of the internal and external carotid arteries in the neck, level with the thyroid cartilage and two finger breadths below the angle of the jaw. Firm pressure for 5–10 seconds is recommended.

It is important to carry out simultaneous heart rate and beat-to-beat blood pressure recording during CSM in order to capture both the cardioinhibitory and vasodepressor components. An abnormal heart rate response is always immediate whereas there is a lag phase in the blood pressure response—both in patients with exaggerated vasodepressor responses and in normal controls—of approximately 18 ± 3 seconds after cessation of CSM (van Dijk et al. 1993). In a study measuring simultaneous intraneural recording of sympathetic nerve traffic, although arterial pressure started to decline abruptly with complete sympathetic withdrawal from peripheral vasculature, the nadir was delayed, suggesting that arterial dilatation is not instantaneous. Furthermore, arterial pressure rebounded slowly, suggesting latency between the neural reflex and vascular compliance (Luck et al. 1996). Because of these observations, an interval of one minute is recommended between episodes of CSM to facilitate stabilization of the baroreflex response.

In a third of symptomatic patients with CSS the response is only positive when patients are in the upright position—highlighting the importance of conducting CSM both supine and upright (Parry et al. 2000). Our recommendation is to tilt the patient head up to 70° (O'Shea et al. 2001). The sensitivity of the response to CSM is increased by 51% and the diagnosis enhanced by 38% when CSM is performed in the upright position (Morillo et al. 1999). The positive cardioinhibitory response is right-sided in 70%, and bilateral or left-sided in the remainder. The vasodepressor response is predominantly seen during left-sided CSM (O'Shea et al. 2001).

Complications as a result of CSM occur in 0.17–0.9% of patients, most of which are transient neurological complications; only one study reported persistent neurological complications in 0.05% (Table 59.3).

A total of 70% of hypersensitive responses are represented by sinoatrial arrest and atrioventricular block, the remainder are sinoatrial arrest (Madigan et al. 1984). The pattern of response is not always consistent, thus dual rather than single chamber pacing is mandatory for treating the cardioinhibitory or mixed subtype.

The prevalence of head-up tilt induced vasovagal reactions is also higher in CSH cases compared with controls (Kenny et al. 1987). In one study of isoprenaline induced vasovagal responses during head-up tilt, 25% of CSH cases had a positive response

Table 59.3 Complications during carotid sinus massage.

Author	Journal	N	Age	F	CI	VD	N complications	Type	Time
Richardson et al.	Age & Ageing 2000	1000	69/10	68%	16%	13%	9 (0.9%)	Hemiplegia 2 Hemiparesis 1 Nonspecific 6	X 5 minutes 20 s to 24 hours
Rosenbaum	J Cardiovasc Electrophysiol 2001	1	78	1	1	—	55 s asystole	Cardiac arrest	Immediate
Davies and Kenny	Am J Cardiol 1998	4000	74/14	—	—	—	11 (0.28%)	Hemiparesis 10 Dysphasia 3 Hemianopia 1	X 5 minutes 5 minutes to 2 hours Two persistent hemiparesis
Puggioni et al.	Am J Cardiol 2002	1719	63/16	44%	46%	43%	3 (0.17%)	Neurological	Recovery within 1 hour
Kumar et al.	Age & Ageing 2003	266	79	—	22%	43%	0	—	—

CI, cardioinhibitory; VD, vasodepressor

compared with 6.6% of controls (Morillo et al. 1999). On average, 30% of patients with CSH also have underlying sick sinus syndrome or atrioventricular block as defined by electrophysiological studies (Blanc et al. 1984, Huang et al. 1988).

The prevalence of CSH is remarkably high in neurodegenerative disorders, in particular dementia with Lewy bodies and Parkinson's disease, both of which are associated with neurodegenerative processes in the brainstem and with other features of autonomic dysfunction. In one series, cardioinhibitory CSH was evident in 48% of patients who had a diagnosis of diffuse Lewy body disease (DLBD). Furthermore, the degree of CSM-induced hypotension correlated with the severity of cognitive impairment and with the intensity of white matter lesions (Kenny et al. 2002, Ballard et al. 1998, Kenny et al. 2004). It remains to be seen whether early detection of CSH and intervention for symptomatic CSH influences long-term outcome in patients with cognitive impairment and dementia. Furthermore, the prevalence of cognitive impairment and dementia was significantly higher, during an average of 5 years follow-up, in symptomatic patients with CSH than in case controls (Kenny et al. in preparation). The profile of cognitive impairment reflected that of watershed or hypoperfusion, suggesting that repeated hypotension may ultimately result in sustained cognitive dysfunction.

Clinical presentation

The commonest clinical presentations of CSH are dizziness, presyncope, falls or syncope.

Rarely patients may present with epileptic features (McCrea and Findley 1994). Head movement provokes syncope in 47% and vagal type triggers provoke syncope in 73% (Hampton and Kenny 2005). Episodes are unwitnessed in two thirds (McIntosh et al. 1993b). Therefore, if patients have amnesia for loss of consciousness, which is the case in a minimum of a third of patients (Kumar et al. 2003), these patients will present with falls and not syncope. It is important to be aware of CSH as a possible attributable cause of non-accidental falls.

In a review of 1504 cases for whom CSH was the attributable cause of falls, syncope or dizziness, 27% had a mixed response, 28% had a cardio-inhibitory response and 45% vasodepressor CSH (Hampton and Kenny 2005). The average age at presentation was 75±10 years, less than 5% of cases were under 50 years of age. CSH was marginally more common in men up to 65 years, but

thereafter CSH was two-fold more common in females. The type of presentation—falls, dizziness or syncope—was similar for the cardioinhibitory, vasodepressor or mixed subtypes; overall 45% had syncope, 27% falls, 44% dizziness and 38% had a combination of these symptoms.

Co-morbidity, such as hypertension, ischaemic heart disease, diabetes, atrial fibrillation, cerebral vascular disease, peripheral vascular disease, heart failure or arthritis was also similarly distributed for the subtypes with the exception of hypertension which was more common in the vasodepressor subtype. Medication use (i.e. cardiovascular or psychotropic medication), was also similarly distributed across subtypes. From this series, during an average follow up of 5±2 years, patients with CSH were twice as likely to be in institutional care compared with age and sex-matched cases from same the region and four times more likely to have cognitive impairment and dementia. It is, as yet, unclear whether symptomatic CSH is a risk factor for or indicator of cognitive decline and physical frailty in older persons.

Treatment

Before the advent of cardiac pacing, surgical innervation of the affected CS was the treatment of choice; this has now been superseded by cardiac pacing for mixed and cardioinhibitory components. However, there have been reports addressing successful surgical treatment of the vasodepressor component (Mathias et al. 1991). In one series, 5 of 7 patients derived benefit from CS denervation (3-year follow-up) with negligible reported adverse events (Schellack et al. 1986). In another series, transection of the glossopharyngeal nerve and upper rootlets of the vagus nerve at their exit from the brainstem improved symptoms in 3 patients (Simpson et al. 1987).

Other recommended treatments for the vasodepressor components are ephedrine alone or a combination or ephedrine and propranol (to induce unopposed alpha stimulation) (Almquist et al. 1985). More recently, midodrine—an alpha-agonist—demonstrated benefit in 10 patients with vasodepressor CSH (Moore et al. 2005).

Many studies have reported benefit from cardiac pacing intervention (Brignole et al. 1988). Because 70% of patients with mixed or cardio-inhibitory CSH have associated atrioventricular block during CS stimulation, a ventricular lead is necessary

(Madigan et al. 1984), and because most have preserved retrograde atrioventricular conduction (thus enabling retrograde conduction from the ventricle to the atrium during ventricular stimulation and possible pacemaker syndrome), a dual chamber pace maker system (with leads pacing and sensing in the atrium and ventricle) is recommended (McIntosh et al. 1997, Gregoratos et al. 1998). At least 20% will continue to experience dizziness after pacing despite cure of syncopal episodes because of persistent vasodepression. Further syncope is experienced in a small proportion generally due to other causes of syncope—such as orthostatic hypotension and vasovagal syncope (Mitchell et al. 2002; Chapter 22).

Conclusion

In summary, CSH/CSS is a common cause of symptoms of syncope and falls in older persons. The underlying mechanism for the high prevalence of this altered baroreflex response both in symptomatic and in asymptomatic elderly is unknown. Emerging evidence suggests an association with underlying neurodegenerative pathology. This emphasizes the importance of future long-term follow-up studies of asymptomatic positive responders to determine whether CSH is a risk factor for cognitive impairment, and dementia, a surrogate marker for underlying neurodegeneration or an incidental finding. Cardiac pacing will abolish syncope in most patients with cardioinhibitory responses.

References

Allcock, L. M., O'Shea, D. (2000). Diagnostic yield and development of a neurocardiovascular investigation unit for older adults in a district hospital. *J Gerontol. A Biol. Sci. Med. Sci.* **55**(8), M458–462.

Almquist, A., Gornick, C., Benson, W., Jr, Dunnigan, A., Benditt, D. G. (1985). CS hypersensitivity: evaluation of the vasodepressor component. *Circulation* **71**(5), 927–36.

Aronow, W. S., Ahn, C. (1994). Postprandial hypotension in 499 elderly persons in a long-term health care facility. *J Am. Geriatr. Soc.* **42**, 930–32.

Ballard, C., Shaw, F., McKeith, I., Kenny, R. (1998). High prevalence of neurovascular instability in neurodegenerative dementias. *Neurology* **51**(6), 1760–62.

Blanc, J. J., Boschat, J. Penther, P. (1984). CS hypersensitivity. Median-term development as a function of treatment and symptoms. [French]. *Archives des Maladies du Coeur et des Vaisseaux* **77**(3), 330–36.

Blanc, J. J., L'Heveder, G., Mansourati, J., Tea, S. H., Guillo, P., Mabin, D. (1997). Assessment of a newly recognized association. CS hypersensitivity and denervation of sternocleidomastoid muscles. *Circulation* **95**(11), 2548–51.

Brignole, M., Menozzi, C., Gianfranchi, L., Oddone, D., Lolli, G., Bertulla, A. (1991). CS massage, eyeball compression, and head-up tilt test in patients with syncope of uncertain origin and in healthy control subjects. *American Heart Journal* **122**(6), 1644–51.

Brignole, M., Menozzi, C., Lolli, G., Sartore, B., Barra, M. (1988). Natural and unnatural history of patients with severe CS hypersensitivity: a preliminary study. *PACE: Pacing and Clinical Electrophysiology* **11**(11:Pt 2), 1628–35.

Brignole, M., Alboni, P., Benditt, D., *et al.* (2001). Guidelines on management (diagnosis and treatment) of syncope. *European Heart Journal* **22**(15), 1256–1306.

Brignole M., Alboni P., Benditt D. G., *et al.* (2004). Guidelines on management (diagnosis and treatment) of syncope—update 2004. *Europace* **6**(6), 467–537.

Chimenti C., Kajstura J., Torella D. *et al.* (2003). Senescence and death of primitive cells and myocytes lead to premature cardiac aging and heart failure. *Circ. Res.* **93**(7). 604–13

Cummings, S. R., Nevitt, M. C., Kidd, S. (1988). Forgetting falls. The limited accuracy of recall of falls in the elderly. *J Am. Geriatr. Soc.* **36**, 613–616.

Davies, A. J., Kenny, R. A. (1996). Falls presenting to the accident and emergency department: Types of presentation and risk factor profile. *Age Ageing* **25**, 362–66.

Davies A. J., Kenny R. A. (1998). Frequency of neurologic complications following CS massage. *Am J Cardiol* **81**(10):1256–57

Eltrafi, A., King, D., Silas, J. H., Currie, P., Lye, M. (2000). Role of CS syndrome and neurocardiogenic syncope in recurrent syncope and falls in patients referred to an outpatient clinic in a district general hospital. *Postgrad. Med. J* **76**(897), 405–408.

Gregoratos, G., Cheitlin, M. D., Conill, A., *et al.* (1998). ACC/AHA guidelines for implantation of cardiac pacemakers and antiarrhythmia devices. *Journal of the American College of Cardiology* **31**, 1175–1209.

Hampton, J., Kenny, R. (2005). Clinical characteristics of patients with CS hypersensitivity. In Preparation.

Huang, S. K., Ezri, M. D., Hauser, R. G., Denes, P. (1988). CS hypersensitivity in patients with unexplained syncope: clinical, electrophysiologic, and long-term follow-up observations. *Heart* **116**(4), 989–96.

Hudson, W. M., Morley, C. A., Perrins, E. J., Chan, S. L., Sutton, R. (1985). Is a hypersensitive CS reflex relevant? *Clin. Progress* **3**(2), 155–59.

Jeffreys, M., Wood, D. A., Lampe, F., Walker, F., Dewhurst, G. (1996). The heart rate response to carotid artery massage in a sample of healthy elderly people. *PACE: Pacing and Clinical Electrophysiology* **19**(10), 1488–92.

Kaufman, D. W., Kelly, J. P., Rosenberg, L., Anderson, T. E., Mitchell, A. A. (2002). Recent patterns of medication use in the ambulatory adult population of the United States: The Slone Survey. *JAMA* **287**, 337–44.

Kenny, R. A., Lyon, C. C., Ingram, A. M., Bayliss, J., Lightman, S. L., Sutton, R. (1987). Enhanced vagal activity and normal arginine vasopressin response in CS syndrome: implications for a central abnormality in CS hypersensitivity. *Cardiovascular Research* **21**(7), 545–50.

Kenny, R. A., Richardson, D. A. (2001). CS syndrome and falls in older adults. *American Journal of Geriatric Cardiology* **10**(2), 97–99.

Kenny, R. A., Richardson, D. A., Steen, N., Bexton, R. S., Shaw, F. E., Bond, J. (2001). CS syndrome: a modifiable risk factor for nonaccidental falls in older adults (SAFE PACE). *Journal of the American College of Cardiology* **38**(5), 1491–96.

Kenny, R. A., Kalaria, R., Ballard, C. (2002). Neurocardiovascular instability in cognitive impairment and dementia. *Ann. N Y Acad. Sci.* **977**, 183–95.

Kenny, R. A., Shaw, F. E., O'Brien, J. T., Scheltens, P. H., Kalaria, R., Ballard, C. (2004). CS syndrome is common in dementia with Lewy bodies and correlates with deep white matter lesions. *J Neurol. Neurosurg. Psychiatry* **75**(7), 966–71.

Kenny, R. A., Pearce, M., Pearce, R., Brayne, C. Cognitive impairment in CSH (in prep)

Kerr, S., Pearce, M., Brayne, C., Davis, R., Kenny, R. (2005). CS hypersensitivity is a common finding in asymptomatic older persons—implications for diagnosis of syncope and falls. *Ann. Intern. Med.* (In Press).

Kumar, N. P., Thomas, A., Mudd, P., Morris, R. O., Masud, T. (2003). The usefulness of CS massage in different patient groups. *Age and Ageing* **32**(6):666–9.

Lempert, T., Bauer, M., Schmidt, D. (1994). Syncope: Avideometric analysis of 56 episodes of transient cerebral hypoxia. *Ann. Neurol.* **36**, 233–37.

Lipsitz, L. A. (1989). Altered blood pressure homeostasis in advanced age: Clinical and research implications. *J Gerontol.* **44**, M179–83.

Lipsitz, L. A., Wei, J. Y., Rowe, J. W. (1985). Syncope in an elderly, institutionalised population: prevalence, incidence, and associated risk. *QJM* **55**, 45–54.

Luck, J. C., Hoover, R. J., Biederman, R. W., *et al.* (1996). Observations on CS hypersensitivity from direct intraneural recordings of sympathetic nerve traffic. *American Journal of Cardiology* **77**(15), 1362–65.

Madigan, N. P., Flaker, G. C., Curtis, J. J., Reid, J., Mueller, K. J., Murphy, T. J. (1984). CS hypersensitivity: beneficial effects of dual-chamber pacing. *American Journal of Cardiology* 53(8), 1034–40.

Mankikar, G. D., Clark, A. N. (1975). Cardiac effects of CS massage in old age. *Age and Ageing* 4(2), 86–94.

Mathias, C. J., Armstrong, E., Browse, N., Chaudhuri, K. R., Enevoldson, P., Russell, R. W. (1991). Value of non-invasive continuous blood pressure monitoring in the detection of CS hypersensitivity. *Clinical Autonomic Research* 1(2), 157–59.

McCrea, W., Findley, L. J. (1994). CS hypersensitivity in patients referred with possible epilepsy. *British Journal of Clinical Practice* 48(1), 22–24.

McGlinchey, P. G., Armstrong, L., Spence, M. S., Roberts, M. J, PP. M. (2002). Effect of CS massage and tilt-table testing in a normal, healthy older population (The Healthy Ageing Study). *American Journal of Cardiology* 90(9), 1015–1017.

McIntosh, S. J., da Costa, D., Kenny, R. A. (1993a). Outcome of an integrated approach to the investigation of dizziness, falls and syncope in the elderly referred to a syncope clinic. *Age Ageing* 22, 53–58.

McIntosh, S. J., Lawson, J., Kenny, R. A. (1993b). Clinical characteristics of vasodepressor, cardioinhibitory, and mixed CS syndrome in the elderly. *Am. J Med.* 95, 203–208.

McIntosh, S. J., Lawson, J., Kenny, R. A. (1994). Heart rate and blood pressure responses to CS massage in healthy elderly subjects. *Age and Ageing* 23(1), 57–61.

McIntosh, S. J., Lawson, J., Bexton, R. S., Gold, R. G., Tynan, M. M., Kenny, R. A. (1997). A study comparing VVI and DDI pacing in elderly patients with CS syndrome. *Heart* 77(6), 553–57.

Miller, V., Kenny, R. A., Kalaria, R. N. (2004). Medullary pathology in patients with CS syndrome. *Clinical Autonomic Research* 14(5), Abstr.

Mitchell, L. E., Richardson, D. A., Davies, A. J., Bexton, R. S., Kenny, R. A. (2002). Prevalence of hypotensive disorders in older patients with a pacemaker in situ who attend the Accident and Emergency Department because of falls or syncope. *Europace* 4(2), 143–7.

Moore, A., Watts, M., Sheehy, T., Hartnett, A., Clinch, D., Lyons, D. (2005). Treatment of vasodepressor CS syndrome with midodrine: A randomized, controlled pilot study. *Journal of the American Geriatrics Society* 53(1), 114–118.

Morillo, C. A., Camacho, M. E., Wood, M. A., Gilligan, D. M., Ellenbogen, K. A. (1999). Diagnostic utility of mechanical, pharmacological and orthostatic stimulation of the CS in patients with unexplained syncope. *Journal of the American College of Cardiology* 34(5), 1587–94.

Murphy, A. L., Rowbotham, B. J., Boyle, R. S., Thew, C. M., Fardoulys, J. A., Wilson, K. (1986). CS hypersensitivity in elderly nursing home patients. *Australian and New Zealand Journal of Medicine* 16(1), 24–27.

Nathanson, M. H. (1946). Hyperactive cardioinhibitory CS reflex. *Archives of Internal Medicine* 77, 491–502.

O'Mahony, D., Foote, C. (1998). Prospective evaluation of unexplained syncope, dizziness and falls among community-dwelling elderly adults. *Journals of Gerontology Series a-biological Sciences and Medical Sciences* 53(6), M435–40.

O'Mahony, D. (1995). Pathophysiology of CS hypersensitivity in elderly patients. *Lancet* 346(8980), 950–52.

O'Shea, D., Parry, S. W., Kenny, R. A. (2001). The Newcastle protocol for CS massage. *Journal of the American Geriatrics Society* 49(2):236–37.

Ogawa, T., Spina, R. J., Martin, W. H. 3rd, *et al.* (1992). Effects of aging, sex, and physical training on cardiovascular responses to exercise. *Circulation* 86(2), 494–503.

Parry, S., Steen, N., Baptist, M., Fiaschi, K., Parry, O., Kenny, R. (2005). Cerebral autoregulation is impaired in cardioinhibitory CS syndrome. *Heart* (In Press).

Parry, S. W., Kenny, R. A. (2005). Drop attacks in older adults: Systematic assessment has a high diagnostic yield. *Journal of the American Geriatrics Society* 53(1), 74–78.

Parry, S. W., Richardson, D. A., O'Shea, D., Sen, B., Kenny, R. A. (2000). Syncope and drop attacks in older adults: cardiovascular testing in the upright position is essential. *Heart* 83(1), 22–23.

Parry, S. W., Steen, I. N., Baptist, M., Kenny, R. A. (2005). Amnesia for loss of consciousness in CS syndrome: implications for presentation with falls. *J Am. Coll. Cardiol.* 45(11), 1840–3.

Puggioni, E., Guiducci, V., Brignole, M., *et al.* (2002). Results and complications of the CS massage performed according to the 'method of symptoms'. *Am. J Cardiol.* 89(5), 599–601.

Richardson, D. A., Bexton, R. S., Shaw, F. E., Kenny, R. A. (1997). Prevalence of cardioinhibitory CS hypersensitivity in patients 50 years or over presenting to the accident and emergency department with 'unexplained' or 'recurrent' falls. *PACE: Pacing and Clinical Electrophysiology* 20(3:Pt 2), 820–23.

Richardson, D. A., Bexton, R., Shaw, F. E., Steen, N., Bond, J., Kenny, R. A. (2000). Complications of CS massage—a prospective series of older patients. *Age Ageing* 29(5), 419–24.

Rosenbaum, D. S. (2001). T wave alternans: a mechanism of arrhythmogenesis comes of age after 100 years. *J Cardiovasc. Electrophysiol.* 12(2), 207–9.

Schellack, J., Fulenwider, J. T., Olson, R. A., Smith, R. B., Mansour, K. (1986). The CS syndrome: a frequently overlooked cause of syncope in the elderly. *Journal of Vascular Surgery* 4(4), 376–83.

Simpson, R. K., Jr, Pool, J. L., Grossman, R. G., Rose, J. E., Taylor, A. A. (1987). Neurosurgical management of CS hypersensitivity. Report of three cases. *Journal of Neurosurgery* 67(5):757–59.

Smiddy, J., Lewis, H. D. J., Dunn, M. (1972). The effect of carotid massage in older men. *Journal of Gerontology* 27(2), 209–211.

Tea, S., Mansourati, J., L'Heveder, G., Mabin, D., Blanc, J. (1996). New insights into the pathophysiology of CS syndrome. *Circulation* 93(7), 1411–1416.

Tsioufis, C. P., Kallikazaros, I. E., Toutouzas, K. P., Stefanadis, C. I., Toutouzas, P. K. (2002). Exaggerated CS massage responses are related to severe coronary artery disease in patients being evaluated for chest pain. *Clinical Cardiology* 25(4), 161–66.

van Dijk, P. T., Meulenberg, O. G., van de Sande, H. J., Habbema, J. D. (1993). Falls in dementia patients. *Gerontologist* 33(2), 200–4.

Volkmann, H., Schnerch, B., Kuhnert, H. (1990). Diagnostic value of CS hypersensitivity. *PACE: Pacing and Clinical Electrophysiology* 13(13:Pt 2), 2065–70.

Ward, C., Kenny, R. A. (1996). Reproducibility of orthostatic hypotension in symptomatic elderly. *Am. J Med.* 100, 418–22.

Ward, C., McIntosh, S. J., Kenny, R. A. (1994). The prevalence of CS syndrome in elderly patients with fractured neck of femur. *Age and Ageing* 23(Suppl 1), A16.

Wentink, J. R. M., Jansen, R. W. M. M., Hoefnagels, W. H. L. (1993). The influence of age on the response of blood pressure and heart rate to CS massage in healthy volunteers. *Cardiology in the Elderly* 1, 453–59.

Youde, J., Ruse, C., Parker, S., Fotherby, M. (2000). A high diagnostic rate in older patients attending an in older patients attending an integrated syncope clinic. *J Am. Geriatr. Soc.* 48(7), 783–87.

CHAPTER 60

Situational syncope

C.T. Paul Krediet and Wouter Wieling

Introduction

Neurally (autonomic) mediated syncope refers to a heterogeneous group of conditions in which cardiovascular reflexes that are normally useful in controlling the circulation, become overactive, resulting in loss of vasoconstrictor tone and/or bradycardia and thereby in a fall of arterial blood pressure and cerebral perfusion (Chapter 65). A prerequisite for neurally (autonomic) mediated syncope is therefore the presence of an intact autonomic nervous system.

With a limited fall in blood pressure, the patient experiences light-headedness or visual blackout, but if it is considerable, the individual loses consciousness (Wieling et al. 2009). Not only reflex mediated effects are involved but also internal, patient related and external, environmental physical factors inducing systemic hypotension and diminished cerebral blood flow. Examples of internal factors are straining and hyperventilation. A physical factor is heat exposure, which contributes to hemodynamic stress. Often there is a combination of reflex and both internal and external physical factors (Tables 60.1 and 60.2) (Sharpey-Schafer et al. 1958, Wayne 1961, Johnson et al. 1984, Van Lieshout et al. 1991b).

The terminology of syncope and its related disorders is diverse and if used imprecisely may easily become misleading (Thijs et al. 2004, Thijs et al. 2005). 'Transient loss of consciousness' covers all syncopal, epileptic, metabolic, and psychogenic forms of loss of consciousness. 'Syncope' refers to transient loss of consciousness caused by hypoperfusion of the brain resulting in hypoxia, due to disturbances in blood pressure control either from 'cardiac syncope' (arrhythmias, structural heart disease) or neurally (autonomic) mediated mechanisms (as described above). The majority of neurally mediated syncopes are 'vasovagal syncope' (see dedicated paragraph). 'Faint' is a lay term for transient loss of consciousness, whereas 'the common faint' refers to vasovagal syncope. For the latter 'vasovagal fainting' may be a useful synonym.

Situational syncope is a subclass of neurally (autonomic) mediated syncope (Table 60.1). Kapoor coined the term 'situational syncope' in the late 1980s (Kapoor 1990) and used it as a *toto pro pars* for syncope related to micturition, defecation and cough. In a later publication Kapoor emphasized that vasovagal syncope and other conditions that cause syncope, often share a situational

component as well. Occurrence of a common faint during blood drawing, prolonged motionless standing or after exhaustive exercise are typical examples (Table 60.2)(Kapoor 1994). In concurrence with this, in this chapter the term 'situational syncope' is used in a wider sense than in most literature, applying it to all forms of neurally (autonomic) mediated syncope that have well defined situational triggers or predisposing factors.

After discussing the epidemiology of neurally mediated syncope, the first part of this chapter reviews vasovagal syncope, some of its situational types, initial orthostatic hypotension and the carotid sinus syndrome. The second part focusses on situational syncopes as traditionally described in the literature (cough, defecation, micturition syncope). The third part of the chapter considers some miscellaneous causes of syncope with situational triggering.

Pattern recognition in the patient's history by the attending physician aids to correctly diagnose situational syncope. Questioning (and listening—the proces known as 'narrative medicine' [Haidet and Paterniti 2003]) is therefore directed towards the detection of typical triggers and predisposing factors that elicit situational syncope. The common forms of situational syncope are listed in Table 60.1.

Epidemiology of neurally mediated syncope

Syncope in the general population is extremely common. Almost everybody seems to have either experienced or witnessed an episode. Syncopal events often do not reach medical attention, particularly in the young in whom most episodes are considered to be innocent neurally mediated events (Soteriades et al. 2002, Colman et al. 2004a, Olde Nordkamp et al. 2009).

Studies in teenagers, adolescents and young adults show a strikingly high incidence of syncope. Two recent surveys of the frequency of syncope in medical students demonstrated that 20–25% of males and 40–50% of females report to have experienced at least one such episode (Ganzeboom et al. 2003, Serletis et al. 2006). Most syncope triggers identified in these students involved stresses or conditions that affect orthostatic blood pressure control. Neurally mediated syncope was therefore a likely cause of the symptoms in these young subjects. The incidence peak of presumed neurally mediated syncope around the age of 15 years and the much higher incidence in young females is a consistent finding (Fig. 60.1) (Ganzeboom et al. 2003, Colman et al. 2004a,

Table 60.1 Classification of neurally (autonomic) mediated syncope based on triggers

Vasovagal syncope
Orthostasis induced
Pain/invasive instrumentation (venipunctures, arterial punctures, fractures)
Emotionally induced (e.g. sight of blood or injury)
Post-exercise
Sleep vasovagal syncope
Initial orthostatic hypotension
Carotid sinus syncope
Trigeminal 'reflex' syncope
Ocular syncope
Trigeminal neuralgia syncope
Gastrointestinal
Swallow syncope (glossopharyngeal neuralgia, oesophageal syncope) defecation syncope; gastrointestinal tract instrumentation; rectal examination
Urogenital
(Post)-micturition syncope, urogenital tract instrumentation, prostatic massage
Increased intrathoracic pressure
Cough and sneeze syncope; singer's/wind instrument player's syncope; weight-lifter's syncope, mess trick and fainting lark stretch syncope
Miscellaneous causes (not neurally mediated)
Diving and swimming; subclavian steal syndrome; acceleration induced syncope

Table 60.2 Predisposing factors for neurally (autonomic) mediated syncope

High ambient temperature, confined spaces or crowding
Emotional circumstances, pain
Menstrual period
Hypocapnia
Hypoxia
Fever
Rapid weight loss
Alcohol
Insufficient food intake, starvation (e.g. anorexia nervosa)
Sleep deprivation, tiredness
Prolonged bed rest or weightlessness
After strenuous exercise
During exposure to multiple G-forces
Medications influencing cardiovascular control (e.g. diuretics, beta-blockers)

From Colman et al. 2004b.

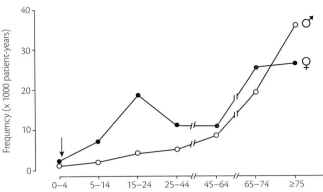

Fig. 60.1 Frequency of the complaint 'fainting' as reason for encounter in general practice in the Netherlands. It concerns an analysis of 93,297 patient-years. The arrow around 1 year is to indicate that a small peak occurs between 6–18 months (breath-holding spells) (Chapter 62). With permission from Wieling et al. 2003.

Ganzeboom et al. 2006, Serletis et al. 2006, Sheldon et al. 2006). A family history of presumed neurally mediated syncope in the first degree relatives is often present in young fainting subjects (Mathias et al. 1998, Serletis et al. 2006). Compared with the 30% prevalence of presumed neurally mediated syncope in young medical students, the prevalence of epileptic seizures in a similar young age group is much lower (<1%) (Wallace et al. 1998) and syncope from cardiac arrhythmias or structural heart disease (i.e. cardiac syncope) is even less common (Colman et al. 2004a).

A first neurally mediated syncopal episode is rare in adults of 30–50 years of age. About 80% of the syncope patients in this age group have experienced presumed neurally mediated episodes as teenagers and adolescents, which may be of help in establishing a diagnosis (Ganzeboom et al. 2006, Serletis et al. 2006).

Patients with presumed neurally mediated syncope present themselves to general practitioners according to a bimodal age distribution, with a first peak at the age of 15 years, and a second peak in older adults and the elderly (Fig. 60.2) (Colman et al. 2004a).

Typical vasovagal syncope is less common in senior persons. It is not unusual that the episodes of vasovagal syncope which a senior patient experiences are far less typical than vasovagal syncope at younger age. Thus, neurally mediated syncope may be considered as a chronic life-long condition, with different clinical presentation and triggers among episodes (Kurbaan et al. 2003, Colman et al. 2004a, Sheldon et al. 2006).

In senior subjects cardiac causes of syncope, orthostatic and postprandial hypotension and carotid sinus hypersensitivity are more frequent (Kapoor 1994, Youde et al. 2000, Mukai and Lipsitz 2002). This can be attributed to diminished efficiency of cardiovascular regulatory systems, to medications affecting orthostatic blood pressure control and to increased prevalence of organic disease (e.g. structural heart disease, cardiac arrhythmia's) (Brady and Shen 1999). In the elderly, multiple causes of syncope are often present and the medical history may be less reliable than in the young, for example syncope may be erroneously reported as a fall (McIntosh et al. 1993, Kapoor 1994, Benke et al. 1997, Kenny 2003).

In large clinical series of patients with transient loss of consciousness 'situational syncope' accounts for about 5% of cases of

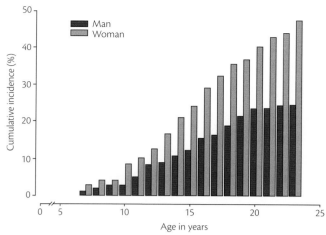

Fig. 60.2 Cumulative incidence of syncope according to age in medical students in the Academic Medical Center at the University of Amsterdam: 118 females (of 252, 47%) with at least one episode of syncope and 30 males (of 124, 24%) with at least one episode of syncope. Reprinted from *American Journal of Cardiology*, **91**, Ganzeboom, K. S. et al., Prevalence and triggers of syncope in medical students, pp. 1006–1008, Copyright 2003, with permission from Elsevier.

transient loss of consciousness (Ammirati et al. 2000, Blanc et al. 2002, Van Dijk et al. 2008). Most forms of situational syncope seem to have their typical age distribution (e.g. initial orthostatic hypotension in the young and swallow syncope in the elderly).

Situational vasovagal syncope

Recognized triggers for vasovagal syncope are prolonged orthostatic stress, blood drawing, instrumentation (see dedicated paragraph) and psychological stressors (Cotton and Lewis 1918, Lewis 1932, Stevens 1966, Van Lieshout et al. 1991b, Van Dijk et al. 2001) (Figs. 60.3 and 60.4).

Psychological stressors include stirring emotional news or witnessing a distressing accident (Lewis 1932, Engel et al. 1944) and unexpected pain or threat (Lewis 1932, Greenfield 1951, Sharpey-Schafer 1956b). Unpleasant smells may trigger vasovagal syncope (Engel and Romano 1947, Ganzeboom et al. 2003). During blood

drawing, vaccination (Braun et al. 1997) or instrumentation, pain of the procedure may contribute to vasovagal syncope. Sharp pain is reported to be an important factor during arterial blood sampling (Rushmer 1944). However, in a patient with blood phobia just thinking or talking about blood drawing may elicit a common faint (Van Dijk et al. 2001). Interestingly blood phobia is the only phobia that can induce vasovagal syncope. Other phobias usually cause arousal with tachycardia and an increased systemic blood pressure (Marks 1988).

There are several situational factors that, by themselves do not trigger syncope, but can act as predisposing factors, such as a high ambient temperatures (Table 60.2) (Graham and Kenny 2001, Wilson et al. 2006). Other environmental factors include confined spaces or crowding ('church syncope' and 'rock concert syncope') (Lewis 1932, Sharpey-Schafer et al. 1958, Moss and McEvedy 1966, Lempert and Bauer 1995, Graham and Kenny 2001), stopping of strenuous exercise ('post exercise vasovagal syncope') (Krediet et al. 2004b), staying at high altitude (Douglas et al. 1913, Westendorp et al. 1997), presence of fever (Kopp 1937) or migraine (Thijs et al. 2006), recent illness or ill health (Cotton and Lewis 1918, Lewis 1932, Wayne 1961), lack of sleep (Ganzeboom et al. 2003), menstruation (Graham and Kenny 2001), rapid weight loss, prolonged bed rest or after weightlessness (space travel) (Buckey, Jr et al. 1996, Gisolf et al. 2005), any form of nausea (Sharpey-Schafer et al. 1958) or motion sickness (Bosser et al. 2006), presence of fatigue (Graham and Kenny 2001), period of fasting and starvation (Bennett et al. 1984, Graham and Kenny 2001) and the use of alcohol (Narkiewicz et al. 2000) and illicit drugs. Witnessing a faint may trigger vasovagal fainting in the witness himself, mass vasovagal fainting can be the result (Moss and McEvedy 1966, Lempert and Bauer 1995). All the factors mentioned here typically affect young, rather than older subjects (over 50 years of age).

Details of presentation, pathophysiology, diagnosis and treatment of vasovagal syncope are given in Chapter 65.

Vasovagal syncope during medical instrumentation

The proneness to vasovagal fainting is strongly increased by the use of intravascular, especially intra-arterial instrumentation (Rushmer 1944, Stevens 1966). Whereas in general, syncope is typically

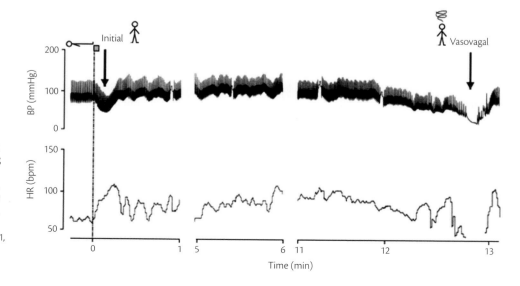

Fig. 60.3 Vasovagal faint in a healthy 22-year-old male. Note the pronounced, but still normal initial heart rate and blood pressure response and marked increase in heart rate after 6 minutes standing. After about 11 minutes of standing, blood pressure and heart rate start to decrease to very low values during syncope, the heart rate tracing during syncope is interrupted by a period of asystole of 7 seconds. On lying down, heart rate and blood pressure recover quickly. Reproduced with permission, from Van Lieshout, J. J., Wieling, W., Karemaker, J. M., and Eckberg, D. L. 1991, *Clinical Science*, vol. **81**, pp. 575–586, © the Biochemical Society.

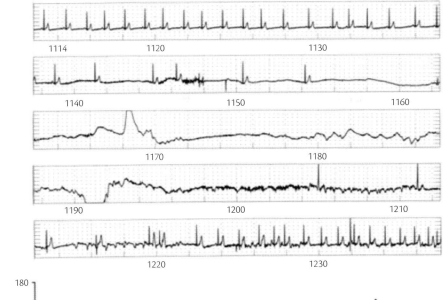

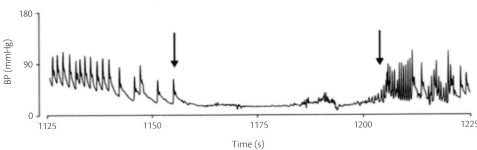

Fig. 60.4 Electrocardiography and continuous blood pressure recordings during 50 seconds of asystole in a 17-year-old male with blood phobia. This vasovagal syncope was elicited by talking about his phobia. Time (s) is taken from the original recording. With permission from Van Dijk, N., et al. 2001, *Pacing and Clinical Electrophysiology*, Wiley.

associated with a standing or sitting position, syncope associated with medical instrumentation may also occur while supine (Verrill and Aellig 1970). Examples are syncope occurring during or shortly after vaccination (Braun et al. 1997), rectal examination (Scott and Sancetta 1950), colonoscopy (Selleger et al. 1988, Herman et al. 1993, Newton et al. 2001), cardiac catheterization (Landau et al. 1994), prostate examination (Bilbro 1970), hysteroscopy (Agostini et al. 2004) and intrauterine device insertion (Menzies 1978).

Another typical example is iatrogenic syncope during pharyngo-oesophageal-gastric manipulations such as during laryngoscopy or gastroscopy (Palmer 1976). Special attention should be given to tetraplegic patients with high cervical spinal cord lesions who are in spinal shock and unable to breathe spontaneously. They are prone to bradycardia and cardiac arrest during tracheal suction (Mathias 1976), which is more likely to occur when they are hypoxic. This bradycardia appears to be due to a vago-vagal reflex similar to that in swallow syncope. A number of factors may play a role including absent sympathetic activity, airway receptor stimulation, hypoxia and the inability to breathe spontaneously. The bradycardia in response to tracheal suction can be prevented by adequate oxygenation, or if this cannot be achieved, by repeated atropine or even a cardiac demand pacemaker (Mathias 1976) (see also Chapter 70).

Vasovagal syncope after exercise

Syncope *after* exercise is often neurally mediated, i.e. post-exercise vasovagal syncope. This condition is typically diagnosed in young fit, furthermore healthy young patients. Foremost, the diagnostic workup of all patients presenting with exercise-related syncope is aimed at excluding dangerous cardiac conditions and includes echocardiography and exercise testing (Krediet et al. 2004b).

During exercise, rhythmically contracting skeletal muscles in the lower part of the body reduce the degree of venous pooling by squeezing veins, thereby increasing the venous return of blood to the heart. This phenomenon is known as the 'muscle pump'. The sudden removal of the muscle pump after stopping exercise decreases cardiac preload, which in combination with a rapid return of vagal tone may promote vasovagal syncope. Characteristically, syncope may occur while the individual is standing motionless during the first five to ten minutes after exercise (Bjurstedt et al. 1983). Especially athletes in the (ultra) endurance sports are at risk for post-exercise vasovagal syncope, for example after marathon swimming (Finlay et al. 1995) or marathon running (Tsutsumi and Hara 1979, Levine et al. 1991, Holtzhausen and Noakes 1995).

Vasovagal syncope after routine treadmill testing is rare (estimated 0.2%(Schlesinger 1973)). However, when treadmill testing is immediately followed by passive head-up tilt testing, this percentage can increase up to 50–70% (Bjurstedt et al. 1983). Vasovagal syncope after exercise is considered to be a benign occurrence (Krediet et al. 2004b).

Vasovagal syncope in airliners

Vasovagal episodes are the most common in-flight medical events, and may affect patients of all ages (Gendreau and DeJohn 2002). In addition to prolonged motionless sitting, the use of alcohol, anxiety and mild hypoxia during air travel all may predispose to vasovagal faints (Sutton 1999). Cabin pressure in commercial aircraft is usually adjusted to the equivalent of an altitude of 1500–2500 metres above sea level. It appears that hypoxic syncope results from the superimposed vasodilator effects of hypoxia on the cardiovascular system (Halliwill and Minson 2005).

Patients who otherwise never experienced a (severe) vasovagal episode may suffer from convulsive syncope during air travel (Wieling et al. 2006). These patients should be advised to have a high salt intake in the days prior to travelling by plane, reducing antihypertensive medication—if feasible—and drinking non-alcoholic beverages galore during the trip. Especially during long flights (> 2 hours) they should perform in-chair muscle tensing exercise and have a regular walk through the aisle. In recurrent cases midodrine prior to flying or supportive stockings can be considered.

Sleep vasovagal syncope

Sleep vasovagal syncope is defined as loss of consciousness in a non-intoxicated adult occurring during the night (e. g. 10:00 pm to 7:00 am), in which the patient wakes up with pre-syncopal and abdominal symptoms (i.e. an urge to defecate) and loses consciousness in bed or immediately upon standing (Krediet et al. 2004a, Marrison and Parry 2007, Jardine et al. 2009). Tongue biting or postictal confusion have not been reported. There is usually a history of daytime vasovagal syncope and there seems to be a more pronounced fear of blood and medical procedures than in other syncope patients (Jardine et al. 2009). Physical examination, electrocardiography (ECG) and electroencephalography (EEG) are within normal limits. Sleep vasovagal syncope is diagnosed by excluding beyond reasonable doubt the hereafter mentioned disorders (Jardine et al. 2006). During syncope there may be a profound sinus-bradycardia or prolonged asystoles (Krediet et al. 2004a). Vasovagal sleep syncope occurs at all ages. The vasovagal reaction

is thought to start while asleep (Krediet et al. 2004a, Jardine et al. 2006), and continuing after waking up, hence the name.

The two foremost diagnoses to exclude are epilepsy and cardiac disorders. Complex partial, generalized tonic-clonic and myoclonic epilepsy may occur during sleep and can imitate syncope when causing cause sinus-bradycardia (Tinuper et al. 2001). Repeated EEG testing may be indicated (Tinuper et al. 2001). Occasionally cardiac disorders may cause cardiac arrhythmias during sleep. Most of these are unlikely if the 12-lead ECG is normal, but in some patients long-term ambulatory ECG monitoring is required (Brierley et al. 2001). The differential diagnosis of sleep vasovagal syncope after excluding epilepsy and cardiac disorders has been discussed elsewhere (Jardine et al. 2006).

Some patients with a diagnosis of defecation syncope (see p.737) described abdominal and pre-syncopal symptoms that started simultaneously during sleep (Pathy 1978, Fisher 1979), there may be some overlap between this condition and sleep syncope (Jardine et al. 2006).

Initial orthostatic hypotension after arising from supine or squatting

Most teenagers and adolescents are familiar with a brief feeling of light-headedness and some visual blurring within a few seconds of standing up quickly (de Marées 1976). Symptoms typically resolve spontaneously within 20 seconds. Such complaints are most common upon arising suddenly after prolonged supine rest or after arising from the squatted position (Figs. 60.5 and 60.6) (Wieling et al. 2007). In some the symptoms are severe and syncope may occur upon standing in otherwise healthy subjects (Wieling et al. 2007). In a recent study in 394 medical students standing up was reported as the trigger for transient loss of consciousness in 8% (Ganzeboom et al. 2003).

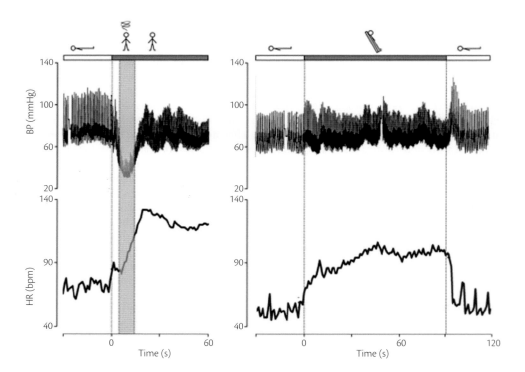

Fig. 60.5 Changes in heart rate and blood pressure in a 20-year-old male with an asthenic habitus (197 cm, 73 kg) and a 10-year history of almost daily near-syncope and occasional syncope upon standing up. Note the marked initial fall in finger blood pressure accompanied by light-headedness upon active standing, but not upon passive head-up tilt. With permission from Van Dijk, Harms, and Wieling 2000.

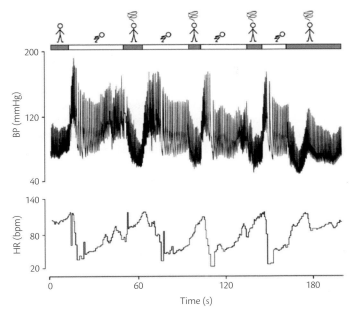

Fig. 60.6 Continuous recording of blood pressure and heart rate during four squat-to-stand manoeuvres in a 37-year-old female referred for evaluation of severe light-headedness and occasional syncope after such manoeuvres. The patient reported that before the loss of consciousness she saw black spots and felt light-headed. Each time she stood up, she complained of the same symptoms that she had originally experienced (light-headedness and seeing 'black spots'). Reproduced with permission of the publisher from Krediet 2002.

The initial orthostatic complaints originate from a transient rapid fall in arterial pressure occurring upon active standing. This fall in blood pressure is a physiological response (Sprangers et al. 1991, Thomas et al. 2009). However, normally blood pressure does not drop for more than 40 mm Hg systolic and 20 mm Hg diastolic (Chapter 23). The onset of symptoms between 5–10 seconds and disappearance within 20 seconds after standing up is typical for this condition. The diagnosis can only be confirmed by a stand test with continuous beat-to-beat blood pressure monitoring (Figs. 60.5 and 60.6) (Wieling et al. 2007). The test is specific, but in our experience not sensitive. Because initial orthostatic hypotension is associated with 'active' arising (Fig. 60.5), tilt testing (i.e. head-up tilting) is not a proper provoking test.

An abnormally large initial fall in blood pressure also occurs in a variety of conditions that affect arterial baroreflex control of sympathetic activation of resistance vessels (Wieling et al. 2007). Examples are patients with de-afferentiated carotid sinus baroreceptors after neck surgery (impairment of afferent pathways) (Smit et al. 2002), subjects receiving clonidine (blockade of central pathways) (Coupland et al. 1995), α-antagonists for prostate hyperplasia, or heterocyclic antidepressants (blockade of efferent pathways) (Schlingemann et al. 1996, Wieling et al. 2001, Wilt et al. 2003).

Rising from squatting encompasses a greater orthostatic stress than rising from supine (Sharpey-Schafer 1956a, Rossberg and Penáz 1988) (see paragraph on the 'fainting lark'). On average blood pressure in healthy young adults falls transiently by 60 mm Hg systolic and 40 mm Hg diastolic with a nadir about 7 seconds after rising (Rossberg and Penáz 1988). Mild symptoms of transient light-headedness are often present. Rising from squatting is a recognized trigger for syncope in daily life (Fig. 60.6). Arising after

prolonged squatting during gardening or household activities is a common scenario (Sharpey-Schafer 1956a).

The squat-stand test with continuous blood pressure measurement can be a helpful tool in documenting this form of situational syncope (Barbey et al. 1966, de Marées 1976, Convertino et al. 1998, Rickards and Newman 2003).

Treatment of initial orthostatic hypotension is symptomatic. The goal is to diminish the drop in blood pressure after standing up. A clear explanation of the underlying mechanism and avoidance of the main triggers (rapid rise) are the main treatment options. A novel approach is training in blood pressure rising manoeuvres. Tensing of leg, abdominal and buttock muscles for 20–40 seconds at maximal voluntary force immediately after standing up may be an effective manoeuvre to decrease the fall in pressure (Krediet et al. 2007). In addition volume expansion can be applied by raising water and salt intake (Shichiri et al. 2002, Wieling et al. 2004).

Carotid sinus syndrome

This syndrome was first described by the Prague physiologist J.N. Czermak (1828–1873) in 1866. Using E.-J. Marey's (1830–1904) wrist sphygmograph (the first practical instrument to record the arterial pulse wave, continuously and non-invasively) (Marey 1860) he documented carotid sinus hypersensitivity in himself while rubbing his right carotid artery (Czermak 1866). Contrary to current insight he assumed that he was directly stimulating the vagus nerve being unaware of the existence of carotid baroreceptors, only to be discovered in 1927 (Hering 1927). The definition of carotid sinus hypersensitivity from the 1930s (Weiss and Baker 1933) includes asystole lasting > 3 seconds (cardio-inhibitory type), or systolic blood pressure falls > 50 mmHg (vasodepressor type), or both (mixed type) in response to carotid sinus massage for 5–10 seconds (Moya et al. 2009). Carotid sinus hypersensitivity is almost exclusively diagnosed in patients over 50 years of age (Franke 1963).

The prevalence of spontaneous carotid sinus syndrome induced by everyday manipulations like wearing a tight collar, shaving, head turning or stretching the neck is unknown, but likely to be rare, since its occurrence is reported as only ~1% of causes of syncope in clinical settings (for review see Colman et al. 2004a). However in a series of 33 cases of carotid sinus hypersensitivity (among a total of 130 consecutive syncope patients) Kenny reported head-turning as a trigger in 52% of cases (Kenny and Traynor 1991). Most syncopal episodes attributed to carotid sinus hypersensitivity after laboratory testing occur apparently spontaneously.

Since the reflex can be triggered in otherwise healthy elderly without a history compatible with the carotid sinus syndrome (i.e. falls, dizziness and light-headedness) (Humm and Mathias 2006, Kerr et al. 2006) the true clinical importance of carotid sinus hypersensitivity remains unclear (Krediet et al. 2011).

In the older literature the clinical presentations of this disorder are reported to be heterogeneous. In the vasodepressor type patients would be likely to have a prodrome pattern as in classical vasovagal syncope, whereas the cardio-inhibitory type could occur without warning and present as a clinical Adams–Stokes attack. In the latter, on regaining consciousness typically there is a facial flush (Franke and Bracharz 1956). However even under standardized laboratory conditions both types often cannot be distinguished on clinical grounds.

Cardiac pacing is the therapy of choice in syncope patients with documented asystole in response to carotid sinus massage, or on ambulatory ECG recording (Kenny et al. 2001, Brignole et al. 2006). Since loss of consciousness seldom occurs with asystolic episodes lasting < 6 s, the duration of asystole that warrants pacemaker therapy is debated (Krediet et al. 2011). The vasodepressor type is likely to benefit from general orthostatic tolerance enhancing measures such as salt and volume loading, and there is some evidence that fludrocortisone may be effective (Hussain et al. 1996). However up to date there are no adequately powered clinical trials on the subject.

Trigeminal 'reflex' syncopes

Ocular syncope

Sudden pressure on the eyeball and orbital contents, including extraocular muscles can induce syncope by the oculocardiac reflex (Wieling and Khurana 2006). This reflex was first described in 1908 by Bernard Aschner (1883–1960) and Guiseppe Dagnini (1866–1928) in almost simultaneous reports (Aschner 1908, Dagnini 1908). The strength of the oculocardiac reflex diminishes with age (Arnold et al. 1991). It is a trigeminal-brainstem-vagal reflex that can elicit pronounced bradycardia or asystole and thereby syncope. An example is syncope immediately after being hit by a tennis ball on the eye (Wieling and Khurana 2006), which leads instantaneously to syncope (i.e. loss of consciousness in such cases does not necessarily point to cerebral concussion). This reflex may also cause bradycardia during eye surgery (Brocklin et al. 1982). The oculocardiac reflex has been employed to differentiate between syncopal and epileptic seizures in infants (Stephenson 1978) and has also been reported to be beneficial in aborting or attenuating attacks of paroxysmal atrial tachycardia (Wieling and Khurana 2006). Some of the reported cases of bradycardia in response to ocular stimulation like placing a contact lens are not due to the activation of the oculocardiac reflex but belong to vasovagal type of situational syncope (Khurana 2002).

Syncope from trigeminal neuralgia

Only four case reports (the first by Kapoor in 1984) describe syncope triggered by trigeminal neuralgia (Kapoor and Jannetta 1984,

Arias 1985, Bonamico and Celnik 1995, Gottesman et al. 1996), often with a profound reflex asystole. Trigeminal neuralgia is a pain syndrome with episodes of shooting facial pain (Burchiel and Slavin 2000). This pain may be triggered by chewing and syncope is a rare complication (Rushton et al. 1981). Trigeminal neuralgia is thought to be based on micro-injuries to the nerve root and may occur in combination with glossopharyngeal neuralgia (Rushton et al. 1981). Syncope from trigeminal neuralgia is thought to be based on a trigeminal-brainstem-vagal reflex, similar to that of ocular syncope. Treatment focuses on the pain syndrome.

Gastrointestinal syncope

Swallow syncope

Swallow syncope incorporates two separate conditions:

♦ a pharyngeal form, which is usually associated with pain ('syncopal glossopharyneal neuralgia')

♦ an oesophageal variety, also known as 'oesophageal' or 'deglutition syncope' (Fig. 60.7) (Deuchar and Trounce 1960, Basker and Cooper 2000).

The first isolated case description dates to 1906 (Mackenzie 1906). Based on the fact that up to that date only about sixty single cases have been reported (Deuchar and Trounce 1960, Basker and Cooper 2000), swallow syncope is probably rare. A systematic case series does not exist. Typically deglutition syncope occurs in older subjects (over 50 years of age), but it has also been reported in children (Basker and Cooper 2000).

The clinical presentation of glossopharyngeal neuralgia is a patient with (seemingly) spontaneous overwhelming pain in a jaw, tongue or throat. In some patients, this pain can be triggered by touching a certain spot in the oral cavity, or by talking or swallowing. Among all patients with glossopharyngeal neuralgia, syncope seems a rare complication (Rushton et al. 1981).

In the oesophageal variety, syncope typically occurs during or shortly after swallowing. Several reports point especially to cold drinks as the culprit (Rainford 1975, Brick et al. 1978, Olshansky 1999). Syncope triggered by belching has been reported (Kim et al. 2005). There are some reports that mention retro-sternal pain induced by swallowing as a trigger (Basker and Cooper 2000).

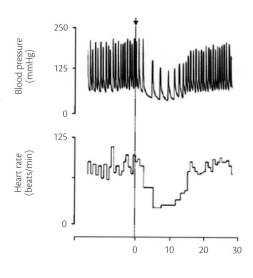
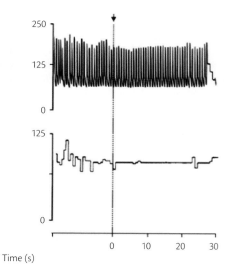

Fig. 60.7 Effects of swallowing (arrow) on blood pressure and heart rate in a 78-year-old male with syncope induced by swallowing before (left panel) and after (right panel) installation of an external on demand pacemaker. With permission from Piek, Imholz, Duren, and Wieling, 1988.

Time (s)

Several cases report oesophageal syncope during recovery from myocardial infarction (Basker and Cooper 2000). Swallowing syncope is characterized by a slow or absent pulse.

The pathophysiology of both entities is poorly understood. The possible neurological pathways and mechanisms that might be involved in swallow syncope cannot be explained on the basis of any known normal reflex (Basker and Cooper 2000). Oesophageal syncope is often ascribed to a vago-vagal reflex (i.e. both afferent and efferent stimulus through the vagus nerve) (Piek et al. 1988), however this merely describes part of the peripheral functional anatomy. Antihypertensive medications are considered to contribute to the proneness for this type of syncope in some patients (Basker and Cooper 2000).

In many cases of oesophageal syncope functional, endoscopic and radiological studies reveal oesophageal abnormalities including diverticulum, hiatal hernia, achalasia, stricture and neoplasms (Basker and Cooper 2000). Although such co-morbidity may be over-reported, this may be an argument to commence an in-depth gastro-oesophageal evaluation.

There are several therapeutic options. In case of overt oesophageal lesions, these should be treated. Management of persisting neuralgia is symptomatic. Modification of antihypertensive drugs should be considered. Based on predominantly positive therapeutic response in over a dozen cases, the treatment of choice of oesophageal syncope is insertion of a cardiac demand pacemaker (Piek et al. 1988, Basker and Cooper 2000). Surgical or pharmacological destruction of (the oesophageal branches of) the vagus nerve is considered obsolete (Basker and Cooper 2000).

Defecation syncope

'Defecation syncope' was first reported in 1978 (Pathy 1978). This series counted 9 patients (63–78 years of age, 7 women). The only other (isolated) series counted 20 subjects (mean age 59 years, 13 women) and dates from 1986 (Kapoor et al. 1986). Epidemiological data from the general population do not exist. There are few case reports that focus on the disorder, often in concurrence with other pathology. Typically episodes occur in the early morning after patients have got out of bed with an urge to defecate. There may be an overlap with nocturnal vasovagal syncope (Krediet et al. 2004a, Jardine et al. 2006) (for details see p.734).

Defecation syncope has been attributed to the raised intrathoracic and intra-abdominal pressure which can accompany bowel movements (Pathy 1978). Moreover reflex mechanisms from the rectum are likely to be involved (Pathy 1978). In a heroic paper by George L. Engel (1913–1999) and John Romano (1908–1994), reflex bradycardia (with sinus arrest and idioventricular rhythm) in one of the authors was documented, triggered by inflating a colon balloon with about 3 litres of air up to 40 cm H_2O pressure (Engel et al. 1944).

In Kapoor's series, diagnostic evaluation revealed an underlying cardiovascular (arrhythmias), gastrointestinal (neoplasmatic) or neurological illness in 50% of the cases (10 from 20) (Kapoor et al. 1986). Furthermore defecation is a known trigger for acute pulmonary thromboembolism (Yamada et al. 2005, Culic 2006). Patients with defecation syncope should undergo careful evaluation to exclude such underlying illness. As management, patients are instructed to avoid straining during defecation. Documented asystoles may be an indication for cardiac pacing.

Micturition syncope

The original reports described the condition in healthy young men, mostly military personnel (Proudfit and Forteza 1959, Lyle Jr et al. 1961) whereas later reports focus on older subjects (Kapoor et al. 1985). Preceding supine rest is typical but not obligatory (Haldane 1969). Cases of women with micturition syncope are rare (Gastaut 1956). Recently an episode during pregnancy was reported (Gastaut 1956, Sherer et al. 2005).

Typically the patient is a healthy male adult who in the early morning hours after waking rises to urinate and loses consciousness during or immediately after standing urination. There may be few or no warning symptoms (Johnson et al. 1984). Predisposing factors include reduced food intake, and/or ingestion of alcohol the night before (Lyle Jr et al. 1961). In particular large quantities of beer may provide both alcohol and sufficient bladder distension (Johnson et al. 1984). Predisposing factors in older subjects include the use of antihypertensive medications (Lyle Jr et al. 1961, Johnson et al. 1984). Daytime episodes are only reported in the elderly (Kapoor et al. 1985), but may also happen to the young. Recurrences of micturition syncope do occur (Kapoor et al. 1985).

Probably a combination of physiological changes during micturition after waking act together leading to syncope. Firstly, sleep is associated with a low arterial blood pressure (Veerman et al. 1995), and the warm bed may facilitate additional cutaneous vasodilatation (Johnson et al. 1984). Secondly, during micturition, sudden emptying of the full bladder causes acutely withdrawal of sympathetic tone (Fagius and Karhuvaara 1989). The hyper-lordotic posture that some men attain when urinating may increase pressure on the lower vena cava (Haldane 1969), thus further compromising the normal circulation. In the elderly straining (e.g. in the presence of bladder outflow obstructions) (Prozan and Litwin 1961), the use of medications that interfere with blood pressure control and pre-existent orthostatic hypotension (Kapoor et al. 1985) or cardiac conductance disorders may be contributing factors (Kapoor et al. 1985).

In the evaluation of elderly patients, factors influencing bladder filling (i.e. prostatic hyperplasia) should be sought. Patients should be advised to sit during micturition and medications interfering with normal blood pressure control are to be avoided.

Syncope from increased intrathoracic pressure

Cough syncope

This type of syncope typically occurs in middle-aged and senior, muscularly built men with a history of chronic obstructive lung disease (Sharpey-Schafer 1953b, Bonekat et al. 1987). The syndrome was first described by J.-M. Charcot (1825–1893) in 1879 (Charcot 1879). Originally cough syncope was thought to be a form of epilepsy (Charcot 1879) and only in the 1940s it was recognized to be of syncopal nature (Rook 1946, McCann and Bruce 1949). Typically syncope occurs after coughing, but it has also been reported interrupting a cough (Fig. 60.8) (Sharpey-Schafer 1953b, Mattle et al. 1995). Cough syncope usually occurs while sitting or standing, but may also occur supine (McIntosh et al. 1956). Consciousness rapidly recovers, typically with few vasomotor or other sequelae (McIntosh et al. 1956).

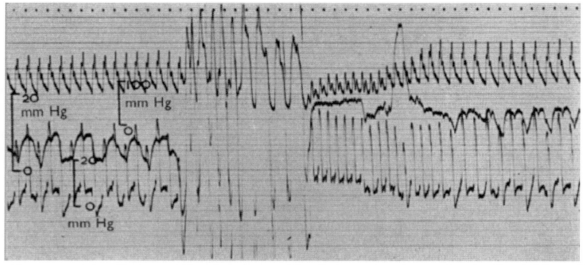

Fig. 60.8 Arterial pressure record of coughing. Large arterial cough transients were followed by hypotension and syncope. Reproduced from *BMJ*, Sharpey-Schafer E. P., **4841**, pp. 860–863, Copyright 1953 with permission from BMJ Publishing Group Ltd.

Three main mechanisms have been postulated to be involved in cough syncope. Firstly, muscularly built males with obstructive lung disease are capable of building up the high intrathoracic pressures that trigger cough syncope (300–450 mmHg compared with less than 100 mmHg in healthy young subjects (Sharpey-Schafer 1953a, Sharpey-Schafer 1965, Van Lieshout et al. 1989). These abrupt very high intra thoracic pressures diminish venous return and cardiac filling and thereby cardiac output (Sharpey-Schafer 1953a). On the arterial side, the abruptly increased intrathoracic pressure is transferred to the systemic circulation, causing vasodilatation (Sharpey-Schafer 1953a, Krediet and Wieling 2008). As in other forms of syncope the mean arterial pressure at which loss of consciousness occurs in cough syncope is about 50 mmHg (Sharpey-Schafer 1953a, Sharpey-Schafer 1965). Sharpey-Schafer considered cough syncope an exaggeration of the post cough fall in blood pressure observed in middle aged and elderly males. In young adults this fall is small, even if coughing is performed in the standing position (Van Lieshout et al. 1989). Up to date, the potential contribution of functional changes in the pulmonary vasculature in obstructive lung disease to the development of cough syncope, have not been studied.

Secondly, the increased intrathoracic pressure is also transmitted to the cerebral spinal fluid (McIntosh et al. 1956), causing an acute pressure increase in the skull, compromising cerebral perfusion (McIntosh et al. 1956, Mattle et al. 1995). In addition, the combination of increased venous pressure in the skull (by the increased intrathoracic pressure (Sharpey-Schafer 1953a)) and the lowered arterial pressure results in perfusion stand-still or even back-flow in the brain (Mattle et al. 1995). This cerebral ischemia mechanism is based on observations in few patients and remains to be better defined. Thirdly, 'cough concussion' has been suggested as a potential mechanism which holds that during coughing the combination of acute increases of arterial, venous and cerebrospinal fluid pressures in the skull, directly compromise cerebral functions (Kerr, Jr and Eich 1961). The importance of 'cough concussion' is also based on observations in a mere few patients and is unclear.

Cough syncope is rarely observed in women (Kerr, Jr and Derbes 1953, Sharpey-Schafer 1953b, Bonekat et al. 1987). In children it may accompany asthmatic attacks and whooping cough (Haslam and Freigang 1985). Occasionally cough syncope may be associated with carotid sinus hypersensitivity (McIntosh et al. 1956, Wenger et al. 1980), cardiomyopathy (White et al. 1975), sick sinus syndrome (Choi et al. 1989), stenoses of cerebral arteries (Linzer et al. 1992) and herniated cerebral tonsils (Larson et al. 1974).

The diagnosis of cough syncope may be confirmed by having the patient cough while sitting up-right, and continuously measuring blood pressure and heart rate. This may also provide an opportunity to show the patient that avoiding violent coughing may prevent syncope (Sharpey-Schafer 1953b). Further treatment focuses on diminishing cough (i.e. symptomatic therapy) and cessation of smoking (Bonekat et al. 1987).

Based on similar pathophysiology as during cough, syncope can also occur after sneezing or laughter (Cox et al. 1997, Bloomfield and Jazrawi 2005). In narcoleptic patients cataplexy may present as transient loss of consciousness after laughing.

Trumpet playing, singing and weight lifting

In trumpet playing prolonged high notes are accompanied by high intrathoracic pressure. This may cause loss of consciousness after about 12 seconds (Faulkner and Sharpey-Schafer 1959). In the (partial) absence of a normal autonomic nervous system singing a scale is another provocation that may provoke (near)syncope. The influence of straining during singing is illustrated by the effect of these manoeuvres in a patient with a high spinal cord lesion (Fig. 60.9) (Van Lieshout et al. 1991a). In the absence of such lesions, singing standing in a choir is a typical orthostatic stress that may predispose to vasovagal syncope.

There is one report that weight-lifters are liable to syncope when performing a 'clean-and-jerk' lift. This is thought to be caused by unintentional hyperventilation before making the lift, a raised intrathoracic pressure while pushing the bar, combined with rising from squatting (Compton et al. 1973) (see paragraph

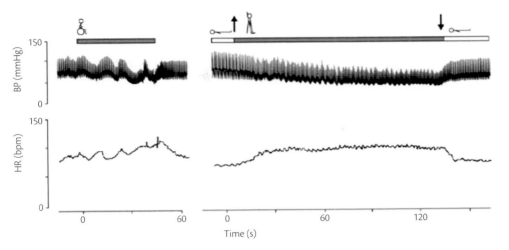

Fig. 60.9 Cardiovascular responses to singing (left) and head-up tilt (right) in a patient with a high spinal cord lesion. On singing a scale, blood pressure drops sharply at high pitched notes, this is comparable to the circulatory effects of about 10 mmHg of Valsalva straining. Reproduced with permission of the publisher from Van Lieshout et al. 1991a.

'fainting lark'). Recent work has confirmed that cerebral perfusion during intense static two-legged exercise is dominated by a (non-intentional) Valsalva manoeuvre (Pott et al. 2003) which may, in combination with standing up from squatting, elicited syncope in some.

Fainting lark

The 'fainting lark' is a self-applied manoeuvre that induces syncope (Howard et al. 1951, Lamb et al. 1960, Wieling and Van Lieshout 2002). Self-induced fainting has been used by children, high school students and military recruits as entertainment for their friends and for more practical purposes such as avoiding imminent examinations (Howard et al. 1951, Lamb et al. 1960, Johnson et al. 1984). Lempert documented the sequence of events during abrupt onset syncope in young subjects using this manoeuvre (Lempert et al. 1994). The procedure consists of squatting in a full knee bend and over-breathing by taking about 20 deep breaths. The subject then stands up suddenly and performs a forced expiration against a closed glottis (Fig. 60.10).

The fainting lark combines the effects of systemic arterial hypotension induced by acute vasodilatation of the lower limbs (post-ischaemic effect of squatting and hypocapnia) and decreased cardiac output (effects of arising and raised intrathoracic pressure [Pott et al. 2000]) and cerebral vasoconstriction induced by hyperventilation driven hypocapnia (Howard and Leathart 1951). This hypocapnia has a differential effect on muscle (vasodilatation, in autonomic failure patients hyperventilation leads acutely to an invalidating hypotension) versus brain (vasoconstriction) vasculature (Howard and Leathart 1951, Brown, Jr 1953) (Chapter 56). In healthy subjects hyperventilation alone is not a trigger strong enough to thus elicit syncope, however in syncope patients diminished vasoconstrictor reserve may give a more profound response.

The high venous cerebral venous pressure induced by straining can be expected to play an important adjunctive role in the effectiveness of the fainting lark to induce syncope (Gastaut and Fischer-Williams 1957). The fainting lark can trigger syncope in almost everyone. Myoclonic jerks directly after falling down are observed in most of the subjects (Howard et al. 1951, Lempert et al. 1994).

Other manoeuvres that are applied to induce syncope are the mess trick (Howard et al. 1951) recently described as suffocation roulette (Shlamovitz et al. 2003). During the latter trick, subjects

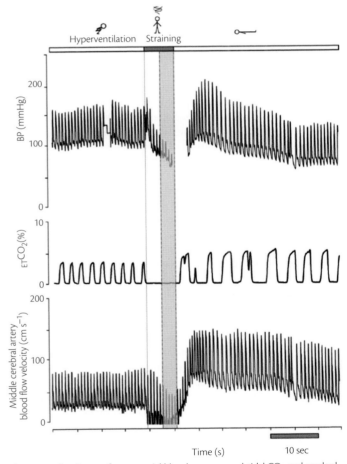

Fig. 60.10 Continuous finger arterial blood pressure, end-tidal CO_2 and cerebral blood flow velocity induced by the fainting lark in a 55-year-old male. Note the precipitous and deep fall in arterial pressure and cerebral blood flow. After a short period of light-headedness (grey area), the subject blacked out and lost consciousness briefly (2–3 seconds). Note the overshoot in blood pressure after lying down. Reproduced with permission of the publisher from Wieling and Van Lieshout 2002.

are instructed to take a deep breath and a companion grasps the subject unexpectedly from behind around the chest and squeezes it as hard as he can. The subject automatically closes his glottis, the intrathoracic pressure is raised and the subject looses consciousness. This is liable be done as entertainment, usually with the effects of alcohol are added to the mechanical effects. Self-induced syncope is reported to be safe, but injuries may occur by falling. Moreover, severe complications, even lethal, have been described (Rumball 1963, Chow 2003).

Stretch syncope

Stretch syncope may occur during stretching with the neck hyperextended while standing. It is reported to occur in teenage boys with a familial tendency to faint. It has been attributed to the effects of straining (which decreases systemic blood pressure) in combination with decreased cerebral blood flow caused by mechanical compression of the vertebral arteries (Pelekanos et al. 1990, Sturzenegger et al. 1995). The lordotic posture during stretching may play an additional role by external pressure on the inferior vena cava (Sharpey-Schafer 1965).

Miscellaneous causes of syncope

Diving and swimming

Several factors should be considered when a patient presents after near-drowning related to diving or swimming.

In the first place diving and swimming are established triggers for ventricular arrhythmias in patients with long QT-syndrome and cathecholamine-induced polymorphic ventricular tachycardia or fibrillation (Ackerman 2005, Tester et al. 2005). The mechanism underlying both conditions constitutes of a heterogeneous group of pathological polymorphisms of proteins involved in ventricular repolarization, that during concomitant activation of both the sympathetic and parasympathetic autonomic pathways facilitate ventricular arrhythmias in affected patients (Viskin and Belhassen 1998, Choi et al. 2004, Ackerman 2005). Since such abnormalities may not always be self-evident on a resting ECG, a clinical suspicion of a long QT-syndrome should warrant genetic counselling regardless of the baseline QT-time (Ackerman 2005).

Secondly, in an attempt to swim a maximum distance under water or to a maximum depth such as in competitive breath-hold diving, swimmers may voluntary hyperventilate before going into the water. This is a dangerous practice that kills medically fit and experienced swimmers (Edmonds and Walker 1999). The underlying mechanism is that hyperventilation lowers $PaCO_2$ and thereby reduces cerebral blood flow considerably, the effects on PaO_2 are however negligible. Swimmers may lose consciousness due to hypoxia before the hypercapnia urges them to surface (Dumitru and Hamilton 1964, Craig, Jr 1976, Fitz-Clarke 2006). In addition, when returning to the surface partial oxygen pressure halves over every 10 metres of ascend (Boyle's law) leading 'ascend hypoxia'. This may result in loss of consciousness and subsequent drowning (Edmonds and Walker 1999).

Furthermore, an exaggerated diving bradycardia has been implicated as a contributing factor to underwater syncope (Landsberg 1975). Breath holding with submersion of the head in cold water produces multiple effects including an almost instantaneous vagally induced bradycardia, peripheral vasoconstriction, decreased cardiac output with increased stroke volume and an increase in mean arterial blood pressure (Ferrigno et al. 1997). These cardiovascular alterations act in a manner which conserves oxygen for the heart and the brain. Facial receptors sensitive to cold play an important role in producing this response (Foster and Sheel 2005). Although an exaggerated diving response has been hypothesized as a causal factor in underwater syncope (Landsberg 1975), it is unclear how this reflex that normally increases arterial pressure and enhances cerebral blood flow (Brown et al. 2003) would lead to syncope. Most literature that focuses on this potential relationship dates from the era before the establishment of the Long QT syndrome. Since then there have been no case reports on the diving response as an isolated mechanism causing underwater syncope.

In cardiac unfit persons, especially middle aged men with preexisting ischemic heart disease the physical effort involved in the (under)water sports as well as some of the factors above may lead to cardiac events (Edmonds and Walker 1999). In scuba-diving, problems with the diving equipment or new procedures should be considered first (Edmonds and Walker 1989).

Occurrence of syncope almost immediately after getting out of a swimming pool is very likely to be due to a transient large fall in blood pressure, similar to that in initial orthostatic hypotension on arising from the supine or squatted position (Wieling et al. 2007).

Syncope during arm exercise: the subclavian steal syndrome

In case of syncope induced by exercise involving the arms a subclavian seal syndrome should be considered. The syndrome was first described in the 1960s (Reivich et al. 1961, Patel and Toole 1965). The condition refers to the circumstance in which a luminal stenosis occurs at or near the origin of the subclavian artery (usually on the left), proximal to the origin of the vertebral artery. If the stenosis is sufficiently severe, exercise of the affected limb may cause reversal of flow in that side's vertebral artery, which is redirected to the post-stenotic subclavian artery. Reversal of flow pulls ('steals') blood from the circle of Willis due to exercise induced low resistance of the arm vasculature.

The early descriptions include syncope and near-syncope during arm exercise accompanied by such diverse neurological symptoms as vertigo, ataxia and diplopia suggestive of vertebrobasilar insufficiency (Taylor et al. 2002). The patients are reported to have arm weakness and arm pain during arm exercise and a marked (> 20 mmHg) difference in blood pressure between both arms. The initial reports suggested that most patients with an angiographic subclavian steal were symptomatic (Taylor et al. 2002). However, the current opinion about subclavian steal markedly differs from the early views. Subclavian steal during angiography is now considered to be most commonly a marker for generalized atherosclerotic vascular disease, and although it may be associated with arm claudicatio, it is rarely the causative factor for symptoms of cerebral ischemia (Taylor et al. 2002).

Another example of syncope associated with arm exercise is a faint during shamming the windows or white-washing a ceiling. In the absence of orthostatic hypotension, kinking of cerebral vessels or carotid sinus hypersensitivity should be considered.

Syncope induced by acceleration

Aerial manoeuvres of military combat aircrafts may result in acceleration-induced loss of vision and consciousness caused by a head-level, hypotensive mediated and critical reduction in retinal and cerebral blood flow. Acceleration induced loss of vision secondary to reduced blood flow to the retina has been reported since the 1920s, when high-speed aircrafts were first developed (Burton 1988). Human centrifuges were designed to reproduce realistic simulations of in-flight, high G profiles on the ground under accurately controlled conditions. Milestone experiments with a human centrifuge were performed during World War II by investigators at the Acceleration laboratory of Mayo Clinic (Lambert and Wood 1946, Wood et al. 1946). Cerebral hypoperfusion triggered by application of accelerations in cranio-caudal direction of increasing magnitude (+ 3G to 6G) was found to induce a characteristic sequence of clinical events just prior to abrupt onset loss of consciousness. They consist of dimming and then loss of peripheral vision ('greyout' or 'brownout'), darkening of the visual fields (black out) without loss of hearing or consciousness, a brief period of staring appearance, fixed eyes and inability to move, followed by drooping of the head and loss of consciousness (Lambert et al. 1945, Lambert and Wood 1946). With a systolic pressure greater than 50 mm Hg at eye level no disturbance of vision occurs. Complete loss of vision occurs at a systolic pressure of less than 20 mm Hg. When unconsciousness occurs, the systolic pressure has fallen to zero at *cerebral level*. This is in sharp contrast to relatively little fall of arterial pressure at *heart level* at this instance (Wood et al. 1946). (When accelerating in the caudial-cranial direction the opposite of blackout may occur. Blood is then pushed toward the head and venous return from the head is diminished. This can cause visual sequelae known as 'redout', possibly caused by transient accumulation of red cells in the retinal vasculature or by retinal haemorrhages. This and the risk of hemorrhagic stroke has limited the research on this subject.)

Conclusions

Situational syncope encompasses a heterogeneous group of disorders. The traditional definition of situational syncope excludes many forms of neurally (autonomic) mediated syncope with clear situational patterns and may therefore not be useful.

The epidemiology of most forms of situational syncope is not or hardly known, but most forms seem to have a typical age distribution (e.g. initial orthostatic hypotension in the young and carotid sinus syndrome in the elderly). Diagnosing situational syncope is based on a detailed medical history, recognizing typical situational patterns and if indicated excluding potentially life-threatening disorders or comorbidity. Treatment focuses on patient education, if feasible the avoidance of triggering action or circumstance, and general measures that increase orthostatic tolerance. In patients with documented bradyarrhythmias pacemaker therapy may be indicated.

References

Ackerman, M. J. (2005). Cardiac causes of sudden unexpected death in children and their relationship to seizures and syncope: genetic testing for cardiac electropathies. *Seminars in Pediatric Neurology* 12(1), 52–58.

Agostini, A., Bretelle, F., Ronda, I., Roger, V., Cravello, L., and Blanc, B. (2004). Risk of vasovagal syndrome during outpatient hysteroscopy. *Journal of the American Association of Gynecologic Laparoscopists* 11(2), 245–47.

Ammirati, F., Colivicchi, F., and Santini, M. (2000). Diagnosing syncope in clinical practice. Implementation of a simplified diagnostic algorithm in a multicentre prospective trial—the OESIL 2 study (Osservatorio Epidemiologico della Sincope nel Lazio). *European Heart Journal* 21(11), 935–40.

Arias, M. J. (1985). Postural syncope and trigeminal neuralgia relieved by percutaneous rhizotomy with glycerol. *Neurosurgery* 17(5), 826–28.

Arnold, R. W., Dyer, J. A., Gould, A. B., Jr., Hohberger, G. G., and Low, P. A. (1991). Sensitivity to vasovagal maneuvers in normal children and adults. *Mayo Clinic Proceedings* 66(8), 797–804.

Aschner, B. (1908). Ueber einen bisher noch nicht beschrieben Reflex vom Auge auf kreislauf and Atmung. Verschwinden des Radialpulsen bei Druck aut des auge. *Wiener Klinische Wochenschrift* 21, 1529–30.

Barbey, K., Brecht, K., and Kutschka, W. (1966). Über die orthostatische Sofortreaktion. *Medizinische Welt* 17, 1648–53.

Basker, M. R. and Cooper, D. K. (2000). Oesophageal syncope. *Annals of the Royal College of Surgeons of England* 82(4), 249–53.

Benke, T., Hochleitner, M., and Bauer, G. (1997). Aura phenomena during syncope. *European Neurology* 37(1), 28–32.

Bennett, T., Macdonald, I. A., and Sainsbury, R. (1984). The influence of acute starvation on the cardiovascular responses to lower body subatmospheric pressure or to standing in man. *Clinical Science* 66(2), 141–46.

Bilbro, R. H. (1970). Syncope after prostatic examination. *New England Journal of Medicine* 282(3), 167–68.

Bjurstedt, H., Rosenhamer, G., Balldin, U., and Katkov, V. (1983). Orthostatic reactions during recovery from exhaustive exercise of short duration. *Acta Physiologica Scandinavica* 119(1), 25–31.

Blanc, J. J., L'Her, C., Touiza, A., Garo, B., L'Her, E., and Mansourati, J. (2002). Prospective evaluation and outcome of patients admitted for syncope over a 1 year period. *European Heart Journal* 23(10), 815–20.

Bloomfield, D. and Jazrawi, S. (2005). Shear hilarity leading to laugh syncope in a healthy man. *Journal of the American Medical Association* 293(23), 2863–64.

Bonamico, L. and Celnik, P. (1995). Syncope and seizure-like activity secondary to acute herpes zoster infection of the trigeminal nerve. *Cephalalgia.* 15(3), 241–42.

Bonekat, H. W., Miles, R. M., and Staats, B. A. (1987). Smoking and cough syncope: follow-up in 45 cases. *International Journal of the Addictions* 22(5), 413–419.

Bosser, G., Caillet, G., Gauchard, G., Marcon, F., and Perrin, P. (2006). Relation between motion sickness susceptibility and vasovagal syncope susceptibility. *Brain Research Bulletin* 68(4), 217–26.

Brady, P. A. and Shen, W. K. (1999). Syncope evaluation in the elderly. *American Journal of Geriatric Cardiology* 8(3), 115–24.

Braun, M. M., Patriarca, P. A., and Ellenberg, S. S. (1997). Syncope after immunization. *Archives of Pediatrics and Adolescent Medicine* 151(3), 255–59.

Brick, J. E., Lowther, C. M., and Deglin, S. M. (1978). Cold water syncope. *Southern Medical Journal* 71(12), 1579–80.

Brierley, E. J., Jackson, M. J., Clark, R. S., and Kenny, R. A. (2001). Alarming asystole. *Lancet* 357(9274), 2100.

Brignole, M., Sutton, R., Menozzi, C. et al. (2006). Early application of an implantable loop recorder allows effective specific therapy in patients with recurrent suspected neurally mediated syncope. *European Heart Journal* 27(9), 1085–92.

Brocklin, V., Hirons, R. R., and Yolton, R. L. (1982). The oculocardiac reflex: a review. *Journal of the American Optometric Association* 53(5), 407–413.

Brown, C. M., Sanya, E. O., and Hilz, M. J. (2003). Effect of cold face stimulation on cerebral blood flow in humans. *Brain Research Bulletin* 61(1), 81–86.

Brown, E. B., Jr. (1953). Physiological effects of hyperventilation. *Physiological Reviews* 33(4), 445–71.

Buckey, J. C., Jr., Lane, L. D., Levine, B. D. et al. (1996). Orthostatic intolerance after spaceflight. *Journal of Applied Physiology,* 81(1), 7–18.

Burchiel, K. J. and Slavin, K. V. (2000). On the natural history of trigeminal neuralgia. *Neurosurgery* **46**(1), 152–54.

Burton, R. R. (1988). G-induced loss of consciousness: definition, history, current status. *Aviation Space and Environmental Medicine* **59**(1), 2–5.

Charcot, M. (1879). Du vertige laryngé. *Progrès Médical* **7**(17), 317–319.

Choi, G., Kopplin, L. J., Tester, D. J., Will, M. L., Haglund, C. M., and Ackerman, M. J. (2004). Spectrum and frequency of cardiac channel defects in swimming-triggered arrhythmia syndromes. *Circulation* **110**(15), 2119–24.

Choi, Y. S., Kim, J. J., OH, B. H., Park, Y. B., Seo, J. D., and Lee, Y. W. (1989). Cough syncope caused by sinus arrest in a patient with sick sinus syndrome. *Pacing and Clinical Electrophysiology* **12**(6), 883–86.

Chow, K. M. (2003). Deadly game among children and adolescents. *Annals of Emergency Medicine* 42(2), 310.

Colman, N., Nahm, K., Ganzeboom, K. S. *et al.* (2004a). Epidemiology of reflex syncope. *Clinical Autonomic Research* **14** Suppl 1, 9–17.

Colman, N., Nahm, K., Van Dijk, J. G., Reitsma, J. B., Wieling, W., and Kaufmann, H. (2004b). Diagnostic value of history taking in reflex syncope. *Clinical Autonomic Research* **14** Suppl 1, 37–44.

Compton, D., Hill, P. M., and Sinclair, J. D. (1973). Weight-lifters' blackout. *Lancet*, **2**(7840), 1234–37.

Convertino, V. A., Tripp, L. D., Ludwig, D. A., Duff, J., and Chelette, T. L. (1998). Female exposure to high G: chronic adaptations of cardiovascular functions. *Aviation Space and Environmental Medicine* **69**(9), 875–82.

Cotton, Th. F. and Lewis, Th. (1918). Observations upon fainting attacks due to inhibitory cardiac impulses. *Heart* **7**, 23–34.

Coupland, N. J., Bailey, J. E., Wilson, S. J., Horvath, R., and Nutt, D. (1995). The effects of clonidine on cardiovascular responses to standing in healthy volunteers. *Clinical Autonomic Research* **5**(3), 171–77.

Cox, S. V., Eisenhauer, A. C., and Hreib, K. (1997). 'Seinfeld syncope'. *Catheterization and Cardiovascular Diagnosis* **42**(2), 242.

Craig, A. B., Jr. (1976). Summary of 58 cases of loss of consciousness during underwater swimming and diving. *Medicine and Science in Sports*, **8**(3), 171–75.

Culic, V. (2006). Triggering of cardiovascular incidents by micturition and defecation. *International Journal of Cardiology* **109**(2), 277–79.

Czermak, J. (1866). Ueber mechanische Vagus-Reizung beim Menschen. *Jenaische Zeitschrift fuer Medizin und Naturwissenschaft* **2**, 384–86.

Dagnini, G. (1908). Interno ad un riflesso provocato in alcuni emiplegici colla stimulo della corneae colo pressione sul bulbo oculare. *Bollettino delle Scienze Mediche* **8**, 380.

Deuchar, D. C. and Trounce, J. R. (1960). Syncopal dysphagia. *Guys Hospital Reports* **109**, 29–41.

Douglas, C. G., Haldane, J. S., Henderson, Y., and Schneider, E. C. (1913). Physiological observations made on Pike's Peak Colorado, with special reference to adaptation to low barometric pressures. *Philosophical Transactions of the Royal Society of London.Series B: Biological Sciences* **B203**, 185–381.

Dumitru, A. P. and Hamilton, F. G. (1964). Underwater blackout- a mechanism of drowning. *GP* **29**, 123–25.

Edmonds, C. W. and Walker, D. G. (1999). Snorkelling deaths in Australia, 1987–1996. *Medical Journal of Australia* **171**(11–12), 591–94.

Edmonds, C. and Walker, D. (1989). Scuba diving fatalities in Australia and New Zealand. *South Pacific Underwater Medicine Society Journal* **19**(3), 94–104.

Engel, G. L., Romano, J., and McLin, T. R. (1944). Vasodepressor and carotid sinus syncope—clinical, eletroencephalographic and electrocardiographic observations. *Archives of Internal Medicine* **74**, 100–119.

Engel, G. L. and Romano, J. (1947). Studies of Syncope: IV. Biologic interpretation of vasodepressor syncope. *Psychosomatic Medicine* **9**(5), 288–94.

Fagius, J. and Karhuvaara, S. (1989). Sympathetic activity and blood pressure increases with bladder distension in humans. *Hypertension* **14**(5), 511–517.

Faulkner, M. and Sharpey-Schafer, E. P. (1959). Circulatory effects of trumpet playing. *British Medical Journal* **15**(5123), 685–86.

Ferrigno, M., Ferretti, G., Ellis, A. *et al.* (1997). Cardiovascular changes during deep breath-hold dives in a pressure chamber. *Journal of Applied Physiology* **83**(4), 1282–90.

Finlay, J. B., Hartman, A. F., and Weir, R. C. (1995). Post-swim orthostatic intolerance in a marathon swimmer. *Medicine and Science in Sports and Exercise* **27**(9), 1231–37.

Fisher, C. M. (1979). Syncope of obscure nature. *Canadian Journal of Neurological Sciences* **6**(1), 7–20.

Fitz-Clarke, J. R. (2006). Adverse events in competitive breath-hold diving. *Undersea and Hyperbaric Medicine* **33**(1), 55–62.

Foster, G. E. and Sheel, A. W. (2005). The human diving response, its function, and its control. *Scandinavian Journal of Medicine and Science in Sports* **15**(1), 3–12.

Franke, H. (1963). *Über das Karotissinus-Syndrom und den sogenannten hyperaktiven Karotissinus-Reflex (book)*. Schattauer, Stuttgart.

Franke, H. and Bracharz, H. (1956). [Clinical manifestation, incidence and pathogenesis of the so-called hypersensitive carotid sinus syndrome.]. *Ärztliche Wochenschrift* **11**(14–15), 306–312.

Ganzeboom, K. S., Colman, N., Reitsma, J. B., Shen, W. K., and Wieling, W. (2003). Prevalence and triggers of syncope in medical students. *American Journal of Cardiology* **91**(8), 1006–1008.

Ganzeboom, K. S., Mairuhu, G., Reitsma, J. B., Linzer, M., Wieling, W., and Van Dijk, N. (2006). Lifetime cumulative incidence of syncope in the general population: a study of 549 Dutch subjects aged 35–60 years. *Journal of Cardiovascular Electrophysiology* **17**(11), 1172–76.

Gastaut, H. (1956). [Nocturnal syncope of patients of hypervagotonia, differentiation from nocturnal epilepsy.] *Revue Neurologique*, **95**(5), 420–21.

Gastaut, H. and Fischer-Williams, M. (1957). Electro-encephalographic study of syncope, its differentiation from epilepsy. *Lancet* **273**(7004), 1018–25.

Gendreau, M. A. and DeJohn, C. (2002). Responding to medical events during commercial airline flights. *New England Journal of Medicine* **346**, 1067–73.

Gisolf, J., Immink, R. V., Van Lieshout, J. J., Stok, W. J., and Karemaker, J. M. (2005). Orthostatic blood pressure control before and after spaceflight, determined by time-domain baroreflex method. *Journal of Applied Physiology* **98**(5), 1682–90.

Gottesman, M. H., Ibrahim, B., Elfenbein, A. S., Mechanic, A., and Hertz, S. (1996). Cardiac arrest caused by trigeminal neuralgia. *Headache* **36**(6), 392–94.

Graham, L. A. and Kenny, R. A. (2001). Clinical characteristics of patients with vasovagal reactions presenting as unexplained syncope. *Europace* **3**(2), 141–46.

Greenfield, A. D. (1951). An emotional faint. *Lancet* **1**(24), 1302–1303.

Haidet, P. and Paterniti, D. A. (2003). 'Building' a history rather than 'taking' one: a perspective on information sharing during the medical interview. *Archives of Internal Medicine* **163**(10), 1134–40.

Haldane, J. H. (1969). Micturition syncope: two case reports and a review of the literature. *Canadian Medical Association Journal* **101**(12), 53–54.

Halliwill, J. R. and Minson, C. T. (2005). Cardiovagal regulation during combined hypoxic and orthostatic stress: fainters vs. nonfainters. *Journal of Applied Physiology* **98**(3), 1050–56.

Haslam, R. H. and Freigang, B. (1985). Cough syncope mimicking epilepsy in asthmatic children. *Canadian Journal of Neurological Sciences* **12**(1), 45–47.

Hering, H. E. (1927). Ueber die Blutdruckregulierung bei Aenderung der Körperstellung vermittels der Blutdruckzügler und das Zustandekommen der Ohnmacht beim plötzlichen Uebergang vom

Liegen zum Stehen. *Münchener Medizinische Wochenschrift* **74**(38), 1611–1613.

Herman, L. L., Kurtz, R. C., McKee, K. J., Sun, M., Thaler, H. T., and Winawer, S. J. (1993). Risk factors associated with vasovagal reactions during colonoscopy. *Gastrointestinal Endoscopy* **39**(3), 388–91.

Holtzhausen, L. M. and Noakes, T. D. (1995). The prevalence and significance of post-exercise (postural) hypotension in ultramarathon runners, *Medicine and Science in Sports and Exercise* **27**(12), 1595–1601.

Howard, P., Leathart, G. L., Dornhorst, A. C., and Sharpey-Schafer, E. P. (1951). The mess trick and the fainting lark. *British Medical Journal.* **4728**, 382–84.

Howard, P. and Leathart, G. L. (1951). Changes of pulse pressure and heart rate induced by changes of posture in subjects with normal and failing hearts. *Clinical Science* **10**(4), 521–27.

Humm, A. M. and Mathias, C. J. (2006). Unexplained syncope—is screening for carotid sinus hypersensitivity indicated in all patients aged over 40 years? *Journal of Neurology, Neurosurgery and Psychiatry* **77**(11), 1267–70.

Hussain, R. M., McIntosh, S. J., Lawson, J., and Kenny, R. A. (1996). Fludrocortisone in the treatment of hypotensive disorders in the elderly. *Heart* **76**(6), 507–509.

Jardine, D. L., Krediet, C. T., Cortelli, P., Frampton, C., and Wieling, W. (2009). Sympatho-vagal responses in patients with sleep and typical vasovagal syncope. *Clinical Science,* **117**(10), 345–53.

Jardine, D. L., Krediet, C. T., Cortelli, P., and Wieling, W. (2006). Fainting in your sleep? *Clinical Autonomic Research,* **16**(1), 76–78.

Johnson, R. H., Lambie, D. G., & Spalding, J. M. (1984). Syncope without heart disease, in *Neurocardiology—the interrelationship between dysfunction in the nervous and cardiovascular systems,* 1st edn, vol. **13**. R. H. Johnson, D. G. Lambie, & J. M. Spalding, eds., W.B. Saunders Company, London, pp. 159–83.

Kapoor, W. N. (1990). Evaluation and outcome of patients with syncope. *Medicine (Baltimore)* **69**(3), 160–75.

Kapoor, W. N. (1994). Syncope in older persons. *Journal of the American Geriatrics Society* **42**(4), 426–36.

Kapoor, W. N., Peterson, J. R., and Karpf, M. (1985). Micturition syncope. A reappraisal. *Journal of the American Medical Association* **253**(6), 796–98.

Kapoor, W. N., Peterson, J. R., and Karpf, M. (1986). Defecation syncope. A symptom with multiple etiologies. *Archives of Internal Medicine* **146**(12), 2377–79.

Kapoor, W. N. and Jannetta, P. J. (1984). Trigeminal neuralgia associated with seizure and syncope. Case report. *Journal of Neurosurgery* **61**(3), 594–95.

Kenny, R. A. (2003). Syncope in the elderly: diagnosis, evaluation, and treatment. *Journal of Cardiovascular Electrophysiology* **14**(9) Suppl, S74–77.

Kenny, R. A., Richardson, D. A., Steen, N., Bexton, R. S., Shaw, F. E., and Bond, J. (2001). Carotid sinus syndrome: a modifiable risk factor for nonaccidental falls in older adults (SAFE PACE). *Journal of the American College of Cardiology* **38**(5), 1491–96.

Kenny, R. A. and Traynor, G. (1991). Carotid sinus syndrome—clinical characteristics in elderly patients. *Age and Ageing* **20**(6), 449–54.

Kerr, A., Jr. and Derbes, V. J. (1953). The syndrome of cough syncope. *Annals of Internal Medicine* **39**(6), 1240–53.

Kerr, A., Jr. and Eich, R. H. (1961). Cerebral concussion as a cause of cough syncope. *Archives of Internal Medicine* **108**, 248–52.

Kerr, S. R., Pearce, M. S., Brayne, C., Davis, R. J., and Kenny, R. A. (2006). Carotid sinus hypersensitivity in asymptomatic older persons: implications for diagnosis of syncope and falls. *Archives of Internal Medicine* **166**(5), 515–20.

Khurana, R. K. (2002). Eye examination-induced syncope Role of trigeminal afferents. *Clinical Autonomic Research* **12**(5), 399–403.

Kim, B. J., Sung, K. C., Kim, B. S., Kang, J. H., Lee, M. H., and Park, J. R. (2005). Situational syncope induced by belching. *Pacing and Clinical Electrophysiology* **28**, 458–60.

Kopp, J. (1937). Effect of fever on postural changes in blood pressure and pulse rate. *American Heart Journal* **13**, 114–20.

Krediet, C. T. (2002). Initial orthostatic hypotension in a 37-year old horse rider. *Clinical Autonomic Research* **12**(5), 404.

Krediet, C. T., Go-Schön, I. K., Kim, Y. S., Linzer, M., Van Lieshout, J. J., and Wieling, W. (2007). Management of initial orthostatic hypotension: lower body muscle tensing attenuates the transient arterial blood pressure decrease upon standing from squatting. *Clinical Science* **113**(10), 401–407.

Krediet, C. T., Jardine, D. L., Cortelli, P., Visman, A. G., and Wieling, W. (2004a). Vasovagal syncope interrupting sleep? *Heart* **90**(5), e25.

Krediet, C. T., Wilde, A. A., Wieling, W., and Halliwill, J. R. (2004b). Exercise related syncope, when it's not the heart. *Clinical Autonomic Research* **14** Suppl 1, 25–36.

Krediet, C. T., Parry, S. W., Jardine, D. L., Benditt, D., Brignole, M., and Wieling, W. (2011). The history of diagnosing carotid sinus hypersensitivity: why are the current criteria too sensitive. *Europace* **13**(1), 14–22.

Krediet, C. T. and Wieling, W. (2008). Edward P. Sharpey-Schafer was right: evidence for systemic vasodilatation as a mechanism of hypotension in cough syncope. *Europace* **10**(4), 486–88.

Kurbaan, A. S., Bowker, T. J., Wijesekera, N. *et al.* (2003). Age and hemodynamic responses to tilt testing in those with syncope of unknown origin. *Journal of the American College of Cardiology* **19**(6), 1004–1007.

Lamb, L. E., Green, H. C., Combs, J. J., Cheesman, S. A., and Hammond, J. (1960). Incidence of loss of consciousness in 1,980 Air Force personnel. *Aeromedica Acta* **31**, 973–88.

Lambert, E. H., Hallenbeck, G. A., Baldes, E. J., Wood, E. H., and Code, C. F. (1945). The symptoms which occur in man during exposure to positive acceleration. *Federation Proceedings* **4**, 43.

Lambert, E. H. and Wood, E. H. (1946). The problem of blackout and unconsciousness in aviators. *Medical Clinics of North America* **30**, 833–44.

Landau, C., Lange, R. A., Glamann, D. B., Willard, J. E., and Hillis, L. D. (1994). Vasovagal reactions in the cardiac catheterization laboratory. *American Journal of Cardiology* **73**(1), 95–97.

Landsberg, P. G. (1975). Bradycardia during human diving. *South African Medical Journal* **49**(15), 626–30.

Larson, S. J., Sances, A., Jr., Baker, J. B., and Reigel, D. H. (1974). Herniated cerebellar tonsils and cough syncope. *Journal of Neurosurgery* **40**(4), 524–28.

Lempert, T., Bauer, M., and Schmidt, D. (1994). Syncope: a videometric analysis of 56 episodes of transient cerebral hypoxia. *Annals of Neurology* **36**(2), 233–37.

Lempert, T. and Bauer, M. (1995). Mass fainting at rock concerts. *New England Journal of Medicine* **332**(25), 1721.

Levine, B. D., Lane, L. D., Buckey, J. C., Friedman, D. B., and Blomqvist, C. G. (1991). Left ventricular pressure-volume and Frank-Starling relations in endurance athletes. Implications for orthostatic tolerance and exercise performance. *Circulation* **84**(3), 1016–23.

Lewis, Th. (1932). A lecture on vasovagal syncope and the carotid sinus mechanism with comments on Gowers' and Nothnagel's syndrome. *British Medical Journal* **1**, 873–76.

Linzer, M., McFarland, T. A., Belkin, M., and Caplan, L. (1992). Critical carotid and vertebral arterial occlusive disease and cough syncope. *Stroke* **23**(7), 1017–20.

Lyle Jr., C. B., Monroe, J. T., Jr., Flinn, D. E., and Lamb, L. E. (1961). Micturition syncope. Report of 24 cases. *New England Journal of Medicine* **265**, 982–86.

Mackenzie, J. (1906). Definition of the term 'heart-block'. *British Medical Journal* **2**, 1107–1111.

de Marées, H. (1976). [Orthostatic immediate regulation]. *Cardiology* **61** suppl 1, 78–90.

Marey, E.-J. (1860). *Recherches sur le pouls au moyen d'un nouvel appareil enregistreur, le sphygmographe.* Thunot, Paris.

Marks, I. (1988). Blood-injury phobia: a review. *American Journal of Psychiatry* **145**(10), 1207–1213.

Marrison, V. K. and Parry, S. W. (2007). A case of nocturnal fainting: supine vasovagal syncope. *Europace* **9**(9), 835–36.

Mathias, C. J. (1976). Bradycardia and cardiac arrest during tracheal suction—mechanisms in tetraplegic patients. *European Journal of Intensive Care Medicine* **2**(4), 147–56.

Mathias, C. J., Deguchi, K., Bleasdale-Barr, K., and Kimber, J. R. (1998). Frequency of family history in vasovagal syncope. *Lancet* **352**(9121), 33–34.

Mattle, H. P., Nirkko, A. C., Baumgartner, R. W., and Sturzenegger, M. (1995). Transient cerebral circulatory arrest coincides with fainting in cough syncope. *Neurology* **45**(3 Pt 1), 498–501.

McCann, W. S. and Bruce, R. A. (1949). Tussive syncope, observations on the disease formerly called laryngeal epilepsy, with report of two cases. *Archivio di Medicina Interna* **84**(6), 845–56.

McIntosh, H. D., Estes, E. H., and Warren, J. V. (1956). The mechanism of cough syncope. *American Heart Journal* **52**(1), 70–82.

McIntosh, S. J., Lawson, J., and Kenny, R. A. (1993). Clinical characteristics of vasodepressor, cardioinhibitory, and mixed carotid sinus syndrome in the elderly. *American Journal of Medicine* **95**(2), 203–208.

Menzies, D. N. (1978). Vasovagal shock after insertion of intrauterine device. *British Medical Journal* **1**(6108), 305.

Moss, P. D. and McEvedy, C. P. (1966). An epidemic of overbreathing among schoolgirls. *British Medical Journal* **2**(525), 1295–1300.

Moya, A., Sutton, R., Ammirati, F. *et al.* (2009). Guidelines for the diagnosis and management of syncope (version 2009): the Task Force for the Diagnosis and Management of Syncope of the European Society of Cardiology (ESC). *European Heart Journal* **30**(21), 2631–71.

Mukai, S. and Lipsitz, L. A. (2002). Orthostatic hypotension. *Clinics in Geriatric Medicine* **18**(2), 253–68.

Narkiewicz, K., Cooley, R. L., and Somers, V. K. (2000). Alcohol potentiates orthostatic hypotension: implications for alcohol-related syncope. *Circulation* **101**(4), 398–402.

Newton, J. L., Allan, L., Baptist, M., and Kenny, R. (2001). Defecation syncope associated with splanchnic sympathetic dysfunction and cured by permanent pacemaker insertion. *American Journal of Gastroenterology* **96**(7), 2276–78.

Olde Nordkamp, L. R., van, D. N., Ganzeboom, K. S. *et al.* (2009). Syncope prevalence in the ED compared to general practice and population: a strong selection process. *American Journal of Emergency Medicine* **27**(3), 271–79.

Olshansky, B. (1999). A Pepsi challenge. *New England Journal of Medicine* **340**(25), 2006.

Palmer, E. D. (1976). The abnormal upper gastrointestinal vagovagal reflexes that affect the heart. *American Journal of Gastroenterology* **66**(6), 513–22.

Patel, A. and Toole, J. F. (1965). Subclavian steal syndrome—reversal of cephalic blood flow. *Medicine* **44**, 289–303.

Pathy, M. S. (1978). Defecation syncope. *Age and Ageing* **7**(4), 233–36.

Pelekanos, J. T., Dooley, J. M., Camfield, P. R., and Finley, J. (1990). Stretch syncope in adolescence. *Neurology* **40**(4), 705–707.

Piek, J. J., Imholz, B. P., Duren, D. R., and Wieling, W. (1988). [Swallowing syncope, a vagovagal reaction]. *Nederlands Tijdschrift voor Geneeskunde* **132**(5), 215–218.

Pott, F., Van Lieshout, J. J., Ide, K., Madsen, P., and Secher, N. H. (2000). Middle cerebral artery blood velocity during a valsalva maneuver in the standing position. *Journal of Applied Physiology* **88**(5), 1545–50.

Pott, F., Van Lieshout, J. J., Ide, K., Madsen, P., and Secher, N. H. (2003). Middle cerebral artery blood velocity during intense static exercise is dominated by a Valsalva maneuver. *Journal of Applied Physiology* **94**(4), 1335–44.

Proudfit, W. L. and Forteza, M. E. (1959). Micturition syncope. *New England Journal of Medicine* **260**(7), 328–31.

Prozan, G. B. and Litwin, A. (1961). Post-micturition syncope. *Annals of Internal Medicine* **54**, 82–89.

Rainford, D. J. (1975). Letter: Syncope after a cold drink. *Lancet* **1**(7904), 463.

Reivich, M., Holling, H. E., Roberts, B., and Toole, J. F. (1961). Reversal of blood flow through the vertebral artery and its effect on cerebral circulation. *New England Journal of Medicine* **265**, 878–85.

Rickards, C. A. and Newman, D. G. (2003). A comparative assessment of two techniques for investigating initial cardiovascular reflexes under acute orthostatic stress. *European Journal of Applied Physiology and Occupational Physiology* **90**(5–6), 449–57.

Rook, A. F. (1946). Coughing and unconsciousness: the so-called laryngeal epilepsy. *Brain* **69**, 138–48.

Rossberg, F. and Penáz, J. (1988). Initial cardiovascular response on change of posture from squatting to standing. *European Journal of Applied Physiology and Occupational Physiology* **57**(1), 93–97.

Rumball, A. (1963). Pulmonary oedema with neurological symptoms after the fainting lark and mess trick. *British Medical Journal* **5349**, 80–83.

Rushmer, R. F. (1944). Circulatory collapse following mechanical stimulation of arteries. *American Journal of Physiology* **141**, 722–29.

Rushton, J. G., Stevens, J. C., and Miller, R. H. (1981). Glossopharyngeal (vagoglossopharyngeal) neuralgia: a study of 217 cases. *Archives of Neurology* **38**(4), 201–205.

Schlesinger, Z. (1973). Life-threatening 'vagal reaction' to physical fitness test. *Journal of the American Medical Association* **226**(9), 1119.

Schlingemann, R. O., Smit, A. A., Lunel, H. F., and Hijdra, A. (1996). Amaurosis fugax on standing and angle-closure glaucoma with clomipramine. *Lancet* **347**(8999), 465.

Scott, R. W. and Sancetta, S. M. (1950). Stokes-Adams attacks induced by rectal stimulation in a patient with complete heart block. *Circulation* **2**(6), 886–89.

Selleger, C., Adamec, R., Morabia, A., and Zimmermann, M. (1988). Vasovagal syncope during rectosigmoidoscopy: report of a case. *Pacing and Clinical Electrophysiology* **11**(3), 346–48.

Serletis, A., Rose, S., Sheldon, A. G., and Sheldon, R. S. (2006). Vasovagal syncope in medical students and their first-degree relatives. *European Heart Journal* **27**(16), 1965–70.

Sharpey-Schafer, E. P. (1953a). Effects of coughing on intrathoracic pressure, arterial pressure and peripheral blood flow. *Journal of Physiology* **122**(2), 351–57.

Sharpey-Schafer, E. P. (1953b). The mechanism of syncope after coughing. *British Medical Journal* **4841**, 860–63.

Sharpey-Schafer, E. P. (1956a). Effects of squatting on the normal and failing circulation. *British Medical Journal* **4975**, 1072–74.

Sharpey-Schafer, E. P. (1956b). Syncope. *British Medical Journal* **1**(4965), 506–509.

Sharpey-Schafer, E. P. (1965). Effects of respiratory acts on the circulation, in *Handbook of physiology section 2: Circulation*, vol. **III**. W. F. Hamilton & F. Dow, eds., American Physiological Society, Washington, pp. 1875–86.

Sharpey-Schafer, E. P., Hayter, C. J., and Barlow, E. D. (1958). Mechanism of acute hypotension from fear or nausea. *British Medical Journal* **2**(5101), 878–80.

Sheldon, R. S., Sheldon, A. G., Connolly, S. J. *et al.* (2006). Age of first faint in patients with vasovagal syncope. *Journal of Cardiovascular Electrophysiology* **17**(1), 49–54.

Sherer, D. M., Santoso, P., Russell, B. A., and Abulafia, O. (2005). Micturition syncope during pregnancy. *Obstetrics and Gynecology* **105**(3), 485–86.

Shichiri, M., Tanaka, H., Takaya, R., and Tamai, H. (2002). Efficacy of high sodium intake in a boy with instantaneous orthostatic hypotension. *Clinical Autonomic Research* **12**(1), 47–50.

Shlamovitz, G. Z., Assia, A., Ben Sira, L., and Rachmel, A. (2003). 'Suffocation roulette': a case of recurrent syncope in an adolescent boy. *Annals of Emergency Medicine* **41**(2), 223–26.

Smit, A. A., Timmers, H. J., Wieling, W. *et al.* (2002). Long-term effects of carotid sinus denervation on arterial blood pressure in humans. *Circulation* **105**(11), 1329–35.

Soteriades, E. S., Evans, J. C., Larson, M. G. *et al.* (2002). Incidence and prognosis of syncope. *New England Journal of Medicine* **347**(12), 878–85.

Sprangers, R. L., Wesseling, K. H., Imholz, A. L., Imholz, B. P., and Wieling, W. (1991). Initial blood pressure fall on stand up and exercise explained by changes in total peripheral resistance. *Journal of Applied Physiology* **70**(2), 523–30.

Stephenson, J. B. P. (1978). Two types of febrile seizure: anoxic (syncopal) and epileptic mechanisms differentiated by oculocardiac reflex. *British Medical Journal* **2**, 726–28.

Stevens, P. M. (1966). Cardiovascular dynamics during orthostasis and the influence of intravascular instrumentation. *American Journal of Cardiology* **17**(2), 211–218.

Sturzenegger, M., Newell, D. W., Douville, C. M., Byrd, S., Schoonover, K. D., and Nicholls, S. C. (1995). Transcranial Doppler and angiographic findings in adolescent stretch syncope. *Journal of Neurology, Neurosurgery and Psychiatry* **58**(3), 367–70.

Sutton, R. (1999). Vasovagal syncope: prevalence and presentation. An algorithm of management in the aviation environment. *European Heart Journal*, vol. **1** Suppl, D109–D113.

Taylor, C. L., Selman, W. R., and Ratcheson, R. A. (2002). Steal affecting the central nervous system. *Neurosurgery* **50**(4), 679–88.

Tester, D. J., Kopplin, L. J., Creighton, W., Burke, A. P., and Ackerman, M. J. (2005). Pathogenesis of unexplained drowning: new insights from a molecular autopsy. *Mayo Clinic Proceedings* **80**(5), 596–600.

Thijs, R. D., Benditt, D. G., Mathias, C. J. *et al.* (2005). Unconscious confusion—a literature search for definitions of syncope and related disorders. *Clinical Autonomic Research* **15**(1), 35–39.

Thijs, R. D., Kruit, M. C., van Buchem, M. A., Ferrari, M. D., Launer, L. J., and Van Dijk, J. G. (2006). Syncope in migraine: the population-based CAMERA study. *Neurology* **66**(7), 1034–37.

Thijs, R. D., Wieling, W., Kaufmann, H., and Van Dijk, G. (2004). Defining and classifying syncope. *Clinical Autonomic Research* **14** Suppl 1, 4–8.

Thomas, K. N., Cotter, J. D., Galvin, S. D., Williams, M. J., Willie, C. K., and Ainslie, P. N. (2009). Initial orthostatic hypotension is unrelated to orthostatic tolerance in healthy young subjects. *Journal of Applied Physiology* **107**(2), 506–517.

Tinuper, P., Bisulli, F., Cerullo, A. *et al.* (2001). Ictal bradycardia in partial epileptic seizures: Autonomic investigation in three cases and literature review. *Brain* **124**(12), 2361–71.

Tsutsumi, E. and Hara, H. (1979). Syncope after running. *British Medical Journal* **2**(6203), 1480.

Van Dijk, N., Boer, K. R., Colman, N. *et al.* (2008). High diagnostic yield and accuracy of history, physical examination, and ECG in patients with transient loss of consciousness in FAST: the Fainting Assessment study. *Journal of Cardiovascular Electrophysiology* **19**(1), 48–55.

Van Dijk, N., Harms, M. P., and Wieling, W. (2000). [Three patients with unrecognized orthostatic intolerance]. *Nederlands Tijdschrift voor Geneeskunde* **144**(6), 249–54.

Van Dijk, N., Velzeboer, S. C., Destree-Vonk, A., Linzer, M., and Wieling, W. (2001). Psychological treatment of malignant vasovagal syncope due to bloodphobia. *Pacing and Clinical Electrophysiology* **24**(1), 122–24.

Van Lieshout, E. J., Van Lieshout, J. J., Ten Harkel, A. D., and Wieling, W. (1989). Cardiovascular response to coughing: its value in the assessment of autonomic nervous control. *Clinical Science* **77**(3), 305–310.

Van Lieshout, J. J., Imholz, B. P., Wesseling, K. H., Speelman, J. D., and Wieling, W. (1991a). Singing-induced hypotension: a complication of a high spinal cord lesion. *Netherlands Journal of Medicine* **38**(1–2), 75–79.

Van Lieshout, J. J., Wieling, W., Karemaker, J. M., and Eckberg, D. L. (1991b). The vasovagal response. *Clinical Science* **81**(5), 575–86.

Veerman, D. P., Imholz, B. P., Wieling, W., Wesseling, K. H., and Van Montfrans, G. A. (1995). Circadian profile of systemic hemodynamics. *Hypertension* **26**(1), 55–59.

Verrill, P. J. and Aellig, W. H. (1970). Vasovagal faint in the supine position. *British Medical Journal* **4**(731), 348.

Viskin, S. and Belhassen, B. (1998). Polymorphic ventricular tachyarrhythmias in the absence of organic heart disease: classification, differential diagnosis, and implications for therapy. *Progress in Cardiovascular Diseases* **41**(1), 17–34.

Wallace, H., Shorvon, S., and Tallis, R. (1998). Age-specific incidence and prevalence rates of treated epilepsy in an unselected population of 2,052,922 and age-specific fertility rates of women with epilepsy. *Lancet* **352**(9145), 1970–73.

Wayne, H. H. (1961). Syncope. Physiological considerations and an analysis of the clinical characteristics in 510 patients, *American Journal of Medicine* **30**, 418–38.

Weiss, S. and Baker, J. P. (1933). The carotid sinus reflex in health and disease: its role in the causation of fainting and convulsions. *Medicine* **12**, 297–354.

Wenger, T. L., Dohrmann, M. L., Strauss, H. C., Conley, M. J., Wechsler, A. S., and Wagner, G. S. (1980). Hypersensitive carotid sinus syndrome manifested as cough syncope. *Pacing and Clinical Electrophysiology* **3**(3), 332–39.

Westendorp, R. G., Blauw, G. J., Frolich, M., and Simons, R. (1997). Hypoxic syncope. *Aviation Space and Environmental Medicine* **68**(5), 410–414.

White, C. W., Zimmerman, T. J., and Ahmad, M. (1975). Idiopathic hypertrophic subaortic stenosis presenting as cough syncope. *Chest* **68**(2), 250–53.

Wieling, W. & Khurana, R. K. (2006). Syncope and the eye, in *Syncope cases*, R. Garcia-Civera *et al.*, eds., Blackwell Futura, Oxford, pp. 74–75.

Wieling, W., Colman, N., Krediet, C. T., and Freeman, R. (2004). Nonpharmacological treatment of reflex syncope. *Clinical Autonomic Research* **14** Suppl 1, 62–70.

Wieling, W., Ganzeboom, K. S., Krediet, C. T., Grundmeijer, H. G., Wilde, A. A., and Van Dijk, J. G. (2003). [Initial diagnostic strategy in the case of transient losses of consciousness: the importance of the medical history]. *Nederlands Tijdschrift voor Geneeskunde* **147**(18), 849–54.

Wieling, W., Harms, M. P., Kortz, R. A., and Linzer, M. (2001). Initial orthostatic hypotension as a cause of recurrent syncope: a case report. *Clinical Autonomic Research* **11**(4), 269–70.

Wieling, W., Krediet, C. T., Van Dijk, N., Linzer, M., and Tschakovsky, M. E. (2007). Initial orthostatic hypotension: review on a forgotten condition. *Clinical Science* **112**(3), 157–65.

Wieling, W., Remme, C. A., & Van Dijk, J. G. (2006). Syncope during air travel, in *Syncope cases*, R. Garcia-Civera *et al.*, eds., Blackwell Futura, Oxford, pp. 12–13.

Wieling, W., Thijs, R. D., van, D. N., Wilde, A. A., Benditt, D. G., and Van Dijk, J. G. (2009). Symptoms and signs of syncope: a review of the link between physiology and clinical clues. *Brain*.

Wieling, W. and Van Lieshout, J. J. (2002). The fainting lark. *Clinical Autonomic Research* **12**(3), 207.

Wilson, T. E., Cui, J., Zhang, R., and Crandall, C. G. (2006). Heat stress reduces cerebral blood velocity and markedly impairs orthostatic tolerance in humans. *American Journal of Physiology* **291**(5), R1443–1448.

Wilt, T. J., Mac, D. R., and Rutks, I. (2003). Tamsulosin for benign prostatic hyperplasia. *Cochrane Database of Systematic Reviews* no. 1, p. CD002081.

Wood, E. H., Lambert, E. H., Baldes, E. J., and Code, C. F. (1946). Effects of acceleration in relation to aviation. *Federation Proceedings* **3**, 327–44.

Yamada, N., Nakamura, M., Ishikura, K. *et al.* (2005). Triggers of acute pulmonary thromboembolism developed in hospital, with focusing on toilet activities as triggering acts. *International Journal of Cardiology* **98**(3), 409–411.

Youde, J., Ruse, C., Parker, S., and Fotherby, M. (2000). A high diagnostic rate in older patients attending an integrated syncope clinic. *Journal of the American Geriatrics Society* **48**(7), 783–87.

CHAPTER 61

Postural orthostatic tachycardia syndrome

Phillip A. Low

Postural orthostatic tachycardia syndrome (POTS) is a syndrome comprising specific symptoms and signs. Symptoms are those of cerebral hypoperfusion and/or autonomic overactivity, which develop while the subject is standing but are relieved by recumbency. Symptoms of hypoperfusion include light-headedness, dizziness, diminished concentration, and syncope; those of autonomic overaction include palpitations, tremulousness, nausea, and syncope. The essential finding is a heart rate (HR) increment of 30 beats/minute or greater within 5 minutes of standing up or on head-up tilt (HUT). Some investigators require an absolute orthostatic HR greater than 120 beats/minute and/or standing plasma norepinephrine ≥ 600 pg/ml.

The prevalence of these conditions is not known precisely. Syncope is common. From 10% to 20% of the population have had a syncopal episode at some time (Allen et al. 1945, Shen and Gersh 1993). The prevalence of POTS is known even less well; it probably is about five to ten times that of neurogenic orthostatic hypotension. Orthostatic intolerance is under-recognized and typically misdiagnosed.

Some patients with chronic fatigue syndrome have orthostatic intolerance with tilt-induced syncope, and a subset has a response to treatment directed at syncope (Bou-Holaigah et al. 1995); however, most patients with chronic fatigue syndrome do not have POTS so that, from the diagnostic and management standpoint, it is best to consider the conditions as separate disorders that sometimes coexist.

Clinical features

There have been recent and alternative views about the abbreviation of the Postural Tachycardia Syndrome, e.g., PoTS (Mathias et al. 2012). This particular abbreviation (PoTS) has been used throughout the book (Introduction and Chapters 12, 22 and 29). The age at presentation most commonly is between 15 years and 50 years of age (Low et al. 1997b). Most patients that we have evaluated have had the symptoms for about 4 years. The orthostatic symptoms consist of light-headedness, visual blurring or tunnelling, palpitations, tremulousness, and weakness (especially of the legs). Less frequent symptoms are those of hyperventilation, anxiety, chest wall pain, nausea, acral coldness or pain, and headaches. The symptoms these patients experience differ from those of patients with orthostatic hypotension in that there are pronounced symptoms of sympathetic activation. Approximately one in two to

one in four of the patients have an antecedent, presumably viral, illness (Low et al. 1994, Schondorf and Low 1993). Some patients with POTS have a cyclical exacerbation of symptoms. The symptoms deteriorate considerably in some women at certain stages of the menstrual cycle, associated with marked weight and fluid changes. Typically, these patients have large fluctuations in their weight, sometimes up to 5 lb. Others have cycles of several days of intense orthostatic intolerance, followed by a similar period when the symptoms are less. Patients may have episodic symptoms at rest associated with changes in blood pressure and HR unrelated to arrhythmias. Typically, the HR alteration is sinus tachycardia, although bradycardia may occur. Fatigue can be a problem during these episodes. The relationship of orthostatic intolerance to anxiety and panic is complex. Patients with typical anxiety-panic disorder are easy to differentiate from those with POTS, and the orthostatic 'anxiety' symptoms are easy to differentiate from an anxiety disorder in most patients. However, the relationship can be more complicated because many of the symptoms of anxiety are mediated by the autonomic nervous system. Orthostatic stress can evoke anxiety-panic symptoms in predisposed subjects. Patients with panic disorders and those with POTS share such clinical features as discomfort at the onset of symptoms, shortness of breath with hyperventilation, dizziness or faintness, palpitations, trembling, numbness or tingling sensations, flushes or chills, chest pain, and generalized weakness. In a small proportion of patients, the two disorders appear to coexist. The proposed central mechanisms for POTS and panic disorders may overlap. The noradrenergic system is involved in both disorders (Uhde and Trancer 1988). Other central neurotransmitters that potentially affect the production of panic disorders include γ-aminobutyric acid (Insel et al. 1984), serotonin (Wise et al. 1972), and adenosine (Boulenger et al. 1984). Their role in POTS needs to be evaluated. Also, both conditions currently have certain treatments in common, including treatment with phenobarbital, benzodiazepines, beta-blockers (Tyrer 1988), and clonidine (Uhde et al. 1989).

Fatigue is commonly present in patients with POTS. Some patients have an extended period of exhaustion following a bout of symptoms. This period may last anywhere from hours to days. In some patients, overwhelming fatigue can be a more chronic and persistent symptom. They described a very low energy level. The autonomic basis for this fatigue is unknown.

Clinical examination demonstrates an excessive HR increment. Pulse pressure may be excessively reduced. One clinical correlate is the difficulty in palpating the radial pulse with continued standing of the patient or with the performance of a Valsalva manoeuvre (Flack sign). Another clinical sign is the development of acral coldness. With continued standing, there may be venous prominence, resulting in blueness and even swelling of the feet (Streeten 1987).

Aetiology

The aetiology and pathophysiology of POTS appears to be heterogeneous. The major categories are:

- POTS due to limited autonomic neuropathy
- POTS due to hypovolaemia
- hyperadrenergic POTS.

Autonomic neuropathy: Some patients clearly have a limited autonomic neuropathy (Shen and Gersh 1993). Evidence for autonomic neuropathy includes the following features. Some patients develop the disorder after an infection, presumably viral in 25–50% of instances. Some of these postviral cases are positive of A_3 acetylcholine receptor (AChR) autoantibody (Rosen and Cryer 1982). There is often evidence of C-fibre denervation. This can be manifest as sudomotor denervation as indicated by the absence of distal responses on the quantitative sudomotor axon reflex test (QSART) and anhidrosis of the feet on the thermoregulatory sweat test (Schondorf and Low 1993a, Schondorf and Low 1993b). There is excellent agreement between sweat loss on thermoregulatory sweat test and QSART loss, indicative of postganglionic cholinergic sudomotor C-fibre loss. There is also evidence of peripheral adrenergic denervation, with cardiovascular changes of absent late phase II, failure of systemic peripheral resistance to increment on head-up tilt (Low et al. 1994, Schondorf and Low 1993b, Stewart 2002), and reduced norepinephrine release in the lower as compared with the upper extremity. Leg arteriolar vasoconstriction is impaired (Schondorf and Low 1993b, Stewart 2002), due to this reduced lower extremity secretion of norepinephrine when compared with the upper extremity (Jacob et al. 2000). There is often a modest gradual fall in BP associated with excessive tachycardia (Fig. 61.1). Perivascular round cell infiltration is sometimes seen on nerve biopsy (Schondorf and Low 1993a), and ganglionic antibody is positive in about 10%, especially in the more severely affected patients (Vernino et al. 2000). Loss of epidermal fibres is sometimes seen on skin biopsy, indicating that C-fibre involvement can spread to involve somatic C fibres (Singer et al. 2004). As a result of

peripheral denervation, and a reduced oedema threshold, venous pooling and leg swelling can occur (Stewart 2002, Stewart 2003), and hypovolaemia can develop with continued standing. Pooling may occur in the splanchnic-mesenteric bed (Novak et al. 1998), and possibly the legs, although the latter observation has been questioned in some studies (Low et al. 1997a). Norepinephrine spillover in the legs of POTS was reduced in response to sympathetic stimulation, in contrast to a normal response in the arm. These findings suggest a length-dependent sympathetic denervation (Jacob et al. 2000).

Hyperadrenergic state: Some patients have apparent resting excessive sympathetic activity manifest as resting tachycardia, sweating, and tremulousness. Some of these patients have episodic 'storms', when they become hypertensive, tachycardic, sweating and are sometimes flushed. There is some support for this concept, evidenced by an excessive fall in blood pressure following ganglion blockade (Jacob et al. 2000, Jordan et al. 2002). Other manifestations include a rise rather than fall in systolic blood pressure during tilt and excessive plasma norepinephrine response to head-up tilt.

Hypovolaemia: Another mechanism seen in some patients is hypovolaemia, reported by some investigators (Fouad et al. 1986, Khurana 1995, Rosen and Cryer 1982). Venous pooling in the limbs (Low et al. 1994, Streeten 1988, Streeten 1987), or splanchnic-mesenteric bed (Tani et al. 1999), is another abnormality. Either or both of these mechanisms or deconditioning, as might occur with bed rest exceeding one week, result in reduced preload and a secondary excessive increase in norepinephrine levels, typically to levels greater than 600 pg/mL (Jacob et al. 1998), resulting in a hyperadrenergic state.

Secondary POTS refers to patients who have a known autonomic disorder with peripheral denervation and relative preservation of the autonomic innervation of the heart. Causes include autonomic neuropathies (e.g. diabetic, amyloid, idiopathic); less commonly, it is a stage in the evolution of pure autonomic failure or multiple system atrophy. Patients who have a length-dependent autonomic neuropathy with sparing of cardiac vagal and sympathetic fibres can have marked orthostatic tachycardia (Fig. 61.2).

Many patients appear to have β-receptor supersensitivity. The excessive HR response to isoproterenol correlates with the HR response to head-up tilt (Low et al. 1997b). Another mechanism is central (presumably brainstem) dysfunction. These patients have spontaneous episodes of tachycardia, and on head-up tilt, they have an exaggerated diastolic blood pressure response (an

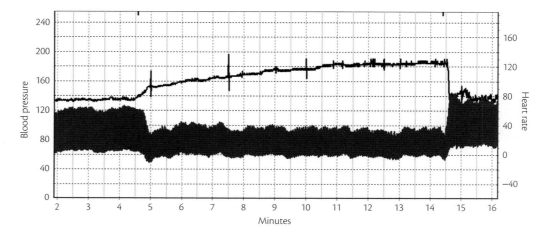

Fig. 61.1 Exaggerated heart rate response in a patient with postural orthostatic tachycardia syndrome without orthostatic hypotension in response to head-up tilt. Filled bar indicates period of tilt.

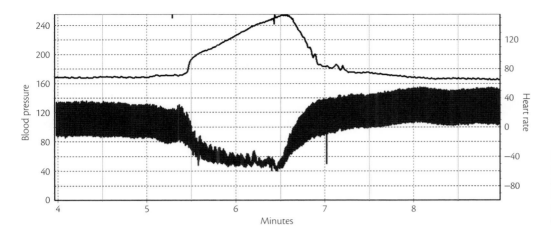

Fig. 61.2 Exaggerated heart rate response in a patient with postviral autonomic neuropathy, orthostatic hypotension, and orthostatic tachycardia. Filled bar indicates duration of head-up tilt.

increase >20 mmHg). Their 24-hour blood pressure recordings are characterized by large oscillations in blood pressure. It has been suggested that these oscillations may have a brainstem origin. There is some evidence that, in the frequency domain, the ultraslow rhythms that modulate the electroencephalogram (EEG) might reflect brainstem function, which might be impaired in POTS (Lagerlund et al. 2005).

Cerebral hypoperfusion occurs in POTS in response to HUT (Jacob et al. 1999, Novak et al. 1998). This occurs due to an alteration in cerebral vasoconstrictor tone, in part due to hypocapnia (Novak et al. 1998).

Changes in venous capacitance of leg veins and splanchnic-mesenteric bed have been described, although some of the data is conflicting. Increased limb venous capacitance has been reported or assumed by a number of investigators (Streeten 1988, Streeten and Scullard 1996). However, in a careful study, Freeman et al. (1996) found reduced capacitance in leg veins of POTS. We measured blood flow and tone in superior mesenteric artery and reported increased resting flow and reduced vascular resistance in POTS when compared with controls supporting the notion that there is excessive splanchnic capacity (pooling) at rest in POTS (Tani et al. 2000). There are also reports of excessive capillary transudation with continued standing, demonstrated by plethysmographic studies (Stewart 2003). The orthostatic intolerance with prolonged standing can be associated with a progressive reduction in plasma volume, suggesting that the transcapillary flux is substantive. The apparent conflict likely reflects heterogeneity of POTS.

β_2-receptor polymorphisms may be responsible for alterations in venomotor tone, resulting in increased capacity and failure of accommodation. β_2-receptor polymorphisms may explain some of the heterogeneity of results. In a recent study (Nicklander and Low 2003), HR and blood pressure changes were correlated to β_2AR genotypes. Orthostatic HR increment was significantly greater in patients with Glu27. The greater orthostatic venodilation that occurs in these patients could account for the excessive HR response to continued standing in some patients with POTS (Nicklander and Low 2003).

Diagnosis

The diagnosis of POTS is based on the presence of orthostatic symptoms associated with unexplained excessive orthostatic tachycardia. Thus, conditions that can result in tachycardia, such as thyrotoxicosis, cardiac rhythm abnormalities, phaeochromocytoma, hypoadrenalism, dehydration, and medications (vasodilators, diuretics, β-agonists) need to be excluded. The presence of a defined autonomic neuropathy (diabetes, amyloidosis, inherited) needs to be sought and could cause secondary POTS. Table 61.1 summarizes the differences between POTS and neurogenic orthostatic hypotension. The role of the laboratory is to confirm orthostatic intolerance and to demonstrate evidence of autonomic denervation. Approximately one-half of the patients have a restricted autonomic neuropathy, typically a length-dependent type (Low et al. 1994, Schondorf and Low 1993a). *Length-dependent neuropathy* refers to a neuropathy in which the ends of the longer fibres are affected before the shorter fibres. In the autonomic nervous system, the postganglionic sympathetic adrenergic fibres to the limbs and splanchnic-mesenteric bed are the longest fibres; next are the vagal fibres to the heart, which have a long preganglionic path. The cardiac adrenergic fibres, in contrast, are relatively short.

The anhidrosis on QSART and the thermoregulatory sweat test has a neuropathic distribution. Sweating is impaired in the lower extremities to varying degrees: the feet typically are anhidrotic and the legs are involved to different extents. The distribution of anhidrosis can be patchy or more widespread. Khurana (1995) reported segmental or patchy anhidrosis in six of the eight patients studied. Skin potential abnormalities, with a loss of skin potentials in the lower extremity, have also been described (Hoeldtke and Davis 1991). The HR response to deep breathing and the Valsalva ratio are usually normal and often large (Khurana 1995, Low et al. 1997a, Low et al. 1994).

The beat-to-beat blood pressure responses to the Valsalva manoeuvre are abnormal in about two-thirds of patients (Low et al. 1997a, Low et al. 1994). The pulse pressure often decreases by more than 50%. Early phase II is exaggerated, and late phase II may be reduced or absent. Phase IV is normal but, more often, excessively large. The cardiovascular responses to tilt-up are abnormal. The HR response varies from 120 to 170 beats/minute on head-up tilt typically by 2 minutes. The HR response may oscillate excessively; in patients with marked peripheral denervation, the variability may be reduced. The blood pressure responses occur in several patterns. Patients who have prominent venous pooling may have an excessive decrease in pulse pressure. Some have a prominent hypertensive response, with increases in diastolic blood pressure by up to 50 mmHg, with large fluctuations. Some patients

Table 61.1 Comparison of patients with generalized autonomic neuropathy and those with postural orthostatic tachycardia syndrome (POTS)

Variable	Neurogenic orthostatic hypotension	POTS
Orthostatic dizziness	Variably present	Present
Orthostatic tremulousness	Absent	Common
Orthostatic palpitations	Absent	Common
Orthostatic hypotension	Consistent	Usually absent
Orthostatic tachycardia	Reduced	Exaggerated
Supine norepinephrine	Usually reduced	Normal or increased
Standing norepinephrine	Reduced	Increased
HR response to deep breathing	Reduced	Normal
Valsalva ratio	Reduced	Normal or increased
BP_{BB} to Valsalva manoeuvre		
Early phase II	Markedly increased	Increased
Late phase II	Absent	Normal or reduced
Phase IV	Absent	Increased

BP_{BB}, beat-to-beat blood pressure; HR, heart rate.

have relatively normal blood pressure responses but have tachycardia and symptoms. The pattern of responses with peripheral sudomotor deficits, absent late phase II with intact phase IV, and normal forced respiratory sinus arrhythmia are consistent with length-dependent autonomic neuropathy. Patients with secondary POTS can have orthostatic hypotension and POTS (Fig. 61.2). The plasma level of norepinephrine is normal with the patient supine and excessive with the patient erect (Low et al. 1997a, Streeten et al. 1988), likely because of increased baroreceptor unloading.

Differential diagnosis

The main differential diagnosis of POTS includes neurogenic orthostatic hypotension, other causes of orthostatic intolerance, and anxiety-panic attacks. Differentiating POTS from neurogenic orthostatic hypotension is straightforward by excluding the presence of orthostatic hypotension. The symptoms of orthostatic hypotension are similar, but symptoms of sympathetic overactivity, such as tremulousness, anxiety, nausea, sweating, and acral vasoconstriction, occur in POTS and not in neurogenic orthostatic hypotension. In the latter, orthostatic hypotension and evidence of generalized autonomic failure (cardiovagal, adrenergic, sudomotor) are found. It is more difficult to differentiate POTS from other causes of orthostatic intolerance. Mild orthostatic intolerance due to an illness that requires prolonged bed rest, dehydration, hypovolaemia, or a medication effect usually is readily recognized. A related condition is constitutional orthostatic intolerance. Patients with this always had some degree of orthostatic intolerance. In their youth, they may have had syncopal episodes in response to prolonged standing or syncope in response to pain or the sight of blood. They may have had transient light-headedness on standing up suddenly. These patients are more prone to develop a greater degree of orthostatic intolerance after a period of bed rest

or a viral illness. The condition may be familial. POTS is differentiated from chronic fatigue syndrome by the predominance of orthostatic symptoms. Chronic fatigue affects the sexes less unevenly, is dominated by non-orthostatic symptoms, and has many quasi-infectious symptoms. However, some of the patients have orthostatic intolerance, including tachycardia. In both POTS and chronic fatigue syndromes, patients have marked worsening of symptoms after syncope or presyncope, perhaps because non-orthostatic symptoms are a continuation of postsyncopal symptoms. We recommend that when the feature of fatigue predominates, the condition should be designated as *POTS associated with chronic fatigue syndrome*. Similarly, orthostatic intolerance should not be considered an integral part of mitral valve prolapse. When orthostatic intolerance is a feature of mitral valve prolapse, the condition should be recognized as orthostatic intolerance or *POTS associated with mitral valve prolapse*. Chronic fatigue syndrome and mitral valve prolapse are described in greater detail below.

Chronic fatigue syndrome

Currently, chronic fatigue syndrome is defined by the Centers for Disease Control and Prevention as fatigue of at least 6 months' duration seriously interfering with the patient's life and without evidence of various organic or psychiatric illnesses that can produce chronic fatigue. The criteria include myalgias, postexertional malaise, headaches, and a group of infectious-type symptoms (chronic fever and chills, sore throat, lymphadenopathy). These criteria appear to distinguish patients with chronic fatigue syndrome from healthy control subjects and from the comparison groups with multiple sclerosis and depression (Komaroff et al. 1996). In addition to chronic fluctuating fatigue, patients have somatic, cognitive, depressive, and sleep dysfunction. The patients often are separated into those with postviral and those with nonpostviral fatigue syndrome. The relationship to orthostatic intolerance is inconstant. Patients may have orthostatic intolerance and some amelioration of their symptoms with treatment of orthostatic intolerance (Bou-Holaigah et al. 1995).

Mitral valve prolapse, the most common human abnormality of heart valves, affects about 4% of the population (Devereux et al. 1989). The term *mitral valve prolapse syndrome* is applied loosely to patients who have several somatic and autonomic symptoms. The autonomic symptoms described in the literature are those of POTS in patients with mitral valve prolapse. Whether patients with mitral valve prolapse are excessively prone to the development of POTS is not known.

Prognosis of POTS

Little information is available on prognosis. Our own early experience has been analysed (Sandroni et al. 1999). We used a structured questionnaire focused on autonomic status at follow-up: the ability to remain on the feet, degree of improvement, standing time, ability to work at the patient's occupation or at home, ability to withstand orthostatic stressors, weight gain or loss, and most beneficial treatment. Follow-up (mean, 67±52 months) has been completed for 40 patients. Overall, at follow-up, 80% of patients had improvement and 60% were functionally back to normal; 67% were able to stand for longer than 30 minutes without symptoms, and 90% were able to work. However, these patients were not entirely asymptomatic. Symptoms may be provoked by meals (30% of patients), exercise (69% of patients), and heat exposure (77% of patients). Patients with an antecedent event appeared to have a better response than those with spontaneous POTS (90% vs 70% had improvement; 84% vs 50% were able to stand >30 minutes). Most commonly, patients continued salt supplementation. Among medications, beta-blockers were the most efficacious. Khurana (1995) reported on the follow-up of 6 patients 8–17 years after autonomic evaluation: 2 patients had spontaneous and complete improvement, 1 had partial improvement, and 3 had persistence of symptoms.

Management

The patient with suspected POTS should have a detailed history, and general and neurological examination, seeking especially evidence of neuropathy. The patient with significant impairment should be evaluated further and treated. Many patients with mild orthostatic intolerance have a recognizable mechanism for orthostatic deconditioning (e.g. confined to bed for more than a few days, debilitating illness, hypovolaemia) and may not need an extensive evaluation.

After the decision has been made to evaluate the patient, the study should include cardiac and autonomic laboratory evaluations. The cardiac evaluation usually includes a cardiac interview and examination, electrocardiography (ECG), chest radiography, and 24-hour Holter monitoring, and the decision is made whether to perform cardiac electrophysiological studies. Electrophysiological testing is most useful in patients with heart disease manifested as:

- abnormal ventricular function (decreased ejection fraction),
- abnormal ECG (conduction defect, ischaemia, arrhythmia, multifocal ventricular ectopic beats)
- cardiac arrhythmia on Holter monitoring (Kapoor et al. 1989).
- As true for patients with syncope, it is likely that electrophysiological studies will be least useful in patients without heart disease, with an ejection fraction greater than 50%, and with normal findings on ECG and Holter monitoring (Shen and Gersh 1993).
- The neurological evaluation comprises a neurological history, examination, and tests seeking evidence for autonomic neuropathy. The autonomic laboratory evaluation follows and comprises a modified (10 minutes or longer head-up tilt) autonomic reflex screen and thermoregulatory sweat test. The 24-hour urinary sodium concentration should be measured. Normal subjects should excrete more than 170 mmol/24 hours (El-Sayed and Hainsworth 1996). Plasma catecholamines should be measured; they typically have an orthostatic value greater than 600 pg/mL.

The findings of the cardiac and autonomic evaluations are synthesized, and treatment is planned. POTS is best considered a syndrome of orthostatic intolerance rather than a disease sui generis. It is reasonable to document the presence and severity of POTS and to seek evidence of associated autonomic neuropathy, mitral valve prolapse, deconditioning, or history of vasovagal syndrome. The severity of POTS, the plasma volume, the degree of vagotonia (degree and duration of reflex bradycardia with the Valsalva manoeuvre and tilt back, Valsalva ratio, and HR range), β-adrenergic supersensitivity (HR increment, anxiety, tremor, and

reduction of muscle peripheral resistance), and central integration (blood pressure and HR oscillations) are determined. The patient's disorder is classified according to the pathophysiological mechanism, and treatment is individualized.

A patient with deconditioning and hypovolaemia should sleep with the head of the bed elevated 4 inches. Also, the plasma volume should be expanded with generous intake of salt and fludrocortisone (sleeping with the head of the bed elevated may expand plasma volume). The salt intake should be 150–250 mEq of sodium (10–20 g of salt). Patients who are intensely sensitive to salt intake can fine-tune their plasma volume and blood pressure control with salt intake alone. Foods that have a high salt content include fast foods such as hamburgers, hot dogs, chicken pieces, French fries, and fish fries. Canned soup, chilli, ham, bacon, sausage, additives such as soya sauce, and commercially processed canned products also have a high sodium content. The patient should have at least one glass or cup of fluids at mealtime and at least two at other times each day to obtain 2–2.5 litres/day. Fludrocortisone, 0.1–0.4 mg/day, can be prescribed if salt supplementation alone is ineffective.

A different approach to treatment is needed for patients who have venous pooling. Body stockings may be beneficial as a temporary measure. Several approaches appear to be effective for some of these patients, including physical countermanoeuvres (Bouvette et al. 1996, van Lieshout et al. 1992), and a 3-month programme of graduated training. Resistance training may be more beneficial than endurance training (Hakkinen and Hakkinen 1995).

The best treatment for patients who have peripheral adrenergic failure manifested as a loss of late phase II or frank orthostatic hypotension is fludrocortisone and an α-agonist. Midodrine appears to have the best absorption, predictable duration of action, and lack of central nervous system side-effects. The recommended dose is 5 mg three times daily. Some patients, at least in the short term appear to respond to the cholinesterase inhibitor, pyridostigmine (Singer et al. 2002). Typical dose is 30 mg three times daily, increasing if necessary to 60 mg three times daily.

Patients with florid POTS who have β-receptor supersensitivity tend to have a response to β-antagonists, but they sometimes are exquisitely sensitive to these agents. At conventional doses, fatigue is a major problem. We prescribe propranolol (Inderal), which may be more efficacious than β-selective non-lipophilic agents at a dose of 10 mg/day, increasing the dose over 2–3 weeks to 30–60 mg/day. The aim is to maintain the HR increment at about 50% of the pretreatment level. For patients with bronchospasm, a β-selective lipophilic agent such as metoprolol (Lopressor) can be given at a beginning dose of 25 mg/day and increased to the typical dose of 50 mg twice daily. For patients who have central side-effects, including lethargy or depression, a non-lipophilic agent is preferred. Nadolol, at a beginning dose of 10 mg/day and increased to 40 mg as needed, is a useful non-selective agent. β-selective agents such as atenolol (Tenormin), betaxolol (Kerlone), and acebutolol (Sectral) can be prescribed. The beginning doses of atenolol, betaxolol, and acebutolol are 25 mg, 10 mg, and 200 mg, respectively.

Treatment is particularly difficult if patients have unstable hypertensive responses to tilt. Some of these patients have a blood pressure response as high as 250/150 mm Hg on standing. In some of these patients, the autonomic instability responds to oral phenobarbital, with a beginning dose of 60 mg at night and 15 mg every morning. An alternative treatment is clonidine or another α2-agonist. Clonidine is given at a dose of 0.1 mg twice daily and increased to the maximally tolerated dose. Autonomic instability reportedly responds to microvascular decompression of the brainstem, but the role of surgical therapy has not been defined.

Occasionally, patients are evaluated during the acute postviral phase of the illness. For these patients, treatment with plasma exchange or intravenous gammaglobulin may be considered, especially if there is additional evidence of acute autonomic neuropathy. Recently, dramatic improvement in autonomic function has been reported following intravenous immunoglobulin treatment.[45–47] Autonomic recovery was well documented in the case of Smit et al. (1995). Improvement has also been reported in a case associated with a lung carcinoma (Bohnen et al. 1997).

References

Allen, S. C., Taylor, C. L., Hall, V. E. (1945). A study of orthostatic insufficiency by the tiltboard method. *Am. J Physiol.* **143**, 11–20.

Bohnen, N. I., Cheshire, W. P., Lennon, V. A., Van Den Berg, C. J. (1997). Plasma exchange improves function in a patient with ANNA-1 seropositive paraneoplastic autonomic neuropathy. *Neurology* **48**, A131.

Bou-Holaigah, I., Rowe, P. C., Kan, J., Calkins, H. (1995). The relationship between neurally mediated hypotension and the chronic fatigue syndrome. *JAMA* **274**, 961–67.

Boulenger, J. P., Uhde, T. W., Wolff, E. A., III, Post, R. M. (1984). Increased sensitivity to caffeine in patients with panic disorders. Preliminary evidence. *Arch. Gen. Psychiatry* **41**, 1067–71.

Bouvette, C. M., McPhee, B. R., Opfer-Gehrking, T. L., Low, P. A. (1996). Role of physical countermaneuvers in the management of orthostatic hypotension: Efficacy and biofeedback augmentation. *Mayo Clin. Proc.* **71**, 847–53.

Devereux, R. B., Kramer-Fox, R., Kligfield, P. (1989). Mitral valve prolapse: causes, clinical manifestations, and management. *Ann. Intern. Med.* **111**, 305–317.

El-Sayed, H., Hainsworth, R. (1996). Salt supplementation increases plasma volume and orthostatic tolerance in patients with unexplained syncope. *Heart* **75**, 134–40.

Fouad, F. M., Tadena Thome, L., Bravo, E. L., Tarazi, R. C. (1986). Idiopathic hypovolemia. *Ann. Intern. Med.* **104**, 298–303.

Freeman, R., Young, J., Landsberg, L., Lipsitz. L. (1996). The treatment of postprandial hypotension in autonomic failure with 3,4-DL-threo-dihydroxyphenylserine. *Neurology* **47**, 1414–20.

Hakkinen, K., Hakkinen, A. (1995). Neuromuscular adaptations during intensive strength training in middle-aged and elderly males and females. *Electromyogr. Clin. Neurophysiol.* **35**, 137–47.

Heafield, M. T., Gammage, M. D., Nightingale, S., Williams, A. C. (1996). Idiopathic dysautonomia treated with intravenous gammaglobulin. *Lancet* **347**, 28–29.

Hoeldtke, R. D., Davis, K. M. (1991). The orthostatic tachycardia syndrome: evaluation of autonomic function and treatment with octreotide and ergot alkaloids. *J Clin. Endocrinol. Metab.* **73**, 132–39.

Insel, T. R., Ninan, P. T., Aloi, J., Jimerson, D. C., Skolnick, P., Paul, S. M. (1984). A benzodiazepine receptor-mediated model of anxiety. Studies in nonhuman primates and clinical implications. *Arch. Gen. Psychiatry* **41**, 741–50.

Jacob, G., Atkinson, D., Jordan, J., *et al.* (1999). Effects of standing on cerebrovascular resistance in patients with idiopathic orthostatic intolerance. *Am. J Med.* **106**, 59–64.

Jacob, G., Biaggioni, I., Mosqueda-Garcia, R., Robertson, R. M., Robertson, D. (1998). Relation of blood volume and blood pressure in orthostatic intolerance. *Am. J Med. Sci.* **315**, 95–100.

Jacob, G., Costa, F., Shannon, J. R., *et al.* (2000). The neuropathic postural tachycardia syndrome. *N Engl. J Med.* **343**, 1008–1014.

Jordan, J., Shannon, J. R., Diedrich, A., Black, B. K., Robertson, D. (2002). Increased sympathetic activation in idiopathic orthostatic intolerance: role of systemic adrenoreceptor sensitivity. *Hypertension* **39**, 173–78.

Kapoor, W. N., Hammill, S. C., Gersh, B. J. (1989). Diagnosis and natural history of syncope and the role of invasive electrophysiologic testing. *Am. J Cardiol.* **63**, 730–34.

Khurana, R. K. (1995). Orthostatic intolerance and orthostatic tachycardia: a heterogeneous disorder. *Clin. Auton. Res.* **5**, 12–18.

Komaroff, A. L., Fagioli, L. R., Geiger, A. M., *et al.* (1996). An examination of the working case definition of chronic fatigue syndrome. *Am. J Med.* **100**, 56–64.

Lagerlund, T. D., Low, P. A., Novak, V., *et al.* (2005). Spectral analysis of slow modulation of EEG amplitude and cardiovascular variables in subjects with postural tachycardia syndrome. *Auton. Neurosci.* **117**, 132–42.

Low, P. A., Opfer-Gehrking, T. L., Textor, S. C., *et al.* (1994). Comparison of the postural tachycardia syndrome (POTS) with orthostatic hypotension due to autonomic failure. *J Auton. Nerv. Syst.* **50**, 181–88.

Low, P. A., Gilden, J. L., Freeman, R., Sheng, K. N., McElligott, M. A. (1997a) Efficacy of midodrine vs placebo in neurogenic orthostatic hypotension. A randomized, double-blind multicenter study. Midodrine Study Group. *JAMA* **277**, 1046–51.

Low, P. A., Schondorf, R., Novak, V., Sandroni, P., Opfer-Gehrking, T. L., Novak, P. (1997b). Postural tachycardia syndrome. In: Low, P. A. ed. Clinical Autonomic Disorders: Evaluation and Management. 2 ed. Philadelphia: Lippincott-Raven, pp. 681–97.

Mathias, C. J., Low, D. A., Iodice, V., Owens, A. P., Kirbiš, M., and Grahame, R . (2012). The Postural Tachycardia Syndrome (PoTS) – Current experiences and concepts. *Nature Neurology Reviews* **8**, 22–34.

Mericle, R. A., Triggs, W. J. (1997). Treatment of acute pandysautonomia with intravenous immunoglobulin. *J Neurol. Neurosurg. Psychiatry* **62**, 529–31.

Nickander, K. K., Low, P. A. (2003). Characterization of molecular alterations in postural orthostatic tachycardia syndrome. *Clin. Auton. Res.* **13**, 385.

Novak, V., Spies, J. M., Novak, P., McPhee, B. R., Rummans, T. A., Low, P. A. (1998). Hypocapnia and cerebral hypoperfusion in orthostatic intolerance. *Stroke* **29**, 1876–81.

Rosen, S. G., Cryer, P. E. (1982). Postural tachycardia syndrome. Reversal of sympathetic hyperresponsiveness and clinical improvement during sodium loading. *Am. J Med.* **72**, 847–50.

Sandroni, P., Opfer-Gehrking, T. L., McPhee, B. R., Low, P. A. (1999). Postural tachycardia syndrome: Clinical features and follow-up study. *Mayo Clin. Proc.* **74**, 1106–1110.

Schondorf, R., Low, P. A. (1993a). Idiopathic postural orthostatic tachycardia syndrome: an attenuated form of acute pandysautonomia? *Neurology* **43**, 132–37.

Schondorf, R., Low, P. A. (1993b). Idiopathic postural tachycardia syndrome. In: Low, P. A. ed. *Clinical Autonomic Disorders: Evaluation and Management.* Boston: Little, Brown and Company: 641–52.

Shen, W. K., Gersh, B. J. (1993). Syncope: Mechanisms, Approach, and Management. In: Low, P. A. ed. *Clinical Autonomic Disorders: Evaluation and Management.* 1 ed. Boston: Little, Brown and Company: 605–40.

Singer, W., Nickander, K. K., Hines, S. M., Opfer-Gehrking, T. L., Low, P. A. Acetylcholinesterase inhibition: a new therapeutic approach in patients with orthostatic intolerance. *Neurology* **58** (Suppl 3), A346.

Singer, W., Spies, J. M., McArthur, J., *et al.* (2004). Prospective evaluation of somatic and autonomic small fibers in selected autonomic neuropathies. *Neurology* **62**, 612–618.

Smit, A. A. J., Vermeulen, M., Koelman, J. H. T. M., Wieling, W. (1995). An unusual recovery in a patient with acute pandysautonomia after intravenous immunoglobulin therapy. *Clin. Auton. Res.* **5**, 323A.

Stewart, J. M. (2002). Pooling in chronic orthostatic intolerance: arterial vasoconstrictive but not venous compliance defects. *Circulation* **105**, 2274–81.

Stewart, J. M. (2003). Microvascular filtration is increased in postural tachycardia syndrome. *Circulation* **107**, 2816–22.

Streeten, D. H. P. (1987). *Orthostatic Disorders of the Circulation, Mechanisms, Manifestations and Treatment.* New York: Plenum Press.

Streeten, D. H., Anderson, G. H., Jr., Richardson, R., Thomas, F. D. (1988). Abnormal orthostatic changes in blood pressure and heart rateHR in subjects with intact sympathetic nervous function: evidence for excessive venous pooling. *J Lab. Clin. Med.* **111**, 326–35.

Streeten, D. H. P., Scullard, T. F. (1996). Excessive gravitational blood pooling caused by impaired venous tone is the predominant non-cardiac mechanism of orthostatic intolerance. *Clin. Sci.* **90**, 277–85.

Tani, H., Singer, W., McPhee, B. R., Opfer-Gehrking, T. L., Low, P. A. (1999). Splanchnic and systemic circulation in the postural tachycardia syndrome. *Clin. Auton. Res.* **9**, 231–32.

Tani, H., Singer, W., McPhee, B. R., *et al.* (2000). Splanchnic-mesenteric capacitance bed in the postural tachycardia syndrome (POTS). *Auton. Neurosci.* **86**, 107–113.

Tyrer, P. (1988). Current status of beta-blocking drugs in the treatment of anxiety disorders. *Drugs* **36**, 773–83.

Uhde, T. W., Tancer, M. (1988). Chemical models of panic: A review and critique. In: Tyrer, P., ed. *Psychopharmacology of Anxiety*. New York: Oxford University Press: 110–31.

Uhde, T. W., Stein, M. B., Vittone, B. J., *et al.* (1989). Behavioral and physiologic effects of short-term and long-term administration of clonidine in panic disorder. *Arch. Gen. Psychiatry* **46**, 170–77.

van Lieshout, J. J., ten Harkel, A. D., Wieling, W. (1992). Physical manoeuvres for combating orthostatic dizziness in autonomic failure. *Lancet* **339**, 897–98.

Vernino, S., Low, P. A., Fealey, R. D., Stewart, J. D., Farrugia, G., Lennon, V. A. (2000). Autoantibodies to ganglionic acetylcholine receptors in autoimmune autonomic neuropathies. *N Engl. J Med.* **343**, 847–55.

Wise, C. D., Berger, B. D., Stein, L. (1972). Benzodiazepines: anxiety-reducing activity by reduction of serotonin turnover in the brain. *Science* **177**, 180–83.

CHAPTER 62

Circulatory shock

Niels H. Secher and Johannes J. Van Lieshout

Introduction

Circulatory shock is characterized by limited tissue perfusion including cerebral blood flow (CBF) and may be loss of consciousness. Monitoring of the critically ill does not regularly include an evaluation of CBF or cerebral oxygenation but management of the circulation can favourably be directed to control of flow-directed variables (Bundgaarsd-Nielsen et al. 2007) or cerebral oxygenation (Murkin and Arango, 2009). With typical monitoring of heart rate (HR) and blood pressure, however, circulatory shock remains largely defined by a low arterial pressure and that is the case although an apparently normal blood pressure may be preserved at the expense of flow and, conversely, flow may be maintained at a low blood pressure. A definition of shock based on blood pressure is, therefore, not adequate or satisfactory and for example anaesthesia can be planned to lower blood pressure and such 'hypotensive anaesthesia' is a standard procedure for reducing the surgical blood loss.

This chapter describes circumstances during which CBF and cerebral oxygenation become affected, illustrating that the lower level of cerebral autoregulation depends critically on cardiac output (CO) and therefore on the central blood volume (CBV) since when CO is limited by CBV, even a minimal reduction in arterial pressure affects CBF and cerebral oxygenation (Madsen and Secher 1999, Van Lieshout et al. 2003), while cerebral oxygenation is maintained at a low blood pressures when CBV is secured (Nissen et al. 2009).

Classification of circulatory shock

As indicated, a definition of circulatory shock depends on what is measured but from the perspective of this chapter situations that limit CO are of particular interest. The blood available to the heart (its preload) is important for CO, but heart function may also limit CO and thereby oxygenation of the tissues as is the case following a large anterior myocardial infarction. Conversely, poisons and drugs, including anaesthetics, may affect (baroreceptor) control of blood pressure and induce hypotension by loss of peripheral resistance if translocation of blood to the periphery is not compensated and CBV maintained (Crandall et al. 2008, Bundgaard-Nielsen et al. 2010). For example, endotoxin in septic shock, accumulation of (maybe) ammonium in liver failure, and

heat stress or fever induces peripheral vasodilatation by loss of sympathetic control of vascular tone (*sympatholysis*). In other words, flow to the brain depends on whether CO is elevated to match the reduced peripheral resistance, but for some patients diastolic heart function limits the ability to raise CO adequately.

Accordingly, any evaluation of circulatory shock needs to ascertain whether CBV is maintained or, in other words, the diagnosis of shock is related intimately to the therapeutic strategy since an evaluation of whether CBV is limiting CO is the key to understand why the circulation fails.

Haemorrhage is obviously an important reason for *hypovolaemic shock*, but a reduced CBV may also be provoked by *dehydration* (e.g. by diabetes insipidus, by glucosuria in untreated diabetes mellitus, or by cholera), by loss of plasma (e.g. in response to injury including burns), and probably most often by a reduced venous return to the heart by accumulation of blood in dependent parts of the body. During gravitational stress, the response to a reduced CBV is described in terms of *fainting* or *a vasovagal syncope*, but the cardiovascular manifestations are similar to those presenting during haemorrhage and may be equally fatal if not corrected promptly.

When standing up CBV is reduced by some 500 ml, and in order to maintain the upright position, humans possess a blood volume that allows for a blood loss of about 1 litre when supine. However, the challenge to CBF can obviously, both in consequence of gravity and in response to haemorrhage, become significant and CBV reduced to a critical level (by ~30%) that results in a vasovagal syncope as described in detail by Barcroft et al. (Fig. 62.1). For humans the influence of gravity on distribution of blood volume is critical since, in contrast to most animals, when we sit or stand up, the major part of the vasculature is positioned below the level of the heart. It is a further problem that venous return is not secured by autonomic reflexes including sympathetic activation and the veno-arterial reflex. Venous return to the heart dependents critically on the 'muscle pump' in the legs: muscle contractions squeeze blood out of the muscle and the venous valves replace its transport to the heart.

Even a small reduction in CO may be critical for humans since as much as ~15% of CO is directed to the brain. For example, when a person stands still, as when a student is attending surgery or when a soldier stands in line, the muscle pump may be inoperative and

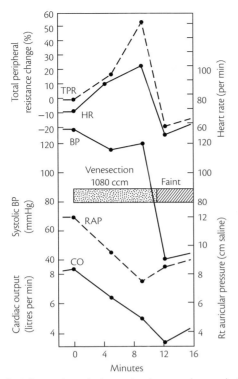

Fig. 62.1 Biphasic haemodynamic changes in a human volunteer during venesection of 1080 ml. RAP, right arterial pressure; CO, cardiac output; BP, systolic blood pressure; TPR, total peripheral resistance; HR, heart rate. Reprinted from *The Lancet*, **243**, Barcroft H, Edholm OG, McMichael J, and Sharpey-Schafer EP, Posthaemorrhagic fainting. Study by cardiac output and forearm flow, 489–91, Copyright (1944), with permission from Elsevier.

blood accumulates in the lower parts of the body and the person faints when the critical reduction in CBF is reached. Also following instrumentation, subjects or patients tend to sit or to stand still, promoting accumulation of blood in lower parts of the body, and they should be encouraged to move their legs (e.g. students may be encouraged to stand on the their toes when attending their first operation or, for patients going through surgery in an upright position, mast trousers or a seat with elevated knees should be applied to ensure that CBV is not critically challenged.

Following a vasovagal syncope, venous return is restored if the person falls and recovery is rapid if there is no injury associated with the fall. But patients with sympathetic failure (e.g. due to anaesthesia) are sensitive to even a small change in body position. A critical reduction in CBV may be provoked simply by raising the head-end of the bed if the legs or the knees are not raised to a position that simulates that used by astronauts when travelling through the atmosphere. The postoperative patient is vulnerable to even minimal orthostatic stress because of drowsiness and also because partial neuromuscular blockade or regional anaesthesia immobilize the legs.

The surgical patient also becomes vulnerable when required to remain motionless if the intervention is carried out in a position that compromises venous return. Vasovagal episodes are regular during procedures on the shoulder using local anaesthesia with the patient sitting up. Similarly, syncope and death in the dental chair were eliminated only by letting the patient lay down (Sharpey-Schafer 1956). For operations carried out with the patient supine, a large abdominal content (fat, ascites or the pregnant uterus) may

obstruct the lower caval vein, but adopting the left lateral tilted position promotes venous return and prevents shock (Brigden et al. 1950).

Accumulation of blood in dependent parts of the body also becomes a problem when regional anaesthesia paralyses venous tone during procedures that squeeze the lower caval vein as with lower abdominal surgery requiring an extended body position. Therefore, regional anaesthesia for postoperative pain treatment should be activated only when the supine position is re-established by the end of surgery or a transverse abdominal plan block should be used. Conversely, CBV is preserved by providing a knee support or by application of a moderate Trendelenburg's position, not only during surgery but also during, for example, a scanning procedure.

Regional anaesthesia as a paradigm of an inability to provide adequate vasoconstriction illustrates the problem affecting patients with autonomic dysfunction or paraplegia as well as tetraplegic patients who add an inability to recruit blood from the splanchnic area (Welply et al. 1975). In these patients, orthostatic intolerance is improved by sleeping in the head-up position (MacLean and Allen 1940) and by volume loading (Wieling et al. 2002) and, as in patients with orthostatic intolerance, until it provokes peripheral oedema. For patients exposed to a transient inability to vasoconstrict, as seen with regional anaesthesia, it is, however, more desirable to provide pharmacological vasoconstriction.

Anaphylactic shock may carry some element of a reduced CBV by peripheral vasodilatation with concomitant reduction in HR and arterial pressure besides bronchospasm, rashes, and swelling. However, CBV has not been measured in anaphylactic shock and there may be an increase in pulmonary vascular pressures.

In addition to hypovolaemia and peripheral vasodilatation, circulatory shock may develop in response to restricted inflow to the heart. Pericardial tamponade and enlarged pressure in the thoracic cavity provoked by pressure breathing, positive end-expiratory ventilation (PEEP), or a pressure pneumothorax is characterized by central hypovolaemia and filled neck veins. A similar situation develops with accumulation of fluid or blood within the mediastinum resulting, for example, from a displaced central venous catheter. With elevated central vascular pressures, venous return and in turn CO are jeopardized, as exemplified during the transient changes that take place during coughing or a Valsalva manoeuvre, illustrating that central vascular pressures can be interrogated in regard to filling of the heart only when it is known whether a change is caused by factors outside or inside the vessels.

Cardiovascular manifestations during hypovolaemic shock

The cardiovascular responses to a reduced CBV are mimicked by prolonged active or passive orthostatic stress. However, in contrast to head-up tilt (HUT) and haemorrhage, assuming the standing position is associated with marked fluctuation in blood pressure with the combined effects of a reduced CBV and the use of the muscles to raise the body (Chapter 20). With haemorrhage or passive HUT, or other means of reducing CBV (e.g. application of negative pressure to the lower body (LBNP), pressure breathing, regional anaesthesia, or exposure to large G-forces as in fighter pilots performing a loop), HR increases to 90–100 bpm, while blood pressure is maintained or, in the case of HUT, slightly

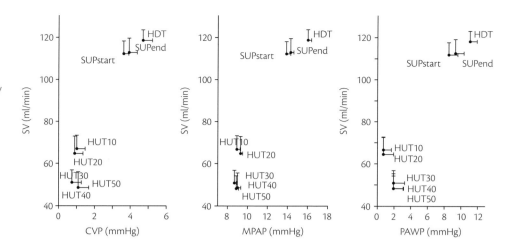

Fig. 62.2 Stroke volume of the heart (SV) related to the thoracic fluid content as expressed by central venous pressure (CVP), mean pulmonary artery pressure (MPAP), and pulmonary artery wedge pressure (PAWP) during head-up (HUT) and head-down tilt. Values are mean ± SE for 9 subjects. With permission from Van Lieshout JJ, MPM Harms, F Pott, M Jenstrup, and NH Secher (2005). Stroke volume of the heart and thoracic fluid content during head-up and head-down tilt. *Acta Anaesthesiologica Scandinavica.* **49**, 1287–92, Wiley.

elevated (Fig. 62.1). As CBV is reduced, stoke volume of the heart and eventually also CO become preload dependent. Central venous pressure, pressure in the pulmonary artery and its wedge pressure also decrease, but while stroke volume and CO continue to decrease over time, central pressures stabilize and for pulmonary pressures there may be some recovery (Fig. 62.2).

During this initial response to a reduced CBV (*Stage I of hypovolaemic shock; preshock*), arterial baroreceptor control of blood pressure is maintained, with a larger gain in the untrained than in endurance trained subjects (Ogoh et al. 2003). However, with a reduction of CBV by ~30%, a vasovagal episode develops with no effective baroreceptor control of HR or blood pressure (*Stage II of hypovolaemic shock*). Thus, blood pressure decreases abruptly due to loss of sympathetic activity to vascular wall smooth muscles and, as parasympathetic activity increases, HR decreases (Fig. 62.1). How profound HR is affected depends on the reduction in CBV. If the patient is provided with intravenous fluid or if the intervention that reduces CBV is terminated when the patient or subject feels ill, then HR is 40–60 bpm. However, if hypovolaemia persists, the vasovagal response continues with extreme bradycardia. Yet, the episode is reversed immediately when CBV is restored by terminating the intervention that reduced CBV, by raising the legs, or by administration of volume.

With even a modest reduction in CBV and CO, CBF and oxygenation of the brain becomes affected, even though arterial pressure is maintained within the range that is considered to secure CBF autoregulation (van Lieshout et al. 2003). During a vasovagal episode, patients feel ill because CBF is reduced by ~50% with a ~15% decrease in cerebral oxygenation at a mean arterial pressure of 80 mmHg (Fig. 62.3). The visual prodromal sensation accompanying cerebral hypoperfusion is the loss of colour vision ('grey out') eventually followed by black out by a progressive reduction in blood supply to the retina because the intra-ocular pressure makes its perfusion the most vulnerable part of the central nervous system.

In contrast, oxygenation of skeletal muscles increases in stage II of shock. Muscle blood flow doubles because muscular sympathetic nerve activity (MSNA) is eliminated, vascular resistance abruptly decreases, and the patient may be comfortable as heat spreads throughout the body. Sympathetic activity is often considered to be uniform, but that is not the case during this stage of shock. As expected, plasma noradrenalin decreases with some delay

in regards to MSNA, while plasma adrenaline increases indicating enhanced adrenal sympathetic activity (Fig. 62.4). The patient also becomes pale giving the impression of peripheral vasoconstriction, but that results from an increase in plasma antidiuretic hormone to a level where it reduces skin blood flow (i.e. it acts as vasopressin) and diuresis. The increase in angiotensin II also reduces subcutaneous blood flow, but angiotensin II does not provoke a similar pale skin. Other manifestations include sweating and, occasionally, peripheral cyanosis although arterial oxygenation is maintained. Increased vagal activity explains nausea and, with the consequent relaxation of the stomach lasting for an hour or more, intake of, for example, water may provoke vomiting.

The bradycardic response to a ~30% reduced CBV does, however, not always manifest. Even in healthy people, HR may not decrease upon a marked reduction in CBV underscoring the priority of the changes indicated by Lewis (1932) when he termed such episodes as vasovagal syncope. Obviously, a lowering of HR cannot manifest when diabetes affects vagal function. Equally important, bradycardia does not develop if haemorrhage is associated with pain as in some trauma. In addition, it is difficult to demonstrate a reduction in HR upon haemorrhage in an acute animal preparation but in chronically instrumented animals, a reduction in CBV is

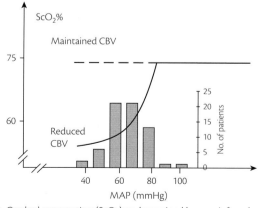

Fig. 62.3 Cerebral oxygenation (ScO₂) as determined by near infrared spectroscopy in relation to mean arterial pressure (MAP) with reduced central blood volume (CBV) by head-up tilt and with maintained CBV during propofol-fentanyl anaesthesia. With permission from Nissen P, JJ Van Lieshout, HB Nielsen, and NH Secher (2009). Frontal lobe oxygenation is maintained during hypotension following propofol-fentanyl anesthesia. *AANA J* **77**, 271–6.

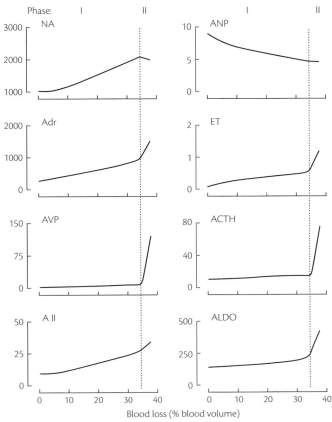

Fig. 62.4 Biphasic changes of plasma concentrations of hormones during progressive central hypovolaemia in humans. NA, noradrenaline; Adr, adrenaline; AVP, arginine vasopressin; AII, angiotensin II; ANP, atrial natriuretic peptide; ET, endothelin; ACTH, adrenocorticotropic hormone; ALDO, aldosterone. All units in pg/litre. Reprinted from Ludbrook J. Haemorrhage and shock. In R. Hainsworth and AL Mark, ed. *Cardiovascular Reflex Control in Health and Disease* pp. 463–90. Copyright (1993).

associated with bradycardia (Schadt and Ludbrook 1991). Conversely, sympathetic activation may be used clinically to accelerate HR and increase blood pressure by peripheral vasoconstriction (Brignole et al. 2002), that is to restore baroreceptor circulatory control. The patient who develops presyncopal symptoms is asked to squeeze ones hand or to lift one or both legs. Similarly, patients suffering from orthostatic intolerance improve blood pressure by performing a leg crossing manoeuvre and fighter pilots use mast trousers and leg contractions not only to prevent accumulation of blood in leg veins, but also to enhance sympathetic activity when they perform a loop.

If CBV is not restored immediately in stage II of hypovolaemic shock, the patient either dies or HR increases again and then to higher values than in Stage I (i.e. to ~125 bpm), while arterial pressure remains low (*Stage III of hypovolaemic shock*). In that situation it is difficult to stabilize the circulation even after apparently adequate volume administration and re-establishment of blood pressure (i.e. stage III represents a transition to *an irreversible stage (IV) of hypovolaemic shock* [Wiggers 1951] or *multiple organ failure*). Such failing circulatory control underscores the importance of continuous and accurate monitoring of CBV and of aggressive volume treatment to prevent organ hypoperfusion. Thus upon

immediate intervention, all patients in stage II, but not in stage III of hypovolaemic shock recover.

Cardiovascular control during hypovolaemic shock

The mechanisms that determine the stage of hypovolaemic shock are not clear, but the initial increase in HR upon a reduced CBV is by vagal withdrawal rapidly replaced by sympathetic activation, which is also responsible for the increase in total peripheral resistance. With central integration in the *n. tractus solitarius* sympathetic activation is via unloading myelinated stretch or pressure sensitive nerve fibres distributed throughout the central circulation, which allow the baroreceptors to maintain blood pressure in spite of a reduced CO. In contrast, the vasovagal response is elicited by activation of unmyelinated (C) fibres equally distributed throughout the central circulation as well as in the pericardium, with the predominance in the posterior wall of the left ventricle of the heart (Öberg and Thorén 1972). Stimulation of any or all of these areas may elicit a *Bezold-Jarish-like reflex* characterized by a simultaneous decrease in HR and blood pressure as originally demonstrated with administration of veratrum alkaloids. The final tachycardic response to haemorrhage could result from a cerebral ischemic reflex with a rise in plasma catecholamines to high levels that, however, do not affect total peripheral resistance. Failing cerebral perfusion explains a transition to an irreversible stage of shock.

It is often considered a paradox that haemorrhage elicits bradycardia and sympathetic inhibition, manifestations not included in many textbooks. In parallel with the reduction in bleeding induced by hypotensive anaesthesia, it may be an advantage to acutely lower blood pressure and reduce bleeding before it becomes fatal. Thus, tolerance to haemorrhage is reduced when the heart is denervated. Whatever the reason for the reduction in HR and total peripheral resistance, if it is present, concealed or delayed haemorrhage in regard to a trauma, as seen with rupture of the spleen should be considered (Secher and Bie 1985).

Central blood volume

With the manifestations of a failing circulation often representing an inadequate CBV or preload to the heart, it is important how CBV is defined. The diastolic volume of the heart is the most rigorous definition of CBV in that other definitions, depending on one of several methods to determine the blood volume within the lungs and the heart, relate to their relevance for filling of the heart. Thus the function of the heart is described by the (Frank-)Starling 'law of the heart' (Fig. 62.2) with hypovolaemia representing a diastolic volume that is smaller than that needed to provide a maximal stroke volume, CO, or venous oxygen saturation (SvO$_2$; Harms et al. 2003). Inherent to that definition is that it does not relate to the total blood volume or to the fluid balance of the patient. This is indicated, for example with standing, which may provoke a hypovolaemic shock by pooling of blood in dependent parts of the body.

In contrast, stroke volume, CO or SvO$_2$ do not increase during head-down tilt although the pulmonary artery mean and wedge pressures do increase as does filling of the heart, i.e. a supine human is *normovolaemic*, in that the flat part of the Starling curve is reached (Fig. 62.2). The classic Starling curve indicates a reduction in contractile function with further filling of the heart. Whether a failing circulation may be provoked by expanding the heart remains

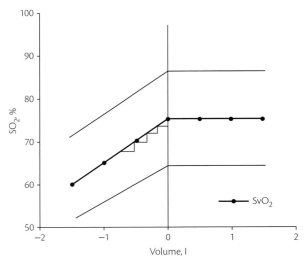

Fig. 62.5 Venous or tissue oxygen saturation related to changes in blood volume. Hypovolaemia represents a preload to the heart that limits oxygen transport; normovolaemia a volume that does not affect oxygen transport, and hypervolaemia a central blood volume that is larger than what provides for a maximal venous or tissue oxygenation. Curves drawn for patients with different cardiac outputs.

unsettled, but the heart may become distended when it is vulnerable, as following heart surgery.

Cardiac output and venous oxygen saturation

In cases of pure hypovolaemic shock (haemorrhage, dehydration, or orthostatic stress), CO and mixed (from the pulmonary artery) or central (from a central venous catheter) SvO_2 decrease. As a rule, a reduction of the circulating blood volume by 100 ml results in a reduction in SvO_2 by 1% in adults (Fig. 62.5). In a supine resting healthy person SvO_2 is ~75%, meaning that for a SvO_2 of 65%, a first approximation is that the patient has a volume deficit of one litre.

However, for many patients there is no single origin of the shock. Often there is some component of vasodilatation (by endotoxaemia, regional or general anaesthesia, or by fever) and the arterial baroreceptors have lost some ability to elicit vasoconstriction. Then maintenance of CBF requires that CBV is large enough to allow CO to increase considerably (e.g. to more than 10 litres/minute) and equally SvO_2 increases (e.g. to 85% for a normal person during heating, during anaesthesia or for liver failure patients) (Fig. 62.5). Consequently, during such circumstances a reduction of CBV provokes fainting at a CO of, e.g. 5 litres/minute and a SvO_2 of, for example, 75% that are quite sufficient under normal conditions.

Administration of fluid and blood

With a reduced circulating blood volume, the body has a substantial capacity to restore the circulating blood volume by recruitment of fluid (the capillary fluid shift). The increase in plasma adrenaline (Fig. 62.4) raises the blood glucose level and because of the osmotic effect, fluid is recruited to the circulation. However, there may be

more subtle adrenergic reflexes in play as the recruitment of fluid is attenuated by beta-adrenergic blockade. Independently of the mechanism responsible for recruitment of fluid from the interstitial space, the added volume resides within the blood vessels for the time it is needed. For example, in patients developing hypotension following spinal anaesthesia, the drop in haematocrit is larger for a given administered volume than for those patients who maintain blood pressure. Furthermore, and as previously mentioned, administration of fluid enhances orthostatic tolerance not only in subjects but also in patients affected by orthostatic intolerance.

With fluid administration the oxygen carrying capacity of blood does not become limited until haemoglobin reaches very low levels (< 4 mM) because of the increase in CO with haemodilution and a reduction in haematocrit to ~30% is accepted (Table 62.1). Saline or lactated Ringer is eventually supplemented by plasma expanders and only when the blood loss is > 1 litre, blood is substituted. With haemorrhage exceeding 1–1.5 times the estimated blood volume, fresh frozen plasma is also provided to maintain the ability to form a clot. With an even larger loss, there is a need to provide platelets and, for example with reperfusion of organs, there is a large use of platelets, and they are administered before such events. Eventually clot formation may be secured by, for example, aprotenin or by recombinant factor VII, but maintenance of body temperature and plasma calcium despite the use of cold and citrated blood products

Table 62.1 Blood volume expanders for the emergency treatment of acute hypovolaemia; 1898 to present

Era	Blood volume expander
Spanish—American War (1898)	Subcutaneous or rectal saline
Pre-First World War	Intravenous physiological saline, direct blood transfusion
First World War (1914–18)	Fresh citrated blood, concentrated albumin
Spanish Civil War (1936–39)	Citrated bank blood
Second World War (1939–45)	Large-pool citrated plasma, concentrated albumin
Korean War (1950–53)	Unmatched O-negative blood, citrated small pool plasma
1950–53	Polyvinylopyrrilidone (PVP)
1950 to present	Modified gelatine solutions
	Hydroxyeethylo starch solutions
	Dextrane solutions of varying molecular weight
1970 to present	Liquid or lyophilized 5% pasteurized human albumin
	Pasteurized plasma protein solutions (PPS)
1970 to present	Balanced electrolyte solutions including lactated Ringer
1980 to present	Hypertonic NaCl solutions (7.5%)
Present	Lactated Ringer followed by plasma expanders,
Unmatched	O-negative blood followed by matched blood, fresh frozen plasma and platelets

Modified from Ludbrook, 1997.

that binds calcium is essential not only for coagulation but also, with respect to calcium, for blood pressure.

It is important not only to secure CBV, but also to assess when to stop an infusion. With volume administration likely to induce haemodilution and with an inverse relationship between CO and haematocrit, volume administration may increase CO beyond what is needed. It is an advantage, therefore, to focus on SvO_2 or on tissue oxygenation. With haemodilution, the oxygen carrying capacity of blood decreases, but that is compensated for by the increase in CO. In other words, whatever fluid is used for volume replacement, volume is administered until a maximal SvO_2 or tissue oxygenation is established (Fig. 62.5).

Monitoring the central blood volume

While central vascular pressures provide a recording of acute changes in CBV (Fig. 62.2), they stabilize quickly and over time there is no association between these variables and CBV, stroke volume or CO, in either an experimental setting or in clinical practice. Ideally the filling of the heart can be followed by echocardiography, but that is not established for routine monitoring. Alternatively, changes in CBV can be monitored accurately with ECG electrodes detecting a small electrical current provided to the thoracic region of the body. These then record changes in impedance or, more conveniently, in admittance. Thus changes in thoracic admittance are reported with correlations to other estimates of CBV or fluid balance with r-values > 0.9 and often with perfection (r > 0.98) (Krantz et al. 2000).

Cerebral blood flow and oxygenation

The relation between CBF and arterial pressure is described by the cerebral autoregulatory curve (i.e. CBF is considered to remain stable within a pressure range of 60 to 140 mmHg) (Fig. 62.3). At lower pressures CBF decreases, defining the lower limit of cerebral autoregulation, while CBF increases at a high blood pressure. However, in stage II of hypovolaemic shock CBF and cerebral oxygenation decrease at a remarkably high blood pressure of 80 mmHg and, as mentioned, even with the reduced CBV induced by standing, there is a small reduction in both variables.

Such reductions in CBF are in sharp contrast to what is experienced when blood pressure is reduced while CBV is maintained, e.g. during anaesthesia induced by drugs that do not influence cerebral autoregulation (Fig. 62.3). Conversely, when haemorrhage reduces blood pressure during anaesthesia, then cerebral oxygenation also decreases. The implication is that unless CBV or, ideally, CBF or oxygenation of the brain, are monitored it remains unknown whether a given blood pressure is of consequence for the brain, possible explaining why some patients feel less alert following anaesthesia.

However, preservation of CBF during states of shock is even more complicated. Because of the lack of elimination of ammonium during liver failure, CBF may double and causes haemorrhage or ischemia following brain oedema, i.e. death from acute liver failure is often due to a cerebral catastrophe (Larsen et al. 1996). Similarly, the inhalation agents used for anaesthesia affect cerebral autoregulation and episodes of cerebral hyperperfusion resulting in formation of oedema are likely to explain the associated postoperative nausea and vomiting.

Cardiogenic shock

The role of the heart in shock is complex. In stage II of hypovolaemic shock the load on the heart is small due to the concomitant decrease in HR and blood pressure and there is detected no ECG signs of ischaemia. An obvious reason for circulatory shook is an inability of the heart to contract brought on by a myocardial infarction or pericardial tamponade. Pump failure develops when an infarct covers a large part of the myocardium, typically the anterior wall of the left ventricle. Under such circumstances, the patient is pale and sweating, but these signs of a limited CO do not necessary manifest with a posterior or an inferior infarct. In the latter case hypotension may be associated with relative wellbeing in spite of bradyarrhythmia suggesting that CO is preserved. Hypotension then develops in response to a decrease in peripheral resistance that, together with the arrhythmia, indicates an activation of C-fibres within the heart. Equally, a Bezold–Jarish like reflex may be provoked by intracoronary injections of a contrast media for angiography and then more likely with administration to the posterior rather than to the anterior coronary artery. Whatever the reason for the failing heart, the well-being of the patient is closely related to oxygenation of the brain.

Fainting and sudden death threat to patients developing a high left ventricular pressure in response to aortic stenosis. Their failing circulation is provoked by stimulation of myocardial C-fibres because in animals, these fibres are identified by their response of clamping of the aorta (Öberg and Thorén 1972). Experimentally, a Bezold–Jarish-like reflex may be demonstrated with the increased load on the heart during exercise, since patients with aortic stenosis react with vasodilatation rather than with vasoconstriction to resting skeletal muscles.

Neurogenic shock

While most situations that provoke a vasovagal syncope are associated with accumulation of blood in the lower parts of the body, a similar reaction can develop in supine humans (e.g. during blood sampling, catheterization), or by exposure to certain smells or pain. Such episodes indicate that circulatory shock may also originate from the central nervous system and may be analogous to the '*playing dead*' reaction seen in animals placed in a dangerous situation. One advantage of such a reaction is that the eye is more sensitive to motion than it is to recognizing shapes. Thus the pray may be left to itself when sitting still (with a low HR and blood pressure). Only when it resumes consciousness and tries to escape, the hunting animal becomes interested and, in the end, makes the kill. In some situations it may be a survival strategy to faint and hope that the threat has gone away when normal baroreceptor control of the circulation is re-established, or in the words of Jarisch (1941) 'als Totstell Reflex in einer Situation, in der es besser ist tot zu scheinin, als es zu sein'.

References

Barcroft, H., Edholm, O. G., McMichael, J., and Sharpey-Schafer, E. P. (1944). Posthaemorrhagic fainting. Study by cardiac output and forearm flow. *Lancet*, i, 489–91.

Brigden, W., Howarth, S., and Sharpey-Schafer, E. P. (1950). Postural changes in the peripheral blood-flow of normal subjects with observations on vasovagal fainting reactions as a result of tilting, the lordotic posture, pregnancy and spinal anaesthesia. *Clinical Science*, **9**, 79–90.

Brignole, M., Croci, F., Menozzi, C., *et al.* (2002). Isometric arm counter-pressure maneuvres to abort impending vasovagal syncope. *Journal of the American College of Cardiology* **40**, 2053–9.

Bundgaard-Nielsen, M., Holte, K., Secher, N. H., and Kehlet H. (2007). Monitoring of peri-operative fluid administration by individidualized goal-directed therapy. *Acta Anaesthesiologica Scandinavica.* **51**, 331–40.

Bundgaard-Nielsen, M., Wilson, T. E., Seifert, T., Secher, N. H., and Crandall, C. G. (2010). Effect of volume loading on the Frank-Starling relation during reductions in central blood volume in heat-stressed humans. *Journal of Physiology* **588**, 3333–9.

Crandall, C. G., Wilson, T. E., Marving, J., Vogelsang, T. W., Kjaer, A., Hesse, B., Secher, N. H. (2008). Effect of passive heating on central blood volume and ventricular dimensions in humans. *Journal of Physiology.* **586**, 293–301.

Harms, M. P., Van Lieshout, J. J., Jenstrup, M., Pott, F., and Secher, N. H. (2003). Postural effects on cardiac output and mixed venous saturation in humans. *Experimental Physiology,* **88**, 611–6.

Jarisch, A. (1941). Vasovagale Synkope. *Zeitscrift für Kreislauf Forschungen* **23**, 267–79.

Krantz, T., Laurizen, T., Cai, Y., Warberg, J., and Secher, N. H. (2000). Accurate monitoring of a blood loss: thoracic electrical impedance during hemorrhage in the pig. *Acta Anaesthesiologica Scandinavica,* **44**, 598–604.

Larsen, F. S., Hansen, B. A., Pott, F., Poulson, O., Ejlersen, E., Secher, N. H., and Knudsen, G. M. (1996). Dissociated cerebral vasoparalysis in acute liver failure: a hypothesis of gradual cerebral hyperaemia. *Journal of Hepatology,* **25**, 145–51.

Lewis, T. (1932). Vasovagal syncope and the carotid sinus mechanism with comments on Grower's and Nothnagel's syndrome. *Br. Med. J,* **i**, 873–6.

Ludbrook, J. (1993). Haemorrhage and shock. In R. Hainsworth and A. L. Mark, ed. *Cardiovascular Reflex Control in Health and Disease* pp. 463–90. WB Saundres, London.

Ludbrook, J. (1997). Shock and its management. In C. Mathias and R. Bannister, ed. *Autonomic Failure: A Textbook of Clinical Disorders of the Autonomic Nervous System* pp. 461–7. Oxford University Press, London.

MacLean, A. R. and Allen, E. V. (1940). Orthostatic hypotension and orthostatic tachycardia; treatment with the 'head-up' bed. *JAMA,* **115**, 2162–7.

Madsen, P. L. and Secher, N. H. (1999). Near infrared spectroscopy of the brain. *Progress in Neurobiology* **58**, 541–60.

Murkin, J. M. and Arango, M. (2009). Near-.ifrared spectroscopy as an index of brain and tissue oxygenation. *British Journal of Anaesthesia* **103**(Suppl 1), 3–13.

Nissen, P., Van Lieshout, J. J., Nielsen, H. B., and Secher, N. H. (2009). Frontal lobe oxygenation is maintained during hypotension following propofol-fentanyl anesthesia. *AANA J* **77**, 271–6.

Öberg, B. and Thorén (1972). Increased activity in left ventricular receptors during hemorrhage or occlusion of caval veins in the cat. A possible cause of the vaso-vagal reaction. *Acta Physiologica Scandinavica,* **85**, 164–73.

Ogoh, S., Volianitis, S., Nissen, P., Wray, D. W., Secher, N. H., and Raven, P. B. (2003). Carotid baroreflex responsiveness to head-up tilt induced central hypovolaemia: effect of aerobic fitness. *Journal of Physiology,* **55**, 601–8.

Schadt, J. C. and Ludbrook, J. (1991) Hemodynamic and neurohumoral responses to acute hypovolaemia in conscious animals. *American Journal of Physiology,* **260**, H305–18.

Secher, N. H., Jacobsen, J., Friedman, D. B., and Matzen, S. (1992). Bradycardia during reversible hypovolaemic shock: associated neural reflex mechanisms and clinical implications. *Clinical and Experimental Pharmacology and Physiology,* **19**, 733–43.

Secher, N. H. and Bie, P. (1985). Bradycardia during reversible hypovolaemic shock—a forgotten observation? *Clinical Physiology* **5**, 315–23.

Sharpey-Schafer, E. P. (1956). Emergencies in general practice. Syncope. *Br. Med. J,* **1**, 506–9.

Van Lieshout, J. J., Harms, M. P. M., Pott, F., Jenstrup, M., and Secher, N. H. (2005). Stroke volume of the heart and thoracic fluid content during head-up and head- down tilt. *Acta Anaesthesiologica Scandinavica.* **49**, 1287–92.

Van Lieshout, J. J., Wieling, W., Karemaker, J. M. and Secher, N. H. (2003). Syncope, cerebral perfusion and oxygenation. *Journal of Applied Physiology,* **94**, 833–48.

Welply, N. C., Mathias, C. J., and Frankel, H. L. (1975). Circulatory reflexes in tetraplegics during artificial ventilation and general anaesthesia. *Paraplegia,* **13**, 172–82.

Wieling, W., Van Lieshout, J. J., and Hainsworth, R. (2002). Extracellular fluid volume expansion in patients with posturally related syncope. *Clinical Autonomic Research,* **12**, 242–9.

Wiggers, C. J. (1950). *Physiology of Shock.* The Commonwealth Fund, New York.

CHAPTER 63

Cardiac failure and the autonomic nervous system

Gary S. Francis and Jay N. Cohn

Introduction

Congestive heart failure has emerged as a highly lethal, major epidemic over the past two decades (Tang and Francis, 2003). In its broadest terms, it is fundamentally a clinical syndrome, characterized by symptoms of shortness of breath and fatigue at rest or with exercise. In some, but not all cases, there is tissue congestion. In all cases there is underlying structural and/or functional heart disease. Any form of heart disease can eventually lead to heart failure. Twenty years ago or more, the primary research focus was on muscle mechanics and mechanisms of left ventricular dysfunction. Since then there has been a much more expansive understanding of this complex syndrome, with a clear recognition that the sympathetic and renin-angiotensin-aldosterone systems have a major role in the progression of the disorder. Along with this came the realization that abnormal reflex control mechanisms contributed importantly to the pathophysiology of heart failure. This is especially true of the autonomic nervous system.

Knowledge that the autonomic nervous system is abnormal in heart failure goes back to and before the time of Starling (Starling 1897). Excess sympathetic nervous system activity is a hallmark of the disorder. By the middle part of the last century it was clear that despite an overly active sympathetic nervous system, there was only limited further activation of the sympathetic nervous system in response to up-right posture in such patients (Brigden and Sharpey-Schafer 1950). Since then there have been hundreds of published studies demonstrating the presence of abnormal reflex control mechanisms and excessive sympathetic drive in patients and experimental animal models with heart failure. Not surprisingly, both the sympathetic and the parasympathetic arms of the autonomic nervous system are abnormal in heart failure. Among the many abnormalities demonstrated are:

- increased plasma levels of plasma noradrenaline (NA)
- reduced density of myocardial β-adrenoceptors
- blunted cardiac baroreceptor responses
- reduced heart rate variability
- reduced chronotropic response to exercise
- reduced heart rate recovery after exercise
- blunted arterial baroreflex abnormalities.

Many investigators have demonstrated that the function of both arterial and cardiac baroreceptors are abnormal in the syndrome of heart failure. These reflex systems operate normally to regulate short-term control of arterial pressure, heart rate, and peripheral vascular resistance. They also modulate the sympathetic nervous system, which in turn can activate the renin-angiotensin-aldosterone and other neuroendocrine systems. When dysfunctional, these perturbed reflex control mechanisms can alter the regional distribution of cardiac output, thus redirecting flow to more vital organs. This may provide a short-term survival advantage, but it has long-term consequences for circulatory homeostasis. For example, renal function may deteriorate at the expense of somewhat improved cerebral blood flow. Additional problems such as reduced heart rate variability may ensue, setting the stage for arrhythmias. There can be reduced blood flow to skeletal muscles, leading to poor exercise tolerance, abnormal glucose metabolism and hyperglycaemia. The failing heart is 'bathed' in excessive NA, making it less sensitive to catecholamines. Plasma NA levels rise, and these higher levels are associated with a poor prognosis (Cohn et al. 1984). Excessive NA activates the renin-angiotensin-aldosterone system, as does a 'perceived' reduction in effective circulating volume (an unmeasurable but generally agreed upon physiological parameter), leading to further vasoconstriction, myocardial remodelling, salt and water retention, and progression of heart failure.

Increased plasma levels of noradrenaline

Patients with left ventricular dysfunction appear to activate the sympathetic nervous system early, even prior to the onset of signs and symptoms (Francis et al. 1990). The same is true for plasma renin activity, plasma arginine vasopressin and B-type natriuretic peptide, but to a lesser extent. These neurohormones progressively rise over time as the natural history of heart failure unfolds. Of some interest, even though there are increased levels of NA in the regional synaptic clefts of the cardiac sympathetic nerves of patients with heart failure (Hasking et al. 1986), the failing myocardial tissue is deplete of NA (Braunwald et al. 1966). Using the radioenzymatic technique, normal plasma NA levels are in the range of 150–300 pg/ml. Patients with heart failure have plasma NA levels in the range of 300–3000 pg/ml, but usually average about 500–600 pg/ml.

It is still not entirely clear how the sympathetic nervous system is activated in patients with heart failure. There may be a 'perceived' need to protect cardiac output and flow to vital organs by sympathetic stimulation of heart rate, force of contractility and peripheral vasoconstriction (Francis et al. 1984), but the nature of the signal and how it is processed is not clear. Some, but not all, of the excessive sympathetic nervous system activity in heart failure is a consequence of impaired reflex control mechanisms. There is also increased 'spillover' of NA from sympathetic neurons and delayed clearance of NA from the circulation in the syndrome of heart failure (Hasking et al. 1986).

Augmented sympathetic nervous system activity contributes to many of the features of heart failure, and is directly toxic to myocardial cells. Blocking β-adrenoceptors with specific beta-blocking drugs (i.e. bisoprolol, metoprolol succinate, and carvedilol) consistently improves survival of patients with heart failure. Utilization of beta-blocking drugs also raises the ejection fraction by 5–7 units on average, re-enforcing the importance of the sympathetic nervous system in the pathophysiology of heart failure.

Sympathetic nervous system 'traffic' can be directly measured using microneurographic techniques (Valbo et al. 1979). Leimbach and colleagues (1986) used this technique to measure sympathetic nervous system activity in patients with heart failure, confirming that there is excessive, unrelenting activity. As with plasma NA, there is a general inverse relation between microneurographically measured sympathetic activity and left ventricular performance. However, the correlations are not close for all human hemodynamic variables. Plasma NA and microneurographic measurements have largely remained research tools rather than clinically relevant laboratory tests (Ferguson et al. 1990).

In 1984, Cohn et al. reported that plasma NA levels provide a better guide to prognosis in patients with heart failure than other more commonly measured indices of cardiac performance. Plasma NA was the best independent prognostic survival guide among several haemodynamic and biochemical measurements as determined by multivariable regression analysis. In an update, this same laboratory (Rector et al. 1987) found that a cut-off value of 600 pg/ml provides the most prognostic information. A recent analysis by this laboratory of both plasma NA and plasma BNP indicated that BNP had a stronger association with morbidity and mortality than plasma NA (Anand et al. 2003). Changes in both neurohormones over time are associated with corresponding increases in mortality and morbidity. Plasma NA remains a more powerful predictor of mortality than more conventionally measured hemodynamic measurements such as left ventricular ejection fraction, supporting the importance of the autonomic nervous system dysfunction in the pathophysiology of heart failure. Very high levels of plasma NA (i.e. >1000 pg/ml) consistently predict a very poor prognosis.

Reduced density of β-adrenoceptors

The membrane-bound β-adreno-G-protein-adenyl cyclase complex regulates myocardial contractility and heart rate in both the normal and failing heart (Fig. 63.1). Both the β_1 and β_2 receptors are engaged by NA released into synaptic clefts. The β receptor is coupled to the stimulatory guanine-nucleotide-finding protein (G_i), which mediates the production of adenylate cyclase. Cyclic adenosine monophosphate (cAMP) is then generated from adenosine

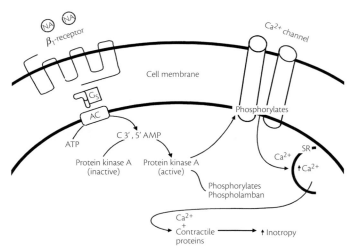

Fig. 63.1 The membrane-bound β-adrenergic receptor-G-protein-adenylate cyclase complex. The signal (i.e. noradrenaline) engages the membrane-bound β1-receptor, which is coupled to a guanine nucleotide regulatory protein (G_S-protein). The G_S-protein dissociates from the receptor and activates the enzyme adenylate cyclase (AC). Adenosine triphosphate (ATP) is converted to cyclic 3', 5' AMP, which in turn catalyses inactive protein kinase A to active protein kinase A (PKA). PKA then phosphorylates a number of highly specialized proteins, including membrane-bound calcium channels to allow the influx of Ca^{2+} into the cell. Ca^{2+} is transported into the intracellular Ca^{2+} storage depots called sarcoplasmic reticulae (SR). The SR then provides Ca^{2+} for interaction with contractile proteins. Contractions of the myofilaments is dependent on phosphorylation by PKA of phospholamban, a specialized protein.

triphosphate (ATP) via adenylate cyclase. cAMP in turn catalyses a number of phosphorylation reactions mediated by protein kinase A, including Ca^{2+} channels and phospholamban, thus allowing for more Ca^{2+} to interact with myofilaments. About 80% of the β-adrenoceptors are β_1 and the remaining are β_2 receptors. The β_2 receptors generate much less cAMP.

It is now clear that the density of β-adrenoceptors is substantially reduced early in the heart failure syndrome (Fig. 63.2),

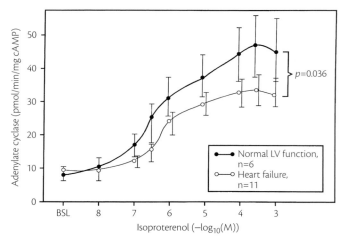

Fig. 63.2 The influence of L-isoproterenol on myocardial tissue isolated from the left ventricles (LV) of patients with severe congestive heart failure who later received a heart transplant (open circles) and from normal hearts of potential heart donors (closed circles). The failing myocardial tissue is unable to generate a normal amount of adenylate cyclase in response to L-isoproterenol. BSL, baseline. With permission from Bristow, M. R. et al., 1982, Copyright MMS.

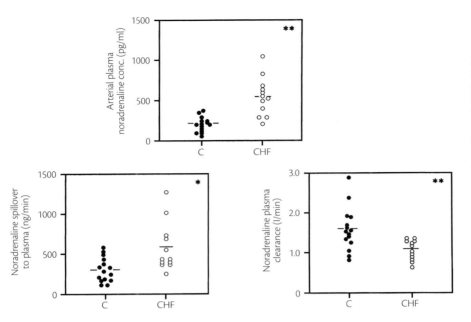

Fig. 63.3 Plasma noradrenaline concentration and its determinants in subjects with and without congestive heart failure (CHF). *, *P* < 0.02; **, *P* < 0.002. Using radioactive tracer techniques, patients with CHF demonstrate enhanced 'spillover' of NAd from synaptic clefts into plasma and reduced clearance of NAd from the circulation. Both mechanisms could contribute to increased plasma concentrations of NAd in patients with CHF. C, controls. With permission from Hasking GL, Esler MD, Jennings GL, Bartow D and Korner PI (1986). Norepinephrine spillover to plasma in patients with congestive heart failure: evidence of increased spillover and cardiorenal sympathetic nervous activity. *Circulation* **73**(4):615–621.

(Bristow et al. 1982). β_2 receptor density may actually increase, but the β_2 receptor becomes more uncoupled from the G protein, and G_i (G inhibitory) may increase, thus inhibiting the release of cAMP. The reduced β-receptor density in the heart and the up-regulation of Gi protein likely contributed to impaired myocardial performance in heart failure, but many other mechanisms are also operative.

The process of down-regulation of β-adrenoceptors in failing human hearts has been studied by Fowler and colleagues (1986). Using myocardial biopsies, they demonstrated that myocardial β-adrenoceptor down-regulation begins with mild to moderate left ventricular dysfunction, is related to the degree of heart failure, and is associated with pharmacologically specific impairment of the β-agonist-mediated contractile response. There appears to be a stepwise reduction in myocardial β-adrenoceptor density as heart failure progresses. The decreased β-adrenoceptor density compromises the ability of catecholamines to support cardiac function, especially endogenous NA. Myocardial β-adrenoceptor down-regulation is likely to be partially responsible for reduced chronotropic and inotropic responses to peak exercise (White et al. 1995). There is also a natural loss of β-adrenoceptors in older patients that is accentuated by heart failure (White et al. 1994). The mechanism of β-adrenoceptor down-regulation is complex, but is likely a reversible phenomena. The widely-used β-blocker metoprolol tartrate appears to up-regulate β-adrenoceptors in the heart, but this is not true of carvedilol, a highly effective β-blocker that is known to improve survival. It is possible that the ability to down regulate the β-adrenoceptors afforded an evolutionary survival advantage by protecting the heart from excessive catecholamine bombardment, but in heart failure this phenomenon becomes a distinct disadvantage. Excessive sympathetic activity, especially increased NA levels in the synapse due to greater 'spillover' (Fig. 63.3) (Hasking et al. 1986), likely initiates the down regulation problem. The high systemic NA values are associated with a poor prognosis (Fig. 63.4) (Rector et al. 1987).

Blunted cardiac baroreceptor responses in heart failure

Normal subjects develop a marked increase in sympathetic activity in response to the vasodilation imposed by nitroprusside. It is characterized by an increase in heart rate and plasma NA levels (Olivari et al. 1983). This sympathetic response is markedly attenuated in patients with heart failure during exercise, upright tilt and acute vasodilation. Those patients with the most dramatic attenuation of sympathetic response have more advanced disease and a more unfavourable prognosis. Similar to acute vasodilation,

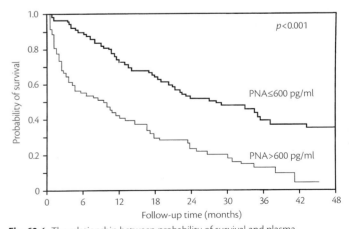

Fig. 63.4 The relationship between probability of survival and plasma noradrenaline (PNA) in 217 patients with congestive heart failure. A cutoff value of 600 pg/ml provides the most prognostic information as determined by multivariate regression analysis of survival times. Reprinted from *Am Heart J*, **114**, Rector TS, Olivari MT, Levine TB, Francis GS, and Cohn JN, Predicting survival for an individual with congestive heart failure using plasma norepinephrine concentration, 148–152, Copyright (1987), with permission from Elsevier.

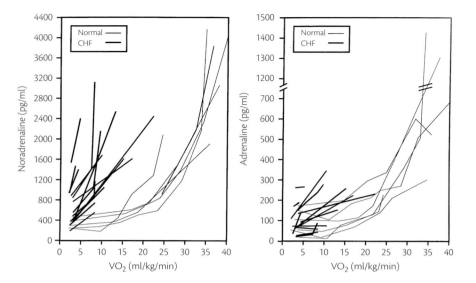

Fig. 63.5 Plasma noradrenaline response to exercise during graded bicycle ergometry is shown in thin lines for normal subjects and in thick lines for patients with congestive heart failure (CHF). VO$_2$, total body oxygen consumption. Reprinted from *Am. J. Cardiol.* **49**, Francis G.S., Goldsmith S.R., Ziesche, S.M., and Cohn, J.N. Response of plasma norepinephrine and epinephrine to dynamic exercise in patients with congestive heart failure, 1152–6, Copyright (1982), with permission from Elsevier.

patients with heart failure who suffer acute blood loss fail to mount an appropriate increase in heart rate. Patients essentially fail to peripherally vasoconstrict in response to a diminishment in cardiac filling pressures. Sometimes there is even paradoxical vasodilation. Lowering blood pressure by applying lower body negative pressure also fails to provoke an expected increase in peripheral vasoconstriction in patients with heart failure. Although the absolute levels of plasma NE rise abruptly during exercise in patients with heart failure (Fig. 63.5) (Francis et al. 1982), there is a relative diminishment in the NA response to exercise when one corrects for the intensity of exercise (Fig. 63.6) (Francis et al. 1985). An abnormal response to upright tilt is characteristic of heart failure (Fig. 63.7) (Levine et al. 1983). The lack of a brisk response of plasma NA to acute vasodilation (nitroprusside) predicts a poor prognosis (Figs 63.8 and 63.9) (Oliveri et al. 1983). Impairment of cardiopulmonary baroreceptor function may also lead to the non-osmotic release of arginine vasopressin, provoking further vasoconstriction and hyponatraemia. Plasma arginine vasopressin levels are increased in patients with heart failure (Goldsmith et al. 1983), and may be important in the pathophysiology of heart failure.

Unloading the baroreceptors with orthostatic stress from lower body negative pressure induces paradoxical vasodilation in patients with heart failure (Fig. 63.10) (Ferguson et al. 1984). This abnormal response to unloading the cardiac baroreceptors can be reversed to some extent by an angiotensin converting enzyme inhibitor (Cody et al. 1982). Acute digitalization also tends to restore normalization of cardiopulmonary baroreceptor reflexes, and reduces excessive sympathetic activity measured microneurographically from desensitized arterial baroreceptors (Ferguson et al. 1989). Experimental animal models of heart failure have consistently demonstrated depressed left atrial stretch receptor discharge sensitivity. Moreover, neural discharge rate from left atrial receptors is reduced during volume expansion. In summary, both loading and unloading of cardiopulmonary baroreceptors is dysfunctional in heart failure, (Fig. 63.11) (Hirsch et al. 1987) and such changes appear to be only partially reversible in response to pharmacological interdiction.

Reduced heart rate variability

The use of power spectral analysis to measure heart rate variability (HRV) (Saul et al. 1988) allowed investigators to study a variety of patients, including those who were post-myocardial infarction and those with heart failure. Abnormal HRV became synonymous with heart disease, and heart failure is a classic example whereby HRV is consistently abnormal and is associated with a poor prognosis. HRV is measured by analyzing the variation between each beat. This is

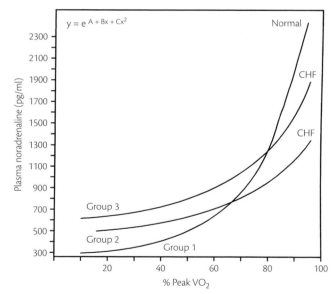

Fig. 63.6 The plasma noradrenaline response to dynamic upright exercise is plotted as a function of relative work intensity, expressed by per cent peak oxygen uptake (% peak VO$_2$). There is no difference in slope between group 2 (mild heart failure) and group 3 (severe heart failure). Group 1 (normal) has a steeper slope than that in groups 2 and 3 ($P = 0.002$), indicating that, at relative work intensities, normal subjects have augmented sympathetic drive. Reprinted from *J. Am. Coll. Cardiol.* **5**, Francis G.S., Goldsmith S.R., Ziesche, S., Nakajima, H., and Cohn, J.N., Relative attenuation of sympathetic drive during exercise in patients with congestive heart failure, 832–9, Copyright (1985), with permission from Elsevier.

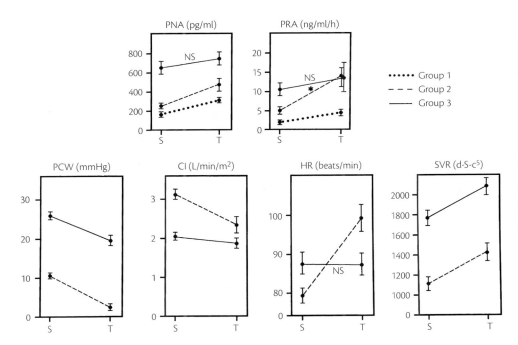

Fig. 63.7 Measurements of plasma noradrenaline (PNA) and plasma renin activity (PRA) during supine rest (S) and 60° orthostatic tilt (T) in normal subjects (group 1), patients with symptoms of heart failure but normal resting haemodynamics (group 2), and patients with heart failure and abnormal resting haemodynamics (group 3). The haemodynamic responses to tilt for groups 2 and 3 are shown in the lower panel. Pulmonary capillary wedge pressure (PCW), cardiac index (CI), and systemic vascular resistance (SVR) all changed significantly. Heart rate (HR) increased significantly in group 2, but did not change in group 3. With permission from Levine TB, Francis GS and Cohn JN (1983). The neurohumoral and hemodynamic response to orthostatic tilt in patients with congestive heart failure. *Circulation* **67**(5):1070–1075.

then compared to the instantaneous heart rate and the so-called normal-to-normal (NN) interval calculated over 24 hours, and its standard deviation (SDNN). Various techniques have been used to measure HRV, and reliability and reproducibility have at times been a problem (Sanderson JE 1998). In general, a reduction in SDNN identifies patients at higher risk for death (Nolan et al. 1998). In heart failure, it is likely that the absent low-frequency component reflects impaired baroreceptor function. The estimation of HRV by ambulatory monitoring provides prognostic information beyond that of traditional risk factors (Tsuji et al. 1996).

HRV is influenced by many physiologic conditions. A low SDNN (≤ 70 ms) carries a significant risk of cardiac mortality in patients with a recent acute myocardial infarction (La Rovere et al. 1998). The autonomic nervous system has been extensively implicated in triggering sudden death. Conditions that reduce vagal activity and increase the relative dominance of the sympathetic nervous system set the stage for arrhythmias. Abnormal HRV is a marker of these conditions.

Inherited factors may explain a substantial proportion of the variance in heart rate (Singh et al. 1999). It may also be that HRV can be altered by treatment. Beta-blockers, which are known to reduce mortality in patients with heart failure and in patients following acute myocardial infarction, may work by improving HRV (Baron and Viskin 1998). Beta-blockers improve HRV in patients with heart failure (Lin et al. 1999) and are well known to improve survival. Some drugs, such as low dose scopolamine, improve baroreceptor sensitivity without reducing the risk of death (Hull et al. 1995). Daily exercise improves both baroreceptor sensitivity and outcomes in patients following myocardial infarction. Nearly all studies indicate that HRV is markedly reduced in patients with heart failure, and the reduction in HRV is related to the severity of heart failure (Sanderson 1998).

The standard deviation of 5-minute median atrial-atrial intervals (SDAAM) can now be continuously measured from an implanted cardiac resynchronization device (Adamson et al. 2004). SDAAM is reduced in patients with heart failure who are at high risk for death or hospitalization. It remains to be seen if such a device becomes a useful clinical tool.

Reduced chronotropic response to exercise

Robinson et al. (1966) described that cardioacceleration during exercise results from release of parasympathetic inhibition at low exercise levels, and from both parasympathetic withdrawal and sympathetic activation at more moderate intensities. The autonomic nervous system's contributions to cardiodeceleration immediately after exercise are less well understood. The chronotropic response to exercise provides important information in

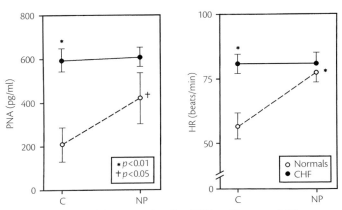

Fig. 63.8 Response of plasma noradrenaline (PNA) and heart rate (HR) to nitroprusside infusion (NP) in five normal subjects (open circles) and 46 patients with congestive heart failure (CHF) (closed circles). Symbols above the control columns (C) indicate significant difference between normal subjects and patients with congestive heart failure; symbols in NP columns indicate significant changes from control during nitroprusside infusion. *, P (probability) < 0.01; †, P < 0.05. Mean values ± standard error of the mean are shown. Reprinted from *J Am Coll Cardiol*, **2**, Olivari MT, Levine TB and Cohn JN, Abnormal neurohumoral response to nitroprusside infusion in congestive heart failure. 411–417, Copyright (1983), with permission from Elsevier.

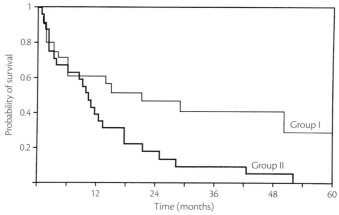

Fig. 63.9 Wilcoxon life table analysis of 21 patients in group I and 25 in group II. Group I and group II denote patients with and without a rise in plasma noradrenaline, respectively, during nitroprusside infusion. Reprinted from *J Am Coll Cardiol*, **2**, Olivari MT, Levine TB and Cohn JN, Abnormal neurohumoral response to nitroprusside infusion in congestive heart failure. 411–417, Copyright (1983), with permission from Elsevier.

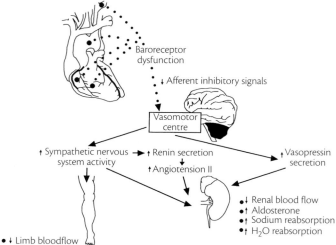

Fig. 63.11 Relationship of abnormal baroreceptor function in neurohormonal activation and regional blood flow in congestive heart failure. Increases in artrial and ventricular filling pressures and increased mean arterial or pulse pressure normally stimulate cardiopulmonary and arterial baroreceptors. Baroreceptor activation sends inhibitory signals to the medullary vasomotor centre, with suppression of sympathetic efferent activity and increased vagal efferent activity (not shown). Baroreflex inhibition is blunted in heart failure, with consequent increased activation of sympathetic and renin-angiotensin systems, and with increased neurohypophyseal release of vasopressin. Limb and renal vasoconstriction ensue, as well as renal retention of sodium and water. (Taken with permission from Hirsch *et al.* (1987).)

patients with heart disease, including those with heart failure. Chronotropic incompetence is generally defined as failure to reach 85% of the age-predicted maximal heart rate during maximal exercise, or failure to reach 80% of the heart rate reserve. It is common in patients with heart disease. Chronotropic incompetence is a proven predictor of a poor prognosis (Lauer et al. 1999).

The attenuated heart rate response to exercise in patients with heart failure has been extensively studied (Colucci et al. 1989). There appears to be a desensitization of post-synaptic β-adrenoceptors and their downstream pathways in patients with

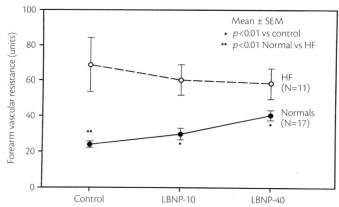

Fig. 63.10 Responses of normal subjects and patients with heart failure (HF) to unloading (deactivation) of baroreceptors with orthostatic stress produced by lower-body negative pressure (LBNP) at −10 mmHg (LBNP, −10) and at −40 mmHg (LBNP, −40). Control forearm vascular resistance (venous occlusion plethysmography) was significantly higher in the heart failure patients than in the normal subjects. Normal subjects developed significant forearm vasoconstriction during LBNP (manifested by an increase in forearm vascular resistance). In contrast, patients with heart failure failed to vasoconstrict and tended to experience paradoxical vasodilation during LBNP. With permission from Ferguson DW, Abboud FM and Mark AL (1984). Selective impairment of baroreflex mediated vasoconstrictor responses in patients with ventricular dysfunction. *Circulation* **69**(3):451–460.

heart failure. Comparing isoproterenol and milrinone, Colucci and colleagues postulated that desensitization of β-adrenoceptors in sinoatrial tissue may have an important effect on exercise capacity in patients with heart failure. Just as reduced HRV is associated with adverse outcomes, attenuated heart rate response to exercise is also predictive of risk. It is likely that chronotropic incompetence is a marker of the dysautonomia of heart failure, but also likely contributes to diminished quality and quantity of life in some patients.

Reduced heart rate recovery following exercise

The parasympathetic effect during maximal exercise is rather minimal, reducing heart rate around 3–6 beats per minute (Kannankeril et al. 2004). During the exercise recovery period, however, the parasympathetic response is profound, averaging a reduction in heart rate of 23 beats per minute in the first minute after exercise. This strong vagal affect normally increases for about 4 minutes after stopping maximal exercise and remains stable for at least 10 minutes. Patients with heart disease fail to recover their baseline resting heart rate in a prompt manner.

Cole and colleagues (1999) have analysed the large Cleveland Clinic exercise data base, primarily patients being evaluated for coronary artery disease, and correlated reduced heart rate recovery with survival. They defined an abnormal heart rate recovery as ≤ 12 beats per minute 1 minute after cessation of exercise, and found it to be a strong independent predictor of survival in patients referred for exercise testing. An abnormal heart rate recovery is due to impaired return of vagal activity following exercise. It is a powerful marker of prognosis, even more powerful than exercise workload, extent of coronary disease, severity of left ventricular dysfunction or myocardial perfusion defects on thallium scintigraphy. Even increased fasting plasma glucose at non-diabetic levels is strongly and independently associated with abnormal heart rate recovery (Panzer et al. 2002). The normal heart demonstrates an exquisite balance between parasympathetic and sympathetic activity, and there are serious consequences for circulatory homeostasis when this balance is upset. Patients who demonstrate increased ventricular ectopy in the recovery period following exercise are more likely to have a poor long-term outcome when followed for 5.3 years (Frolkis et al. 2003). In general, normal vagal input to heart provides a safety margin against a poor outcome, and impaired vagal input is associated with underlying heart disease and is a marker for a poor prognosis. Abnormal heart rate recovery, however, does not appear to identify patients that are likely to benefit from early coronary revascularization (Chen et al. 2004).

Blunted arterial baroreceptor abnormalities in heart failure

Studies from humans (Eckberg et al. 1971) and animal models (Wang et al. 1990) have demonstrated that the carotid sinus baroreceptor sensitivity is diminished in the setting of heart failure. Eckberg and colleagues produced transient elevation in blood pressure with an infusion of phenylephrine in a small group of patients with various forms of heart disease. The reflex fall in heart rate was monitored. The results were compared with a group of normal subjects. There was a consistent and remarkably greater slowing of heart rate in normal subjects in response to the pressor effects of phenylephrine than in patients with heart disease. This difference could be abolished with atropine, pointing to a profound abnormality in parasympathetic cardiovascular regulation in patients with heart disease. By implication, there is likely a major abnormality of arterial baroreceptor function in patients with heart failure, and it likely resides at the afferent baroreceptor endings. The arterial baroreceptors are less sensitive to heightened pressure, and this is manifested as less bradycardia.

Patients with heart failure are also unable to raise blood pressure during carotid sinus baroreceptor unloading (Creager and Creager 1994). It is postulated that a reduction in inhibitory signals from arterial baroreceptors may contribute to the heightened state of sympathetic activity found in patients with heart failure. Normally, stimulation of arterial baroreceptors by increased blood pressure reduces efferent sympathetic activity (Sanders 1988), more so in the aorta than in the carotid sinus. Both unloading of the arterial baroreceptors (such as with nitroprusside), and loading the baroreceptors with enhanced blood pressure (phenylephrine) are impaired in patients with heart failure (Ferguson et al. 1992). During heightened blood pressure, patients with heart failure exhibit little reduction in heart rate. Unloading the arterial baroreceptors with nitroprusside leads to little or no change in heart rate or change in skeletal muscle sympathetic tone as measured by microneurography. The impaired response of vagal and sympathetic inhibitory reflexes parallels clinical and hemodynamic deterioration and can be associated with a foreshortened survival. Animal models of heart failure likewise demonstrate altered reflex control mechanisms (Dibner-Dunlap and Thames 1992), although it remains somewhat unclear if the lesion is in the receptors themselves, or in the central nervous system. The fact that heart transplantation does not completely reverse the abnormal reflex control mechanisms suggests that the central nervous system is somehow involved.

Autonomic dysfunction following cardiac transplantation

Following heart transplantation there is usually normalization of resting plasma NA levels and reversal of some but not all baroreceptor reflex abnormalities. However, disturbances in sensitivity to catecholamines persist and cardiopulmonary baroreflex control of forearm vascular resistance remains impaired. Experimental chronic denervation in dogs results in 'up-regulation' of β-adrenoceptors and 'down-regulation' of muscarinic receptors. A 'supersensitivity' to catecholamines develops. The major mechanism of denervation supersensitivity to NA appears to involve lack of neuronal NA reuptake. Despite animal data to the contrary, data from human orthotopic cardiac allografts indicate that myocardial β-adrenergic receptors are not increased. Moreover, there is no direct evidence of β-receptor-mediated supersensitivity of postsynaptic origin in patients. The β-adrenergic supersensitivity is likely presynaptic in origin.

Patients with heart transplants generally exhibit a relative resting tachycardia (90–110 beats per minute) and demonstrate little or no increase in heart rate within 30 seconds of standing up. There is also a characteristic delayed rate of acceleration during dynamic and isometric exercise, and also a delayed deceleration at the end of exercise. Carotid sinus massage and the Valsalva manoeuvre do not affect the heart rate in the donor heart. Of interest, heart-transplant patients do demonstrate a marked tachycardia (130–140 beats per minute) in response to fever (Francis and Cohn, personal observations).

There has been a general consensus that the human donor heart is not reinnervated. Histochemical studies have failed to demonstrate reinnervation beyond the suture line following transplantation. In contrast with humans, the transplanted hearts of experimental animals have been shown to exhibit functional extrinsic reinnervation. The distinction between reinnervation in humans and animals may represent either a species difference or variations between allografts and autografts, since many of the animal experiments involved autotransplantation. Following human heart transplantation, myocardial catecholamines are undetectable in tissue biopsies up to five years, indicating that, at least soon after transplantation, the adrenergic responses of these hearts probably depend mainly on variations in plasma catecholamines or presynaptic supersensitivity.

Evidence suggests that some patients have functional reinnervation developing 2 or more years following heart transplantation. Wilson and colleagues (1991) have demonstrated clear increases in NA flowing from the coronary sinus of orthotopically transplanted human hearts when tyramine is given systematically or directly into the coronary arteries. Tyramine is known to displace NA from sympathetic neurons, and should increase NA efflux only if there is functional reinnervation. Moreover, evidence is now accumulating that functional reinnervation may occur in a minority of heterotopic allografts. A recent study identified one case out of nine in which electrocardiographic and indirect clinical evidence of functional reinnervation was obtained 33 months after orthotopic cardiac transplantation. We have seen occasional patients with orthotopic cardiac transplantation who have developed severe coronary artery disease and classic angina pectoris, although, typically, coronary disease remains clinically silent in the transplant population.

In summary, heart transplantation and heart–lung transplant will reverse some of the autonomic deficiencies observed in preceding severe heart failure, but patients may continue to demonstrate some autonomic abnormalities including presynaptic supersensitivity to catecholamines, a blunted response to upright posture and exercise, and reduced heart rate variation. These persistent abnormalities do not keep them from leading a nearly normal lifestyle. Although mainly dependent soon after transplantation on circulating catecholamines, new data are emerging suggesting that reinnervation occurs in some cases.

Role of the autonomic nervous system in the clinical syndrome in heart failure

Still unresolved is whether the protean abnormalities in afferent and efferent sympathetic nervous system function in heart failure are fundamental to the clinical manifestations of the syndrome or are merely epiphenomena indicative of the severity of the physiological derangement. It is clear that at least some of the clinical signs of severe heart failure—tachycardia, cool extremities, diaphoresis—are at least in part due to sympathetic activation. Other manifestations—renal sodium conservation, ventricular arrhythmia—are probably also aggravated by heightened sympathetic nervous system activity. Other important complications of heart failure—exercise intolerance, sudden death, ventricular hypertrophy and remodelling, atrial fibrillation, renin stimulation, etc—are likely in part related to autonomic dysfunction, but the evidence is in some cases rather indirect.

Attempts to block the enhanced sympathetic nervous system activity represent an interesting and provocative approach to long-term therapy of heart failure. α-adrenoceptor blockade, as a means of producing systemic vasodilation, exerts a favourable acute haemodynamic effect, but produces no evidence for a long-term survival benefit, whereas β-adrenoceptor blockade exerts a long-term favourable effect on survival in patients with heart failure. The mechanism of the survival benefit may be related to inhibition of myocardial remodelling and subsequent slowing of disease progression.

The autonomic nervous system is abnormal in human and experimental heart failure. This perturbation likely contributes to excessive sympathetic activity, leading to progressive myocardial remodelling, arrhythmias and foreshortened survival. We are now more aware of the importance of the dysautonomia of heart failure, and our understanding has led to new and improved treatment strategies.

References

Adamson, P. B., Smith, A. L., Abraham, W. T. et al. (2004). Continous autonomic assessment in patients with symptomatic heart failure. Prognostic value of heart rate variability measured by an implanted cardiac resynchronization device. *Circulation* **110**, 2389–94.

Anand, I. S., Fisher, L. D., Chiang, Y-T. et al. (2003). Changes in brain natriuretic peptide and norepinephrine over time and mortality and morbidity in the Valsartan Heart Failure Trial (Val-HeFT). *Circulation* **107**, 1278–83.

Barron, H. V. and Viskin, S. (1998). Autonomic markers and prediction of cardiac death after myocardial infarction (editorial). *Lancet* **351**, 461–62.

Braunwald, E., Chidsey, C. A., Pool, P. E. et al. (1966). Congestive heart failure: biochemical and physiological considerations. *Ann. Int. Med.* **64**, 904–41.

Brigden, W. and Sharpey-Shafer, E. P. (1950). Postural changes in peripheral blood flow in cases with left heart failure. *Clinical Science* **9**, 93–100.

Bristow, M. R., Ginsburg, R., Minobe, W. et al. (1982). Decreased catecholamine sensitivity and B-adrenergic-receptor density in failing human hearts. *N Engl. J Med.* **307**, 205–211.

Chen, M. S., Blackstone, E. H., Pothier, C. E., Lauer, M. S. (2004). Heart rate recovery and impact of myocardial revascularization on long-term mortality. *Circulation* **110**, 2851–57.

Cody, R. J., Kenneth, W. F., Kluger, J. and Laragh, J. H. (1982). Mechanisms governing the postural response and baroceptor abnormalities in chronic congestive heart failure: effect of acute and long-term converting enzyme inhibition. *Circulation* **66**, 135–42.

Cohn, J. N., Levine, T. B., Olivari, M. T. et al. (1984). Plasma norepinephrine as a guide to prognosis in patients with chronic congestive heart failure. *N Engl J Med.* **311**, 819–23.

Cole, C. R., Blackstone, E. H., Pashkow, F. J., Snader, C. E., Lauer, M. S. (1999). Heart rate recovery immediately after exercise as a predictor of mortality. *N Engl. J Med.* **341**, 1351–57.

Cole, C. R., Foody, J. M., Blackstone, E. H., Lauer, M. S. (2000). Heart rate recovery after submaximal exercise testing as a predictor of mortality in a cardiovascular healthy cohort. *Ann. Intern. Med.* **132**, 552–55.

Colucci, W. S., Ribeiro, J. P., Rocco, M. B. et al. (1989). Impaired chronotropic response to exercise in patients with congestive heart failure. Role of postsynaptic B-adrenergic desensitization. *Circulation* **80**, 314–23.

Creager, M. A. and Creager, S. L. (1994). Arterial baroreflex regulation of blood pressure in patients with congestive heart failure. *J Am. Coll. Cardiol.* **23**, 401–405.

Dibner-Dunlap, M. E. and Thames, M. D. (1992). Control of sympathetic nerve activity by vagal mechano-reflexes is blunted in heart failure. *Circulation* **86**, 1929–34.

Eckberg, D. L., Drabinsky, M. and Braunwald, E. (1971). Defective cardiac parasympathetic control in patients with heart disease. *N Engl. J Med.* **285**, 877–83.

Ferguson, D. W., Abboud, F. M. and Mark, A. L. (1984). Selective impairment of baroreflex mediated vasoconstrictor responses in patients with ventricular dysfunction. *Circulation* **69**, 451–60.

Ferguson, D. W., Berg, W. J., Roach, P. J. et al. (1992). Effects of heart failure on baroreflex control of sympathetic neural activity. *Am. J Cardiol.* **69**, 523–31.

Ferguson, D. W., Berg, W. J., Sanders, J. S., Roach, P. J., Kempf, J. S. and Kienzle, M. G. (1989). Sympathoinhibitory response to digitalis glycosides in heart failure patients. *Circulation* **80**, 65–77.

Ferguson, D. W., Berg, W. J., Sanders, J. S., and Kempf, S. J. (1990). Clinical and hemodynamic correlates of sympathetic nerve activity in normal humans and patients with heart failure: evidence from direct microneurographic recordings. *J Am. Coll. Cardiol.* **16**, 1125–34.

Fowler, M. B., Laser, J. A., Hopkins, G. L., Minobe, W., and Bristow, M. R. (1986). Assessment of the B-adrenergic receptor pathway in the intact failing heart: progressive receptor down-regulation and subsensitivity to agonist response. *Circulation* **74**, 1290–1302.

Francis, G. S., Benedict, C., Johnstone, D. E. et al. (1990). Comparison of neuroendocrine activation in patients with left ventricular dysfunction with and without congestive heart failure. *Circulation* **82**, 1724–29.

Francis, G. S., Goldsmith, S. R., Levine, T. B., Olivari, M. T. and Cohn, J. N. (1984). The neurohumoral axis in congestive heart failure. *Ann. Int. Med.* **101**, 370–77.

Francis, G. S., Goldsmith, S. R., Ziesche, S., Nakajima, H., and Cohn, J. N.. (1985). Relative attenuation of sympathetic drive during exercise in patients with congestive heart failure. *J. Am. Coll. Cardiol.* **5**, 832–9.

Francis, G. S., Goldsmith, S. R., Ziesche, S., and Cohn, J. N. (1982). Response of plasma norepinephrine and epinephrine to dynamic exercise in patients with congestive heart failure. *Am. J. Cardiol.* **49**, 1152–6.

Frolkis, J. P., Pothier, C. E., Blackstone, E. H., Lauer, M. S. (2003). Frequent ventricular ectopy after exercise as a predictor of death. *N Engl. J Med.* **348**, 781–90.

Goldsmith, S. R., Francis, G. S., Cowley, A. W., Levine, T. B. and Cohn, J. N. (1983). Increased plasma vasopressin levels in patients with congestive heart failure. *J Am. Coll. Cardiol.* **1**, 1385–90.

Hasking, G. L., Esler, M. D., Jennings, G. L., Bartow, D. and Korner, P. I. (1986). Norepinephrine spillover to plasma in patients with congestive heart failure: evidence of increased spillover and cardiorenal sympathetic nervous activity. *Circulation* **73**, 615–21.

Hirsch, A. T., Dzau, V. J., Creager, M. A. (1987). Baroreceptor function in congestive heart failure: effect on neurohumoral activation and regional vascular resistance. *Circulation* **75**, (Suppl. IV), IV-36–IV-38.

Kannankeril, P. J., Le, F. K., Kadish, A. H., Goldberger, J. J. (2004). Parasympathetic effects on heart rate recovery after exercise. *J Investigative Med.* **52**, 394–401.

La Rovere, M. T., Bigger, T. J. Jr., Marcus, F. I. *et al.* (1998). Baroreflex sensitivity and heart rate variability in prediction of total cardiac mortality after myocardial infarction. *Lancet* **351**, 461–78.

Lauer, M. S., Francis, G. S., Okin, P. M. *et al.* (1999). Impaired chronotropic response to exercise stress testing as a predictor of mortality. *JAMA* **281**, 524–29.

Leimbach, W. N., Wallin, G., Victor, R. G., Aylward, P. E., Sundolf, G., and Mark, A. L. (1986). Direct evidence from intraneural recordings for increased central sympathetic outflow in patients with heart failure. *Circulation* **73**, 913–19.

Levine, T. B., Francis, G. S. and Cohn, J. N. (1983). The neurohumoral and hemodynamic response to orthostatic tilt in patients with congestive heart failure. *Circulation* **67**, 1070–75.

Lin, J-L., Chan, H-L., Du, C-C. *et al.* (1999). Long-term B-blocker therapy improves autonomic nervous regulation in advanced congestive heart failure: a longitudinal heart rate variability study. *Am. Heart J* **137**, 658–65.

Nolan, J., Batin, P. D., Andrews, R. *et al.* (1998). Prospective study of heart rate variability and mortality in chronic heart failure. Results of the United Kingdom Heart Failure Evaluation and Assessment of Risk Trial (UK-Heart). *Circulation*, 1510–1516.

Olivari, M. T., Levine, T. B. and Cohn, J. N. (1983). Abnormal neurohumoral response to nitroprusside infusion in congestive heart failure. *J Am. Coll. Cardiol.* **2**, 411–417.

Panzer, C., Lauer, M. S., Brieke, A., Blackstone, E., Hoogwerf, B. (2002). Association of fasting plasma glucose with heart rate recovery. A population based study. *Diabetes* **51**, 803–807.

Porter, T. R., Eckberg, D. L., Fritch, J. M. *et al.* (1990). Autonomic pathophysiology in heart failure patients-sympathetic-cholinergic interrelations. *J Clin. Invest.*, 1362–71.

Rector, T. S., Olivari, M. T., Levine, T. B., Francis, G. S., and Cohn, J. N. (1987). Predicting survival for an individual with congestive heart failure using plasma norepinephrine concentration. *Am. Heart J* **114**, 148–52.

Robinson, B. F., Epstein, S. E., Beiser, G. D. and Braunwald, E. (1966). Control of heart rate by the autonomic nervous system. *Circ. Res.* **29**, 400–411.

Sanders, J. S., Ferguson, D. W. and Mark, A. L. (1988). Arterial baroreflex control of sympathetic nerve activity during elevation of blood pressure in normal man: Dominance of aortic baroreflexes. *Circulation* **77**, 279–88.

Sanderson, J. E. (1998). Heart rate variability in heart failure. *Heart Fail. Rev.* **2**, 235–44.

Saul, J. P., Arai, Y., Berger, R. D., Lilly, L. S., Colucci, W. S., Cohen, R. J. (1988). Assessment of autonomic regulation in chronic congestive heart failure by heart rate spectral analysis. *Am. J Cardiol.* **61**, 1292–99.

Schrier, R. W. and Abraham, W. T. (1999). Hormones and hemodynamics in heart failure. *N Engl. J Med.* **341**, 577–85.

Singh, J. P., Larson, M. G., O'Donnell, C. J. *et al.* (1999). Heritability of heart rate variability. The Framingham Heart Study. *Circulation* **99**, 2251–54.

Starling, E. H. (1897). Points on pathology of heart disease. *Lancet*, **1**, 569–72.

Tang, W. H. W. and Francis, G. S. (2002). Natural history of heart failure. In: *Oxidative stress and heart failure*. Futura pp. 3–47. Eds. Kukin, M. and Fuster, V. Armonk, New York.

Tsuji, H., Larson, M. G., Venditti, F. J. *et al.* (1996). Impact of reduced heart rate variability on risk factors for cardiac events. The Framingham Heart Study. *Circulation* **94**, 2850–55.

Valbo, A. B., Hagbarth, K. E., Torebjork, H. E. and Wallin, B. G. (1979). Somatosensory, proprioceptive, and sympathetic activity in human peripheral nerves. *Physiol. Rev.* **59**, 919–67.

Wang, W., Chen, J. and Zucker, I. H. (1990). Carotid sinus baroreceptor sensitivity in experimental heart failure. *Circulation* **81**, 1959–66.

White, M., Roden, R., Minobe, W. *et al.* (1994). Age-related changes in B-adrenergic neuroeffector systems in human heart. *Circulation* **90**, 1225–38.

White, M., Yanowitz, F., Gilbert, E. M. *et al.* (1995). Role of beta-adrenergic receptor down regulation in the peak exercise response to patient with heart failure due to idiopathic dilated cardiomyopathy. *Am. J Cardiol.* **76**, 1271–76.

Wilson, R. F., Christensen, B. V., Simon, A., Olivari, M. T., White, C. W., and Laxson, D. D. (1991). Evidence for structural sympathetic reinnervation after orthotopic cardiac transplantation in humans. *Circulation* **83**, 1210–20.

CHAPTER 64

Phaeochromocytoma: a clinical chameleon

Graeme Eisenhofer, Jacques W.M. Lenders, William M. Manger and Karel Pacak

Key points

- Phaeochromocytomas are rare catecholamine-producing tumours, frequently searched for, rarely found and often overlooked or mistaken for other conditions.

- Clinical presentation is highly variable, can include sustained or paroxysmal hypertension, normotension and, in up to 71% of patients, orthostatic hypotension.

- Up to 30% of phaeochromocytomas have a hereditary basis and are also increasingly being discovered incidentally during imaging procedures for unrelated conditions—such patients are often normotensive and asymptomatic.

- Secretion of catecholamines by phaeochromocytomas is often episodic and variable, whereas metabolism to metanephrines is a continuous process that occurs within tumour cells independently of catecholamine release.

- Measurements of plasma free or urinary fractionated metanephrines provide more reliable and accurate methods to diagnose phaeochromocytoma than measurements of the parent amines or other metabolites (e.g. vanillylmandelic acid).

- Computerized tomography or magnetic resonance imaging provide sensitive methods for localization of adrenal tumours, but are less reliable than functional imaging (e.g. meta-iodobenzyl guanidine scintigraphy) for locating extra-adrenal disease or metastases or identifying lesions as phaeochromocytomas.

- Most phaeochromocytomas can be cured by surgical removal, but a small and important proportion manifest or recur as malignant disease—for these, there is currently no effective cure.

Introduction

There is perhaps no more treacherous and deceptive disease than phaeochromocytoma. It has been likened to a 'pharmacological bomb', since its release of catecholamines into the circulation can cause a very sudden or 'explosive' appearance of clinical manifestations and disastrous or lethal complications. If this tumour is not recognized, it will almost invariably be fatal.

Patients with high blood pressure and symptoms of catecholamine excess are those in whom the tumour is most frequently suspected. The prevalence of the tumour among hypertensive patients tested at general outpatient clinics is about 0.2–0.6% (Anderson et al. 1994, Ariton et al. 2000, Omura et al. 2004). Phaeochromocytomas represent a dangerous yet mostly curable cause of secondary hypertension that due to the high prevalence of hypertension in the general population are frequently searched for, but rarely found. Unfortunately, phaeochromocytomas are also often missed. Autopsy studies, while showing a drop in the prevalence of undiagnosed tumours, from 0.12% in the 50 year period before 1982 (Sutton et al. 1981), to 0.05% in the period following 1980 (Lo et al. 2000, McNeil et al. 2000), continue to indicate that many phaeochromocytomas remain undetected throughout life, contributing to premature death.

Phaeochromocytomas occur at any age, but mostly in the fourth and fifth decades (Manger and Gifford 1996). About 80–85% of phaeochromocytomas arise in adrenal medullary chromaffin cells, and 15–20% arise in extra-adrenal chromaffin cells in the abdomen, pelvis, and rarely in the chest or neck. Those arising from extra-adrenal tissue are commonly known as paragangliomas. Paragangliomas that develop from parasympathetic-associated tissues, mainly along the cranial nerves and vagus (e.g. glomus tumours, chemodectomas, carotid body tumours), often do not produce catecholamines. Those developing from sympathetic-associated chromaffin tissue are usually designated extra-adrenal phaeochromocytomas, invariably produce catecholamines, and develop mainly in the abdomen, less commonly in the pelvis, and rarely in the mediastinum and neck.

Most phaeochromocytomas are benign and curable by surgical resection, but some are malignant and not effectively cured (Lehnert et al. 2004). Although the prevalence of malignant phaeochromocytoma is commonly cited at about 10%, other estimates suggest higher rates (up to 26%) depending on how malignancy is defined, with even higher or lower rates in certain patient groups depending on the underlying mutation (Edstrom Elder et al. 2003, Gimenez-Roqueplo et al. 2003).

Clinical presentation

Although the presence of signs and symptoms of catecholamine excess remains the principal reason for clinicians to suspect a phaeochromocytoma, this does not imply that all phaeochromocytomas exhibit such manifestations. Increasing proportions of phaeochromocytomas are being discovered incidentally during imaging procedures for unrelated conditions or during routine periodic screening in patients with identified mutations that predispose to the tumour. In such patients the clinical presentation may differ considerably from those in whom the tumour is suspected based on signs and symptoms.

Signs and symptoms

The clinical manifestations of phaeochromocytoma are diverse and highly variable (Table 64.1). They largely result from the haemodynamic and metabolic actions of circulating catecholamines, or less commonly, due to effects of other amines or co-secreted neuropeptides (Manger and Gifford 1996). Hypertension may be sustained or more usually paroxysmal. Paroxysmal hypertension may occur on a background of normal blood pressure or sustained hypertension. Some patients also present with periods of hypotension and a

Table 64.1 Signs and symptoms characteristic of phaeochromocytoma

Signs	Percentage*
Hypertension	>98
Sustained	50–60
Paroxysmal	60
Orthostatic hypotension	12–71
Pallor	30–60
Flushing	18
Fever	up to 66
Hyperglycaemia	42
Vomiting	26–43
Convulsions	3–5
Symptoms	**Percentage***
Headache	70–90
Palpitations/tachycardia	50–70
Diaphoresis	60–70
Anxiety	20
Nervousness	35–40
Abdominal/chest pain	20–50
Nausea	26–43
Fatigue	15–40
Dyspnoea	11–19
Dizziness	3–11
Heat intolerance	13–15
Pain/Paraesthesias	up to 11
Visual symptoms	3–21
Constipation	10
Diarrhoea	6

* Percentages are for patients with phaeochromocytoma investigated because of signs and symptoms and do not reflect values for patients investigated because of an adrenal incidentaloma or a hereditary condition, who are often normotensive and asymptomatic.
Adapted from Manger and Gifford 1996.

significant proportion with orthostatic hypotension (Streeten and Anderson 1996).

Examination of 24-hour blood pressure profiles in patients with phaeochromocytoma has generally indicated a blunting of the normal nocturnal decrease in blood pressure (Middeke and Schrader 1994; Zelinka et al. 2004). Inversion of the normal diurnal rhythm in some patients with phaeochromocytoma was ascribed to a tendency to daytime orthostatic hypotension, with a normal baroreflex (Zelinka et al. 2004).

Orthostatic hypotension was first described as an important clue to the diagnosis of phaeochromocytoma by Smithwick and colleagues (1950). More recently orthostatic hypotension and orthostatic tachycardia have been shown to occur in 58–71% of patients with phaeochromocytoma (Streeten and Anderson 1996, Munakata et al. 1999). Several mechanisms may explain the phenomenon, including decreased intravascular volume and desensitization of α-adrenoceptors due to sustained increases in circulating catecholamines.

The most frequent symptoms of phaeochromocytoma, such as severe headaches, generalized inappropriate sweating, and palpitations (with tachycardia or occasionally bradycardia) are almost invariably paroxysmal in nature. The presence of this 'classic triad' has a reported specificity of more than 90% (Plouin et al. 1981). However, only about 24–36% of patients with phaeochromocytoma report the complete triad of symptoms (Mannelli et al. 1999, Baguet et al. 2004). Nevertheless, if a patient presents with spells of these symptoms, the possibility of a phaeochromocytoma should be strongly considered. Other symptoms include severe anxiety (fear of death), tremulousness, pain in the chest and/or abdomen, nausea, vomiting, weakness, fatigue, prostration, weight loss, visual disturbances (occasionally acute blindness), severe constipation (occasionally pseudo-obstruction), paraesthesias, face pallor (occasionally flushing), and hypertensive retinopathy when hypertension is severe and sustained.

Attacks usually occur weekly, but may occur several times daily or once every few months; 80% last less than an hour but occasionally they last for several days. Attacks may be precipitated by palpitation of the tumour, postural changes, exertion, anxiety, trauma, pain, ingestion of foods or beverages containing tyramine (certain cheeses, beers, and wines), use of certain drugs (histamine, glucagon, tyramine, phenothiazine, metoclopramide), intubation, induction of anaesthesia, chemotherapy, and micturition or bladder distention (with bladder tumours).

The nature of catecholamine secretion by phaeochromocytomas varies considerably, accounting in part for variable clinical presentations. Signs and symptoms such as palpitations, anxiety, dyspnoea, pulmonary oedema, hyperglycaemia and paroxysmal hypertension are more common in patients with phaeochromocytomas producing substantial amounts of adrenaline (Aronoff et al. 1980, Ito et al. 1992, Eisenhofer et al. 2001). In part, this difference likely reflects the more potent β$_2$-adrenergic effects of adrenaline than noradrenaline.

The more often paroxysmal nature of hypertension in patients with adrenaline-producing tumours and more sustained hypertension in patients with high circulating levels of noradrenaline may also reflect underlying differences in the nature of catecholamine secretion among tumours with different biochemical phenotypes. Noradrenaline-producing tumours show larger and more consistent increases in plasma and urinary catecholamines than adrenaline-producing tumours (Eisenhofer et al. 2005c). This has been proposed to lead to down-regulation of adrenoceptors, and consequently a lower incidence of hypertension and other symptoms of catecholamine excess in patients with noradrenaline-producing than adrenaline-producing tumours.

Phaeochromocytomas that produce predominantly dopamine are rare, occurring mainly as paragangliomas (Proye et al. 1986, Eisenhofer et al. 2005a). Carotid body or glomus tumours, in particular, are often noted for production of dopamine. Patients with predominantly dopamine-producing tumours are usually normotensive and do not present with the classic symptoms of phaeochromocytoma. Nausea has been reported in several patients with dopamine-producing tumours (Awada et al. 2003, Eisenhofer et al. 2005a), this presumably related to the emetic effects of dopamine. Presence of orthostatic hypotension has also been reported, which might reflect the vasodilatory actions of dopamine and reduced blood volume secondary to dopamine-induced natriuresis.

Highly variable symptoms in patients with phaeochromocytoma, in addition to variations in catecholamine secretion, can also reflect co-secretion of neuropeptides. The classic examples are phaeochromocytomas with ectopic secretion of corticotrophin or corticotrophin-releasing factor, resulting in the presentation of Cushing's syndrome (Jessop et al. 1987, O'Brien et al. 1992). In patients with such tumours, hypertension may be due to both hypersecretion of cortisol and catecholamines. Phaeochromocytomas have also been described that secrete vasoactive intestinal peptide, this resulting in presentation of watery diarrhoea and hypokalaemia (Viale et al. 1985, Smith et al. 2002).

Differential diagnosis

Since the clinical presentation of phaeochromocytoma can be highly variable, with similar signs and symptoms produced by numerous other clinical conditions (Table 64.2), phaeochromocytomas are often referred to as the 'great mimic'. As discussed in detail elsewhere (Manger and Gifford 1996), distinguishing phaeochromocytoma from these and other less common conditions challenges the diagnostic acumen of the clinician.

Among disorders that may be encountered by specialists in the dysautonomias, baroreflex failure and postural tachycardia syndrome are perhaps the most obvious requiring discrimination from phaeochromocytoma. Baroreflex failure is characterized by volatile hypertension and hypotension, tachycardia and emotional instability (Robertson et al. 1993). Clinically, baroreflex failure may closely resemble phaeochromocytoma, commonly presenting with hypertensive crises and include symptoms of diaphoresis and headache (Manger 1993, Ketch et al. 2002). Confounding differential diagnosis, some patients may present with substantial elevations of plasma noradrenaline, occasionally reaching the range (> 12 nmol/L) considered diagnostic of phaeochromocytoma (Phillips et al. 2000). The underlying pathology in baroreflex failure can usually, however, be traced to denervation of carotid baroreceptors following carotid body tumour resection, carotid artery surgery, neck irradiation or neck trauma (Timmers et al. 2004).

Systemic mastocytosis (mast cell disease) and carcinoid syndrome are two conditions with manifestations that sometimes mimic those of phaeochromocytoma (Young and Maddox 1995, Kuchel 1998). The most frequent symptom in both conditions is flushing, resulting from vasodilatory actions of histamine or prostaglandins in the former condition, and serotonin in the latter.

Table 64.2 Conditions to consider in the differential diagnosis of phaeochromocytoma

| **Autonomic or neurological** |
| Baroreflex failure** |
| Postural tachycardia syndrome* |
| Orthostatic hypotension |
| Stroke* |
| Cerebrovascular insufficiency |
| Seizure disorders |
| Diencephalic (autonomic) epilepsy |
| Migraine or cluster headaches |
| **Cardiovascular** |
| Labile essential hypertension* |
| Therapy-resistant hypertension |
| Hypertension due to obstructive sleep apnoea* |
| Pre-eclampsia and eclampsia |
| Cardiomyopathy (with heart failure**) |
| Pulmonary oedema |
| Hyperdynamic β-adrenergic circulatory state |
| Unexplained shock** |
| Renovascular disease and endstage kidney failure* |
| **Neuropsychiatric or pharmacologic** |
| Anxiety, panic attacks |
| Factitiously-produced hypertension (e.g. self-injection of adrenaline)** |
| Monoamine oxidase inhibitors and tyramine (in food) |
| Illicit drugs (e.g. amphetamines, cocaine)* |
| Over-the-counter sympathomimetics (e.g. ephedrine)* |
| Acrodynia ('Pink disease'—mercury poisoning)* |
| **Miscellaneous** |
| Carcinoid syndrome |
| Systemic mastocytosis |
| Menopause |
| Hyperthyroidism |
| Adrenal medullary hyperplasia* |
| Hypoglycaemia (e.g. due to insulinoma)* |
| Hyper-adrenaline states (e.g. Dumping syndrome)* |
| Neuroblastoma, ganglioneuroma, ganglioneuroblastoma |

Conditions associated with mild to moderate* or occasionally severe** increases in catecholamines.

In contrast, flushing in phaeochromocytoma is less common than appearance of pallor, the latter occurring secondary to catecholamine-induced vasoconstriction. Both mastocytosis and carcinoid syndrome may also present with haemodynamic instability, mainly involving hypotension, but also occasionally hypertension. Systemic mastocytosis appears responsible for the underlying pathology in a subset of patients with postural tachycardia syndrome associated with flushing episodes (Shibao et al. 2005).

Several neurological disorders may mimic a phaeochromocytoma, the most well known being migraine or cluster headaches (Thomas et al. 1966). Less commonly, stroke, epilepsy or cerebral tumours may arouse diagnostic confusion. Symptoms of stroke or seizures may also occur as the presenting manifestation of a phaeochromocytoma (Lehmann et al. 1999, Leiba et al. 2003). Diencephalic autonomic epilepsy represents another neurological condition causing paroxysms of hypertension and tachycardia—sometimes with flushing, diaphoresis, and other autonomic disturbances—that may masquerade as phaeochromocytoma (Metz et al. 1978, Freeman and Schachter 1995). The condition may be diagnosed if symptoms subside after anticonvulsant therapy.

Elevations of plasma adrenaline may occur during attacks in patients with panic disorder (Wilkinson et al. 1998), which also often require discrimination from phaeochromocytoma. Elevations of plasma adrenaline have also been described repeatedly in patients with symptoms mimicking phaeochromocytoma, but without the tumour (Streeten et al. 1990). In some patients the findings may reflect adrenal medullary hyperplasia (Rudy et al. 1980, Dupont et al. 1985).

Resistance to antihypertensive medications or paroxysmal blood pressure increases during treatment with beta-blockers, or marked pressure increases by conditions known to precipitate attacks (mentioned above), should suggest phaeochromocytoma (Sheaves et al. 1995, Martell et al. 2003).

Obstructive sleep apnoea can cause hypertension with sympathetic nervous system activation resulting in increases in urinary catecholamines and O-methylated metabolites (Elmasry et al. 2002). Several cases have been reported with clinical features of phaeochromocytoma, including labile or drug-resistant hypertension, headaches and other symptoms, complicated by findings of increase urinary outputs of noradrenaline (Hoy et al. 2004).

Unrecognized phaeochromocytoma during pregnancy carries a high risk of maternal and fetal mortality (Mannelli and Bemporad 2002). Manifestations may first appear in pregnancy, remit after delivery, and return in a subsequent pregnancy. Phaeochromocytoma attacks may be aggravated during pregnancy and can be confused with preeclampsia or eclampsia. However, pre-eclampsia usually occurs after 20 weeks of pregnancy and is accompanied by modest hypertension, periorbital and ankle oedema, proteinuria, and an elevated blood uric acid—manifestations atypical for phaeochromocytoma. It is always crucial and may be lifesaving to consider phaeochromocytoma as a possible cause of hypertension developing during pregnancy.

It is extremely important for clinicians to appreciate that congestive heart failure may be caused by catecholamine myocarditis and cardiomyopathy secondary to phaeochromocytoma (Garcia and Jennings 1972). Prompt recognition is crucial since appropriate treatment may return even severely depressed cardiac function to normal, avoiding unnecessary heart transplant (Wilkenfeld et al. 1992, Quigg and Om 1994).

Endstage renal failure is often associated with significant haemodynamic instability, with episodes of hypertension and symptoms that can mimic phaeochromocytoma (Stumvoll et al. 1995, Box et al. 1997). Numerous case reports of phaeochromocytoma in patients with renal insufficiency, including some where the tumour contributed to impaired kidney function, attest to the importance of differential diagnosis in such patients. Diagnosis can be complicated by several factors: urine collections may be impossible or

inappropriate, there is often sympathetic activation so that plasma catecholamines are usually elevated, and circulatory accumulation of blood-borne substances can interfere with biochemical analyses performed on blood samples (Eisenhofer et al. 2005b).

Phaeochromocytoma should be considered in unexplained shock, especially if accompanied by abdominal pain, pulmonary oedema, and pronounced mydriasis unreactive to light (Bergland 1989). Another rare presentation is multisystem organ failure accompanied by severe hypertension or hypotension, encephalopathy, hyperpyrexia, and lactic acidosis (i.e. phaeochromocytoma multisystem crisis) (Newell et al. 1988). Occasionally, haemorrhagic necrosis in a phaeochromocytoma presents as an acute abdomen or cardiovascular crisis. Only rarely will prompt recognition and immediate intervention reverse these conditions, which are usually lethal.

Many of the above conditions can be excluded clinically. Judging the likelihood of phaeochromocytoma can also benefit from consideration of clinical clues (Table 64.3), but usually requires confirmation or exclusion by biochemical testing. It is, however, always important to recognize that some of the above conditions and many types of stress (e.g. strenuous exercise, myocardial infarction, congestive heart failure, hypoglycaemia, increased intracranial pressure, hypoxia, acidosis, surgery, trauma) may elevate plasma and urinary catecholamines and their metabolites. Where this presents a problem for differential diagnosis, phaeochromocytoma is most reliably distinguished from other conditions using

Table 64.3 Clues helpful in identifying patients with phaeochromocytoma

---

◆ Hyperglycaemia without a history of diabetes. Elevated catecholamines (especially adrenaline) can cause hyperglycaemia in at least 40% of patients with phaeochromocytoma.

◆ Transitory tachycardia may suddenly appear because of a sudden release of catecholamines from a phaeochromocytoma; however, subsidence of the tachycardia is gradual, unlike the abrupt cessation of tachycardia that occurs with paroxysmal atrial tachycardia.

◆ Although hyperthyroidism may clinically be very similar to phaeochromocytoma, depression of thyroid stimulating hormone is diagnostic of hyperthyroidism.

◆ Evidence of familial disease (e.g. von Hippel-Lindau syndrome, medullary thyroid cancer, hyperparathyroidism, mucosal neuromas, thickened corneal nerves, intestinal ganglioneuromatosis, neurofibromatosis), especially if hypertension exists.

◆ Orthostatic hypotension in patients with hypertension who are not on antihypertensive medication and do not have diabetes or autonomic dysfunction.

◆ Severe constipation accompanying hypertension, since excess circulating catecholamines can inhibit intestinal peristalsis.

◆ Cardiomyopathy with hypertension and sometimes with congestive heart failure can result from excess circulating catecholamines, but is frequently thought to have another aetiology.

◆ Hypertension with micturition or bladder distension (from delayed urination) frequently accompanied by haematuria—this suggests a urinary bladder phaeochromocytoma.

◆ On rare occasions patients with excess circulating catecholamines may develop hyperpyrexia accompanied by a markedly elevated white blood count (adrenaline-provoked), erroneously suggesting an infection.

the clonidine suppression test (see description under biochemical diagnosis).

All of the rare and unusual presentations of phaeochromocytoma require clinical acumen and knowledge of the vagaries of phaeochromocytoma. Above all, the key is to first think of it! Failure to consider phaeochromocytoma in the differential diagnosis may be fatal.

Hereditary phaeochromocytoma

Although most cases of phaeochromocytoma are sporadic, a significant proportion occur secondary to several hereditary syndromes (Table 64.4): von Hippel-Lindau (VHL) disease due to mutations of the VHL gene, multiple endocrine neoplasia type 2A and 2B (MEN 2) due to germline mutations of the RET gene, neurofibromatosis type 1 (NF 1) due to mutations of the NF 1 gene, and familial paragangliomas and phaeochromocytomas caused by mutations of genes for members of the succinate dehydrogenase family (SDHD and SDHB). All are autosomal dominant disorders, usually indicated by a syndrome with a family history and presentation of specific clinical manifestations according to the underlying mutation.

MEN 2 (Sipple's syndrome), affecting about one in 25,000 individuals, is characterized by medullary thyroid carcinoma (MTC) and phaeochromocytoma; additional parathyroid neoplasia occurs in MEN 2A form, whereas multiple mucosal neuromas and a Marfinoid habitus occur in MEN 2B form (Gagel 1998). At least 70% of phaeochromocytomas are bilateral, and are usually preceded by medullary thyroid cancer. Adrenomedullary hyperplasia precedes phaeochromocytoma, which manifests in about 50% of MEN 2A patients at a peak age of about 40 years (Gagel et al. 1988, Nguyen et al. 2001). However, tumours may occur as early as 10 years of age, particularly in the more aggressive, but less common, MEN 2B form.

Clear cell renal carcinomas and cysts, central nervous system and retinal hemiangioblastomas, phaeochromocytomas, pancreatic tumours and cysts, endolymphatic sac tumours, and epididymal cysts are clinical manifestations of VHL syndrome, which has an incidence of about one in 36,000 births (Lonser et al. 2003). The presentation

of these manifestations can be variable, thought to depend on the particular mutation and functional effects in specific tissues (Hes et al. 2003). In some VHL kindreds phaeochromocytomas are common, but the overall penetrance of phaeochromocytomas in VHL syndrome is only 10–20% (Lonser et al. 2003). When present, the tumours may be bilateral or extra-adrenal. The mean age at presentation is about 30 years of age (Walther et al. 1999b). Screening of affected families may detect tumours in children as early as 5 years of age (Weise et al. 2002).

Neurofibromatosis is a relatively common inherited disorder affecting one in 3000 individuals (Friedman 1999). Common clinical manifestations on which the diagnosis of NF 1 is made include café au lait spots, neurofibromas, axillary or inguinal freckling, optic glioma, Lisch nodules, and osseous lesions (Friedman and Birch 1997). NF 1 is associated with a higher prevalence than normal of neoplasms such as carcinoids and phaeochromocytomas. Nevertheless, the penetrance of phaeochromocytoma in NF 1 is relatively low (< 2%), and unlike other hereditary conditions, usually occurs after the 5th decade (Riccardi 1991, Friedman and Birch 1997, Walther et al. 1999a). Routine screening for phaeochromocytoma in patients with NF 1 is therefore not generally recommended unless hypertension is present (Kalff et al. 1982).

Hereditary paragangliomas result from mutations of three of the four subunits of the succinate dehydrogenase gene family (SDHB, SDHC and SDHD), presenting either as hormonally silent head and neck tumours or catecholamine-producing extra-adrenal and adrenal tumours (Baysal et al. 2002). While mutations of SDHB, SDHC and SDHD genes all may lead to head and neck paragangliomas, only mutations of SDHB and SDHD genes appear to show any significant association with catecholamine-producing phaeochromocytomas. Most head and neck paragangliomas do not produce significant amounts of catecholamines and are often only detected due to the space-occupying effects of lesions (Erickson et al. 2001). Accurate estimates of the true incidence of paragangliomas, including hereditary tumours, have been difficult to obtain.

Identification of genes responsible for hereditary phaeochromocytoma now makes it possible to routinely test for underlying mutations. The contribution of hereditary factors to phaeochromocytoma is consequently becoming more widely recognized, expanding to cases where there is no obvious syndrome. In a population-based series of 271 patients with non-syndromic phaeochromocytoma, Neumann et al. (Neumann et al. 2002) reported that 24% had disease-causing germline mutations. Based on a review of the literature, Bryant et al. (2003) estimated the frequency of mutations among patients with non-syndromic phaeochromocytoma to be 19%. From the above estimates, and the traditional but now defunct rule-of-10 (where 10% of phaeochromocytomas were considered hereditary) it now seems likely that close to 30% of all phaeochromocytomas may have a hereditary basis.

Realization of the significant hereditary contribution to phaeochromocytoma is leading to recommendations for widening testing of disease-causing genes to patients with tumours who do not have any clear family history or associated syndrome (Neumann et al. 2002, Bryant et al. 2003). Conversely, patients significantly at risk for phaeochromocytoma due to mutations of RET, VHL and succinate dehydrogenase genes are now being encouraged to undergo routine periodic screening for the tumour. Consequently, phaeochromocytomas are being detected at an earlier stage in

Table 64.4 Hereditary phaeochromocytoma

Gene	RET	VHL	NF 1	SDHD	SDHB
Gene location	10q11.2	3p25–26	17q11.2	11q23	1p36
Non-syndromic frequency*	1–5%	6–10%	unknown	2–8%	4–5%
Catecholamine phenotype†	A	NA	A	NA	NA
Adrenal location	++	++	++	+	+
Extra-adrenal location	–	+	+	++	++
Frequency of malignancy§	3%	5%	11%	<3%	66–83%

* Frequencies of germline mutations in non-syndromic (apparently sporadic) phaeochromocytoma are derived from several published studies (Neumann et al. 2002, 2004, Bryant et al. 2003, Dannenberg et al. 2005).

† Tumour catecholamine phenotypes are designated as either predominantly noradrenaline-producing (NA) or noradrenaline and adrenaline-producing (A).

§ Frequencies of malignancy are derived from several published studies (Casanova et al. 1993, Walther et al. 1999a).

patients who are often normotensive and asymptomatic (Neumann et al. 1993, Eisenhofer et al. 2001).

In addition to the variable tumour syndromes associated with disease-causing mutations, there is also heterogeneity in the clinical manifestations of phaeochromocytomas dependent on the underlying mutation (Table 64.4). In MEN 2, almost all tumours are confined to the adrenals. Tumour cells express phenylethanolamine-N-methyltransferase (PNMT), the enzyme that converts noradrenaline to adrenaline (Eisenhofer et al. 2001). Consequently, phaeochromocytomas in patients with MEN 2 produce both noradrenaline and adrenaline. In contrast, phaeo-chromocytomas in VHL syndrome do not express PNMT and thus only produce noradrenaline.

Phaeochromocytomas in patients with SDHD and SDHB mutations show closer phenotypic features to VHL than MEN 2 tumours, possibly reflecting activation of hypoxia-associated pathways of tumourigenesis (Baysal 2003, Favier et al. 2005). Similar to VHL tumours, tumours in patients with SDHD and SDHB mutations are highly vascularized and produce noradrena-line, but not adrenaline. A major difference among these tumours, however, is predisposition to malignancy (Table 64.4). In MEN 2 and VHL patients, malignant phaeochromocytoma is rare. In contrast, patients with SDHB mutations have a high risk of malig-nant disease (Gimenez-Roqueplo et al. 2003, Neumann et al. 2004).

Adrenal incidentalomas

Adrenal incidentalomas are clinically unapparent adrenal masses discovered inadvertently during diagnostic imaging for other con-ditions unrelated to adrenal disease. Improvements in imaging technologies and their increasing use in diagnosis and manage-ment of disease has led to gaining recognition of adrenal incidenta-lomas as a public health problem (Aron 2001, Grumbach et al. 2003). Prevalence of adrenal incidentalomas discovered during computerized abdominal imaging procedures increases with age from as low as 0.2% in the young (< 30 years) to 6.9% or more in the elderly (> 70 years) (Young 2000).

Most adrenal incidentalomas are benign non-functional adeno-mas, requiring little more than periodic follow-up to assess for increased size. An important proportion, however, are highly malignant adrenocortical carcinomas or functional endocrine tumours, these requiring immediate attention. Among the latter, phaeochromocytomas represent a frequent cause of clinically unapparent adrenal masses, literature reviews indicating a fre-quency of 5.1–8.0% (Young 2000, Mansmann et al. 2004). The proportion of cases of phaeochromocytoma discovered inciden-tally during imaging studies for unrelated conditions has increased over time. In one series of patients, 41% of all phaeochromocyto-mas diagnosed between 1986 and 1995 were discovered inciden-tally compared with only 2.0% during 1957–1985 (Noshiro et al. 2000). In another series, close to half of all tumours were found incidentally during imaging studies (Baguet et al. 2004).

Patients with phaeochromocytomas found as adrenal incidenta-lomas are often normotensive and usually do not display the classic symptoms of catecholamine hypersecretion (Bernini et al. 1997, Mannelli et al. 1999, Mantero et al. 2000). Urinary or plasma cate-cholamines are often normal, making diagnosis difficult. Despite the often-asymptomatic nature of such tumours, they remain a time bomb capable of releasing catecholamines in large and dangerous amounts. All patients with adrenal incidentalomas should therefore be tested for phaeochromocytoma. As discussed below and recommended in a consensus report (Grumbach et al. 2003), improved diagnosis may be facilitated by measurements of plasma free metanephrines.

Biochemical diagnosis and tumour localization

Phaeochromocytomas are catecholamine-metabolizing tumours

Phaeochromocytomas are usually described as tumours that pro-duce, store, and secrete catecholamines. It is rarely appreciated that phaeochromocytomas also metabolize catecholamines, and that this is a more consistent process than that of catecholamine secre-tion (Eisenhofer et al. 2003a). Failure to recognize this key feature is probably due to the misconception that metabolism occurs mainly after release of catecholamines. Catecholamines are in fact mainly metabolized within the same cells where they are synthe-sized, mostly following passive leakage of the amines from storage granules into the cytoplasm, a process that is independent of catecholamine release.

Phaeochromocytoma tumour cells, like adrenal medullary cells, contain catechol-O-methyltransferase, the enzyme that converts noradrenaline to normetanephrine, adrenaline to metanephrine, and dopamine to methoxytyramine (Eisenhofer et al. 1998). The adrenal glands, not the more commonly considered liver and kidneys, represent the single largest site of catecholamine O-methylation, accounting for over 90% of all circulating metane-phrine and about 23% of normetanephrine (Eisenhofer et al. 1995). Normally this O-methylation pathway represents a minor route of catecholamine metabolism; deamination of noradrenaline within sympathetic nerves is the major pathway (Fig. 64.1). Intraneuronal deamination is followed by O-methylation of the deaminated metabolite in extraneuronal tissues, and finally oxidation in the liver to vanillylmandelic acid (VMA), the major urinary metabolite of noradrenaline and adrenaline.

In patients with phaeochromocytoma, intra-tumoural O-methylation becomes a dominant pathway of catecholamine metabolism. Consequently, the presence of the tumour leads to relatively large increases in production of the O-methylated metab-olites, compared with minor increases in deaminated metabolites. Due to the continuous high rate of intra-tumoural catecholamine O-methylation, and because some tumours secrete catecholamines episodically or in low amounts, patients with phaeochromocytoma usually have relatively larger and more consistent increases of plasma normetanephrine or metanephrine than of the parent catecholamines.

The normetanephrine and metanephrine produced in adrenal medullary or phaeochromocytoma tumour cells are either deami-nated or converted to sulphate-conjugated metabolites. The sulphate-conjugated O-methylated metabolites are cleared from the circulation by the kidney, and thus represent the major forms of normetanephrine and metanephrine excreted in urine. The enzyme responsible for sulphate conjugation is present in high concentrations in digestive tissues where it functions to inactivate dietary amines and conjugate the large amounts of noradrenaline, dopamine, and their metabolites produced locally.

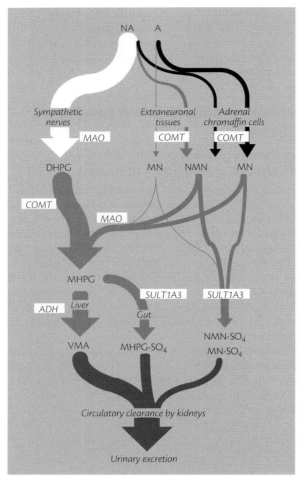

Fig. 64.1 Diagram showing the main pathways for metabolism of the noradrenaline and adrenaline derived from sympathoneuronal or adrenal-medullary sources. Deamination in sympathetic nerves (white) is the major pathway of catecholamine metabolism and involves intraneuronal deamination of noradrenaline leaking from storage granules or of noradrenaline recaptured after release by sympathetic nerves. Metabolism in adrenal chromaffin cells (black) involves O-methylation of catecholamines leaking from storage granules into the cytoplasm of adrenal-medullary cells. The extraneuronal pathway (grey) is a relatively minor pathway of metabolism of catecholamines released from sympathetic nerves or the adrenal medulla, but is important for further processing of metabolites produced in sympathetic nerves and adrenal chromaffin cells. The free metanephrines produced in extraneuronal tissues or adrenal chromaffin cells are either further metabolized by deamination or sulphate conjugation. Abbreviations: NA, noradrenaline; A, adrenaline; DHPG, 3,4-dihydroxyphenylglycol; MN, metanephrine; NMN, normetanephrine; MHPG, 3-methoxy-4-hydroxyphenylglycol; VMA, vanillylmandelic acid; MHPG-SO$_4$, 3-methoxy-4-hydroxyphenylglycol sulphate; NMN-SO$_4$, normetanephrine-sulphate; MN-SO$_4$, metanephrine-sulphate; MAO, monoamine oxidase; COMT, catechol-O-methyltransferase; ADH, alcohol dehydrogenase; SULT1A3, phenolsulfotransferase type 1A3.

Initial biochemical testing

Because missing a phaeochromocytoma can have deadly consequences, one of the most important considerations in the choice of an initial test is a high level of reliability that the test will provide a positive result in that rare patient with the tumour. This conversely also provides confidence that a negative result reliably excludes the tumour, thus avoiding the need for multiple or repeat biochemical

tests or even costly and unnecessary imaging studies to rule out the tumour. Therefore, the initial work-up of a patient with suspected phaeochromocytoma should include a suitably sensitive biochemical test.

Independent studies from three centres have established that measurements of plasma free metanephrines (normetanephrine and metanephrine) provide the most sensitive biochemical test for diagnosis of phaeochromocytoma (Raber et al. 2000, Lenders et al. 2002, Sawka et al. 2003). In the largest of these studies (Lenders et al. 2002), involving over 200 patients with phaeochromocytoma and more than 600 patients in whom the tumour was excluded, measurements of plasma free metanephrines and urinary fractionated metanephrines provided the most sensitive diagnostic tests, urinary and plasma catecholamines offered intermediate sensitivity, while urinary total metanephrines and VMA were the least sensitive (Table 64.5). Receiver-operating characteristic curves showed that at equivalent levels of sensitivity, the specificity of plasma metanephrines was higher than that of all other tests and that at equivalent levels of specificity, the sensitivity of plasma metanephrines was also higher than that of other tests.

Plasma free and urinary fractionated metanephrines offer similarly high diagnostic sensitivity so that negative results for either test appear equally effective for excluding phaeochromocytoma (Lenders et al. 2002). However, because urinary fractionated metanephrines have lower specificity, tests of plasma free metanephrines exclude phaeochromocytoma in more patients without the tumour than do tests of urinary fractionated metanephrines. Initial biochemical testing for phaeochromocytoma should therefore include measurements of plasma free metanephrines or measurements of urinary fractionated metanephrines as the next best test. Additional measurements of catecholamines may also be carried out, but are unlikely to lead to detection of additional tumours not indicated by elevated levels of normetanephrine or metanephrine (Lenders et al. 2002). Exceptions include rare tumours that produce exclusively dopamine. As outlined above, such patients usually have an atypical presentation. The tumours can be identified biochemically by measurements of plasma concentrations of methoxytyramine or dopamine (Eisenhofer et al. 2005a).

Table 64.5 Sensitivities and specificities of biochemical tests for diagnosis of phaeochromocytoma

	Sensitivity	**Specificity**
Plasma free metanephrines	99% (211/214)	89% (575/644)
Urine fractionated metanephrines	97% (102/105)	69% (310/452)
Urine catecholamines	86% (151/175)	88% (471/535)
Plasma catecholamines	84% (178/212)	81% (523/643)
Urine total metanephrines	77% (88/114)	93% (170/183)
Urine vanillylmandelic acid	64% (96/151)	95% (442/465)

The sensitivities of tests of plasma and urinary fractionated metanephrines or plasma and urinary catecholamines were determined as the percentage of patients with phaeochromocytoma with positive test results for either normetanephrine or metanephrine (i.e. for tests of plasma or urinary metanephrines) or with positive test results for either noradrenaline or adrenaline (i.e. for tests of plasma or urinary catecholamines). The sensitivities of tests of urinary total metanephrines reflect tests of urinary total metanephrines (i.e. the combined sum of free plus conjugated normetanephrine and metanephrine). Adapted from Lenders et al. 2002.

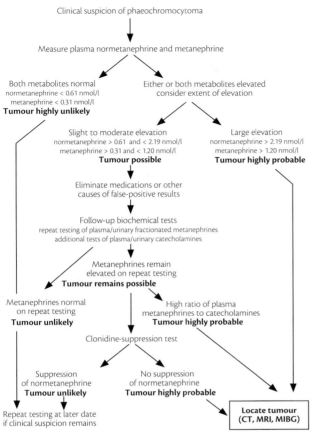

Fig. 64.2 Algorithm for biochemical diagnosis of phaeochromocytoma.

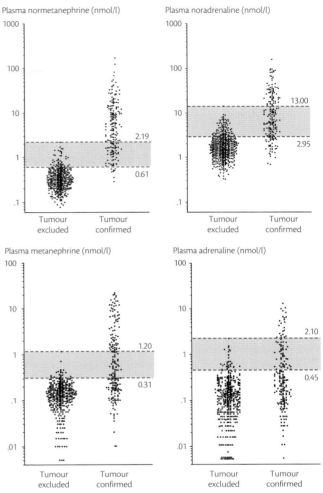

Fig. 64.3 Dot plots showing distributions of concentrations of plasma free metanephrines and catecholamines in patients with (Tumour Confirmed) and without (Tumour Excluded) phaeochromocytoma. The lower dashed horizontal lines show the upper reference limits of normal for each test in nmoles per litre. The upper dashed horizontal lines show the upper limit of values for patients in whom the tumour was excluded. Values above this line indicate a high probability of phaeochromocytoma (e.g. specificity = 100%), whereas values below this line and in the grey area above the upper reference limits of normal indicate a positive result that may or may not reflect a phaeochromocytoma and for which further follow-up testing is required (see diagnostic algorithm in Fig. 64.2). Note the relatively larger and more consistent increases above the upper reference limits for plasma normetanephrine than for plasma norepinephrine and for plasma metanephrine than for plasma epinephrine. Data are from 648 patients in whom phaeochromocytoma was excluded and 208 patients in whom the tumour was confirmed as published elsewhere (Lenders et al. 2002).

Follow-up biochemical testing

Apart from a few rare exceptions, findings of normal plasma concentrations of normetanephrine and metanephrine rule out phaeochromocytoma. In such patients no further testing for the tumour should usually be necessary (Fig. 64.2). Exceptions include patients at high risk for phaeochromocytoma because of a hereditary syndrome or a previous tumour, where small tumours or recurrences may be found during routine screening that do not produce signs and symptoms or a positive result by any biochemical test. In such patients, positive results will likely follow enlargement of tumours.

With the above exceptions in mind, follow-up testing for phaeochromocytoma should be necessary only in patients with positive results of initial measurements of plasma free or urinary fractionated metanephrines. The need for follow-up testing depends on the likelihood that positive results indicate a tumour, best assessed from the magnitude of elevation of test results (Fig. 64.3). For example, increases in plasma concentrations of normetanephrine above 2.19 nmol/L (400 ng/L) or of metanephrine above 1.20 nmol/L (236 ng/L) are extremely rare in patients without phaeochromocytoma, but occur in about 80% of patients with the tumour (Lenders et al. 2002). Providing biochemical test results are accurate, the likelihood of phaeochromocytoma in such patients is so high that the immediate task is to locate the tumour.

The remaining problem is to confirm or exclude phaeochromocytoma in patients with positive results in the equivocal range (Fig. 64.3). Due to the rarity of phaeochromocytoma in patients tested for the tumour, false-positive results in this range can be expected to far outnumber true-positive results. Thus, although a tumour is possible, the likelihood is low. Follow-up tests are required for an equivocal test results when diagnosis is uncertain.

When there is concern about the analytical accuracy or validity of a positive result for measurements of plasma metanephrines, this can be checked by follow-up measurements of urinary fractionated metanephrines, and vice versa when there is concern about an initial urinary test result. Similar patterns of increases of both urinary and plasma metabolites not only help confirm accuracy of results, but also increase the likelihood of a tumour.

Before follow-up testing is initiated, consideration should be given to sources of false-positive results, including as detailed elsewhere (Eisenhofer et al. 2003b), inappropriate sampling conditions, dietary factors, clinical conditions, and medications likely to interfere with analytical results or increase levels of normetanephrine or metanephrine. Tricyclic antidepressants and phenoxybenzamine (dibenzyline) in particular can be frequent causes of false-positive elevations of plasma and urinary noradrenaline and normetanephrine.

Patterns of follow-up test results for plasma catecholamines and free metanephrines can provide additional information about the likelihood of phaeochromocytoma (Eisenhofer et al. 2003b). Relatively larger increases in plasma normetanephrine than of noradrenaline or of metanephrine than of adrenaline are more consistent with phaeochromocytoma than sympathoadrenal activation. Conversely, an activated sympathetic nervous system is usually associated with relatively larger increases of noradrenaline than of normetanephrine. False-positive elevations of plasma noradrenaline or normetanephrine can be further identified using the clonidine-suppression test (Bravo et al. 1981). Clonidine activates alpha$_2$-adrenoceptors in the brain and on sympathetic nerve endings, thereby suppressing sympathoneural release of noradrenaline. The drug, however, does not affect release of catecholamines from a phaeochromocytoma.

Lack of suppression of noradrenaline provides strong evidence for a phaeochromocytoma; however, normal suppression does not exclude phaeochromocytoma or reliably identify patients with false-positive results. The test has particularly limited utility in patients with phaeochromocytoma who have normal or mildly elevated levels of noradrenaline. In such patients only small amounts of circulating noradrenaline are derived from the tumour; most originates from sympathetic nerves and is responsive to clonidine.

The above problem with the clonidine suppression test is largely overcome using measurements of plasma normetanephrine (Eisenhofer et al. 2003b). Similar to noradrenaline, clonidine consistently decreases plasma levels of normetanephrine in patients without phaeochromocytoma. Thus, if measurements are accurate, elevated levels and lack of suppression of plasma normetanephrine after clonidine indicate a high probability of phaeochromocytoma. More importantly, because elevations of normetanephrine are more consistent and relatively larger than those of noradrenaline, very few patients with phaeochromocytoma show normal suppression of normetanephrine. Thus, measurements of normetanephrine after clonidine confirm more cases of phaeochromocytoma and are more effective for excluding the tumour than measurements of noradrenaline.

Additional interpretative considerations

Phaeochromocytomas are highly heterogeneous tumours with diverse phenotypes. Although the tumours are characterized by production of catecholamines, the nature of this can vary considerably, accounting in part for variable clinical presentation (Ito et al. 1992). About one half of adrenal tumours produce almost exclusively noradrenaline and the other half a variable mixture of noradrenaline and adrenaline (Kimura et al. 1992, Eisenhofer et al. 2005c). In contrast, extra-adrenal tumours produce near exclusively noradrenaline. Differences in plasma concentrations of normetanephrine and metanephrine reflect underlying differences in tumour catecholamine phenotype better than do differences in plasma or urinary

noradrenaline and adrenaline (Eisenhofer et al. 2005c). Thus, the nature of increases in urinary or plasma metanephrines can provide information about tumour location that may be useful during follow-up imaging studies. Although exclusive increases of normetanephrine occur in both adrenal and extra-adrenal tumours, the presence of additional or exclusive increases in metanephrine reliably indicates an adrenal location or a recurrence of a previous adrenal tumour (Fig. 64.4).

A consequence of the considerable variation in catecholamine release among patients with phaeochromocytoma is that plasma concentrations or urinary excretion of catecholamines are poorly correlated with tumour size (Crout and Sjoerdsma 1964, Lenders et al. 1995). In contrast, and as shown in Fig. 64.4, due to metabolism of catecholamines within tumours and the independence of this process on catecholamine release, urinary excretion or plasma concentrations of metanephrines show strong positive correlations with tumour size (Stenstrom and Waldenstrom 1985, Lenders et al. 1995). The magnitude of the increase in metanephrines above normal can therefore be useful in predicting extent and progression of disease (Eisenhofer et al. 2005c).

Finally, patterns of biochemical test results can provide some information about presence of malignant disease; noradrenaline is usually the predominant catecholamine produced, with occasionally significant increases in plasma and urinary levels of L-3,4-dihydroxyphenylalanine (L-DOPA) and dopamine, the immediate precursors of noradrenaline, and of methoxytyramine, the O-methylated metabolite of dopamine (Eisenhofer et al. 2005a). Elevations of plasma or urinary dopamine and methoxytyramine are not in themselves particularly sensitive or specific markers of metastatic phaeochromocytoma. However, when accompanied by elevations in plasma noradrenaline or other clinical evidence of phaeochromocytoma, such elevations should arouse immediate suspicion of metastatic disease.

Tumour localization

Tumour localization depends primarily on anatomic imaging using computerized tomography (CT) or magnetic resonance imaging (MRI), and secondly on functional imaging, mainly with meta-iodobenzyl guanidine (MIBG). There are now also a variety of other functional ligands that may be used in conjunction with single photon emission computed tomography (SPECT) or positron emission tomography (PET) (Table 64.6).

Studies aimed at localizing a phaeochromocytoma should ideally only be implemented after biochemical testing indicates a high probability of the tumour. Most tumours have an adrenal location, but a possible extra-adrenal location should not be overlooked. CT has good sensitivity for detecting adrenal phaeochromocytomas, but sensitivity is lower (~90%) for extra-adrenal tumours (Mannelli et al. 1999). The high spatial resolution of CT, particularly with helical scanning using 3–5 mm thick slices, allows detection of small adrenal lesions that may not be so readily detected by MRI (Lockhart et al. 2002). MRI, however, is superior for detection of extra-adrenal tumours (Goldstein et al. 1999). Due to issues of radiation, MRI is also preferred over CT for locating tumours during pregnancy and in children.

There are differing opinions about use and choice of functional imaging modalities once CT or MRI has been used to locate a suspected phaeochromocytoma. Some authorities have indicated that MIBG scintigraphy offers little additional help in guiding operative

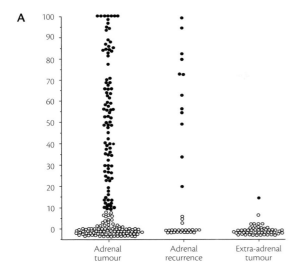

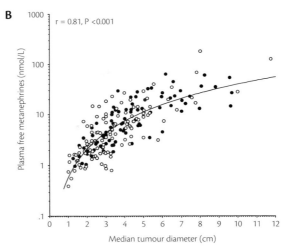

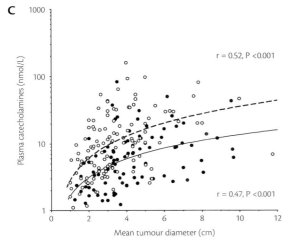

Fig. 64.4 Distributions of adrenergic and noradrenergic tumours according to adrenal or extra-adrenal location **(A)** and relationships of tumour diameter with plasma concentrations of free metanephrines **(B)** or catecholamines **(C)**. The predominantly noradrenaline-producing noradrenergic tumours (O) and adrenaline-producing adrenergic tumours (●) in panel **A** are distinguished by the increases in plasma free metanephrine (MN), expressed as a percent of combined increases of metanephrine and normetanephrine (MN plus NMN). Note the noradrenergic biochemical profile of extra-adrenal tumours compared with the mixed adrenergic and noradrenergic profiles of adrenal tumours or recurrences. Relationships of plasma metanephrines and catecholamines with tumour diameter in panels **B** and **C** are shown using a logarithmic scale and represent summed plasma concentrations of normetanephrine and metanephrine **(B)** or noradrenaline and adrenaline **(C)**. Data for adrenergic tumours (●) and noradrenergic tumours (O) are shown separately. Note that relationships of tumour diameter with plasma metanephrines are stronger than relationships with plasma catecholamines. The different relationships of tumour diameter with plasma catecholamines for patients with noradrenergic (dashed regression lines) compared with adrenergic tumours (solid regression lines) reflect greater secretion of catecholamines in noradrenergic than adrenergic tumours. With permission from Eisenhofer G, Lenders JW, Goldstein DS et al. (2005c), American Association for Clinical Chemistry.

management once an adrenal mass and suspected phaeochromocytoma has been located by CT or MRI (Miskulin et al. 2003). In line with this, others have advocated diagnostic imaging algorithms where MIBG should only be used if CT or MRI fails to locate a suspected phaeochromocytoma (Sawka et al. 2004). The capability of whole body imaging with MIBG certainly offers an advantage for locating extra-adrenal tumours not detected by CT or MRI. Nevertheless, MIBG is often over-used in these circumstances and is best restricted to cases where the biochemical evidence of a catecholamine-producing tumour is compelling (Clesham et al. 1993, Noblet-Dick et al. 2003).

Provided pathological uptake of MIBG is distinguished from physiological uptake, the main advantage of MIBG imaging lies in the high specificity of the method, this dependent on the presence of uptake and storage mechanisms for concentrating the imaging agent in phaeochromocytoma tumour cells (Pacak et al. 2004). Adrenal tumours visualized by MIBG may thereby be correctly identified as phaeochromocytomas. This specificity, together with the capability of whole body imaging also make MIBG particularly useful for locating multifocal tumours or metastases (Sisson et al. 1981). Such additional findings of MIBG-positive multifocal disease or metastases can impact importantly on subsequent medical and surgical management (Taieb et al. 2004).

While MIBG offers high specificity, sensitivity of the method is limited at about 80 to 88% in sporadic phaeochromocytoma, and as low as 60% in smaller hereditary tumours (Berglund et al. 2001, Taieb et al. 2004). MIBG labelled with iodine-123 (^{123}I) (offers improved sensitivity over ^{131}I-labelled MIBG for localization of phaeochromocytoma, and also allows use of SPECT for improved spatial resolution (Shapiro and Gross 1987). Nevertheless, a negative scan using either ^{131}I-MIBG or ^{123}I-MIBG does not reliably exclude phaeochromocytoma. There is a variety of medications (e.g. labetolol, tricyclic antidepressants) that may also interfere with tumour uptake or retention of MIBG (Solanki et al. 1992). Temporarily withholding such drugs may avoid some false-negative results of MIBG imaging.

Other functional imaging approaches with high specificity for diagnostic localization of phaeochromocytomas include PET utilizing 6-[^{18}F]fluorodopamine, ^{11}C-adrenaline, ^{11}C-hydroxyephedrine, or 6-[^{18}F]fluorodopa as imaging agents (Pacak et al. 2001a, Hoegerle et al. 2002). Although presently not widely available, these approaches have some advantages over MIBG imaging. PET involves less radiation exposure and requires a shorter duration of scanning, which can be carried out immediately after administration of the imaging agent rather than days later. There is also no need to block exposure of the thyroid to

Table 64.6 Radioligands used for functional imaging of phaeochromocytoma

Radioligand	Uptake and imaging mechanism	Imaging technique	$T_{1/2}$ (hours)
[123I]-MIBG	Noradrenaline analogue; actively transported into neurosecretory granules via catecholamine transporters	Planar, SPECT	13
[131I]-MIBG	Noradrenaline analogue; actively transported into cells and neurosecretory granules via catecholamine transporters	Planar	196
[11C]-epinephrine	Catecholamine; actively transported into cells and neurosecretory granules via catecholamine transporters	PET	0.34
[11C]-hydroxyephedrine	Catecholamine analogue; actively transported into cells and neurosecretory granules via catecholamine transporters	PET	0.34
[11C]-DOPA	Catecholamine precursor; transported into cells, converted to dopamine and stored in neurosecretory vesicles	PET	0.34
[18F]-DA	Catecholamine; actively transported into cells and neurosecretory granules via catecholamine transporters	PET	1.83
[18F]-DOPA	Catecholamine precursor; transported into cells, converted to dopamine and stored in neurosecretory vesicles	PET	1.83
[18F]-FDG	Glucose analogue; uptake and intracellular accumulation dependent on glucose utilization/energy requirements of tumour cells.	PET	1.83
[123I]-tyr3-DTPA octreotide	Somatostatin analogue acting on somatostatin cellular membrane receptors; undergoes receptor-mediated endocytosis but because of its polarity does not cross the lysosomal and cell membranes	Planar, SPECT	13
[111In]-DTPA octreotide	Somatostatin analogue acting on somatostatin cellular membrane receptors; undergoes receptor-mediated endocytosis but because of its polarity does not cross the lysosomal and cell membranes	Planar, SPECT	68

PET, positron emission tomography; SPECT, single photon emission computed tomography; MIBG, meta-iodobenzyl guanidine; DOPA, dihydroxyphenylalanine; DA, dopamine; FDG, fluorodeoxyglucose; DTPA, diethylenetriamine pentaacetic acid.

radioactive iodine. More importantly, PET provides superior resolution than SPECT or planar scintigraphy. 6-[18F]fluorodopamine PET offers improved diagnostic sensitivity compared with 131I-MIBG scintigraphy, particularly in metastatic phaeochromocytoma where the agent localizes many more foci than possible with 131I-MIBG (Ilias et al. 2003). The new generation of combined PET/CT scanners promises both good resolution and specificity for accurately locating tumours and identifying masses as phaeochromocytomas using functional imaging ligands (Fig. 64.5).

Occasional inability to locate or confirm a phaeochromocytoma by some of the above functional imaging approaches probably reflects loss of expression of the catecholamine uptake mechanisms in dedifferentiated tumours. In such cases, 2-[18F]deoxyglucose PET scanning or 111In-octreotide scintigraphy may prove

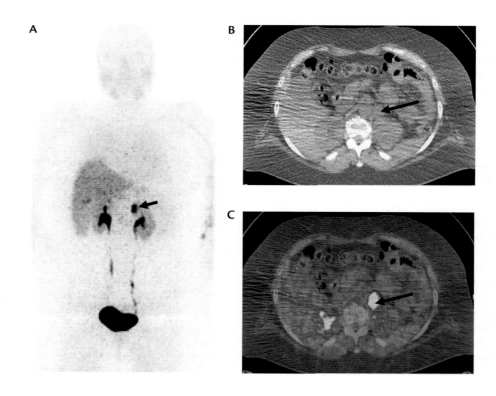

Fig. 64.5 6-[18F]Fluorodopamine positron emission tomography (PET) scan **(A)**, computerized tomography **(B)** 6-[18F]Fluorodopamine PET/computerized tomography in a patient with a left adrenal phaeochromocytoma (arrow).

useful due to increased glucose metabolism or expression of somatostatin receptors on tumour cells (van der Harst et al. 2001, Pacak et al. 2004).

Disease management

Preoperative management

Cure for phaeochromocytoma requires total surgical removal. Endotracheal intubation, anaesthesia, and surgical manipulation of the tumour can provoke massive release of catecholamines with potentially fatal consequences (Manger and Gifford 1996). Thus, once a phaeochromocytoma is located, there is a need for prompt and appropriate medical treatment to minimize complications before and during surgery.

The goal for preoperative management of patients with phaeochromocytoma is relaxation of the constricted vasculature, expansion of the reduced plasma volume, and normalization of blood pressure for about 2 weeks before operation. Returning blood volume to normal minimizes the possibility of shock resulting from sudden diffuse vasodilation at the time of tumour removal. Because of the dangers of a hypertensive crisis, appropriate preoperative preparation is called for regardless of whether patients are consistently normotensive or hypertensive (Manger and Gifford 1996).

The α-adrenoceptor blocker, phenoxybenzamine (Dibenzyline), was introduced in the 1950s for preoperative control of blood pressure, an advance credited for significantly reducing operative mortality and morbidity. Subsequently introduced alternatives to phenoxybenzamine for preoperative blockade of catecholamine-induced vasoconstriction include calcium channel blockers and selective α_1-adrenoceptor blocking agents, such as terazosin (Hytrin) and doxazosin (Cardura) (Proye et al. 1989, Prys-Roberts and Farndon 2002). Compared with phenoxybenzamine, these drugs have advantages of fewer side-effects and are less likely to cause false-positive elevations of plasma and urinary levels of noradrenaline and noradrenaline metabolites (Prys-Roberts 2000, Eisenhofer et al. 2003b). Nevertheless, phenoxybenzamine remains the most commonly used drug for preoperative blood pressure control.

Additional administration of alpha-methyl-*para*-tyrosine (metyrosine, Demser™) to block catecholamine synthesis may improve control of blood pressure compared with that achieved by α-adrenoceptor blockade alone (Perry et al. 1990, Steinsapir et al. 1997). Nevertheless, this combined drug regimen remains part of the standard of care at only a few centres and may be most suitable in patients with highly active tumours where blood pressure remains poorly controlled with α-blockers.

A β-adrenoceptor blocker may be used for preoperative control of arrhythmias, tachycardia or angina (Prys-Roberts 2000). However, loss of β_2-adrenoceptor-mediated vasodilatation in a patient with unopposed catecholamine-induced vasoconstriction can result in dangerous increases in blood pressure (Manger and Gifford 1996). Therefore, β-adrenoceptor blockers should never be used without first blocking α-adrenoceptor mediated vasoconstriction. The combined α- and β-adrenoceptor blocker, labetalol, does not provide a useful solution due to more potent effects on β- than α-adrenoceptors, which in a patient with phaeochromocytoma may lead to severe hypertension. Additionally, the drug can interfere with some diagnostic tests, including MIBG localization studies (Solanki et al. 1992).

Surgery and intraoperative management

Induction of anaesthesia and surgical removal of phaeochromocytoma may cause considerable cardiovascular instability, even after appropriate preoperative control of blood pressure (Manger and Gifford 1996). In addition to standard anaesthetic monitoring, an arterial line is required for blood pressure monitoring.

The laparoscopic approach for tumour removal is now largely replacing laparotomy as the method of choice for surgical resection of most abdominal phaeochromocytomas (Thompson et al. 1997, Vargas et al. 1997). Operative times, blood loss, and complications are similar by both open and laparoscopic approaches, but advantages of the latter include less postoperative pain, a shortened hospital stay and convalescent period, and improved cosmetic result.

Maintenance of cardiovascular stability is a challenge for the anaesthetist that requires availability of specific drugs (Prys-Roberts 2000). Since episodes of cardiovascular instability can be extreme, rapid, and unexpected, with hypertension alternating with hypotension, these agents should ideally be quick acting and have short durations of effect. Intravenous phentolamine (Regitine) and nitroprusside provide effective short-term control of intraoperative hypertension. Control of arrythmias can be achieved using lidocaine or the short-acting β-adrenoceptor blocker esmolol (Brevibloc). Profound hypotension can be a problem, particularly at the time of venous clamping and tumour isolation and removal. This is most appropriately corrected using intravenous fluids, with pressor agents, such as phenylephrine, if needed.

In patients with hereditary phaeochromocytoma there is a high probability of bilateral adrenal disease. Complete surgical removal of both adrenals with ensuing loss of adrenal cortical function and requirement for life-long hormone replacement therapy is associated with significant morbidity. Partial adrenalectomies are therefore often carried out, but in such patients the benefits of preserving adrenocortical function should be weighed against the risk of further disease (Walther et al. 2000).

Postoperative care and follow-up

Although some patients remain hypertensive in the immediate post-operative period, most require treatment for hypotension, which is best remedied by administration of fluids. Hypoglycaemia after tumour removal is a problem best prevented by infusion of 5% dextrose starting immediately after tumour removal and continuing for several hours thereafter. Postoperative hypoglycaemia is transient, whereas low blood pressure and orthostatic hypotension may persist for up to a day or more after surgery and require care with assumption of sitting or upright posture.

Despite successful surgery, up to 50% of patients with previous high blood pressure remain hypertensive (Plouin et al. 1997). Completeness of tumour resection should be confirmed three to six weeks after surgery by biochemical testing with a return of previously abnormally elevated test results to normal. Five year post-surgical survival for patients with sporadic phaeochromocytoma who have no evidence of metastatic disease is about 95%. However, about 17% of patients operated for phaeochromocytoma develop recurrent disease, and about half of these have evidence of malignancy (Amar et al. 2005). Due to this relatively high risk, biochemical testing should continue at yearly intervals irrespective of the absence of signs and symptoms.

Malignant phaeochromocytoma

There are currently no reliable histopathological methods for distinguishing benign from malignant phaeochromocytoma; only the presence metastases at sites where no chromaffin tissue should be expected establishes a definitive diagnosis of malignant phaeochromocytoma (Eisenhofer et al. 2004). The most frequent sites of metastases are the bones, liver, lungs and lymph nodes.

Although there are no markers for reliably predicting development of malignant phaeochromocytoma, there are several factors associated with increased risk of malignancy. Rates of malignancy tend to be higher for large tumours and those that have an extra-adrenal location (John et al. 1999). Paragangliomas in patients with mutations of the SDHB gene have a particularly high rate of malignancy (Gimenez-Roqueplo et al. 2003). As reviewed earlier, the biochemical profile of plasma or urinary test results can also provide some limited information about likelihood of malignancy.

There continues to be no effective cure for malignant phaeochromocytoma. Once malignancy is confirmed, the 5-year survival rate is about 50% (John et al. 1999). The natural clinical course is, however, highly variable, with occasional patients living more than 20 years after diagnosis (van den Broek and de Graeff 1978).

Most treatments for malignant phaeochromocytoma are palliative, with therapy generally directed at controlling blood pressure and symptomatology. α- and β-adrenoceptor blockers provide the accepted method for controlling symptoms and treating high blood pressure.

Surgery in patients with metastatic phaeochromocytoma is rarely curative, but resection of a primary mass or metastases can reduce exposure of the cardiovascular system to high toxic levels of catecholamines (Mishra et al. 2000). External beam radiation, cryoablation, radiofrequency ablation, transcatheter arterial embolization may offer alternative treatments, but only after appropriate medical blockade (Takahashi et al. 1999, Pacak et al. 2001b).

Chemotherapy with a combination of cyclophosphamide (Cytoxan), vincristine (Oncovin), and dacarbazine (DTIC-Dome) provides partial remission and improvement of symptoms in up to 50% of patients with malignant phaeochromocytoma (Averbuch et al. 1988). Radiopharmaceutical therapy using high doses of ^{131}I-MIBG, which is transported into phaeochromocytoma tumour cells via the cell membrane noradrenaline transporter, provides an alternative palliative therapy that can also be effective in temporarily reducing tumour burden and symptoms (Shapiro et al. 1991, Rose et al. 2003). About 75% of patients treated with ^{131}I-MIBG show improvement in symptoms, 50% have reductions in hormonal activity, and 22% show objective tumour responses. Complete remissions are rare and progressive disease following ^{131}I-MIBG treatment is common.

References

Amar, L., Servais, A., Gimenez-Roqueplo, A. P., Zinzindohoue, F., Chatellier, G. and Plouin, P. F. (2005). Year of diagnosis, features at presentation, and risk of recurrence in patients with pheochromocytoma or secreting paraganglioma. *Journal of Clinical Endocrinology and Metabolism* **90**, 2110–6.

Anderson, G. H., Jr., Blakeman, N. and Streeten, D. H. (1994). The effect of age on prevalence of secondary forms of hypertension in 4429 consecutively referred patients. *Journal of Hypertension* **12**, 609–15.

Ariton, M., Juan, C. S. and AvRuskin, T. W. (2000). Pheochromocytoma: clinical observations from a Brooklyn tertiary hospital. *Endocrine Practice* **6**, 249–52.

Aron, D. C. (2001). The adrenal incidentaloma: disease of modern technology and public health problem. *Reviews of Endocrine and Metabolic Disorders* **2**, 335–42.

Aronoff, S. L., Passamani, E., Borowsky, B. A., Weiss, A. N., Roberts, R. and Cryer, P. E. (1980). Norepinephrine and epinephrine secretion from a clinically epinephrine-secreting pheochromocytoma. *American Journal of Medicine* **69**, 321–4.

Averbuch, S. D., Steakley, C. S., Young, R. C., *et al.* (1988). Malignant pheochromocytoma: effective treatment with a combination of cyclophosphamide, vincristine, and dacarbazine. *Annals of Internal Medicine* **109**, 267–73.

Awada, S. H., Grisham, A. and Woods, S. E. (2003). Large dopamine-secreting pheochromocytoma: case report. *Southern Medical Journal* **96**, 914–7.

Baguet, J. P., Hammer, L., Mazzuco, T. L., *et al.* (2004). Circumstances of discovery of phaeochromocytoma: a retrospective study of 41 consecutive patients. *European Journal of Endocrinology* **150**, 681–6.

Baysal, B. E. (2003). On the association of succinate dehydrogenase mutations with hereditary paraganglioma. *Trends in Endocrinology and Metabolism* **14**, 453–9.

Baysal, B. E., Willett-Brozick, J. E., Lawrence, E. C., *et al.* (2002). Prevalence of SDHB, SDHC, and SDHD germline mutations in clinic patients with head and neck paragangliomas. *Journal of Medical Genetics* **39**, 178–83.

Bergland, B. E. (1989). Pheochromocytoma presenting as shock. *American Journal of Emergency Medicine* **7**, 44–8.

Berglund, A. S., Hulthen, U. L., Manhem, P., Thorsson, O., Wollmer, P. and Tornquist, C. (2001). Metaiodobenzylguanidine (MIBG) scintigraphy and computed tomography (CT) in clinical practice. Primary and secondary evaluation for localization of phaeochromocytomas. *Journal of Internal Medicine* **249**, 247–51.

Bernini, G. P., Vivaldi, M. S., Argenio, G. F., Moretti, A., Sgro, M. and Salvetti, A. (1997). Frequency of pheochromocytoma in adrenal incidentalomas and utility of the glucagon test for the diagnosis. *Journal of Endocrinological Investigation* **20**, 65–71.

Box, J. C., Braithwaite, M. D., Duncan, T. and Lucas, G. (1997). Pheochromocytoma, chronic renal insufficiency, and hemodialysis: a combination leading to a diagnostic and therapeutic dilemma. *American Surgeon* **63**, 314–6.

Bravo, E. L., Tarazi, R. C., Fouad, F. M., Vidt, D. G. and Gifford, R. W., Jr. (1981). Clonidine-suppression test: a useful aid in the diagnosis of pheochromocytoma. *New England Journal Medicine* **305**, 623–6.

Bryant, J., Farmer, J., Kessler, L. J., Townsend, R. R. and Nathanson, K. L. (2003). Pheochromocytoma: the expanding genetic differential diagnosis. *Journal of the National Cancer Institute* **95**, 1196–204.

Casanova, S., Rosenberg-Bourgin M., Farkas D., *et al.* (1993). Phaeochromocytoma in multiple endocrine neoplasia type 2 A: survey of 100 cases. *Clinical Endocrinology* **38**, 531–7.

Clesham, C. J., Kennedy, A., Lavender, J. P., Dollery, C. T. and Wilkins, M. R. (1993). Meta-iodobenzylguanidine (MIBG) scanning in the diagnosis of phaeochromocytoma. *Journal of Human Hypertension* **7**, 353–6.

Crout, J. R. and Sjoerdsma, A. (1964). Turnover and metabolism of catecholamines in patients with pheochromocytoma. *Journal of Clinical Investigation* **43**, 94–102.

Dannenberg, H., van Nederveen, F. H., Abbou, M., Verhofstad, A. A., Komminoth, P., de Krijger, R. R., Dinjens, W. N. (2005). Clinical characteristics of pheochromocytoma patients with germline mutations in SDHD. *Journal of Clinical Oncology* **23**, 1894–901.

Dupont, A. G., Vanderniepen, P. and Gerlo, E. (1985). A case of unilateral adrenal epinephrine excess: adrenal medullary hyperplasia? *Acta Clinica Belgium* **40**, 230–5.

Edstrom Elder, E., Hjelm Skog, A. L., Hoog, A. and Hamberger, B. (2003). The management of benign and malignant pheochromocytoma and abdominal paraganglioma. *European Journal of Surgical Oncology* **29**, 278–83.

Eisenhofer, G., Bornstein, S. R., Brouwers, F. M., *et al.* (2004). Malignant pheochromocytoma: current status and initiatives for future progress. *Endocrine Related Cancer* **11**, 423–36.

Eisenhofer, G., Goldstein, D. S., Kopin, I. J. and Crout, J. R. (2003a). Pheochromocytoma: rediscovery as a catecholamine-metabolizing tumour. *Endocrine Pathology*, **14**, 192–212.

Eisenhofer, G., Goldstein, D. S., Walther, M. M., *et al.* (2003b). Biochemical diagnosis of pheochromocytoma: How to distinguish true-from false-positive test results. *Journal of Clinical Endocrinology and Metabolism* **88**, 2656–66.

Eisenhofer, G., Goldstein, D. S., Sullivan, P., *et al.* (2005a). Biochemical and clinical manifestations of dopamine-producing paragangliomas: utility of plasma methoxytyramine. *Journal of Clinical Endocrinology and Metabolism* **90**, 2068–75.

Eisenhofer, G., Huysmans, F., Pacak, K., Walther, M. M., Sweep, F. C. G. J. and Lenders, J. W. M. (2005b). Plasma metanephrines in renal failure. *Kidney International* **67**, 668–77.

Eisenhofer, G., Lenders, J. W., Goldstein, D. S., *et al.* (2005c). Pheochromocytoma catecholamine phenotypes and prediction of tumour size and location by use of plasma free metanephrines. *Clinical Chemistry* **51**, 735–44.

Eisenhofer, G., Keiser, H., Friberg, P., *et al.* (1998). Plasma metanephrines are markers of pheochromocytoma produced by catechol-O-methyltransferase within tumours. *Journal of Clinical Endocrinology and Metabolism* **83**, 2175–85.

Eisenhofer, G., Rundquist, B., Aneman, A. *et al.* (1995). Regional release and removal of catecholamines and extraneuronal metabolism to metanephrines. *Journal of Clinical Endocrinology and Metabolism* **80**, 3009–17.

Eisenhofer, G., Walther, M. M., Huynh, T. T. *et al.* (2001). Pheochromocytomas in von Hippel-Lindau syndrome and multiple endocrine neoplasia type 2 display distinct biochemical and clinical phenotypes. *Journal of Clinical Endocrinology and Metabolism* **86**, 1999–2008.

Elmasry, A., Lindberg, E., Hedner, J., Janson, C. and Boman, G. (2002). Obstructive sleep apnoea and urine catecholamines in hypertensive males: a population-based study. *European Respiratory Journal* **19**, 511–7.

Erickson, D., Kudva, Y. C., Ebersold, M. J., *et al.* (2001). Benign paragangliomas: clinical presentation and treatment outcomes in 236 patients. *Journal of Clinical Endocrinology and Metabolism* **86**, 5210–6.

Favier, J., Briere, J. J., Strompf, L., *et al.* (2005). Hereditary Paraganglioma/Pheochromocytoma and Inherited Succinate Dehydrogenase Deficiency. *Hormone Research*, **63**, 171–79.

Freeman, R. and Schachter, S. C. (1995). Autonomic epilepsy. *Seminars in Neurology* **15**, 158–66.

Friedman, J. M. (1999). Epidemiology of neurofibromatosis type 1. *American Journal of Medical Genetics* **89**, 1–6.

Friedman, J. M. and Birch, P. H. (1997). Type 1 neurofibromatosis: a descriptive analysis of the disorder in 1,728 patients. *American Journal of Medical Genetics* **70**, 138–43.

Gagel, R. F. (1998). Multiple endocrine neoplasia. In J. D. Wilson, D. W. Foster, H. M. Kronenberg & P. R. Larsen, ed. *Williams Textbook of Endocrinology*, 9th edn, pp. 1627–49. WP Saunders Company, Philadelphia, PA.

Gagel, R. F., Tashjian, A. H., Jr., Cummings, T., *et al.* (1988). The clinical outcome of prospective screening for multiple endocrine neoplasia type 2a. An 18-year experience. *New England Journal Medicine* **318**, 478–84.

Garcia, R. and Jennings, J. M. (1972). Pheochromocytoma masquerading as a cardiomyopathy. *American Journal of Cardiology* **29**, 568–71.

Gimenez-Roqueplo, A. P., Favier, J., Rustin, P., *et al.* (2003). Mutations in the SDHB gene are associated with extra-adrenal and/or malignant phaeochromocytomas. *Cancer Research* **63**, 5615–21.

Goldstein, R. E., O'Neill, J. A., Jr., Holcomb, G. W., 3rd, *et al.* (1999). Clinical experience over 48 years with pheochromocytoma. *Annals of Surgery* **229**, 755–64; discussion 64–6.

Grumbach, M. M., Biller, B. M., Braunstein, G. D., *et al.* (2003). Management of the clinically inapparent adrenal mass ('incidentaloma'). *Annals Internal Medicine* **138**, 424–9.

Hes, F. J., Hoppener, J. W. and Lips, C. J. (2003). Clinical review 155: Pheochromocytoma in Von Hippel-Lindau disease. *Journal of Clinical Endocrinology and Metabolism* **88**, 969–74.

Hoegerle, S., Nitzsche, E., Altehoefer, C., *et al.* (2002). Pheochromocytomas: detection with 18F DOPA whole body PET—initial results. *Radiology* **222**, 507–12.

Hoy, L. J., Emery, M., Wedzicha, J. A., *et al.* (2004). Obstructive sleep apnea presenting as pseudopheochromocytoma: a case report. *Journal of Clinical Endocrinology and Metabolism* **89**, 2033–8.

Ilias, I., Yu, J., Carrasquillo, J. A., *et al.* (2003). Superiority of 6-[18F]-fluorodopamine positron emission tomography versus [131I]-metaiodobenzylguanidine scintigraphy in the localization of metastatic pheochromocytoma. *Journal of Clinical Endocrinology and Metabolism* **88**, 4083–7.

Ito, Y., Fujimoto, Y. and Obara, T. (1992). The role of epinephrine, norepinephrine, and dopamine in blood pressure disturbances in patients with pheochromocytoma. *World Journal of Surgery* **16**, 759–63.

Jessop, D. S., Cunnah, D., Millar, J. G., *et al.* (1987). A phaeochromocytoma presenting with Cushing's syndrome associated with increased concentrations of circulating corticotrophin-releasing factor. *Journal of Endocrinology* **113**, 133–8.

John, H., Ziegler, W. H., Hauri, D. and Jaeger, P. (1999). Pheochromocytomas: can malignant potential be predicted? *Urology* **53**, 679–83.

Kalff, V., Shapiro, B., Lloyd, R., *et al.* (1982). The spectrum of pheochromocytoma in hypertensive patients with neurofibromatosis. *Archives of Internal Medicine* **142**, 2092–8.

Ketch, T., Biaggioni, I., Robertson, R. and Robertson, D. (2002). Four faces of baroreflex failure: hypertensive crisis, volatile hypertension, orthostatic tachycardia, and malignant vagotonia. *Circulation* **105**, 2518–23.

Kimura, N., Miura, Y., Nagatsu, I. and Nagura, H. (1992). Catecholamine synthesizing enzymes in 70 cases of functioning and non-functioning phaeochromocytoma and extra-adrenal paraganglioma. *Virchows Archiv. A, Pathological anatomy and histology* **421**, 25–32.

Kuchel, O. (1998). Increased plasma dopamine in patients presenting with the pseudopheochromocytoma quandary: retrospective analysis of 10 years' experience. *Journal of Hypertension* **16**, 1531–7.

Lehmann, F. S., Weiss, P., Ritz, R., Harder, F. and Staub, J. J. (1999). Reversible cerebral ischemia in patients with pheochromocytoma. *Journal of Endocrinological Investigation* **22**, 212–4.

Lehnert, H., Mundschenk, J. and Hahn, K. (2004). Malignant pheochromocytoma. *Frontiers of Hormone Research* **31**, 155–62.

Leiba, A., Bar-Dayan, Y., Leker, R. R., Apter, S. and Grossman, E. (2003). Seizures as a presenting symptom of phaeochromocytoma in a young soldier. *Journal of Human Hypertension* **17**, 73–5.

Lenders, J. W., Keiser, H. R., Goldstein, D. S., *et al.* (1995). Plasma metanephrines in the diagnosis of pheochromocytoma. *Annals of Internal Medicine* **123**, 101–9.

Lenders, J. W., Pacak, K., Walther, M. M., *et al.* (2002). Biochemical diagnosis of pheochromocytoma: which test is best? *Journal of the American Medical Association* **287**, 1427–34.

Lo, C. Y., Lam, K. Y., Wat, M. S. and Lam, K. S. (2000). Adrenal pheochromocytoma remains a frequently overlooked diagnosis. *American Journal of Surgery* **179**, 212–5.

Lockhart, M. E., Smith, J. K. and Kenney, P. J. (2002). Imaging of adrenal masses. *European Journal of Radiology* **41**, 95–112.

Lonser, R. R., Glenn, G. M., Walther, M., *et al.* (2003). von Hippel-Lindau disease. *Lancet* **361**, 2059–67.

Manger, W. M. (1993). Baroreflex failure—a diagnostic challenge. *New England Journal Medicine* **329**, 1494–5.

Manger, W. M. and Gifford, R. W. (1996). *Clinical and Experimental Pheochromocytoma*. Blackwell Science, Cambridge, MA.

Mannelli, M., Ianni, L., Cilotti, A. and Conti, A. (1999). Pheochromocytoma in Italy: a multicentric retrospective study. *European Journal of Endocrinology* **141**, 619–24.

Mannelli, M. and Bemporad, D. (2002). Diagnosis and management of pheochromocytoma during pregnancy. *Journal of Endocrinological Investigation* **25**, 567–71.

Mansmann, G., Lau, J., Balk, E., Rothberg, M., Miyachi, Y. and Bornstein, S. R. (2004). The clinically inapparent adrenal mass: update in diagnosis and management. *Endocrine Reviews* **25**, 309–40.

Mantero, F., Terzolo, M., Arnaldi, G., *et al.* (2000). A survey on adrenal incidentaloma in Italy. Study Group on Adrenal Tumours of the Italian Society of Endocrinology. *Journal of Clinical Endocrinology and Metabolism* **85**, 637–44.

Martell, N., Rodriguez-Cerrillo, M., Grobbee, D. E., *et al.* (2003). High prevalence of secondary hypertension and insulin resistance in patients with refractory hypertension. *Blood Press* **12**, 149–54.

McNeil, A. R., Blok, B. H., Koelmeyer, T. D., Burke, M. P. and Hilton, J. M. (2000). Phaeochromocytomas discovered during coronial autopsies in Sydney, Melbourne and Auckland. *Australian and New Zealand Journal of Medicine* **30**, 648–52.

Metz, S. A., Halter, J. B., Porte, D., Jr. and Robertson, R. P. (1978). Autonomic epilepsy: clonidine blockade of paroxysmal catecholamine release and flushing. *Annals of Internal Medicine* **88**, 189–93.

Middeke, M. and Schrader, J. (1994). Nocturnal blood pressure in normotensive subjects and those with white coat, primary, and secondary hypertension. *British Medical Journal* **308**, 630–2.

Mishra, A. K., Agarwal, G., Kapoor, A., Agarwal, A., Bhatia, E. and Mishra, S. K. (2000). Catecholamine cardiomyopathy in bilateral malignant pheochromocytoma: successful reversal after surgery. *Internal Journal of Cardiology* **76**, 89–90.

Miskulin, J., Shulkin, B. L., Doherty, G. M., Sisson, J. C., Burney, R. E. and Gauger, P. G. (2003). Is preoperative iodine 123 meta-iodobenzylguanidine scintigraphy routinely necessary before initial adrenalectomy for pheochromocytoma? *Surgery* **134**, 918–22; discussion 22–3.

Munakata, M., Aihara, A., Imai, Y., Noshiro, T., Ito, S. and Yoshinaga, K. (1999). Altered sympathetic and vagal modulations of the cardiovascular system in patients with pheochromocytoma: their relations to orthostatic hypotension. *American Journal of Hypertension* **12**, 572–80.

Neumann, H. P., Bausch, B., McWhinney, S. R., *et al.* (2002). Germ-line mutations in nonsyndromic pheochromocytoma. *New England Journal Medicine* **346**, 1459–66.

Neumann, H. P., Berger, D. P., Sigmund, G., *et al.* (1993). Pheochromocytomas, multiple endocrine neoplasia type 2, and von Hippel-Lindau disease. *New England Journal Medicine* **329**, 1531–8.

Neumann, H. P., Pawlu, C., Peczkowska, M., *et al.* (2004). Distinct clinical features of paraganglioma syndromes associated with SDHB and SDHD gene mutations. *Journal of the American Medical Association* **292**, 943–51.

Newell, K. A., Prinz, R. A., Pickleman, J., *et al.* (1988). Pheochromocytoma multisystem crisis. A surgical emergency. *Archives of Surgery* **123**, 956–9.

Nguyen, L., Niccoli-Sire, P., Caron, P., *et al.* (2001). Pheochromocytoma in multiple endocrine neoplasia type 2: a prospective study. *European Journal of Endocrinology* **144**, 37–44.

Noblet-Dick, M., Grunenberger, F., Brunot, B., Jaeck, D. and Schlienger, J. L. (2003). Pheochromocytoma in internal medicine: distinctive features and place of 123I MIBG scintigraphy. *La Revue de Medecine Interne* **24**, 358–65.

Noshiro, T., Shimizu, K., Watanabe, T., *et al.* (2000). Changes in clinical features and long-term prognosis in patients with pheochromocytoma. *American Journal of Hypertension* **13**, 35–43.

O'Brien, T., Young, W. F., Jr., Davila, D. G., *et al.* (1992). Cushing's syndrome associated with ectopic production of corticotrophin-releasing hormone, corticotrophin and vasopressin by a phaeochromocytoma. *Clinical Endocrinology* **37**, 460–7.

Omura, M., Saito, J., Yamaguchi, K., Kakuta, Y. and Nishikawa, T. (2004). Prospective study on the prevalence of secondary hypertension among hypertensive patients visiting a general outpatient clinic in Japan. *Hypertension Research* **27**, 193–202.

Pacak, K., Eisenhofer, G., Carrasquillo, J. A., Chen, C. C., Li, S. T. and Goldstein, D. S. (2001a). 6-[18F]fluorodopamine positron emission tomographic (PET) scanning for diagnostic localization of pheochromocytoma. *Hypertension* **38**, 6–8.

Pacak, K., Fojo, T., Goldstein, D. S., *et al.* (2001b). Radiofrequency ablation: a novel approach for treatment of metastatic pheochromocytoma. *Journal of the National Cancer Institute* **93**, 648–9.

Pacak, K., Eisenhofer, G. and Goldstein, D. S. (2004). Functional imaging of endocrine tumours: role of positron emission tomography. *Endocrine Reviews* **25**, 568–80.

Perry, R. R., Keiser, H. R., Norton, J. A., *et al.* (1990). Surgical management of pheochromocytoma with the use of metyrosine. *Annals of Surgery* **212**, 621–8.

Phillips, A. M., Jardine, D. L., Parkin, P. J., Hughes, T. and Ikram, H. (2000). Brain stem stroke causing baroreflex failure and paroxysmal hypertension. *Stroke* **31**, 1997–2001.

Plouin, P. F., Chatellier, G., Fofol, I. and Corvol, P. (1997). Tumour recurrence and hypertension persistence after successful pheochromocytoma operation. *Hypertension* **29**, 1133–9.

Plouin, P. F., Degoulet, P., Tugaye, A., Ducrocq, M. B. and Menard, J. (1981). Screening for phaeochromocytoma: in which hypertensive patients? A semiological study of 2585 patients, including 11 with phaeochromocytoma. *La Nouvelle Presse Medicale* **10**, 869–72.

Proye, C., Fossati, P., Fontaine, P., *et al.* (1986). Dopamine-secreting pheochromocytoma: an unrecognized entity? Classification of pheochromocytomas according to their type of secretion. *Surgery* **100**, 1154–62.

Proye, C., Thevenin, D., Cecat, P., *et al.* (1989). Exclusive use of calcium channel blockers in preoperative and intraoperative control of pheochromocytomas: hemodynamics and free catecholamine assays in ten consecutive patients. *Surgery* **106**, 1149–54.

Prys-Roberts, C. (2000). Phaeochromocytoma—recent progress in its management. *British Journal of Anaesthesiology* **85**, 44–57.

Prys-Roberts, C. and Farndon, J. R. (2002). Efficacy and safety of doxazosin for perioperative management of patients with pheochromocytoma. *World Journal of Surgery* **26**, 1037–42.

Quigg, R. J. and Om, A. (1994). Reversal of severe cardiac systolic dysfunction caused by pheochromocytoma in a heart transplant candidate. *Journal of Heart and Lung Transplantation* **13**, 525–32.

Raber, W., Raffesberg, W., Bischof, M., *et al.* (2000). Diagnostic efficacy of unconjugated plasma metanephrines for the detection of pheochromocytoma. *Archives of Internal Medicine* **160**, 2957–63.

Riccardi, V. M. (1991). Neurofibromatosis: past, present, and future. *New England Journal Medicine* **324**, 1283–5.

Robertson, D., Hollister, A. S., Biaggioni, I., Netterville, J. L., Mosqueda-Garcia, R. and Robertson, R. M. (1993). The diagnosis and treatment of baroreflex failure. *New England Journal Medicine* **329**, 1449–55.

Rose, B., Matthay, K. K., Price, D., *et al.* (2003). High-dose 131I-metaiodobenzylguanidine therapy for 12 patients with malignant pheochromocytoma. *Cancer* **98**, 239–48.

Rudy, F. R., Bates, R. D., Cimorelli, A. J., Hill, G. S. and Engelman, K. (1980). Adrenal medullary hyperplasia: a clinicopathologic study of four cases. *Human Pathology* **11**, 650–7.

Sawka, A. M., Gafni, A., Thabane, L. and Young, W. F., Jr. (2004). The economic implications of three biochemical screening algorithms for pheochromocytoma. *Journal of Clinical Endocrinology and Metabolism* **89**, 2859–66.

Sawka, A. M., Jaeschke, R., Singh, R. J. and Young, W. F., Jr. (2003). A comparison of biochemical tests for pheochromocytoma: Measurement of fractionated plasma metanephrines compared with the combination of 24-hour urinary metanephrines and catecholamines. *Journal of Clinical Endocrinology and Metabolism* **88**, 553–8.

Shapiro, B., Sisson, J. C., Wieland, D. M., *et al.* (1991). Radiopharmaceutical therapy of malignant pheochromocytoma with [131I]metaiodobenzylguanidine: results from ten years of experience. *Journal of Nuclear and Biological Medicine* **35**, 269–76.

Shapiro, B. and Gross, M. D. (1987). Radiochemistry, biochemistry, and kinetics of 131I-metaiodobenzylguanidine (MIBG) and 123I-MIBG: clinical implications of the use of 123I-MIBG. *Medical and Pediatric Oncology* **15**, 170–7.

Sheaves, R., Chew, S. L. and Grossman, A. B. (1995). The dangers of unopposed beta-adrenergic blockade in phaeochromocytoma. *Postgraduate Medical Journal* **71**, 58–9.

Shibao, C., Arzubiaga, C., Roberts, L. J., 2nd, *et al.* (2005). Hyperadrenergic postural tachycardia syndrome in mast cell activation disorders. *Hypertension* **45**, 385–90.

Sisson, J. C., Frager, M. S., Valk, T. W., *et al.* (1981). Scintigraphic localization of pheochromocytoma. *New England Journal of Medicine* **305**, 12–7.

Smith, S. L., Slappy, A. L., Fox, T. P. and Scolapio, J. S. (2002). Pheochromocytoma producing vasoactive intestinal peptide. *Mayo Clinic Proceedings* **77**, 97–100.

Smithwick, R. H., Greer, W. E., *et al.* (1950). Pheochromocytoma; a discussion of symptoms, signs and procedures of diagnostic value. *New England Journal of Medicine* **242**, 252–7.

Solanki, K. K., Bomanji, J., Moyes, J., Mather, S. J., Trainer, P. J. and Britton, K. E. (1992). A pharmacological guide to medicines which interfere with the biodistribution of radiolabelled meta-iodobenzylguanidine (MIBG). *Nuclear Medicine Communications* **13**, 513–21.

Steinsapir, J., Carr, A. A., Prisant, L. M. and Bransome, E. D., Jr. (1997). Metyrosine and pheochromocytoma. *Archives of Internal Medicine* **157**, 901–6.

Stenstrom, G. and Waldenstrom, J. (1985). Positive correlation between urinary excretion of catecholamine metabolites and tumour mass in pheochromocytoma. Results in patients with sustained and paroxysmal hypertension and multiple endocrine neoplasia. *Acta Medica Scandinavica* **217**, 73–7.

Streeten, D. H., Anderson, G. H., Jr., Lebowitz, M. and Speller, P. J. (1990). Primary hyperepinephrinemia in patients without pheochromocytoma. *Archives of Internal Medicine* **150**, 1528–33.

Streeten, D. H. and Anderson, G. H., Jr. (1996). Mechanisms of orthostatic hypotension and tachycardia in patients with pheochromocytoma. *American Journal of Hypertension* **9**, 760–9.

Stumvoll, M., Radjaipour, M. and Seif, F. (1995). Diagnostic considerations in pheochromocytoma and chronic hemodialysis: case report and review of the literature. *American Journal of Nephrology* **15**, 147–51.

Sutton, M. G., Sheps, S. G. and Lie, J. T. (1981). Prevalence of clinically unsuspected pheochromocytoma. Review of a 50-year autopsy series. *Mayo Clinic Proceedings* **56**, 354–60.

Taieb, D., Sebag, F., Hubbard, J. G., Mundler, O., Henry, J. F. and Conte-Devolx, B. (2004). Does iodine-131 meta-iodobenzylguanidine (MIBG) scintigraphy have an impact on the management of sporadic and familial phaeochromocytoma? *Clinical Endocrinology* **61**, 102–8.

Takahashi, K., Ashizawa, N., Minami, T., *et al.* (1999). Malignant pheochromocytoma with multiple hepatic metastases treated by chemotherapy and transcatheter arterial embolization. *Internal Medicine* **38**, 349–54.

Thomas, J. E., Rooke, E. D. and Kvale, W. F. (1966). The neurologist's experience with pheochromocytoma. A review of 100 cases. *Journal of the American Medical Association* **197**, 754–8.

Thompson, G. B., Grant, C. S., van Heerden, J. A., *et al.* (1997). Laparoscopic versus open posterior adrenalectomy: a case-control study of 100 patients. *Surgery* **122**, 1132–6.

Timmers, H. J., Wieling, W., Karemaker, J. M. and Lenders, J. W. (2004). Baroreflex failure: a neglected type of secondary hypertension. *Netherlands Journal Medicine* **62**, 151–5.

Vargas, H. I., Kavoussi, L. R., Bartlett, D. L., *et al.* (1997). Laparoscopic adrenalectomy: a new standard of care. *Urology* **49**, 673–8.

Viale, G., Dell'Orto, P., Moro, E., Cozzaglio, L. and Coggi, G. (1985). Vasoactive intestinal polypeptide-, somatostatin-, and calcitonin-producing adrenal pheochromocytoma associated with the watery diarrhea (WDHH) syndrome. First case report with immunohistochemical findings. *Cancer* **55**, 1099–106.

Walther, M. M., Herring, J., Choyke, P. L. and Linehan, W. M. (2000). Laparoscopic partial adrenalectomy in patients with hereditary forms of pheochromocytoma. *Journal of Urology* **164**, 14–7.

Walther, M. M., Herring, J., Enquist, E., Keiser, H. R. and Linehan, W. M. (1999a). von Recklinghausen's disease and pheochromocytomas. *Journal of Urology* **162**, 1582–6.

Walther, M. M., Reiter, R., Keiser, H. R., *et al.* (1999b). Clinical and genetic characterization of pheochromocytoma in von Hippel-Lindau families: comparison with sporadic pheochromocytoma gives insight into natural history of pheochromocytoma. *Journal of Urology* **162**, 659–64.

Weise, M., Merke, D. P., Pacak, K., Walther, M. M. and Eisenhofer, G. (2002). Utility of plasma free metanephrines for detecting childhood pheochromocytoma. *Journal of Clinical Endocrinology and Metabolism* **87**, 1955–60.

Wilkenfeld, C., Cohen, M., Lansman, S. L., *et al.* (1992). Heart transplantation for end-stage cardiomyopathy caused by an occult pheochromocytoma. *Journal of Heart and Lung Transplantation* **11**, 363–6.

Wilkinson, D. J., Thompson, J. M., Lambert, G. W., *et al.* (1998). Sympathetic activity in patients with panic disorder at rest, under laboratory mental stress, and during panic attacks. *Archives of General Psychiatry* **55**, 511–20.

Young, W. F., Jr. (2000). Management approaches to adrenal incidentalomas. A view from Rochester, Minnesota. *Endocrinology and Metabolism Clinics of North America* **29**, 159–85, x.

Young, W. F., Jr. and Maddox, D. E. (1995). Spells: in search of a cause. *Mayo Clinic Proceedings* **70**, 757–65.

Zelinka, T., Strauch, B., Pecen, L. and Widimsky, J., Jr. (2004). Diurnal blood pressure variation in pheochromocytoma, primary aldosteronism and Cushing's syndrome. *Journal of Human Hypertension* **18**, 107–11.

van den Broek, P. J. and de Graeff, J. (1978). Prolonged survival in a patient with pulmonary metastases of a malignant pheochromocytoma. *Netherlands Journal Medicine* **21**, 245–7.

van der Harst, E., de Herder, W. W., Bruining, H. A., *et al.* (2001). [(123)I]metaiodobenzylguanidine and [(111)In]octreotide uptake in benign and malignant pheochromocytomas. *Journal of Clinical Endocrinology and Metabolism* **86**, 685–93.

CHAPTER 65

Sympathetic neural mechanisms in hypertension

Krzysztof Narkiewicz and Virend K. Somers

Key points

- The sympathetic nervous system plays a key role in acute changes in blood pressure.

- Sympathetic activation may contribute to chronic blood pressure elevation by effects on the kidney, on blood vessel structure, and by resetting the baroreflex.

- Obstructive sleep apnoea is an important identifiable cause of hypertension.

- Increases in sympathetic activation with age, and its effects on blood pressure, may be especially marked in women.

- Adrenaline may contribute importantly to maintenance of hypertension, through enhanced noradrenaline release.

- Insulin and leptin are important potential mediators of higher blood pressures in patients with the metabolic syndrome.

- Hypertension is a multifactorial disorder, and no single mechanism has been identified as the dominant aetiology factor.

The sympathetic nervous system is an integral mechanism in the overall regulation of blood pressure. While sympathetic contributions to acute blood pressure increases are well established, the role of sympathetic activation in chronic hypertension is less clear-cut. This is due to several factors, including the heterogeneity of characteristics of essential hypertension, the evolution of the haemodynamics of hypertension from the 'early' to the 'established' phase, and the multiple other aetiological mechanisms that have been implicated in the genesis of hypertension. This review examines first, the potential importance of the sympathetic nervous system in hypertension; second, the evidence that hypertension is accompanied by sympathetic activation; third, the mechanisms by which sympathetic activity may be increased in hypertension; and fourth, the importance of humoral and metabolic mechanisms in sympathetic activation. The review focuses primarily on human hypertension. Emphasis is placed on more recent findings, particularly those involving microneurography, noradrenaline 'spillover', and studies examining central neural mechanisms in hypertension. Because of the breadth of the subject matter and space limitations, only a few references to the various topics are cited.

Potential importance of the sympathetic nervous system

The sympathetic nervous system can acutely increase peripheral vascular resistance and cardiac output to raise blood pressure. Arteriolar vasoconstriction, as well as sympathetic mediated veno-constriction (with consequent central redistribution of blood and increased cardiac output), both act to enable acute blood pressure increases. Cardiac sympathetic chronotropic and inotropic effects also increase blood pressure, particularly in the setting of increased vascular resistance. Thus, sympathetic traffic to the peripheral vasculature and sympathetic discharge to the heart have complementary effects on blood pressure. In normotensive subjects, muscle sympathetic nerve activity (MSNA) and heart rate have an interactive effect on systolic blood pressure and pulse pressure (Narkiewicz 1999c). No relationship between MSNA and blood pressure is evident in subjects with slower heart rates (Fig. 65.1). However, in subjects with faster heart rates, higher levels of MSNA are associated with higher systolic and pulse pressures.

The sympathetic nervous system may also contribute to blood pressure levels in the long term by other mechanisms, by its effects on the kidney, on blood vessel growth, and via resetting of the arterial baroreflex.

First, increased renal efferent sympathetic traffic promotes sodium retention and renin release, in the absence of any effects on renal blood flow or glomerular filtration (DiBona 2004). Furthermore, while increases in arterial pressure promote natriuresis, even low levels of renal sympathetic activity attenuate the natriuretic response to an increase in arterial or renal perfusion pressure. This sympathetic mediated shift in the pressure–natriuresis curve could favour the maintenance of hypertension by interfering with the ability of renal homeostatic mechanisms to compensate for an increase in blood pressure through pressure natriuresis. The renal effects of increased sympathetic activity also include decreased renal blood flow and glomerular filtration rate with renal vasoconstriction, and increased renin release leading to angiotensin II production (DiBona 2004). The role of the sympathetic nervous system in the pathogenesis of hypertension has been recently supported by studies documenting a significant blood pressure-lowering effect of renal sympathetic denervation in patients with resistant hypertension (Esler 2010).

Second, the sympathetic nervous system, like the renin-angiotensin system, promotes growth of vascular muscle.

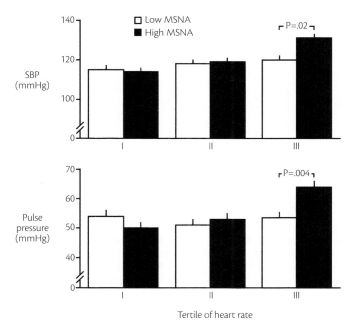

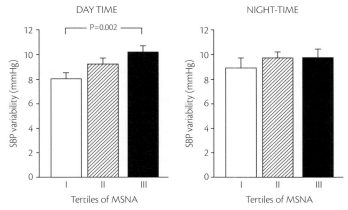

Fig. 65.1 Systolic blood pressure (SBP) and pulse pressure in male subjects grouped according to the tertiles of heart rate (HR) and to the level of muscular sympathetic nerve activity (MSNA). Within each tertile of HR, subjects were subdivided into those with MSNA lower than average (open bars) and those with MSNA higher than average (solid bars) for the given tertile. HR and MSNA had interactive effect on both SBP (p = 0.007) and pulse pressure (p = 0.001). With permission from Narkiewicz, K., Somers,V.K. (1999c). Interactive effect of heart rate and muscle sympathetic nerve activity on blood pressure. *Circulation*, **100**(25): 2514–2518.

Fig. 65.2 Systolic blood pressure (SBP) variability during daytime (left) and night-time (right) in 69 normal subjects grouped according to tertiles of muscle sympathetic nerve activity (tertile I: <18 bursts/minute; tertile II: 18–25 bursts/minute; tertile III: >25 bursts/minute). SBP variability was significantly different across the MSNA tertiles during daytime (p = 0.002 by analysis of variance), but not during night-time (p = 0.60). With permission from Narkiewicz K. et al. (2002), Relationship between muscle sympathetic nerve activity and diurnal blood pressure profile. *Hypertension*, **39**(1):168–72.

The effects of sympathetic activity on vascular growth are independent of haemodynamic effects. These trophic effects on blood vessels appear to be greatest during growth and development. This may be important because sympathetic overactivity appears to occur particularly during the early stages of hypertension, when it is most likely to influence the structure of vessels and, thus, the long-term regulation of arterial pressure. Structural changes in blood vessels increase vascular resistance and the response to vasoconstrictor stimuli so that the effects of the sympathetic nervous system on vasomotor tone and vascular structures interact to increase vascular resistance and arterial pressure.

Third, sustained sympathetic induced increases in blood pressure may contribute to baroreflex resetting. Increases in arterial pressure activate baroreceptors located in the carotid sinuses and aortic arch, triggering reflex inhibition of sympathetic activity, causing vasodilation and bradycardia, which oppose the rise in pressure. An important mechanism that allows sympathetic and arterial pressure to increase is baroreflex resetting (Chapleau and Abboud 1993). Baroreflex resetting refers to a shift in the relationship between blood pressure changes and the efferent autonomic response (e.g. sympathetic nerve activity or heart rate). Sustained increases in pressure cause a resetting of the operating point of the reflex to a higher level of pressure (i.e. the baroreflex loses much of its ability to buffer the rise in pressure and actually functions to maintain pressure at the higher level). Hypertension-induced resetting of the baroreflex may be caused by both 'baroreceptor resetting' (shift in pressure-afferent baroreflex activity relationship) and by 'central resetting' (shift in afferent baroreflex-efferent autonomic relationship) (Chapleau and Abboud 1993).

Thus sympathetic mediated pressor responses, for example in situations of environmental stress, may, by resetting of the arterial baroreflexes, allow the development of higher long-term blood pressure levels.

Sympathetic neural mechanisms may contribute importantly to daytime blood pressure variability and the diurnal blood pressure profile (Narkiewicz 2002). Higher sympathetic traffic is associated with increased daytime blood pressure variability (Fig. 65.2) and greater day-night blood pressure differences.

Evidence for sympathetic hyperactivity in hypertension

Essential hypertension

Tachycardia

Early hypertension is characterized by tachycardia and increased cardiac output (Julius 1968). Using adrenergic blocking agents to probe the role of the sympathetic nervous system, Julius and Esler (Julius 1975) found that autonomic blockade normalized the elevated heart rates and stroke volumes of young mildly hypertensive patients.

Faster heart rate predicts the development of sustained hypertension in subjects with borderline elevated blood pressure values (Palatini and Julius 2003). Furthermore, tachycardia is associated with increased risk of cardiovascular morbidity and mortality (Palatini and Julius 2004).

Catecholamine measurements

Numerous studies have evaluated sympathetic activity in human hypertension using measurements of plasma catecholamines. Goldstein (1983) has reviewed many of the studies of plasma catecholamine levels in normal subjects and patients with essential hypertension and concluded that most studies demonstrated elevated plasma noradrenaline levels in young hypertensive patients.

In a combined study of plasma catecholamines and responses to adrenergic antagonists and agonists, mildly hypertensive individuals had elevated plasma noradrenaline levels, augmented decreases in vascular resistance in response to α-adrenergic blockade, and no increase in α-receptor sensitivity as assessed by responses to noradrenaline (Egan 1987). This study demonstrated augmented sympathetic vasoconstrictor activity in young mildly hypertensive humans, suggesting that increased sympathetic vasoconstriction results from enhanced sympathetic neural release of noradrenaline, and not from augmented α-adrenergic responses to the neurotransmitter.

The sympathetic nervous system has the capacity for selective increases in efferent discharge to different subdivisions. Wallin et al. (1996) have demonstrated, however, that in healthy human subjects, resting sympathetic nerve traffic is similar or proportional in sympathetic nerves to both muscle blood vessels and the kidney.

There is evidence of uniformity of sympathetic activation to the heart and kidney in early hypertension. Using measurements of norepinephrine spillover, Esler et al. (1989) found that norepinephrine was elevated in hypertensive patients, particularly in young hypertensives, and that the increased spillover emanated mainly from the heart and kidneys. There is also functional evidence for heightened sympathetic neural influences on the kidney in essential hypertension (Oparil 1986, DiBona 2003). These observations may help explain the haemodynamic profile of the 'hyperdynamic circulation' of early human hypertension, which is characterized by increased heart rate, cardiac output, and renal vasoconstriction. Recent evidence suggests that neuronal reuptake of noradrenaline in the heart of hypertensives is impaired (Rumantir 2000b). This abnormality might amplify the sympathetic neural signal by impairing removal of noradrenaline from the synaptic cleft, and contribute to maintenance of increased blood pressure and to progression of hypertension (Esler 2003).

Microneurographic recordings

Microneurographic recordings of resting sympathetic nerve activity to muscle blood vessels in humans have provided conflicting evidence for increased sympathetic neural activity in human essential hypertension. In early studies, Wallin and Sundlof (1979) reported no increase in muscle sympathetic nerve activity in hypertensive versus normotensive individuals after accounting for age (sympathetic nerve activity increases with age). Several other authors (Somers et al. 1988, Rea and Hamdan 1990) also did not detect elevated resting muscle sympathetic nerve activity in hypertensive humans. In contrast, other studies have found an increased level of resting muscle sympathetic nerve activity in humans with essential hypertension (Fig. 65.3) (Anderson et al. 1989, Miyajima et al. 1991, Grassi et al. 1998). For example, Anderson et al. (1989) found an increased level of muscle sympathetic nerve activity in young mildly hypertensive men. A high-salt diet reduced muscle sympathetic nerve activity in both groups, but on both low-salt and high-salt diets, sympathetic nerve activity was higher in the mildly hypertensive group than in the normotensive group.

In a study of patients with accelerated hypertension, Matsukawa et al. (1993) have shown an increase in muscle sympathetic nerve activity, compared to patients with benign hypertension. This increase appeared to be closely related to activation of the renin-angiotensin system. In these patients, who had diastolic blood pressures of >130 mmHg, accompanied by retinal changes, treatment with angiotensin converting enzyme inhibitors lowered blood pressure and decreased muscle sympathetic activity. Thus, interactions between the renin-angiotensin system and the

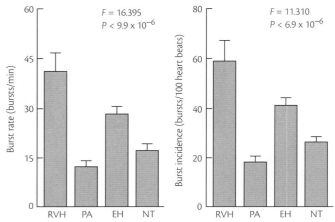

Fig. 65.3 Muscle sympathetic nerve activity in normotensive subjects (NT) and in patients with renovascular hypertension (RVH), primary aldosteronism (PA), and essential hypertension (EH). Sympathetic burst frequency was higher in both renovascular hypertension and essential hypertension than in normal individuals. Sympathetic activity was, however, decreased in patients with primary aldosteronism. With permission from Miyajima, E. et al. (1991). Muscle sympathetic nerve activity in renovascular hypertension and primary aldosteronism. *Hypertension,* **17**(6):1057–62.

sympathetic nervous system may be implicated in the rapid progression of hypertension severity.

The explanation for the finding of high levels of resting muscle sympathetic nerve activity in hypertensives in some, but not all, studies is not clear, but several factors may be pertinent. The first is sodium intake, which has a profound influence on sympathetic nerve activity. Grassi and colleagues (1997) suggested that sodium restriction not only increases resting sympathetic activity, but may also impair baroreflex sensitivity in hypertension. Second, obesity may contribute to increased sympathetic neural activity by promoting insulin resistance and hyperinsulinaemia. The third factor is a buffering influence of cardiopulmonary baroreceptors. Rea and Hamdan (1990) suggested that elevated levels of sympathetic neural drive in human mild hypertensives might be partially masked in the supine position because of a heightened sympathetic-inhibitory influence originating in cardiopulmonary baroreceptors.

In summary, neurochemical, neurophysiological, and haemodynamic studies indicate heightened sympathetic neural activity in human essential hypertension. This is particularly notable in young mildly hypertensive individuals and may contribute to the haemodynamic profile of early human hypertension. The heightened sympathetic drive also appears to involve the kidney, and could thereby contribute to long-term elevation of arterial pressure and to accelerated hypertension.

Secondary hypertension

The most obvious sympathetic mediated form of secondary hypertension is that due to phaeochromocytoma, where the hypertension is principally due to intermittent release of catecholamines. Sympathetic neural mechanisms may, however, also contribute to chronic mild elevations of blood pressure in patients with phaeochromocytoma due to sustained adrenaline-mediated facilitation of noradrenaline release from peripheral adrenergic nerve terminals.

Heightened sympathetic activation may also be a factor in secondary hypertension. Increases in plasma renin activity and angiotensin II are accompanied by a striking increase in muscle sympathetic nerve activity in patients with renal vascular hypertension (Miyajima 1991). Renal-sympathetic interactions may also contribute to hypertension associated with renal failure. In patients receiving haemodialysis, in whom the native kidneys were still present, sympathetic nerve traffic was double the levels recorded in haemodialysis patients who had undergone bilateral nephrectomy (Converse 1992). Thus, it is conceivable that afferent signals from the native kidneys may act centrally to increase sympathetic outflow.

An iatrogenic form of secondary hypertension associated with cyclosporine therapy may also involve increased levels of sympathetic nerve activity (SNA). Patients receiving cyclosporine as immunosuppressive therapy have a high incidence of hypertension. Scherrer et al. (1990) have shown an impressive association between direct measurements of sympathetic nerve traffic and hypertension in these patients. The hypertensive effects of increased SNA would be potentiated by cyclosporine-mediated augmentation of noradrenaline-induced vasoconstriction. Kaye and colleagues (1993), however, in studies utilizing combined measurements of renal blood flow, renal and whole body norepinephrine spillover, and microneurography, have reported that while cyclosporine therapy in humans causes acute renal vasoconstriction, these effects were not due to increased sympathetic activation. In their subjects, cyclosporine A did not cause an increase in either muscle sympathetic activity or in total body or renal norepinephrine spillover rates. Hausberg et al. (2005) have also not found any evidence for cyclosporine-induced sympathetic activation in transplant recipients. Reasons for the controversy regarding cyclosporine effects on sympathetic activity are not clear.

Schobel et al. (1996) have provided important new information regarding the role of the sympathetic nervous system in pre-eclampsia. Patients with pre-eclampsia had higher blood pressures and vascular resistance than normal pregnant women and had sympathetic nerve traffic three times greater than that seen in control subjects (Fig. 65.4). Sympathetic activity was also twice that seen in non-pregnant women with hypertension. After delivery, both blood pressure and sympathetic activity decreased towards normal levels in the patients with pre-eclampsia. Obstructive sleep apnoea (OSA) is emerging as an important secondary cause of hypertension. Patients with sleep apnoea have very high resting daytime sympathetic activity, even in normoxic awake conditions and independent of obesity (Somers et al, 1995). They also have faster heart rates, diminished heart rate variability and increased blood pressure variability (Narkiewicz et al. 1998), all of which would be expected to increase the risk of future hypertension. Data from the Wisconsin cohort study (Peppard et al. 2000) have suggested that in normotensive subjects with moderate to severe sleep apnoea, there is a three-fold increase in risk of incident hypertension at 4 years of follow-up. Recent data employing randomized placebo control designs suggest that treatment of OSA with continuous positive airway pressure (CPAP) may significantly reduce daytime blood pressure (Pepperell et al. 2000; Becker et al. 2000). In light of these and other data, the most recent recommendations of the Joint National Committee on Prevention, Detection, Evaluation, and Treatment of High Blood Pressure (JNC) (Chobanian et al. 2003) have listed sleep apnoea as first of the identifiable causes of hypertension. The acute chemoreflex-mediated effects of sleep apnoea are discussed later.

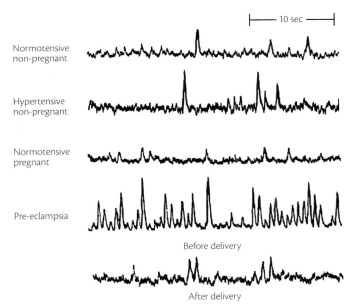

Fig. 65.4 Recordings of sympathetic nerve activity in a normotensive non-pregnant woman, a hypertensive non-pregnant woman, a normotensive pregnant woman, and a woman with pre-eclampsia (before and after delivery). Sympathetic nerve activity was similar in the two non-pregnant women and the normotensive pregnant woman, but was much higher in the patient with pre-eclampsia. After delivery blood pressure and sympathetic activity returned towards baseline in this patient. With permission from Schobel, H. P., et al. (1996). *New England Journal of Medicine*, Copyright MMS.

Sympathetic overactivity and target organ damage

There is growing evidence that sympathetic overactivity may be implicated in the development of structural cardiovascular changes. For example, Greenwood et al. (2001) have demonstrated that the presence of left ventricular hypertrophy (LVH) is associated with higher sympathetic discharge in subjects with moderate to severe hypertension. However, whether LVH per se, in part due to altered cardiac afferent activity, may contribute to increased sympathetic drive, is not known.

Mechanisms of increased sympathetic activity—implications for hypertension

Arterial baroreflex

Probably the most extensively studied of the possible aetiologies of sympathetic overactivity in hypertension are depressor and pressor autonomic reflexes (Mancia 1997). The traditional concepts hold, first, that arterial baroreflexes are abnormal in hypertension with a higher threshold for activation and a reduction in sensitivity and, second, that these alterations result from chronic increases in arterial pressure. In recent years, two new concepts have emerged regarding alterations in arterial baroreflexes in hypertension. First, it has been found that alterations in arterial baroreflexes in hypertension could be related to genetic abnormalities that precede and are independent of the increase in arterial pressure. Second, it is now known that abnormalities in baroreflex control of parasympathetic activity (heart rate) do not necessarily predict alterations in baroreflex control of sympathetic nerve activity and vascular resistance (Rea and Hamdan 1990). Indeed, there is evidence from both experimental animals and humans that baroreflex control of sympathetic activity, vascular resistance and arterial pressure may be preserved in early or mild hypertension despite impairment of baroreflex control of heart rate. This dissociation appears to result from a greater central nervous system 'reserve' for maintaining baroreflex control of sympathetic versus parasympathetic activity. Insofar as hypertension is concerned, the baroreflex-mediated sympathetic and vascular resistance responses to blood pressure changes are obviously of greater haemodynamic significance than the heart rate responses.

Cardiopulmonary baroreflex

Patients with borderline hypertension, with a family history of hypertension, show an augmented increase in sympathetic activity and vascular resistance in response to lower body negative pressure (simulating orthostatic stress) (Rea and Hamdan 1990). These findings may help explain the exaggerated diastolic blood pressure increase with upright tilt in borderline hypertension. Importantly, this sympathetic hyperreactivity to non-hypotensive lower body negative pressure occurred despite no detectable abnormality in arterial baroreflex regulation of sympathetic nerve responses to rising and lower blood pressure. In addition, the augmented sympathetic nerve response to orthostatic stress occurred in the absence of an increased baseline sympathetic activity in the borderline hypertensives in the supine position. Two conclusions emerge

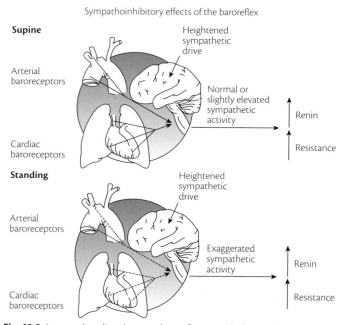

Fig. 65.5 Increased cardiopulmonary baroreflex control of sympathetic activity and its interaction with heightened central sympathetic drive may explain the reflex adjustment to changes in posture in mild hypertensive individuals. The heightened central neural sympathetic drive is attenuated by cardiopulmonary baroreflex activation when subjects are in the supine position, so that sympathetic activity, plasma renin levels, and vascular resistance may be normal or only slightly increased. When subjects are standing, however, decreased cardiac filling pressure eliminates that cardiopulmonary baroreflex buffering, allowing the heightened central sympathetic drive to manifest itself as exaggerated reflex increases in sympathetic nerve activity, plasma renin levels, and vascular resistance. With permission from Mark, A. L. (1990). Regulation of sympathetic nerve activity in mild human hypertension. *Journal of Hypertension*, **8**, S67–75.

from these studies. First, the exaggerated sympathetic response to simulated orthostatic stress suggests that mild hypertensives have a potentiated sympathetic neural drive, but in the supine position this elevated drive is masked by an augmented sympathoinhibitory effect of the cardiopulmonary baroreflex (Fig. 65.5). Second, the heightened sympathetic neural drive in mild hypertensives can occur in the absence of impairment of arterial baroreflex modulation of sympathetic activity. This strengthens the view that central neural mechanisms may be responsible for enhanced sympathetic nerve activity in early or mild hypertension.

Chemoreflex

The role of the chemoreceptors in determining sympathetic nerve discharge as well as ventilation has recently received considerable attention. Hypoxic stimulation of the peripheral chemoreceptors triggers sympathetic excitation (Somers et al. 1989a). This chemoreceptor reflex may be exaggerated in spontaneously hypertensive rats and hypertensive humans. Young human hypertensives have an increased inspiratory drive when exposed to hypoxic conditions (Trzebski et al. 1982). Sympathetic nerve discharge during hypoxia is enhanced in both borderline hypertensive men (Somers et al. 1988) and patients with obstructive sleep apnoea (Narkiewicz et al. 1999a). Concomitant hypercapnia during OSA may potentiate the sympathetic response to hypoxia (Somers et al. 1989b). This potentiation is especially marked during voluntary apnoea, when the sympathetic-inhibitory influence of breathing and thoracic afferent activity is eliminated. These findings have two important implications. First, heightened resting sympathetic discharge in early hypertension may be explained by an augmented tonic chemoreflex-mediated sympathetic excitation even during normoxia. Second, the strong association between hypertension and sleep apnoea may be explained by chronic sympathetic excitation and consequent blood pressure elevation during sleep, triggered by episodes of hypoxia, hypercapnia, and apnoea. These frequent elevations in sympathetic nerve activity and blood pressure during episodes of sleep apnoea may have functional and structural consequences and may contribute to daytime sympathetic excitation and blood pressure elevation. Indeed, chemoreflex deactivation by 100% oxygen in sleep apnoea patients elicits decreases in sympathetic drive, as well as in blood pressure and heart rate, suggesting that increases in tonic chemoreflex gain may contribute to daytime sympathetic drive in OSA (Narkiewicz et al. 1989c).

In studies of patients with sleep apnoea, we have shown that even though these patients have high sympathetic activity when awake (Fig. 65.6), sympathetic activity increases even further during sleep (Fig. 65.7) (Somers et al. 1995). In contrast to sleep in normal subjects, blood pressure does not fall during sleep in patients with obstructive sleep apnoea. Treatment with continuous positive airway pressure prevents apnoea, and reduces sympathetic activity and blood pressure during sleep (Fig. 65.7).

Central mechanisms

Oparil et al. (1995) and Esler and colleagues (1995) have reviewed the evidence for central causes of excessive sympathetic discharge in hypertension. There may be a subgroup of hypertensive patients in whom the posterior inferior cerebellar artery and/or the vertebral artery causes compression of cardiovascular regulatory centres in the region of the ventrolateral medulla. Microvascular decompression

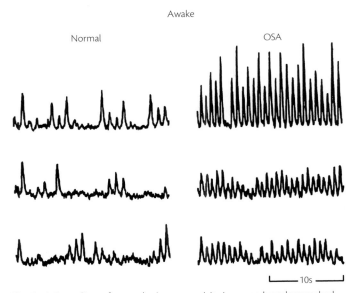

Fig. 65.6 Recordings of sympathetic nerve activity in age and gender matched normal subjects compared with patients with obstructive sleep apnoea. Sympathetic nerve recordings were obtained when subjects were awake, in the absence of any breathing abnormalities or oxygen desaturation. Sympathetic activity even during wakefulness was much greater in patients with obstructive sleep apnoea. With permission from Somers, V. K., Dyken, M. E., Clary, M. P., and Abboud, F. M. (1995), American Society for Clinical Investigation.

of this region has been reported to decrease blood pressure significantly.

Using jugular vein noradrenaline spillover measurements, Ferrier et al. (1992) have reported that higher sympathetic activity in hypertension may be explained by increased cerebral noradrenaline release. These investigators subsequently reported that subcortical noradrenaline release was linked with both total body noradrenaline spillover as well as renal noradrenaline spillover.

Chronic stress

There is increasing evidence that behavioural and psychological factors play an important role in the pathogenesis of human hypertension and might contribute to increased cardiovascular risk. Environmental or behavioural factors may be involved in the initiation and maintenance of sympathetic overactivity in hypertension (Esler 2003). Chronic stress may be related to the onset of hypertension. During mental challenge, the increase in norepinephrine spillover into arterial blood is increased in patients with essential hypertension, as compared to normotensive control subjects.

Experimental studies indicate that environmental stress increases renal sympathetic nerve (DiBona 2003). Chronic or repetitive stressful stimuli may conceivably result in sustained sympathetic activation and hypertension in susceptible persons. This response may be augmented by baroreflex resetting and by the sustained sympathetic neural effects of adrenaline uptake by nerve terminals during stressful stimuli, as discussed later.

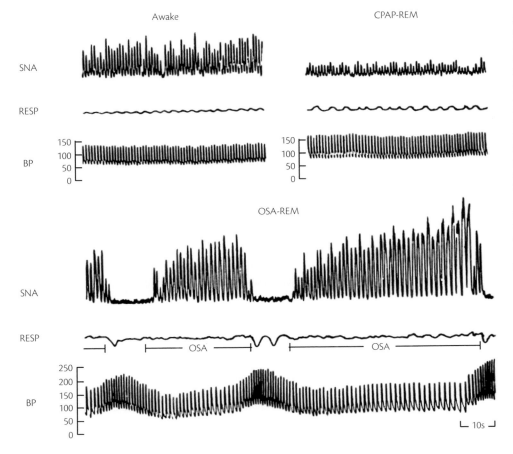

Fig. 65.7 Recordings of sympathetic activity, respiration and intra-arterial blood pressure in a patient with sleep apnoea on no medications and free of other diseases. Measurements were obtained during wakefulness (top left), during obstructive sleep apnoea in rapid eye movement (REM) sleep (bottom), and during REM sleep after treatment of obstructive sleep apnoea with continuous positive airway pressure (CPAP). During wakefulness sympathetic activity was high and blood pressure was approximately 130/60. During REM sleep, repetitive apnoeas resulted in hypoxia and chemoreflex stimulation with consequent sympathetic activation. The vasoconstriction resulting from sympathetic activation causes marked surges in blood pressure, to levels as high as 250/110 mmHg at the end of apnoea, because of increases in cardiac output at termination of apnoea. Treatment of sleep apnoea and elimination of apnoeic episodes by CPAP resulted in stabilization and lower levels of both blood pressure and sympathetic activity during REM sleep. With permission from Somers, V. K., Dyken, M. E., Clary, M. P., and Abboud, F. M. (1995), American Society for Clinical Investigation.

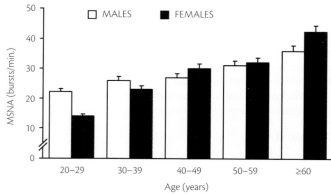

Fig. 65.8 Muscular sympathetic nerve activity (MSNA) per decade in male and female subjects. The age-related increase in MSNA was strikingly greater in female subjects. There was a significant interaction of gender with age (p = 0.02), indicating that the effect of age on MSNA is gender-dependent. With permission from Narkiewicz K. et al. (2005). Gender-selective interaction between aging, blood pressure, and sympathetic nerve activity. *Hypertension*, **45**(4): 522–5.

Ageing

In younger subjects, MSNA is lower in females than males. Sympathetic activity increases progressively with ageing (Ng 1993, Matsukawa 1998). However, ageing has a more striking effect on increasing sympathetic traffic in women than in men (Matsukawa 1998, Narkiewicz 2005) (Fig. 65.8) and blood pressure is higher for a given increase in sympathetic activation in older women compared with older men (Narkiewicz 2005). The findings of a more striking age-related increase in sympathetic activation in women parallel epidemiological data indicating a higher prevalence of hypertension in women by 60 years of age.

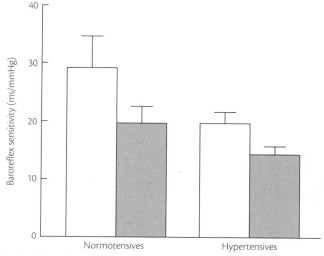

Fig. 65.9 Baroreflex sensitivity measured using phenylephrine bolus injections in normotensive and hypertensive subjects stratified by the presence (shaded bars) or absence (open bars) of family history of hypertension. Both hypertension and a family history of hypertension were associated with significant reductions in baroreflex sensitivity. With permission from Parmer R. J., Cervenka, J. H. and Stone, R. A. (1992). Baroreflex sensitivity and heredity in essential hypertension. *Circulation*, **85**(2):497–503.

Genetic factors

While the genetic contribution to essential hypertension is widely recognized, there is surprisingly little information on the heritability of sympathetic neural outflow and the factors which regulate sympathetic drive.

For example, alterations in arterial baroreflexes in hypertension could be related to genetic abnormalities that precede, and are independent of, the increase in arterial pressure. Parmer et al. (1992) measured baroreflex control of heart rate in patients with essential hypertension and in normotensive humans, grouped by the presence or absence of family history of hypertension (Fig. 65.9). Analysis of variance showed significant effects on baroreflex sensitivity of blood pressure status and of family history of hypertension. After controlling for effects of age, mean arterial pressure, and body weight, the effect of family history of hypertension and baroreflex sensitivity was still highly significant, suggesting that impairment in baroreflex sensitivity in humans is, in part, genetically determined and may represent a hereditary component in the pathogenesis of essential hypertension.

With respect to sympathetic activity itself, Williams et al. (1993) in a study of over 100 twin pairs, concluded that genetic influences contributed to more than half the variability in norepinephrine levels. In a study using microneurography, Wallin et al. (1993) found that levels of sympathetic traffic were very similar in monozygotic twins, as compared to unrelated controls subjects. Thus, the heritability of blood pressure may be explained, in part, by the heritability of levels of sympathetic nerve traffic and/or the factors which govern it.

Environmental factors

A number of risk factors frequently associated with hypertension may influence sympathetic activity. These include cigarette smoking and alcohol consumption. While smoking increases blood pressure and heart rate, there is a significant reduction in muscle sympathetic nerve activity. Increased blood pressure in response to smoking, acting via the baroreflexes, may itself elicit sympathetic inhibition, and may thus obscure any sympathetic excitatory property of cigarette smoke. Indeed, when the blood pressure increase in response to cigarette smoking is blunted by simultaneous infusion of sodium nitroprusside, there is a striking increase in sympathetic nerve traffic (Narkiewicz et al. 1998a). Sympathetic activity may reach levels two-fold to three-fold higher than is seen prior to smoking. A similar response is seen in young healthy subjects exposed to chewing (spit) tobacco or placebo in a double blind study (Wolk et al. 2005). In these subjects, both blood pressure and heart rate increased strikingly in response to the spit tobacco, but sympathetic nerve traffic was not reduced. Furthermore, spit tobacco elicited a 50% increase in plasma adrenaline levels (Wolk. 2005).

Importance of humoral and metabolic mechanisms in sympathetic activation

Adrenaline

In linking the sympathetic system and hypertension, neural actions of adrenaline have been proposed. Circulating adrenaline is taken up by adrenergic nerve terminals, with subsequent sustained neural release as a cotransmitter with noradrenaline. Neurally released adrenaline stimulates prejunctional β-receptors on adrenergic nerve terminals, thereby facilitating further release of neural noradrenaline. Several studies have reported increased levels of plasma adrenaline in hypertensive patients. Infusion of adrenaline for 6 hours can result in a sustained elevation of ambulatory blood pressure for up to 18 hours after the infusion (Blankestijn et al. 1988). Floras et al. (1990) have demonstrated that intra-arterial infusion of adrenaline facilitates neurogenic vasoconstriction in borderline hypertensive humans. Tachycardia after adrenaline infusion persists even when plasma adrenaline levels return to normal. Pretreatment with desipramine, which inhibits neuronal uptake of adrenaline, prevents the tachycardia. Thus, uptake and subsequent release of adrenaline, with facilitation of noradrenaline release at the level of the adrenergic nerve terminals may contribute to increases in sympathetic activity and reflex responsiveness in hypertensive patients, and to a 'hyperkinetic' circulatory state. It may be that repetitive adrenomedullary stimulation and adrenaline release during stress in subjects prone to developing hypertension could promote a sustained facilitation in neurally released noradrenaline which, over many years, could contribute to sustained hypertension. Rumantir et al. (2000a) have shown that adrenaline is released from cardiac sympathetic nerves in patients with essential hypertension and might enhance cardiac noradrenaline release.

Renin-angiotensin system

The interactions between the renin-angiotensin system and the sympathetic nervous system are considerable, and may be especially important in renal and renovascular hypertension as discussed earlier. Angiotensin II acts on the sympathetic nervous system at the central, ganglionic, and nerve terminal levels, as well as at the adrenal medulla to increase sympathetic nerve activity. Angiotensin II also facilitates release of noradrenaline, reduces its reuptake, and sensitizes blood vessels to the effects of noradrenaline. Infusion of exogenous angiotensin II in humans augments sympathetic mediated vasoconstriction. The reduced sympathetic nerve traffic and heart rate observed when blood pressure is increased by infusions of angiotensin II is significantly less than that seen with equivalent blood pressure elevations using phenylephrine (Matsukawa et al. 1988), suggesting that angiotensin II inhibits baroreflex control of both sympathetic activity as well as heart rate in humans. Conversely, angiotensin-converting enzyme inhibition in animals blunts the vascular responses to exogenous noradrenaline as well as to electrical stimulation of the sympathetic nerves. Acute angiotensin-converting enzyme inhibition in hypertensive humans is associated with arterial baroreceptor resetting and facilitation of parasympathetic reflex responsiveness. These angiotensin-autonomic-baroreflex interactions may explain the ability of angiotensin-converting enzyme inhibitors to reduce both vascular resistance and blood pressure without any reflex increase in heart rate.

In studies in patients with heart failure, Dibner-Dunlap et al. (1996) report that angiotensin converting enzyme inhibition reduced blood pressure, central venous pressure and muscle sympathetic nerve activity, and enhanced the sensitivity of arterial and cardiopulmonary baroreflexes. Thus, the renin-angiotensin system may influence sympathetic activity by actions at a central and ganglionic level, by increasing noradrenaline release, by potentiating the vasoconstrictor effects of noradrenaline, and by modulating important reflex mechanisms; angiotensin may also influence the

relative balance between vagal and sympathetic drives. In patients with chronic and renal failure, Ligtenberg et al. (1999) demonstrated that treatment with enalapril normalized blood pressure and muscle sympathetic-nerve activity. The MSNA decrease could not be attributed solely to blood pressure reduction since amlodipine treatment, despite similar lowering of blood pressure, increased muscle sympathetic-nerve activity.

Insulin

The importance of insulin in sympathetic activation and hypertension has aroused great interest. Obesity, particularly upper body obesity, is associated with insulin resistance and hyperinsulinaemia. Hypertension is also associated with a state of insulin resistance and hyperinsulinaemia, independent of obesity or diabetes mellitus. Interestingly, the insulin resistance which occurs in obesity and hypertension affects actions of insulin on glucose uptake in skeletal muscle, but actions of insulin on the sympathetic nervous system and the kidney are preserved (Mark 1990). Thus, it has been postulated that the hyperinsulinemia which occurs in insulin resistance causes renal sodium retention, heightened sympathetic activity, and increased vascular resistance and arterial pressure. Euglycaemic hyperinsulinaemia (insulin <400 μU/m) results in increases in plasma noradrenaline and modest increases in blood pressure in normotensive humans. Lower levels of insulin (approximately 75–150 μU/m), within the physiological postprandial range, result in increases in muscle sympathetic nerve activity, but produce vasodilation (not the expected sympathetic vasoconstriction), and do not increase blood pressure in normal humans (Anderson et al. 1991). Thus, it appears that insulin elicits both pressor (sympathetic-excitatory) and depressor (vasodilator) actions. At high levels of plasma insulin, exceeding the physiological range, the pressor effect is predominant. However, with physiological levels in normal humans the sympathetic-excitatory and vasodilator actions are balanced and blood pressure does not increase. It is possible that the presence of other factors, such as structural vascular changes, insulin resistance, or genetic predisposition to hypertension, could augment the sympathetic (pressor) action of insulin or attenuate the vasodilator (depressor) action, thereby permitting insulin to produce a sympathetically mediated increase in arterial pressure.

Hausberg et al. (1997) provide precedent for this concept of differential responses in their recent study of the effects of insulin in young versus elderly healthy subjects. While insulin caused the expected vasodilation in young subjects, elderly subjects responded to insulin by vasoconstriction (Fig. 65.10). This vasoconstriction was not explained by greater sympathetic activation, since the increase in sympathetic activity in the elderly subjects was less than that seen in the young subjects.

Leptin

Leptin acts in the central nervous system to decrease appetite and increase energy expenditure. There is growing evidence that leptin may have effects beyond control of body fat, and may importantly influence cardiovascular structure and function. Leptin receptors are widely distributed in central neural regions involved in cardiovascular regulation (Tartaglia 1995). In animals, acute administration of leptin, acting probably via the hypothalamus, increases sympathetic traffic to brown adipose tissue and to the kidney, hindlimb and adrenal gland (Haynes 1997); chronic leptin infusion

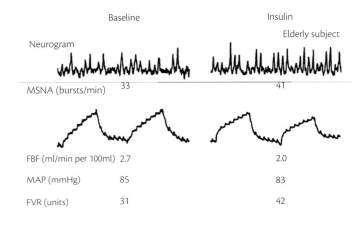

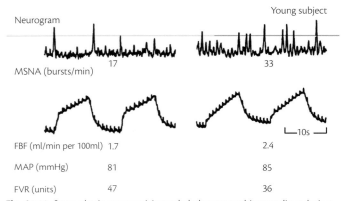

Fig. 65.10 Sympathetic nerve activity and plethysmographic recordings during baseline and after 90 minutes of insulin infusion in an elderly subject (top) and in a young subject (bottom). Baseline sympathetic activity (MSNA) was higher in the elderly subject but the insulin induced increase was smaller than in the young subject. Forearm flow (FBF) decreased in the elderly subject whereas FBF increased in the young subject with insulin. Since mean arterial pressure (MAP) did not change significantly in either subject, forearm vascular resistance (FVR) increased with insulin in the elderly and decreased in the young subject. With permission from Hausberg M et al. (1997), Contrasting autonomic and hemodynamic effects of insulin in healthy elderly versus young subjects, *Hypertension* **29**(3):700–5.

increases blood pressure and heart rate (Shek EW). Leptin has also been implicated in metabolic factors contributing to cardiovascular risk (Levya 1998) as well as to poorer cardiovascular outcomes (Wolk et al. 2004).

While several studies have shown a correlation between leptin and blood pressure, this relationship appears to be secondary to higher leptin levels in patients with increased body mass index. Nevertheless, more recent data suggest an independent link between leptin and haemodynamics in humans. In untreated patients with essential hypertension, heart rate is linked to plasma leptin levels (Narkiewicz et al., 1999b). This relationship is independent of age, body mass index, blood pressure level, smoking status and physical activity. Heart rate is fastest in those hypertensives in whom leptin levels are higher than would be expected based on body mass index. Thus, the heart rate effects of leptin may contribute to the haemodynamic profile of early hypertension, and to the development of sustained hypertension. Even in cardiac transplant recipients, higher leptin levels are associated

with faster heart rates (Winnicki et al. 2001). Plasma leptin has also been shown to correlate with renal norepinephrine spillover (Eikelis 2003).

Possible interactions between sympathetic activation and metabolic abnormalities in hypertension

While studies of cardiovascular regulation in hypertension have focused primarily on neural and vascular structural and functional changes, there is increasing evidence that metabolic abnormalities may play an important role in the pathophysiology of essential hypertension. These metabolic abnormalities have been alluded to above. They include abnormalities in glucose tolerance, hypetriglyceridaemia and dyslipidaemia. Insulin and leptin and their mutual interactions may be relevant to these metabolic abnormalities that characterize hypertension. Interestingly, the influence of insulin and leptin, first on sympathetic activation, and second on metabolism, makes them potentially important variables in understanding the complex interrelationships involved in the pathophysiology of the metabolic syndrome. Indeed, it was recently demonstrated that metabolic syndrome is a state of sympathetic nerve hyperactivity even in non-diabetic subjects, and that the additional presence of hypertension further intensifies this hyperactivity (Huggett 2004). The combination of hypertension and overt Type 2 diabetes mellitus may result in the greatest sympathetic hyperactivity (Hugget 2003).

Summary and conclusion

While we have provided extensive evidence to support a potential role for the sympathetic nervous system in essential hypertension, it is clear that this is a multifactorial disorder and at this time no single mechanism can be identified as the dominant aetiological factor. It is likely that the multiple possible causative mechanisms interact, possibly to potentiate their individual effects in raising blood pressure.

The weight of evidence strongly suggests that sympathetic overactivity is important in the aetiology and maintenance of hypertension. This appears to be especially true for the early stages of hypertension. In the later stages of hypertension, the sympathetic nervous system may continue to be important in augmenting the vascular and myocardial dysfunction and structural damage that ensue from chronic elevations in arterial pressure.

Acknowledgements

The authors were supported by NIH HL61560, HL65176, HL14388, R03 TW0 1148, 3F05 TW05200, MO1-RR00059, MO1-RR00585 and NIH Sleep Academic Award.

References

Anderson, E. A., Hoffman, R. P., Balon, T. W., Sinkey, C. A., and Mark, A. L. (1991). Hyperinsulinemia produces both sympathetic neural activation and vasodilation in normal humans. *J Clin. Invest.*, **87**, 2246–52.

Anderson, E. A., Sinkey, C. A., Lawton, W. J., and Mark A. L. (1989). Elevated sympathetic nerve activity in borderline hypertensive humans: evidence from direct intraneural recordings. *Hypertension* **14**, 177–83.

Becker, H. F., Jerrentrup, A., Ploch, T., Grote, L., Penzel, T., Sullivan, C. E., Peter, J. H. (2003). Effect of nasal continuous positive airway pressure treatment on blood pressure in patients with obstructive sleep apnoea. *Circulation* **107**, 68–73.

Blankestijn, P. J., Man in't Veld, A. J., Tulen, J., van de Meiracker, *et al.* (1988). Support for adrenaline-hypertension hypothesis: 18 hour pressor effect after 6 hours adrenaline infusion. *Lancet*, **2**, 1386–9.

Chapleau, M. W., and Abboud, F. M. (1993) Mechanism of adaptation and resetting of the baroreceptor reflex. In *Cardiovascular reflex control in health and disease* (ed. R.. Hainsworth and A.L. Mark), pp.165–93. W.B. Saunders, London.

Chobanian, A. V., Bakris, G. L., Black, H. R., *et al.*; Joint National Committee on Prevention, Detection, Evaluation, and Treatment of High Blood Pressure. (2003). National Heart, Lung, and Blood Institute; National High Blood Pressure Education Program Coordinating Committee. Seventh report of the Joint National Committee on Prevention, Detection, Evaluation, and Treatment of High Blood Pressure. *Hypertension*. **42**(6), 1206–52.

Converse, R. L., Jacobsen, T. N., Toto, R. D., Jost, C. M. T., Cosentino, F., Fouad-Tarazi, F., and Victor, R. G. (1992). Sympathetic overactivity in patients with chronic renal faiulre. *N Engl. J Med.*, **327**, 1912–8.

DiBona, G. F. (2003). Neural control of the kidney: past, present, and future. *Hypertension*, **41**, 621–24.

DiBona, G. F. (2004). The sympathetic nervous system and hypertension: recent developments. *Hypertension*, **43**, 147–50.

Dibner-Dunlap, M. E., Smith, M. L., Kinugawa, T., Thames, M. D. (1996) Enalaprilat augments arterial and cardiopulmonary control of sympathetic nerve activity in patients with heart failure. *Journal of the American College of Cardiology*, **27**, 358–64.

Egan, B., Panis, R., Hinderliter, A., Schork, N., and Julius, S. (1987). Mechanism of increased alpha adrenergic vasoconstriction in human essential hypertension. *Journal of Clinical Investigation*, **80**, 812–7.

Eikelis, N., Schlaich, M., Aggarwal, A., Kaye, D., Esler, M. (2003). Interactions between leptin and the human sympathetic nervous system. *Hypertension*, **41**, 1072–9.

Esler, M. D., Lambert, G. W., Ferrier, C., *et al.* (1995). Central nervous system noradrenergic control of sympathetic outflow in normotensive and hypertensive humans. *Clinical and Experimental Hypertension*, **17**, 409–23.

Esler, M., Jennings, G., and Lambert, G. (1989). Noradrenaline release and the pathophysiology of primary human hypertension. *American Journal of Hypertension*, **2**, 140S–46S.

Esler, M. D., Krum, H., Sobotka, P. A., Schlaich, M. P., Schmieder, R. E., and Bohm, M. (2010). Renal sympathetic denervation in patients with treatment-resistant hypertension (The Symplicity HTN-2 Trial): a randomised controlled trial. *Lancet*, **376**(9756), 1903–9.

Esler, M., Lambert, G., Brunner-La Rocca, H. P., Vaddadi, G., Kaye, D. (2003). Sympathetic nerve activity and neurotransmitter release in humans: translation from pathophysiology into clinical practice. *Acta Physiologica Scandinavica* **177**, 275–84.

Ferrier, C., Essler M. D., Eisenhofer, G., *et al.* (1992). Increased norepinephrine spillover into the jugular veins in essential hypertension. *Hypertension*, **19**, 62–9.

Floras, J. S., Aylward P. E., Mark, A. L., and Abboud, F. M. (1990). Adrenaline facilitates neurogenic vasocontriction in borderline hypertensives. *Journal of Hypertension*, **8**, 443–8.

Goldstein, D. S. (1983). Plasma catecholamine and essential hypertension: an analytical review. *Hypertension*, **5**, 86–99.

Grassi, G., Cattaneo, B. M., Seravalle, G., Lanfranchi, A., Bolla, G., and Mancia, G. (1997). Baroreflex impairment by low sodium diet in mild or moderate essential hypertension. *Hypertension*, **29**, 802–7.

Grassi, G., Cattaneo, B. M., Seravalle, G., Lanfranchi, A., Mancia, G. (1998). Baroreflex control of sympathetic nerve activity in essential and secondary hypertension. *Hypertension*, **31**, 68–72.

Grassi, G., Esler, M. (1999). How to assess sympathetic activity in humans. *Journal of Hypertension*, **17**, 719–34.

Greenwood, J. P., Scott, E. M., Stoker, J. B., Mary, D. A. (2001). Hypertensive left ventricular hypertrophy: relation to peripheral sympathetic drive. *Journal American College of Cardiology*. **38**, 1711–7.

Hausberg, M., Hoffman, R. P., Somers, V. K., Sinkey C. A., Mark, A. L., and Anderson, E. A. (1997). Contrasting autonomic and hemodyanmic effects of insulin in healthy elderly versus young subjects. *Hypertension*, **29**, 700–5.

Hausberg, M., Lang, D., Levers, A., Suwelack, B., Kisters, K. and Kosch, M. (2005). Sympathetic nerve activity in renal transplant patients before and after withdrawal of cyclosporine. *Circulation* (in press).

Haynes, W. G., Morgan, D. A., Walsh, S. A., Mark, A. L., Sivitz, W. I. (1997). Receptor-mediated regional sympathetic nerve activation by leptin. *Journal Clinical Investigation*, **100**, 270–78.

Huggett, R. J., Burns, J., Mackintosh, A. F., Mary, D. A. (2004). Sympathetic neural activation in nondiabetic metabolic syndrome and its further augmentation by hypertension. *Hypertension*, **44**, 847–52.

Huggett, R. J., Scott, E. M., Gilbey, S. G., Stoker, J. B., Mackintosh, A. F., Mary, D. A. (2003). Impact of type 2 diabetes mellitus on sympathetic neural mechanisms in hypertension. *Circulation*, **108**, 3097–3101.

Julius, S., Conway, J. (1968). Haemodynamic studies in patients with borderline blood pressure elevation. *Circulation, 38*, 282–88.

Julius, S. and Esler, M. (1975) Autonomic nervous cardiovascular regulation in borderline hypertension. *American Journal of Cardiology*, **36**, 685–96.

Kaye, D., Thompson, J., Jennings, G., and Esler, M. (1993). Cyclosporine therapy after cardiac transplantation and renal vasoconstriction without sympathetic activation. *Circulation*, **88**, 1101–9.

Levya, F., Godsland, I. F., Ghatei, M., *et al.* (1998). Hyperleptinemia as a component of a metabolic syndrome of cardiovascular risk. *Arteriosclerosis Thrombosis and Vascular Biology*, **18**, 928–33.

Ligtenberg, G., Blankestijn, P. J., Oey, P. L., *et al.* (1999). Reduction of sympathetic hyperactivity by enalapril in patients with chronic renal failure. *N Engl. J Med*, **340**, 1321–8.

Mancia, G. Bjorn Folkow Award Lecture. (1997). The sympathetic nervous system in hypertension. *Journal of Hypertension*, **15**, 1553–65.

Mark, A. L. (1990). Regulation of sympathetic nerve activity in mild human hypertension. *Journal of Hypertension*, **8**, S67–75.

Mark, A. L. (1991). Sympathetic neural contribution to salt induced hypertension in Dahl rats. *Hypertension*, **17**, 186–90.

Matsukawa, T., Gotoh, E., Miyajima, E., Yamada, Y., Shionoiri, H., Tochikubo, O., and Ishii, M. (1988). Angiotensin II inhibits baroreflex control of muscle sympathetic nerve activity and the heart rate in patients with essential hypertension. *Journal of Hypertension*, **6**, S501–S504.

Matsukawa, T., Mano, T., Gotoh, E., and Ishii, M. (1993). Elevated sympathetic nerve activity in patients with accelerated essential hypertension. *Journal of Clinical Investigation*, **92**, 25–8.

Matsukawa, T., Sugiyama, Y., Watanabe, T., Kobayashi, F., Mano, T. (1998). Gender differences in age-related changes in muscle sympathetic nerve activity in healthy subjects. *American Journal Physiology (Regulatory Integrative Comparative Physiology)*, **275**, R1600–R1604.

Miyajima, E., Yamada, Y., Yoshida, Y., Matsukawa, T., Shionoiri, H., Tochikubo, O., and Ishii, M. (1991). Muscle sympathetic nerve activity in renovascular hypertension and primary aldosteronism. *Hypertension*, **17**, 1057–62.

Narkiewicz, K., Montano, N., Cogliati, C., van de Borne, P. J., Dyken, M. E., Somers, V.K. (1998b). Altered cardiovascular variability in obstructive sleep apnoea. *Circulation* **98**, 1071–77.

Narkiewicz, K., Phillips, B. G., Kato, M., Hering, D., Bieniaszewski, L., Somers, V. K. (2005). Gender-selective interaction between aging, blood pressure, and sympathetic nerve activity. *Hypertension*, **45**. 522–5.

Narkiewicz, K., Somers, V.K. (1999c). Interactive effect of heart rate and muscle sympathetic nerve activity on blood pressure. *Circulation*, **100**, 2514–2518.

Narkiewicz, K., Somers, V.K., Mos, L., Kato, M., Accurso, V., and Palatini, P. (1999b). An independent relationship between plasma leptin and heart rate in untreated patients with essential hypertension. *Journal of Hypertension*, **17**, 245–49.

Narkiewicz, K., Winnicki, M., Schroeder, K., Phillips, B. G., Kato, M., Cwalina, E., Somers, V. K. (2002). Relationship between muscle sympathetic nerve activity and diurnal blood pressure profile. *Hypertension*, **39**, 168–72.

Narkiewicz, K., van de Borne, P. J. H., Hausberg, M., Cooley, R. L., Winniford, M. D., and Somers, V. K. (1998a). Cigarette smoking increases sympathetic outflow. *Circulation*, **98**, 528–34.

Narkiewicz, K., van de Borne, P. J., Pesek, C. A., Dyken, M. E., Montano, N., and Somers, V. K. (1999a). Selective potentiation of peripheral chemoreflex sensitivity in obstructive sleep apnoea. *Circulation*, **99**, 1183–89.

Narkiewicz, K., van de Borne, P. J., Montano, N., Dyken, M. E., Phillips, B. G., Somers, V. K. (1998c). Contribution of tonic chemoreflex activation to sympathetic activity and blood pressure in patients with obstructive sleep apnoea. *Circulation*, **97**, 943–45.

Ng, A. V., Callister, R., Johnson, D. G., Seals, D. R. (1993). Age and gender influence muscle sympathetic activity at rest in healthy humans. *Hypertension*, **21**, 498–503.

Oparil, S. (1986). The sympathetic nervous system in clinical and experimental hypertension. *Kidney International*, **30**, 4437–52.

Oparil, S., Chen, Y., Berecek, K. H., Calhoun, D. A., and Wyss, J. M. (1995). The role of the central nervous system in hypertension. In *Hypertension: pathophysiology, diagnosis, and management* (ed. J.H. Laragh and B.M. Brenner), pp. 713–40. Raven Press, New York.

Palatini, P., Julius, S. (1997). Heart rate and cardiovascular risk. (1997). *Journal of Hypertension*, **15**, 3–17.

Palatini, P., Julius, S. (2004). Elevated heart rate: a major risk factor for cardiovascular disease. *Clinical and Experimental Hypertension*, **26**, 637–44.

Parmer R. J., Cervenka, J. H. and Stone, R. A. (1992). Baroreflex sensitivity and heredity in essential hypertension. *Circulation*, **85**, 497–503.

Peppard, P. E., Young, T., Palta, M., Skatrud, J. (2000). Prospective study of the association between sleep-disordered breathing and hypertension. *N Engl. J Med.*, **342**, 1378–84.

Pepperell, J. C., Ramdassingh-Dow, S., Crosthwaite, N., *et al.* (2002). Ambulatory blood pressure after therapeutic and subtherapeutic nasal continuous positive airway pressure for obstructive sleep apnoea: a randomised parallel trial. *Lancet*, **359**, 204–210.

Rea, R. F. and Hamdan, M. (1990). Baroreflex control of muscle sympathetic nerve activity in borderline hypertension. *Circulation*, **82**, 856–62.

Rumantir, M. S., Jennings, G. L., Lambert, G. W., Kaye, D. M., Seals, D. R., Esler, M. D. (2000a). The 'adrenaline hypothesis' of hypertension revisited: evidence for adrenaline release from the heart of patients with essential hypertension. *Journal of Hypertension*, **18**, 717–23.

Rumantir, M. S., Kaye, D. M., Jennings, G. L., Vaz, M., Hastings, J. A., Esler, M. D. (2000b). Phenotypic evidence of faulty neuronal norepinephrine reuptake in essential hypertension. *Hypertension*. **6**, 824–9.

Scherrer, U., Vissing, S. F., Morgan, B.J., *et al.* (1990). Cyclosporine-induced sympathetic activation and hypertension after heart transplantation. *N Engl. J Med.*, **323**, 693–9.

Schobel, H. P., Fischer, T., Heuszer, K., Geiger, H., and Schmieder, R. E. (1996). Preeclampsia—a state of sympathetic overactivity. *N Engl. J Med.*, **335**, 1480–5.

Shek, E. W., Brands, M. W., Hall, J. E. (1998). Chronic leptin infusion increases arterial pressure. *Hypertension,* **31**, 409–414.

Somers, V. K., Dyken, M. E., Clary, M. P., and Abboud, F. M. (1995). Sympathetic neural mechanisms in obstructive sleep apnoea. *Journal of Clinical Investigation*, **96**, 1897–904.

Somers, V. K., Mark, A. L., and Abboud, F. M. (1988). Potentiation of sympathetic nerve responses to hypoxia in borderline hypertensive subjects. *Hypertension*, **11**, 608–12.

Somers, V. K., Mark, A. L., Zavala, D. C., Abboud, F. M. (1989b). Contrasting effects of hypoxia and hypercapnia on ventilation and sympathetic activity in humans. *Journal of Applied Physiology* **67**, 2101–2106.

Somers, V. K., Mark, A. L., Zavala, D. C., Abboud, F. M. (1989a). Influence of ventilation and hypocapnia on sympathetic nerve responses to hypoxia in normal humans. *Journal of Applied Physiology*, **67**, 2095–2100.

Tartaglia, L. A., Dembski, W., Weng, X., *et al.* (1995). Identification and expression of a leptin receptor, OB-R. *Cell*, **83**, 1263–71.

Trzebski, A., Tafil, M., Zoltowski, M., and Przybylski, J. (1982). Increased sensitivity of the arterial chemoreceptor drive in young men with mild hypertension. *Cardiovascular Research*, **16**, 163–72.

Wallin, B. G., Kunimoto, M. M., and Sellgren, J. (1993). Possible gentic influence on the strength of human muscle nerve sympathetic activity at rest. *Hypertension*, **22**, 282–4.

Wallin, B. G., Thompson, J. M., Jennings, G. L., and Esler M. D. (1996). Renal noradrenaline spillover correlates with muscle sympathetic activity in humans. *Journal of Physiology*, **491**, 881–7.

Wallin, B. G. and Sundlof, G. (1979). A quantitative study of muscle nerve sympathetic activity in resting normotensive and hypertensive subjects. *Hypertension*, **1**, 67–77.

Williams, P. D., Puddey, I. B., Beilin, L. J., and Vandongen, R. (1993). Genetic influences on plasma catecholamines in human twins. *Journal of Clinical Endocrinology and Metabolism*, **77**, 794–9.

Winnicki, M., Phillips, B. G., Accurso, V., *et al.* (2001). Independent association between plasma leptin levels and heart rate in heart transplant recipients. *Circulation*, **104**, 384–86.

Wolk, R., Berger, P., Lennon, B. J., Brilakis, E. S., Somers, V. K. (2004). Plasma leptin and prognosis in patients with established coronary atherosclerosis. *Journal American College Cardiology*, **44**(9), 1819–24.

Wolk, R., Shamsuzzaman, A. S. M., Svatikova, A., Deml, C. M., Huck, C., Narkiewicz, K., Somers, V. K. (2005). Haemodynamic and autonomic effects of smokeless tobacco in healthy young men. *Journal American College Cardiology*, **45**, 910–914.

CHAPTER 66

Autonomic disturbances in spinal cord lesions

Christopher J. Mathias, David A. Low and
Hans L. Frankel

Introduction

The integrity of the spinal cord is of particular importance to the normal functioning of the autonomic nervous system, as the entire sympathetic outflow (from Tl to L2/3) and a proportion of the parasympathetic outflow (the sacral parasympathetic) traverse and synapse in the spinal cord before they supply their target organs. In patients with spinal cord injuries (SCI), therefore, there are varying degrees of autonomic involvement, depending upon the site and extent of the lesion. In patients with cervical cord transection, if complete, the entire sympathetic and sacral parasympathetic outflow is separated from cerebral control. This results in a variety of abnormalities affecting the cardiovascular, thermoregulatory, gastrointestinal, urinary, and reproductive systems (Mathias and Low 2011). In patients with transection, which is common after traumatic injuries to the spinal cord, despite destruction of one or more segments, the distal portion of the spinal cord often retains function, although independently of the brain. This results, in certain situations, in additional autonomic abnormalities. In incomplete lesions the functional deficits will vary. This chapter will concentrate on patients with cervical and high SCI, as these patients often have major clinical problems resulting from autonomic dysfunction. The principles apply to other diseases affecting the spinal cord, such as due to syringomyelia or transverse myelitis, with the autonomic impairment depending on the site and extent of the lesion.

Recently injured versus chronically injured

There are differences between the autonomic problems affecting recently and chronically injured patients following a spinal lesion. Soon after transection there is initially a transient state of hypoexcitability of the isolated cord, described as 'spinal shock' (Ditunno et al. 2004). This is partially analogous to cerebral shock, as observed in the early stages after a hemisphere lesion. In spinal shock there is flaccid paralysis of the muscles, with lack of tendon reflexes. Spinal autonomic function is also impaired; the urinary bladder and large bowel are usually atonic, there is dilatation of blood vessels particularly in the skin, and spinal autonomic reflexes cannot be elicited. This stage of spinal cord depression may last from a few days to a few weeks, after which isolated activity of the spinal cord usually returns. This heralds the onset of a different range of autonomic abnormalities, which are often the result of autonomic reflex activity at a spinal level, without the normal control from higher centres in the brain.

The biochemical and molecular basis of spinal shock is not known. A range of possibilities has been proposed over the years, ranging from alterations in monoamine and neuropeptide transmitters, to abnormalities involving free oxygen radicals, lipid peroxidation, and calcium ions. Previously promising work in animals using the opiate antagonist, naloxone, and the endogenous antagonist, thyrotrophin-releasing hormone, have not been fulfilled in man. Some benefit has been shown with methylprednisolone, raising a number of possibilities, which include the deleterious effects of lipid peroxidation and hydrolysis, and breakdown of cell membranes. This, however, is more likely to be related to neuronal damage and its prevention, rather than to the understanding of the mechanisms of spinal shock. The reversal of the processes causing spinal shock is of clinical importance, as a reduction in skeletal muscle flaccidity and neural activation of the vasculature is probably beneficial in preventing deep venous thrombosis; furthermore, postural hypotension, which occurs in the early stages, is less likely to be a problem and the return of activity to the urinary bladder and bowel should help speed up the overall rehabilitation process.

The descriptions below largely relate to the chronic stage of spinal cord injuries, unless specifically stated. They will apply to both tetraplegics and high thoracic spinal cord lesions, unless otherwise indicated.

Cardiovascular system

Basal blood pressure and heart rate

The recently injured

The basal supine blood pressure in recently injured tetraplegics in spinal shock is usually lower than normal, and this applies particularly to the diastolic blood pressure (57 mm Hg in tetraplegics and 82 mmHg in normal subjects) (Mathias et al. 1979a). The extent and the duration of the hypotension varies, as it is dependent upon a number of factors including complicating trauma and drug therapy. A subnormal basal blood pressure and low levels of both plasma noradrenaline and adrenaline (Fig. 66.1) may occur from the second day after injury. It is likely that the level of blood pressure is secondary to the marked diminution in sympathetic nervous

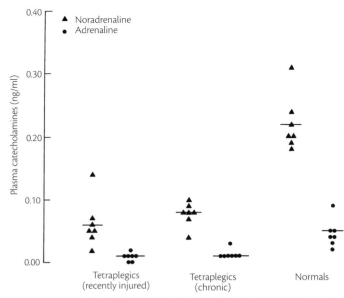

Fig. 66.1 Resting levels of plasma noradrenaline and adrenaline in recently injured tetraplegics in spinal shock, in chronic tetraplegics, and in normal age-matched subjects. The horizontal bar indicates the mean value. Basal catecholamines in both recently injured and chronic tetraplegics are a third or less than normal levels. From Mathias et al. 1979a, with permission.

activity, which normally accounts for about 20% of vascular tone. It is unlikely that skeletal muscle paralysis alone contributes, as patients with tetraplegia due to poliomyelitis often have normal or even higher levels of blood pressure.

In tetraplegics in spinal shock, the basal heart rate is usually below 100 beats/minute, unlike in patients with low spinal cord injuries, in whom the heart rate is often higher. This is probably due to a reduction in neural and hormonal sympathetic-mediated chronotropic influences in the tetraplegics. The efferent cardiac parasympathetic pathways, however, are intact and the absence of sympathetic activation may predispose susceptible patients to vagal overactivity. This may result in bradycardia and cardiac arrest, as has been noted during tracheal stimulation.

The chronically injured

In the chronic stage, the basal level of both systolic and diastolic blood pressure in high lesions is lower than in normal subjects (Fig. 66.2) (Frankel et al. 1972, Mathias et al. 1976a). Non-invasive

ambulatory 24-hour recordings indicate loss of the nocturnal circadian fall in blood pressure, as occurs normally (Nitsche et al. 1996) (Fig. 66.3). Basal levels of plasma noradrenaline and adrenaline in tetraplegics, in the absence of stimulation from below the lesion, remain low as in the stage of spinal shock, reflecting absent tonic supraspinal sympathetic impulses and diminished peripheral sympathetic activity. This has been confirmed in tetraplegics using microneurography to detect skin and muscle sympathetic nerve activity (Stjernberg et al. 1986). Patients with spinal cord injury, however, are prone to renal damage and renal failure which may account for sustained hypertension in some.

In the absence of adequate resting sympathetic tone, a number of secondary mechanisms, particularly hormonal, attempt to compensate for and help maintain blood pressure. An important component is the renin–angiotensin–aldosterone system, which through the direct pressor effects of angiotensin II and the salt-retaining effects of aldosterone, helps raise blood pressure. This is particularly evident when drugs that interfere with the system are used; the angiotensin-converting enzyme inhibitor, captopril, substantially lowers supine blood pressure in tetraplegics. Even small doses of diuretics, which cause salt loss and lower intravascular fluid volume, may cause a catastrophic fall in supine blood pressure. A low salt diet lowers blood pressure, despite the ability of tetraplegics to reduce salt excretion as do normal subjects (Sutters et al. 1992). In tetraplegics, recumbency itself may induce a diuresis but not a natriuresis; this differs from patients with primary autonomic failure, who also have nocturnal polyuria (Chapter 19), and in whom recumbency causes both diuresis and natriuresis (Kooner et al. 1987). The difference may relate to the ability of the tetraplegics to mount an adequate hormonal response to oppose natriuresis, unlike the autonomic failure patients in whom these responses are often muted (Chapter 16). These observations have practical importance, as a period of recumbency in high spinal lesions will often result in accentuation of postural hypotension. This may be reduced or prevented by head-up tilt.

In chronic high lesions, the basal heart rate may be marginally lower than, or no different from, that of normal subjects. Twenty-four-hour ambulatory recordings of heart rate indicate preservation of the circadian fall at night (Nitsche et al. 1996). Power spectral analytical techniques in tetraplegics indicate a diminished low-frequency (presumed sympathetic) component with preservation of the high frequency (presumed parasympathetic) component (Inoue et al. 1991) (Fig. 66.4). There are changes in heart rate and RR intervals (heart periods) which occur when baroreceptor

Fig. 66.2 Relationship between systolic and diastolic blood pressure in male patients with spinal cord lesions at differing levels. Tetraplegics have the lowest resting blood pressure. Reprinted by permission from Macmillan Publishers Ltd: *Spinal Cord*, Frankel, H. L., Michaelis, L. S., Golding, D. R., and Beral, V., The blood pressure in paraplegia-1, **10**, 193–8, Copyright 1972.

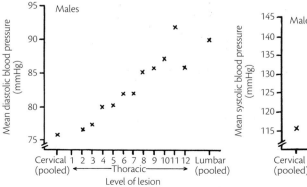

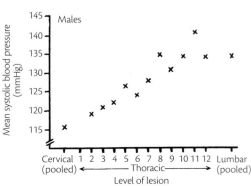

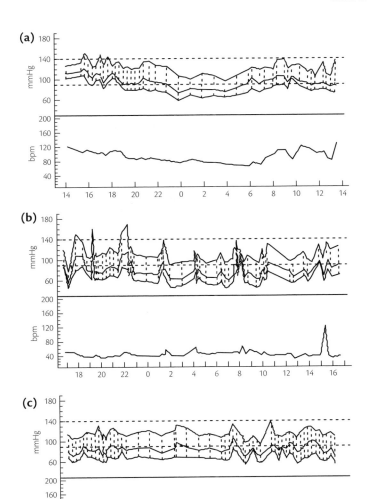

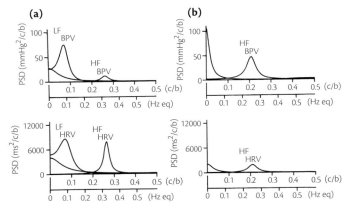

Fig. 66.4 Individual autoregressive power spectral density (PSD) components showing systolic blood pressure variabilities (BPV) (upper panel) and heart rate period as R-R interval variabilities (HRV) (lower panel) in a healthy subject **(a)** and a complete tetraplegic **(b)** at rest while supine. In the healthy male **(a)** there were two major spectral components; the low-frequency (LF; LF_{BPV} or LF_{HRV}) component and the high-frequency (HF; HF_{BPV} or HF_{HRV}) component. In the tetraplegic **(b)**, the HF (HF_{BPV} and HF_{HRV}) component was present, but there was no LF (LF_{BPV} or LF_{HRV}) component. From Inoue, K., Miyake, S., Kumashiro, M., Ogata, H., Ueta, T., and Akatsu, T. (1991). *Am. J. Physiol.*, Am Physiol Soc, used with permission.

Fig. 66.3 Ambulatory blood pressure measurements demonstrating **(a)** a normal profile with a preserved physiological fall in blood pressure at night between midnight and 04.00 hours, **(b)** multiple episodes of autonomic dysreflexia in a complete tetraplegic, and **(c)** the same patient as in **(b)** after effective treatment of autonomic dysreflexia with the antihypertensive drug nifedipine. Despite improvement in **(c)**, the loss of the circadian regulation of blood pressure persists. Reproduced from *J. Neurol. Neurosurg. Psychiat.*, Curt, A., Nitsche, B., Rodic, B., Schurch, B., and Dietz, V., Assessment of autonomic dysreflexia in patients with spinal cord injury. **62**, 473–7, Copyright 1997 with permission from BMJ Publishing Group Ltd.

afferents are influenced either by a rise or a fall in blood pressure (such as by phenylephrine or nitroprusside respectively; Fig. 66.5), that results in reciprocal changes in vagal efferent activity (Koh et al. 1994). Various observations, therefore, suggest preservation of cardiac vagal function.

Cardiovascular responses to physiological stimuli

In tetraplegics with physiologically complete transection the brain is functionally separated from the peripheral sympathetic nervous system. This may cause a number of abnormalities, when cardiovascular responses are the result of cerebral initiation or modulation.

Depending on the level and extent of the lesion, there are varying disturbances.

Postural change

Patients with high spinal cord lesions are prone to hypotension, which commonly occurs during postural change from the horizontal to the upright position (Illman et al. 2000). This occurs in both recently injured patients in spinal shock and in chronically injured patients, especially in the early stages during rehabilitation. Their mobility, even in a wheelchair, can be considerably impeded (Chelvarajah 2009). The fall in blood pressure is accompanied by symptoms mainly related to diminished cerebral perfusion (Table 66.1). The symptoms can vary in nature and intensity and are not necessarily related to the degree of hypotension.

During head-up postural change, as on a tilt table, there is usually an immediate fall in both systolic and diastolic blood pressure. The pressure may fall to extremely low levels, but usually there is no loss of consciousness except in recently injured tetraplegics or in chronic tetraplegics following a period of recumbency. This tolerance to a low cerebral perfusion pressure is similar to that of patients with chronic autonomic failure, who are also able to autoregulate their cerebral circulation despite an extremely low perfusion blood pressure (Chapter 13). The precise mechanisms responsible for this are unclear.

Following the initial fall in blood pressure, the subsequent responses vary. In some patients, especially in the early stages, blood pressure continues to fall (Fig. 66.6a). There is no rise in levels of plasma noradrenaline in the early phases following head-up postural change (Fig. 66.7), consistent with their inability to reflexly increase sympathetic nervous activity in response to postural change, as occurs normally. In many chronically injured patients, however, if tilt is prolonged, the blood pressure tends to partly recover, often with oscillations (Fig. 66.6b). This recovery may be related to activation of the renin–angiotensin–aldosterone system. The release of renin appears to be independent of

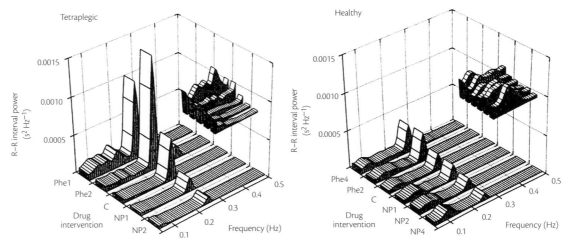

Fig. 66.5 Heart period (R-R interval) power spectrum in a tetraplegic patient (left) and healthy subject (right) in the control (C) phase and during drug intervention with increasing doses of phenylephrine (Phe 1 and Phe 2) to raise blood pressure, and sodium nitroprusside (NP1, NP2 and NP4) to lower blood pressure. There is a rise in the high-frequency spectrum after phenylephrine and an increase in blood pressure in both subjects; the rise is greater in the tetraplegic. With a fall in blood pressure after nitroprusside, the low-frequency (presumed sympathetic) spectrum is elevated in the normal subject but not in the tetraplegic patient. The insets represent low-frequency (0.05–0.15 Hz) R-R interval spectral power displayed at identical high gains. With permission from Koh, J., Brown, T. E., Beighton, L. A., Ha, C. Y., and Eckberg, D. L., Human autonomic rhythms: vagal cardiac mechanisms in tetraplegic subjects, *J. Physiol.*, Wiley.

sympathetic stimulation and may be secondary to renal baroreceptor stimulation from the fall in renal perfusion pressure (Fig. 66.8a). Renin results in the formation of the peptide angiotensin II, which has powerful direct vasoconstrictor effects, may facilitate peripheral noradrenaline release and activity, and also stimulates the release of aldosterone from the adrenal cortex (Fig. 66.8b). The salt- and water-retaining effects of aldosterone have slower but important effects in increasing intravascular volume. These various actions of the renin–angiotensin–aldosterone system help to raise blood pressure. A further mechanism contributing to blood pressure recovery during tilt is the activation of spinal reflexes either from stimulation of the skin, the skeletal muscles, or the viscera. This is more likely to account for the reduction in peripheral blood flow and rise in occluded venous pressure observed during head-up tilt in tetraplegics than the spinal postural reflexes that were previously proposed. Local sympathetic reflexes (venoarteriolar reflexes) may operate in high lesions during postural change.

During head-up postural change the fall in blood pressure is accompanied by a reduction in central venous pressure, stroke volume, and cardiac output, which is probably the result of venous pooling, diminished venous return, reduced skeletal muscle pumping activity and the inability to increase sympathetic cardiac

Table 66.1 Clinical manifestations of postural hypotension*

◆ Giddiness, buzzing, and ringing in ears
◆ Blurring, greying out, and loss of vision
◆ Facial pallor
◆ Syncope
◆ Hypotension and elevation in heart rate
◆ Venous pooling and cyanotic discoloration of lower limbs
◆ Reduced urine secretion

* Other symptoms as described in autonomic failure (Mathias 1995) may also occur.
  (See Chapter 22)

(a)

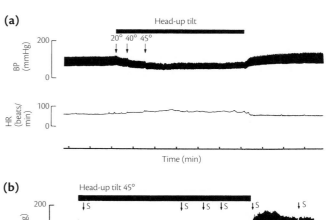

(b)

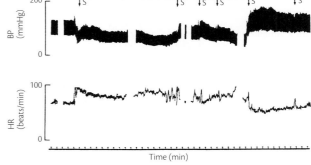

Fig. 66.6 **(a)** Blood pressure (BP) and heart rate (HR) in a tetraplegic patient before and after head-up tilt, in the early stages of rehabilitation, when there were few muscle spasms and minimal autonomic dysreflexia. From Mathias and Frankel 1992, with permission. **(b)** Blood pressure (BP) and heart rate (HR) in a tetraplegic patient before, during and after head-up tilt to 45°. Blood pressure promptly falls but with partial recovery, which in this case is linked to skeletal muscle spasms (S) inducing spinal sympathetic activity. Some of the later oscillations may be due to the rise in plasma renin, which was measured where there are interruptions in the intra-arterial record. In the later phases of tilt, skeletal muscle spasms occur more frequently, and further elevate the blood pressure. On return to the horizontal, blood pressure rises rapidly above the previous level, and then slowly returns to the horizontal. Heart rate usually moves in the opposite direction, except during muscle spasms, where there is an increase. With permission from Mathias, C. J. and Frankel, H. L. (1988). Cardiovascular control in spinal man. *Ann. Rev. Physiol.* **50**, 577–92.

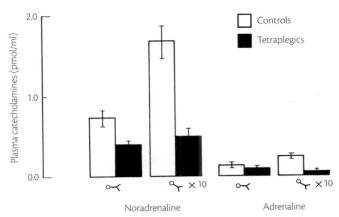

Fig. 66.7 Plasma noradrenaline and adrenaline levels in controls (normal subjects) and chronic tetraplegic patients at rest and during head-up tilt to 45° to 10 minutes. There is a rise in plasma noradrenaline in the control subjects but little change in the tetraplegics. The bars indicate ± SEM.

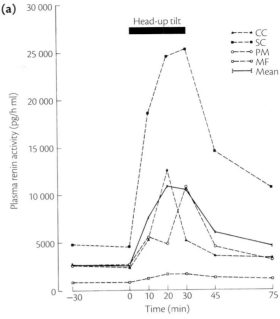

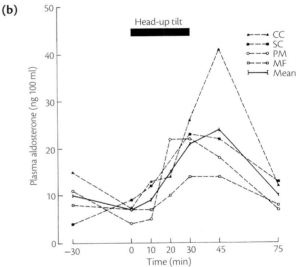

Fig. 66.8 **(a)** Plasma renin activity levels in four chronic tetraplegic patients before, during, and after head-up tilt to 45°. In three patients there was pronounced hypotension and a marked rise in plasma renin activity levels. Patient MF had minimal changes in blood pressure during head-up tilt and the smallest rise in plasma renin activity. From Mathias et al. 1975, with permission. **(b)** Plasma aldosterone levels before, during, and after head-up tilt to 45° in the same four patients as in **(a)**. The rise in plasma aldosterone levels is later in timing to that of plasma renin activity. Reproduced with permission, from Mathias, C. J., Christensen, N. J., Corbett, J. L., Frankel, H. L., Goodwin, T. J., and Peart, W. S. (1975). *Clin. Sci. Mol. Med.* **49**, 291–9, © the Biochemical Society.

inotropic activity (Claydon et al. 2006). Venous pooling often causes cyanotic discoloration of the legs and may account for ankle oedema, as observed in these with high lesions and in wheelchairs. Urine volume is usually reduced, often to extremely low levels, which occasionally raises the question of whether there may be obstruction to the urinary outflow tract. Oliguria may be due to a combination of causes; these include a fall in blood pressure, thus reducing renal plasma flow and glomerular filtration rate, and an elevation in levels of the antidiuretic hormone, vasopressin. In high spinal lesions there is an exaggerated rise in vasopressin levels during head-up tilt compared with normal individuals.

During head-up postural change there is often a rapid rise in heart rate, which is inversely related to the fall in blood pressure. This is likely to be due to withdrawal of vagal tone in response to unloading of baroreceptor afferents, as it is markedly attenuated, although not abolished, by atropine. Propranolol also reduces the heart rate rise during tilt, suggesting that β-adrenoceptor stimulation also partially contributes. In the majority of patients, heart rate does not usually rise above 100 beats/minute even during a marked fall in blood pressure. This therefore is different from the situation in patients with an intact sympathetic nervous system, who are in 'shock' with a similarly low level of blood pressure.

The clinical problems resulting from postural hypotension in high spinal lesions are not usually as severe and prolonged as those in patients with primary autonomic failure. Clinical observations indicate that the symptoms of postural hypotension are often diminished with frequent postural change to the head-up position, along with elevation of the head end of the bed at night. The activation of the renin–angiotensin–aldosterone axis, with both early and longer-acting effects resulting from vasoconstriction and plasma volume expansion, probably helps buffer the fall in blood pressure during head-up postural change. Another possibility is an improved ability to autoregulate cerebral blood flow, which such patients often can do at lower perfusion pressures than normal subjects. It is not known whether changes in other circulating and locally produced hormones acting on the cerebral vasculature and oxygenation levels (Houtman et al. 2000, 2001) also contribute.

A variety of physical methods have been used to prevent postural hypotension; these include abdominal binders and thigh cuffs,

upper body exercise, and functional electrical stimulation applied to the legs that aim to prevent pooling (Gillis et al. 2008). Activation of spinal sympathetic reflexes, by induction of muscle spasms or tapping of the anterior abdominal wall suprapubically to activate the urinary bladder, may be of value in some patients by causing autonomic dysreflexia and thus elevating blood pressure.

A range of drugs, as used in patients with autonomic failure (Chapter 47), may alleviate postural hypotension in high spinal cord lesions. Such spinal patients, unlike patients with autonomic failure, are, however, prone to paroxysms of hypertension, which may be severe and exacerbated by such drugs. Usually, the need for drugs is for limited periods, when postural hypotension is a particular problem, as in the early stages of rehabilitation and after prolonged recumbency. If neither of these factors is responsible, other causes of orthostatic hypotension (especially non-neurogenic causes) need to be sought (Chapter 22). Ephedrine, in a dose of 15 mg half-an-hour before postural change, is often of value. Its ability to act directly on adrenoceptors and indirectly by releasing noradrenaline is probably the basis of its efficacy. Dihydroergotamine and other α-adrenoceptor agonists may have a role, especially if they have short-lived effects. Indomethacin, a prostaglandin synthetase inhibitor, also elevates basal blood pressure and reduces the blood pressure fall during postural change but has potential side-effects. In most patients, however, drugs are not needed.

Valsalva manoeuvre

In high spinal lesions the responses to the Valsalva manoeuvre are abnormal because the baroreceptor reflex is impaired due to the disruption of sympathetic efferent pathways through the cervical and thoracic spinal cord. When intrathoracic pressure is elevated there is a fall in blood pressure, despite a fairly modest increase in intrathoracic pressure that is often difficult to achieve and maintain because of the inability to activate intercostal muscles. There is no recovery in blood pressure while the intrathoracic pressure is elevated. Heart rate rises with the fall in blood pressure because the cardiac vagi respond to the fall in blood pressure. On reducing the elevated intrathoracic pressure, there is a gradual recovery of blood pressure with a reduction in heart rate that does not fall below the basal level.

The blood pressure may fall to extremely low levels during the Valsalva manoeuvre if intrathoracic pressure is elevated to 20–30 mmHg, as demonstrated in a tetraplegic who suffered severe dizziness while singing, which raised her intrathoracic pressure (van Lieshout et al. 1991) (Fig. 66.9). This ability to lower blood pressure has also been used to the benefit of patients, to prevent hypertension during urological surgery by increasing positive pressure during assisted ventilation.

Pressor stimuli originating above the lesion

Pressor stimuli dependent on sympathetic activation that either originate in, or are modulated by, the brain do not raise blood pressure in patients with complete cervical cord transaction. Stimuli such as mental arithmetic, a loud noise, and cutaneous stimulation by either pain or cold in areas above the lesion have no effect in tetraplegics, unlike in normal subjects in whom they elevate blood pressure. The lack of response to these stimuli provides evidence of severance of sympathetic pathways descending within the cervical spinal cord.

Pressor stimuli originating below the lesion: 'autonomic dysreflexia'

The reverse, an exaggerated rise in blood pressure, occurs in high spinal lesions when stimuli originate below the level of the lesion, predominantly, but not always, through noxious stimuli (Burton et al. 2008). Stimulation of the skin, abdominal and pelvic viscera, or skeletal muscles, can cause a paroxysmal rise in blood pressure (Fig. 66.10), which usually is accompanied by a fall in heart rate because of increased vagal activity. In recently injured tetraplegics in spinal shock there is often no change in blood pressure or heart rate during such stimulation (Fig. 66.11). This differs markedly from the chronic stage when there is increased activity in a number of target organs supplied by the sympathetic and parasympathetic nerves. These effects, in combination, contribute to the syndrome of autonomic dysreflexia (Table 66.2). Detailed observations were made by Head and Riddoch (1917) who described sweating around and above the level of the lesion, with evacuation of the urinary bladder and rectum, penile erection, and seminal fluid emission, together with skeletal muscle spasms—components of the 'mass reflex' in response to cutaneous stimulation below the lesion or during bladder and bowel evacuation. The cardiovascular changes, however, were not described until 1947, when Guttmann and Whitteridge reported their observations during urinary bladder stimulation. The cardiovascular responses to stimuli below the lesion include a rise in both systolic and diastolic blood pressure. There is a marked reduction in peripheral blood flow (Fig. 66.12)

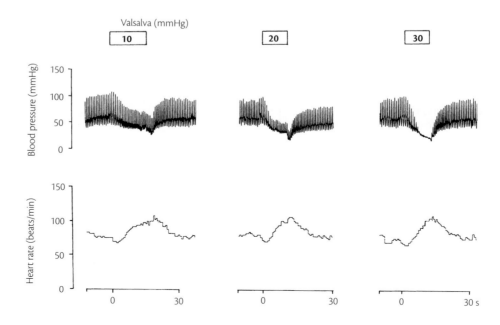

Fig. 66.9 Blood pressure and heart rate responses to the Valsalva manoeuvre in a tetraplegic patient. With increasing degrees of intrathoracic pressure there is a progressively greater fall in blood pressure in phase II. There is virtually no blood pressure recorded when intrathoracic pressure is raised to 30 mmHg. Blood pressure has been measured non-invasively with the Finapres. With permission from, van Lieshout, J. J., Imholz, B. P. M., Wesseling, K. H., Speelman, J. D., and Wieling, W. (1991). Singing-induced hypotension: a complication of high spinal cord lesion. *Neth. J. Med.* **38**, 75–9, Van Zuiden Communications.

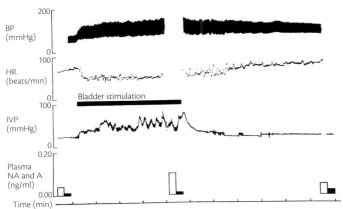

Fig. 66.10 Blood pressure (BP), heart rate (HR), intravesical pressure (IVP), and plasma noradrenaline (NA) and adrenaline (A) levels in a tetraplegic patient before, during, and after bladder stimulation induced by suprapubic percussion of the anterior abdominal wall. The rise in BP is accompanied by a fall in heart rate as a result of increased vagal activity in response to the rise in blood pressure. Level of plasma NA (open histograms), but not A (filled histograms) rise, suggesting an increase in sympathetic neural activity independently of adrenomedullary activation. This figure was published in *J. Autonom. Nerv. Syst. Suppl.*, Mathias, C. J., Frankel, H. L., The neurological and hormonal control of blood vessels and heart in spinal man, 457–64, Copyright Elsevier (1986).

Table 66.2 Clinical manifestations of autonomic dysreflexia

- ◆ Paraesthesiae in neck, shoulders, and arms
- ◆ Fullness in head
- ◆ Hot ears
- ◆ Throbbing headache, especially in the occipital and frontal regions
- ◆ Tightness in chest and dyspnoea
- ◆ Hypertension and bradycardia
- ◆ Occasionally cardiac dysrythmias
- ◆ Pupillary dilatation
- ◆ Above lesion—pallor initially, followed by flushing of face and neck and sweating in areas above and around the lesion
- ◆ Below lesion—cold peripheries; piloerection
- ◆ Contraction of urinary bladder and large bowel[a]
- ◆ Penile erection and seminal fluid emission[a]

[a] May occur as part of the 'mass reflex'.

which may result in cold limbs, thus accounting for poikilothermia spinalis, one of the original terms used to describe autonomic dysreflexia. In addition to constriction of resistance vessels, there is also a rise in occluded venous pressure, indicating contraction of capacitance vessels. There is an elevation in both stroke volume and cardiac output, suggestive of activation of spinal cardiac reflexes. These changes occur soon after stimulation, the rapidity indicating that they are of neurogenic origin and likely to be due to

reflex sympathetic activity through the isolated spinal cord. Biochemical evidence of increased sympathoneural activity has been obtained from levels of plasma noradrenaline, which are closely correlated with the blood pressure changes (Fig. 66.13a,c). Plasma dopamine beta hydroxylase levels rise later (Fig. 66.13b) and are not related to the rise in blood pressure (Mathias et al. 1976b) (Fig. 66.13d). Plasma adrenaline levels do not change, indicating that adrenomedullary secretion does not contribute to the elevation in blood pressure. However, plasma noradrenaline levels, even at the height of hypertension and despite their increasing by two-fold to three-fold, are only moderately above the resting basal levels of normal subjects. This differs markedly from the extremely high levels of plasma catecholamines often found in patients with a phaeochromocytoma (Chapter 64). During autonomic dysreflexia,

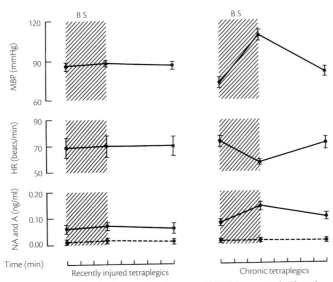

Fig. 66.11 Average levels of mean blood pressure (MBP), heart rate (HR), and plasma noradrenaline (NA, continuous line) and adrenaline (A, interrupted line) in recently injured and chronic tetraplegics, before, during, and after bladder stimulation (BS). The bars indicate ± SEM. No changes occur in the recently injured tetraplegics, unlike the chronic tetraplegics in whom MBP and plasma NA levels rise and HR falls. There are no changes in plasma A levels. From Mathias et al. 1979a, with permission.

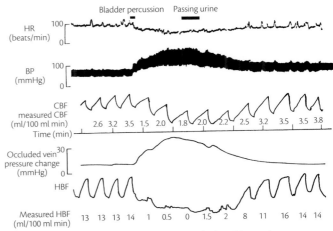

Fig. 66.12 The effects of bladder percussion and micturition on heart rate (HR), blood pressure (BP), calf blood flow (CBF), occluded vein pressure, and hand blood flow (HBF) in a chronic tetraplegic with a physiologically complete transaction of the cervical spinal cord. The rise in blood pressure is accompanied by a fall in heart rate (after an initial transient rise), a marked reduction in both calf and hand blood flow, and a rise in occluded vein pressure. With permission from Corbett, J. L., Frankel, H. L., and Harris, P. J. Cardiovascular reflex responses to cutaneous and visceral stimuli in spinal man. *J. Physiol.*, Wiley.

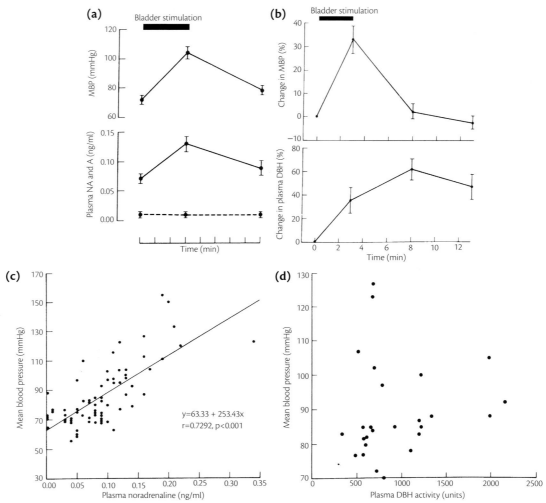

Fig. 66.13 (a), (b) Changes in mean blood pressure (MBP) in tetraplegic patients before, during, and after bladder stimulation. **(a)** Plasma noradrenaline (NA, continuous line) levels rise with the blood pressure and fall as the pressor effects wane. There is no change in plasma adrenaline (A, dashed line) levels. **(b)** Levels of plasma dopamine-beta-hydroxylase (DBH) rise slowly and remain elevated for a longer period. The bars indicate ± SEM. **(c)** There is a strong relationship between mean blood pressure and plasma noradrenaline levels, which is not observed for **(d)** plasma DBH. In short-term studies, plasma noradrenaline levels appear to be a better indicator of sympathoneural activation than plasma DBH levels. With permission from Mathias, C. J. (1976a). *Neurological disturbances of the cardiovascular system*. D. Phil. thesis, University of Oxford, and also Mathias, C. J., Christensen, N. J., Corbett, J. L., Frankel, H. L., and Spalding, J. M. K. (1976). Plasma catecholamines during paroxysmal neurogenic hypertension in quadriplegic man, *Circulation Res.* **39**, 204–8.

levels of other vasoconstrictor substances in plasma, such as renin (and by inference angiotensin II levels), aldosterone, vasopressin, and atrial natriuretic peptide remain unchanged or fall (Mathias et al. 1981, Krum et al. 1992). Whether levels of other vasoconstrictor peptides, such as neuropeptide Y (NPY) and endothelin, rise in man is not known. These are, however, more likely to play a local role than through circulating levels. In spinal animal models, plasma NPY levels do not rise during autonomic dysreflexia (Santajuliana et al. 1995); however, there is evidence that NPY spillover may increase markedly in certain regions, including the hepatomesenteric vascular bed, without plasma levels changing substantially (Morris et al. 1997). The sympathetic skin response in complete tetraplegia is present in the feet during urinary bladder contraction but this does not occur with incomplete lesions (Previnaire et al. 1993); also, sweating does not occur in the feet during autonomic dysreflexia (Guttmann and Whitteridge 1947) and reasons for the dissociation are unclear.

The rise in blood pressure and the widespread involvement of the vasculature below the lesion, despite a modest and often localized stimulus only involving a few segments, suggest the spread of neuronal impulses intraspinally and/or extraspinally. In tetraplegics, microneurography indicates only a moderate and transient rise in muscle sympathetic nerve activity during autonomic dysreflexia (Stjernberg et al. 1986) with no association between the cardiac cycle and muscle sympathetic nerve discharge as occurs normally (Fig. 66.14). There is evidence of hyperactivity of target organs innervated by the autonomic nervous system; as has been demonstrated in the dorsal foot vein of tetraplegics in response to local intravenous noradrenaline (Arnold et al. 1995). The exaggerated blood pressure response to various stimuli suggests supersensitivity of adrenoceptors, or that other mechanisms are responsible for the enhanced vascular response. The contribution of sympathetic nonadrenergic transmission to increases in vascular resistance during autonomic dysreflexia has recently been proposed

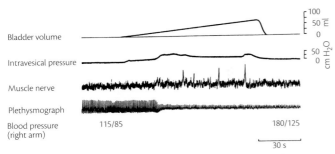

Fig. 66.14 Mean voltage neurogram record of sympathetic activity in a peroneal muscle nerve fascicle obtained while filling the urinary bladder with carbon dioxide (CO_2) at 50 cm³/minute in a patient with a C5 lesion. There is an increase in intravesical volume and pressure associated with marked cutaneous vasoconstriction, as indicated by the photoelectrical pulse plethysmograph. Blood pressure is markedly elevated despite only a moderate increase in sympathetic nerve activity. From Stjernberg et al. 1986, with permission.

(Groothius et al. 2010). Experimental studies also indicate the importance of certain neuronal cells with activated nerve growth factors (NGF); furthermore neutralizing intraspinal NGF prevents the development of autonomic dysreflexia (Krenz et al. 1999, Krenz and Weaver 2000). Overall, the result of the physiological and pharmacological studies, in conjunction with the neurohormonal

observations, suggest that the term 'autonomic hyperreflexia' is erroneous and should not be used. In contrast, however, reports of a marked (15-fold) increase in noradrenaline spillover in the leg during bladder stimulation, suggest that in high lesions greater quantities of noradrenaline may be released per impulse than previously recorded (Karlsson 1997) (Fig. 66.15).

Increased pressor responses to stimuli do not occur in patients with lesions below the fifth thoracic segment (Fig. 66.16), indicating that the sympathetic neural outflow above that level is of major importance in blood pressure homeostasis. It is likely that in the lesions below T5 there is sparing of the neural control of the large splanchnic circulatory bed. In high lesions, stimuli causing autonomic dysreflexia unmask primary cutaneovascular, viscerovascular, and somatovascular reflexes; these primary effects appear to be modulated by the brain in both normal subjects and in patients with lesions below T5, thus preventing hypertension. Indirect evidence for the role of descending cerebral pathways in preventing autonomic dysreflexia has emerged from measurement of the sympathetic skin response that tests integrity of sympathetic cholinergic pathways. In complete tetraplegics the response was absent in the hands and feet; however, in incomplete tetraplegics autonomic dysreflexia occurs only in those with an absent response, while in those with a response dysreflexia did not occur (Curt et al. 1996).

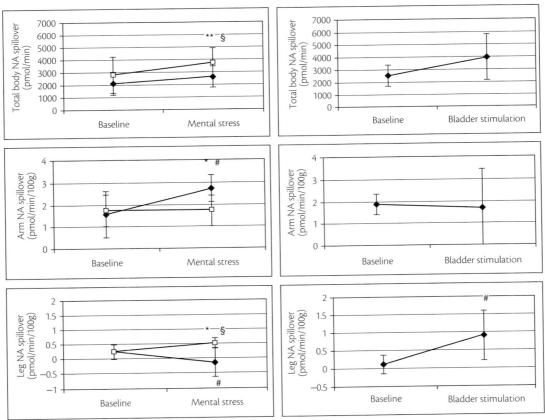

Fig. 66.15 Total body, arm and leg noradrenaline (NA) spillover (upper middle and lower panels, respectively) during mental stress (left panels) and bladder stimulation (right panels) in patients with high spinal-cord injuries (filled symbols) and in control subjects (open symbols; only in left panel). With mental stress, total and leg NA spillover increases in the controls, with an increase in arm NA spillover only in the spinal are indicated by * p < 0.05 and ** p < 0.01 and patients. With bladder stimulation (only in the spinal injured), leg NA spillover only increases. Significant differences between groups between baseline and stimulation by patients in patients and 8 controls (§). Values are means with 95% confidence interval. With permission from Karlsson, A.-K. (1997). *Metabolism and sympathetic function in spinal cord injured subjects.* PhD Thesis, University of Gothenburg, Sweden.

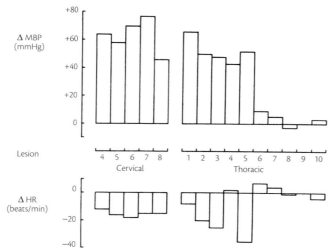

Fig. 66.16 Changes in mean blood pressure (Δ MBP) and heart rate (Δ HR) in patients with spinal cord lesions at different levels (cervical and thoracic) after bladder stimulation induced by suprapubic percussion of the anterior abdominal wall. In the cervical and high thoracic lesions there is a marked elevation in blood pressure and a fall in heart rate. In patients with lesions below T5 there are minimal cardiovascular changes. With permission from *J. Autonom. Nerv. Syst. Suppl.*, Mathias, C. J., Frankel, H. L., The neurological and hormonal control of blood vessels and heart in spinal man, 457–64, Copyright Elsevier (1986).

In high lesions, the heart rate may rise transiently with the elevation in blood pressure, presumably because of sympathetic stimulation of the heart as a result of spinal cardiac reflexes. There is usually a subsequent fall in heart rate because of stimulation of sinoaortic baroreceptors and increased vagal efferent activity. This may help dampen the rise in blood pressure during autonomic dysreflexia, as parasympathetic blockade with atropine or other anticholinergic agents that prevents this reflexly induced fall in heart rate often results in an even greater rise in blood pressure. During autonomic dysreflexia there is often facial vasodilatation accompanied by sweating, which may be profuse above the level of the lesion (Fig. 66.17). Sweating below the level of the lesion may be minimal. The precise mechanisms responsible are not known.

Autonomic dysreflexia is of major clinical importance. Mild episodes probably occur intermittently through the day, often are not noticed, and may be of little consequence. Hypertension, especially linked to bladder contractions and voiding, may not be accompanied by symptoms (silent autonomic dysreflexia; Linsenmeyer et al. 1996). When autonomic dysreflexia is prolonged, there may be considerable morbidity, as a result of excessive sweating over the head and neck, and a throbbing headache. The latter is often, but not always, related to the level of blood pressure and may be dependent on distension of pain-sensitive cranial blood vessels. With recurrent episodes of dysreflexia, headache may be particularly severe, despite later but only modest elevations in blood pressure. This may be due to increased sensitivity of afferent nerves on blood vessels caused by the formation or release of substances including substance P, calcitonin-gene-related peptide, and prostaglandins. Other complications of the vasospasm and hypertension accompanying autonomic dysreflexia include myocardial failure and neurological deficits such as epileptic seizures, visual defects, and cerebral haemorrhage. These may result in extensive and permanent neurological deficits or death.

Whether these cardiovascular abnormalities may become an even greater problem as patients grow older, and they become more vulnerable to cardiac and vascular damage, remains to be determined.

The key factor in the management of autonomic dysreflexia is prevention. It is necessary to determine the provoking cause and to rectify it (Table 66.3). To lower blood pressure rapidly, head-up tilt (which causes venous pooling) may be used initially, although occasionally a fall in blood pressure may induce autonomic dysreflexia and in particular hyperhidrosis (Khurana 1987). A variety of drugs are helpful (Krassioukov et al. 2010), and their actions are related to the postulated mechanisms responsible for autonomic dysreflexia (Table 66.4). Preventing afferent stimulation, for instance by the use of a local anaesthetic, such as lignocaine in the urinary bladder, can be effective. Drugs that act partially (reserpine) or entirely (spinal anaesthetics) on the spinal cord are particularly useful especially in severe episodes of dysreflexia. The ganglionic blocker, hexamethonium, was used successfully in the past but, like other drugs that reduce sympathetic efferent activity, is likely to cause profound postural hypotension. The α_2-adrenoceptor agonist, clonidine, does not lower supine blood pressure but reduces hypertension during autonomic dysreflexia (Mathias et al. 1979c). Drugs acting directly on blood vessels, such as glyceryl trinitrate and calcium-channel blockers, such as nifedipine (Thyberg et al. 1994), are also effective and have the advantage of being given sublingually. They also have the potential to cause severe hypotension (Fig. 66.18).

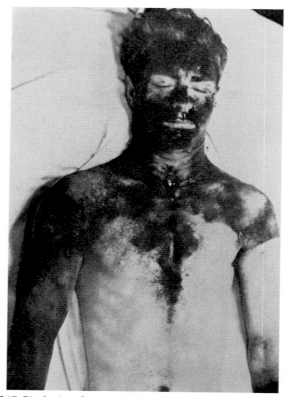

Fig. 66.17 Distribution of sweating, indicated by darker areas covered by quinizarine dye, in a tetraplegic patient during bladder distension. The band over the left arm indicates the site of the sphygmomanometer cuff. From Guttmann, L., Spinal cord injuries. *Comprehensive management and research* (2nd ed), Wiley.

Table 66.3 Causes of autonomic dysreflexia

Abdominal or pelvic visceral stimulation

- Ureter
- Calculus
- Urinary bladder
- Distension by blocked catheter or discoordinated bladder
- Infection
- Irritation by calculus, catheter, or bladder washout
- Rectum and anus
- Enemas
- Faecal retention
- Anal fissure
- Gastrointestinal organs
- Gastric dilatation
- Gastric ulceration
- Cholecystitis or cholelithiasis
- Uterus
- Contraction during pregnancy
- Menstruation, occasionally

Cutaneous stimulation

- Pressure sores
- Infected in-growing toenails
- Burns

Skeletal muscle spasms

- Especially in limbs with contractures

Miscellaneous

- Intrathecal neostigmine
- Electroejaculatory procedures
- Ejaculation
- Vaginal dilatation
- Urethra—insertion of catheter or abscess
- Fractures of bones

The α-adrenoceptor blockers theoretically should be highly effective in autonomic dysreflexia. Phenoxybenzamine, and the selective blockers prazosin and terazosin are useful in autonomic dysreflexia due to bladder outflow obstruction, as they relax the smooth muscle of the urinary sphincter (Chancellor et al. 1994). α-adrenoceptor blockers such as phentolamine may not prevent the paroxysmal surges in blood pressure during autonomic dysreflexia (Fig. 66.19). The reasons for this are unclear, but could include inadequate entry and disposition of the α-adrenoceptor blocker at postsynaptic sites, thus enabling the trans-synaptic actions of noradrenaline to continue. Furthermore, secretion from sympathetic nerve endings of non-adrenergic substances, such as NPY or adenosine triphosphate (ATP), can cause vasoconstriction during autonomic dysreflexia and are not affected by α-adrenoceptor blockers (Groothius et al. 2010). Preventing release, or depleting tissue levels of such substances, may explain

Table 66.4 Some of the drugs used in the management of autonomic dysreflexia classified according to their major site of action on the reflex arc and target organs

Afferent		Topical lignocaine
Spinal cord		Clonidine[a]
		Reserpine[a]
		Spinal anaesthetics
Efferent	Sympathetic ganglia	Hexamethonium
	Sympathetic nerve terminals	Guanethidine
	α-adrenoceptors	Phenoxybenzamine
Target organs	Blood vessels	Glyceryl trinitrate
		Nifedipine
	Sweat glands	Pro-Banthine®

[a] Clonidine and reserpine have multiple effects, some of which are peripheral.

the greater benefit provided by drugs such as reserpine and guanethidine in severe cases of dysreflexia, when other agents have failed.

In some patients, autonomic dysreflexia may be a major and recurring problem because of difficulty in either defining or resolving the precipitating cause. More unusual examples of the former are gastric ulceration or cholecystitis, which are difficult to detect because of lack of pain. A more common example, which may easily be missed, is an anal fissure. Despite recognizing the cause, it may be extremely difficult to resolve problems, which include severe skeletal muscle spasms or recurrent urinary bladder infection. Long-term drug therapy for autonomic dysreflexia in such patients is often only partially successful and may result in undesirable side-effects. In severe cases, surgical procedures on the spinal cord, such as rhizotomy and cordotomy, or peripheral procedures, such as sacral and hypogastric neurotomy, may need to be considered. Non-surgical approaches, such as a subarachnoid block with alcohol or phenol, have also been utilized. However, these procedures usually abolish spinal reflex activity and result in flaccidity of skeletal muscles and bladder and bowel atony, with their attendant disadvantages.

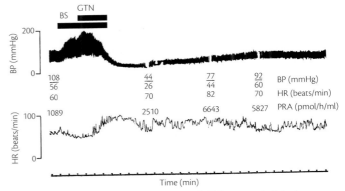

Fig. 66.18 Blood pressure (BP) and heart rate (HR) in a tetraplegic in the supine position before, during, and after bladder stimulation (BS) by suprapubic percussion of the anterior abdominal wall, which induces hypertension. Sublingual glyceryl trinitrate (GTN) (0.5 mg for 3.5 minutes) rapidly reverses the hypertension, elevates the heart rate, and then causes substantial hypotension. Levels of plasma renin activity (PRA) rise as a result of the fall in blood pressure. With permission from Mathias, C. J. and Frankel, H. L. (1988).

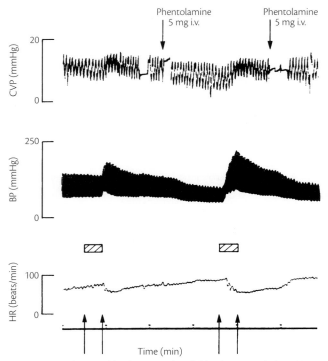

Fig. 66.19 Central venous blood pressure (CVP), blood pressure (BP), and heart rate (HR) in a tetraplegic patient undergoing electroejaculation with stimuli given per rectum over the seminal vesicles during the times indicated by arrows and hatched areas. The α-adrenoceptor blocker phentolamine, even after a total close of 10 mg, did not suppress the paroxysmal rise in blood pressure during stimulation when reassessed latter (not shown in figure).

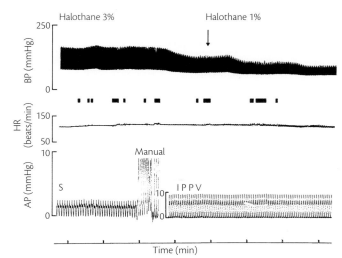

Fig. 66.20 Changes in blood pressure (BP) and heart rate (HR) of a chronic tetraplegic patient undergoing transurethral resection. The dark blocks indicate where resection and diathermy were performed. Airway pressure (AP) is also indicated when the patient was breathing spontaneously, was manually ventilated, and no intermittent positive pressure ventilation (IPPV). The blood pressure has been satisfactorily controlled on 3% halothane. Increasing airway pressure reduces blood pressure and enables the use of a lower concentration of halothane (1%), which successfully maintains the blood pressure during operative procedures that would otherwise greatly elevate it. Reprinted by permission from Macmillan Publishers Ltd: *Paraplegia*, Welply et al., copyright 1975.

Autonomic dysreflexia can be a particular problem during surgery, especially if the urinary bladder or the large bowel is involved. In these patients either spinal anaesthesia or a general anaesthetic, such as halothane, along with an increase in positive pressure ventilation, is often successful in controlling the hypertension (Fig. 66.20). Short-acting ganglionic blockers, such as trimethaphan, have been used successfully during surgery. The management of autonomic dysreflexia during pregnancy is discussed later.

Tracheal stimulation and intubation

Recently injured tetraplegics with high cervical lesions involving spinal segments that supply the phrenic nerves are dependent on artificial respiration because of diaphragmatic paralysis. In these patients bradycardia and cardiac arrest may occur during tracheal suction, especially when they are hypoxic (Fig. 66.21). The bradycardia is effectively prevented by atropine, which confirms the role of vagal efferent pathways in the response. The mechanisms by which tracheal suction and hypoxia contribute to bradycardia in these patients are outlined in Table 66.5. These stimuli activate vagal and glossopharyngeal afferents that increase vagal efferent activity. This is opposed by a number of factors, including the pulmonary inflation vagal reflex, which normally raises heart rate, as is observed in spontaneously breathing tetraplegics when exposed either to hypoxia or to tracheal suction (Fig. 66.22). Other factors include the inability to activate sympathetic nerves, which are normally stimulated by tracheal suction or hypoxia.

The management of bradycardia and cardiac arrest during tracheal suction is directly related to knowledge of the mechanisms involved. Reconnecting the patient to the respirator will

activate the pulmonary inflation vagal reflex, and the addition of oxygen will reverse hypoxia. External cardiac massage may be needed, along with intravenous atropine. Precipitant factors often include respiratory infection and pulmonary emboli. Both cause hypoxia, which initially may be difficult to reverse. Such patients may need maintenance atropine, in a dose of 0.3 mg or 0.6 mg either subcutaneously or intramuscularly at 4-hourly intervals. Parasympathomimetic agents such as neostigmine and carbachol, which reverse bladder and bowel atony in spinal shock, should be avoided or used with caution. Heart rate may be increased also by the use of β-adrenoceptor agonists, but drugs such as isoprenaline also have actions on vasodilatatory β₂-adrenoceptors, which may lower blood pressure further, as in chronic tetraplegics (Chapter 22). Temporary demand pacemakers have also been used.

In chronic tetraplegics, bradycardia and cardiac arrest may also occur when the trachea is stimulated while respiration is prevented, despite the potential presence of opposing sympathetic cardiac reflexes operating at a spinal level. This may occur during endotracheal intubation after the use of skeletal muscle relaxants such as suxamethonium (Fig. 66.23). The mechanisms of this vagal reflex appear to be similar to those described in recently injured tetraplegics, with afferent vagal stimulation causing an increase in vagal efferent activity that is not opposed by the pulmonary inflation reflex because of respiratory paralysis. An important practical point is to administer an adequate amount of atropine prior to intubation, especially in patients who are at greater risk from autonomic dysreflexia and increased cardiac vagal activity, such as during urological surgery.

Food ingestion

In tetraplegics, unlike patients with chronic primary autonomic failure (Chapter 28), ingestion of either a balanced meal, an equivalent liquid meal (Baliga et al. 1997), or an isocaloric solution of

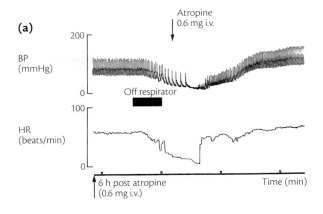

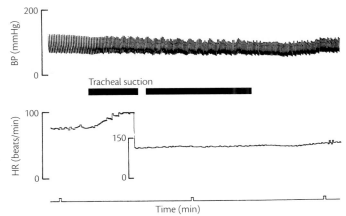

Fig. 66.22 Effect of tracheal suction on blood pressure (BP) and heart rate (HR) of a chronic tetraplegic patient 7 months after injury when he had recovered spontaneous respiration and isolated reflex spinal cord sympathetic activity. Tracheal suction performed through an indwelling tracheostomy tube caused hyperventilation, tachycardia, and a fall in blood pressure. The heart rate scale alters as shown. With kind permission from Springer Science+Business Media: *Eur. J. Intensive Care Med.*, Bradycardia and cardiac arrest during tracheal suction mechanisms in tetraplegic patients, **2**, 1976, 147–56, Mathias, C. J.

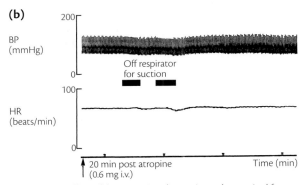

Fig. 66.21 (a) The effect of disconnecting the respirator (as required for aspirating the airways) on the blood pressure (BP) and heart rate (HR) of a recently injured tetraplegic patient (C4/5 lesion) in spinal shock, 6 hours after the last dose of intravenous atropine. Sinus bradycardia and cardiac arrest (also observed on the electrocardiograph) were reversed by reconnection, intravenous atropine, and external cardiac massage. From Frankel et al. 1975, with permission. **(b)** The effect of tracheal suction, 20 minutes after atrophine. Disconnection from the respirator and tracheal suction did not lower either heart rate or blood pressure. With kind permission from Springer Science+Business Media: *Eur. J. Intensive Care Med.*, Bradycardia and cardiac arrest during tracheal suction mechanisms in tetraplegic patients, **2**, 1976, 147–56, Mathias, C. J.

glucose does not result in a substantial fall in supine blood pressure. The modest fall in blood pressure is accompanied by an elevation in heart rate. Levels of forearm venous plasma noradrenaline do not change, excluding a generalized increase in sympathetic nerve activity. The mechanisms responsible for preventing a substantial fall in blood pressure in tetraplegics are unclear; these could include the stimulation of reflexes from the gastrointestinal tract and mesentery (Chapter 28).

Hypoglycaemia

In normal individuals, hypoglycaemia results in a marked rise in plasma adrenaline levels and a modest rise in plasma noradrenaline levels. The clinical manifestations include anxiety, tremulousness,

Table 66.5 The major mechanisms contributing to bradycardia and cardiac arrest in recently injured tetraplegics in spinal shock during tracheal suction and hypoxia

	Tracheal suction	**Hypoxia**
Normal	Increased sympathetic nervous activity causes tachycardia and raises blood pressure	Bradycardia is the primary response opposed by the pulmonary (inflation) vagal reflex, resulting in tachycardia
Tetraplegics	No increase in sympathetic nervous activity, therefore no rise in heart rate or blood pressure. Vagal afferent stimulation may lead to unopposed vagal efferent activity	The primary response, bradycardia, is not opposed by the pulmonary (inflation) vagal reflex, because of disconnection from respirator or 'fixed' respiratory rate
	↘	↙
	Increased vagal cardiac tone	
	↓	
	Bradycardia and cardiac arrest	

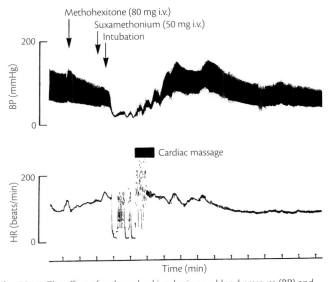

Fig. 66.23 The effect of endotracheal intubation on blood pressure (BP) and heart rate (HR) of a chronic tetraplegic patient being anaesthetized for urological surgery. Intubation was followed by cardiac arrest, which was reversed by oxygen and external cardiac massage. Reprinted by permission from Macmillan Publishers Ltd: *Paraplegia*, Welply et al., copyright 1975.

hunger, sweating, and tachycardia. There is little change in mean blood pressure as systolic blood pressure often rises and there is a small fall in diastolic blood pressure. Microneurography studies indicate that both muscle and skin sympathetic nerve activity increase during insulin hypoglycaemia, indicating that the response in normal individuals is not entirely due to adrenal stimulation and release of adrenaline. Similar or even greater increases in integrated muscle sympathetic nerve activity occur in adrenalectomized patients, in whom there is no rise in plasma adrenaline levels (Chapter 22). In tetraplegics, insulin-induced hypoglycaemia does not raise levels of plasma adrenaline or noradrenaline (Fig. 66.24). There is a fall in systolic blood pressure, along with a rise in heart rate. There are no symptoms of hypoglycaemia except for sedation, which is readily reversed with intravenous hypertonic glucose. If rapidly injected, however, this may cause a marked fall in blood pressure, as has been observed in patients with primary autonomic failure (Chapter 28). The symptoms accompanying hypoglycaemia in normal individuals, therefore, appear to be largely dependent upon an elevation in adrenaline levels and intact sympathetic nervous pathways. In tetraplegics and high thoracic lesions, the lack of warning signs accompanying neuroglycopenia are similar to observations made in some patients with diabetes mellitus and complicating autonomic neuropathy, or patients on non-selective β-adrenergic blockers.

Cardiovascular responses to pharmacological stimuli

Centrally acting agents—clonidine

Clonidine is an α_2-adrenoceptor agonist, which has a number of actions that include cerebral effects, predominantly on the brainstem.

In normal individuals this results in a withdrawal of sympathetic tone and a fall in blood pressure. Effects on the medullary vagal centres result in a fall in heart rate. In tetraplegics, intravenous clonidine (150 μg) transiently raises blood pressure, consistent with its peripheral agonist effects on postsynaptic α_1 and α_2-adrenoceptors. Neither intravenous (150 μg) nor oral (300 μg) clonidine lowers supine basal levels of blood pressure in tetraplegics (Fig. 66.25a) because of the disruption of descending sympathetic pathways. The heart rate, however, falls, in keeping with its vagal effects. Clonidine has additional effects, either on sympathetic neurones within the spinal cord or on peripheral presynaptic α_2-adrenoceptors which inhibit noradrenaline release. These may explain its partial ability to prevent hypertension during autonomic dysreflexia, as demonstrated during bladder stimulation (Fig. 66.25b) (Mathias et al. 1979c). Clonidine is also able to

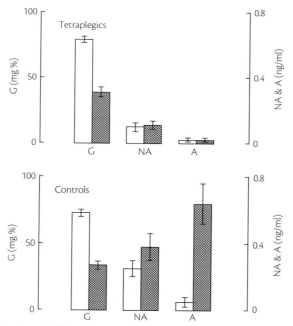

Fig. 66.24 Levels of blood glucose (G), plasma noradrenaline (NA), and adrenaline (A) before (blank histograms) and during (hatched histograms) insulin-induced hypoglycaemia in chronic tetraplegics (upper panel) and normal subjects (controls, lower panel). In the controls hypoglycaemia caused a small rise in plasma noradrenaline and a marked elevation in plasma adrenaline levels. A similar degree of hypoglycaemia did not change the low plasma noradrenaline and adrenaline levels in the tetraplegics. The bars indicate ± SEM. Reprinted by permission from Macmillan Publishers Ltd: *Spinal Cord*, Mathias et al., copyright 1979.

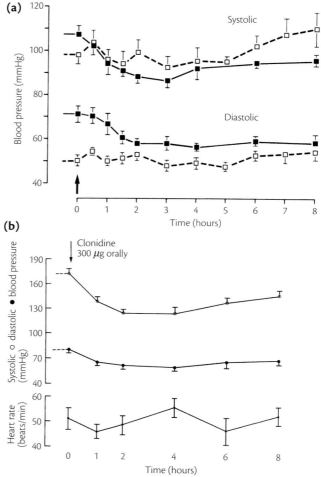

Fig. 66.25 (a) The effect of 300 g of oral clonidine (at time 0, arrow) on systolic and diastolic blood pressure of normal subjects (filled squares, continuous line) and chronic tetraplegics (open squares, dashed line). There is a substantial fall in both systolic and diastolic blood pressure in the normal subjects but no fall in blood pressure in the tetraplegics. The bar indicate ± SEM. Reprinted by permission from Macmillan Publishers Ltd: *Clin. Pharmacol. Therapeut.* (Reid et al.), copyright 1977. **(b)** Systolic and diastolic blood pressure and heart rate recorded at the end of 3 minutes of bladder stimulation in a group of chronic tetraplegics before and after 300 μg of clonidine. There is a marked attenuation of the pressor response, with the largest reductions in the second and fourth hours. Effects persist even 8 hours after clonidine. The bars indicate ± SEM.

reduce muscle spasticity and pain, as has been demonstrated also with intrathecal administration (Middleton et al. 1996). These actions may explain its value in the management of autonomic dysreflexia in high spinal-cord lesions.

Peripherally acting vasopressor agents

An increased pressor response to intravenously infused noradrenaline occurs in both recently injured and chronic tetraplegics (Fig. 66.26). This was originally considered to be a clinical manifestation of denervation hypersensitivity, as relating to Canon's law that denervated organs are supersensitive to their neurotransmitter. In classical denervation hypersensitivity, however, impairment of function of postganglionic sympathetic nerve terminals results in reduction in the neuronal uptake of noradrenaline. This inability to clear noradrenaline increases its synaptic concentration and results in a greater target organ response. In tetraplegics, however, there is histochemical evidence of intact adrenergic nerve terminals (Norberg and Normell 1974) and functional evidence during autonomic dysreflexia (as based on the rise in plasma noradrenaline, blood pressure, reflex increase in resistance and capacitance vessels, and increase noradrenaline spillover) of the integrity of postganglionic sympathetic nerves. Circulating levels of noradrenaline in tetraplegics and normal subjects are similar after identical intravenous infusions of noradrenaline, although the pressor responses are markedly different (Mathias et al. 1976c). Impaired clearance

and higher levels of noradrenaline thus do not appear to account for the increased pressor responses in tetraplegics.

The lesion in tetraplegics and high thoracic lesions is effectively preganglionic, which is more proximal to the experimental lesions of immediately preganglionic nerves that also can cause an enhanced response to noradrenaline (decentralization hypersensitivity). This is thought to be due to an increase in receptor population, an improvement of the functional link between receptor activation and the final response, or both factors. Although tetraplegics have a low background level of sympathetic activity, this is punctuated by repeated episodes of autonomic dysreflexia, which ensure that sympathetic nerve terminals and receptors and target organs are intermittently kept active and stimulated. There is indirect evidence, based on *in vitro* studies of platelet α_2-adrenoceptor binding, that tetraplegics have a normal population of α-adrenoceptors (Davies et al. 1982). Microneurography studies, however, indicate a modest increase in muscle sympathetic nerve activity during autonomic dysreflexia when there is a pronounced vascular response (Stjernberg et al. 1986), suggesting that decentralization supersensitivity, for reasons that are currently unclear, may contribute to the enhanced pressor response to noradrenaline.

A further possibility includes the impairment of baroreflex pathways that descend through the cervical spinal cord and are normally concerned with buffering a rise in blood pressure. This would explain the elevated pressor response during autonomic dysreflexia and the clearly defined relationship between these hypertensive responses and the segmental level of the lesion at T5. In normal subjects it is likely that, despite a substantial rise in sympathoneural activity induced by a range of stimuli, blood pressure is maintained at near normal levels by efferent baroreflex activity, partly through the vagal efferents and predominantly by descending nerve tracts within the spinal cord, which selectively inhibit sympathetic vasoconstrictor activity, and may even cause vasodilatation by mechanisms that are yet to be clearly defined in humans. The only intact efferent component of the baroreflex pathways in tetraplegics is the vagal outflow; this slows the heart but is clearly inadequate in controlling the rise in blood pressure during autonomic dysreflexia. It is possible, therefore, that the absence of blood pressure restraining reflexes descending through the cervical and upper thoracic spinal cord down to the level of T5 may be a major factor accounting for the enhanced pressor responses to noradrenaline. This may also explain the observations that exaggerated pressor responses are not specific to α-adrenoceptor agonists but occur in response to agents with different structures and properties, ranging from phenylephrine to prostaglandin $F_{2\alpha}$, and angiotensin II. The low circulating levels of adrenaline and noradrenaline may not be major contributory factors, as there is a similar degree of pressor sensitivity to angiotensin II (Fig. 66.27), despite normal or elevated circulating levels of renin and angiotensin II. This argues strongly against receptor up-regulation alone being a factor.

The enhanced responses to pressor agents are of clinical importance, as the five to tenfold increase in sensitivity should be borne in mind if drugs with pressor actions are used in high spinal lesions.

Peripherally acting vasodepressor agents

Enhanced depressor responses to a range of vasodilatory substances also occur in high spinal-cord lesions. Bolus injections and intravenous infusion of isoprenaline lower blood pressure

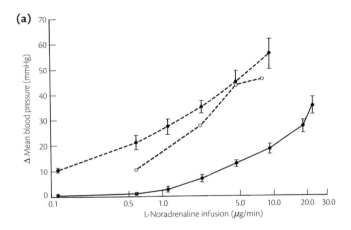

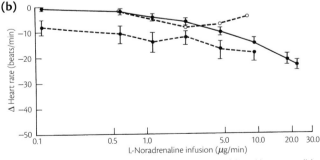

Fig. 66.26 Changes (Δ) in average mean blood pressure (a) and heart rate (b) during different dose infusion rates of noradrenaline in three recently injured tetraplegics (open circles, dashed line), five chronic tetraplegics (filled circles, dashed line), and 10 control subjects (filled circles, continuous line). The bars indicate ± SEM. There is an enhanced pressor response to noradrenaline in both groups of tetraplegics over the entire dose range studied. From Mathias et al. 1976c, 1979a, with permission.

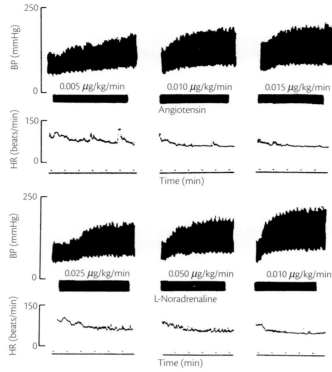

Fig. 66.27 Blood pressure (BP) and heart rate (HR) effects of different dose infusion rates of angiotensin II (upper panels) and L-noradrenaline (lower panels) given intravenously to a chronic tetraplegic patient. These doses of angiotensin II and noradrenaline cause only small blood pressure changes in normal subjects. With permission from *J. Autonom. Nerv. Syst. Suppl.*, Mathias, C. J., Frankel, H. L., The neurological and hormonal control of blood vessels and heart in spinal man, 457–64, Copyright Elsevier 1986.

substantially (Chapter 22). Indirect evidence from *in vitro* β-adrenoceptor binding studies on lymphocytes exclude up-regulation of these receptors. In high lesions isoprenaline will stimulate both β_1- and β_2-adrenoceptors; it is likely that stimulation of the latter causes vasodilatation which would normally stimulate the baroreflex pathways, increase sympathetic activity, and prevent a substantial fall in blood pressure. This would not occur in high lesions and may account for the fall in blood pressure. The increase in heart rate, which is often exaggerated, is likely to be a combination of the vagal response to the fall in blood pressure and the direct β_1 effects of isoprenaline.

Enhanced vasodepressor responses occur to a variety of drugs, including intravenous prostaglandin E2 and sublingual glyceryl trinitrate and nifedipine. The last two may be used to advantage in high lesions, as they can be taken readily and can substantially lower blood pressure in autonomic dysreflexia. The risk of extreme hypotension should be kept in mind (Fig. 66.18).

Cutaneous circulation

The skin is innervated by the sympathetic nervous system and changes may occur both in recently injured and in chronic tetraplegics. Soon after injury there is often vasodilatation in the periphery, as the skin below the level of the lesion is often warmer and veins appear dilated. It is not clear whether this may lead to extravasation of fluid into subcutaneous tissue and contribute to skin breakdown and pressure sores, which is a major problem in recently

injured patients. The vasodilatation may also involve mucosal tissues such as the nose, and result in nasal congestion, a problem seen in patients with high lesions who often have to breathe through their mouth. This has been referred to as Guttmann's sign, and is similar to the nasal vasodilatation after α-adrenoceptor blockade induced by either phenoxybenzamine or guanethidine, both previously used in the management of patients with hypertension.

The cutaneous Lewis or triple response varies in the different stages. In the stage of spinal shock, responses above and below the lesion are similar. This differs from the later phases, with return of isolated spinal-cord reflex activity, when stimulation of skin below the lesion results in cutaneous vasoconstriction, leading to skin pallor which may last for a prolonged period—hence the term 'dermatographia alba', as compared to 'dermatographia rubra' in the stage of spinal shock. In chronic high lesions, autonomic dysreflexia may result in marked constriction of cutaneous blood vessels (causing cold peripheries; poikilothermia spinalis) and activation of piloerector muscles (causing goose skin and pimples; cutis anserina) below the level of the lesion.

Thermoregulation

The autonomic nervous system plays an important role in the regulation of body temperature, which may be seriously deranged in tetraplegics.

Hypothermia

On exposure to cold a number of mechanisms are activated, which are dependent initially on appreciation of the temperature change and then on the ability to increase heat production and gain. Cold appreciation is dependent upon activation of both cutaneous and also central temperature receptors, which may explain why tetraplegics, although they have only a limited area of intact sensation, can still detect body cooling.

One of the major mechanisms responsible for heat production is shivering thermogenesis, which depends upon activation of skeletal muscles and shivering. In tetraplegics and those with high thoracic spinal cord lesions, a major proportion of skeletal muscle mass is not directly under voluntary control; this is a particular problem in spinal shock when there is skeletal muscle flaccidity. Hypothermia may therefore readily occur in such patients, as it does in other groups without autonomic lesions who have extensive paralysis either due to drugs or to poliomyelitis (Fig. 66.28). Tetraplegics and those with high thoracic lesions have the ability to shiver in innervated areas as the body temperature falls, but this often results only in a small increase in metabolism which, dependent upon the external temperature, may be inadequate for body temperature homeostasis. An additional problem in recently injured tetraplegics in spinal shock is cutaneous vasodilatation, and the inability to appropriately vasocon- strict. This enhances heat loss, lowers body temperature further, and can be a particular problem in causing hypothermia especially in temperate climates (Fig. 66.29). A low-reading rectal thermometer is essential in the assessment and management of hypothermia. The patient should be warmed, externally with care taken to prevent skin damage, and internally using warm drinks or infusion of warm saline. Drugs (including alcohol), which cause cutaneous vasodilatation and increase heat loss therefore should be strictly avoided.

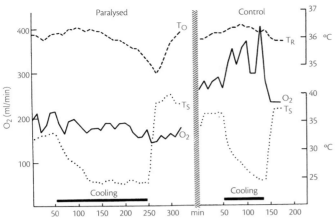

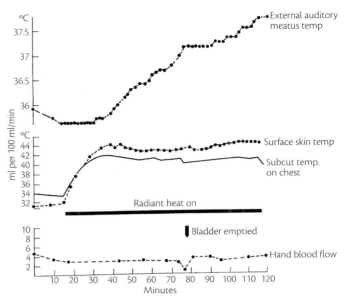

Fig. 66.28 The effect of body cooling on oesophageal (T_o), rectal (T_R), and skin (T_s) temperature and oxygen consumption (O_2) of a severely paralysed patient with poliomyelitis and a normal subject (control). The lack of shivering in the patient causes no rise in oxygen consumption and heat production, which leads to a fall in central temperature, unlike the normal subject. With permission from Johnson, R. H., Smith, A. C. and Spalding, J. M. K., Oxygen consumption of paralysed men exposed to cold, *J. Physiol.*, Wiley.

Fig. 66.30 Pronounced rise in both skin and core temperature (measured as external auditory meatus temperature) during application of radiant heat to the trunk of a tetraplegic patient. Hand blood flow does not rise, indicating lack of vasodilatation, as would occur normally during an elevation in temperature. From Johnson 1965, with permission.

Hyperthermia

Hyperthermia may occur particularly in tetraplegics and high spinal-cord lesions when environmental temperature is elevated, or in response to infection. Heat loss is dependent on two major mechanisms, vasodilatation and sweating, both of which are impaired in spinal lesions (Price 2006). Vasodilatation normally occurs during warming, and is dependent on a rise in central temperature. It may occur passively as a result of withdrawal of sympathetic vasoconstrictor tone, or actively. Both components are dependent on neural pathways within the cervical spinal cord, which are involved in high spinal-cord lesions (Fig. 66.30). Vasodilatation may also occur following application of radiant or

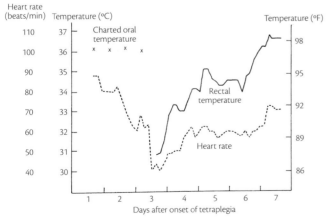

Fig. 66.29 Fall in central temperature (measured as rectal temperature) and heart rate in a recently injured tetraplegic in a temperate climate. Hypothermia is best monitored with a low-reading rectal thermometer and as indicated, may be missed if oral temperature is recorded. Reproduced with permission and copyright © of the British Editorial Society of Bone and Joint Surgery, Pledger HG. Disorders of temperature regulation in acute traumatic tetraplegia. *J Bone Joint Surg [Br]* 1962;**44**-B:110–13 (Figure 1).

local heat to tetraplegics; this is more likely to be a direct effect than due to reflexes via the isolated spinal cord.

Sweating normally causes heat loss by evaporation, and is dependent upon a rise in central temperature and activation of sudomotor fibres within the sympathetic nervous system. Thermoregulatory sweating in large areas below the lesion is impaired in high spinal lesions, and is a further reason for these patients being prone to hyperthermia. The sympathetic skin response (SSR), a technique that records neurogenic activation of sweat glands, is abnormal in spinal injuries, depending on the level of lesion (Cariga et al. 2002). Activation of supraspinal centres and descending sudomotor neural pathways in the spinal cord are necessary for the SSR, which is absent in the plantar region in low injuries, and absent in the palmar region in high spinal injuries. Importantly, the presence or absence of the SSR can be a useful marker of spinal cord autonomic involvement, in addition to motor and sensory evaluation, and may improve classification of the extent of spinal functional deficits (Nicotra et al. 2005). The studies also exclude spinal cord sudomotor centres, isolated from the brain stem, that are capable of generating an SSR (Cariga et al. 2002).

The maintenance of a suitable environmental temperature is of importance in the prevention of hyperthermia in high spinal lesions. When hyperthermia occurs, cooling with the aid of tepid sponging and increased airflow with a fan accelerates heat loss by a combination of evaporation, conduction, and convection. In severe cases, ice-cooled saline by intravenous infusion or urinary bladder irrigation and in extreme cases immersion of the whole body in an ice bath may be necessary. In hyperpyrexia associated with infection, drugs such as aspirin and paracetamol appear to be effective in lowering body temperature. The mechanisms by which they do this are unclear. Chlorpromazine is also effective, but has the potential to induce hypotension.

Gastrointestinal system

The autonomic nervous system richly innervates the gastrointestinal tract which is often affected especially in the early stages, after spinal cord lesions.

Upper gastrointestinal bleeding

There is a high incidence of upper gastrointestinal bleeding in the early stages following spinal-cord injury. The incidence is greater in those with higher lesions. It is often unrelated to a previous history of peptic ulceration and may not be related to concomitant drug therapy, such as dexamethasone and analgesics. In such patients there is evidence of increased vagal activity, which may cause hyperacidity, along with high gastrin levels which also may contribute to gastric hypersecretion and ulceration.

The lesions may be either patchy or extensive and affect the oesophagus, stomach, or the duodenum. Erosions and ulceration may occur. Abdominal pain is usually absent. Shoulder-tip pain, accentuated by abdominal palpation, may indicate perforation. Autonomic dysreflexia may occur (Bar-On and Ohry 1995). There may be haematemesis or melaena. Fibreoptic endoscopy is probably the investigation of choice, the major limitation being the restriction to cervical spine mobility. Atropine may be needed to prevent vagal reflexes and bradycardia. The management consists of the administration of H_2 receptor antagonists (such as cimetidine or ranitidine), antacids, and fluid and blood replacement where relevant. The role of newer drugs such as omeprazole and orally active prostaglandin analogues, has not been clearly defined. Occasionally, surgery may be needed.

Paralytic ileus

This often occurs in spinal shock and may be accompanied by gastric dilatation. The mechanisms remain unclear as the motor innervation of the stomach and small intestines is by the vagus nerves, which are intact and often hyperactive in this phase. Paralytic ileus usually occurs a few days after injury and may be induced by solid food, which should therefore be avoided in the immediate period following a cervical or high thoracic SCI.

Paralytic ileus results in meteorism, which is a particular problem as it interferes with the movement of the diaphragm, often the only major functional muscle of respiration in these patients. It may be particularly prolonged in patients with intercurrent infection. The management consists of gastrointestinal aspiration to prevent further dilatation, the administration of intravenous fluids, and, if necessary, intravenous alimentation. Parasympathomimetic agents such as neostigmine are occasionally used to activate the bowel but carry the risk of potentiating bradycardia and cardiac arrest, especially in patients with high cervical lesions on artificial respiration. The dopamine antagonist, metoclopramide, which enhances gastric emptying, may be of value in some cases. It may be that newer drugs that increase gastrointestinal motility, such as the prodrug, cisapride and the cholecystokinin antagonist, loxeglumide, will be of value. Once spinal shock has subsided small intestine function often returns to normal. Tetraplegics and high thoracic lesions are, however, prone to paralytic ileus even in the chronic stage, especially after undergoing general anaesthesia and abdominal surgery.

Large bowel dysfunction

In spinal shock, paralysis of the sacral parasympathetic results in atony of the colon and rectum. Voluntary or reflexly induced defecation does not occur and this results in faecal retention. Digital evacuation is often necessary in the early stages.

After the stage of spinal shock, autonomous function of the lower bowel returns and is regulated at a spinal level, as it is abolished by intrathecal block with alcohol. The stimulus to bowel activity appears to be increased volume and distension, which then causes relaxation of the external anal sphincter and evacuation of contents. This stimulus is utilized in the reconditioning of lower bowel function. Adequate training, together with the use of an appropriate diet, e.g. high residue foods, mild laxatives and stool softeners may be needed to ensure regular bowel evacuation (Chung and Emmanuel 2006). This is an important part of the management, as regular bowel movement prevents faecal retention, which predisposes patients with high lesions to autonomic dysreflexia for a variety of reasons. These include distension of the lower bowel and the predisposition to haemorrhoids and anal fissures.

Urinary system

Function of the urinary bladder is dependent upon higher centres in the brain and the sympathetic and parasympathetic nerves, and is therefore affected in varying degrees in patients with spinal cord lesions. In the chronic stage complications to the ureters and kidneys, such as infection, calculi, urinary reflux, hydroureters, and hydronephrosis, may lead to renal damage, resulting in chronic renal failure, which largely stems from this basic dysfunction.

In spinal shock there is usually complete paralysis of bladder function with retention of urine followed by distension and urinary overflow after excessive intravesical pressure has developed. This should be avoided, as it often impedes functional return of detrusor muscle activity once spinal shock has subsided. Bladder paralysis is invariable in most adult Europeans, but does not usually occur in children and adult Afro-Caribbeans. The management in spinal shock consists of drainage using an indwelling catheter, or preferably intermittent catheterization, which causes fewer complications.

With the return of parasympathetic activity within the isolated sacral cord, there is detrusor muscle contraction, which occurs in response to filling of the urinary bladder, or following stimuli such as tapping of the anterior abdominal wall suprapubically. This is the automatic reflex bladder, or neurogenic bladder. During detrusor contraction there is a need for simultaneous relaxation of the sphincters and pelvic floor to allow the free passage of urine. Training is needed to achieve coordination of these components of bladder function, and if this is successful male patients may be catheter-free, using a condom and receptacle to collect urine. In some patients, however, detrusor contraction is not accompanied by simultaneous relaxation of the bladder outlet, and in high lesions the resultant discoordinated bladder can cause marked autonomic dysreflexia. Retained urine often results in infection, which can involve the kidneys, especially when there is retrograde pressure in the urinary tract. In such patients an indwelling catheter, or various forms of urological and neurological surgery (Hohenfellner et al. 1996), may be needed to relieve the functional obstruction and prevent autonomic dysreflexia. The α-adrenoceptor blockers, phenoxybenzamine and prazosin, may be of value in some patients as the bladder outlet is relaxed. In low lesions there may be a flaccid bladder even in the chronic stage. Manual compression using Credé's manoeuvre is needed to ensure complete emptying, along with the other aids for urine collection.

In female patients, the bladder can be trained to empty in response to distension and external stimuli. Because of the lack of suitable collecting systems, there may be incontinence, which is often not helped by an indwelling catheter. In some, an ileal conduit may be the most practical outcome.

Reproductive system

In the male reproduction and sexual function is dependent on the interrelationship between parasympathetic and sympathetic nerve function and therefore is usually impaired. Few changes occur in the female with SCI.

Male

Penile erection is dependent largely upon the sacral parasympathetic nerves with ejaculation dependent upon the sympathetic nerves. In spinal shock there is an absence of both erectile and ejaculatory function. In some patients, however, passive penile enlargement and priapism may occur, probably due to paralytic dilatation resulting in engorgement of the corpora cavernosa. Following the return of isolated spinal cord reflex activity, penile erection may occur if the glans penis is stimulated, or as part of autonomic dysreflexia. Ejaculation, however, seldom occurs per urethra and is usually retrograde, as the associated contraction of muscles at the bladder neck which prevents seminal fluid flowing back into the bladder does not usually occur. In spinal-cord injuries, therefore, procreation in the male is largely dependent on the collection of seminal fluid for artificial insemination using various approaches (Consortium for Spinal Cord Medicine 2010). The original technique involved intrathecal neostigmine which caused skeletal muscle depression followed by penile erection and ejaculation. In high lesions, side-effects such as vomiting and severe autonomic dysreflexia often occurred, and in one patient this resulted in cerebral haemorrhage and death. In addition to vibrator techniques, electroejaculation also is used, although this may result in severe hypertension, and careful monitoring of blood pressure is necessary in those with high lesions, especially when seminal emission occurs. Many of the drugs that are often used to lower blood pressure in autonomic dysreflexia are not the ideal ones to use during such procedures as they interrupt sympathetic pathways and have the potential to interfere with ejaculation. The phosphodiesterase inhibitor sildenafil (Viagra) is an effectively used drug in spinal injuries; whether it also lowers blood pressure excessively, as it does in other groups with autonomic failure, such as multiple system atrophy, is not known (Hussain et al. 2001).

Female

In women transient disruption of the menstrual cycle is often observed after spinal lesions, as occurs during other traumatic conditions or illnesses. There is usually a return to normal menstrual periods within a year. Successful pregnancies have been reported in both tetraplegics and paraplegics. In those with high lesions a particular problem is severe autonomic dysreflexia and paroxysmal hypertension (Fig. 66.31) which may be accompanied by cardiac dysrhythmias, especially during uterine contractions. Such patients are particularly prone to epileptic seizures and cerebral haemorrhage and it is essential to lower their blood pressure. Anticonvulsants such as phenytoin may be needed. Spinal anaesthesia appears to be a satisfactory method of preventing the hypertension without interfering with uterine contraction. This often

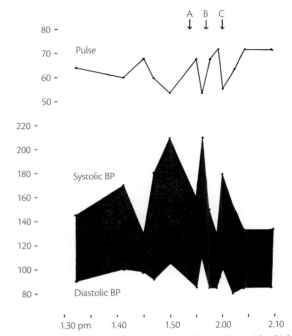

Fig. 66.31 Blood pressure and pulse rate in a paraplegic patient with a high thoracic lesion (T5) during (A) application of forceps, (B) completion of delivery, and (C) placental delivery. The hypertension is closely followed by bradycardia. Reprinted by permission from Macmillan Publishers Ltd: Nature Publishing Group, Guttmann, Frankel and Paeslack, copyright 1965.

allows progression of a normal delivery and avoids a Caesarean section.

Rehabilitation interventions

Recent developments in clinical practice and scientific research have led to interventions that may facilitate recovery from SCI (Ellaway et al. 2004). Functional recovery from SCI could be achieved by interventions that re-innervate disconnected systems or promote the natural plasticity of the central nervous system to facilitate the actions of surviving neurons that have retained axonal connections with their targets (Ellaway et al. 2011). Interventions to produce functional improvements in SCI include repetitive transcranial magnetic stimulation to the motor cortex (Belci et al. 2004), tele-rehabilitation using functional electrical stimulation together with exercise and weight-assisted treadmill walking therapy (Popovic et al. 2006, Dobkin et al. 2007), which result in improved functional outcome of upper limb function and changes to sensorimotor systems.

References

Arnold, J. M., Feng, Q. P., Delaney, G. A., and Teasell, R. W. (1995). Autonomic dysreflexia in tetraplegic patients: evidence for alpha-adrenoceptor hyper-responsiveness. *Clin. Auton Res.* **5**, 267–70.

Belci, M., Catley, M., Husain, M., Frankel, H. L. and Davey, N. J. (2004). Magnetic brain stimulation can improve clinical outcome in incomplete spinal cord injured patients. *Spinal Cord.* **4**, 417–9.

Baliga, R. R., Catz, A. B., Watson, L. P., Short, D. J., Frankel, H. L., and Mathias, C. J. (1997). Cardiovascular and hormonal responses to food ingestion in humans with spinal cord transection. *Clin. Auton Res.* **7**, 137–41.

Bar-On, Z. and Ohry, A. (1995). The acute abdomen in SCI individuals. *Paraplegia* 33, 704–6.

Burton, A. R., Brown, R., Macefield, V. G. (2008). Selective activation of muscle and skin nociceptors does not trigger exaggerated sympathetic responses in spinal-injured subjects. *Spinal Cord.* 46, 660–65.

Cariga P., Catley, M., Savic, G., Frankel, H. L., Mathias, C. J., Ellaway, P. H. (2002). Organisation of the sympathetic skin response in SCI. *J Neurol. Neurosurg. Psychiatry* 72, 356–60.

Chancellor, M. B., Erhard, M. J., Hirsch, I. H., and Stass, W. E. (1994). Prospective evaluation of terazosin for the treatment of autonomic dysreflexia. *J. Urol.* 151, 111–13.

Chelvarajah, E. (2009). Orthostatic hypotension following SCI: Impact on the use of standing apparatus. *NeuroRehabilitation.* 24:3, 237–42.

Chung, E. A., Emmanuel, A. V. (2006). Gastrointestinal symptoms related to autonomic dysfunction following SCI. *Prog Brain Res.* 152, 317–33.

Claydon, V. E., Steeves, J. D. and Krassioukov, A. (2006). Orthostatic hypotension following SCI: understanding clinical pathophysiology. *Spinal Cord*, 44, 341–51.

Consortium for Spinal Cord Medicine. (2010). Sexuality and reproductive health in adults with SCI: a clinical practice guideline for health-care professionals. *J Spinal Cord Med.* 33, 281–336.

Corbett, J. L., Frankel, H. L., and Harris, P. J. (1971). Cardio-vascular reflex responses to cutaneous and visceral stimuli in spinal man. *J. Physiol.* 215, 395.

Curt, A., Nitsche, B., Rodic, B., Schurch, B., and Dietz, V. (1997). Assessment of autonomic dysreflexia in patients with SCI. *J. Neurol. Neurosurg. Psychiat.* 62, 473–7.

Curt, A., Weinhardt, C., and Dietz, V. (1996). Significance of sympathetic skin response in the assessment of autonomic failure in patients with spinal injury. *J. Autonom. Nerv. Sys.* 61, 175–80.

Davies, I. B., Mathias, C. J., Sudera, D., and Sever, P. S. (1982). Agonist regulation of alpha-adrenergic receptor responses in man. *J. Cardiovasc. Pharmacol.* 4, s139–44.

Ditunno, J. F., Little, J. W., Tessler, A., Burns, A. S. (2004). Spinal shock revisited: a four-phase model. *Spinal Cord.* 42, 383–95.

Dobkin, B., Barbeau, H., Deforge D., *et al.*, (2007). The evolution of walking related outcomes over the first 12 weeks of rehabilitation for incomplete traumatic SCI: the multicenter randomized SCI trial. *Neurorehabil. Neural Rep.* 21, 25–35.

Ellaway, P. H., Anand, P., Bergstrom, E. M., *et al.* (2004). Towards improved clinical and physiological assessments of recovery in SCI: a clinical initiative. *Spinal Cord.* 42, 325–37.

Ellaway, P. H., Kuppuswamy, A., Balasubramaniam, A. V., *et al.* (2011). Development of quantitative and sensitive assessments of physiological and functional outcome during recovery from SCI: A Clinical Initiative. *Brain Res. Bull.* 84, 343–57.

Frankel, H. L., Mathias, C. J., and Spalding, J. M. K. (1975). Mechanisms of reflex cardiac arrest in tetraplegic patients. *Lancet* ii, 1183–5.

Frankel, H. L., Michaelis, L. S., Golding, D. R., and Beral, V. (1972). The blood pressure in paraplegia-1. *Spinal Cord* 10, 193–8.

Gillis, D. J., Houda, W. and Hjeltness, N. (2008). Non-pharmacological management of orthostatic hypotension after SCI: a critical review of the literature. *Spinal Cord*, 46, 652–59.

Groothuis, J. T., Rongen, G. A., Deinum, J., *et al.* (2010). Sympathetic nonadrenergic transmission contributes to autonomic dysreflexia in spinal cord-injured individuals. *Hypertension.* 55, 636–43.

Guttmann, L. (1976). *SCI. Comprehensive management and research* (2nd edn). Blackwell Scientific, Oxford.

Guttmann, L., Frankel, H. L., and Paeslack, V. (1965). Cardiac irregularities during labour in paraplegic women. *Paraplegia* 3, 144–51.

Guttmann, L. and Whitteridge, D. (1947). Effects of bladder distension on autonomic mechanisms after SCI. *Brain* 70, 361–404.

Head, H. and Riddoch, G. (1917). The autonomic bladder, excessive sweating and some other reflex conditions in gross injuries of the spinal cord. *Brain* 40, 188–263.

Hohenfellner, M., Fahle, H., Dahms, S., Linn, J. F., Hutschenreiter, G., and Thuroff, J. W. (1996). Continent reconstruction of detrusor hyperreflexia by sacral bladder denervation combined with continent vesicostomy. *Urology* 47, (6), 930–1.

Houtman, S., Colier, W. N. J. M., Oeseburg, B. and Hopman, M. T. E. (2000). Systemic circulation and cerebral oxygenation during head-up tilt in spinal cord injured individuals. *Spinal Cord*, 38, 158–163.

Houtman, S., Serrador, J. M., Colier, W. N. J. M., Strijbos, D. W., Shoemaker, K. and Hopman, M. T. E. (2001). Changes in cerebral oxygenation and blood flow during LBNP in spinal cord-injured individuals. *J Appl Physiol*, 91, 2199–2204.

Hussain, I. F., Brady, C., Swinn, M. J., Mathias, C. J., Fowler, C. (2001). Treatment of erectile dysfunction with sildenafil citrate (Viagra) in parkinsonism due to Parkinson's disease or multiple system atrophy with observations on orthostatic hypotension. *J Neurol, Neurosurg, Psychiatry* 71, 371–4.

Illman, A., Stiller, K., Williams, M. (2000). The prevalence of orthostatic hypotension during physiotherapy treatment in patients with an acute SCI. *Spinal Cord* 38, 741–747.

Inoue, K., Miyake, S., Kumashiro, M., Ogata, H., Ueta, T., and Akatsu, T. (1991). Power spectral analysis of blood pressure variability in traumatic quadriplegic humans. *Am. J. Physiol.* H842–4.

Johnson, R. H. (1965). Neurological studies in temperature regulation. *Ann. Roy. Coll. Surg.* 36, 339–52.

Johnson, R. H., Smith, A. C. and Spalding, J. M. K. (1963). Oxygen consumption of paralysed men exposed to cold *J. Physiol.* 169, (3) 584–91.

Karlsson, A.-K. (1997). Metabolism and sympathetic function in spinal cord injured subjects. PhD Thesis, University of Gothenburg, Sweden.

Khurana, R. K. (1987). Orthostatic hypotension-induced autonomic dysreflexia. *Neurology* 37, 1221–4.

Koh, J., Brown, T. E., Beighton, L. A., Ha, C. Y., and Eckberg, D. L. (1994). Human autonomic rhythms: vagal cardiac mechanisms in tetraplegic subjects. *J. Physiol.*, London 474, 483–95.

Kooner, J. S., da Costa, D. F., Frankel, H. L., Bannister, R., Peart, W. S., and Mathias, C. J. (1987). Recumbency induces hypertension, diuresis and natriuresis in autonomic failure, but diuresis alone in tetraplegia. *J. Hypertension* 5, (Suppl. 5), 327–9.

Krassioukov, A., Warburton, D. E., Teasell, R., Eng, J. J. (2009). A systematic review of the management of autonomic dysreflexia after SCI. *Arch Phys Med Rehabil.* 90, 682–95.

Krenz, N. R., Meaking, S. O., Krassioukov, A. V., Weaver, L. C. (1999). Neutralizing intraspinal nerve growth factor blocks autonomic dysreflexia caused by SCI. *J Neurosci* 19, 7405–14.

Krenz, N. R., Weaver, L. C. (2000). Nerve growth fact in glia and inflammatory cells of the injured rat spinal cord. *J Neurochem.* 74, 730–9.

Krum, H., Louis, W. J., Brown, D. J., Clarke, S. J., Fleming, J. A., and Howes, L. G. (1992). Cardiovascular and vasoactive hormone responses to bladder distension in spinal and normal man. *Paraplegia* 30, 348–54.

Linsenmeyer, T. A., Campagnolo, D. I., and Chou, I. H. (1996). Silent autonomic dysreflexia during voiding in men with SCI. *J. Urol.* 155, (2), 519–22.

Mathias, C. J. (1976a). Neurological disturbances of the cardiovascular system. D. Phil. thesis, University of Oxford.

Mathias, C. J. (1976b). Bradycardia and cardiac arrest during tracheal suction mechanisms in tetraplegic patients. *Eur. J. Intensive Care Med.* 2, 147–56.

Mathias, C. J. (1995). Orthostatic hypotension causes, mechanisms and influencing factors. *Neurology* 45, (suppl 5) 56–11.

Mathias, C. J., Christensen, N. J., Corbett, J. L., Frankel, H. L., Goodwin, T. J., and Peart, W. S. (1975). Plasma catecholamines, plasma renin activity and plasma aldosterone in tetraplegic man, horizontal and tilted. *Clin. Sci. Mol. Med.* 49, 291–9.

Mathias, C. J., Christensen, N. J., Corbett, J. L., Frankel, H. L., and Spalding, J. M. K. (1976a). Plasma catecholamines during paroxysmal neurogenic hypertension in quadriplegic man, *Circulation Res.* 39, 204–8.

Mathias, C. J., Christensen, N. J., Frankel, H. L., and Spalding, J. M. K. (1979a). Cardiovascular control in recently injured tetraplegics in spinal shock. *Q. J. Med.,* NS **48**, 273–87.

Mathias, C. J., Frankel, H. L. (1986). The neurological and hormonal control of blood vessels and heart in spinal man. *J. Autonom. Nerv. Syst. Suppl.* 457–64.

Mathias, C. J., Frankel, H. L., Christensen, N. J., and Spalding, J. M. K. (1976c). Enhanced pressor response to noradrenaline in patients with cervical spinal cord transection. *Brain* **99**, 757–70.

Mathias, C. J., Frankel, H. L., Davies, I. B., James, V. H. T., and Peart, W. S. (1981). Renin and aldosterone release during sympathetic stimulation in tetraplegia. *Clin. Sci.* **60**, 399–604.

Mathias, C. J., Frankel, H. L., Turner, R. C., and Christensen, J. N. (1979b). Physiological responses to insulin hypoglycaemia in spinal man. *Paraplegia* **17**, 319–26.

Mathias, C. J. and Low, D. A. (2011). Autonomic Disturbances in Spinal Cord Injuries. In: D. Robertson, I. Biaggioni, G. Burnstock, P.A. Low and J. Paton (eds). *Primer on the Autonomic Nervous System.* 3rd Edition. Amsterdam: Elsevier.

Mathias, C. J., Reid, J. L., Wing, L. M. H., Frankel, H. L., and Christensen, N. J. (1979c). Antihypertensive effects of clonidine in tetraplegic subjects devoid of central sympathetic control. *Clin. Sci.* **57**, 425–8s.

Mathias, C. J., Smith A. D., Frankel, H. L., and Spalding, J. M. K. (1976b).Release of dopamine B-hydroxylase during hypertension from sympathetic over-activity in man. *Cardiovascular Res.* **10**, 176–81.

Mathias, C. J. and Frankel, H. L. (1988). Cardiovascular control in spinal man. *Ann. Rev. Physiol.* **50**, 577–92.

Mathias, C. J. and Frankel, H. L. (1992). The cardiovascular system in tetraplegia and paraplegia. Ins. *Handbook of Clinical Neurology,* vol 17, Spinal Cord Trauma, (ed. H. L. Frankel) pp. 435–56. Elsevier Science Publishers B. V., Netherlands.

Middleton, J. W., Siddall, P. J., Walker, S., Molloy, A. R., and Rutkowski, S. B. (1996). Intrathecal clonidine and baclofen in the management of spasticity and neuropathic pain following SCI: a case study. *Arch. Phys. Med. Rehabil.* **77**, 824–6.

Morris, M. J., Cox, H. S., Lambert, G. W., *et al.* (1997). Region-specific neuropeptide Y overflows at rest and during sympathetic activation in humans. *Hypertension.* **29**, 137–43.

Nicotra, A., Catley, M., Ellaway, P. H., Mathias, C. J. (2005). The ability of physiological stimuli to generate the sympathetic skin response in human chronic SCI. *Restor. Neurol. Neurosci.* **23**(5–6), 331–39.

Nitsche, B., Perschak, H., Curt, A., and Dietz, V. (1996). Loss of circadian blood pressure variability in complete tetraplegia. *J. Hum. Hypertens.* **10**, 311–17.

Norberg, K. A. and Normell, L. A. (1974). Histochemical demonstration of sympathetic adrenergic denervation in human skin. *Acta Neurol. Scand.* **50**, 261.

Pledger, H. G. (1962). Disorders of temperature regulation in acute traumatic paraplegia. *J. Bone Joint Surg.* **44B**, 110–13.

Popovic, M. R., Thrasher, T. A., Adams, M. E., Takes, V., Zivanovic, V. and Tonack, M. I. (2006). Functional electrical therapy: retraining grasping in SCI, *Spinal Cord.* **44**, 143–51.

Previnaire, J. G., Soler, J. M., and Hanson, P. (1993). Skin potential recordings during cystometry in spinal cord injured patients. *Paraplegia* **31**, 13–21.

Price, M. J. (2006). Thermoregulation during exercise in individuals with SCI. *Sports Med.* **36**(10), 863–79.

Reid, J. L., Wing, L. M. H., Mathias, C. J., Frankel, H. L., and Neill, E. (1977). The central hypotensive effect of clonidine: studies in tetraplegic subjects. *Clin. Pharmacol. Therapeut.* **21**, 375–81.

Santajuliana, D., Zukowska-Grojec, Z., and Osborn, J. W. (1995). Contribution of alpha- and beta-adrenoceptors and neuropeptide Y to autonomic dysreflexia. *Clin. Auton Res.* **5**, 91–7.

Stjernberg, L., Blumberg, H., and Wallin, B. G. (1986). Sympathetic activity in man after SCI: outflow to muscle below the lesion. *Brain* **109**, 695–715.

Sutters, M., Wakefield, C., O'Neil, K., *et al.* (1992). The cardiovascular, endocrine and renal response of tetraplegic and paraplegic subjects to dietary sodium restriction. *J. Physiol., London* **457**, 515–23.

Thyberg, M., Ertzgaard, P., Gylling, M., and Granerus, G. (1994). Effect of nifedipine on cystometry-induced elevation of blood pressure in patients with a reflex urinary bladder after a high level SCI. *Paraplegia* **32**, 308–13.

Welply, N. C., Mathias, C. J., and Frankel, H. L. (1975). Circulatory reflexes in tetraplegics during artificial ventilation and general anaesthesia. *Paraplegia* **13**, 172–82.

van Lieshout, J. J., lmholz, B. P. M., Wesseling, K. H., Speelman, J. D., and Wieling, W. (1991). Singing-induced hypotension: a complication of high spinal cord lesion. *Neth. J. Med.* **38**, 75–9.

CHAPTER 67

Autonomic disorders affecting cutaneous blood flow

Peter D. Drummond

Key points

- Cutaneous blood flow is regulated by sympathetic vasoconstrictor and vasodilator reflexes, parasympathetic vasodilator reflexes in the forehead and lips, and local autoregulatory mechanisms that involve sensory nerves and the vascular endothelium.

- Nerve injury or dysfunction triggers compensatory adjustments (e.g. supersensitivity in vascular smooth muscle to neurotransmitters), and provokes sprouting of collateral fibres that sometimes make functional but inappropriate connections with denervated tissue. One unfortunate outcome of these compensatory adjustments may be to compromise nutritive flow through superficial cutaneous vessels.

- Cutaneous vasomotor disturbances that disrupt nutritive flow contribute to a range of disorders (e.g. erythromelalgia, painful diabetic neuropathy, complex regional pain syndrome, and Raynaud's syndrome).

- Parasympathetic cross-innervation of sympathetically denervated facial blood vessels mediates aberrant facial flushing and sweating in various disorders associated with peripheral cervical sympathetic deficit (e.g. cluster headache and Frey's syndrome), whereas cross-innervation in the sympathetic chain probably accounts for the development of aberrant facial flushing and sweating after more proximal injury or disease.

Introduction

In addition to supplying nutrients and removing waste products, the cutaneous blood supply helps to regulate core and local temperature and is a major conduit of the neuroimmune defence system. Broad adjustments to thermal conditions and to exercise are coordinated by sympathetic vasodilator and constrictor nerves. In the lips and forehead, a parasympathetic vasodilator supply adds another layer of control. At the local level the cutaneous blood supply is fine-tuned by autoregulatory mechanisms, driven to a large extent by the vascular endothelium and by local neural activity. When this complex regulatory system fails, the body attempts to restore function by repairing faulty connections or by increasing vascular sensitivity to depleted neurotransmitters. In this chapter, the normal control of skin blood flow is outlined briefly, followed by examples of what can happen after normal control fails.

Normal control of skin blood flow

Cutaneous vasomotor reflexes help to regulate body temperature during the extremes of heat and cold, contribute to the maintenance of blood pressure during changes of posture and loss of blood volume, participate in fight–flight responses, and help to dissipate body heat produced during exercise. In the glabrous (hairless) skin of the hands, feet and face, sympathetic vasoconstrictor discharge closes high-capacity arteriovenous shunts during pain, cold and stress. This is adaptive in the short term, as it helps to conserve body heat, reduces blood loss to superficial injuries, and directs blood to the muscles during exercise. However, persistence of this response over long periods may lead to nutritive insufficiency in the skin and evoke or aggravate inflammation.

To protect against frostbite, the sympathetic vasoconstrictor influence lifts periodically during prolonged cold, perhaps due to cold-induced paralysis of adrenergic nerves (Daanen 2003). Elsewhere in the skin, sympathetic vasoconstrictor nerves apply a weak tonic vasoconstrictor influence on arterioles and veins that intensifies in cold surroundings. The vasoconstrictor response appears to involve co-release of noradrenaline and neuropeptide Y from sympathetic nerve terminals (Stephens et al. 2004). This response is attenuated in older people, due to loss of the non-adrenergic component of vasoconstriction, a probable reduction in sympathetic neural discharge and noradrenaline release, and desensitization of postjunctional α-adrenoceptors (Seals and Dinenno 2004, DeGroot and Kenney 2007, Thompson-Torgerson et al. 2008). This loss of reflex vasoconstriction increases the likelihood of excessive heat loss and, ultimately, hypothermia in elderly people.

Direct application of a cold stimulus to the skin induces cold-sensitive sensory nerves to trigger the local release of noradrenaline from sympathetic vasoconstrictor nerves. The adrenergic vasoconstriction masks a non-neural vasodilatation that precedes non-neural vasoconstriction (Johnson et al. 2005), mediated by direct effects of cold on the vascular endothelium and smooth muscle. This involves an inhibition of the nitric oxide vasodilator system (Hodges et al. 2006) and movement of α_{2C}-adrenoceptors from the Golgi apparatus to the surface membrane of vascular smooth muscle cells (Johnson 2007, Thompson-Torgerson et al. 2007a). The adrenergic component of vasoconstriction to local cooling decreases with advancing age (Thompson et al. 2005) whereas non-neural vasoconstriction intensifies (Thompson-Torgerson et al. 2007b), thereby becoming increasingly dependent on intracellular pathways associated with vascular disease (Thompson-Torgerson et al. 2008).

Before and during the early stages of exercise, an increase in sympathetic adrenergic vasoconstrictor tone moves blood away from the skin to exercising muscles (Kenney and Johnson 1992). Cutaneous blood vessels in non-glabrous (hairy) skin then dilate actively when skin and internal body temperature rise (Kamijo et al. 2005, Kellogg 2006). Botulinum toxin blocks increases in cutaneous blood flow during body heating (Kellogg et al. 1995), implying that active sympathetic vasodilatation is mediated by a neurotransmitter released from cholinergic nerves. Full expression of the response appears to involve several vasodilator agents, including neuronal nitric oxide (Kellogg et al. 2003, Kellogg et al. 2008a), vasoactive intestinal polypeptide (VIP) (Bennett et al. 2003, Kellogg et al. 2010, but see Wilkins et al. 2005), prostanoids (McCord et al. 2006), histamine (Wong et al. 2004), and a neurokinin receptor agonist (e.g. substance P) (Wong and Minson 2006). In addition, acetylcholine may contribute to the early phase of active vasodilatation (Shibasaki et al. 2002). Sequential delineation of this response is difficult, because relationships between many of the agents are reciprocal or redundant (e.g. between substance P and histamine, histamine and prostaglandins, and prostaglandins and nitric oxide). However, it could entail discharge of acetylcholine, VIP and nitric oxide from sympathetic cholinergic nerves that innervate the vasculature of sweat glands. This may liberate histamine from nearby tissue (e.g. mast cells) which, in turn, increases endothelial nitric oxide synthesis (Wilkins et al. 2004), prostaglandin production (McCord et al. 2006), and substance P release (Wong and Minson 2006).

Central and systemic influences affect the threshold and gain of active sympathetic vasodilatation. For example, nocturnal increases in melatonin (Aoki et al. 2006) and fluctuations in sex hormones during menopause (Charkoudian 2003) may lower the threshold for the response, so that flushing is initiated at comparatively low body temperatures. Conversely, active sympathetic vasodilatation is attenuated by exercise, orthostasis, and dehydration, and is impaired in diseases such as essential hypertension and diabetes (Charkoudian 2010).

Local warming of the skin induces direct and substantial increases in cutaneous blood flow at the site of warming (Johnson and Kellogg 2010). The initial response is mediated by an axon reflex that involves heat-sensitive vanilloid type-1 receptors on sensory nerves (Minson et al. 2001), and possibly also endothelial nitric oxide provoked by release of noradrenaline and neuropeptide Y from sympathetic vasoconstrictor nerves (Houghton et al. 2006, Yamanaka et al. 2007, Hodges et al. 2008, Hodges et al. 2009). The subsequent vasodilator response is maintained by local endothelial nitric oxide production (Kellogg et al. 2008b), independent of sensory nerve activity (Minson et al. 2001) or histamine or prostaglandin release (Wong et al. 2006, Gooding et al. 2006).

Like responses to cooling, reflex sympathetic vasodilatation and the local dilator response to heat decrease markedly with age (Pierzga et al. 2003, Holowatz and Kenney, 2010), due to structural changes in blood vessels associated with ageing, attenuated synthesis and release of neurotransmitters during active sympathetic vasodilatation (Holowatz et al. 2003, Holowatz and Kenney, 2010),

and decreased production or response to nitric oxide (Minson et al. 2002). An increase in oxidative stress with ageing may also contribute to the decline in active sympathetic vasodilatation (Holowatz and Kenney, 2010). The attenuated cutaneous vasodilator response increases the incidence of heat-related illness and death in the elderly. Fortunately, however, undertaking exercise training or maintaining a high level of fitness prevents the age-related decline in the local vasodilator response to heat (Black et al. 2008).

The deficit in cutaneous vasodilatation associated with normal ageing appears to intensify in Alzheimer's disease. For example, increases in skin blood flow during isometric exercise were smaller in patients with probable Alzheimer's disease than in age-matched controls (Kalman et al. 2002). Similarly, cutaneous vasodilatation to acetylcholine and isoprenaline (a β-adrenergic agonist), introduced into the skin by iontophoresis, was diminished in patients with probable Alzheimer's disease (Algotsson et al. 1995). The vasodilator response to acetylcholine was recently found to be attenuated not only in patients with early clinically confirmed Alzheimer's disease but also in other forms of dementia and in healthy elderly people with signs of mild cognitive impairment (Khalil et al. 2007). Thus, it might prove to be a useful indicator of cognitive decline. The abnormal regulation of cutaneous blood flow suggests that systemic factors that contribute to circulatory disturbances play a role in cognitive decline in Alzheimer's disease and other forms of dementia.

Injury or painful stimulation of the skin initiates local neurogenic vasodilatation via an axon reflex mechanism that discharges neuropeptides such as substance P and calcitonin-gene-related peptide from the cutaneous terminals of unmyelinated and thinly myelinated nociceptive fibres. Among other functions, neuropeptides increase the calibre and permeability of blood vessels, thereby releasing plasma proteins and white blood cells into the extracellular fluid to combat infection and to begin repair. In certain circumstances neuropeptides may also provoke mast cell degranulation, thus amplifying local neurogenic inflammation and sensitivity to noxious thermal stimuli (Drummond, 2004). Conversely, painless heat stimulation evokes axon reflexes in nociceptive afferents (Magerl and Treede 1996), suggesting that axon reflexes help to protect the skin by dispersing heat or by diluting potentially harmful substances. Curiously, stimulation of adrenergic receptors evokes axon reflex vasodilatation in the skin (Drummond and Lipnicki 1999, Drummond 2009), possibly due to an accumulation of inflammatory agents at the site of iontophoresis or via direct stimulation of these receptors on nociceptive afferents. Adrenergic mediation of axon reflexes could play a role in aberrant sensory-sympathetic coupling in neuroinflammatory diseases of the kidney and lower urinary tract (Trevisani et al. 2007, Kopp et al. 2007).

The vascular endothelium produces vasodilating and vasoconstricting substances in response to local physiological and chemical factors (e.g. changes in blood flow and oxygenation, neurotransmitters, hormones, and products of inflammation). These endothelial substances orchestrate a local inflammatory response that includes chemotactic attraction, infiltration and activation of white blood cells, immunoglobulin and cytokine production, phagocytosis, and mast cell degranulation (Lindsey et al. 2000). Local release of opioid peptides from white blood cells appears to fine-tune cutaneous vasodilatation and other components of the inflammatory response by balancing mast cell degranulation against neural discharge and neurogenic inflammation (Drummond 2000).

Autonomic control of the facial circulation

Facial blood vessels participate in the preliminary stages of food digestion, help to protect the membranes of the eyes, nose, and mouth against injury and infection, take part in thermoregulation and, by adding colour to emotional reactions, shape social behaviour. Sympathetic vasoconstrictor tone is greatest in the most exposed parts of the face, such as the ears, nose and lips (Fig. 67.1). Active sympathetic vasodilatation predominates in other parts of the face when body temperature rises during exercise (Drummond 1997a) (Fig. 67.2) and during passive heating (Drummond and Finch 1989). Bursts of sympathetic activity in the supraorbital nerve precede vasodilator and galvanic skin responses (a sign of sweating) in the forehead during body heating, mental stress, and arousal stimuli (Nordin 1990). Competition between adrenergic vasoconstriction and active sympathetic vasodilatation during emotional reactions may account for the spectrum of colour change ranging from the pallid face of fear through to the blush of embarrassment, and the flush of rage. The vasodilator response could be more prominent in the face than elsewhere in the body because of the density and proximity of blood vessels to the skin surface.

Parasympathetic vasodilator fibres regulate the supply of blood to the lacrimal and salivary glands, and the secretory glands of the nose, to enable the rapid production of secretory products. This vasodilator supply extends beyond the secretory glands to include the cutaneous circulation of the lips and forehead (Fig. 67.1). The primary stimulus for parasympathetic vasodilatation in the face seems to be irritation of the mucosal lining of the eyes, nose, and mouth (Drummond 1992, Drummond 1995a, Drummond 1997b). The glandular secretions help to dilute and remove potentially harmful substances. More broadly, stimulation of capsaicin-sensitive nociceptive afferents in the mouth (e.g. by eating food

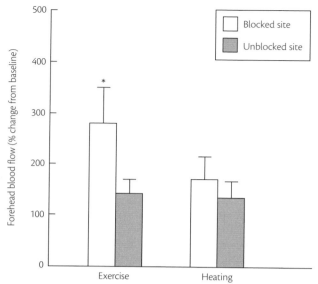

Fig. 67.2 Effect of α-adrenergic blockade with phentolamine on forehead blood flow during exercise and body heating. Phentolamine was administered by iontophoresis to a small area of the forehead before exercise. Skin blood flow was monitored at this site and at a similar site on the other side of the forehead with laser Doppler flow probes. Subjects pedalled as fast as they could for 1 minute on an exercise bicycle, then pedalled at 50% of this rate for the next 10 minutes. Subjects were then wrapped in blankets and heated with hot air for 5 minutes. Blood flow measured during the last 2 minutes of exercise and the last 3 minutes of heating was expressed as the percentage change from baseline flow. During exercise, increases in flow were greater at the blocked site than at the unblocked site (*p < 0.05), indicating that an increase in vasoconstrictor tone during exercise normally opposes facial flushing. Bars represent the standard error of responses. With permission from Drummond PD (1997a), *Psychophysiology*, Wiley.

spiced with chilli peppers) triggers facial sweating and flushing as well as salivation. Curiously, gustatory sweating in the forehead is mediated by sympathetic sudomotor discharge whereas gustatory flushing is due to trigeminal-parasympathetic vasodilatation (Drummond 1995a).

The major sensory nerve of the face, the trigeminal nerve, innervates extracranial and intracranial blood vessels and probably initiates neurogenic and parasympathetic vasodilatation in these vessels and in the facial microcirculation during migraine and cluster headache (Drummond 2006a). Cutaneous vasodilatation to painful stimulation of the face (Drummond 1997b) and limbs (Drummond and Granston 2003, Drummond and Granston 2004) is greater in migraine sufferers than controls, possibly due to amplification of the extracranial vasodilator component of the fight–flight (defence) response. On the other hand, trigeminal-parasympathetic vasodilatation to ocular irritation appears to be smaller in migraine sufferers than controls (Avnon et al. 2003), more so in patients with right-sided than left-sided migraine (perhaps reflecting an asymmetric hypothalamic influence on trigeminal-parasympathetic reflexes) (Avnon et al. 2004).

Remarkably, the extracranial vasodilator response to limb pain is greater ipsilaterally than contralaterally (Drummond and Granston 2003). The response is inhibited by pretreatment with guanethidine, an agent that displaces noradrenaline from sympathetic nerve terminals (Drummond 2006b) (Fig. 67.3), suggesting that limb pain provokes ipsilateral release of sympathetic vasoconstrictor

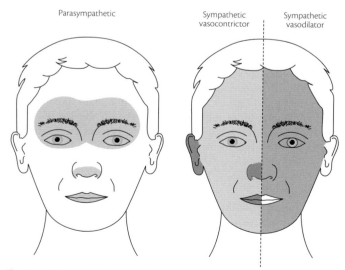

Fig. 67.1 Distribution of sympathetic vasoconstrictor nerves and sympathetic and parasympathetic vasodilator nerves in the face. Vasoconstrictor innervation is greatest in the lips, ears, eyes, and nose, whereas active sympathetic vasodilatation predominates in other parts of the face. Parasympathetic vasodilator fibres supply the respiratory and gastrointestinal tracts and large cranial blood vessels, and spills over to the facial circulation in the lips, nostrils, and forehead.

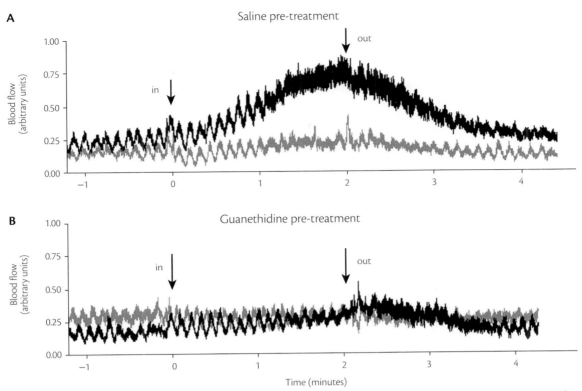

Fig. 67.3 Effect of immersing the right hand in 2°C water for 2 minutes on blood flow in the right temple (black waveform) and left temple (grey waveform) after bilateral saline pre-treatment **(A)**, and after guanethidine pretreatment to the right temple (to block adrenergic vasoconstriction) and saline pretreatment to the left temple **(B)**. The right hand was immersed in the water at the arrow marked 'in', and removed from the water at the arrow marked 'out'. The cold-pain-induced increase in blood flow in the right temple after saline pretreatment was inhibited by guanethidine pretreatment, indicating that the vasodilator response was mediated by release of adrenergic vasoconstrictor tone. Pulse amplitude (indicated by the thickness of the blood flow signal) also increased in the right temple after saline pretreatment, and this response was inhibited by guanethidine pretreatment. Reprinted from *Autonomic Neuroscience,* **128**, Drummond PD. Immersion of the hand in ice water releases adrenergic vasoconstrictor tone in the ipsilateral temple, 70–5, Copyright (2006), with permission from Elsevier.

tone in the face. These observations imply that sympathetic reflexes are more tightly controlled than previously thought, with some capacity to differentiate between stimulated and unstimulated sides of the body. This could be important in unilateral autonomic disorders such as migraine headache and complex regional pain syndrome.

Effects of nerve injury

After peripheral nerve injury, many neurons with injured or transected fibres die. This triggers a regenerative response in surviving neurons (Navarro et al. 2007) that is modulated by an inflammatory cytokine-neurotrophin axis (Hendrix and Peters 2007). The injured fibres of surviving neurons attempt to grow back to their original destination but sometimes cannot because the perineurial sheath has been damaged or destroyed. In such circumstances, collateral twigs sprout from nearby fibres in response to the high concentration of trophic agents produced by the injured and denervated tissue (Diamond et al. 1992). These collateral sprouts occupy the empty perineurial sheath and can eventually make functional connections with the denervated tissue. Because sympathetic, parasympathetic, and sensory fibres compete for trophic agents such nerve growth factor, injury to one category of nerve fibre can cause sprouting from other nerve fibre categories (Kessler 1985). However this cross-innervation is sometimes quite inappropriate.

In addition, supersensitivity to local neurotransmitters often develops in denervated tissue, either through the removal of prejunctional constraints (e.g. presynaptic autoreceptors or neurotransmitter enzymes) or through the development of postjunctional supersensitivity (Fleming and Westfall 1988, Tripovic et al. 2010). Supersensitivity may also develop if neurotransmitter release is disrupted due to some cause other than nerve injury (e.g. pharmacological depletion or receptor blockade) (Lipnicki and Drummond 2001). As described below, neurovascular disturbances, resulting from nerve injury or dysfunction, contribute to a variety of cutaneous autonomic disorders.

Disturbances in cutaneous blood flow in the limbs

Erythromelalgia refers to painfully hot, swollen, red hands or feet. In familial cases erythromelalgia is associated with mutation of a gene that encodes a voltage-gated sodium channel ($Na_v1.7$) in primary afferent nociceptors and sympathetic efferent fibres (Waxman and Dib-Hajj 2005, Choi et al. 2006, Fischer and Waxman 2010). In other cases, erythromelalgia is associated with degeneration of small-fibre nerve endings in the skin (Paticoff et al. 2007), high red blood cell and platelet counts, or diabetic autonomic neuropathy. The burning pain of erythromelalgia appears to result from cutaneous hypoxia, despite increased flow through arteriovenous shunts rendered immobile by loss of sympathetic vasoconstrictor function (Mork et al. 2002a). The pain is relieved by cooling the symptomatic part, consistent with sensitization of cutaneous nociceptors. Between episodes of burning pain, skin blood flow in symptomatic limbs appears to be lower than normal, and vasoconstrictor reflexes are impaired (Mork et al. 2002b). More broadly, autonomic function tests are abnormal in most patients with erythromelalgia (Davis et al. 2003). One explanation for these findings is that sympathetic nerve dysfunction triggers an increase in adrenoceptor sensitivity. Hyperexcitability in the cutaneous sensory C-fibres of patients with erythromelalgia might account for ongoing pain and tenderness, and might trigger axon reflex vasodilatation (Orstavik et al. 2003). Conduction slowing in these fibres is consistent with small-fibre neuropathy (Orstavik et al. 2003), presumably resulting from the sodium channelopathy or cutaneous ischaemia. Thus, the mechanism of erythromelalgia may involve adrenergic supersensitivity in superficial resistance vessels, chronic neurogenic vasodilatation with sensitization of nociceptors, and perhaps small-fibre neuropathy maintained in a vicious circle by nutritional insufficiency in superficial vessels.

Parallels between the symptoms of erythromelalgia and those of complex regional pain syndrome (CRPS, causalgia and reflex sympathetic dystrophy) make one wonder whether similar mechanisms might underlie vascular disturbances and pain in these conditions. In the warm stage of CRPS, the increase in blood flow through the pain-affected extremity is associated with signs of sympathetic dysfunction (Kurvers et al. 1994, Wasner et al. 2001, Gradl and Schurmann, 2005), and these signs may persist at later stages of the disease (Vogel et al. 2010). At least a subgroup of CRPS patients also have symptoms and histological signs of small-fibre neuropathy (Oaklander et al. 2006, Oaklander and Fields 2009), signs of cutaneous hypoxia, elevated levels of inflammatory mediators, and enhanced axon-reflex vasodilatation (Koban et al. 2003, Huygen et al. 2002, Weber et al. 2001, Schinkel et al. 2006). Skin lactate levels are high (Birklein et al. 2000) and oxygen consumption is low in the affected limb (Koban et al. 2003), even in the presence of an adequate blood oxygen supply. Antioxidants such as vitamin C (Zollinger et al. 1999, Zollinger et al. 2010) and dimethyl sulphoxide (Perez et al. 2003) are beneficial in CRPS, suggesting that the production of oxygen-derived free radicals in hypoxic tissue might prevent normal healing. Autonomic disturbances in CRPS range from signs of sympathetic deficit (a warm, dry limb) to signs of sympathetic overactivity (a cool, sweaty limb). One explanation for this variation is that in the later stages of CRPS an adrenergic supersensitivity overcompensates for an underlying sympathetic deficit (Drummond 2010). Indeed, levels of noradrenaline are lower in the affected than unaffected limbs of CRPS patients (Drummond et al. 1991, Harden et al. 1994), and the cutaneous blood vessels of patients with long-standing pain are supersensitive to noradrenaline (Arnold et al. 1993). Perhaps an adrenoceptor disturbance that increases the excitability of cutaneous nociceptors (Drummond et al. 1996) contributes to burning pain and vascular disturbances both in erythromelalgia and CRPS.

In some respects Raynaud's phenomenon is the antithesis of erythromelalgia, but in other respects the similarities are striking. Raynaud's phenomenon is characterized by episodic vasospasm in the fingers or toes in response to cold, vibration or emotion. Occasionally it is associated with occlusive arterial disease or connective tissue diseases such as scleroderma which narrow the lumen of digital arteries and decrease capillary blood flow (Bakst et al. 2008). During attacks, the affected digits turn white then cyanotic,

and feel numb. However, later on during the stage of reactive hyperaemia, throbbing pain may develop in flushed skin as sensation returns (Herrick 2005, Cooke and Marshall 2005). Erythromelalgia and Raynaud's phenomenon occasionally co-exist (Berlin and Pehr 2004), implying a shared mechanism (e.g. superficial ischaemia due to shunting of blood through arteriovenous anastomoses). Sensitivity to adrenergic agents (particularly α_2-adrenoceptor agonists) is increased in the digital arteries of patients with Raynaud's phenomenon (Freedman et al. 1989), possibly because of redistribution of α_{2C}-adrenoceptors to the surface of vascular smooth muscle cells (Flavahan 2008). Similarly, adrenergic supersensitivity might contribute to vascular disturbances in erythromelalgia (Mork et al. 2002b). Since the burning phase of erythromelalgia is often preceded by a vasoconstrictive phase, perhaps Raynaud's phenomenon is an acute variant of erythromelalgia.

Painful sensitivity to cold can also develop after peripheral nerve injury. Ochoa and Yarnitsky (1994) identified the coexistence of impaired cold perception with pain to more intense cold in patients with peripheral nerve disease from various causes. In addition, the symptomatic skin was abnormally cold in most patients. They suggested that partial loss of cold-specific afferent fibres releases inhibition of nociceptor input centrally, so that cold induces burning pain. Ochoa and Yarnitsky postulated that sympathetic denervation resulting from the peripheral neuropathy provokes denervation supersensitivity and vasospasm to circulating catecholamines. The cold skin might then activate nociceptors and cause pain.

Hyperglycaemia evokes autonomic disturbances and pain in diabetic neuropathy (Lefrandt et al. 2003, Wigington et al. 2004), and the associated microvascular disturbances increase the risk of impaired wound healing, ulceration and subsequent amputation of affected limbs (Chao and Cheing 2009). Moreover, endothelial function is compromised (Veves et al. 1998, Quattrini et al. 2007) possibly even in diabetic patients without neuropathy (Sokolnicki et al. 2007). Pain in diabetic neuropathy is associated with raised cutaneous thermal thresholds (a sign of small-fibre neuropathy) (Kramer et al. 2004) and an impaired vasoconstrictor response to an inspiratory gasp (Quattrini et al. 2007). Loss of sympathetic tone in patients with diabetic neuropathy may disrupt normal capillary permeability (Lefrandt et al. 2003), perhaps due to enhanced flow through arteriovenous anastomoses. The resulting microcirculatory changes might impair nutritive capillary function in the skin (Chao and Cheing 2009), thereby worsening peripheral neuropathy and contributing to pain. Similar autonomic and nutritive disturbances may develop in other forms of peripheral neuropathy.

Disturbances in facial blood flow

The ocular, sudomotor, and vasomotor deficit that results from injury to the sympathetic innervation of the face is known as Horner's syndrome. The injury blocks sweating, blushing and thermoregulatory flushing on the affected side of the face (Drummond and Lance 1987, Drummond and Lance 2002), sometimes producing a striking line of demarcation between flushing and sweating on the unaffected side and pallor on the affected side after strenuous exercise or heating.

Overactivity in cervical sympathetic pathways may also result in unusual facial symptoms. Parry–Romberg syndrome is characterized by slowly progressive but self-limited wasting of subcutaneous tissues in the distribution of a branch of the trigeminal nerve. This tissue destruction might be due to chronic sympathetic hyperactivity

(Wartenberg 1945), possibly involving a trophic disturbance triggered by inflammation of cranial blood vessels and nerves (Cory et al. 1997). In support of this hypothesis, facial flushing developed rapidly during body heating in the symptomatic region of the face in a patient with Parry–Romberg syndrome (Drummond et al. 2006). The broader implications of this finding for sympathetic regulation of subcutaneous fat deposits need to be investigated.

Since most sympathetic oculomotor fibres leave the spinal cord before vasomotor and sudomotor fibres, hemifacial loss of sweating and flushing without ocular signs of sympathetic deficit indicates an injury of preganglionic sympathetic fibres below the first

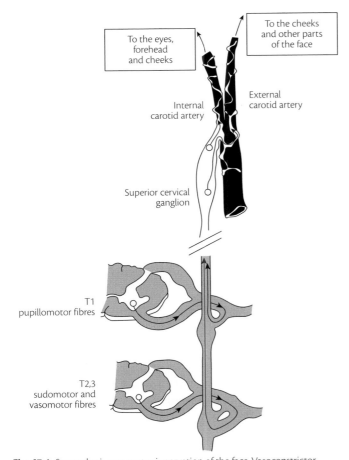

Fig. 67.4 Sympathetic vasomotor innervation of the face. Vasoconstrictor, vasodilator, and sudomotor fibres probably all follow much the same course to the face because injury affects all functions simultaneously. The development of excessive sweating on the paralysed side of the body after a stroke indicates the presence of a central inhibitory contralateral influence on sweating; however, a similar inhibitory influence on vasomotor reactions has not been described. Sympathetic vasomotor neurons projecting from the hypothalamus and higher centres synapse ipsilaterally with preganglionic neurons in the thoracic region of the spinal cord. Most preganglionic sudomotor and vasomotor fibres leave the cord in the second, third, and fourth thoracic roots, and then synapse with postganglionic neurons in the superior cervical ganglion. Fibres from the rostral part of the ganglion follow the internal carotid artery and cranial nerves to be distributed to the forehead and sometimes the cheek. Fibres from the caudal part of the ganglion follow the external carotid artery before projecting to the cheeks and other parts of the face. With kind permission from Springer Science + Business Media: *Clinical Autonomic Research*, Sweating and vascular responses in the face: normal regulation and dysfunction in migraine, cluster headache and harlequin syndrome, **4**, 1994, 273–85, Drummond PD.

thoracic root (Fig. 67.4). This pattern of sympathetic deficit, termed harlequin syndrome by Lance et al. (1988) and reviewed recently by Willaert et al. (2009), occasionally develops after surgery to the thoracic roots, mass lesions in the neck or mediastinum (e.g. Pancoast's tumour) or spinal cord pathology but typically develops without obvious trauma to spinal nerve roots (Drummond and Lance 1993, Tascilar et al. 2007). The condition is generally thought to be benign. However, Bremner and Smith (2008) reported recently that hemifacial flushing preceded general autonomic failure by years in a patient with multiple system atrophy and in another with pure autonomic failure.

Despite the grossly normal appearance of the pupils in harlequin syndrome, patients often show pupillary signs of denervation supersensitivity to sympathetic and parasympathetic agonists (Drummond and Lance 1993). Occasionally, tonic pupils and diminished tendon reflexes (termed Holmes–Adie syndrome) are associated with segmental sympathetic deficit in the face and elsewhere (termed Ross's syndrome). A pathological process that attacks parasympathetic ciliary ganglia, sympathetic ganglia and/or dorsal root ganglia might account for the spectrum of autonomic and motor disturbances in harlequin, Holmes–Adie and Ross's syndrome (Shin et al. 2000, Kalapesi et al. 2005, Nolano et al. 2006, Bremner and Smith 2008). The nature of the pathogen is uncertain, but might be a slow virus or an autoimmune reaction.

Harlequin colour changes are also associated with paroxysmal extreme pain disorder, a rare familial condition resulting from a mutation that impairs fast inactivation of $Na_v1.7$ channels (Fertleman et al. 2007). The mechanism of the one-sided facial flushing in this syndrome is unknown, but presumably is due to asymmetric impairment of cervical sympathetic pathways to the face.

Painful gustatory stimulation normally induces parasympathetic vasodilatation in the forehead which is opposed by sympathetic vasoconstrictor activity (Fig. 67.5). After injury to preganglionic or postganglionic sympathetic fibres, stimuli that induce salivation can provoke facial sweating and flushing in the distribution of sympathetic denervation. In the *preganglionic syndrome*, aberrant connections may develop between salivatory fibres and denervated vasomotor and sudomotor neurones in the superior cervical ganglion (Fig. 67.5), cross-innervation lower down in the stellate ganglion can also produce autonomic disturbances in the sympathetically denervated arm (e.g. gustatory piloerection). Cross-innervation in the sympathetic chain probably mediates aberrant gustatory flushing and sweating in Ross's syndrome and harlequin syndrome (Lance et al. 1988, Drummond and Edis 1990, Drummond and Lance 1993). In the *postganglionic syndrome*, collateral sprouts from sympathetic or parasympathetic salivatory fibres make functional connections with sympathetically denervated sweat glands and blood vessels (Fig. 67.5). Consequently, salivation is accompanied by flushing and sweating in the sympathetically denervated region of skin (often termed Frey's syndrome). This mechanism is also likely to mediate aberrant facial flushing and sweating to gustatory stimulation in cluster headache (Drummond and Lance 1987, Drummond and Lance 1992).

Botulinum toxin inhibits pathological gustatory flushing and sweating (Tugnoli et al. 2002, de Bree et al. 2007), implying that these responses are mediated by cholinergic neurons. The neurotransmitter responsible for pathological gustatory flushing is unlikely to be acetylcholine, because flushing persists after sweating has been blocked by atropine (Uprus et al. 1934). VIP co-exists with

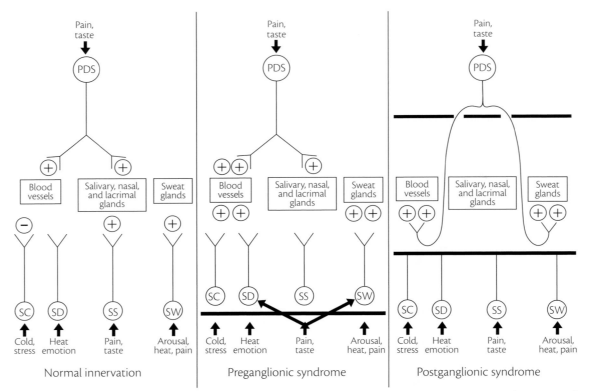

Fig. 67.5 Mechanisms of normal and pathological gustatory flushing. SC, sympathetic postganglionic vasoconstrictor neuron; SD, sympathetic postganglionic vasodilator neuron; SS, sympathetic postganglionic secretory neuron; SW, sympathetic postganglionic sudomotor neuron; PDS, parasympathetic postganglionic vasodilator and secretory neurons. In *normally innervated skin*, gustatory flushing to painful stimulation of the mouth is mediated by parasympathetic vasodilator neurons and inhibited by sympathetic vasoconstrictor discharge. Sweating during painful gustatory stimulation is mediated by sympathetic sudomotor fibres. In the *preganglionic syndrome*, connections develop between preganglionic secretory fibres and postganglionic sympathetic vasodilator and sudomotor neurons in the superior cervical ganglion. Denervation supersensitivity may also develop to neurotransmitters (e.g. vasoactive intestinal peptide) released from postganglionic sympathetic vasodilator and sudomotor fibres (shown as + +). In the *postganglionic syndrome* (e.g. Frey's syndrome and cluster headache), collateral sprouts from parasympathetic fibres occupy vacant sympathetic pathways to super-sensitive sweat glands and blood vessels. Nerve injury is shown as a solid line that cuts across the normal pathway of the nerve.

acetylcholine in cranial parasympathetic ganglia (Leblanc et al. 1987), and nerve fibres containing VIP congregate around large proximal arteries that supply muscles, glands, the mucous membranes of the face, and the supraorbital skin (Zhu et al. 1997). Similarly, sweat glands are surrounded by a dense network of nerve fibres containing VIP (Eedy et al. 1990, Nolano et al. 2006). Thus, the release of VIP from the collateral sprouts of parasympathetic fibres could contribute to pathological gustatory flushing and sweating by acting on sensitized receptors that previously mediated sweating and active sympathetic vasodilatation in the facial skin.

A similar mechanism, this time involving cross-innervation of sympathetically denervated forehead sweat glands and blood vessels by parasympathetic lacrimal fibres, may induce sweating and flushing in response to stimuli that induce lacrimation. This mechanism may account for aberrant facial sweating in sympathetically-denervated skin during attacks of cluster headache (Drummond and Lance 1992, Drummond 2006a). The mirror-image of this response develops in patients with a preganglionic lesion of parasympathetic fibres supplying the lacrimal gland. The dry eye of these patients waters during body heating, presumably because of cross-innervation of denervated parasympathetic neurons in the sphenopalatine ganglion by sympathetic sudomotor and vasomotor fibres that pass through the ganglion on their way to the forehead (Drummond 1995b).

Pathological gustatory sweating and flushing can be painful. In a recent case report, acetylcholine and an acetylcholinesterase inhibitor provoked pain and sweating whereas topical application of an anticholinergic drug blocked these responses (Goldstein et al. 2004). The efferent pathway appeared to involve parasympathetic rather than sympathetic nerves because strong gustatory stimulation provoked episodes of burning pain, sweating and flushing in the forehead and cheeks whereas exercise evoked sweating without pain. The patient may have sustained injury to cutaneous nerves when facial warts were removed 15 years previously. Thus, aberrant crosstalk might occasionally develop between parasympathetic cholinergic nerves and trigeminal nociceptive afferents.

Vasomotor disturbances in the face may result in localized flushing (as in the read ear syndrome) or more widely distributed symptoms (as in rosacea). Red ear syndrome consists of intermittent attacks of redness and burning in one or both ears that can be precipitated by touching or exposure to cold or warmth. It may be associated with migraine, glossopharyngeal or trigeminal neuralgia, or cervical disorders (Lance 1996), and could be mediated by an axon reflex with antidromic discharge of neuropeptides from the fibres of the third cervical nerve root. An alternate explanation was recently put forward by Brill et al. (2009), who drew parallels between the symptoms of red ear syndrome and those of auricular erythromelalgia.

Table 67.1 Some causes of facial flushing

Stimulus	Postulated mechanism
Emotion	Active sympathetic vasodilatation, and activation of vascular adrenoceptors by circulating catecholamines
Indirect heat and exercise	Active sympathetic vasodilatation mediated by vasoactive intestinal polypeptide, histamine and nitric oxide, and release of sympathetic vasoconstriction. Fluctuations in sex hormones during menopause may lower the hypothalamic set-point for thermoregulatory flushing
Direct heat	Axon reflex vasodilatation, succeeded by non-neural vasodilatation mediated by nitric oxide
Endogenous vasodilators	These include vasoactive substances (e.g. serotonin, bradykinin, prostaglandins, histamine) synthesized during inflammation or by carcinoid tumours, neuropeptides (e.g. substance P, calcitonin-gene-related peptide, vasoactive intestinal peptide) secreted during neurogenic inflammation, and nitric oxide released from the vascular endothelium
Facial pain	Local neuropeptide release from peripheral nociceptor terminals supplements parasympathetic vasodilatation in response to ocular, nasal, or oral pain (e.g. dental pain). Sympathetic denervation supersensitivity may augment facial flushing during attacks of cluster headache
Drugs	Direct vasodilatation (e.g. calcium-channel antagonists), or indirect vasodilatation (e.g. to metabolites of alcohol)
Taste, ocular pain	Postganglionic parasympathetic secretory fibres cross-innervate denervated sympathetic pathways after local injury to sympathetic nerves (e.g. in Frey's syndrome and cluster headache), or preganglionic sympathetic secretory fibres cross-innervate denervated sympathetic neurons in the superior cervical ganglion (e.g. in preganglionic Horner's syndrome, harlequin syndrome, and Ross's syndrome)

Rosacea is associated with flushed skin, oedema and burning pain in the central part of the face, and can be separated into several subtypes: prolonged flushing associated with stinging and burning pain and with dilated superficial blood vessels (telangiectasia), persistent cutaneous inflammation associated with papules and pustules, and the rhinophyma and ocular subtypes (Crawford et al. 2004, Powell 2005). Based on histological findings, Aroni et al. (2008) suggested that ultraviolet radiation (e.g. from prolonged sun exposure) increases vulnerability to rosacea by damaging the elastin and collagen fibre network that supports cutaneous lymph and blood vessels. This may trigger a chronic inflammatory process that involves mast cell accumulation, granuloma formation and angiogenesis. Little else is known about the pathophysiology of facial flushing or other cutaneous disturbances in rosacea, but a recent report suggests that the inflammation evoked by innate immune responses might drive abnormal generation of the pro-inflammatory antimicrobial peptide cathelicidin (Yamasaki et al. 2007). This could establish a positive loop that augments inflammation and that triggers features of rosacea such as hyperplasia and angiogenesis (Yamasaki and Gallo 2009). Involvement of antimicrobial peptides in other inflammatory skin disorders could be worth exploring.

In conclusion, some of the causes of normal and pathological facial flushing are summarized in Table 67.1. Investigating each of these triggers and pathways may help to identify the basis of abnormal facial flushing in individual cases.

References

Algotsson, A., Nordberg, A., Almkvist, O. and Winblad, B. (1995). Skin vessel reactivity is impaired in Alzheimer's disease. *Neurobiology of Ageing* **16**, 577–82.

Aoki, K., Stephens, D. P., Zhao, K., Kosiba, W. A. and Johnson, J. M. (2006). Modification of cutaneous vasodilator response to heat stress by daytime exogenous melatonin administration. *American Journal of Physiology: Regulatory, Integrative and Comparative Physiology* **291**, R619–624.

Arnold, J. M. O., Teasell, R. W., MacLeod, A. P., Brown, J. E. and Carruthers, S. G. (1993). Increased venous alpha-adrenoceptor responsiveness in patients with reflex sympathetic dystrophy. *Annals of Internal Medicine* **118**, 619–21.

Aroni, K., Tsagroni, E., Kavantzas, N., Patsouris, E. and Ioannidis, E. (2008). A study of the pathogenesis of rosacea: how angiogenesis and mast cells may participate in a complex multifactorial process. *Archives of Dermatological Research* **300**, 125–31.

Avnon, Y., Nitzan, M., Sprecher, E., Rogowski, Z. and Yarnitsky, D. (2003). Different patterns of parasympathetic activation in uni- and bilateral migraineurs. *Brain* **126**, 1660–70.

Avnon, Y., Nitzan, M., Sprecher, E., Rogowski, Z. and Yarnitsky, D. (2004). Autonomic asymmetry in migraine: augmented parasympathetic activation in left unilateral migraineurs. *Brain* **127**, 2099–108.

Bakst, R., Merola, J. F., Franks, A. G., Jr., Sanchez, M. (2008). Raynaud's phenomenon: pathogenesis and management. *Journal of the American Academy of Dermatology* **59**, 633–53.

Bennett, L. A., Johnson, J. M., Stephens, D. P., Saad, A. R. and Kellogg, D. L. Jr (2003). Evidence for a role for vasoactive intestinal peptide in active vasodilatation in the cutaneous vasculature of humans. *Journal of Physiology* **552**, 223–32.

Berlin, A. L. and Pehr, K. (2004). Coexistence of erythromelalgia and Raynaud's phenomenon. *Journal of the American Academy of Dermatology* **50**, 456–60.

Birklein, F., Weber, M. and Neundorfer, B. (2000). Increased skin lactate in complex regional pain syndrome: evidence for tissue hypoxia? *Neurology* **55**, 1213–15.

Black, M. A., Green, D. J. and Cable, N. T. (2008). Exercise prevents age-related decline in nitric-oxide-mediated vasodilator function in cutaneous microvessels. *Journal of Physiology* **586**, 3511–24.

Bremner, F., Smith, S. (2008). Pupillographic findings in 39 consecutive cases of harlequin syndrome. *Journal of Neuro-ophthalmology* **28**, 171–77.

Brill, T. J., Funk, B., Thaci, D., Kaufmann, R. (2009). Red ear syndrome and auricular erythromelalgia: the same condition? *Clinical and Experimental Dermatology* **34**, e626–628.

Chao, C. Y., Cheing, G. L. (2009). Microvascular dysfunction in diabetic foot disease and ulceration. *Diabetes Metabolism Research Reviews* **25**, 604–614.

Charkoudian, N. (2003). Skin blood flow in adult human thermoregulation: how it works, when it does not, and why. *Mayo Clinic Proceedings* **78**, 603–12.

Charkoudian, N. (2010). Mechanisms and modifiers of reflex induced cutaneous vasodilation and vasoconstriction in humans. *Journal of Applied Physiology*, **109**, 1221–8.

Choi. J. S., Dib-Hajj, S. D. and Waxman, S. G. (2006). Inherited erythermalgia: limb pain from an S4 charge-neutral Na channelopathy. *Neurology* **67**, 1563–67.

Cooke, J. P. and Marshall, J. M. (2005). Mechanisms of Raynaud's disease. *Vascular Medicine* **10**, 293–307.

Cory, R. C., Clayman, D. A., Faillace, W. J., McKee, S. W., Gama, C. H. (1997). Clinical and radiologic findings in progressive facial hemiatrophy (Parry-Romberg syndrome). *American Journal of Neuroradiology* **18**, 751–7.

Crawford, G. H., Pelle, M. T. and James, W. D. (2004). Rosacea: I. Etiology, pathogenesis, and subtype classification. *Journal of the American Academy of Dermatology* **51**, 327–41.

Daanen, H. A. (2003). Finger cold-induced vasodilation: a review. *European Journal of Applied Physiology* **89**, 411–26.

Davis, M. D., Sandroni, P., Rooke, T. W. and Low, P. A. (2003). Erythromelalgia: vasculopathy, neuropathy, or both? A prospective study of vascular and neurophysiologic studies in erythromelalgia. *Archives of Dermatology* **139**, 1337–43.

Degroot, D. W. and Kenney, W. L. (2007). Impaired defense of core temperature in aged humans during mild cold stress. *American Journal of Physiology: Regulatory, Integrative and Comparative Physiology* **292**, R103–108.

Diamond, J., Holmes, M. and Coughlin, M. (1992). Endogenous NGF and nerve impulses regulate the collateral sprouting of sensory axons in the skin of the adult rat. *Journal of Neuroscience* **12**, 1454–66.

Drummond, P. D. (1992). The mechanism of facial sweating and cutaneous vascular responses to painful stimulation of the eye. *Brain* **115**, 1417–28.

Drummond, P. D. (1994). Sweating and vascular responses in the face: normal regulation and dysfunction in migraine, cluster headache and harlequin syndrome. *Clinical Autonomic Research* **4**, 273–85.

Drummond, P. D. (1995a). Mechanisms of physiological gustatory sweating and flushing in the face. *Journal of the Autonomic Nervous System* **52**, 117–24.

Drummond, P. D. (1995b). Lacrimation induced by thermal stress in patients with a facial nerve lesion. *Neurology* **45**, 1112–14.

Drummond, P. D. (1997a). The effect of adrenergic blockade on blushing and facial flushing. *Psychophysiology* **34**, 163–8.

Drummond, P. D. (1997b) Photophobia and autonomic responses to facial pain in migraine. *Brain* **120**, 1857–64.

Drummond, P. D. (2000). The effect of peripheral opioid block and body cooling on sensitivity to heat in capsaicin-treated skin. *Anesthesia and Analgesia* **90**, 923–27.

Drummond, P. D. (2004). The effect of cutaneous mast cell degranulation on sensitivity to heat. *Inflammation Research* **53**, 309–15.

Drummond, P. D. (2006a). Mechanisms of autonomic disturbance in the face during and between attacks of cluster headache. *Cephalalgia* **26**, 633–41.

Drummond, P. D. (2006b). Immersion of the hand in ice water releases adrenergic vasoconstrictor tone in the ipsilateral temple. *Autonomic Neuroscience* **128**, 70–5.

Drummond, P. D. (2009). Alpha-1 adrenoceptor stimulation triggers axon-reflex vasodilatation in human skin. *Autonomic Neuroscience: Basic and Clinical* **151**, 159–63.

Drummond, P. D. (2010). Sensory disturbances in complex regional pain syndrome: clinical observations, autonomic interactions and possible mechanisms. *Pain Medicine,* **11**, 1257–66.

Drummond, P. D., Finch, P. M. and Smythe, G. W. (1991). Reflex sympathetic dystrophy: the significance of differing plasma catecholamine concentrations in affected and unaffected limbs. *Brain* **114**, 2025-2036.

Drummond, P. D., Hassard, S. and Finch, P. M. (2006). Trigeminal neuralgia, migraine and sympathetic hyperactivity in a patient with Parry-Romberg syndrome. *Cephalalgia* **26**, 1146–9.

Drummond, P. D., Lipnicki, D. M. (1999). Noradrenaline provokes axon reflex hyperaemia in the skin of the human forearm. *Journal of the Autonomic Nervous System* **77**, 39–44.

Drummond, P. D., Skipworth, S. and Finch, P. M. (1996). α_1-Adrenoceptors in normal and hyperalgesic skin. *Clinical Science* **91**, 73–7.

Drummond, P. D. and Edis, R. H. (1990). Loss of facial sweating and flushing in Holmes-Adie syndrome. *Neurology* **40**, 847–9.

Drummond, P. D. and Finch, P. M. (1989). Reflex control of facial flushing during body heating in man. *Brain* **112**, 1351–8.

Drummond, P. D. and Granston, A. (2003). Facilitation of extracranial vasodilatation to limb pain in migraine sufferers. *Neurology* **61**, 60–3.

Drummond, P. D. and Granston, A. (2004). Facial pain increases nausea and headache during motion sickness in migraine sufferers. *Brain* **127**, 526–34.

Drummond, P. D. and Lance, J. W. (1987). Facial flushing and sweating mediated by the sympathetic nervous system. *Brain* **110**, 793–803.

Drummond, P. D. and Lance, J. W. (1992). Pathological sweating and flushing accompanying the trigeminal–lacrimal reflex in patients with cluster headache and in patients with a confirmed site of cervical sympathetic deficit: evidence for parasympathetic cross-innervation. *Brain* **115**, 1429–45.

Drummond, P. D. and Lance, J. W. (1993). Site of autonomic deficit in harlequin syndrome. *Annals of Neurology* **34**, 814–19.

Eedy, D. J., Shaw, C., Armstrong, E. P., Johnston, C. F. and Buchanan, K. D. (1990). Vasoactive intestinal peptide (VIP) and peptide histidine methionine (PHM) in human eccrine sweat glands: demonstration of innervation, specific binding sites and presence in secretions. *British Journal of Dermatology* **123**, 65–76.

Fertleman, C. R., Ferrie, C. D., Aicardi, J., *et al.* (2007). Paroxysmal extreme pain disorder (previously familial rectal pain syndrome). *Neurology* **69**, 586–95.

Fischer, T. Z., Waxman, S. G. (2010). Familial pain syndromes from mutations of the NaV1.7 sodium channel. *Annals of the New York Academy of Sciences* **1184**, 196–207.

Flavahan, N. A. (2008). Regulation of vascular reactivity in scleroderma: new insights into Raynaud's phenomenon. *Rheumatic Disease Clinics of North America* **34**, 81–7.

Fleming, W., Westfall, D. P. (1988). Adaptive supersensitivity. In: Trendelenberg U, Weiner N (Eds), Catecholamines. I. *Handbook of Experimental Pharmacology* **90**, 509–59.

Freedman, R. R., Sabharwal, S. C., Desai, N., Wenig, P. and Mayes, M. (1989). Increased α-adrenergic responsiveness in idiopathic Raynaud's disease. *Arthritis and Rheumatism* **32**, 61–5.

Goldstein, D. S., Pechnik, S., Moak, J. and Eldadah, B. (2004). Painful sweating. *Neurology* **63**, 1471–5.

Gooding, K. M., Hannemann, M. M., Tooke, J. E., Clough, G. F. and Shore, A. C. (2006). Maximum skin hyperaemia induced by local heating: possible mechanisms. *Journal of Vascular Research* **43**, 270–77.

Gradl, G. and Schurmann, M. (2005). Sympathetic dysfunction as a temporary phenomenon in acute posttraumatic CRPS I. *Clinical Autonomic Research* **15**, 29–34.

Harden, R. N., Duc, T. A., Williams, T. R., Coley, D., Cate, J. C. and Gracely, R. H. (1994). Norepinephrine and epinephrine levels in affected versus unaffected limbs in sympathetically maintained pain. *Clinical Journal of Pain* **10**, 324–30.

Hendrix, S., Peters, E. M. (2007). Neuronal plasticity and neuroregeneration in the skin—the role of inflammation. *Journal of Neuroimmunology* **184**, 113–26.

Herrick, A. L. (2005). Pathogenesis of Raynaud's phenomenon. *Rheumatology (Oxford)* **44**, 587–96.

Hodges, G. J., Kosiba, W. A., Zhao, K., Johnson, J. M. (2009). The involvement of heating rate and vasoconstrictor nerves in the cutaneous vasodilator response to skin warming. *American Journal of Physiology: Heart and Circulatory Physiology* **296**, H51–56.

Hodges, G. J., Kosiba, W. A., Zhao, K. and Johnson, J. M. (2008). The involvement of norepinephrine, neuropeptide Y, and nitric oxide in the cutaneous vasodilator response to local heating in humans. *Journal of Applied Physiology* **105**, 233–40.

Holowatz, L. A., Houghton, B. L., Wong, B. J. *et al.* (2003). Nitric oxide and attenuated reflex cutaneous vasodilation in aged skin. *American Journal of Physiology: Heart and Circulatory Physiology* **284**, H1662–7.

Holowatz, L. A., Kenney, W. L. (2010). Peripheral mechanisms of thermoregulatory control of skin blood flow in aged humans. *Journal of Applied Physiology*, **109**, 1538–44.

Houghton, B. L., Meendering, J. R., Wong, B. J. and Minson, C. T. (2006). Nitric oxide and noradrenaline contribute to the temperature threshold of the axon reflex response to gradual local heating in human skin. *Journal of Physiology* **572**, 811–20.

Huygen, F. J., De Bruijn, A. G., De Bruin, M. T., Groeneweg, J. G., Klein, J. and Zijistra, F. J. (2002). Evidence for local inflammation in complex regional pain syndrome type 1. *Mediators of Inflammation* **11**, 47–51.

Johnson, J. M. (2007). Mechanisms of vasoconstriction with direct skin cooling in humans. *American Journal of Physiology: Heart and Circulatory Physiology* **292**, H1690–1691.

Johnson, J. M., Kellogg, D. L., Jr. (2010). Local thermal control of the human cutaneous circulation. *Journal of Applied Physiology,* **109**, 1229–38.

Johnson, J. M., Yen, T. C., Zhao, K. and Kosiba, W. A. (2005). Sympathetic, sensory, and nonneuronal contributions to the cutaneous vasoconstrictor response to local cooling. *American Journal of Physiology: Heart and Circulatory Physiology* **288**, H1573–9.

Kalapesi, F. B., Krishnan, A. V. and Kiernan, M. C. (2005). Segmental facial anhidrosis and tonic pupils with preserved deep tendon reflexes: a novel autonomic neuropathy. *Journal of Neuro-ophthalmology* **25**, 5–8.

Kalman, J., Szakacs, R., Torok, T., *et al.* (2002). Decreased cutaneous vasodilatation to isometric handgrip exercise in Alzheimer's disease. *International Journal of Geriatric Psychiatry* **17**, 371–4.

Kamijo, Y., Lee, K. and Mack, G. W. (2005). Active cutaneous vasodilation in resting humans during mild heat stress. *Journal of Applied Physiology* **98**, 829–37.

Kellogg, D. L. Jr (2006). In vivo mechanisms of cutaneous vasodilation and vasoconstriction in humans during thermoregulatory challenges. *Journal of Applied Physiology* **100**, 1709–1718.

Kellogg, D. L. Jr, Pergola, P. E., Piest, K. L., *et al.* (1995). Cutaneous active vasodilation in humans is mediated by cholinergic nerve cotransmission. *Circulation Research* **77**, 1222–8.

Kellogg, D. L. Jr, Zhao, J. L., Friel, C. and Roman, L. J. (2003). Nitric oxide concentration increases in the cutaneous interstitial space during heat stress in humans. *Journal of Applied Physiology* **94**, 1971–7.

Kellogg, D. L., Jr., Zhao, J. L., Wu, Y., Johnson, J. M. (2010). VIP/PACAP receptor mediation of cutaneous active vasodilation during heat stress in humans. *Journal of Applied Physiology,* **109**, 95–100.

Kellogg, D. L., Jr., Zhao, J. L. and Wu, Y. (2008a). Neuronal nitric oxide synthase control mechanisms in the cutaneous vasculature of humans in vivo. *Journal of Physiology* **586**, 847–57.

Kellogg, D. L., Jr., Zhao, J. L. and Wu, Y. (2008b). Endothelial nitric oxide synthase control mechanisms in the cutaneous vasculature of humans in vivo. *American Journal of Physiology: Heart and Circulation Physiology* **295**, H123–9.

Kenney, W. L. and Johnson, J. M. (1992). Control of skin blood flow during exercise. *Medicine and Science in Sports and Exercise* **24**, 303–12.

Kessler, J. A. (1985). Parasympathetic, sympathetic, and sensory interactions in the iris: nerve growth factor regulates cholinergic ciliary ganglion innervation *in vivo*. *Journal of Neuroscience* **5**, 2719–25.

Khalil, Z., LoGiudice, D., Khodr, B., Maruff, P., Masters, C. (2007). Impaired peripheral endothelial microvascular responsiveness in Alzheimer's disease. *Journal of Alzheimers Disease* **11**, 25–32.

Koban, M., Leis, S., Schultze-Mosgau, S. and Birklein, F. (2003). Tissue hypoxia in complex regional pain syndrome. *Pain* **104**, 149–57.

Kopp, U. C., Cicha, M. Z., Smith, L. A., Mulder, J., Hokfelt, T. (2007). Renal sympathetic nerve activity modulates afferent renal nerve activity by PGE2-dependent activation of alpha1- and alpha2-adrenoceptors on renal sensory nerve fibers. *American Journal of Physiology: Regulatory, Integrative and Comparative Physiology* **293**, R1561–1572.

Kramer, H. H., Rolke, R., Bickel, A. and Birklein, F. (2004). Thermal thresholds predict painfulness of diabetic neuropathies. *Diabetes Care* **27**, 2386–91.

Kurvers, H. A. J. M., Jacobs, M. J. H. M., Beuk, R. J. *et al.* (1994). Reflex sympathetic dystrophy: result of autonomic denervation? *Clinical Science* **87**, 663–9.

Lance, J. W. (1996). The red ear syndrome. *Neurology* **47**, 617–20.

Lance, J. W., Drummond, P. D., Gandevia, S. C. and Morris, J. G. L. (1988). Harlequin syndrome: the sudden onset of unilateral flushing and sweating. *Journal of Neurology, Neurosurgery and Psychiatry* **51**, 635–42.

Leblanc, G. G., Trimmer, B. A. and Landis, S. C. (1987). Neuropeptide Y-like immunoreactivity in rat cranial parasympathetic neurons: coexistence with vasoactive intestinal peptide and choline acetyltransferase. *Proceedings of the National Academy of Sciences U S A* **84**, 3511–15.

Lefrandt, J. D., Bosma, E., Oomen, P. H., *et al.* (2003). Sympathetic mediated vasomotion and skin capillary permeability in diabetic patients with peripheral neuropathy. *Diabetologia* **46**, 40–7.

Lindsey, K. Q., Caughman, S. W., Olerud, J. E., Bunnett, N. W., Armstrong, C. A. and Ansel, J. C. (2000). Neural regulation of endothelial cell-mediated inflammation. *Journal of Investigative Dermatology: Symposium Proceedings* **5**, 74–8.

Lipnicki, D. M. and Drummond, P. D. (2001). Vascular and nociceptive effects of localized prolonged sympathetic blockade in human skin. *Autonomic Neuroscience* **88**, 86–93.

Magerl, W. and Treede, R. D. (1996). Heat-evoked vasodilatation in human hairy skin: axon reflexes due to low-level activity of nociceptive afferents. *Journal of Physiology* **497**, 837–48.

McCord, G. R., Cracowski, J. L. and Minson, C. T. (2006). Prostanoids contribute to cutaneous active vasodilation in humans. *American Journal of Physiology: Regulatory, Integrative and Comparative Physiology* **291**, R596–602.

Minson, C. T., Berry, L. T. and Joyner, M. J. (2001). Nitric oxide and neurally mediated regulation of skin blood flow during local heating. *Journal of Applied Physiology* **91**, 1619–26.

Minson, C. T., Holowatz, L. A., Wong, B. J., Kenney, W. L. and Wilkins, B. W. (2002). Decreased nitric oxide- and axon reflex-mediated cutaneous vasodilation with age during local heating. *Journal of Applied Physiology* **93**, 1644–49.

Mork, C., Kvernebo, K., Asker, C. L. and Salerud, E. G. (2002a). Reduced skin capillary density during attacks of erythromelalgia implies arteriovenous shunting as pathogenetic mechanism. *Journal of Investigative Dermatology* **119**, 949–53.

Mork, C., Kalgaard, O. M. and Kvernebo, K. (2002b). Impaired neurogenic control of skin perfusion in erythromelalgia. *Journal of Investigative Dermatology* **118**, 699–703.

Navarro, X., Vivo, M., Valero-Cabre, A. (2007). Neural plasticity after peripheral nerve injury and regeneration. *Progress in Neurobiology* **82**, 163–201.

Nolano, M., Provitera, V., Perretti, A., *et al.* (2006). Ross syndrome: a rare or a misknown disorder of thermoregulation? A skin innervation study on 12 subjects. *Brain* **129**, 2119–31.

Nordin, M. (1990). Sympathetic discharges in the human supraorbital nerve and their relation to sudo- and vasomotor responses. *Journal of Physiology* **423**, 241–55.

Oaklander, A. L., Fields, H. L. (2009). Is reflex sympathetic dystrophy/ complex regional pain syndrome type I a small-fiber neuropathy? *Annals of Neurology* **65**, 629–38.

Oaklander, A. L., Rissmiller, J. G., Gelman, L. B., Zheng, L., Chang, Y. and Gott, R. (2006). Evidence of focal small-fiber axonal degeneration in complex regional pain syndrome-I (reflex sympathetic dystrophy). *Pain* **120**, 235–43.

Ochoa, J. L. and Yarnitsky, D. (1994). The triple cold syndrome: cold hyperalgesia, cold hypoaesthesia and cold skin in peripheral nerve disease. *Brain* **117**, 185–97.

Orstavik, K., Weidner, C., Schmidt, R., *et al.* (2003) Pathological C-fibres in patients with a chronic painful condition. *Brain* **126**, 567–78.

Paticoff, J., Valovska, A., Nedeljkovic, S. S. and Oaklander, A. L. (2007). Defining a treatable cause of erythromelalgia: acute adolescent autoimmune small-fiber axonopathy. *Anesthesia and Analgesia* **104**, 438–41.

Perez, R. S., Zuurmond, W. W., Bezemer, P. D., *et al.* (2003). The treatment of complex regional pain syndrome type I with free radical scavengers: a randomized controlled study. *Pain* **102**, 297–307.

Pierzga, J. M., Frymoyer, A. and Kenney, W. L. (2003). Delayed distribution of active vasodilation and altered vascular conductance in aged skin. *Journal of Applied Physiology* **94**, 1045–53.

Powell, F. C. (2005). Clinical practice. Rosacea. *New England Journal of Medicine* **352**, 793–803.

Quattrini, C., Harris, N. D., Malik, R. A. and Tesfaye, S. (2007). Impaired skin microvascular reactivity in painful diabetic neuropathy. *Diabetes Care* **30**, 655–59.

Schinkel, C., Gaertner, A., Zaspel, J., Zedler, S., Faist, E. and Schürmann, M. (2006). Inflammatory mediators are altered in the acute phase of posttraumatic complex regional pain syndrome. *Clinical Journal of Pain* **22**, 235–39.

Seals, D. R. and Dinenno, F. A. (2004). Collateral damage: cardiovascular consequences of chronic sympathetic activation with human ageing. *American Journal of Physiology: Heart and Circulatory Physiology* **287**, H1895–1905.

Shibasaki, M., Wilson, T. E., Cui, J. and Crandall, C. G. (2002). Acetylcholine released from cholinergic nerves contributes to cutaneous vasodilation during heat stress. *Journal of Applied Physiology* **93**, 1947–51.

Shin, R. K., Galetta, S. L., Ting, T. Y., Armstrong, K. and Bird, S. J. (2000). Ross syndrome plus: beyond horner, Holmes-Adie, and harlequin. *Neurology* **55**, 1841–6.

Sokolnicki, L. A., Roberts, S. K., Wilkins, B. W., Basu, A. and Charkoudian, N. (2007). Contribution of nitric oxide to cutaneous microvascular dilation in individuals with type 2 diabetes mellitus. *American Journal of Physiology: Endocrinology and Metabolism* **292**, E314–318.

Stephens, D. P., Saad, A. R., Bennett, L. A., Kosiba, W. A. and Johnson, J. M. (2004). Neuropeptide Y antagonism reduces reflex cutaneous vasoconstriction in humans. *American Journal of Physiology: Heart and Circulatory Physiology* **287**, H1404–1409.

Tascilar, N., Tekin, N. S., Erdem, Z., Alpay, A., Emre, U. (2007). Unnoticed dysautonomic syndrome of the face: Harlequin syndrome. *Autonomic Neuroscience: Basic and Clinical* **137**, 1–9.

Thompson, C. S., Holowatz, L. A. and Kenney, W. L. (2005). Attenuated noradrenergic sensitivity during local cooling in aged human skin. *Journal of Physiology* **564**, 313–319.

Thompson-Torgerson, C. S., Holowatz, L. A., Flavahan, N. A. and Kenney, W. L. (2007a). Cold-induced cutaneous vasoconstriction is mediated by Rho kinase in vivo in human skin. *American Journal of Physiology: Heart and Circulatory Physiology* **292**, H1700–1705.

Thompson-Torgerson, C. S., Holowatz, L. A., Flavahan, N. A. and Kenney, W. L. (2007b). Rho kinase-mediated local cold-induced cutaneous vasoconstriction is augmented in aged human skin. *American Journal of Physiology: Heart and Circulatory Physiology* **293**, H30–36.

Thompson-Torgerson, C. S., Holowatz, L. A. and Kenney, W. L. (2008). Altered mechanisms of thermoregulatory vasoconstriction in aged human skin. *Exercise and Sport Sciences Review* **36**, 122–7.

Trevisani, M., Campi, B., Gatti, R., *et al.* (2007). The influence of alpha1-adrenoreceptors on neuropeptide release from primary sensory neurons of the lower urinary tract. *European Urology* **52**, 901–908.

Tripovic, D., Pianova, S., McLachlan, E. M., Brock, J. A. (2010). Transient supersensitivity to alpha-adrenoceptor agonists, and distinct hyper-reactivity to vasopressin and angiotensin II after denervation of rat tail artery. *British Journal of Pharmacology* **159**, 142–53.

Tugnoli, V., Marchese Ragona, R., Eleopra, R., *et al.* (2002). The role of gustatory flushing in Frey's syndrome and its treatment with botulinum toxin type A. *Clinical Autonomic Research* **12**, 174–8.

Uprus, V., Gaylor, J. B. and Carmichael, E. A. (1934). Localized abnormal flushing and sweating on eating. *Brain* **57**, 443–53.

Veves, A., Akbari, C. M., Primavera, J., *et al.* (1998). Endothelial dysfunction and the expression of endothelial nitric oxide synthetase in diabetic neuropathy, vascular disease, and foot ulceration. *Diabetes* **47**, 457–63.

Vogel, T., Gradl, G., Ockert, B., Pellengahr, C. S., Schurmann, M. (2010). Sympathetic dysfunction in long-term complex regional pain syndrome. *Clinical Journal of Pain* **26**, 128–31.

Wartenberg, R. (1945). Progressive facial hemiatrophy. *Archives of Neurology and Psychiatry* **54**, 75–96.

Wasner, G., Schattschneider, J., Heckmann, K., Maier, C. and Baron, R. (2001). Vascular abnormalities in reflex sympathetic dystrophy (CRPS I): mechanisms and diagnostic value. *Brain* **124**, 587–99.

Waxman, S. G. and Dib-Hajj, S. D. (2005). Erythromelalgia: a hereditary pain syndrome enters the molecular era. *Annals of Neurology* **57**, 785–88.

Weber, M., Birklein, F., Neundorfer, B. and Schmelz, M. (2001). Facilitated neurogenic inflammation in complex regional pain syndrome. *Pain* **91**, 251–57.

Wigington, G., Ngo, B. and Rendell, M. (2004). Skin blood flow in diabetic dermopathy. *Archives of Dermatology* **140**, 1248–50.

Wilkins, B. W., Chung, L. H., Tublitz, N. J., Wong, B. J. and Minson, C. T. (2004). Mechanisms of vasoactive intestinal peptide-mediated vasodilation in human skin. *Journal of Applied Physiology* **97**, 1291–8.

Wilkins, B. W., Wong, B. J., Tublitz, N. J., McCord, G. R. and Minson, C. T. (2005). Vasoactive intestinal peptide fragment VIP_{10-28} and active vasodilation in human skin. *Journal of Applied Physiology* **99**, 2294–2301.

Willaert, W. I., Scheltinga, M. R., Steenhuisen, S. F., Hiel, J. A. (2009). Harlequin syndrome: two new cases and a management proposal. *Acta Neurologica Belgica* **109**, 214–20.

Wong, B. J., Wilkins, B. W. and Minson, C. T. (2004). H1 but not H2 histamine receptor activation contributes to the rise in skin blood flow during whole body heating in humans. *Journal of Physiology* **560**, 941–8.

Wong, B. J., Williams, S. J. and Minson, C. T. (2006). Minimal role for H1 and H2 histamine receptors in cutaneous thermal hyperemia to local heating in humans. *Journal of Applied Physiology* **100**, 535–40.

Wong, B. J. and Minson, C. T. (2006). Neurokinin-1 receptor desensitization attenuates cutaneous active vasodilatation in humans. *Journal of Physiology* **577**, 1043–51.

Yamanaka, Y., Asahina, M., Mathias, C. J., Akaogi, Y., Koyama, Y. and Hattori, T. (2007). Skin vasodilator response to local heating in multiple system atrophy. *Movement Disorders* **22**, 2405–8.

Yamasaki, K., Di Nardo, A., Bardan, A., *et al.* (2007). Increased serine protease activity and cathelicidin promotes skin inflammation in rosacea. *Nature Medicine* **13**, 975–80.

Yamasaki, K., Gallo, R. L. (2009). The molecular pathology of rosacea. *Journal of Dermatological Science* **55**, 77–81.

Zhu, B. S., Blessing, W. W. and Gibbins, I. L. (1997). Parasympathetic innervation of cephalic arteries in rabbits: comparison with sympathetic and sensory innervation. *Journal of Comparative Neurology* **389**, 484–95.

Zollinger, P. E., Tuinebreijer, W. E., Kreis, R. W. and Breederveld, R. S. (1999). Effect of vitamin C on frequency of reflex sympathetic dystrophy in wrist fractures: a randomised trial. *Lancet* **354**, 2025–8.

Zollinger, P. E., Unal, H., Ellis, M. L., Tuinebreijer, W. E. (2010). Clinical Results of 40 Consecutive Basal Thumb Prostheses and No CRPS Type I After Vitamin C Prophylaxis. *The Open Orthopaedics Journal* **4**, 62–66.

de Bree, R., van der Waal, I. and Leemans, C. R. (2007). Management of Frey syndrome. *Head and Neck* **29**, 773–78.

CHAPTER 68

Autonomic aspects of migraine: pathophysiology and treatment

Lars Lykke Thomsen and Jes Olesen

Key points

- Migraine is considered a neurovascular disorder.

- Cerebrovascular regulatory dysfunction may be implicated in migraine pathophysiology.

- Cerebrovascular regulation is complex and involves autonomic, trigeminovascular, endothelial, and humoral factors.

- Some studies of autonomic regulation in migraine suggest parasympathetic hypofunction.

- NO and calcitonin-gene-related peptide may be important transmitters in migraine.

- A further understanding of autonomic involvement and the molecular mechanisms of migraine seems near and new therapies are likely to evolve.

Introduction

There are two main types of migraine—migraine with aura and migraine without aura. In migraine with aura, the attacks are initiated by 'marching' neurological symptoms—the aura—which typically affects one or more of the following in the order of frequency: vision, speech, sensation, and strength, either alone or in combination. Apart from these aura symptoms, the attacks are the same as in migraine without aura and are characterized by severe pulsating headaches, lasting 4–72 hours, often unilateral and accompanied by nausea and hypersensitivity to light and sounds.

Migraine headache is a very common complaint affecting up to 16% of the adult population. The burden on society, in terms of workdays lost, healthcare costs, and the amount of suffering by affected individuals, is enormous (Rasmussen 1995).

The mechanisms of migraine are complex and still not fully understood. However, an impressive advance in basic and clinical headache research over the past decades has markedly improved our understanding. As a consequence, the therapeutic strategies have become more specific. In fact, migraine became one of the first neurological conditions to be treated successfully with a receptor-selective drug (the 5-hydroxytryptamine receptor 1D [5-HT$_{1D}$] agonist, sumatriptan). Studies of the cephalic vascular system and its regulation have markedly contributed towards this development. This regulation is complex and involves autonomic, trigeminovascular, endothelial, and humoral factors. The present review focuses on these aspects of migraine pathophysiology. In addition, links are drawn between autonomic and cerebrovascular aspects of migraine and the mechanism of action of specific antimigraine therapy, and potential targets for new drug development in migraine.

Blood flow and large artery dynamics in migraine

Cerebral blood flow in migraine

Clinical studies of regional cerebral blood flow (rCBF) in migraine with aura have shown a hypoperfusion, usually not reaching ischaemic thresholds, in the posterior part of the brain at the onset of the aura. This hypoperfusion gradually spreads forward to contiguous areas not respecting the territories of supply of the major arteries. The hypoperfusion lasts throughout the aura phase and well into the headache phase, after which hyperperfusion develops (Olesen et al. 1990). The relation between the usual unilateral aura symptoms and unilateral rCBF changes suggests that in most patients the aura symptoms originate from the hemisphere affected by hypoperfusion (see Olesen 1991). The characteristic spreading rCBF changes suggest that the migraine aura may be due to a so-called cortical spreading depression (Lauritzen 1994). This phenomenon consists of a depolarization of neurons and glial cells that spreads slowly across the cortical surface and which is associated with changes in blood flow similar to rCBF changes during migraine with aura (Table 68.1). Thus, the basis of the migraine aura seems to be neuronal in nature and rCBF changes seem to be secondary phenomena. In addition the timing between rCBF changes and headache in migraine with aura suggests that these events are not causally related.

Several previous single photon emission computed tomography (SPECT) and positron emission tomography (PET) studies suggest that the cortical perfusion is unchanged during attacks of migraine without aura and also at the very beginning of provoked attacks (Olesen 1991). A study applying PET did, however, show spreading cortical changes in blood flow in a patient with symptoms not typical for a migraine aura as the patient mentioned only vague visual problems (Woods et al. 1994). Based on the clinical description, it cannot be ruled out that the patient actually suffered an

Table 68.1 Similarities between migraine aura and spreading depression

Factor	Migraine	Spreading depression
Site of origin	Primary visual cortex	High neuron density
Way of spread	Contiguous cortical	Contiguous cortical
Excitation/depression	Yes	Yes
Rate of spread	2–6 mm/minute	2–6 mm/minute
Unilateral	Yes	Yes
Repeated waves		Yes
Hypoperfusion lasting	Hours	Hours
Initial hyperperfusion	?	Yes
Autoregulation	Preserved	Preserved
CO_2 reactivity	Impaired	Impaired

Modified from Olesen 1993, with permission.

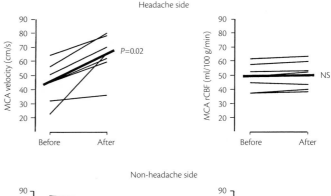

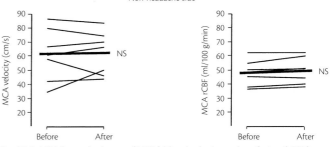

Fig. 68.1 Middle cerebral artery (MCA) blood velocity and perfusion (rCBF) during unilateral migraine headache. Responses before and after treatment with sumatriptan (2 mg intravenously). Sumatriptan induced a reversal of a decreased MCA velocity on the headache side whereas rCBF was unchanged. At the same time headaches disappeared (not shown on figures). These findings suggests that the mechanism of action of sumatriptan involves contraction of pathologically dilated large intracranial arteries. Reprinted from *The Lancet* **338**, Friberg, L., Olesen, J. , Iversen, H. K., and Sperling, B., Migraine pain associated with middle cerebral artery dilatation: reversal by sumatriptan, 13–17, Copyright (1991), with permission from Elsevier.

attack of migraine without aura and despite the prominence of studies suggesting normal rCBF during migraine without aura more studies seem necessary before this question can be regarded as settled.

A PET scan study showed an ipsilateral centre of increased blood flow in the brainstem, which persisted after successful treatment of headache with sumatriptan. The findings were made in nine patients studied within 6 hours of onset of right-sided migraine without aura. These changes were absent in a headache-free interval 3 days to 4 months later (Diener and May 1996).

Cranial arteries during migraine pain

Whereas changes in blood flow and therefore changes of arteriolar diameter seem unrelated to migraine pain, dilatation of the large cranial arteries has long been suspected to be a mechanism of migraine pain.

A study using high-frequency ultrasound demonstrated dilatation of the superficial temporal artery on the headache side during unilateral migraine attacks (Iversen et al. 1990). This dilatation was, however, small (9%) and relative to a generalized vasoconstriction. Unfortunately, the diameter of the intracranial arteries is difficult to measure directly *in vivo*. However, the ultrasound technique, transcranial Doppler (TCD), provides measurements of the velocity of circulating blood in the large intracranial arteries at the base of the brain. Since changes in blood velocity in situations of unchanged blood flow are inversely related to changes in the cross-sectional vessel area, the TCD method provides an indirect way of estimating large intracranial artery diameter changes. Friberg and colleagues used a combination of TCD and SPECT, and measured middle cerebral artery (MCA) blood velocity and rCBF simultaneously in the supply area of the MCA during unilateral migraine headache. TCD recordings showed reduced velocity on the headache side compared with the non-headache side. No such difference was found in rCBF in the MCA territory, a finding that suggests that the MCA was dilated on the headache side. In addition to this finding, evidence was provided showing that the 5-HT$_1$ receptor agonist sumatriptan (2 mg intravenously), returned blood velocity to normal without affecting rCBF, and at the same time ameliorated the headache (Friberg et al. 1991) (Fig. 68.1). Not all TCD studies have confirmed the presence of ipsilateral large artery dilatation (reviewed by Thomsen et al. 1995a). However, in a study

focusing exclusively on MCA side-to-side asymmetry in patients suffering from half-sided migraine without aura, reduced velocity was again demonstrated on the headache side (Thomsen et al. 1995a). Although these studies suggest an association between migraine pain and dilatation of the large cranial arteries, this does not necessarily imply that the pain is elicited by simple mechanical force caused by arterial dilatation. The magnitude of cranial arterial dilatation found in previous studies is most likely too small (9%) (Iversen et al. 1990, Thomsen et al. 1995a) to be the only cause of pain. Also migraine has been induced experimentally without concomitant changes in MCA diameters (Kruuse et al. 2003).

Regulation of vascular tone in migraine

Due to this vascular involvement, a possible dysregulation of vascular tone in migraine has long been a subject of considerable interest. Based on cardiovascular tests, vasomotor reactions to temperature changes, and responses to pharmacological tests, as well as changes in biochemical parameters, hypofunctioning as well as hyperfunctioning of both the sympathetic and parasympathetic nervous system has been suggested (Thomsen and Olesen 1995). Based on experimentally induced migraine attacks, a key role of the vasodilator molecule, nitric oxide (NO), has been suggested and based on an animal model of so-called neurogenic inflammation and clinical studies of plasma levels of vasoactive neuropeptides during migraine headache involvement of the trigeminovascular system has been suggested.

Cardiovascular reflexes

A number of studies have focused on sympathetically mediated cardiovascular reflexes, as elicited by the orthostatic test, the cold pressor test, and the isometric work test. An extensive series of studies has been published by Havanka-Kanniainen and colleagues. They found no evidence of disturbances in young migraineurs outside the attack (11–22 years of age) compared with a control group. Significant abnormalities suggesting sympathetic hypofunction were, however, found interictally in older migraineurs (23–50 years of age) (Havanka- Kanniainen et al. 1986). No difference was found between these responses in migraineurs suffering from migraine with and without aura. During attacks a decreased blood pressure response to an isometric work test was found to be more pronounced than between attacks. Based on decreased R-R variation during normal and deep breathing, and a decreased Valsalva ratio in migraineurs, the same authors concluded that parasympathetic hypofunction was present in migraine. Gotoh and collaborators (1984) compared responses to a Valsalva manoeuvre, an orthostatic test, and Achner's test (reflex bradycardia induced by pressure on the eyeballs) interictally in migraine patients suffering from migraine either with or without aura to age-matched healthy controls. In addition, a noradrenaline bolus injection and eye installation tests were evaluated. Sympathetic hypofunction, with denervation hypersensitivity and parasympathetic hyperfunction was suggested. In contrast to this suggested sympathetic hypofunction other studies using similar cardiovascular tests have shown either sympathetic hyperfunction or normal sympathetic function, including a recent study in which normal cardiovascular responses to cognitive stress in migraine was found (Leistad et al. 2007). Furthermore, normal parasympathetic function has also been described, based on cardiovascular tests. In our own experience migraine is not associated with disturbed cardiovascular tests reflecting sympathetic function, whereas a mild parasympathetic hypofunction seems to be present (Thomsen and Olesen 1995). The latter has also been found in a study focusing on baroreflex-mediated cardiovascular responses (Sanya et al. 2005).

Arterial and arteriolar vasomotor reactivity

Reduced vasodilatation in the forehead and hands of migraineurs after heating has been reported. In another study an increase of digital blood volume during heating was only absent in male migraineurs. In contrast, a peripherally applied cold stimulus failed to induce decreased hand blood flow in migraineurs. Finally, normal peripheral vasomotor reactivity in migraineurs has also been described (Thomsen and Olesen 1995).

Local autonomic control regarding the cranial arterial bed is obviously more relevant than studies of systemic vascular reactivity, but is more difficult to investigate. Using TCD, a recent study showed no differences in MCA blood velocity responses in migraineurs studied during tests of cardiovascular sympathetic function both during and between attacks (Thomsen et al. 1995b). This suggests normal MCA reactivity during increased sympathetic drive. In the temporal region, extracranial blood-flow responses to an orthostatic test have been studied during and between migraine attacks. This study revealed no statistical difference between the attack and the attack-free state, apart from a slightly decreased response on the headache side as compared to the non-headache side during attack (Jensen 1987). Interestingly other studies suggest that cranial parasympathetic function seems to differ among patients with unilateral and bilateral migraine pain as assessed by vasodilator response of forehead skin using photoplethysmography (Avnon et al. 2003, Avnon et al. 2004).

Cerebral blood-flow responses to functional tests such as speech, reading, listening, and arm work have been studied during attacks of migraine with aura. These activation procedures were not accompanied by the usual increase in rCBF in low-flow areas, whereas a normal, focal rCBF increase was observed in the non-affected parts of the brain. It is most likely, but not definitely established, that autoregulation is normal during attacks of both migraine with and without aura (Olesen 1991). Several studies have focused on cerebrovascular reactivity to alterations in PaCO2. During attacks of migraine with aura, PaCO2 reactivity seems to be impaired or abolished, whereas PaCO2 reactivity seems to be normal during attacks of migraine without aura. Interictally an exaggerated PCO2 reactivity during hyperventilation has been reported but only in migraine with aura (Thomsen and Olesen 1995). The interictal response to CO_2 inhalation may, however, be exaggerated both in migraine with and without aura, and more studies are needed to establish whether interictal differences in cerebrovascular reactivity exist between migraine with and without aura.

Pupillometry

Autonomic function may be studied by pupillometry. Such results generally suggest sympathetic or parasympathetic hypofunction in migraine. Interictally the mydriatic response to tyramine, phenylephrine, guanethidine, and adrenaline was enhanced in adult migraineurs but not in children. Furthermore, pupillometric data have suggested α-receptor supersensitivity of the iris (for review see Thomsen and Olesen 1995).

Central sympathetic function and conclusions on functional studies of the autonomic nervous system in migraine

It has been suggested that the contingent negative variation (CNV)—a slow cerebral potential elicited by a reaction task with a warning and an imperative stimulus—is modulated by catecholamine afferents to the frontal cortex. If this is so, studies of CNV in migraine may indicate a central sympathetic involvement (Maertens de Noordhout et al. 1986). However, at present this possibility remains hypothetical. As mentioned, changes in blood flow in certain areas of the brainstem may be present during attacks (Diener and May 1996). This may be a visualization of a dysfunction of the locus coeruleus in migraine as previously suggested (Lance 1993).

Thus it may be concluded that brainstem activity involving the locus coeruleus, which utilizes noradrenaline as a transmitter and which is involved in anti-nociception, and extracranial and intracranial vascular control, may be present in migraine. However, a clear dysfunction of the sympathetic nervous system still remains to be shown. If sympathetic dysfunction is involved, most studies suggest hypofunction. However, considering that several studies, applying different methods, have been inconclusive and that the response of cranial arteries is normal during increased sympathetic activity, it seems unlikely that a sympathetic dysfunction plays any major role. Mild parasympathetic hypofunction with denervation supersensitivity may be present in migraine. The origin of such disturbances are unknown and it remain to be demonstrated whether large cranial artery parasympathetic responses are abnormal and which transmitters or modulators may be involved.

Vasoactive neurotransmitters in migraine

5-HT and catecholamines

Plasma levels and urinary excretion of catecholamines and their metabolites have often been studied, but with contradicting results (Lance 1993, Thomsen and Olesen 1995). Indirect evidence points towards a role for the vasoactive amine 5-HT in migraine. In humans 5-HT is found in the brain, the pineal gland, the blood, platelets, and blood vessels, including the circle of Willis. There is a close interaction between the central 5-HT system and the central noradrenergic system, but it is unknown whether this interaction plays a role in migraine. During attacks of migraine without aura the platelet content of 5-HT is decreased, but not during attacks of migraine with aura. 5-HT in platelet-free plasma, on the other hand, shows similar changes in migraine with and without aura. Thus, interictally migraineurs have lower 5-HT and higher 5-hydroxyin-doleacetic acid (5-HIAA, the main metabolite of 5-HT) compared with controls. During attacks, the plasma level of 5-HT increases significantly compared with outside of attack, whereas 5-HIAA levels fall. This could imply a release of 5-HT from platelets during attack and/or an increased metabolic turnover of 5-HT outside of attack (Ferrari and Saxena 1995).

Neuropeptides and trigeminovascular mechanisms

Neuropeptide Y (NPY), vasoactive intestinal peptide (VIP), and substance P in blood from the external and internal jugular vein were normal during migraine attacks. However, increased levels of calcitonin-gene-related peptide (CGRP) in blood from the external jugular vein has been demonstrated during migraine attacks (Table 68.2) (Goadsby et al. 1990). Interestingly CGRP infused intravenously in patients with migraine was able to induce headache in a great majority of patients which in some patients fulfilled all diagnostic criteria for migraine without aura (Lassen et al. 2002). Antidromic activity in perivascular nerve endings of trigeminal origin releases neurotransmitters, which in turn induce vasodilatation and plasma extravasation as part of a so-called neurogenic inflammation. A series of experimental studies in rats has

Table 68.2 Calcitonin-gene-related peptide (CGRP) and substance P (SP) during migraine headache

	CGRP	SP
Migraine with aura		
Site		
◆ External jugular vein	92 (±11)*	5 (±2)
◆ Cubital fosa	40 (±6)	5 (±3)
Control values	<40	<4
Migraine without aura		
Site		
◆ External jugular vein	86 (±4)*	6 (±2)
◆ Cubital fosa	43 (±6)	4 (±1)
Control values	<40	<4

*, p > 0.001. Modified from Goadsby et al. 1990, with permission.

shown alterations in vascular permeability and ultrastructural changes in the dura mater associated with stimulation of the trigeminal ganglion (Moskowitz 1993). Trigeminal ganglion stimulation has been shown to be associated with a release of CGRP and substance P in the rat and in humans. It remains to be demonstrated whether neurogenic inflammation takes place during migraine attacks.

NO and cGMP

NO is not only a transmitter in parasympathetic perivascular nerves, it is also the main endothelium-derived relaxant factor (EDRF). NO is liberated from the endothelium upon stimulation of several receptors and also by shear stress phenomena. Endothelial receptor stimulation may occur from the luminal side and perhaps also from the abluminal side. Thus, relevant transmitters may be released from perivascular nerve endings in the adventitia, diffuse to the endothelium, and stimulate the release of NO. NO is a gas that easily crosses membranes. It thus enters smooth muscle cells and causes relaxation via activation of soluble guanylate cyclase hence causing accumulation of cyclic guanosine monophosphate (cGMP). Glyceryl trinitrate (GTN)—which has been systematically validated as an experimental headache-inducing substance—is a NO donor, and hypersensitivity to NO has been shown indirectly in migraineurs by means of intravenous infusion of GTN. Interestingly, increased sensitivity to GTN in migraine has been shown both for the induction of pain and for dilatation of the MCA (Olesen et al. 1995).

The nitric oxide pathway and the triggering of migraine pain

Not only has hypersensitivity to pain and arterial dilatation induced by GTN been demonstrated in migraine but this NO donor also triggers delayed genuine migraine attacks in migraineurs which are almost identical to spontaneous attacks. Based on these observations, hypotheses have been made stating that release of NO provides a common final pathway for several substances that trigger migraine pain (Olesen et al. 1995). Beside the NO donor, GTN, other substances which have been shown to reliably cause more headache than placebo in single-dose experiments include histamine, reserpine, and *meta*-chloro-phenylpiperazine (m-CPP). Interestingly, migraineurs have been described to be hypersensitive to these substances regarding headache development, which in migraineurs resembles migraine attacks, in controlled trials (Olesen et al. 1995). In a double-blind controlled trial, migraineurs were randomized to pretreatment with either mepyramine or placebo before histamine infusion. Half of the placebo pretreated patients developed a migraine attack. The mepyramine pretreated patients only developed a very mild headache, if any. Activation of endothelial H_1-receptors induces the formation of endogenous NO. Thus, as with GTN, the increased sensitivity to histamine in migraineurs may also be explained by hypersensitivity to activation of the NO pathway.

In migraineurs, reserpine causes headache with some features of migraine. Reserpine depletes not only platelets but also presynaptic nerve terminals of their content of monoamines. Substances released include 5-HT. The 5-HT_{2B} (formerly called 5-HT_{1C} and 5-HT_{2C}) receptor has been suggested to play a crucial role in the initiation of spontaneous migraine attacks. 5-HT caused an endothelium-dependent relaxing response in a number of vessels from different species, and this effect was mediated via the

5-HT$_{2B}$ receptor. The vascular response to 5-HT$_{2B}$ activation, at least in the pig, is primarily a consequence of the release of NO. Interestingly, in this context m-CPP is a direct agonist at the 5-HT$_{2B}$ receptor and, therefore, is likely to cause vascular headache via NO synthesis. Thus, NO may be a common denominator for headaches induced by GTN, histamine, reserpine, and m-CPP. In addition, the 5HT$_{2B}$ receptor may provide a link between the suggested biochemical changes in 5-HT metabolism during spontaneous migraine attacks and the NO pathway in migraine. In theory, formation of NO relevant for the triggering of spontaneous migraine may be elicited by fluctuations in numerous neurotransmitters, both in the blood and/or the brain, as part of pathological reactions such as spreading depression, activation of the trigeminovascular system with liberation of, for example, substance P, fever, and inflammation, via interleukins and histamine, etc. (Olesen et al. 1995).

Further support for implication of the NO-cGMP pathway comes from a study where migraine was induced in migraineurs with Sildenafil which increases cGMP levels by selective inhibitor of phosphodiesterase 5 (PDE5) (Kruuse et al. 2003). As mentioned previously the latter study also demonstrated that these migraines were induced without initial dilatation of the middle cerebral artery

Therapeutic implications

Mechanisms of action of acute migraine therapy

Traditionally the mechanism of action of acute migraine therapy (except generally acting analgesics) has been ascribed to constriction of pathologically dilated cranial arteries. Thus, intravenous administration of the effective antimigraine drug, ergotamine, was long ago shown to reduce temporal artery pulsations in parallel with a decrease in headache intensity. It has been suggested that one important action of ergotamine may be the inhibition of antidromic release of trigeminal neuropeptides as part of a neurogenic inflammation (Moskowitz 1993). Ergotamine interacts with 5-HT, dopamine and noradrenaline receptors. Thus, elucidation of a specific receptor involvement requires more specific pharmacological tools. So far the most specific and highly effective acute migraine treatment available is the 5-HT$_{1D}$ receptor agonists—the triptans. Several mechanisms of action of triptans have been proposed. A direct pain-modulating effect in the central nervous system is unlikely since one of the triptans—sumatriptan—is soluble in water and crosses the blood–brain barrier very slowly. One possibility is that constriction of dilated large intracranial arteries provides the causative mechanism (Friberg et al. 1991). However, as with ergotamine, another possible mechanism of action is blockade of the release of sensory neuropeptides as part of a neurogenic inflammation (Moskowitz 1993). Since these neuropeptides also induce vasodilatation, the observed vasoconstrictive effect may be a secondary phenomenon. Thus, despite that current specific drugs used in the acute treatment of migraine interact with vascular receptors, this may not be the primary mechanism of action but certainly has cardiovascular safety implications. It is interesting, therefore, that recent studies have shown that CGRP antagonist (BIBN 4096 BS and MK 0974), which seem to have no constrictor effect on the middle cerebral or on regional cerebral blood flow, are effective in the treatment of acute migraine headache (Olesen et al. 2004, Petersen et al. 2005, Ho et al. 2008).

Interaction with the nitric oxide cascade provides a possible mechanism of action of existing prophylactic migraine therapy

Regarding drugs with established prophylactic effect in migraine, their mechanism of action has for long been an enigma. These drugs include β-adrenergic blocking drugs without partial agonist activity (i.e. propranolol, metroprolol, atenol, nadolol, and timolol), antiserotonergic drugs (i.e. methysergide, pizotifen), and calcium antagonists (i.e. flunarizine and verapamil). Many observations suggest that all of these drugs interact with the NO-triggered cascade of reactions. Thus, calcium antagonists block non-adrenergic non-cholinergic perivascular nerves by inhibiting calcium ion channels and therefore the activation of neuronal NOS (Toda, personal communication). Methysergide and pizotifen are 5-HT antagonists that do not discriminate between the 5-HT$_1$ and the 5-HT$_2$ receptors. It has recently been suggested that their effect is via 5-HT$_{2B}$ (formerly 5-HT$_{2C}$) receptor antagonism. 5-HT$_{2B}$ receptor stimulation liberates NO. Thus, amine antagonists may well exert their action by reducing NO production. Propranolol blocks isoprenaline-induced relaxation of rat thoracic aorta in an endothelium-dependent fashion. The response is also blocked by the NOS inhibitor L-NOARG. The prophylactic effect of β-adrenergic blockers in migraine may thus result from blockade of β-adrenoceptor-induced NO production. Propranolol also antagonizes the 5-HT$_{2B}$ receptor on the endothelium. This is another mechanism whereby it may reduce endothelial NO production. In contrast to propranolol, pindolol, which is ineffective in migraine, lacks affinity to the 5-HT$_{2B}$ receptor (Olesen et al. 1995).

Novel targets for drug development in migraine

Based on the elevated plasma levels of CGRP during migraine attacks, CGRP antagonists are currently in clinical development and seem to be of importance as future antimigraine drugs. In fact it has recently been demonstrated that two CGRP antagonist (BIBN4096BS and MK 0974), which as previously mentioned seems to have no direct contractile effects on human cerebral vasculature, alleviate acute migraine attacks without significant side-effects (Olesen et al. 2004, Ho et al. 2008). In addition, the central role of NO in migraine pain is also likely to offer future therapeutic possibilities. Thus, drugs which directly counteract the NO-activated cascade (NOS inhibitors, NO scavengers, guanylate cyclase inhibitors, etc.) may be effective in migraine. A study actually suggests that the nonspecific NOS inhibitor L-N^G-methylarginine hydrochloride (546C88) is effective in the acute treatment of migraine headache (Lassen et al. 1997). The more specific these drug become the more effective they are likely to be, and the fewer side-effects they are likely to induce. Thus, a further understanding of the molecular mechanisms of the neurovascular mechanisms of migraine seems near and new therapies are likely to evolve.

References

Avnon, Y., Nitzan, M., Spercher, E., Rogowski, Z. and Yarnitsky, D. (2003). Different patterns of parasympahathetic acitivation in uni- and bilateral migraineurs. *Brain* **126**, 1660–70.

Avnon, Y., Nitzan, M., Spercher, E., Rogowski, Z. and Yarnitsky, D. (2004). Autonomic asymmetry in migraine: augmented parasympathetic acitivation in left unilateral migraineurs. *Brain* **127**, 2099–2108.

Diener, H. C. and May, A. (1996). Positron emission tomography studies in acute migraine attacks. In *Migraine pharmacology and genetics* (ed. M. Sandler, M. Ferrari, and S. Harnett), pp. 109–14. Chapman & Hall, London.

Ferrari, M. D. and Saxena, P. (1995). 5-HT$_1$ receptors in migraine pathophysiology and treatment. *Eur. J. Neurology*, **2**, 5–21.

Friberg, L., Olesen, J., Iversen, H. K., and Sperling, B. (1991). Migraine pain associated with middle cerebral artery dilatation: reversal by sumatriptan. *Lancet* **338**, 13–17.

Goadsby, P. J., Edvinsson, L., and Ekman, R. (1990). Vasoactive peptide release in the extracerebral circulation of humans during migraine headache. *Ann. Neurol.* **28**, 183–7.

Gotoh, F., Komatsumota, S., Araki, N., and Gomi, S. (1984). Noradrenergic nervous activity in migraine. *Arch. Neurol.* **41**, 951–5.

Havanka-Kanniainen, H., Tolonen, U., and Myllyla, V. V. (1986). Autonomic dysfunction in adult migraineurs. *Headache* **26**, 425–30.

Ho T. W., Mannix L. K., Fan X., *et a.l* (2008). Randomized controlled trial of an oral CGRP receptor antagonist, MK-0974, in acute treatment of migraine. *Neurology.* **15**, 1304–12.

Iversen, H. K., Nielsen, T. H., Olesen, J., and Tfelt-Hansen, P. (1990). Arterial responses during migraine headache. *Lancet* **336**, 837–9.

Jensen, K. (1987). Subcutaneous blood flow in the temporal region of migraine patients. *Acta Neurol. Scand.* **72**, 561–70.

Kruuse, C. Thomsen, L. L. Birk, S. and Olesen, J. (2003). Migraine can be induced by sildenafil without changes in middle cerebral artery dimater. Brain **126**, 241–47.

Lance, J. W. (1993). *Mechanism and management of headache*, (5th edn). Butterworth-Heinemann, Oxford.

Lassen, L. H., Ashina, M., Christiansen, I., Ulrich, V., and Olesen, J. (1997). NO synthase inhibition in migraine. *Lancet* **349**, 401–2.

Lassen, L. H., Haderslev, P. A. Jacobsen, T. B., Iversen, H. K. Sperling, B. and Olesen, J. (2002). CGRP may play a causative role in migraine. *Cephaalgia* **22**, 54–61.

Lauritzen, M. (1994). Pathophysiology of the migraine aura. The spreading depression theory. *Brain* **117**, 199–210.

Leistad, R. B., Sand. T., Nilsen K. B. Westgaard R. H. and Stovner L. J. (2007). Cardiovascular responses to cognitive stress in patients with migraine and tension- type headache. BMC Neurology, **7**, 1–12.

Maertens de Noordhout, A., Timsit-Berthier, M., and Schoenen, J. (1986) Contigent negative variation in headache. *Ann. Neurol.* **19**, 78–80.

Moskowitz, M. A. (1993). Neurogenic inflammation in the pathophysiology and treatment of migraine. *Neurology* **43** (Suppl. 3), S16–20.

Olesen, J. (1991). Cerebral and extracranial circulatory disturbances in migraine: pathophysiological implications. *Cerebrovasc. Brain Metab. Rev.* **3**, 1–28.

Olesen, J. (1993). Hemodynamics. In *The headaches*, (ed. J. Olesen, P. Tfelt-Hansen, and K. M. A. Welch), pp. 209–22. Raven Press, New York.

Olesen, J., Diener, H. C., Husstedt, P. J., *et al.* (2004). Calcitonin gene-related peptide receptor antagonist BIBN4096BS for the acute treatment of migraine. *N Eng J Med* **350**, 1104–10.

Olesen, J., Friberg, L., Oslen, T. S., *et al.* (1990). Timing and topography of cerebral blood flow and headache during migraine attacks. *Ann. Neurol.* **28**, 791–8.

Olesen, J., Iversen, H. K., and Thomsen, L. L. (1993). NO supersentivity: a possible molecular mechanism of migraine pain. *Neuroreport* **4**, 1027–30.

Olesen, J., Thomsen, L. L., Lassen, L. H., and Jansen-Olesen, I. (1995). The NO hypothesis of migraine and other vascular headaches. *Cephalalgia* **15**, 94–100.

Petersen K. A., Lassen L. H., Birk S., Lesko L. and Olesen J. (2005). BIBN4096BS on human-alpha–calcitonin Gene Related Peptide—induced headache and Extracerebral Artery dilatation. *Clinical Pharmacology and Therapeutics* **23**, 725.

Rasmussen, B. K. (1995). Epidemiology of headache. Thesis. *Cephalalgia* **15**, 45–68.

Sanya, E. O. Brown, C. M. Wilmowsky, C. Neundorfer, B. and Hilz, M. J. (2005). Impairments of parasympathetic baroreflex responses in migraine patients. *Acta Neurol Scand* **111**, 102–7,

Thomsen, L. L., Iversen, H. K., Boesen, F., and Olesen J. (1995*b*). Transcranial Doppler and cardiovascular responses during cardiovascular autonomic tests in migraineurs during and outside of attacks. *Brain* **118**, 1319–27.

Thomsen, L. L., Iversen, H. K., Brinck, T. A., and Olesen, J. (1993). Arterial supersensitivity to NO (nitroglycerin) in migraine sufferes. *Cephalagia* **13**, 395–9.

Thomsen, L. L., Iversen, H. K., and Olesen, J. (1995*a*). Cerebral blood flow velocities are reduced during attacks of unilateral migraine without aura. *Cephalalgia* **15**, 109–16.

Thomsen, L. L. and Olesen, J. (1995). The autonomic nervous system and the regulation of arterial tone in migraine. *Clin. Auton. Res.* **5**, 243–50.

Woods, R. P., Iacoboni, M., and Mazziotta, J. C. (1994). Bilateral spreading cerebral hypoperfusion during spontaneous migraine headache. *New Engl. J. Med.* **331**, 1689–92.

CHAPTER 69

Mechanisms underlying complex regional pain syndrome

Role of the sympathetic nervous system

Ralf Baron and Wilfrid Jänig

Introduction

For almost a century it is discussed that activity in the sympathetic nervous system may be involved in the generation of pain (e.g. in causalgia and reflex sympathetic dystrophy). This assumption is based mainly upon two observations:

◆ The pain is spatially correlated with signs of autonomic dysfunction (i.e. with abnormalities in blood flow and sweating), as well as with trophic changes.

◆ Blocking the efferent sympathetic supply to the affected part relieves the pain.

In 1995 the terminology of these pain syndromes was changed. The term reflex sympathetic dystrophy was thought to be not appropriate as a clinical designation because it has been sloppily used to describe an extensive range of clinical presentations. Moreover, since the pathophysiological mechanisms underlying these syndromes are poorly understood it is probably premature to use terms like 'reflex' and 'sympathetic'. Therefore, the new terminology is based entirely on elements of history, symptoms, and findings on clinical examination with no implied pathophysiological mechanism (Stanton-Hicks et al. 1995). According to the International Association for the Study of Pain (IASP) *Classification of Chronic Pain* reflex sympathetic dystrophy and causalgia are now called complex regional pain syndromes (CRPS). In CRPS type I (reflex sympathetic dystrophy) minor injuries at the limb or lesions in remote body areas precede the onset of symptoms. CRPS type II (causalgia) develops after injury of a major peripheral nerve (Merskey and Bogduk 1994).

Furthermore, it was recognized that patients with CRPS presenting with exactly the same clinical signs and symptoms can be divided into two groups by the negative or positive effect of sympathetic blockade. The pain component that is relieved by specific sympatholytic procedures is considered 'sympathetically maintained pain' (SMP). Thus, SMP is now defined to be a *symptom* and *not a clinical entity*. *The positive effect of a sympathetic blockade is not essential for the diagnosis* of CRPS. On the other hand, the only possibility to differentiate between SMP and sympathetically independent pain (SIP) is the efficacy of a correctly applied sympatholytic intervention (Stanton-Hicks et al. 1995).

Despite the extensive body of clinical experience, it remains controversial whether and in which way the sympathetic nervous system plays a causal role in the generation of pain. The lack of well-controlled clinical studies has been accompanied by extensive speculations about the underlying pathophysiology. We will first present a hypothesis stating that CRPS is a disorder of the central nervous system (CNS) and then argue on which clinical and experimental data this hypothesis is based with special focus on the sympathetic nervous system. In Chapter 20 of this volume pathophysiological mechanisms underlying the role of the sympathetic nervous system in the generation of pain are discussed.

Diagnostic criteria for complex regional pain syndrome

The clinical phenomena of CRPS are described in detail in Baron (2006, 2009). The diagnosis of CRPS is mainly based on clinical criteria because there are no gold standards to compare with and no absolute diagnostic tests that are specific for CRPS. It is difficult to distinguish CRPS from other extremity pain syndromes. Furthermore it is difficult, if not impossible, to predict acutely after a trauma at an extremity who is going to develop a CRPS and who not. Thus, we have no predictor for CRPS. This is not very surprising in view of the hypothesis that CRPS is a disease of the CNS (see p.836) and cannot be causally related in its development to a distinct group of traumatic events as outlined below.

An extended diagnostic algorithm that is at least to some extend anchored in mechanisms has recently been proposed (Table 69.1). Several procedures are often used to support the clinical diagnosis of CRPS, such as plain radiograph, three-phase bone scan, quantitative

Table 69.1 Criteria for clinical diagnosis of complex regional pain syndromes

Categories of clinical signs or symptoms
Positive sensory abnormalities
◆ Spontaneous pain
◆ Mechanical hyperalgesia
◆ Thermal hyperalgesia
◆ Deep somatic hyperalgesia
Vascular abnormalities
◆ Vasodilation
◆ Vasoconstriction
◆ Skin temperature asymmetries
◆ Skin colour changes
Oedema, sweating abnormalities
◆ Swelling
◆ Hyperhidrosis
◆ Hypohidrosis
Motor (M) and trophic changes (T)
◆ Motor weakness (M)
◆ Tremor (M)
◆ Dystonia (M)
◆ Coordination deficit (M)
◆ Nail or hair changes (T)
◆ Skin atrophy (T)
◆ Joint stiffness (T)
◆ Soft tissue changes (T)

Interpretation

Clinical use	Research use
≥1 symptoms of ≥3 categories each	≥1 symptoms in each of the 4 categories
AND ≥1 signs at the time of evaluation	AND ≥1 signs at the time of evaluation in
in ≥2 categories each	≥2 categories each
sensitivity 0.85, specificity 0.60	*sensitivity 0.70, specificity 0.96*

These diagnostic criteria have been modified compared to the original criteria as defined by Stanton-Hicks et al. (1995) by Harden et al. (2007) in order to obtain a higher specificity for clinical use (to avoid overdiagnosis of CRPS) and a higher sensitivity for research use. This table was published in *Wall and Melzacks Textbook of Pain* (5th edn.), ed. S.B. McMahon and M. Koltzenburg, Complex regional pain syndromes, Baron, R. pp. 1011–1027, Copyright Elsevier (2006). From Baron (2006).

sensory testing, temperature difference between right and left hand or foot, and magnetic resonance imaging (for discussion see Baron 2006, 2009). In addition to the improved clinical categories it became clear to distinguish between criteria for clinical use and a classification for research purposes. For the clinician, and in particular for the patients, it is important to have a high sensitivity value combined with a fair specificity (e.g. 0.85 vs 0.60, Table 69.1). For research purposes, however, it is much more important to have a high specificity in order to perform studies in a precisely diagnosed population (e.g. 0.7 vs 0.96, Table 69.1).

Harden et al. (2007) have modified these diagnostic criteria compared with the original criteria as defined by Stanton-Hicks et al.

(1995) in order to obtain a higher specificity for clinical use (to avoid over diagnosis of CRPS) and a higher sensitivity for research use.

Complex regional pain syndrome type I is a neuronal disease involving the central nervous system

Here we hypothesize that the sensory, sympathetic, somatomotor, and trophic changes (including swelling), observed in variable combinations in patients with CRPS, in particular those with CRPS type I, are the results of changes and distorted processing of information in the CNS involving the somatosensory non-nociceptive and nociceptive systems, the endogenous neuronal systems controlling nociceptive impulse transmission, the sympathetic systems as well as the somatomotor system. Various levels of integration probably are involved such as spinal cord, brainstem, diencephalon (hypothalamus, thalamus), and telencephalon (cortex and limbic system). A key player in generation and maintenance of CRPS is most likely the nociceptive system. However, this system must not be seen to *cause* CRPS in the sense that CRPS can be reduced to the malfunctioning of the nociceptive system. Furthermore, although the sympathetic nervous system is important, CRPS cannot be reduced to a malfunctioning of this system or components of it. In the following sections we will discuss the arguments supporting that CRPS is a central nervous system disorder. The upper part in Table 69.2 lists clinical and experimental observations made on patients with CRPS that clearly support this contention. The lower part in Table 69.2 lists the peripheral changes observed in patients with CRPS that are also related in some yet unknown way to the central changes.

Fig. 69.1 outlines a general heuristic explanatory hypothesis that has been developed in the past 25 years (Jänig 1985, Jänig and Stanton-Hicks 1996) and goes back to Livingston (1976). This hypothesis puts the clinical findings observed in patients with CRPS in relation to the changes in the somatosensory, autonomic, and somatomotor systems, and postulates that changes in the central representations of these systems must occur in order to explain the clinical findings. The events initiating the clinical symptoms are mostly associated with a trauma in the somatic domains at the extremities, but sometimes also with trauma in the viscera or in the CNS. The changes developing after these triggering events usually outlast the trauma by orders of magnitude. It is unknown whether neuroendocrine systems are involved too.

An important component of the hypothesis for patients with CRPS with sympathetically maintained pain (SMP) is postulated to be a positive feedback circle consisting of afferent neurons, central neurons (spinal circles and their supraspinal controls), sympathetic neurons, and sympathetic-afferent coupling (see Chapter 20). This circle would maintain spontaneous pain (sympathetically maintained), hyperalgesia and allodynia and the associated changes (Harden et al. 2001, Jänig and Stanton-Hicks 1996). It is important to emphasize that this positive feedback circle does not explain the (peripheral and central) mechanisms in detail and fails to explain the central changes which must occur in CRPS in view of the clinical changes observed in these patients (Table 69.2). Furthermore, it fails to explain why CRPS I without SMP is clinically entirely indistinguishable from CRPS I with SMP although we do not know whether this loop plays a role in the generation of other peripheral phenomena observed in patients with CRPS.

Table 69.2 Arguments for central and for peripheral changes in complex regional pain syndromes

Central changes

Changes of regulation by sympathetic systems (1 in Fig. 69.1)

- Thermoregulatory reflexes in cutaneous vasoconstrictor neurons reduced
- Respiration elicited reflexes (generated by deep inspiration and expiration) in cutaneous vasoconstrictor neurons reduced
- Changes of activity in sudomotor neurons (sweating)
- Swelling reduced by sympathetic blocks

Sensory changes (2 in Fig. 69.1)

- Mechanical allodynia (quadrant, hemisensory)
- Hypoaesthesias (mechanical, cold, warm; hemisensory, quadrant)
- Bilateral distribution of hypoaesthesias and hyperaesthesias (mechanical, cold, warm, heat)

Somatomotor changes (3 in Fig. 69.1)

- Active motor force and active range of motion reduced
- Physiological tremor increased
- Poor motor control and coordination of movement; altered gait and posture
- Dystonia
- Sensory-motor body perception disturbance

Initiating events (4 in Fig. 69.1)

- Out of proportion to pain disease (minor trauma)
- Events remote from affected extremity (e.g. in the visceral domain)
- Central (e.g. after stroke; related to endogenous control systems?)

Pain relief by sympathetic blocks with local anaesthetics (5 in Fig. 69.1)

- Relief of pain *outlasts conduction block* by an order of magnitude, (i.e. a temporary block is followed by a *long-lasting* pain relief)
- A few temporary blocks are sometimes sufficient to generate permanent pain relief
- *Sympathetic activity maintains a positive feedback circle (?)*

Peripheral changes

Sympathetic-afferent coupling (6 in Fig. 69.1)

- After nerve lesion via noradrenaline and adrenoceptors (CRPS II)
- Indirectly via vascular bed and other mechanisms (CRPS I; deep somatic?)
- [Indirectly via inflammatory mediators and neurotrophic factors]
- [Mediated by the adrenal medulla (adrenaline)]

Inflammatory changes and oedema (7 in Fig. 69.1)

- Neurogenic inflammation (precapillary vasodilation, venular plasma extravasation), involvement of peptidergic afferents (?)
- Sympathetic fibres mediating effects of inflammatory mediators (e.g. bradykinin) to venules leading to plasma extravasation (?)
- Involvement of inflammatory cells and immune system (?)
- Change of capillary filtration pressure (?)

Trophic changes (8 in Fig. 69.1)

- Long-range consequences of inflammatory changes and oedema (?)
- Direct (trophic?) effect of sympathetic and afferent fibres on tissue (?)
- Endothelial damage (?)

Modified from Jänig and Baron (2003).

Therefore, as fascinating and attractive the idea of a positive feedback circle via the efferent sympathetic outflow may be, from the scientific and the clinical point of view, we should be careful reducing the mechanisms operating in CRPS to this positive feedback circle, although its interruption may lead in some patients to complete relief of pain and to the disappearance of other changes observed in CRPS patients. In this context it has been shown in patients with CRPS, using microneurographic recording from postganglionic fibres or measurement of noradrenaline overflow, that the activity in sympathetic neurons innervating skin of the affected extremity is not increased and spillover of noradrenaline is not increased but decreased (Baron 2006, 2009). These findings are not at variance with the idea of a positive feedback circle. In fact, the activity in cutaneous sympathetic vasoconstrictor neurons seem to be decreased in those CRPS patients who have warm skin and are successfully treated by sympathetic blocks.

Sympathetic systems supplying skin

Cutaneous vasoconstrictor neurons and blood flow through skin

Thermoregulatory reflexes to whole body heating and cooling are changed in the distal parts of the affected extremity of CRPS I patients. During whole body cooling, activity in the vasoconstrictor neurons supplying skin is increased leading to decrease of blood flow through the hand and decrease of skin temperature. Patients with CRPS I exhibit three different pathophysiological patterns of behaviour of the cutaneous vasoconstrictor neurons supplying the hand of the affected extremity during thermoregulatory load (whole body cooling and warming). Whole body cooling generates:

- a weaker than normal activation or no activation,
- a stronger than normal activation, or
- an intermediate response pattern,

leading to the expected difference in temperature and blood flow through acral skin between the affected side and the contralateral (control) side.

At extreme thermoregulatory states (maximal cooling and maximal warming), when the cutaneous vasoconstrictor activity is either maximal or absent, the temperature difference (and cutaneous blood flow difference) between affected and non-affected (control) extremity is small or absent; at thermoregulatory states in between the difference in cutaneous temperature (and cutaneous blood flow) is maximal and can reach values up to 10°C (● in Fig. 69.2). These differences never occur in healthy control subjects and in patients with pain of another aetiology (e.g. pain in patients with traumatic mononeuropathy)(■ and ▲ in Fig. 69.2). Weaker than normal activations of the cutaneous vasoconstrictor system to whole body cooling are usually observed in patients with CRPS early after the initiating trauma and stronger than normal responses particularly in chronic CRPS patients (Wasner et al. 2001).

In the early stages of CRPS type I, cutaneous vasoconstriction and vasodilation in fingers elicited by deep inspiration (and expiration) is attenuated (Fig. 69.3A) (Wasner et al. 1999). This lack of respiratory modulation of vascular perfusion is not due to damage of the cutaneous vasoconstrictor neurons since the modulation returned after successful treatment of the CRPS in the patient (Fig. 69.3B). The respiration-induced vasoconstriction of the

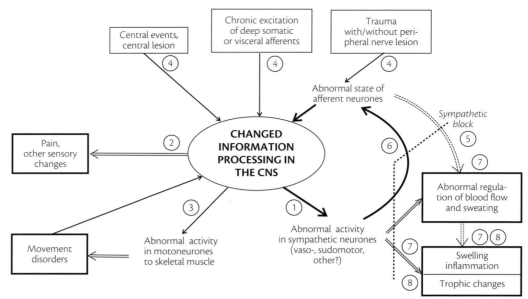

Fig. 69.1 General explanatory hypothesis about the neural mechanisms of generation of complex regional pain syndrome types I and II (CRPS I and I) following peripheral trauma with and without nerve lesions, chronic stimulation of deep somatic afferents or occasionally visceral afferents (e.g. during angina pectoris, myocardial infarction) or, occasionally, central trauma. The clinical observations are put in bold lined boxes. Note the vicious circle (arrows in bold). An important component of this circle is the excitatory influence of postganglionic sympathetic axons on primary afferent neurons. The numbers indicate the changes occurring potentially in patients with CRPS that have been quantitatively measured or postulated on the basis of clinical observations (see Table 69.2): **1**: changes in sympathetic neurons; **2**: pain, somatosensory changes; **3**: changes in somatomotoneurons; **4**: initiating events; **5**: consequences of sympathetic blocks or sympathectomy (dotted line); **6**:, sympathetic-afferent coupling (positive vicious feedback circle [in bold]); **7**: 'antidromically' conducted activity in peptidergic afferent C-fibres (double dotted arrow) leading to increase of blood flow (arteriolar vasodilation) and venular plasma extravasation, both hypothetically contributing to increase in blood flow, swelling/inflammation and trophic changes. **8**: sympathetic postganglionic fibres hypothetically contributing to swelling/inflammation and trophic changes. For details see text. Modified from Jänig (1985) and Jänig and Stanton-Hicks (1996).

cutaneous vascular blood vessels of the hand is generated by activation of cutaneous vasoconstrictor neurons. The basis of this activation is the coupling between the neuronal network regulating respiration and the neuronal network regulating the cardiovascular system in the lower brain stem (pons and medulla oblongata [for review see Jänig 2006]). The central command that activates the respiratory network and leads to deep inspiration and expiration would modulate, via the respiratory network, the activity in the cutaneous vasoconstrictor system.

The changes occurring in cutaneous blood flow and temperature during these interventions can only be attributed to central changes, which are reflected in changes of activity in cutaneous vasoconstrictor neurons innervating the distal parts of the affected extremity. These observations are fully consistent with experiments on cats showing that nerve lesions lead to changes of chemoreceptor, baroreceptor and nociceptor reflexes in cutaneous vasoconstrictor neurons but not in muscle vasoconstrictor neurons. The differentiation in reflex pattern between muscle and cutaneous vasoconstrictor neurons (Jänig 2006; Chapter 1 of this volume) disappears and cutaneous vasoconstrictor neurons tend to exhibit reflexes that are identical to those in muscle vasoconstrictor neurons. These reflex changes are chronic, being present months and possibly years after nerve lesion (Blumberg and Jänig 1985; Jänig and Koltzenburg 1991).

For most sympathetic systems the organization of the central circuits that regulate the activity in the final sympathetic pathways are largely unknown (Jänig 2006). Some central pathways linked, on the output side, to vasoconstrictor systems regulating resistance vessels in skeletal muscle or viscera and, on the afferent side, to arterial baroreceptors, arterial chemoreceptors or other receptors

related to regulation of cardiovascular system and respiration, were successfully worked out in the last 20 years (Jänig 2006, Llewellyn-Smith et al. 2011; see Chapter 1). However, in which way these circuits in lower brain stem (pons and medulla oblongata) are integrated with the circuits regulating respiration, with spinal reflex pathways, with circuits in the mesencephalon and hypothalamus, and with central commands originating in the telencephalon is still very much unknown. We hypothesize that the central changes which are reflected in the changed reflexes in cutaneous vasoconstrictor neurons may at least in part occur at the level of the spinal cord. Integration between supraspinally generated signals (e.g. in the hypothalamus and in the respiratory network) and signals in spinal circuits may have changed. This change is possibly induced and maintained by the nociceptive afferent input from the periphery, either directly at the spinal cord level or indirectly via the hypothetical supraspinal changes in the representations of the sensory system and in the endogenous control system. This idea is consistent with the observation that the thermoregulatory changes in patients with CRPS are only present in the affected extremity but not in the contralateral one (Fig. 69.2).

Sudomotor neurons and sweating

Clinical observations described in the literature show that sweating is changed in the affected extremity (hypohidrosis or hyperhidrosis) in patients with CRPS. Activation of sweat glands always occurs only by its cholinergic innervation and not by circulating substances or local mechanisms. These changes can therefore only be attributed to central changes, which then lead to changes of activity in sudomotor neurons. There is compelling evidence from

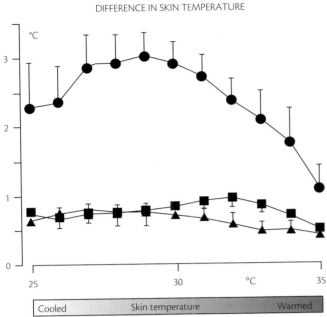

DIFFERENCE IN SKIN TEMPERATURE

Fig. 69.2 Average absolute side differences in skin temperature in 25 patients with complex regional pain syndrome (●), in 20 age-matched healthy control subjects (■), and in 15 control patients with extremity pain of other origin (▲) during a controlled thermoregulatory cycle (controlled alteration in cutaneous vasoconstrictor activity). Patients and control subjects were lying in a thermal suit supplied by tubes that were perfused by water of 12°C and 50°C respectively (inflow temperature) in order to cool or warm the whole body, leading to increase or decrease of activity in cutaneous vasoconstrictor neurons. The level of the overall cutaneous sympathetic vasoconstrictor activity was estimated indirectly by using the skin temperature on the unaffected side (or right side in healthy controls) as reference value. A skin temperature on the healthy side of 25°C indicates a high level, a temperature of 30°C an intermediate level and a temperature of 35°C a complete inhibition of sympathetic vasoconstrictor activity to the skin. Mean + S.E.M. From Wasner et al. (2001), with permission.

experimentation on cats and humans that central regulation of activity in cutaneous vasoconstrictor neurons and sudomotor neurons are closely linked to each other. Reflex inhibition in cutaneous vasoconstrictor neurons induced by peripheral or central (warm) stimuli is always accompanied by reflex activation of sudomotor neurons. This reciprocal reflex organization is based on the organization of both systems in the spinal cord, brainstem and hypothalamus (Jänig 2006). However, during mental/emotional stimulation both systems are activated simultaneously in humans, this being related to the control of both systems by the telencephalon. In regard of these results is it not surprising that the sudomotor system is affected in CRPS patients. Systematic experimentation on patients with CRPS should test whether the central coupling between both sympathetic systems during thermoregulatory, mental and other stimuli is qualitatively and quantitatively changed.

Sympathetic neurons and oedema, inflammation and trophic changes

Oedema

Based on observations following sympathetic blocks, it is a long-standing assumption that swelling (oedema) in the affected limb of patients with CRPS is dependent on activity in sympathetic neurons.

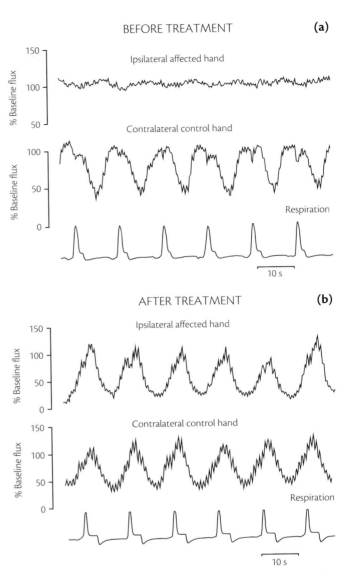

Fig. 69.3 Changes of cutaneous blood flow through the index finger tips of the affected (right) arm (upper trace) and the contralateral (control) arm (second trace) during deep inspiration (5/min, lower trace) in a patient (**a**) 2 weeks after onset of complex regional pain syndrome type I (CRPS I) before treatment and (**b**) 5 weeks after successful treatment and clinical improvement. CRPS I developed after right radius fracture. The treatment consisted of repeated sympatholytic procedures using regional guanethidine blocks combined with the application of a non-steroidal anti-inflammatory drug and later with physiotherapy. The regional sympathetic blocks significantly reduced the pain, showing that the patient had sympathetically maintained pain. Five weeks after start of treatment the typical symptoms of CRPS I were significantly reduced but still present. Blood flow was measured by laser Doppler flowmetry. Inspiration was measured by electronic spirometry. Deep inspiration causes phasic activation of cutaneous vasoconstrictor neurons and decrease of cutaneous blood flow. There was a complete loss of function of the cutaneous vasoconstrictor neurons early after onset of CRPS I (no inspiration-induced vasoconstriction) and a complete functional recovery after successful treatment. The loss of function of the cutaneous vasoconstrictor system was central and not due to lesion of the peripheral vasoconstrictor pathway. Modified from Wasner et al. (1999).

Spinal anaesthesia may be followed by a decrease of the oedema. This decrease starts within 1–2 hours and the oedema may disappear within days (Fig. 69.4). Whether this dependence of the oedema on the sympathetic innervation is related to changes of rate and pattern of activity in sympathetic neurons innervating blood vessels (and/or lymph vessels) or also related to changes in neurovascular transmission is unknown. Furthermore, it cannot be excluded that the oedema is also related to antidromic activity in peptidergic afferent neurons with unmyelinated (C) or small-diameter myelinated (Aδ) fibres (see interrupted arrow in Fig. 69.1). It has been proposed that: *first*, persistent activation of nociceptors generates strong primary afferent depolarization of the central terminals of these peptidergic afferent neurons in the superficial horn of the spinal cord via GABAergic interneurons, *second*, that this depolarization generates impulses in these afferent neurons travelling antidromically to the periphery, and, *third*, that these antidromically conducted impulses produce arteriolar vasodilation in peripheral tissues and are possibly involved in inflammatory processes (i.e. venular plasma extravasation) (for review see Willis 1999). However, it must be kept in mind that the swelling is present in many CRPS patients in the entire distal extremity (i.e. far beyond the territory of the site of the trauma). In view of the prominence of the oedema in many patients with CRPS (in particular type I) the lack of knowledge about its underlying mechanism is surprising.

An important point is that *temporary* blockade of the sympathetic activity (and/or possibly of the antidromically conducted activity in afferent neurons) appears to interrupt a vicious circle that maintains the oedema (see 6 in Fig. 69.1). The mechanism underlying this vicious circle is unknown.

Inflammation

The idea that CRPS I patients undergo *inflammatory processes* in the affected extremity, in particular in the deep somatic tissues

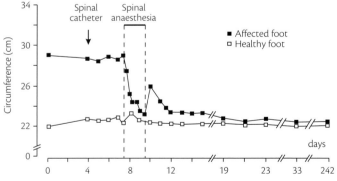

Fig. 69.4 Spinal anaesthesia reduces severe oedema in a patient with complex regional pain syndrome type I (CRPS I). Female patient, 15 years, 3 months after trauma on foot. No spontaneous pain, cutaneous hyperalgesia or allodynia, but deep hyperalgesia. Implantation of a spinal catheter at thoracic level T10 on day 4. Spinal anaesthesia for 43 hours starting on day 7 with 1.4 ml 0.5% bupivacaine/hour. Increase of skin temperature of foot to 36°C (indicating complete decrease of activity in cutaneous vasoconstrictor neurons). Significant decrease of oedema in one day and its complete disappearance with time after termination of the spinal anaesthesia together with other symptoms of CRPS I. The decrease of the oedema was considered to be due to decrease of activity in sympathetic neurons. However, it cannot be excluded that antidromically conducted activity in peptidergic primary afferent neurons with unmyelinated axons was blocked. For details see text. Ordinate scale, circumference of affected foot and contralateral healthy foot. Modified from Blumberg et al. (1994).

including bones, goes back to Sudeck who believed that this syndrome is an inflammatory bone atrophy ('entzündliche Knochenatrophie'). Accordingly, bone scintigraphy demonstrates periarticular tracer uptake in acute CRPS, and synovia biopsies and scintigraphic investigations with radiolabelled immunoglobulins show protein extravasation, hypervascularity and neutrophil infiltration. Furthermore, in the fluid of artificially produced skin blisters significantly higher cytokine levels (interleukin-6, tumour necrosis factor-alpha) as well as tryptase (a measure of mast cell activity) were observed in the involved extremity as compared with the uninvolved extremity (Jänig and Baron 2003). This is supported by animal studies showing that the sympathetic nervous system can influence the intensity of an inflammatory process and clinical studies showing that sympatholytic procedures can ameliorate pain, inflammation, and oedema in human beings (Jänig et al. 1996; Jänig and Levine 2006). The mechanisms of initiation and maintenance of inflammatory processes occurring in early CRPS and the role of sympathetic postganglionic neurons in it are unclear and remain to be worked out.

Trophic changes

The underlying mechanisms of trophic changes, as prominent as they may be, are entirely unclear. However, based on the observation that these changes may ameliorate after sympathetic blocks, argues that they are related to the sympathetic innervation.

Sensory systems of the skin

Up to 50% of patients with chronic CRPS I develop hypoaesthesia and hypoalgesia on the whole half of the body or in the upper quadrant ipsilateral to the affected extremity, showing that these patients have increased thresholds to mechanical, cold, warm and heat stimuli compared with the responses generated from the corresponding contralateral healthy body side. Patients with these extended sensory deficits have longer illness duration, greater pain intensity, a higher frequency of mechanical allodynia, and a higher tendency to develop changes in the somatomotor system than do patients with spatially restricted sensory deficits (Rommel et al. 1999, 2001). These findings have considerable implications:

- The anatomical distribution of the changed painful and non-painful somatosensory perceptions observed in CRPS patients are likely due to changes in the central representation of somatosensory sensations in the thalamus and cortex. Magnetic encephalographic (MEG) and functional magnetic resonance imaging (fMRI) studies revealed a shortened distance between little finger and thumb representations in the primary somatosensory (SI) cortex contralateral to the painful body side. The MEG responses in the SI cortex were increased on the affected side, indicating processes of central sensitization. fMRI studies indicate that frontal and parietal cortical networks are involved in generating movement disorders in patients with CRPS (Baron 2009; Maihöfner et al. 2007). We do not know the extent to which these central changes depend on continuous nociceptive input from the affected extremity, although it has been shown that they may disappear after successful treatment of the pain. Finally, it is unclear to what degree these changes are specific for CRPS, or also occur in other chronic pain states or after immobilization.

- Generalized sensory deficits are particularly found in patients with chronic CRPS I. If these central changes, that are reflected in the generalized sensory deficits, are permanent and irreversible it would be the first documented case of such irreversible changes in the brain that is triggered by trauma with minor or no nerve lesion (i.e. under conditions in which the peripheral and central nociceptive system are intact).

- It is worthwhile to investigate the question whether the generalized sensory changes are correlated with neglect-like phenomena in these CRPS patients, whether the generalized sensory changes are also present in patients with disuse syndrome following immobilization of an extremity (see Harden et al. 2001), or whether the common denominator of generalized sensory changes, neglect-syndrome and disuse syndrome is the changed or absent input in afferent neurons from deep somatic tissues (skeletal muscles, joints, fascia) to the central body representations leading to a mismatch between somatosensory input and central somatosensory and motor body representations. This would then be reflected in a body perception disturbance (Lewis et al. 2007). This idea is fully supported by the finding that viewing visual illusions causes enhanced pain, abnormal autonomic responses and abnormal motor responses (dystonia) in some patients with CRPS but not in healthy controls (Cohen et al. 2012).

- Patients with CRPS I mostly locate their spontaneous pain into deep somatic structures of the affected extremity. They have furthermore deep somatic mechanical hyperalgesia/allodynia. This raises the question whether the non-painful sensations elicited from muscle and joints are changed too.

Somatomotor changes

About 50% of patients with CRPS I show a decrease of active range of motion, increased amplitude of physiological tremor, and reduced active motor force in the affected extremity (Deuschl et al. 1991; Harden et al. 2001). Fig. 69.5 demonstrates, in a patient with CRPS I, increased physiological tremor amplitude of the affected hand compared with the normal tremor amplitude of the contralateral unaffected hand. The inset in Fig. 69.5 shows the maximal tremor amplitudes in 18 CRPS patients (most of them with type I), 12 of them having a pathological tremor. Other observations include associated movement disorders (myoclonus, dystonia) (Bhatia et al. 1993; Schwartzman and Kerrigan 1990; Harden et al. 2001). It is unlikely that these motor changes are related to a peripheral process (e.g. influence of the sympathetic nervous system on neuromuscular transmission and/or contractility of skeletal muscle [see Chapter 20]). These somatomotor changes are more likely generated by changes of activity in the motoneurons (i.e. they have a central origin) and are possibly related to plastic changes in the somatosensory, motor and premotor cortices (Maihöfner et al. 2007).

With kinematic analysis of target reaching, grip force analysis and fMRI to quantitatively assess motor deficits in CRPS patients, abnormalities in the cerebral motor processing were revealed. A pathological sensorimotor integration located in the parietal cortex may induce an abnormal central programming and processing of motor tasks (Harden et al. 2001; Maihöfner et al. 2007). According to this view, a neglect-like syndrome was clinically described to be involved in the disuse of the extremity. Furthermore, incongruence between central motor output and sensory input (body perception disturbance) was hypothesized as underlying

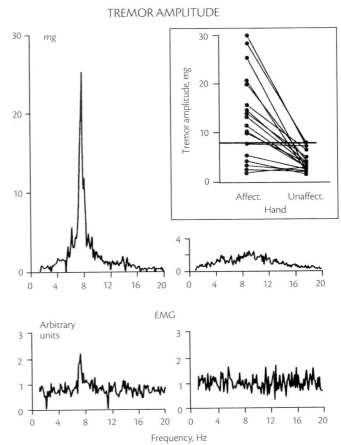

Fig. 69.5 Increased physiological tremor in a patient with complex regional pain syndrome type I (CRPS I) on the (left) affected side (left) and its absence on the (right) unaffected side (right). The amplitude of the physiological tremor was determined using an accelerometer (amplitude in milligravity [*mg*], upper records); in parallel the electromyogram (EMG, lower records) was measured. Power spectra of hand acceleration and of EMG of the extensor muscles. **Inset**: Peak amplitude of tremor of the affected hand and of the contralateral hand in 18 CRPS patients. The horizontal bar represents the 99% confidence limit of healthy subjects. Amplitudes above that limit were pathological. Modified from Deuschl et al. (1991).

mechanism in CRPS (Lewis et al. 2007). Using the method of graded motor imagery followed by mirror visual feedback from a moving unaffected limb can reduce pain and swelling in patients with chronic CRPS and re-establish the pain-free relationship between sensory feedback and motor execution (Moseley 2004; see Baron 2009).

Initiating events

The clinical signs and symptoms in CRPS I are disproportionate to the traumatic events initiating or triggering this syndrome. The local changes generated by the trauma often disappear, yet the syndrome persists. Furthermore, CRPS I in an extremity may be triggered by remote events (e.g. in the viscera) or by events in the CNS (e.g. central lesions) (Fig. 69.1). In fact it has been proposed that processes in the prefrontal, frontal and parietal cortices that are related to psychosocial changes enhance the clinical signs and symptoms in CRPS or even may initiate them. These clinical observations argue that mechanisms operating in CRPS I cannot simply be explained to be caused by events in the periphery of the body related to the trauma (e.g. sympathetic-afferent coupling or persistent activation of nociceptive afferents).

Complex regional pain syndrome and sympathetically maintained pain

The sympathetic nervous system may be involved in the *generation* of pain under certain pathophysiological conditions yet not under physiological conditions (Chapter 12). Pain dependent on activity in the sympathetic neurons called sympathetically maintained pain (SMP) (Baron 2006; Stanton-Hicks et al. 1995) usually includes both spontaneous and evoked pain (i.e. allodynia evoked by mechanical or cold stimuli). It is present in about 60% of patients with acute CRPS and sometimes in other neuropathic pain syndromes and can persist for years. The concept that the (efferent) sympathetic nervous system is involved in the generation of pain is based on long-standing clinical observations (Baron 2006). Three groups of experimental studies on patients with CRPS are representative for this extensive work:

◆ In CRPS patients with SMP (CRPS I, II) it has been shown that spontaneous pain, mechanical allodynia and cold allodynia in the hand, that are alleviated by stellate ganglion block, can be rekindled, under the condition of proximal sympathetic block, or enhanced by injection of noradrenaline into the skin area that is painful or was painful before sympathetic blockade (Fig. 69.6). Intradermal injection of noradrenaline, in physiological concentrations (0.1–1 μM) in the unaffected contralateral limb or in limbs of healthy subjects does not elicit pain. Furthermore, SMP is significantly reduced by the α-adrenoceptor blocker phentolamine infused intravenously (Ali et al. 2000; Torebjörk et al. 1995).

Spontaneous pain, mechanical allodynia and cold allodynia develop or are enhanced ≥ 20 minutes after intradermal injection of noradrenaline (Fig. 69.6). This long time delay is difficult to reconcile with the idea that noradrenaline directly excites nociceptors (Chapter 12). It may be hypothesized that a state of central sensitization requires a continuous low-frequency excitation of nociceptive afferent fibres produced by noradrenaline and that the central sensitization outlasts the activation of nociceptive neurons up to several tens of minutes. We have no models to explain the long time course of central sensitization.

◆ The intensity of spontaneous pain and the area of mechanical hyperalgesia/allodynia (punctate/dynamic) increase during selective activation of the cutaneous vasoconstrictor outflow to the painful extremity by whole body cooling in CRPS I patients with SMP but not in CRPS I patients without SMP (i.e. having SIP)(Baron et al. 2002; Fig. 69.7). In the CRPS patients with SMP, the relief of spontaneous and evoked pain after sympathetic blockade is significantly more pronounced than the change in pain generated experimentally by change of the activity in cutaneous vasoconstrictor neurons from the thermoregulatory hot state (vasoconstrictor activity absent or low) to the thermoregulatory cold state (vasoconstrictor activity high) (44.0±9.1% vs 16.0±0.05%). This difference in reduction of pain is explained as follows: a complete sympathetic block affects *all* sympathetic outflow channels projecting to the affected extremity whereas the physiological interventions as used in Fig. 69.7 change only the sympathetic activity to the skin. Thus, sympathetic-afferent coupling may particularly occur in the *deep somatic tissues* such as *skeletal muscle, joint* or *bone*, and less so in the skin. Supporting this view, especially the deep somatic

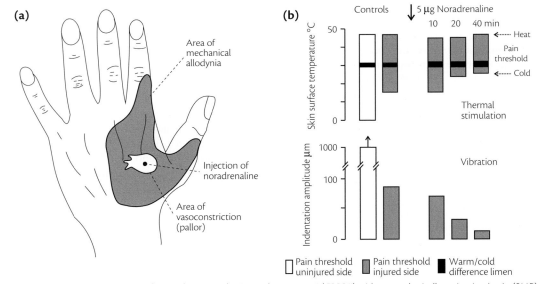

Fig. 69.6 Mechanical and cold allodynia in patients with complex regional pain syndrome type II (CRPS II) with sympathetically maintained pain (SMP) elicited or enhanced by intradermal injection of noradrenaline. Noradrenaline was injected at the site of mechanical and cold allodynia. **(a)** Area of pallor and mechanical allodynia 20 minutes following intradermal injection of 2 μg noradrenaline in a patient temporarily relieved from his pain by a stellate ganglion block. **(b)** Sequential quantitative sensory testing of a patient before and after intradermal injection of 5 μg noradrenaline during a time without blockade of the stellate ganglion. This patient had mechanical allodynia (indentation amplitude of a mechanical vibration stimulus to evoke pain about 90 μm, lower panel) and cold hyperalgesia/allodynia (cold pain threshold about 15°C, upper panel). The mechanical allodynia (further decrease of indentation amplitude to elicit pain) and cold allodynia (further decrease of cold-pain threshold) progressively worsened starting approximately 20 minutes after intradermal injection of noradrenaline. Note that the heat pain threshold did not change. Modified with permission from Torebjörk, E., Wahren, L.K., Wallin, B.G., Hallin, R. and Koltzenburg, M. (1995). Noradrenaline-evoked pain in neuralgia. *Pain* **63**, 11–20. This figure has been reproduced with permission of the International Association for the Study of Pain ® (IASP®). The figure may not be reproduced for any other purpose without permission.

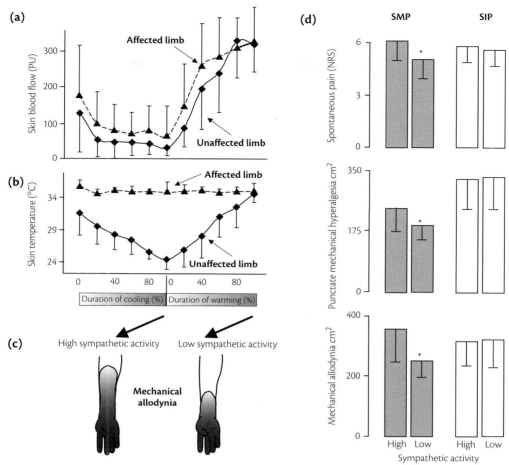

Fig. 69.7 Modulation of spontaneous pain, punctate mechanical hyperalgesia and mechanical allodynia by activity in cutaneous vasoconstrictor neurons in patients with complex regional pain syndrome type I (CRPS I) and sympathetically maintained pain (SMP). With the help of a thermal suit, whole-body cooling or warming were performed to alter sympathetic skin nerve activity. The subjects were lying in a suit supplied by tubes, in which running water of 12°C and 50°C, respectively (inflow temperature) was used to cool or warm the whole body. By these means activity in cutaneous vasoconstrictor neurons can be switched on and off. **(a, b)** Cooling of the patients lowers core temperature and increases activity in cutaneous vasoconstrictor neurons with decrease of skin temperature (◆ in **b**) and skin blood flow (hand; ▲, ◆ in **a**). Warming of the patients increases core temperature with decrease of activity in cutaneous vasoconstrictor neurons and increase of skin temperature (◆ in **b**) and skin blood flow (▲, ◆ in **a**). On the affected side the forearm temperature was clamped at 35°C by a feed-back-controlled heat lamp to exclude temperature effects on the sensory receptors. Measurements of blood flow and skin temperature were taken at 5 minute intervals (mean + SD), thus the whole cycle lasted 50 minutes. **(c)** Effect of cutaneous vasoconstrictor activity on mechanical allodynia in one CRPS I patient with SMP. Activation of sympathetic neurons (during cooling) leads to an increase of the area of mechanical allodynia. **(d)** Spontaneous pain (upper; numerical rating scale [NRS]), area of punctate mechanical hyperalgesia (middle; in cm²; stimulation of skin with a nylon filament of 250 mN bending force) and area of mechanical allodynia (lower; in cm²; stimulation of skin with a cotton swab) during high sympathetic activity to the skin (whole body cooling) or low sympathetic activity to skin (whole body warming) in CRPS I patients with SMP (N = 7) and CRPS I patients without SMP (sympathetically independent pain [SIP], N = 6). Mean + 1 SD. *, p<0.05 (Wilcoxon´s paired test). Modified from Baron et al. (2002).

structures are extremely painful in many CRPS patients. Based on quantitative measurements in CRPS patients with SMP about a third of SMP is related to the sympathetic innervation of the skin and two thirds to the sympathetic innervation of deep somatic tissues. Furthermore, the SMP component is quantitatively higher in early CRPS than in chronic CRPS (Fig. 69.8; Schattschneider et al. 2006).

◆ Blockade of sympathetic activity to the affected extremity by a local anaesthetic applied to the appropriate sympathetic paravertebral ganglia generates pain relief in the affected extremity for significantly longer time periods compared with saline injected close to the same site in the same group of CRPS patients with SMP (Fig. 69.9; Price et al. 1998). Thus the pain relief generated

by blockade of sympathetic activity exceeds that produced by a similar placebo 'block'. The duration of pain relief greatly outlasts the duration of conduction block generated by the local anaesthetic, arguing that the pain-relieving effect of sympathetic blocks observed in CRPS patients with SMP cannot be explained simply by temporary blockade of activity in the sympathetic neurons. No animal model can explain this long-lasting pain-relieving effect of sympathetic blocks nor have we an animal model for the positive feedback circle via the primary afferent neurons (see 6 in Fig. 69.1). The long-lasting pain-relieving effects of sympathetic blocks clearly argue that activity in sympathetic neurons, which is of *central origin*, maintains a positive feedback circle via the primary afferent neurons. We hypothesize that activity in sympathetic neurons maintains a central state of hyperexcitability (e.g. of neurons in the spinal dorsal horn), via excitation of afferent neurons (Fig. 69.1), which may be initiated by an intense noxious event or by other central events. The rate of persistent afferent activity that maintains the central state of hyperexcitability is probably low. This central state of hyperexcitability is switched off during a temporary block of conduction in the sympathetic chain lasting only for a few hours and cannot be switched on again when the block wears off and the sympathetic activity, and therefore also the sympathetically induced activity in afferent neurons, comes back again. The experiment shown in Fig. 69.8 strongly argues that this positive feedback mechanism involving the sympathetic outflow mainly acts via the deep somatic tissues.

These experiments on human patients clearly argue that, in some patients with CRPS:

◆ activity in sympathetic neurons is involved in generating pain

◆ blockade of the sympathetic activity relieves the pain

◆ noradrenaline injected intracutaneously rekindles the pain.

The mechanisms of the sympathetic-afferent coupling leading to SMP are discussed in Chapter 20 (Figs. 20.1 to 20.7) and elsewhere (Jänig 2009). We do not know whether the abnormal communication between sympathetic and afferent neurons leading to SMP only involves nociceptive afferent neurons or also other groups of afferent neurons (e.g. mechanosensitive ones with myelinated axons). Furthermore, whether SMP depends on special functional constellations of the sympathetic nervous system that are clinically expressed in other phenomena, particularly in CRPS I patients (changes of blood flow in skin and deep somatic tissues, changes of sweating, oedema, trophic changes of tissues) is unclear.

Conclusion

Clinical observations, experimentation on humans, and experimentation on animals argue that CRPS is primarily a disorder of the CNS.

◆ Patients with CRPS exhibit alterations of the somatosensory system, the sympathetic nervous system, and the somatomotor system. These alterations are reflected in multiple somatosensory changes (including the perception of tactile, thermal, and

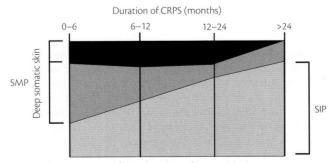

Fig. 69.8 The component of pain that depends on activity in cutaneous sympathetic noradrenergic neurons (skin sympathetically maintained pain [SMP]) or on activity in sympathetic noradrenergic neurons innervating deep somatic tissues (deep SMP) or is independent of activity in sympathetic neurons (sympathetically independent pain [SIP]) over the course of complex regional pain syndrome (CRPS). Modified from Schattschneider et al. (2006).

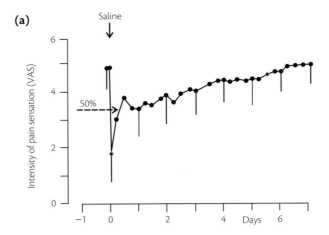

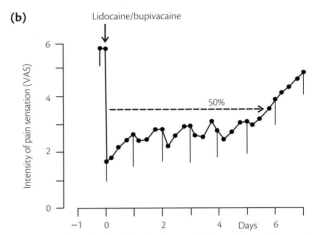

Fig. 69.9 Sympathetic blocks with a local anaesthetic in patients with complex regional pain syndrome type I (CRPS I) with sympathetically maintained pain (SMP) leads to a long-lasting significant reduction of pain. The local anaesthetic or saline (control) were injected close to the corresponding paravertebral sympathetic ganglia (stellate ganglion in 4 patients, lumbar sympathetic ganglia in 3 patients) in the same group of 7 CRPS I patients. Double-blind crossover study. Pain was measured repeatedly using the visual analogue scale (VAS) on the day of the injection and on 7 days after the injection. Both interventions produced pain relief (see 50% value of pain relief). However, the duration of the mean relief of pain to injection of the local anaesthetic lasted for 6 days and was significantly longer than the mean pain relief following local injection of saline, which lasted for 6 hours (placebo block). The initial maximal peaks of relative analgesia were statistically not different. Means + SEM. Modified from Price et al. (1998).

noxious stimuli), in changes of blood flow and sweating, and in movement disorders indicating that the central representations of these systems are changed (see dots in Fig. 69.10 and bold-lined boxes in Fig. 69.1). Thus, CRPS appears to be a disorder involving these neuronal systems and their central representations (Cohen et al. 2012).

◆ The peripheral changes (sympathetic-afferent coupling, vascular changes, inflammation, oedema, trophic changes) cannot be seen independently of the central ones. CNS and peripheral body tissues interact with each other via afferent and efferent signals. Although the nature of this interaction is still a puzzle we postulate that it is the mismatch between the afferent and efferent signals, occurring on different levels of integration in the afferent and efferent body maps in the CNS, that cause the changed autonomic, sensory and somatomotor reactions.

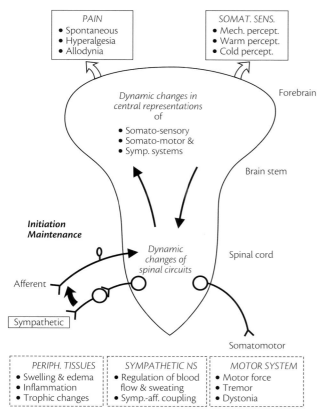

Fig. 69.10 Development of complex regional pain syndrome (CRPS) as a disease of the central nervous system (CNS): a hypothesis. Schematic diagram summarizing the sensory, autonomic and somatomotor changes in CRPS I patients. The figure symbolizes the CNS (forebrain, brainstem and spinal cord). Changes occur in the central representations of the somatosensory, somatomotor and sympathetic nervous system (which include spinal circuits) and are reflected in the changes of perception of painful and non-painful stimuli, of cutaneous blood flow and sweating, and of motor performances. They are triggered and possibly maintained by nociceptive afferent inputs from the somatic and visceral body domains. It is unclear whether these central changes are reversible in chronic CRPS I patients. The central changes possibly also affect the endogenous control system of nociceptive impulse transmission. Coupling between sympathetic neurons and afferent neurons in the periphery (see bold closed arrow) is one component of pain in CRPS I patients with SMP. However, it seems to be unimportant in patients with CRPS I without SMP. Modified from Jänig and Baron (2002, 2003).

◆ This way of looking at CRPS shifts the attention away from interpreting this syndrome conceptually in a narrow manner and to reduce it to *one* system or to *one* mechanism only, centrally or peripherally. This view will further our understanding why CRPS I may be triggered after a trivial trauma, after a trauma being remote from the affected extremity exhibiting CRPS, after immobilization of an extremity, or following processes in the cerebral hemispheres. It will explain why, in CRPS patients with SMP, a few temporary blocks (and sometimes only one block!) of the sympathetic supply to an affected extremity sometimes lead to a long-lasting (even permanent) pain relief and to resolution of the other changes present in CRPS.

◆ Using imaging techniques we will learn which central (cortical and subcortical) changes are specific for CRPS and how these central changes are expressed in the efferent (somatomotor

and autonomic) systems and the distorted sensory perceptions of the body.

◆ This changed view will bring about a diagnostic reclassification and redefinition of CRPS, will lead to new mechanism-based therapeutic approaches, and will shift the focus of our research efforts.

Acknowledgement

This work was supported by the Deutsche Forschungsgemeinschaft (DFG Ba 1921/1-2), the German Ministry of Research and Education within the German Research Network on Neuropathic Pain (BMBF, 01EM01/04) and an unrestricted educational grant of Pfizer (Germany).

References

Ali, Z., Raja, S.N., Wesselmann, U., Fuchs, P.N., Meyer, R.A., and Campbell, J.N. (2000). Intradermal injection of norepinephrine evokes pain in patients with sympathetically maintained pain. *Pain* **88**, 161–68.

Baron, R. (2006). Complex regional pain syndromes. In *Wall and Melzack's Textbook of Pain* (5th edn.)(ed. S.B. McMahon and M. Koltzenburg), pp. 1011–27. Elsevier Churchill Livingstone, Edinburgh.

Baron, R. (2009) Complex regional pain syndromes. In *Science of pain* (ed. A.I. Basbaum, M.C. Bushnell), pp. 909–918. Academic Press, San Diego.

Baron, R., Schattschneider, J., Binder, A., Siebrecht, D., and Wasner, G. (2002). Relation between sympathetic vasoconstrictor activity and pain and hyperalgesia in complex regional pain syndromes: a case-control study. *Lancet* **359**, 1655–60.

Bhatia, K.P., Bhatt, M.H., and Marsden, C.D. (1993). The causalgia-dystonia syndrome. *Brain* **116**, 843–51.

Blumberg, H., Hoffmann, U., Mohadjer, M., and Scheremet, R. (1994). Clinical phenomenology and mechanisms of reflex sympathetic dystrophy: emphasis on edema. In: *Proceedings of the 7th World Congress on Pain.* (ed. G.F. Gebhart, D.L. Hammond and T.S. Jensen), pp. 455–81. IASP Press, Seattle.

Blumberg, H., and Jänig, W. (1985). Reflex patterns in postganglionic vasoconstrictor neurons following chronic nerve lesions. *J Auton Nerv Syst* **14**, 157–80.

Cohen, H.E., Hall, J., Harris, N., McCabe, C.S., Blake, D.R., and Jänig, W. (2012). Enhanced pain and autonomic responses to ambiguous visual stimuli in chronic Complex Regional Pain Syndrome (CRPS) type I. *Eur. J. Pain* **16**, 182–195.

Deuschl, G., Blumberg, H., and Lücking, C.H. (1991). Tremor in reflex sympathetic dystrophy. *Arch. Neurol.* 48, 1247–52.

Harden, R.N., Baron, R., and Jänig, W. (eds.)(2001). *Complex regional pain syndrome.* Progress in Pain Research and Management, Vol. 22. IASP Press, Seattle.

Harden, R.N., Bruehl, S., Stanton-Hicks, M., and Wilson, P.R. (2007). Proposed new diagnostic criteria for complex regional pain syndrome. *Pain Med* **8**, 326–31.

Jänig, W. (1985). Causalgia and reflex sympathetic dystrophy: in which way is the sympathetic nervous system involved? *Trends Neurosci.* **8**, 471–477.

Jänig, W. (2006). *The integrative action of the autonomic nervous system. Neurobiology of homeostasis.* Cambridge University Press, Cambridge, New York

Jänig, W. (2009) Autonomic nervous system and pain. In *Science of pain* (ed. A.I. Basbaum, M.C. Bushnell), pp. 193–225. Academic Press, San Diego.

Jänig, W., Levine, J.D., and Michaelis, M. (1996). Interaction of sympathetic and primary afferent neurons following nerve injury and tissue trauma. *Progr. Brain Res.* **112**, 161–84.

Jänig, W. and Baron, R. (2002). Complex regional pain syndrome is disease of the central nervous system. *Clin. Auton. Res.* **12**, 150–64.

Jänig, W. and Baron, R. (2003). Complex regional pain syndrome: a mystery explained? *The Lancet Neurol.* **2**, 687–97.

Jänig, W. and Koltzenburg, M. (1991). Plasticity of sympathetic reflex organization following cross-union of inappropriate nerves in the adult cat. *J. Physiol.* **436**, 309–23.

Jänig, W. and Levine, J.D. (in press). Autonomic-endocrine-immune responses in acute and chronic pain. In *Wall and Melzack´s Textbook of Pain* (6th edn.)(ed. S.B. McMahon and M. Koltzenburg), Elsevier Churchill Livingstone, Edinburgh.

Jänig, W. and Stanton-Hicks, M. (eds.) (1996). *Reflex sympathetic dystrophy—a reappraisal.* Seattle, IASP Press, Vol. 6.

Lewis, J.S., Kersten, P., McCabe, C.S., McPherson, K.M., and Blake, D.R. (2007). Body perception disturbance: a contribution to pain in complex regional pain syndrome (CRPS). *Pain* **133**, 111–119.

Livingston, W.K. (1943/1976). *Pain mechanisms. A physiological iterpretation of causalgia and its related states.* Plenum Press, New York London.

Llewellyn-Smith, I.J. and Verbene, A.J.M. (eds.) (2011). *Central regulation of autonomic functions.* 2nd edition. Oxford University Press, New York.

Maihöfner, C., Baron, R., DeCol, R., Binder, A., Birklein, F., Deuschl, G., Handwerker, H.O., and Schattschneider, J. (2007). The motor system shows adaptive changes in complex regional pain syndrome. *Brain* **130**, 2671–87.

Merskey, H. and Bogduk, N. (1994). *Classification of chronic pain: description of chronic pain syndromes and definition of terms.* IASP Press, Seattle.

Moseley, G.L. (2004) Graded motor imagery is effective for long-standing complex regional pain syndrome: a randomized controlled trial. *Pain* **108**, 192–98.

Price, D.D., Long, S., Wilsey, B., and Rafii, A. (1998). Analysis of peak magnitude and duration of analgesia produced by local anesthetics injected into sympathetic ganglia of complex regional pain syndrome patients. *Clin. J. Pain* **14**, 216–26.

Rommel, O., Gehling, M., Dertwinkel, R., Witscher, K., Zenz, M., Malin, J.-P., and Jänig W. (1999). Hemisensory impairment in patients with complex regional pain syndrome. *Pain* **80**, 95–111.

Rommel, O., Malin, J.-P., Zenz, M., and Jänig, W. (2001). Quantitative sensory testing, neurophysiological and psychological examination in patients with complex regional pain syndrome and hemisensory deficits. *Pain* **93**, 279–93.

Schattschneider, J., Binder, A., Siebrecht, D., Wasner, G., and Baron, R. (2006). Complex regional pain syndromes. The influence of cutaneous and deep somatic sympathetic innervation on pain. *Clin. J. Pain* **22**, 240–44.

Schwartzman, R.J. and Kerrigan, J. (1990). The movement disorder of reflex sympathetic dystrophy. *Neurol* **40**, 57–61.

Stanton-Hicks, M., Jänig, W., Hassenbusch, S., Haddox, J.D., Boas, R., and Wilson, P. (1995). Reflex sympathetic dystrophy: changing concepts and taxonomy. *Pain* **63**, 127–33

Torebjörk, E., Wahren, L.K., Wallin, B.G., Hallin, R., and Koltzenburg, M. (1995). Noradrenaline-evoked pain in neuralgia. *Pain* **63**, 11–20.

Wasner, G., Heckmann, K., Maier, C., and Baron, R. (1999). Vascular abnormalities in acute reflex sympathetic dystrophy (CRPS I): complete inhibition of sympathetic nerve activity with recovery. *Arch. Neurol.* **56**, 613–20.

Wasner, G., Schattschneider, J., Heckmann, K., Maier, C., and Baron, R. (2001). Vascular abnormalities in reflex sympathetic dystrophy (CRPS I): mechanisms and diagnostic value. *Brain* **124**, 587–99.

Willis, W.D. (1999). Dorsal root potentials and dorsal root reflexes: a double-edged sword. *Exp. Brain Res.* **124**, 395–421.

CHAPTER 70

Ageing and the autonomic nervous system

Lewis A. Lipsitz and Vera Novak

Introduction

Normal human ageing is associated with changes in the autonomic control of several bodily functions that may affect adaptation to activities of daily living. For example, regulatory changes affecting the cardiovascular and cerebrovascular systems may have broad impact on adaptation to orthostatic stress. Common clinical manifestations of autonomic dysfunction in elderly patients include orthostatic hypotension (OH), postprandial hypotension, hypothermia, and heat stroke. These are rarely problematic in healthy elderly individuals under the usual demands of life, but may become clinically significant during exposure to a variety of external influences, such as medications, changes in fluid intake, or relatively hot or cold environmental temperatures. Other geriatric problems such as constipation, urinary incontinence and sexual dysfunction may mimic autonomic insufficiency, but are usually caused by conditions outside of the autonomic nervous system. For example, sexual dysfunction in old age is more likely due to vascular disease, diabetes, depression, or medications, than it is to age-associated autonomic dysfunction.

Normal ageing also predisposes people to the onset of diseases that may affect the autonomic nervous system. It is important to differentiate physiological changes due to ageing from those due to age-associated diseases, or medications to treat these diseases. For example, increased blood pressure variability may be a manifestation of age-related impairments in parasympathetic and baroreflex heart rate control or be a result of antihypertensive medications or be a presentation of autonomic failure. By recognizing this, clinicians can identify and treat the underlying disease or age-related condition and potentially improve the quality of life of their elderly patients.

Several methodological problems confound the interpretation of research data in the area of ageing and autonomic function. Research findings are often influenced by the presence of occult disease, making it inappropriate to attribute them to normal ageing. Furthermore, since clinical tests of autonomic function rely on reflex responses to specific stimuli, the actual level of abnormality is difficult to ascertain unless subjects of different ages receive identical stimuli. This may be difficult to achieve if, for example, the level of blood pressure, sympathetic arousal, intrathoracic pressure, core body temperature, or cooperation with a test differs as a function of age. In addition, most previous human studies have not been adequately controlled for the presence of cardiovascular and behavioural risk factors, body composition, physical exercise, and diet. Moreover, in elderly people who are physically active, decline in aerobic capacity may be reduced and adaptation to everyday stress may be better than predicted for on age (Byrne et al. 2005). Therefore, many of the reported autonomic nervous system changes with advancing age are probably due to a sedentary lifestyle and decrease in lean body mass, rather than ageing per se.

Animal studies also must be interpreted with caution because of considerable differences in autonomic responses among different animal species. Some studies do not compare mature and senescent animals but, rather, look at the differences between young and mature animals. This approach may lead to confusion between true age-related changes and those that occur as a result of growth and development. Despite these complexities, accumulated evidence suggests that some deterioration in selected areas of autonomic nervous system function occurs with normal ageing.

This chapter will review age-related physiological changes in the autonomic nervous system that impair an older person's ability to adapt to stress, as well as common pathological conditions in advanced age that further impair autonomic function. The chapter will focus on those functions most commonly associated with autonomic changes in elderly individuals, namely thermoregulation, blood pressure regulation, cerebral blood flow regulation, control of respiration and gastrointestinal, urinary tract, and sexual function.

Thermoregulation

Thermoregulation requires sensory systems that detect temperature, central connections in the anterior hypothalamus, efferent autonomic pathways to the sweat glands and vasculature, metabolic processes that generate heat, and behavioural responses that enable an individual to adjust the temperature in their external environment. Efferent autonomic signals are transmitted primarily via the sympathetic nervous system from the brain to receptors in the sweat glands and vasculature, which function to preserve or dissipate heat. Impairments of thermoregulation in elderly persons due to autonomic dysfunction or complications of diseases and medications increase their vulnerability to hypothermia or hyperthermia (Wongsurawat et al. 1990). Peripheral vasoconstriction in response to exposure to cold or even face cooling in winter results in physiological shift of fluids from vascular to interstitial compartments. Sweating at higher temperatures may also contribute to intravascular hypovolaemia, posing a risk of increased blood viscosity and cardiovascular/cerebrovascular accidents (Vogelaere and Pereira 2005). The sections that follow summarize age-related and disease-related alterations in heat generation, conservation, and dissipation; temperature perception; and behavioral responses to ambient temperature changes. This material ends with a brief review of the common geriatric problems of hypothermia and heat stroke.

Heat generation

Basal metabolic rate

Ageing is accompanied by a gradual decrease in basal metabolic rate (BMR), due in large part to a reduction in skeletal muscle mass. The reduction in BMR is evident at thermoneutral temperatures and in response to cold environments (Collins et al. 1981). Ageing is also associated with a blunted thermic response to feeding (Schwartz et al. 1990). Deconditioned sedentary individuals with muscle atrophy, and malnourished patients with inadequate energy stores, may not be able to generate sufficient heat to protect them from hypothermia when exposed to the cold.

Shivering

Shivering is an important mechanism of muscular heat production that is mediated through central hypothalamic pathways. Healthy elderly individuals exhibit delayed and less intense shivering on exposure to cold (Collins and Exton-Smith 1981). The mechanism of this alteration in shivering response is not known.

Heat conservation via vasoconstriction

Peripheral vasoconstriction in response to cold exposure is an important mechanism of heat conservation. Elderly individuals demonstrate considerable variability in their capacities to respond to cold exposure. However, in general, older people exhibit delayed and reduced cutaneous vasoconstriction after cold exposure (Collins and Exton-Smith 1981, Richardson et al. 1992, Khan et al. 1992).

Heat dissipation via vasodilatation and sweating

Sweating and vasodilatation normally occur in response to elevations in environmental temperature to prevent an excessive rise in core body temperature. Skin atrophy, which accompanies normal ageing, results in a loss of skin small nerve fibres and sympathetic innervation to sweat glands (Periquet et al. 1999). Therefore, the sweating response and ability to vasodilate to heat may be reduced. Elderly people show greater metabolic heat for a given body mass, as well as higher heat gain from the environment production, but reduced sweating efficiency, and therefore may be more prone to elevate their core temperatures in hot environment (Inbar et al. 2004). The elderly have a higher core temperature threshold for the onset of sweating and vasodilatation (Ryan and Lipsitz 1995, Novak et al. 2001b). Some studies have shown that the age-related impairment in sweating follows the pattern of a length-dependent small fibre neuropathy and is localized to certain regions, such as the feet, legs, and thighs (Inoue et al. 1991).

Vasodilatory responses to radiant heat on the forearm have been investigated using Doppler skin blood flow velocity measurements (Richardson 1989). Young subjects demonstrate an increase in forearm cutaneous blood flow in response to local heat, while elderly subjects have an attenuated response. It is not clear whether this is secondary to reduced vasodilatation or less recruitment of capillary vessels. When the effect of age, cholesterol, and plasma glucose on cutaneous blood flow response to ambient heat was investigated, age was the most important variable (Richardson 1989).

The thermoregulatory response to cold exposure is also impaired in elderly people. Although muscle sympathetic nerve activity is generally greater in elderly subjects compared with middle-aged or young subjects, skin sympathetic nerve activity induced by cold exposure is significantly smaller in elderly subjects (Grassi et al. 2003).

Temperature perception

Young individuals are able to discriminate temperature differences of 1–2°C. In contrast, many elderly people are unable to detect differences in temperature closer than 2–4°C (Collins et al. 1981). Alterations in temperature perception with ageing may result in part from changes in the peripheral temperature receptors. These receptors are highly dependent on oxygen and therefore may be affected by diminished peripheral blood flow. Also, age-related alterations in skin collagen and elastic tissue may influence receptor function. The potential role of the hypothalamus on temperature perception and behaviour is not well elucidated.

Behavioural responses to ambient temperature

Elderly individuals with poor temperature discrimination also have less ability to regulate their ambient temperature. This was demonstrated in a study by Collins et al. (1981) in which subjects were asked to regulate room temperature by adjusting a thermostat. Elderly individuals with poor temperature discrimination lacked precision in adjusting the temperature, possibly due to impaired perception of ambient room temperature. This notion is supported by reports that elderly persons are less uncomfortable than the young when exposed to a cold environment, and require a more intense thermal stimulus to elicit a behavioural response (Taylor et al. 1995).

Clinical syndromes

Hypothermia

Hypothermia is defined as a decrease in core body temperature (oesophageal, rectal, or tympanic) below 35°C or 95°F. In UK surveys in 1975, 3.6% of individuals over 65 years of age admitted to the hospital were hypothermic. Unfortunately, prevalence data on hypothermia can be difficult to interpret as much of it relies on death certificate information, which may under-report the incidence of hypothermia. Incidence of and mortality from hypothermia doubled with each 4°C fall in temperature and most deaths and hospital admissions occurred between October and March. Incidence and mortality increased with age, and men had 30% higher case fatality than women (Herity et al. 1991). Elderly people in warm climates are also at risk of hypothermia (Kramer et al. 1989). In Israel, despite a warm climate, one-third of patients developed hypothermia even in the warm season (Kramer et al. 1989). Disorders that contribute to the development of hypothermia are listed in Table 70.1. These conditions may predispose elderly people to hypothermia even under relatively mild cold stress. Diseases such as Parkinson's disease and severe arthritis can immobilize the older person and thereby impair heat production. Malnutrition—by itself or in association with dementia, poor

Table 70.1 Causes of hypothermia

- Cold exposure
- Medications
- Phenothiazines
- Narcotics
- Vasodilators
- Barbiturates

Drugs and alcohol

Diseases

- Inflammatory skin conditions
- Paget's disease
- Endocrine disorders
- Hypothyroidism
- Hypopituitarism
- Adrenal insufficiency
- Diabetes mellitus
- Cardiovascular diseases
- Congestive heart failure
- Myocardial infarction
- Hepatic failure
- Neurological diseases
- Stroke
- Parkinson's disease
- Hypothalamic tumours or strokes
- Wernicke's encephalopathy
- Spinal cord lesions

Metabolic, biochemical and systemic abnormalities

- Hypoglycaemia
- Sepsis
- Malnutrition/starvation
- Uraemia

living conditions, cancer, or other conditions—can result in a lowered basal metabolic rate and reduced heat production. Neuroleptic medications impair central heat regulation. Sepsis is frequently observed among elderly patients admitted with hypothermia. It appears that underlying medical conditions predisposing to hypothermia are more common than autonomic dysfunction per se. Mortality in elderly persons with hypothermia is high and ranges from 30% to 80%. Mortality from hypothermia in association with myxoedema is particularly high.

Heat stroke

Heat stroke also appears to be more prevalent in the elderly. This may be attributable to poor temperature perception and a lack of protective behavioural responses, or impairments in sweating and vasodilatation. Comorbidity, such as dementia and neuroleptic medications, also impair the elderly person's capacity to detect and respond appropriately to elevated ambient temperatures.

Associated conditions

Abnormalities in temperature regulation are frequently seen in individuals with other symptoms of autonomic dysfunction. OH may be more common in elderly people with a history of hypothermia. Temperature dysregulation may be due to a number of autonomic nervous system diseases that commonly occur in elderly persons. These include diabetes, strokes, dementia, multiple systems atrophy, Parkinson's disease, and other conditions that are reviewed extensively in other chapters.

Blood pressure regulation

One of the most important, and most widely studied, functions of the autonomic nervous system is the maintenance of an adequate blood pressure to assure vital organ perfusion. Blood pressure is the product of heart rate, stroke volume, and systemic vascular resistance. These physiological parameters are regulated on a beat-to-beat basis by the baroreflexes and both sympathetic and parasympathetic limbs of the autonomic nervous system. Normal human ageing is associated with several changes in autonomic regulation of blood pressure. The superimposition of cardiovascular diseases and the medications used to treat them in elderly patients, further alter autonomic control, and manifest as hypotension and syncope. This section will review physiological and pathological changes in autonomic cardiovascular regulation associated with ageing, and the common geriatric syndromes that often result.

Baroreflex mechanisms

The baroreflex maintains a normal blood pressure by increasing heart rate and vascular resistance in response to transient reductions in stretch of arterial baroreceptors, and by decreasing these parameters in response to an increase in stretch of baroreceptors. Normal human ageing is associated with a reduction in baroreflex sensitivity. This is evident in the blunted cardioacceleratory response to stimuli such as upright posture, nitroprusside infusion and lower body negative pressure, which lower arterial pressure, as well as a reduced bradycardic response to drugs such as phenylephrine that elevate pressure. Furthermore, baroreflex impairment manifests as an increase in blood pressure variability, often with potentially dangerous blood pressure reductions during hypotensive stresses such as upright posture or meal digestion.

Age-associated elevations in blood pressure have been considered to be both a possible cause and consequence of baroreflex impairment. Both normal ageing and hypertension exert independent effects on baroreflex sensitivity. It has been suggested that the decrease in arterial distensibility that accompanies ageing and hypertension results in diminished baroreceptor stretch, less tonic inhibition of the brainstem vasomotor centre, and increased sympathetic outflow. Increased sympathetic outflow results in increased circulating noradrenaline, which in turn may result in further vasoconstriction, blood pressure elevation, and baroreflex impairment. Elevated basal plasma noradrenaline levels and muscle sympathetic nerve activity, as well as a heightened plasma noradrenaline response to baroreceptor unloading in elderly subjects support this hypothesis. Furthermore, in healthy young individuals carotid artery distensibility or stiffness correlates with baroreflex sensitivity (Lipsitz et al. 2005) (Fig. 70.1). The baroreflex may be impaired at any of multiple sites along its arc, including carotid and cardiopulmonary pressure receptors, afferent neuronal pathways, the

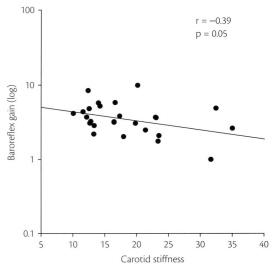

Fig. 70.1 The linear relationship between carotid stiffness and baroreflex gain among healthy elderly subjects. From Mukai et al. 2003, with permission.

brainstem (nucleus tractus solitarius) and higher regulatory centres, efferent sympathetic and parasympathetic neurons, postsynaptic cardiac β-receptors, or intracellular signal transduction G proteins. Several lines of evidence discussed below localize the defect to the β-receptor and signal transduction pathways within myocardial cells.

Sympathetic nervous system

Basal sympathetic nerve activity

Much of our current knowledge about age-related changes in sympathetic nervous system function is derived from studies of circulating plasma catecholamine levels, norepinephrine kinetics, and microneurographic recordings from sympathetic nerves to skeletal muscle. Significant evidence suggests that basal plasma noradrenaline levels increase with age. Age-related elevations in plasma noradrenaline may be due to many factors, including increased appearance at the synapse, increased spillover into the systemic circulation, decreased reuptake by presynaptic neurons, decreased local metabolism, and decreased systemic clearance. To determine whether elevations in plasma noradrenaline levels reflect heightened sympathetic nervous system activity, or merely decreased clearance, recent investigations have used radiotracer methods to examine noradrenaline kinetics. Using tritiated noradrenaline infusions and a two-compartment model to estimate noradrenaline disposition, Veith et al. (1986) demonstrated a 32% increase in arterialized noradrenaline appearance, and 19% decrease in clearance in healthy elderly subjects compared with young individuals. Studies of sympathetic nervous system activity measured by microelectrode recordings from the peroneal nerve in healthy subjects demonstrate an age-related increase in muscle sympathetic nerve activity (Ng et al. 1993). Sympathetic nerve activity is higher in males than females. Furthermore, venous plasma noradrenaline levels appear to correlate with muscle sympathetic nerve activity. Increases of sympathetic activity appear to specifically target skeletal and smooth muscle, but not kidney. These data lend further support to the notion that healthy ageing is associated with elevated basal sympathetic nervous system activity. It is not known whether this is related to arterial stiffness that may attenuate the

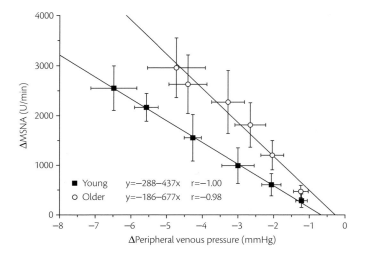

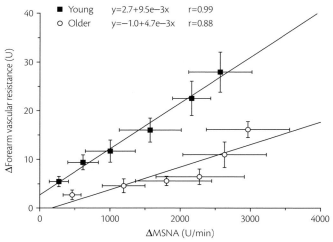

Fig. 70.2 Top panel: The change in muscle sympathetic nerve activity (MSNA) during reductions in peripheral venous pressure induced by lower body suction in healthy young and elderly subjects. **Bottom panel:** The corresponding change in forearm vascular resistance in response to induced changes in MSNA in the same subjects. Note the increase in MSNA, but reduction in forearm vascular response in older versus young subjects. With permission from Davy, K.P., Seals, D.R., and Tanaka, H. (1998) Augmented cardiopulmonary and integrated baroreflexes but attenuated peripheral vasoconstriction with age. *Hypertension* **32**, 298–304.

stretch of baroreceptors in the carotid arteries and aortic arch, or whether it is due to alterations in central sympathetic outflow.

Therefore, increases in muscle sympathetic activity during reductions in peripheral venous pressure are associated with reduced peripheral vasoconstriction in elderly individuals compared with young people (Fig. 70.2).

In contrast to noradrenaline, adrenaline is released directly into the bloodstream from the adrenal medulla in response to sympathetic stimulation, and is then transported via the circulation to target organs. Adrenaline is removed through non-neuronal uptake and metabolism. In contrast to sympathetic activity, tonic adrenaline (epinephrine) secretion from the adrenal medulla is reduced with age. Plasma levels may not be affected because of reduced clearance.

Circadian rhythm of catecholamine levels

Catecholamines exhibit diurnal variation that is preserved during ageing. Plasma noradrenaline levels are highest during the late morning to early afternoon and fall gradually during the night. Elderly subjects have higher noradrenaline levels during a 24-hour period than young subjects. This elevation is most pronounced during the night and is associated with increased nocturnal wakefulness and less stage 4 sleep in elderly subjects (Prinz et al. 1979) and reduced nocturnal dipping in blood pressure.

Stimulated catecholamine levels

Postural stress induced by active standing and head-up tilt results in an exaggerated increase in plasma noradrenaline in old subjects compared with the young. Furthermore, the time required for plasma noradrenaline levels to return to baseline is prolonged in elderly subjects (Young et al. 1980). The prolongation of noradrenaline response to sympathetic nervous system stimulation may be misinterpreted as elevated supine resting level if subjects are not given a sufficient length of time to achieve truly basal conditions. Plasma noradrenaline responses to isometric exercise, the cold pressor test, psychological stimuli, and graded levels of cardiac work, are all increased in old compared with young healthy subjects (Ryan and Lipsitz 1995).

β-Adrenergic activity

The fact that plasma noradrenaline levels are heightened and prolonged during hypotensive stress, but heart rate responses are blunted in elderly subjects, suggests that ageing results in impaired β-mediated adrenoceptor responses to sympathetic activation. This notion is further supported by the findings that infusions of β-adrenergic agonists result in smaller increases in heart rate, left ventricular ejection fraction, cardiac output, and vasodilatation in older compared with younger men (Lakatta 1993).

β$_1$-Adrenoceptors

In normal individuals stimulation of β$_1$-receptors using intravenous infusions of sympathetic agonists such as isoproterenol results in cardioacceleration. The dose of isoproterenol required to raise the heart rate is increased with ageing in humans and animals. The normal increase in heart rate induced by isoproterenol may also be due to a reflex cardioacceleratory response to the vasodilatation produced by simultaneous activation of β$_2$-receptors. Evidence discussed below indicates that β$_2$-adrenoceptor function is impaired with senescence.

In the heart the blunted cardioacceleratory response to β-adrenergic stimulation has been attributed to multiple molecular and biochemical changes in β-receptor coupling and post-receptor events. The number of β-receptors on cardiac myocytes is unchanged with advancing age, but the affinity of β-receptors for agonists is reduced. Post-receptor changes with ageing include a decrease in the activity of G$_s$-proteins and the adenylate cyclase catalytic unit, and a decrease in cAMP-dependent phosphokinase-induced protein phosphorylation (Lakatta 1993). As a result of these changes, G protein-mediated signal transduction is impaired. Although a recent study suggests that exercise training by treadmill running may increase β-adrenergic signal transduction in senescent rats (Scarpace et al. 1994), endurance exercise does not appear to improve the cardiac response to β-adrenergic stimulation in elderly humans (Stratton et al. 1992).

The decrease in cardiac contractile response to β-adrenergic stimulation has been studied in rat ventricular myocytes, where it appears to be related to decreased influx of calcium ions via sarcolemmal calcium channels, and a reduction in the amplitude of the cytosolic calcium transient. These changes are similar to those seen in receptor desensitization due to prolonged exposure of myocardial tissue to β-adrenergic agonists. Thus, age-associated alterations in β-adrenergic response may be due to desensitization of the adenylate cyclase system in response to chronic elevations of plasma catecholamine levels (Lakatta 1993).

β$_2$-Adrenoceptors

Several studies suggest that β$_2$-mediated vasodilatation is also impaired in elderly individuals. In order to study β$_2$-adrenergic effects in isolation from baroreflex responses to systemic vasodilators, Pan et al. (1986) infused isoproterenol directly into the dorsal hand vein of healthy young and old subjects. Isoproterenol-mediated vascular relaxation was impaired in elderly individuals. In contrast, nitroglycerine-mediated relaxation was normal in both young and elderly subjects. Since nitrate-induced vasodilatation was intact, the impairment in β-agonist response was probably not due to structural alterations in the vessel wall. This finding supports an age-related decline in β$_2$-mediated vasodilatation in the elderly.

α-Adrenergic activity

Current evidence also suggests that α-adrenergic responsiveness decreases with normal human ageing. Several studies have shown that the α$_1$-adrenergic vasoconstrictor response to noradrenaline infusion (Hogikyan and Supiano 1994), phenylephrine infusion (Dinenno et al. 2002), or endogenous norepinephrine release by tyramine (Dinenno et al. 2002) or sympathetic activation by lower body negative pressure (see Fig. 70.2) (Davy et al. 1998) are reduced in the forearm of healthy elderly subjects. The fact that this impairment can be reversed by suppression of sympathetic nervous system activity with guanadrel (Hogikyan and Supiano 1994), suggests that it is due to receptor desensitization in response to heightened sympathetic nervous system activity. This remarkable observation indicates that some of the autonomic nervous system changes associated with ageing may be reversible.

Since ageing is associated with blood pressure elevation, it is important to distinguish the effects of ageing from those of hypertension. In contrast to the previous findings of attenuated vasoconstriction, which was observed predominantly in normotensive elderly men, hypertensive elderly women have enhanced systemic vasoconstriction in response to sympathetic activation during head-up tilt (Lipsitz et al. 2006). This exaggerated response was reversed after 6 months of antihypertensive therapy. Enhanced vasoreactivity may contribute to excessive cardiovascular morbidity and mortality in elderly hypertensive women.

Parasympathetic nervous system

Age-related alterations in the parasympathetic nervous system are difficult to evaluate. Most of the currently available clinical evidence for a decline in parasympathetic function with ageing is derived from studies of heart rate variability. Previous studies demonstrating age-related reductions in overall heart rate variability in response to respiration, cough, and the Valsalva manoeuvre suggest that ageing is associated with impaired vagal control of heart rate. Elderly patients with unexplained syncope have even greater impairments in heart rate responses to cough and deep breathing than elderly subjects without syncope (Maddens et al. 1987).

The ratio of R-R intervals during expiration and inspiration is a standard method of evaluating autonomic function and reflects primarily parasympathetic influences on the heart rate. The difference between R-R interval prolongation during expiration and shortening during inspiration is reduced with ageing. However, many physiological changes associated with ageing may influence this finding. Impaired baroreflex function, decreased cardiac responsiveness to sympathetic and parasympathetic input, and changes in lung and chest wall compliance—which affect intrathoracic pressures and venous return to the heart during deep breathing—all may influence heart rate variability. Furthermore, the reflex responses to respiratory manoeuvres are dependent on the extent of blood pressure change, and therefore may vary from one individual to the next depending on the performance of the test and the associated blood pressure response. Therefore, R-R variability during respiration cannot be considered a pure test of parasympathetic function (Fig. 70.3).

Recently, the technique of frequency domain (spectral) analysis has been used to quantify the relative contributions of sympathetic and parasympathetic nervous systems to heart rate or interbeat interval variability. The power spectrum produced by this technique can be divided into low and high frequency components. Previous pharmacological blocking studies using beta-blockade and/or atropine suggest that the low frequency oscillations (0.06–0.12 Hz) represent baroreflex-mediated sympathetic and parasympathetic influences on heart period variability, while the high frequency portion at breathing frequency, typically 0.15–0.5 Hz, represents the respiratory sinus arrhythmia and is under parasympathetic control (Pagani et al. 1986). When studying parasympathetic

modulation to the heart, it is important to take into account that breathing frequencies may vary from fast to very slow over a wide range of 0.05–2 Hz (Novak et al. 1993) and that the amplitude of respiration-induced R-R interval fluctuations increases exponentially as breathing frequency slows down from 2 Hz to 0.1 Hz. Frequency domain analysis techniques have confirmed that healthy ageing is associated with reductions in both baroreflex and parasympathetic modulation of heart rate, with a relatively greater loss of the high frequency parasympathetic component (Lipsitz et al. 1990). Furthermore, there may be gender differences in heart rate variability, with relatively greater high frequency variability in healthy women compared with men across all ages (Ryan et al. 1994). Given the known inverse relationship between heart rate variability and cardiovascular mortality, this finding may reflect healthier cardiovascular function in women compared with men.

It is important to recognize that frequency domain analyses yield different results depending on whether heart rate or interbeat interval (R-R) are used as the unit of measure. R-R interval is linearly related to cardiac vagal outflow, while heart rate is inversely related to R-R interval and reflects minute-to-minute systemic hemodynamic adjustments to physiological stimuli. Therefore, R-R interval spectra are probably best suited for the evaluation of parasympathetic influences on the heart.

The age-related attenuation of autonomic, neurohumoral, and other influences on the heart results not only in a reduction in heart rate variability, but also in a marked change in the dynamics of beat-to-beat heart rate fluctuations. As shown in Fig. 70.3, the highly irregular, complex dynamics of heart rate variability that is characteristic of healthy young individuals, is lost with healthy ageing, resulting in a more regular and predictable heart rate time series. This loss of complexity in heart rate dynamics appears to be generalizable to the fluctuating output of many different physiological processes as they age (Lipsitz and Goldberger 1992, Lipsitz 2002). For example, measurements of continuous blood pressure, electroencephalographic waves, frequently sampled thyrotropin or luteinizing hormone levels, and centre-of-pressure changes during quiet stance all show more regular, less complex behaviour with ageing. This apparent loss of dynamic range in physiological functions may be due to fewer regulatory influences as an individual ages, thus leading to an impaired capacity to adapt to stress (Lipsitz 2002).

Cardiac ventricular function

The maintenance of a normal blood pressure also depends on the ability to generate an adequate cardiac output. Cardiac output tends to decrease with normal ageing, both at rest and with exercise. This is due not only to a reduction in heart rate response to β-adrenergic stimulation, as mentioned above, but also to changes in systolic and diastolic myocardial performance that influence stroke volume.

Diastolic function

As a result of several structural and functional changes in the myocardium, the aged heart stiffens and early diastolic ventricular filling becomes impaired. These changes include an increase in cross-linking of myocardial collagen and prolongation of ventricular relaxation time. The latter may be due in part to reduction in the active uptake of calcium into the sarcoplasmic reticulum after ventricular contraction, as a consequence of reduced oxygen tension in the coronary circulation, decreased oxidative phosphorylation, and cumulative mitochondrial peroxidation.

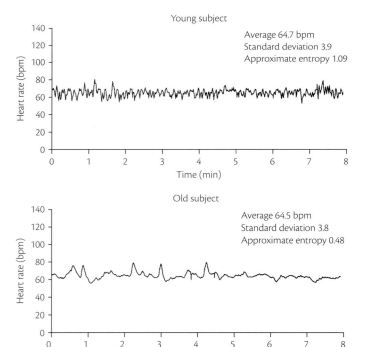

Fig. 70.3 Continuous 8-minute heart rate time series for a healthy young subject (upper panel) and healthy elderly subject (lower panel). Note that the average and standard deviation of heart rate over 8 minutes are nearly identical, but the dynamics are very different. The dynamics can be quantified by the statistic Approximate Entropy, which measures the regularity of the signal. With permission from Lipsitz, L. and Goldberger, A. L. (1992) Loss of "complexity" and aging. Potential applications of fractals and chaos theory to senescence. *J Am Med Assoc* **267**, 1806–1809. Copyright 1992 American Medical Association. All rights reserved.

The age-related impairment in early ventricular filling makes the heart dependent on adequate preload to fill the ventricle, as well as on atrial contraction during late diastole to maintain stroke volume. Thus, OH and syncope occur commonly in older people because of volume contraction or venous pooling which reduce cardiac preload, or at the onset of atrial fibrillation when the atrial contribution to cardiac output is suddenly lost.

Systolic function

With ageing there is preservation of myocardial contractile strength, but a decrease in left ventricular ejection fraction in response to exertion. This is due to both reduced β-adrenergic responsiveness, as well as an increase in afterload. Afterload, which represents opposition to left ventricular ejection, increases progressively with ageing due to stiffening of the ascending aorta, and narrowing of the peripheral vasculature. These changes result in an increase in systolic blood pressure. They also decrease the maximum cardiac output during exercise.

The cardiac response to exercise differs between healthy young and old subjects. While the young increase cardiac output via increases in heart rate and decreases in end systolic volume (greater contractility), the healthy elderly do so by increasing end diastolic volume (cardiac dilatation) (Rodeheffer et al. 1984). Thus, the elderly rely on the Frank–Starling relationship to achieve an increase in stroke volume during exercise. A similar mechanism can be demonstrated in young subjects in the presence of β-adrenergic blockade, suggesting that the age effect is due to reduced β-adrenergic responsiveness.

Recent data suggest that the decrease in maximal cardiac output during exercise observed in the elderly, may in large part be related to a sedentary lifestyle and consequent cardiovascular deconditioning. A 6-month training program of endurance exercise training has been shown to enhance end-diastolic volume and contractility, thereby increasing ejection fraction, stroke volume, and cardiac output at peak exercise in elderly men (Stratton et al. 1994). Thus, the elderly may be able to compensate for age-associated physiological changes, by using alternate mechanisms (such as the Frank–Starling relationship) to maintain cardiac function at times of stress.

Intravascular volume regulation

An adequate blood pressure also depends on the maintenance of intravascular volume. Ageing is associated with a progressive decline in plasma renin, angiotensin II, and aldosterone levels, and elevations in atrial natriuretic peptide, all of which promote salt wasting by the kidney. Furthermore, healthy elderly individuals do not experience the same sense of thirst as younger subjects when they become hyperosmolar during water deprivation (Phillips et al. 1984). Thus, dehydration and hypotension may develop rapidly during conditions such as an acute illness, preparation for a medical procedure, or exposure to a warm climate when insensible fluid losses are increased and/or access to oral fluids is limited. The interaction between volume contraction and impaired diastolic function may threaten cardiac output, and result in hypotension and organ ischaemia.

Regulation of organ blood flow

Age-related changes in vascular response to sympathetic nervous system activity have been described above. However, the regulation of blood flow to various circulatory beds also depends on complex interactions at the cellular level between the endothelium, local vasoactive peptides, neuroendocrine influences, and mechanical factors, few of which have been studied as a function of ageing in humans. In angiographically normal coronary arteries (Egashira et al. 1993) and the brachial artery (Gerhard et al. 1996), the endothelium-dependent vasodilatory response to acetylcholine or methacholine is reduced with ageing. In contrast, endothelium-independent vasodilation by nitroprusside is not affected by ageing.

Normal human ageing is also associated with a reduction in cerebral blood flow, which is further compromised by the presence of risk factors for cerebrovascular disease (Meyer and Shaw 1984). Although it is not clear whether the decline in cerebral blood flow is due to reduced supply or demand, it is likely that elderly individuals, particularly those with cerebrovascular disease, have a resting cerebral blood flow that is closer to the threshold for cerebral ischemia (Figure 70.4). Consequently, relatively small, short-term reductions in blood pressure may produce cerebral ischaemic symptoms.

The brain normally maintains a constant blood flow over a wide range of perfusion pressures through the process of autoregulation. During reductions in blood pressure resistance vessels in the brain dilate to restore blood flow to normal. Although the effects of

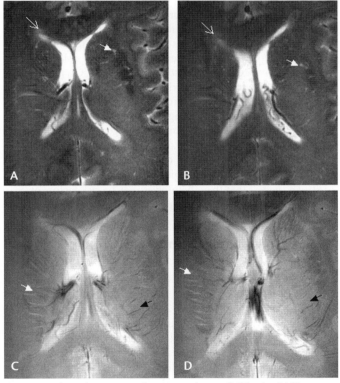

Fig. 70.4 High resolution magnetic resonance images (MRI) using RARE sequence (rapid acquisition with relaxation enhancement) images at 8 Tesla at the levels of the ventricles **(A, B)** show high signal intensity white matter changes adjacent to the ventricles (white empty arrows) and punctuate white matter lesions in basal ganglia and periventricular white matter (white arrows). MRI gradient echo images at 8 Tesla **(C, D)** at the level of the ventricles show normal appearing medullary veins as signal voids. Microvessels with high signal intensity are seen distally to the normal vasculature (white arrows). Reprinted from *Magnetic Resonance Imaging* **19**, Novak, V., et al. Intracranial ossifications and micronagiopathy at 8 Tesla MRI, 1133–1137. Copyright 2001, with permission from Elsevier, and also Novak, V., et al. Autonomic impairment in painful neuropathy, *Neurology*, 56/7/861.

ageing on cerebral autoregulation have received very little attention, limited data suggest that the autoregulation of cerebral blood flow is preserved into old age. However, patients with symptomatic OH appear to have a reduction in cerebral blood flow in response to decreased perfusion pressure (Wollner et al. 1979).

The decline in cerebral blood flow that occurs with normal ageing is further potentiated by the presence of risk factors for cerebrovascular disease such as hypertension (Meyer and Shaw 1984). It has been well established that hypertension is associated with an increase in cerebral vascular resistance and reduction of cerebral blood flow in addition to any age effect (Shenkin et al. 1953). Dysfunction of the arterial endothelium with ageing and age-related disorders (Volpe et al. 1996) may affect arteriolar reactivity and contribute to reduction in cerebral blood flow (Samdani et al. 1997). Vascular reactivity to hypercapnia, a measure of the vasodilatatory response of cerebral arterioles (Chimowitz et al. 1993, Bullock et al. 1985) is diminished with ageing and is further reduced with hypertension (Lipsitz 1985, Lipsitz et al. 2000). Cerebral oxygenation in the frontal lobes, measured by near infrared spectroscopy, is reduced during active standing in the healthy elderly people (Mehagnoul-Schipper et al. 2001). Common features of ageing and hypertension are their effects on microvessels with concentric thickening of vessel walls of small arteries and penetrating arterioles (Mejia et al. 1990, Julius et al. 1991). There is an increasing evidence that white matter hyperintensities that are seen on magnetic resonance (MR) images, reflect areas of silent hypoperfusion. White matter changes may arise as a consequence of the long-standing effects of age, hypertension and other risk factors on cerebral microvasculature (Marstrand et al. 2002). On pathological specimens, periventricular hyperintensities are correlated with the severity of demyelination, astrocytic gliosis, and dilatation of perivascular spaces. These findings support the notion that arteriolosclerosis is the primary factor in the pathogenesis of diffuse white matter changes in the elderly (van Swieten et al. 1991, Roob et al. 1999). The strong relationship of MR hyperintensities with age (Wahlund et al. 2001), neurological slowing and other risk factors for stroke suggest that they themselves may be risk factors or even manifestations of clinically important cerebrovascular disease (Desmond et al. 1993).

Clinical manifestations of impaired autonomic control of blood pressure

Two of the most common age-associated manifestations of autonomic nervous system impairment are orthostatic and postprandial hypotension, defined as a 20 mmHg or greater decline in systolic blood pressure upon assumption of the upright posture, or within one hour of eating a meal, respectively. These are two distinct conditions which may or may not occur together in the same patient. Both are related to a reduction in venous blood return to the heart due to blood pooling in the lower extremities or splanchnic circulation, and inadequate baroreflex compensation. Several of the physiological abnormalities that may predispose elderly people to hypotension are summarized in Table 70.2. The onset of diseases in old age, such as diabetes, cerebrovascular disease, Parkinson's disease, malignancy, and amyloidosis, as well as the medications used to treat them, may have additional adverse effects on autonomic function (Table 70.3). Therefore, hypotensive syndromes in old age may be considered due to physiological changes that accompany usual ageing, and pathological conditions that

Table 70.2 Age-related physiological changes predisposing to hypotension

Decreased baroreflex sensitivity
◆ Diminished heart rate response to hypotensive stimuli
◆ Impaired α-adrenergic vascular responsiveness
Impaired defence of intravascular volume
◆ Reduced secretion of renin, angiotensin, and aldosterone
◆ Increased atrial natriuretic peptide, supine and upright
◆ Decreased plasma vasopressin response to orthostasis
◆ Reduced thirst after water deprivation
Impaired early cardiac ventricular filling (diastolic dysfunction)

become more prevalent with advancing age. In addition, several abnormal reflexes may precipitate hypotension in elderly people. These three classifications of the hypotensive syndromes are summarized in Table 70.4.

Orthostatic hypotension

OH is increasingly more common with ageing and is a marker of general frailty. OH occurs in 5–18% of elderly people (Rutan

Table 70.3 Disease-related causes of orthostatic and postprandial hypotension

Central nervous system disorders
Multiple system atrophy
Brainstem lesions
Multiple cerebral infarctions
Parkinson's disease
Myelopathy
Peripheral and autonomic neuropathies
Pure autonomic failure
Diabetes
Amyloidosis
Tabes dorsalis
Alcoholic and nutritional
Paraneoplastic syndromes
Prolonged immobility
Medications
Phenothiazines and other neuroleptics
Monoamine oxidase inhibitors
Tricyclic antidepressants
Antihypertensives and diuretics
L-DOPA
Vasodilators
Beta-blockers
Calcium-channel blockers
ACE inhibitors

ACE, angiotensin-converting enzyme; L-DOPA, L-3,4-dihydroxyphenylalanine.

Table 70.4 Mechanisms of hypotension in the elderly

Physiological	Pathological	Reflex
Impaired adaptive capacity	**Disease-related**	**Health and cardiovascular disease**
Associated with HTN	Blunted noradrenaline response to posture or meals	Sudden bradycardia and/or hypotension
Increased noradrenaline response to posture	Causes:	Causes:
Precipitants of hypotension:	◆ CNS: strokes, MSA, Parkinson's	◆ Carotid sinus hypersensitivity
◆ Hypovolaemia	◆ Peripheral nervous system: diabetes mellitus, EtOH, nutritional, amyloid	◆ Neurally mediated syncope
◆ Preload reduction	◆ Pure autonomic failure	◆ Micturition, cough, swallow syncope
◆ Inactivity	◆ Salt-wasting: renal disease, Addison's disease	
◆ Other drugs		

et al. 1992) and in as many as 30% of those over 75 years of age with multiple pathological conditions, particularly hypertension. Blood pressure decline greater than 20 mm Hg systolic or 10 mm Hg diastolic within the first minute of standing up may occur in up to 50% of the seniors (Chokroverty et al. 1969). The reported prevalence differs according to the population studied, the subject's position (supine to sitting or standing), and the time measurements are taken (standing blood pressure is generally lower 1 minute after posture change than at 3 minutes). In cross-sectional studies, postural hypotension was associated with cerebrovascular disease, neurological symptoms and transient ischaemic attacks and falls (Dobkin 1989). A cross-sectional nursing home study identified OH as an independent risk factor for stroke, falls and cognitive decline (Hussain et al. 2001). The prospective Atherosclerosis Risk in Communities (ARIC) study (Eigenbrodt et al. 2000) has identified OH as an independent predictor of the first ischaemic stroke regardless OH type (systolic vs diastolic blood pressure drop) and baseline blood pressure. With OH, cerebral perfusion in the upright position critically depends on cerebral vasodilatory response. Stereotyped transient ischaemic attacks that were triggered by postprandial hypotension in an elderly hypertensive patient, serve as an example of OH-associated cerebral hyperperfusion (Kamata et al. 1994).

In a study of 911 long-stay nursing home residents whose supine, 1-minute, and 3-minute standing blood pressures were taken four times during the day (before and after breakfast, and before and after lunch) by trained nurses using random zero sphygmomanometers, three patterns of OH were defined: isolated (occurring once, 18% of subjects), variable (2–3 times, 20%), and persistent (4 or more times, 13%) (Ooi et al. 1997). The presence of OH was associated with elevated supine systolic blood pressure before breakfast, dizziness or light-headedness upon standing, male gender, medication for Parkinson's disease, time of day (before breakfast), greater independence in activities of daily living, and low body mass index. Therefore, ambulatory residents with hypertension, or those taking antiparkinsonian medications, may be at greatest risk of falls due to hypotension, particularly in the early morning when they first get out of bed.

Although OH is a cardinal feature of autonomic dysfunction in a young individual—often heralding the onset of autonomic failure—in the older person it is more likely to result from comorbidity and medication usage (Table 70.3) than from a syndrome of pure autonomic failure.

On assumption of the upright posture, approximately 500 cc of blood pools in the lower extremities and splanchnic circulation,

thereby reducing venous return to the heart. The consequent unloading of cardiopulmonary and carotid baroreceptors reduces tonic inhibitory input to brainstem vasomotor centres in the nucleus tractus solitarius and results in efferent sympathetic activation and parasympathetic withdrawal. Within 10 seconds of standing, the healthy young subject demonstrates a brisk heart rate response due to vagal inhibition. The systolic blood pressure falls transiently for 10–20 seconds, but is rapidly restored by sympathetically mediated cardioacceleration and vasoconstriction. Blood pressure may continue to fall if there is an excessive reduction in blood volume which is not counteracted by these normal physiological responses.

In the aged individual, the early baroreflex-mediated cardioacceleration observed in young people is blunted. This is probably due to defective cardiac β-receptor responsiveness discussed above. Despite the lack of heart rate acceleration on standing, most normotensive elderly persons are probably protected from OH by α-mediated vasoconstriction. However, when vasoconstriction is compromised by vasodilator medications or intravascular volume is reduced by diuretics, many elderly individuals lack the physiologic reserve to guard against hypotension. These individuals have age-related impairments in cardioacceleration and heightened plasma noradrenaline responses to postural stress (Table 70.4); they are often asymptomatic.

In contrast, elderly persons with severe symptomatic OH have a 'pathological' condition due to specific diseases, which impair autonomic function (Tables 70.3 and 70.4). These patients have symptoms of autonomic insufficiency and subnormal plasma noradrenaline responses to upright posture. They are chronically disabled by orthostatic symptoms, in contrast to individuals with physiological OH who become symptomatic only during periods of excessive haemodynamic stress.

Postprandial hypotension

The epidemiology of postprandial hypotension is unknown, but it is particularly common in the nursing home population, and in elderly patients with unexplained syncope (Jansen and Lipsitz 1995). In one report, 67% of elderly patients admitted to two Dutch hospitals (aged 60–98 years) had postprandial hypotension; 37% had both orthostatic and postprandial hypotension. A majority (65%) of patients with postprandial hypotension were symptomatic with syncope or sleepiness following a meal (Vloet et al. 2005). Like OH, postprandial hypotension is a condition commonly seen in patients with autonomic failure as well as in multiply-impaired and elderly people. In ways similar to OH, postprandial hypotension may also be viewed as a consequence of either age-related physiological changes or pathological abnormalities in autonomic function. Although the mechanisms of postprandial hypotension are unknown, asymptomatic elderly persons with the 'physiological' variant appear to have inadequate cardiovascular compensation for splanchnic blood pooling during food digestion. This is evident in the moderate decline in blood pressure after a meal and a blunted heart rate increase that is unable to compensate for reduced blood pressure. These individuals may become symptomatic if hypotensive medications are taken before a meal, or in the setting of volume contraction.

Elderly patients with pathological postprandial hypotension have marked, symptomatic reductions in blood pressure that may result in syncope. These patients demonstrate an initial increase in plasma noradrenaline following a meal, but a subsequent inappropriate decline at the time that blood pressure is falling.

Previous studies have examined the potential role of various gut peptides, including insulin in the pathophysiology of postprandial hypotension. Insulin may play a significant role, since fructose, fat and protein meals that fail to increase insulin concentration do not result in blood pressure reduction (Jansen and Hoefnagles 1990). Furthermore, when insulin is given with a high fat meal blood pressure falls and calf vascular resistance fails to increase (Kearney et al. 1998).

In autonomic failure, caffeine and somatostatin analogues have proven beneficial in preventing postprandial hypotension. These agents may work by preventing splanchnic vasodilation, although the exact mechanisms are not fully understood. There is some evidence that walking exercise after a meal may restore blood pressure to its baseline, and thus prevent postprandial hypotension.

Reflex causes of hypotension

Hypotension may also result from neurally mediated (vasovagal) syncope; the sudden triggering of vagal reflexes during micturition, defecation, or swallowing; or the stimulation of a hypersensitive carotid sinus reflex (Table 70.4). One probable mechanism of neurally mediated syncope is provocation of the Bezold–Jarisch reflex by marked sympathetic stimulation of a relatively empty cardiac ventricle, during upright posture. Stimulation of vagal C-fibres in the ventricular wall by vigorous cardiac contraction results in reflex hypotension and bradycardia. This reflex may be less common in elderly patients due to age-related reductions in sympathetic and vagal control of heart rate.

In contrast, ageing is associated with an increased prevalence of carotid sinus hypersensitivity, probably due to dropout of sinus node pacemaker cells and the onset of ischemic heart disease, rather than enhanced vagal outflow. However, the frequently observed hypotensive and bradycardic response to a Valsalva maneuver while straining to overcome fecal impaction during defecation, or to overcome prostatic obstruction in men during micturition, suggests that vagal reflexes remain an important cause of hypotension, even in advanced age.

Control of respiration

Autonomic control of pulmonary and circulatory systems are closely linked, so that adjustments in heart rate, cardiac output, blood pressure, and organ flow can be made in response to changing demands for oxygen. Ageing is associated with a reduction in the partial pressure of oxygen in the blood, primarily due to a mismatch of ventilation and perfusion in the dependent portions of the lungs. This results from a reduction in lung compliance, which causes airways to close prematurely at higher lung volumes (increased closing volume), within the range of vital capacity. It has been thought that the relative hypoxemia in advanced age is offset by a reduced tissue demand for oxygen (reduced maximal oxygen uptake or VO_2max). However, much of the reduction in VO_2max is attributable to reduced muscle mass, and is reversible with endurance exercise training.

Chemoreceptors located in brainstem respiratory centres adjust respiratory amplitude and frequency on a moment-to-moment basis, in order to assure adequate oxygen availability and carbon dioxide clearance from the blood. Longer-term changes in oxygen supply and demand are matched by finely tuned adjustments in the sensitivity (gain) of chemoreceptors. With advancing age, there is a decline in chemosensitivity to oxygen and carbon dioxide tension, resulting in relative hypoventilation in response to hypoxemia or hypercarbia. Thus, older individuals may be more vulnerable to vital organ ischemia during stresses such as surgery, acute pulmonary infections, or high altitude, when oxygen availability is reduced.

Gastrointestinal function

Many of the common gastrointestinal symptoms experienced by elderly people, including heartburn, constipation, diarrhoea, and faecal incontinence, suggest that ageing is associated with impaired autonomic control of the gastrointestinal tract. However, in the absence of disease, ageing is associated with only minor alterations in gastrointestinal function. Early studies of elderly people demonstrated frequent non-propulsive tertiary contractions of the oesophagus, impaired lower oesophageal sphincter relaxation, and delayed oesophageal emptying. This constellation of findings was called 'presbyoesophagus' because the abnormalities were thought to be due to ageing. However, many of the subjects of previous studies had medical and neurological conditions, including diabetes mellitus, which may have been responsible for these findings. More recent studies in healthy elderly people have revealed a small decrease in the amplitude of oesophageal contractions, a slight increase in the frequency of simultaneous contractions in the upper and lower oesophagus, and a decrease in the regularity of peristaltic waves after a swallow. These physiological changes may be due to a decrease in myenteric ganglion cells per unit area and thickening of the smooth muscle layer of the oesophagus. In healthy elders, however, these changes are usually asymptomatic.

In the stomach, basal and maximal gastric acid output decreases with normal ageing, probably as a result gastric mucosal atrophy and drop-out of parietal cells. There also may be a minor delay in liquid emptying from the stomach. The role of the autonomic nervous system in these changes is not known.

There have been very few human studies of age-related changes in small and large bowel function. Although there is a significant slowing of colonic transit time in senescent rats due to decreased responsiveness to neurotransmitters and progressive denervation, both small and large intestinal motility are probably unchanged with normal human ageing. Constipation in elderly people is probably related more to a decrease in faecal water content and laxative abuse than to age-related changes in intestinal transit time. In the anorectal area, an increase in resting sphincter tone and decrease in maximal contractile pressure have been observed in some healthy elders. Resting tone may be influenced by increases in collagenous connective tissue that replaces anal smooth muscle, while muscle loss may account for a reduction in the generation of anal squeeze pressure.

Urinary tract function

Alterations in lower urinary tract function that mimic autonomic insufficiency, particularly urinary incontinence, become increasingly prevalent with ageing. However, urinary symptoms are due primarily to age-associated diseases that affect autonomic nervous system control of the urinary tract, rather than ageing per se. Little is known about the effects of healthy human ageing on voiding function. Current evidence suggests that there are functional and structural changes in the lower urinary tract outside of the autonomic nervous system that may predispose elderly people to urinary incontinence (Resnick 1995). These include declines in bladder capacity, contractility, and the ability to postpone voiding in both sexes, and decreases in urethral length and closing pressure in women. The prevalence of involuntary bladder contractions and the post-voiding residual bladder volume increase with age. Ultrastructurally, bladders of healthy elderly people with normal contractility show a normal configuration of muscle cells and cell junctions, but dominant dense bands and depleted caveolae in muscle cell membranes. In contrast, aged bladders with impaired contractility have widespread degeneration of muscle cells and axons superimposed on the 'dense band pattern'. These histopathological changes may be responsible for the age-related change in bladder contractility.

One of the most common causes of established incontinence in elderly people is detrusor overactivity. This may be associated with central nervous system disease (e.g. stroke), normal ageing, or local urinary tract abnormalities (e.g. prostatic obstruction). Ultrastructurally, the bladder demonstrates replacement of normal muscle junctions with 'protrusion junctions', which may facilitate propagation of heightened smooth muscle activity, causing involuntary bladder contractions. The role of the autonomic nervous system in these changes is not clear.

Sexual function

Normal sexual function is dependent on the complex integration of endocrine, autonomic, and vascular systems. The sympathetic nervous system innervates blood vessels in the reproductive organs; erectile tissue in the penis, clitoris, and bulbs of the vestibule; and smooth muscle in the seminal vesicles, prostate, vagina, and uterus. The parasympathetic nervous system also innervates erectile tissue in the penis and clitoris, as well as smooth muscle in the urethra, seminal vesicles, prostate, vagina, and uterus. In addition, parasympathetic nerves innervate glandular tissue and secretory epithelium in these structures. Although sexual dysfunction becomes more common with advancing age, ageing per se is not associated with impairments in autonomic control of genital function. Diseases such as diabetes, peripheral vascular disease, neuropathies, spinal cord lesions, and uraemia, as well as alcohol and drugs are most frequently implicated.

In women, reproductive capacity ends in mid-life at the time of menopause and levels of 17-beta-oestradiol, the predominant circulating oestrogen during reproductive life, declines. This subsequently predisposes women to the development of pathological conditions such as cardiovascular disease and osteoporosis. Men do not experience as abrupt a change in reproductive function as women do, but undergo gradual alterations in sex steroid metabolism that predispose them to prostate enlargement and bone loss. In men normal ageing probably results in a modest degree of primary testicular failure, characterized by a decrease in testicular size. The age-related decline in testicular function is highly variable and its clinical implications have not been well established. It may contribute to a decline in the frequency of sexual activity, but probably plays a secondary role to social, psychological, and medical factors that have the greatest influence on sexual dysfunction in late life. Although both healthy men and women may experience changes in sexual performance with advancing age, their capacity to enjoy sexual activity remains intact.

References

Bullock, R., Mendelow, A. D., Bone, I., Patterson, J., Macleod, W. N., and Allardice, G. (1985). Cerebral blood flow and CO_2 responsiveness as an indicator of collateral reserve capacity in patients with carotid artery disease. *Br. J. Surg.* **72**, 348–51.

Byrne, N. M., Hill, A. P., Hunter, G. R., and Schutz, Y. (2005). Metabolic equivalent: one size does not fit all. *J Appl. Physiol.* **99**, 1112–1119.

Chimowitz, M. I., Furlan, A. J., Jones, S. C., Sila, C. A., Lorig, R. L., Parandi, L., and Beck, G. J. (1993). Transcranial Doppler assessment of cerebral perfusion reserve in patients with carotid occlusive disease and no evidence of cerebral infarction. *Neurology* **43**, 353–57.

Chokroverty, S., Barron, K. D., Katz, F. H., Del Greco, F., and Sharp, J. T. (1969). The syndrome of primary OH. *Brain* **92**, 743–68.

Collins, K. J., Easton, J. C., and Exton-Smith, A. N. (1981). Shivering thermogenesis and vasomotor responses with convective cooling in the elderly. *J Physiol. London* **320**, 76.

Collins, K. J. and Exton-Smith, A. N. (1981). Urban hypothermia: preferred temperature and thermal perception in old age. *Br. Med. J.* **282**, 175–77.

Davy, K. P., Seals, D. R., and Tanaka, H. (1998). Augmented cardiopulmonary and integrated baroreflexes but attenuated peripheral vasoconstriction with age. *Hypertension* **32**, 298–304.

Desmond, D. W., Tatemichi, T. K., Myunghee, P., and Stern, Y. (1993). Risk factors for cerebrovascular disease as correlate of cognitive function in a stroke-free cohort. *Arch. Neurol.* **50**, 162–66.

Dinenno, F., Dietz, N., and Joyner, M. (2002). Ageing and forearm postjunctional α-adrenergic vasoconstriction in healthy men. *Circulation* **106**, 1349–54.

Dobkin, B. H. (1989). OH as a risk factor for symptomatic occlusive cerebrovascular disease. Neurology **34**.

Egashira, K., Inou, T., Hirooka, Y., *et al.* (1993). Effects of age on endothelium-dependent vasodilation of resistance coronary artery by acetylcholine in humans. *Circulation* **88**, 77–81.

Eigenbrodt, M. L., Rose, K. M., Couper, D. J., Arnett, D. K., Smith, R., and Jones, D. (2000). OH as a risk factor for stroke. The Atherosclerosis Risk in Communities (ARIC) Study, 1987–1996. *Stroke* **31**, 2307–2313.

Gerhard, M., Roddy, M. A., Creager, S. J., and Creager, M. A. (1996). Ageing progressively impaires endothelium-dependent vasodilation in forearm resistance vessels of humans. *Hypertension* **27**, 849–53.

Grassi, G., Seravalle, G., Turri, C., Bertinieri, G., Dell'Oro, R., and Mancia, G. (2003). Impairment of thermoregulatory control of skin sympathetic nerve traffic in the elderly. *Circulation* **108**, 729–35.

Herity, B., Daly, L., Bourke, G. J., and Horgan, J. M. (1991). Hypothermia and mortality and morbidity. An epidemiological analysis. *J. Epidemiol. Community Health* **45**, 19–23.

Hogikyan, R. V. and Supiano, M. A. (1994). Arterial α–adrenergic responsiveness is decreased and SNS activity is increased in older humans. *Am. J Physiol.* **266**, E717–24.

Hussain, M., Ooi, W. L., and Lipsitz, L. A. (2001). Intra-individual postural blood pressure variability and stroke in elderly nursing home residents. *Journal of Clinical Epidemiology* **54**, 488–94.

Inbar, O., Morris, N., Epstein, Y., and Gass, G. (2004). Comparison of thermoregulatory responses to exercise in dry heat among prepubertal boys, young adults and older males. *Exp. Physiol.* **89**, 691–700.

Inoue, Y., Nakao, M., Araki, T., and Murakami, H. (1991). Regional differences in the sweating responses of older and younger men. *J Appl. Physiol.* **71**, 2453–59.

Jansen, R. W. and Hoefnagles, W. H. (1990). Postprandial blood pressure reduction. *Netherlands Journal of Medicine* **37**, 80–88.

Jansen, R. W. and Lipsitz, L. (1995). Postprandial hypotension: epidemiology, pathophysiology, and clinical management. *Ann. Intern. Med.* **122**, 286–95.

Julius, S., Jones, K., Schork, N., Johnson, E., Krause, L., Nazzaro, P., and Zemva, A. (1991). Independence of pressure reactivity from pressure levels in Tecumseh, Michigan. *Hypertension* **17**, III12–21.

Kamata, T., Yokota, T., Furukawa, T., and Tsukagoshi, H. (1994). Cerebral ischemic attack caused by postprandial hypotension. *Stroke* Feb 25, 511–513.

Kearney, M. T., Cowley, A. J., Stubbs, T. A., Evans, A., and MacDonald, A. (1998). Depressor action of insulin on skeletal muscle vasculature: a novel mechanism for postprandial hypotension in the elderly. *J Am. Coll. Cardiol.* **31**, 209–216.

Khan, F., Spence, V. A., and Belch, J. J. F. (1992). Cutaneous vascular responses and thermoregulation in relation to age. *Clin. Sci.* **82**, 521–28.

Kramer, M. R., Vandijk, J., and Rosin, A. J. (1989). Mortality in elderly patients with thermoregulatory failure. *Arch. Intern. Med.* **149**, 1521–253.

Lakatta, E. G. (1993). Deficient neuroendicrine regulation of the cardiovascular system with advancing age in healthy humans. *Circulation* **87**, 1806–1809.

Lipsitz, L. A. (1985). Intraindividual variability in postural blood pressure in the elderly. *Clin. Sci.* **69**, 337–41.

Lipsitz, L. A. (2002). Dynamics of stability: The physiological basis of functional health and frailty. *Journal of Gerontol. Biol. Sciences* **57A**, B115–25.

Lipsitz, L. A., Gagnon, M., Vyas, M., *et al.* (2005). Antihypertensive therapy increases cerebral blood flow and carotid distensibility in hypertensive elderly subjects. *Hypertension* **45**, 216–21.

Lipsitz, L. A., Iloputaife, I., Gagnon, M., and Serrador, J. M. (2006). Enhanced vasoreactivity and its response to antihypertensive therapy in hypertensive elderly women. *Hypertension* **47**.

Lipsitz, L. A., Mietus, J., Moody, G. B., and Goldberger, A. L. (1990). Spectral characteristics of heart rate variability before and during postural tilt. Relations to ageing and risk of syncope. *Circulation* **81**, 1803–1810.

Lipsitz, L. A., Mukai, S., Hammer, J., Gagnon, M., and Babikian, V. L. (2000). Dynamic regulation of middle cerebral artery blood flow velocity in ageing and hypertension. *Stroke* **31**, 1897–1903.

Lipsitz, L. and Goldberger, A. L. (1992). Loss of 'complexity' and ageing. Potential applications of fractals and chaos theory to senescence. *J Am. Med. Assoc.* **267**, 1806–1809.

Maddens, M. E., Lipsitz, L., Wei, J. Y., Pluchino, F. C., and Mark, R. (1987). Impared heart rate responses to cough and deep breathing in elderly patients with unexplained syncope. *Am. J Cardiol.* **60**, 1368–72.

Marstrand, J. R., Garde, E., Rostrup, E., Ring, P., Rosenbaum, S., Mortensen, E. L., and Larsson, H. B. (2002). Cerebral perfusion and cerebrovascular reactivity are reduced in white matter hyperintensities. *Stroke* **34**, 972–76.

Mehagnoul-Schipper, D. J., Colier, W. N., and Jansen, R. W. (2001). Reproducibility of orthostatic changes in cerebral oxygenation in healthy subjects aged 70 years and older. *Clin. Physiol.* **21**, 77–84.

Mejia, A. D., Julius, S., Jones, K. A., Schork, N. J., and Kneisley, J. (1990). The Tecumseh Blood Pressure Study. Normative data on blood pressure self-determination. *Archives of Internal Medicine* **150**, 1209–1213.

Meyer, J. S. and Shaw, T. G. (1984). Cerebral blood flow in ageing. In *Clinical Neurology of Ageing.* (Edited by Albert, M. L.) pp. 178–96. Oxford University Press, New York.

Mukai, S., Gagnon, M., Iloputaife, I., Hamner, J. W., Lipsitz, L. A. (2003). Effect of systolic blood pressure and carotid stiffness on baroreflex gain in elderly subjects. *J Gerontol.* **58A**(7), 626–30.

Ng, A. V., Callister, R., Johnson, D. G., and Seals, D. R. (1993). Age and gender influence muscle sympathetic nerve activity at rest in healthy humans. *Hypertension* **21**, 498–503.

Novak, V., Abduljalil, A. M., Kangarlu, A., *et al.* (2001a). Intracranial ossifications and micronagiopathy at 8 Tesla MRI. *Magnetic Resonance Imaging* **19**, 1133–37.

Novak, V., Freimer, M. L., Kissel, J. T., *et al.* (2001b). Autonomic impairment in painful neuropathy. *Neurology* In press.

Novak, V., Novak, P., de Champlain, J., Le Blanc, A. R., Martin, R., and Nadeau, R. (1993). Influence of respiration on heart rate and blood pressure fluctuations. *J Appl. Physiol.* **74**, 617–26.

Ooi, W. L., Barrett, S., Hossain, M., Kelley-Gagnon, M., and Lipsitz, L. (1997). Patterns of orthostatic blood pressure change and their clinical correlates in a frail, elderly population. *J Am. Med. Assoc.* **277**, 1299–1304.

Pagani, M., Lombardi, F., Guzzetti, S., *et al.* (1986). Power spectral analysis of heart rate and arterial pressure variabilities as a marker of sympatho-vagal interaction in man and conscious dog. *Circulation Research* **59**, 178–93.

Pan, H. Y. M., Hoffman, B. B., Pershe, R. A., and Blaschke, T. F. (1986). Decline in beta adrenergic receptor-mediated vascular relaxation with agen in men. *J Pharmacol. Exp. Ther.* **239**, 802–807.

Periquet, M. I., Novak, V., Collins, M. P., *et al.* (1999). Painful sensory neuropathy. Prospective evaluation using skin biopsy. *Neurology* **53**, 1641–47.

Phillips, P. A., Phil, D., Rolls, B. J., *et al.* (1984). Reduced thirst after water deprivation in healthy elderly men. *N Engl. J Med.* **311**, 753–59.

Prinz, P.N., Halter, J., Benedetti, C., and Raskind, M. (1979). Circadian variation of plasma catecholamines in young and old men: relation to rapid eye movement and slow wave sleep. *J Clin. Endocrin. Metab.* **49**, 300–304.

Resnick, N. (1995). Urinary incontinence. *Lancet* **346**, 94–99.

Richardson, D. (1989). Effects of age on cutaneous circulatory response to direct heat on the forearm. *J Gerontol.* **44**, M189–94.

Richardson, D., Tyra, J., and McCray, A. (1992). Attenuation of the cutaneous vasoconstrictor response to cold in elderly men. *J Gerontol.* **47**, M211–M214.

Rodeheffer, R. J., Gerstenblith, G., Becker, L. C., Fleg, J. L., Weisfeldt, M. L., and Lakatta, E. G. (1984). Exercise cardiac output is maintained with advancing age in healthy human subjects: cardiac dilation and increased stroke volume compensate for a diminished heart rate. *Circulation* **69**, 203–213.

Roob, G., Schmidt, R., Kappeller, P., Lechner, A., Hartung, H. P., and Fazekas, F. (1999). MRI evidence of past cerebral microbleeds in a healthy elderly population. *Neurology* **52**, 991–94.

Rutan, G. H., Hermanson, B., Bild, D. E., Kittner, S. J., LaBaw, F., and Tell, G. S. (1992). OH in older adults. The Cardiovascular Health Study. CHS Collaborative Research Group. *Hypertension* **19**, 508–519.

Ryan, S. M., Goldbeger, A. L., Pincus, S. M., Meitus, J., and Lipsitz, L. (1994). Gender- and age-related differences in heart rate dynamics: are women more complex than men? *J Am. Coll. Cardiol.* **24**, 1700–1707.

Ryan, S. M. and Lipsitz, L. (1995). Age-related changes in the autonomic nervous system. In *Disorders of the Autonomic Nervous System* (Edited by Robertson, D. and Biaggioni, I.) pp. 61–82. Hardwood Academic Publishers, Luxembourg.

Samdani, A. F., Dawson, T. M., and Dawson, V. L. (1997). Nitric oxide synthase in models of focal ischemia. *Stroke* **28**, 1283–8.

Scarpace, P. J., Shu, Y., and Tumer, N. (1994). Influence of exercise training on myocardial -adrenergic signal transduction: differential regulation with age . *J Appl. Physiol.* **77**, 737–41.

Schwartz, R. S., Jaeger, L. F., and Veith, R. C. (1990). The thermic effect of feeding in older men: the importance of the sympathetic nervous system. *Metabolism* **39**, 733–37.

Shenkin, H. A., Novak, P., Goluboff, B., Soffe, A. M., Bortin, L., Golde, D., and Batson, P. (1953). The effects of ageing, arteriosclerosis, and hypertension upon the cerebral circulation. *J. Clin. Invest.* **32**, 459–65.

Stratton, J. R., Cerqueira, M. D., Schwartz, R. S., Levy, W. C., Veith, R. C., Kahn, S. E., and Abrass, I. B. (1992). Differences in cardiovascular responses to isoproterenol in relation to age and exercise training in healthy men. *Circulation* **86**, 504–512.

Stratton, J. R., Levy, W. C., Cerqueira, M. D., Schwartz, R. S., and Abrass, I. B. (1994). Cardiovascular responses to exercise. Effects of ageing and exercise training in healthy men. *Circulation* **89**, 1648–55.

Taylor, N. A., Allsopp, N. K., and Parkes, D. G. (1995). Preferred room temperature of young vs aged males: the influence of thermal sensation, thermal comfort, and affect. *J Gerontol.* **50**, M216–22.

Veith, R. C., Featherstone, J. A., Linares, O. A., and Halter, J. B. (1986). Age differences in plasma norepinephrine kinetics in humans. *J Gerontol.* **41**, 319–24.

Vloet, L., Pel-Lillte, R., Jansen, P., and Jansen, R. W. (2005). High prevalence of postprandial and OH among geriatric patients admitted to Dutch hospitals. *J Gerontol.* **60A**, 1271–77.

Vogelaere, P. and Pereira, C. (2005). Thermoregulation and ageing. *Rev. Port. Cardiol.* 747–61.

Volpe, M., Laccarino, G., Vecchione, C., *et al.* (1996). Association and cosegregation of stroke with impaired endothelium-dependent vasorelaxation in stroke-prone, spontaneously hypertensive rats. *J. Clinical Investigations* **98**, 256–61.

Wahlund, L. O., Barkhof, F., Fazekas, F., *et al.* (2001). A new rating scale for age-related white matter changes applicable to MRI and CT. *Stroke* **32**, 1318–22.

Wollner, L., McCarthy, S. T., Soper, N. D. W., and Macy, D. J. (1979). Failure of cerebral autoregulation as a cause of brain dysfunction in the elderly. *Br. Med. J.* **1**, 1117–1118.

Wongsurawat, N., Davis, B. B., and Morley, J. E. (1990). Thermoregulatory failure in the elderly. *J Am. Geriatr. Soc.* **38**, 899–906.

Young, J. B., Rowe, J. W., Pallotta, J. A., Sparrow, D., and Landsberg, L. (1980). Enhanced plasma norepinephrine response to upright posture and oral glucose administration in elderly human subjects. *Metabolism* **29**, 532–39.

van Swieten, J. C., van den Hout, J. H., van Ketel, B. A., Hijdra, A., and van Gijn, J. (1991). Periventricular lesions in the white matter on magnetic resonance imageing in the elderly. A morphometric correlation with arteriolosclerosis and dilated perivascular spaces. *Brain* **114**, 761–74.

CHAPTER 71

Drugs, chemicals, and toxins that alter autonomic function

Anne L. Tonkin and Derek B. Frewin

Introduction

Many drugs, chemicals, and toxins are capable of interacting with the autonomic nervous system to alter autonomic function in humans (Fig. 71.1). While acute exposure may cause autonomic overactivity, the chronic effect of most such compounds is a reduction in autonomic activity. This chapter will focus primarily on drugs and other chemicals that reduce autonomic activity, either directly by inhibiting the activity of otherwise functional autonomic nerve fibres and/or receptors, or indirectly by causing an autonomic neuropathy. It will conclude with a brief discussion of compounds, including naturally occurring toxins and venoms, that cause an abnormal increase in autonomic activity.

Direct reduction of autonomic activity

Therapeutic drugs

Drugs whose pharmacodynamic effects depend on direct antagonism of autonomic neurotransmission are very widely used in clinical cardiovascular medicine. Examples include antagonists at alpha- or beta-adrenoceptors, centrally acting antihypertensive drugs, and ganglion blockers, all of which have been clinically important at various times, particularly in the management of hypertension. In general, their effects on autonomic function are well known and underpin their therapeutic efficacy. These drugs are described fully in pharmacological textbooks and will not be discussed in detail here.

It is also important to recognize those drugs that have antagonist activity within the autonomic nervous system in addition to their primary pharmacodynamic effect. These drugs often cause anticholinergic or alpha-antagonist adverse effects. Common examples are listed in Table 71.1.

In practice, the drugs that most commonly lead to clinical presentations suggesting autonomic dysfunction are those that have widespread use amongst the elderly. Both sympathetic and parasympathetic inhibition are generally more likely to cause clinically significant sequelae in the elderly than in younger individuals. Some important examples are discussed here.

Sympathetic inhibitors

The clinical effects of sympathetic inhibition depend upon the balance of inhibition of alpha- and beta-adrenoceptors produced by the particular drug. Drugs with alpha-antagonist properties (such as the phenothiazines and tricyclic antidepressants) commonly cause orthostatic hypotension, particularly when more than one of these drugs are used in combination in an elderly individual. A less common but very important complication of alpha-receptor antagonism is reversible urinary incontinence (Marshall and Beevers, 1996), caused by antagonism of sympathetic activity in the internal bladder sphincter. This is seen most commonly in elderly women and may have significant consequences, including institutionalization if the causative agent is not identified and removed.

An alpha-receptor blocking agent (tamsulosin) which has a high affinity for the alpha-1_A receptor sub-type (predominantly present in human prostatic tissue) is often used in the treatment of lower urinary tract symptoms in men with benign prostatic hyperplasia. This receptor type is also present in the iris, and intra-operative "Floppy Iris syndrome" has been observed during cataract surgery in patients treated with alpha-1 adrenoceptor antagonists, particularly tamsulosin (Cantrell et al. 2008). The resultant billowing of the iris and its prolapse towards the phaco-emulsification incisions can lead to significant complications. Ophthalmologists undertaking cataract surgery in patients taking alpha-receptor blockers should be prepared to modify their surgical technique to accommodate this possibility.

Beta-blocker drugs are well known to have negative inotropic effects, leading occasionally to significant exacerbations of cardiac failure. In addition, they have negative chronotropic effects, the latter being a particular risk when a beta-blocker is administered in conjunction with other drugs that slow atrioventricular nodal conduction, such as digoxin or verapamil. Such a combination may cause clinically significant atrioventricular conduction delay, even in individuals with normal baseline ECGs. Exacerbation of symptoms of obstructive airways disease is also well recognized as a complication of the use of beta-blockers in susceptible people.

Local administration of drugs with autonomic effects may also cause systemic symptoms. A well-recognized example of this phenomenon is the local instillation of timolol to the eye for the treatment of glaucoma, with subsequent exacerbation of bronchospasm or cardiac insufficiency due to its systemic beta-adrenoceptor antagonist effect. A recent report documents the occurrence of severe depression in a patient with a past history of depression who received ocular timolol for glaucoma (Schweitzer et al. 2008).

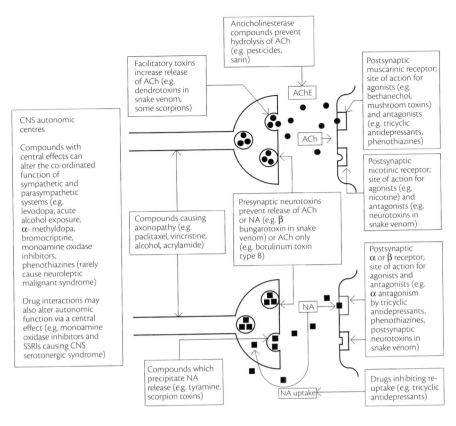

Fig. 71.1 Schematic representation of a cholinergic (upper) and noradrenergic (lower) autonomic synapse showing potential sites of action of drugs and toxins that influence autonomic function.

Treatment of the depression may be unsuccessful until the timolol is ceased.

Parasympathetic inhibitors

Parasympathetic inhibition, particularly peripheral muscarinic receptor antagonism, occurs during treatment with many therapeutic drug groups whose primary mechanism of action does not involve the parasympathetic system (Table 71.1). Class I antiarrhythmic agents such as quinidine and disopyramide have significant antimuscarinic effects in addition to their sodium channel blocking activity. Protriptyline and amitriptyline are the most potent muscarinic receptor antagonists amongst the tricyclic antidepressants, and should be considered as possible contributors to presentations such as urinary retention or constipation. An advantage of the newer, non-tricyclic antidepressant drugs, such as fluoxetine and venlafaxine, is that they do not have clinically important antagonistic effects at alpha- and muscarinic receptors.

Anticholinergic drugs are sometimes given specifically to produce muscarinic antagonism. Examples are the use of benztropine in the management of Parkinson's disease or the movement disorders associated with antipsychotic use, and the use of oxybutynin in the management of overactive bladder, which is more common in the elderly. In all of these cases the drug is administered systemically and can be expected to have widespread autonomic effects. These include blurred vision due to cycloplegia (which is more symptomatic in young people with preserved lens accommodation), dry mouth, severe constipation, and urinary retention, particularly in the elderly male with prostatic hypertrophy. At very high doses, gastric emptying and gastric secretion may also be inhibited, leading to epigastric discomfort. Cognitive dysfunction is also common in elderly patients receiving antimuscarinic drugs, particularly non-selective drugs which readily cross the blood-brain barrier, such as oxybutynin (Kay and Granville, 2005).

Drugs with anticholinergic activity should be avoided in patients with dementia as they have been implicated in cognitive deterioration and delirium in the elderly. There is also evidence that anticholinergic drugs can lead to significant impairment of verbal

Table 71.1 Drugs with autonomic antagonist effects unrelated to their main therapeutic use

Autonomic effect	Drug/drug group	Clinical manifestations
α-adrenoceptor antagonism	Phenothiazines	Orthostatic hypotension
	Tricyclic antidepressants	Nasal stuffiness
	Antihistamines	Urinary incontinence (especially in elderly women)
	Quinidine	
β-adrenoceptor antagonism	Sotalol	Bronchospasm
		Negative inotropic and chronotropic effects
Muscarinic receptor antagonism	Phenothiazines	Urinary obstruction (especially in elderly men)
	Tricyclic antidepressants	Dry mouth and eyes
	Antihistamines	Blurred vision (less troublesome in elderly)
	Quinidine, disopyramide	Sinus tachycardia
	Antispasmodics	Constipation
		Confusion, memory impairment, hallucinations

memory encoding in patients with schizophrenia (Brebion et al. 2004), and the use of anticholinergics as a routine prophylactic measure in schizophrenic patients receiving antipsychotic drugs is no longer recommended.

Centrally acting drugs

Many centrally acting drugs have autonomic effects, the pathogenesis of which remains poorly understood. Levodopa and dopamine D2 receptor agonists, such as bromocriptine and pergolide, have been suspected as primary causes of orthostatic hypotension, particularly in the early phase of therapy of Parkinson's disease. However, studies of Parkinsonian patients with and without orthostatic hypotension have not supported this view (Goldstein 2003) and it is now postulated that peripheral dopaminergic stimulation, together with augmentation of natriuresis and diuresis, results in orthostatic intolerance only in the presence of the abnormal baroreflex and sympathoneural pathophysiological processes that commonly occur in Parkinson's disease.

Other centrally acting drugs that reduce sympathetic activity include the centrally acting antihypertensive drugs such as alpha-methyldopa and clonidine, and the imidazoline receptor agonists, moxonidine and rilmenidine, all of which lower blood pressure by reducing tonic sympathetic outflow (recently reviewed by Sica, 2007). Rilmenidine lowers blood pressure, baseline sympathetic activity and peripheral resistance, but does not suppress reflex sympathetic responses to stimuli such as mental stress and head-up tilt (Esler et al. 2004). Postural hypotension, dry mouth, somnolence and constipation occur more frequently during treatment with alpha-methyldopa and clonidine than with the imidazoline agonists. Guanfacine is another centrally acting alpha2-adrenoreceptor agonist which was initially used as an antihypertensive but is now being used for the suppression of tics, the treatment of attention-deficit hyperactivity disorder, generalized anxiety disorder and post-traumatic stress disorder. A recent case report describes an overdose with this agent, which resulted in intial hypertension followed by delayed onset and persistent orthostatic hypotension (Minns et al. 2010).

Other drugs and toxins

A wide variety of non-therapeutic naturally occurring and synthetic compounds also interact with neurotransmission, thereby influencing autonomic function.

Nicotine

Nicotine has a variety of pharmacological actions in the central and peripheral nervous systems (Swan and Lessove-Schlaggar, 2007). It has recently been recognized that short-term administration enhances several cognitive functions, including attention and working memory. It may also have central neuroprotective effects, for example in Parkinson's disease. In the periphery, nicotine binds to nicotinic receptors in autonomic ganglia, as well as at neuromuscular junctions, and stimulates them. Acute autonomic effects include increased heart rate, blood pressure, and cutaneous vasoconstriction (Hanna 2006). Exposure to toxic doses (e.g. in tobacco workers or those exposed to nicotine-containing pesticides) can result in ganglionic paralysis with bradycardia, hypotension, coma, and eventual respiratory muscle paralysis. The role of nicotine itself, apart from the other components of tobacco, in the pathogenesis of the known toxic effects of long-term tobacco smoking remains unclear.

Long-acting anticholinesterase compounds

Compounds with anticholinesterase activity, such as organophosphorus esters and carbamate compounds, are commonly used in agriculture as insecticides. Acute ingestion by humans causes increased activity at autonomic ganglia and parasympathetic terminals (discussed later). In some circumstances, however, they may reduce autonomic function. Observations on workers involved in handling similar compounds during the Second World War have indicated that autonomic dysfunction may persist for years after acute exposure. Long-term chronic exposure to organophosphorus ester insecticides may also produce persistent autonomic dysfunction, although the literature in this area is controversial. The evidence in favour of this proposal has been summarized by Jamal et al. (2002). Organophosphorus compounds bind to acetylcholinesterase for a much longer period than the more recently developed carbamate compounds, and there is little evidence of prolonged toxicity with the latter group.

Herbal remedies

Many freely available proprietary herbal remedies contain alkaloids such as atropine and scopolamine and there have been case reports of anticholinergic poisoning resulting in confusion, dry mouth, tachycardia, and dilated pupils (Chan et al. 1994).

Illicit drugs

The first report of amphetamine-induced suppression of vasomotor outflow was published in 1996 (Smit et al. 1996), although this phenomenon has been observed previously in animal models. The clinical presentation occurred 10 hours after ingestion, and included pronounced drowsiness and severe orthostatic hypotension which was due, on formal baroreflex function testing, to suppression of vasomotor outflow with preservation of normal vagal function. Spontaneous recovery occurred over 3 days. This is a potential differential diagnosis in cases of acute autonomic neuropathy.

Contamination of illicit drugs may also lead to acute autonomic dysfunction. During the period 1996–97 a number of cases of acute anticholinergic poisoning were reported in individuals who had self-administered material sold as street 'heroin', but which had been mixed with scopolamine. The clinical picture of hallucinations, tachycardia, pupillary dilatation, dry skin and mucous membranes, and urinary retention responds rapidly to treatment with the anticholinesterase compound, physostigmine.

Snake venoms

Much progress has been made over recent years in understanding the molecular structure and mechanisms of toxicity of snake venoms (reviewed by Koh et al. 2006 and Kang et al. 2011). Apart from the therapeutic implications of these investigations, neurotoxins derived from snake venoms are becoming scientifically important as laboratory probes for the study of neural mechanisms. There is great variability in the neurotoxic components of venoms from various species of snake, but some generalizations can be made. Postsynaptic neurotoxins (also called α-neurotoxins) have an action similar to curare in that they bind with high specificity to the nicotinic acetylcholine receptor on the postsynaptic membrane of the neuromuscular junction, causing flaccid paralysis and respiratory arrest. Nicotinic receptors in autonomic ganglia are less affected by α-neurotoxins, but are blocked by other neurotoxins, such as κ-bungarotoxin and κ-flavitoxin, both of which produce complete and long-lasting autonomic ganglion blockade at low doses. Other snake venom toxins are known to bind selectively to subtypes of muscarinic receptors, and have been used as pharmacological tools for investigating the functional role of these receptors, and may prove to have therapeutic efficacy in diseases such as Alzheimer's disease and Parkinson's disease.

The β-neurotoxins, including β-bungarotoxin and crotoxin, act on presynaptic neurones to inhibit the release of acetylcholine and thus cause paralysis. Crotoxin is currently in clinical trials as an anti-cancer agent.

Reduction of autonomic activity due to autonomic neuropathy

Drug- or toxin-induced autonomic neuropathy is an important differential diagnosis in the assessment of patients with evidence of subacute or chronic autonomic dysfunction. It is important to note that many neurotoxic compounds have selective effects on particular components of the nervous system, and not all compounds that cause peripheral neuropathy affect the autonomic system. An example is arsenic, which causes a primarily sensory neuropathy but has not been reported to cause autonomic dysfunction. Other examples include lead neurotoxicity, which commonly causes motor neuropathy and central nervous system effects (encephalopathy, behavioural changes) with little, if any, effect on autonomic function.

In specific clinical situations, damage to the autonomic nervous system can be induced for therapeutic purposes by introduction of neurolytic agents into specific regions. Agents such as phenol are used for this purpose, and the resulting autonomic dysfunction includes the intended effect (e.g. in sympathectomy for peripheral vascular disease or hyperhidrosis) in addition to any unintended sequelae. More commonly, autonomic neuropathy is an unintended complication of exposure to drugs or chemicals in a therapeutic or occupational context.

Therapeutic drugs

Cytotoxic agents used in cancer chemotherapy

The vinca alkaloids, vincristine and vinblastine, are commonly used in the chemotherapy of haematological malignancies such as lymphomas and leukaemias. Vincristine, and to a lesser extent, vinblastine, can cause a dose-dependent peripheral sensory neuropathy due to axonal degeneration. Both drugs bind to the protein tubulin, preventing its polymerization into microtubules that form the spindle apparatus essential for mitosis in both normal and malignant cells. In neurones, these microtubules appear to be involved in the rapid transport of essential proteins from the cell body to the axon, and interruption of the transport process results in axonal degeneration. In this form of neuropathy, longer fibres are more susceptible to damage, thus explaining the distal distribution of sensory loss and the particular susceptibility of the vagus nerve to damage.

This neurotoxic effect extends to autonomic neuropathy, and there have been many case reports of orthostatic hypotension, constipation, paralytic ileus, and urinary retention following treatment with vinca alkaloids, suggesting both sympathetic and parasympathetic involvement. Studies using formal tests of autonomic function have had varying results. Some studies have indicated that

vincristine therapy is associated with abnormalities of both sympathetic and parasympathetic efferent activity (Hirvonen et al. 1989). In contrast, a prospective study of 10 patients receiving a mean cumulative dose of 15.2 mg of vincristine, which caused peripheral sensorimotor neuropathy in all of them, showed no effect on Valsalva ratio, heart rate variability with deep breathing, or systolic blood pressure response to head-up tilt (Lahtinen et al. 1989). A long-term follow-up study in young patients treated for sarcoma has indicated that vinca alkaloids are not associated with persistent autonomic abnormalities at 8 months of follow-up (Earl et al. 1998). The clinical significance of vinca alkaloid-induced autonomic neuropathy remains controversial, and the cause of the apparently autonomic symptoms described in the case reports remains in some doubt.

Doxorubicin may rarely have toxic effects on peripheral neurones, particularly those in the dorsal root ganglia and autonomic ganglia. The toxicity takes the form of a neuronopathy and results in degeneration of the entire neurone, including its axonal processes.

Although cisplatin frequently causes a predominantly sensory peripheral neuropathy, it also appears to affect the autonomic nervous system although only relatively rarely. A prospective clinical study assessed 28 patients receiving cisplatin, vinblastine, and bleomycin and showed that two of them had abnormal heart rate responses to both the Valsalva manoeuvre and deep breathing, indicating parasympathetic dysfunction (Hansen 1990). Whether or not these patients, most of whom also had peripheral sensory neuropathy, were affected by cisplatin, vinblastine, or the combination of the two could not be determined. The follow-up study by Earl et al. (1998) in young patients treated for sarcoma indicated that cisplatin was the only drug that was common to the small proportion of patients who had persistent mild autonomic dysfunction at 8 months after combination chemotherapy.

Paclitaxel, a chemotherapeutic agent with activity against breast and ovarian cancer, causes a peripheral sensory neuropathy, probably by preventing the normal dissociation of axonal microtubles. This action interferes with fast axonal transport, which appears to require repeated association and dissociation of microtubules. Paclitaxel has also been reported to cause acute severe orthostatic hypotension (Jerian et al. 1993) associated with abnormalities in heart rate response to the Valsalva and deep breathing manoeuvres (parasympathetic dysfunction) and a loss of the normal pressor response to isometric hand grip (sympathetic dysfunction). However, detailed measurement of cardiovascular autonomic reflex responses before and after paclitaxel-based chemotherapy in 18 women with breast or ovarian cancer showed a decrease in diastolic blood pressure variability, but no detectable differences in responses to deep breathing, Valsalva manoeuvre or orthostasis (Eckholm et al. 1997). It seems likely that there is considerable inter-individual variability in susceptibility to taxane-induced autonomic dysfunction. When it does occur, paralytic ileus and orthostatic hypotension appear to be the most common manifestations, and patients with diabetes mellitus may be more susceptible to this complication.

Other therapeutic drugs

Perhexiline, used as a last-line agent in the management of refractory angina, is known to cause a peripheral sensorimotor neuropathy. In a few of these cases the neurotoxicity extends to the autonomic nervous system, causing postural hypotension and abnormal heart rate control.

Chronic treatment of cardiac arrhythmias with amiodarone causes peripheral neuropathy (predominantly sensory) in a small proportion of patients. In some of these there may also be autonomic dysfunction, manifested as orthostatic hypotension, although the evidence for this to date is not definitive.

Pentamidine, used in the management of *Pneumocystis carinii* pneumonia secondary to AIDS, has been associated with acute autonomic insufficiency manifested as severe orthostatic hypotension with a fixed heart rate, and complete loss of heart rate responsiveness to deep breathing and the Valsalva manoeuvre (Siddiqui and Ford 1995).

Occupational exposure

Organic solvents

Neuropsychiatric disorders associated with exposure to organic solvents have been reported frequently, although there are relatively few reports of objective autonomic dysfunction in this group of patients. Long-term exposure to low levels of carbon disulphide, for example in the viscose/rayon industry, may cause autonomic effects. Average cumulative exposure of 213 p.p.m.-years over 20 years resulted in parasympathetic dysfunction on formal testing (Ruijten et al. 1993), although the effects were very small and not associated with any clinical sequelae. Styrene monomer, an aromatic solvent used in the manufacture of polystyrene, resins, rubber, plastic, and fibreglass products, is known to cause acute neurotoxic effects following high-intensity exposure. The effect, if any, of low-level exposure is unclear.

Parasympathetic function (measured as changes in heart rate variability and heart rate responses to deep breathing and the Valsalva manoeuvre) appears to be disturbed in some workers exposed to a variety of other organic solvents, including hydrocarbons, alcohols, ketones, esters, and ethers, but the clinical sequelae are uncertain (Matikainen and Juntunen 1985). Few recent data are available.

Acrylamide

Acrylamide, which is widely used in paper manufacture, water treatment, building construction, and laboratory research, is known to cause a distal symmetrical axonopathy which affects somatic and autonomic nerves. The underlying mechanism of toxicity may be interference with fast axonal transport. As is the case for other causes of axonal degeneration (including alcohol and other toxins), longer fibres are most susceptible to damage. In the autonomic nervous system the vagus nerve is the initial site of dysfunction, so that heart rate control and gastrointestinal function are impaired before blood pressure regulation becomes involved. Autonomic disturbances are uncommon in humans but have been studied extensively in experimental animals, in which damage to sympathetic vasomotor nerves as well as parasympathetic fibres has been demonstrated, both neuro-physiologically and histologically.

Heavy metals

Chronic exposure to lead is known to cause a peripheral neuropathy with axonal degeneration, particularly affecting motor fibres. Whether or not the autonomic nervous system is also involved is controversial. Workers with mixed exposure to lead, zinc, and copper have been studied using heart rate variability techniques (Murata and Araki 1991) and were found to have reduced median nerve conduction velocities in addition to reduced RR variability, particularly in relation to respiratory variation (mediated by the vagus nerve). Lead exposure more commonly causes a predominantly motor peripheral neuropathy.

Pesticides

Most insecticides in common use in agricultural, industrial, or domestic settings are neurotoxic to the target organisms. In general they are not species-selective, and can also affect mammalian nervous systems, the outcome depending on the level of exposure in relation to body size. Organochlorine insecticides (such as DDT) affect sensory and motor nerves with few, if any, autonomic effects after acute or chronic exposure.

Organophosphorus compounds (discussed earlier in relation to their acute anticholinesterase activity) may also cause various subacute or chronic neuropathies. These have been reported following a single high-intensity exposure, as in the case of the use of organophosphorus-based chemical weapons in warfare, or during chronic exposure, for example in manufacturing processes.

Much interest in recent years has centred around the possible contribution of organophosphorus compounds, including sarin gas, to the peripheral neuropathies that have been demonstrated in veterans of the Persian Gulf war. Sarin is a highly toxic cholinesterase inhibiting organophosphorus compound originally developed during the Second World War and more recently used in the Gulf War and in terrorist attacks in Japan. A factor analysis of symptoms reported by veterans with Gulf War syndrome found that many common symptoms had autonomic features (Haley et al. 1997), and a subsequent study examining cardiovascular autonomic regulation has found a loss of the normal parasympathetically-mediated nocturnal reduction in heart rate in ill veterans compared with controls (Haley et al. 2004), suggesting that subtle autonomic (particularly parasympathetic) dysfunction may contribute to this condition. The cause of this remains unknown.

Polycyclic Aromatic Hydrocarbons

Benzo(a)pyrene (B(a)P) is an industrial and environmental pollutant which belongs to this class of chemicals. Industries emitting this agent include the production of coke, asphalt and tar, as well as aluminium electrolysis, with occupational exposure occurring mainly through inhalation of particulates in the ambient air of the operation areas. Zhang et al. (2008) have observed that B(a)P affects the autonomic function of coke oven workers by 'downregulating' the activity of the parasympathetic nervous system.

Other forms of exposure

Alcohol

Alcohol ingestion has both acute and chronic effects on autonomic function in humans. Acute exposure of healthy volunteers to alcohol reduces parasympathetic modulation of heart rate, measured by power spectral parameters of heart rate variability (Murata et al. 1994). The mechanism of this effect is uncertain, but may involve alterations in central cardiovascular control centres rather than a direct effect on vagal function.

Chronic alcohol abuse causes an axonal neuropathy, affecting both somatic (sensory and motor) and autonomic, predominantly vagal, function. Approximately 25 per cent of chronic alcohol abusers have detectable abnormalities in the parasympathetic control of heart rate (Monforte et al. 1995), while sympathetic function may become affected at a later stage, resulting in orthostatic hypotension and anhidrosis. Sympathetically-mediated blood pressure responses to pressor stimuli, including the cold pressor test and sustained isometric exercise, as well as phase IV of the Valsalva manoeuvre, are reduced in alcoholics compared with age-matched controls (Chida et al. 1994). Both somatic and autonomic nerve damage appear to be correlated to total lifetime ethanol intake (Monforte et al. 1995), and in some cases abstinence may result in an improvement over months to years. Long-term follow-up of chronic alcohol abusers suggests that the presence of autonomic abnormalities on clinical testing is associated with an increased mortality.

Botulinum toxin

Although rare, poisoning with botulinum toxin (type B) is an important differential diagnosis for the presentation of acute autonomic neuropathy, particularly when there is predominant parasympathetic dysfunction. The toxin acts on cholinergic synapses to prevent the calcium-mediated release of acetylcholine from the presynaptic terminal. Its effects are seen primarily at neuromuscular junctions and at autonomic ganglia where the effect is to block autonomic transmission acutely. There have been reports of dysautonomia, particularly involving cholinergic pathways, occurring in the absence of the typical motor abnormalities (Freeman, 2007).

Stimulation of excess autonomic activity

Excessive autonomic activity is frequently seen in individuals with denervation hypersensitivity (e.g. due to pre-existing autonomic neuropathy) during treatment with autonomic agonists. Examples include the use of sympathetic alpha-adrenoceptor agonists in orthostatic hypotension, and the parasympathomimetic agent, bethanechol, in the management of bladder atony. The effects are predictable from the pharmacological action of the agonist. In other situations, a toxic compound may cause abnormally increased autonomic activity in an individual with previously normal autonomic function.

Acute parasympathetic overactivity occurs following anticholinesterase poisoning with agricultural chemicals such as organophosphorous compounds, which inhibit acetylcholinesterase. The inhibition results in the typical picture of increased secretions, bronchoconstriction, miosis, abdominal cramps, and bradycardia (all related to muscarinic receptor stimulation) and hypertension, muscle fasciculations, tremor and eventual muscle paralysis (due to nicotinic receptor stimulation at autonomic ganglia and at neuromuscular junctions).

Therapeutic drugs

Sympathetic stimulation

Hyperactivity of the sympathetic division of the autonomic nervous system is seen occasionally as a consequence of exposure to psychoactive drugs, both therapeutic and illicit. Neuroleptic malignant syndrome is a syndrome thought to be mediated by changes in central dopaminergic transmission causing increased sympathetic outflow manifested as hyperthermia, muscle rigidity, and unstable blood pressure and heart rate. It occurs in fewer than

1 per cent of patients receiving antipsychotic drugs, but can be fatal if untreated. A similar clinical picture, with occasional fatalities, occurs in some individuals who ingest the so-called 'designer drug' Ecstasy (3,4-methylenedioxymethamphetamine [MDMA]) and other amphetamine derivatives.

An interaction between antidepressant drugs, which inhibit noradrenaline and/or serotonin reuptake from the synapse, and tyramine, which releases catecholamines from storage vesicles, can result in a marked increase in neurotransmitter concentrations within sympathetic synapses. Clinically there is marked sympathetic hyperactivity with sweating, tachycardia, and severe hypertension, which may lead to intracranial haemorrhage. A similar picture can be seen following the use of the combination of a monoamine oxidase inhibitor and a serotonin uptake inhibitor (such as fluoxetine). Known as the 'CNS serotonergic syndrome', it comprises general CNS overactivity, muscle spasms, hyperthermia, and autonomic instability, resulting in hyper- or hypotension, tachycardia, and profuse sweating. Fatalities have been reported (Flanagan, 2008). The mechanism is believed to be an increase in serotonergic activity, particularly involving 5-HT1A receptors in the brainstem and spinal cord.

The neurolept anaesthetic/analgesic agent, ketamine, has an interesting combination of stimulatory and inhibitory cardiovascular and respiratory effects. In isolated organ experiments, in the absence of an intact autonomic nervous system, it has a direct negative inotropic effect on the myocardium. However, in the intact animal or human, this is counterbalanced by a central stimulatory effect, probably mediated by increased sympathetic outflow, which results in an elevation in blood pressure, heart rate and cardiac output, and bronchodilatation.

Parasympathetic stimulation

A case has been described in which significant cholinergic toxicity was induced by the use of bethanechol in a patient with diabetic autonomic neuropathy. The patient suffered shivering, salivation, dyspnoea, profuse sweating and pinpoint pupils, requiring treatment with atropine (Caraco et al. 1990). Denervation hypersensitivity was presumed to be the underlying mechanism for the exaggerated response to usual therapeutic doses.

The short-acting cholinesterase inhibitors (donepezil, galantamine and rivastigmine) are being increasingly used in the treatment of Alzheimer's disease to increase cholinergic transmission in the cortex and improve cognitive function. These agents do not alter the pathology of Alzheimer's disease but at best delay progression and improve symptoms according to subjective measurements and cognitive assessment tools. Gastrointestinal side effects such as diarrhoea are common at the onset of treatment and following escalation of the dose. Other peripheral effects of the increased cholinergic activity include nausea and vomiting, which are common in patients receiving anticholinesterase treatment (Cummings, 2003).

Other substances

Sympathetic stimulation

Some venomous creatures, including snakes and scorpions, cause prominent sympathetic hyperactivity, resulting in the potentially fatal clinical syndrome sometimes known as 'autonomic storm'. In the case of stings from some scorpion species which are common in India and the Middle East, the major problem is uncontrolled catecholamine release from sympathetic nerve endings and the adrenals, with acute hypertension and hypertensive encephalopathy, best treated with prazosin. In many instances the precise mechanism of action remains unknown. Some snake and scorpion venoms are known to contain dendrotoxin, which can augment sympathetic activity by stimulating catecholamine release from nerve endings, while others have direct effects on alpha-adrenoceptors (Gwee et al. 2002).

Parasympathetic stimulation

Muscarinic stimulatory effects are seen after poisoning with wild mushroom species that contain neurotoxins with muscarinic agonist activity. The effects occur rapidly and, predictably, include lacrimation, salivation, nausea, vomiting, abdominal pain, bronchospasm, headache, miosis, blurred vision, bradycardia, and hypotension. Some herbal remedies contain alkaloids that have cholinomimetic activity and can lead to papillary constriction, vomiting, diarrhoea, salivation, sweating, lacrimation, rhinorhoea, bradycardia and hypotension.

Less common causes of this constellation of features include acute exposure to sarin gas, for example in terrorist attacks. Long-term follow-up of the survivors exposed to high levels of sarin in Japan in the mid-1990s has shown that none had detectable anticholinesterase effect at three weeks after the incident, although psychological recovery was much slower (Yamagisawa et al. 2006). Snake venom toxins known as fasciculins also have anticholinesterase activity, both at neuromuscular junctions, where they produce a prolonged muscular contraction, and at autonomic ganglia, where they increase autonomic transmission. These toxins have a synergistic effect with dendrotoxins, also found in some snake venoms, which act presynaptically to increase the release of acetylcholine (Koh et al. 2006). Some scorpion toxins have a similar effect, probably by binding to neuronal voltage-sensitive sodium channels and increasing the spontaneous release of acetylcholine, while also blocking potassium channels and thus prolonging action potentials. In addition there are some that have been shown to have direct agonist actions on post-synaptic muscarinic receptors (Gwee et al. 2002). Such venoms continue to be explored as possible sources of pharmacologically active agents interacting with the autonomic nervous system.

Conclusion

While the mechanisms of action of drugs which interact reversibly with autonomic nerve fibres or receptors as part of their pharmacodynamic activity are well known, much remains to be established about the effect of drugs and other compounds causing autonomic neuropathy. Drugs, chemicals, and toxins should always be considered as a possible cause of autonomic neuropathy in patients presenting with the clinical manifestations of either sympathetic or parasympathetic dysfunction, or both.

References

Brebion, G., Bressan, R. A., Amador, X., Malaspina, D., and Gorman, J. M. (2004). Medications and verbal memory impairment in schizophrenia: the role of anticholinergic drugs. *Psychol. Med.* **34**, 369–74.

Cantrell, M. A., Bream-Rouwenhorst, H. R., Steffensmeier, A. Hemerson, P., Rogers, M. and Stamper, B. (2008). Intraoperative floppy iris syndrome associated with alpha1-adrenergic receptor antagonists. *Ann. Pharmacother.* **42**, 558–63.

Caraco, Y., Arnon, R., and Raz, I. (1990). Bethanecol-induced cholinergic toxicity in diabetic neuropathy. *Ann. Pharmacother.* **24**, 327.

Chan, J. C. N., Chan, T. Y. K., Chan, K. L., Leung, N. W., Tomlinson, B., and Critchley, J. A. (1994). Anticholinergic poisoning from Chinese herbal medicines. *Aust. N. Z. J. Med.* **24**, 317–18.

Chida, K., Tkasu, T., Mori, N., Tokujnaga, K., Komatsu, K., and Kawamura, H. (1994). Sympathetic dysfunction mediating cardiovascular regulation in alcoholic neuropathy. *Funct. Neurol.* **9**, 65–73.

Cummings, J. L. (2003). Use of cholinesterase inhibitors in clinical practice; evidence-based recommendations. *Am. J. Geriatr. Psychiatry* **11**, 131–145.

Earl, H. M., Connolly, S., Latoufis, C., Eagle, K., Ash, C. M., Fowler, C., and Souhami, R. L. (1998) Long-term neurotoxicity of chemotherapy in adolescents and young adults treated for bone and soft tissue sarcomas. *Sarcoma* **2**, 97–105.

Eckholm, E., Rantanen, V., Antila, K., and Salminen, E. (1997). Paclitaxel changes sympathetic control of blood pressure. *Eur. J. Cancer* **33**, 1419–24.

Esler, M., Lux, A., Jennings, G., Hastings, J., Socratous F., and Lambert, G. (2004) Rilmenidine sympatholytic activity preserves mental stress, orthostatic sympathetic responses and adrenaline secretion. *J. Hypertens.* **22**, 1529–34.

Flanagan, R. J. (2008). Fatal toxicity of drugs used in psychiatry. *Hum. Pscychopharmacol.* **23**, 43–51.

Freeman, R. (2007). Autonomic peripheral neuropathy. *Neurol. Clin.* **25**, 277–301.

Goldstein, D. S. (2003). Dysautonomia in Parkinson's disease: neurocardiological abnormalities. *Lancet Neurol*, 669–76.

Gwee M. C. E., Nirthanan, S., Khoo, H-E., Gopalahrihnakone P., Kini R. M., and Cheah, L-S. (2002). Autonomic effects of some scorpion venoms and toxins. *Clin Exp. Pharmacol. Physiol.* **29**, 795–801.

Haley, R. W., Kurt, T. M, and Hom, J. (1997). Is there a Gulf War syndrome? Searching for syndromes by factor analysis of symptoms. *JAMA* **277**, 215–22.

Haley, R. W., Vongpatanasin, W., Wolfe, G.I., *et al.* (2004). Blunted circadian variation in autonomic regulation of sinus node function in veterans with Gulf War syndrome. *Am. J. Med.* **117**, 469–78.

Hanna, S. T. (2006). Nicotine effect on cardiovascular system and ion channels. *J. Cardiovasc. Pharmacol.* **47**, 348–58.

Hansen, S. W. (1990). Autonomic neuropathy after treatment with cisplatin, vinblastine, and bleomycin for germ cell cancer. *BMJ.* **300**, 511–12.

Hirvonen, H. E., Salmi, T. T., Heinonen, E., Antila, K. J., and Välimäki, I. A. (1989). Vincristine treatment of acute lymphoblastic leukaemia induces transient autonomic cardioneuropathy. *Cancer* **64**, 801–5.

Jamal, G. A., Hansen, S., and Julu, P. O. O. (2002). Low level exposures to organophosphorus esters may cause neurotoxicity. *Toxicol.* **181–182**, 23–33.

Jerian, S. M., Sarosy, G. A., Link, C. J., Fingert, H. J., Reed, E., and Dohn, E. C. (1993). Incapacitating autonomic neuropathy precipitated by taxol. *Gynecol. Oncol.* **51**, 277–80.

Kang, T. S., Georgieva, D., Genov, N., *et al.* (2011). Enzymatic toxins from snake venom: structural characterization and mechanism of catalysis. *FEBS Journal* **278**, 4544–76.

Kay, G. G. and Granville, L. J. (2005). Antimuscarinic agents: implications and concerns in the management of overactive bladder in the elderly. *Clin. Ther.* **27**, 127–38.

Koh, D. C. I., Armugam, A., and Jeyaseelan, K. (2006). Snake venom components and their applications in biomedicine. *Cell. Mol. Life Sci.* **63**, 3030–41.

Lahtinen, R., Koponen, A., Mustonen, J., *et al.* (1989). Discordance in the development of peripheral and autonomic neuropathy during vincristine therapy. *Eur. J. Haematol.* **43**, 357–8.

Marshall, H. J. and Beevers, D. G. (1996) -adrenoceptor blocking drugs and female urinary incontinence: prevalence and reversibility. *Br. J. Clin. Pharmacol.* **42**, 507–9.

Minns, A. B., Clark, R. F, and Schneir, A. (2010). Guanfacine overdose resulting in initial hypertension and subsequent delayed, persistent orthostatic hypotension. *Clin. Toxicol.* **48**, 146–8.

Matikainen, E., and Juntunen, J. (1985). Autonomic nervous system dysfunction in workers exposed to organic solvents. *J. Neurol. Neurosurg. Psychiat.* **48**, 1021–4.

Monforte, R., Estruch, R., Valls-Sole, J., Nicolas, J., Villalta, J., and Urbano-Marquez, A. (1995). Autonomic and peripheral neuropathies in patients with chronic alcoholism. A dose-related toxic effect of alcohol. *Arch. Neurol.* **52**, 45–51.

Murata, K. and Araki, S. (1991). Autonomic nervous system dysfunction in workers exposed to lead, zinc, and copper in relation to peripheral nerve conduction: a study of R–R interval variability. *Am. J. Ind. Med.* **20**, 663–71.

Murata, K., Araki, S., Yokoyama, K., and Ono, Y. (1994). Autonomic neurotoxicity of alcohol assessed by heart rate variability. *J. Autonom. Nerv. Syst.* **48**, 105–11.

Ruijten, M. W. M. M, Salle, H. J. A., and Verberk M. M. (1993). Verification of effects on the nervous system of low level occupational exposure to CS$_2$. *Br. J. Ind. Med.* **50**, 301–7.

Schweitzer, I., Maguire, K., and Ng, C. H. (2008) A case of melancholic depression induced by β-blocker antiglaucoma agents. *Med J. Aust.* **189**, 406–7.

Sica, D. A. (2007). Centrally acting antihypertensive agents: an update. *J. Clin. Hypertens. (Greenwich)* **9**, 399–405.

Siddiqui, M. A. and Ford, P. A. (1995). Acute severe autonomic insufficiency during pentamidine therapy. *Southern Med. J.* **88**, 1087–8.

Smit, A. A. J., Wieling, W., Voogel, A. J., Koster, R. W., and van Zwieten, P. A. (1996). Orthostatic hypotension due to suppression of vasomotor outflow after amphetamine intoxication. *Mayo Clin. Proc.* **71**, 1067–70.

Swan, G. E. and Lessove-Schlaggar, C. N. (2007) The effects of tobacco smoke and nicotine on cognition and the brain. *Neuropsychol. Rev.* **17**, 259–273.

Yamagisawa, N., Morita, H., and Nakajima, T. (2006). Sarin experiences in Japan: acute toxicity and long-term effects. *J. Neurolog. Sci.* **249**, 76–85.

Zhang, H. M., Nie, J. S., Wang, F., et al. (2008). Effects of benzo(a)pyrene on autonomic nervous system of coke oven workers. *J. Occup. Health.* **50**, 308–16.

CHAPTER 72

Surgery and the autonomic nervous system

Omer Aziz, Marios Nicolaou and Ara W. Darzi

Introduction

By the late 18th century, the anatomy of the sympathetic nervous system had been described (Royle 1999), yet despite this its role as part of a wider 'autonomic' nervous system was not clearly understood. In 1852 autonomic physiology and function began to be appreciated, with Claude Bernard noting that cervical sympathetic denervation resulted in an increased skin temperature of the ipsilateral side of the head (Hashmonai and Kopelman 2003). Around the same time, Brown–Séquard reported that stimulation of sympathetic nerves resulted in vasoconstriction. The leap from delineation of anatomy and physiology to performing targeted sympathetic surgery was first taken by Alexander in 1889 to treat epilepsy, and led others to perform sympathetic surgery for a variety of indications ranging from exophthalmic goitre and idiocy, to glaucoma, all of which are now obsolete. In addition to this, before arterial surgery and angiography were possible, sympathectomy was the only surgical treatment option for peripheral vascular disease and angina pectoris (Jonnesco 1920). This latter indication has now started to re-emerge for the treatment of refractory, endstage, cardiovascular disease.

Surgery for hyperhidrosis was first described in 1920 by Kotzareff, who performed open removal of the upper sympathetic chain via a dorsal paravertebral incision under local anaesthetic in a woman with severe unilateral facial hyperhidrosis (Kotzareff 1920). The procedure was a success and the patient was satisfied despite suffering from Horner's syndrome. Since that original report multiple open surgical approaches have been developed including the anterior supraclavicular (Keaveny et al. 1977), posterior paravertebral (Golueke et al. 1988), posterior midline (Cloward 1969), anterior thoracic (Palumbo 1988), axillary thoracic (Atkins 1954), and the axillary extrathoracic with first rib resection (Campbell et al. 1982). The initial limitation of these procedures was that although symptomatic relief from hyperhidrosis was good, most of the open techniques were associated with a significant morbidity and therefore were abandoned. Thoracoscopic sympathectomy as first described by Hughes in 1942, has revolutionized targeted sympathetic surgery for hyperhidrosis, greatly reducing the morbidity associated with the open procedure (Doolabh et al. 2004). The first large series reporting the use of this procedure for the treatment of palmar hyperhidrosis was published by Kux in 1978, and since then technological advances in video optics and specialized instrumentation have meant that the sympathetic trunk can now be easily identified through the parietal pleura thoracoscopically and surgical division of the trunk can be performed safely.

Historically subtotal gastrectomy was considered optimal for the elective management of duodenal and gastric ulcers until Dragstedt's description of vagotomy (interrupting vagal innervation and its impact on ulcer healing and recurrence (Dragstedt and Lulu 1974). During the past 20 years, however, medical therapy of peptic ulcer disease has dramatically improved, and the recognition of *Helicobacter pylori* together with results of its effective eradication have meant that vagotomy (both truncal and highly selective) for peptic ulcer disease is rarely performed, and is now of only historical interest.

Despite this long and diverse history, there are now a few areas where surgery on the autonomic system is commonly indicated, namely hyperhidrosis, facial blushing, and chronic regional pain syndrome. For other conditions such as angina pectoris, cardiac arrhythmias, peripheral vascular disease, and Raynaud's syndrome, surgery for autonomic denervation is being used more and more frequently, particularly in the case of chronic refractory disease. Finally the use of agents such as botulinum toxin A, as later described in this text, has meant that targeted sympathetic inactivation therapy can be delivered without the need for invasive surgery. This chapter aims to outline the conditions for which autonomic surgery is currently indicated, highlighting the benefits, risks, and prognostic outcomes from these techniques.

Hyperhidrosis

Definition

'Primary hyperhidrosis' is a chronic idiopathic disorder characterized by excessive sweating that is bilateral and relatively symmetric in its distribution (Chapter 32). Commonly affected areas include the axillae, palms, soles or craniofacial region (Naumann et al. 2003). This should be differentiated from 'physiological hyperhidrosis', which is a normal thermoregulatory response to exertion, hot climates or spicy food (gustatory sweating). 'Secondary hyperhidrosis' is generalized excessive sweating caused by an underlying pathological process, as outlined in Table 72.1. It is important to

Table 72.1 Causes of secondary hyperhidrosis

Aetiology	Clinical condition causing hyperhidrosis
Endocrine	Hyperthyroidism, diabetes mellitus, hyperpituitarism, gout, menopause, acromegaly
Neoplasia	Hodgkin's disease, carcinoid tumour, phaeochromocytoma
Infection	Chronic and acute infection
Neurological	Riley–Day syndrome, irritative hypothalamic lesions, syringomyelia
Pharmacotherapy	Antidepressants: tricyclics, selective serotonin reuptake inhibitors, reboxetine, venlafaxine
	Anti-hypertensives: telmisartan, enalapril, nifedipine
	Analgesics: morphine, nefopam
	Other: pilocarpine, levodopa, ciprofloxacin, anti-retrovirals
Other	Shock, syncope, anxiety, pain, alcohol ingestion, drug withdrawal, pachydermoperiostosis

identify and exclude such pathology prior to offering treatment for primary hyperhidrosis (Chapter 32).

Relevant pathophysiology

Eccrine sweat glands found in high concentrations in the palms, soles, and axillae, are skin appendages embryonically derived from surface epithelium. The secretory portion, located deep within the dermis, consists of a single layer of simple cuboidal or columnar cells arranged in a coil surrounded by myoepithelial cells. Perspiration occurs when these cells contract following cholinergic stimulation by sympathetic nerves. In primary hyperhidrosis the sweat glands are morphologically normal but their neurological stimulation is exaggerated (Lowe et al. 2004).

Clinical presentation

A recent survey in the USA estimates that hyperhidrosis affects up to 2.8% of the population, with an average age of onset at 25 years, equal sex distribution (Strutton et al. 2004), and positive family history in 57% of patients (Doolabh et al. 2004). The main complaint is the excessive production of odourless sweat, with the axilla being the most commonly affected site (Strutton et al. 2004). Importantly, this is different from 'bromidrosis', which involves the production of malodorous sweat. Occasionally, the profuse sweating in hyperhidrosis can result in skin maceration (particularly in the axillae or soles), with subsequent secondary bacterial or fungal infection (Lowe et al. 2004). The excessive volume of sweat produced often compels patients to change clothes several times a day and avoid physical contact particularly in the case of palmar hyperhidrosis, where the hands are cold, wet, and slippery. It is important, therefore, to appreciate the social stigmatization that can result from this condition as well as the psychological effects of impaired occupational and physical activity, which may lead the patient to seek professional help (Hornberger et al. 2004, Strutton et al. 2004).

Diagnosis

A diagnosis of primary hyperhidrosis can be made if there is at least a 6-month history of visible, focal, and excessive sweating without other apparent cause, affecting at least one of the axillae, palms,

soles or craniofacial region. In addition, the sweating must also have two of the following features (Hornberger et al. 2004):

- bilateral and relatively symmetric
- impairs daily activities
- frequency of at least one episode per week
- age of onset less than 25 years
- positive family history
- cessation of focal sweating during sleep.

The affected areas can be localized with Minor's Iodine starch testing, where 5% potassium iodide solution in alcohol is applied to the skin surface and allowed to dry, followed by the application of powdered starch, which is subsequently brushed off after a few minutes. Excessive sweating results in a blue/black discoloration of the starch as demonstrated in Fig. 72.1, allowing identification of the affected site for further localization of therapy. Laboratory tests such as gravimetry or evaporimetry are used for research purposes to accurately quantify the production of sweat before and after treatment, and are not routinely used to make a diagnosis.

Non-surgical treatment

Treatment for hyperhidrosis aims to reduce the volume of sweat produced to an acceptable level, and ultimately prevent the social stigmatization suffered by the patient (Chapter 32). Before considering interventional and surgical options that achieve this, it is important to appreciate conservative and medical measures that may be of benefit.

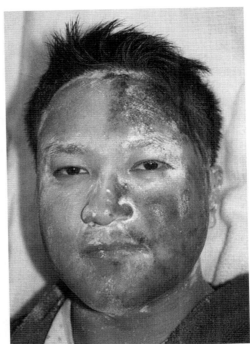

Fig. 72.1 A positive left-sided Minor's iodine test demonstrating hemi-facial hyperhidrosis. The patient was anhidrotic on the right following previous right thoracoscopic sympathectomy. Reproduced from *Postgraduate Medical Journal*, Swan MC, Nicolaou M and Paes TR, **79**, 278–594, Copyright (2003), with permission from BMJ Publishing Group Ltd.

Education

Patients should be educated on simple general measures that can help with management of this condition. These include frequent changing of socks and clothes, using absorbent powders or insoles and wearing dark clothes to conceal stains.

Topical agents

Over-the-counter antiperspirants based on aluminium compounds (such as 25% aluminium chloride hexahydrate in absolute alcohol or in salicylic acid gel) work by mechanically obstructing the eccrine sweat ducts at the level of the acrosyringium (Benohanian 2001), and may be of benefit not only in axillary hyperhidrosis but also for use on palms and soles. Disadvantages include the need for application several times a day and the potential to cause skin irritation, which may be unacceptable to the patient (Horneberger et al. 2004).

Pharmacotherapy

Anticholinergic drugs such as glycopyrolate reduce perspiration by blocking the stimulatory effect of acetylcholine on the sweat gland. Unfortunately, they tend to be poorly tolerated due to systemic side-effects such as dry mouth, blurred vision, and constipation (Nyamekye 2004). Beta-blockers and benzodiazepines are also used to reduce anxiety induced hyperhidrosis.

Iontophoresis

Iontophoresis was first described in 1952 by Bouman and Grunewald-Lentzer, and involves immersing the affected areas (hands and/or feet) in a solution of water and passing low intensity current (8–20 mA) from a DC generator via metal electrodes for 20 minutes. The procedure is repeated 3–4 times per week and euhidrosis is usually achieved after 10–15 sessions (Togel et al. 2002) but requires a maintenance session every about 4 weeks. The exact mechanism of action is unknown, although it is believed that the ionic changes temporarily disrupt the function of the sweat glands in the treated areas. Iontophoresis works well for palmar and plantar hyperhidrosis and is the treatment of choice for the latter, although it is infrequently used to treat axillary hyperhidrosis as it is difficult to administer and can cause skin irritation (Hornberger et al. 2004). There have been recent reports using either botulinum toxin A (Kavanagh et al. 2004) or glycopyrolate (Dolianitis et al. 2004) in the iontophoresis solution, with the former reported to result in 70% reduction in sweating within 48 hours.

Botulinum toxin

Since first being described to treat hyperhidrosis in 1996 (Bushara 1996), botulinum neurotoxin type A (BoNT/A) injection has now become the first-line licensed treatment for axillary hyperhidrosis. Produced by the Gram-positive spore forming anaerobic bacterium clostridium botulinum, the toxin reduces sweating by irreversibly inhibiting the release of acetylcholine from overactive cholinergic sudomotor nerve fibres which innervate eccrine sweat glands (Naumann et al. 2001). The toxin is administered in the affected areas (identified using Minor's starch-iodine test) by intradermal injection, with for example 50–60 mouse units used in each axilla (Naumann et al. 2003). Evidence of euhidrosis appears within 24 hours and peaks at one week (Glogau 2002), with up to 96% of patients reporting reduction in sweating after 4 weeks (Naumann et al. 2003). Unfortunately the effect is temporary with repeat injections required after approximately 7 months, with evidence of reduced efficacy thereafter, probably due to antibody formation against the toxin (Lowe et al. 2004). Adverse effects from BoNT/A are rare, and include perceived increase in non-axillary sweating as well as pain at the injection sites (Naumann et al. 2003). Overall, the treatment is well tolerated by patients and has been showed to significantly improve their quality of life (Campanati et al. 2003, Swartling et al. 2001). BoNT/A has also been used with good results in the treatment of frontal (Kinkelin et al. 2000), palmar (Hornberger et al. 2004) and plantar hyperhidrosis (Vadoud-Seyedi, 2004) although complication such as pain at injection sites, and transient muscular weakness in the hand have made it less popular here.

Finally there is recent evidence suggesting high efficacy of botulinum toxin type B (BoNT/B) for treating axillary and palmar hyperhidrosis (Dressler et al. 2002, Baumann and Halem 2004), with anhidrosis being reported to occur more rapidly and evenly in comparison with BoNT/A (Glogau 2002). It is important to appreciate, however, that unlike BoNT/A, BoNT/B is not currently licensed for the treatment of hyperhidrosis, with more evidence in its efficacy and safety profile awaited.

Behavioural treatments

Although techniques such as biofeedback, cognitive behavioural therapy and hypnotherapy have been described, their efficacy in reducing symptoms of hyperhidrosis are not yet clear (Shenefelt 2003).

Surgical treatment

A potential disadvantage of the non-surgical treatments for hyperhidrosis is that they have temporary effect, requiring repeated administration in order to maintain a euhidrotic state. Surgical intervention has the advantage of providing a potentially permanent cure, but not without the potential risk of complications. Both local surgery and surgical sympathectomy for hyperhidrosis should therefore only be considered after failure of non-surgical treatment, with the patient fully aware of the potential post operative complications.

Local surgery for hyperhidrosis is only suitable for axillary disease, and aims to reduce the population of the eccrine sweat glands in the axilla. This can be achieved by either skin excision, curettage of the underlying subcutaneous tissue through small incisions, or liposuction, all performed under local/tumescent anaesthesia. Complications such as scarring, contractures, and infection, together with a long recovery time have meant that skin excision is now rarely performed (Lowe et al. 2004, Nyamekye 2003), with curettage and liposuction being favoured due to better patient acceptance (Breach 1979, Rompel and Scholz 2001).

Surgical anatomy of the sympathetic trunk

The sympathetic division of the autonomic nervous system arises from pre-ganglionic cell bodies located in the intermediolateral cell columns of the 12 thoracic and the upper two lumbar segments of the spinal cord. They form the white communicating rami (myelinated) and reach the sympathetic trunk on the lateral surfaces of the thoracic and lumbar vertebrae. Upon entering the ganglia, the fibres may synapse with a number of ganglion cells, pass up and down the sympathetic trunk to synapse with ganglion cells at higher or lower level, or pass through the trunk ganglia and out

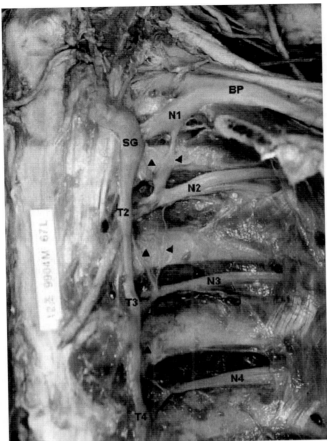

Fig. 72.2 An anatomical dissection of the rami communicantes of the thoracic sympathetic ganglia. See also Plate 21. Reprinted from *European Journal of Cardio-thoracic Surgery*, **27**, Cho HM, Lee DY and Sung SW, Anatomical variations of rami communicantes in the upper thoracic sympathetic trunk, 320–324, Copyright (2005), with permission from Elsevier.

to one of the intermediary sympathetic ganglia. Postganglionic fibres form the gray (unmyelinated) communicating rami and may join a somatic nerve to reach the sweat glands around the body (Waxman 1996). Fig. 72.2 shows an anatomical dissection of the rami communicantes of the thoracic sympathetic ganglia.

There are wide anatomical variations of the sympathetic trunk and many aberrant pathways have been described (Cho et al. 2005). The most common of these pathways is the nerve of Kuntz, which connects the second intercostal to the ventral ramus of the first thoracic nerve (Ramsaroop et al. 2001). There is evidence that despite having a normal anatomical sympathetic trunk, physiologically this is overactive in patients with hyperhidrosis (Noppen et al. 1996). Surgery interrupts the sudomotor innervation of the sweat glands by the resection, ablation or clamping the part of the sympathetic trunk responsible. Any aberrant sympathetic pathways should also be carefully destroyed as failure to do so may result in persistent symptoms (Cho et al. 2005). A sympathectomy can be performed via the open approach, endoscopically or percutaneously.

With regards to the level of sympathectomy, there is good evidence to support that the second thoracic sympathetic ganglion (T2) is primarily responsible for the sympathetic innervation of the hand (Hashmonai 1994). Based on this, most surgeons treat palmar hyperhidrosis with either denervation at the T2 level only

(Lin et al. 1998), or from T2 to T3 (Licht and Pilegaard 2004). Similarly facial hyperhidrosis and blushing are treated by denervation of T2 (Drott et al. 2002), with axillary hyperhidrosis requiring a more extensive denervation (T2–T4 or T2–T5) (Drott 2003).

Indications for endoscopic transthoracic sympathectomy

The main indication for endoscopic transthoracic sympathectomy (ETS) is palmar hyperhidrosis refractory to the non-surgical treatments previously mentioned in this chapter. ETS is also indicated for the treatment of hyperhidrosis in more than one area (e.g. the palms, axillae, and face) or in cases of severe isolated or concomitant facial blushing. For isolated facial or axillary hyperhidrosis, ETS should only be considered when other measures have failed particularly as for mild disease post-operative complications carry the potential to cause more morbidity than the disease itself.

Procedure for endoscopic transthoracic sympathectomy

Although several modifications exist, we present a technique commonly used to perform ETS. The patient is usually anaesthetized with a double lumen endotracheal tube, and positioned in a supine cruciate position, with arms abducted to an angle of approximately 80 degrees. The anterior surface of the thorax is exposed and prepared with aqueous iodine, and two small incisions made in the anterior axillary line over the 3rd or 4th intercostal spaces, through which two disposable 5 mm ports are inserted, with the lung on that side temporarily deflated. A 5 mm 80° thoracoscope is then placed through one of the ports into the pleural cavity, and the sympathetic chain identified. Fig. 72.3 shows a typical thoracoscopic view of the sympathetic chain. The appropriate ganglia are then dissected and either transected using scissors, destroyed with low power coagulating current diathermy, or clipped. Extreme care must be taken not to destroy the inferior cervical (stellate) ganglion as this will result in Horner's syndrome. If the nerve of Kuntz or any other aberrant sympathetic pathway is identified, it should also be carefully divided over a rib. A pleural chest drain connected to an under-water seal may be left *in situ* for 3–4 hours postoperatively to ensure full lung re-expansion. The wounds are then closed

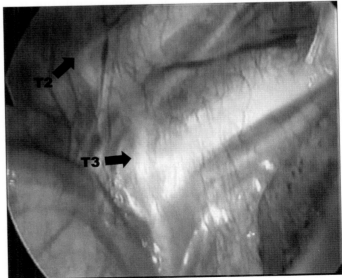

Fig. 72.3 A view of the sympathetic chain through the thoracoscope demonstrating the second and third sympathetic ganglia (arrows). See also Plate 22. Photograph courtesy of Mr Trevor Paes, FRCS.

and the procedure repeated on the opposite side. A chest radiograph may be taken several hours postoperatively to exclude any significant residual pneumothorax and patients discharged usually within the next 24 hours. They are also advised to refrain from vigorous physical activity, use regular oral analgesia, and not to fly for at least 2 weeks postoperatively due to the theoretical risk of a pneumothorax (Cheatham and Safcsak 1999).

Morbidity associated with endoscopic transthoracic sympathectomy

In experienced hands, ETS is known to be a safe procedure with a relatively low morbidity. Patients should be warned that almost one third of those undergoing ETS for hyperhidrosis experience a transient recurrence of sweating within a few days of surgery, which is usually self-limiting (Ojimba and Cameron 2004). Short-term complications include pain, either at the port site or neuralgia along the ulnar aspect of the arm and along the rib. The former can be reduced by oral analgesics or perioperative intercostal nerve block (Rennie 2003), and the latter usually resolves within 6 weeks. Persistent pneumothorax and pleural effusion is uncommon and may require pleural chest drain insertion for a longer period. Finally surgical emphysema is occasionally noted, although this is usually self-limiting and requires no specific treatment (Ojimba and Cameron 2004).

The most common long-term complication of ETS is compensatory sweating, defined as increased abnormal perspiration in other areas of the body, occurring in some form or other in 67–100% of patients (Schick and Horbach 2003) but severe in only 1–2% (Ojimba and Cameron 2004). Areas commonly involved include the upper back, thighs and anterior chest wall, although the face, buttocks, popliteal fossa, and feet can all be affected. The mechanism by which compensatory sweating occurs is poorly understood, with one theory suggesting it is a thermoregulatory response to compensate for the loss of sweating on both the hands and face following sympathectomy (Drott 2003). Improvement is spontaneous in up to 94% of patients within 3–9 months of surgery (Chiou and Chen 1999), but in the case of severe focal sweating, botulinum toxin A injections can be administered (Huh et al. 2002), and where sweating is more generalized anticholinergic drugs such as glycopyrolate may be prescribed to the patient.

Other well-recognized long-term complications include gustatory sweating and Horner's syndrome. The former, reported as occurring in anywhere from 3% to 51% of patients (Doolabh et al. 2004, Herbst et al. 1994), is characterized by excessive perspiration on the forehead, upper lip, and perioral region subsequent to gustatory stimuli (Schick and Horbach 2003). The latter results from injury to the stellate ganglion, although fortunately full Horner's syndrome post sympathectomy is now a rare phenomenon due to a more accurately targeted surgical technique around the stellate ganglion. It is important to appreciate that up to 1% of patients have a degree of ptosis after ETS which resolves over weeks or months (Ojimba and Cameron 2004). Finally, ETS has also been linked with a reduction of the resting and maximal heart rates, although this has not been shown to affect the maximal workload (Kingma et al. 2002), and phantom sweating where the patient has the feeling of perspiration without hidrosis (Ojimba and Cameron 2004).

The reversibility of sympathectomy performed with clips has been described in some isolated reports, suggesting that sympathetic re-activation can be achieved by removing the clips (Lin et al. 1998). Although this concept is interesting particularly for patients who suffer some of the long-term complications such as compensatory sweating as well as for patients who have been clipped at the wrong level, such reports are as yet mostly isolated with little objective evidence to support nerve recovery after unclipping (Drott 2003).

Prognosis

On the whole, ETS is thought to be a successful operation particularly in the case of palmar hyperhidrosis with experienced surgeons reporting a cure rate of 95–100% (Rex et al. 1998), recurrence rate of only 0–4% (Hashmonai et al. 1992), and overall patient satisfaction rate of up to 95% (Loscertales et al. 2004). In isolated axillary or facial hyperhidrosis euhidrosis rates of up to 95% have been reported but with a satisfaction rate of 68% and 76% for axillary and facial hyperhidrosis respectively (Rex et al. 1998). Paradoxically, up to 58% of patients with concomitant plantar hyperhidrosis being treated for upper limb or facial hyperhidrosis report improvement in symptoms following ETS (de Campos et al. 2003). Plantar hyperhidrosis can also be treated by a lumbar sympathectomy, but this procedure is only rarely performed due to the risk of sexual dysfunction post operatively (Tseng and Tseng 2001).

Facial blushing

Definition

'Blushing' or 'flushing' is characterized by episodic attacks of facial erythema, often also involving the ears and the neck, usually accompanied by the feeling of warmth or burning. Occasionally the erythema may extend down to the chest, abdomen and limbs. Blushing can also be caused by a number of physiological and pathological processes as demonstrated in Table 72.2, which again must be excluded before a diagnosis can be made.

Pathophysiology

Blushing occurs due to increased blood flow through the skin resulting in an increased temperature and the engorgement of the subpapillary venous plexus causing erythema (Greaves 1998). The exact mechanism for blushing is complex and poorly understood but it is believed that unlike other areas, the dominant mechanism

Table 72.2 Non-emotional causes of blushing

Aetiology	Clinical condition causing blushing
Physiological	Exercise or hot environment
Infection	Acute or chronic, febrile illness
Hormonal	Post-menopausal
Drugs	Nitrites and nitrates, calcium-channel blockers, ephedrine, irbesartan, propantheline, sumatriptan, quinine sulphate, niacin, danazol, prostaglandins, desmopressin, disulfiram, levodopa, adenosine and others
Neoplastic	Carcinoid syndrome, phaeochromocytoma, vipoma
Immunological	Acute allergic reaction
Dermatological	Rosacea, mastocytosis
Other	Alcohol, spicy foods, scombroid fish poisoning, opioid intoxication

for vasomotor control in the face is for vasodilatation (Fox et al. 1962). This is mediated by both cholinergic (via bradykinin) and β-adrenergic stimulation as well as relaxation of sympathetic vasoconstrictor tone. In addition, the release of vasoactive intestinal peptide (VIP) from reflexly activated trigeminal pathways and the release of substance P or serotonin from trigeminal terminals contribute to this mechanism (Sterodimas et al. 2003). Since autonomic nerve fibres also supply sweat glands, blushing is frequently associated with facial hyperhidrosis.

Clinical presentation

Darwin characterized blushing as 'the most peculiar and most human of all expressions' (Darwin 1979). It is involuntary, uncontrollable, cannot be inhibited, and can be triggered by the mildest of emotions. It is an exaggerated response and should not to be confused with the slight facial reddening seen when a person becomes ashamed. In a small minority of individuals it is severe enough to become debilitating, with devastating consequences socially and at work (Gawande 2002). The age of onset is usually adolescence and despite popular belief that women blush more than men, the prevalence may be similar (Nicolaou et al. 2003). It is also seen in all races, although those with darker skin types have less of a problem as the visible changes are less striking. The main problem in these patients is not the redness itself but rather the associated fear, known as eythrophobia (Drummond 2003). This often leads to avoidant behaviour and social isolation and in a few cases it may even cause suicidal thoughts and alcoholism (Savin 2002).

Diagnosis

The diagnosis of emotionally induced blushing is clinical and can be made by taking a careful history. Specific questions should be asked on the frequency and circumstances in which the patient blushes as well as other explainable cause (as listed in Table 72.2). The severity of blushing is subjective, can only be defined by the patient and may not correlate with the intensity of redness. There are therefore no quantitative laboratory tests that are required for diagnosis, although facial blood flow measurements can be made using photoplethysmography, Doppler, and temperature measurement.

Non-surgical treatment

At present, several treatment options for emotionally induced blushing exist, although physicians tend to be ill informed of these, considering blushing as a condition that patients will 'grow out of' and for which nothing can be done. Fortunately, with the increased availability of the internet there is a growing awareness among patients and doctors about the problems of and treatments available for blushing (Nicolaou et al. 2003).

General measures

Some patients choose simply to use camouflaging make up or high necked clothing to conceal any embarrassing facial erythema. There are also isolated accounts reporting the use of cognitive and behavioural therapies to treat blushing, although these techniques remain as yet largely unsubstantiated (Scholing and Emmelkamp 1993, Mulken et al. 2001).

Pharmacotherapy

Whereas drugs such as beta-blockers can reduce blushing, propranolol has been found to reduce the intensity and duration of the blush in many patients (Drott 2003). Clonidine is licensed for use in post-menopausal flushing, with anxiolytics and antidepressants (such as serotonin reuptake inhibitors) used to help alleviate the anxiety associated with the colour change. A third of patients admit to ingesting alcohol for alleviation of the associated anxiety, leaving themselves vulnerable to alcohol abuse (Drott et al. 2002).

Botulinum toxin

BoNT/A as described earlier in this chapter, has recently been used to successfully treat patients with facial and neck blushing (Tugnoli et al. 2002, Sterodimas et al. 2003, Yuraitis and Jacob 2004). Although treatment with BoNT/A is not permanent (typically lasting for 9–12 months), it can be repeated.

Surgical treatment

The only surgical option available to treat blushing is the bilateral ETS of the second thoracic sympathetic ganglion (T2), as described earlier in the chapter. First reported by Wittmoser in 1985, this has since been confirmed by several subsequent large series, showing benefit in over 90% of patients and a satisfaction rate of up to 85% (Drott et al. 2002). Although extremely effective for this indication, ETS should only be offered if other treatment modalities have been exhausted and in severely debilitated patients. The reason for this is that ETS is effectively an irreversible procedure which is again not without complications such as those previously mentioned (compensatory sweating). Other specific complications include phantom blushing which is characterized by the feeling of going red with no associated colour change. Reassurance and teaching them to ignore this by behaviour modification often helps. It is paramount therefore that patients undergoing ETS for facial blushing are adequately informed prior to surgery.

Frey's syndrome

Frey's syndrome is characterized by gustatory facial sweating, erythema and/or general discomfort about an area of skin in front of the ear and on the cheek, and is reported to occur in up to 30% of patients following parotid gland surgery (Linder et al. 1997), although it may also occur following facial injuries, syringomyelia, tuberculous lymphadenitis, dorsal sympathectomy, and radical neck dissection (Birch et al. 1999). It is thought to be caused by the regeneration of damaged neurons whereby postganglionic parasympathetic fibres from the otic ganglion reach the damaged fibres of the auriculotemporal nerve supplying sympathetic innervation to sweat glands and subcutaneous vessels over the distribution of the nerve. This results in the formation of a new reflex at the time of mastication. The true incidence of the syndrome may indeed be higher (up to 96%) as suggested by performing Minor's starch iodine test on asymptomatic patients following parotid surgery (Kornblut et al. 1977).

Treatment options for Frey's syndrome range from medical, with the use of antiperspirants and anti-cholinergic preparations, to injection of botulinum toxin over the affected area. Naumann et al. (1997) investigated the action of intracutaneous botulinum toxin injections in 45 patients with gustatory sweating, finding a 93% reduction in the area of sweating following treatment. Half the patients rated gustatory sweating subjectively as completely abolished, and the remainder felt pronounced improvement, with no recurrence noted over a 6-month follow-up period. A more radical approach to the prevention of this syndrome is the use of a sternocleidomastoid muscle flap rotated into the area of parotid resection at the time of initial surgery in order to separate the skin from secretomotor nerve fibres (Sood et al. 1999).

Chronic regional pain syndrome

Chronic regional pain syndrome (CRPS) is a term used to describe the constellation of conditions previously known as 'Sudeck's atrophy', 'causalgia', reflex sympathetic dystrophy, and 'mimio-causalgia' (Pather et al. 2004). The theory that this syndrome results from an abnormal hyperactive sympathetic tone stems from the observation that sympathetic blockade in these patients results in an alleviation of their symptoms (Buckley et al. 1990). Despite this, the exact pathophysiology behind CRPS remains poorly understood. The International Association for the Study of Pain has further defined and classified CRPS into type I and II (Stanton-Hicks et al. 1995). In order for a patient to be diagnosed with CRPS type I, three of the following four criteria must be fulfilled:

1 the presence of an initiating even or cause for immobilization

2 continuous (disproportionate) pain, allodynia, or hyperalgesia

3 oedema, changes in skin blood flow or sudomotor activity in the region of pain

4 exclusion of conditions that would otherwise account for degree of pain.

In order to de diagnosed with CRPS type II, the patient has to fulfill 2–4 and also have a peripheral nerve injury as the initiating factor.

Because of this poor understanding of the mechanisms underlying CRPS, management of the condition is non-uniform across centres, and is based largely on personal clinical experience. Current treatment options consist of psychosocial counselling (pain coping skills, relaxation techniques), combination pharmacological therapy (non-steroidal anti-inflammatory agents, corticosteroids, bisphosphonates, calcitonin, antidepressants, anticonvulsants, opioids, and/or sympatholytics), and regional sympathetic blocks. The goal in the treatment of CRPS is attempting to relieve pain whilst attempting to restore functional outcome to the limb by encouraging physical therapy (Stanton-Hicks et al. 1998). Selective sympathetic blockade can be used by the treating physician in determining whether the pain experienced by the patient is 'sympathetically maintained' and therefore potentially responsive sympathectomy, a process that should be undertaken before considering any surgical sympathectomy (Bandyk et al. 2002).

In the case of upper limb CRPS that is refractory to medical treatment, alleviation or improvement of symptoms following stellate ganglion blockade is used to determine whether the pain is 'sympathetically maintained' and therefore predict whether cervical sympathectomy will be successful. Although several approaches for this have been described, the most widely used of these is the paratracheal or anterior approach (Guntamukkala and Hardy 1991). If positive, the stellate ganglion block results in a transient Horner's syndrome with alleviation of upper limb pain. Recent evidence suggests however that stellate ganglion block is a poor predictor of determine success from cervical sympathectomy, although it may prove useful as a therapeutic method with analgesia noted to extend beyond the duration of the block itself (Singh et al. 2003). Authors suggest that early identification of the disease is a crucial factor in achieving a good prognostic outcome, and

advocate a 6-week trial of medical treatment following which stellate ganglion block may be undertaken as both a diagnostic and therapeutic tool. Following this thoracoscopic sympathectomy limited to the second thoracic ganglion (interrupting sympathetic outflow to alternative pathways such as the nerve of Kuntz) may be performed, with Sing et al. reporting an overall success rates of up to 76%. Dorsal sympathectomy from below the stellate ganglion to the third or fourth thoracic ganglion has also been reported with a similar success rate (72%) and minimal patient morbidity (Bandyk et al. 2002).

Lumbar sympathectomy for lower limb CRPS, non-reconstructable arterial occlusive disease, and symptomatic vasospasm using a retroperitoneal approach has been shown to result in an overall pain reduction and patient satisfaction of up to 84% (Bandyk et al. 2002). Here, a transverse skin incision is made lateral to the rectus sheath midway between the costal margin and iliac crest. This muscle-splitting incision is used to gain access to the retroperitoneum, and once the peritoneum is retracted medially, the psoas muscle and genital-femoral nerve visualized. The sympathetic chain can then be palpated and dissected on the vertebral column, and the first to fourth lumbar ganglia subsequently excised. Percutaneous lumbar sympathectomy using phenol or alcohol injections, and radiofrequency ablation have all been used with some success, but a limitation these minimally invasive procedures is incomplete sympathectomy, return of sympathetic tone, and thereby symptoms (Cotton and Cross 1985). Laparoscopic lumbar sympathectomy through both retroperitoneal and transperitoneal approaches is a relatively new technique for which more long-term follow-up data is required before its efficacy for CRPS can be accurately determined (Watarida et al. 2002).

It is important to bear in mind that despite this reported success, sympathectomy in patients with CRPS is not without its complications. Post-sympathectomy syndromes such as neuralgia or sympathalgia can develop in up to 20% of patients following lumbar and thoracic sympathectomy for CRPS, requiring further pharmacotherapy, sympathetic blockade, and transcutaneous electrical nerve stimulation (Bandyk et al. 2002). Other adverse sequelae include compensatory sweating, and chronic neurological pain, although these tend to occur less frequently.

Angina pectoris

In the early 1920s, at a time when cardiac pharmacology was in its infancy, and interventions such as angioplasty yet undeveloped, Jonnesco first described the open thoracic sympathectomy for angina pectoris (Lingren 1950). This was followed by a series of 88 cases by Kux, reporting good results for relief on angina pain, but with some mortality (Kux 1950). In the early 1960s, advances in pharmacology (namely β-adrenergic blockers) and revascularization procedures such as percutaneous transluminal coronary angioplasty (PTCA), and coronary artery bypass grafting (CABG) resulted in the procedure being abandoned. More recently, advances in thoracoscopy and minimally invasive surgery have resulted in the renaissance of thoracic sympathectomy, with ETS being performed in those with severe angina pectoris who are already on maximal pharmacotherapy, and in whom further invasive intervention is not possible (Claes 2003).

In a study by Wettervik et al. (1995) 24 patients ineligible for CABG or angioplasty underwent bilateral endoscopic transthoracic sympathectomy through a single port inserted in each axillary fossa, pneumoperitoneum induced, and an electroresectoscope used to divide the sympathetic chain overlying the first to fourth costovertebral joints. A favourable outcome was reported with the frequency of anginal attacks significantly reduced, maximal exercise capacity significantly increased, and no major surgical complications reported by the authors. A later study by the same group in 43 patients suggests similarly positive results with 49% of patients completely symptom free at months, and the remaining 51% reporting significantly fewer and milder attacks (from 18 to 5 per week) (Claes et al. 1996). Complications reported included unilateral Horner's syndrome in one patient (2.3%) and air leak resulting in pneumothorax requiring drainage for 24 hours longer in two patients (4.7%). Khogali et al. (1999).have reported the use of video-assisted thoracoscopic sympathectomy (VATS) in 10 patients in whom PTCA or CABG was not possible. They describe a 3-incision technique on each side to access the second to fourth ganglia bilaterally, reporting marked improvement in angina frequency, intensity of symptoms, and exercise tolerance on treadmill at a mean follow-up of 11.5 months. It should be noted, however that ETS for angina pectoris is a technically demanding operation not only because of the presence of multiple pleural adhesions from previous surgery, but also because these patients are often obese, with co-existing lung disease, and unable to tolerate partial lung collapse (Drott 2003).

The mechanism by which transthoracic sympathectomy acts to relieve anginal symptoms is unclear, although its effect on heart rate variability is may provide a clue. Heart rate variability is thought by some to reflect the heart's autonomic responsiveness, with a shift towards parasympathetic dominance (and increased variability) thought to be beneficial, potentially reducing ventricular fibrillation in the ischaemic heart (Kleiger et al. 1987, Podrid et al. 1990, Kolman et al. 1975). In a study of 57 patients, pre- and post- sympathectomy 24-hour Holter electrocardiographic (ECG) measurements were taken, showing a significant increase in the mean R-R interval (923 and 1006 ms respectively) following sympathectomy, suggesting increased parasympathetic tone. The authors did however identify limitations such as small study size, measurement inaccuracies, and changes in drug therapy (β-adrenergic blockers) as factors that may have affected their outcome (Tygesen et al. 1997). In a later study, the same authors used similar measurement up to 2 years following ETS for severe angina pectoris, suggesting that global heart rate variability increased with time in these patients (Tygesen et al. 1999). Other mechanisms by which sympathectomy is thought to alleviate anginal symptoms include a protective effect against vasoconstriction, and finally the interruption of afferent pain fibres that pass through the sympathetic chain (Claes et al. 1996). This latter effect has been demonstrated by performing repeated unilateral left Stellate ganglion local anaesthetic blockade in a patient with end stage coronary artery disease and chronic refractory angina, with the effect lasting almost 6 weeks, and markedly improving quality of life (Chester et al. 2000).

Cardiac arrhythmias

Chronic atrial fibrillation (AF) is known to affect up to 2% of the general population at some point during their lives (Kannel et al. 1982), with an incidence increasing dramatically with age

(Go 2005). The role of parasympathetic innervation in the generation of paroxysmal AF has been investigated with circumferential pulmonary vein ablation and complete vagal denervation used as a both treatment and preventative measures (Pappone et al. 2004). AF has in the past been shown to be induced and maintained using parasympathetic stimulation in experimental protocols (Wang et al. 1992). The mechanism for this is thought to be related to a shortening of the atrial effective refractory period (Smeets et al. 1986), decreasing the wavelength of atrial excitation wave fronts, and increasing the probability of multiple re-entrant circuits and thereby atrial fibrillation (Allessie 1998). Schauerte et al. (2000) successfully identified and ablated parasympathetic atrial innervation in an experimental dog model, by transvenous catheter stimulation and radiofrequency current catheter ablation techniques. They were able to show that after this ablation technique atrial fibrillation was no longer inducible by vagal verve stimulation, concluding that such ablative could potentially abolish vagally mediated atrial fibrillation and may form part of the treatment options for this common arrhythmia.

The importance of autonomic innervation has also been observed following surgery for CABG, where postoperative AF is the most common arrhythmia with an incidence ranging from 19% to 27% (Melo et al. 2004). The role of autonomic imbalance in the generation of AF has therefore been appreciated by cardiac surgeons, with ventral cardiac denervation being used as a method of preventing postoperative AF following CABG. In a prospective randomized study of 426 patients (207 undergoing ventral cardiac denervation vs 219 control subjects), Melo et al. found an AF incidence of 7% in the denervated group versus 27% in the control group, a difference that was statistically significant. They found ventral cardiac denervation to be the most significant predictor of postoperative atrial fibrillation following CABG.

Finally, congenital long QT syndrome, an electrophysiological disorder manifest by frequent syncopal attacks and cardiac arrest. Although first line treatment consists of oral β-adrenergic blockers, failure of patient to respond to this medication (partially due to non-compliance) has led some to suggest left cardiac sympathetic denervation as a second line treatment (Wang et al. 2004). The procedure seems to be effective in reducing the syncopal, and cardiac arrest events, without significantly affecting heart rate or left ventricular dysfunction (Schwartz et al. 1991). One of the options available for performing this procedure is the left cervicothoracic sympathectomy (total left stellectomy and removal of first 4–5 left thoracic sympathetic ganglia). Although this produces adequate cardiac sympathetic blockade, it is also associated with Horner's syndrome. More recently, the high thoracic left sympathectomy has been preferred, where the lower part of the left stellate ganglion and the first 4–5 left thoracic ganglia are removed (Schwartz et al. 2002). The incidence of Horner's syndrome is low with this procedure due to sparing of ocular sympathetic fibres whilst producing adequate cardiac sympathetic denervation.

Raynaud's syndrome

Operative intervention forms the last line of treatment for patients suffering from Raynaud's syndrome, characterized by episodic vascular spasm resulting in digital ischaemia in response to cold or emotional stimuli, and ultimately painful digital ulceration. Obliteration of the sympathetic innervation by thoracic sympathectomy in patients who have failed medical therapy carries with it the theoretical advantage of increasing skin circulation, temperature, and ulcer resolution. In the pre-endoscopic surgery era, however, invasiveness of transthoracic procedures and their associated complication, prevented the use of thoracic sympathectomy to treat Raynaud's syndrome. ETS carries with it a much lower complication profile, and has since been used to treat the condition, but with mixed results. Although initial improvement is often dramatic, with the patient's hand becoming warm, this benefit has been noted to reduce dramatically over the next six months (Claes 2003). In a study by Matsumoto et al. (2002), 28 patients with Raynaud's phenomenon presenting with severe chronic symptoms or non-healing digital ulceration refractory to intensive medical therapy underwent ETS. Initial resolution or improvement of symptoms was achieved in 93% of patients, but recurred in 82% at a follow-up of 62.5 months. Despite this, digital ulceration did not recur, and 89.3% of patients reported overall improvement in the frequency and severity of their symptoms. A proposed mechanism for the recurrence of symptoms in Raynaud's syndrome treated with ETS is hypersensitivity of noradrenergic receptors regulating the pre-capillary sphincters, which then react on very small amounts of circulating catecholamines (Lowell et al. 1993). Other proposed mechanisms include incomplete sympathectomy, and nerve fibre regeneration. These mixed results have led to endoscopic thoracic sympathectomy for Raynaud's syndrome no longer being offered at many centres. ETS has also been described for Buerger's disease in patients presenting with ischaemic pain, ulcers and gangrene, with encouraging results (Chander et al. 2004). Finally the technique may also be used to treat patients with upper limb distal vascular disease (either traumatic, atherosclerotic, or due to cytotoxic drug treatment) presenting with fingertip ulcers (Claes, 2003).

Key points

◆ Surgery on the autonomic nervous system has been performed since the late 19th century for a range of indications but is now used to treat certain conditions with relatively low morbidity.

◆ Endoscopic transthoracic sympathectomy is the best surgical option for the treatment of refractory palmar hyperhidrosis and severe facial blushing, carrying with it relatively low associated morbidity.

◆ Compensatory sweating is an important complication following endoscopic thoracic sympathectomy that patients and their clinicians should be aware of.

◆ Sympathectomy to relieve symptoms from chronic regional pain syndromes may be used following failure of other treatment options, and is most effective when treated early.

◆ Autonomic surgery is also used for refractory conditions such as angina, Raynaud's syndrome, Frey's syndrome, and cardiac arrhythmias.

Acknowledgements

The authors would like to thank Mr Trevor Paes (FRCS) for his contribution to the hyperhidrosis and facial blushing sections of this chapter.

References

Allessie, M. A. (1998). Atrial electrophysiologic remodeling: another vicious circle? *J Cardiovascular Electrophysiology* **9**, 1378–93.

Atkins, H. J. (1954). Sympathectomy by the axillary approach. *Lancet* **266**, 538–39.

Bandyk, D. F., Johnson, B. L., Kirkpatrick, A. F., Novotney, M. L., Back, M. R. and Schmacht, D. C. (2002). Surgical sympathectomy for reflex sympathetic dystrophy syndromes. *Journal of Vascular Surgery* **35**, 269–77.

Baumann, L. S., Halem, M. L. (2004). Botulinum toxin-B and the management of hyperhidrosis. *Clinics in Dermatology* **22**, 60–65.

Benohanian, A. (2001). Antiperspirants and deodorants. *Clinics in Dermatology* **19**, 398–405.

Birch, J. F., Varma, S. K. and Narula, A. A. (1999). Botulinum toxoid in the management of gustatory sweating (Frey's syndrome) after superficial parotidectomy. *Br J Plast. Surg* **52**, 230–1.

Breach, N. M. (1979). Axillary hyperhidrosis: surgical cure with aesthetic scars. *Annals of the Royal College of Surgeons of England* **61**, 295–97.

Buckley, F. P., Morricca, G. and Murphy, T. (1990). Neurolytic blockade and hypophysectomy. In: Bonnica, J. J. *The Management of Pain* 2nd ed, vol 11, Lea & Febiger, Philadelphia, pp. 2012–2014.

Bushara, K. O., Park, D. M., Jones, J. C. and Schutta, H. S. (1996). Botulinum toxin—a possible new treatment for axillary hyperhidrosis. *Clinical and Experimental Dermatology* **21**, 276–78.

Campanati, A., Penna, L., Guzzo, T., *et al.* (2003). Quality-of-life assessment in patients with hyperhidrosis before and after treatment with botulinum toxin: results of an open-label study. *Clinical Therapeutics* **25**, 298–308.

Campbell, W. B., Cooper, M. J., Sponsel, W. E., Baird, R. N. and Peacock, J. H. (1982). Transaxillary sympathectomy—is a one-stage bilateral procedure safe? *The British Journal of Surgery* **69** Suppl, S29–31.

Chander, J., Singh, L., Lal, P., Jain, A. and Ramteke, V. K. (2004). Retroperitoneoscopic lumbar sympathectomy for buerger's disease: a novel technique. *Journal of the Society of Laparoscopic Surgeons* **8**, 291–6.

Cheatham, M. L. and Safcsak, K. (1999). Air travel following traumatic pneumothorax: when is it safe? *The American Surgeon* **65**, 1160–64.

Chester, M., Hammond, C. and Leach, A. (2000). Long-term benefits of stellate ganglion block in severe chronic refractory angina. *Pain* **87**, 103–5.

Chiou, T. S. and Chen, S. C. (1999). Intermediate-term results of endoscopic transaxillary T2 sympathectomy for primary palmar hyperhidrosis. *The British Journal of Surgery* **86**, 45–47.

Cho, H. M., Lee, D. Y. and Sung, S. W. (2005). Anatomical variations of rami communicantes in the upper thoracic sympathetic trunk. *European Journal of Cardio-thoracic Surgery* **27**, 320–24.

Claes, G. (2003). Indications for endoscopic thoracic sympathectomy. *Clinical Autonomic Research* **13** Suppl 1, I16–9.

Claes, G., Drott, C., Wettervik, C., Tygesen, H., Emanuelsson, H., Lomsky, M. and Radberg, G. (1996). *Cardiovascular Surgery* **4**, 830–1.

Cloward, R. B. (1969). Hyperhydrosis. *Journal of Neurosurgery* **30**, 545–51.

Cotton, L. T. and Cross, F. W. (1985). Lumbar sympathectomy for arterial disease. *British Journal of Surgery* **72**, 678–83.

Darwin, C. (1979). Expression of emotions in man and animals-1872. In Porter, D. M. and Graham, P. W., ed. *The Portable Darwin*, pp. 364–93. Penguin Books, New York.

Dolianitis, C., Scarff, C. E., Kelly, J. and Sinclair, R. (2004). Iontophoresis with glycopyrrolate for the treatment of palmoplantar hyperhidrosis. *The Australasian Journal of Dermatology* **45**, 208–212.

Doolabh, N., Horswell, S., Williams, M., *et al.* (2004). Thoracoscopic sympathectomy for hyperhidrosis: indications and results. *The Annals of Thoracic Surgery* **77**, 410–4.

Dragstedt, L. R., 2nd and Lulu, D. J. (1974). Truncal vagotomy and pyloroplasty. Critical evaluation of one hundred cases. *American Journal of Surgery* **128**, 344–6.

Dressler, D., Adib Saberi, F. and Benecke, R. (2002). Botulinum toxin type B for treatment of axillar hyperhidrosis. *Journal of Neurology* **249**, 1729–32.

Drott, C. (2003). Results of endoscopic thoracic sympathectomy (ETS) on hyperhidrosis, facial blushing, angina pectoris, vascular disorders and pain syndromes of the hand and arm. *Clinical Autonomic Research* **13** Suppl 1, I26–30.

Drott, C., Claes, G. and Rex, L. (2002). Facial blushing treated by sympathetic denervation-long lasting benefits in 831 patients. *Journal of Cosmetic Dermatology* **1**, 115–119.

Drummond, P. D. (2003). Endoscopic thoracic sympathectomy for blushing. *Journal of Cosmetic Dermatology* **2**, 45–6.

Fox, R. H., Goldsmith, R. and Kidd, D. J. (1962). Cutaneous vasomotor control in the human head, neck and upper chest. *The Journal of Physiology* **161**, 298–312.

Gawande, A. (2002). Crimson Tide. In A. Gawande, ed. *Complications: a surgeon's notes on an imperfect science*, pp. 146. Profile Books, London.

Glogau, R. G. (2002). Review of the use of botulinum toxin for hyperhidrosis and cosmetic purposes. *The Clinical Journal of Pain* **18**, S191–97.

Go, A. S. (2005). 1. Go AS. The epidemiology of atrial fibrillation in elderly persons: the tip of the iceberg. *American Journal of Geriatric Cardiology* **14**, 56–61.

Golueke, P. J., Garrett, W. V., Thompson, J. E., Talkington, C. M. and Smith, B. L. (1988). Dorsal sympathectomy for hyperhidrosis—the posterior paravertebral approach. *Surgery* **103**, 568–72.

Greaves, M. W. (1998). Flushing and flushing syndromes. In Champion RH, Rook A,

Guntamukkala, M. and Hardy, P. A. (1991). Spread of injectate after stellate ganglion block in man: an anatomical study. *British Journal of Anaesthesia* **66**, 643–4.

Hashmonai, M., Kopelman, D., Kein, O. and Schein, M. (1992). Upper thoracic sympathectomy for primary palmar hyperhidrosis: long-term follow-up. *The British Journal of Surgery* **79**, 268–71.

Hashmonai, M., Kopelman, D. and Schein, M. (1994). Thoracoscopic versus open supraclavicular upper dorsal sympathectomy: a prospective randomised trial. *The European Journal of Surgery*, 13–16.

Hashmonai, M. and Kopelman, D. (2003). History of sympathetic surgery. *Clinical Autonomic Research* **13** Suppl 1, I6–I9.

Herbst, F., Plas, E. G., Függer, R. and Fritsch, A. (1994). Endoscopic thoracic sympathectomy for primary hyperhidrosis of the upper limbs. A critical analysis and long-term results of 480 operations. *Annals of Surgery* **220**, 86–90.

Hornberger, J., Grimes, K., Naumann, M., *et al.* (2004). Recognition, diagnosis, and treatment of primary focal hyperhidrosis. *Journal of the American Academy of Dermatology* **51**, 274–86.

Huh, C. H., Han, K. H., Seo, K. I. and Eun, H. C. (2002). Botulinum toxin treatment for a compensatory hyperhidrosis subsequent to an upper thoracic sympathectomy. *The Journal of Dermatological Treatment* **13**, 91–93.

Jonnesco, T. (1920). Angine de poitrine guérie par la résection du sympatique cervicothoracique. *Bull. Acad. Med. Paris* **4**, 479–96.

Kannel, W. B., Abbott, R. D., Savage, D. D. and McNamara, P. M. (1982). Epidemiologic features of chronic atrial fibrillation: the Framingham study. *New England Journal of Medicine* **306**, 1018–22.

Kavanagh, G. M., Oh, C. and Shams, K. (2004). BOTOX delivery by iontophoresis. *The British Journal of Dermatology* **151**, 1093–95.

Keaveny, T. V., Fitzgerald, P. A., Donnelly, C. and Shanik, G. D. (1977). Surgical management of hyperhidrosis. *The British Journal of Surgery* **64**, 570–71.

Khogali, S. S., Miller, M., Rajesh, P. B., Murray, R. G. and Beattie, J. M. (1999). Video-assisted thoracoscopic sympathectomy for severe intractable angina. *European Jounal of Cardiothoracic Surgery* **16** Suppl 1, S95–8.

Kingma, R., TenVoorde, B. J., Scheffer, G. J., *et al.* (2002). Thoracic sympathectomy: effects on hemodynamics and baroreflex control. *Clinical Autonomic Research* **12**, 35–42.

Kinkelin, I., Hund, M., Naumann, M. and Hamm, H. (2000). Effective treatment of frontal hyperhidrosis with botulinum toxin A. *The British Journal of Dermatology* **143**, 824–27.

Kleiger, R. E., Miller, J. P., Bigger, J. T., Jr. and Moss, A. J. (1987). Decreased heart rate variability and its association with increased mortality after acute myocardial infarction. *American Journal of Cardiology* **59**, 256–62.

Kolman, B. S., Verrier, R. L. and Lown, B. (1975). The effect of vagus nerve stimulation upon vulnerability of the canine ventricle: role of sympathetic-parasympathetic interactions. *Circulation* **52**, 578–85.

Kornblut, A. D., Westphal, P. and Miehlke, A. (1977). A reevaluation of the Frey syndrome following parotid surgery. *Archives of Otolaryngology* **103**, 258–61.

Kotzareff, A. (1920). Résection partielle de tronc sympathique cervicale droit pour hyperhidrosis unilatérale. *Revue medicale de la Suisse romande*, **40**, 111–113.

Kux, E. and Vetter, R. (1950). Endoscopic sympathectomy in angina pectoris. Deutsche Schwesternzeitung, **75**, 747–51.

Licht, P. B. and Pilegaard, H. K. (2004). Severity of compensatory sweating after thoracoscopic sympathectomy. *The Annals of Thoracic Surgery* **78**, 427–31.

Lin, C. C., Mo, L. R., Lee, L. S., Ng, S. M. and Hwang, M. H. (1998). Thoracoscopic T2-sympathetic block by clipping—a better and reversible operation for treatment of hyperhidrosis palmaris: experience with 326 cases. *The European Journal of Surgery* 13–16.

Linder, T. E., Huber, A. and Schmid, S. (1997). Frey's syndrome after parotidectomy: a retrospective and prospective analysis. *Laryngoscope* **107**, 1496–501.

Lindgren, I. (1950). Angina pectoris; a clinical study with special reference to neurosurgical treatment. *Acta Medica Scandinavica Supplement* **243**, 1–203.

Loscertales, J., Arroyo Tristán, A., Congregado Loscertales, M., *et al.* (2004). [Thoracoscopic sympathectomy for palmar hyperhidrosis. Immediate results and postoperative quality of life]. *Archivos de bronconeumologia* **40**, 67–71.

Lowe, N., Campanati, A., Bodokh, I., *et al.* (2004). The place of botulinum toxin type A in the treatment of focal hyperhidrosis. *The British Journal of Dermatology* **151**, 1115–22.

Lowell, R. C., Gloviczki, P., Cherry, K. J., Jr., Bower, T. C., Hallett, J. W., Jr., Schirger, A. and Pairolero, P. C. (1993). Cervicothoracic sympathectomy for Raynaud's syndrome. *Int. Angiol.* **12**, 168–72.

Matsumoto, Y., Ueyama, T., Endo, M., Sasaki, H., Kasashima, F., Abe, Y. and Kosugi, I. (2002). Endoscopic thoracic sympathicotomy for Raynaud's phenomenon. *Journal of Vascular Surgery* **36**, 57–61.

Melo, J., Voigt, P., Sonmez, B., *et al.* (2004). Ventral cardiac denervation reduces the incidence of atrial fibrillation after coronary artery bypass grafting. *Journal of Thoracic and Cardiovascular Surgery* **127**, 511–6.

Mulken, S., Bögels, S. M., de Jong, P. J. and Louwers, J. (2001). Fear of blushing: effects of task concentration training versus exposure in vivo on fear and physiology. *Journal of Anxiety Disorders* **15**, 413–32.

Naumann, M., Lowe, N. J., Kumar, C. R., Hamm, H. (2003). Botulinum toxin type a is a safe and effective treatment for axillary hyperhidrosis over 16 months: a prospective study. *Archives of Dermatology* **139**, 731–36.

Naumann, M., Zellner, M., Toyka, K. V. and Reiners, K. (1997). Treatment of gustatory sweating with botulinum toxin. *Annals of Neurology* **42**, 973–5.

Naumann, M. and Lowe, N. J. (2001). Botulinum toxin type A in treatment of bilateral primary axillary hyperhidrosis: randomised, parallel group, double blind, placebo controlled trial. *British Medical Journal* **323**, 596–99.

Nicolaou, M., Sterodimas, A., Swan, M. C. and Paes, T. R. (2003). Is the internet the best resource for blushers? *Clinical Autonomic Research* **13** Suppl 1, I71–73.

Noppen, M., Dendale, P., Hagers, Y., *et al.* (1996). Changes in cardiocirculatory autonomic function after thoracoscopic upper dorsal sympathicolysis for essential hyperhidrosis. *Journal of the Autonomic Nervous System* **60**, 115–20.

Nyamekye, I. K. (2004). Current therapeutic options for treating primary hyperhidrosis. *European Journal of Vascular and Endovascular Surgery* **27**, 571–76.

Ojimba, T. A. and Cameron, A. E. (2004). Drawbacks of endoscopic thoracic sympathectomy. *The British Journal of Surgery* **91**, 264–69.

Palumbo, L. T. and Lulu, D. J. (1966). Anterior transthoracic upper dorsal sympathectomy; current results. *Archives of Surgery* **92**, 247–57.

Pappone, C., Santinelli, V., Manguso, F., *et al.* (2004). Pulmonary vein denervation enhances long-term benefit after circumferential ablation for paroxysmal atrial fibrillation. *Circulation* **109**, 327–34.

Pather, N., Singh, B., Partab, P., Ramsaroop, L. and Satyapal, K. S. (2004). The anatomical rationale for an upper limb sympathetic blockade: preliminary report. *Surg. Radiol. Anat.* **26**, 178–81.

Podrid, P. J., Fuchs, T. and Candinas, R. (1990). Role of the sympathetic nervous system in the genesis of ventricular arrhythmia. *Circulation* **82**, I103–13.

Ramsaroop, L., Partab, P., Singh, B. and Satyapal, K. S. (2001). Thoracic origin of a sympathetic supply to the upper limb. *Journal of Anatomy* **199**, 675–82.

Rennie, J. A., Lin, C. C. and Cameron, A. E. (2003). The technique of endoscopic thoracic sympathectomy: resection, clipping and cautery. *Clinical Autonomic Research* **13** Suppl 1, I22–25.

Rex, L. O., Drott, C., Claes, G., Göthberg, G. and Dalman, P. (1998). The Borås experience of endoscopic thoracic sympathicotomy for palmar, axillary, facial hyperhidrosis and facial blushing. *The European Journal of Surgery*, 23–26.

Rompel, R. and Scholz, S. (2001). Subcutaneous curettage vs. injection of botulinum toxin A for treatment of axillary hyperhidrosis. *Journal of the European Academy of Dermatology and Venereology* **15**, 207–211.

Royle, J. P. (1999). A history of sympathectomy. The Australian and New Zealand Journal of Surgery **69**, 302–307.

Savin, J. (2002). Blushing unseen. *J Cosmet. Dermatol.* **1**, 227.

Schauerte, P., Scherlag, B. J., Pitha, J., Scherlag, M. A., Reynolds, D., Lazzara, R. and Jackman, W. M. (2000). Catheter ablation of cardiac autonomic nerves for prevention of vagal atrial fibrillation. *Circulation* **102**, 2774–80.

Schick, C. H. and Horbach, T. (2003). Sequelae of endoscopic sympathetic block. *Clinical Autonomic Research* **13** Suppl 1, I36–39.

Scholing, A. and Emmelkamp, P. M. (1993). Cognitive and behavioural treatments of fear of blushing, sweating or trembling. *Behaviour Research and Therapy* **31**, 155–70.

Schwartz, P. J., Locati, E. H., Moss, A. J., Crampton, R. S., Trazzi, R. and Ruberti, U. (1991). Left cardiac sympathetic denervation in the therapy of congenital long QT syndrome. A worldwide report. *Circulation* **84**, 503–11.

Schwartz, P. J., Priori, S. G. and Napolitano, C. (2002). Cardiac Electrophysiology: From Cell to Bedside, Zipes D. P., Jalife J. pp. 597–610.

Shenefelt, P. D. (2003). Biofeedback, cognitive-behavioral methods, and hypnosis in dermatology: is it all in your mind? *Dermatologic Therapy* **16**, 114–22.

Singh, B., Moodley, J., Shaik, A. S. and Robbs, J. V. (2003). Sympathectomy for complex regional pain syndrome. *Journal of Vascular Surgery* **37**, 508–11.

Smeets, J. L., Allessie, M. A., Lammers, W. J., Bonke, F. I. and Hollen, J. (1986). The wavelength of the cardiac impulse and reentrant arrhythmias in isolated rabbit atrium. The role of heart rate, autonomic transmitters, temperature, and potassium. *Circulation Research* **58**, 96–108.

Sood, S., Quraishi, M. S., Jennings, C. R. and Bradley, P. J. (1999). Frey's syndrome following parotidectomy: prevention using a rotation sternocleidomastoid muscle flap. *Clinical Otolaryngology* **24**, 365–8.

Stanton-Hicks, M., Baron, R., Boas, R., *et al.* (1998). Complex Regional Pain Syndromes: guidelines for therapy. *Clinical Journal of Pain* **14**, 155–66.

Stanton-Hicks, M., Janig, W., Hassenbusch, S., Haddox, J. D., Boas, R. and Wilson, P. (1995). Reflex sympathetic dystrophy: changing concepts and taxonomy. *Pain* **63**, 127–33.

Sterodimas, A., Nicolaou, M. and Paes, T. R. (2003). Successful use of Botulinum toxin-A for the treatment of neck and anterior chest wall flushing. *Clinical and Experimental Dermatology* **28**, 592–94.

Strutton, D. R., Kowalski, J. W., Glaser, D. A. and Stang, P. E. (2004). US prevalence of hyperhidrosis and impact on individuals with axillary hyperhidrosis: results from a national survey. *Journal of the American Academy of Dermatology* **51**, 241–48.

Swan, M. C., Nicolaou, M. and Paes, T. R. (2003). Iatrogenic harlequin syndrome. *Postgraduate Medical Journal* **79**, 278–594.

Swartling, C., Naver, H. and Lindberg, M. (2001). Botulinum A toxin improves life quality in severe primary focal hyperhidrosis. *European Journal of Neurology* **8**, 247–52.

Togel, B., Greve, B. and Raulin, C. (2002). Current therapeutic strategies for hyperhidrosis: a review. *European Journal of Dermatology* **12**, 219–23.

Tseng, M. Y. and Tseng, J. H. (2001). Endoscopic extraperitoneal lumbar sympathectomy for plantar hyperhidrosis: case report. *Journal of Clinical Neuroscience* **8**, 555–56.

Tugnoli, V., Marchese Ragona, R., Eleopra, R., *et al.* (2002). The role of gustatory flushing in Frey. *Clinical Autonomic Research* **12**, 174–78.

Tygesen, H., Claes, G., Drott, C., *et al.* (1997). Effect of endoscopic transthoracic sympathicotomy on heart rate variability in severe angina pectoris. *American Journal of Cardiology* **79**, 1447–52.

Tygesen, H., Wettervik, C., Claes, G., *et al.* (1999). Long-term effect of endoscopic transthoracic sympathicotomy on heart rate variability and QT dispersion in severe angina pectoris. *International Journal of Cardiology* **70**, 283–92.

Vadoud-Seyedi, J. (2004). Treatment of plantar hyperhidrosis with botulinum toxin type A. *International Journal of Dermatology* **43**, 969–71.

Wang, Z., Page, P. and Nattel, S. (1992). Mechanism of flecainide's antiarrhythmic action in experimental atrial fibrillation. *Circulation Research* **71**, 271–87.

Watarida, S., Shiraishi, S., Fujimura, M., Hirano, M., Nishi, T., Imura, M. and Yamamoto, I. (2002). Laparoscopic lumbar sympathectomy for lower-limb disease. *Surgical Endoscopy* **16**, 500–3.

Waxman, S. G. (1996). The Autonomic Nervous System. In Waxman, S. G., ed. *Correlative Neuroanatomy*, pp. 259–74. Appleton & Lange, Connecticut.

Wettervik, C., Claes, G., Drott, C., Emanuelsson, H., Lomsky, M., Radberg, G. and Tygesen, H. (1995). Endoscopic transthoracic sympathicotomy for severe angina. *Lancet* **345**, 97–8.

Wilkinson, D. S. and Ebling, F. J., ed. Rook, Wilkinson, Ebling. *Textbook of Dermatology*, pp. 2099–2107. Blackwell Science, Oxford, Malden, MA.

Yuraitis, M. and Jacob, C. I. (2004). Botulinum toxin for the treatment of facial flushing. *Dermatologic Surgery* **30**, 102–104.

de Campos, J. R., Kauffman, P., Werebe Ede, C., *et al.* (2003). Quality of life, before and after thoracic sympathectomy: report on 378 operated patients. *The Annals of Thoracic Surgery* **76**, 886–91.

Index